Leading Causes of Childhood[a] Deaths: 1950, 1979, and 1985

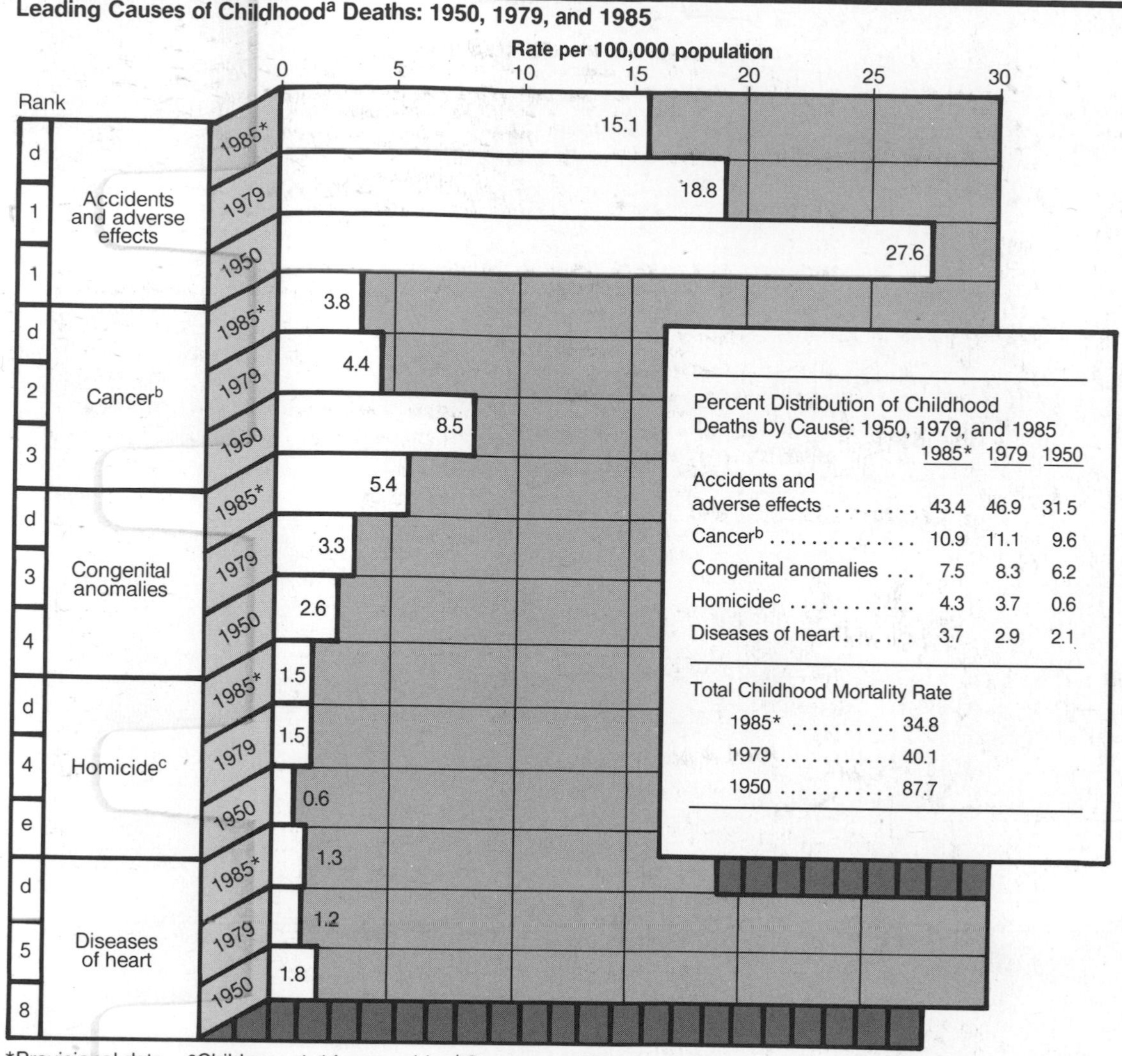

Percent Distribution of Childhood Deaths by Cause: 1950, 1979, and 1985

	1985*	1979	1950
Accidents and adverse effects	43.4	46.9	31.5
Cancer[b]	10.9	11.1	9.6
Congenital anomalies	7.5	8.3	6.2
Homicide[c]	4.3	3.7	0.6
Diseases of heart	3.7	2.9	2.1

Total Childhood Mortality Rate

1985*	34.8
1979	40.1
1950	87.7

*Provisional data. [a]Children = 1-14 years old. [b]Cancer = malignant neoplasms, including neoplasms of lymphatic and hematopoietic tissues. [c]Homicide = homicide and legal intervention. [d]Rank not available for 1985 provisional data. [e]Not ranked in the first 10 leading causes of death.

Note: This figure shows rates for leading causes of childhood deaths in 1979 and comparable rates and ranks for 1950 and 1985.

Source: National Center for Health Statistics.

Reprinted from *Prevention '86/'87: Federal Programs and Progress.* Washington, D.C., U.S. Department of Health and Human Services.

Leading Causes of Childhood[a] Deaths: 1950, 1979, and 1985

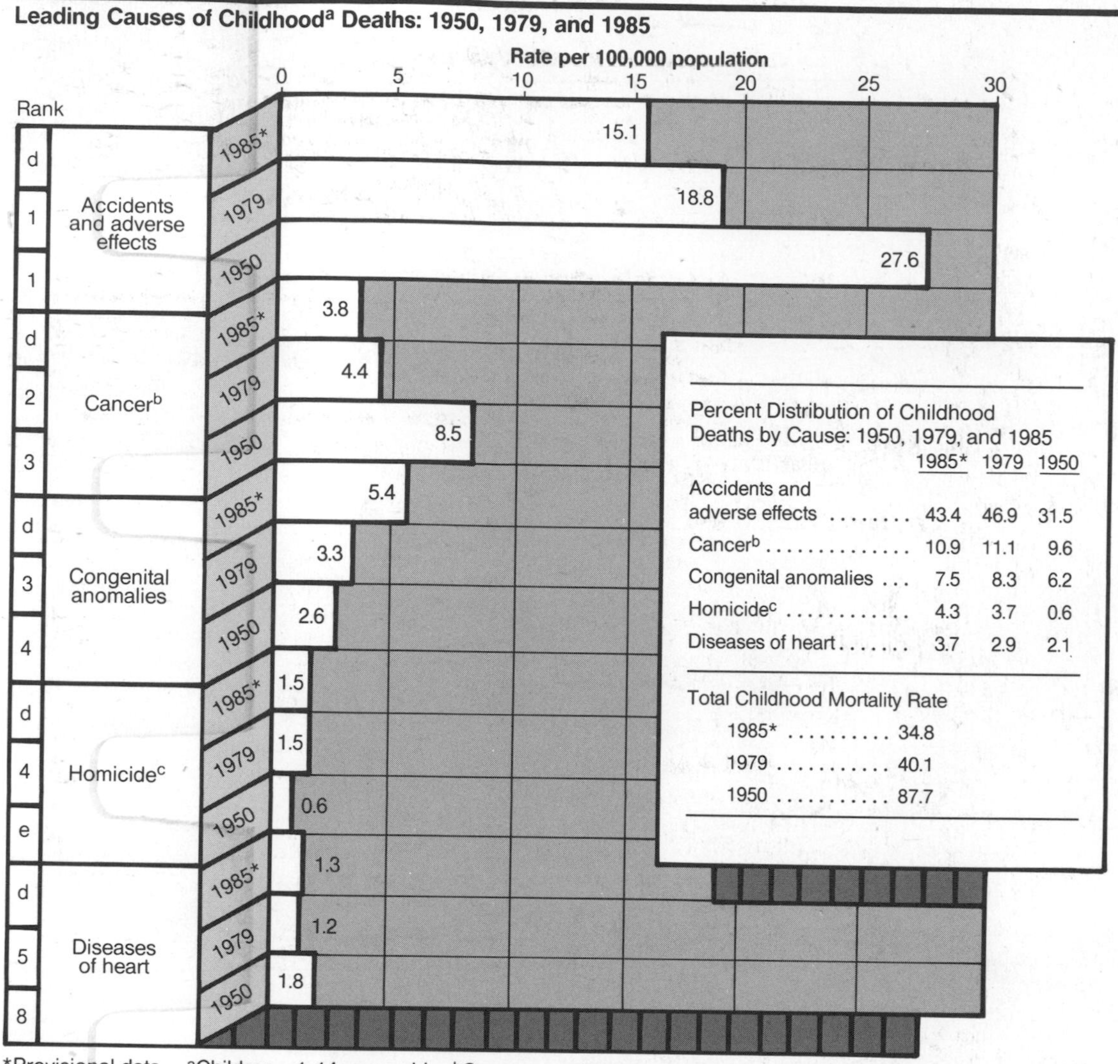

Percent Distribution of Childhood Deaths by Cause: 1950, 1979, and 1985

	1985*	1979	1950
Accidents and adverse effects	43.4	46.9	31.5
Cancer[b]	10.9	11.1	9.6
Congenital anomalies	7.5	8.3	6.2
Homicide[c]	4.3	3.7	0.6
Diseases of heart	3.7	2.9	2.1

Total Childhood Mortality Rate

1985*	34.8
1979	40.1
1950	87.7

*Provisional data. [a]Children = 1-14 years old. [b]Cancer = malignant neoplasms, including neoplasms of lymphatic and hematopoietic tissues. [c]Homicide = homicide and legal intervention. [d]Rank not available for 1985 provisional data. [e]Not ranked in the first 10 leading causes of death.

Note: This figure shows rates for leading causes of childhood deaths in 1979 and comparable rates and ranks for 1950 and 1985.

Source: National Center for Health Statistics.

Reprinted from *Prevention '86/'87: Federal Programs and Progress.* Washington, D.C., U.S. Department of Health and Human Services.

PEDIATRIC MEDICINE

EDITED BY

Mary Ellen Avery, M.D.
Thomas Morgan Rotch Professor of Pediatrics
Harvard Medical School
Senior Associate in Medicine
The Children's Hospital
Boston, Massachusetts

Lewis R. First, M.D.
Instructor in Pediatrics
Harvard Medical School
Associate in Medicine
The Children's Hospital
Boston, Massachusetts

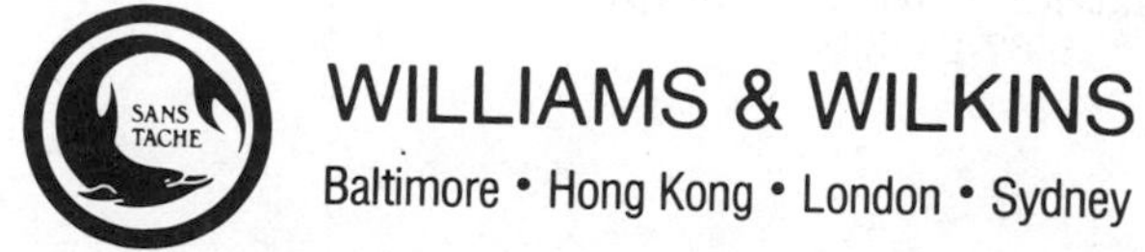

WILLIAMS & WILKINS
Baltimore • Hong Kong • London • Sydney

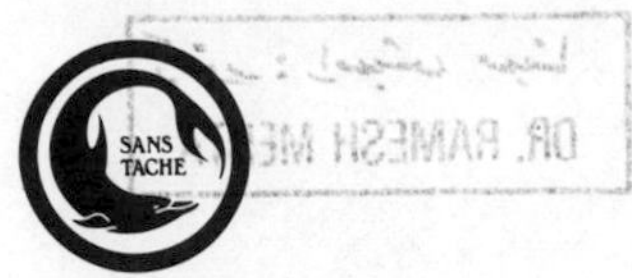

Editor: Carol-Lynn Brown
Associate Editor: Linda Napora
Copy Editor: Shelley Potler
Design: JoAnne Janowiak
Illustration Planning: Wayne Hubbel
Production: Anne G. Seitz

Williams & Wilkins
428 East Preston Street
Baltimore, MD 21202, USA

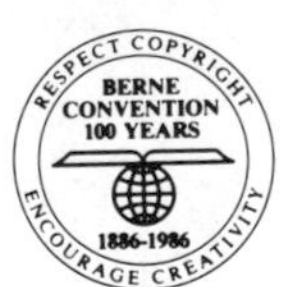

Accurate indications, adverse reactions, and dosage schedules for drugs are provided in this book, but it is possible that they may change. The reader is urged to review the package information data of the manufacturers of the medications mentioned.

Printed in the United States of America

Library of Congress Cataloging-in-Publication Data

Pediatric medicine.

Includes bibliographies and index.
1. Pediatrics. I. Avery, Mary Ellen, 1927—.
II. First, Lewis. [DNLM: 1. Pediatrics. WS 200 P3713]
RJ45.P394 1988 618.92 87-29433
ISBN 0-683-00294-5

89 90 91 92 93
1 2 3 4 5 6 7 8 9 10

To the medical house staff of
The Children's Hospital, Boston
whose observations and questions were the stimulus for this book

Preface

"Everything should be made as simple as possible, but not simpler."
Attributed to Albert Einstein by Marvin Minsky

Pediatric Medicine has been designed to meet the needs of the clinician today. It is a textbook of pediatrics for the 1980s and 1990s, written from the perspective of those who serve as attending pediatricians at The Children's Hospital, Boston, and who work closely with medical students, residents, and colleagues on day-to-day pediatric problem solving.

This book is organized by organ system, which is a very traditional but ever useful approach. Presentations of symptoms are often discussed within the context of the most likely system responsible, but we will sometimes refer the reader to other chapters. Most sections begin with one or more introductory topics designed to facilitate or gain a knowledge base for the general subject under study. Following this introductory material, almost all subsequent chapters within a section are structured with the subheadings that follow:

Definition: A description of relevant terms to be used in the chapter.

Basic Science: What the clinician needs to know to understand a disease or formulate an approach to its diagnosis and treatment. We have tried to include the most recent information, although we acknowledge that in rapidly moving fields we cannot be up-to-the month by date of publication.

Epidemiology: Important statistics and epidemiologic descriptions regarding the occurrence of the topic of interest.

Natural History: A description of the course of an illness and its associated complications.

Diagnosis: Useful clinical and laboratory studies as well as a comparison of their diagnostic efficacy when relevant.

Treatment: An approach to and description of relevant treatment modalities with comparisons of effectiveness.

Prognosis and Prevention: Issues related to follow-up as well as preventive health care for the illness under study.

In some sections we have included two additional subheadings when appropriate: New Developments and Controversies. In this way clinical issues not universally accepted (but important nonetheless) are highlighted.

We have included some current illustrations to involve the reader in problem-solving. They have been chosen to bring up interesting twists or dilemmas, or to underscore important considerations. As is our custom in everyday activities, we rely on a computerized data system for the most recent publications to bring a larger experience to our teaching and patient care. We have cited references to document specific points and, sometimes, we have included either classic descriptions of disease or definitive review articles that will guide the reader to information too detailed for inclusion in a textbook. We have deliberately not explored basic science in depth, nor have we devoted much space to embryology, pathology, or any of the surgical specialties since excellent books exist in those areas and, for the most part, the pediatrician depends on colleagues for relevant expert opinions.

We have enjoyed launching this book and hope our readers will find it instructive. We welcome all comments and suggestions, recognizing that a first edition of a totally new textbook with the scope of this one will probably have some significant omissions. We are ready to try to improve it on the basis of feedback from our readers.

Mary Ellen Avery, M.D.
Lewis R. First, M.D.

The Children's Hospital
Boston, Massachusetts

Acknowledgments

We, the editors, have written much of this book, even though we do not qualify as experts in many of the topics we discuss. We have tried to pose the questions that we encounter on the wards and in the clinics, and have asked our consultants to review our chapters. In some sections, we have felt inadequate to produce a contemporary or authoritative approach and have asked colleagues in Boston to become the principal authors, and we have then served as their editors to provide a reasonably uniform approach. Cardiology, neurology, behavioral pediatrics, and gynecology are subspecialties so outside our area of expertise that we sought primary authors from specialists. The fields of genetics, endocrinology, immunology, and hereditary metabolic disorders have so much new and exciting basic science that is relevant to clinical problems that we sought as authors colleagues who are deeply engaged in research and practice in those disciplines.

The question of specific doses of drugs was considered, with concern that any attempt to be comprehensive would be futile. We left it to each contributor to decide when specific recommendations were deemed appropriate. We assumed our readers would have access to other sources of updated information.

We wrestled with the question of "inclusive language" to avoid repetition of *he* when we could just as well say *she* or *he/she*. The English language and its usage does not make it easy to change without a sense of awkwardness, even in the 1980s. We, therefore, chose not to intrude this issue into this text. We hope the reader will interpret he in the sense of humankind and forgive us for not alternating *he* and *she*.

We elected to highlight the mortality figures from the United States on the inside covers because of the major reductions in infant and childhood deaths that have occurred over the past few decades. These reductions have been due largely to innovations in diagnostic and therapeutic modalities that are discussed in our text. The five leading causes of infant deaths (for those less than 1 year of age) on the inside front cover show that in each category there has been a reduction. The major reduction in deaths from congenital anomalies can be attributed in large part to increasing use of prenatal diagnosis and elective abortion. The five leading causes of childhood deaths (for those ages 1–14 years) are shown on the inside back cover. By 1984, the total population of children in that age group was about 48 million, or one-fifth of the total. It is satisfying to see the 60% reduction in the overall rate, but worrisome to note the increase in homicide, which in 1985 was the fourth leading cause of death.

Mary Ellen Avery wishes to acknowledge the teaching and invaluable clinical experiences at the Harriet Lane Home of the Johns Hopkins Hospital, the Montreal Children's Hospital, and the Children's Hospital, Boston. Interactions with medical students and house staff have inspired this work as a thank you for making learning and teaching so pleasurable.

Lewis First, as a house officer, chief medical resident, and now faculty member at The Children's Hospital, Boston, conceived the format of the book as a way to be helpful to those on the front lines, where he continues to spend much of his time.

Rita Teele, our consulting editor in radiology, wrote the sections on imaging, and provided the radiographs throughout the text. All of us recognize that a completely new textbook will have imbalances and imperfections, points of view not universally held (although we have tried to highlight controversies) and probably recommendations that may be outdated by expanding new knowledge by the date of publication. We have tried to "tell it as it is" in Boston at least in 1985–1988 when the book was written.

Among those to whom we are especially grateful for assisting this book to publication are Dr. Dorothy Villee, who not only wrote the section on endocrinology, but reviewed the other sections as well. We are grateful to former Children's Hospital residents who contributed many of the clinical histories; they include Drs. Paul Cotran, William Gerson, George Hoffman, Jane Neuberger, Jonathan Rome, Norman Rosenblum, and Evan Snyder. We are most indebted to Dr. Pamela Talalay who translated much of our writing into respectable English, and the editors at Williams & Wilkins who carried out the innumerable tasks that moved manuscript to publication. To Ellen Collins, who typed all the manuscript, some of it dictated, much of it poorly handwritten, we extend sympathy and heartfelt thanks. And finally, Florence Avitabile provided advice and encouragement at all stages of writing this textbook.

Contributors

EDITORS

Mary Ellen Avery, M.D.
Thomas Morgan Rotch Professor of Pediatrics, Harvard Medical School; Senior Associate in Medicine, The Children's Hospital, Boston, Massachusetts

Lewis R. First, M.D.
Instructor in Pediatrics, Harvard Medical School; Associate in Medicine, The Children's Hospital, Boston, Massachusetts

Consultant Editor, Radiology

Rita L. Teele, M.D.
Associate Professor of Radiology, Harvard Medical School; Radiologist, The Children's Hospital, Boston, Massachusetts

Section 1: WELL CHILD CARE

CONTRIBUTORS

MARY ELLEN AVERY, M.D.

ROBERT MASLAND, M.D.
Associate Professor of Pediatrics, Harvard Medical School Chief, Division of Adolescent/Young Adult Medicine, The Children's Hospital, Boston, Massachusetts

RICHARD FERBER, M.D.
Instructor in Neurology, Harvard Medical School; Assistant in Neurology, The Children's Hospital, Boston, Massachusetts

JANICE WARE, Ph.D.
Instructor in Psychiatry, Harvard Medical School; Developmental Psychologist, Infant Follow-up Program, The Children's Hospital, Boston, Massachusetts

LEWIS R. FIRST, M.D.

Consultants

H. Burtt Richardson, M.D.
Pediatrician
Winthrop Family Pediatrics Center, Winthrop, Maine

Gerald Hass, M.D.
Assistant Clinical Professor of Pediatrics, Harvard Medical School; Senior Associate in Medicine, The Children's Hospital, Boston; Physician-in-Chief, South End Community Health Center, Boston, Massachusetts

John Robey, M.D.
Assistant Clinical Professor of Pediatrics, Harvard Medical School; Senior Associate in Medicine, The Children's Hospital, Boston, Massachusetts

Section 2: BEHAVIORAL PEDIATRICS

GORDON HARPER, M.D.
Assistant Professor of Psychiatry, Harvard Medical School; Director of Inpatient Psychiatry, The Children's Hospital, Boston, Massachusetts

Section 3: NUTRITION

CONTRIBUTORS

MARY ELLEN AVERY, M.D,

DOROTHY VILLEE, M.D.
Assistant Clinical Professor of Pediatrics, Harvard Medical School; Associate in Endocrinology, The Children's Hospital, Boston, Massachusetts

SUSAN BAKER, M.D.
Assistant Professor of Pediatrics; Co-director, Pediatric GI/ Nutrition; University of Massachusetts Medical School, Worcester, Massachusetts

ROBERT WHARTON, M.D.
Instructor in Pediatrics, Harvard Medical School; Assistant in Medicine, The Children's Hospital; Director of Pediatrics, Spaulding Rehabilitation Hospital, Boston, Massachusetts

Section 4: NEONATOLOGY

CONTRIBUTORS

MARY ELLEN AVERY, M.D.

HEIDELISE ALS, Ph.D.
Associate Professor of Pediatrics (Psychology), Harvard Medical School; Associate in Psychiatry and Director of Neurobehavioral Infant and Child Studies, The Children's Hospital, Boston, Massachusetts

Consultants

Michael F. Epstein, M.D.
Associate Professor of Pediatrics, Harvard Medical School; Chief, Division of Newborn Medicine, The Children's Hospital, Boston, Massachusetts

David Schiff, M.D., Ph.D., FRCP(C)
Professor of Pediatrics, Obstetrics and Gynecology; University of Alberta; Director, Newborn Nurseries, University of Alberta Hospitals; Edmonton, Alberta, Canada

Helen G. Liley, M.B., ChB.
Instructor in Pediatrics, Harvard Medical School, Boston, Massachusetts

Janice Ware, Ph.D.

Section 5: PULMONOLOGY

MARY ELLEN AVERY, M.D.

Consultants

Raif Geha, M.D.
Professor of Pediatrics, Harvard Medical School; Chief, Allergy-Immunology, The Children's Hospital, Boston, Massachusetts

Mary Ellen Wohl, M.D.
Associate Professor of Pediatrics, Harvard Medical School; Chief, Division of Respiratory Diseases, The Children's Hospital, Boston, Massachusetts

Raezelle Zinman, MDCM
Assistant Professor of Pediatrics, Faculty of Medicine, McGill University, Montreal, Canada

Section 6: CARDIOLOGY

DONALD C. FYLER, M.D.
Professor of Pediatrics, Harvard Medical School; Associate Chief, Cardiology Department, The Children's Hospital, Boston, Massachusetts

ALEXANDER S. NADAS, M.D.
Professor of Pediatrics, Harvard Medical School; Chief Emeritus, Cardiology Department, The Children's Hospital, Boston, Massachusetts

Section 7: GASTROENTEROLOGY

LEWIS R. FIRST, M.D.

Consultant

John Snyder, M.D.
Assistant Professor of Pediatrics, Harvard Medical School; Associate in Gastroenterology, The Children's Hospital, Boston, Massachusetts

Section 8: HEMATOLOGY

LEWIS R. FIRST, M.D.

Consultants

Orah S. Platt, M.D.
Associate Professor of Pediatrics, Harvard Medical School; Associate in Hematology/Oncology, The Children's Hospital; Associate in Pediatric Oncology, Dana Farber Cancer Institute, Boston, Massachusetts

David G. Nathan, M.D.
Robert A. Stranahan Professor of Pediatrics, Harvard Medical School; Physician-in-Chief, The Children's Hospital, Boston, Massachusetts

Section 9: ONCOLOGY

CONTRIBUTORS

LEWIS R. FIRST, M.D.

CHARLES BERDE, M.D., Ph.D.
Assistant Professor of Anesthesia, Harvard Medical School; Associate in Anesthesia, The Children's Hospital, Boston, Massachusetts

ALAN L. SCHWARTZ, M.D., Ph.D.
Professor of Pediatrics and Pharmacology; Director Pediatric Hematology-Oncology; Washington University School of Medicine; The Children's Hospital, St. Louis, Missouri

GARRETT M. BRODEUR, M.D.
Associate Professor of Pediatrics and Genetics; Washington University School of Medicine; The Children's Hospital, St. Louis, Missouri

Consultants

Howard Weinstein, M.D.
Associate Professor of Pediatrics, Harvard Medical School; Associate in Hematology/Oncology, The Children's Hospital, Boston, Massachusetts

David G. Nathan, M.D.

Section 10: NEPHROLOGY

CONTRIBUTORS

MARY ELLEN AVERY, M.D.

JAMES MANDELL, M.D.
Assistant Professor of Surgery (Urology), Harvard Medical School; Attending Physician, The Children's Hospital, Boston, Massachusetts

CHARLES SIMMONS, M.D.
Instructor in Medicine, Harvard Medical School; Assistant in Medicine, The Children's Hospital, Boston, Massachusetts

WILLIAM HARMON, M.D.
Associate Professor of Pediatrics, Harvard Medical School; Chief, Division of Nephrology, The Children's Hospital, Boston, Massachusetts

LEWIS R. FIRST, M.D.

Consultants

Jean M. Smellie, DM, FRCP, DCH
Senior Lecturer in Paediatrics, University College Hospital, London, England

Julie R. Ingelfinger, M.D.
Associate Professor of Pediatrics, Harvard Medical School; Director of Hypertension Clinic, The Children's Hospital, Boston, Massachusetts

Section 11: GYNECOLOGY

S. JEAN EMANS, M.D.
Assistant Professor of Pediatrics, Harvard Medical School; Associate Chief, Division of Adolescent/Young Adult Medicine, The Children's Hospital, Boston, Massachusetts

Section 12: NEUROLOGY

CONTRIBUTORS

DAVID K. URION, M.D.
Instructor in Neurology, Harvard Medical School; Assistant in Neurology, The Children's Hospital, Boston, Massachusetts

MARY ELLEN AVERY, M.D.

JAMES H. SABRY, M.D.
Clinical Fellow in Neurology, Harvard Medical School; Resident in Neurology, The Children's Hospital, Boston, Massachusetts

BRUCE R. KORF, M.D., Ph.D.
Assistant Professor of Neurology, Harvard Medical School; Director, Clinical Genetics Section, Division of Genetics; The Children's Hospital, Boston, Massachusetts

Consultant

H. Burtt Richardson, M.D.

Section 13: GENETICS

DIANA W. BIANCHI, M.D.
Instructor in Pediatrics, Harvard Medical School; Assistant in Medicine, The Children's Hospital, Boston, Massachusetts

Consultant

Samuel Latt, M.D., Ph.D.
Professor of Pediatrics and Genetics, Harvard Medical School; Chief, Genetics Division, The Children's Hospital, Boston, Massachusetts

Section 14: ENDOCRINOLOGY

DOROTHY VILLEE, M.D.

Section 15: HEREDITARY METABOLIC DISEASES

CONTRIBUTORS

HARVEY LEVY, M.D.
Associate Professor of Neurology, Harvard Medical School; Director, Biochemical Genetics, The Children's Hospital, Boston, Massachusetts

MIRA IRONS, M.D.
Clinical Associate in Pediatrics, Massachusetts General Hospital, Boston, Pediatric Geneticist, Prenatal Diagnostic Center, Lincoln, Massachusetts

MARY ELLEN AVERY, M.D.

DOROTHY VILLEE, M.D.

Section 16: IMMUNOLOGY

CONTRIBUTORS

RAIF S. GEHA, M.D.

DALE T. UMETSU, M.D., Ph.D.
Assistant Professor of Pediatrics, Stanford University School of Medicine; Division of Allergy and Pulmonary Disease, The Children's Hospital at Stanford, Palo Alto, California

RICHARD B. JOHNSTON, JR., M.D.
William H. Bennett Professor and Chairman; Department of Pediatrics, University of Pennsylvania, School of Medicine; Physician-in-Chief, The Children's Hospital of Philadelphia, Philadelphia, Pennsylvania

LEWIS R. FIRST, M.D.

Consultant

Fred S. Rosen, M.D.
James Gamble Professor of Pediatrics, Harvard Medical School; President, The Center for Blood Research, The Children's Hospital, Boston, Massachusetts

Section 17: INFECTIOUS DISEASES

CONTRIBUTORS

MARY ELLEN AVERY, M.D.

LEWIS R. FIRST, M.D.

ALICE HUANG, Ph.D.
Professor of Microbiology and Molecular Genetics; Harvard Medical School; Director, Laboratories of Infectious Diseases, The Children's Hospital, Boston, Massachusetts

Consultants

Kenneth McIntosh, M.D.
Professor of Pediatrics, Harvard Medical School; Chief, Clinical Infectious Diseases, The Children's Hospital, Boston, Massachusetts

Donald Goldmann, M.D.
Associate Professor in Pediatrics, Harvard Medical School; Senior Associate in Medicine, The Children's Hospital, Boston, Massachusetts

Edward O'Rourke, M.D.
Assistant Professor in Pediatrics, Harvard Medical School; Associate in Medicine, The Children's Hospital, Boston, Massachusetts

Thomas Weller, M.D.
Emeritus Professor of Tropical Public Health; Harvard School of Public Health, Boston, Massachusetts

Melvin Marks, M.D.
Professor of Pediatrics, University of California, Irvine; Medical Director, Miller Children's Hospital, Memorial Medical Center, Long Beach, California

Donna Ambrosino, M.D.
Assistant Professor of Pediatrics, Assistant in Medicine, The Children's Hospital, Boston, Massachusetts

Section 18: DERMATOLOGY

MARY ELLEN AVERY, M.D.

Consultant

Arthur Rhodes, M.D.
Assistant Professor of Dermatology, Harvard Medical School; Assistant Dermatologist, Massachusetts General Hospital, Boston, Massachusetts

Rita Berman, M.D.
Associate Professor of Pediatrics, Harvard Medical School; Acting Director, Division of Dermatology, The Children's Hospital, Boston, Massachusetts

Section 19: OTOLARYNGOLOGY

MARY ELLEN AVERY, M.D.

Consultant

Gerald Healy, M.D.
Associate Professor of Otolaryngology, Harvard Medical School; Otolaryngologist-in-Chief, The Children's Hospital Boston, Massachusetts

Section 20: OPHTHALMOLOGY

MARY ELLEN AVERY, M.D.

Consultant

Richard Robb, M.D.
Associate Professor of Ophthalmology, Harvard Medical School; Ophthalmologist-in-Chief, The Children's Hospital, Boston, Massachusetts

Section 21: DENTISTRY

CONTRIBUTORS

HOWARD L. NEEDLEMAN, D.M.D.
Assistant Clinical Professor of Pediatric Dentistry, Harvard School of Dental Medicine; Associate Dentist-in-Chief, The Children's Hospital, Boston, Massachusetts

STEPHEN SHUSTERMAN, D.M.D.
Assistant Clinical Professor of Pediatric Dentistry, Harvard School of Dental Medicine; Dentist-in-Chief, The Children's Hospital, Boston, Massachusetts

Section 22: RHEUMATOLOGY

JANE G. SCHALLER, M.D.
David and Leona Karp Professor and Chairman; Department of Pediatrics, Tufts University School of Medicine; Pediatrician-in-Chief, Floating Hospital for Infants and Children, New England Medical Center Hospitals, Boston, Massachusetts

Section 23: ORTHOPEDICS

CONTRIBUTORS

MICHAEL MILLIS, M.D.
Assistant Clinical Professor Orthopaedic Surgery; Harvard Medical School; Associate in Orthopaedics, The Children's Hospital, Boston, Massachusetts

FRANK RAND, M.D.
Instructor in Orthopaedic Surgery, Harvard Medical School; Assistant in Orthopaedics, The Children's Hospital, Boston, Massachusetts

MARY ELLEN AVERY, M.D.

LEWIS R. FIRST, M.D.

Consultant

Kenneth R. First, M.D.
Instructor in Orthopaedics, Harvard Medical School; Assistant in Orthopaedics, Massachusetts General Hospital, Boston, Massachusetts

Section 24: INJURIES

CONTRIBUTORS

ALAN WOOLF, M.D., M.P.H.
Instructor in Pediatrics, Harvard Medical School; Assistant in Medicine, Director, Young Adult Team, Associate Director, Community Services Program, The Children's Hospital, Boston, Massachusetts

LEWIS R. FIRST, M.D.

Section 25: TOXICOLOGY

ALAN WOOLF, M.D., M.P.H.

Contents

SECTION 5
PULMONOLOGY

SECTION 6
CARDIOLOGY

SECTION 7
GASTROENTEROLOGY

SECTION 8
HEMATOLOGY

SECTION 9
ONCOLOGY

SECTION 10
NEPHROLOGY

SECTION 11
GYNECOLOGY

SECTION 12
NEUROLOGY

SECTION 13 GENETICS

SECTION 14 ENDOCRINOLOGY

SECTION 15
HEREDITARY METABOLIC DISEASES

SECTION 16 IMMUNOLOGY

SECTION 17 INFECTIOUS DISEASES

SECTION 18
DERMATOLOGY

SECTION 19
OTOLARYNGOLOGY

SECTION 20 OPHTHALMOLOGY

SECTION 21 DENTISTRY

SECTION 22 RHEUMATOLOGY

SECTION 23 ORTHOPEDICS

SECTION 24
CHILDHOOD INJURIES

SECTION 25
TOXICOLOGY

PEDIATRIC MEDICINE

Section 1

Well Child Care

Overview of Well Child Care

1

GUIDELINES

The primary role of the pediatrician is to assume responsibility for working with parents to assure the normal growth and development of the infant, child, and adolescent and to screen for and identify any physical or psychosocial abnormalities that require treatment or counseling. This is an enormous responsibility, requiring education about the stages of normal growth and development, as well as knowledge of the myriad disorders that may afflict children.

No topic could be more relevant to the practice of pediatrics than its preventive arm, well child care. This section is designed to highlight some of the developmental considerations. It could well be expanded to a monograph or an encyclopedia of normal values. We have tried to abstract only the most salient issues, although we feel somewhat presumptuous in doing so. We hope that the references will be helpful to those who seek more complete discussions.

These guidelines were assembled in 1979–1988 by residents and their preceptors, Gerald Hass and John Robey, to assist in formalizing some aspects of well child care. They are issued to The Children's Hospital house staff each year and have provided a helpful introduction to this all-important aspect of pediatrics. To Mark Lerner who coordinated much of the material and to the many house officers who have contributed to it, we are grateful for their thoughtful insight. We present this modified format in the hope that it will prove useful to future students of clinical pediatrics.

Prenatal Visit

The prenatal visit is unlike all other well child visits in that the emphasis of the interview is on the parents rather than the child. The goals of the visit are:

1. to establish a relationship with the parents which is caring and supportive;
2. to inquire about family history;
3. to aid in decision-making regarding feeding and circumcision;
4. to anticipate specific concerns about the new baby—such as a congenital deformity in a child with a family history of heart disease; what are the family's expectations for this child?
5. to allow time for discussion about the couple's feelings and fears about their new role as parents.

It is a privilege to establish a relationship early in the child-rearing process. During this visit, the pediatrician can discuss style and approach to health care and the couple has an opportunity to know the pediatrician as well. Do not miss this chance for physician-family attachment.

Hospital Visit

History

The history should include the pregnancy, labor, and delivery. Here the skill of the pediatrician is evident in the ability to assimilate a tremendous amount of information and its relevance to the individual baby. Some of the high points in the history are discussed.

Subject

PREGNANCY

1. General health, adequacy of prenatal care
2. Specific disease—chronic or acute; inquire about "viral illnesses" for evidence of particular disease; for known chronic diseases such as diabetes, renal disease, collagen vascular disease, and cardiopulmonary disease, determine the stage of involvement, and how the disease was controlled during pregnancy
3. Medications, hormones, vitamins, diets, unusual food practices during pregnancy, alcohol, smoking
4. Exposures—radiation, toxic, environmental

LABOR

1. Onset—spontaneous or induced; gestational age
2. Fetal heart monitoring
3. Anesthesia
4. Duration
5. Medications

DELIVERY

1. Method—vaginal or cesarean
2. Presentation
3. Complications
4. Condition of infant
5. Birth weight and gestational age

Physical Examination of the Infant

The evaluation of the newborn is a process of several exams: from the initial inspection and Apgar scoring in the delivery room to the complete examination in the nursery to the demonstration of the physical examination and behavioral observations to the parents in their room. There is hardly a more important examination that this new person will have, especially from the parents' perspective. New parents want to know "is my baby normal?"

DELIVERY ROOM EXAMINATION

1. Apgar scoring
2. Congenital anomaly search
3. Besides making sure that the baby makes the transition from the uterine environment to the outside world, the pediatrician communicates the news of how the baby is doing in that transition period

NEWBORN EXAMINATION (NURSERY)

1. General appearance—features of a syndrome, appropriateness of weight for gestational age, cry: vigorous vs. lethargic
2. Skin color (early jaundice), skin quality, cyanosis, plethora, rashes
3. Measurements: height, weight, head circumference
4. Head, eyes, ears, nose, throat: fontanelles, sutures, birth trauma, scalp electrode mark, ear shape, position, abnormal eye movements (VI nerve palsy is common), red reflex, cataracts, conjunctivae, nose patency, bridge, septum, oropharynx palate, Epstein pearls, "natal" teeth, ranula, tongue, frenulum, uvula
5. Neck: trachea midline, masses, clefts, goiter, torticollis
6. Chest: conformation, clavicles, respiratory efforts, breath sounds, breasts, cardiac impulse, murmurs, heart sounds
7. External genitalia: male—phallus length, meatal opening, testes; female—clitoral size, virilization, introitus
8. Abdomen: distention, bowel sounds, anus (patency and position), palpation of liver edge, umbilicus, presence of palpable spleen, bimanual palpation of kidneys
9. Spine: flexibility, sinuses, hairy patch, defects
10. Extremities: anomalies, movement, in utero positional deformity vs. fixed deformity (clubfeet)
11. Neurologic: overall state of alertness, vigor of cry, weakness, tone, reflexes (DTRs and primitive), suck, response to light and voice
12. Behavioral control of state (alertness), response to holding, feeding, voice, overall degree of activity and ability to stimulate interactions

DEMONSTRATION EXAMINATION TO THE PARENTS

1. Point out any unusual features that are obvious and explain the significance to the parents, i.e., hemangioma, pigmentation over dorsal aspect of trunk (Mongolian spot).
2. Answer any questions about features with which the parents show concern and reassure them if normal.
3. Explain appearance of cord and cord care.
4. Explain about jaundice.
5. Discuss how feeding is progressing and reassure them if they are concerned about the intake.
6. Anticipate the problems in certain risk situations, i.e., maternal illness or drug exposure, difficult delivery, or antenatal problem.
7. Wherever possible, facilitate parent-infant bonding by demonstrating the infant's own behavioral characteristics.
8. Be sensitive to the stresses of the birth process for the mother and the father and the children at home. Be as supportive as necessary.

The challenge of the newborn period for the pediatrician stimulates all aspects of expertise, scientific and humanistic. Time spent in careful examination and thorough explanation is an investment in the future relationship with the child and the parents.

Preventive Screening

ROUTINE SCREENING

1. PKU (phenylketonuria), other aminoacidurias
2. Congenital hypothyroidism
3. Galactosemia

ROUTINE PROPHYLAXIS

1. Silver nitrate drops (1%) or antibiotic erythromycin ophthalmic ointment
2. Vitamin K_1 oxide, 0.5–1.0 mg (intramuscular)
3. Bathing with nonmedicated, nonabrasive soap

Anticipatory Guidance

1. Infant seats: car safety devices can be rented inexpensively at some hospitals
2. Umbilical cord slough at about 10 days; dangers of erythema at base; granulomas
3. Bathing
4. Encourage telephone calls before first visit; because going home can initiate parental stress, make yourself easily accessible to the family at this time

Routine Follow-up

Ten days to 3 weeks (child's age).

First Office Visit

The first visit between pediatrician, parents, and infant is of crucial importance. It is to be hoped that this is not the first time they have met (ideally, they would already have met in a prenatal and/or newborn visit), but if it is a first visit, it is even more important that a favorable rapport be established. The development of good rapport can be fostered by a caring, empathic attitude on the part of the pediatrician.

The timing of this visit is usually when the baby is between 1 and 4 weeks of age, with 2 weeks being the most common, especially if the parents are young and/or inexperienced. A wealth of data should be obtained at the visit and the pediatrician should be prepared to listen to the parents without hurrying. Thus, it is probably wise to set aside 30–45 minutes of nursing or physician time in order to accomplish these tasks.

History

Topics under these headings may have already been covered during the newborn visit.

PREGNANCY

Elicit previous pregnancy history. Was this pregnancy planned, difficult? Was there any bleeding, illness, hospitalization; were there infections or restrictions? What medications, alcohol, or street drugs were taken and when?

LABOR AND DELIVERY

Date and location of birth. Length and character of labor. Type of delivery, anesthesia. Were there any problems (did the baby cry right away?) Did the doctors comment on the baby's Apgar scores or birth weight?

NEWBORN

Were there any problems with breathing, feeding, jaundice? Did the baby go home from the hospital with the mother? What was the discharge weight?

FAMILY HISTORY

Specifically ascertain the age and health status of parents, siblings, and grandparents. Elicit any family history of inherited disease, early infant death, malformations, allergies, asthma, early heart attacks, hypertension, diabetes mellitus.

INTERVAL HISTORY

Always begin with an open-ended question such as, "How are you and the baby doing?" Ask about interaction with siblings.

DIET

In general, inquire what the baby is eating, how frequently, how much at a time, and are there any problems such as poor sucking, spitting up, etc? For breast-fed babies, specifically ask how long the baby spends at the breast, elicit maternal perceptions of the experience, and ask about specific problems such as cracked nipples, engorgement, soreness. For formula-fed babies, find out which formula is being used, how it is being mixed up, how long it takes to finish a can, whether the formula contains iron, and who else feeds the baby. Ask about other foods (such as solids), whether they are being given, as well as vitamins, fluoride, and iron.

ELIMINATION

Stools: color, consistency, frequency; urine: force of stream (especially for males), frequency.

Anticipatory Guidance

NORMAL INFANT BEHAVIOR

If not already discussed, go over normal patterns of eating, sleeping, crying, and elimination as well as the usual infant repertoire of reflexes (startle, sneeze, hiccough, pushing with defecation). Encourage parents *not* to sleep with the baby in their bed.

SAFETY

Car seats: If parents travel with the baby in a car, use of a car seat should be introduced now. If finances are a problem, rental is often available. Remind the parents not to leave the infant unsupervised on a table (i.e., possibility of rolling off).

Routine Follow-up

Next visit at age 2 months. Make sure that the parents know how to get in touch with you and encourage them to do so.

Two-Month Visit

The 2-month visit often marks a time of changing emphasis, away from concerns regarding basic body functions (eating, sleeping, elimination, etc) and toward a recognition of the child as a growing and developing individual. Beginning perhaps with the baby's first smile, and recognizing an increasing responsiveness by the child to sensory cues, parents sense an exciting progression in a child's development. Thus, the pediatrician should emphasize the child's growing awareness for his surroundings, and explore parental concerns and coping strategies as they emerge in the family.

History

INTERVAL HISTORY

Begin in an open-ended fashion by asking "How are things going?", or "How is the baby doing?" Determine primary parental concerns at the start of the visit, without making parents wait through a specific agenda.

DIET

Is the mother breast-feeding? Are there problems? Is mother feeling pressure to stop? By 2 months, although the technique is usually established, some mothers feel restricted by their situation, or have little energy for nursing (particularly if the child is temperamentally difficult). Is the child taking supplementary bottles? One bottle per day of formula or expressed breast milk may aid a mother and/or enable a father to participate in feedings.

What is the feeding schedule? By 2 months, most mothers can organize some routine such as at 8:00, 12:00, 4:00, and 7:00 with one night feeding. The details are less important than consistency.

For bottle-fed children, ask about the details of formula preparation.

A 2-month-old needs an average 120 cal/kg/day or 150 ml/kg/day.

Is the child taking vitamins? Breast-fed children require vitamins containing fluoride (TriViFlor, fluoride drops) to provide 0.25 mg of elemental fluoride daily, if there is no fluoride in the maternal diet. Vitamin D is also needed (400 IU daily), and can be provided by vitamin preparations. Iron is probably not necessary as a supplement for breast-fed children unless other foods are added to the diet that reduce absorption of iron from breast milk. Then the requirement is 7 mg/day. Infants receiving evaporated milk formulas need vitamin C (40 mg) and iron (7 mg) supplements. Most prepared formulas do not require supplementation.

ELIMINATION

A wide range of bowel function is considered normal at this age. Unless the stools are hard or bloody, most can be assumed to be normal provided that the child is growing and gaining well. Breast-fed children tend to have more frequent stools, but frequency ranges from one every few days to 6–10/day. Blood is most often from anal fissures. Hard stools may be managed by removing iron, by adding carbohydrate (such as Karo syrup), or by adding extra water to the formula.

COLIC

Is the child straining, crying excessively? When does crying occur?

DEVELOPMENTAL

Is the child smiling responsively, cooing, gurgling? Does the baby follow an object with his eyes? Does he raise his head from the prone position?

Physical Examination

VITAL SIGNS

Plot weight, height, head circumference. The full term infant's head grows 2.5 cm per month in circumference, in the premature infant, it may be as fast as 1 cm per week (see appropriate charts).

GENERAL MEDICAL EXAMINATION

The posterior fontanelle is usually closed. Careful cardiovascular, pulmonary, and abdominal examinations are important. Check for hernias, and for testicular descent in boys. A careful hip examination is needed, as congenital dislocation may not be evident at birth. Is a tibial torsion or metatarsus adductus present? If the foot can be maneuvered to neutral, massage and re-evaluation may be the only treatment required.

Preventive/Screening

IMMUNIZATIONS

Most children receive the first diphtheria, tetanus, pertussis and oral polio vaccines (OPV) at this time. It is generally accepted that 2 months chronologic age is appropriate as well for prematures. Contraindications are febrile illness, immunosuppression (consider postponement for siblings of children with hereditary immunologic deficiencies) or evolving neurologic disease.

TEMPERATURE

A significant number of children will experience their first fever after the DTP. Do the parents have a thermometer? Do they know how to use one? Do they know how to respond to an elevation in temperature?

Routine Follow-up

Next visit at age 4 months.

Four-Month Visit

At this age, the infant is often "delightful" in that schedules of sleeping and feeding become more fixed, and the child is growing more sociable.

History

INTERVAL HISTORY

How are things going? Has the child been well since the last visit? Do you have any concerns?

DIET

If the mother is breast-feeding, have there been any problems? What are both parents' attitudes about plans for continuing or stopping this approach. It may be necessary to discuss the positive and negative attributes of substitutes when converting to the bottle which may occur over the next few months. For bottle-fed children, ask about possible formulas or milk switches. Review plans for additions to the diet if the child is not yet taking them (or what factors led to their addition against your advice). Cereals, fruits, and vegetables may be introduced between 4 and 6 months, usually in that order. Fruit juices permit a nursing mother to omit a feeding.

ELIMINATION

Ask about changes in these functions or related parental concerns.

SLEEP

By 4 months some babies may sleep through the night. If not, a review of the child's other schedules, temperament, and familial factors and responses is appropriate.

DEVELOPMENT

Do the parents have questions about the baby's progress?

SOCIAL/BEHAVIORAL

What are the parents' perceptions of their baby's temperament? How does the child respond to change, such as new food or surroundings? Is the child easy or difficult to manage?

Physical Examination

VITAL SIGNS

Plot the height, weight, and head circumference, with attention to the velocity of growth.

GENERAL EXAMINATION

A full physical examination is done, with particular attention to areas of parental concern, or of risk (based on the history). Specific features for attention include: the ability of a child to follow an object 180° in the horizontal plane, an assessment of the hip regarding adductor tone, penile and labial adhesions.

DEVELOPMENTAL

Does the child manage tasks relating to functions including:

1. fine motor—hands to midline, reaches for/grasps items
2. gross motor—good head control (steady with sitting), rolling over (front to back precedes back to front)
3. language—squeals and laughs may be present; a child begins to turn to sounds and voices

Preventive/Screening

VISION

Observe ability to follow objects, and look for constant strabismus.

HEARING

Note the child's response to soft voices, or a ringing bell.

IMMUNIZATION

Give the child's second DTP and oral polio immunizations barring contraindications. Inquire about specific reactions to the first shot, for both minor and major responses.

Anticipatory Guidance

SAFETY

Safety concerns should be highlighted as the baby's motor skills increase. Baby can now roll over and roll off beds, sofas, changing tables, etc. The ability to reach for and grasp objects in this ever-expanding space makes a "baby-proof" house imperative. Beware of small object ingestion. Re-emphasize the use of car seat.

INFANT ACTIVITY

With head held erect the child may now use jumpers, walkers, and high chairs, with appropriate warnings about potential hazards, especially with walkers.

DENTAL

Teething questions arise, though time of first tooth eruption is very variable. Drooling may be a sign of developing salivary glands and does not necessarily mean baby is teething.

ILLNESS

Discuss upper respiratory infections. Baby's immunity is near low point because of a decrease in mother's passively transmitted immunoglobulins.

Routine Follow-up

Next visit at age 6 months.

Six-Month Visit

This is a period of considerable social development and should be an enjoyable time for the family.

History

DIET

What is the child eating? Most are taking several different types of fruits and vegetables. At the 6-month visit, families may wish to switch to whole cow's milk, but formula is less likely to contribute to iron loss from the bowel and is generally recommended until 9–12 months. Discuss weaning with breast-feeding mothers; some may want to wait until 1 year of age before weaning and others want to start now. Parents may start baby on baby meats. Parents should start baby on supplemental iron—1 mg/kg/24 hr (Fer-in-Sol); fortified cereal is another source of iron.

ELIMINATION

The gastrocolic reflex is decreased by 6 months. How are the bowels and bladder functioning?

SLEEP

Baby may be sleeping through the night at this time, however, some infants may start awakening in the night, and need reassurance. A simple stroking (not a bottle) should be enough. Parents may be encouraged to leave the child with a sitter while they go out by themselves. It is best if the baby has seen the sitter before.

BEHAVIOR

Infants begin to differentiate themselves from the outer world and become "persons." With a more acute awareness of differences in people, a child may experience the beginning of stranger anxiety, recognizing parents as different from all others. The sucking need is less and it is time to attempt withdrawing a pacifier. Teething is in progress. Suggest a teething ring; one filled with liquid that may be refrigerated (cold feels better) may be preferred.

DEVELOPMENT

No head lag when pulled to sitting. Sits without support. Not present in all 6-month-olds, but should be assessed from this age. Turns to sounds; rolls over; reaches for objects; pincer grasp beginning; babbles; puts objects in mouth.

INTERCURRENT ILLNESS

Discuss any intercurrent illnesses.

LIVING SITUATION

Discuss home environment. Is living space restricted so that the baby has to sleep in same room as parent? Is current dwelling suitable for a baby who will soon be exploring the environment? Does family need help with housing?

Preventive/Screening

IMMUNIZATIONS

Time for third immunization (DTP, OPV). Ask about previous fevers with DTP. Child may be given acetaminophen (Tylenol) liquid. Fever should not last more than 24 hours; if very high or does not resolve, parents should call pediatrician.

Physical Examination

Check weight, height, head circumference.

AGE-SPECIFIC ITEMS

Head:	Anterior fontanelle may start to close.
Mouth:	Central incisors may be starting to come in.
Eyes:	Any strabismus by 6 months is abnormal; if present, should see ophthalmologist.
Ears:	Check hearing by seeing if baby turns to sound.
Genitourinary:	Inquire (if observation not possible) about adequacy of urinary stream.
Neurologic:	Reflexes: Moro and tonic neck reflexes should not be present; Babinski—normal until 1 year; parachute reflex begins; weight-bearing on lower extremities.

Anticipatory Guidance

Review issues regarding diet, accidents, family adjustment. Many developments occur at this age. Discuss plans for another baby, and the need to space pregnancies. It is best to wait 2 years to permit adequate parenting of the older child and lessen risk of preterm birth.

Routine Follow-up

Next visit at age 9 months.

Nine-Month Visit

History

INTERVAL HISTORY: RECENT ILLNESS

May need to explain the "normal" number of respiratory infections.

NUTRITION

An accurate dietary history is important at this age when solid food intake is increasing, weaning is being entertained. Ask about special diets: vegetarian; any pica? Begin to wean off bottle.

ELIMINATION

Any problems?

SLEEP

There may be difficulty putting the child to bed; bedtime rituals may help in this regard.

DEVELOPMENT

1. Gross motor—Can the child crawl, "cruise," stand holding on or pull to stand? Inability to sit without support indicates a delay.
2. Fine motor—Thumb-finger grasp should be becoming secure. Does the baby transfer block hand to hand, or feed self with cracker?
3. Language—Does the baby babble, jabber, and imitate speech sound? Say Mama and Dada?
4. Personal/social—Plays peek-a-boo (and maybe pat-a-cake). Looks for fallen object. Resists toy being pulled away.

SOCIAL/BEHAVIORAL

Inquire about playing with siblings or other children.

Physical Examination

Height, weight, and head circumference. NOTE: many normal children will drop a few percentiles between 6 and 12 months; this may be due to decreased milk intake associated with increased intake of solids. Check eruption of teeth. Check for strabismus. Check the developmental points noted above. Carry out a complete physical examination, and discuss the findings with the parents.

Prevention

May do at 1 year.

SCREENING TESTS

Hematocrit (optional, desirable if receiving cow's milk). Free erythrocyte protoporphyrin (FEP) (optional). Sickle cell screen, if indicated. Consider the formal administration of the Denver Development Screen, at 9 or 12 months for all children.

Anticipatory Guidance

PHYSICAL HEALTH ISSUES

1. The child is becoming increasingly mobile, so "baby-proofing" the house should be emphasized, with specific recommendations for cabinet locks, keeping poisons out of reach, and electric socket safety. However, the child should have areas of the house which are safe, so that normal exploration can be allowed.
2. Ipecac should be prescribed and parents instructed in its use to induce vomiting after ingestion of poisons, other than caustic substances. Parents should be told to call pediatrician or poison center before giving ipecac.
3. Help prevent caries by encouraging brushing or cleaning of the child's new teeth, and strongly discouraging bedtime bottles, unless only water is given.
4. Discuss diet, and the importance of maintaining adequate milk, formula, or breast milk intake as the intake of solid foods increases. Sweets should be discouraged. The cup may be introduced, but not yet relied upon for milk intake.

About this time, a normal decrease in appetite begins.

DEVELOPMENTAL ISSUES

1. This can be a peak age for the infant to have feelings of anxiety about separation from family and exposure to strangers. Related to this is a strong need for affection.
2. The child must be able to satisfy his normal curiosity. Saying "no" and other disciplinary actions should be reserved for dangerous situations, not for normal exploration. The child will enjoy large boxes to crawl in, large balls or blocks, and hide-and-seek games.

PARENTING ISSUES

1. Discuss the importance of responding to the child's initiatives with peek-a-boo or imitating sounds.
2. Explore with the parents their feelings about weaning, toilet training, and discipline. If the parents are being pressured about toilet training, "let them off the hook" by explaining that most children are not ready for toilet training until after 18 months.
3. As usual, reassure the parents that they are doing a good job.

Routine Follow-up

Next visit at age 1 year.

One-Year Visit

The child and family are emerging from a period of considerable adjustment (sleep, diet, activity, temperament). This visit can be an important time for guidance on unresolved issues.

History

INTERVAL HISTORY

How are things going? Any problems or illnesses since the last visit?

DIET

The child should be managing to feed himself. Is table behavior excessively disruptive? How often is he being fed? Most (90%) can manage with three meals a day at this stage. The child should have all classes of foods except those that could be easily aspirated (peanuts and popcorn). Some authorities recommend 1 year as a time of conversion from formula to whole milk.

ELIMINATION

Any problems?

SLEEP

Is the child going to sleep without resistance? Rocking, head banging, and finger sucking are normal. Most children are awakening by 5:00–6:00 AM, and will nap in the afternoon.

DEVELOPMENTAL

Can the child hold on to furniture, or stand alone for 2–3 seconds (gross motor); bang blocks together (fine motor); imitate vocalizations (language); or play patty cake (social)? More than 90% of 1-year-olds can perform these activities. The child often manages 3–4 words with meaning at 1 year.

Physical Examination

Height and weight should be obtained, including head circumference. A complete physical should be done, with attention to strabismus, hernia, muscle tone, lower extremity problems (torsions, etc).

Preventive/Screening

At 1 year, the following studies can be obtained.

1. A PPD or tine test (9 or 12 months); this should be done before measles, mumps, rubella vaccinations, to avoid anergy;
2. Hemoglobin or hematocrit;
3. Urinalysis;
4. Lead screening (FEP or blood lead) (in locations of likely exposure);
5. Sickle cell screen (if indicated by ethnicity).

Anticipatory Guidance

Parents sharing discipline.

Fifteen- and 18-Month Visits

These months mark a period of intense social growth for the child, when many variations are seen among children.

History

INTERVAL HISTORY

1. Identify any problems for the child (i.e., crying, sleep patterns, feeding, vomiting, sphincter control), and review family and social history. This history should include who is responsible for child care (i.e., mother-father, day care, babysitter).
2. Nutrition—inquire about appetite, milk intake.
3. Developmental—12 months and up—sits on floor with no support; chews (7 months); bye-bye, patty-cake, crawls on abdomen (9 months); helps dress, creeps (hands and knees) (10 months); walks (holding on) (11 months); words with meaning (12 months).
4. Social—interactions at home with family.

Physical Examination

General physical examination includes growth paramaters (do not forget teeth). Developmental and neurological—full examination with a special emphasis on the child's interest, alertness, responsiveness. Tone reflexes and strength (by 18 months, all children should be able to go from sitting to standing without holding on). Check hearing. Can child secure grasp with both hands? Gait—does the child walk well? Can he stoop to pick up a toy? Speech—this is usually examined by history because many children will not speak in the doctor's office. Can the child roll or toss ball back to examiner? At 15 months, can the child build a tower of two 1-inch cubes? Manage a cup without help? At 18 months, can the child create a tower of three to four 1-inch cubes? Point to two to three body parts?

IMMUNIZATIONS

At 15 months—should have had DTP/OPV three times; tuberculin (tine) test one time. At 15 months—measles, mumps, rubella vaccine (MMR). At 18 months—DTP/OPV, *H. influenzae* B vaccine.

Counseling

Any specific concerns? Review areas that should have been covered before, but are still important.

1. Make sure all dangerous substances are out of reach. Parents have ipecac at home and know how to use it.
2. No bottle to bed, except with water if necessary.
3. Car seat.

Continuing discussion:

1. Beginning of toilet training.
2. Methods for dealing with negativism and behavior problems (i.e., obedience and temper tantrums).

Anticipatory Guidance

Review accident prevention, ipecac, car seat, weaning, night bottles.

TOILET TRAINING

Discuss benefits of waiting for the child to mature regarding possible success and problems (i.e., until at least 18 months). Then, a nonpressured, step-by-step, behavioral approach can be instituted.

DISCIPLINE

Discuss coping strategies for dealing with negativism and behavior problems (obedience and tantrums). Treat child with respect at all times.

Routine Follow-up

Next visit at age 18 months, then 24 months.

Two- and 2½-Year Visits

This age marks a period of personality and cognitive growth for children when parenting issues are often prominent. Issues of control become central, and should be appreciated as a child's striving for independence. The 30-month visit is considered optional by some doctors, especially for children at low risk.

History

INTERVAL HISTORY

Recent illnesses should be reviewed. Problems and concerns for the child or family should be identified. Caretaking arrangements can be discussed.

DIET

Ask about the child's habits and preferences, with a review of dietary balance and calories, as well as any parental concerns.

ELIMINATION

Inquire as to the status of the training process. Bowel control often precedes control of urine and by 30 months, 75% of boys and 90% of girls will have established bowel control.

SLEEP

Review parental concerns, pattern, location (with parents?).

DEVELOPMENTAL

Use the following "tasks" guidelines with the categories of:

1. Gross motor—24 months—kicks a ball without support for balance, walks up steps; 30 months—jumps with both feet in place, throws overhead.
2. Fine motor—24 months—dumps raisins from jar, scribbles spontaneously; 30 months—stacks more than four cubes, copies a horizontal and vertical line within 30 degrees of standard.

SOCIAL

Helps put things away, assists with dressing and does most of undressing. At 24 months, the child points correctly to body parts.

LANGUAGE

At 30 months, the child uses phrases and "I". Repeats a sequence of two digits, follows two of three simple instructions "Give block to . . . Mom; table; floor."

SOCIAL/BEHAVIORAL

At 24 months, a child often cannot share, or take turns. Stubbornness, tantrums, and aggression are all common issues. By the mid-2s, a child's attention is turning toward peers as well as mother, and conversations as well as activities. Exploration of object qualities and mastery of simple skills remain active pursuits. A child manages best near one or two other children, who may be watched more than played with directly. Also, children may show their first interest in TV. Other activities enjoyed include climbing, swings, blocks, clay, and very simple puzzles.

Physical Examination

Height and weight should be obtained, with an attempt at obtaining the child's blood pressure. At age 2 years, perform a full examination. At 30 months, a full physical examination is optional, but can be directed at interval problems, parental concerns, or chronic disease issues.

Preventive/Screening

Thirty months is usually the time for the first formal vision screening with picture cards. Normal vision is 20/30–20/40 at this age. Of five cards, three should be identified at a distance of 15 feet. *Haemophilus influenzae* type B (Hib) immunization is advised (even if given at 18 months). Urinalysis/culture, hematocrit/lead, and PPD may be checked for high-risk groups.

Anticipatory Guidance

HANDEDNESS

A child usually shows hand preference by 1–2 years and it is firmly established by 3–5 years of age. Because lateralization is likely to reflect brain development, it is not surprising that delay in its development is associated with other developmental delays. By contrast, about half of very low birth weight infants (under 1 kg) are left-handed or ambidextrous. About 90% of people are right-handed. Left-handedness tends to be familial, with males more prone to it than females. Thus, left-handed fathers have a greater likelihood of a left-handed son than a daughter (Longstreth, 1980).

On the average, the ability to distinquish left from right is achieved by age 6 years, and the added ability to identify the examiner's left from right side is evident by age 9 or 10 years. Left to right reversal of letters is very common when the child first begins to write, and almost always changes to normal writing without intervention.

Topics

Many behavior problems are precipitated by significant change in the family (new school, move, marital problems, siblings). A bedtime routine is important, and should not be too stimulating. Parents should support each other in setting firm appropriate limits, or seek help if problems escalate.

TODDLER BEHAVIOR—SAFETY

This may be a time of increased genital manipulation and parental attitudes should be addressed. Major concerns are falls (stairs, windows), ingestion of foreign bodies or poisons, foot injuries (stings, cuts), and, especially, (a) water safety (pools, tubs) and (b) street safety. A 30-month-old cannot maintain satisfactory limits, and environmental management is essential. Use parks, playgrounds, or fenced-in areas.

TELEVISION

Suggestions concerning selective time with television: use and limits for toddlers should be discussed.

NURSERY SCHOOLS

These often have long waiting lists, so, if appropriate for the child and family, guidance and registration should be considered now.

Routine Follow-up

Next visit at age 3 years.

Three-Year Visit

History

INTERVAL HISTORY

There are no specific questions for this age group. Ask questions as to general status of mother/child/family and include recent (or interval) illnesses, accidents, and injuries.

DIET

Ascertain whether the diet is: (a) adequate in calories and (b) well balanced. Ask what role the child is playing in feeding himself and how problems of over-, under-, and inappropriate eating are dealt with by parents. NOTE: Parents may misinterpret the normal decrease in calorie requirement, and hence focus on appetite, rather than body weight, when suggesting a problem with undereating.

ELIMINATION

Focus on the status of toilet training. Ask about bowel and bladder control, both during the day and at night. Also ask if new problems have arisen as the 3-year-old begins to assert control over his body (and with this new ability, over the family as well). (See discussion of toilet training in 2-year visit.) One can reassure parents with the statistics that: 10% of 3-year-olds lack bowel control; 15% of 3-year-olds lack daytime bladder control; 33% of 3-year olds lack nighttime bladder control. Hence, failure to achieve control by age 3 years is not unusual.

SLEEP

Determine the child's pattern, i.e., bedtime, waking hour, naps. Ask about difficulties in getting child to bed, awakening during the night and how these problems are approached by parents.

DEVELOPMENTAL

Use the following tasks as guidelines in assessing development in the four categories.

1. Gross motor—pedals tricycle, goes upstairs one foot per step, stands on one foot for a few seconds.
2. Fine motor—copies a circle, begins to button/unbutton.
3. Language—uses plurals; uses four-word sentences; beginning to understand use of prepositions "in," "on," "under"; knows some nursery rhymes.
4. Social/personal—feeds self, takes off shoes and jacket, washes and dries hands; knows own sex; beginning to play with other children.

SOCIAL/BEHAVIORAL

Discuss behavior that is prominent at this age: resolution of the negativism; able to understand some logic and is almost conversational; tries to do what is expected of him; constantly questioning; sometimes has unreasonable fears; discovers sexual differences. Ask about plans for nursery school and readiness as judged by ability to be separated from home.

Physical Examination

Complete examination should be possible at this age; use of puppet as "patient" may be helpful; blood pressure (should be measured now if not earlier). Hearing assessment—reaction to or repetition of whispered speech.

VISUAL ACUITY

Age 3 years is probably the earliest age at which assessment of visual acuity can be performed reliably. Vision is tested by use of a Snellen Chart at 20 feet. "E" figures are preferable. Children should be taken up to the chart so they can examine the figures at close range and learn to indicate the direction of the "E" before formal testing. If testing is not successful, mother can teach the child the procedure at home before the next visit. Use of figures depicting familiar objects is an alternative to their names. Referral to an ophthalmologist should be made if vision in either eye (when tested separately) is unequal. An assessment of whether gaze is conjugate can be made with cover tests.

Preventive/Screening

No immunizations necessary, unless missed at an earlier age. Laboratory testing of hematocrit/hemoglobin (Hct/Hgb) as part of lead (Pb) screen. Urine culture in girls (optional). Skin testing—tine (in regions where exposure is likely). If result equivocal, PPD (purified protein derivative). Dental appointments should be started.

Anticipatory Guidance

Parents should be advised about the following areas:

1. Accident update—guard against falls, drowning, motor vehicle accidents, ingestions of foreign objects, and burns. (Check on car seats and seat belts.) It is still necessary to lock doors and windows, review cars and street crossing, and teach about sharp objects.
2. Nutrition—ensure adequate calorie intake and balanced diet; avoid faddism.
3. Disciplinary issues—emphasize need for consistency and agreement between parents; use of removal of wanted object and beginning use of logic in explaining wrongdoing.
4. Emphasize need for dental care with visit to dentist soon after this visit.
5. Straightforward approach to sexual discovery—tolerance of some degree of sexual play and certainly no use of punishment. Instruction about sexual molestation.

Routine Follow-up

Next visit at age 4 years.

Four-Year Visit

This visit marks a period of transition for most children as the time when growth and developmental gains are more steadily accomplished, and when traditional medical concerns become less prominent.

History

INTERVAL HISTORY

Questions regarding the interval health history are asked as well as information about the condition of the family.

DIET

Ask about eating habits and preferences, with attention to balance and quantity. It is important to identify children at risk from unusual or bad diets. Is the child receiving an excess of sweets? Dental checkups every 6 months should be encouraged, as children experience their greatest period of carious activity at 4–8 years. Watch for obesity, as success in treatment often depends on early intervention.

ELIMINATION

Is the child experiencing bed wetting (about one-third of 4-year-olds do), or daytime enuresis? What are the child's and parents' attitudes and responses? Has the child experienced constipation or soiling (encopresis)?

BEHAVIOR

Is the child lying, overly stubborn, or destructive? Ask about excessive shyness, clinging, jealousy, selfishness, and temper.

DEVELOPMENTAL

Do the parents have specific concerns about the child's progress?

Physical Examination

SENSORY

Vision and hearing screens are important for all children. Most children can use an E chart. Immunizations are not required if currently up to date.

Anticipatory Guidance

NORMAL CHILD

Normal behavior at this age is characterized by shyness, short attention span, and distractibility. There may be a persistence of negativism seen earlier. This is a consideration in the assessment of a child's performance or when advising parents. An increase in socialization and peer activity occurs, and many problems may be manifested at this age. The process of socialization may be aided by nursery school and more outside excursions.

SAFETY

Four-year-olds should be taught how to respond to the home smoke alarm, to buckle their seat belts, and to avoid eating berries, plants, etc, outside. Continued monitoring of home safety by the parents should be encouraged.

Routine Follow-up

Next visit at age 5 years.

Five-Year (Preschool) Visit

This examination is an important contact point for pediatricians, as preparation for school entry requires completion of the basic immunizations at this time, as well as a general examination before the start of school. It is a time which is well-suited for a full developmental assessment, and sensory screenings, as a determination of school readiness.

History

INTERVAL HISTORY

Ask about illnesses, injuries, or major changes for the child or family since the last visit. If desired, address general parental and child concerns via open-ended questions.

DIET

Continue to review the child's eating style and habits, with special regard to snacks, and excessive intake of any given food.

ELIMINATION

Ask about patterns of stool frequency and nature as well as control of bladder and bowel functions. Also consider latent urinary tract symptoms.

DEVELOPMENT

Are there specific concerns about the child's rate of progress?

SOCIAL/BEHAVIORAL

Ask about the child's social interaction in regard to separation, sharing, etc. How is the child's attention span? Is the child's activity level a major disruption at home or school?

Physical Examination

GENERAL

Focus attention on speech rhythm, articulation, tone, clarity.

VITAL SIGNS

Plot height, weight, and blood pressure.

GENERAL MEDICAL EXAMINATION

Areas of emphasis include funduscopy; the cover test for heterophorias; dental hygiene. Check for scoliosis or flat pronated feet.

Preventive/Screening

PROCEDURES

Check a urinalysis for protein, glucose, cells. Obtain a clean-voided specimen for all girls.

IMMUNIZATIONS

Give an OPV/DTP vaccination, providing the child's previous shots were up to date and no untoward reactions have been noted.

DEVELOPMENTAL SCREENING FOR SCHOOL READINESS

Consider results of locally administered developmental screens (available in many towns) and/or perform a full screen. Pediatric examination of educational readiness (Levine or other—Denver) (see pp. 44–46).

Social—separates easily from mother, dresses without supervision

Fine motor—picks longer line (three of three times); copies +

Gross motor—balances on one foot 5 seconds (two of three times); hops on one foot

Language—recognizes colors (three of four); opposite analogies (two of three) fire/hot/ice— mother/woman/dad.

Anticipatory Guidance

ACCIDENT PREVENTION

Issues include seat belt use, burns, falls, poisons.

SCHOOL PLACEMENT ISSUES

Anticipate separation problems, assess parental attitudes and plans.

Routine Follow-up

Next visit at age 6 years, and annually or biannually thereafter.

Visit for the School-Age Child

During the school years, children establish more independence and autonomy. Acute illnesses are much less frequent than during early childhood years, and school, behavioral and emotional complaints predominate. For generally healthy children, yearly visits are recommended during this time although there are few data to support the benefit of these visits when only medical outcomes are measured. Visits are encouraged to maintain contact, assess adjustment to school, peers, and family, and provide a chance to observe "the whole child."

History

In earlier years, the child's parents are the chief source of history, but now the physician may prefer to interview and examine children without their parents present in the room. This demonstrates to the child that the physician sees him as independent from his parents and allows the child to express things to the physician that he may not express with his parents present. Many physicians also prefer to interview parents alone before they meet with the child so that parents may freely discuss issues to which their child may not be particularly sensitive. Optimally, this should be done while he is getting his height and weight measured. Meeting with the parents alone after the child has been seen should be avoided because children often feel excluded from discussions and may fantasize about what is being said about them. In addition, children usually do recognize any problems that they have, even though they may not express them verbally. During interviews with both the parents and child present, the physician should make a point of addressing the child as well as the parents.

A general medical history is required for any new patient. For patients who have been seen previously, an interval medical history is sufficient. In addition, school performance, development, relationships with peers, relationships at home, interval events, and any behavioral concerns should be investigated.

Self-administered questionnaires can be used for screening to identify problem areas. Often a parent will identify specific areas of concern more readily on a questionnaire (by circling a word or marking a box) than with an open-ended question. However, it is important in every interview to leave some time open for discussion.

Physical Examination

When school is entered, every child should have a complete physical examination. If it is entirely normal, a complete physical does not need to be repeated every year. However, every year the following should be checked.

VISUAL SCREEN

1. Visual acuity should be tested by use of a Snellen chart with each eye individually and both together.
2. Strabismus should be screened for. This is most easily done by having a child focus on an object, alternately covering each eye, and watching for a compensatory shift of the covered eye when the cover is removed.
3. Color vision should be tested at the time school is entered by using specially designed charts.

Children with problems of visual acuity or strabismus should be referred to an ophthalmologist for further evaluation. If a child has impaired color vision, no referral is necessary, but it will help a child to be aware of color vision deficits.

HEARING SCREEN

Pure tone audiometric screening can be done by referring patients to an audiology department, or may be performed in a pediatrician's office.

HEIGHT AND WEIGHT

Height and weight should be plotted on a growth chart each year. Deviations from normal are often hard to assess because there is so much individual variation. However, changes in growth pattern may be helpful in detecting underlying otherwise subtle abnormalities including endocrine and gastrointestinal disorders.

BLOOD PRESSURE

It is adequate to check blood pressure every 2 years. However, it should be checked yearly in children with positive family history, obesity, or other risk factors.

SCOLIOSIS

The back should be checked each year for early signs of scoliosis, especially in girls. The spine should be examined from the back while the child stands in front of the examiner. The child should then bend forward, flexing 90° at the waist. The scapulae should remain level at all times. Any child with abnormalities should be referred to an orthopedic surgeon (see Section 23).

PSYCHOMOTOR ASSESSMENT

Time does not usually permit detailed psychomotor assessment. Problem areas can usually be identified by asking about school performance and sports participation and examination and/or appropriate referrals can be done in accordance with identified problem areas.

Preventive/Screening

LABORATORY

1. The value of laboratory assessment in this age group is controversial. Between the ages of 4 and 10 years, Hgb and Hct determination is not thought to be necessary if previous tests have been normal.
2. Some recommend that urine should be "dipsticked" at least once during the school years to look for proteinuria and glycosuria. Girls should be screened for asymptomatic bacteriuria at least once during the school years. Those with a history of urinary tract infection should be screened more often.

DENTAL CARE

Every child should have regular dental checkups.

IMMUNIZATIONS

If immunizations have been up-to-date previously, DTP and OPV are necessary on admission to school. Td should be repeated every 10 years. Tetanus toxoid should be repeated if there is a contaminated injury more than 5 years after the last dose.

Anticipatory Guidance

ACCIDENTS

Accidents are the leading cause of death in this age group. Parents and children should be instructed to: (a) use seat belts when riding in cars; (b) obey traffic rules when riding bicycles; (c) keep firearms locked up and away from children; (d) children should be taught to swim and should be properly supervised when around water; (e) the seriousness of burns should be emphasized; (f) sports should be properly supervised.

NORMAL BEHAVIOR

Parents should be warned that this is a time when children become increasingly independent from their parents. Some children will have anxiety reactions during this process of separation. This is a time when children need consistent limit setting. They will also challenge limits and guidelines. Age-appropriate sex education should be encouraged.

School years are exciting times. Children are verbal enough to communicate readily with adults. Their individual personalities become more apparent and there is often a vitality which has not yet been inhibited by the stresses of the adult world.

BODY/SOMATIC CONCERNS

Many anxieties may become manifested by somatic complaints such as abdominal pain and headache.

Adolescent Visit

Adolescence is a period in life when good health is the rule rather than the exception. Trauma, acute infectious disease, and routine school, job, or camp physical examinations are the most frequent reasons given for adolescent medical visits and care. In large pediatric medical centers, adolescents are cared for with a wide variety of medical problems that are often complex and chronic. The growth and development issues, both physical and psychological, become an integral part of the physician's management of the presenting problem. When one adds the social pressures imposed by the adolescent's environment in the family, school, and community it is readily apparent that adolescent health care has the potential to become a significant portion of pediatric practice.

It is useful to consider the developmental tasks an adolescent must achieve to become a mature adult.

1. Achieve identity/self-esteem/self-image
2. Acceptance of change within themselves
3. Strength to achieve independence
4. Relationships with the opposite sex
5. Relationships with peers
6. Cognitive and vocational achievement
7. Ability to control periods of depression

While not all inclusive, this list is a starting point in the evaluation of adolescent complaints. The inability to achieve any one or more of these goals may bring about behavior problems, poor school performance, and disruption of communication patterns with parents and peers. These young people in distress may be unable to function adequately in society. When these conflicts are expressed as somatic complaints the patient may be referred to a pediatrician who is known to have an interest in adolescent medicine. To diagnose correctly and then to manage and treat appropriately, the adolescent with a psychosomatic problem requires extraordinary skill on the part of the pediatrician. Patients and their parents can and do resist the notion that the somatic complaints are but a reflection of the turmoil in the adolescent's life. Hence the need for the pediatrician to remain medically vigilant throughout the period of sorting out the emotional conflicts. Occasionally, a referral for psychotherapy is appropriate and should be directed not only to meet the patient's needs, but also to support the parents.

History

Although most adolescent patients will be able to furnish reasonably accurate past medical information, it is advisable for the physician to check with the parents regarding early development, injuries, illnesses, surgery, and immunizations.

When taking the history from the adolescent, it is imperative that the adolescent be seen alone. A brief visit with parents and adolescent is satisfactory only when it is designed to gain general information and not sensitive material which requires a confidential relationship between physician and patient. Clearly the adolescent patient should be treated more as an adult than a child. Special subjects must be covered.

SUBSTANCE USE

Tobacco, alcohol, drugs (street and over the counter), and prescribed medications must be discussed.

SEXUAL ACTIVITY

This information will not be difficult to obtain when the inquiry is made in a professional manner which is both thoughtful and considerate of the patient's feelings.

SCHOOL

School level, attendance, and performance must be ascertained. Are there any learning problems, tutoring, or special classes?

SOCIAL

Relationship with parents, siblings, peers, relatives, teachers, and others in the community may be elicited in the course of the history taking.

CAREER GOALS

A specific answer may not be forthcoming but the patient will be able to tell the physician about areas of special interest and talent, i.e., sports, music, drama, etc. After school and summer jobs should be explored.

REVIEW OF SYSTEMS

In addition to the traditional system review, for the adolescent female the menarchal history must be obtained. For both sexes, when appropriate (and it often is), inquiry as to sexually transmitted disease is important.

Physical Examination

The physical examination need not be supervised by either a parent or nurse. Should the parent insist on being in the examining room, it is advisable to do a limited examination and not an examination which would embarrass the adolescent. Pelvic and rectal examinations on female patients when the physician is a male will require the presence of a nurse or nursing assistant in the room. The decision as to whether or not to do a pelvic and rectal examination will be determined by the patient's complaints and whether or not she is sexually active. A rectal examination for either a male or female adolescent is not routine, but may become a part of the regular physical examination when the patient reaches 18 years of age. It is always important to inspect the genitalia and determine the Tanner stage of sexual development (see pp. 872).

Height and weight should be noted and recorded as part of the record on a growth chart. Earlier heights and weights should be obtained from the parents or the previous pediatrician.

Breast examination with Tanner staging should be done. Male gynecomastia, when present, should be noted and discussed with the patient. Invariably, the young male (typically in the 13- to 16-year age range) with gynecomastia will have two major concerns. Am I growing a female breast or do I have cancer? Clearly the physician's input at this time is critical for the patient's well-being.

Preventive/Screeening

1. PPD yearly (depends on prevalence of tuberculosis)
2. Tetanus-diptheria booster at approximately 15 years of age or 10 years after the last booster
3. Urinalysis
4. Hematocrit
5. Rubella titers for the females; if negative, then immunize
6. Fasting cholesterol and triglycerides for adolescents with a positive family history of atherosclerotic disease and coronary artery disease in early and middle adult years

Routine health care for adolescents who are not seen frequently can be accomplished by means of a medical examination every 2 years through high school. The opportunity for the physician to develop a relationship in this manner is self-evident. The meeting for a checkup should lead to a discussion that will include the topics already listed as part of the history taking. The time given for this visit need not be lengthy. Adolescents will appreciate the physician's willingness and interest to help them then or in the future (Fig.1.1).

ACCIDENT PREVENTION

Throughout these guidelines we have listed under anticipatory guidance the topic of accident prevention

GUIDELINES FOR HEALTH SUPERVISION

Each child and family is unique; therefore these **Guidelines for Health Supervision of Children and Youth**[1] are designed for the care of children who are receiving competent parenting, have no manifestations of any important health problems, and are growing and developing in satisfactory fashion. **Additional visits may become necessary** if circumstances suggest variations from normal. These guidelines represent a consensus by the Committee on Practice and Ambulatory Medicine, in consultation with the membership of the American Academy of Pediatrics through the Chapter Chairmen.

The Committee emphasizes the great importance of **continuity of care** in comprehensive health supervision[2] and the need to avoid **fragmentation of care**[3].

A **prenatal visit** by the parents for anticipatory guidance and pertinent medical history is strongly recommended.

Health supervision should begin with medical care of the newborn in the hospital.

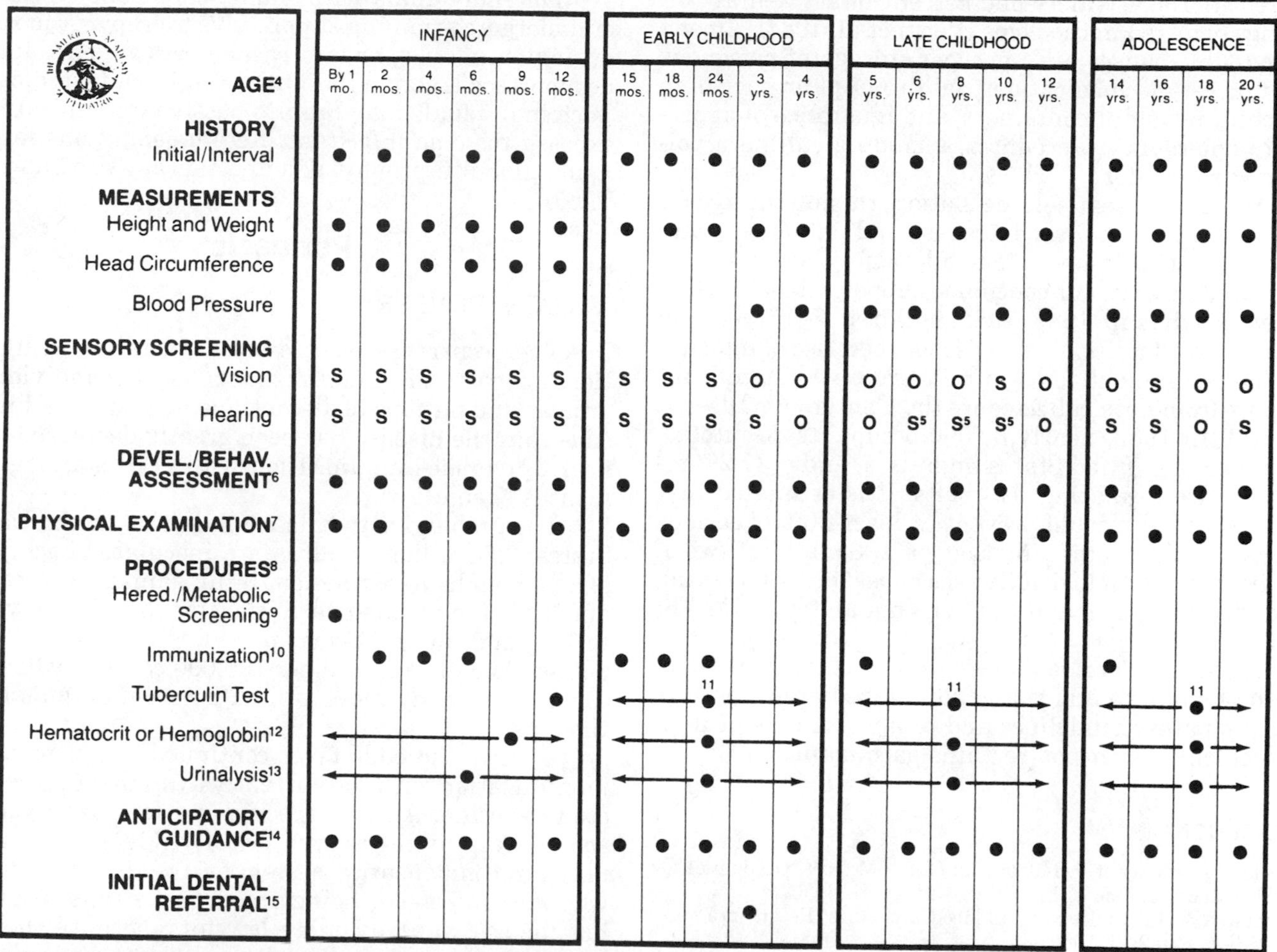

	INFANCY						EARLY CHILDHOOD					LATE CHILDHOOD					ADOLESCENCE			
AGE[4]	By 1 mo.	2 mos.	4 mos.	6 mos.	9 mos.	12 mos.	15 mos.	18 mos.	24 mos.	3 yrs.	4 yrs.	5 yrs.	6 yrs.	8 yrs.	10 yrs.	12 yrs.	14 yrs.	16 yrs.	18 yrs.	20+ yrs.
HISTORY Initial/Interval	●	●	●	●	●	●	●	●	●	●	●	●	●	●	●	●	●	●	●	●
MEASUREMENTS Height and Weight	●	●	●	●	●	●	●	●	●	●	●	●	●	●	●	●	●	●	●	●
Head Circumference	●	●	●	●	●	●														
Blood Pressure										●	●	●	●	●	●	●	●	●	●	●
SENSORY SCREENING Vision	S	S	S	S	S	S	S	S	S	O	O	O	O	O	S	O	O	S	O	O
Hearing	S	S	S	S	S	S	S	S	S	S	O	O	S[5]	S[5]	S[5]	O	S	S	O	S
DEVEL./BEHAV. ASSESSMENT[6]	●	●	●	●	●	●	●	●	●	●	●	●	●	●	●	●	●	●	●	●
PHYSICAL EXAMINATION[7]	●	●	●	●	●	●	●	●	●	●	●	●	●	●	●	●	●	●	●	●
PROCEDURES[8] Hered./Metabolic Screening[9]	●																			
Immunization[10]		●	●	●			●	●	●			●					●			
Tuberculin Test						●	←	←	●[11]	→	→	←	←	●[11]	→	→	←	←	●[11]	→
Hematocrit or Hemoglobin[12]	←	←	←	←	●	→	←	←	●	→	→	←	←	●	→	→	←	←	●	→
Urinalysis[13]	←	←	←	●	→	→	←	←	●	→	→	←	←	●	→	→	←	←	●	→
ANTICIPATORY GUIDANCE[14]	●	●	●	●	●	●	●	●	●	●	●	●	●	●	●	●	●	●	●	●
INITIAL DENTAL REFERRAL[15]										●										

1. Committee on Practice and Ambulatory Medicine, 1981.
2. Statement on Continuity of Pediatric Care, Committee on Standards of Child Health Care, 1978.
3. Statement on Fragmentation of Pediatric Care, Committee on Standards of Child Health Care, 1978.
4. If a child comes under care for the first time at any point on the Schedule, or if any items are not accomplished at the suggested age, the Schedule should be brought up to date at the earliest possible time.
5. At these points, history may suffice; if problem suggested, a standard testing method should be employed.
6. By history and appropriate physical examination; if suspicious, by specific objective developmental testing.
7. At each visit, a complete physical examination is essential, with infant totally unclothed, older child undressed and suitably draped.
8. These may be modified, depending upon entry point into schedule and individual need.
9. PKU and thyroid testing should be done at about 2 wks. Infants initially screened before 24 hours of age should be rescreened.
10. Schedule(s) per Report of Committee on Infectious Disease, ed. 18, 1982.
11. The Committee on Infectious Diseases recommends tuberculin testing at 12 months of age and every 1-2 years thereafter. In some areas, tuberculosis is of exceedingly low occurrence and the physician may elect not to retest routinely or to use longer intervals.
12. Present medical evidence suggests the need for reevaluation of the frequency and timing of hemoglobin or hematocrit tests. One determination is therefore suggested during each time period. Performance of additional tests is left to the individual practice experience.
13. Present medical evidence suggests the need for reevaluation of the frequency and timing of urinalyses. One determination is therefore suggested during each time period. Performance of additional tests is left to the individual practice experience.
14. Appropriate discussion and counselling should be an integral part of each visit for care.
15. Subsequent examinations as prescribed by dentist.

N.B.: **Special chemical, immunologic, and endocrine testing** are usually carried out upon specific indications. Testing other than newborn (e.g., inborn errors of metabolism, sickle disease, lead) are discretionary with the physician.

Key: ● = to be performed; **S** = subjective, by history; **O** = objective, by a standard testing method.

Figure 1.1. Guidelines for routine health care. (Courtesy of American Academy of Pediatrics.)

safety. It is of such overriding importance, added emphasis and further information seem relevant here.

Despite a gratifying reduction in childhood deaths from poisoning, attributable, in part, to poison control networks, hospitalizations remain at about 20,000 per year in the United States. According to the Association of Poison Control Centers, 1,400,000 calls were answered in 1983. Ninety-one percent of accidental poisonings occurred in the home (Veltri et al, 1984). Among the possible causes are improper storage of poisonous substances and medications, failure of pharmacists to use child-resistant containers, and ignorance of appropriate emergency procedures, including calling a poison control center.

Mandatory seat belt legislation, raising the age for purchase of alcoholic beverages, and intensive campaigns in schools on automobile safety seem worthwhile and deserve our continued support. It is startling to realize that in 1980–1981, children 6–16 years of age missed 14 million days of school because of injuries.

The argument for seat belts received significant support from data collected by the Centers for Disease Control. In 1983, nearly 30,000 occupants of automobiles died on United States highways, and only 2% reportedly were wearing seat belts. It is estimated that use of seat belts could prevent at least 60% of serious injuries. It is encouraging that, in 1985, all but two of the 49 states with legislative sessions were considering at least one bill to make seat belts mandatory (MMWR, 1985).

As long as accidents remain the leading cause of death of children and young adults, pediatricians' role in anticipatory guidelines and promotion of education on accident prevention remains paramount.

REFERENCES

American Academy of Pediatrics: In: Green M (ed): "Guidelines for Health Supervision." Elk Grove Village, IL 60007.

Feldman KW: Prevention of childhood accidents: Recent progress. *Pediatr Rev* 2:75, 1980.

Frankenburg WK, Fandal AW, et al: The newly abbreviated and revised Denver Developmental Screening Test. *J Pediatr* 99:995, 1981.

Galaburda AM, LeMay M, Kemper FL, Geshchwind N: Right-left asymmetries in the brain: Structural differences between the hemispheres may underlie cerebral dominance. *Science* 199:852, 1978.

Hockelman RA, Blatman S, Friedman S, et al: *Primary Pediatric Care*. St. Louis, CV Mosby, 1987.

Levine M, Carey WB, Crocker AC, et al: *Developmental-Behavioral Pediatrics*. Philadelphia, WB Saunders, 1983.

Longstreth LE: Human handedness: More evidence for genetic involvement. *J Genetic Psych* 137:275, 1980.

MMWR: State Legislative activities concerning use of seat belts—United States 1985. 34:505, 1985.

Veltri JC, Litovitz TL: 1983 Annual Report of the American Association of Poison Control Centers National data collection system. *Am J Emerg Med* 2:420, 1984.

IMMUNIZATIONS

Some aspects of immunization are discussed in the sections on Infectious Diseases and Immunology. A review of the essentials of immunization of well children is pertinent in this overview because it is such an essential aspect of preventive pediatrics.

The recommended schedule for active immunization is shown in Table 1.1. This same schedule applies to premature infants who have an adequate serological response after the second immunization.

For individuals with immunodeficiency disorders or undergoing immunosuppressive therapy, or mothers during pregnancy, or family members who are immunosuppressed, active immunization is contraindicated. Such individuals may require passive immunization if exposed to some infections. Recommendations for immune globulin prophylaxis and therapy are shown in Table 1.2.

Pertussis

CONTROVERSY

The occurrence of rare but devastating complications of pertussis immunization has led individuals, groups, and nations to discontinue it, even with knowledge that the disease has been greatly decreased since near-universal immunization with DTP starting at 2 months (Table 1.3).

The problem is to balance the risks. In the United States, 3.5 million children are inoculated each year, 50 of whom have permanent brain damage as a result, and 5 to 20 have died each year, for the past 10 years. In England, in one 2-year period, when DTP fell into disuse, 36 children died per 100,000 cases of whooping cough, and many more will suffer from chronic bronchiectasis.

Clearly the odds favor continued use of pertussis immunization with the currently available *B. pertussis* crude vaccine. A more specific and less toxic vaccine should be a high research priority. Meanwhile, some national compensation system for the unfortunate few who were affected is being urged, as a means of spreading the costs and avoiding lawsuits, because these so intimidate manufacturers that shortages of vaccines may become serious.

Haemophilus influenzae Vaccine

Recently published data (*MMWR*: 37:13, 1988) regarding vaccine efficacy and the risk of Hib disease among young children strongly support the use of Hib vaccine in the United States in high-risk persons for whom efficacy has been established. Specific recommendations are as follows.

A vaccine from *Haemophilus* B capsular polysaccharide was licensed in the United States in April 1985 and was recommended for infants at 24 months of age. A more immunogenic vaccine conjugated with diphtheria toxoid (conjugate vaccine) is available in 1988.

Immunization of Children at 18 Months of Age, Particulary Those in Known High-Risk Groups, is Recommended. Although the precise efficacy of the vaccine among children 18–23 months of age is not known, this age group accounts for approximately 12%

Table 1.1a
Recommended Schedule for Active Immunization of Normal Infants and Children, Including Prematures[1]

Recommended Age	Vaccine [2]	Comments
2 months	DTP, OPV	Can be initiated earlier in areas of high endemicity
4 months	DTP, OPV	2-month interval desired for OPV to avoid interference
6 months	DTP (OPV)	OPV optional for areas where polio might be imported
15 months	Measles, mumps, rubella (MMR) DTP, OPV	DTP, OPV may be given at 15 months or 18 months if desired
24 months	*Haemophilus influenzae B*	18 months in groups at risk as in day care
4–6 years [3]	DTP, OPV	Preferably at or before school entry
14–16 years	Td	Repeat every 10 years for lifetime

[1]Adapted from the CDC: *Morbidity and Mortality Weekly Report* 35:577, 1986.
[2]Note: For all products used, consult manufacturer's brochure for instructions for storage, handling, and administration. Abbreviations: DTP = diptheria and tetanus toxoids with pertussis vaccine absorbed; OPV = oral, attenuated poliovirus vaccine which contains poliovirus, Types 1, 2, and 3; MMR = live measles, mumps,and rubella viruses in a combined vaccination; Td = adult tetanus toxoid (full dose) and diptheria (reduced dose) in combination.
[3]Up to seventh birthday.

Table 1.1b
Recommended Immunization Schedules for Children Not Immunized in First Year of Life [1]

Recommended Time	Immunization(s)	Comments
	Less Than 7 Years Old	
First visit	DTP, OPV, MMR	MMR if child ≥ 15 months old; tuberculin testing may be done (see Tuberculosis)
Interval after first visit		
1 month	HBPV[2]	For children 24–60 months
2 month	DTP, OP	
4 month	DTP (OPV)	OPV is optional (may be given in areas with increased risk of poliovirus exposure)
10–16 month	DTP, OPV	PV is not given if third dose was given earlier
Age 4–6 yr (at or before school entry)	DTP, OPV	DTP is not necessary if the fourth dose was given after the fourth birthday; OPV is not necessary if recommended OPV dose at 10–16 months following first visit was given after the fourth birthday
Age 14–16 yr	Td	Repeat every 10 yr throughout life
	7 Years Old and Older	
First visit	Td, OPV, MMR	
Interval after first visit		
2 month	Td, OPV	
8–14 month	Td, OPV	
Age 14–16 yr	Td	Repeat every 10 yr throughout life

[1]Reproduced with permission from the *Report of the Committee on Infectious Diseases*. American Academy of Pediatrics, 20th edition, 1986.
[2]*Haemophilus b* vaccine can be given, if necessary, simultaneously with DTP (at separate sites). The initial three doses of DTP can be given at 1- to 2-month intervals; so, for the child in whom immunization is initiated at 24 months old or older, one visit could be eliminated by giving DTP, OPV, MMR at the first visit; DTP and HBPV at the second visit (1 month later); and DTP and OPV at the third visit (2 months after the first visit). Subsequent DTP and OPV 10 to 16 months after the first visit are still indicated.

of all invasive Hib disease among children under 5 years of age, and Hib vaccine has been shown by serologic methods to be immunogenic in most children of this age group. These children may need a second dose of vaccine at age 24 months to ensure protection. Additional data regarding the duration of the antibody response are needed to define the timing of a second dose more precisely.

Children who received the polysaccharide vaccine before 24 months of age, should be vaccinated with a single dose of conjugate vaccine. Children who had invasive *H. influenzae* at less than 24 months of age should still be given the vaccine.

Vaccination does not inhibit asymptomatic carriage of *H. influenzae* B. Therefore, rifampin is recommended for chemoprophylaxis of close contacts.

Table 1.2
Immune Globulin Prophylaxis and Therapy [1]

Disorder	Value	Purpose	Dose	Comment
Standard Human Immune Globulins				
Measles	Proved	Modification	0.5 ml/kg	Rarely indicated
		Prevention	0.25 ml/kg	Given immediately on exposure to unvaccinated children
			0.50 ml/kg (maximum 15 ml)	For immunosuppressed patients
Varicella [2]	Limited	Modification	0.6-1.2 ml/kg	Give immediately at exposure if VZIG not available; see indications for use in the text
Rubella	Limited	Prevention	20 ml	For pregnant women in the first trimester who will not consider abortion
Special Human Immune Globulins				
Tetanus (TIG)	Proved	Prevention	250-500 U	For contaminated wounds in individuals not fully immunized
		Treatment	3000-6000 U	
Rabies (RIG)	Proved	Prevention	20 U/kg	Give with human diploid rabies vaccine
Varicella-zoster (VZIG)	Proved	Prevention	1 complete vial/10 kg (maximum 5 vials)	Give to exposed immunodeficient individuals; give within 96 hours of exposure
Pertussis	Unproved	Prevention Treatment		Protection not reliable
Mumps	Unproved	Prevention		No evidence that orchitis is prevented
Special Animal Immune Serums [3]				
Botulism (trivalent ABE)	Proved	Treatment		As soon as possible—testing for sensitivity to serum
Diptheria	Proved	Treatment	20,000–120,000 U	As soon as clinical diagnosis is made; high doses for more extensive disease
Gas gangrene (polyvalent Clostridial antitoxin)	Unproved	Treatment		No longer commerically available

[1]Reproduced with permission from Graef, JW, Cone TE: *Manual of Pediatric Therapeutics,* 3rd edition. Boston, Little, Brown & Co., 1985.
[2]Zoster immune plasma (ZIP) from patients convalescing from herpes zoster may also modify illness but carries the risk of hepatitis. The dose is 10 ml/kg/ IV.
[3]Detailed information about indications, source of supply, and dosage can be obtained from the Centers for Disease Control (404) 639–3311 (8:00 AM–5:00 PM weekdays) and (404) 639–2888 (off-duty hours).

Children who attend day care facilities are at particular risk of acquiring systemic Hib disease. Initial vaccination at 18 months of age for this high-risk group is essential.

Children with chronic conditions known to be associated with increased risk for Hib disease should receive the vaccine, although only limited data on immunogenicity and clinical efficacy in this group are available. These conditions include anatomic or functional asplenia, such as sickle cell disease or splenectomy, and malignancies associated with immunosuppression.

Immunization of Individuals Over 24 Months of Age Who Have Not Yet Received Hib Vaccine Should be Based on Risk of Disease. The risk of invasive Hib disease decreases with increasing age over the age of 2 years. Because the vaccine is safe and effective between 2 years and 5 years of age, the potential benefit of immunization declines with increasing age of the child. Therefore, children 2–3 years of age who attend day care facilities should be given a higher priority than day care attendees who are 4–5 years old.

Insufficient Data are Available on Which to Base a Recommendation Concerning Use of the Vaccine in Older Children and Adults with the Chronic Conditions Associated with an Increased Risk of Hib Disease.

Vaccine is not Recommended for Children Under 18 Months of Age.

Table 1.3
Adverse Events Occurring Within 48 Hours of DTP Immunizations [1]

Event	Frequency [2]
Local	
Redness	1/3 doses
Swelling	2/5 doses
Pain	1/2 doses
Mild/moderate systemic	
Fever > 38°C (100.4°F)	1/2 doses
Drowsiness	1/3 doses
Fretfulness	1/2 doses
Vomiting	1/15 doses
Anorexia	1/5 doses
More serious systemic	
Persistent, inconsolable crying duration > 3 hours	1/100 doses
High-pitched, unusual cry	1/900 doses
Fever > 40.5°C (105°F)	1/330 doses
Collapse (hypotonic-hyporesponsive episode)	1/1750 doses
Convulsions (with or without fever)	1/1750 doses
Acute encephalopathy [3]	1/110,000 doses
Permanent neurologic deficit	1/310,000 doses

[1]Modified from Cody CL, et al: *Pediatrics* 68:650, 1981
[2]Number of adverse events per total number doses regardless of dose number in DTP series.
[3]Occurring within 7 days of DTP immunization.

Simultaneous Administration of Hib and DTP Vaccines at Separate Sites Can Be Performed, Because No Impairment of the Immune Response to the Individual Antigens Occurs Under These Circumstances.

Side Effects and Adverse Reactions. Polysaccharide vaccines are among the safest of all vaccine products. To date, over 60,000 doses of the Hib polysaccharide vaccine have been administered to infants and children, and several hundred doses have been given to adults. Only one serious systemic reaction has been reported thus far—a possible anaphylactic reaction that responded promptly to epinephrine. High fever (38.5°C [101.3°F] or higher) has been reported in fewer than 1% of Hib vaccine recipients. Mild local and febrile reactions were common, occuring in as many as half of vaccinated individuals in the Finnish trial. Such reactions appeared within 24 hours and rapidly subsided. Current preparations appear to result in fewer such local reactions. Simultaneous administration with DTP does not result in reaction rates above those expected with separate administration.

Precautions and Contraindications. Because the vaccine will not protect against nontypeable strains of *Haemophilus influenzae,* recurrent upper respiratory diseases, including otitis media and sinusitis are not considered indications for vaccination.

New Vaccine Development. New vaccines, such as the Hib polysaccharide-protein conjugate vaccines, are being developed and evaluated and may prove to be efficacious for children under 18 months of age.

Poliomyelitis, Measles, Mumps, and Rubella

Contraindications To Live Virus Vaccines

In general, live virus vaccines are contraindicated in patients who are pregnant, immunosuppressed, or immunodeficient. Other considerations include the following:

1. A diagnosis of immunodeficiency in a child should prompt a screening of the immunocompetency of all siblings before any immunizations are given. Normal siblings of immunosuppressed or immunodeficient patients should receive killed poliomyelitis vaccine (IPV).
2. It is permissible to give rubella vaccine to the child of a pregnant woman.
3. Do not immunize if immune globulin has been given in the preceding 8 weeks.
4. When a primary series of OPV is completed at or beyond the 4th birthday, a booster dose is not required. Children who have received primary immunization with IPV should receive a booster dose of IPV every 5 years until the age of 18 years unless a primary series of OPV is completed. Routine primary poliomyelitis virus vaccination of adults (19 years and older) residing in the United States is not necessary (see *MMWR* 31:22-33, 1982).
5. Children with static, unchanging neurologic disorders may be immunized against poliomyelitis, pertussis, measles, mumps, and rubella. These vaccines afford protection against even more damaging neurologic sequelae.

Side Effects

The side effects of immunizations may be local or systemic but are usually mild and self-limited. Fever and/or minor erythema or swelling in the extremity used for the injection are the most common. Parents should be advised that such reactions may occur, but that the incidence and severity of these reactions are far exceeded by the risks and dangers of the diseases against which they afford protection (Table 1.3).

Recommendations for Specific Nonroutine Immunizations

Smallpox

In the United States, routine vaccination of children or adults, including health workers, has been discontinued.

Pneumococcal Vaccine

A vaccine containing polysaccharide antigens from the pneumococcal serotypes most prominent in human disease (American types 1–4, 6, 8, 9, 12, 14, 19, 23, 51, and 56) has been licensed in the United States. Infants and toddlers may have a poor or unpredictable antibody response; hence, the vaccine is not recommended for children under age 2 years. Patients with splenic dysfunction (e.g., sickle hemoglobinopathies or splenectomy patients) and those whose chronic diseases have an increased susceptibility to pneumococcal infection (e.g., patients with diabetes, hepatic disease, cardiopulmonary disease, and chronic renal failure and hemodialysis patients) should receive the accepted single dose injection of pneumococcal vaccine and should, in addition, be maintained on daily antibiotic prophylaxis with penicillin, ampicillin, or erythromycin.

The clinical efficacy is 85–95% for at least 1 year with protection achieved 1–2 weeks after immunization.

Meningococcal Polysaccharide Vaccines

A serospecific quadrivalent meningococcal vaccine is currently licensed in the United States for the following indications: (a) travel to countries having epidemic meningococcal disease; (b) as an adjunct to antibiotic prophylaxis for household contacts of a person with meningococcal disease caused by serogroup A or C; (c) control of epidemic meningococcal disease caused by serogroup A or C; (d) asplenic children over 2 years old; (e) children with terminal complement component deficiencies. The duration of protection has not been established as of 1988.

Hepatitis B

Children at substantial risk of hepatitis B should be immunized on a case by case basis. Those at risk are: (a) residents of institutions; (b) children on hemodialysis; (c) homosexually active males; (d) drug abusers (by injection); (e) recipients of blood products (such as hemophiliacs); (f) household contact with carriers; (g) infants of mothers who are chronic carriers.

Influenza

Vaccination with killed virus vaccine is recommended for those at high risk of severe influenzal illness because of underlying cardiac, renal, or pulmonary disease, diabetes, sickle cell anemia, or malignancy. Allergy to previous influenza vaccinations or hypersensitivity to eggs or egg products is a contraindication to immunization. At present, the subvirion (split virus) preparation is recommended for persons less than 12 years old.

Adolescence

Robert Masland, M.D.

That period during life covering the span of 12–21 years is known as adolescence. The word adolescence is derived from the Latin "adolescere" which means grow into maturity. From a biologic standpoint, adolescence may begin as early as 8 years for the female and 10 years for the male. These early maturers may complete their physical growth and sexual development well before their 16th birthday. Still within the normal range for the onset of puberty will be females who enter puberty at age 14 and males as late as age 16. These so-called late maturers will complete their physical growth in the 19- to 21-year range. These are important age spans to consider when caring for adolescent patients. The dilemma for physicians and indeed all adults, including parents, is how to treat these young people. Do we react to their chronologic age or to their biologic development? The answer is never clear, which enhances the mystery of adolescence. What does the expression mean, "to act your age?"

The transition from child to adult, marked as it is by profound physical and psychologic changes, has been given special attention by most primitive cultures in the world. These "rites" of puberty are significant in all cultures. In our society, the young people compete in the classroom, on the athletic field, and in areas of artistic and creative endeavors. The pressure to perform can be intense. Peer pressure leads to experimentation with adult activities, heretofore forbidden. The litany is familiar. Tobacco, drugs, and alcohol are the perennial favorites. In a society which seems to be better informed about sexual matters, our adolescent boys and girls appear to be just as confused as their parents were (and are) about sex. Throughout adolescence, the separation process ("striving for independence") is a constant source of pain for both the adolescent and the parents. There are many tasks for the adolescent to discover and complete. One's identity in a situation where role confusion prevails is a matter which Erikson speaks to in eloquent fashion in "*Childhood and Society.*"

It is impossible to separate the physical from the emotional when discussing adolescence. However, the endocrinology of adolescence is special and will be addressed in Section 14, Endocrinology.

Psychologic Growth and Development

Keeping in mind that the age of onset for puberty has a wide range of normal for girls and boys, we arbitrarily consider grades 6–9, ages 11–15 years, as the early adolescent period. Middle adolescence describes individuals in grades 10–12, (ages 15–18 years). Late adolescence is the time when young people attend college or university, work, marry, join the military service or do nothing. This is the age group 18–21 years.

Early Adolescence

Physical proportion (height and weight) and sexual maturation are the all consuming interests for the early adolescent girl and boy. Thoughts and conversation constantly play on these subjects. For the most part, the thinking process is concrete making it difficult to engage in any conversation which requires that one relate to abstract material.

These young people are the quintessential pragmatists. The time is now; do it now. Impulse control is poor, hence, the tendency to act in a fashion that is self-centered with little regard for the consequences or the effect on others. Adults, and especially parents, bewildered by what appears to be aberrant adolescent behavior may react to their seeming lack of parental authority by becoming more authoritarian. If rules and sanctions are imposed which are not enforceable, the adolescent can become confused and sometimes rebellious.

Middle Adolescence

By midadolescence one can expect increasing anxiety from both parent and adolescent on the critical issue of sexuality. Who I am and what I am are not merely career-oriented statements; they are statements which involve gender preference and identity. Society is more open about sexual lifestyles. Most adolescents yearn to be accepted by their peers and shun behavior which might subject them to ridicule. For this reason, sexual intimacy during the middle adolescent years is predominantly heterosexual. However, in today's sexual climate, it is not unusual to have a parent or an adolescent seek professional advice about homosexuality. One must remember that experimentation continues throughout adolescence, experimentation which may be sexual. Decisions with regard to sexual preference need not be considered irrevocable. Conversation that leads to understanding is preferable to criticism which creates an atmosphere of distrust and hostility.

These young people are able to marshall thoughts in a more logical manner. Abstract reasoning is not just a possibility, it is a reality. Connections are made between facts and acts. Few, if any subjects should be avoided in adult-adolescent conversation. Adolescents should be encouraged to take more control. Study habits, recreation time, and home chores are negotiable, with the expectation that the adolescent will cooperate when given the opportunity to be responsible. Control can be a problem when an eating disorder is present or the youngster denies the presence of a disease which requires daily medication and refuses to follow the doctor's orders. (For additional information and discussion on Eating Disorders, refer to pp. 67.)

Late Adolescence

Graduation from secondary school heralds the beginning of the third period of adolescence. Growth and sexual maturation are complete for most adolescents. The difficulties encountered during early and middle adolescence may not be resolved completely, but they tend to pale somewhat in the presence of the final challenge for the late adolescent. This challenge is the looming separation from friends, family, and long-cherished childhood surroundings.

For perhaps the first time the adolescent may experience the ultimate loss, the death of a friend or a member of the family. Although the loss may have come earlier than this period, divorce and the attendant reaction, which may have been delayed or denied, can cause considerable discomfort for the adolescent seeking to gain independence. The small world the adolescent lives in is falling apart when the outside world must be met and subdued.

Academic failure, job loss, and marital problems may represent the fallout for the adolescent unable to deal successfully with separation. Increased alcohol and/or drug use are inappropriate means employed by the distressed adolescent attempting to cope with a seemingly unfriendly environment. The resulting depression is the most serious complication one may anticipate, a depression which may be masked by somatic complaints. These young people may say, "I am depressed." The threat of a suicide attempt cannot be underestimated. At this point, it is imperative that a medical/psychiatric evaluation be carried out.

Patient/Doctor Visit

Privacy is all-important for the adolescent, as indeed it is for every patient. The concern should dictate the site of the interview and examination. A professional, not a social, setting is an absolute requirement. Establishing a relationship based on mutual respect leading to confidentiality may be done by inquiring about things other than medical, such as friends, social and athletic activities, hobbies, and music. Open-ended questions can define cognitive level, and may even reveal hidden anxieties.

Confidential information may be shared with the parents only with the permission of the adolescent. Of course, when the adolescent presents a problem which is potentially dangerous for the patient and/or other individuals, then the physician must inform the parents, with the patient knowing that this is the only course of action possible. A meeting with the patient and the parents is clearly indicated in such a case.

Legal Rights of Minors

Patients over 18 years of age are considered adults and are able to consent to their own health care. For patients over 18 who may not be functionally competent by reason of mental retardation or mental illness, parents must obtain legal guardian status from the court in order to approve medical care for these special patients. Local or state laws may differ, hence, it is important for the physician to have awareness of the proper procedure to follow.

In general, adolescent patients under age 18 years require parental consent for treatment with the following exceptions:

1. The patient is married, widowed, or divorced.
2. The patient is a parent, a member of the Armed Forces, or living separate and apart from parents or legal guardian and managing his own financial affairs.
3. The patient has a disease dangerous to the public health (sexually transmitted disease).
4. The patient has an alcohol and/or substance abuse problem and consents to treatment.
5. The patient is pregnant. She may consent to the management of the pregnancy. Consenting to an abortion is another matter. The state laws vary and must be followed by the patient and the physician.
6. The patient is deemed a mature minor by the physician, using the following criteria:
   a. The nature of the health care needs.
   b. The capacity of the patient not only to understand these health needs, but also the ability and desire to act in a responsible manner.
   c. The relationship and involvement with the parents.

Prescribing contraceptives is a good example of an instance when the physician might wish to consider the adolescent to be a mature minor.

One caveat bears repeating. The physician must involve the parents or legal guardians when the patient's situation is life-threatening or life-endangering to self and/or others.

Adolescent Pregnancy

Important data regarding teenage pregnancy in developed countries have been reported from the Alan Guttmacher Institute. In the United States in 1982, the survey revealed that 50% of all 16-year-old females were sexually active (sexual intercourse). Contraceptive use was at the lowest level in the United States compared to the other nations. Teenage mothers acquire less education, tend to have larger families, and are over-represented on the welfare lists. The risks of infant morbidity seem to be more related to poor maternal health habits in pregnancy than to inherent biologic factors.

Support for the young mother and assuring her of care appears to decrease developmental and social morbidity. In our Out-Patient Department we have a Young Parent Program, in which both the teenage mother and her infant receive periodic care provided by the same physician or nurse practitioner. We have noted that in this setting the mothers often show more concern for their babies than they do for themselves. Serving both at the same visit enhances health education, compliance, and the ultimate goal of better health for the mother and child.

SCREENING PROGRAMS

Definition

Screening is the process of performing a diagnostic test in an otherwise healthy population with the intent of identifying those with an illness or at risk of subsequently developing an illness. The ideal screening test should be simple, low in cost, acceptable to the patient, and both sensitive and specific. In other words, it should identify most individuals who have the disorder and not those who do not have it. It should be reliable so that it can be repeated in the same individual with the same results, and it should provide an accurate measurement.

Sensitivity is the percentage of those detected by the test who truly have the disease. *Specificity* is the percentage of those without the disease who are correctly identified by the test as not having a disease. *The predictive value positive* of a screening test is the percentage of those identified as being positive by the test who actually have the disease. *The predictive value negative* provides the percentage of those who are identified as negative on screening and do not have the disease. The predictive value, therefore, depends not only on the test's sensitivity and specificity, but also on the prevalence of the disorder—the lower the prevalence, the higher the number of over-referrals for further work-up. Useful guidelines for a good screening test are as follows: (a) there must be a consensus for criteria for diagnosis of the condition; (b) the potential condition must be of sufficient importance or if it is infrequent, of significant severity; (c) the problem can be assessed and treated more effectively in the asymptomatic phase (and there should be an effective treatment for that disease once it has been detected); (d) treatment facilities should be available once the disease has been detected and a connection should be set up between the screening program and that treatment facility; (e) the cost should be known and acceptable to all involved with the test; (f) parental explanation and consent should be obtained before a child is screened to allay alarm at information that may require further evaluation.

This chapter will focus on the screening tests considered basic in a well child visit and will raise some of the more controversial issues regarding their effectiveness.

Physical Examination

Perhaps there is no better method of screening than a complete examination of the structure and function of the human body. During this examination, judgments are made as to the normality or abnormality of numerous measurements and observations because they can be compared with predetermined standards. The most useful components of the physical examination, in terms of detecting an abnormality, are the measurements of height, weight, head circumference, and vital signs. When screening the presumably well newborn or child, certain components of the physical examination need to be performed only once to ascertain the presence or absence of a specific disease, whereas other abnormalities require repeated evaluation. The possibility of detecting a disorder by repetition of physical examination determines the frequency with which such examinations are done in well children.

Hoekelman (1984), for example, cites 10 conditions detectable on physical examination in seemingly normal infants and children that may not be detectable by any other means. These are: cataract, congenital dislocated hip, congenital heart disease, cryptorchidism, some genetic syndromes, glaucoma, lymphadenopathy, scoliosis, strabismus, and tumors and masses.

CONTROVERSIES

Although the physical examination remains a strong tool in the screening armamentarium, studies have shown that the yield of abnormal findings detected on a routine well child examination is extremely small. Abnormal findings of 1.9% have been detected in infants during their first year, 2.6% in preschool children, and 4% in primary school and high school students (Hoekelman, 1984). Because of its small yield, the physical examination could be an inefficient use of medical manpower if it is done too frequently, or of little value if it is done even less frequently than it is now. The number of examinations that a well child should undergo with the intent of detecting an abnormality remains arbitrary. For the well child at low risk, however, screening physical examinations should probably be performed at birth, 2 weeks, 2 months, 4 months, 6 months, 1, 2, 5, 10, and 14 years of age at a minimum. Some pediatricians would argue that a yearly physical, at least until school age, is necessary in order to screen for growth disorders, but no studies document that frequent visits result in better detection of abnormalities.

Screening for Genetic Disorders

Screening for hereditary metabolic diseases or chromosomal disorders is now recognized to be an important aspect of prenatal care and will be discussed in Section 4 (Neonatology) and under the relevant diseases.

Neonatal screening for PKU, galactosemia, hypothyroidism, and branch-chain ketoaciduria is routine in most nurseries in North America, Europe, and many other parts of the world. Early treatment is of unquestionable benefit in each of these disorders.

CONTROVERSIES

While there are a number of other genetic disorders for which screening is possible, such as homocystinuria, histidinemia, hyperlipoproteinemia, and tyrosinemia, the cost-effectiveness of these screening tests remains to be established. Tests for neonatal screening for cystic fibrosis remain controversial (see pp. 255, Section 15).

Tuberculosis Skin Testing

The incidence and prevalence of tuberculosis in the United States is declining. Nonetheless, evidence suggests that the treatment of those whose skin tests have recently become positive significantly reduces the chance of developing a more severe active disease. Therefore, the standardized dose of purified protein derivative (PPD) is used for antigen skin testing. The addition of an antiabsorbant called Polysorbate-80 (TWEEN-80) to the PPD has resulted in a more stable preparation which allows uniformity of dose. The standard test dose is best administered by the Mantoux intracutaneous injection which will detect 99% of proven active tuberculosis cases (Bailey, 1975).

False-negative results may occur in patients with certain systemic diseases, such as sarcoidosis, malignancy, measles, chickenpox, uremia, and generalized tuberculosis. In addition, patients on immunosuppressive therapy, and those who have been recently immunized, may have false-negative skin tests. Moreover, even with good planning of a tubercular screening program, poor compliance in reporting test results may still occur. Even when prepaid postcards are provided, no more than 70% of parents in a clinic setting may respond (see Section 5).

Anemia

Screening for anemia is done primarily to reveal nutritionally correctable anemias, such as iron deficiency, as well as to identify other anemias that are genetically determined or secondary to a generalized disorder. The measurement by a microhematocrit is a simple, inexpensive, and reliable measure for anemia. Measurement of hemoglobin is also appropriate although it is more expensive than the microhematocrit because it requires more expensive capillary pipettes, standards, and a photometer. The best way to screen for anemia is by measuring multiple hematological parameters with use of an electronic counter. Although this is more expensive, it is advantageous in that it not only identifies an anemia but also provides some clues as to its etiology. For example, if iron deficiency anemia is suspected, an electronic Coulter counter will usually reveal a low mean corpuscular volume consistent with the microcytic hypochronic anemia due to inadequate iron stores. Once an anemia is detected, it is necessary to search further for its etiology and then begin appropriate treatment. For example, a deficiency in iron may represent blood loss as well as a nutritional problem.

All children should be screened for anemia between 9 and 12 months when the majority of congenital anemias become apparent. They should be screened once more between the ages of 1 and 2 years when a nutritional anemia may become manifest in the absence of other symptoms. If there is no evidence of anemia by age 2 years, no data support the advantage of doing yearly hematocrit screens unless the child is at risk for nutritional anemia. Otherwise, repeat hemoglobin or microhematocrit can be determined during adolescence, another period of active growth. If an anemia is detected by the screen, it must be re-emphasized that further work-up will be indicated (as discussed in the chapter on anemias) to determine the appropriate etiology.

Lead Screening

Because subtle neurologic and intellectual damage has been attributed to an excessive body burden of lead, even in the absence of demonstrable clinical symptoms, it is important that asymptomatic children be screened periodically for lead toxicity. A complete discussion of the signs and symptoms of lead poisoning and their treatment are included in Toxicology, Section 25, pp. 1339.

The screening test involves either measurement of blood lead or evidence of metabolic effects of lead overload by measurement of the free erythrocyte porphyrins (FEP level). Because the measurement of blood lead is difficult and expensive, the FEP is adequate for determining those at risk, as long as this is followed by a blood lead level. Elevation of FEP can result not only from lead poisoning, but from iron deficiency anemia, and sometimes, although rarely, from a genetic disorder, and from erythropoietic protoporphyria which can also be asymptomatic in childhood. Moreover, the FEP test has a lower sensitivity relative to a serum lead level and if lead intoxication is suspected, despite a negative FEP, a blood lead test should be obtained. Because the age group at highest risk is from 9 months to 5 years, screening should be conducted during this period. Current recommendations suggest that an FEP be obtained beginning at 1 year of age, unless it is thought the infant is at risk before that time. Subsequent checks should be made every year until age 5 years. Lead poisoning may develop over a period of 2–3 months, despite a previously negative screen. Thus, if a history is suspicious, a repeat screen should be obtained.

Sickle Cell Anemia

The question may be asked why screen for sickle cell disease? No established procedures exist to prevent the episodic complications or progressive damage that can result from sickle cell disease in children. Nonetheless, identification of diseased children can create parental awareness of early signs and symptoms of crises, splenic sequestration, or overwhelming infection and lead to earlier medical care, including penicillin prophylaxis. Identification of the child with sickle cell trait is also useful for initiating genetic counseling so that before conception information can be provided regarding: the nature of sickle cell disease, the risk of having a child with the disease, and options available to the parents who carry this trait, such as prenatal diagnosis. Therefore, screening programs for prevention of sickle cell disease are performed in newborn infants who are considered at risk, as well as in adolescent adults to permit genetic counseling.

A complete discussion of sickle cell disease as well as the implications of carrying sickle cell trait are discussed in Section 8, Hematology (pp. 511–514).

Urinalysis Screening

Urinalysis is one of the more widely recommended screening tests in childhood. In light of studies that suggest the possibility of renal parenchymal damage identified with the first clinically evident urinary tract infection, and suggestive of previous asymptomatic infections, screening for occult bacteria is recommended in girls, age 2–3 years (Smellie et al, 1981). If a dipstick is positive, a suprapubic tap (or clean-voided specimen) and culture are indicated to confirm the diagnosis. The prevalence of urinary tract infections in male children who are otherwise healthy remains too low to justify periodic testing for bacteriuria in boys of the same age.

A screening urinalysis can detect glycosuria and proteinuria as well as bacteriuria. The need for evaluating a child with proteinuria is related to the concentration of urinary protein found on "dipstick" analysis. Children with a urinary protein of 50 mg/dl or more have been shown to be 1.6 times as likely to have persistent proteinuria, as those with protein of 10–45 mg/dl. The prevalence of proteinuria increases from infancy to adolescence and is greater in girls at all ages. It also increases to a prevalence of about 6% in children with febrile illnesses (Marks, 1970).

Auditory Screening

Between 15 and 30 children per 1000 have some degree of hearing impairment (Public Health Service Monograph, no. 7, 1968). This fact combined with the evidence that the first 2 years of life are critical for acquisition of normal language development suggest that undetected hairing loss in this period may lead to severe language and speech disabilities. Even mild hearing loss from active middle ear disease has been found to delay language growth and development such that screening beyond infancy becomes important in children who have a history suggestive of a hearing disorder.

In 1973, a Committee from the American Speech and Hearing Association, the American Academy of Pediatrics, and the American Academy of Ophthalmology and Otolaryngology defined the following criteria for high-risk infants suspected of having hearing loss: Children with: (a) a family member with a history of congenital hearing loss in a first cousin or closer relative; (b) a history of having a bilirubin level greater than or equal to 20 mg/dl; (c) a history of congenital rubella, or other viral intrauterine infection; (d) congenital defects of the ear, nose, and throat; (e) small size for gestational age with a birthweight less than 1500 g. In addition, recent studies suggest that patients who have had multiple apneic spells in the nursery, treatment with furosemide, an exchange transfusion, an episode of meningitis, or an Apgar of 5 or less are also thought to be at risk. For these high-risk infants, screening consists of stimulating the infant with 100 decibels of sound at a pitch level of 3000 Hz for a duration of 2 seconds and watching the child for movement consistent with an arousal response. A child with a profound hearing loss will not be aroused by the stimulus. Auditory evoked potentials are useful if risk factors are present. For a child not at risk, hearing should be evaluated at the 6- to 9-month visit, at which point standardized sounds can be made behind and to the side of the infant, who should turn the head 45° and begin to localize the sound. If this does not occur, a more formal audiometric testing should be given. A complete discussion of audiometry appears in the chapter on Hearing Loss.

In preschoolers who are less anxious to cooperate, audiometry requires trained examiners, time, and environmental conditions which makes it impractical as a screening device in office or clinic. When a child is ready to enter school, however, pure tone audiometry is the recommended screening test because children are far more cooperative at this stage. If mild conductive hearing loss is detected, tympanometry should be performed in addition to audiometry and is also discussed in Section 19.

Of note, despite routine screenings in infancy, preschool, and during school age checks, usually in kindergarten, first, third, fifth, and seventh grade, any evidence of aberrant language or behavioral development or parental concern with these matters should be considered seriously as evidence of perhaps inadequate hearing and should be evaluated.

Vision Screening

Because 5% of preschool children have one or more visual defects and the vast majority of these defects are correctable, vision screening becomes an important component of preventive pediatrics (Bailey, 1975). Vision screening begins in infancy, by observing pupillary reaction and the blink response to light in the newborn examination. "Following" movements should be detectable within 4–6 weeks after birth. After that the method used to detect abnormalities in visual acuity depends upon the age and cooperation of the child. For example, between the ages of 1 and 4 years, visual acuity may be assessed and compared by the ability to recognize familiar toys at a distance of 10 feet (Stycar miniature toy test). Such a test allows detection of visual acuity and of strabismus as well.

Preschool and school-age children can be tested by use of the Snellen Chart, whereby the child is directed toward identifying either pictures, a letter "E" in various directions or letters of the alphabet. Visual acuity is indicated by the smallest line in which more than one-half of the letters can be seen at a distance of 20 feet.

An additional test for strabismus is the Hirshberg test in which the light reflex from an otoscope is observed on the subject's pupil with his eyes focusing on the light. Any deviation of the light reflected from the center of the pupils indicates strabismus. This test can only be done if the infant is old enough to be cooperative. Strabismus can be detected by the cover/uncover test, in which each eye is alternately covered and movement of the eye after removing the cover is observed. Again, cooperation of the infant is required. As noted above, because this abnormality can be diagnosed early and can be treated, there is benefit to screening for an eye movement disorder as well as acuity.

Current recommendations include: screening at birth and at all well baby visits; checking for strabismus and acuity; assessing visual acuity on a yearly basis, during the preschool and early school years, and again at early adolescence when the incidence of myopia is at its peak. Any further screens should be done when symptoms suggest (see Section 19).

Developmental Screening

In common with any of the screening tests discussed, the decision to screen for developmental abnormalities should be based upon the availability of diagnostic and therapeutic services for children who are identified as being developmentally delayed. Inasmuch as some studies suggest that intervention before the age of 2 years may significantly improve the intelligence quotient of high-risk children, it is all the more important that developmental screening be integrated into the routine, well child pediatric examination (Bailey et al, 1975). For adequate developmental screening, a pediatrician must be familiar with normal development and developmental milestones. A developmental history should be a requirement of each routine well child examination, whether or not a formal screening test is used. Moreover, pediatricians should not overinterpret the results of such a developmental screening, but rather should be prepared either to perform further developmental tests themselves or refer these children on for formal testing by experts. It is important that this be done before the child is labeled developmentally delayed.

Although a variety of developmental tests exist, the most efficient assessment can be made by obtaining a good history, performing a careful physical examination, and focusing on such entities as motor and language skills as well as by screening vision and hearing. Delayed or atypical socialization and communication behavior can be highly significant in identifying children at risk for developmental abnormalities. Moreover, if an abnormality is suspected, at least two similar abnormal observations should be made at two different times to ensure that the abnormality really exists and to determine the rate at which development is occurring. This can be useful to rule out a transient deficit that may be an acute illness or simply fatigue from the overall examination. Parents can also aid in evaluating the validity and reliability of the observations made during the visit in terms of the child's behavioral pattern.

If a formal developmental screening test is required, the Denver Developmental Screening Test is the most extensively used in this country (see pp. 46).

Of note, a Denver Prescreening Developmental Questionnaire has been constructed that consists of 10 age-appropriate questions derived from the Denver Developmental Screening Test. When administered at periodic intervals on routine visits, it can identify those infants and children who might require more thorough screening beginning with a complete Denver Developmental Screening Test. It is currently recommended that the Denver Developmental Screening Test be performed at the 9-month visit, and the Denver Prescreening Developmental Questionnaire be given at the 18- and 24-month visit, and again at the 4-year visit. If any abnormalities are detected at this time, a full Denver should be performed on a yearly basis for the higher risk group (Frankenburg and Camp,1975).

Developmental screening can be useful in assessing school readiness in the preschool child. There is, however, no formal readiness test available for the pediatrician that has been adequately validated at this time. The overall assessments made during the previous 5 years, including routine history, physical examination, and developmental assessment, are the most useful tools for aiding the decision whether a child should begin school.

Blood Pressure Screening

Screening for high blood pressure in children is based on the assumption that early detection and treatment of high blood pressure can provide a more favorable prognosis. It is important to use the appropriate cuff and to assess blood pressure readings according to criteria of the American Academy of Pediatrics Task Force on Blood Pressure Control in Children. Nonetheless, most hypertensive children detected on initial screening examinations are found to have reverted to normal blood pressure on second testing. In fact, the American Academy of Pediatrics School Health Committee no longer recommends screening school children for hypertension because of the low yield of cases that require treatment. Blood pressure measurement should be included as part of a routine physical examination in childhood, however, in order to establish baseline values to allow the child to become accustomed to the procedure, and to discover the occasional child with secondary hypertension of known organic etiology.

Scoliosis

Scoliosis can appear in early childhood in association with musculoskeletal disease, which usually involves more than back muscles. Adolescent idiopathic scoliosis can have an insidious onset and may result in a crippling deformity that can be prevented if detected early (see Section 23).

Screening programs in schools can focus on children who are at greatest risk, namely those with a family history of scoliosis and those who are subject to rigorous diet and exercise such as ballet dancers. Screening consists of asking the child to stand and bend at the hips in such a way as to produce a right angle. The observer examines the back for any asymmetry or spinal deviation. Only if an abnormality is found on inspection should radiographs be made.

About 2% of children will have some degree of scoliosis (if minor curves of 5–10° are included). Curves under 20° are considered benign. Progressive curvature in growing adolescents is amenable to therapy with braces. About 15–20% will progress even with braces and require surgery.

CONTROVERSY

The argument for screening by physical examination is that scoliosis can be detected in time to correct it or at least prevent progression. Opponents argue that screening in schools will lead to overdiagnosis and require unnecessary radiation in follow-up. They also fear overtreatment with braces. The best judge of the need for radiation or orthopedic referral should be the primary pediatrician who can follow the adolescent with photographs. Radiographs in children with scoliosis can be as few as two to three a year during the adolescent growth spurt (Winter, 1986).

REFERENCES

American Academy of Pediatrics: Report of the Committee on Infectious Diseases. Evanston, IL, 1984, p. 3.

Bailey EN, Kiehl PS, et al: Screening in pediatric practice. *Pediatr Clin North Am* 21:1, 1975.

Bernbaum J, Anolik R, Polin RA, et al: Development of the premature infant's host defense system and its relationship to routine immunizations. *Clin Perinatol* 11:73, 1984.

Erikson E: *Childhood and Society*. New York, Norton, 1950, 1963.

Frankenburg WK, Camp B: *Pediatric Screening Tests*. Springfield, IL, Charles C Thomas, 1975.

Frankenburg WK, Sciarillo W, Burgess D: The newly abbreviated and revised Denver Developmental Screening Test. *J Pediatr* 99:995, 1981.

Graef J, Cone TE (eds): *Manual of Pediatric Therapeutics*, 3rd edition. Boston, Little, Brown & Co., 1985.

Green M, Haggerty R, et al: *Ambulatory Pediatrics*. Philadelphia, WB Saunders, 1984, pp. 32–33, 70–72, 81–83.

Hoekelman RA: Screening programs. In Frankenburg W (ed): *Screening Programs, Principles of Pediatrics*. Philadelphia, WB Saunders, 1984, pp. 181–215.

Human Communication: The public health aspects of hearing, language, and speech disorders. US Department of HEW, PHS NINDB Monograph 2, 1968.

Jones EF, Forest JD, Goldman N, et al: Teenage pregnancy in developed countries: Determinants and policy implications. *Fam Plann Perspect* 17:2, 1985.

Koshland DE: Benefits, risks, vaccines, and the courts. *Science* 227: (editorial), 1985.
Kunin CM: Current status of screening children for urinary tract infections. *Pediatrics* 54:619, 1974.
Levy H, Mitchell M: The current status of newborn screening. *Hosp Prac* 1982.
Marks MJ, McLaine PN, Drummond KN: Proteinuria in children with febrile illnesses. *Arch Dis Child* 45:256, 1970.
Rapp CE: The adolescent patient. *Ann Intern Med* 99:52, 1983.
Reeves J: Iron deficiency anemia: Cost effective screening and management. *Contemp Pediatr* 1:10, 1984.
Smellie JM, Edwards D, Normand ICS, et al: Effect of vesicoureteric reflux on renal growth in children with urinary tract infection. *Arch Dis Child* 56:593, 1981.
Sun M: Whooping cough vaccine research revs up. *Science* 227:1184, 1985.
Tanner J: *Growth at Adolescence*. Oxford, Blackwell, 1955, 1962.
Thorpe HS, Werner EE: Developmental screening of preschool children. A review of inventories used in health and education programs. *Pediatrics* 53:362, 1974.
Winter RB: Adolescent idiopathic scoliosis (editorial). *N Engl J Med* 314:1379, 1986.
Zuckerman BS, Walker DK, Frank DA, et al: Adolescent pregnancy: Biobehavioral determinates of outcome. *J Pediatr* 105:857, 1984.

Aspects of Nutrition 2

In this chapter, we have selected those topics in infant nutrition that are a prominent part of well child care. The reader is referred to Section 3 for a fuller discussion, and to Howard and Winter: *Nutrition and Feeding of Infants and Toddlers*. Boston, Little, Brown & Co., 1984.

BREAST-FEEDING

The purpose of all infant feeding is to provide the required nutrients in a way that optimizes growth and development. Infants grow the fastest during the first 4–6 months of life, a period over which many nursing mothers elect to provide their own milk as the exclusive food for the infant. When adequate amounts of human milk are ingested, the nutritional status of the infant is considered to be optimal; in fact, it is the reference standard against which growth on all modified cow's milk formulas is compared.

The normal infant in a temperate environment adjusts intake to achieve on the average 100–120 kcal/kg body weight per day, and 120–180 ml/kg/day. Supplemental water or solids are not required and, indeed, may interfere with the needed stimuli for maternal milk production.

Nursing

Successful breast-feeding requires milk production which is stimulated by sucking and emptying the breast. This process is mediated by prolactin. Transport of milk to the nipple area (milk letdown) is mediated by oxytocin acting on myoepithelial cells in the breast. The "letdown" milk has a higher fat content than the initial or "fore" milk from the ductules.

Nursing can begin whenever mother and infant are alert and ready, usually 4–8 hours after birth. Initially, the infant should be limited to 5 minutes per breast to avoid irritation of the nipples. The usual interval between feedings is 3–4 hours, although many mothers prefer to nurse "on demand," which can alter the duration of the intervals by an hour or two. By the end of the first week, the infant usually empties a breast in 10–15 minutes. Most mothers allow the infant to empty both breasts at each feeding, but alternate the starting breast.

Trends

One can assume that for millennia in the past, human milk was the universal food for the infant. One can hope it becomes nearly so in the future.

When it became possible to provide clean cow's milk, and add carbohydrate to it, many physicians encouraged development of "formulas" for infants who for a variety of reasons were not breast-fed. Through the years modification of the cow's milk made it well tolerated, it was widely available, necessary vitamins were added, and by 1955 fewer than 30% of mothers in the United States nursed for longer than 1 week. With increasing awareness that even the best prepared formula did not have all the additional non-nutritive advantages of human milk, a shift in practice occurred over the next 25 years, so that by 1984 about 65% of mothers nursed their infants in hospital, but only 29% were nursing at 5–6 months (see Table 1.4 for comparison composition of human milk and formulas and Table 1.5 for nursing demographics).

Table 1.4
Comparison of Composition of Human Milk and Selected Formulas

Approximate Analyses Per Liter: Values calculated from nutrient values per 100 Calories

	Mature Human Milk[1,9a]	Similac® and Similac® With Iron 20	Enfamil® and Enfamil® With Iron 20	SMA® and SMA® Lo-Iron 20	Similac® PM 60/40 20	Enfamil® Premature Formula® 20	Isomil® 20	ProSobee® 20	Progestimil® 20	Nutramigen® 20
ENERGY, Cal	**730**	**676**	**670**	**676**	**676**	**670**	**676**	**670**	**670**	**670**
PROTEIN, g	**11**	**15.0**	**15**	**15**	**15.8**	**20**	**18.0**	**20**	**19**	**22**
% of total Calories	6	9	9	8.9	9	12	11	12	11	13
Source	Mature Human Milk	Cow's Milk	Reduced Minerals Whey and Nonfat Milk	Nonfat Milk and Demineralized Whey	Whey and Caseinate	Demineralized Whey and Nonfat Milk Solids	Soy Protein Isolate	Soy Protein Isolate	Casein Hydrolysate, Cystine, Tryosine and Tryptophan	Casein Hydrolysate
Amino Acids, mg										
Histidine	240	310	290	380	380	390	450	460	570	660
Isoleucine	580	730	910	1030	950	1160	800	920	1140	1340
Leucine	1000	1410	1560	1850	1620	1940	1440	1520	1940	2230
Lysine	710	1070	1040	1560	1360	1510	1060	1200	1630	1890
Tryptophan	180	190	230	270	230	310	190	240	640	240
Phenylalanine	480	730	590	800	600	760	950	980	910	1060
Threonine	480	640	740	1050	940	1100	650	640	930	1080
Valine	660	810	930	1090	990	1220	830	920	1420	1680
Methionine	220	420	290	340	410	450	360	360	590	680
Cystine	200	130	180	280	260	220	170	180	300	90
FAT, g	**45**	**36.3**	**38**	**36**	**37.6**	**34**	**36.9**	**36**	**27**	**22**
% of total Calories	55	48	50	48.2	50	44	49	48	35	35
Source	Mature Human Milk	Soy and Coconut Oils	Coconut and Soy Oils	Oleo, Coconut, Oleic and Soy Oils	Soy and Coconut Oils	Medium-Chain Triglycerides, Soy and Coconut Oils	Soy and Coconut Oils	Coconut and Soy Oils	Corn Oil and Medium-Chain Triglycerides	Corn Oil
Fatty Acids										
Polyunsaturated, g	7[10b]	14	11.1	4.9	12	7.8	13	10.1	9.7	15.7
Saturated, g	17[10b]	15	17.9	15.0	18	22.3	16	19.4	12.7	3.5
Monounsaturated, g	19[10b]	5	5.9	14.0	6	3.7	6	5.4	4.6	6.9
Linoleic acid, mg	550	8790	7400	3300	8790	7170	8790	6700	9110	13,400
E:PUFA Ratio	0.3	1.0	1.3	1.3	1.1	1.0	1.0	1.3	1.1	0.45
CARBOHYDRATE, g	**71**	**72.3**	**69**	**72**	**69.0**	**74**	**68.3**	**68**	**91**	**88**
% of total Calories	39	43	41	42.9	41	44	40	40	54	35
Source	Lactose	Lactose	Lactose	Lactose	Lactose	Corn Syrup Solids, Lactose	Corn Syrup and Sucrose	Corn Syrup Solids	Corn Syrup Solids and Modified Tapioca Starch	Sucrose and Modified Tapioca Starch

MINERALS	Mature Human Milk	mEq	Similac® 20	mEq	Enfamil® 20	mEq	SMA® 20	mEq	Similac® PM 60/40 20	mEq	Enfamil® Premature Formula® 20	mEq	Isomil® 20	mEq	ProSobee® 20	mEq	Progestimil® 20	mEq	Nutramigen® 20	mEq
Calcium, mg	330	17	510	25	460	23	420	21	380	19	790	40	710	35	630	32	630	32	630	32
Phosphorus, mg	150		390		320		280		190		400		510		500		420		480	
Magnesium, mg	40[10c]		41		52		45		41		33		51		74		74		74	
Iron, mg	0.22[10d]		12[2]		12.6[3]		12.0[4]		1.5		1.7		12		12.7		12.7		12.7	
Zinc, mg	1.5[10d]		5.1		5.2		5		5.1		7		5.1		5.3		4.2		4.2	
Manganese, mcg	7–15[10c]		34		105		150		34		88		200		210		200		210	
Copper, mcg	240[10c]		610		630		470		610		1080		510		630		600		600	
Iodine, mcg	30[10c]		100		68		60		41		53		100		69		48		48	
Sodium, mg	180	8	220	10	180	8	150	7	160	7	260	11	320	14	290	13	320	14	320	14
Potassium, mg	530	14	810	21	720	18	560	14	580	15	750	19	950	24	780	20	740	19	690	18
Chloride, mg	390[10c]	11	510	15	420	12	375	11	400	11	570	16	440	12	550	16	580	16	480	14

VITAMINS										
Vitamin A, IU	2500	2030	2100	2000	2030	8100	2030	2100	2100	1690
Vitamin D, IU	22[10c]	410	420	400	410	2230	410	420	420	420
Vitamin E, IU	1.8(mg)[10c]	20	21	9.5	20	31	20	21	15.9	10.6
Vitamin K, mcg	20[10c]	54	58	55	54	88	100	106	106	106
Thiamine (Vitamin B_1), mcg	140	680	520	670	680	1690	410	530	500	500
Riboflavin (Vitamin B_2), mcg	370	1010	1050	1000	1010	2370	610	630	600	600
Vitamin B_6, mcg	110	410	420	420	410	1690	410	420	400	400
Vitamin B_{12}, mcg	0.4	1.7	1.5	1.3	1.7	2.0	3.0	2.1	2.1	2.1
Niacin, mcg	1830	7100	8400	5000	7100	27,040	9130	8380	8500	8500
Folic acid (Folacin), mcg	50	100	105	50	100	240	100	106	106	106
Pantothenic acid, mcg	2300	3040	3100	2100	3040	8110	5070	3200	3200	3200
Vitamin C (Ascorbic acid), mg	50	60	54	55	60	240	60	55	55	55
OTHER NUTRIENTS										
Cholesterol, mg	145	11	<5.3	33	22	<10	0	0	trace	<10
Taurine, mg	42[10e]	45	40	40	45	40	45	40	40	40
Water, g	910	900	900	904	910	902	900	900	900	900
OSMOTIC CHARACTERISTICS										
Renal Solute Load, ** mosm	77	105	98	91	95	126	122	129	126	134
Osmolality, mosm/kg water	300[10f]	290	300	300	260	244	250	200	350	480
Osmolarity, mosm/liter	270[10f]	260	270	271	240	220	230	180	310	430

[1]Composition of human milk varies with the stage of lactation and from mother to mother.
[2]Similac® Low-Iron Infant Formula 20 contains 1.5 mg iron/liter.
[3]Enfamil® Low-Iron Infant Formula 20 contains 1.1 mg iron/liter.
[4]SMA® Low-Iron 20 contains 1.5 mg iron/liter.
[5]Similac® Low-Iron Infant Formula 24 contains 1.8 mg iron/liter.
[6]Similac® Low-Iron Infant Formula 13 contains 1 mg iron/liter.
[7]Values listed are for Similac® Natural Care® only; designed for use as a human milk fortifier.
[8]Values listed are for 1:1 dilution with water. However, standard dilution is one part formula base to one part prescribed carbohydrate and water solution.

[9]References:
[a]*Composition of Foods.* Agriculture Handbook No. 8-1. US Dept of Agriculture. Agricultural Research Service, rev. 1976, item no. 01-107
[b]Guthrie HA, Picciano MF, Sheehe D. Fatty acid patterns of human milk. *J Pediatr* 90:39, 1977.
[c]Fomon SJ, Filer LJ Jr. Milks and formulas, in Fomon SJ *Infant Nutrition*, ed 2 Philadelphia: WB Saunders Co., 1974, p 363.
[d]Picciano MF, Guthrie HA: Copper, iron and zinc content of mature human milk. *Am J Clin Nutr* 29:242, 1976.
[e]Rassin D, Gaull G: Taurine and other free amino acids in milk of man and other animals. *Early Hum Dev* 2:1–13, 1978.
[f]Tomarelli RM: Osmolality, osmolarity and renal solute load of infant formulas. *J Pediatr* 88:454, 1976.

Table 1.5
Infants Breast-Feeding in Hospital and at 5 and 6 Months by Selected Demographic Characteristics—Revised Weights [1,2]

	In Hospital			At 5 and 6 Months		
Characteristic	1983	1984	% Point Change 1983–1984	1983	1984	% Point Change 1983–1984
Ethnicity						
White	64.4	65.0	0.6	28.9	28.6	(0.3)
Black	29.8	33.3	3.5	9.7	11.7	2.0
Maternal age (yr)						
<20	39.3	36.8	(2.5)	8.7	10.2	1.5
20–24	55.5	58.0	2.5	19.1	19.7	0.6
25–29	65.3	66.6	1.3	31.1	30.6	(0.5)
30–34	67.8	69.4	1.6	38.0	39.1	1.1
≥35	60.7	64.7	4.0	34.9	38.5	3.6
Family income						
<$7,000	36.2	36.6	0.4	12.3	12.4	0.1
$7,000–14,999	54.0	54.5	0.5	20.4	21.1	0.7
$15,000–24,999	63.8	64.8	1.0	29.2	29.2	0.0
≥$25,000	71.3	71.8	0.5	33.9	33.4	(0.5)
Maternal education						
Noncollege	49.1	50.7	1.6	17.8	19.2	1.4
College	76.7	77.5	0.8	39.8	38.8	(1.0)
Maternal employment						
Employed full-time	55.5	56.2	0.7	12.2	12.3	0.1
Employed part-time	65.9	67.6	1.7	26.8	28.9	2.1
Total employed	59.3	60.3	1.0	17.5	18.2	0.7
Not employed	58.0	58.6	0.6	29.0	29.2	0.2
US census region						
New England	57.8	58.5	0.7	27.4	25.8	(1.6)
Middle Atlantic	48.9	50.9	2.0	23.1	23.4	0.3
East north central	57.1	57.7	0.6	24.1	24.9	0.8
West north central	62.3	66.0	3.7	26.9	28.2	1.3
South Atlantic	50.2	50.5	0.3	20.2	20.2	0.0
East south central	42.7	45.9	3.2	16.1	17.3	1.2
West south central	55.4	55.9	0.5	20.0	20.2	0.2
Mountain	75.8	77.6	1.8	36.4	37.6	1.2
Pacific	77.4	77.7	0.3	34.8	36.0	1.2

[1] All point changes are positive unless enclosed in parentheses, which indicates negative.
[2] Reproduced with permission from Martinez, GA, Krieger, FW: 1984 Milk-feeding patterns within United States. *Pediatrics* 76:1004, 1985.

Advantages of Human Milk

It has been possible to modify the protein, carbohydrate, fat, and minerals in cow's milk to make it very close to human milk in food value. Some differences persist, however. For example, calcium absorption is superior in human milk so that artificial formulas require enrichment in calcium. Human milk contains inadequate amounts of fluoride, so breast-fed infants require 0.25–0.5 mg of fluoride daily if maternal intake is low.

The initial colostrum is cloudy, relatively low in fat, and significantly enriched with secretory IgA. This antibody is critical to the development of local gastrointestinal immunity in many mammals and clearly has a role in the human, although it is probably less critical than in other mammals. Some local production of IgM, IgG_4 and IgD occurs. IgG groups are found in milk, presumably by passive transfer from the mother (Ogra and Ogra, 1978; Keller et al, 1985).

In human milk, other factors also probably protect against enteric infection. Macrophages found in human milk are capable of killing bacteria in vitro. Their antibacterial activity withstands 24 hours of refrigeration, but not freezing or sterilizing.

Although the published evidence from developed and developing countries supports fewer serious gastrointestinal illnesses in infants fed human milk, the question of protection from respiratory illness is less clear (Kovar et al, 1984). One of the most impressive studies is that of Saarinen (1982) who followed prospectively 256 healthy term infants for a year and correlated episodes of otitis media with breast-feeding versus bottle feeding. The incidence of otitis was inversely associated with the duration of breast-feeding. The frequency of upper respiratory infections was the same in each group, which led the authors to speculate that the result may have been from bottle feeding while supine (positional otitis media) rather than any attribute of human milk.

The question of any continuing protection from infection after discontinuing breast milk has not been answered adequately by any well-controlled studies.

The possible protective effect of human milk on development of allergic diseases has been studied prospectively in a number of settings, but the evidence is not convincing (Hide and Guyer, 1985). Clearly individuals raised exclusively on human milk for the first 6 months may develop eczema, rhinitis, or asthma. In one retrospective study, increasing duration of breast-feeding was associated with increased likelihood of eczema, which raised the possibility of contaminants or allergens in human milk (Taylor et al, 1983).

There is no convincing support for a protective effect of human milk on the likelihood of cow's milk allergy at a later age.

The psychologic advantages to the mother can be observed and readily documented. Klaus and others have shown that early and extended physical contact between mother and infant enhanced later "mothering" behavior. Clearly, physical contact can also be a prominent part of formula feeding, but breast-feeding guarantees it.

Contraindications: Not every mother wants to nurse her infant, especially if she is sick, or the infant is to be adopted. The pediatrician has an obligation to be sure the maternal choice is well-considered, and not based on misinformation.

Some maternal medications may have an adverse effect on the infant; these include most cancer chemotherapy, lithium chloride, radioactive compounds, isoniazid, and chloramphenicol. It seems wise to avoid nursing when the mother requires those drugs.

Sometimes the composition of maternal milk is inappropriate. An illustration of this problem is presented below.

CASE ILLUSTRATION

A 16-day-old white male presented with dehydration and constipation. The baby was the 3.0-kg product of a 42-week gestation to a 27-year-old primagravida mother whose pregnancy was essentially uncomplicated. The baby was started on breast-feeds and did "well" feeding 10–12 minutes on each breast every 3–4 hours. Discharge weight was 2.75 kg.

Over the next 2 weeks the baby was felt to continue to "feed well" with the only problem being mother's complaint of some breast discomfort, but no obvious mastitis. On the night before admission, the father, a physician, noted that the baby looked somewhat "dry" and had not passed stools in several days, prompting the first visit to their pediatrician and a quick referral to our emergency room.

The baby appeared cachectic and irritable with significant muscle wasting. Temperature was 35°, HR 90, RR 50, BP 80/P, and weight 2.8 kg. Examination was notable for poor skin turgor and tenting, a markedly depressed fontanel and no obvious focus for infection. Initial laboratory results revealed a serum sodium of 155 mEq/L, K 6.1 mEq/L, C1 118 mEq/L, HCO_3 16, BUN 111 mg/dl, and Cr 8.9 mg/dl. Total protein was 6.7 g and albumin 4.0 gms. Hct was 57.5, WBC 9,900 with a normal differential, and urine specific gravity 1.021 with a benign sediment. A full septic work-up was performed and all cultures were negative. (i.e., blood, urine, and cerebrospinal fluid.)

QUESTION AND COMMENT

What is the mechanism for the hypernatremic dehydration?

Although hypernatremic dehydration can occur in infants secondary to excessive fluid losses (e.g., gastroenteritis, diabetes insipidus, or feeding of high solute diet), we do not believe that this patient's clinical presentation suggested such an etiology. Instead we believe this baby's symptoms were secondary to inadequate breast-feeding (despite the benign feeding history), a rarely considered cause for hypernatremic dehydration and malnutrition, but one that has been recently reported in the literature, particularly with primagravida mothers.

The mechanism for hypernatremia is thought to be a combination not only of diminished fluid intake by the baby but also excess sodium load. In this patient's mother's milk, the sodium concentration was 35 mEq/L (compared with the normal 7 mEq/L). Previously reported cases of hypernatremia secondary to breast feeding also showed high sodium content in milk. Why the sodium concentration was elevated in this mother's milk is not clear, although inadequate early lactose production has been found to cause elevations in sodium levels in breast milk. Mastitis may also contribute.

Whether inadequate breast milk volume was secondary to the mother's inability to produce enough or baby's inability to suck properly is also not clear, although both may play a role. In addition to hypothermia and bradycardia (seen in our patient), convulsions, hyperglycemia, focal and generalized seizures and DIC have all been reported in dehydrated infants fed only on breast milk. Our patient responded to appropriate oral rehydration and parental education. Breast milk was restarted without further problems once the infant was well hydrated.

CASE ILLUSTRATION

A 24-year-old mother wanted to nurse her firstborn, a daughter, and started at about 2 hours after birth. She fed the infant on breast milk on frequent demand until 6 months; no formula or other supplements were given. Some table food was introduced gradually over the next 6 months. The mother's periods returned at 9 months and at 12 months after the first birth she conceived. She continued to nurse her firstborn throughout the pregnancy, noting only that the color of the milk was "more orange" starting at the 3rd month.

A son was born at term and nursed. The firstborn now 21 months old was reluctant to give up the breast, so the mother succeeded in nursing both infants, sometimes at the same time. She commented that the force of sucking of the new baby brought on a large letdown of milk that had reverted to normal color and consistency. The daughter was weaned at age 34 months forcibly, and the son at 27 months.

QUESTIONS AND COMMENTS

Should this mother have breast-fed her children beyond the first year of life?

In many parts of the world, mothers do nurse infants for several years, even as long as 5 years. It is unusual to find a mother willing to nurse two at the same time. She hoped the firstborn would want to wean during pregnancy, but this did not happen, and it seemed unwise to produce sibling rivalry when the new baby arrived, so the mother decided to nurse both. She found support from La Leche League during those years and, in retrospect, felt rewarded for giving her children a foundation of security that she hopes will promote their later independence. Most mothers are reluctant to be so continuously available to their infants over so long a period. When they choose to do so, it can be rewarding. Exclusive breast-feeding for more than 6 months is associated with a decrease in linear growth (Salmenpera et al, 1985).

How effective a contraceptive is nursing?

Obviously in this case it was ineffective. It has long been assumed that postpartum amenorrhea is associated with absent ovulation, although it is known that women can ovulate before their first menstruation after a birth (Anderson et al, 1984). For women who do not nurse, the average duration of amenorrhea is 2 months; for those who do, amenorrhea usually persists throughout the period of nursing. Thus, prolonged nursing is sometimes advocated to lengthen the interval between births. The relationship between birth interval and infant health has been studied with some evidence that neonatal death rates are slightly higher in pregnancies conceived within 6 months of the birth of the previous infant. Probably the most serious aspect of short intervals between pregnancies is the dilution of parenting of the previously born infant, and in developing countries, the risk of malnutrition.

For a comprehensive review of "Current Issues in Feeding the Normal Infant," the reader is referred to a series of papers on the topic in a supplement to *Pediatrics* Vol. 75, Part 2. Jan. 1985 pages 135–215, and "Report of the Task Force on Assessment of the Scientific Evidence Relating to Infant Feeding Practices and Infant Health," Supplement *Pediatrics* 74 Part 2:579, 1984.

SOLID FOODS

The time of introduction of solid foods is arbitrary and can be individualized within limits. No nutritional need dictates the average time that is currently widely recommended, between 4 and 6 months. Socially it is deemed advisable to wean then (or later) and to give the infant experience with food other than milk. Less dependency on cow's milk for protein, and more on solids in particular, during the second 6 months is advisable to lessen the irritation to the gastrointestinal tract commonly seen with more than a pint (500 ml) of cow's milk a day. Because solid foods may impair bioavailability of iron, iron supplements will be required. (See Table 1.6 for recommendation on solid food introduction during the first year.)

VITAMINS

Breast-fed infants require 400 IU of vitamin D per day. They tolerate well an added 1500 IU vitamin A and 50 mg vitamin C per day.

Infants fed on modified cow's milk will need added vitamins only if they are not present in suitable concentration in the prepared formula, or the infant consumes less milk than needed to supply the recommended quantities. (See Table 3.7 [Nutrition, Section 3] for Recommended Daily Allowances, from Food and Nutrition Board, National Academy of Sciences, Revised 1980.)

FLUORIDE

Fluoride prevents dental decay by becoming incorporated into the structure of teeth as they are forming during infancy and childhood. The mineral literally enhances the strength of the tooth and makes it more resistant to decay. It has been known for decades that a naturally occurring fluoride level of one part per million parts of water, is associated with less tooth decay in the population. When levels in drinking water are below this amount and supplemental fluoride is not entering into the food chain, the prevalence of cavities is much higher.

Table 1.6
Solid Food Introductions During the First Year[1]

Food	Age (months) 0–2	2–4	4–6	6–8[2]	8–10[2]	10–12[2]
Breast milk or iron fortified formula	5–9 feedings (16–32 oz)	4–7 feedings (20–36 oz)	4–6 feedings (24–40 oz)	3–4 feedings (24–32 oz)	3–4 feedings (16–32 oz)	3–4 feedings (16–32 oz)
Grains			Infant cereal,[3] single grain (i.e., rice, barley, oatmeal)	Infant cereal, all varieties	Infant cereals, plain hot cereal (adult type), plain crackers, toast	Infant cereal, cooked cereal, bread products, rice, pasta
Vegetables				Strained or mashed vegetables (plain)	Cooked, mashed table vegetables	Cooked vegetable pieces, raw vegetables (finger foods)
Fruit			Fruit juice (from cup)	Strained fruit, applesauce, mashed bananas, fruit juice (from cup)	Soft peeled fruit (i.e., banana, pear, apple, peach), fruit juice (from cup)	Fresh fruits (peeled), canned fruits (packed in own juice), fruit juice (from cup)
Protein foods				Plain yogurt, strained meats, egg yolk, tofu, cottage cheese	Strained meats, egg yolk, tofu, cottage cheese, legumes (sieved)	Small pieces of chicken or meat (tender), whole egg, cooked dry beans (mashed), peanut butter

[1]Reprinted with permission from Howard RB, Winter HS: *Nutrition and Feeding of Infants and Toddlers*. Boston, Little, Brown & Co., 1984.
[2]This is a time when the sodium content of the infant's diet can increase greatly; highly processed, canned,and salted foods should be avoided.
[3]Iron-fortified dry, boxed cereals are better sources of iron and protein than jarred cereals mixed with fruit.

In 1985, about 60% of communities in the United States had adequate fluoride levels in their drinking water, either from natural sources or as an additive. For the 40% of American children who reside in areas where fluoride levels are low, fluoride supplements are available either in the form of drops or tablets.

The recommendation of the American Dental Association is that children living in areas with less than 0.7 part per million of fluoride be given supplements from birth to 13 years of age. Inasmuch as the actual dose of sodium fluoride required depends on the concentration in the drinking water, it is well to consult your local water department to ascertain the situation where you live.

Breast-fed babies in some communities should receive 0.25 mg of supplemental fluoride each day, according to the recommendations of the American Academy of Pediatrics. Human milk contains very little fluoride (Table 1.7). However, current practice varies; not all doctors begin fluoride supplements at birth, and many delay until about 6 months. The data are not adequate to make a strong recommendation for either position.

Table 1.7
Supplemental Fluoride Dosage Schedule (mg/day[1])[2]

Age	Concentration of Fluoride in Drinking Water (ppm) <0.3	0.3–0.7	>0.7
2 weeks–2 yr	0.25	0	0
2–3 yr	0.50	0.25	0
3–16 yr	1.00	0.50	0

[1]Fluoride content of 2.2 mg of sodium fluoride is 1 mg fluoride.
[2]Adapted (with permission) from *Pediatric Nutrition Handbook*, Evanston IL, Academy of Pediatrics, 1985, p. 171.

It is possible to have an overdose of fluorides because of a high level in the drinking water and excessive supplemental doses. Although this is not a major health concern, the teeth can become discolored with some white spots; this condition of tooth mottling is termed fluorosis (see pp. 1233).

REFERENCES

American Academy of Pediatrics: *Pediatric Nutrition Handbook,* 2nd edition Committee on Nutrition. Elk Grove, IL, American Academy of Pediatrics, 1985.

Anderson JE, Marks JS, Park TK: Breast-feeding, birth interval, and infant health. *Pediatrics* 74 part 2:695, 1984.

Arnand SK, Sandborg C, Robinson RG, et al: Neonatal hypernatremia associated with elevated sodium concentration of breast milk. *J Pediatr* 96:66, 1980.

Hide DW, Guyer BM: Clinical manifestation of allergy related to breast and cow's milk feeding. *Pediatrics* 76:973, 1985.

Howard RB, Winter HS: *Nutition and Feeding of Infants and Toddlers.* Boston, Little, Brown & Co., 1984.

Keller, MA, Heiner DC, Myers AS, et al: IgD in human colostrum. *Pediatr Res* 19:122, 1985.

Kovar MO, Serdula MK, Marks JS, et al: Review of the epidemiologic evidence for an association between infant feeding and infant health. *Pediatrics* 74, Part 2:615, 1984.

Nichols BL, Nichols VN: Lactation. *Adv Pediatr* 26:137, 1979.

Ogra SS, Ogra PL: Immunologic aspects of human colostrum and milk: 1. Distribution characteristics and concentrations of immunoglobulins at different times after the onset of lactation. *J Pediatr* 92:546, 1978.

Rowland TW, et al: Malnutrition and hypernatremic dehydration in breast-fed infants. *JAMA* 247:1016, 1982.

Saarinen UM: Prolonged breastfeeding as prophylaxis for recurrent otitis media. *Acta Paediatr Scand* 71:567, 1982.

Salmenpera L, Perheentupa J, Simes MA: Exclusively breast-fed healthy infants grow slower than reference infants. *Pediatr Res* 19:307, 1985.

Taylor B, Wadsworth J, Golding J, et al: Breast-feeding eczema, asthma and hay fever. *J Epidemiol Commun Health* 37:95, 1983.

Behavioral Issues 3

The overview of Well Child Care (Chapter 1) highlights some of the questions that will illuminate behavioral issues for each age. Whereas no general textbook can do justice to the rapidly expanding field of developmental-behavioral pediatrics, such a textbook would not serve its purpose unless some key topics are at least summarized, and references are provided for more complete discussions. We have drawn on the writings of Levine and colleagues in their book, *Developmental Behavioral Pediatrics* (Philadelphia, WB Saunders, 1983), and recommend it to those of our readers who want more than we can provide.

INFANCY SLEEP-WAKE DEVELOPMENT

In the newborn, sleep and wakefulness are distributed as intervals of 3–4 hours of sleep punctuated by 1–2 hours of wakefulness throughout the 24-hour cycle. By the end of the first month, there is more sleep at night and subsequent months are characterized by the infant's ability to sustain relatively more sleep during the night and more wakefulness during the daylight hours. By 5 months of age, most infants are able to sustain 7 hours of sleep at night.

By 1 year of age, most children sleep for one long period at night and have one or two daytime naps, with a total of 14 hours of sleep per day. After infancy, the amount of sleep decreases to about 12–13 hours during the second year, with one daytime nap, and between 2 and 5 years the daytime nap is usually given up and total sleep is reduced to about 11 hours. Koch et al (1984) report a negative correlation between duration of day sleep and night sleep. The decline is gradual until the adult level of 7–8 hours is reached in late adolescence.

In the early 1950s, Kleitman and associates described two distinct states of sleep; one characterized by rapid eye movements (called REM sleep), the other quiet sleep. The REM state represents considerable physiological activation and loss of motor neuron reflexes. Cardiac and respiratory activity are also irregular and periodic breathing and apneic spells are most common during REM sleep. The non-REM or quiet state is characterized by slower cardiac and respiratory rates and infrequent body movements. The electroencephalogram (EEG) is synchronous with slow frequency and high voltage, unlike the low amplitude fast frequency characteristics of the EEG during REM sleep.

An inability to sleep well is rare in infants and toddlers without other illness.

APPROACH TO COLIC

Definition

Colic has always been, and still remains, a confusing problem for the pediatrician, to some extent because no standard definition exists at the present time. The most objective definition is that used by Wessel et al (1954) in which colic is defined as "paroxysms of irritability, fussing, or crying, lasting for a total of more than 3 hours a day and occurring on more than 3 days in any week" in a young infant less than 3 months of age.

CASE ILLUSTRATION

A 6-week-old female infant, born after an uncomplicated pregnancy and delivery, was doing well in all respects except she would waken several times each night and seemed unconsolable. She was nursing every 4 hours during the day, but more frequently at night in an attempt to quiet her.

COMMENT

This infant was normal on physical examination and gaining weight appropriately. The reason for the night waking was assumed to be excessive fluid intake and the hypothesis tested by advising gradual reduction in time on breast and lengthening the interval between feedings at night. Finally nighttime feedings were stopped after 10 days, and the infant slept well. This most common problem sets up the vicious cycle of increased urine output, wet diapers, and often diaper rashes. Moreover, the gastrointestinal tract is stimulated by nutrients so that stools are also more frequent.

CASE ILLUSTRATION

A 4-year-old boy began to snore at night and seemed to have difficulty breathing. He was asymptomatic during the day and had no other problems. On physical examination, the tonsils nearly met in midline, although they were not inflamed. Radiographs of the upper airways showed adenoid hypertrophy but no other lesions. A chest radiograph showed a normal cardiac silhouette, and clear lungs. The electrocardiagram was normal.

COMMENT

Snoring may be the most prominent symptom of obstructive sleep apnea. In this instance, a recording of respiration during sleep (sleep pneumogram), revealed respiratory irregularities and apneic episodes. The enlarged tonsils and adenoids were assumed to be the obstruction. After resection, the snoring disappeared.

When tonsillar and adenoidal hypertrophy is severe and persists, alveolar ventilation may be compromised in the same manner seen in infants with relative macroglossia (such as Down syndrome, Pierre Robin syndrome, etc). The resulting chronic disturbance in blood gases is thought to be the cause of pulmonary hypertension, and eventually right heart failure. The cardiopulmonary changes reverse when the upper airway obstruction is removed.

Basic Science

The pathophysiology underlying colic remains poorly understood. Crying patterns as documented by parental report remain an inaccurate and biased method by which to quantify the frequency, duration, or intensity of crying episodes. Nevertheless, a number of theories have been proposed to describe the etiology for colic. These include problems in feeding techniques or dietary intolerance to some formula preparations. However, in a survey by questionnaire, parents reported that 35% of infants had moderate to severe feeding and crying problems regardless of breast- or formula feeding (Forsyth et al, 1985). Other theories suggest that there are extrinsic problems in an infant's environment contributing to excessive crying such as overstimulation or exposure to noxious stimuli. A third theory points to intrinsic problems in the infant, such as immaturity of the GI tract or the CNS. Another view holds that all three simple hypotheses interact to produce excessive crying in the infant. Intrinsic factors such as a milk protein allergy might be combined with the extrinsic factor of a parent handling the child inappropriately, such that the crying behavior of the child is exacerbated and colic results.

Epidemiology

About 10% of the population between ages 1 and 3 months experiences colic (Carey, 1984).

Natural History

Most cases persist until age 3–4 months when, for unexplained reasons, the frequency of crying episodes begins to diminish. Apparently, in settings where inappropriate care or attention is given to the excessive crying, the symptom may persist even longer.

Diagnosis

Colic is a diagnosis that is reached by excluding other organic possibilities for excessive crying. The intensity, duration, and frequency of crying should be noted. Associated symptoms reflecting neurologic or GI abnormalities should also be elicited to avoid missing another treatable ailment. A detailed narration of a typical day allows insight into the infant's behavior. If the infant cries during the visit, observation of the way in which the parent tries to soothe the infant may be helpful in instituting treatment. Parental concerns about the pregnancy and about the baby as well as possible sources of stress or lack of support in the family also should be examined.

Physical examination is rarely useful if the child is crying excessively, although it can be useful to rule out other potential diagnoses, such as neurologic abnormalities and GI disorders including intermittent obstruction and intussusception. If there is no suspicion of a surgical, GI, or neurologic disability, laboratory tests are seldom indicated.

Treatment

Treatment is primarily directed toward counseling the parents about their infant's behavior. First, they should be reassured that the examination does not reveal a significant organic problem in the child's physical or neurologic well-being. It is possible that the parent's perception of crying is at fault and that it really conforms to that of a normal infant. A colicky infant cries an average of 2.6±1.1 hours/day as compared with 1.0±0.5 hours/day for normal infants (Taubman, 1984). Counseling for psychosocial stresses involving the parents or the parent-child interaction should also be discussed. Some parents tend to overstimulate a crying infant rather than soothing him, and placing him with a pacifier in a quiet environment, with a minimum of unnecessary handling. Not every crying baby wants to be picked up. Parents should be encouraged to distinguish when a baby cries for food or for attention, and when a baby calls for help (Taubman, 1984).

Antispasmodic agents to treat overfeeding or gas have not been found beneficial in the treatment of colic and are not recommended.

Finally, the apparently optimistic statement that this behavior pattern is only temporary may be less beneficial to the parents if 5–6 more weeks of colicky behavior are predicted. On the other hand, frequent follow-up of the family is important and phone calls every several days will provide the family with a support network. Formula changes are seldom appropriate and, in fact, any feeding change probably acts more as a placebo than as a therapeutic maneuver.

Prognosis

Colicky behavior rarely continues beyond 3 or 4 months of age. If the children have a neurologic disability, a more difficult temperament, or a lower sensory threshold, it is possible that these characteristics will continue to affect the way the infant and older child interacts with the environment. This has yet to be documented. No longitudinal studies of the eventual outcome of colicky infants have been made.

Prevention

The best method of prevention is to alert the parents about the possibility and reasons for excessive crying: hunger, fatigue, overstimulation, or calling for assistance. Being available to a family of a colicky infant is probably the best preventive measure that a pediatrician has to offer in ensuring that a successful interaction between parents and their infant will occur.

NIGHTMARES AND NIGHT FEARS

Probably all children experience fears or even panic at some time, but for the most part, they are short lasting and the child can be readily consoled.

Frequent recurrent nightmares should be taken more seriously on the assumption that they are a symptom of ongoing conflict.

Sometimes sleepwalking or inappropriate urination may occur during a period of partial arousal, usually 1–3 hours after sleep onset. Some children are terrified during these arousals. When thrashing behavior or sleep walking occurs at ages 5 or 6 years, it will probably be outgrown. When it occurs in adolescence, underlying psychologic disorders may be present and deserve exploration.

NARCOLEPSY

Excessive or inappropriate sleepiness deserves evaluation. Sometimes it is the sole sign of hepatitis or infectious mononucleosis. If persistent, an evaluation of thyroid function and glucose metabolism is in order. It rarely appears before 10 years of age, and more often the onset is adolescence.

When the condition is clearly persistent, and not a transient response to being overtired, it is considered narcolepsy. The condition is characterized by sudden, irresistible attacks of sleep, loss of muscle tone after laughter or fright, and visual or auditory hallucinations on falling asleep or wakening.

The diagnosis depends on awake-asleep EEG studies. The affected individual requires brief daytime naps, and then feels refreshed. The diagnosis is one of exclusion and treatment requires counseling about this lifelong problem. Medications such as dimenhydrinate or meclizine are often helpful, but should be individualized.

REPETITIVE BEHAVIOR PATTERNS

Repetitive movements are characteristic of all infants and children at certain stages of development. Infants have startle reactions or myoclonic jerks, and bursts of non-nutritive sucking which may last a month or more. Most infants indulge in some thumb, toe, or lip sucking during the first year, and head banging is not uncommon. Attempts to stop these behaviors should not be undertaken before age 4 years. After a year of age, nail-biting is common and, of course, may persist to adulthood although usually children stop by 4 or 5 years.

Habit spasms or tics are manifest in many different ways, from eye-blinking, facial grimaces, swallowing, throat clearing, or jerking movements of shoulders or neck. Up to 10% of the population has some kind of tic for periods of at least a month (Schowalter, 1980).

Any of these transient repetitive behaviors can become chronic and very troublesome. One of the most debilitating is Gilles de la Tourette syndrome which manifests with motor and vocal tics such as barks, yelps, or echolalia or coprolalia (an irresistible tendency to utter profanities.) Self-abusive behavior may occur. The condition occurs in families with a history of tics. Sometimes "soft" neurological signs are evident. Haloperidol is sometimes therapeutic (2–6 mg /day) but has side-effects, such as parkinsonian symptoms, weight gain, and intellectual blunting. Clonidine hydrochloride has been of benefit (see Section 12, Neurology).

No single approach has been uniformly beneficial to individuals with troublesome tics. The pediatrician's role is to identify any underlying cause, and in its absence to be supportive of the individual and reassuring that most tics will disappear.

BREATH-HOLDING SPELLS

Definition

Breath-holding spells (BHS) are a response to frustration or pain or fear, and usually follow violent crying.

Basic Science

Little is known about the reasons why some children will go to the extreme of unconsciousness from voluntary breath holding. No physiologic difference between those with spells and those without has been reported. Extensive studies of ventilatory responses to carbon dioxide and hypoxia have failed to show depressed chemosensitivity in those prone to hold their breath. In the absence of measured differences in ventilatory control, we assume the cause is emotional or behavioral.

Epidemiology

They are most common between ages 6 months and 6 years. The incidence is unknown.

CONTROVERSY

We should admit we do not understand this phenomenon. No treatment is known. Difficult as it may seem, all we find appropriate to offer is reassurance that we are unaware of any late, adverse effects.

ENURESIS

Definition

Enuresis literally means the voiding of urine; it is applied to situations in which voiding is uncontrollable and inappropriate by usual standards. Primary enuresis refers to prolonged bedwetting or daytime voiding after the age when most children stop. Secondary enuresis is the recurrence of uncontrollable voiding after a period of dryness of more than 3 months at least, and usually 6 months.

Basic Science

Mature bladder function requires awareness of fullness, ability to postpone initiation of micturition, and ability to sustain voiding until the bladder empties. All these functions require a degree of maturation of the nervous system which on average is achieved between 18 and 30 months.

Epidemiology and Natural History

The incidence depends on definition, and is very difficult to ascertain, although most accounts of the achievement of bladder control are similar. The percentage of children who attain dryness rises steeply between 1 and 3½ years. The sequence of control is first bowel, then bladder by day, and finally bladder at night.

In a Scandinavian study, 12% of males and 7% of females had nocturnal enuresis at 4–4½ years, and in 8% of males and 6% of females, this persisted through 7–8 years of age. Enuresis is more common in the United States. It is more likely in blacks than whites and more common among lower socioeconomic classes and households of three or more children (Hallgreen, 1956).

Diagnosis

Bedwetting is one of the most common conditions discussed during well-child visits. A careful history to distinguish dribbling from enuresis, consideration of organic causes (such as diabetes) and urinalysis are all essential to be certain the condition is primary.

Differences in temperament have been described in enuretic children, such as "high-strung," afraid of the dark, and not very well liked by other children. They may be less attentive at school and perform less well on achievement tests. Enuresis may be associated with stressful events such as hospitalization or parental separation.

Treatment

Treatment must be appropriate for the age of the individual and the severity of the problem. Sometimes counseling against too early toilet training and reassurance that enuresis is self-limited is sufficient.

A search for problems that coexist with enuresis often directs attention to adverse environmental factors that may be remedied.

Urine alarms are widely used among children old enough to understand their purpose (5–6 years). This is essentially behavioral therapy. A few drops of urine activate the alarm which wakens the child and permits him to get up and urinate. With respect to drugs, for about half of the enuretic children, tricyclic antidepressants (imipramine, amitriptyline) are effective, often within 1–2 weeks. The mechanism of action is not understood. The most common side effect is dryness of the mouth, but drowsiness, dizziness, cardiac arrhythmias, and nightmares may occur. Only the rare child should be treated with drugs, and preferably for a short period, such as at summer camp, during visits to other houses or on trips.

ENCOPRESIS

Encopresis, lack of bowel control, is a distressing problem that deserves the attention and intervention of a physician.

Definition

As with enuresis, primary encopresis defines continuous lack of bowel control, and secondary implies a period of control followed by loss of control.

Epidemiology

Encopresis or daytime soiling occurs in 1–2% of second graders, six times more commonly in boys.

Natural History

Most encopretics have some degree of constipation. Although many defecate daily, they do not empty the colon. Gradual distention and blunting of sensory input starts a vicious cycle of less bowel tone, further constipation and fecal impaction. In this respect, they mimic youngsters with Hirschsprung disease.

Table 1.8
Management of Encopresis [1, 2]

Treatment Phase	Treatment Program	Comments
Initial counseling	1. Education and "demistification" of the problem 2. Removal of blame 3. Establishment and explanation of treatment plan	Include diagram, review of colonic function, shared observaton and x-ray views. Emphasize need for intestinal "musclebuilding"
Initial catharsis Inpatient	1. High normal saline enemas (750 cc. b.i.d.), 3–7 days 2. Bisacodyl (Dulcolax) suppositories b.i.d. 3–7 days 3. Use of bathroom for 15 minutes after each meal	Patient admitted when: Retention is very severe Home compliance likely to be poor Parents prefer admission Parental administration of enemas is inadvisable psychologically
At home	1. For moderate to severe retention, 3–4 cycles as follows: Day 1: hypophosphate enemas (Fleet Adult) twice Day 2: bisacodyl (Dulcolax) suppositories twice Day 3: bisacodyl (Dulcolax) tablet once 2. For mild retention senna or danthron, one tablet daily 1–2 weeks	1. Dosages or frequency may need alteration if child experiences excessive discomfort 2. Admission should be considered if there is inadequate yield 3. No lubricant during this phase
	Follow-up abdominal x-ray examination to confirm adequate catharsis	
Maintenance regimen	1. Child sits on toilet twice a day at same times each day for 10 minutes each time 2. Light mineral oil (at least 2 tablespoons) twice a day for at least 4–6 months 3. Multiple vitamins, two a day, between mineral oil doses 4. High roughage diet: bran, cereal, vegetables, fruits 5. Use of an oral laxative (senna or danthron) for 2–3 weeks, then alternate days for 1 month (given between mineral oil doses); then laxative is discontinued; lubricant is continued.	1. A kitchen timer may be helpful 2. A chart with stars for sitting may be good for children under 7 years of age 3. Bathroom reading encouraged 4. Mineral oil may be put in juice or Coke or any other medium 5. Vitamins to compensate for alleged problem with absorption secondary to mineral oil 6. Diet should be applied but not to the point of coercion
Follow-up pattern	1. Visits every 4 to 10 weeks, depending on severity, need for support, compliance, and associated symptoms 2. Telephone availability to adjust doses when needed 3. In case of relapse: Check compliance Use of oral laxative (e.g. Senokot) for 1–2 weeks Adjust dosage of mineral oil 4. Counseling or referral for associated psychosocial and developmental issues 5. Continuing use of demystificaton diagram to document progress	1. Duration of treatment program may be as long as 2–3 years or as short as months 2. Signs of relapse: Excessive oil leaks Large caliber stools Abdominal pain Decreased frequency of defecation Soiling 3. Physician should spend time alone with child 4. In patients who are slow to respond, physician should sustain optimism; persistence cures almost all cases (eventually)

[1] Reproduced with permission from Levine MD: In Levine, Carey, Crocker, et al: *Developmental Behavioral Pediatrics*. Philadelphia, WB Saunders, 1983.
[2] All dosages and frequencies are for an average-sized 7-year-old-child. Appropriate adjustments should be made for smaller and larger patients.

In the presence of a predisposition to constipation, many psychosocial factors can aggravate the problem. These include, for example, parental overreaction, punishment, or excessive use of enemas or other laxatives.

Diagnosis

Diagnostic studies include a thorough physical examination to ascertain the degree of constipation and any anorectal abnormalities. A plain radiograph of the abdomen is very useful. If Hirschsprung disease is suspected, anal manometry is helpful. (Encopresis is uncommon in Hirschsprung disease, but a paradoxical diarrhea may occur.) Encopretic stools are of large caliber, in contrast to those in patients with aganglionosis in which there is a constricted segment.

Treatment

Levine's approach to management has been very effective. It is outlined in detail in Table 1.8.

REFERENCES

Anas NG, McBride JT, Boettrich C, et al: Ventilatory chemosensitivity in subjects with a history of childhood cyanotic breath-holding spells. *Pediatrics* 75:76, 1985.

Anders T: Night waking in infants during the first year of life. *Pediatrics* 63:860, 1979.

Anders T, Weinstein P: Sleep and its disorders in infants and children. *Pediatrics* 90:312, 1972.

Aserinsky E, Kleitman N: Regularly occurring periods of eye motility and concomitant phenomena during sleep. *Science* 118:243, 1953.

Brazelton TB: A child-oriented approach to toilet training. *Pediatrics* 29:121, 1962.

Brazelton TB: Crying in infancy. *Pediatrics* 29:579, 1962.

Brazelton TB. Neonatal behavior and its significance. In Avery ME, Taeusch HW (eds): *Diseases of the Newborn.* Philadelphia, WB Saunders, 1984, p.68.

Carey WB: "Colic" or excessive crying in young infants. In Levine M, Carey, Archer, et al (eds): *Developmental Behavioral Pediatrics.* Philadelphia, WB Saunders, 1983.

Carey WV: "Colic"—primary excessive crying as an infant environment interaction. *Pediatr Clin North Am* 31:993, 1984.

Cohen DJ, Detlor J, Young JG, et al: Clonidine ameliorates Gilles de la Tourette syndrome. *Arch Gen Psychiatry* 37:1350, 1980.

Engen T, Lipsett LP, Kaye H: Olfactory responses in adaptation in the human neonate. *J Comp Physiol Psychol* 56:73, 1963.

Ferber R: *Solve Your Child's Sleep Problems.* New York, Simon & Schuster, 1985.

Forsyth BWC, Leventhal JM, McCarthy PL: Mothers' perceptions of problems of feeding and crying behaviors. *Am J Dis Child* 139:269, 1985.

Gross RT, Dornbusch SM: Enuresis. In Levine M, Carey, Archer, et al (eds): *Developmental Behavioral Pediatrics.* Philadelphia, WB Saunders, 1983, pp. 573–586.

Hallgreen B: Enuresis: A study with reference to morbidity risk and symptomatology. *Acta Psychol Neurol Scand* 31:379, 1956.

Hoder EL, Cohen DJ: Repetitive behavior patterns of childhood. In Levine, Carey, Archer, et al (eds): *Developmental Behavioral Pediatrics.* Philadelphia, WB Saunders, 1983.

Illingsworth RS: Evening colic in infants. A double blind trial of dicyclomine hydrochloride. *Lancet* 2:1119, 1959.

Klaus MH, Kennell JH: Mothers separated from their newborn infants. *Pediatr Clin North Am* 17:1015, 1970.

Koch P, Soussignan R, Montager H: New data on wake-sleep rhythm of children aged from 2½–4½ years. *Acta Paediatr Scand* 73:667, 1984.

Kravitz H, Boehm JJ: Rythymic habit patterns in infancy: Their sequence, age of onset and frequency. *Child Dev* 42:399, 1971.

O'Donovan C, Bradstock AS: The failure of conventional drug therapy in the management of infantile colic. *Am J Dis Child* 133:999, 1979.

Parmelee AH: Sleep patterns in infancy. A study of one infant from birth to eight months of age. *Acta Paediatr Scand* 50:150, 1961.

Schowalter JE: Tics. *Pediatr Rev* 2:55, 1980.

Taubman B: Clinical trial of the treatment of colic by modification of parent-infant interaction. *Pediatrics* 74:998, 1984.

Wessel M, Cobb A, Jackson JC, et al: Paroxysmal fussing in infants, sometimes called "colic." *Pediatrics* 14:421, 1954.

Widmayer SM, Field TM: Effects of Brazelton demonstrations for mothers on the development of preterm infants. *Pediatrics* 67:711, 1981.

Mental Handicaps

4

OVERVIEW

Definition

Mental retardation is a syndrome, because it represents a constellation of behavioral findings which result from many different causes. The two symptoms that define mental retardation are significant impairment in intelligence as measured by a test of intelligence quotient (IQ) and an inability to adapt to the expectations of the environment which, for young children, is principally school. The arbitrary point of demarcation between the retarded and the nonretarded has been set at 2 standard deviations from the mean or at an IQ of 70. With this definition, it is estimated that 3% of the population of the United States are retarded. These definitions are hazardous, however, because it is manifestly ridiculous to describe anything as complex as a human being by 2 digits or even 3 digits. The IQ tests tend to define areas of weakness in performance and often overlook many areas of great strength. Nonetheless, it is true that individuals who deviate significantly from their peer group in any area of performance may deserve special attention, extra education, or if the deviation is toward the side of unusual competence in some area, positive reinforcement to achieve satisfaction from that strength.

Organic causes of mental deficiency can include gross anatomic lesions such as agenesis of portions of the brain or changes in cell architecture produced by viral illnesses or in trisomies, such as Down syndrome.

A wide variation in the incidence of visible anatomic defects in the brains of mentally deficient individuals has been described. Other lesions are molecular or, in other words, are not readily apparent anatomically. More than 50 molecular diseases have been identified in which a specific enzyme defect is associated with an alteration in metabolism and in turn with mental dysfunction. Illustrative of this group of diseases are maple syrup disease and phenylketonuria (see section on Inborn Errors of Metabolism).

APPROACHES

Major changes in our expectations of life of a retarded child have been brought about in the last few decades. The concept of university-affiliated programs for evaluation of handicapped individuals has expanded facilities for treatment programs. Before they were initiated, large state institutions were the only major service resource and few trained professionals were available to assist the individual child. Now multidisciplinary teams of physicians, dentists, social workers, anthropologists, and educators have learned to work together to develop means for assessing the strengths and weaknesses of the individual and to work out prescriptions for remedial care and stimulation. As a result, the number of these individuals who are now in large institutions has decreased dramatically in recent years and their placement in special programs in the public school systems has been a major advance. It is clear that the needs of the individual must be met, which depends on community resources and the willingness of parents to work with their handicapped child. Some, mainly the most profoundly handicapped, will probably always require custodial care in institutions. This should be a small proportion, however, of the number of individuals with either known or unknown causes of mental deficiency (for details of the natural history of given conditions, please refer to the appropriate sections).

Diagnosis

When a delay in motor development or acquisition of skills or language is first noted, what investigations are appropriate? Obviously, when major neurologic deficits become evident in infancy, full work-up for possible correctable causes is required. This section concerns the child without neurological deficits whose development is delayed, and includes those whose problems are first encountered on entry to preschool or school environments. In general, the physician should consider genetic causes or environmental insults, which can be revealed by appropriate history-taking. Among adverse environmental influences would be: malnutrition (from whatever cause), severe electrolyte imbalance such as hypernatremia, a systemic infection that could involve the CNS, an exposure to environmental toxins, such as lead, and the possibility of psychosocial deprivation.

The laboratory studies will depend on the information obtained through careful history-taking. Any findings suggestive of seizures would mandate neurologic evaluation and an electroencephalogram. Most probably, a cranial CT scan would be undertaken to search for relevant anatomic lesions. For infants, but also for children of most any age, it is useful to have a full psychologic evaluation administered by an experienced psychologist. The value of these tests is to specify in more detail than a simple IQ the areas of adequate or excellent performance as well as the areas of deficiency (see Table 1.9).

Table 1.9
Suggestions for Evaluation of a Child With Mental Retardation [1]

Chromosomal karyotype, if abnormal features
Aminoaciduria
Urinary mucopolysaccharides
Urinary reducing substances
Urinary ketoacids
Blood lead level (if pica present)
Skull radiographs (if head abnormal)
CT scan (if focal seizures present, or head abnormal)
Serum uric acid (if self-mutilation or choreoathetosis is present)
Serum ammonia
Serum neuroenzymes or skin biopsy, if loss of milestones
Skin histamine test if autonomic dysfunction is present

[1]Modified from Taft L: In: *Nelson's Textbook of Pediatrics*, 12th edition. Philadephia, WB Saunders, 1983.

Treatment

Appropriate treatment of an anatomic problem or neurological deficit depends on its definition and will be discussed elsewhere. The approach to the nearly 90% of mentally retarded persons with no demonstrable neurological defect involves full and open discussion with the parents or other caretakers, including teachers, to provide full description of the individual's problem. Because mentally retarded individuals are disproportionately represented among poor people, psychologists and pediatricians have begun to evaluate the role of early intervention with preschool programs to try to overcome the adverse effects of an unstimulating or otherwise oppressive home environment, or simply to give added support to those in this group.

The best known of these programs has been "Head Start," launched in the United States in the 1960s, and continuing until now (mid-1980s). Although findings on follow-up are controversial, the conclusion that intervention has at least a temporary positive effect on learning is supported, and the earlier the program is started, the greater the benefit.

In 1972, Ramey et al initiated a very early intervention program (Day Care for high-risk infants in the first years of life). The program involved social service support for the families, nutritional supplements, medical care, and a learning curriculum administered by experienced teachers. On testing at 18 months, the infants in the program scored higher than those not enrolled. These preliminary results have stimulated a national collaborative program to test the applicability of such intervention in a larger and more diverse sample of infants (Infant Health and Development Program, Robert Wood Johnson Foundation, Princeton, New Jersey).

Learning Abilities and Disabilities

Janice Ware

DEFINING INTELLIGENCE

The practical value for early characterization of intellectual abilities is apparent, yet controversial. There are many definitions and theoretically derived models of intelligence. Spearman's original conception of intelligence as a unitary "g" (general intelligence) factor was followed by the multifactored models of Guilford and Cattell. Within the last decade all of these models have made way for the currently predominant information processing model which regards cognition as a kind of computer program with powerful input and output components. Thus, current attempts to measure intelligence rely heavily on techniques that describe an individual's ability to process different types of information across a variety of sensory modalities.

TESTING CONSIDERATIONS

Regarding intelligence as primarily a neurologic function, however, fails to explain the large body of dramatic findings demonstrating the powerful effects of socioeconomic (or social/emotional) influences. The best model of intellectual functioning recognizes and accounts for the complex transactional nature of both biology and environment in shaping what is ultimately described as an individual's cognitive ability. Sternberg's (1985) thoughtful review on human intelligence defines intelligence as those mental functions employed for purposes of adaptation to and shaping and selection of real-world environments.

Understanding these models has relevance for deciding how best to measure intelligence in a standardized way. Just as controversy has always surrounded the nature of intelligence so has it challenged the theory and practice of intelligence testing. Proponents of intelligence tests praise their sound statistical properties while opponents of testing express serious concerns about their role in perpetuating social and economic injustice as well as perpetuating myths about the nature of intellectual functioning.

MEASURING INTELLIGENCE

Intelligence tests emphasize language development, problem-solving, and abstract reasoning abilities. Psychometricians have long since recognized that 'intelligence is what the test measures.' Well-standardized and well-administered intelligence tests are excellent means to describe reliably a variety of behaviors linked together to represent one or more aspects of intellectual functioning. For example, an individual's verbal intelligence would typically be measured by his ability to speak spontaneously and fluently and to understand the content and structure of language. Testing of this sort samples only part of the wide domain of abilities most people label as intelligence. Intelligence tests are used across age levels from infancy through adult life. The ability of the tests to predict development accurately improves as the child matures.

Many characteristics that play a major role in determining test outcome are assessed subjectively by the examiner and influence scoring of the test. Most notable among these characteristics are attention, persistence, responsiveness to the test situation, and motivation. Impairments in motor and/or sensory ability also will directly affect test performance. Other important influences often implicated in cognitive status include a variety of maternal and family characteristics including socioeconomic status, life stress, and amount and type of environmental stimulation available to the child. This combination of multiple factors along with the child's actual pass-fail performance on individual test items is often defined as cognition.

IDENTIFYING LEARNING DISABILITIES

Increased interest in early detection and treatment of learning disabilities has made the subject a topical one for parents of young children. Although the prevalence of learning disabilities in the United States was estimated at 2% by the National Center for Educational Statistics in 1970, estimates vary *widely* depending on the definition applied to the term "learning disability." There is widespread confusion among parents and professionals about what the term learning disability means and the potential impact of such a label. To some, the term learning disabilities includes notions of brain damage, hyperactivity, mild forms of retardation, social-emotional adjustment problems, language difficulties, subtle forms of deafness, perceptual problems, motor problems, and most commonly, reading disorders. In the broad sense, they can refer to learning difficulties that can be associated with any type of factor, including mental retardation, brain injury, sensory difficulties, or emotional disturbance. Others restrict the term to the failure to learn an academic skill by a child who has adequate intelligence, maturational level, and cultural background. The narrower definition is termed "specific learning disability."

The most common learning disability is reading disability (frequently called dyslexia). Other learning disabilities are associated with writing, spelling, and arithmetical skills. According to learning-disability specialists, the five disabilities that best differentiate learning-disabled children are disabilities in reading comprehension, attention, auditory-visual-coordination, writing, and auditory speed of perception.

The term learning disability sidesteps the previously used term, minimal brain dysfunction (MBD), to describe learning problems. The label MBD is currently regarded as stigmatic. However, there is now a tendency for every kind of school problem to be called a learning disability. Levine's description of a learning disability as a term used to describe a handicap that interferes with someone's ability to store, process, or produce information seems appropriate.

It is sometimes difficult to distinguish limited general intelligence from cognitive dysfunctions related to specific types of processing or organizing difficulties within the child. This distinction does not rule out the possibility that children who are functioning in below-average intellectual ranges also have processing difficulties that impede their learning ability.

Levine's ANSER system contains a series of age-specific neurodevelopmental examinations for the evaluation and interpretation of learning problems. The Pediatric Early Elementary Examination (PEEX) is the most well-known portion of this system. The PEEX evaluates neurodevelopmental status for the first, second, and third grades. These grades correspond to the ages in which learning disabilities are most frequently diagnosed. Table 1.10 displays the developmental areas assessed by the PEEX.

CONTROVERSY

In response to the well-recognized deficiencies of intelligence tests some theorists call for the use of social competence measures as opposed to measures of intelligence. Included in their definition of social competence are four categories of behavior: physical health, formal cognitive ability, achievement in school, and motivational-emotional variables. Their work is consistent with the growing interest in minimizing the use of a single developmental test score to characterize a child's level of functioning and maximizing the use of qualitative and descriptive assessments of the child's abilities.

The broader perspective of intellectual functioning calls for the examiner to have a clear understanding

Table 1.10
Areas and Test Items on a School-Age Neurodevelopmental Examination (PEEX) [1]

Area	General Description	Items [2]
Minor neurologic indicators	Various signs thought to be associated with developmental dysfunction and learning problems	Visual tracking Stimulus extinction Left-to-right discrimination Rapid pronation-supination Imitative finger movement Finger differentiation Associated movements
Temporal-sequential organization	Tasks that assess a child's knowledge of everyday sequences and time relationships as well as ability to understand and remember new data in the correct order	Digit spans Word spans Imitative block tapping Count forward and backward Days of week, telling time Gross and fine motor sequence Understand temporal prepositions
Visual-spatial orientation	Tasks that reveal a child's ability to appreciate spatial relationships and visual detail, to integrate such inputs with motor responses, and to remember visual configurations	Connect dots to imitate design Copy designs (direct and from memory) Matching designs Visual recognition Visual retrieval Object spans
Auditory-language function	Exercises tapping a child's understanding and use of language	Comprehension of oral directions Comprehension of complex sentences Confrontation naming test finding (word-finding and expressive vocabulary)
Fine motor function	Activities entailing eye-hand coordination, finger localization, neuromotor speed, pencil control, and fine motor pattern mastery	Finger opposition (simple and sequential) Sentence copying (legibility) and speed Pencil control Motor speed test Imitiative finger movements Finger differentiation
Gross motor function	Exercises requiring motor praxis, inhibition, rhythm, body positon sense, and eye–upper limb coordination	Hopping in rhythm Tandem gait Catch a ball Sustained stance (eyes closed) Associated movements
Memory	Ability to recall at end of PEEX certain stimuli presented near the beginning	Object recall, other visual recall Form copying (revisualization) Word recall

[1]Reproduced with permission from Levine MD, et al: *Developmental Behavioral Pediatrics*. Philadelphia, WB Saunders, 1983, p. 946.
[2]Certain items are listed in more than one area because they entail several developmental components.

about what is being assessed, to think through what is to be learned as a result of the cognitive evaluation, and, further, to consider what decisions about the child's life will be affected by the knowledge from the testing.

Despite the limitations of standardized intelligence tests they continue to be the best available long-term predictor of developmental outcome and adjustment using the common language of standardized scores. These scores can be readily communicated across disciplines for purposes of appropriate educational planning. Formal intelligence tests also allow for the measurement of changes over time in order to evaluate the effects of remediation.

Instruments

Screening Tools

Because pediatricians have frequent contact with children and their families during the formative years, they are well placed to assist in the earliest possible detection of intellectual handicaps. Early detection is critical in intellectual impairment because early recognition and appropriate intervention can improve the prognosis. Another important task of the pediatrician is to ascertain whether the child has any physical problems that require medical attention, especially disorders of hearing and vision. One cost-effective and practical means of doing this is by utilizing screening techniques as a means to identify individuals in need of further more comprehensive diagnostic testing. The goal of an effective screening tool is to maximize the identification of those individuals who, as a result of further diagnostic testing, turn out to be impaired while minimizing the number of both false-positives (individuals whose screening results indicate impairment but who subsequently turn out not to be impaired) while at the same time minimizing the number of false-negatives (the number of impaired individuals who fail to show up as such as a result of the screening test). This balance requires both a reliable screening tool and experienced test administrators. One positive feature of many pediatric screening tools is their ability to be effectively utilized across disciplines by individuals with a sound working knowledge of child development rather than specific intelligence testing training.

Gesell Developmental Schedules

Gesell and his colleagues at Yale were the original pioneers of mental testing for infants (Knobloch et al, 1980). Gesell's first scale was published in 1925. Gessell conceived of his scale as a global index of development rather than as a test of mental abilities or IQ. The purpose of his test was to describe an infant's overall developmental status in order to detect atypical infants in need of special services. The scale is used clinically to assign developmental levels or calculate a rough Developmental Quotient (DQ) by dividing the child's mental age by his chronologic age. The abilities tested by the original Gesell included motor, language, adaptive, and personal-social behaviors. The recent revision of the schedules includes items appropriate for use with 1- to 36-month-old children. The original ability areas defined by Gesell remain the same with the exception of the motor scale, which now distinguishes between fine and gross motor behavior.

The Gesell Schedules have been criticized over the years for having inadequate norms and little available information on reliability and validity. Because of these limitations, the Gesell is used primarily by pediatricians as a screening tool rather than as a diagnostic instrument. The scales are most noteworthy for their historical significance and the important role they have played in stimulating the development of other standardized infant assessments.

Denver Developmental Screening Test

The purpose of the Denver Developmental Screening Test (DDST) is to provide a quick, easily administered, nontechnical screening instrument for identification of significant delays in children (Frankenburg et al, 1981). The test was developed for children aged birth to 6 years but is generally considered to be most effective with infants and very young children. Administration and scoring time for the test is about 15–20 minutes. Test performance is not scored numerically but described as "normal," "abnormal," or "questionable" based on a comparison to the performance of the norm group (Fig. 1.2). Thus, results from the test can serve only as a broad screening. Children identified as having abnormal or questionable DDST results need further indepth diagnostic testing. Many items on the DDST are taken directly from the Gesell including the four general ability areas comprising the scale (personal/social, fine motor/adaptive, language, and gross motor). Although early reports indicated that it was an effective tool for identifying developmental problems requiring diagnostic testing, more recent evidence with the British Griffith Scale indicates that it may not be as useful as previously assumed, particularly with premature infants (Elliman et al, 1985). The extent to which these findings can be generalized to premature infants in the United States is not certain at this time.

Diagnostic Tools

Bayley Scales of Infant Development

Bayley's infant scale (Bayley, 1969) has been developed, adapted, and refined over a period of 40 years. It is now accepted as the best available measure of infant developmental status. The scales yield standard scores (Mean = 100, SD = 16) for the Mental and Motor portions. Percentile ranks are available for each of the 24 ratings of the Infant Behavior Record. The Bayley has excellent psychometric properties including highly representative standardization procedures. In addition to standard scores, developmental age levels can also be computed for a more meaningful clinical description of a child's performance on the test. The scale is designed to be used with infants 1 month to 2½ years but is most typically and reliably used from 3 months to 2½ years.

The scale was originally intended to be a measure of infant intelligence. Prediction studies quickly dispelled the notion that scores from the Bayley were highly correlated with intelligence at older ages. Rather, the test has come to be recognized as an accurate, reliable, and valid measure of current developmental status with increasingly impressive predictive properties after the age of 18 months.

The Bayley Scales are comprised of three separate scales: Mental, Motor, and Infant Behavior Record. Among these three, the Mental Scale is the most widely used.

Stanford-Binet Intelligence Scale

The Stanford-Binet was the first global intelligence test ever designed and continues to be widely used as a general measure of intelligence (Terman and Merrill, 1972). The Stanford-Binet scales begin with tests at the 2-year level and continue to the adult level. The Binet scales represent the only standardized global intelligence test available for very young children. The test yields standard scores based on a mean of 100 and a standard deviation of 16. The Binet has sound statistical value. The test is frequently criticized because

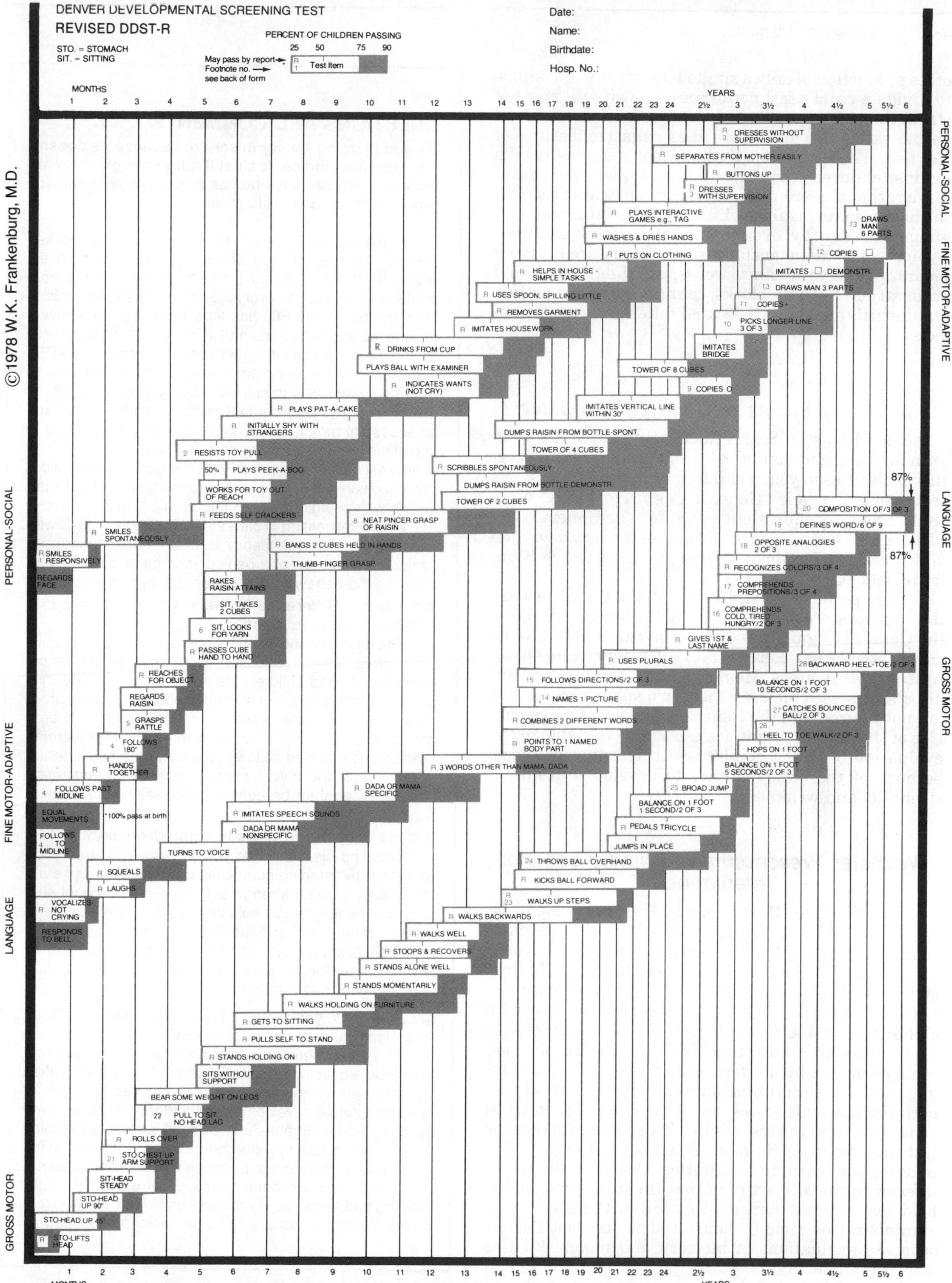

Figure 1.2. Denver Developmental Screening Test—Revised.

of its production of only a single IQ score and its failure to divide a child's test performance down into areas of strengths and weaknesses. Its reliance on memory and verbal skills also are regarded as negative features of the test. These test construction features bias results against children who respond to test questions in creative rather than routine ways. Similarly, it is thought to discriminate against children with bilingual language barriers by overemphasizing verbal abilities. Typical test items include naming pictures, giving meanings for vocabulary words, building towers and other structures with blocks, counting and calculating, and identifying similarities and differences among objects.

McCarthy Scales of Children's Abilities

The McCarthy Scales (McCarthy, 1972) are well-standardized and statistically sound measures of cognitive abilities in young children aged 2½–8 years. The test yields a single "General Cognitive Index" score that is roughly equivalent to an IQ. The General Cognitive Index has a mean of 100 and a standard deviation of 16, making it numerically equivalent to the Stanford-Binet IQ.

The special strength of the McCarthy Scales are the subtest scores (mean = 50, SD = 10) which allows the General Cognitive Index performance to be broken down into Verbal, Perceptual/Performance and Quantitative ability areas. Memory and Motor development are also assessed yielding their own subtest scores, but are not figured into the General Cognitive Index score. Use of the subtest scores are especially valuable in the evaluation of young children with learning problems because of the scale's ability to develop a profile of strengths and weaknesses.

Wechsler Preschool and Primary Scale of Intelligence

The Wechsler Preschool and Primary Scale of Intelligence (WPPSI, Wechsler, 1967) is the preschool counterpart of the Wechsler scales originally developed for adults (WAIS) and later revised for older children (WISC-R). It is a well-standardized test with good statistical properties. The test is designed for use with children aged 4–6½ years. The WPPSI is composed of 11 subtests grouped into a Verbal Scale (verbal comprehension) and a Performance Scale (perceptual organization). Individual subtest scores, verbal and performance scale scores, and a full-scale IQ can all be generated from the test results. This feature makes the test superior to the Stanford-Binet because of its utility in detecting learning disabilities. However, the test is inferior to the McCarthy in that the test items tend to hold less interest for small children, there is a long administration time (1 hour) and it does not include separate evaluations of memory and motor skills as does the McCarthy.

QUESTIONS AND COMMENTS

My son is doing poorly in school because he doesn't pay attention and can't sit still long enough to do his work. His teacher says he has a hyperactive behavior problem. What does this mean?

Hyperactivity is an old term and a catch-all phrase used to describe children who suffer from motoric overactivity to the extent that it interferes with their school productivity and behavioral adjustment. The term minimal brain dysfunction (MBD) has also been used extensively to describe this behavioral profile in children. Most professionals now use the term attention deficit disorder (ADD) to describe children who are not appropriately attentive or who are excessively impulsive. ADD with hyperactivity is a subtype of this disorder that refers to children who have an excess of motor activity for their age. This subtype is one of the most common types of learning disability. Prevalence estimates range 1–20% in the general population. The condition is much more likely to be found in boys than in girls with boy/girl ratio ranging from 3:1 to 8:1.

One complication in differential diagnosis of ADD with hyperactivity is the tendency to misinterpret normal behavior characteristic of a particular stage of development (such as the behavior of a 2-year-old) with hyperactivity.

What is the difference between being learning disabled and being retarded?

The term learning disability refers to deficits in specific ability areas rather than deficiencies in global intelligence. Mentally retarded children, particularly those in the mild and moderate range, can also have specific learning problems. In fact, reading problems in this group of children are common. Decisions about how to improve learning problems in retarded children are reliant on accurate assessments of the child's learning potential. Intervention strategies can then be adapted to developmental limitations.

Will my child outgrow his learning disability?

Learning disabilities do not go away. Children cope with them by learning compensatory strategies while utilizing other existing strengths. Prognosis for school success and healthy social adjustment strongly relate to the severity of the learning disabilities. Mild learning problems in a single ability area are much less likely to be associated with social-emotional problems. Long-term follow-up data about diagnosis and treatment are not available.

My child is 4½ years old and reverses his letters. Does this mean he is learning disabled?

Parents sometimes confuse immature responses with fears about developmental difficulties. This problem often occurs when parents compare their children to others or to some external developmental standards they have fixed in their minds. Emphasis should be placed on helping parents appreciate the wide range of normal in achieving development milestones. Because preschool children are not usually expected to read, write, or calculate math, early learning problems usually present as either deficits in language abilities or visual perceptual-motor functioning.

CASE ILLUSTRATION

A 2.2-kg child was born at 36 weeks' gestation. He had severe streptococcal Group B pneumonia followed by bronchopulmonary dysplasia. The child was hospitalized for most of the first 7 months of life. He was discharged home on oxygen by nasal cannula and weaned off the oxygen at 2 years. As he matured, he continued to have chronic pulmonary problems. He also developed a severe feeding problem involving frequent gagging and vomiting of food.

He was the first child born into a stable two-parent professional family. The pregnancy was planned and desired. The child's early medical course and continuing requirements for care proved to be an extreme stress for his parents. Parental reactions to his birth and illness included virtual social isolation of the child during the first years of life in order to protect him from exposure to viral infections. Despite the fact that he was born in a teaching hospital with a well-established developmental follow-up program, the parents chose to travel several hundred miles to Boston for monitoring of the child's developmental progress.

We evaluated his developmental progress from 18 months to 6 years of age using standardized psychological tests including cognitive assessments.

His cognitive assessments consistently revealed overall developmental functioning and IQs in high-average range. At the age of 3 years, test results indicated continuing difficulties with gross motor coordination activities. In addition, multiple anxious behaviors such as nail biting and eye blinking as well as moderate levels of motoric overactivity and distractibility were noted. Recommendations were made for a physical therapy evaluation and referral for family counseling. The family complied with the physical therapy recommendation but did not pursue the psychotherapy recommendation.

At the age of 5½ years he was reevaluated in our clinic. Referral for this evaluation again came from his parents because of the school's recommendation that he be retained in kindergarten the following year. The school's recommendation was based on their concern with his inability to do age-level work. At his parent's insistence the school had repeatedly and frequently retested his cognitive abilities in attempts to understand better his school difficulties and to reassure the parents about the validity of the test results. The parents, however, were convinced that the school psychologist had failed to detect the presence of major learning disabilities. His parents were alarmed by increasing hyperactive behavior and inability to pay attention and sit still for even brief periods of time. They wished to have the child's hyperactivity problems treated with amphetamine therapy and wanted our evaluation to include a recommendation for this treatment.

Our test results were remarkably consistent with the many evaluations completed by the child's school showing above-age level cognitive abilities with no evidence of specific learning disabilities. His attentional difficulties were considered to be secondary to his excessive fearfulness and anxious preoccupation with several themes in his life. Psychotherapeutic treatment was strongly recommended to the family.

QUESTIONS AND COMMENTS

Why were this child's cognitive abilities tested so much?

His complex medical history and neonatal high risk status warranted monitoring of his developmental progress. However, by any standard, he was *overtested.* This overtesting may well have contributed to his anxiety.

Why was drug treatment for his hyperactive behavior not recommended?

Treating a young child with amphetamines for an attention deficit disorder would have been wrong for numerous reasons. Drug treatment would have further supported the parent's avoidance of the emotional issues involved. Other less aggressive management techniques based on behavioral treatment of the problem should be employed first.

Parental request for treatment of "hyperactive" behavior with drugs has become increasingly common. Unfortunately, some parents think of drug treatment as a cure-all rather than a single component of a comprehensive treatment strategy with a strong emphasis on family involvement in treatment.

What was the outcome for the child?

The child entered therapy after a period of considerable procrastination by his parents. Not unexpectedly, the parents needed time to process findings very different from their expectations. The parents initiating contact with the psychotherapist was enormously important in recognizing and accepting the child's diagnosis, and tackling the underlying emotional problems.

How could this case have been managed better?

In retrospect, it was a mistake to follow this child medically from such a long distance. This type of management supported his parents in not establishing more effective working relationships with resources closer to home. He needed to have developmental evaluation services that would also serve as a liaison between the parents and the community agencies.

Wechsler Intelligence Scale for Children—Revised

The Wechsler Intelligence Scale for Children—Revised (WISC-R, Wechsler, 1974) almost completely dominates intelligence testing among school-age children aged 6–16 years. The WISC-R is organized in the same manner as both the preschool (WPPSI) and adult (WAIS) versions of the Wechsler scales. Subtest scores, verbal and performance IQ's, and a full-scale IQ has excellent psychometric properties. Individual subtests (such as the child's score on the vocabulary or block design) are short and, therefore, unreliable for use as independent ability measures. Significant differences between verbal and performance scale scores are used to differentiate learning disabilities from mental retardation.

REFERENCES

Bayley N: *Manual for the Bayley Scales of Infant Development.* New York, Psychological Corporation, 1969.

Caldwell BM (ed): *Group Care for Young Children. A Supplement to Parental Care* Lexington Books. DC Heath and Co., Lexington, MA, 1987.

Coplan J: Wrongful life and wrongful birth: New concepts for the pediatrician. *Pediatrics* 75:65, 1985.

Elliman AM, Bryan EM, Elliman AD, et al: Denver Developmental Screening Test and preterm infants. *Arch Dis Child* 60:233, 1985.

Farnham-Diggory S: *Learning Disabilities.* Cambridge, MA, Harvard University Press, 1978.

Frankenburg WK, Fandal AW, Sciarillo W, et al: The newly abbreviated and revised Denver Developmental Screening Test. *J Pediatr* 99:995, 1981.

Knobloch H, Stevens F, Malone AF: *Manual of Development Diagnosis: The Administration and Interpretation of the Revised Gesell and Amatruda Developmental and Neurologic Examination.* New York, Harper and Row, 1980.

Levine MD: The developmental assessment of the school age child. In Levine MD, Carey WB, Crocker AC, et al (eds): *Developmental-Behavioral Pediatrics.* Philadelphia, WB Saunders, 1983.

McCarthy D: *Manual for the McCarthy Scales of Children's Abilities.* New York, Psychological Corporation, 1972.

Ramey CT, Smith BJ: Assessing the intellectual consequences of early intervention with high-risk infants. *Am J Mental Deficiency* 81:318, 1976.

Rosenblith JF, Sims-Knight JE: *In the Beginning: Development in the First Two Years.* Monterey CA, Brooks/Cole Publishing Co, 1985.

Sattler JS: *Assessment of Children's Intelligence and Special Abilities,* 2nd edition. Boston, Allyn and Bacon, 1982.

Scarr S: Testing for children: Assessment and the many determinants of intellectual competence. *Am Psychol* 36:1159, 1981.

Sternberg RJ: Human intelligence: The model is the message. *Science* 230:1111, 1985.

Tarnopol L: *Learning Disorders in Children: Diagnosis, Medication, Education.* Boston, Little, Brown & Co, 1971.

Terman LM, Merrill MA: *Stanford-Binet Intelligence Scale: Manual for the Third Revision.* Boston, Houghton Mifflin, 1973.

Thorndike RL, Hagen EP, Sattler JM: *Stanford-Binet Intelligence Scale,* 4th edition. Chicago, Riverside Publishing Co., 1986.

Wechsler D: *Manual for the Wechsler Preschool and Primary Scale of Intelligence.* New York, Psychological Corporation, 1967.

Wechsler D: *Manual for the Wechsler Intelligence Scale for Children—Revised.* New York, Psychological Corporation, 1974.

Wodrich DL: *Children's Psychological Testing: A Guide for Nonpsychologists.* Baltimore, Paul H. Brooks, 1984.

Family Issues 5

We include in this section brief comments and selected references on some important family issues with which pediatricians should be concerned. This chapter is a synopsis of the extensive literature on these topics in journals of psychology and sociology. The textbooks by Levine et al (*Developmental Behavioral Pediatrics,* Philadelphia, WB Saunders, 1983) and Hoekelman et al (*Pediatric Care,* St. Louis, CV Mosby, 1987) are valuable general resources.

DIVORCE

The impact of parental separation or divorce on children is a topic of enormous importance to the physicians of more than one million children whose parents divorce each year (1.2 million in 1980–1981) in the United States. About three-fourths of all women and five-sixths of all divorced men remarry.

The acute phase of a divorce may lead to unusual behavior on the part of parents that can be upsetting to children. Angry outbursts and accusations may be expressed in a setting previously characterized by a routine calm. Financial concerns, new babysitters, and new homes may escalate in ways that create more anxiety in the child. Not infrequently, deterioration in school performance is noticed. Children may feel neglected or lonely. Recruitment of grandparents, close friends, and others to give the child special attention has been suggested. The pediatrician may, if an opportunity presents itself, become the central support figure. Continued relationship of the child with both parents correlates with the best outcome.

When to Tell the Child

A child needs to be told of an impending divorce before a parent leaves the house. Full discussion with both parents is appropriate as long as each (in the presence of the other) can assure the child of their love. If amid the tensions of the time, such a meeting is not possible, meeting with a counselor or a physician present may be useful. Details of arrangements for visits with both parents can be reassuring.

Parents are often apprehensive and uncomfortable about telling of the separation. It is best not to arrange a single time for communication, but rather to have an initial conversation with scheduled time for answering questions that arise later. The child's most important need is to know that the relationship with both parents will endure. If that cannot be achieved, the custodial parent must make a special effort to be available, and to avoid details of reasons for marital failure such as sexual infidelity.

Divorce may be particularly upsetting to adolescents, who project concerns about their own future marriages. The physician needs to be alert to signs of depression or suicidal tendencies in this age group, and should initiate direct contact with the adolescent.

SINGLE PARENT

Over 1 million pregnancies occur annually in this country among teenagers, many of whom are not married. Whereas some young mothers relinquish their children for adoption, more and more are embarking on single parenthood. Some drop out of school, marry, and establish a home. Others try to raise their babies in the household of their own parents. Grandmothers may assume complete responsibility for rearing the child which may set up difficult competition between mother and daughter. The pediatrician has a role in listening to both sides and helping to work out ways in which each can contribute appropriately to the care of the child without hostility or anger. If the father is available, it is also important to involve him in some arrangements.

Because the one-parent family has become an acceptable lifestyle in this society, there is considerable interest in a single parent adopting an infant. The relatively few babies or young children available for adoption make this an unusual circumstance, but it has occurred, particularly in the placement of older children. Many of these children require an intense relationship to compensate for early deprivation, abandonment, or abuse. The single adoptive parent may be preferred for some children.

WORKING PARENTS

No discussion of family issues can ignore one of the major changes of our times, that is, the increase in the number of mothers who have part-time or full-time employment (Table 1.11) (Klein, 1985). The employment rate for mothers of children under 1 year old was 33.7% in 1982. The implications of this fact on child rearing are widely discussed in many settings, including women's magazines, and innumerable studies in the psychologic and sociologic literature, although far fewer in the pediatric literature. The topic is of great concern to the ever-increasing proportion of women in medicine, whose working days are often (in fact, usually) greater than the traditional 8 hours.

Are children being deprived and likely to suffer in academic achievement or socialization from less time with their mothers? Are they enriched by day care or babysitting, or by greater independence as adolescents? Are the implications the same for all races and social classes? How important is the working mother's extra contribution to the family income? Is the issue the quality of time with children or its quantity? Are there critical periods at which a mother's presence is irreplaceable? Is the nature of the parents' work important in the sense that prestige or achievement of either parent is a source of pride? Is an achieving parent so preoccupied with creative work that little time is left to relate to the child's own achievements? Are children frustrated because they may feel they cannot match the expectations of parents who measure success by income or recognition in the professions or market place?

No one of these questions can be viewed as unimportant. A few moments of reflection, or even hours in the library lead to the same answer. The variables are so great that no study can be viewed as conclusive, and no answer completely satisfactory.

It appears that work itself is not the central issue. Parenting can be shared; surrogate caregivers can provide the necessary love and support to a child. Family size, birth order, socioeconomic status, neighborhood, and school support can be over-riding variables. Arguments can be made (and defended by one or another study), that a woman's place is in the home with a central concern for mothering. Equally compelling arguments with equally impressive data can be made for women to participate in the excitement and stimulation of the workplace and bring to the children the wisdom from their wider experiences.

Table 1.11
Employment Status of Women With Children Under 5 Years Old: 1977 and 1982 [1]

	Age of Youngest Child [2]				
% Employed	<1	1	2	3	4
1977	24.0	31.0	39.7	39.2	45.7
1982	33.7	40.4	44.1	43.1	47.3
Increase 1977–1982	40.4	30.3	11.1	10.0	3.5

[1] Data from O'Connell and Rogers 1983, cited by Klein RP: *Dev Psychol*, 21:403, 1985.
[2] In years.

It is no longer acceptable to assume that paternal unemployment and maternal employment are necessarily problems for children. Each family has to resolve the complex issues that arise in the context of their family in their social milieu. It is our view that continuing attention to these issues is the responsibility of families, and pediatricians to whom they turn for advice. As in so many aspects of medicine, this one demands individualization. For those who feel the need for more data in order to be knowledgeable counselors, the reader is referred to a thoughtful and comprehensive review of existing studies, published by the National Research Council.

CASE ILLUSTRATION

A working mother brings her 1-year-old child into the office and asks for advice. Because of the financial stresses of needing to return to work, she had stopped breastfeeding when the child was 4 months of age and placed him into a day care center that contained 30 other children. Since then the child has experienced frequent colds and ear infections requiring the mother to miss more work days than she had ever missed before, so she could take care of the child at home. She asked if she should quit her job, since she feels that the combination of stopping the breastfeeding and placing the child with other "sick children" in day care has resulted in the child's more frequent illnesses. She smoked a pack of cigarettes a day and wondered if it posed any hazard for the child.

QUESTIONS AND COMMENTS

What should the mother be told?

The decision as to who should benefit from placement in a day care setting is a complex one that needs to be individualized to a family's needs. The pediatrician needs to have an understanding of not only the child's needs for growth and development but also a knowledge of parental needs and of the day care center or home setting into which the child is to be placed.

No child should be placed into a day care setting where the care is purely custodial, and no effect is made to provide a comprehensive approach to the child's physical, cognitive, and emotional development. The ratio of trained and experienced care providers to infants should be 1:3 if children are less than age 2 years old, and no more than 1:5 for older children. Children should not be initially placed into a day care environment during times of family stress, such as a move, parental separation, parental illness, or birth of a sibling.

If the child is to start day care at age 8–9 months when stranger-anxiety begins to evolve, or at 17–18 months when dependency on parents can be most notable, the children may have difficulty adjusting to a day care center with multiple providers and children. Nonetheless, given the ever-increasing number of dually employed parents or working single parents, the need to enroll children in day care programs is ever increasing. The impact of these centers has yet to be fully assessed; nonetheless, no prospective study proves they are harmful to development or that they increase the overall frequency of illness, although they have been shown to decrease the age of onset of common childhood illnesses. Some surveys report a 60% increase in risk of upper respiratory infection (Fleming et al, 1987). However, children who are disadvantaged and/or disabled may benefit from specialized, high-quality day care environments, and may be less likely to have problems in coping with their disabilities or disadvantages.

Center size is important. It has been shown that the larger the center the higher the risk in developing the more common infectious diseases. For example, the larger day care centers containing 12 or more children show an increased risk for development of illness from *Haemophilus influenzae* infection, diarrhea, hepatitis, and possible cytomegalovirus exposure. The smaller day care centers for 6 or fewer children may have less compliance with health regulations and be less specific in their requirements for immunizations and personnel training. If that is the case, the child may be exposed to a variety of diseases through lack of hand-washing and/or understanding of the mechanisms of disease spread (Gessert et al, 1980, Aronson and Aiken, 1980).

Regardless of whether or not a child should be placed in a day care center, the pediatrician's role is to make certain that parents do not feel guilty about their choice. It helps to educate families as to what diseases and behavioral adjustments to expect in the day care centers before enrolling a child. It is also useful to acquaint the parents with a variety of day care choices ranging from the small family care for up to 6 children in a home, to large often corporate-sponsored day care centers supervising the needs of dozens of children. Whether the child was breast-fed or not, one needs to inform the parent that, most likely, the child will pick up his first infections at a much earlier period than usual, and the overall number of infant infections will be slighly greater than that of a child who has not been placed in a day care setting at an early age.

Since most day care infections are mild and self-limited, and since the family needed the mother's income, the recommendation for this mother was to keep the child in day care but place him in an alternate care setting with fewer children and, hence, less chance of spread of infection, (assuming that the care providers were knowledgeable in disease control as well as developmental issues).

The most important advice to the mother was to stop smoking. In the survey in Atlanta, Fleming et al (1987) found that maternal smoking was associated with a 70% increase in a child's likelihood of an upper respiratory tract infection. In other words, smoking posed a slightly greater hazard than day care.

With an estimated 11 million children in the United States attending some kind of day care center, it is obvious such centers are here to stay. Pediatricians have an important role in understanding the issues involved and in monitoring illness in children in their care.

ADOPTION

Adoption is widely accepted in our society and, in fact, is considered desirable, not only for infants, but for any child who has no other family with which to relate. Children with special needs or handicaps may be difficult to place, although some couples are particularly anxious to take on the responsibility of a child with problems.

When adopted children are compared with children who remain with their single mothers, adopted children seem to have less educational failure and fewer psychiatric disorders (Wolff, 1974). Therefore, many pediatricians and social workers make every effort to place a child in a family setting.

Even so, there is a significant incidence of behavioral problems in adopted children and the problems are indeed very complex. It is generally considered that the difficulties are somewhat greater the older the child at the time of adoption although this assumption has been challenged (Eldred et al, 1976).

Medical Evaluation of the Newborn Adoptee

This is a time for the pediatrician to investigate as thoroughly as possible the family history for genetic illnesses, alcohol or drug abuse during pregnancy, health of the parents, and any difficulties encountered in the perinatal period. The medical evaluation, which should be as objective and complete as possible, should be shared fully with the adopting parents.

When to Tell the Child of Adoption

Most professionals working in the adoption field believe that the fact of adoption should be revealed at 2–4 years of age to avoid the child's learning of it for the first time from other sources. The depth of the discussion can be adjusted to the child's ability to comprehend it and, clearly, time should be given for full answers to any questions from the child. The facts about adoption may need to be discussed on multiple occasions as the child's awareness of family structure matures. It is generally assumed that the parents will emphasize the fact that, whatever the reason, the child was chosen by these parents and this may provide an extra measure of assurance that he was, indeed, wanted.

Adolescence

It is not unusual for an adoptee to have more concerns about his own identity around the time of adolescence and want to know about his parents. There is often a great interest in whether the biologic parents were married, whether there are other children, and whether specific familial diseases are present.

In a sense, an adoptee adolescent who is striving to achieve independence from his parents reflects on two sets of parents from which to separate. A lingering concern about the unknown biologic parents may become an obsession. For this reason, the maximum amount of biological information that can be obtained at the time of adoption should be made available to the adolescent if he cannot contact the biologic parents.

Adoption Process

The adoption process in the United States has been designed to safeguard the rights of adoptive parents and makes access to original birth certificates and official documents impossible. In a few states, however, there are provisions for opening records on demand of the adoptee, but only as an adult. It is inappropriate for adolescents to have access to such information, because it is not clear that they are mature enough to handle it. The pediatrician is in a strong position to become the child's advocate and to provide as much information and reassurance as possible.

DEATH

Parents often ask what a child comprehends about death and what should be communicated in the event of death of a close friend, sibling, or parent. Conceptions of death vary depending on the family's religion, their sociocultural status, and maturity. A child's first experience may be the death of a pet, which may be helpful in underscoring its irreversibility. The impact of death as seen by a child who views television is hard to assess, but it is difficult for a child to go through a day without seeing death on the screen at some time.

Vaughan suggests that sharing with a child what we do not know about death is preferable to some "protective" fantasies. He further advises in the face of serious illness in a parent, that the child be told in a way compatible with his level of understanding. Visiting the terminally ill can be helpful, but need not be forced, and the decision must be individualized. After death, the child should be assured of other support systems, to transfer the interactions and expectations previously invested in the departed parent to another person.

The pediatrician has an important role in reassuring the child about his own health and allowing time for questions. Some children feel guilty after death of a parent or sibling, or try to compensate by overachieving. It is particularly distressing to a child to be asked to take on the role of the deceased. An opportunity for full discussion with the physician of the child's fears and feelings can be helpful.

TELEVISION

Many studies have linked television viewing with aggressive behavior. The Surgeon General's report in 1972 concluded that TV violence is harmful to the viewer, and this point of view was reaffirmed in 1982 by the National Institute of Mental Health. More than 96% of American homes have at least one television set. The average American child is said to watch television 3–4 hours each day, and sees 20,000 commercials each year. By graduation from high school, Rothenberg (1975) estimates an individual will have seen 18,000 television murders. To what extent this blurs the distinction between reality and fantasy is unclear. Furthermore, television is a significant source of information and misinformation about normal and abnormal sexual behavior. The effect of this exposure on the young child is of concern.

One way children can be victimized by violence on television is through imitative behaviors of parents. Vulnerable, socially isolated parents may abuse their own children after seeing abusive behavior on television (Wharton and Mandell, 1985).

The tradeoffs are obvious. Many programs on television are informative and entertaining, whereas others may show violence in all its phases. Most television programs use rapid shifts in visual images to hold attention. The question remains, does this reduce attention span and interfere with more thoughtful processing of information?

Parents have a responsibility to establish limits for television viewing and encourage alternate activities.

Zuckerman and Zuckerman (1985) suggest that the pediatrician discuss television-viewing and parental attitudes toward it. Even a 1-year-old may be entertained by children's programs that can also be instructive. It is extremes that should be avoided. For example, no time to watch TV can be counterproductive, in that it encourages children to watch neighbor's programs. Too much time watching TV is at the expense of exercise, reading and more creative activities and acquisition of skills. For more specific information, the reader is referred to: Action for Children's Television, 20 University Rd, Cambridge, MA 02138.

PARENT EDUCATION

We think it appropriate to offer some advice about approaches to patient education. A supplement to *Pediatrics* (Vol. 74, 1984) has some useful comments. A patient or parent is apprehensive about something, otherwise they would not seek help. Even though the condition may be trivial, an effort has been made to make contact with another individual who is presumed to be in a position to shed light on the problem, and try to solve it.

The first rule of a physician should be to establish a relationship with the parent and child. Everyone has his own techniques to accomplish this. A relaxed demeanor, such as sitting and listening is essential.

The nature of the problem dictates the time required for its resolution. A chronic problem should not be reviewed in an emergency room; rather, an appointment for its careful review is more appropriate. On the other hand, an emergency requires only enough history to permit appropriate action, with a careful follow-through in a more relaxed setting.

The issue of lack of patient compliance with physician's instructions has plagued us all. The reasons are multiple, but for the most part preventable. A little thought will underline the obvious issues. Are we listening to the patient's real concerns, or are we diverted by our own assessment of the problem, which we then fail to communicate? Are our suggestions for therapy practical in the context of the patient's socioeconomic status, or are we operating in ignorance of the environment to which the patient returns? A prescription for an expensive but necessary antibiotic will go unfilled if the patient does not have the cash to pay for it. Careful observation at home may be neither achievable in some settings, nor the ideal recommendation in others.

Have we been mindful of the comfort of the child or are we so concerned with differential diagnosis that we subject a sick and often tired child to multiple examinations and tests done rapidly to shorten the duration of the visit or hospitalization? The same concerns relate to the parents, who may have had sleepless nights and considerable disruption of their personal life as they care for their child. Six hours of waiting in an emergency room can be an eternity for both child and parent. Much testing and consulting is tiring for both.

We hope that students, residents, and pediatricians who read this text for guidance will also remember that their effectiveness as physicians depends on their sensitivity to the needs of the child and parent, not only for an appropriate diagnosis and therapy, but also for their humanity.

REFERENCES

American Academy of Pediatrics, Committee on Infant and Preschool Child: Recommendations for day care centers for infants and children. Evanston, IL, 1980

Aronson SS, Aiken LS: Compliance of child care programs with health and safety standards: Impact of program evaluation and advocate training. *Pediatrics* 65:318, 1980.

Caldwell BM (ed): *Group Care for Young Children. A Supplement to Parental Care.* Lexington Books, Lexington, MA, DC Heath and Co., 1987.

Eldred CA, Rosenthal D, Wender PH, et al: Some aspects of adoption and selected samples of adult adoptees. *Am J Orthopsychiatry* 46:279, 1976.

Fleming DW, Cochi SL, Hightower AW, et al: Childhood upper respiratory tract infections: To what degree is incidence affected by day-care attendance? *Pediatrics* 79:55, 1987.

Furman E: *A Child's Parent Dies.* New Haven, Yale University Press, 1974.

Gessert C, Granoff DM, Gilsdorf J: Comparison of rifampin and ampicillin in day care center contacts of *Haemophilus influenzae* type B disease. *Pediatrics* 66:1, 1980.

Kamerman SB, Hayes CD (eds): *Families that Work: Children in a Changing World.* Commission on Behavioral and Social Sciences and Education. National Research Council, 1982. 2101 Constitution Avenue, NW, Washington DC 20418.

Klein RP: Caregiving arrangements by employed women with children under 1 year of age. *Dev Psychol* 21:403, 1985.

National Institute of Mental Health: Television and Behavior. Rockville, MD, NIMH, 1982.

Rothenberg MB: Effects of television violence on children and youth. *JAMA* 234:1043, 1975.

Rutter M: Social-emotional consequences of day care for preschool children. *Am J Orthopsychiat* 51:4, 1981.

Scarr S: *Mother Care Other Care.* New York, Warner Books, 1985.

Sokolff BZ: Adoption and foster care. In Levine MD, et al (eds): *Developmental Behavioral Pediatrics.* Philadelphia, WB Saunders, 1983.

Vaughan V: In Levine MD, et al (eds): *Developmental-Behavioral Pediatrics.* Philadelphia, WB Saunders, 1983.

Wallerstein, JS: Separation, divorce and remarriage. In Levine M, et al (eds): *Development-Behavioral Pediatrics.* Philadelphia, WB Saunders, 1983.

Wharton R, Mandell F: Violence on television and imitative behavior: Impact on parenting practices. *Pediatrics* 75:1120, 1985.

Wolff S: The fate of the adopted child. *Arch Dis Child* 49:165, 1974.

Zuckerman DM, Zuckerman BS: Television's impact on children. *Pediatrics* 75:233, 1985.

Travel

6

MOTION SICKNESS

Definition

Motion sickness refers to nausea and vomiting elicited by certain kinds of motion, particularly swaying or rolling encountered on the sea and, sometimes, in automobiles or other vehicles. It is more prominent in children and tends to diminish with age, but can be elicited by the appropriate stimuli at any age. The condition is often familial and has been found to be associated with both adult and childhood migraine (Barabas, 1983).

Basic Science

Motion sickness is aggravated by visual stimuli that induce a shifting lateral gaze. Sometimes sitting in the front seat and focusing straight ahead lessens the problem. Even with the eyes closed, however, the rolling or rocking motions can stimulate receptors in the labyrinth and initiate impulses that are transmitted either directly or by way of the vestibular nuclei into the cerebellum. After passing through the uvula and nodule of the cerebellum, the signals are believed to go to the chemoreceptor trigger zone in the medulla and induce vomiting.

Neurotransmitters appear also to be involved in the mechanism of motion sickness. This can be inferred from the fact that parasympatholytic agents, such as scopolamine and atropine have been found to be effective in preventing motion sickness. In addition, on the basis of their anticholinergic effect, antihistamines are frequently used to protect against motion sickness. Whereas stimulation of cholinergic neurons appears to be involved in the pathogenesis of motion sickness, adrenergic systems are inhibitory because sympathomimetic agents such as amphetamines and ephedrine have effectively suppressed motion sickness (Wood et al, 1981).

Natural History and Epidemiology

The highest incidence of motion sickness occurs in persons who experience turbulence at sea; approximately one-quarter will become seasick (Barabas, 1983). Estimates for the prevalence of carsickness range 3–4%, with the lowest occurring on trains (0.13%). Air travelers have a much lower prevalence as well, with fewer than 1% reporting symptoms.

Motion sickness has been found to be an associated feature in 45% cases of childhood migraine, in contrast to a 5–7% incidence in children with nonmigraine headaches, seizure disorders, or learning disabilities (Barabas, 1983).

Diagnosis

As described above, disturbances of the vestibular system result in a spectrum of symptoms that include predominantly nausea, vomiting, dizziness, and loss of appetite. The presence of these symptoms while on a moving vehicle should make the diagnosis obvious.

Treatment

The old adage to the seamen to focus on the distant horizon is good advice. This can be achieved in an automobile if an infant is in a car seat where attention can be drawn to objects out of the window rather than those within reach. Some cars are built to absorb bumps and convert them into a rolling motion, which can be a more serious instigator of motion sickness than the more tightly built cars in which every shock is felt.

The essentials of treatment are to plan to travel when well-rested, stop frequently for rest periods, and remain well-hydrated. Shorten intervals between meals so that the traveller has neither an over-full nor an empty stomach.

When motion sickness occurs despite the simple preventive measures, some drugs are available. Dramamine (dimenhydrinate) is effective and safe when given in the recommended dose of 1–1.5 mg/kg/dose every 6 hours as needed. It is helpful to begin treatment 1–2 hours before travel.

Many other drugs have been evaluated in adults. Scopolamine given in a disc applied to the skin behind the ear is one of the latest additions. We do not recommend this method for children because of uncertainty of amount absorbed and potential toxicity.

TRAVELER'S DIARRHEA

Definition

Traveler's diarrhea (TD) is usually defined as being three or more loose or watery bowel movements per day, experienced while traveling or shortly after returning home. The onset of the acute diarrhea is uncommon before the third day of a visit, with the frequency and the number of attacks being a function of exposure and duration of stay in a different environment.

Basic Science

Over one-half to two-thirds of traveler's diarrhea in high-risk nations, is due to *Escherichia coli* strains that produce heat stable and/or heat-labile enterotoxins. Remaining cases are caused by a variety of other microorganisms, particularly *Shigella* which accounts for 10–20% of episodes. In the setting of an enterotoxigenic strain of *E. coli,* stool electrolytes have been found to be compatible with a secretory diarrhea, with recovery of normal fluid electrolyte absorption via the jejunum and ileum, usually by 6–8 days after the onset of the disease (Banwell et al, 1971). The most common complication is dehydration and in rare circumstances, depending on the etiology, bacteremia may develop. More serious complications are an abscess in the liver (amebiasis), or significant weight loss and malabsorption (giardiasis). The most common viral agent for traveler's diarrhea is rotavirus, which contributes to 5–10% of the cases (Feldman, 1984).

The most likely source of enteric pathogens is food. Food becomes contaminated when pathogens are not killed during food preparation or when food handlers expose a food preparation to feces, because of poor sanitation habits. The most commonly contaminated foods include meats and other foods served buffet style that are not steaming hot, uncooked green vegetables and salads, hot sauces left in open containers, and fresh cheese and milk served in less than sanitary eating establishments. Contaminated water is an uncommon source of enteric infection, although giardiasis and viruses may be contracted in this way.

Epidemiology

Men and women are affected equally (Feldman, 1984). Young adults and children, however, are more likely to develop diarrhea than older adults. The attack rate in Americans is highly dependent upon the country being visited, with highest incidence after visits to Mexico and the Latin American countries, and the lowest incidence in European countries.

Tropical and subtropical countries, particularly those where sanitation is poor, are the high-risk areas for developing the illness. In addition, risk of developing diarrhea is maximized when visitors from a low-risk country travel to a high-risk area (Steffen et al, 1983). The risk of illness in these high-risk countries is greater in summer than in winter.

Diagnosis

The diagnosis of traveler's diarrhea is most easily made when there is the history of travel, particularly travel to a high-risk area. The symptom-complex is nonspecific, but consists primarily of abdominal pain and cramping, nausea, and anorexia. Only rarely is there blood in the stools or a high fever (Gorbach and Hoskins, 1980).

Diagnostic procedures are usually unnecessary because the syndrome is usually self-limited. Moreover, even if a diagnosis of an enteric organism is made, these infections usually resolve spontaneously without need of specific therapy (see below). Only if therapy is to be instituted or altered is a further diagnostic work-up warranted. Such a situation would occur if the diarrhea has lasted longer than 1–2 weeks, or if high fever, chills, or bloody diarrhea are present. In this case, diagnostic work-up should consist of examination of the stools under the microscope for the presence or absence of polys and microorganisms; stool cultures and sensitivity; proctosigmoidoscopy for colitis or evidence of entameba; duodenal aspirate by string test for giardiasis if the history is suspicious.

Treatment

Traveler's diarrhea is usually such a mild illness that no specific therapy is required beyond the reduction in food intake and increased oral intake of clear liquids only. If dehydration is significant, oral rehydration solutions may be needed (see pp. 601). Only in settings where patients are unable to drink fluid is it necessary to administer fluids via nasogastric tube or intravenously. If fever is not present, a nonspecific agent such as bismuth subsalicylate may be effective by inhibiting the ability of an *E. coli* enterotoxin to induce fluid secretion from the small bowel. If the diarrhea is profuse or protracted and associated with fever, trimethoprim sulfamethoxazole has been found to allay symptoms in more than 90% of patients (Weiss, 1983). This drug should treat almost all pathogenic organisms except *Campylobactor, Giardia,* or rotavirus. It is rarely indicated for young children and is not recommended for prophylaxis.

Drugs that slow intestinal transit time are often used for older children and adults. Although drugs that slow peristalsis are effective in relieving the symptoms, they may delay recovery from diarrhea. Inasmuch as diarrhea is a best defense against irritating toxins and microorganisms, it should be allowed to "run" its course. Bismuth mixtures, Kaopectate, and other agents advocated to lessen symptoms are not advised for children, and are contraindicated in infants. Maintenance of hydration, preferably orally, is the treatment of choice.

Prevention

Hand-washing before eating and avoidance of food that is likely to be contaminated is helpful. In the developing world, drinking water may not be safe. The prudent traveler inquires about it, or restricts fluids to bottled beverages. Chemoprophylaxis is not indicated in children (Johnson et al, 1985).

REFERENCES

Banwell JG, Gorbach SL, Pierce NF, et al: Acute undifferentiated human diarrhea in the tropics. II Alterations in intestinal fluid and electrolyte movements. *J Clin Invest* 50:890, 1971.

Barabas G, Matthews WS, Ferrari M: Childhood migraine and motion sickness. *Pediatrics* 72:188, 1983.

Borison HL, Borison R, McCarthy LE: Role of the area postrema in vomiting and related functions. *Fed Proc* 43:2955, 1984.

Clements NL, Levine MM, Black RE, et al: Lactobacillus prophylaxis for diarrhea due to enterotoxigenic *E. coli. Antimicrob Agents Chemother* 20:104, 1981.

Feldman M: Traveler's diarrhea. *Am J Med Sci* 288:136, 1984.

Gorbach SL, Edelman R: Traveler's diarrhea: Introduction. *Rev Infect Dis* 8 (Suppl 2): 1986.

Gorbach SL, Hoskins DW: Traveler's diarrhea. *Disease-a-Month* 27:1, 1980.

Guyton AC: *Textbook of Medical Physiology*, 2nd edition. Philadelphia, WB Saunders, 1961.

Johnson PC, DuPont HL, Ericsson CD: Chemoprophylaxis and chemotherapy of traveler's diarrhea in children. *Pediatr Infect Dis* 4:620, 1985.

Money KE: Motion sickness. *Physiol Rev* 50:1, 1970.

Noy S. Shapria S, et al: Transdermal therapeutic system scopalamine (TSSS), dimenhydrinate and placebo 55:—a comparative study at sea. *Aviat Space Environ Med* 1051, 1984.

Steffen R, VanderLinde F, Gyr K, et al: Epidemiology of diarrhea in travelers. *JAMA* 249:1176, 1983.

Talbot JM, Fisher KD: Space sickness. *Physiologist* 27:423, 1984.

Toscano WB, Cowings PS:. Reducing motion sickness: A comparison of autogenic-feedback training and an alterntive cognative task. *Aviat Space Environ Med* 53:449, 1982.

Weiss BD: Traveler's diarrhea: Update 1983. *Am J Fam Prac* 27:193. 1983.

Wood CD, Cramer VB, Graybiel A: Antimotion sickness drug efficacy. *Otolaryngol Head Neck Surg* 89:1041, 1981.

Mary Ellen Avery
Richard Ferber
Lewis R. First
Robert Masland
Janice Ware

Consultants
Gerald Hass
H. Burtt Richardson
John Robey

Section 2

Behavioral Pediatrics

Developmental Assessment—Considerations at Any Age

1

At all ages and developmental levels, the overall situation of child and parent must be assessed. The "phase-specific" aspects of development are dealt with in Section 1, Well Child Care, Chapters on Infancy, Middle Childhood, and Adolescence. This section discusses the "nonphase-specific aspects."

How much *vigor* does the child show for life in general and for development in particular? Is the child moving ahead in motor, language, and psychosocial development, or is he plateauing or "stuck"? The clinician making this assessment must remember the "two-steps forward, one-step back" pattern of development, that is, the tendency for periods of rapid progress to alternate with periods of consolidation or even regression; one must not confuse a period of consolidation with a developmental arrest. Nonetheless, the child who persistently is unable to reach out and grasp the opportunities which life offers vigorously and with pleasure should be identified and assessed further.

In particular, the child's *play*—as reported by parents and teachers, and as observed by the doctor in the office—is a good reflection of the developmental state. One is interested in the spirit of the child at play, the content of the play, and the variability, or, conversely, the monotony or "stuckness" of the play. Many pediatricians bring a bright ball, puppets, or small wind-up toys, as well as stethoscopes and otoscopes, to their examinations. They use them both to build rapport with the child and to assess the child's ability to play.

Similarly, the child's *relating to people* is a critical dimension at all ages, though the expectations of what the child will do obviously change from the infant's first social smile to the complex relationship of the older child or adolescent. What remains constant is that the child is expected *at all ages* to care about relating to people, to communicate in some way, to be able to attend to the other person, and to modulate his own behavior in response to that of the other person.

A particular aspect of relatedness is the management of *separation*. At any age, the child has the task of managing separation experiences while staying connected. A developmental line of separation extends from infancy through early and middle childhood to adolescence. At each age there are specific milestones. These include allowing the parent to be away but nearby; accomodating to a babysitter; playing at friends' houses; entering playgroups and school without the parent; sleeping over at friends'and going away to camp; and eventually, moving into the "away-from-home" educational, occupational, and marital experiences of young adulthood. Managing separation does not mean having no reaction to it; to have no reaction to separation is as pathologic as to remain at home, frozen by fear.

One of the places, at all ages, in which unspoken developmental stress may be seen, is that of eating, sleeping, and overall energy level, the *vegetative functions* which are always sensitive measures of the child's overall adaptation. In assessing them, the physician must keep in mind that reports about eating and sleeping are always filtered through the parent's own expectations. Those expectations may derive more from the parent's own needs, than from an appreciation of the child's own individuality and developmental needs.

Finally, and most complex, the assessment of *mutuality* is relevant at all ages. Mutuality refers to the reciprocal facilitation of development by parent and child. It has three components: the parent's (parents') providing what the child needs to move ahead in development; the child's facilitating the parent's development as a parent by "growing in grace" and appearing to be able to manage emerging capacities; and the degree of mutual pleasure or fun which parents and child enjoy. This is clearly a complicated subject: it requires definition of the child's developmental needs (both those shared by all children and those specific to a given child), a concept of parental development, again in its universal and particular aspects, and of the ways that children aid or complicate it, and an assessment of the mix of pleasure and frustration which a given family enjoys. Most pediatricians develop an intuitive sense for each of these. We are not trying here to explicate them fully, but rather to encourage the physician to take that intuition seriously as a part of developmental assessment.

Diagnosis—Considerations with Any Disease

2

In addition to diagnosing the biologic aspects of a child's disease, the pediatrician must assess dimensions of the child's and family's life which apply whether the child is well or sick, and regardless of the disease. They are considered "non-disease-specific" or "generic."

Whatever the disease, diagnosis includes attention to possible *precipitants*. Epidemiology demonstrates that the incidence of nearly all disease, from respiratory infection to malignancy, increases after stress. Stressors include both discrete life-events (deaths, births, moves), both "positive" and "negative," and larger developmental events—like separation milestones or the onset of adolescence. With a particular patient, the goal is not to "prove" etiology, but to develop as broad a view as possible of the context in which a child has become sick as a basis both for understanding and for treatment planning.

For any child, from any family, regardless of the disease, assessment of how they are *coping with illness* will aid diagnosis and treatment planning. One is interested in how a family copes in general, including the uses they make of information and of action, and in how they are coping with this particular illness. In the case of any serious or chronic illness or condition, where are they in the process of *adaptation*? Adaptation, like grieving, proceeds from shock and denial through anger and bargaining to mature adaptation. In most chronic disorders, the child's adaptation is correlated less with physiologic limitations than with how child and family understand and are coping with the disorder.

Assessment of the *developmental* aspects of disease includes both consideration of the *developmental biology of disease* (the biological basis for the specific age at which a specific infection or chronic disorder occurs) and of the *impact of illness on development*—especially, where disability is chronic, its impact on education, self-concept, and peer relationships.

An important aspect of the family's adaptation to illness consists of the *models of attribution* the parents use. These are the "explanatory models," compounded of folklore, medical information, and idiosyncratic beliefs, which parents use to "make sense" of their children's illness. Doctors usually overestimate the extent to which parents' models conform to medical models. Nonmedical factors of great force in parents' "explanatory models" range from "fate" and "bad genes" to actual or presumed accidents of gestation or development to evil eyes or other forms of interpersonal malevolence. These models of attribution help the physician to understand the child's and parents' worlds. They are of immediate practical importance with regard to *treatment compliance*: failure to elicit the *parents'* ways of understanding disease makes it less likely that the doctor's treatment plan will be carried out.

Consideration of compliance with treatment leads to consideration of the family's *relationship to the network of medical care,* an assessment which includes both the pattern of use of care (episodic or sustained), the relationships with individual physicians and other treaters, and the child's and parents' feelings about their care.

Finally, consideration of the perspective of *family development* will be of use to the physician in understanding the impact of illness on the family and in planning treatment. One will consider the maturity of both parents and the nature of their relationship. What is their relationship to grandparents and other extended family members? How is this family, as a new family, struggling with the tasks of family development, from planning (or not planning) the arrival of new children, to providing food, shelter, clothing and privacy, to deciding anew such age-old questions as "How do we organize the work of the home?" "How do we feel about rights and responsibilities of the young versus the old?" "How shall we discipline?" and "How shall we relate to the faith(s) of our fathers?"

Approach to the Difficult-to-Manage Child 3

A behavioral problem frequently brought to pediatricians is that of the "difficult-to-manage child." Evaluation of this problem requires asking three questions:

What is the endowment of this particular child? (and the parents' understanding of it?)

What are the parents' expectations of the child? (compared to which, the child is "difficult")

What are the parents' and child's needs for help? (put differently, what is the level of pathology?)

ASSESSMENT OF ENDOWMENT

The pediatrician's assessment of the difficult-to-manage child begins with a review of possible gestational, perinatal and early developmental events which may have contributed to current adaptive problems. Shifting to the present, what is the child's current ability to take in sensory input, to integrate data from multiple domains, including state and affect regulation, and to coordinate output? One must assess the integrity of hearing, vision, and language; the child's ease in managing arousal, state transitions, and intense affects; and the coordination of verbal, motor, and social outputs. Problems in the control of activity level (see Hyperactivity and Attention Deficit Disorder, Chapter 6) are symptoms which parents bring to medical attention; they represent a final common pathway for a variety of neurological, emotional, and situational problems. For example, undiagnosed seizures or hypoglycemia, or an undiagnosed language problem, may present in the form of a difficult-to-manage child.

Specific developmental assessment, including psychological, audiological, or language testing, may be indicated as part of this assessment.

Assessment of the *parents' understanding of the child's endowment* follows. Many parents, in the absence of professional help in understanding the nature of the child, will react with hurt and frustration to behavior different from what they expect. Parents may inappropriately attribute the behavior to oppositional motivation ("He could calm down if he wanted to"; "She can remember if she just makes up her mind to do it"). They may also put attributions of motivation in pejorative terms ("She's just doing it to get attention").

PARENTAL EXPECTATIONS

One next reviews the parents' expectations of the child. Some inappropriate expectations are the result of misinformation about child development in general: for example, expectations that the 3-month-old will sleep through the night, that the 1-year-old will eat as passively and as nonselectively as the 6-month-old, or that the 18-month-old will be ready for toileting "on schedule." Other expectations do not fit the individual child—for example, regarding their activity level, academic ability, or particular interests. Still other parents may have expectations which do not take into consideration special needs of the individual child: for example, difficulty in organizing themselves, trouble in following complex auditory instructions, or a need for more-than-average "lead time," help with transitions, or anticipatory explanations. Finally, some expectations may be seen to have arisen out of an "impasse" in family life which needs to be addressed.

NEEDS FOR HELP

Regarding treatment, the reader is referred to the introductory chapters in the first section of this book, discussing infancy, early childhood, middle childhood, and adolescence, and to the references at the end of this section. Here we present principles to use in assessing and planning treatment regardless of the child's age or developmental level.

> **CASE ILLUSTRATION**
>
> A mother sought consultation because of her 3-year-old daughter's daytime tantrums and frequent night waking, at which times she was inconsolable unless given a bottle of juice. Her pediatrician noted that the child had always had a difficult temperament and that the parents by now were exhausted and feeling unable to cope. Referral was made to a behavior therapist. Treatment began with discussion of development in general and of the child's needs in particular, then specifically on behavior management, focused, at the parents' request, on the daytime tantrums. Interventions included efforts to minimize the situations which precipitated tantrums, positive reinforcement for the child for not screaming, and a specific form of "time-outs" for tantrums. Parents learned to chart the frequency of the tantrums and of nighttime waking. Tantrums decreased and ceased in 3 weeks, night-waking, though not directly targeted, soon after. Follow-up after some months showed these gains were sustained.

Hierarchy of Disorders

When parents complain that the child is difficult-to-manage, the child may have no disorder, the child-and-parents together may have reached an impasse in living together, or the child (or parent) may have a disorder requiring major psychiatric treatment. These possibilities, and the corresponding hierarchy of interventions, may be arranged as follows:

Level of Pathology	*Intervention*
Child has no disorder; parental expectations need modification	*Pediatric assessment and counseling*, with clarification of developmental needs in general, and of the needs of this child in particular, to enhance parents' understanding of the child and modify their expectations
Child has undiagnosed adaptive problems or there is a mismatch between child's needs and current services	*Compensatory help* (refraction, language therapy, anticonvulsants), a modified school program, modified management at home
Child has undiagnosed activity level problems (hyperactivity)	Trial of *stimulant medication*, preferably as part of a total program, not a single intervention
Child and parents together have a disorder	Systematic *modification of child management*, including identification of target behaviors, analysis of reinforcers, and contingency manipulation (this may be undertaken by some pediatricians; others will refer to a child psychologist or psychiatrist)
An "internalized" disorder in child (or parent), that is, a problem not responding to changed expectations or reinforcement, but representing a developmental bind	*Referral for psychotherapy* for child (or parent), with object of "unsticking" the developmental process

REFERENCES

Academy of Pediatrics: Guidelines for Health Supervision.

Clark L: *SOS: Help for Parents.* Bowling Green, KY, Parents Press, 1985.

Dreikurs R: *Discipline without Tears.* New York, Dutton (Hawthorn Book), 1975.

Dreikurs R, Soltz V: *Children: The Challenge.* New York, Dutton (Hawthorn Book), 1964.

Ginott HG: *Between Parent and Child.* New York, MacMillan, 1965.

Patterson GR: *Living with Children: New Methods for Parents and Teachers.* Champagne, IL, Research Press, 1976.

Audiocassettes

Patterson GR, Forgatch MS: Family living audio cassette series, Parts I and II. Champagne, IL, Research Press, 1975–1976.

Mood Disorders: Depression and Suicide 4

Definition

The mood disorders[1] are those in which a disturbance of mood is the essential feature. These disorders were formerly called "affective disorders," reflecting the use of the ambiguous word "affect" to mean "mood." (Affect also means "expressiveness" [as in the term, "he displayed flat affect"] and "specific emotion" [as in the phrase, "he could not tolerate the *affects* of sadness and fear"]).

"Depression" may refer to *depressed mood*, a normal and transient phenomenon in children as in adults, which may be a symptom of, but is not the same as any of the disorders listed below. It is, however, often confused with them. A *major depressive disorder* is an illness characterized by dysphoric mood, anhedonia (loss of ability to have pleasure), depressed mood, and somatic, social, and mental symptoms (for example, poor appetite, sleep disturbance, social withdrawal, im-

[1]In this chapter, diagnostic terminology generally follows that used in *DSM-III-R, the Diagnostic and Statistical Manual of Mental Disorders (Third Edition—Revised)*, of the American Psychiatric Association, Washington, D.C., 1987.

paired concentration, feelings of worthlessness, and thoughts of death), lasting at least 2 weeks. *Dysthymia* is a chronic, low-grade depression. *Adjustment disorder with depressed mood* is a reaction to a specific life event, with variable symptoms prominent among which is depressed mood, but not as severe as in major depressive disorder. *Juvenile manic-depressive disorder* is diagnosed when children (rarely) and adolescents (more commonly) show a disorder characterized by elevated mood, hyperexcitability, and lability, and thought to be the precursor of manic-depressive disorder in the adult.

Similarly, in using the term "suicide," referring to actual suicide, one must differentiate between *suicidal ideation* (thoughts about one's death, both passive thoughts, as in "I wish I were dead," and active thoughts, as in "I think about killing myself"), *suicidal gestures* (suicidal talk or behavior felt to reflect a communicative purpose as opposed to a wish to die), *suicide attempts* (or "parasuicide"), that is, deliberate self-injury with the intent to die but not resulting in death, and *completed suicidal acts*.

Basic Science

The biologic basis of the mood disorders has been clarified through family and cross-fostering studies and by psychophysiologic studies of depressed children (especially disturbances of endocrine function and sleep architecture). These distinguish major depressive disorder from the other mood disorders. Psychologically, controversy exists about the primary or secondary role of impaired self-esteem, identification with depressed parents, and intrapsychic conflict in depression; that is, are these manifestations of an underlying biologic disorder, or are they primary mediating factors? Socially, the effect of peer culture and of the degree to which a child feels himself socially isolated or integrated are evident, particularly in the epidemics of teenage suicide in which psychosocial "contagion" and the role of television and newspaper reporting seem important. Other environmental factors, including specific traumata, such as the loss of a parent or other trauma including sexual abuse, must be considered in the evaluation of the depressed child and not lost sight of in the contemporary enthusiasm for understanding the biology of the disorder.

Epidemiology

The incidence of recognized depression in children is rising, but this is probably due as much to increased recognition as to true increase in occurrence. Low population estimates include those of Rutter in 1970 in England, 0.2%, but higher estimates more recently, 1.9–8 or 9% appear more accurate (Rutter et al, 1985). The incidence of suicide in the young has been rising rapidly, including the appearance of clusters of suicide among high school students. Evidence suggests that media events about suicide contribute to such clustering (Phillips and Carstensen, 1986; Gould and Shaffer, 1986).

Natural History

Kovacs et al (1984) established the average length of major depressive disorder to be 9 months, with a range of 3–18 months. Adjustment disorder with depressed mood averaged 6 months. Dysthymia ran a more chronic course, with average length of 3 years. The course of juvenile manic-depressive disorder is highly variable.

Diagnosis

Like the recognition of child abuse, the recognition of depression in children has to overcome the reluctance of the observer to perceive a child in emotional pain. One manifestation of this reluctance is the tendency to answer the question, is the child depressed? by reference, not to how the child is feeling or behaving, but to life events which the adult believes might "cause" depression. For example, one says, "he is depressed; his grandfather died 2 months ago," as opposed to, "he is depressed: he has depressed mood, anhedonia, difficulty concentrating, sleeplessness, and hopelessness about the future." Puig-Antich (1985) cautions against the following errors in assessing depression in children: use of abstract language; assuming a word means the same to child and to interviewer, failing to appreciate the child's different sense of time; failing to ask repetitive questions; disbelieving the child because his statement is troubling to the adult; and minimization of a symptom because of adult preconception about its meaning to the child.

Treatment

The relative roles of biologic and psychologic treatments in mood disorders are controversial. The controversy derives from divergent opinion about the etiologic roles played by biologic and psychologic factors. In major depressive disorder and juvenile manic-depressive disorder, the strongest case is made for biologic treatment, with tricyclic antidepressants for depression and neuroleptics or lithium carbonate for mania. In dysthymia and adjustment disorder with depressed mood, the role of medication is not well established.

In all cases, one must understand the child's situation from three points of view: empathically, in terms of their painful feelings, usually shared with no one; developmentally, in that the depressed child has usually not adequately integrated some of his needs, and remains unconsciously opposed to them, with consequent self-deprivation and depletion; and ecologically, that is, in terms of frustrations, deprivations, or abuse actually occurring at home or in school. All of these—current painful feelings, distortions of development, and current stressors—when identified, require attention. Treatment must provide protection for children who might harm themselves; treatment of the biologic depression; evaluation and intervention in the internal and external factors precipitating or perpetuating the depression, as outlined above; and assessment, once the depression has lifted, of the psychologic and social problems which remain.

Of the tricyclic antidepressants, imipramine has been most used in children. Doses as high as 6 mg/kg/day are used, most often in a single nighttime dose. The drug is started at a lower level, say 1.5 mg/kg/day, and raised by stages every few days. Pulse rate (PR), blood pressure (BP), and ECG are monitored before starting and while increasing the dose; resting pulse over 130/min, PR interval of .22 sec, QRS interval 30% over baseline, BP greater than 140/90 mm Hg, or other intolerable side effects lead to holding or decreasing slightly the dose. The goal is a serum level in the therapeutic range (imipramine plus desipramine, the principal metabolite, between 150 and 250 ng/ml). Therapeutic response may occur in 7–10 days, but may take 3 or 4 weeks.

CONTROVERSY

As indicated, we now have consensus about the seriousness of childhood and adolescent depression and suicide as biopsychosocial disorders but no consensus yet about the relative roles of psychologic, social, and biologic processes either in pathogenesis or in treatment. While children have benefited from the recognition of a condition which results in immense suffering and premature deaths, clarification is still needed as to which interventions are most indicated in each disorder. In the meantime, prudent care requires giving each child that combination of treatments which clinical experience suggests he needs.

NEW DEVELOPMENTS

Clinical trials and long-term follow-up now under way will answer many of the questions alluded to above. In addition, increasing interest in the biology of the mood disorders will probably produce specific tests to define therapeutically relevant subgroups within the larger population of depressed children.

Prognosis

The mood disorders carry high risk: 10% of children and adolescents admitted to hospital after a suicidal attempt will die by suicide within the next five years. Children with a major depressive disorder are likely at risk for recurring depressions throughout life.

CASE ILLUSTRATION: MAJOR DEPRESSIVE DISORDER

A 9-year-old girl presented for evaluation because of irritability and decreased school performance over the previous 3 months. Parents and teacher had attributed these symptoms to "manipulativeness" and "attention-seeking." Her symptoms had begun after her mother's increased hours of work. This had coincided with the beginning of a new school year with a teacher who was very unlike the previous year's teacher, to whom the patient had been very close. Family history was notable for maternal history of depression during college and for a strained relationship between mother and this child. Further history revealed that the patient had also had initial and some middle insomnia, loss of appetite, secret periods of crying, and thoughts that she should never have been born. She denied suicidal plan, but became silent when asked whether she had ever contemplated suicide. She had a weary and sad look on her face and showed psychomotor slowing. When the examining physician mentioned that children often find it hard to share painful and sad feelings, though they want to, she cried. Treatment consisted of sharing the diagnosis of depression with child and parents, showing the parents how depressed their daughter was feeling, despite the criticism and exhortation she tended to elicit, and providing weekly "talking sessions" for child (in which she ventilated, both directly and indirectly, her frustration with mother and teacher), for mother (in which her own frustrations were identified), and for them together (focusing on improving communication and finding ways to have special times together, to compensate for mother's increased time at work). Because of the prominent disturbance of mood and vegetative function, imipramine was also prescribed. Over the course of a month, the patient brightened considerably, she became more pleasant to be with and her schoolwork improved, and it was possible to address and work through long-standing grievances between mother and daughter.

CASE ILLUSTRATION: JUVENILE MANIC-DEPRESSIVE DISORDER

A 16-year-old male, with a history of oppositional and limit-testing behavior, over several months underwent a change in behavior. While he continued to test family rules with late nights out and schoolwork done irregularly, he now talked much faster, seemed to be sleeping even less than before, and was even more intolerant of parental advice or criticism, bursting out at any suggestion that he slow down or examine how he was living, with vituperative denunciations of his parents. Attending counseling sessions with his father and mother (she had a history of bipolar illness, manic-depressive disorder, treated with lithium), he agreed to a trial of lithium, but failed to take it regularly, and he was hospitalized. In the hospital, he was constantly moving, talking fast and interrupted both other patients and staff, and disclosed that his thoughts were going too fast for him to be able to pay attention to them. "Slowed down" in the hospital ward and reaching lithium levels in the 1.0–1.2 mEq/L range, he became able to sit in meetings and allow others to talk, though he was still the most garrulous (and the most frequently interrupting) patient on the ward. While he noticed he could think more clearly, he remained suspicious that the medication would "change" him, take away "parts of myself that I don't want to give up," and considerable work was required over time to support his identifying with the goals of treatment.

After discharge, on maintenance lithium therapy, he was in many ways "his old self again," resuming school and activities with peers. Over the long run, lithium will decrease, but not eliminate, the risk of repeated manic episodes.

The same applies to juvenile manic-depressive disorder.

REFERENCES

Childhood depression and sexual abuse. Editorial. *Lancet* 1:196, 1986.
Cytryn L, McKnew DH: Treatment issues in childhood depression. *Pediatr Ann* 15:856, 1986.
Gould MS, Schaffer D: The impact of suicide in television movies. *N Engl J Med* 315:690, 1986.
Kovacs M, Feinberg T, Crouse MA, et al: Depressive disorders in childhood: I. A longitudinal prospective study of characteristics and recovery. *Arch Gen Psychiatry* 41:229, 1984.
Phillips DP, Carstensen LL: Clustering of teenage suicides after television news stories about suicide. *N Engl J Med* 315:685, 1986.
Poznanski E: Affective disorders. In Michels R and Cavenar JO (eds): *Psychiatry*. Chap 30, Vol 2. Philadelphia, Lippincott, 1985.
Poznanski E: The clinical phenomenology of childhood depression. *Am J Orthopsychiatry* 52:308, 1982.
Puig-Antich J: Affective disorders. In Kaplan HI, Sadock BJ (eds): *Comprehensive Textbook of Psychiatry*, 4th edition, Section 41.10. Baltimore, Williams & Wilkins, 1985.
Puig-Antich J: Biological factors in prepubertal major depression. *Pediatr Ann* 15:867, 1986.
Rutter M, Izard CE, Read PB: *Depression in Young People*. New York, Guilford Press, 1985.
Weller EB, Weller RA: Clinical aspects of childhood depression. *Pediatr Ann* 15:843, 1986.

5 Eating Disorders (Anorexia Nervosa and Bulimia Nervosa)

Definition

Anorexia nervosa[2] is a chronic eating disorder characterized by loss of 15% of body weight (or weight proportionately below ideal weight), characteristic psychologic changes (preoccupation with food and appetite, fear of appetites, body image distortion, relentless pursuit of thinness), and (in females) amenorrhea, all in the absence of another medical or psychiatric disorder to account for these findings. *Bulimia nervosa* is a chronic eating disorder characterized by episodic dyscontrol, with gorging on food followed by exhaustion or vomiting or both, which may occur in patients at normal, low, or high body weight. The existence of these two names should not suggest two discrete disorders: there is considerable overlap between these two disorders and many patients with anorexia nervosa go on to develop bulimia nervosa. The term "bulimarexia" has been used for patients with symptoms of both disorders.

Basic Science

Pathogenesis of these disorders involves sociocultural factors operating on psychologically vulnerable individuals, probably from culturally or psychologically vulnerable families, with the setting-in-motion through the disease of self-sustaining changes mediated through the endocrinologic, hypothalamic, and psychological systems. Epidemiologic studies indicate a true increase in prevalence, probably responsive to cultural changes regarding roles and identities available to women, the ecology of food and eating, and the values placed on food, consumption, and the thin female body. Familial risk factors appear to include family history of affective or addictive disorders, family preoccupation with food and thinness, and rigidity in problem-solving. Psychologically, affected individuals lack a deep sense of their own worth and do not believe they can truly affect their environment; they experience themselves as complying with others' wishes. Whether these traits are primary or secondary remains controversial. Endocrinologically, anorexia nervosa produces amenorrhea and estrogen deficiency, a reversion of gonadotropin secretion to prepubertal levels (which is reversible upon provision to the pituitary of exogenous releasing factors), the "euthyroid sick" picture characterized by decreased peripheral conversion of T4 to T3, elevated growth hormone, and sluggish hypothalamic function, reflected in erratic vasopression response to osmotic challenge and in poor defense of body temperature in response to environmental heat and cold. Gastroenterologically, patients with anorexia nervosa have slowed gastric emptying, subjective bloating, abdominal pain, and constipation. Bulimia nervosa produces a host of medical complications of recurrent vomiting, from esophagitis to dental erosion and sialoadenitis to hypochloremic alkalosis and life-threat-

[2] In this chapter, diagnostic terminology generally follows that used in *DSM-III-R, the Diagnostic and Statistical Manual of Mental Disorders (Third Edition—Revised),* of the American Psychiatric Association, Washington, D.C., 1987.

ening potassium deficiency. Both disorders produce psychologic chronicity through poorly understood perpetuating mechanisms, some of which may be similar to those involved in the addictive disorders.

Epidemiology

Incidence of both disorders appears to be rising. One study found an increase in one decade from 0.35 to 0.64 new treated cases of anorexia nervosa per year per 100,000 population. Another found an increase in two decades from 0.38 to 1.12/100,000. In a high-risk group, a British secondary school population, Crisp estimated prevalence rate to be 1%. Females outnumber males by nearly 10:1. In contrast to severe anorexia nervosa, which usually comes to medical attention, bulimia nervosa, even of severe degree, may be concealed for decades. Despite this tendency to secrecy, estimates of the lifetime prevalence of bulimia nervosa have been made, and range from 4–20%.

Natural History

Both disorders may begin benignly, in the context of group pressure to lose weight. For many, an initial "volitional" phase of weight reduction or self-induced vomiting ("I'm doing what I want to do") soon shifts to a "dysvolitional" phase ("I can't stop") in which compulsive weight reduction and/or vomiting appears to have become autonomous, as in an addiction. Course is extremely variable, ranging from single episodes with apparently good recovery, to relapsing courses in which chronic eating dysfunction (inability to eat in company, or persisting bingeing and vomiting) may persist even when weight recovery has occurred. More than half the patients have the latter course. Suicide has occurred in 2–5% of patients with chronic anorexia nervosa, and the overall death rate in some series is as high as 9%.

Diagnosis

Not many years ago, diagnosis was often delayed while emaciated patients underwent extensive gynecologic or gastroenterologic investigations for amenorrhea or abdominal pain, the physician being unaware that an eating disorder accounted for the chief complaint. With patients and physicians more aware of the eating disorders today, this pattern is now less likely. Inflammatory bowel disease, malabsorption syndromes, or thyroid or adrenal disorders can usually be ruled out clinically or with routine laboratory tests. Careful initial (and, with refractory cases, serial) neurologic exams will identify the occasional case of primary neurologic disorder, such as diencephalic syndrome, presenting as a disorder of eating and inanition. Obstacles to diagnosis of the eating disorder include patients' secretiveness and the difficulty of differentiating depression from eating disorders, particularly in patients with medical disorders complicating their eating, such as diabetes mellitus.

Treatment

Treatment is not satisfactory in either disorder. Regarding anorexia nervosa, it is clear that nutritional rehabilitation must precede meaningful change on the individual or family level, but such change is by no means guaranteed once weight and eating have been restored and therapy initiated. The obvious physiologic derangements in the disorder, and the many affinities between anorexia nervosa and the mood disorders, have stimulated interest in pharmacotherapeutic approaches which have, as yet, not produced a magic bullet. Antidepressants are used when patients are symptomatically depressed, but with variable results. Most experienced clinicians feel that recovery is most likely when the family can make changes which allow the patient new room for growth, and when the patient, over time, can identify for herself her true inner experiences, in contrast to looking for, and fighting off, others' wishes for her.

CASE ILLUSTRATION

Nancy was a 17-year-old college freshman who was 172 cm tall and had weighed 70 kg when she graduated from high school. Over the summer before starting college, she was concerned about being overweight and started to restrict calories and to exercise excessively (2 hours jogging each morning) in an effort to lose weight.

She sought medical attention at the college health service because of amenorrhea. There she appeared well and active but thin (weighing 52 kg), with dry skin and hands and feet colder than expected. Her pulse was 56. The rest of the physical examination was normal. She did not feel that she was underweight, declined to pursue psychiatric referral, but compliantly promised to try to gain weight, to which end she was advised to increase her caloric intake and to reduce her exercising.

Two months later, she had lost further weight (to 45 kg), had a low body temperature (35.5° rectal), pulse of 46, and BP of 80/50. She had become much less active and acknowledged dysphoria. Hospitalization was indicated.

During 4 weeks in the hospital, she initially denied strenuously that she had an eating disorder, and was panicky as she gained 5 kg on a fixed amount of prescribed calories per day. With psychiatric interviews and through groups on the ward with other patients with eating problems, she began to find ways to talk about her chronic self-doubts and the crisis which the move to college had precipitated. Discharge was followed by continued individual and group counseling and by careful medical supervision to support continued weight gain. She remained underweight, but was able to resume college.

COMMENT

It is not unusual to have anorexia nervosa develop in overweight adolescents whose legitimate desire to lose weight becomes pathologic. The delay in diagnosis in this patient was in the context of her denial that she was underweight.

Bulimia nervosa treatment is also frustrating. Despite some enthusiasm for pharmacotherapy, especially with tricyclic and monoamine oxidase inhibiting antidepressants, most patients do not respond to these drugs. Treatment programs use combinations of habit training and stress identification, along with exploratory individual therapy, to attempt to help the individual recover a sense of control over her eating. Abstinence from bingeing, analogous to the use of sobriety in the treatment of alcoholism, is achieving considerable popularity, and a network of self-help groups modeled on Alcoholics Anonymous has spread across the country.

In both disorders, it is tempting to prescribe oral potassium supplements to replace gastric and renal potassium losses secondary to vomiting. This practice is ill-advised and dangerous, because the physician usually has no way of knowing to what use the patient will put the supplements, which can cause gastric and metabolic complications in their own right and mask the severity of a patient's metabolic compromise, and because doctor and patient may acquire through the act of prescribing a misleading sense that a life-threatening situation is under control.

Prognosis

As indicated, for both bulimia nervosa and anorexia nervosa, prognosis is guarded.

REFERENCES

Crisp AH, Norton KR, Jurczak S, et al: A treatment approach to anorexia nervosa—25 years on. *J Psychiatr Res* 19:393, 1985.

Crisp, AH, Palmer RL, Kalucy RS: How common is anorexia nervosa? A prevalence study. *Br J Psychiatr* 128:549, 1976.

Gold PW, Gwirtsman H, et al: Abnormal hypothalamic-pituitary-adrenal function in anorexia nervosa. *N Engl J Med* 314:1335, 1986.

Herzog DB, Copeland PM: Eating disorders. *N Engl J Med* 313: 295, 1985.

Hsu LKG: Treatment of anorexia nervosa. *Am J Psychiatry* 143: 573, 1986.

Swift WF, Andrews D, Barklage NE: The relationship between affective disorder and anorexia nervosa: A review of the literature. *Am J Psychiatry* 143:290, 1986.

Disruptive Behavior Disorders 6

CONDUCT DISORDER AND DELINQUENCY

Definition

Conduct disorder[3] is the current term for repetitive behavior which violates others' rights. Conduct disorder is further classified as solitary aggressive, group, or undifferentiated. Many youth with conduct disorder are labeled delinquent, delinquency being a social and judicial label, not a medical diagnosis.

Basic Science

Youths with conduct disorders are a heterogeneous group, though they have not always been seen in such terms. Nineteenth century medicine, exemplified by the work of Lombroso, emphasized presumed biologic degeneracy; earlier in this century, psychologists and sociologists aspired to find *the* crucial determinants of delinquent behavior. In contrast, the contemporary view of delinquency emphasizes the heterogeneity of a group united more by the social fact of being caught and labeled than by any intrinsic features. This heterogeneity applies to medical, neuropsychiatric, and psychoeducational findings. Medically, history of excess perinatal problems, head and face injuries, and physical abuse are noted, as are current abnormal neurologic findings including lags in coordination, positive Babinskis, and deficits in short-term memory and mental arithmetic. History of seizures is more common than in the general population and in one study of incarcerated youths, 18% actually suffered from psychomotor seizures, which occurs in 0.5–1.0% of the general population. Psychiatrically, many delinquent youth are on the borders of paranoia and depression. Psychoeducationally, deficits both in academic achievement and overall intellectual ability, and specific learning disabilities, once attributed to the so-called "basic" personality problem, are now seen as independent risk factors contributing to the youth's poor adjustment.

[3]In this chapter, diagnostic terminology generally follows that used in *DSM-III-R, the Diagnostic and Statistical Manual of Mental Disorders (Third Edition—Revised),* of the American Psychiatric Association, Washington, D.C., 1987.

Epidemiology

Children and youth contribute significantly to the total amount of crime in society. In the United States in 1981, 18% of all arrests for violent crimes and 39% of arrests for property crimes were of youths below the age of 18 years. Furthermore, 5% of arrests for violent crimes were of youths below the age of 15 years. Preponderance of males is noted, at a ratio of 8:1 for violent crimes and 4:1 for property crimes. Geographic differences in rate are large, with urban areas registering 10 times the crime seen in rural areas, and 5 times as much as in the suburbs. A population study in Philadelphia attempted to determine arrest rates in boys followed through adolescence: 35% were arrested at least once before the age of 18 years, and nearly one-fifth of these became chronic offenders (West, 1985).

Natural History

Follow-up studies have supported the idea that delinquent youth are a heterogeneous group with multiple diagnosable problems beside their delinquency. Robins' (1966) follow-up of children with antisocial behavior showed that nearly 40% were afflicted in adulthood with a variety of disturbances, including psychosis, depression, anxiety, and conversion disorder, in addition to conduct disorder.

Diagnosis

The social and judicial part of ascertaining a conduct disorder is usually done by nonclinicians, in the police or court systems. The role of the medical diagnostician evaluating a child or adolescent with conduct disorder is to detect the medical, psychiatric, and learning problems associated with the conduct problem. It is emphasized that many factors, in the child, the examiner, and the community reaction to the offenses committed, make it easy to overlook significant problems with, for example, hearing, untreated infections, coordination problems, learning disabilities, depression or paranoia, and that contact with the physician is the most likely place for these factors to be detected.

Treatment

Treatment follows from diagnosis as defined above.

CONTROVERSY

Many aspects of the social and legal management of delinquent youth are controversial. The actual parts played in a given case by a host of personal, familial, and social factors remain undefined. About the need to respond medically to identified medical, psychiatric, and psychoeducational problems, once detected, there is more agreement.

Prognosis

Identified delinquents are at risk for continued antisocial behavior as adults (20% or more) as well as for a host of associated personal, social, and psychiatric disabilities. Early recognition and intervention is indicated, including advocacy for youths who face stigmatization and discrimination in adolescence in addition to the environmental deprivations they have faced in earlier life.

FIRE-SETTING

Definition

Fire-setting is a symptom seen in a variety of disorders. When a pattern of fire-setting behavior is not associated with psychosis, retardation, other conduct disorder symptoms, or a specific wish for revenge, the term *pyromania* is used.

Basic Science

The psychological determinants of fire-setting appear to include covert permission from the family (often impulse-dominated itself) for the child to set fires and the child's failure to integrate aggressive and sexual drives into his overall development. The overwhelming male predominance is unexplained, but doubtless implicates the mediating biologic, psychologic, and social mechanisms.

Epidemiology

There are no reliable figures on incidence. The overwhelming majority of fire-setters, up to 90%, are male. Two periods of peak incidence in childhood are noted, one in 4- to 6-year olds, the other in early to midadolescence.

Natural History

Course depends on the larger disorder—psychosis, retardation, conduct disorder—in which the firesetting occurs. A triad of symptoms—firesetting, enuresis, cruelty to animals—was formerly believed to be predictive of serious impulse control problems, but controlled studies have indicated these symptoms to be equally prevalent in other psychiatric populations.

Diagnosis

Diagnosis must be directed at identifying the larger disorder—retardation or psychosis in the child, pathologic stimulation from the family—in which the firesetting is occurring, and then identifying the factors supportive of control in the child—usually responsible, caring adult males—which can be identified and mobilized.

Treatment

First intervention is directed at protecting the child and his surroundings. This requires both psychologic assessment of child and family assessment, mobilization of needed supports (including adults who can spend time with the child), and psychologic intervention to help the child identify with the forces for control available to him.

Prognosis

No data exist on prognosis.

HYPERACTIVITY (ATTENTION DEFICIT HYPERACTIVITY DISORDER)

Definition

Hyperactivity in popular usage may mean little more than "overactivity" (and the reference criterion for "normal" activity varies greatly from family to family and from context to context). As a medical diagnosis, "hyperactivity" in the sense of poor regulation of activity level is linked to poor regulation of attention, called "attention-deficit." Our understanding of the relationship between these two is still evolving. While the old DSM-III called the syndrome "attention deficit disorder with/without hyperactivity;" the new DSM-III-R (revision), reflecting recent work which focuses equally on both impairments, uses the term "attention-deficit hyperactivity disorder (ADHD)."

Weiss and Hechtman (1986) summarized the syndrome as follows. "Hyperactive children have a short attention span, high distractibility, and an inability to cut out extraneous stimuli when trying to attend to a task. They are impulsive in behavior and on cognitive tasks, they do not 'stop, look and listen,' and they jump in where angels fear to tread. They speak out of turn and impulsively interrupt adults. They have a hard time regulating their activity to conform with expected social norms, and may be actually overactive or inappropriately active. They tend to have poor frustration tolerance and are often poor at losing games, waiting in line, or obeying rules of a game."

Basic Science

Despite many attempts at identification of precursors of ADHD, no single event or correlation is uniformly present. Thus the conclusion is that some as-yet-undefined biologic dysfunction and some psychosocial antecedents contribute to the syndrome. Hyperactive behavior in general (as opposed to the ADHD syndrome) may be due to specific toxins, like lead (and treatable by chelation) or to behavioral trauma, especially child abuse.

Patients with ADHD usually have academic underachievement, lowered performance on standard IQ tests, and a group of them have prenatal and perinatal risk factors.

An increased prevalence of psychiatric problems in parents of hyperactive children, and hyperactivity in the parents support the view that sometimes, at least, a genetically determined predisposition is present (Cantwell, 1975).

Epidemiology

The prevalence of hyperactive syndromes in children depends on the definition. Hyperactivity is a frequent reason for referral to child psychiatrists. In a survey in the East Bay area near San Francisco, Lambert et al (1978) found 1.2% of 5000 children were hyperactive when diagnosed by the parents and the teacher and the physician.

Natural History

The core symptoms of "inappropriate restlessness, attentional difficulties, and impulsivity manifest themselves in different ways at different ages" (Weiss and Hechtman, 1986). Most children with ADHD continue as adolescents to have the core symptoms, though they may decrease somewhat. They have the most trouble with academic underachievement, poor peer relationships, and oppositional or delinquent behavior (seen in one-quarter to one-half of the group). In adulthood, one-third may "outgrow" the syndrome, but another one-third to one-half of the group have adaptive problems due to their impulsivity (poor work records, frequent job changes, unstable personal relationships).

Diagnosis

The diagnosis depends on recognition of the core features of the syndrome, which are usually present from early childhood. Symptoms vary with context (home, school, office); normal behavior in the office does not rule out ADHD. The lack of normal standards complicates the use of any list of criteria, and makes diagnosis controversial.

Diagnostic Criteria (Adapted from DSM-III-R)

Use only behaviors clearly more frequent than age-expectations.

A. For 6 months or more, child does 8 or more of the following:

(1) fidgets or squirms
(2) can't stay seated
(3) easily distracted
(4) can't wait his turn
(5) blurts out answers before question done
(6) doesn't follow-through on instructions
(7) can't sustain work or play
(8) shifts from one thing to another, none finished
(9) can't play quietly
(10) talks excessively
(11) interrupts or butts into others' talk or games
(12) appears not to listen
(13) loses things at school or home
(14) is reckless

B. Onset before age 7 years.

C. Does not have a pervasive development disorder (see p. 75).

The pediatrician's first responsibility, as usual, is to obtain a careful history and perform a thorough physical examination (including testing of hearing and vision) to identify any physical or situational problems that should be treated. Persistence of symptoms in the absence of identified and remedial underlying cause is reason for psychiatric referral.

Treatment

Counseling and medication are the mainstays of treatment. Counseling helps parents to understand the nature of the problem and to modify expectation of the child. Stimulant drugs are beneficial in childhood, but not in adults. Dextroamphetamine and methylphenidate improve symptoms in about 70% of children. Side effects of headaches, stomach aches, reduced appetite, and urticaria are managed by adjusting the dose. If there is no response to the short-acting stimulants, a trial with a tricyclic antidepressant, such as imipramine, may be worthwhile.

CONTROVERSY

The biologic bases of ADHD remain obscure. Because many children with ADHD also come from depriving or traumatic backgrounds, it is often difficult to assess how much overactivity and distractibility is the result of ADHD per se, and how much is the result of psychologic trauma and anxiety. Secondary prevention of poor life adaptation and social deviancy in adults with ADHD is a major unmet challenge; ADHD clearly adversely affects a child's chances for normal socialization. For a full discussion of the socialization process, the reader is referred to the chapter by Offord DR and Waters GBH: Socialization and its failure. In Levine MD, Carey WB, Crocker AC, Gross RT (eds): *Developmental Behavioral Pediatrics*. Philadelphia, WB Saunders Co, 1983.

REFERENCES

Cantwell DP: Genetics of hyperactivity. *J Child Psychol Psychiatry* 16:261, 1975.

Lambert NM, Sandoval J, Sassone D: Prevalence of hyperactivity in elementary school children as a function of social system definers. *Am J Orthopsychiatry* 48:446, 1978.

Lewis DO: Conduct disorder. In Michels R, Cavenar JO (eds): *Psychiatry*. Vol 2, Chapt 36. Philadelphia, Lippincott, 1986.

Lombroso, C: *Crime: Its Causes and Remedies*. Boston, Little, Brown and Co., 1911.

Robins L: *Deviant Children Grown Up*. Baltimore, Williams & Wilkins, 1966.

Rutter M: Syndromes attributed to "minimal brain dysfunction" in childhood. *Am J Psychiatry* 139:21, 1982.

Weiss G, Hechtman LT: *Hyperactive Children Grown-up*. New York, Guilford Press, 1986.

West D: Delinquency. In Rutter M, Hersov L (eds): *Child and Adolescent Psychiatry: Modern Approaches*, 2nd edition. Boston and Palo Alto, Blackwell Scientific Publications, 1985.

Wherry JS: Drugs and learning. *J Child Psychol Psychiatry* 22:283, 1981.

Wolff S: Non-delinquent disorders of conduct: In Rutter M, Hersov L (eds): *Child and Adolescent Psychiatry: Modern Approaches*, 2nd edition. Boston and Palo Alto, Blackwell Scientific Publications, 1985.

Drug Abuse 7

Definition

The definition of drug abuse differs according to the context, legal or medical. Legally, any use of a nonprescribed or illegal drug is considered abuse, while injudicious use of prescribed medicines or of legal psychoactive drugs such as nicotine and ethanol is not. From a medical point of view, abuse occurs when any drug is used for nontherapeutic purposes or when a legal "recreational" drug like nicotine or ethanol is used in a way which injures health or which interferes with normal life. The principal drugs of abuse in the pediatric age population are ethanol, nicotine, cannabis, heroin, and cocaine.

CONTROVERSY

The search for psychologic factors which "predispose" to the development of addiction has given rise to considerable controversy. The study of alcoholism is relevant. Those working with patients with late-stage alcoholism often are impressed with similar personality traits among such patients, which they presume to have been predisposing to the development of the addiction. Vaillant's work (1983), among others, has refuted such a hypothesis, by showing that such traits do not antedate, but follow the development of the alcoholism, and are probably an effect of the illness itself, especially its effects on the brain.

A recent study for the National Academy of Sciences reviewed data on the role of personality in addictions and concluded that there is no single set of psychological characteristics common to all addictions. Significant contributing factors, however, were felt to include impulsivity, nonconformity, social alienation, and a heightened sense of stress. Deykin et al (1987) found that major depression usually preceded, rather than followed, alcohol and other substance abuse, which they considered supportive of the hypothesis that much substance abuse begins as self-medication for undiagnosed depression.

In contrast to the uncertain state of our knowledge regarding individual predisposing characteristics, there is little doubt about the powerful role which social context plays in the development both of drug use and of addiction. For instance, many Vietnam veterans with experience with illegal drugs, including opiates, in Vietnam, did not continue such use after the war in the changed context of being back home. Similarly, the large numbers of youths using alcohol, cannabis, opiates and cocaine in groups are in situations where group mores and pressures appear to play as powerful a role in shaping use patterns as individual characteristics.

Treatment

The traditional debate in the drug treatment field has focused on whether the rehabilitating addicted person should be "drug-free" or should use medically prescribed agents to stable himself physically while addressing larger life problems. With regard to the opiates, in which the physiologic withdrawal syndrome is unmistakable, the debate has centered on the role of methadone maintenance versus the use of drug-free residential treatment communities. This debate, largely ideologic in the absence of cogent data supporting the superiority of either approach, now involves the investigational use of the antidepressants to treat cocaine addiction. Some investigators have reported good recovery and lessened relapse rates with the use of imipramine and desipramine; those representing the drug-free tradition feel any such drug trials are inevitably "merely" palliative and fail to help the addicted person confront his personal and existential dilemmas. Clinical trials will be necessary to settle this (at present) largely ideologic controversy.

REFERENCES

Deykin EY, Levy JC, Wells V: Adolescent depression, alcohol and drug abuse. *Am J Public Health* 77:178, 1987.

Vaillant GE: *The Natural History of Alcoholism.* Cambridge, Harvard University Press, 1983.

Factitious Illness in the Child 8

MUNCHAUSEN SYNDROME BY PROXY (MEADOW SYNDROME)

Definition

Munchausen syndrome by proxy (MBP) is a form of child abuse in which a parent (almost always, the mother) creates the impression that a child is ill, either by presenting false information to doctors or by actually inflicting harm on the child. The name derives from Baron Munchhausen, an 18th century German author of fantastic stories. In adult psychiatry, the term Munchausen syndrome (with this spelling), meaning "chronic factitious illness with physical symptoms," is used for patients who lie about symptoms in order to obtain unneeded medical care. The term MBP was suggested by Meadow for parents who fabricate history, or induce signs of disease, in their children. In England, MBP is known as Meadow syndrome. (The term Polle syndrome has been used by some for this disorder, based on the inaccurate belief that Baron Munchhausen had a son named Polle, but this use is not recommended.)

Basic Science

Several aspects of the psychology of parent (and child) in MBP are relevant. First, although MBP behavior involves gross distortion of reality, the perpetrating parents are not psychotic—that is, in other areas of their lives they perceive the environment accurately. Second, the parent, when presented with undeniable evidence, may or may not be able to acknowledge what he/she has been doing. Third, MBP behavior is on a continuum with less malignant forms of inaccurate perception of the child's needs, a spectrum with which all pediatricians are familiar, in which anxiety or other factors interfere with accurate perception of the child's state of health. MBP differs from "ordinary" parental overperception of child illness because of its tenacity (parents will not accept reassuring information) and because harm is actually done to the child (sometimes fatally) to simulate illness. Fourth, the child may also participate in deceiving the doctors, either out of fear or out of loyalty to the parent.

Epidemiology

No figures on prevalence in populations exist; diagnosis depends greatly on clinician readiness to consider the possibility of this disorder. In pediatric hospitals, as many as 2% of all inpatients at a given time may have this disorder. The ease with which MBP is missed must be kept in mind; it was first described only in 1977, although it certainly existed before.

Natural History

Waller (1983) reported a 30% mortality rate on follow-up of MBP patients. No other studies have followed these children longitudinally.

Diagnosis

Because of the threat to the life and health of the child in MBP, much effort has been devoted to making the diagnosis and to recognizing the obstacles to that diagnosis. The feigned illness may take many forms: reported respiratory symptoms or passage of blood from any orifice (including blood-stained diapers—the blood coming from child, parent, or an animal), reported seizures or apnea spells; unexplained apnea spells occurring only when the child is alone with the parent; induced infections, as through the cutaneous injection of saliva; intractable diarrhea from administration of laxatives (Epstein et al, 1987) and induced drug toxicity. The parent's evident behavior may be exemplary, the parent caring lovingly for the sick child. Physicians, social agencies, and courts may be extremely reluctant to consider the possibility of child-harming behavior by a parent. And parents usually react with great indignation (and often with threats) when the possibility of MBP is raised. Diagnosis depends on critical thinking and ingenuity in evaluating all reported symptoms and any signs of illness which could be induced; on alertness to the nature of the parent-child and the parent-doctor relationship; and, mostly, on the physician's willingness to consider the possibility of MBP. Persistent and pathologic lying on the parent's part; a highly dramatic presentation of the symptoms; and the willingness to hurt the child in order to persuade the physician that the child is sick all make the diagnosis of MBP likely.

The possibility in some cases of using covert high-tech methods (e.g., a hidden video camera) to "trap" the perpetrator should not distract the physician from using clinical observation, especially of parent-physician behavior, as a basis for assessment (Epstein et al, 1987).

Treatment

Treatment begins with unequivocal demonstration of the nature of the threat (or lack thereof) to the child. Protective measures (including hospitalizing the child, restriction of unsupervised parental visiting with the child, and appropriate reporting of suspected child abuse) must be instituted. At the same time that one recognizes the possibility of parentally inflicted harm to the child and takes protective action, a supportive relationship must be offered to the parent, in a nonpunitive way, offering help in dealing with a situation which has clearly been beyond the parent's ability to cope. According to the parent's ability to respond realistically and join in working to make life safe for the child, the child may continue living with the parent, or may require placement elsewhere.

CASE ILLUSTRATION

Two sisters, aged 2 and 4 years, were brought to hospital for evaluation of combined medical and behavioral problems. The older was said to have multiple food allergies, previously confirmed during evaluation at another referral center in the area, which, despite elimination diets, continued to cause behavioral symptoms (tantrums, fighting with sister, lack of cooperation). The younger was said to have had seizures and was on anticonvulsants. The mother requested joint admission for both, for further treatment of the medical problems and because she, partly out of her efforts at caring for them, was on the point of emotional collapse. Observation in hospital revealed no medical or behavioral symptoms, even when food challenges were introduced and anticonvulsants withdrawn. The findings at the other hospital, the team learned, had been misrepresented: the physicians there felt there was *no* food allergy and recommended against food restrictions. Confronted with these findings, the mother abruptly left town, and the father, previously uninvolved, took them home. Six years later, the parents, long since divorced, were still involved in custody battles. The mother attributed her long history of behavioral lability to a recently diagnosed food allergy. The children were physically healthy, in the father's custody, but the older girl had multiple anxiety symptoms.

COMMENT

This case is unusual in that the psychologic distress of the mother was evident from the beginning; most cases in the literature are remarkable for the calm with which mothers negotiate their children's frightening illnesses and the long and frustrating diagnostic and therapeutic efforts of the doctors. These children were also lucky in undergoing no worse trauma than elimination diets, anticonvulsant therapy, and invasive diagnostic tests; others have undergone surgery and others have died. Characteristic is the mother's long-term involvement with medicine in one form or another, and the "low-profile" role of a potentially interested and helpful father while the mother carries the child from doctor to doctor, inducing symptoms of varying severity.

CONTROVERSY

Controversy usually occurs when MBP is diagnosed for several reasons. Apart from the few cases in which incontrovertible proof may be generated, some ambiguity usually attends the diagnosis. The parent usually elicits outraged sympathy from some of the professionals (in or out of hospital) in the case, and clinicians in general are reluctant to acknowledge something as violating of society's basic rules as harming a child and lying to doctors. Controversy also attends the question of whether and under what circumstances the child may return to be with parents.

NEW DEVELOPMENTS

Increasing professional recognition of MBP and increasing public awareness of it as a disorder are leading to earlier diagnosis of MBP.

Prognosis

As noted, Waller (1983) found a 30% mortality rate in MBP. Data are not available about developmental or behavioral outcome in those who survive. Because of the known high proportion of history of previous abuse in abusive adults, children with MBP must be considered at high risk for serious behavior problems as adults and as parents.

REFERENCES

Epstein MA, Markowitz RL, Gallo DM, et al: Munchausen syndrome by proxy: Considerations in diagnosis and confirmation by video surveillance. *Pediatrics* 80:220, 1987.

Guandolo VL: Munchausen syndrome by proxy: An outpatient challenge. *Pediatrics* 75:526, 1985.

Malatack JJ, Wiener ES, Gartner JC, et al: Munchausen syndrome by proxy: A new complication of central venous catheterization. *Pediatrics* 75:523, 1985.

Meadow R: Munchausen syndrome by proxy. *Arch Dis Child* 57:92, 1982.

Meadow R: Munchausen syndrome by proxy: The hinterland of child abuse. *Lancet* 2:343, 1977.

Waller DA: Obstacles to the treatment of Munchausen by proxy syndrome. *J Am Acad Child Psychiatry* 22:80, 1983.

Pervasive Developmental Disorders 9

INFANTILE AUTISM

Definition

The pervasive developmental disorders (PDDs), the most severe behavioral disorders in children, are marked by "qualitative impairment in the development of reciprocal social interaction, in the development of verbal and nonverbal communication skills, and in imaginative activity" (*DSM-III-R*). Affected children vary greatly in the types and degrees of impairments they suffer; they comprise a heterogeneous group. Mental retardation and a multitude of medical diagnoses are often seen in association with the PDDs. The *DSM-III-R* notes the variety of diagnostic terms (atypical development, symbiotic psychosis, childhood psychosis, childhood schizophrenia, etc) used in the past to describe these children. These terms, and the term "psychosis" in general, have been discarded in favor of the pervasive developmental disorder rubric, in order to emphasize the variety of developmental abnormalities these children suffer (social, language, motor, cognitive) and the difference between these disorders and psychosis in adolescents or adults. In this heterogeneous group, the only discrete syndrome is that of infantile autism (IA) or autistic disorder, which is also called Kanner syndrome.

Associated features include abnormal development of cognitive skills, abnormal posture and motor behavior, hyper- or hyposensitivity to certain stimuli, abnormal eating, sleeping, or drinking, emotional lability or absence of emotional reactions, and self-harming behavior, often severe, such as finger- or hand-biting.

Basic Science

Much evidence points to an underlying biologic defect in the PDDs, but the precise nature of the defect is undefined. By many criteria, no brain pathology is demonstrable. Except in the few cases associated with specific dysmorphic, metabolic, or infectious disorders such as tuberous sclerosis, congenital rubella or phenylketonuria, gross and microscopic brain morphology is unremarkable. In contrast to children with mental retardation, children with PDDs generally have unremarkable, even handsome physiognomies.

But there is clearly something wrong with the brain, particularly in IA and childhood-onset PDD (COPDD). Up to 30% of children with IA have enlarged ventricles by CT scan. One-third of those with IA develop seizures by adolescence. They move awkwardly and perform stereotypies (flapping, rocking, spinning objects). Overall cognitive level is significantly impaired in children with PDDs, with 70% of children with IA having IQs below 70, and with wide scatter on subtests. Older children or adolescents with psychosis are more likely to have IQ in the normal or low-normal range. Historically, a higher incidence of perinatal complications is seen in children with PDDs than in the general population. On the environmental side, parents of children with PDDs do not differ from the general population. From a genetic point of view, IA is more common than expected among the siblings of children with IA. Monozygotic twins are more often concordant for IA than dizygotic twins. Physiologically, considerable overlap is seen in EEG findings among children with PDDs and aphasia; nonetheless, specific low amplitude waves, especially when focused attention is required, are seen in autistic children, consistent with the clinical impression that they have impaired ability to concentrate. Neurochemical studies indicate elevated blood serotonin in about one-third of children with IA; interventions which increase central dopamine concentrations worsen symptoms in IA.

Epidemiology

The pervasive developmental disorders are much rarer than psychosis in adulthood. PDDs occur in 10–15/10,000 children; IA in 4–5/10,000 children. In all these disorders, males outnumber females, by as much as 4:1. The PPDs appear to occur to the same extent in all social classes.

Natural History

From birth, children with IA relate and respond to people differently, even in their postural anticipation of being held. Despite this, the age at which diagnosis occurs depends on the degree of the child's impairment, on parental sensitivity and on physician alertness; it may come early in infancy when parents realize a baby is not looking back and smiling; it may come only later when language fails to appear or much later when nursery school entrance makes the extent of the child's handicap apparent to others. Other children appear to regress after what appears to have been a period of normal development, possibly after encephalitis or another insult to the brain.

With all of these disorders, prognosis is poor. Most children require increasing support and specialized care as they grow larger and stronger and as the difference between their abilities and social expectations increases. Only 1–2% of autistic persons, notably some with better language and higher IQ, appear "normal" as adults; one in six sustains gainful employment, and another one in six can work in a sheltered and supervised workshop. Two-thirds need constant supervision and support throughout life.

Diagnosis

As in all areas of child development, two distinct aspects of diagnosis must be stressed: *syndromic* diagnosis, that is, fitting a child as best one can into one of the syndromes listed here, and *developmental* diagnosis, in which one is concerned less with the syndrome than with the pattern of developmental strengths and weaknesses shown by a particular child, with the goal of identifying capacity for growth along each affected developmental line. Using both approaches to diagnosis is important in all areas of pediatrics and child psychiatry, but is essential with regard to the more severely impaired child for two reasons. First, children with PDDs are defined in terms of gross behavioral symptoms, and not in terms of etiology nor of underlying pathologic processes nor of treatment outcome. Second, our treatments are specific to a child's capacity, not to a particular diagnosis; that is, a child needs speech therapy, behavioral shaping, haloperidol to control agitation, instructions to his parents about how to manage frustrating situations, or empathic understanding of his situation, not because he has a PDD, but because he has particular needs which may respond to these interventions. The remarks about syndromic classification which follow should not diminish the need for this kind of developmental diagnosis.

IA is diagnosed when a child, before the age of 2½, shows pervasive lack of responsiveness to other people, gross deficits in language development, peculiar speech (echolalia, pronoun reversals, failure to appreciate social implications of language), resistance to change, and absence of delusions or hallucinations. Other children with impaired reciprocal social interaction, communication and imaginative development are considered to have pervasive development disorder, not otherwise specified.

Treatment

Treatment is not satisfactory for any of the PDDs. What can be done should be undertaken by mental health and educational specialists. The physician managing a child with autism will find it useful, for himself and for the parents, to develop a relationship with the local chapter of the National Society for Children and Adults with Autism (national office: 1234 Massachusetts Avenue, NW, Suite 1017, Washington, DC 20005).

Children with IA and the other PDDs are managed by behavioral techniques to decrease symptoms and increase ability to attend and respond; parental guidance attempts to increase the range of empathic responses to the child and decrease frustration-generating encounters. Trials of a variety of pharmacologic agents have yielded little evidence of sustained and replicable benefit; haloperidol may have a role in IA in managing agitation and difficulty attending. No pharmacologic treatment affects the underlying disorder. Higher functioning children with IA and other PDDs benefit from attempts to talk about the predicaments they find themselves in, having to deal with people in a variety of bewildering contexts where they do not understand what is going on nor what is expected of them.

CONTROVERSY

While earlier theories that the PDDs, especially IA, were the result of environmental failure (specifically, unresponsive parenting) have been discarded in favor of a more biologic model, there is still no consensus about the nature of the fundamental defect or defects. Similarly, treatment is a matter of controversy, especially concerning the role of pharmacologic intervention.

Controversy concerning the use of severely aversive or punitive reinforcements in the management of severe self-harming behavior reached the public arena when the State of Massachusetts tried unsuccessfully to close, and parents came to the defense of, a residential program for older adolescents and adults with IA. This program uses aversive reinforcements (very loud sounds, dousing with water) to decrease severe self-mutilating behaviors (chewing one's hands, tearing out one's hair). Litigation and public debate resulted in continued operation of the program, under strict guidelines for such treatment.

Several principles are relevant. First, aversive reinforcement has a place, but only when less drastic approaches fail—a criterion which immediately raises a value judgment, since the alternative to severe aversion is vigorous pharmacotherapy. Parents and physicians must choose between two approaches, either of which may be effective, but neither of which is wholly benign. Second, thorough documentation is required with the use of any extraordinary treatment, whether pharmacological or behavioral. Documentation may include videotaping the patient with and without treatment and recording of parents' observations of the patient in both conditions. Third, any aversives used must be introduced by plan, and not on the spur of the moment, nor their use left to the discretion of the direct care staff. Finally, each program using such procedures should establish an institutional Human Rights Committee, to which oversight responsibility is given, and on which serve members from outside as well as from within the institution.

NEW DEVELOPMENTS

Progress is occurring and is expected to continue in delineating the brain defects in these disorders, especially using noninvasive techniques such as magnetic resonance imaging and positron-emission tomography.

Prognosis

As indicated, prognosis in children with PDDs is poor, with two-thirds of those with IA requiring long-term supervision and support.

CASE ILLUSTRATION: INFANTILE AUTISM

Born after a benign pregnancy and a delivery during which anoxic stress may have occurred, Frank, as an infant, was quiet and undemanding; as the first year of life progressed, his self-absorption and lack of interest in social play with his parents were noted. Speech was slow to appear, but motor development was quite appropriate and made parents and pediatrician play down the increasingly obvious abnormalities in social and language development. By age 4 years, Frank had language, but it was odd, with pronoun reversals, literalness, and echolalia. Socially, he preferred solitary play to any activity with children or adults. He had self-stimulatory motor behaviors, including flapping, bouncing up and down while sitting, and staring at his hands. In the next few years he became rigid about any change from the usual routine (such as a guest in the house, or places at table not set in the usual way) but impressed parents and visitors with his great memory for numbers and for songs heard on the radio, the social meaning of which he did not understand. Specialized school was sought while he continued living at home, but by adolescence his bizarre and, at times, aggressive behavior required placement in a residential facility for children with pervasive developmental disorders.

COMMENT

Usually no positive family history, no clear adverse events in pregnancy (or even putative ones as in this case) can be mobilized to "explain" the bizarre lack of affect and of capacity to relate to others that is seen very early in autistic infants. Lack of appropriate parenting, once proposed, is clearly not the explanation for autistic behavior.

Placement in supportive residential facilities is the humane approach. Unfortunately, most autistic infants remain compromised and require life-long care.

REFERENCES

American Psychiatric Association: *Diagnostic and Statistical Manual, Third Edition, Revised,* (DSM-III-R). Washington, DC: American Psychiatric Association, 1987.

Kanner L: Autistic disturbance of affect contact. *Nervous Child* 2:217, 1943.

Nasarallah HA, Weinberger DW (eds): *Handbook of Schizophrenia.* Amsterdam, Elsevier, 1986.

Schopler E, Mesibov GB (eds): *The Effects of Autism on the Family.* New York, Plenum Press, 1984.

Schopler E, Mesibov GB, Baker A: Evaluation of treatment for autistic children and their parents. *J Am Child Psychiatry* 21:262, 1982.

GORDON HARPER

Section 3

Nutrition

The nutritional status of an individual is an important aspect of the maintenance of good health. This is particularly true for infants and children who require balanced nutrients for growth and development and who are dependent on parents and caretakers for their diet. Because the pediatrician plays such an important role in maintaining appropriate nutrition we include a separate section on this topic, even though many of the conditions which may be considered to be related to nutrition are described in detail in other sections. Aspects of nutrition require consideration in a variety of emotional and somatic disorders as well as many inborn errors of metabolism and probably as yet undiscovered genetic disorders. The importance of understanding the basis of these disorders and, thus, the ability to alleviate them by relatively simple dietary maneuvers is exemplified by the dramatic effects of eliminating gluten in the diet of patients with celiac disease and of phenylalanine in the diet of phenylketonurics. Because these are not strictly nutritional disorders, however, these and other problems, such as obesity in endocrine disease, for instance, are discussed in their respective sections.

The present section will focus on disorders that are related specifically to under- and overnutrition (including malnutrition and obesity), to inappropriate amounts of specified dietary components (vitamin deficiencies and hypervitaminosis), to the mechanics of parenteral nutrition, and, briefly, to adverse reactions to food.

For more detailed information of food composition and selected diets the reader is referred to dietary manuals such as, Kelts DG, Jones EG: *Manual of Pediatric Nutrition.* Boston, Little, Brown & Co., 1984, and textbooks: Howard RB, Winter HS: *Nutrition and Feeding of Infants and Toddlers.* Boston, Little, Brown & Co., 1984; American Academy of Pediatrics: *Pediatric Nutrition Handbook,* 2nd edition. Elk Grove Village, IL, 1985; Walker WA, Watkins JB: *Nutrition in Pediatrics, Basic Science and Clinical Application.* Boston, Little, Brown & Co., 1985; and Grand RJ, Sutphen JL, Dietz WH: *Pediatric Nutrition.* Stoneham, MA, Butterworths, 1987.

Energy Balance and Its Regulation

1

Living cells require a constant supply of energy to drive activities such as muscle contraction, protein synthesis, active transport, and cell division. The source of this energy is the food we eat which is metabolized to release chemical energy in the form of ATP (adenosine triphosphate).

FOODS

Each of the major kinds of food (carbohydrate, fat, protein) is broken down to its constituent calorigenic substrates: glucose, free fatty acids, and amino acids. Each substrate can be metabolized within the cell to yield ATP. The energy value of each food is expressed in terms of calories: 4 kcal/g for protein and carbohydrate, 9 kcal/g for fat. Generally, roughly 50% of calories is used for basal energy requirements, 30% for growth requirements, and 15–20% for normal variations in activity.

Carbohydrate

The term originates from the chemical structure shared by all of the members of this family of organic molecules. The formula ($C[H_20]$) signifies that any carbohydrate can be accurately described as a multiple of the basic $C\text{-}H_20$ "carbohydrate" moiety. Within the carbohydrate family are the simple sugars (monosaccharides and the complex carbohydrates (di- and polysaccharides). The latter are hydrolyzed to simple sugars within the gut. These sugars are a main source of energy for the body.

Protein

Vital molecules including enzymes, hormones, and antibodies are protein and along with nucleic acids require nitrogen and/or amino acids obtained from ingested protein for their synthesis. The protein which is consumed must offer adequate amounts of methionine, phenylalanine, threonine, tryptophan, and valine, which are the traditional "essential" amino acids for the adult, the full-term infant also needs tyrosine, cystine, and histidine. Protein deficiency is likely to occur when protein intake accounts for less than 6% of the total caloric intake. Protein itself is a costly and inefficient source of energy. Its main role is in biosynthesis of critical nitrogen-containing molecules; however, certain amino acids can be converted to glucose when necessary (gluconeogenesis). Utilization of protein for biosynthesis requires energy; therefore, adequate amounts of carbohydrate are essential to provide ATP for the biosynthetic reactions.

Fat

Lipids (fat) are nonwater-soluble organic compounds which are vital to cell structure and whole body function. The major lipids in the human body are the fats (triglycerides and fatty acids), phospholipids (principally lecithin), cholesterol, and fat-soluble vitamins. Triglyceride constitutes the major calorie storage in the body. Adipose cells contain 90% triglyceride with only 3% water. Two types of fatty acids exist: saturated and unsaturated. Animal triglyceride contains mostly saturated fatty acids (palmitic, stearic). Vegetable oils contain fatty acids with two (linoleic) or more (arachidonic) unsaturated bonds. The term polyunsaturated fatty acid refers to two or more such bonds.

Essential fatty acids (linoleic, linolenic, and arachidonic) are integral components of the phospholipid structure of all cell membranes. Arachidonic and linolenic acids can be synthesized from linoleic; therefore, only linoleic is a nutritional essential fatty acid. The recommended minimum requirement for linoleic acid in infant formulas is 300 mg/100 kcal.

Fiber

This term designates the complex of carbohydrates and other substances that are present mainly in the cell walls of the plants used as foods. Fiber includes cellulose, hemicelluloses, gums, mucilages, pectic substances, and lignin. These substances are poorly digested by humans and have little nutritional value. However, fiber aids in gastrointestinal motility and helps ensure regularity of bowel movements.

GASTROINTESTINAL TRACT

The gastrointestinal (GI) tract has an essential role in providing energy for the body. Taste and smell activate the parasympathetic system to anticipate nutrients. Chewing stimulates salivation to hydrate solid foods and the tongue guides food bits into a position for swallowing. The bolus of food is thrust into the esophagus wherein peristaltic waves carry it into the stomach. Prior psychic stimulation as well as distention of the stomach with food causes certain cells to secrete the hormone gastrin which, in turn, stimulates other cells in the stomach to secrete acid and pepsin for digestion of the food (Lebenthal and Siegel, 1985).

Most absorption occurs in the small intestine, where digestive enzymes from both the pancreas and cells lining the small intestine break down food components. Digested food molecules are absorbed into the bloodstream from the intestine and then pass directly into the liver by way of the hepatic portal vein. Within the liver these molecules are processed. Lipids are handled differently in the GI tract. Fatty acids, cholesterol, and fat-soluble vitamins are packaged into chylomicrons within the enterocyte and channeled into vessels called lacteals which are part of the lymphatic system. The chylomicrons travel through the lymphatic system to reach the systemic blood circulation instead of going directly to the liver.

METABOLISM OF FOOD

Absorption after ingestion of mixed meal elevates blood glucose concentration and triggers insulin release from the pancreas (Fig. 3.1). Insulin enhances the extraction of glucose by certain cells for energy utilization. The RQ (respiratory quotient) approaches 1.0 because all lean body systems metabolize glucose in the fed state. Insulin also reduces the release of free fatty acids from adipocytes by inhibiting hormone-sensitive lipase. In addition, the liver replenishes glycogen and packages excess calories into very low density lipoprotein (VLDL), while adipocytes clear chylomicron triglyceride and later VLDL triglyceride for storage. Over 90% of excess energy is stored as triglycerides in adipose tissue.

In the fasting state, glycogen is broken down under the influence of glucagon and epinephrine to provide glucose for energy. In the chronic calorie-deprived state, glucocorticoids and growth hormone enhance the breakdown of protein and fat, respectively, to release substrates for generation of energy. Thyroid hormone causes an increase in metabolic rate and increased energy consumption, except in the chronically malnourished.

ENERGY BALANCE

Basal metabolism is the level of energy expended during the resting state after an overnight fast. It increases with body weight, but changes less with surface area (see Table 3.1). There is an approximately 20% variation around median figures which explains the wide descrepancy between individual food intake and weight gain. During fasting, triiodothyronine output falls, with a decrease in resting metabolism and activity of the sympathetic nervous system is lowered.

Measurements of metabolic rate for several minutes are widely used to describe the energy expenditure of an individual. Extrapolation to 24 hours from brief observations is clearly hazardous, as noted by Schulze et al (1986). Their measurements of oxygen consumption and carbon dioxide production in healthy growing low birth weight infants were made over eight consecutive 3-hour periods between feedings. Mean oxygen

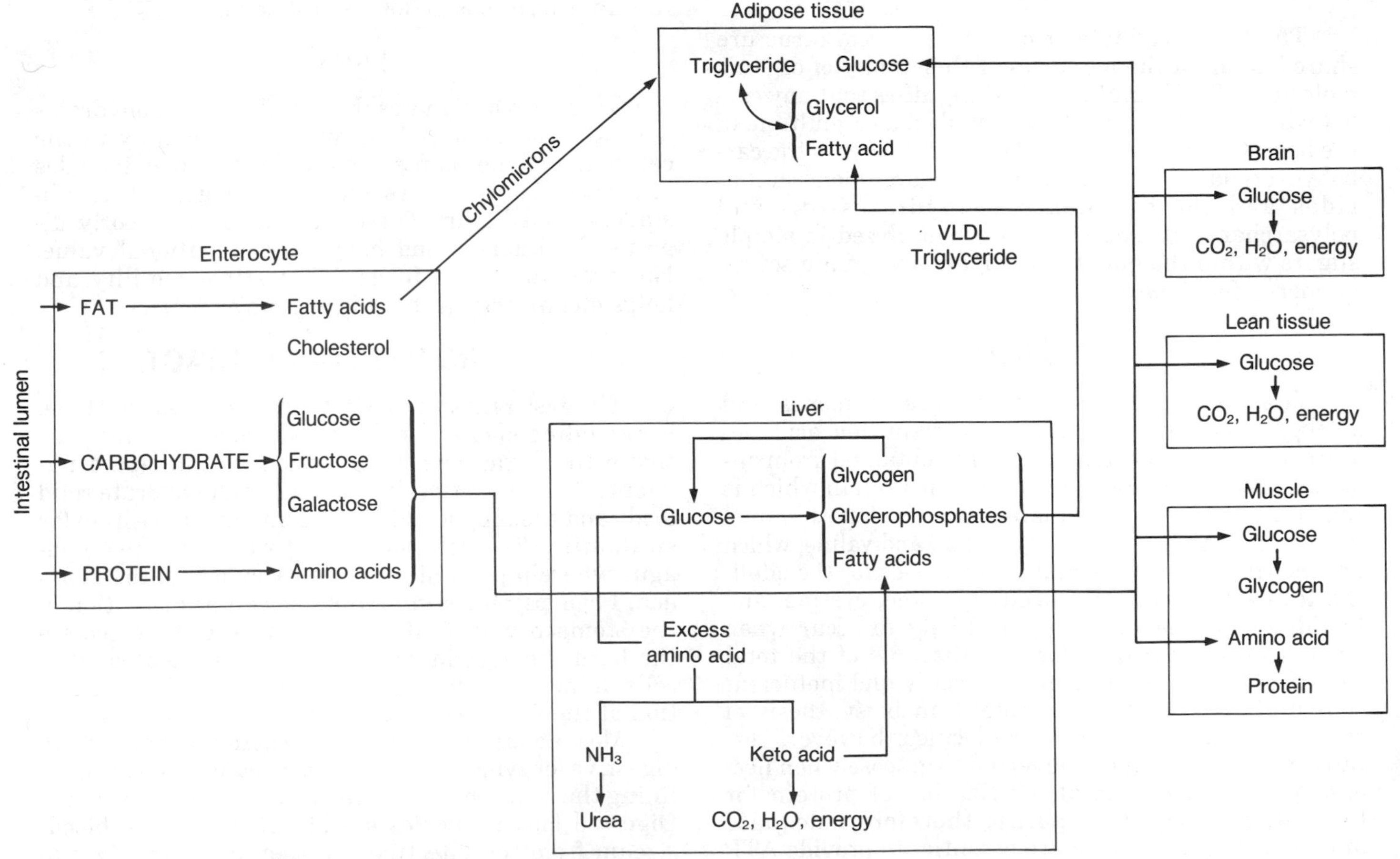

Figure 3.1. Metabolism of food energy sources.

Table 3.1
Estimating Energy Needs Using Basal Metabolic Rate (BMR)[1,2]

	Kcal/24 hours			Kcal/24 hours	
Body Weight (kg)	Males	Females	Body Weight (kg)	Males	Females
3.0	150	136	36.0	270	1173
4.0	210	205	38.0	1305	1207
5.0	270	274	40.0	1340	1241
6.0	330	336	42.0	1370	1274
7.0	390	395	44.0	1400	1306
8.0	445	448	46.0	1430	1338
9.0	495	496	48.0	1460	1369
10.0	545	541	50.0	1485	1399
11.0	590	582	52.0	1505	1429
12.0	625	620	56.0	1580	1487
13.0	665	655	54.0	1555	1458
14.0	700	687	58.0	1600	1516
15.0	725	718	60.0	1630	1544
16.0	750	747	62.0	1660	1572
17.0	780	775	64.0	1690	1599
18.0	810	802	66.0	1725	1626
19.0	840	827	68.0	1765	1653
20.0	870	852	70.0	1785	1679
22.0	910	898	72.0	1815	1705
24.0	980	942	74.0	1845	1731
26.0	1070	984	76.0	1870	1756
28.0	1100	1025	78.0	1900	1781
30.0	1140	1063	80.0		1805
32.0	1190	1101	82.0		1830
34.0	1230	1137	84.0	2000	1855

[1]Basal metabolic rate (BMR), or the energy required to maintain basic body function of a fasted subject at rest in a thermal neutral environment, may also be used as a means to determine energy needs. NOTE: Not applicable to obese weight. *Maintenance Energy Requirements (MER) refers to neutral energy balance in a state without stress and near total inactivity. In contrast to BMR, the MER allows for the specific dynamic action (SDA) of food ingested. MER = BMR × 1.5.*

[2]Reproduced from *Handbook for Nutrition Services of The Dietary Department*, The Children's Hospital, Boston, 1982.

consumption (ml/kg/min) was 8.41 ± 0.50 (SD). Carbon dioxide production (ml/kg/min) was 8.24 ± 0.45. The mean energy expenditure per day (kcal/kg) was 60.6 ± 3.4. The variability would have been even greater if measurements were made during crying, feeding, or other activity.

Energy requirements for normal infants, children, and young adults are shown in Table 3.2. In the first year of life, energy is mostly directed to maintenance and growth. By the time the infant crawls—toward the end of the first year—about 15% of total energy is required for physical activity. The average requirements, based on studies of healthy children in the United States and United Kingdom are 90–103 kcal/kg/day for ages 1–4 years; about 90 kcal/kg/day for ages 4–6 years and 78 kcal/kg/day for ages 7–9 years. Requirements gradually fall with age so that by 16–19 years, 49 kcal/kg/day are appropriate. No changes are seen in the metabolism of individual tissues, but rather in the proportion of tissues with differing metabolic rates. The infant has relatively more visceral mass, which has a high metabolic rate, and the adult more musculoskeletal mass, with lower resting metabolic rate.

Resting metabolic rates vary greatly among individuals who are ill. In general, septicemia increases metabolism 25–55%. Infections of many types, even without fever, are associated with a metabolic rate about 10% above normal. Patients with congenital heart disease have increased metabolic rates, which can be increased over 50% in congestive failure. Severe trauma or burns increase protein turnover in proportion to the extent of the injury, reaching levels of 2.5 times normal (Kien, 1985).

Central Nervous System

The hypothalamus is the central integration station. Experimental insult to regions of the ventromedial aspect can produce hyperphagia in animals. The effects are mediated through the vagus nerve and can be reversed with vagotomy. Destruction of regions of the lateral hypothalamus reduces hunger, and destroys components of the dopaminergic system. Hypothalamic centers regulate trophic hormones which in turn affect metabolism. Thyroid, adrenal, and gonadal steroids modulate energy balance (Bray, 1985).

Finally, the individual has cortical control over intake and expenditure. Restraint in intake and increase in utilization through exercise are within the control of children and adults.

Table 3.2
Estimating Energy and Protein Needs Recommended Dietary Allowance (RDA), Considered Adequate to Meet the Needs of Practically All Healthy Children [1,2]

Age	Kcal/kg	Protein	
		gm/kg	% Kcal
Males and Females			
0–6 mo.	115	2.2	7.6
6–12 mo.	105	2.0	7.6
1–3 yrs.	100	1.8	7.0
4–6 yrs.	85	1.5	7.2
7–10 yrs.	86	1.2	5.6
Males			
11–14 yrs.	60	1.0	6.6
15–18 yrs.	42	.85	8.0
19–22 yrs.	41	.80	7.7
23–50 yrs.	39	.80	8.3
Females			
11–14 yrs.	48	1.0	8.4
15–18 yrs.	38	.84	8.8
19–22 yrs.	38	.80	8.4
23–50 yrs.	36	.80	8.8

[1]*ENERGY*: Energy allowances for children through age 18 are based on MEDIAN energy intakes of children these ages followed on longitudinal growth studies. More appropriate *individual* allowances are based on observation of appetite, activity growth and weight gain.
PROTEIN: RDA guidelines for infants are based on amount of milk protein known to insure a satisfactory rate of growth. For ages 1–18 years, a maintenance level based on body weight is supplemented to satisfy growth requirements based on a 75% efficiency of utilization.
NOTE: Estimates of protein requirements are valid only when energy requirements are fully met.
[2]Reproduced from *Handbook for Nutrition Services of the Dietary Department*, The Children's Hospital, Boston, 1982, p. 6.

Table 3.3
Recommended Caloric Distribution [1,2]

Population	Recommended % Distribution		
	4 kcal/g		9 kcal/g
	CHO	PRO	FAT
Full-term normal infant	35–65	7–16	30–55
> 1 year—for individual consideration (particularly with diets <2000 kcal)—if at high risk for coronary artery disease or with chronic disease considered to have risk factors which include diet	56–58	7–9	35 (PUFA should not exceed 10% of cal)

[1]Demand for energy will take first priority in metabolism; insufficient intake of CHO and fat will promote catabolism of dietary and body protein in an effort to satisfy energy needs.
[2]Reproduced from *Handbook for Nutrition Services of the Dietary Department*, Children's Hospital, Boston, 1982, p.6.

DIETARY RECOMMENDATIONS

The distribution of calories recommended for children is given in Table 3.3. The caloric demands on infants suggest that restriction of calories will promote breakdown of protein to satisfy energy needs. In children over 2 years of age, reduced intake of fat may be advisable, particularly in the child at risk for coronary heart disease or hyperlipidemia.

Many physicians believe that dietary recommendations consistent with the guidelines of the Nutrition Committee of the American Heart Association, the Senate Select Committee on Nutrition and Human Needs and the recent National Institutes of Health Consensus Development Statement should be implemented for children over 2 years of age. The evidence that atherosclerosis probably begins early in life, that nutritional habits are formed in early life, and that children in a number of modern-day societies do well on such diets are facts in favor of adopting certain dietary fat, cholesterol, salt, and sugar restrictions. These recommendations include a fat intake of 30% of total calories with restriction of saturated fat to 10% of total calories. Cholesterol intake of less than 300 mg/day, protein at 15–20% of calories, and carbohydrate (primarily complex) at 50–55% of calories are also recommended. Such a diet would emphasize lean meat, fish, and poultry with decreased use of fatty meats and eggs. Consumption of whole grain breads and cereals, fruits and vegetables is encouraged. Consumption of sweets and salty high fat snack foods is discouraged. At all times, the calories provided must be adequate for normal growth and development (Committee on Nutrition, 1986).

REFERENCES

Bray GA: Regulation of energy balance. *Physiologist* 28:186, 1985.

Committee on Nutrition, American Academy of Pediatrics: Prudent life-style for children: Dietary fat and cholesterol. *Pediatrics* 78:521, 1986.

Kien CL: Energy metabolism and requirements in disease. In Walker WA, Watkins JB(eds): *Nutrition in Pediatrics.* Boston, Little, Brown & Co., 1985.

Lebenthal E, Siegel M: Understanding gastric emptying: Implications for feeding the healthy and compromised infants. *J Pediatr Gastroenterol Nutr* 4:1, 1985.

Schulze K, Stefanski M, Masterson J, et al: An analysis of the variability in estimates of bioenergetic variables in preterm infants. *Pediatr Res* 20:422, 1986.

Malnutrition and Starvation

2

Optimal nutrition of all children is a basic expectation of physicians and others who carry responsibility for their health. In most of the Western world and among affluent individuals in other areas, adequate nutrition has come to be taken for granted as appropriate foods are usually readily available. Even in such settings, however, dietary idiosyncracies, cultural dictates, and illnesses such as anorexia nervosa or chronic diarrhea (malabsorption) can produce specific deficiency states or even starvation.

Premature infants are devoid of much muscle mass or subcutaneous tissue, and thus, can show signs of "starvation" if adequate nutrients are not provided at frequent intervals. Similarly, older children with chronic illness and increased metabolic demands associated with chronic infection (as in cystic fibrosis) are often lean and prone to some of the metabolic consequences of starvation if deprived of food during acute exacerbations of illness.

Among the poorer people of the world where undernutrition is common, short stature is prevalent and listlessness and apathy caused by inadequate food intake can be attributed mistakenly to laziness or even retardation. In times of famine induced by droughts, wars, or overpopulation, deaths from starvation continue to occur, particularly among children who are often underfed when limited food supplies are distributed first to adults. It has been stated that half the world's children go to bed hungry every night. This staggering and depressing fact is often suppressed by those who have abundant food available. It becomes manifestly clear on inspection of village life, or in the urban slums of many parts of the world, such as Central and South America, parts of Africa, Asia, Indonesia, and parts of the United States.

For these reasons, it seems pertinent to summarize some of the massive amount of information that describes the sequence of metabolic events in human malnutrition.

Basic Science

The three main classes of nutrients, carbohydrates, proteins, and fats, are metabolized in ways that permit breakdown products of one class to regulate flux in the metabolism of another. For example, the liver is primarily concerned with maintenance of normal blood glucose levels, but amino acids such as alanine and glutamine that are needed for gluconeogenesis come mainly from muscle. During food deprivation, there is a change in the regulation of metabolic events.

The initial need of the starving individual is to maintain blood glucose levels for energy, particularly for cerebral metabolism. (The brain consumes 60–70% of total circulatory glucose.) Liver glycogen stores are depleted first, usually within a few hours. Thus, the liver must have substrates from other tissues, particularly amino acids from muscle.

After a few days of fasting, fat stores are recruited to supply energy. Both glycerol and free fatty acids are released from the fat cells. The glycerol is metabolized mainly in the kidney and liver, where it is phosphorylated by glycerol kinase and either reutilized for triglyceride formation or used for gluconeogenesis. The fatty acids circulate as complexes with albumin. Some are oxidized in muscle and other tissues. Those taken up by the liver are activated by reaction with ATP and CoA to form acyl CoA. During fasting, the flow of free fatty acids to the liver is greatly increased and acetyl CoA accumulates. In the presence of glucose and insulin the acetyl CoA is converted primarily to triglyceride; however, in conditions of decreased availability of glucose and insulin (fasting, diabetes mellitus) the pathway is blocked and acetyl CoA accumulates within liver cells, condensing to form acetoacetyl CoA and hydroxymethylgutaryl CoA. The latter is cleaved to yield acetoacetate and acetyl CoA. The free acetoacetate can be reduced to form β-hydroxybutyrate or it can decompose spontaneously to form acetone. All three molecules (acetoacetate, β-hydroxbutyrate, acetone), called ketone bodies, are released by the liver. They can be metabolized by the brain and the heart; however, in large amounts they accumulate in plasma lowering the plasma pH. Their effect is buffered by bicarbonate, by the release of carbon dioxide which is exhaled. As predicted by the Henderson-Hasselbalch equation, when bicarbonate levels fall below the level at which respiratory compensation is possible, a metabolic acidosis results. Most individuals with prolonged or severe ketoacidosis have lowered total body CO_2 content and chronic acidemia.

MALNUTRITION AND HOST DEFENSES

Undernutrition compromises host defenses and contributes to deaths from respiratory and diarrheal diseases in particular. Infection, in turn, may impair food intake and, thus, aggravate the malnutrition.

The cell-mediated immune response is most profoundly affected. Atrophy of lymphoid tissues may be evident on physical examination. Tonsils and lymph nodes are reduced, and on chest radiographs, the thymus appears shrunken. Delayed hypersensitivity is impaired so that responses to tuberculin testing are unreliable. T4 helper lymphocytes are reduced relatively more than is the T8 suppressor population.

Other components of host defense are also impaired. Secretory IgA levels are low. Other immunoglobulins may be elevated from repeated infections or depressed, especially in low birth weight infants.

Polymorphonuclear leukocytes (polys) can ingest bacteria and fungi, but intracellular killing is reduced.

All of these abnormalities are reversible with the assumption of adequate nutrition (Chandra, 1985).

Diagnosis

Aspects of diagnosis in malnourished infants are discussed in the context of the following cases.

CASE ILLUSTRATION

A 10-month-old black female infant was brought to the emergency room because of diarrhea. It was immediately evident that the infant, who weighed only 6 kg, was profoundly malnourished. On examination, temperature was 35°C, pulse 80, respirations 16, blood pressure 70/0. The head appeared large with respect to the rest of the infant, but was only on the third percentile for age. The eyes were sunken and glazed. The infant was hypotonic and only minimally responsive to stimuli. Skin was dry and subcutaneous tissue was nonexistent. Bowel patterns could be seen on the abdominal wall, but the abdomen was not distended, and liver and spleen were not enlarged. The kidneys were readily felt and of normal size and position. Extremities were marked by gross demarcation in muscle mass and minimal pitting edema of the dorsa of the feet.

Further history established that the stools were small, and consisted of mucus with a water ring on the diaper. The mother of this child was 16 years old and the pregnancy was unplanned. The father was not identified. The mother had delivered at term a 3.5-kg infant and nursed the infant for about 2 weeks. After that, she was employed as a clerk and delegated care of the infant to her sister who had three children of her own. The baby had been to a neighborhood health center at 3 months, when the weight was 4.5 kg and had received the first round of immunizations. No subsequent visits were made. The mother was prompted to bring the child to hospital for "diarrhea" which was not of recent origin, but was recently seen by her as a problem.

QUESTIONS AND COMMENTS

What are the first steps in elucidating the cause of the infant's marasmus?

Although the provocative social history immediately suggested the possibility of child neglect, chronic diarrhea and the associated malabsorption could lead to marasmus even with adequate food intake. Against this possibility was the initial period of well-being, which eliminates some of the most serious types of diarrhea such as secretory diarrhea of infancy or chronic postinfectious diarrhea of the newborn. Even more telling was the absence of a history of excessive stools.

Other conditions that can lead to wasting are cystic fibrosis, uremia, liver disease, and inborn errors of carbohydrate or amino acid metabolism. Chronic infections or malformations of the gastrointestinal tract also should be considered.

Before undertaking extensive diagnostic studies, many of which deprive the infant of much needed rest and blood, we admit such infants to hospital and observe for 1–2 weeks on graduated food intake.

A child this malnourished should be nursed in a thermoneutral environment and unnecessary exposure to infectious agents should be minimized. Initial evaluation should include serum glucose, electrolytes, calcium, phosphorus, magnesium, and albumin. Initially, small frequent milk feeds, 60 ml/kg/day increased by 20 ml/kg/day, are offered. If they are not tolerated, lactose-free formula is tried. If vomiting or diarrhea ensue, intravenous alimentation may be required.

During refeeding, blood glucose should be monitored with Dextrostix every 4 hours until stable (usually 48–72 hours). Deficiencies of elecrolytes or calcium, phosphorus, and magnesium are common and should be corrected. A serum phosphorus measurement should be repeated as feeding is initiated because glucose will drive phosphorus into cells and serum inorganic phosphorus, on which energy metabolism depends, could be depleted to dangerously low levels. Potassium supplements, 4 mEq/kg/day are required for about 2–3 weeks, even if serum potassium is normal inasmuch as in most patients total body potassium is depleted.

In a situation as chronic as this one, there is usually no urgency for a specific diagnosis. Weight gain over a period of several weeks with adequate intake may in itself make a diagnosis of inadequate food provided in the past, as was the case in our 10-month-old patient. Meanwhile, with social service support, and interactions among parent and physicians and nurses, the pathogenesis of child neglect can be established and appropriate interventions can be recommended. If there is likely to be a recurrence because mother is hostile, refractory to suggestions, or fails to show an interest in the child, it is useful to report such child neglect to the appropriate authorities.

If it is ascertained that inadequate intake is not the problem, and the child fails to gain weight in a hospital setting, systematic pursuit of hormonal or metabolic abnormalities, anatomic defects in the intestinal tract, or chronic infection is necessary (Table 3.4). On admission, a chest radiograph, blood count, urinalysis, and blood electrolytes, albumin and total proteins, glucose, and urea nitrogen should be obtained. Further investigations could be deferred pending results of refeeding or information that could emerge from a more extended family and social history, and ongoing examination.

A common error in management of a child with marasmus and an adverse social history is a desire to rule out the many possible organic causes of malnutrition as soon as possible. Inasmuch as a number of tests may be slightly abnormal, this may lead to further testing and exacerbation of the problem. For example, liver function tests may be mildly abnormal and blood gases will probably show a metabolic acidosis. Thyroid function may be de-

***Case Illustration**—continued*

pressed, aminoaciduria could be present and a megaloblastic anemia may be found. (Iron deficiency anemia would be improbable in the absence of much growth in the first 10 months, although it could be present in a mild degree.) If each derangement becomes the object of confirmation and additional tests, significant amounts of blood may be drawn, and transfusions may be required. Most of the chemical abnormalities will be corrected by adequate food intake and will not require specific intervention individually. A malnourished child needs food, affection, mild stimulation and rest to avoid unnecessary mobilization of limited or nearly nonexistent reserves, which sets up further metabolic derangements. Even the most profoundly marasmic children are capable of rapid catch-up growth and full recovery given appropriate intake.

Table 3.4
Gastrointestinal Cause of Malnutrition

- Swallowing dysfunction (often in association with other neurologic problems)
- Esophageal abnormalities
  - After repair of esophageal atresia
  - Gastroesophageal reflux
- Anatomic abnormalities
  - Small stomach
  - Congenital partial obstruction (stenoses or bands)
- Defective assimilation
  - Pancreatic insufficiency
  - Bile salt insufficiency
  - Intestinal mucosal abnormalities
- Fecal loss
  - Chronic diarrhea (any cause)

KWASHIORKOR

Protein Malnutrition

A particular kind of malnutrition, protein malnutrition or *kwashiorkor* occurs when the diet is inadequate in essential amino acids required for growth, or there is intestinal malabsorption as in chronic diarrhea, or abnormal losses occur as with proteinuria or severe burns, or chronic liver disease is present (Table 3.5).

The name, first applied to this most common form of malnutrition, was used by Dr. Cicely Williams (1963) to describe African children who were "deposed," or no longer nursed because of the birth of another child, or

CASE ILLUSTRATION

This 2-year-old black female from a rural slum in Africa was the third child born to a 22-year-old mother who delivered at home after 35 weeks of gestation. The infant was approximately 2 kg at birth, was nursed for 1 year, and was said to have grown well with normal developmental milestones. Thereafter, the mother had a fourth pregnancy, delivered another infant at term, and nursed the new baby.

Gradually, the patient failed to gain weight and grow, despite availability of some food such as grains and maize and some fruit. No milk was provided, and meat was nonexistent. The neighborhood had chickens and abundant coconuts, but neither eggs nor coconut milk were considered good food for children and this child had none.

When seen at the clinic, the child was apathetic and unable to sit or walk. Height was under the third percentile; weight was at the third percentile. The skin was grossly edematous, with pigmentation in some areas of irritation and loss of pigment in others. The hair was sparse and streaky red or blond. The child had bilateral otitis media and watery nasal discharge with breakdown of skin around the nares. The muscles were atrophied, but subcutaneous fat was present. The abdomen was distended and the liver was enlarged and firm.

Laboratory data showed a normal blood count, ketonuria, and total proteins of 3.2 g with 1.8 g of albumin. She was able to tolerate oral feedings of simple carbohydrates, followed by elemental formulas with amino acids. Eventually she recovered completely.

COMMENT

The diagnosis of kwashiorkor was made on physical examination and finding of low serum albumin. Extensive studies of biochemical derangements in protein energy malnutrition have confirmed low blood glucose, decreased essential amino acids and low levels of potassium and magnesium. Serum cholesterol is low, as are most enzymes such as amylase, transaminase, and alkaline phosphatase (Waterlow, 1984).

Malnutrition is associated with a suppression in cell-mediated immunity. Measles can be lethal in such a setting and is one of the leading contributors to death. Other common infections include impetigo, chronic infectious diarrhea, and parasitic infestations.

The most common form of malnutrition in underdeveloped countries, and among the poor of developed ones, is chronic undernutrition with short stature and proportionately low weight, so that the weight for height relationship is normal. These children are best identified when height and weight are measured at intervals and plotted on a growth chart. They may otherwise escape detection because they can look normal. They are, nonetheless, at risk of serious, even overwhelming and fatal infection.

Table 3.5
Differences Between Marasmus and Kwashiorkor (Both Defined as Having an Actual Weight for Age That is Less Than 60% of Expected)

Characteristic	Marasmus	Kwashiorkor (protein malnutrition)
Age of peak incidence	6–18 months	12–48 months
Serum albumin	Normal	Low
Edema	No	Yes
Fatty liver	No	Yes
Response to therapy	Slow	Rapid (diuresis) then slow weight gain

weaned for other reasons in both instances on to a low-protein, relatively high-carbohydrate, diet. The onset is gradual, after weaning, usually between ages 4 months to 5 years. Mortality is high; in some areas, mortality rates are 10–70%. Even with appropriate treatment, the rate remains about 5%.

Treatment

Initial treatment of kwashiorkor requires management of shock if present, then feedings with gradual increases in calories of simple carbohydrates, followed by addition of elemental formulas with amino acids. If the latter are not available, small frequent feedings with milk are appropriate as with marasmic infants. Time is required to correct the profound metabolic derangements, and slow introduction of protein-containing foods is advisable. Daily vitamin requirements can be met with water-miscible vitamin supplements, which should be started immediately and then given daily. Weight loss after initiation of treatment is expected, as edema fluid is mobilized and excreted. If the malnutrition has been severe over a prolonged period into childhood, normal stature and mental function would be permanently compromised.

Prevention

For the clinician, education of parents is a high priority. Sometimes starvation occurs in surroundings where food is abundant, but is not made available to children out of ignorance. Simple messages are often effective, such as encouragement of breast-feeding, appropriate vitamins and iron intake, need for solid foods after 6–9 months, importance of dairy products to supply calcium and protein to growing children, and that readily available foods including whole grain bread, beans, coconuts, rice, bananas, and eggs are nutritious. Melons and other fruits are a good source of clean water in unhygienic environments. This is not the place to discuss the details of diets. The overriding principle is to identify which foods are available and affordable, and make certain that mothers or other caretakers understand how to provide a balanced daily intake for every child. Food supplements will be needed in circumstances of extreme poverty or if available foods are not nutritious.

Pediatricians have an essential role to advocate for adequate food supplies for whatever group of patients comes under their care.

REFERENCES

Cahill GF: Starvation in man. *N Engl J Med* 282:668, 1970.

Chandra RK: Nutrition and host defenses. In Walker WA, Watkins JB(eds): *Nutrition in Pediatrics*. Boston, Little, Brown & Co., 1985, p.309.

Frisancho AR: New norms of upper limb fat and muscle areas for assessment of nutritional status. *Am J Clin Nutr* 34:2540, 1981.

Hamilton JR: Gastrointestinal disease: an important cause of malnutrition in childhood. In Suskind R (ed): *Textbook of Pediatric Nutrition*. New York, Raven Press, 1981.

Kerr DS, Stevens MCG, Robinson HM: Fasting metabolism in infants. I. Effect of severe undernutrition on energy and protein utilization. *Metabolism* 27:411, 1978.

Montgomery R, Dryer RL, Conway TW, et al: *Biochemistry A Case-Oriented Approach,* 4th edition. St. Louis, CV Mosby Co., 1983.

Waterlow JC: Kwashiorkor revisited: The pathogenesis of oedema in Kwashiorkor and its significance. *Trans Roy Soc Trop Med J Hygiene* 78:436, 1984.

Williams CD: The story of Kwashiorkor. Courrier (Centre International de L'Enfance) XIII:361, 1963.

Obesity

3

Definition

Being overweight depends on the definition of upper limit of normal variability for height. The usual definition is weight/height greater than 120% of standards for age and sex. The concept of obesity also depends on the sociocultural milieu of the family. Thus, a chubby child at the 90th percentile for weight, in a family whose members are all heavy for their height may not be perceived as overweight, whereas the same child in another weight-conscious family whose members are slender may be perceived as obese and become the victim of excessive worry about overeating.

Basic Science

Physicians' concern for obesity arises not only from a response to the patient's complaint, but with the knowledge that an overweight child has greater likelihood of being overweight at maturity with all its associated problems (Charney et al, 1976). Many studies have been directed toward elucidating the relationship of infantile or childhood obesity to adult obesity. About one-third of obese adults were overweight as children. Notably, two-thirds were not. The study by Charney et al (1976) was based on records of practicing pediatricians; infants whose weights were over 90% for age in the first 6 months were more than twice as likely as others to become overweight children. Knittle (1972) found the adipose tissue of overweight children had an increased cell number as well as cell size, whereas adult obesity was predominantly an increase in cell size.

The nature versus nurture issue in the pathogenesis of obesity has attracted the interest of many investigators through the years who have based their often conflicting findings on studies in twins and adoptees. The most extensive study was reported on a sample of 540 Danish adults who had been adopted within the first year of life. Their adult weight was more closely related to that of their biologic parents than their adoptive parents. The relationship was strongest for maternal weight (Stunkard et al, 1986). Although this study lends strong support for genetic influences, it remains within the control of the individual to avoid excess intake, especially with knowledge of parental weights.

The question of why some individuals overeat is not answered in a simple way. In fact, the answer may be dictated by the training of the specialist who is posing the question. The geneticist will inquire into family nutritional status, the psychologist will explore eating habits and their possible response to emotional need, the gastroenterologist may explore abnormal function of the GI tract or hyperinsulinism, and the cell biologist will study the metabolic state of fat cells. The final common pathway to weight reduction may lead to the nutritionist who can prescribe the quantity of foods of appropriate quality that will satisfy without providing excessive calories.

Experience with hospitalization for weight reduction establishes that obese people can achieve normal weight. Unfortunately, they are not normal in that they require fewer calories to maintain a normal weight than do individuals of the same weight who were never obese. After major weight reduction, women may have low levels of thyroid hormone, low pulse rates and blood pressure, and often do not menstruate. Leibel and others (cited by Kolata, 1985) have studied the cellular basis of these phenomena and note that formerly obese individuals have up to three times as many fat cells as do normal people. In the obese individual, the fat cells reesterified fatty acids at the same rate as did normal individuals; after weight reduction, re-esterification was decreased. They postulate this phenomenon may make formerly-obese-now-normal weight adults behave as if starved, and drive them to regain their former steady state of overweight.

The pathophysiology of obesity must relate to altered stimuli to the appetite centers of the hypothalamus. Hormonal influences are sometimes at fault, as in hyperadrenocorticism, hypothyroidism, and hyperinsulinism. The Prader-Willi syndrome is associated with hypotonia, hypogonadism, and latent diabetes as well as obesity. Contrary to widely held opinions, no evidence exists to suggest nutrients are metabolized in an abnormal fashion, or that the laws of conservation of energy are defied. Obesity represents the imbalance between food intake and energy expenditure.

Epidemiology

About 10% of Americans are at least 20% over their desirable weight.

Natural History

The consequences of obesity affect many organ systems as summarized by Dietz (1985).

I. Psychosocial dysfunction
II. Growth
    Increased height, advanced bone age, early menarche.
III. Respiratory disorders
    Increased prevalence of infections
    Hypoventilation (Pickwickian syndrome)
    Sleep apnea
IV. Orthopedic disorders
    Slipped capital femoral ephiphysis
    Blount disease (tibial deformity)

V. Abnormal carbohydrate metabolism
 Increased basal insulin levels
 Abnormal glucose tolerance curves
VI. Hypertension—seven times more frequent in obese children
VII. Persistence into adulthood
 Gallbladder disease
 Hypertension
 Diabetes mellitus
 Sudden death

Obesity can occur in association with some congenital and acquired syndromes which, as a group, are responsible for less than 1% of cases.

Prader-Willi syndrome, mentioned previously, is associated with hypotonia in infancy, and a central distribution of fat. Short stature and hypogonadism are characteristic. Affected children have ravenous appetites. Some patients have a deletion of chromosome 15 (Ledbetter et al, 1981).

Laurence-Moon-Bardet-Biedl syndrome is characterized by mental retardation, retinal degeneration with retinitis pigmentosa, polydactyly, and hypogonadism.

Children with myelodysplasia are often obese, probably because of reduced energy expenditure.

Although endocrinopathies are considered as possible causes of obesity, probably Cushing disease is the only serious candidate. The central distribution of fat, hirsutism, striae and hypertension distinguish this condition (see pp. 861–863). Nevertheless, mild Cushing syndrome may be difficult to differentiate from exogenous obesity.

Rarely, a hypothalamic tumor is present (Frohlich syndrome). The condition should be considered in the presence of obesity and signs of increased intracranial pressure.

Diagnosis

Despite the difficulty of precise definitions, the complaint of being overweight must be taken seriously, for it indicates concern with self-image and is, for the most part, based on a difference in appearance in comparison with peers, or with a desired appearance.

In this setting, a detailed history is the most important part of the encounter. Listening to both parents and child reveals their reasons for concern, their perception of the cause and severity of the problem, the habits of other family members, parents' weights at the same age as the child, ethnic background, and culturally influenced dietary habits.

The personality of the child is an issue as well. Overeating (and undereating as well) can be signs of depression. Is the child withdrawn, more at ease in front of television than on the playing fields, the focus of jokes about weight? Is overeating an attention-getting gesture for a child who has been deprived of demonstrated parental affection? Is the child as concerned about obesity as the parents, or more or less so?

The diet history and pattern of eating require detailed documentation. This can be done by asking the parents or child to answer a dietary questionnaire, to be followed by a prospective record of total intake for several typical days, including weekdays and weekends.

The adjective "junk" refers to foods high in refined carbohydrate, salt, fat, and low in protein and vitamins. Typically, they are popcorn, candy bars, fried potatoes, and soda drinks consumed in large quantities by children and many adults. They, of course, contain calories and supply energy, so can hardly be written-off with a pejorative adjective. The concern is that intake of such foods may be excessive and at the exclusion of vegetables, fruits, meats, and cereals that supply necessary vitamins, minerals, protein, and fiber. A balanced diet can contain "junk" food, but in moderation.

The physical diagnosis of obesity demands careful serial measurements of height and weight (and plotting of weight: height ratios). Measurement of a double layer of skin and subcutaneous tissue at midtriceps by use of calipers is useful, although not very reproducible (Tanner et al, 1975; Fig. 3.2). Serial photographs of the standing nude child documents both weight distribution and the changes with puberty.

Treatment

The treatment of obesity depends on the environmental setting and the severity. When obesity is severe (over 180% of ideal body weight) and the social setting is disturbed, psychiatric help may be more important than emphasis on dietary changes. Hilde Bruch (1957) pointed out that overeating may be a balancing factor in the adjustment to life; deprivation of the comfort of eating may precipitate mental illness.

In less severe situations, the pediatrician can set goals, establish programs of eating that optimize the

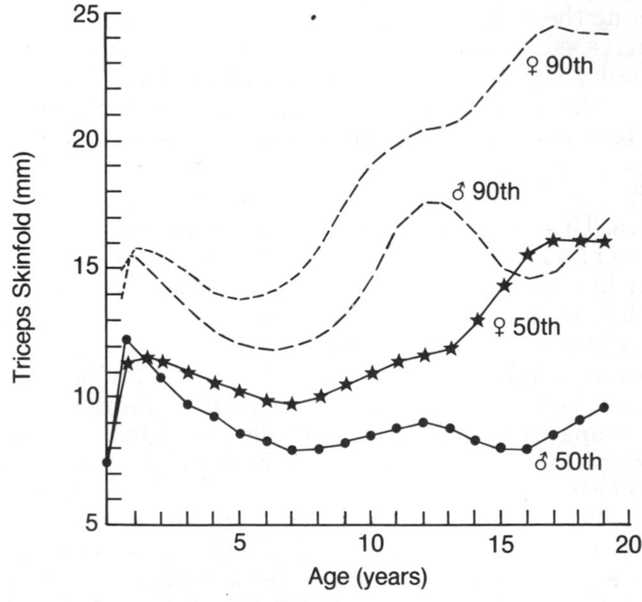

Figure 3.2. Age changes on subcutaneous fat. Median and 90th percentile values for triceps skinfold thickness (redrawn from Tanner and Whitehouse). Reproduced with permission from *Pediatric Nutrition Handbook,* 2nd edition. Evanston, IL, American Academy of Pediatrics, 1985.

child's comfort, but maintain intake at an appropriate level, advise on filling but low calorie foods and beverages, and work out a regular regimen of exercise. Parental involvement should be encouraged to foster the concept that the problem is shared by the family and that the child is not being selectively punished. Behavior modification may be helpful within the framework of this treatment. It is essential to avoid use of drugs to suppress appetite or increase metabolism, to maintain food requirements, to provide the youngster with his or her favorite foods, but in controlled amounts, and to discourage crash programs. The loss of 1 pound per week for adolescents is sufficient to show rewarding results by month's end.

Mechanical approaches to treating obesity include intestinal bypass, stapling of the stomach, insertion of balloons into the stomach, and even wiring the jaw to prevent the possibility of eating solid foods. None of these are appropriate in growing children. In some adolescents with morbid obesity, a surgical approach might be considered if all other methods of weight reduction have failed.

CONTROVERSY

Should the level of cholesterol intake for children be controlled? The major attention given to the role of dietary cholesterol in serum lipid levels and risk of myocardial infarction in adults provides pediatricians with concern for what age child, and which child should have limited cholesterol intake. Recommendations have been made for children based on extrapolations from studies on adults; no data were available on risk factors in normal children as of December 1984 (Mauer, 1985).

NEW DEVELOPMENTS

Serum levels of apolipoproteins A-I and B in children may be more strongly related to clinical disease

CASE ILLUSTRATION (courtesy of Dr. R. Wharton)

B.H. was a 9-year-old boy who had been obese for 3 years. Although his weight had been steadily increasing for 5 years, his parents decided to seek help at this time because they felt he was having trouble physically keeping up with his peers. They were concerned about a possible medical reason for his weight gain because he did not appear to eat more than his peers and was constantly active. He had been growing well. There was no history of constipation, lethargy, or hair loss. His birth history and developmental milestones were normal.

A 72-hour dietary history revealed that he ate appropriate amounts of food at mealtimes, but preferred fried foods and other foods of high caloric density. The boy tended to drink 6–8 large glasses of whole milk a day. He also ate frequent snacks and was constantly being rewarded with food by his grandparents who lived next door.

Family history was significant for maternal obesity; starting after the last pregnancy; this had become a source of friction between the parents. In addition, the mother had worked outside the home for the past 3 years. Father was not obese. There was a strong family history of diabetes, heart disease, and gout.

The child was in the third grade and was described as quiet. His work was average. He was well-behaved and cooperative. At home, he was described as moody with frequent outbursts of temper. Mother stated that she could not get her son to listen to her and that the father was the disciplinarian.

On examination, B.H. was a shy boy who separated from his mother with difficulty. He was growing well with a height at the 75th percentile; his weight was 70 kg (greater than 2 SD above the 95th percentile). He was 180% ideal body weight. Blood pressure was 100/70. He had a prominent "buffalo hump." There was no thyroidomegaly, no dysmorphic features, and neurological examination was normal. Laboratory data showed a cholesterol of 225 mg/dL (2 SD greater than 95th percentile for age) with normal high density lipoprotein (HDL) 42 mg/dl. Triglycerides were elevated to 280 mg/dl (4 hours postprandial). During the physical examination, which was conducted without the parents, the boy indicated that he was frequently teased by other children. Further interview with the parents revealed that there was considerable marital strain centered around the boy's obesity. They stated that the resolution of the child's problems was their first priority. It was the father's view that the boy's behavior was becoming difficult and that the mother could not discipline him. Father also felt that he was being excluded from his wife and son's close relationship. Mother's view was that father undertook little family responsibility and the onus of raising the children was on her.

The medical impression was of exogenous obesity caused by excessive dietary intake. Additionally, the patient had hypercholesterolemia. Fasting triglycerides were normal. Persistence of obesity was seen as evidence of poor limit-setting and mild family dysfunction. The child was placed on a balanced calorie deficit diet with reduction in total dietary fat intake to 30% of total daily calories. In addition, the diet was designed to attain a polyunsaturated to saturated fat ratio of 1.0 and to limit dietary cholesterol to 10 mg/1000 cal/day. Parents were advised to generate together a plan for improved behavioral and dietary compliance with supervision by both parents. A reward system for appropriate eating behavior was also introduced for positive reinforcement. Child and parents were seen at 2-week intervals to reinforce parental involvement and to evaluate progress. At the end of six visits, the child had lost 15 kg. Cholesterol was 180 mg/dl. Everyone was encouraged and follow-up was spaced to 3 months to permit continued reinforcement and encouragement. One year later, he was 150% of ideal body weight because of linear growth and no further weight gain.

CASE ILLUSTRATION (Courtesy of Dr. R. Wharton)

A.H., a 14-year-old white female, was referred for weight reduction after discovery of high blood pressure on a routine before-school physical. Subsequent medical evaluation of her hypertension was negative and she was diagnosed as having obesity-related hypertension. The patient stated that she had been overweight all her life. She believed she had never before been motivated to lose weight but was now becoming interested in boys and nice clothes and thought her weight was excluding her from social activities. Her parents were quite concerned about her hypertension.

A 72-hour dietary history revealed excess intake at meals plus frequent high-carbohydrate snacks. There was no other specific inappropriate eating behavior. She was said to be physically inactive. Family history revealed that both the mother (who was a lawyer) and the father (who was in business) were obese. Moreover, the mother had several other obese relatives. There were two younger siblings, one of whom was overweight. The patient was in the ninth grade and was described as an average student, with many friends. She had no headaches, joint pain, nocturia, or sleep problems. Examination revealed a pleasant cheerful adolescent. Height was greater than 85th percentile. She weighed 101 kg (175% ideal body weight). Blood pressure was 150/95. The rest of the physical examination was normal. Laboratory data revealed normal cholesterol, HDL, and triglycerides, and a normal urinalysis. An additional interview with the parents and the patient disclosed that the parents disagreed about the daughter's weight problem with mother ambivalent about weight loss and father somewhat noncommittal but appearing to want weight loss. Daughter expressed confusion and lack of motivation.

The medical impression was of exogenous obesity caused by excessive dietary intake with minimal activity in an individual predisposed to accelerated weight gain due to hereditary factors. Persistence of obesity was caused by family dysfunction in which the daughter's weight was used as core of family conflict. The daughter was placed on a balanced calorie deficit diet with no added salt. She was also given an exercise program that included 20 minutes of sustained exercise per day. After an initial 6 sessions with no sustained weight loss for the daughter, parents agreed to become involved with the program but to be seen separately from her. Six sessions later, modest weight reduction had begun, and blood pressure was 130/85. The daughter's visits continued closely spaced for 3 months with parents being seen less frequently. Weight loss continued for 2 months but 6 months after the start of the program patient had regained her former weight and she was subsequently lost to follow-up.

QUESTIONS AND COMMENTS (Courtesy of Dr. R. Wharton)

Does obesity in infancy cause adult obesity?

This persistent and important question has paralleled the long debate concerning the role of fat cell hypertrophy versus fat cell hyperplasia in obesity. While it has been observed that obese infants develop fat cell hyperplasia and obese adults develop fat cell hypertrophy, there is as yet no proven correlation between obesity in infancy and later obesity. In fact, recent longitudinal studies that have tracked infants through early childhood have demonstrated that obese infants are no more likely to become obese children than are their nonobese counterparts (Shapiro et al, 1984). As noted earlier, however, about one-third of obese adults were overweight as children. Although these studies may be reassuring, they were performed without attention to family variables. Parental obesity, if factored into these studies, could be a reliable and valid predictor of childhood obesity (Stunkard et al, 1986).

Are laboratory tests or radiographs useful?

Disorders of lipid metabolism are quite prevalent in obese children and all obese children should have careful family history taken followed by measurement of cholesterol, HDL, and triglycerides. Other laboratory tests should be based on particular signs and symptoms, such as those required to assess bone age, thyroid, or adrenal status.

Do obese children become obese adults?

Although obesity in infancy does not predict obesity in childhood, two important features of childhood obesity are useful in predicting obesity in adulthood. First, it has been demonstrated that severity of obesity is highly correlated with its persistence. In one Swedish study of 7-year-old boys followed for 7 years, of those boys more than 180% of ideal body weight, none had remission of obesity during the study period (Borjeson, 1962). Second, there is considerable documentation linking obesity in late childhood and adolescence with obesity in adulthood. Obese adolescents have an 80% likelihood of becoming obese adults, a statistic that must encourage the exploration of methods for prevention.

in adults than serum cholesterol or lipoproteins. These tentative findings were based on reported histories of myocardial infarction in parents in a survey of black and white school-age children (Freedman et al, 1986).

REFERENCES

Börjeson M: Overweight children. *Acta Pediatr* 51(Suppl 132):1, 1962.

Bray GA: Adolescent obesity. In Kretchmer N (ed): *Frontiers in Clinical Nutrition,* Rockville, MD, Aspen Publications, 1986, pp. 153–183.

Bruch H: Psychiatric aspects of obesity. *Metabolism* 6:461,1957.

Charney E, Goodman HC, McBride M, et al: Childhood antecedents of obesity: Do chubby infants become obese adults? *N Engl J Med* 295:6,1976.

Dietz WH: Childhood and adolescent obesity. In Walker WA, Watkins JB (eds): *Nutrition in Pediatrics.* Boston, Little, Brown & Co., 1985, p.769.

Forbes GB: Obesity. In *Pediatric Nutrition Handbook.* Evanston, IL, American Academy of Pediatrics, 1979, p. 322.

Freedman DS, Srinivasan SR, Shear CL, et al: The relation of apolipoproteins A-I and B in children to parental myocardial infarction. *N Engl J Med* 315:721, 1986.

Howard RB, Winter HS (eds): *Nutrition and Feeding of Infants and Toddlers*. Boston, Little, Brown & Co., 1984.
Knittle JL: Obesity in childhood: A problem in adipose tissue cellular development. *J Pediatr* 81:1048, 1972.
Ledbetter DH, Riccardi VM, Airhart SD, et al: Deletions of chromosome 15 as a cause of the Prader-Willi syndrome. *N Engl J Med* 304:325, 1981.
Leibel R (cited by Kolata G): Why do people get fat? Commentary. *Science* 227:1327, 1985.
Mauer AM: A pediatrician attends the National Institutes of Health concensus conference on lowering blood cholesterol. *Pediatrics* 76:125, 1985.
Shapiro LR, Crawford PB, Clark MJ, et al: Obesity prognosis: A longitudinal study of children from the age of 6 months to 9 years. *Am J Public Health* 74:968, 1984.
Stunkard AJ, Sorenson TIA, Hanis C, et al: An adoption study of human obesity. *N Engl J Med* 314:193, 1986.
Tanner JM, Whitehouse RH: Revised standards for triceps and subscapular skinfolds in British children. *Arch Dis Child* 50:142, 1975.

Vitamins 4

This chapter presents a review of some of the disorders associated with deficiencies and excesses of each of the vitamins, their pathophysiology and treatment. Full-blown deficiency states are uncommon in societies that have fortified formulas for infants and vitamin supplements. Nonetheless, vigilance is required for supervision of infant feeding (see Well Child Care, Chapter 1) and for recognition of deficiencies that can develop in children whose parents seek special natural diets for themselves, and may inadvertently deprive their young children of necessary vitamins. In areas of the underdeveloped world, or wherever undernutrition is common, vitamin deficiencies may accompany and exacerbate other nutritional inadequacies.

Inadequate intake is the first and obvious cause of deficiencies, but other possibilities should be considered. Steatorrhea from any cause impairs absorption of fat-soluble vitamins A, D, E, and K. Liver disease can impair conversion of the vitamins to their active metabolites, so that vitamin K and D deficiencies are seen in infants with biliary atresia who are not given appropriate supplements. Renal disease can affect vitamin D metabolism, causing renal rickets with its attendant problems. Compensatory hyperparathyroidism occurs and may cause cyst formation in bones (osteitis fibrosa cystica) see page 642. Other causes of vitamin deficiencies include impaired absorption in infants with gastric or intestinal resections who will need supplemental parenteral vitamin B_{12}, thiamine, and folic acid to achieve normal serum levels.

Certain vitamin-drug interactions may be detrimental (see Table 3.6). In particular, some anticonvulsants such as phenytoin affect vitamin D metabolism. Children who receive diphenylhydantoin or related compounds for control of seizures should have serum levels of the drug measured to prevent excess. Rickets is unlikely if vitamin D intake is adequate and phenytoin levels are between 15–30 μg/ml.

Recommended vitamin requirements are estimates, based on experience, of amounts that are sufficient to prevent deficiencies and are not toxic in a general population; (Table 3.7). Optimal vitamin intakes are not known. As in most areas of medicine, some individuals will have special needs. Those with inborn errors of metabolism, for example, may show a vitamin dependency, and require many times the usual intake (see pp. 849).

The diet itself can alter vitamin requirements. With increased carbohydrate content, the thiamin requirement increases. As protein content rises, B_6 requirement increases, but pantothenic acid and niacin requirements are reduced. Recommendations for vitamin and mineral supplementation from the Committee on Nutrition, American Academy of Pediatrics (1985) are as follows:

All newborn infants: vitamin K_1 at birth.

Breast-fed infants of well-nourished mothers: fluoride if water supply has less than 0.3 ppm.

Formula-fed infants: no additional supplements needed if commercial formulas have vitamins and iron and water supply has fluoride.

After age 1 year: adequate food intake, including fresh fruits or juices provides vitamin and mineral requirements.

Exceptions: children on dietary regimens for obesity, pregnant teenagers, and individuals on vitamin B_{12}- and vitamin D-deficient vegetarian diets.

Table 3.6
Vitamin-Drug Interactions[1]

Vitamin	Drug	Interaction
Folic acid	Phenytoin	Decreased phenytoin effect; decreased dietary folate absorption
	Sulfasalazine	Decreased dietary folate absorption
Niacin	Isoniazid	Niacin requirement may be increased
Pyridoxine	Barbiturates	Decreased barbiturate effect
	Contraceptives, oral	May increase pyridoxine requirement
	Hydralazine	May increase pyridoxine requirement
	Isoniazid	May increase pyridoxine requirement
	Levodopa	Decreased levodopa effect (but not with carbidopa)
	Penicillamine	May increase pyridoxine requirement
	Phenytoin	Decreased phenytoin effect
Vitamin A	Anticoagulants, oral	Increased anticoagulant effect with large doses of Vitamin A
Vitamin C	Anticoagulants, oral	Occasional decreased anticoagulant effect
	Contraceptives, oral	Increased serum concentration and possibly adverse effects of estrogen with 1 g/day of vitamin C
	Estrogens	Increased serum concentration and possibly adverse effects of estrogens with 1 g/day of vitamin C
	Phenothiazines	Decreased phenothiazine effect after vitamin C deficiency corrected
Vitamin D	Phenytoin	Decreased activity of vitamin D
	Phenobarbital	Decreased activity of vitamin D
Vitamin E	Oral anticoagulants	Increased anticoagulant effect
Vitamin K	Oral anticoagulants	Decreased anticoagulant effect
Vitamins, fat-soluable	Cholestyramine	Decreased vitamin absorption
	Colestipol	Decreased vitamin absorption
	Neomycin	Decreased vitamin absorption

[1]Reproduced with permission from *The Medical Letter* 27:68, 1985.

VITAMIN A

Definition

Vitamin A (retinol) is a fat-soluble member of a family of compounds called retinoids, which affect cell differentiation and proliferation. Vitamin A is essential for growth, vision, reproduction, maintenance of epithelial cell integrity, and secretion of mucus.

Basic Science

The major dietary sources are β-carotene found in carrots and other yellow vegetables, eggs and liver. The ingested esters are hydrolyzed in the intestinal lumen, absorbed in the mucosal cell, and esterified with long-chain fatty acids. They are associated with chylomicrons and transported via lymph to blood and then to the liver. Uptake of chylomicrons by liver parenchymal cells is by receptor-mediated endocytosis with participation of apolipoprotein E. The parenchymal cells are believed to be sites of storage of the vitamin, although other fat storage cells are present. Parenchymal cells synthesize and secrete a retinol-binding protein, molecular weight 21,000, with one binding site. This protein interacts with another protein, transthyretin, and circulates as a complex. In the presence of liver disease, the levels of binding proteins may be low.

Epidemiology

Vitamin A deficiency defined as serum retinol less than 10 μg/dl is rare in the United States except among individuals with malabsorption or low birth weight infants who are not provided with water-miscible vitamin supplements. Worldwide, it is a problem wherever undernutrition is present. It is estimated that half a million new cases of xerophthalmia occur annually in southeast Asia (Goodman, 1984).

Among infants in North Thailand, vitamin A levels in serum were below 20 μg/dl in 56% of 144 patients with protein-calorie malnutrition admitted to hospital (Clinical Nutrition Cases, 1985).

Natural History

The most important manifestation of vitamin A deficiency is xerophthalmia, or dry eye. Initially night

Table 3.7
Food and Nutrition Board, National Academy of Sciences-National Research Council
Recommended Daily Dietary Allowances, Revised 1980 [1]
Designed for the maintenance of good nutrition of practically all healthy people in the U.S.A.

	Age (years)	Weight		Height		Protein (g)	Fat-Soluble Vitamins			Water-Soluble Vitamins							Minerals					
		(kg)	(lb)	(cm)	(in)		Vitamin A (μg RE)[2]	Vitamin D (μg)[3]	Vitamin E (mg α TE)[4]	Vitamin C (mg)	Thiamin (mg)	Riboflavin (mg)	Niacin (mg NE)[5]	Vitamin B-6 (mg)	Folacin (μg)[6]	Vitamin B-12 (μg)	Calcium (mg)	Phosphorus (mg)	Magnesium (mg)	Iron (mg)	Zinc (mg)	Iodine (μg)
Infants	0.0-0.5	6	13	60	24	kg × 2.2	420	10	3	35	0.3	0.4	6	0.3	30	0.5[7]	360	240	50	10	3	40
	0.5-1.0																					
	0.5-1.0	9	20	71	28	kg × 2.0	400	10	4	35	0.5	0.6	8	0.6	45	1.5	540	360	70	15	5	50
Children	1-3	13	29	90	35	23	400	10	5	45	0.7	0.8	9	0.9	100	2.0	800	800	150	15	10	70
	4-6	20	44	112	44	30	500	10	6	45	0.9	1.0	11	1.3	200	2.5	800	800	200	10	10	90
		28	62	132	52	34	700	10	7	45	1.2	1.4	16	1.6	300	3.0	800	800	250	10	10	120
Males	11-14	45	99	157	62	45	1000	10	8	50	1.4	1.6	18	1.8	400	3.0	1200	1200	350	18	15	150
	15-18	66	145	176	69	56	1000	10	10	60	1.4	1.7	18	2.0	400	3.0	1200	1200	400	18	15	150
	19-22	70	154	177	70	56	1000	7.5	10	60	1.5	1.7	19	2.2	400	3.0	800	800	350	10	15	150
	23-50	70	154	178	70	56	1000	5	10	60	1.4	1.6	18	2.2	400	3.0	800	800	350	10	15	150
	51+	70	154	178	70	56	1000	5	10	60	1.2	1.4	16	2.2	400	3.0	800	800	350	10	15	150
Females	11-14	46	101	157	62	46	800	10	8	50	1.1	1.3	15	1.8	400	3.0	1200	1200	300	18	15	150
	15-18	55	120	163	64	46	800	10	8	60	1.1	1.3	14	2.0	400	3.0	1200	1200	300	18	15	150
	19-22	55	120	163	64	44	800	7.5	8	60	1.1	1.3	14	2.0	400	3.0	800	800	300	18	15	150
	23-50	55	120	163	64	44	800	5	8	60	1.0	1.2	13	2.0	400	3.0	800	800	300	18	15	150
	51+	55	120	163	64	44	800	5	8	60	1.0	1.2	13	2.0	400	3.0	800	800	300	10	15	150
Pregnant						+30	+200	+5	+2	+20	+0.4	+0.3	+2	+0.6	+400	+1.0	+400	+400	+150	h	+5	+25
Lactating						+20	+400	+5	+3	+40	+0.5	+0.5	+5	+0.5	+100	+1.0	+400	+400	+150	[8]	+10	+50

[1]The allowances are intended to provide for individual variations among most normal persons as they live in the United States under usual environmental stresses. Diets should be based on a variety of common foods in order to provide other nutrients for which human requirements have been less well defined. See text for detailed discussion of allowances and of nutrients not tabulated.

[2]Retinol equivalents. 1 retinol equivalent = 1μg β carotene. See text for calculation of vitamin A activity of diets as retinol equivalents.

[3]As cholecalciferol. 10 μg cholecalciferol = 400 IU of vitamin D

[4]α-tocopherol equivalents. 1 mg d-α tocopherol = 1α = TE. See text for variation in allowances and calculation of vitamin E activity of the diet as, α-tocopherol equivalents.

[5]1 NE (niacin equivalent) is equal to 1 mg of niacin or 60 mg of dietary tryptophan

[6]The folacin allowances refer to dietary sources as determined by *Lactobacillus casei assay* after treatment with enzymes (conjugases) to make polyglutamyl forms of the vitamin available to the test organism.

[7]The recommended dietary allowance for vitamin B_{12} in infants is based on average concentration of the vitamin in human milk. The allowances after weaning are based on energy intake (as recommended by the American Academy of Pediatrics) and consideration of other factors, such as intestinal absorption; see text.

[8]The increased requirement during pregnancy cannot be met by the iron content of habitual American diets nor by existing iron stores of many women; therefore the use of 30-60 mg of supplemental iron is recommended. Iron needs during lactation are not substantially different from those of nonpregnant women, but continued supplementation of the mother for 2-3 months after parturition is advisable in order to replenish stores depleted by pregnancy.

blindness is noted, then conjunctival dryness, and finally corneal dryness and ulceration. Loss of taste and smell may occur in older individuals.

Squamous metaplasia of airway epithelium has been found in association with chronic malabsorption of vitamin A in steatorrhea such as occurs in cystic fibrosis or celiac disease. The possibility of low serum retinol levels contributing to the squamous metaplasia in bronchopulmonary dysplasia was raised by Hustead et al (1984), although it remains to be tested.

Retinoids have powerful effects on skin in that they inhibit sebum production, which is involved in the pathogenesis of acne (see pp. 1168).

Diagnosis

Deficiency is defined as a serum retinol concentration of less than 10 μg/dl (normal values in infants are 20–50 μg/dl). Electroretinograms may be abnormal.

Treatment

Administration of water-miscible vitamin A, 5000 IU daily until symptoms are relieved is adequate. For xerophthalmia, larger doses (25,000 IU by intramuscular injection daily) are recommended.

For treatment of severe nodulocystic acne, 13-cis-retinoic acid is now the drug of choice.

The possibility that retinoids may be of value in treatment of cell proliferative diseases, including some forms of cancer, psoriasis, icthyosis, scleroderma and cirrhosis is in the experimental stage (see review by Goodman, 1984).

Toxicity

Vitamin A can be toxic when taken medicinally, as in the treatment of acne, or when taken in excess by those who believe in megavitamin intake for better health. The symptoms include drowsiness in association with increased intracranial pressure, diplopia and papilledema. Cranial nerve palsies may occur. The findings are those of pseudotumor cerebri, the cause of which may be overlooked without a careful nutritional history.

Chronic hypervitaminosis A is associated with anorexia and weight loss, alopecia, fissuring of skin at the corners of the mouth, and desquamation of palms and soles. Radiographs of long bones may show hyperostosis of the midshafts. The changes are reversible when vitamin A excess is discontinued.

Of great concern is the teratogenicity of vitamin A when taken in the first trimester of pregnancy. Although the association of vitamin A excess with craniofacial abnormalities has been known in animals, affected infants have been identified only since high-dose vitamin A has been available for the treatment of acne (Fernhoff et al, 1984). Isotretinoin (Accutane, Roche) was marketed in the United States in September 1982. Since then, at least nine confirmed cases of severe, sometimes fatal malformations involving the skull, face, and cardiovascular systems have been reported. Based on this tragic experience, pediatricians should determine whether an adolescent is sexually active, and not prescribe the drug unless it is certain the patient is not pregnant and that she uses effective forms of birth control, preferably abstinence, while taking isoretinoin.

Prevention

In areas where xerophthalmia is prevalent, large scale intervention programs with 200,000 IU of vitamin A given to children every 6 months have had dramatic results. In Indonesia, not only was xerophthalmia eliminated, but mortality rates in the treated group were lower by about 25%. Presumably hypovitaminosis A predisposes to infection. Nutrition education and increased availability of vitamin-A rich foods are essential in many developing countries (Staff report, Select Committee on Hunger, U.S. House of Representatives. U.S. Government Printing Office, Washington, 1985).

CAROTENEMIA

Definition

Carotenemia, yellow skin pigmentation, is the result of excessive dietary intake of carotene-containing foods, most commonly carrots and carrot-containing products. Carotenemia can occur in association with certain diseases, such as hypothyroidism, diabetes mellitus, and nephrosis, even in the absence of excessive intake of carotene (Lascari, 1981).

Basic Science

Carotene is a pigment normally present in keratin and subcutaneous fat. It can be measured in microgram quantities in circulating blood of normal individuals, and reaches a peak level by about age 5 years. When plasma carotene levels are above 250 μg/dl, yellow pigmentation shows in superficial areas of skin such as face, palms, and soles. It is uncommon in mucosal areas such as the sclerae (Congdon et al, 1981).

β-Carotene is the most important precursor of vitamin A because of its prevalence. One molecule of β-carotene can be cleaved to 2 molecules of retinol (vitamin A). Nevertheless, excessive intake of carotene does not produce symptoms other than yellow skin pigmentation probably because it is not absorbed as well as vitamin A and it is metabolized too slowly to cause hypervitaminosis.

Epidemiology

The condition is common but the prevalence is unknown.

Natural History and Treatment

Children who are on pureed baby foods are most likely to have excess levels of carotene. The peak time for the appearance of carotenemia is 6 months to 5 years of age. It has been seen in breast-fed infants of mothers who consume large quantities of carrots. The skin color will return to normal within 2–6 weeks after discontinuing intake of carrots. The only known hazard to carotenemia is that it could be mistaken for jaundice and stimulate an unnecessary workup for liver disease.

VITAMIN B GROUP

Definition

The five classic deficiency states of vitamins of the B complex are beri-beri (thiamine), ariboflavinosis (riboflavin), pellagra (niacin), vitamin B_6 (pyridoxine) deficiency, and vitamin B_{12} deficiency. Other B vitamins, inositol, choline, and panthothenic acid are not known to be deficient in isolation of other nutritional problems and no specific syndromes are identified with their lack in children.

Epidemiology

Isolated B vitamin deficiencies are rare in the developed countries. The incidence of borderline deficiencies is not known, inasmuch as many are probably not recognized or reported.

Beriberi (Thiamine Deficiency)

Natural History and Diagnosis

Beriberi (thiamine deficiency) is characterized by peripheral neuritis (dry beriberi), congestive heart failure from edematous myocardium, and edema of the extremities with a waxy skin. Laryngeal paralysis may lead to hoarseness. Muscle atrophy, ataxia, and eventually coma can ensue. In alcoholics, the combination of ophthalmoplegia, ataxia and confusion is called Wernicke's syndrome.

Blood lactic and pyruvic acid levels rise in thiamine deficiency. Clinical response to oral thiamine remains the best test for deficiency. For mild disease, 5 mg/day orally is appropriate; 10 mg twice daily is needed for severe forms.

Toxicity

Hypersensitivity or idiosyncratic responses may occur.

Thiamine dependency occurs in some megaloblastic anemias, maple syrup urine disease, and chronic lactic acidosis of infancy.

Vitamin B_2 (Riboflavin Deficiency)

Riboflavin deficiency leads to glossitis (a purple discoloration with a smooth or pebbly surface of the tongue), conjunctivitis, keratitis, photophobia, and even corneal vascularization. Cheilosis is common. Pyruvate kinase deficiency is found and may be associated with hemolysis. Treatment with oral riboflavin, 1 mg three times daily should result in improvement in a few days.

Toxicity

No toxicity has been reported.

Pellagra (Niacin Deficiency)

Pellagra (niacin deficiency) has an insidious onset of anorexia, weakness, numbness, and dizziness. Eventually the classic triad of diarrhea, dermatitis, and dementia follow. Redness and induration of the edges of the tongue may be early signs. Skin lesions are present on exposed surfaces, and are erythematous with sharp borders and may have a "glove" distribution. Vesicles and bullae may develop. Healing is associated with desquamation and pigmentation.

Diagnosis is based on nutritional history, physical findings, and a prompt response to niacin, given as 50–100 mg/day of oral nicotinamide.

Toxicity

Peripheral vasodilation can occur. Nausea, vomiting, and low blood pressure result from niacin excess.

Pyridoxine Deficiency

Pyridoxine deficiency results in seizures and a peripheral neuropathy. In older individuals, dermatitis and anemia are present. One cause of mild pyridoxine deficiency is treatment with INH (isonicotinic acid hydrazide) for tuberculosis, although this problem is rarely encountered in children. An inborn error, pyridoxine dependency, presents as convulsions in infancy.

Treatment with 25–50 mg of pyridoxine leads to a prompt response. If 50 mg of pyridoxine are injected intramuscularly while an electroencephalogram is recorded, improvement can be seen and the diagnosis is confirmed.

Toxicity

None is known at doses up to 50 times the United States' recommended dietary allowance of 2 mg. Higher doses are associated with sensory nervous system dysfunction.

Biotin Deficiency

Biotin deficiency from an inborn error of biotinidase occurs in about 1/48,000 births, and is characterized by seizures, progressive neurological dysfunction, hearing loss, rashes, hair loss, and mental retardation. Symptoms may appear as early as 2 months of age (see pp. 956). Organic aciduria may or may not be present (Wolf et al, 1983). This condition can be screened on the same blood used for screening phenylketonuria. Treatment is 10 mg of biotin added to food or formula each day. No side effects have been reported with this dose.

Pantothenic Acid Deficiency

Naturally occurring pantothenic acid deficiency has not been described in humans, although experimentally, individuals deprived of pantothenic acid show weakness, headache, abdominal cramp and diarrhea, as well as personality changes and ataxia.

Cobalamin (Vitamin B_{12}) Deficiency

Vitamin B_{12} deficiency, secondary to inadequate intake or malabsorption, leads to a megaloblastic anemia (pernicious anemia), and, if long-term, leads to posterior and lateral spinal column disease which presents as a peripheral neuropathy. The absence of cobalamin-binding (R) protein or of gastric intrinsic factor may be congenital or acquired in association with achlorhydria and gastric atrophy. Pernicious anemia may follow gastric resection if vitamin B_{12} supplements are not provided. A rare disorder that leads to vitamin B_{12} deficiency is absence of transcobalamin II (Hakami et al, 1971). Transcobalamin II is a protein that binds cobalamin and delivers it to tissues.

Folic Acid Deficiency

Folic acid deficiency is most commonly the consequence of inadequate intestinal absorption as in celiac disease or in congenital malabsorption. Deficiency leads to a megaloblastic anemia and, in infants, may result in disaccharide deficiency from blunting of the intestinal villi. Therapy with 1–5 mg/day orally results in prompt reversal of the symptoms.

VITAMIN C DEFICIENCY—SCURVY

Definition

Vitamin C deficiency results in impaired incorporation of hydroxyproline into collagen, deficient osteoid production, and painful bone lesions (scurvy).

Basic Science

Water-soluble vitamin C (L-ascorbic acid), a ketolactone, is a potent reducing agent that is essential for hydroxylation of proline in the synthesis of collagen, and for normal function of osteoblasts and odontoblasts. It functions in intermediary metabolism of tryptophan and tyrosine. In premature infants on high protein feedings, deficiency of vitamin C results in significant elevations in tyrosine which recede over time with adequate C intake (transient tyrosinemia) (Avery et al, 1967). Vitamin C participates in synthesis of adrenal steroids and is found in high concentrations in the adrenal cortex and medulla. It is required in vitro to maximize hydroxylation of dopamine to form norepinephrine (Levine, 1986). The half-life of ascorbic acid is 12.8–29.5 days in adults.

Epidemiology

Scurvy is very rare among individuals living in the United States in the 1980s. Only those who are deprived of citrus fruits, fresh vegetables, or vitamins for some cultural or geographic reasons are at risk of scurvy.

Natural History

Scurvy in infants is not usually manifest before 6 months of age. Irritability may be the only sign, but with progression, petechial hemorrhages, especially along the swollen gingivae, may be evident. The infants may show weakness and pseudoparalysis that results in a frog-like position from painful subperiosteal hemorrhages. A costochondral rosary may appear and is distinguished clinically (with difficulty) from that of rickets by sharper angulation of the prominences. Poor wound healing, anemia, possibly from decreased iron absorption or impaired folate metabolism, hematuria, and low-grade fever may be present in severe cases.

Diagnosis

A history of vitamin C deficiency and any of the classic signs should suggest the diagnosis. (An unusual event is to find an infant whose fruit juices were all boiled by a compulsive well-meaning mother who was unaware that boiling inactivates ascorbic acid.)

A fasting vitamin C level of over 0.6 mg/dl excludes the diagnosis, but a lower level does not confirm it. Tissue content or saturation can be estimated by urinary excretion after a test dose of vitamin C.

Treatment

No diagnostic tests are necessary, however, because a therapeutic trial of 100–200 mg ascorbic acid orally produces improvement within a few days. Even fruit juices alone produce prompt improvement.

Prognosis

Untreated patients die of scurvy; treated patients recovery completely.

Prevention

As little as 50 mg of ascorbic acid daily prevents scurvy in otherwise normal infants.

CONTROVERSY

The question of benefit from large doses of vitamin C produced much controversy in the 1970s. Although scorbutic individuals have more than the expected number of respiratory infections, large doses have not been shown to confer protection on normal children. Fueled by the zeal of Nobel Laureate Linus Pauling, the debate captured the headlines and stimulated some parents to give infants excessive amounts of the vitamin or large quantities of fruit juices. The vitamin in large doses (over 4 g/day) may precipitate oxalate stones in kidneys but reports of toxicity in children are unconvincing. However, rarely is any nutrient in excess of benefit to normal individuals.

Although the recommended requirement of 60 mg of ascorbic acid a day is adequate to prevent scurvy and maintain a body pool in adults of 1500 mg, the optimal ascorbic acid intake for human health is unknown. The effects of supplemental ascorbate on wound healing, cold tolerance, allergic responses, and even mental health have been studied, with contradictory results (Levine, 1986).

NUTRITIONAL VITAMIN D DEFICIENCY—RICKETS

Definition

Vitamin D deficiency results in rickets, which is a condition of defective mineralization of growing bone and deformities that result from weight-bearing on structurally soft bones. In nongrowing bones, it produces osteomalacia (DeLuca, 1974; Bell, 1985). For inborn errors of vitamin D metabolism, see page 849.

Basic Science

Vitamin D is a fat-soluble vitamin that is essential for normal absorption of calcium and phosphorus from small intestine, and possibly reabsorption of phosphorus from kidney. Two forms are active in man, vitamin D_2 (calciferol) and vitamin D_3, activated 7-dehydrocholesterol. A provitamin D_3 (7-dehydrocholesterol) is normally found in skin, and is activated by ultraviolet light (296–310 nm) but not by other wave lengths such as those that are transmitted through glass.

Once absorbed, vitamin D is transported to liver where it is converted to 25 hydroxyvitamin D (25 OH-D) then to kidney to be converted to 1,25-dihydroxyvitamin D (1,25-$(OH)_2$D), which is the active metabolite, and the major determinant of intestinal absorption of calcium. The metabolites are bound in the serum to a vitamin D-binding protein of molecular weight 55,000. Serum concentrations of the active form of vitamin D rise with restriction of phosphorus intake, and fall below normal with dietary phosphorus supplements (Portale et al, 1986).

1,25-$(OH)_2$D increases absorption of calcium and phosphate from intestine and enhances skeletal resorption of calcium and phosphate. Receptors for this compound have been identified in nearly all tissues except liver and muscle, which suggests other roles yet to be determined (Avioli et al, 1984). Structural abnormalities in receptors result in rickets and osteomalacia despite increased levels of circulating 1, 25 (OH_2)D (type II vitamin D-dependent rickets) (see pp. 849; Fig. 3.3).

Rickets is characterized by formation of normal osteoid and collagen, but disorganization of growth plate connective tissue and defective calcification of the epiphyses and shafts of growing bone. Infants do not get adequate vitamin D from milk alone, hence the need for vitamin D-fortified formulas or supplementary vitamin D to provide a total of 400 units/day. Maximal calcium absorption requires a dietary calcium/phosphate ratio of about 2:1. In low birth weight infants, daily calcium intake of 220–250 mg/kg and phosphate of 110–125 mg/kg permit normal mineralization of rapidly growing bones.

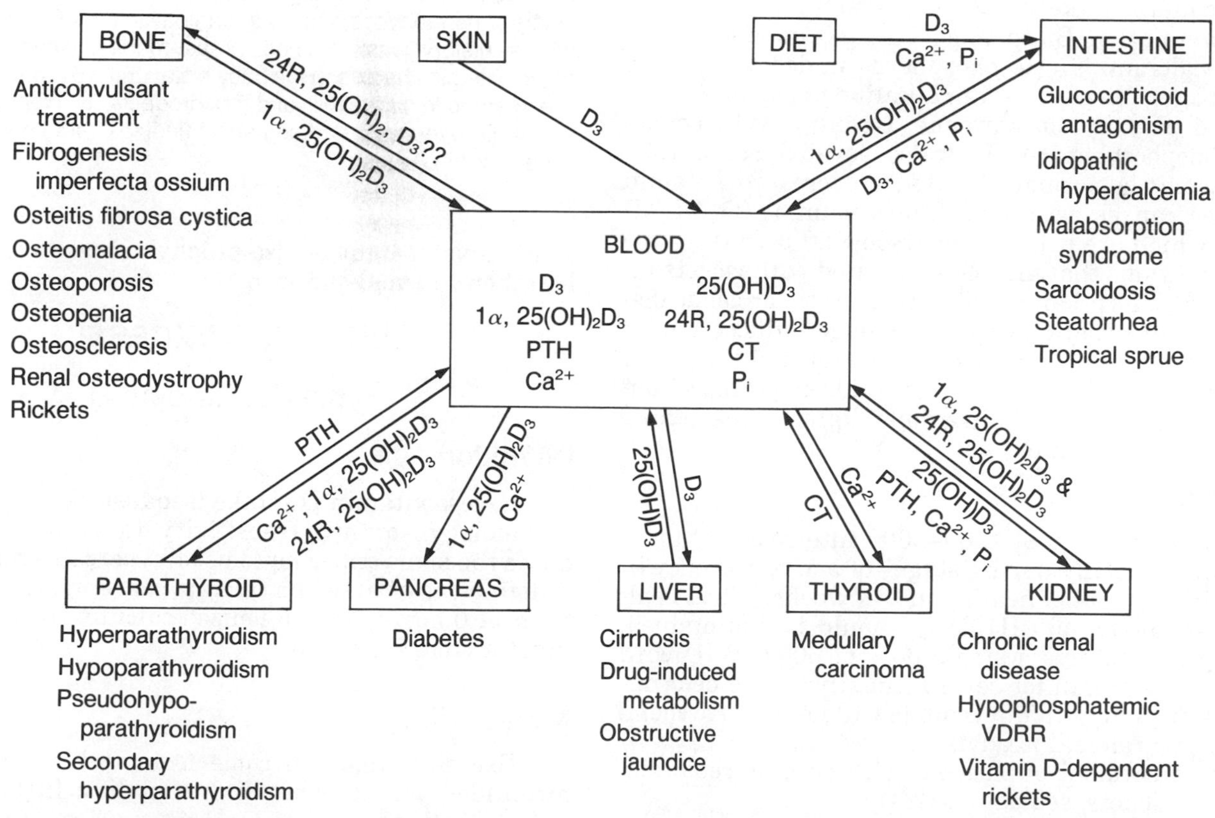

Figure 3.3. Disease states in humans related to vitamin D. Reproduced with permission from Norman AW: The vitamin D endocrine system. *Physiologist* 28:219, 1985.

Epidemiology

Vitamin D deficiency rickets is rare among individuals on a normal diet. Between 1956 and 1960, only 843 cases were recognized among approximately 2,250,000 infants and children admitted to 226 teaching hospitals in the United States (Fomon, 1974). Currently, rickets is seen in infants whose parents are vegetarians and avoid all dairy products and food supplements such as vitamins. The prevalence is not known (Edidin et al, 1980).

Natural History

After several months of vitamin D deficiency, rickets can present as craniotabes in infants. Thinning of the inner table of the skull is evident on pressing firmly over the posterior parietal bones and feeling a ping-pong ball effect. Costochondral junctions enlarge to produce the rachitic rosary. If the infant crawls, weight-bearing on the wrists will produce an enlargement or knobby appearance. With walking, ankles become prominent and limbs may be angulated or bowed. Later scoliosis, lordosis, and failure of the pelvis to grow can produce severe deformities, and potential difficulty with vaginal deliveries. In severe forms, the chest wall is too compliant (flail), and may hinder normal respiration.

Diagnosis

Clinical diagnosis is made on the basis of history of inadequate intake of vitamin D and findings on physical examination. Biochemical changes include normal or low calcium values, phosphorus under 4 mg/dl (or low for age), elevated serum alkaline phosphatase and elevated parathyroid hormone. Urinary cyclic adenosine monophosphate (AMP) is also elevated. Serum 1,25-$(OH)_2D$ may be normal, elevated or decreased. Vitamin D stores can be estimated from serum 1, 25-$(OH)_2D$ levels, which are usually low (below 20 pg/ml).

Conditions that may be associated with rickets include malabsorption, as in cystic fibrosis or celiac disease, severe hepatic disease, prolonged glucocorticoid administration, or kidney disease. Black children are more susceptible than are white children, perhaps from reduced absorption of ultraviolet light in pigmented skin (Fig. 3.4*A* and *B*).

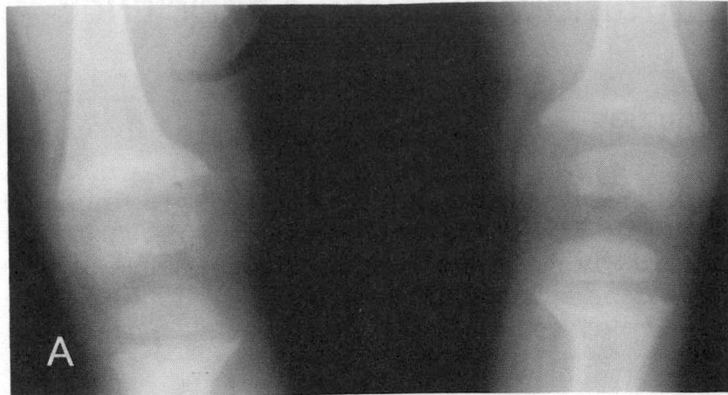

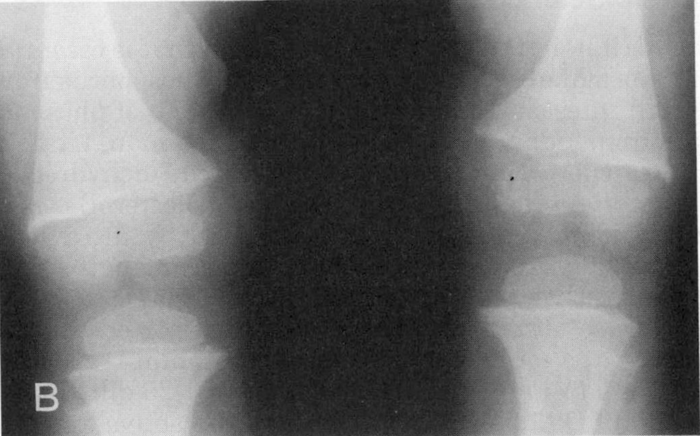

Figure 3.4. A. Radiographs of this 16-month-old girl were obtained after trauma. Obvious changes of unsuspected rickets are present with widened growth plates (physes) cupping and flaring of metaphyses and undeterminalization of bones. A nutritional history was obtained; breast-feeding without supplemental vitamins had been the baby's diet until 15 months of age, She seemed to dislike milk and milk products. **B.** Treatment with vitamin D reversed the radiographic findings with improvement evident within 8 weeks.

Treatment

Administration of 1500–5000 international units of vitamin D daily during stages of active rickets will result in evidence of healing in 2–4 weeks. When healing is complete, 400 IU daily should be maintained. Some prefer to give a single dose of 600,000 IU with no further vitamin for several months. Once deformities are present, vitamin D alone will not reverse them. Orthopedic referral is advised.

For treatment of patients with chronic renal disease and rickets, see page 642.

Prevention

The daily requirement is estimated at 200–400 IU/day, and the latter amount is recommended. Exposure to ultraviolet light is also prophylactic but care must be taken to avoid sunburn.

VITAMIN D EXCESS

Hypervitaminosis D

Definition

Excess vitamin D intake (see also Section 14, Endocrinology), or hypersensitivity to vitamin D, produces the signs and symptoms of hypercalcemia, which is defined as total serum calcium concentration greater than 11.0 mg/dl, and an ionized calcium concentration greater than 5.0 mg/dl.

Natural History

Excess intake can come from well-meaning but misguided parents who think that "if a little is good, more is better."

The clinical manifestations of hypercalcemia include hypotonia, weakness, listlessness, and irritability. Anorexia, headache, weight loss, constipation, vomiting, polydipsia, and polyuria are other common symptoms. Prolonged or severe hypercalcemia can cause nephrocalcinosis and subsequent hypertension and renal failure.

In infants with extensive subcutaneous fat necrosis, particularly resulting from traumatic delivery, hypercalcemia may develop. The necrosis usually involves the areas subjected to greatest pressure. For example, with forceps delivery, the cheeks are affected typically. The signs of hypercalcemia usually occur one or several weeks after birth, with vomiting, lethargy, or irritability, and fever. As the fat necrosis resolves serum calcium levels fall to normal.

Vitamin D sensitivity may be the reason for hypercalcemia in William syndrome. The syndrome is characterized by elfin features, receding mandible and hypertelorism. Craniosynostosis may be present, and supravalvular aortic stenosis and peripheral pulmonic arterial stenoses are common.

Diagnosis

Radiographic findings include dense mineralization at the base of the skull and in the metaphyseal ends of long bones. Extraskeletal calcification, especially nephrocalcinosis, may occur. The levels of inorganic phosphate in serum are not reduced, in contrast to the situation in hyperparathyroidism (see pp. 848).

Treatment

Hypercalcemia is treated with a low calcium (less than 100 mg/day)-low vitamin D diet. Glucocorticoids are recommended in severe cases.

VITAMIN E

Definition

Vitamin E (α-tocopherol) is a fat-soluble vitamin (see also Anemia of Prematurity); its major function is as an antioxidant.

Natural History

Inasmuch as it is widely distributed in food, vitamin E is rarely deficient except in chronic fat malabsorption. Premature infants absorb the vitamin poorly and have a low grade hemolytic anemia if not given supplements (Oski et al, 1967). However, if they receive formulas fortified with vitamin E, or breast milk, no further supplementation is necessary (Zipursky et al, 1987).

Chronic deficiency states have been described in children with cystic fibrosis who may show peripheral nerve dysfunction or cerebellar and posterior column disease, which responds to treatment with vitamin E (Bye et al, 1985).

The role of low levels of vitamin E in the retinopathy of prematurity has been evaluated in prospective controlled trials of administration of the vitamin. Promising results reported by Hittner and associates (1981, 1983) have not been confirmed. Similarly, controlled trials of added vitamin E to prevent bronchopulmonary dysplasia have had early success, which has not been confirmed (Ehrenkranz et al, 1982). Excess vitamin E apparently can interfere with resistance to serious infection in preterm infants. Johnson et al (1985) found significantly more sepsis and necrotizing enterocolitis in infants maintained on pharmacologic doses of vitamin E to maintain serum levels at about 5 mg/dl. (Untreated infants had levels of <1 mg/dl.) Johnson et al speculate that the increased concentration of vitamin E may have compromised the intracellular killing of phagocytes by overly effective destruction of intracellular hydrogen peroxide.

Hepatotoxicity attributed to an intravenous preparation of vitamin E (E-Ferol IV, O'Neal, Jones and Feldman, Pharmaceuticals, Maryland Heights, Missouri) was reported in low birth weight infants (Bove et al, 1985). The findings, which included thrombocytopenia, hepatomegaly, cholestasis, hypotension, and metabolic acidosis were otherwise unexplained. Progressive deterioration and death in at least 38 infants occurred before the symptoms were attributed to the high polysorbate load given with vitamin E. The drug is no longer on the market in the United States.

Treatment

There are inadequate data to specify with confidence the serum levels of vitamin E that are optimal in preterm infants. Clearly too little is associated with hemolytic anemia, and too much may put the infant at risk of sepsis. Johnson et al (1985) suggest that serum concentrations are best kept between 1.0 and 3.0 mg/dl. The requirement is an intake of 0.5 mg of d-α-tocopherol/100 kcal/day. These values are usually achieved in preterm infants with 25 IU by mouth daily until 8–10 weeks of age. No iron supplements should be given during the first 2 months inasmuch as they interfere with vitamin E absorption.

VITAMIN K

Definition

Vitamin K, a naphthoquinone, participates in oxidative phosphorylation and is essential for synthesis of prothrombin (Factor II) and other blood clotting factors (VII, IX, and X), as well as other essential proteins. Vitamin K deficiency is the cause of hemorrhagic disease of the newborn. The natural vitamin is labeled vitamin K_1 to distinguish it from synthetic compounds with similar activity.

Epidemiology

The prevalence of vitamin K deficiency depends on the number of predisposing conditions, such as infants of malnourished mothers who do not receive intramuscular vitamin K soon after birth, individuals with fat malabsorption, and some with liver dysfunction such as biliary atresia or α-1-antitrypsin deficiency. Prolonged oral antibiotic therapy can reduce intestinal flora and lower vitamin K absorption.

In Japan, Motohara et al (1985) reported the presence of a protein in cord blood that is induced by vitamin K deficiency. If not given vitamin K_1 by 3–5 days of age 50–60% of infants had the protein present. Thus, a chemical marker of vitamin K supports the argument that deficiencies are common in newborns.

Natural History

Infants have only 30–60% of adult levels of vitamin K-dependent clotting factors (Factors II, VII, IX, and X). They normally acquire adult levels by 6 weeks. About half the amount of vitamin K absorbed comes from dietary sources; it is present in most prepared formulas, and in small amounts in breast milk. Once intestinal flora are established, the vitamin is synthesized.

Vitamin K deficiency may occur in any condition in which fat malabsorption is present. Another rarer cause of deficiency is use of coumarin anticoagulants such as warfarin. When taken early in pregnancy, serious bone defects are produced in the fetus, presumably because warfarin interferes with the reduction of vitamin K to its active metabolite hydroquinone. Vitamin K-dependent proteins are essential for normal bone growth.

Excess intake is unlikely because vitamin K is not usually added to foods, nor is it generally included in nutrition supplements.

Diagnosis and Treatment

Prothrombin times are prolonged in vitamin K deficiency, although not all hypoprothrombinemic states respond to exogenous vitamin K. Confirmation of the diagnosis depends on a rapid therapeutic response to administration of vitamin K intramuscularly.

Prothrombin deficiency can be treated with 1–2 mg vitamin K daily by mouth. If deficiency is severe, 5 mg intramuscularly are recommended.

Prevention

Vitamin K_1 oxide, 1 mg, administered subcutaneously or intrasmuscularly soon after birth prevents hypoprothrombinemia from the third day of life.

CASE ILLUSTRATION (adapted from Payne and Hasegawa: *Pediatrics* 73:712, 1984).

A 30-day-old female infant suddenly refused feedings, became lethargic, and lapsed into coma. Nothing in the past history was unusual except that the mother requested the infant not receive vitamin K at birth.

On physical examination, the infant had a dilated left pupil, bulging anterior fontanelle, posturing, liver edge palpable 4 cm below right costal margin. The hemogram was normal. Prothrombin time was greater than 120 seconds, and partial thromboplastin time was in excess of 120 seconds. SGOT was 49 IU/ml. Serum bilirubin was 5.4 mg/dl with 2.6 direct. CT scan of the brain showed a 3 × 4 cm left parietal intracerebral hematoma.

The infant was given fresh frozen plasma 10 ml/kg and 5 mg of vitamin K intravenously. Within 18 hours, coagulation studies were normal.

Management of the hematoma required surgical evacuation, with gradual recovery.

QUESTIONS AND COMMENTS

How would you explain the elevated SGOT (normal 0–40), mild hyperbilirubenemia, and enlarged liver at 30 days of age?

Hemorrhagic disease of the newborn more commonly presents with bleeding at under a week of age. If some subclinical bleeding had occurred, prolonged icterus may have followed slow resorption of the heme pigments. The clue that another process was occurring was the direct reacting bilirubin, elevated SGOT, and enlarged liver. Further studies revealed the patient to be homozygous (P_iZZ) for α-1-antitrypsin deficiency.

This infant did not receive prophylactic vitamin K_1 and presumably had decreased absorption of vitamin K synthesized by intestinal bacteria inasmuch as she had cholestatic liver disease. Low oral intake may have tipped the scale inasmuch as she was on breast milk only. Late onset hemorrhagic disease of the newborn should be considered a diagnostic possibility in any infant who may have inadequate vitamin K for whatever reason. Conversely, liver function should be evaluated when late onset hemorrhage occurs.

REFERENCES

Avery ME, Clow C, Menkes J, et al: Transient tyrosinemia of the newborn: Dietary and clinical aspects. *Pediatrics* 39:378, 1967.

Avioli LV, Haddad JG: Editorial retrospective. The vitamin D family revisited. *N Engl J Med* 311:47, 1984.

Bell NH: Vitamin D-endocrine system. *J Clin Invest* 76:1, 1985.

Bove KE, Kosmetatos N, Wedig KE, et al: Vasculopathic hepatotoxicity associated with E-Ferol syndrome in low-birth-weight infants. *JAMA* 254:2422, 1985.

Burman JF, Jenkins WJ, Walker-Smith JA, et al: Absent ileal uptake of IF-bound vitamin B_{12} in vivo in The Imerslund-Gräsbeck syndrome (familial vitamin B_{12} malabsorption with proteinuria). *Gut* 26:311, 1985.

Bye AME, Muller DPR, Wilson J, et al: Symptomatic vitamin E deficiency in cystic fibrosis. *Arch Dis Child* 60:162, 1985.

Clinical Nutrition Cases: Vitamin A deficiency—a global disease. *Nutr Rev* 43:240, 1985.

Congdon PJ, Kelleher J, Edwards P, et al: Benign carotenaemia in children. *Arch Dis Child* 56:292, 1981.

Corrigan JJ: Vitamin K-dependent proteins. *Adv Pediatr* 28:57, 1981.

DeLuca HF: Vitamin D: The vitamin and the hormone. *Fed Proc* 33:2211, 1974.

Edidin DV, Levitsky LL, Schey W, et al: Resurgence of nutritional rickets associated with breast-feeding and special dietary practices. *Pediatrics* 65:232, 1980.

Ehrenkranz RA, Ablow RC, Warshaw JB: Effect of vitamin E on the development of oxygen-induced lung injury in neonates. *Ann NY Acad Sci* 393:452, 1982.

Fernhoff PM, Lammer EJ: Craniofacial features of isoretinoin embryopathy. *J Pediatr* 105:595, 1984.

Fomon SJ: *Infant Nutrition*, 2nd edition. Philadelphia, WB Saunders, 1974.

Forbes GB, Cafarelli C, Manning J: Vitamin D and infantile hypercalcemia. *Pediatrics* 42:203, 1968.

Goodman DS: Vitamin A and retinoids in health and disease. *N Engl J Med* 310:1023, 1984.
Grewar D: Infantile scurvy. *Clin Pediatr* 4:82, 1965.
Hakami N, Neiman PE, Canellos GP, Lazerson J: Neonatal megaloblastic anemia due to inherited transcobalamin II deficiency in two siblings. *N Engl J Med* 285:1163, 1971.
Harrison HE, Harrison HC: Hypercalcemic states. In: *Disorders of Calcium and Phosphate Metabolism in Children and Adolescence.* Philadelphia, WB Saunders, 1979.
Herbert V: Risk of oxalate stone from large doses of vitamin C. *N Engl J Med* 298:856, 1978.
Hittner HM, Godio LB, Rudolph AJ, et al: Retrolental fibroplasia: Efficacy of vitamin E in a double-blind clinical study of preterm infants. *N Engl J Med* 305:1365, 1981.
Hittner HM, Godio LB, Speer ME, et al: Retrolental fibroplasia: Further clinical evidence and ultrastructural support for efficacy of vitamin E in the preterm infant. *Pediatrics* 71:423, 1983.
Hunt AD, Stokes J Jr, McCrory WW, et al: Pyridoxine dependence: Report of a case of intractable convulsions in an infant controlled by pyridoxine. *Pediatrics* 13:140, 1954.
Hustead VA, Gutcher GR, Anderson SA, et al: Relationship of vitamin A (retinol) status to lung disease in the preterm infant. *J Pediatr* 105:610, 1984.
Johnson L, Bowen FW, Abbasi S, et al: Relationship of prolonged pharmacologic serum levels of vitamin E to incidence of sepsis and necrotizing enterocolitis in infants with birth weight 1500 grams or less. *Pediatrics* 75:619, 1985.
Lane PA, Hathaway WE: Vitamin K in infancy. *J Pediatr* 106:351, 1985.
Lane PA, Hathaway WE, Githens JH, et al: Fatal intracranial hemorrhage in a normal infant secondary to vitamin K deficiency. *Pediatrics* 72:562, 1983.
Lascari AD: Carotenemia, a review. *Clin Pediatr* 20:25, 1981.
Levine M: New concepts in the biology and biochemistry of ascorbic acid. *N Engl J Med* 314:892, 1986.
Motohara K, Endo F, Matsuda I: Effect of vitamin K administration on acarboxyprothrombin (PIVKA II) levels in newborns. *Lancet* 2:242, 1985.
Ong DE: Vitamin A-binding proteins. *Nutr Rev* 43:225, 1985.
Oski FA, Barness LA: Vitamin E deficiency: A previously unrecognized cause of hemolytic anemia in the premature infant. *J Pediatr* 70:211, 1967.
Payne NR, Hasegawa DK: Vitamin K deficiency in newborns: A case report in alpha-1-antitrypsin deficiency and a review of factors predisposing to hemorrhage. *Pediatrics* 73:712, 1984.
Portale AA, Halloran BP, Murphy MM, et al: Oral intake of phosphorus can determine the serum concentration of 1,25-dihydroxyvitamin D by determining its production rate in humans. *J Clin Invest* 77:7, 1986.
Scriver CR: Vitamin B_6 deficiency and dependency in man. *Am J Dis Child* 113:109, 1967.
Ware S, Mills M: Vitamin K deficiency causing infantile intracranial haemorrhage after the neonatal period. *Lancet* 1:1439, 1983.
Wolf B, Grier RE, Allen RJ, et al: Phenotypic variation in biotinidase deficiency. *J Pediatr* 103:233, 1983.
Zipursky A, Brown EJ, Watts J, et al: Oral vitamin E supplementation for the prevention of anemia in premature infants: A controlled trial. *Pediatrics* 79:61, 1987.

Minerals 5

Inorganic elements are required for normal growth and biologic function. They may be divided into two classes: those that are required in relatively large quantities, on the order of grams per day, such as calcium, which serves as a structural component of bone mineral and in the form of calcium ions as an important regulatory agent in the cell cytosol; and trace elements, which are required in milligram or microgram quantities and frequently function as cofactors or prosthetic groups for enzymes.

CALCIUM

Calcium (see also pp. 841, Section 14, Endocrinology) is so widely available in milk, dairy products, fish, and green vegetables, that nutritional deficiency is rare unless infants are on strict elimination diets without adequate supplements. Calcium deficiency can occur if chronic diarrhea or fat malabsorption are present and intestinal absorption is impaired.

Calcium is abundant in bones and teeth and plays an essential role in muscle contraction and nerve irritability as well as coagulation of blood. The distribution of calcium in the body is in dynamic equilibrium and mediated by parathyroid hormone, calcitonin, and vitamin D (see pp. 843). The normal serum levels are 9–11 ml/dl of which 60% is ionized. Even when dietary intake is low, the percentage absorbed is high and is usually sufficient (assuming normal parathyroid function and normal vitamin D status).

Deficiency of calcium over a long period leads to poor mineralization of bones and teeth, with osteomalacia and osteopenia. Severe lowering of the serum calcium (below about 7 mg/dl) results in tetany. Reduction in adequate calcium intake in growing children impairs growth and results in rickets (see pp. 99).

Neonatal Hypocalcemia (Tetany)

Definition

Neonatal hypocalcemia is a condition in which levels of circulating calcium are low. Two forms are seen: early onset hypocalcemia is symptomatic before the first feeding; late onset (end of first week) is seen in infants who have a high phosphate intake.

Basic Science

Stressed infants (prematures, infants of diabetic mothers, acidotic and hypoxic infants) are most at risk, possibly from breakdown of intracellular organic phosphate, and subsequent increase in extracellular inorganic phosphate. An imbalance between calcitonin secretion and parathyroid hormone output has been postulated in some infants. Calcitonin levels are high in the fetus, probably to increase the net bone mineral deposition in the growing fetal skeleton.

Early Onset Hypocalcemia

Stressed infants may have serum calcium levels below 7.5 mg/dl (ionized calcium below 2.5 mg/dl) and can be symptomatic in the first day of life. Seizures are very common, and can only be distinguished from seizures of other causes by finding a low serum calcium.

Late Onset Hypocalcemia

Natural History

Neonatal tetany was seen most commonly in the 1950s and 1960s in infants whose initial feedings were delayed 24 hours or longer, and who received evaporated milk formulas that had a relatively high phosphorus content (human milk has 150 mg phosphorus per liter; cow's milk, 1000 mg/L). One of the principal modifications in infant formulas is the removal of phosphorus from cow's milk sufficient so that the levels of phosphorus approximate those in human milk.

The clinical features of neonatal tetany are poor feeding, vomiting, or cyanotic episodes after several days or weeks of feeding. Convulsive twitchings are usually generalized, but may be lateralized. They occur repeatedly and last a few minutes. The infant remains responsive during the seizures. Laryngospasm and apnea may occur.

Diagnosis

Electrocardiographic changes with prolonged Q-T interval may occur, but definitive diagnosis rests on determination of serum calcium concentration.

Treatment

A 10% calcium gluconate solution can be given to the infant intravenously at a dose of 2 ml/kg slowly while the heart rate is monitored. Improvement should be immediate. Infants unresponsive to calcium may have hypomagnesemia, and can be given magnesium sulfate intramuscularly as a 25% solution of the anhydrous salt in a dosage of 0.2 ml/kg.

Prevention

The rarity of transient neonatal hypocalcemia since appropriately prepared infant formulas or breast milk feedings have been widely used establishes that prevention has indeed occurred.

IRON

Source

Iron (see also pp. 504–506, Hematology) is abundant in liver, meats, egg yolks, green vegetables, grains, and nuts.

Function

Iron is a component of hemoglobin and myoglobin. It is found in cytochrome c, catalase, and other oxidative enzymes. It is absorbed in the ferrous form, and absorption is facilitated by ascorbic acid and gastric juices, and inhibited by phytic acid and fiber. It is transported in the ferric state bound to transferrin (a β-1-globulin) and stored in liver, spleen, bone marrow, and kidneys in the form of ferritin and hemosiderin. In normal conditions, about 90% of intake is excreted in stool; iron stores are conserved and reutilized.

Deficiency

Iron deficiency can occur when intake is inadequate during growth. Thus, the most vulnerable individuals are preterm infants who may have rapid postnatal growth with adequate milk, but without iron supplements. Infants and children require about 0.8 mg of iron to be absorbed daily during the first 15 years (dietary intake of 8–15 mg of iron daily).

Iron deficiency in infants can occur from failure to receive placental blood at birth, especially if the cord is clamped before the first breath with the infant held above the level of the uterus, as in cesarean section. A twin can be iron deficient if vascular communications in the placenta favored more blood flowing to the other twin. Blood loss from any cause at any age can result in iron deficiency. Steatorrhea, GI blood loss from excess cow's milk, chronic diarrhea, or infection over a prolonged period can be sufficient to produce the hypochromic microcytic anemia characteristic of iron deficiency. Blood that enters the lung (as in pulmonary hemosiderosis) is broken down and the iron is sequestered in the reticuloendothelial system. Thus, reutilization is minimal and anemia can occur (Table 3.8).

The sequence of events in iron deficiency anemia is a decrease in available iron with a reduction in ferritin levels to less than 10 ng/ml. Serum iron levels fall and total iron binding capacity increases. Free erythrocyte protoporphyrins (FEP) increase. Anemia follows and if severe, iron-containing intracellular enzymes lose

Table 3.8
Considerations of Possible Reasons for Iron Deficiency

Intrauterine	Twin-to-twin placental vascular connection
Perinatal	Loss from baby to placenta by occlusion of umbilical cord before the first breath
Postnatal Iatrogenic	Blood loss from blood sampling for diagnosis during illness
Rapid growth	With inadequate intake of iron
Blood loss	From any site
Pulmonary hemosiderosis	Iron is sequestered in lung
Unmodified cow's milk	Before 4–6 months of age

activity. Thrombocytosis up to 1,000,000 mm^3 may occur.

Excess

Excess intake can lead to hemosiderosis or an accumulation of iron in the reticuloendothelial system. The most common cause of iron overload is from transfusions for hemolytic or refractory anemias. Each 500 ml of blood contains about 250 mg of iron which is stored in the reticuloendothelial system, skin, and myocardium. Cardiomegaly and eventual heart failure are the most feared consequences of iron overload. Chelation therapy with desoxyferramine has been useful in enhancing elimination of iron in transfusion-dependent individuals (see pp. 515).

PHOSPHORUS

Source

Milk, eggs, nuts, meats, vegetables, and grains are sources of phosphorus.

Function

Phosphorus is a constituent of bones and teeth and is widely distributed throughout the body as a key component of ATP. It exists in every cell membrane in the form of phospholipids. About 70% of intake is absorbed as free phosphates. Vitamin D regulates its absorption and renal retention.

Deficiency of phosphorus may be associated with rickets. It occurs in individuals on parenteral alimentation and dialysis unless levels are closely monitored. Deficiency can also follow use of large amounts of antacids. Symptoms include muscle weakness and malaise. An excess of phosphorus can develop in infants on a formula with a low calcium to phosphorus ratio and can produce tetany.

For a more complete discussion of calcium, phosphorus, iron, and iodine refer to other sections.

TRACE ELEMENTS

Trace elements occur in all tissues in minute amounts. Because of low concentrations, measurement was difficult before the development of sensitive analytical technologies suitable for study of biologic materials. The two most widely used techniques are atomic absorption spectrometry and neutron activation analysis. Chemical methods are based on spectrophotometric determination of metal complexes that form in solution after chemical separation of the element from its matrix. Investigation of metabolism of trace metals usually requires use of isotope tracer methods.

Trace elements essential for human nutrition include copper, zinc, cobalt, manganese, and iodine. Those thought to be beneficial are chromium, manganese, selenium, molybdenum, boron, and fluoride. Other trace elements are present and may be required, although no reproducible deficiency states have been described: these include lead, cadmium, tin and mercury. Their toxicity when present in excess is well-known (Table 3.9).

COBALT

Source

Vitamin B_{12} is a source of cobalt.

Function

Cobalt is a component of vitamin B_{12} and also erythropoietin. Absorption decreases with increased iron in the intestine.

There are no known deficiencies of cobalt and no reports of cobalt poisoning in children.

COPPER

Source

Copper is widely distributed in the body and associated with the activity of a number of metallo-enzymes, such as superoxide dismutase and serum amino oxidase. It is also a catalyst in hemoglobin formation. It is transported in plasma mostly bound to ceruloplasmin, but also bound to albumin and metallothionein. The highest concentrations are in the liver and the CNS.

Function

Copper is widely distributed in the body and associated with the activity of a number of metallo-enzymes, such as superoxide dismutase and serum amino oxidase. It is also a catalyst in hemoglobin formation. It is transported in plasma mostly bound to ceruloplasmin, but also bound to albumin and metallothionein. The highest concentrations are in the liver and the CNS.

Deficiency of copper can lead to a refractory anemia and osteopenia. Ceruloplasmin levels are reduced

Table 3.9
Functions and Deficiency States for Inorganic Elements[1]

Inorganic Element	Function	Major Causes of Deficiency	Manifestations of Deficiency
Magnesium [2]	Major constituent of bone; Required for neuromuscular contraction, protein synthesis,and reactions involving ATP	Alcoholism, diuretic use, Kwashiorkor, malabsorption, diabetic ketoacidosis, parenteral nutrition	Muscle irritability and tetany, weakness, confusion, coma, tremor, seizures, arrhythmias (plasma Mg may be normal though tissue levels are low)
Copper [2]	Essential for connective tissue metabolism, heme synthesis, and nerve function; bound to ceruloplasmin and metallothionein; a component of several oxidative enzymes	Nephrotic syndrome, malabsorption, Kwashiorkor, parenteral nutrition, high-fiber diets decrease copper absorption	Pancytopenia; bone marrow shows increased megaloblasts and sideroblasts with maturation arrest
Zinc [2]	Required for normal growth and development; essential component of a number of enzymes and the salivary protein gustin	1. Digests limited largely to whole wheat bread and beans (Dietary phytate binds zinc and decreases its absorption.) 2. Acrodermatitis enteropathica, an autosomal recessive disorder	1. Dwarfed males with hypogonadism, anemia, lethargy, hepatosplenomegaly, geophagia 2. Severe chronic diarrhea; thickened, ulcerated skin on limbs and around mouth and anus Loss of normal taste sensation
Chromium [2]	Glucose tolerance factor, a low-molecular-weight organic complex, is needed in some animal species for normal glucose metabolism; low chromium levels have been reported in some diabetics, but the role of chromium in human diabetes is unclear		
Cobalt	Cobalt is a component of vitamin B_{12}; cobalt deficiency has not been reported in man; cardiomyopathy has resulted from the addition of cobalt to beer; other toxic manifestations of cobalt include nausea, vomiting, diarrhea, tinnitus, and hearing loss		
Fluoride	Fluoride is incorporated into bones and teeth; addition of fluoride to water supplies low in this element reduces the incidence of dental caries; excessive fluoride causes mottling of dental enamel, gastrointestinal symptoms, tetany, and cardiovascular collapse		
Manganese [2]	Manganese is a cofactor for several enzymes and a component of bone and several metalloenzymes; manganese deficiency has not yet been described in humans		
Molybdenum	Molybdenum is a constituent of some oxidases; no deficiency state is known in humans		
Selenium	Selenium is a component of glutathione peroxidaxe and may function, like vitamin E, to protect against intracellular peroxides; a fatal cardiomyopathy in Chinese children has been attributed to selenium deficiency.		

[1]Reproduced with permission from Harvey et al: *The Principles and Practice of Medicine*, 21st edition. Norwalk, CT, Appleton-Century-Croft, 1984.
[2]Inorganic elements commonly included in parenteral nutrition solutions.

and, consequently, oxidation of ferrous to ferric iron does not occur. (Ceruloplasmin is a ferroxidase.) In some infants with chronic malnutrition, anemia, neutropenia, and osteopenia in association with hypocupremia can occur. Symptoms are reversible with copper supplementation. Some individuals on intravenous alimentation with inadequate copper intake have had copper deficiency and developed hypercholesterolemia (Karpel and Peden, 1972). Congenital copper deficiency (Menkes steely hair syndrome) is a defect in release of absorbed copper by intestinal mucosal cells. This severe illness is associated with reduced lysyl oxidase, which is required for collagen cross-linking. The hair is sparse and fragile, leaving short stubbles that feel "steely." The course of progressive neurological deterioration is not altered by parenteral copper administration (see pp. 974).

Excess copper is stored in Wilson disease from impaired copper homeostasis. The pathophysiology is unknown. The dominant manifestation is cirrhosis, but the pigment can be seen in the eyes in Kayser-Fleischer rings. Copper deposition also occurs in brain and kidneys. Urinary copper is increased. Many changes are reversible with chelation therapy (see pp. 476).

There are no known circumstances of excess dietary copper.

IODINE

Source

Iodized salt and seafood are sources of iodine.

Function

Iodides are essential constituents of thyroxine (T_4) and triiodothyronine (T_3) (see pp. 826). Iodides are absorbed from the intestine and selectively concentrated about 25-fold in the thyroid gland where they form part of the thyroglobulin complex. Proteolytic enzymes release T_4 and T_3 into the blood where they are distributed to all cells. The metabolic activity of cells is regulated by levels of thyroid hormones.

Excess

No natural excess occurs. Medicinal excess can lead to iodism. Increased iodine uptake by the thyroid inhibits organic iodide formation and leads to goiter and/or myxedema.

Deficiency

Too little iodine is the cause of simple goiter or endemic cretinism (see pp. 829).

MAGNESIUM

Source

Magnesium is abundant in milk, meat, nuts, and cereals.

Function

Magnesium is important in the structure of bones and teeth. Appropriate intracellular concentrations are essential for many metabolic processes including those that require ATP. It is the second most common intracellular cation, so in a sense is not a trace element.

Excess

Excess magnesium is a sedative and can produce shock. Magnesium excess can occur in infants of preeclamptic mothers who are treated with $MgSO_4$. Serum magnesium levels remain above normal for at least 3 days. Preterm or asphyxiated infants may have even higher levels. No clear symptoms have been defined other than possible hypotonia. Serum calcium levels are elevated and parathyroid hormone is depressed.

Deficiency

Magnesium deficiency is frequently associated with hypocalcemia and may produce convulsions or tetany.

MANGANESE

Source

The normal source is nuts, vegetables, and cereals. Milk contains small amounts of manganese, predominantly bound to lactoferrin, which is also the major iron-binding protein in breast milk.

Function

Manganese is found in bone, liver, retina, and pancreas. It is found in association with mitochondria and is a component of at least two metalloenzymes, pyruvate carboxylase and superoxide dismutase (Doisy, 1974).

Deficiency

Dietary deficiency is unknown. In one experimental situation, an adult volunteer was fed a diet inadvertently deficient in manganese and developed weight loss, reddening of black hair, a transient dermatitis and slow growth of hair and nails. Suboptimal levels have been noted in some children with seizures; treatment reduced their frequency.

Excess

Manganese toxicity from inhalation of metal fumes produces a Parkinson-like syndrome, fever, and pneumonitis.

SELENIUM

Source

Barley and whole wheat are the best sources. Meat and fish have some selenium, as do mushrooms, garlic, and radishes. Human milk selenium content and glutathione peroxidase activity are positively correlated with maternal plasma selenium (Mannan and Picciano, 1987).

Function

Selenium is distributed through all tissues except fat. Glutathione peroxidase is the only known enzyme with a requirement for selenium. The enzyme functions to metabolize hydrogen peroxide as it oxidizes glutathione.

Deficiency

Selenium deficiency leads to reduction in levels of glutathione peroxidase; when levels are 10–15% of normal, diminished killing of bacteria by neutrophils occurs (Serfass and Ganther, 1975). Another manifestation of selenium deficiency is cardiomyopathy, indigenous to selenium poor areas of China. It is preventable when selenium is provided (Chen et al, 1980).

Children on long-term intravenous alimentation may show signs of selenium deficiency, manifested as muscle pain and tenderness and white fingernail beds. Serum creatine kinase and transaminases are elevated.

Excess

Toxicity from excess selenium is not well-documented in man.

ZINC

Source

Zinc is found in colostrum, and in lower concentration in milk and in many meats and vegetables. The availability for absorption is decreased by ferrous iron, calcium, and phytic acid.

Function

Zinc is a constituent of some enzymes, including carbonic acid anhydrase, alkaline phosphatase, and superoxide dismutase. It is widely distributed in the body, being present in red and white cells, liver, muscles, retina, and bones. Congenital deficiency of zinc leads to dwarfism and anemia, and a condition known as acrodermatitis enteropathica. The condition is an autosomal recessive disorder that occurs with normal zinc intake and can be corrected with therapeutic doses of zinc.

Acquired deficiency can occur in individuals of all ages on total parenteral nutrition without supplemental zinc. The requirement for preterm infants is 300 μg/kg/day. Nutritional zinc deficiency leads to impairment of DNA and RNA metabolism with consequent poor growth, anorexia, diminished taste and smell, hypogonadism, dermatitis, and lethargy. Zinc status is best estimated from serum and urinary zinc levels. Normal serum levels in males are 83–88 μg/dl, females 85–91 μg/dl. The activity of alkaline phosphatase, a metalloenzyme, may reflect total body zinc status.

Dietary excess of zinc, or increased absorption is unknown. Inhalation of zinc oxide fumes may cause fever, pneumonitis, headache, and leukocytosis.

CASE ILLUSTRATION (Abstracted from Kumar and Andey, 1984).

A 950-g male infant was born after a 29-week gestation. He had mild respiratory distress syndrome, but no other neonatal problems. Parenteral nutrition was started in the first week of life, along with transpyloric feeds of breast milk alternating with formula. At 8 weeks, the infant weighed 1600 g and was receiving 110 kcal/kg/day. At 9 weeks, periorbital edema developed. Total serum proteins were 3.3 g/dl and albumin 2.3 g/dl. Serum alkaline phosphatase was 49 u/l. Serum zinc was 42 μg/dl.

An elemental zinc supplement, 1 mg/kg/day was started and 5 days later, the edema had resolved, albumin was 3 g/dl, the alkaline phosphatase was 158 u/l, and zinc was 72 μg/dl. After discontinuing zinc supplements 1 month later, neither edema nor hypoproteinemia recurred.

The diagnosis of zinc deficiency was made on the basis of a low plasma zinc level (less than 65 μg/dl), a low serum alkaline phosphatase, and a rapid response to zinc supplementation.

QUESTIONS AND COMMENTS

Why are premature infants at risk of zinc deficiency?

The human fetus accumulates about 70% of zinc stores in the last trimester. Thus, in an infant born after 29 weeks, stores are low, and breast milk does not have enough zinc to prevent a negative balance. Symptoms were evident when the infant was growing well and receiving less than the recommended intake of 3 mg/day. Formulas prepared especially for low birth weight infants are now fortified with zinc to provide 1–1.5 mg/100 kcal. Human milk contains only 0.22 mg/100 kcal.

What is the reason for the hypoproteinemia?

Protein intake was thought to be adequate in this infant. No diarrhea, liver disease, or urinary losses were present. It seems probable that zinc deficiency was responsible for the reduction in serum albumin, because zinc has an important role in protein synthesis (Bates and McLain, 1981).

More prolonged deficiency would probably have produced growth retardation, diarrhea, and cutaneous lesions characteristic of acrodermatitis enteropathica.

REFERENCES

Arlette JP: Zinc and the skin. *Pediatr Clin North Am* 30:583, 1983.

Bates J, McClain CJ: The effect of severe zinc deficiency on serum levels of albumin, transferrin and prealbumin in man. *Am J Clin Nutr* 34:1655, 1981.

Chen X, Yang G, Chen J, et al: Studies on the relations of selenium and Keshan disease. *Biol Trace Elem Res* 2:91, 1980.

Doisy EA Jr.: Effects of deficiency in manganese upper plasma levels of clotting proteins and cholesterol in man. In: Hoekstra WG, Suttie JW, Ganther HE, et al(eds). *Trace Element Metabolism in Animals*. Baltimore, University Park Press, 1974, p.668.

Karpel JT, Peden VH: Copper deficiency in long-term parenteral nutrition. *J Pediatr* 80:32, 1972.

Kien CL, Ganther HE: Manifestations of chronic selenium deficiency in a child receiving total parenteral nutrition. *Am J Clin Nutr* 37:319, 1983.

Kumar SP, Anday EK: Edema, hypoproteinemia and zinc deficiency in low-birth-weight infants. *Pediatrics* 73:327, 1984.

Levander DA: A global view of human selenium nutrition (review). *Ann Rev Nutr* 7:227, 1987.

Mannan S, Picciano MF: Influence of maternal selenium status on human milk selenium concentration and glutathione peroxidase activity. *Am J Clin Nutr* 46:95, 1987.

Prasad AS (ed): Clinical, biochemical and nutritional aspects of trace elements. In: *Current Topics in Nutrition and Disease*. Vol. 6, New York, Alan R. Liss, 1982.

Serfass RE, Ganther HE: Defective microbicidal activity in glutathione peroxidase-deficient neutrophils of selenium-deficient rats. *Nature* 255:640, 1975.

Parenteral Nutrition

6

Parenteral nutrition refers to partial or total intravenous alimentation. Intravenous administration of vitamins dates from the late 1940s; experience with glucose solutions and other amino acid mixtures in an effort to meet nutritional requirements originated in the late 1960s (Dudrick et al, 1968). Partial nutritional support through peripheral veins has been used in small infants since the early 1960s, but total intravenous alimentation in low birth weight infants was not widely used until after the report of Driscoll et al in 1972.

Appropriate mixtures of amino acids, carbohydrates, and fats have been and continue to be sought in ways that will facilitate metabolic utilization of the various constituents, avoid batch to batch variation in composition, lessen the likelihood of hyperammonemia, and minimize the possibility of severe allergic reactions. The composition of intravenous solutions depends on the indication for their use, i.e., in renal failure, it is necessary to provide the essential amino acids but to depend on the patients' utilization of urea for synthesis of nonessential amino acids. If hepatic failure is present, high levels of branched-chain amino acids are required, coupled with a low intake of aromatic amino acids. In the event of trauma, high levels of branched-chain amino acids are preferable; in the case of low birth weight infants, it is necessary to try to mimic the specific postprandial amino acid patterns of the growing infant.

The prevalence of use of intravenous nutrition depends of course on the type of the patients seen in any pediatric service. At The Children's Hospital in Boston, on the average, about 25 patients are receiving total parenteral nutrition each day with a total census of about 280 patients. Almost all infants weighing under 1000 g at birth receive some parenteral nutrition, usually via peripheral veins, during the course of their stay in the intensive care nursery.

Who is a candidate for intravenous alimentation? Any individual who cannot absorb adequate liquids and calories from the intestinal tract for any reason. Excessive losses as in the case of burns or diarrhea can be alleviated with intravenous infusions and should be considered when the patient's condition extends over a period of time when superimposed malnutrition could aggravate the underlying problem.

Intravenous alimentation has been life-saving where there are major anomalies of the GI tract, which require resection (to allow time for the short remaining bowel to grow) and for infants with chronic intractable diarrhea (to permit the intestine to recover). Normal growth and development over several years have been achieved in such patients. More recently, very immature infants who could not absorb enough nutrients for growth through their immature intestinal tracts have been kept alive with total parenteral nutrition. In all instances, there is significant individual variation in the tolerance to different mixtures so that careful monitoring of serum constituents as well as weight gain is essential.

Mechanics of Parenteral Nutrition

If long-term intravenous nutritional support is required, a surgical cut-down on an interior jugular vein is indicated to insert the catheter into the superior vena cava. The reason for the use of a major vein is that the osmolality of any mixture with sufficient nutrients is in the range of 1800 mOsm/kg of water (normal serum osmolality is 300 mOsm/kg water). Smaller vessels tend to sclerose with a high osmolar solution.

The successful use of total parenteral nutrition depends on meticulous attention to the technical details of handling the infusate and the catheter. Infection rates, in our hands, are about 5–6%. They can be much higher in the absence of a team of individuals in charge of the care of the central venous lines, which should be used only for infusions rather than withdrawal of blood samples. Nonetheless, infection that is related to the catheter and dislodgment of the catheter are of sufficient concern that central venous alimentation should not be undertaken lightly.

Guidelines for composition of parenteral feedings, in general, have evolved as experience increased. For preterm infants, a positive nitrogen balance and appropriate growth occur with parenteral lipid and/or glucose intakes of 60 kcal/kg/day and amino acid intakes of 2.5–3.0 g/kg/day, to total approximately 70 kcal/kg/day. The availability of intravenous lipids has permitted a high concentration of calories (1.1 kcal/ml) in 10% solutions that are isosmolar with plasma. Lipids should not be added to the infusate until jaundice has subsided because of their capacity to displace bilirubin from albumin binding-sites and possibly potentiate kernicterus. The recommended amounts are 0.5–1.0 g/kg/day of lipids and increased by 0.5 g daily to a maximum of 3.0 g/kg/day. Triglycerides should be measured at least weekly, and kept under 150 mg/dl.

Calcium and phosphorus requirements are met by intravenous administration of 30–40 mg/kg/day of each.

Recommendations for trace metals are based on intrauterine accretion rates. They are:

Zinc	100–300 μg/kg/day
Copper	20 μg/kg/day
Chromium	0.14–0.2 μg/kg/day
Manganese	2–10 μg/kg/day

Daily vitamin requirements are met with a commercial preparation (MVI, Pediatric) which contains per vial of powder (from Zlotkin et al, 1985):

Vitamin A	2300 IU
Vitamin D	400 IU
Vitamin C	80.0 mg
Vitamin K	0.2 mg
Vitamin E	7.0 IU
Thiamine	1.2 mg
Riboflavin	1.4 mg
Pyridoxine	1.0 mg
Niacin	17.0 mg
B_{12}	1.0 μg
Folic acid	0.14 mg
Pantothemic acid	5.0 mg
Biotin	20 μg

Because metabolic complications can develop, it is important to monitor blood levels as suggested in Table 3.10 (from *Pediatric Nutrition Handbook,* 2nd edition, American Academy of Pediatrics, 1985).

Table 3.10
Suggested Monitoring Schedule During Total Parenteral Nutrition [1]

Variable Monitored	Suggested Frequency	
	Initial Period [2]	Later Period [3]
Serum electrolytes	3–4 times/week	2–3 times/week
Serum urea nitrogen	3 times/week	2 times/week
Serum calcium, magnesium, phosphorus	3 times/week	2 times/week
Serum glucose	[4]	[4]
Serum acid-base status	3–4 times/week	2–3 times/week
Serum ammonia	2 times/week	Weekly
Serum protein (electrophoresis or albumin/globulin)	Weekly	Weekly
Liver function studies	Weekly	Weekly
Hemoglobin	2 times/week	2 times/week
Urine glucose	Daily	Daily
Clinical observations (activity, temperature, etc)	Daily	Daily
WBC count and differential count	As indicated	As indicated
Cultures	As indicated	As indicated
Serum triglyceride	As indicated	As indicated

[1] Reproduced with permission from *Pediatric Nutrition Handbook*, 2nd edition. American Academy Pediatrics, 1985, p.157.
[2] Initial period is period before full glucose intake is achieved, or any period of metabolic instability.
[3] Later period is period during which patient is in a metabolic steady state.
[4] Blood glucose should be monitored closely during the period of glucosuria (to determine the degree of hyperglycemia) and for 2–3 days after cessation of parenteral nutrition (to detect hypoglycemia). In the latter instance, frequent Dextrostix determination constitutes adequate screening.

CONTROVERSY

Cholestasis can be associated with intravenous alimentation. The prevalence varies from center to center, but it is evident that infants who receive intravenous alimentation for more than 2 weeks have about a 33% chance of liver dysfunction. The diagnosis is evident when the direct bilirubin value is over 2 mg/dl. Alkaline phosphatase may be elevated as well as SGOT and SGPT (serum enzymes). The liver dysfunction occurs with and without use of lipid emulsions. Presumably, the high calorie-to-nitrogen ratio leads to increased fatty acid flux into the liver with development of a fatty liver. The abnormalities will persist as long as the intrave-

CASE ILLUSTRATION (abstracted from Case Records Massachusetts General Hospital, *N Engl J Med* 310:774, 1984).

A male infant was born with 2-cm defect to the right of the umbilicus through which several loops of intestine protruded (gastroschisis). At operation, approximately 31 cm of small bowel was present, and a microcolon began as a blind pouch at the hepatic flexure. Protruding bowel was resected and a jejunostomy was placed, and the infant was placed on parenteral nutrition.

On the fifth day, total bilirubin was 13.2 mg/dl and the conjugated fraction was 1.2 mg/dl. Because of bleeding at the jejunostomy site, transfusions were given weekly until day 17. Hyperbilirubinemia persisted and, on day 54, the total was 11.8 mg/dl, conjugated 7.2. Other laboratory studies revealed total protein 5.4 g (albumin 2.6)/dl. SGOT was 86 units (normal 5–30 U) and SGPT 57 U (normal 2–50 U). Alkaline phosphatase was 141 IU (normal up to 104 IU). Serologic tests for hepatitis, and cultures were all negative.

A percutaneous liver biopsy disclosed cholestasis, bile-duct proliferation, and early portal fibrosis. Inasmuch as extrahepatic obstruction was not present, the possibility of cholestasis in association with parenteral nutrition was considered. Nonetheless, total parenteral nutrition was maintained in this infant until a bowel-lengthening procedure was undertaken at 11 months. His subsequent course was complicated by *Pseudomonas* sepsis, pneumonia, and ultimately liver failure. He died at 14 months of age.

QUESTION AND COMMENT

Should intravenous alimentation have been discontinued earlier?

The answer has to be yes because, in general, reversal of cholestasis is possible only before cirrhosis develops. However, some infants with short-bowel syndrome cannot be maintained on oral feeds. Only careful attempts to maximize oral intake and minimize dependency on intravenous feeding have a chance of saving such an infant. We cannot know in retrospect if the liver disease was reversible when discovered. Some oral intake may lessen the risk of cholestatic changes, by increasing the enterohepatic circulation of bile acids and reducing the accumulated sludge in the bile (Merritt, 1986).

nous alimentation is continued, but usually resolve within 2 weeks thereafter. Serial biopsies have shown evidence of some persisting minimal periportal fibrosis. The long-term significance of these findings awaits further study.

The possibility that taurine deficiency is responsible for cholestasis was studied by Heird et al (1987). They reported near elimination of the problem in the short term (10–21 days) when taurine was added to the intravenous solution so that plasma concentrations were within the normal range.

CONTROVERSY

Iron is not usually added to intravenous alimentation solutions because of possible physical incompatibility with other constituents. Experience with low dose ferrous citrate is promising (Sayers et al, 1983). When very low birth weight infants are on long-term parenteral alimentation, iron supplementation is essential. Often, it is tolerated by mouth. When the oral route is not feasible 2 μmol (0.11 mg) iron/kg/day can be given intravenously.

REFERENCES

Clinicopathological Exercises, Massachusetts General Hospital. Cholestasis and portal fibrosis associated with total parenteral nutrition. *N Engl J Med* 310:774, 1984.

Driscoll JM Jr, Heird WC, Schullinger JN, et al: Total intravenous alimentation in low-birth-weight infants: a preliminary report. *J Pediatr* 81:145, 1972.

Dudrick SJ, Wilmore DW, Vars HM, et al: Long-term total parenteral nutrition with growth, development and positive nitrogen balance. *Surgery* 64:134, 1968.

Forbes GB, Woodruff CW: *Pediatric Nutrition Handbook,* 2nd edition. Elk Grove Village, IL, American Academy of Pediatrics, 1985.

Heird WC, Dell RB, Heims RA, et al: Amino acid mixtures designed to maintain normal plasma amino acid patterns in infants and children requiring parenteral nutrition. *Pediatrics* 80:401, 1987.

Merritt RJ: Cholestasis associated with parenteral nutrition. *J Pediatr Gastroenterol Nutr* 5:9, 1986.

Peden VH, Witzleben CL, Skelton MA: Total parenteral nutrition. *J Pediatr* 78:180, 1971.

Postuma R, Trevenen CL: Liver disease in infants receiving total parenteral nutrition. *Pediatrics* 63:110, 1979.

Sayers MH, Johnson DK, Schumann LA, et al: Supplementation of total parenteral nutrition solutions with ferrous citrate. *J Parent Enter Nutr* 7:117, 1983.

Winters RW, Heird WC, Dell RB: History of parenteral nutrition in pediatrics with emphasis on amino acids. *Fed Proc* 43:1407, 1984.

Zlotkin SH, Stallings VA, Pencharz PB: Total parenteral nutrition in children. *Pediatr Clin North Am* 32:381, 1985.

Adverse Reactions to Food 7

Adverse reactions to food or additives are thought to be common, but when not rigorously defined, they probably have more to do with distaste than with abnormal responses or allergies.

Definition

The time-honored criteria for allergy are first, consistent reproduction of symptoms by blinded provocation (neither physician nor patient is told if the substance tested is food or placebo until after the test); second, functional changes or lesions in the target organ; and third, demonstration of an immune mechanism in pathogenesis (Ingelfinger et al, 1949).

Basic Science

Adverse reactions to food can be idiosyncratic meaning, in this instance, by an unknown mechanism, or they can have an immunologic basis. Among classical idiosyncratic reactions are the Chinese restaurant syndrome from monosodium glutamate, headaches after ingestion of cured meat such as hot dogs (sodium nitrite) or wine and cheese (tyramine) (Kerr et al, 1979).

Immunologic responses may be IgE-mediated and show positive skin tests to the offending food. The most notorious foods are fish, shellfish, nuts, eggs, cow's milk, and wheat.

After food challenge, histamine release can be demonstrated in some children with atopic eczema. A rise in circulating neutrophil chemotactic factor can occur after bronchospasm that results from challenge with milk. These observations support an allergic basis for some adverse reactions to food.

Epidemiology

The prevalence of confirmed or documented food allergy in children is unknown, but is probably less than 1%.

Natural History

The complaint of adverse reaction or allergy to food requires a careful medical history. Most convincing are the immediate reactions that are usually IgE-mediated, such as angioedema of the lips, mouth, uvula, or epiglottis, or generalized urticaria. Occasionally, bronchospasm will be precipitated.

Other reactions may be delayed, as in milk allergy, where vomiting, blood-streaked mucoid diarrhea (or occult fecal blood loss) may begin a few hours after ingestion.

Food intolerance from lactase deficiency includes delayed appearance of abdominal pain, distention, and diarrhea.

Treatment

Offending foods should be eliminated. Care must be taken to ensure that the remaining diet is nutritionally adequate. After a few years, cautious refeeding may be undertaken because tolerance develops in time, except with disorders such as gluten-induced celiac syndrome, which is lifelong. Hyposensitization is not advised.

CONTROVERSY

A topic of much interest to pediatricians and parents concerns appropriate time to introduce solids to the diet of normal infants. Can precocious introduction of solids permit absorption of allergens into the circulation and initiate food intolerances? Will delayed introduction deprive the infant of nutrients not available in breast milk or formula? Two questions are posed under the heading of controversy because opinions and practice differ widely.

Conventional wisdom is that at about 4–6 months of age is the right time to introduce solids, which is supported by the willingness of infants of this age to accept them. Single grain cereals, such as rice cereal are well-tolerated. If the infant tolerates cereal, vegetables, egg yolk (not as allergenic as egg white), fruits, and meats are introduced one at a time. Once tolerated, combinations of foods are offered. Juices are offered by cup. Salt and sugar are not added to most commercially available baby foods, and probably should not be added to home-prepared foods.

The scientific basis for introduction of solids at about 4–6 months of age rests on evidence that production of IgA antibodies by the intestinal tract does not reach appreciable levels before that age. IgA antibodies, directed against food protein, could depress the amount of potentially antigenic molecules that pass through the mucosa to the blood stream (Eastham et al, 1978).

No convincing evidence exists to attribute food allergy or the many symptoms attributed to it such as colic, diarrhea, eczema, or poor weight gain to early introduction of solids. Nonetheless, withholding of solids is a common practice when such symptoms occur. The only method of verification of the rare intolerances to food in infants under age 3 years is a food challenge. The putative offending food should be withheld for a week, then reintroduced to see if symptoms reappear. For toddlers over age 3 years, skin tests are available to ascertain if immediate-type hypersensitivity exists. Both false-positive and false-negative reactions can occur. A radioallergosorbent test (RAST) indicates IgE levels in serum, and is useful if skin testing is difficult, as in eczema. Verification with food challenges remains essential.

The question of whether early introduction of solids is dangerous is not clearly answered. Many infants are given solids to thicken feedings in an effort to prevent regurgitation, or to establish the precocious development of a baby by ambitious parents. For the most part, such infants do well (Orenstein et al, 1987). Contradictory findings cloud the picture of the relation of early introduction of solids to later occurrence of eczema (Kramer and Moroz, 1981). Certainly no convincing evidence of a relationship exists.

The question of late adverse effects of infant feeding practices is even more difficult to answer. Many infants have thrived on breast milk, with added iron and vitamins as the only supplements for a year or more. Others have apparently enjoyed and tolerated much earlier introduction of solids.

By 9 or 10 months of age, infants are able to eat and seem to enjoy pieces of fruit and vegetables, cheese, and other finger foods that they can grasp. Nuts, raisins, and popcorn should be avoided because of the risk of aspiration. Avoidance of excessive sodium intake seems prudent because of its possible relationship to later hypertension, although at least one study failed to find such a relationship (Whitten and Stewart, 1980).

For older children, the question of dietary lipids as possible precursors of atherosclerosis is another area of interest and controversy. Abundant evidence exists to show that fatty streaks of atherosclerosis are found in arteries of children and young adults who die of other causes (Newman et al, 1986). A National Institutes of Health Consensus conference (*JAMA* 253:2080, 1985) made the following recommendations:

> It is desirable to begin prevention in childhood because patterns of life-style are developed in childhood. The moderate-fat and moderate-cholesterol diets recommended for the population at large in this report should be suitable for all family members, including healthy children older than 2 years.
>
> Children at "high risk" should be identified primarily by carefully obtained family histories rather than routine screening.
>
> Those children with blood cholesterol levels between the 75th and 90th percentile (170–185 mg/dl) should be counseled regarding diet and other cardiovascular risk factors and then followed up at 1-year intervals. Those with levels above the 90th percentile (>185 mg/dl) require special dietary instruction and close supervision with evaluation of other risk factors. A child with a blood cholesterol level above the 95th percentile (200 mg/dl) on two occasions is in a special category and may have one of the hereditary hypercholesterolemias. Strict dietary intervention is indicated and will be sufficient for many children. Nonresponders should be considered for

CASE ILLUSTRATION

A 4-week-old white female had some blood-flecked "mucousy" stools that progressed to frankly bloody a few days later. Investigation at that time showed bloody stools with sheets of polymorphonuclear cells on microscopic examination. Stool cultures were negative. A complete blood count was normal. The infant was asymptomatic and had a normal physical examination except for rectal mucosa that was friable, red, and edematous.

Further investigation showed a normal upper gastrointestinal series and normal barium enema. When infection with *Salmonella, Shigella, Campylobacter*, and *Yersinia* was ruled out, the question was what else would give a purulent bloody diarrhea? Although the infant was breast-fed, it was noted that the mother drank several glasses of cow's milk each day. Thus, to test the possibility of cow's milk allergy, breast-feeding was discontinued and the infant promptly improved on oral electrolyte solution, followed by elemental formula. After the mother refrained from cow's milk and milk products, breast feeding was carefully and successfully resumed.

treatment with a lipid-lowering agent, e.g., bile-acid sequestrant (such as cholestyramine). All family members should be screened.

The question of lipid screening in childhood is open. High-risk children (based on family history) should be screened for plasma cholesterol and high density lipoprotein. Probably most children approaching adolescence should have a test for blood lipids. The efficacy and safety of cholesterol-lowering regimens deserve continued study (Glueck, 1986).

REFERENCES

Eastham EJ, Lichauco T, Grady MI, et al: Antigenicity of infant formulas: Role of immature intestine on protein permeability. *J Pediatr* 93:561, 1978.
Glueck CJ: Pediatric primary prevention of atherosclerosis. Editorial. *N Engl J Med* 314:175, 1986.
Ingelfinger FJ, Lowell FC, Franklin W: Gastrointestinal allergy. *N Engl J Med* 241:303, 1949.
Kerr GR, Wu-Lee M, et al: Prevalence of the "Chinese restaurant syndrome." *J Am Diet Assoc* 75:29, 1979.
Kramer MS, Moroz B: Do breast-feeding and delayed introduction of solid foods protect against subsequent atopic eczema? *J Pediatr* 98:546, 1981.
Metcalfe DD, Kaliner MA: Editorial "What is food to one is to others bitter poison." *N Engl J Med* 311:399, 1984.
National Institutes of Health Consensus Conference. Lowering blood cholesterol to prevent heart disease. *JAMA* 253:2080, 1985.
Newman WP, Freedman DS, Voors AW, et al: Relation of serum lipoprotein levels and systolic blood pressure to early atherosclerosis. *N Engl J Med* 314:138, 1986.
Orenstein SR, Magill HL, Brooks P: Thickening of infant feedings for therapy of gastroesophageal reflux. *J Pediatr* 110:181, 1987.
Sampson HA, Jolie PL: Increased plasma histamine concentrations after food challenges in children with atopic dermatitis. *N Engl J Med* 311:372, 1984.
Whitten CF, Stewart RA: The effect of dietary sodium in infancy on blood pressure and related factors. *Acta Paediatr Scand* 279 (Suppl)3:1980.

MARY ELLEN AVERY
SUSAN BAKER
DOROTHY VILLEE
ROBERT WHARTON

Section 4

Neonatology

Neonatology, a term first coined by Schaffer in 1960, has come to be a subspecialty of pediatrics, because so many conditions are unique to, or most prominent in neonatal life, defined as the first 28 days. Clearly, many of the disorders of newborn infants also persist or are most problematical in later infancy and childhood. They are also best discussed in the relevant organ-oriented sections of this text.

In this section, we have chosen to focus on some of those problems that confront the physician who assumes responsibility for caring for infants in the first month of life. Although many problems are limited to this period when postnatal adaptations may go awry, others are included because their recognition and treatment must take place in the newborn period.

Infant Mortality

1

One of the major medical and social advances of our time, and perhaps the most significant, has been the reduction in infant mortality (e.g., from over 100/1000 live births in 1900 to about 11/1000 in 1984 in the United States). The lowest infant mortality rates were reported in 1985 from Japan, Finland, Sweden, and Switzerland; with the United States ranking 19th (Wegman, 1987).

Fertility rates decreased in 1983 from 122.7 live births per 1000 women ages 15–44 years in 1957, to 65.4 live births per 1000, which is below that calculated for zero population growth. Approximately 3.7 million babies were born in the United States in 1984, which is about 2% higher than in 1983.

The contribution of low birth weight to continuing infant mortality is significant. Although survival has been improved, the proportion of infants under 2.5 kg has remained about 7% in recent years in the United States. No change has been noted in the proportion of babies weighing less than 1.5 kg at birth, who comprise 1.15% of all births.

In the United States the percentage of infants born weighing less than 2.5 kg to blacks is 12.7%; the percentage in whites is 5.9%. Despite the fact that birth weight specific mortality slightly favors the very low birth weight (VLBW) black who is more mature at a given gestational age, infant mortality values remain nearly double for blacks. At term and in the first year of life, however, the black infant is at a disadvantage. The reasons are complex, but closely linked with poverty. Mortality rates are higher for adolescent mothers,

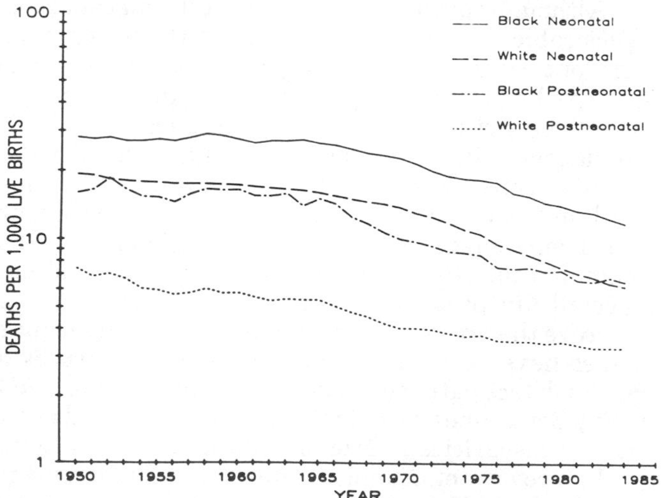

Figure 4.1. Infant mortality rates by race for the United States, 1940–1984. Reproduced with permission from Wegman M: *Pediatrics* 78:983, 1985.

and those with poor education and low income (McCormick, 1985; Wise et al, 1985; Figs. 4.1 and 4.10).

Morbidity among low birth weight survivors is greatest among the smallest. Because many of these infants are also of low birth weight for gestational age and may have several problems, it is difficult to attribute late sequelae to any single perinatal event (McCormick et al, 1980). The interdependence of factors is seen in the observation that low birth weight infants of disadvantaged mothers are more likely to fail in school than those of similar birth weight of advantaged mothers (Ramey et al, 1978). These observations and others have motivated the development of infant stimulation programs, child care centers, and other forms of early intervention.

Apart from prolonged hospitalization at birth (usually until the infant is 38–40 weeks' postconceptual age), readmission among low birth weight infants is frequently significant. Up to 40% of VLBW infants (weighing less than 1.5 kg) have almost two additional admissions in the first year (with an average of 16 days of hospitalization); 19% of all those weighing less than 2.5 kg (average of 12.5 days of hospitalization); and 8.7% of term infants (average of 8 days of hospitalization; McCormick et al, 1980).

GENDER AND PERINATAL MORTALITY

The excess proportion of male deaths in comparison with females is well-documented, about 1.28:1, which differs significantly from the 1.05:1 ratio for live births (Naeye et al, 1971). Conditions in which excess male morbidity has been found include hyaline membrane disease, erythroblastosis, and postnatal infections.

Although the explanations are not obvious, some provocative hypotheses have been proposed. One definite hormonal difference in fetal life is the exposure of the male to testosterone early in gestation. Indeed, the male phenotype is determined by the androgen surge from fetal testes. In a series of experiments in animals in vivo and in tissue culture, Nielsen et al (1982) have provided convincing evidence that testosterone antagonizes the effect of glucocorticoid on development of the surfactant system. These observations are undoubtedly relevant to the excess male morbidity in hyaline membrane disease.

The predisposition of the male to more serious infection may be related to a less mature immune system at term. Geschwind and Behan (1982) in commenting on the association of immune disease, migraine, and developmental learning disorders with left-handedness in males, speculated that testosterone could interfere with development of regions of the cerebral cortex known to be involved with organogenesis of the thymus. The complex interactions between gonadal steroids and the immune system are clearly worthy of further study (Grossman, 1985).

CESAREAN BIRTH

A major change in recent years has been in the number of births by cesarean section in the United States which has more than tripled since the 1950–1965 era when the rate was about 2–5%. In 1981, the cesarean section rate in the United States was 18/100 hospital deliveries (Notzon et al, 1987).

This increase has raised concern in the medical and lay community but it has been associated with a dramatic reduction in maternal mortality from approximately 40/100,000 deliveries in 1955 to about 12/100,000 in 1975. Equally impressive has been the association of a continuing reduction in perinatal mortality.

CONTROVERSY

The major indications for section are dystocia, repeat cesarean section, breech presentation, and fetal distress (Bottoms et al, 1980). Most of the controversy centers around the necessity for a repeat cesarean section, which constitutes about 23% of the increase in cesarean births. A major change has been in the management of breech presentation. In the past, many breech births were difficult vaginal deliveries with forceps extractions. A major reduction in morbidity has occurred as guidelines for cesarean section for breech presentation have become more liberal. Electronic monitoring has provided more insight into the episodes of fetal distress that may previously have been overlooked. The question of the significance of dips in heart rate, or alterations in fetal blood gases as obtained by scalp puncture before delivery, remains controversial. Nevertheless, a significant temporal relationship between the introduction of fetal monitoring and increased operative deliveries suggests that attention should be given to the predictive value of information gained from monitoring.

A reminder: we cannot conclude that high rates of performing cesarean section are solely responsible for the improvement in mortality and morbidity: this comes from experiences in other parts of the world, where major reductions in perinatal mortality have occurred through a reduction in prematurity rates (Papiernik et al, 1985). The 1985 clinical report from Coombe Lying-In Hospital, Dublin, Ireland reveals a perinatal mortality for all infants weighing more than 500 g (including late neonatal deaths) at 14.1/1000, among 6354 births. The cesarean section rate was only 7.8%, and in Japan, with one of the lowest mortality rates, the cesarean section rate in 1981 was about 8%.

The proponents of a more liberal use of delivery by section argue that a number of late obstetric disasters still occur. The combined rates of neonatal death and severe neurological impairment were over 2%, among 45,777 infants born in the 1960s and enrolled in the collaborative perinatal project in the United States (Nelson and Ellenberg, 1984). A report from Stockholm indicated that severe neonatal asphyxia occurred in 2.9% of full-term infants (Ergander et al, 1983). Our own experience is similar.

What can be done to reduce this significant problem? One proposal is to widen the indications for delivery by section when the fetus is mature. Of concern is the risk of maternal death from elective section, quoted as about 1/5000 (Consensus Report, 1980). The currently accepted indications for prophylactic section at term are previous section, breech presentation, and maternal infection with active herpes. The danger inherent in expanding the indications is that some infants will be born prematurely and be at risk of respiratory distress syndrome and other complications of preterm birth. The issue is a complicated one, and no consensus exists at the time of writing (Feldman and Freiman, 1985).

Our view is to urge careful consideration of known risk factors including maternal age, postmaturity, accuracy of dates, and tests of fetal well-being. The institutional section rates (deliveries by section/total delivered) or societal attempts to establish a "norm" should not interfere with the obstetrician's best judgment and, after consultation, with the views of the parents.

CONSIDERATIONS ON AUTOPSIES OF PERINATAL DEATHS

Stillbirths and neonatal deaths may be associated with obvious defects or well-described conditions or, especially in the case of stillborns, may occur without explanation. The pathologist who has specialized in neonatal pathology has much to contribute both from systematic examination of dead infants and of the placenta.

Although routine examination of the placenta may be desirable, few services can support the personnel to carry out careful studies. In general, the obstetrician decides when information might be useful. If guidelines were to be written, we would propose examination of the placentas in all deaths, in all infants admitted to intensive care units (except for observation only), and in all multiple births inasmuch as the information obtained may shed light on the cause of disease. Chorioamnionitis is one of the most common findings, especially in preterm infants, and suggests but does not prove the presence of infection. Possibly inadequate studies have been carried out to search for viruses or hard to detect pathogens such as *Mycoplasma* or *Chlamydia*. Sometimes vascular communications will be the cause of disparities in size and blood volume in twins.

In a review of neonatal autopsies at Duke University, Craft (1985) reported unsuspected or erroneous clinical diagnosis in 40%. These included congenital anomalies, infections, and iatrogenic complications. In our own experience, unanticipated findings at autopsy have included pancreatic lesions consistent with cystic fibrosis, a ruptured hypogastric artery, a chest tube accidentally inserted into the left ventricle, cytomegalovirus disease, pulmonary hypoplasia, and hypoplastic left heart syndrome.

Driscoll (1984) has made the case for routine autopsies of stillbirths by being able to assign a cause of death in 90% of them. Information from the pathologist can be communicated to the family by the attending obstetrician and/or pediatrician with appropriate counseling about subsequent pregnancies.

In summary, we are saddened by the number of infants who die without an autopsy and by stillbirths which probably are not subjected to any medical examination. Factors that were associated with low autopsy rates at Brigham and Women's Hospital, Boston, 1982–1984, included infants weighing less than 700 g (55% autopsied) and race (65% for blacks, 75% for caucasians; Van Marter et al, 1987). Persistence in requesting autopsies for all infants is important to monitor trends in perinatal deaths, to ascertain unsuspected diagnoses, and to permit genetic counseling.

REFERENCES

Bottoms SF, Rosen MG, Sokol RJ: The increase in cesarean birth rate. *N Engl J Med* 302:559, 1980.
Coombe Lying-In Hospital, Clinical Report 1985, Dublin, Ireland.
Craft WH: Neonatal autopsy: An investment with a high rate of return. *Pediatr Res* 19:197A, 1985.
Driscoll S: Autopsy following stillbirth: A challenge neglected. In Ryder OA, Byrd ML (eds): *One Medicine*. Berlin, Spring-Verlag, 1984, pp. 20–31.
Ergander U, Eriksson M, Zetterstrom R: Severe neonatal asphyxia: Incidence and prediction of outcome in the Stockholm area. *Acta Paediatr Scand* 72:321, 1983.
Feldman GB, Freiman JA: Prophylactic cesarean section at term. *N Engl J Med* 312:1264, 1985.
Geschwind N, Behan P: Left-handedness: Association with immune disease, migraine and developmental learning disorder. *Proc Nat Acad Sci* 79:5097, 1982.
Grossman CJ: Interactions between the gonadal steroids and the immune system. *Science* 227:257, 1985.
McCormick MC: The contribution of low birth weight to infant mortality and childhood morbidity. *N Engl J Med* 312:82, 1985.
McCormick MC, Shapiro S, Starfield BH: Rehospitalization in the first year of life for high-risk survivors. *Pediatrics* 66:991, 1980.
Naeye RL, Burt LS, Wright DL, et al: Neonatal mortality, the male disadvantage. *Pediatrics* 48:902, 1971.
National Institute of Child Health and Human Development: Cesarean childbirth: Report of a Consensus Development Conference. Washington, DC, United States Government Printing Office. (DHHS publication—NIH 82–2067), 1980.
Nelson KB, Ellenberg JH: Obstetric complications as risk factors for cerebral palsy or seizure disorders. *JAMA* 251:1843, 1984.
Nielsen HC, Zinman HM, Torday JS: Dihydrotestosterone inhibits fetal rabbit pulmonary surfactant production. *J Clin Invest* 69:611, 1982.
Notzon FC, Planck PJ, Taffel SM: Comparisons of national cesarean section rates. *N Engl J Med* 316:386, 1987.
Papiernik E, Bouyer J, Dreyfus J, et al: Prevention of preterm birth: A perinatal study in Haguenau, France. *Pediatrics* 76:154, 1985.
Ramey CT, Stedman DJ, Borders-Patterson A, et al: Predicting school failure from information available at birth. *Am J Ment Defic* 82:525, 1978.
Van Marter LJ, Taylor F, Epstein MF: Parental and physician-related determinants of consent for neonatal autopsy. *Am J Dis Child* 141:149, 1987.
Wegman ME: Annual summary of vital statisics, 1986. *Pediatrics* 80:817, 1987.
Wise PH, Kotelchuk M, Wilson MC, et al: Racial and socioeconomic disparities in childhood mortality in Boston. *N Engl J Med* 313:360, 1985.

Screening 2

PRENATAL DIAGNOSIS

Overview

(See Section 13, Genetics for specific diseases)

Definition

Examination of fetal cells by biochemical, microscopic, or molecular techniques can permit diagnosis of some hereditary disorders. Examination of the fetus by ultrasonography may allow diagnosis of fetal sex (after 18 weeks) and some structural abnormalities. Samples of maternal blood for α-fetoprotein reflect some fetal abnormalities. Cell-sorting of maternal blood to identify fetal cells that have entered the maternal circulation during pregnancy is promising for future prenatal diagnosis.

Basic Science

Genetic disorders can be categorized into four groups, autosomal dominants, autosomal recessive disorders, polygenic conditions, and chromosomal abnormalities. The first are those transmitted as autosomal dominants, of which more than 1000 are known, but only rarely are they diagnosed prenatally. Fortunately, molecular diagnosis is possible when the basic defect is known, as in α-thalassemia (Rubin and Kan, 1985).

Second, autosomal recessive disorders number about 850, about 100 of which are now diagnosable on the basis of identifiable abnormalities in fetal fibroblasts obtained by amniocentesis or from chorionic villi biopsy. About 150 X-linked disorders are known, and information about fetal sex allows the option of abortion of male fetuses to eliminate all risk. Identification of the biochemical defect is clearly preferable inasmuch as 50% of male fetuses will have the disorder.

A third category of genetic disease is the large group of polygenic conditions. One illustration is open neural tube defects, whose diagnosis depends on assessment of α-fetoprotein in maternal blood or amniotic fluid and confirmation by ultrasonography. Others include cardiac defects, cleft palate, diaphragmatic hernia, polycystic kidneys, and others identifiable with ultrasonography.

The fourth group of disorders, chromosomal abnormalities, accounts for over 90% of all requests for prenatal studies and, of these, trisomy 21 is the most common, occurring in approximately 1 of every 1000 live births. In mothers who are over age 35 years, it is about as great as the risk of the procedure. By age 40 years, maternal risk of Down syndrome is 1/100.

Risks of Procedures

Virtually no risk to mother or infant is involved with the procedure for determination of α-fetoprotein on maternal blood. Nonetheless, the question of the wisdom of universal application of this test is valid on the basis of its interpretation. It leads to the detection of all anencephalic infants, and two-thirds of open spina bifidas. Low levels are found in approximately 20% of Down syndrome infants (Palomaki et al, 1985). The problem is that 2% of all pregnancies have elevated α-fetoprotein levels, and only 10% of these have fetal abnormalities confirmed by ultrasonography. The anxiety, apprehension, and expense of making screening universal needs careful consideration (Milunsky and Haddow, 1985).

Amniocentesis, the aspiration of 15–20 ml amniotic fluid, is the best source of fetal cells for further study. Chromosome analysis depends on dividing cells that appear after 2–3 weeks in culture. The overall accuracy of the test with banding analysis is greater than 99%.

The procedure itself is not useful before about 16 weeks, and given the time for results, puts the decision for abortion close to the 20-week limit, past which time many obstetricians are reluctant to carry out the procedure. A finite risk of fetal death or injury is present with estimates of fetal loss of 1:300 to 1:500 when done with ultrasonographic monitoring for fetal position and electronic monitoring of fetal heart rate.

Chorionic villi have been examined as a source of fetal cells in the first trimester. As of October 1985, more than 8000 procedures have been evaluated with fetal loss of 4.2%. The risk of maternal infection is small, but nonetheless a major consideration. About 10 mg of chorionic tissue are aspirated through a catheter, and permit chromosomal analysis with a report within about 7 days (Personal communication, Frigoletto, 1985). Enzymatic amplification of β-globin target sequences in DNA makes prenatal diagnosis of sickle cell disease possible on less than 1 μg of genomic DNA in less than 1 day (Saiki et al, 1985).

Ultrasonography

Ultrasonographic evaluation of fetal sex and well-being has become an important adjunct to prenatal care and is estimated to be performed in 40% of pregnancies in the United States in 1984. Although probably not indicated in a normal pregnancy, it is widely used when there is a family history of congenital malformations, there are reasons to expect fetal growth retardation, or to assess fetal sex, abnormal amounts of amniotic fluid or edema in the event of isoimmunization, or fetal tachycardia (Birnholz, 1983; Deter et al, 1982).

Ultrasonography can provide the best estimation of fetal dimensions and weight. Birnholz (1980) devised a formula based on measurements of biparietal diameter, cranial occipitofrontal diameter, and average anteroposterior and transverse abdominal diameters. Other formulas have been proposed (Roberts et al, 1985; Jeanty, 1984; Hadlock et al, 1983). Table 4.5 is from the Baylor group (Hadlock) and shows the actual measurements. If computer facilities are available, regression equations that use a combination of measurements have been widely used.

Screening for Hepatitis

Inasmuch as prophylaxis of an exposed newborn infant to hepatitis is so effective, it seems worthwhile to screen mothers whose risk of active infection or car-

Table 4.1
Aspects of Patient History that Indicate a Need for Prenatal HbsAg Screening[1]

I. Asian, Alaskan, or Pacific Island descent
II. Haitian, sub-Saharan African, Eastern European, Middle Eastern, Caribbean, or Central or South American birth
III. History of liver disease
IV. Occupational exposure (including dialysis and medical or dental settings)
V. Intravenous drug abuse
VI. Household contact with a patient with hepatitis B
VII. Rejection as blood donor
VIII. Repeated blood transfusions
IX. Work or residence in an institution for the mentally retarded
X. Multiple episodes of venereal disease

[1]Data adapted from the Centers for Disease Control.

rier state is 1% or higher. In the United States in the 1980s, individuals at risk are listed in Table 4.1. If a mother has a positive HBsAg titer, the infant should receive 0.5 ml immune globulin within 12 hours of birth, and hepatitis B vaccine, 0.5 ml, within 12 hours, and at 1 and 6 months of age (Snydman, 1985).

Controversy exists about prophylaxis of infants with non-B hepatitis exposure. In general, we advise 0.5 ml immune serum globulin at birth for infants whose mothers had active disease in the third trimester. This should be repeated at 28 days (see also pp. 471).

POSTNATAL SCREENING

Routine screening of newborn infants is now an established procedure for the early detection of metabolic disorders for which effective treatment is available. Initiated in 1964, it is now done throughout the United States and in all developed countries of the world (Nyhan, 1985).

The prototype of a disorder for which neonatal screening is of established value is phenylketonuria (PKU). The reason for screening is that the disease is not readily detected on clinical grounds until the damage from the high levels of circulating phenylalanine have become irreversible. The disorder is associated with severe mental retardation in nearly all infants unless phenylalanine is restricted in their diets. Early treatment is compatible with normal growth and development and when monitored carefully has no toxic effects. Consequently, the benefit of early detection to the individual is enormous and the harm to individuals being screened is infinitesimal because it simply requires use of a "heel stick" to obtain a drop of blood on a piece of filter paper. The decision for mandatory screening depends on knowledge of the incidence of the disorder, which is approximately 1 in 15,000 caucasian individuals. PKU is rarely found among blacks and Ashkenazi Jews (see section on Inborn Errors and Meryash and Levy, 1981).

Another condition for which routine screening is of unquestioned value is congenital hypothyroidism. It occurs in 1/4600 live births in New England. Screening more than 700,000 newborn infants over a 5-year period detected hypothyroidism in 146 infants, representing more than 98% of the infants born in the area. Only 10 infants were missed by the screening program either because their initial hormonal values were normal or through human error. In this condition also the methods for detection are precise and specific and only a drop of blood is required. If untreated, the condition is associated with severe mental retardation whereas treatment can restore the infant to normal. A 5-year follow-up of the treated infants showed that their performance on the Stanford Binet IQ test was no different than that of normal children.

These are the only two conditions widely screened in the United States at this time. Other rarer conditions that can be detected include: galactosemia, homocystinuria, maple syrup urine disease, tyrosinemia, and histidinemia. Hemoglobinopathies can sometimes be detected by hemoglobin electrophoresis in blood samples.

For those conditions that might be detected at birth but are clinically benign, screening does not appear to be necessary. Questions remain with respect to those conditions for which screening has been advocated (such as cystic fibrosis) but the tests are not sufficiently specific to detect all affected individuals, and they may be associated with significant numbers of false-positives. Because there is no specific treatment, which, even if begun in the newborn period is known to influence the course of the disease, screening for this condition on a widespread basis does not seem warranted. Siblings of known cases can be given a sweat test to ascertain presence of disease.

Newborn screening is one of those impressive advances in modern medicine that has led to legislation mandating it for all infants. However, this legislation is not without its opponents, some of whom feel that even a heel stick to obtain a drop of blood is unwarranted. This minority view is contradicted by the evidence of safety and efficacy of screening which is now mandated for both PKU and hypothyroidism. Screening is usually done in a central state laboratory which decreases the cost by virtue of a large number of analyses. Obviously prompt feedback to the physician and parents is essential if appropriate therapy is to be initiated early enough to have a beneficial effect. Repeat tests are clearly indicated before therapy is started and confirmatory tests by measurement of blood phenylalanine levels or T-4 and thyroid-stimulating hormone (TSH) levels are essential.

The information obtained from screening does not always provide the anticipated benefit. In a survey of 91 infants identified as having hemoglobin AS or AC (sickle trait) Grossman et al (1985) found that only 35% of the parents responded to an invitation for genetic counseling, and one-quarter of those did not remember information provided at the first interview when seen later. Probably the absence of overt illness and/or any intervention lessened enthusiasm for information.

Because screening detects only a few hereditary metabolic diseases, individuals with signs of a metabolic problem should always have specific blood tests and screening of urine for possible abnormal metabolites.

REFERENCES

Bickel H, Guthrie R, Hammersen G (eds): *Neonatal Screening for Inborn Errors of Metabolism.* Berlin, Springer-Verlag, 1980.

Birnholz JC: Determination of fetal sex. *N Engl J Med* 309:942, 1983.

Birnholz JC: Ultrasound characteristics of fetal growth. *Ultrasonic Imaging* 2:135, 1980.

Committee on Genetics, American Academy of Pediatrics: New issues in newborn screening for phenylketonuria and congenital hypothyroidism. *Pediatrics* 69:104-106, 1982.

Creasy RK, Resnik R: *Maternal-Fetal Medicine: Principles and Practice.* Philadelphia, WB Saunders, 1984.

Deter RL, Harris RB, Hadlock FP, et al: Longitudinal studies of fetal growth with the use of dynamic image ultrasonography. *Am J Obstet Gynecol* 143:545, 1982.

Elias S, Simpson, JL, Martin AO, et al: Chorion villus sampling for

first trimester prenatal diagnosis. *Am J Obstet Gynecol* 152:204, 1985.
Grossman L: Neonatal sickle cell screening. *Am J Dis Child* 139:241, 1985.
Grossman LK, Holtzman NA, Charney E, et al: Neonatal screening and genetic counseling for sickle cell trait. *Am J Dis Child* 139:241, 1985.
Guthrie R, Susi A: A simple phenylalanine method for the detection of phenylketonuria in large populations of newborn infants. *Pediatrics* 32:338, 1963.
Hadlock FP, Deter RL, Harrist RB, et al: Computer assisted analysis of fetal age in the third trimester using multiple fetal growth parameters. *J Clin Ultrasound* 11:313, 1983.
Jeanty P, Cantraine F, Romero R, et al: A longitudinal study of fetal weight growth. *Ultrasound Med* 3:321, 1984.
Klein RZ: Infantile hypothroidism then and now: The results of neonatal screening (entire journal). *Curr Probl Pediatr* 15:1, 1985.
Klein S, Young B, Wilson S, et al: Continuous fetal heart rate monitoring following third trimester amniocentesis. *Obstet Gynecol* 58:444, 1981.
Lau YF, Dozy AM, Huang JC, et al: A rapid screening test for antenatal sex determination. *Lancet* 1:14, 1984.
Meryash DL, Levy HL: Prospective study of early neonatal screening for phenylketonuria. *N Engl J Med* 304:294, 1981.
Milunsky A, Haddow JE: Cautions about maternal serum alpha-fetoprotein screening, Letter to editor. *N Engl J Med* 313:694, 1985.
National Institutes of Health Consensus Development Conference: Consensus statement diagnostic ultrasound in pregnancy. Washington, DC, United States Government Printing Office, 1984.
Nyhan WL: Neonatal screening for inherited disease. *N Engl J Med* 313:43, 1985.
Palomaki GE, Knight GJ, Kloza EM, et al: Maternal weight adjustment and low serum alpha-fetoprotein values. *Lancet* 1:468, 1985.
Roberts AB, Lee AJ, James AG: Ultrasonic estimation of fetal weight: A new predictive model incorporating femur length for the low-birth-weight fetus. *J Clin Ultrasound* 13:555, 1985.
Rubin EM, Kan YW: A simple sensitive prenatal test for hydrops fetalis caused by alpha-thalassemia. *Lancet* 1:75, 1985.
Saiki RK, Scharf S, Faloona F, et al: Enzymatic amplification of B-globin genomic sequences and restriction site for analysis of sickle cell anemia. *Science* 230:1350, 1985.
Snydman DR: Current concepts: Hepatitis in pregnancy. *N Engl J Med* 313:1398, 1985.

Evaluation of the Newborn Infant 3

The newly delivered infant must first be stimulated to breathe, which normally occurs through the naturally stimulating events of delivery. After warming and wrapping the infant in a blanket to permit some stabilization of vital signs, the attendants should communicate with the mother who should see her infant as soon as she wishes. Thereafter, the baby deserves a complete examination, some features of which are described in this chapter.

It is essential to keep the infant warm during the examination. An open incubator or examining surface under radiant heat is ideal and permits the infant to be naked and unrestrained. Warm hands are appreciated. A simple way to know if the infant is in a comfortable environment is to compare temperature of the abdominal wall and of the feet. The infant responds to cold by peripheral vasoconstriction that can be so severe as to make the cool extremities appear dusky or even blue, a condition called acrocyanosis.

PHYSIOLOGIC ADAPTATIONS

It is helpful to recall while carrying out an examination of an infant the remarkable and major physiologic adaptations to extrauterine life that occur within minutes after birth and over the ensuing few hours. Thus, the cord may continue to pulsate after it is clamped because the umbilical arteries do not always constrict immediately. Oxygen mediates constriction, and any delay in aeration of the lungs will prolong the time of pulsation. The number of umbilical arteries should be noted at the initial examination. The ductus arteriosus may not close for some hours after birth. Careful auscultation may reveal a murmur which could reflect continued right-to-left shunting. If marked, the left arm may be blue the right arm pink; even slight differences in color reflect the persistent fetal circulatory pathways that allow venous blood to enter the aorta through the ductus at a site that directs it to the left subclavian artery but not to the right. Normally, however, blood flow is left-to-right through the ductus after birth because aeration of the lung results in a prompt fall in pulmonary vascular resistance and lower pressures than in the systemic circulation. The persistence of a soft systolic murmur localized to the region of the ductus along the left upper sternal border signals the possible patency of the ductus. Such a murmur, heard intermittently by careful auscultation for several days in some infants, should disappear after that time.

The fetal lung at term contains about 40–60 ml of liquid, or an amount equivalent to the functional residual capacity. Aeration of the lung stimulates increased blood flow and resorption of this liquid by the circulation and by lymphatics. The rate at which this occurs is variable; it is not unusual to hear fine crackling rales throughout the lungs before this process is completed. Some of the liquid may persist in interstitial spaces and not be heard as rales, but it will reduce lung compliance with a remitting increase in respiratory rate. Crying during the first minutes of life doubtless facilitates complete aeration of the lung. If the infant does not cry, the respirations will be variable in depth, and at rates of 40–100/minute. As lung liquid is resorbed, the rates fall to a range of 30–50/minute and, by the second day of life, rarely are over 40/minute at rest. Variability in respiratory rates is characteristic of normal postnatal adaptations.

Fortunately for the fetus, peristalsis is absent during intrauterine life so that passage of meconium before birth is abnormal. Soon after birth, or at least by 24 hours, most infants will have passed nearly all of the meconium accumulated during fetal life. The mechanism that controls this remarkable adaptation has not been described. (Conditions responsible for delayed passage of meconium, such as cystic fibrosis, intestinal perforation, and/or obstruction are discussed in other sections of this text.) The examiner should note whether the anus is patent and whether meconium is present on the examining finger. Equally important is observation and notation of urination. Presence of a normal amount of amniotic fluid testifies to kidney and bladder function in fetal life because fetal urine is a major source of amniotic fluid. Most normal infants void soon after delivery, and observation of the stream is a useful part of the physical examination.

Because the postnatal adaptations require different amounts of time to complete, the examiner is required to note with care the precise time of examination. The Apgar score at 1 minute has a different connotation from the score at 5 minutes as the infant begins to establish ventilation with air for the first time (see pp. 156–157). A proper record of the initial examination should include date, time of day, and postnatal age in minutes.

Physical Examination

By systematic organ-oriented approach, the initial examination can proceed quickly. Five minutes is usually ample, particularly if the mother is to be given the opportunity to hold or suckle her infant. A more thorough leisurely examination at a later time can be carried out in the mother's presence so that her inevitable questions about the infant can be answered.

GENERAL STATUS

Gross malformations are evident on inspection. The quality, quantity, and symmetry of movements provide information about the nervous system. Does the infant assume a flexed position reminiscent of the fetal posture? Is the cry vigorous and of unusual intensity?

SKIN

In the initial examination, the infant should be observed rather than manipulated. The infant born at term or preterm will be protected with a white creamy material called vernix caseosa, which accumulates over the entire skin between the sixth and seventh month of gestation. Toward term it becomes less abundant, but is usually present in skin creases. After birth it disappears, and the underlying skin may be wrinkled and even parchment-like in postmature infants.

Vernix is a sebaceous material of high molecular weight fatty acids and esters and contains epithelial cells and lanugo hairs (Karkkainen et al, 1985). Because it protects the fetal skin for months in a liquid environment vernix must be the most effective skin cream ever designed. (We wipe off all excess vernix and bathe the baby with bland soap and water in the first days of life so as to take advantage of the protection. Overzealous bathing of infants, especially with detergent soaps, can cause cracked skin and even bleeding; hexachlorophene is contraindicated because it can be absorbed through the skin of premature infants.)

The skin of all infants is lightly pigmented. Those destined to be pigmented later may show evidence of color only around the genitalia or nail beds. Nonwhite infants often have large irregularly outlined areas of dusky pigmentation over the back and buttocks, which have been given the unfortunate name of Mongolian spots. They occur in more than 90% of black and oriental infants, but in less than 5% of caucasians. Most gradually fade during the first few years. They may be distinguished from bruises mainly by their distribution and the evenness of pigmentation. Nonwhite infants acquire more skin pigmentation during the first few weeks of extrauterine life, regardless of gestational age.

Breast nodules may be evident by 36 weeks' gestational age and can assume considerable enlargement in term and post-term infants. The average size is 6–7 mm diameter. About 6% of normal infants born at term will produce a thin milky discharge, called "witch's milk" in the old literature, and galactorrhea in more scientific terms. The condition probably reflects estrogenation of the infant by maternal hormones or neonatal prolactin and is as common in male as in female infants. Breast discharge usually subsides in a few weeks, but can persist for several months (Madlon-Kay, 1986).

HEAD

Is the head of unusual shape, or molded from a prolonged second stage of labor? Is there soft tissue swelling of the presenting part of the head (caput succedaneum) or a collection of blood in the subperiosteal space and, hence, limited to one side or the other (cephalohematoma)? Are the fontanelles of normal dimension and tension?

If the infant is supported in a sitting or standing position, the eyes should open so that their clarity can be observed. Conjunctival hemorrhages from pressure during delivery are common and usually clear within a few days. The normal infant has an "alert" look within minutes after birth, and in the first days will turn toward a soft voice and appear both to see and to hear. A minimal examination of the eyes should be made before discharge from hospital, including use of ophthalmoscope to elicit a red reflex in each eye, to assess the clarity of the vitreous and the absence of a lesion such as retinoblastoma. Full funduscopic examination is difficult before several days of age.

EARS

The position of the ears should be noted. Normally the pinnae are at the level of the eyes. Low set ears may coexist with malformations of the branchial clefts, or chromosomal abnormalities. Abnormal dimples, tags, or sinuses should be noted. Response to sound is evident in normal infants who are alert and attentive to a human voice, rattle, or bell.

NOSE

The shape of the nose, position of septum, and patency of nares should be observed. Occlusion of one nostril should be tolerated if the other is patent.

MOUTH

Appearance of mucous membranes, alveolar ridge, and palate should be noted and any defects carefully described or documented with photographs. Natal teeth, usually lower central incisors, are present in about 1/3500 live births, and require radiographs to ascertain if they are prematurely erupted decidual teeth or are supernumerary.

NECK

The neck of the newborn is short, and sometimes hard to palpate. The effort should be made to look for congenital cysts, hygromas, thyroid enlargement, and sternocleidomastoid tumors. If the neck has limited mobility, Klippel-Feil syndrome should be considered; if it is webbed, Turner syndrome is a possibility.

CHEST

The clavicles should be felt to ascertain fracture or absence. The shape of the chest is a clue to lung size, and chest circumference is useful if pulmonary hypoplasia is a possibility. Asymmetrical thoraces may result from skeletal disorders, diaphragmatic hernias with bowel in the thorax, overdistended lobes of the lung or intrathoracic masses. Mediastinal shift can occur with effusions, masses, or atelectasis. The position of the maximal cardiac impulse should be noted.

HEART AND LUNGS

Inspection and palpation are most useful to ascertain appropriate air entry, respiratory rates, heart rates, and circulatory adequacy. Percussion and auscultation are of less value, but differences between the left and right lungs can be noted by percussion, and decreased air entry or wheezes may best be noted on auscultation. The quality of heart sounds and presence of murmurs depend on careful auscultation in an infant who is not crying.

ABDOMEN

The important observations are fullness or emptiness, and the integrity of the abdominal wall. The liver edge is usually palpable just below the costal margin with the liver soft and easily pushed back. The spleen is not normally felt. The lower poles of the kidneys can be felt if the abdomen is not distended. Peristaltic waves are not evident unless obstruction is present.

Palpation of the inguinal canals for gonads or hernias is important. This part of the examination should be carried out with the infant crying because many hernias will not be evident at rest. Hernias occur 8–10 times more often in males; they are 10 times more common in infants born before 36 weeks' gestation, and 20 times as common in infants weighing less than 1.5 kg at birth (Broocock and Todd, 1985).

GENITALS

The size, position, and color of the labia, clitoris, vagina, and anus should be noted in females and size of penis, position of meatus, size of scrotum and testes, or hydroceles should be observed in males. It is an advantage to note a urinary stream which is often stimulated by gentle pressure over the bladder.

EXTREMITIES

Most information about the back and extremities is evident from inspection during the examination. Special attention should be given to the hips with the infant supine. Compare leg length, then abduct the thighs from a position of right angle flexion laterally and down to the table top. If one or both hips slip (click) or fail to abduct, subluxation or dislocation may be present (see also pp. 1273–1275).

Distal extremities deserve scrutiny for abnormalities of digits or nails, clubbing, edema, or unusual creases.

The rest of the physical examination, including neurologic evaluation and assessment of gestational age is discussed under the appropriate organ systems in other sections.

Follow-up Observations

Before discharge, a careful set of measurements should be recorded. Birth weight should be accurately measured on well-calibrated scales. Head circumference is best measured after a day or two when molding will decrease. (At term, it should be 33–37 cm.) The head tends to shrink with postnatal water redistribution, so the time of measurement is important. Chest circumference at the nipple line is usually the same as head circumference. A discrepancy of more than 2–3 cm requires serial measurements to determine whether growth of either head or chest is inappropriate. Length is difficult to measure without a device that permits extension and position of feet against a sliding panel. Normal term infants are usually 48–53 cm. Parents should be given a copy of the initial measurements and a growth chart on which to record subsequent ones.

REFERENCES

Broocock GR, Todd PJ: Inguinal hernias are common in preterm infants. *Arch Dis Child* 60:669, 1985.

Karkkainen MD, Nikkari, T, Ruponen MD, et al: Lipids of vernix caseosa. *J Invest Dermatol* 44:333, 1985.

Madlon-Kay DJ: "Witch's milk," galactorrhea in the newborn. *Am J Dis Child* 140:252, 1986.

Neurobehavioral Development of the Premature Infant

4

Heidelise Als

FETAL BRAIN DEVELOPMENT

All the basic divisions of the human brain appear to be in place by 6 weeks' gestation. Although they are relatively undifferentiated, their destinies appear assigned. Each of the millions of cells in the cerebral cortex originates in the germinal layers lining the ventricular system. During the period of maximal productivity, the germinal layer, which is well vascularized, is very active metabolically releasing as many as 10^5 cells per day. Each new brain cell migrates through the cortex to a specific, precise spot. These migrations occur in waves beginning at around 8 weeks and waning at around 26 weeks of pregnancy.

Once in place, each cell puts out hundreds of tiny branched processes called dendrites, which hook up with other cells to bring impulses into the cell. The dendrites are covered with tiny spines that eventually allow each cell to connect to an average of 1000 others. New brain cells are probably formed up until 40 weeks and synapses continue to be established rapidly until age 5 years and, more slowly, at least until age 18. As the cells become larger and more elaborately connected, more and more sulci appear.

The surface of the brain changes from smooth to convoluted as different areas organize for different functions. A marked increase in the number of gyri occurs at the end of the second trimester; a concurrent gain in brain weight and a change in head contour from oval to prominent biparietal bossing takes place. The right side organizes about 2 weeks before the left and asymmetry between the hemispheres is normal (Dooling et al, 1983). The pattern of the later sulci and gyri of the brain surface is as unique as a fingerprint.

Another important developmental process is myelination, in which a fatty sheath is deposited around the axons to allow faster and highly repetitive conduction of impulses. Myelination also seems to proceed in an orderly, hierarchic fashion; peak activity for myelination occurs at around full-term birth, but continues significantly until age 9 years and perceptibly into the 40s (Volpe, 1981).

Passage of impulses or messages from cell to cell is accomplished by chemical neurotransmitters, which often are released only if up to four or five different regulatory systems operate in a proper, specific configuration. More than two dozen neurotransmitters have been identified so far and, no doubt, there are many more. The sensitivities and densities of receptors for certain neurotransmitters vary widely from region to region in the brain, and are influenced by experience because the brain and the sensory organs are in continuous and mutual dependence on each other for normal structural and functional development.

All parts of the brain are interdependent. Areas which are remote from the original focus of insult or scar can show damage or malfunction much later, when certain connections become important in the course of development. Damage in one area may have ripple effects into other areas. Yet compensatory strategies can also be induced, with appropriate developmental support, especially in the very young brain.

Neurobehavioral Evaluation

OBSERVATION

Much can be learned by observation of the preterm newborn in his alien environment. Most babies actively seek contact with a stable surface, including the incubator wall, by either pressing against it with shoulder, head or back, or pushing against it with palms and soles of hands and feet. The infant seems more stable and restful when in contact with a surface than in an open area. This range finding appears to be intentional and actively stimulus-seeking. Another aspect of intentionality is observable in the differential reaction to painful experience, such as blood drawing. The infant responds with tight eye closure, grimace, constriction of arm muscles, and tight flexion. In contrast, being held quietly by the parent elicits open-eyed attention, if not visual engagement, reflecting receptive availability and the beginning of the social communication process.

MONITORING OF OXYGENATION

Transcutaneous oxygen monitoring is a reliable, safe, relatively nonintrusive mode of assessing oxygenation continuously. On the basis of this technique, it has been learned that behavioral changes in the infant and environmental changes around the infant can exacerbate or ameliorate arterial oxygen saturation. Infants have higher arterial oxygen saturation when awake than when asleep. Oxygen saturation falls with feeding and with active sleep (Mok et al, 1986).

Sleep State. The infant in light rapid eye movement (REM) sleep, shows significantly lower arterial oxygen saturation than the infant in deep sleep. Many preterm infants spend prolonged periods in light sleep and do not achieve deep sleep easily in the nursery. Korones (1976) documented 134 interruptions of sleep in the course of a 24-hour period in the neonatal intensive care unit (NICU). This means that many preterm infants spend much time in a state of increased vulnerability for hypoxemia.

Position. Prone positioning improves oxygenation, respiration, and heart rate, in contrast to supine positioning (Martin et al, 1979).

Auditory Environment. Ambient noise such as door and drawer closing, porthole manipulations, or laughter in the nursery significantly reduces the arterial oxygen saturation (Long et al, 1980). The background noise of the incubator itself has been found disturbing to infants (Peltzman et al, 1970); it blocks out the human voice while amplifying mechanical sounds such as door slamming. Infants may be startled from such stimuli.

Gentle Handling and Rest Periods. Continuous transcutaneous oxygen monitoring allows observation of the effects of handling on oxygenation. Gentle handling and appropriate rest periods are associated with fewer episodes of hypoxemia (Long et al, 1980).

Systematic Examination of Behavioral Functioning

Several methods have been developed to assess the behavioral developmental functioning of the preterm newborn (for a review, see Als, 1984). These grew largely out of previously existing assessments of full-term newborns.

The first behavioral examination of the full-term newborn was devised by Graham and her colleagues in the 1950s (Graham, 1956; Graham et al, 1956). Rosenblith (1985) modified the Graham scale by deleting the previous pain threshold test and dividing the rest of the examination into two subsets: a motor score and a tactile adaptive score. Furthermore, two sensory scales were established, one to assess auditory responses and one to assess vision.

Best performance rather than average performance was rated in an effort to overcome behavioral instability in the newborn. Predictive validity studies showed significance to 8-month Bayley measures. Of interest are the very specific relationships that have emerged from Rosenblith's extensive studies, identifying unusual hypersensitivity to light as related to neurologic abnormalities at 3 and 4 years. *Rosenblith has summarized her ongoing work in a recent textbook* (Rosenblith and Sims-Knight, 1985).

The Brazelton Neonatal Behavioral Assessment Scale, referred to as BNBAS or NBAS (Brazelton, 1985), is a comprehensive behavioral assessment of the full-term newborn that incorporates and largely extends functions assessed in the Graham-Rosenblith scales. Its main goal is the assessment of individuality in the spectrum of healthy full-term newborns. Therefore, in addition to assessing in a screening mode the basic reflex repertoire of the organism, it focuses on motoric integration, stage regulation, and attentional, interactive capacities, as well as reactivity and consoling capacities of the organism as measured in cuddliness, consolability, peak of excitement, rapidity of build-up to crying, and irritability. The adequacy of reflex performance is scored on 4-point scales, and the behavioral dimensions are rated on 26 9-point behaviorally defined scales. As in the Graham-Rosenblith scales, the *best* performance of the newborn is sought. Extensive training is required to elicit the newborn's best performance reliably and to score the behavior observed accurately.

The behavioral dimensions assessed are as follows:

1. Response decrement to light
2. Response decrement to rattle
3. Response decrement to bell
4. Response decrement to tactile stimulation of the foot
5. Orientation response—inanimate visual
6. Orientation response—inanimate auditory
7. Orientation response—inanimate visual and auditory
8. Orientation response—animate visual
9. Orientation response—animate auditory
10. Orientation response—animate visual and auditory
11. Alertness
12. General tone—predominant tone

13. Motor maturity
14. Pull-to-sit
15. Cuddliness
16. Defensive movements
17. Consolability with intervention
18. Peak of excitement
19. Rapidity of build-up
20. Irritability
21. Activity
22. Tremulousness
23. Amount of startle during examination
24. Lability of skin color
25. Lability of states
26. Self-quieting activity
27. Hand-to-mouth
28. Smiles

In the recent revision of the BNBAS (Brazelton, 1985), nine supplementary dimensions have been added derived from the work of Als (1984) and Horowitz et al (1978), including:

1. Quality of alert responsiveness
2. Onset of attention
3. Examiner persistence
4. General irritability
5. Robustness and endurance
6. Regulatory capacity
7. State regulation
8. Balance of tone
9. Reinforcement value of the infant's behavior

The Brazelton scale has received much attention and use in clinical and research areas. It provides an interactive approach to the infant, attending to complex organizational parameters of functioning rather than to very specific yes/no reactions.

One aspect of the Brazelton Neonatal Behavioral Assessment Scale that distinguishes it from other newborn assessments concerns its use as an intervention with mothers, fathers, and medical staff. When used in this manner, the BNBAS is intended to improve and enhance the caregiver's attitude to and interaction with the infant.

Several more recent assessments are designed to quantify the behavioral functioning not only of the full-term, but also of the preterm newborn. *The Albert Einstein Neonatal Neurobehavioral Scale* (Daum et al, 1977) is a modified version of the Brazelton Neonatal Behavioral Assessment Scale, with stringent administration criteria and a reduction in score points. *The Neurological Assessment of the Preterm and Fullterm Infant* by Dubowitz and Dubowitz (1981) is designed to be used by any physician without special training and allegedly can be administered even to the sick newborn in an isolette from the first postnatal day.

The *LAPPI* (Longitudinal Neurobehavioral Assessment Procedure for Preterm Infants, Korner et al, 1983), again, a combination of Dubowitz, Brazelton, and Prechtl items, is segmented into portions of least aversiveness for the youngest and sickest babies to increasing demand placed on the infant born healthy and at term. This examination emphasizes ability to establish states of sleep, arousal and wakefulness, ease or difficulty of eliciting certain performances, the speed and vigor of motor activity, amount and quality of crying, quality and duration of alertness, and persistence of performance, all areas of functioning which are likely to be different in preterm compared to full-term infants.

Assessment of Preterm Infants' Behavior (APIB) is currently the most comprehensive neurobehavioral assessment specifically geared to the preterm infant, but also appropriate for evaluating the full-term infant. It is based on detailed behavioral observation and requires extensive training. In 45–60 minutes, it assesses the interaction of autonomic, visceral, motor, state organizational, and attentional functioning via a systematic sequence of manipulations, broadly derived from the Brazelton scale. Table 4.2 gives a list of stress and defense behaviors; Table 4.3 gives a list of self-regulatory and approach behaviors that are evaluated by the APIB.

The APIB shows predictive validity to 9 and 18 months post-term, and to performance at age 5 years. Newborns with a low threshold disorganization and, therefore, presumably hypersensitive, become significantly more disorganized children later on than modulated, well-regulated newborns (Als, 1985). Furthermore, electrophysiologic studies on the same newborns have implicated differential vulnerability of the right hemisphere and the frontal lobe in the behaviorally hypersensitive newborns (Duffy and Als, 1983).

APPROACH TO SUPPORTING BEHAVIORAL DEVELOPMENT—ORGANIZATION OF THE INFANT

The APIB, with its focus on the interplay of autonomic, motoric, and state organizational functioning in the face of environmental demands impinging on the preterm newborn, has provided a framework for the development of a detailed behavioral observation paradigm of the very small baby during medical and caregiving interventions in the NICU. On the basis of the behavioral observations, caregiving modifications are then made in order to reduce the infant's stress behaviors and enhance his self-regulatory behaviors.

Two major areas of caregiving are attended to in this approach:

1. The physical environment around the infant:
   a. location of the infant's crib or isolette: avoidance of proximity to faucets and sinks, radiograph screen, telephone or radio speakers;
   b. bedding and clothing: provision of water mattress, sheepskin, with shielding of isolette or crib; and clothing, hat, and swaddling for the infant;
   c. specific aids to self-regulation: opportunity to suck during and between feedings (gavage feedings); to hold on during manipulations; (e.g., finger rolls or foot rolls to grasp);

Table 4.2
Stress and Defense Behaviors of Preterm Infants

Autonomic and visceral stress signals
- Seizures
- Respiratory pauses, irregular respirations, breath holding
- Color changes to mottled, webbed, cyanotic, or gray
- Gagging, choking
- Spitting up
- Hiccoughing
- Straining as if or actually producing a bowel movement
- Gasping
- Tremors and startling
- Coughing
- Sneezing
- Yawning
- Sighing

Motoric stress signals
- Motoric flaccidity or "tuning out"
  - Truncal flaccidity
  - Extremity flaccidity
  - Facial flaccidity (gape face)
- Motoric hypertonicity
  - With hyperextensions of legs: sitting on air; leg bracing; of arms: airplaning; salutes; of trunk: arching; opisthotonus; fingersplays; facial grimacing; tongue extensions; high guard arm position
  - With hyperflexions of trunk and extremities: fetal tuck; fisting
- Frantic, diffuse activity; squirming
- Frequent twitching

State-related stress signals
- Diffuse sleep or awake states with whimpering sounds, facial twitches
- Eye floating; roving eye movements
- Strained fussing or crying; silent crying
- Staring
- Frequent active averting
- Panicked or worried alertness; hyperalertness
- Glassy-eyed, strained alertness;
- Rapid state oscillations; frequent build-up to arousal
- Irritability and prolonged diffuse arousal
- Crying
- Frenzy and inconsolability
- Sleeplessness and restlessness

d. reduction of stress on treatment table: covering and shielding the infant during procedures;

e. optimal positioning of infant: prone, with supports (e.g., back rolls) to maintain position.

2. Direct caregiving to infant:

a. timing and sequencing of manipulations for care so as to minimize frequent interruptions of sleep state;

b. feeding: gavage feeding inside the shielded isolette; or bottle- or breast-feeding in quiet, shielded corner of room; timing of feeding with natural sleep cycle without interruption of deep sleep and without permitting periods of exhausting crying to precede feeding;

Table 4.3
Self-Regulatory and Approach Behaviors of Preterm Infants

Autonomic stability:
- Smooth respiration
- Pink, stable color
- Normal bowel function

Motor stability:
- Smooth, well-modulated posture
- Well-regulated tone
- Synchronous, smooth movements with efficient motoric strategies: hand clasping,foot clasping, finger folding, hand-to-mouth maneuvers, grasping, suck searching and sucking, handholding, and tucking

State stability and attentional regulation
- Clear sleep states
- Rhythmical crying
- Effective self-quieting
- Reliable consolability
- Robust, focused, shiny-eyed alertness with intent and/ or animated facial expression: frowning, cheek softening, attentional smiling

c. bathing: i.e., soothing effect of immersion versus sponge bathing;

d. transition facilitation: some manipulations which are essential for care are painful and stressful to the infant, e.g., spinal tap, suctioning, etc. Facilitation consists of:

(i) ensuring that conditions are as calm as possible for the infant with minimal interruptions and stresses; providing opportunity for sucking during procedure;

(ii) carrying out the procedure as quickly and efficiently as possible, with second person maintaining infant in comfortable position;

(iii) returning the infant to a prone position in his quiet environment and providing opportunity for him to hold on to the caregiver's finger, continue sucking, and be given containment until relaxation is re-established;

e. sleep organization: attention to the sleep cycle of the infant so that deep sleep is not interrupted. Critical review of the use of the automatic swing is indicated. For some infants it leads to momentary quieting, but does not improve self-regulation stabilization. Soothing, quiet instrumental music, on the other hand, while the baby is contained in flexion and removed from all unnecessary stimulation, is helpful for many babies in increasingly managing transition into restful sleep more effectively

(i) avoidance of bright lighting, shielding of eyes and of isolette, crib;

(ii) avoiding overstimulation both inside and outside the isolette, a cluttered visual environment can be too stimulating;

f. social contact: parent and other family involvement is, of course, a very important ingredient of developmental support. Continuous containment by soothing, quiet inhibition of motor arousal provided by the parent's steady hands and/or body for the hands, feet, and mouth of the baby may be much more productive for the infant's organization and assuring to the parent, than touching, stroking, holding, and talking to the infant. Excessive stimuli may produce apnea and/or other withdrawal behaviors. The individualized careful timing of inputs with the increasing self-regulatory stability and differentiation of the infant needs to be kept in mind.

A third major area of caregiving involves the care of the preterm infant's parents and family, who are themselves premature and need the staff's support in their gradual regaining of their infant and their development of confidence in their own parenting and nurturing abilities.

Controversy: The Issue of Age Correction for Preterm Infants

The postnatal evaluation of the development of preterm infants continues to be important to monitor late effects of perinatal interventions and to provide appropriate ongoing support. The question is by what standard developmental criteria should progress of preterm infants be judged? This was not a major problem when most survivors were more than 1.5 kg in birth weight and had "caught up" with term infants' growth and development by about 1 year of age. The question is more complex with even smaller infants surviving.

The issue is usually simplified to argue the pros and cons of chronologic versus postconceptual or adjusted age. (Adjusted age is calculated by subtracting infant's gestational age from 40 weeks, then subtracting that difference from chronologic age at time of evaluation.) The effect is, of course, relatively greater in the early months, and becomes less significant after a few years.

Several assumptions underlie this approach. One is that development is neither accelerated nor retarded by the fact of extrauterine existence in comparison to that of term infants. Another assumption is that gestational age (dated from onset of last menstrual period) can be known accurately either by history or physical examination. Occasionally, it can be known precisely but, more often, history is unreliable particularly in pregnancies that end preterm in which some vaginal bleeding may occur in the early months. Physical signs can help with assessment of gestational age but are most reliable in infants over 32 weeks' gestational age.

Typically, it has been the practice to correct for the degree of prematurity in, at least, the first 2 years of life, but there is little empirical evidence about whether this is the most appropriate course to take. *Corrected* scores in the first year of life are usually more highly correlated with developmental outcome during later preschool years. From 12 months of age, the *uncorrected* scores are better predicters of subsequent development. Early test scores (<12 months) are significantly influenced by the degree of biologic maturity whereas the impact of environmental influences increases with development. The conservative approaches to correction (i.e., limiting correction to the first 1–2 years of life) are aimed at adjusting for "catch-up" but not "covering-up" dysfunction.

Admitting to possible inaccuracies in the calculation, adjusted age remains useful for the first 2 years at least in evaluation of cognitive function. Similarly, evaluation of motor function with the revised and standardized Peabody Developmental Motor Scales showed that preterm (29–32 weeks' gestational age) infants without neonatal illness scored below term infants at 1 year of age when judged by chronologic age, but were comparable when age was adjusted (Palisano et al, 1985). How long the adjustment is appropriate is not clear, but its impact is proportionately smaller with time.

REFERENCES

Als H: Infant individuality: Assessing patterns of very early development. In Call J, Galenson E (eds): *Frontiers of Infant Psychiatry*. New York, Basic Books, 1983, pp. 363–378.

Als H: Newborn behavior assessment. In Burns WJ, Lavigne JV (eds): *Progress in Pediatric Psychology,* vol. 1. New York, Grune & Stratton, 1984, pp. 1– 46.

Als H: Patterns of infant behavior: Analogs of later organizational difficulties? In Duffy FH, Geschwind N (eds): *Dyslexia: A Neuroscientific Approach to Clinical Evaluation*. Boston, Little, Brown & Co., 1985, pp. 67–92.

Aylward G, Verhulst S, Colliver J: To correct or not to correct: Adjustment for prematurity. Abstract, paper presented at American Psychological Association Meeting, Division 7, August 25, 1985.

Brazelton TB: Neonatal Behavioral Assessment Scale. *Clinics in Developmental Medicine,* No. 50, 1973; 2nd edition, no. 88. Philadelphia, JB Lippincott, 1985.

Daum C, Grellong B, Kurtzberg D, et al: The Albert Einstein Neonatal Neurobehavioral Scale Manual 1977. Bronx, NY, Albert Einstein College of Medicine.

Dooling EC, Chi JG, Gilles FH: Telencephalic development: Changing gyral patterns. In Gilles FH, Leviton A, Dooling EC (eds): *The Developing Human Brain*. Boston, John Wright, 1983.

Dubowitz L, Dubowitz V: The Neurological Assessment of the Preterm and Fullterm Infant. *Clinics in Developmental Medicine,* no. 79, Philadelphia, JB Lippincott, 1981.

Dubowitz L, Dubowitz V, Goldberg C: Clinical assessment of gestational age in the newborn infant. *J Pediatr* 77:1, 1970.

Duffy FH, Als H: Neurophysiological assessment of the newborn: An approach combining brain electric activity mapping (BEAM) with behavioral assessment (APIB). In Brazelton TB, Lester BM (eds): *New Approaches to Developmental Screening of Infants*. New York, Elsevier North Holland, 1983.

Graham F: Behavioral differences between normal and traumatized newborns: I. The test procedures. *Psychol Monogr* 70:1, 1956.

Graham F, Matarazzo R, Caldwell B: Behavioral differences between normal and traumatized newborns: II. Standardization, reliability, and validity. *Psychol Monogr* 70:17, 1956.

Horowitz FD, Sullivan JW, Linn P: Stability and instability in the newborn infant: The quest for elusive threads. *Monographs of the Society for Research in Child Development*. 43:29, 1978.

Hunt JV: Predicting intellectual disorders in childhood for preterm infants with birthweights below 1501 grams. In SI Friedman, M Sigman (eds): *Preterm Birth and Psychological Development*. New York, Academic Press, 1981.

Korner AF, Schneider P, Forrest T: Effects of vestibular-proprioceptive stimulation on the neurobehavioral development of preterm infants: A pilot study. *Neuropediatrics* 14:170, 1983.

Korones SB: Iatrogenic problems in intensive care. In Moor T (ed): *Report of the 1969 Ross Conference on Pediatric Research.* Columbus OH, Ross Laboratories, 1976.

Long FGM, Philip AGS, Lucey JF: Excessive handling as a cause of hypoxemia. *Pediatrics* 65:203, 1980.

Martin RJ, Herrell N, Rubin D, et al: Effect of supine and prone positions on arterial oxygen tension in the preterm infant. *Pediatrics* 63:528, 1979.

Mok JYQ, McLaughlin FJ, et al: Transcutaneous monitoring of oxygenation: What is normal? *J Pediatr* 108:365, 1986.

Palisano RJ, Short MA, Nelson DL: Chronological vs. adjusted age in assessing motor development of healthy twelve-month-old premature and full term infants. *Phys Occup Therap Pediatr* 5:1, 1985.

Peltzman P, Kitterman JA, Ostwald PF, et al: Effects of incubator noise on human hearing. *J Aud Res* 10:335, 1970.

Prechtl H: The neurological examination of the fullterm newborn infant. *Clinics in Developmental Medicine,* no. 63. Philadelphia, JB Lippincott, 1977.

Rosenblith JF, Sims-Knight JE: *In the Beginning. Development in the First Two Years.* Monterey, CA, Brooks/Cole Publishing Co., 1985.

Siegel L: Correction for prematurity and its consequences for the assessment of the very low birthweight infant. *Child Devel* 54:1176, 1983.

Volpe JJ: *Neurology of the Newborn.* Philadelphia, WB Saunders, 1981.

Determinants of Size and Maturity at Birth

5

The principal determinant of size at birth is gestational age. Nevertheless, infants of like gestational age can differ greatly in size as the result of a host of genetic and intrauterine environmental influences.

Assessment of fetal size has attained a new level of accuracy with the advent of ultrasonography. Serial studies of crown-rump length or head diameter allow the obstetrician to assess the appropriateness of placental supply lines as well as of fetal disease (Fig. 4.2). Selection of time of delivery is now aided by knowledge of fetal size as well as degree of lung maturity as determined from surfactant measurements in amniotic fluid.

PRETERM BIRTH

Background

The reduction in mortality and morbidity of infants born before term (37 weeks) or below 2.5-kg birth weight has been one of the major advances of the past few decades. This accomplishment has been the result of improved obstetric care, including referral of high risk pregnancies to medical centers, and improved understanding of the needs of low birth weight infants and methods of providing appropriate neonatal intensive care. Nonetheless, preterm labor remains the most important cause of perinatal mortality and morbidity.

Improving insight into the heterogeneity of the population of premature infants has allowed care tailored to the needs of the individual baby. "Routine orders" have been replaced by specific instructions that are based on the ever-changing status of the infant. Certain principles of care emerge, however, and will be highlighted in this chapter.

Definitions

For comparisons of values obtained at different centers and among different nations, definitions should be agreed-upon. The weight of the infant at birth is most widely accepted as the best index of prematurity, with the acknowledgment that some infants are of normally low birth weight for gestational age (see pp. 146). Worldwide, 2.5 kg is accepted as the weight below which infants are considered premature, even though in some parts of the developing world many term infants are below that weight for a number of reasons, the most obvious of which are chronic malnutrition of the mother, close spacing of births, and twin pregnancies.

Because the outlook for normal survival of most infants with birth weight above 1.5 kg or 2.5 kg is about the same, special attention has been focused on those below 1.5 kg, sometimes referred to as infants of very low birth weight (VLBW). With the outlook for infants weighing more than 1 kg so much better than for those weighing less than 1 kg, this designation should per-

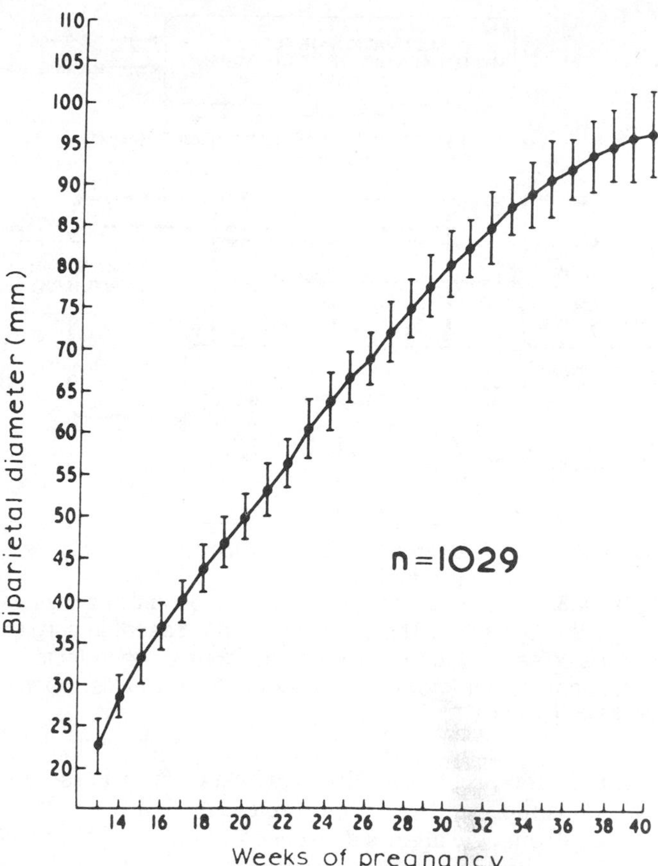

Figure 4.2. Mean fetal biparietal diameter (mm); 2 SD for each week of pregnancy from 13 weeks to term: 1029 individual measurements taken during normal pregnancy. Data of Campbell S: Size at Birth: Ciba Foundation Symposium 27, p. 281, 1974.

Table 4.4
Correlations Between Gestational Length and Embryonic and Fetal Bodily Dimensions[1]

Week of Gestation	Crown-rump Length (cm)	Weight (g)	Biparietal Diameter
6	0.5		
7	0.8	0.07	
8	1.5	0.22	
9	2.5	0.88	
10	3.5	3.5	
11	4.6	6.0	
12	5.7	11.0	
13	6.8	19.0	
14	8.1	33.0	
15	9.4	55.0	
16	10.7	80.0	
17	12.1	120.0	3.7
18	13.6	170.0	4.0
19	15.3	253.0	4.4
20	16.4	316.0	4.8
21	17.5	385.0	5.2
22	18.6	460.0	5.5
23	19.7	542.0	5.75
24	20.8	630.0	5.95
25	21.8	723.0	6.1
26	22.8	823.0	6.2
27	23.8	930.0	6.35
28	24.7	1045.0	6.5
29	25.6	1174.0	6.65
30	26.5	1323.0	6.85
31	27.4	1492.0	7.1
32	28.3	1680.0	7.3
33	29.3	1876.0	7.6
34	30.2	2074.0	7.8
35	31.1	2274.0	8.1
36	32.1	2478.0	8.35
37	33.1	2690.0	8.6
38	34.1	2914.0	8.9
39	35.1	3150.0	9.2
40	36.2	3405.0	9.55
41		3600.0	9.8
42		3650.0	9.85
		3750.0	10.0
		3900.0	10.2
		4000.0	10.3
		4200.0	10.6

[1] Data based on the study of Bartolucci L: *Am J Obstet Gynecol* 122:439, 1975. Courtesy of Iffy L, et al: *Pediatrics* 1975.

haps be changed to refer to those from the 1- to 1.5-kg group, with extremely low birth weight (ELBW) referring to those weighing less than 1 kg at birth. These are usually also less than 28 weeks' gestational age. Infants born before 24 weeks are usually less than 600 g and those born before 20 weeks are most often less than 400 g and are considered previable or abortuses (Tables 4.4 and 4.5).

FETAL GROWTH

Fetal growth is a topic of such enormous complexity that only some of the salient features will be considered in this chapter. Only recently has ultrasonography permitted physicians to view the early stages of morphogenesis during life. In addition, certain indicators of abnormal development can be identified through examination of fetal cells obtained by aspiration of amniotic fluid (amniocentesis). The pediatrician is most concerned with the last trimester of human development because premature birth requires an attempt to provide supports that would normally occur in utero. The greater the insight into late fetal development, the more closely can the challenge be met.

MECHANISMS INVOLVED IN ONSET OF LABOR

Although much has been learned about hormonal changes in pregnancy and the structure of the myometrium and cervix, the precise sequence of events that initiate and sustain labor remains unclear. For example, the relative ratio of circulating estrogens to progesterone increases before labor begins, but does not change abruptly. Fetal cortisol production increases in

Table 4.5
Predicted Fetal Measurements at Specific Menstrual Weeks[1]

Menstrual Age (weeks)	BPD (cm)	Head Circumference (cm)	Abdominal Circumference (cm)	Femur Length (cm)
12	2.0	7.1	5.6	0.8
13	2.3	8.4	6.9	1.1
14	2.7	9.8	8.1	1.5
15	3.0	11.1	9.3	1.8
16	3.3	12.4	10.5	2.1
17	3.7	13.7	11.7	2.4
18	4.0	15.0	12.9	2.7
19	4.3	16.3	14.1	3.0
20	4.6	17.5	15.2	3.3
21	5.0	18.7	16.4	3.6
22	5.3	19.9	17.5	3.9
23	5.6	21.0	18.6	4.2
24	5.8	22.1	19.7	4.4
25	6.1	23.2	20.8	4.7
26	6.4	24.2	21.9	4.9
27	6.7	25.2	22.9	5.2
28	7.0	26.2	24.0	5.4
29	7.2	27.1	25.0	5.6
30	7.5	28.0	26.0	5.8
31	7.7	28.9	27.0	6.1
32	7.9	29.7	28.0	6.3
33	8.2	30.4	29.0	6.5
34	8.4	31.2	30.0	6.6
35	8.6	31.8	30.9	6.8
36	8.8	32.5	31.8	7.0
37	9.0	33.1	32.7	7.2
38	9.1	33.6	33.6	7.3
39	9.3	34.1	34.5	7.5
40	9.5	34.5	35.4	7.6

[1]Reproduced with permission from Hadlock FP, Deter RL, Harrist RB, et al: *J Clin Ultrasound* 11:312, 1983.

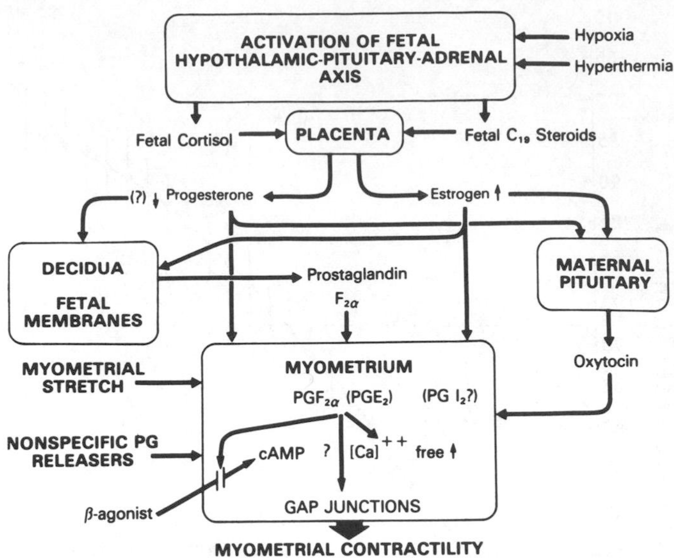

Figure 4.3. A general schema of some mechanisms thought to have a role in labor. The observations are based, in part, on animal studies, and the relative contributions of each factor in the human are not known. Courtesy of Dr. J. Challis. *Perinat Dev Med* 15:8, 1979.

the last trimester of pregnancy and affects the timing of maturation of some fetal organs. In sheep, it can initiate parturition, but cortisol given to human mothers in pregnancy does not promote labor. Oxytocins and prostaglandins are clearly important. Prostaglandin F_2 is known to be produced by fetal membranes, and induces contractions of the myometrium (Fig. 4.3).

It is established that the beginning of pregnancy requires suppression of prostaglandin synthesis and release; termination requires removal of that suppression. As Liggins (1983) noted, prostaglandins are the major hormones that activate parturition. Humans differ significantly from animals in hormonal events surrounding parturition, and uterine connective tissue is more important than formerly thought. In all situations the conceptus determines biochemical events.

One possible trigger for the sequence of events that occur in labor is phospholipase A_2 which is synthesized by many of the bacteria that constitute normal vaginal flora. Arachidonic acid in the fetal membranes becomes available for prostaglandin synthesis when it is split from phospholipid by phospholipase A_2 (Gluck, 1986).

β-Adrenergic agents decrease myometrial contractibility and are the most widely used tocolytic drugs (ritodrine, terbutaline, isoxuprine). At best, these agents can delay delivery by a matter of days, which may be crucial if administration of prenatal glucocorticoids is indicated to accelerate fetal lung maturation and permit postnatal survival (see pp. 166). Magnesium sulfate is an old standby which is administered with or without β-adrenergic agonists. The mechanism of action of magnesium is unknown, but it may reduce calcium influx into smooth muscle, thereby reducing contractility.

At present, according to Huszar and Naftolin (1984), only 30% of patients who arrive at the hospital in preterm labor are candidates for tocolytic therapy. Thus, efforts at prevention must be emphasized. Early recognition of labor, bed rest, and cessation of coitus remain the mainstays of treatment.

EARLY DEVELOPMENT

The fertilized ovum implants in the uterus between days 4 and 7, and thereafter (days 7–12) is called a blastocyst which imbeds more deeply into the myometrium. On days 13–19, chorionic villi branch capillaries proliferate in the villi. A yolk sac is present and a neural plate appears. On days 20–23 the embryo is 1.5–2.0 mm. Crown-rump, head and tail folds are evident and the hind gut appears. After day 24 (embryo 4-mm crown-rump), the neural groove closes and the primitive brain vesicles form, as do the optic and otic vesicles. Limb buds are present, and primordia of lungs, liver, pancreas, heart, and mesonephric tubules appear. The two heart tubes fuse in midline and rhythmic contractions can be seen.

At the beginning of the second month of pregnancy (embryo 7- to 8-mm crown-rump), the cerebral hemispheres enlarge and arm buds divide into a hand segment and arm-shoulder segment. By days 36–38 (embryo 14- to 16-mm crown-rump), the mullerian ducts are present. Other identifiable structures are the tip of the nose, early formation of the external ear, secondary bronchi, and aortic and pulmonary valves.

The end of week 8 marks the end of the embryonic period and the beginning of the fetal period. The fetus undergoes a stage of very rapid growth and differentiation between weeks 9 and 20. The external genitalia are fully differentiated into male or female organs by week 12 (Fig. 4.4).

PLACENTA

The embryo resides in membranes—the amnion, which encloses the cavity in which the fetus develops and an outer surface of extraembryonic mesoderm, which becomes the chorion. The chorion follows the outer suface of the stalk that connects the embryo to the placenta (early stage of umbilical cord). The placenta is composed of multiple projections which invade the myometrium. These villi have a connective tissue core and fetal capillaries develop within them. Eventually, the capillaries lie close to the syncytiotrophoblast and provide the necessary surface to subserve the functions of nutrition, excretion, and gas exchange for the fetus.

The mature placenta, which usually weighs 500 g at birth, is about 20 cm in diameter and 2.5 cm thick. It is normally implanted on the dorsal aspect of the upper part of the uterus, but may be implanted elsewhere, including near the cervical os (placenta praevia). The fetal surface is smooth and glistening and has many blood vessels leading from each segment (cotyledon) of the placenta. The maternal surface is rough and raised by the 10–38 cotyledons, separated by septae.

The umbilical cord at birth is usually about 50 cm long and 12 mm in diameter. It has pronounced spiral twists, with irregular projections of vessels. The cord is stiff during fetal life because the rate of blood flow through two arteries (to the placenta) and one vein (from the placenta) is high. The vessels are surrounded by gelatinous connective tissue derived from the primary mesoderm cells (Wharton jelly) (see also pp. 213).

Placental function during the last trimester is much more difficult to study in the human because manipulations of the placenta tend to induce contractions of the vessels that can be fatal to the fetus. Thus, it is not surprising that much of our understanding of late fetal physiology is inferred from studies on other primates, or the lamb. In lambs, however, the cotyledons of the placenta are separate from each other. The fetus can tolerate being marsupialized or exteriorized without contraction of vessels in the cord, thus, permitting cannulae to be inserted so that blood samples can be withdrawn (Young, 1981). These studies were pioneered by the English physiologists, and described in detail by Sir Joseph Barcroft in his classic "Researches on Prenatal Life."

HORMONAL CONTROL OF FETAL GROWTH

This complex topic has been the subject of many studies but gaps in understanding persist. This is, in part, because lower animals differ significantly from primates and also, the endocrine milieu of the fetus involves maternal, placental, and fetal hormones, which are difficult to separate experimentally (Ciba Foundation Symposium, 1974).

The approaches that have been useful in animals include endocrine ablations, treatment with hormones and measurement of serum hormone concentrations and cell receptors in pregnancy. In the human, some experiments of nature have been very instructive, such as congenital absence of the pancreas that is associated with profound fetal growth retardation. Radioimmunoassays for detection of small amounts of hormones now make possible serial determinations.

Growth hormone apparently has little role in the fetus. Both rabbit and human are independent of their own growth hormone in fetal life. Thyroxine has a role in influencing fetal prolactin secretion. Fetal growth is impaired in athyroid infants.

The principal growth hormone of the fetus is insulin. In those rare instances of congenital absence of the pancreas, fetal growth is profoundly retarded. In hyperinsulin states, the infant is oversize. High affinity insulin receptors are found in higher number on fetal mononuclear leukocytes than on adult cells (Thorsson and Hintz, 1977).

Prolactin is an important hormone of pregnancy in that it alters maternal metabolism to ensure adequate nutrition of the fetus. Its role in fetal growth is not clear because it has been found absent in otherwise normal gestation (Nielsen et al, 1979).

Cellular mechanisms of fetal growth are only beginning to be understood. Initially, studies were concentrated on the classical hormones which act distant from their site of synthesis. It is now apparent that these hormones (thyroxin, glucocorticoids, etc) regulate a host of growth factors whose function is paracrine or autocrine (Table 4.6).

Glucocorticoids rise toward the end of pregnancy in both small and large animals. Their role, first appreciated by Moog (1953), is as a timer of maturation. Prenatal administration to the mother 24–48 hours before preterm delivery allows precocious appearance of some enzymes that are important to extrauterine existence. Examples include enzymes essential to synthesis of the phospholipid components of pulmonary surfactant and intestinal enzymes.

Somatomedins are important regulators of fetal growth. Laron's dwarfs who resemble those with growth hormone deficiency have high levels of growth hormone but have low somatomedin levels and a reduction in bulk weight. The function of these peptide growth factors may be paracrine (on neighboring cells) or autocrine (self-regulatory within a cell; D'Ercole et al, 1986).

Epidermal growth factor, angiogenesis factors, and many other cell products are doubtless among the many players in the orchestra that dictate and regulate growth

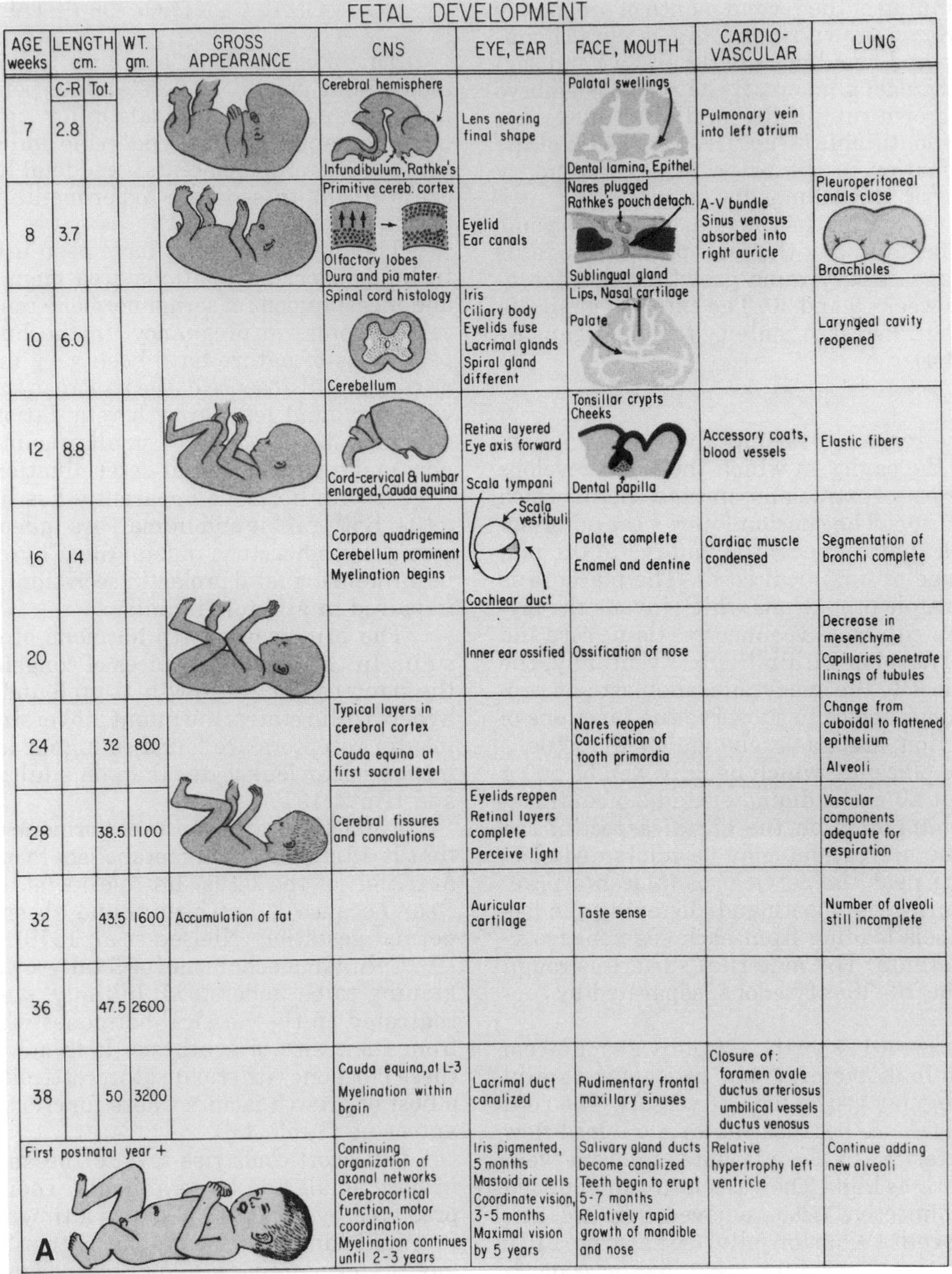

FETAL DEVELOPMENT

AGE weeks	LENGTH cm. C-R	LENGTH cm. Tot.	WT. gm.	GROSS APPEARANCE	CNS	EYE, EAR	FACE, MOUTH	CARDIO-VASCULAR	LUNG
7	2.8				Cerebral hemisphere; Infundibulum, Rathke's	Lens nearing final shape	Palatal swellings; Dental lamina, Epithel.	Pulmonary vein into left atrium	
8	3.7				Primitive cereb. cortex; Olfactory lobes; Dura and pia mater	Eyelid; Ear canals	Nares plugged; Rathke's pouch detach.; Sublingual gland	A-V bundle; Sinus venosus absorbed into right auricle	Pleuroperitoneal canals close; Bronchioles
10	6.0				Spinal cord histology; Cerebellum	Iris; Ciliary body; Eyelids fuse; Lacrimal glands; Spiral gland different	Lips, Nasal cartilage; Palate		Laryngeal cavity reopened
12	8.8				Cord-cervical & lumbar enlarged, Cauda equina	Retina layered; Eye axis forward; Scala tympani	Tonsillar crypts; Cheeks; Dental papilla	Accessory coats, blood vessels	Elastic fibers
16	14				Corpora quadrigemina; Cerebellum prominent; Myelination begins	Scala vestibuli; Cochlear duct	Palate complete; Enamel and dentine	Cardiac muscle condensed	Segmentation of bronchi complete
20						Inner ear ossified	Ossification of nose		Decrease in mesenchyme; Capillaries penetrate linings of tubules
24		32	800		Typical layers in cerebral cortex; Cauda equina at first sacral level		Nares reopen; Calcification of tooth primordia		Change from cuboidal to flattened epithelium; Alveoli
28		38.5	1100		Cerebral fissures and convolutions	Eyelids reopen; Retinal layers complete; Perceive light			Vascular components adequate for respiration
32		43.5	1600	Accumulation of fat		Auricular cartilage	Taste sense		Number of alveoli still incomplete
36		47.5	2600						
38		50	3200		Cauda equina, at L-3; Myelination within brain	Lacrimal duct canalized	Rudimentary frontal maxillary sinuses	Closure of: foramen ovale; ductus arteriosus; umbilical vessels; ductus venosus	
First postnatal year +				A	Continuing organization of axonal networks; Cerebrocortical function, motor coordination; Myelination continues until 2-3 years	Iris pigmented, 5 months; Mastoid air cells; Coordinate vision, 3-5 months; Maximal vision by 5 years	Salivary gland ducts become canalized; Teeth begin to erupt 5-7 months; Relatively rapid growth of mandible and nose	Relative hypertrophy left ventricle	Continue adding new alveoli

Figure 4.4A. Fetal development. Reproduced with permission from Smith DW: *Recognizable Patterns of Human Malformation*, 3rd edition. Philadelphia, WB Saunders, 1982.

and differentiation. The central nervous system and neurohormones probably occupy the first chairs in the orchestra. How the complex performance is conducted remains a mystery.

BODY COMPOSITION

Fetal growth has also been studied by analyses of body composition in infants at different gestational ages. These data are summarized in Table 4.7. Of note is the decrease in water content with increasing gestational age. This is obvious to the clinician based on observations of the gelatinous consistency of the VLBW infant, and the pronounced water losses that occur after birth. The amount of water is relatively greater in the extracellular space, and is excreted in the dilute urine of the neonate, so that 5–8% reduction in body weight occurs in the first week of life. Most of this represents

GUT	UROGENITAL	SKELETAL MUSCLE	SKELETON	SKIN	BLOOD, THYMUS LYMPH	ENDOCRINE
Pancreas, dorsal and ventral fusion	Renal vesicles 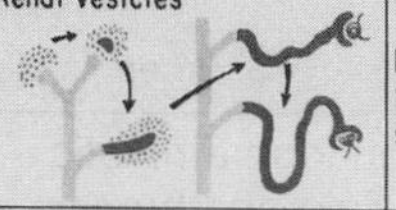	Differentiation toward final shape	Cartilaginous models of bones Chondrocranium Tail regression	Mammary gland 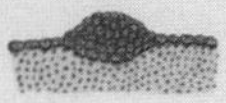		Parathyroid associated with thyroid Sympathetic neuroblasts invade adrenal
Liver relatively large Intestinal villi	Müllerian ducts fusing Ovary distinguishable	Muscles well represented Movement	Ossification center 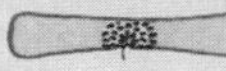 Sternum 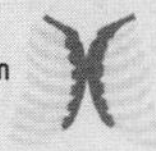	Basal layer 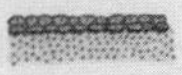	Bone marrow Thymus halves unite Lymphoblasts around the lymph sacs	Thyroid follicles
Gut withdrawal from cord Pancreatic alveoli Anal canal	Renal excretion Bladder sac Müllerian tube into urogenital sinus Vaginal sacs Prostate	Perineal muscles	Joints 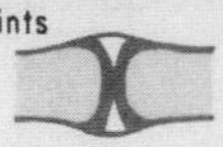	Hair follicles 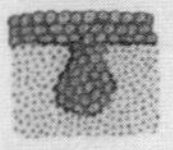 Melanocytes	Enucleated R.B.C.'s Thymus yields reticulum and corpuscles Thoracic duct Lymph nodes; axillary iliac	Adrenalin Noradrenalin
Gut muscle layers Pancreatic islets Bile	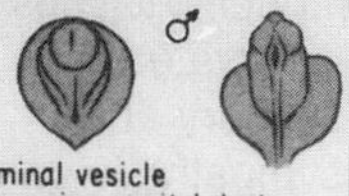 ♀ ♂ Seminal vesicle Regression, genital ducts		Tail degenerated Notochord degenerated	Corium, 3 layers Scalp, body hair Sebaceous glands Nails beginning	Blood principally from bone marrow Thymus-medullary and lymphoid	Testicle-Leydig cells Thyroid-colloid in follicle Anterior pituitary acidophilic granules Ovary-prim. follicles
Omentum fusing with transverse colon Mesoduodenum, asc. & desc. colon attach to body wall. Meconium. Gastric, intest. glands	Typical kidney Mesonephros involuting Uterus and vagina	In-utero movement can be detected	Distinct bones	Dermal ridges hands Sweat glands Keratinization		Anterior pituitary-basophilic granules
Decrease in mesenchyme Capillaries penetrate lining of tubules		No further collecting tubules		Venix caseosa Nail plates Mammary budding	Blood formation decreasing in liver	
						Testes-decrease in Leydig cells
						Testes descend
	Urine osmolarity continues to be relatively low			Eccrine sweat Lanugo hair prominent Nails to fingertips		
			Only a few secondary epiphyseal centers ossified in knee		Hemoglobin 17-18 gm Leukocytosis	
B			Ossification of 2nd epiph. centers-hamate, capitate, proximal humerus, femur New ossif. 2nd epiph. centers till 10-12 yrs. Ossif. of epiphyses till 16-18 yrs.	New hair, gradual loss of lanugo hair	Transient (6 wk) erythroid hypoplasia Hemoglobin 11-12 gm 7S gamma globulin produced by 6 wks. Lymph nodes develop cortex, medulla	Transient estrinization Adrenal-regression of fetal zone Gonadotropin with feminization of ♀ 9-12 yr. (onset); masc. of ♂ 10-14 yr. (onset)

Figure 4.4B.

loss of stores of water, especially from skin, but also from the brain. Head circumferences are smaller when postnatal weight is low (Williams et al, 1977).

Of note also are the small fat stores in infants born prematurely. Most subcutaneous fat is accumulated after 34 weeks' gestation. Fat stores increase 0.1–1.2 g/dl or more than 10-fold, whereas protein accretion at 24–40 weeks increases 8.8–12 g/dl.

ENERGY REQUIREMENTS

Information about energy requirements has been gained by meticulous metabolic balance studies of human infants after birth. The energy requirements before birth are met by the placenta and are estimated by net accretion by the fetus. At the present time, techniques to examine the dynamic situation in the human

Table 4.6
Illustrative Growth Factors[1]

Name	Structure	Action	Sources	Regulation of Tissue Concentrations
Epidermal (EGF)	53-amino-acid peptide	Mitogen for cells of ectodermal and mesodermal origin	Found in amniotic fluid and human milk	Regulated by androgens and thyroxine
Somatomedins (insulin-like growth factors)	Peptides, amino-acid sequence with insulin	Mitogens for a wide variety of cells; cell surface receptors are ubiquitous	Synthesized by many tissues	Regulation by growth hormone postnatally, and placental lactogen prenatally; nutrient supply important
Nerve growth factor	13,259 da peptide 25% homologous	Promotes survival, differentiation and axonal outgrowth of sensory and sympathetic ganglia	Peripheral tissues innervated by sensory and sympathetic ganglia	Regulated, in part, by thyroxine
Fibroblast pneumonocyte factor	Low molecular weight peptide	Stimulates type 2 alveolar cells to make surfactant	Lung fibroblasts	Responds to glucocorticoids
Erythropoietin	Acidic sialoprotein 166 amino acids	Stimulates mitosis and differentiation of red cell precursors	Kidney	Increases in response to hypoxia, androgens, and growth hormone
Interleukins				
1	Group of peptides	Act on T and B lymphocytes	Macrophages	Inflammation
2	15,500 da peptide	Promotes proliferation of T lymphocytes after antigenic stimulation	T lymphocytes	Inflammation
3	28,000 da glycosylated protein	Stimulates growth of immature lymphocytes	T lymphocytes	

[1]Other stimulators of fetal growth include cellular oncogenes, thymosins, and transforming growth factors (TGF).

fetus are not available. Yet knowledge of postnatal needs is essential for any reasonable approach to nutrition. Unfortunately, it is not even possible to duplicate the situation in utero with respect to requirements for weight gain or distribution of amino acids or trace minerals.

Experience with preterm infants has led to the following guidelines. A 1-kg infant requires 60 cal/24 hours to sustain life, and more than 100 kcal/24 hours to grow. The partition of calories measured by Reichman and colleagues in Toronto for infants weighing less than 1.3 kg at about 3 weeks of age was as follows:

	kcal/kg/day
Energy stored in a new tissue	67.8
Thermal effect of food	11.3
Basal metabolism	47.0
Cost of activity	4.3
Stool and urine	18.2

(Based on caloric intake 148 kcal/kg/day, gaining weight at 16.8 g/kg/ day)

TEMPERATURE REGULATION

The fetus in utero has a body temperature about 1°C higher than maternal core (deep body) temperature. After birth, which must be both a stimulating and chilling experience, the infant must regulate body temperature for homeostasis in the face of widely different environmental conditions. Heat losses after delivery at room temperature can be large. They occur by evaporation from the wet skin, convection from circulating air, conduction to surfaces of lower temperatures, and radiation to nearby objects. Because heat production cannot immediately compensate for such losses, most infants have lowered body temperatures in the minutes after birth unless their caretakers provide heated blankets or incubators. Premature infants are at special risk of excess heat loss because of a greater surface-to-volume ratio and poor insulation from small stores of subcutaneous fat.

Most infants attempt to increase metabolism when subjected to cold stress, not by shivering, but by chemical thermogenesis. Skin receptors, concentrated in the face, transmit thermal information to the central ner-

Table 4.7
Body Composition of the Reference Fetus[1]

Gestational Age (weeks)	Body Weight (g)	per 100 g body weight				per 100 g fat-free weight							
		Water (g)	Protein (g)	Lipid (g)	Other (g)	Water (g)	Protein (g)	Ca (mg)	P (mg)	Mg (mg)	Na (mEq)	K (mEq)	Cl (mEq)
24	690	88.6	8.8	0.1	2.5	88.6	8.8	621	387	17.8	9.9	4.0	7.0
25	770	87.8	9.0	0.7	2.5	88.4	9.1	615	385	17.6	9.8	4.0	7.0
26	880	86.8	9.2	1.5	2.5	88.1	9.4	611	384	17.5	9.7	4.1	7.0
27	1010	85.7	9.4	2.4	2.5	87.8	9.7	609	383	17.4	9.5	4.1	6.9
28	1160	84.6	9.6	3.3	2.4	87.5	10.0	610	385	17.4	9.4	4.2	6.9
29	1318	83.6	9.9	4.1	2.4	87.2	10.3	613	387	17.4	9.3	4.2	6.8
30	1480	82.6	10.1	4.9	2.4	86.8	10.6	619	392	17.4	9.2	4.3	6.8
31	1650	81.7	10.3	5.6	2.4	86.5	10.9	628	398	17.6	9.1	4.3	6.7
32	1830	80.7	10.6	6.3	2.4	86.1	11.3	640	406	17.8	9.1	4.3	6.6
33	2020	79.8	10.8	6.9	2.5	85.8	11.6	656	416	18.0	9.0	4.4	6.5
34	2230	79.0	11.0	7.5	2.5	85.4	11.9	675	428	18.3	8.9	4.4	6.4
35	2450	78.1	11.2	8.1	2.6	85.0	12.2	699	443	18.6	8.9	4.5	6.3
36	2690	77.3	11.4	8.7	2.6	84.6	12.5	726	460	19.0	8.8	4.5	6.1
37	2940	76.4	11.6	9.3	2.7	84.3	12.8	758	479	19.5	8.8	4.5	6.0
38	3160	75.6	11.8	9.9	2.7	83.9	13.1	795	501	20.0	8.8	4.5	5.9
39	3330	74.8	11.9	10.5	2.8	83.6	13.3	836	525	20.5	8.7	4.6	5.8
40	3450	74.0	12.0	11.2	2.8	83.3	13.5	882	551	21.1	8.7	4.6	5.7

[1]Data of Ziegler EE, et al: *Growth* 40:329, 1976.

vous system, which activates the autonomic system to release norepinephrine. This in turn promotes peripheral vasoconstriction and displays itself in the blue hands and feet of chilled infants (acrocyanosis). Brown fat, distributed in term infants around the great vessels, the nape of the neck, and in perirenal fat, has a high oxidative capacity and through exothermic reactions produces local heat to the blood going to vital organs (Hull, 1966).

Thermographic studies in term infants with modest cold exposure demonstrate the warmest skin over the central core, mean skin temperatures over upper arm and upper thigh, and coolest temperatures over the distal extremities. The infant is in a thermoneutral environment when oxygen consumption is lowest and all skin surfaces are at the same temperature. When differences in temperature between abdominal wall and distal extremities can be felt by an observer, the infant is subject to cold stress and requires further heating.

The increase in metabolism resulting from cold stress can be assessed by measuring oxygen consumption. In a term infant, a fall in environmental temperature from 33° to 31°C is a sufficient stimulus to double oxygen consumption, which, in turn, requires an approximate doubling of alveolar ventilation. Clearly, the low birth weight infant who may have pulmonary insufficiency may not be able to increase oxygen intake adequately. The consequence is hypoxia, lactic acidemia, and a fall in body temperature. This sequence of events can be lethal if permitted to continue. An arterial oxygen tension of 45–55 torr depresses the infant's capacity to generate heat and a tension of 30 torr abolishes it. Thus, a fall in body temperature is an index of poor blood oxygenation, under circumstances which should be preventable with appropriate application of heat to the infant.

From a practical viewpoint, an optimal skin temperature is 36°–36.5°C. The operative environmental temperatures for infants of different weights and postnatal age have been summarized by Hey (1975). For the very immature infant in the first days of life, incubator temperatures of 37° with over 50% relative humidity are needed (Sauer et al, 1984).

FETAL GAS EXCHANGE

The placenta is the organ of fetal gas exchange, bringing oxygen to the fetus and removing carbon dioxide. It is in a sense the fetal lung. Under conditions where the partial pressure of oxygen is low (i.e., equivalent to life at the summit of Everest) the fetus has adopted at least three adaptations. First, distribution of the fetal circulation is arranged so that the most oxygenated blood is delivered to the myocardium and the brain, and the least oxygenated blood to the "dormant" fetal organs, lung, intestine, and kidney, whose functions are largely subserved by the placenta. The second adaptation is the relatively high volume of red cells (hematocrit) in the fetus (Table 4.8). The oxygen-carrying capacity of the blood is increased by the increase in numbers of red cells, and also by the third adaptation, the increase in oxygen-carrying capacity of fetal hemoglobin (Barcroft, 1946).

Adult hemoglobin is 95% saturated at oxygen tensions of 100 torr; fetal hemoglobin is 95% saturated at oxygen tensions of about 50 torr. The difference depends on the concentration of 2,3-diphosphoglycerate (2,3 DPG). This organic phospate decreases the affinity of hemoblobin A (adult) for oxygen and, thus, promotes its release.

Fetal hemoglobin does not interact significantly with 2,3-DPG; thus, cells with fetal hemoglobin have

Table 4.8
Mean Red Cell Values During Gestation[1]

Age (weeks)	Hb (g/dl)	Hematocrit (%)	RBC (10^6/mm^3)	Mean Corpusc. Volume (fl)	Mean Corpusc. Hb (pg)	Mean Corpusc. Hb Concentration (g/dl)	Nucleated RBC (% of RBCs)	Reticulocytes (%)	Diameter (μ)
12	8.0-10.0	33	1.5	180	60	34	5-0-8.0	40	10.5
16	10.0	35	2.0	140	45	33	2.0-4.0	10-25	9.5
20	11.0	37	2.5	135	44	33	1.0	10-20	9.0
24	14.0	40	3.5	123	38	31	1.0	5-10	8.8
28	14.5	45	4.0	120	40	31	0.5	5-10	8.7
34	15.0	47	4.4	118	38	32	0.2	3-10	8.5

[1]Reproduced with permission from Oski, FA, Naiman JL: *Hematologic Problems in the Newborn*, 3rd edition. Philadelphia, WB Saunders, 1982.

a relative increase in oxygen-carrying capacity. Postnatally, when oxygen delivery to actively metabolizing tissues is essential, and the lung takes over gas exchange, it is an advantage to promote oxygen release with relatively more adult hemoglobin. The changes with postnatal age have been well studied and are illustrated in Figure 4.5.

The Bohr effect also favors gas exchange in the fetus; that is, the influence of Pco_2 on oxygen affinity of hemoglobin. The effect depends on the reduction in Pco_2 as fetal blood gives up CO_2 to the maternal circulation; the rise in Pco_2 in the maternal circulation favors a movement of oxygen to the fetus. The combined effect of the opposite "Bohr shifts" increases the difference in partial pressures of oxygen by about 2 torr (higher in the mother). This effect does not appear to be critically important, however, because infants with Rh incompatibility given adult hemoglobin fare well in utero. (For further details the reader is referred to Strang LB: *Neonatal Respiration. Physiological and Clinical Studies.* Oxford, Blackwell Scientific Publications, 1977).

EXCRETION

In the human fetus, nephrogenesis is complete by the end of the 36th week of gestation. Infants born before then continue nephrogenesis in postnatal life.

Studies on fetal animals confirm that in utero the kidneys (like the intestine and the lungs) are relatively poorly perfused compared to postnatal perfusion. These are the dormant fetal organs whose main functions are served by the placenta. Indeed, infants born without kidneys can be well-developed at birth. Approximately 3–5% of combined ventricular output perfuses fetal kidneys (in contrast to about 50% to the placenta). In neonates, renal blood flow increases with postnatal and postconceptual age. It is estimated to double by 2 weeks of postnatal age, and reaches adult levels by 2 years.

The glomerular filtration rate as measured with inulin clearance in prematures at 28 weeks' gestation is 5 ml/min/m^2, and at 40 weeks, it is 12 ml/min/m^2. It then doubles postnatally by 2 weeks of age (Fawer et al, 1979).

Newborns have a relative inability to excrete promptly a sodium and volume load. The situation improves so that by 1 year, sodium excretion reaches 16 mEq/hour/m^2.

Urine-diluting capacity is well-developed because urine osmolality can be 25–35 mOsm/L. However, the immature kidney has a problem with a hypotonic load because of a low glomerular filtration rate. Urine concentrating ability is limited. When infants were thirsted for the first 72 hours of life in the 1950s, urine osmo-

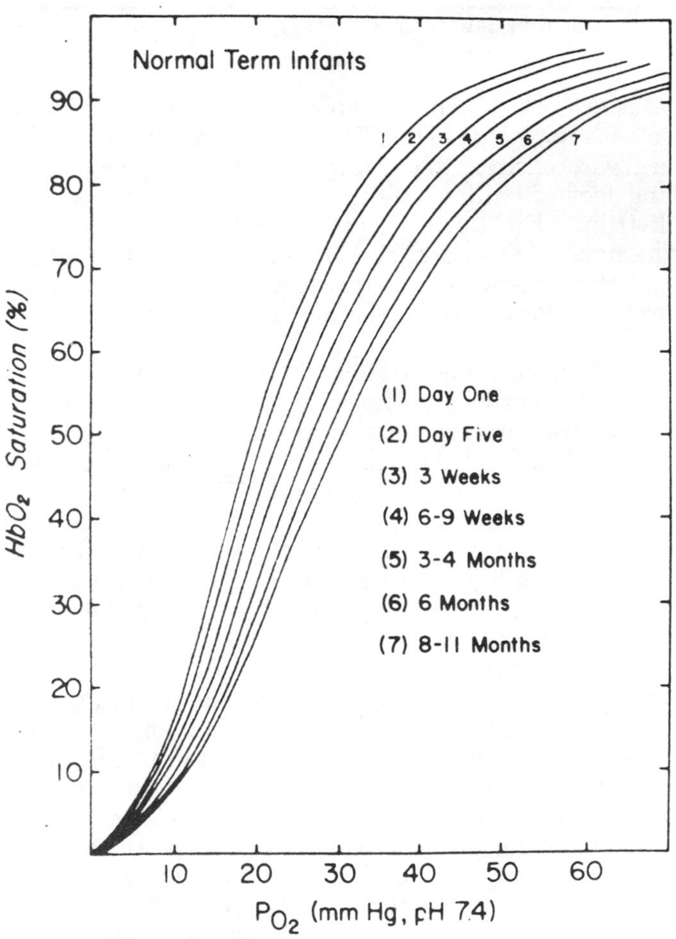

Figure 4.5. The oxygen affinity of blood from term infants at birth and at different postnatal ages. The gradual rightward shift of the oxygen saturation curve indicates increased oxygen release from hemoglobin as infants get older. This decreased oxygen affinity is due to decrease in hemoglobin F and an increase in hemoglobin A. From Oski FA, Delivoria-Papadopoulos M: *J Pediatr* 77:941, 1980.

lality was 680 mOsm/L compared to 1400 mOsm/L in adults under similar circumstances. Presumably the problem relates to low levels of antidiuretic hormone and relative unresponsiveness of the renal distal tubule to the hormone. Low birth weight infants tend to lose sodium through impaired tubular resorption.

Preterm infants are less able to acidify urine than those at term. The urine pH is often over 6. Urine is maximally acidified by 1 month of postnatal age.

Evaluation of Renal Function

URINANALYSIS

In the first days of life, urine specific gravity or osmolarity will reflect fluid intake and can range 1.001–1.021 (50–700 mOsm/kg H_2O). Proteinuria is common and has been detected in about three-fourths of term infants. A concentration greater than 2+ in a qualitative reaction is unusual and deserves repeat quantitative analysis. Tubular resorption of amino acids and phosphate is lower in preterm than term infants.

Uric acid crystals are common in urine specimens especially after stress such as asphyxia or hypoxia. Their red-brown color may be observed in a diaper and can readily be distinguished from blood by a negative heme test. Hyperuricosuria is associated with oliguria.

Cellular elements are similar to those found in urine of older children. Occasional white cells are often seen in a voided specimen. Catheterization or a suprapubic puncture is necessary to evaluate bacteriuria. Hematuria is abnormal (unless introduced at the time of suprapubic puncture).

URINE FLOW RATE

Urine flow can vary widely. The bladder capacity at term is about 30 ml. Urine production in the fetus is about 10 ml/kg/hour so it is clear why many infants void soon after delivery. By 12 hours 50% will have voided and by 24 hours nearly all should have voided. A careful examination is warranted at 24 hours in the absence of voiding, although some normal infants will not void for 48 hours. Postnatal urine flow rates in term infants are variable at 15–60 ml/24 hours. Volume is rarely recorded. Rather specific gravity or osmolality are more appropriate measures of hydration or solute loads.

GLOMERULAR FILTRATION RATE

The plasma creatinine concentration can be used to estimate glomerular filtration rates in infants and children. Plasma creatinine levels are relatively high (1.2 mg/dl) before 34 weeks and fall gradually toward term, then rapidly between 1 and 6 days of life. By 1–2 months of age values are about 0.25 mg/dl. Inasmuch as the range is wide, serial determinations are necessary. A significant increase in plasma creatinine is always abnormal (Stonestreet and Oh, 1978).

RADIOGRAPHY AND ULTRASONOGRAPHY

The success of intravenous urography depends on an adequate glomerular filtration rate and plasma concentration of the contrast material to permit visualization of renal parenchyma and collecting systems. Experience shows poor results in most infants in the first week of life, because of poor visualization of the kidneys. Because of this, ultrasonography has become a popular technique by which to evaluate the urinary tract. The presence of anatomically normal kidneys is established easily as is agenesis, dysplasia, hydronephrosis, polycystic disease, and other more unusual conditions. Ultrasonography aids in selecting the appropriate next study be it voiding cystourethrography, radionuclide scintigraphy, or percutaneous nephrostomy.

BLOOD PRESSURE

In the fetus, mean arterial blood pressure is 25–40 mm Hg. In premature infants it is between 30 and 50 mm Hg and, by term, it is 50–70 mm Hg on the first day of life. It increases to 60–80 mm Hg by the end of the first week even in infants < 34 weeks (Tan, 1988).

Blood pressure in normal infants is not raised by volume expansion. Even 100 ml from the placenta given to the infant before the cord was clamped did not result in an increase in pressure 2 hours later (Oh et al, 1966). If the infant is volume depleted, blood pressure can be raised by restoring volume.

HYPERTENSION

No upper limit of normal blood pressure has been defined for newborn infants, but clearly some have major increases (over 100 mm Hg mean pressure). Investigation into causes usually reveals a renovascular cause, such as renal artery or vein thrombosis, coarctation of aorta, emboli to the kidney (from clots at tip of umbilical catheter) or renal cortical necrosis.

Nutrition

The fundamental nutritional needs of most babies are met by adequate intake of breast milk of healthy mothers (see pp. 29). Modified cow's milk formulas are available in most parts of the world and may be substituted for human milk if mother's milk is not available, or the mother prefers to use a formula. Whole cow's milk is not ideal before about 6 months of age because it has relatively more protein and less carbohydrate than human milk or prepared formulas.

Formulas are modified to produce growth and amino acid profiles comparable to those in human milk fed infants. For preterm infants, the whey-casein ratio is adjusted to provide more whey. For term infants, such adjustments are not required (Raiha, 1985). Other modifications of cow's milk for low birth weight infants include medium-chain triglycerides in addition to coconut and soy bean oils added to nonfat milk to bring the total fat to 4.5 g/dl. Calcium is increased in some preparations and phosphorus is lower than that in cow's milk, but higher than in human milk (Watkins, 1985; Wu et al, 1986).

Taurine has been identified as a "conditionally essential" nutrient because synthesizing capacity is limited. When added to formulas for preterm infants, intestinal fat absorption is increased, (Galeano et al, 1987). When added to parental alimentation solutions of infants and children, cholestasis was nearly eliminated, (Heird et al, 1987). The major metabolic role of taurine is conjugation with bile acids in the liver (Wright et al, 1986).

Calcium and phosphorus requirements are relatively greater in preterm infants who are rapidly growing. Osteopenia, fractures, and rickets were common in low birth weight infants before it was realized that they needed more calcium and phosphorus. When the calcium content of formula is increased to provide 220–250 mg/kg day, and phosphate to 110–125 mg/kg/day bone mineralization proceeds at about the intrauterine rate (Steichen et al, 1980).

Long-term use of furosemide in VLBW infants has resulted in hypercalciuria. Presumably, the daily calcium losses not only contribute to nephrocalcinosis but also depletion of skeletal calcium (Carey and Rowe, 1987).

ELECTROLYTE ABNORMALITIES

Recognition that VLBW infants may have significant hyponatremia and hypocalcemia has made it imperative to measure electrolytes periodically, particularly in infants between 2 and 6 weeks of age.

Hyponatremia (plasma sodium under 120 mEq/L) may be from low intake or increased losses in association with water retention. Some such infants have presented with convulsions from the electrolyte imbalance. With continuing growth, increased amounts of sodium are required not only for normal extracellular concentrations but they also coprecipitate with calcium in bone formation. Added to these problems, the immature kidney is inefficient in retaining calcium and both hyponatremia and hyperkalemia may occur in these VLBW infants. On the basis of balance studies, Day et al (1976) advocate that VLBW infants receive 3 mEq/kg/24 hours of sodium to achieve normonatremia between ages 2 and 5 weeks.

Sodium is 14–16 mEq/L in formulas for preterm infants, which is about double that of human milk to meet their requirements. Diet supplements of calcium and phosphorus are also required to prevent chemical or even radiographic rickets in preterm infants. This condition is widely recognized and occurs even when serum concentrations of vitamin D metabolites are normal or elevated. Laing and colleagues (1985) found that they could prevent elevations in alkaline phosphatase in infants weighing less than 1.5 kg when the mean calcium intake was 4 mMol/kg/day. Although precise nutritional requirements have not been defined for all groups of low birth weight infants, the recommendations of Laing seem appropriate at the present time and such intakes should be ensured to prevent deficiencies.

Most formulas have per liter about 3000 IU of vitamin A, 100–250 mg of vitamin C, 480–1000 IU of vitamin D, 18–25 IU of vitamin E, and minimal amounts of vitamin B group and K. Inasmuch as preterm infants do not consume enough milk to meet their vitamin requirements, vitamin supplements are given.

Trace Elements (see also Section 3)

Deficiencies of zinc, magnesium, and phosphorus can occur in infants on intravenous alimentation with mixtures that are inadequate in these minerals. Rarely are deficiencies encountered in infants on human milk or formula inasmuch as the daily requirements are readily met.

The requirements for trace elements are not well understood for preterm infants. Empirically, deficiencies are prevented by including in intravenous solutions:

Element	Amount/ml
zinc	400 μg
copper	200 μg
fluoride	10 μg
iodide	59 μg
manganese	200 μg

Hyperammonemia

Premature infants have levels of serum ammonia as much as twice that of term infants for the first 6–8

CASE ILLUSTRATION

A 2.2-kg infant was born after 35 weeks' gestation and had Apgar scores of 7 and 8 at 1 and 5 minutes, respectively. Her course was benign until 12 hours of age, when jerking movements of the extremities were noted, followed by lethargy, apnea, and the need for mechanical ventilation. Because septicemia was deemed likely, cultures were taken and antibiotics were given. An electroencephalogram showed generalized depression, with some α wave activity. Plasma ammonia was 2900 μ/dl at 76 hours (normal 5–150). Treatment with exchange transfusion and peritoneal dialysis, and intravenous alimentation with glucose and a fat emulsion was begun. The infant became responsive after 36 hours of dialysis when the plasma ammonia was 200 μ/dl.

Extensive laboratory studies, including liver biopsy at 6 weeks of age, established normal urea-cycle enzyme levels. At 24 months, she was normal in development and neurologic function.

COMMENT

A study of this patient underscores the importance of a search for metabolic derangements in any infant who deteriorates without obvious cause in the first hours or days of life (see Section 15). Transient hyperammonemia is unusual, but the possibility should always be considered in the differential diagnosis.

weeks of postnatal life (Batshaw and Brusilow, 1976). Usually these infants are asymptomatic. An unusual, but severe and potentially fatal elevation in ammonia may appear in the first or second day of life in preterm infants who present with central nervous system symptoms such as seizures, coma, apnea, and circulatory collapse. Some of these infants lack enzymes in the Krebs-Henseleit cycle (see pp. 947). Others have normal enzyme complements and can recover completely if the diagnosis is established and exchange transfusion and peritoneal dialysis is instituted promptly.

Designated transient hyperammonemia of the preterm infant, this condition is probably underdiagnosed and mistaken for sepsis, or intrauterine asphyxia. Ballard et al (1978) described five such infants, the course of one of which is summarized here.

NATURAL HISTORY AND EPIDEMIOLOGY OF LOW BIRTH WEIGHT

The incidence of low birth weight (less than 2.5 kg) varies widely among different populations. In the United States as a whole it is between 6 and 7% of all births, or about 250,000 per year. The variations among regions are significant and correlate in general with differences between the developing countries and the developed countries. For example, in 1982 for the developed countries 6.9% of infants born weighed less than 2500 g. The corresponding figure in the developing countries was 17.6%. The region with the highest rate is 31% in Middle South Asia, 19.7% for Asia as a whole, 14% for Africa, 10% in Latin America, and the lowest rates are in the United States and Europe; 6.8% and 6.5%, respectively. In some parts of India and Africa, it may be as high as 20% of all births. In Scandinavian countries and Japan, it is closer to 4% of births and, in some regions, may be as low as 2%. The incidence of births below 1.25 kg is estimated to be about 0.6–1.0% of births per year and varies less widely among different populations (Figs. 4.6–4.9).

The highest proportion of premature births in the United States is among persons of lower socioeconomic groups. Thus, nonwhite underprivileged groups have nearly twice the prematurity rate as the white race with higher socioeconomic status. Neonatal and infant mortality, whereas decreasing for all infants, remain nearly twice as high among nonwhites (Fig. 4.10). Thespecific mortality rates for the low birth weight infants, on the other hand, are somewhat lower for the nonwhites partly because these infants mature a few weeks ahead of white infants.

The reasons for the differences are perplexing. Miller has approached the problem by analyzing carefully a small cohort of white infants born during a 15-month period in Kansas City. He divided the probable causes of infant mortality (mostly associated with prematurity) into extrinsic and intrinsic causes. Among the extrinsic factors were fetal abnormalities, maternal complications of pregnancy, adverse maternal practices, and environmental factors. Intrinsic causes were race, sex, maternal height and weight parity, and gestational age. He found that in the absence of identifiable extrinsic factors, the number of infants born with a weight below 2.5 kg was 1.8% of 339 pregnancies. Fetal complications were found in 37 pregnancies and 38% of those infants were below 2.5 kg. Medical complications of pregnancy were higher among poorer mothers and, when present, resulted in 18.5% low birth weight infants. When adverse maternal practices were present (smoking, poor prenatal care, etc) 96% of the infants were of low birth weight. These striking results, which are clearly preliminary and based on a small sample, suggest that many events associated with low birth weight are theoretically preventable (Miller, 1983; Naeye, 1981).

One aspect of premature birth is its likelihood to recur. Once a mother has had a preterm birth, the risk of a repeat is about 25%. If two pregnancies have ended spontaneously preterm, the risk of a third similar event is about 70%. Among some of the reasons are uterine anatomy, incompetence of the cervix or abnormal growth of the placenta.

Other known events associated with preterm birth are multiple pregnancy (twins, etc); maternal infection, such as with *Mycoplasma* and *Chlamydia*, which may be subclinical and unknown by mother or obstetrician; maternal hypertension and/or heart disease; abnormal fetuses as in trisomies and other congenital anomalies; and short intervals between births. Sometimes ill-timed cesarean section can lead to unexpected prematurity. It is unfortunate that in at least one-third of pregnancies, no identifiable cause of premature birth is possible (see Table 4.9).

Prevention

The striking differences in the rate of preterm birth cited earlier require consideration of different practices. Overwhelmingly, higher socioeconomic class, and all that accompanies it, remains the most significant condition associated with a low rate of preterm birth.

It is impossible to quantify the impact of interventions, but collectively they can reduce prematurity significantly, as has been shown in recent years in Japan and Sweden. A prevention program in France was associated with a reduction in preterm births from 5.4% in 1971–1974 to 3.7% in 1979–1982 (Papiernik et al, 1985). In general, more attendance at prenatal clinics, obstetric monitoring, and a modest increase in the cesarean section rate, as well as liberalization of abortions as of 1975, could have been important contributions to the reduction in preterm births. Countries with the lowest prematurity rates provide paid absence from work for at least the last month of pregnancy. Avoidance of heavy exercise is thought to be one factor in prolonging pregnancy.

Prognosis

Throughout recorded history, the survival of some very small infants has been noted, although not well-documented because the infants were rarely weighed or measured before the 19th century. According to Cone

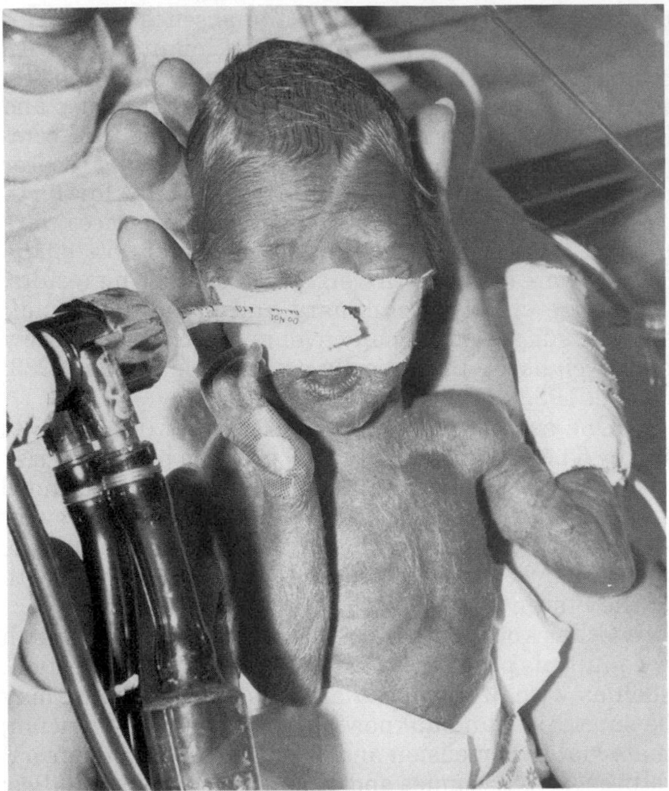

Figure 4.6. A 710-g infant girl born at 25 weeks of gestation because of incompetent cervix. She was vigorous at birth and breathed spontaneously. Because of her extreme prematurity and inevitable need for ventilatory assistance, a nasotracheal tube was inserted and attached to a mechanical ventilator.

Note the very fine hairs over the body (lanugo) which will disappear in a few weeks. The sparse amount of subcutaneous fat at this gestational age gives the infant a wrinkled appearance.

The bandage over the left hand protects the site of an intravenous feeding line. Photo courtesy of Mark Weber.

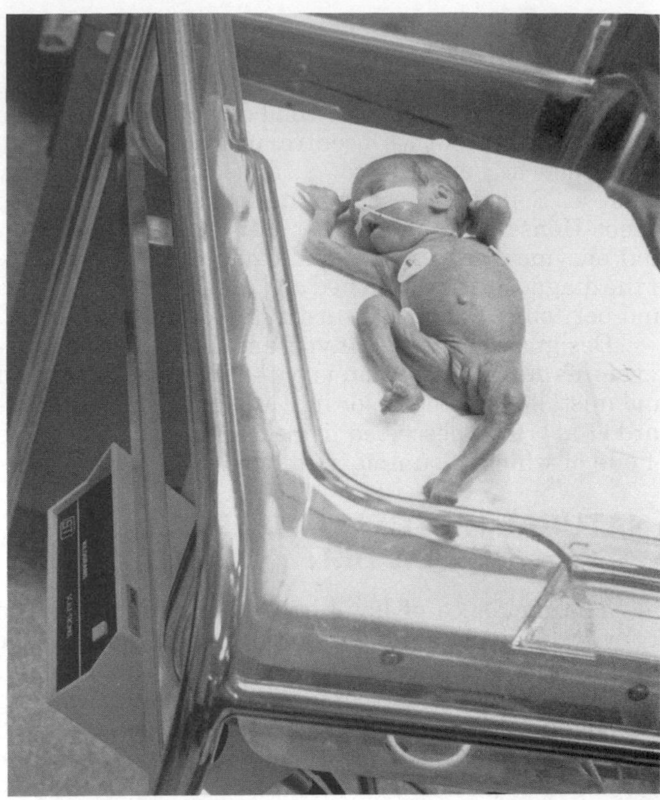

Figure 4.7. Same infant, age 6 weeks. Note the relatively large size of head to body and slightly distended abdomen. These are normal for an infant of such low birth weight at age 6 weeks. She had required ventilatory assistance for 33 days, but by 6 weeks, she maintained normal spontaneous breathing. She was receiving breast milk from her mother (who pumped her breasts every 4 hours). At this time, her weight was 850 g. (Her low weight was 660 g when she was 9 days old.) She was able to take some of her mother's milk from the breast by 2 months of age, but tired easily and was given the remainder by gavage. Photograph courtesy of Georgia Litwack.

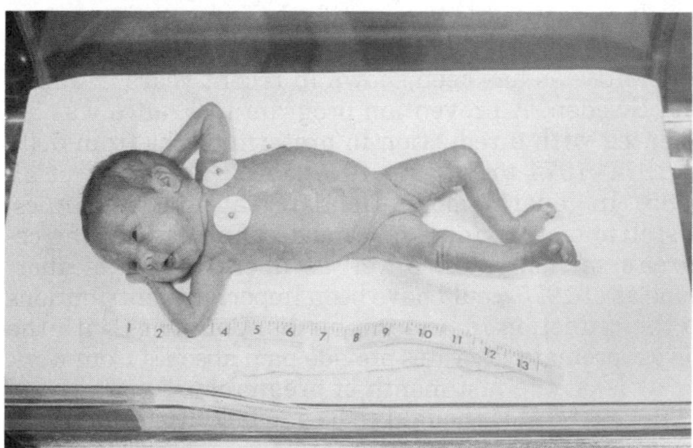

Figure 4.8. At 10 weeks old, the weight is 1 kg. At this stage, she was clearly able to differentiate her mother (who visited daily) from other caretakers, as indicated by eye contact and the hint of a smile. Her total fluid intake was 150 ml/kg/day and 134 cal/kg/day. Her weight gain was a consistent 20 g/kg/day. Photograph courtesy of Georgia Litwack.

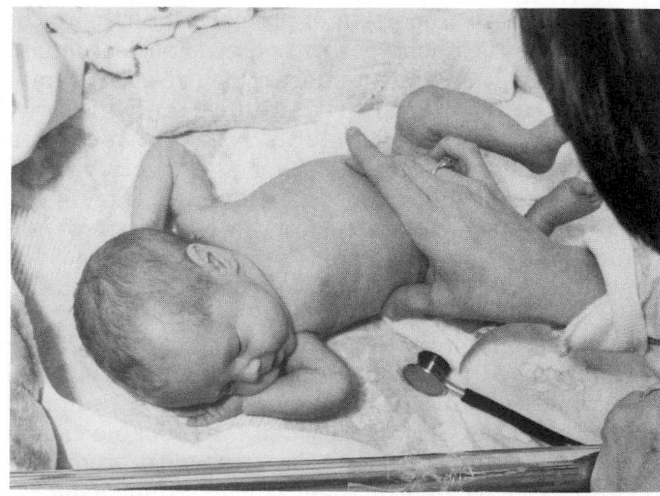

Figure 4.9. At 15 weeks old, or 40 weeks' postconceptual age, she was being prepared for discharge home with a weight of 1960 g. Photograph courtesy of Georgia Litwack.

Table 4.9
Principal Risk Factors for Low Birth Weight[1]

Demographic Risks	Placental problems, such as placenta previa, abruptio placentae
Age (less than 17; over 34)	Hyperemesis
Race (black)	Oligohydramnios/polyhydramnios
Low socioeconomic status	Anemia/abnormal hemoglobin
Unmarried	Isoimmunization
Low level of education	Fetal anomalies
Medical Risks Predating Pregnancy	Incompetent cervix
Parity (0 or more than 4)	Spontaneous premature rupture of membranes
Low weight for height	*Behavioral and Environmental Risks*
Genitourinary anomalies/surgery	Smoking
Selected diseases, such as diabetes, chronic hypertension	Poor nutritional status
Nonimmune status for selected infections, such as rubella	Alcohol and other substance abuse
Poor obstetric history including previous low birth weight infant, multiple spontaneous abortions	DES exposure and other toxic exposures, including occupational hazards
Maternal genetic factors (such as low maternal weight at own birth)	High altitude
Medical Risks in Current Pregnancy	*Health Care Risks*
Multiple pregnancy	Absent or inadequate prenatal care
Poor weight gain	Iatrogenic prematurity
Short interpregnancy interval	*Evolving Concepts of Risk*
Hypotension	Stress, physical and psychosocial
Hypertension/preeclampsia/toxemia	Uterine irritability
Selected infections, such as symptomatic bacteriuria, rubella, and cytomegalovirus	Events triggering uterine contractions
1st or 2nd trimester bleeding	Cervical changes detected before onset of labor
	Selected infections such as *Mycoplasma* and *Chlamydia trachomatis*
	Inadequate plasma volume expansion
	Progesterone deficiency

[1]Reproduced with permission from Summary: Preventing low birthweight. Institute of Medicine. *Nat Acad Sci*, Washington, D.C., 1985.

(1961), the first report of correct measurements on human infants was by Roederer in Gottingen in 1753. It was not until 1835 that Quetelet in Brussels published his studies on physical growth and development through childhood. Among the notables said to have been premature or small were Isaac Newton and Winston Churchill. Thus, it has long been known that premature infants can become normal or even distinguished individuals. The first extremely low birth weight infant whose survival was recorded was a 14-oz (420 g) infant born in Nova Scotia in 1937 (Munro, 1939). The infant was thought to be 2 months premature, which suggested severe intrauterine growth retardation and presumably organ maturation consistent with gestational age. In the absence of an incubator, the infant was kept in a warm oven and fed brandy and corn syrup from a dropper. By 4 months, the infant weighed 6 lb, and at 1 year, 13 lb 12 oz and was 25½ inches long.

Alm's study (1953) of 999 boys with birth weights of less than 2.5 kg, born between 1902 and 1921, was concerned almost exclusively with those weighing 1.75 kg or more. Higher mortality was noted until 2–3 years of age. Among the survivors of the first few years, the premature infants had a higher incidence of disorders attributed to birth injury, and were somewhat smaller at age 20 years.

In modern times, a number of follow-up studies have described the ever-improving outlook for infants of low birth weight, both with respect to mortality and morbidity. Ylppo, writing in 1919 described 323 surviving prematures under 2.5 kg and noted severe abnormalities in 10.5% of them. More than half the infants were dead by the time of follow-up at 7–8 years of age. A much quoted study was that of Drillien in 1948. By use of a questionnaire to obtain information, she compared 103 premature with 174 full-term infants followed for 1–4 years. Although only 40% of replies were received, the 23% of prematures with "behavior disorders" was in contrast to 15% of full-term infants. (These and other pioneering studies are reviewed by Alm I, in a supplement to *Acta Paediatr* 42:1-116, 1953.)

Drillien's later studies, published in 1964, took note of a reduction in the proportion of serious handicaps in the survivors born between 1956 and 1960, although the rate was about 30% among infants who weighed less than 3 lb (1360 g) at birth.

The reports of the outcome of infants born after neonatal intensive care have all been encouraging, when contrasted to findings on infants born before the mid-1960s in the United States, Britain, and Australia. One

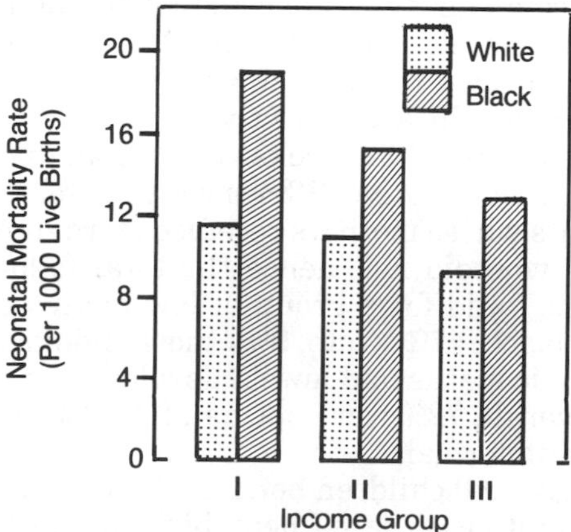

Figure 4.10. Neonatal mortality rates for the city of Boston 1972–1979, according to race and income group. Group 1 is the lowest income group. Reproduced with permission from Wise et al: *N Engl J Med* 313:360, 1985.

Table 4.10
Diagnostic Assessment Timetable[1]

Age of evaluation	Metabolic screening test	Physical growth	Neurological assessment	Ophthalmological assessment	Auditory assessment	Bayley motor mental[2]	Behavioral questions	Zimmerman[3]	Beery visual motor integration[4]	Stanford-Binet,[5] McCarthy,[6] Murphy-Durrell, WISC [7]
Birth	+	+	+	+	+					
6 months [8]						+				
		+	+			+	+			
12 months						+				
		+	+	+	+	+	+			
2 years		+	+			+	+			
3 years										+
		+	+	+			+	+	+	Stanford-Binet
4 years		+	+			+	+	+	+	9 ,10
5 years		+	+			+	+	+	+	9 ,10

[1]Reproduced with permission from *Guidelines for Perinatal Care*. American Academy of Pediatrics American College of Obstetrics and Gynecology, 1983.
[2]Bayley N: Bayley Scale of Infant Development. New York, The Psychological Corp, 1969
[3]Zimmerman JH: Preschool Language Scale. Columbus, OH, Charles E. Merrill, 1969
[4]Beery KE: Developmental Test of Visual Motor Integration. Chicago, Follett Educational Corp. 1967
[5]Terman LM, Merrill MA: Stanford-Binet Intelligence Scale, Boston, Houghton-Mifflin, 1973
[6]McCarthy M: McCarthy Scales of Children's Abilities, New York, The Psychological Corp, 1972
[7]Wechsler Intelligence Scale for Children
[8]Corrected age
[9]Choice of Stanford Binet, McCarthy, or Wechsler
[10]Murphy-Durrell reading readiness analysis (optional)

of the most notable is that of Kitchen et al (1984) from Melbourne, reporting on infants of 500–999 g born in 1979 and 1980. Survival of this group (previously considered negligible) was 29% for those born in major centers, and 25.4% overall. The morbidity was significant among survivors with 22% severely impaired and only 48% normal. Weight-specific survival by 100-g increments is important in interpretation of data because the outlook improves so much with added weight and gestational age.

When the spectrum of low birth weight infants is viewed from a long-range perspective, the overall outlook for normal survival is excellent. The collaborative group on antenatal steroid therapy (National Institutes of Health) in 1984 reported a 3-year follow-up of 739 infants enrolled in a prospective study. Their gestational ages averaged 31 weeks, 12.7% had died; 32.5% were lost to follow-up. No differences were found among those infants whose mothers received steroid compared with those who did not, hence the total follow-up information is valid for a group of low birth weight infants (44% black, 47% white, 9% other). Infants of lowest socioeconomic status had lowest development scores at 3 years. Overall, 72% were normal, 22% "suspect," and 5% clearly abnormal.

A group of 80 children born in 1976 and recipients of neonatal intensive care (mean birth weights 1209 ± 255 g, gestational ages 30.1 ± 2.4 weeks) were evaluated at age 5 years by Klein et al in Cleveland (1985); 65 were neurologically intact with normal IQ. When compared with infants born at term, they were distinguishable only by lower performance on spatial relations testing and on a visual-motor integration test. Of the 15 children with abnormalities, five had neurologic disabilities such as spastic diplegia and 10 had IQs below 85.

This careful evaluation of functional performance should alert families and teachers to the possibility of some visual-motor and visual-perceptual problems that are not accounted for by ocular abnormalities. Others have reported similar findings, and have noted that the development of visual-evoked responses is delayed after preterm birth, and auditory-evoked responses are not. Earlier recognition of these problems and appropriate intervention seems in order. Guidelines for assessment of preterm infants up to 5 years of age are listed in Table 4.10.

Although such data are important to monitor effects of nursery practices, they are of less help to the pediatrician whose patient may be born prematurely because the fetus is abnormal genetically (i.e., it may be trisomic, or because of infection, or for other reasons which have their own prognosis). In general, the more premature the infant, the greater is the likelihood of serious handicap. This is not inevitable, however, and there is reason to struggle for the survival of even these infants provided that major malformations or other potentially lethal problems are not present (Table 4.11).

CONTROVERSY

The increase in survival and decrease in morbidity for infants weighing more than 700 g in most neonatal intensive care centers has been well documented. The

Table 4.11
Variables Associated with Increasing Survival After 24–28 Weeks' Gestation[1]

Variable	Significance
Gestation increasing	p = .001
Hypertension absent	.007
Singleton pregnancy	.007
Prenatal steroids	.018
Tocolytics	NS
Cesarean section	NS
Vertex	NS
Monitored labor	NS
326 infants, 172 discharged alive	

[1]Data from Kitchen et al: *Obstet Gynecol* 66:149, 1985.

outlook for infants weighing less than 700 g is less well documented, although some infants of even 600 g have done well.

The problem is that as VLBW infants are resuscitated and ventilated, many will survive, but with major neurologic disabilities. The trend for even more vigorous intervention on behalf of infants of 500–800 g was described by Hack et al (1986).

At some point, it is evident that an infant is previable, although this may not be predicted precisely by either birth weight or gestational age. Other factors, including sex and race are determinants of the outlook for survival. (Female infants are more mature at a given gestational age than males and black infants are more mature than white.) Perhaps the major determinant of survival of VLBW infants is the condition at birth and the quality of intensive care that is immediately available.

The controversy revolves around the question of when to resuscitate and mobilize intensive care. Some physicians will try to resuscitate an infant with an Apgar score of 0 (no heartbeat at birth is defined as a stillbirth). Some will also try to support life in any infant with a heart beat regardless of gestational age or weight, which highlights the paradox of treating an abortus as an infant. No one to date has undertaken to write guidelines for procedures in the unusual circumstance of a liveborn infant under 500 g, and most countries do not report such infants as liveborn in neonatal statistics.

Our view, as in most difficult decisions, is to ask for individualization by caring physicians and loving parents.

REFERENCES

Alm I: *Acta Paediatr* (Suppl)42:1–116, 1953.

Ballard R, Vincour B, Reynolds JW, et al: Transient hyperammonemia of the preterm infant. *N Engl J Med* 299:920, 1978.

Barcroft J: *Researches on Prenatal Life.* Springfield, IL, Charles C Thomas, 1946.

Batshaw ML, Brusilow SW: Hyperammonemia and hyperglutaminemia in low birth weight infants. *Pediatr Res* 10:405, 1976.

Carey DE, Rowe JC: Metabolic bone disease in premature infants. *Pediatr Ann* 16:947, 1987.

Centers for Disease Control: Update: Incidence of low birth weight. *MMWR* 33:459, 1984.

Ciba Foundation Symposium 27 (new series): Size at birth. Amsterdam, Elsevier Excerpta Medica, Associated Sci Publ, 1974.

Cone TE Jr: De pondere infantum recens natorum: The history of weighing the newborn infant. *Pediatrics* 46:490, 1961.

Cook PS, Nicoll CS: Hormonal control of fetal growth. *Physiologist* 26:317, 1983.

Coulter DM, Avery ME: Paradoxical reduction in tissue hydration with weight gain in neonatal rabbit pups. *Pediatr Res* 114:1122, 1980.

Day GM, Radde IC, Balfe JW, et al: Electrolyte abnormalities in very low birthweight infants. *Pediatr Res* 10:522, 1976.

D'Ercole AJ, Hill DJ, Strain AJ, et al: Tissue and plasma somatomedin-C/Insulin-like growth factor I concentrations in the human fetus during the first half of gestation. *Pediatr Res* 20:253, 1986.

Deter RL, Harrist RB, Hadlock FB, et al: Fetal head and abdominal circumferences ratios. *J Clin Ultrasound* 10:365, 1982.

Drillien CM: Studies in prematurely born children in the preschool period. *Arch Dis Child* 23:69, 1948.

Drillien CM: *The Growth and Development of the Prematurely Born Infant.* Baltimore, Williams & Wilkins, 1964.

England MA: Normal fetal development. In *Color Atlas of Life Before Birth.* Chicago, Year Book Medical Publishers, 1983.

Fawer C, Torredo A, Guignard JP, et al: Single injection clearance in the neonate. *Biol Neonate* 35:321, 1979.

Galeano NF, Darling P, Lepage G, et al: Taurine supplementation of a premature formula improves fat absorption in preterm infants. *Pediatr Res* 22:67, 1987.

Gluck L: The infectious etiology of premature labor. Abstracts. Scientific Presentation at the International Congress of Pediatrics, Honolulu, July 7–12, 1986.

Hack M, Fanaroff AA: Changes in the delivery room care of the extremely small infant (<750 g). Effects on morbidity and outcome. *N Engl J Med* 314:660, 1986.

Hambraeus L, Forsum E, Lonnerdal B: Nutritional aspects of breast versus cow's milk formulas. In McFarlane H, Hambraeus L, Hanson LA (eds): *Food and Immunology Symposium.* Stockholm, Almqvist and Wiskell, 1976.

Heird WC, Dell RB, Helms RA, et al: Amino acid mixture designed to maintain normal plasma amino acid patterns in infants and children requiring parenteral nutrition. *Pediatrics* 80:401, 1987.

Hey E: Thermal neutrality. *Br Med Bull* 31:69, 1975.

Hull D: Brown adipose tissue. *Br Med Bull* 22:92, 1966.

Huszar G, Naftolin F: The myometrium and uterine cervix in normal and preterm labor. *N Engl J Med* 311:571, 1984.

Jones CT, Rolph TP: Metabolism during fetal life. A functional assessment of metabolic development. *Physiol Rev* 65:357, 1985.

Jost A: Fetal hormones and fetal growth. In:Keller P(ed): *Gynecologic and Obstetric Investigation.* vol. 5. Basel, Karger, pp. 1–20.

Katyal SL, Singh G, Silverman J, et al: Deficient lung surfactant apoproteins in amniotic fluid with mature phospholipid profile from diabetic pregnancies. *Am J Obstet Gynecol* 148:118, 1984.

Kitchen W, Ford G, Orgill A, et al: Outcome in infants with birth weight 500 to 999 gm: A regional study of 1979 and 1980 births. *J Pediatr* 104:921, 1984.

Klein N, Hack M, Gallagher J, et al: Preschool performance of children with normal intelligence who were very low-birth-weight infants. *Pediatrics* 75:531, 1985.

Laing IA, Glass EJ, Hendry GMA, et al: Rickets of prematurity: Calcium and phosphorus supplementation. *J Pediatr* 106:265, 1985.

Liggins GC: Initiation of spontaneous labor. *Clin Obstet Gynecol* 26:47, 1983.

Longo LD: Carbon monoxide: Effects on oxygenation of the fetus in utero. *Science* 194:523, 1976.

Longo LD: The biologic effects of carbon monoxide on the pregnant woman, fetus and newborn infant. *Am J Obstet Gynecol* 129:69, 1977.

Lorenz J, Kleinman L, Katagel U, et al: Water balance in very low birth weight infants: Relationship to water and sodium intake and effect on outcome. *J Pediatr* 101:423, 1982.

Mactutus CF, Fechter LD: Prenatal exposure to carbon monoxide: Learning and memory deficits. *Science* 223:409, 1984.

McCormick MC, Shapiro S, Starfield B: High risk young mothers: Infant mortality and morbidity in four areas in the United States. *Am J Publ Health* 74:18, 1984.
McLaurin JC: Changes in body water distribution during the first two weeks of life. *Arch Dis Child* 41:286, 1966.
Miller HC: A model for studying the pathogenesis and incidence of low birth weight infants. *Am J Dis Child* 137:323, 1983.
Mobossaleh M, Montgomery RK, Biller JA, et al: Development of carbohydrate absorption in the fetus and neonate. In: *Current Issues in Feeding the Normal Infant. Pediatrics* (Suppl) 75:160, 1985.
Moog F: The influence of the pituitary-adrenal system of the differentiation of phosphate in the duodenum of the suckling mouse. *J Exp Zool* 124:329, 1953.
Munro JS: A premature infant weighing less than one pound at birth who survived and developed normally. *Can Med Assoc J* 40:69, 1939.
Naeye RL: Influence of maternal cigarette smoking during pregnancy on fetal and childhood growth. *Obstet Gynecol* 57:18, 1981.
Nielsen PV, Pedersen H, Kampmann EM: Absence of human placental lactogen in an otherwise uneventful pregnancy. *Am J Obstet Gynecol* 135:322, 1979.
Oh W, Lind J, Gesner IH: The circulatory and respiratory adaptation to early and late cord clamping in newborn infants. *Acta Paediatr Scand* 55:17, 1966.
Papiernik E, Bouyer J, Dreyfus J, et al: Prevention of preterm births: A perinatal study in Itaguenu, France. *Pediatrics* 76:154, 1985.
Raiha NCR: Nutritional proteins in milk and the protein requirement of normal infants. *Pediatrics* 75(Suppl):136, 1985.
Raiha NCR: Protein quality in feeding the normal infant: Do whey-predominant formulas offer nutritional advantages? Letter to the editor. *Pediatrics* 76:329, 1985.
Reichman BC, Chessex P, Putet G, et al: Partition of energy metabolism and energy cost of growth in the very low birth weight infant. *Pediatrics* 69:446, 1982.
Sauer PJJ, Dane H, Visser HKA: New standards for the neutral thermal environment of healthy very low birth weight infants. *Arch Dis Child* 59:18, 1984.
Schultz FS, Stennart H, Wullbrand W, et al: The ontogeny of sensory perception in preterm infants. *Eur J Pediatr* 126:211, 1977.
Steichen JJ, Gratton TL, Tsang RC: Osteopenia of prematurity: The cause and possible treatment. *J Pediatr* 96:528, 1980.
Stewart AL, Reynolds EOR, Lipscomb AP: Criteria for infants of very low birthweight: Survey of world literature. *Lancet* 2:1038, 1981.
Stonestreet BS, Oh W: Plasma creatinine levels in low birth weight infants during the first 3 months of life. *Pediatrics* 61:788, 1978.
Strang LB: *Neonatal Respiration. Physiological and Clinical Studies.* Oxford, Blackwell Scientific Publications, 1977.
Tan KL: Blood pressure in very low birth weight infants in the first 70 days of life. *J Pediatr* 112:266, 1988
Watkins JB: Lipid digestion and absorption. In: *Current Issues in Feeding the Normal Infant. Pediatrics* (Suppl) 75:151, 1985.
Wigglesworth JS: Fetal growth retardation. *Br Med Bull* 22:13, 1966.
Williams J, Hirsch NJ, Corbet AJS, et al: Postnatal head shrinkage in small infants. *Pediatrics* 59:619, 1977.
Wright CE, Tallan HH, Lin YY, et al: Taurine: Biological update. *Ann Rev Biochem* 55:427, 1986
Wu PYK, Edwards N, Storm MC: Plasma amino acid pattern in normal breast-fed infants. *J Pediatr* 109:347, 1986.
Yared A, Kon V, Ichikawa I: In: Tune BM, Mendoza SA (guest eds): *Pediatric Nephrology*. New York, Churchill Livingstone, 1984.
Ylppo A: Zur physiologie, klinik and zum schicksal der fr[u]ge borenen. *Z Kinderheilk* 24:1–110, 1919.
Young M: Placental factors and fetal nutrition. *Am J Clin Nutr* 34:738, 1981.

INTRAUTERINE GROWTH RETARDATION

Definition

If the fetus is below the 10th percentile for predicted weight for gestational age, or more than 2 SDs from the mean, the condition is defined as intrauterine growth retardation (also called small-for-gestational age, SGA; Fig. 4.11).

Basic Science

When the cause of intrauterine growth retardation is inadequate nutrition in utero, the infant may be at risk of continued growth retardation postnatally. The likelihood of poor postnatal growth is greater if failure to grow began before 26–34 weeks in a pregnancy that goes to term. This is one of the reasons for elective early delivery if sequential ultrasonographic studies document poor fetal growth.

Although long-term adverse effects on the fetus can occur, Warshaw (1985) reminds us that some of the time intrauterine growth retardation can be viewed as an adaptation to reduced availability of nutrients. By a decrease in metabolic demands, the infant may be better able to defend against hypoxic injury than a larger fetus. Surely that is one perspective that prompts caution in attempts to promote fetal growth by increasing maternal intake.

Observations on growth and energy metabolism, reported by Chessex et al (1984), are in Table 4.12.

The major determinants of metabolic rate include age, weight, thermal environment, relative organ size, growth rate, caloric intake, and activity. The hypermetabolism of the undergrown infant is probably at least in part, the result of the relatively larger brain size and higher growth rate. Brain metabolism accounts for about half the energy expenditure of infants. The higher rate of growth of the small infants has an energy cost. The undergrown infants deposit less fat

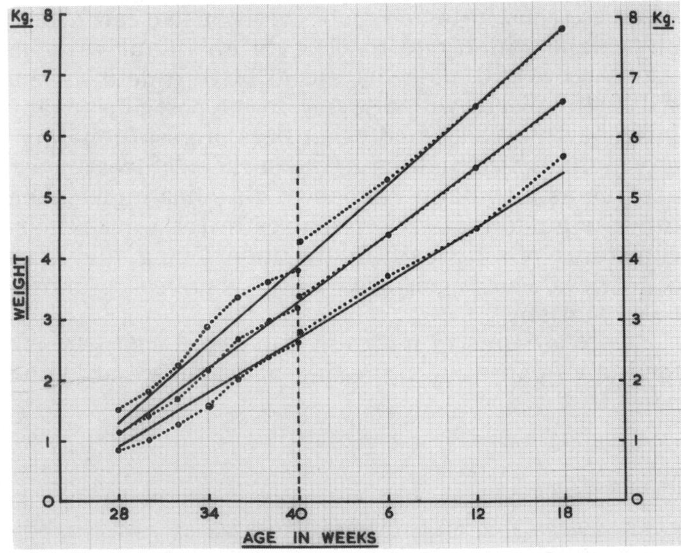

Figure 4.11. Fetal growth curves (10th, 50th, 90th centiles) of Lubchenco et al and early growth curves of Tanner as superimposed on the Bristol Perinatal Growth Chart of Dunn. Illustration courtesy of Dr. Peter Dunn. Originally published in *Acta Paediatr Scand* (Suppl) 319:180, 1985.

Table 4.12
Growth and Energy Metabolism

	Small for Gestational Age (SGA)	Appropriate for Gestational Age (AGA)
Birth weight	1120 ± 30 g	1150 ± 40 g
Gestational age	33.1 ± 0.3	29.3 ± 0.4
Age at study (days)	26 ± 3	21 ± 2
Weight/kg/day (g/kg/day)	19.4 ± 0.9	16.8 ± 1
Length gain (cw/week)	1.25 ± 0.14	1.02 ± 0.1
Head circumference gain (cm/week)	1.16 ± 0.09	0.94 ± 0.08
Metabolic rate (kcal/kg/day)	67.4 ± 1.3	62.6 ± 0.9[1]
Macronutrient		
Fat	4.3 ± 0.4	5.4 ± 0.3[1]
CHO	2.6 ± 0.4	1.8 ± 0.4
Protein	1.57 ± 0.12	1.92 ± 0.08

[1]Results are mean ± SE; $P < 0.05$; Data of Chessex et al: *Pediatr Res* 18:709, 1984.

and protein and have a relatively higher content of total body water.

The pathologic findings include a small placenta, often with infarcts. The lungs, liver, thymus, and adrenals are the organs most reduced in size. Some evidence suggests that even though small, the lung is more mature for gestational age and the infants are less likely to have surfactant deficiency (Gruenwald et al, 1961).

Epidemiology

It is estimated that about one-fourth of low birth weight infants are growth retarded or about 50,000 are born each year in the United States (NIH Workshop on Fetal Growth, Bethesda MD, June 1983).

Natural History

Maternal illness, especially toxemia, should alert one to the possibility of inadequate fetal nutrition from placental dysfunction. Maternal heart disease, chronic hypertension, anemia or severe malnutrition, are all associated with low fetal weight. Infants of mothers who live at high altitude have a slightly lower birth weight than those at sea level.

The adverse effects of maternal cigarette smoking on the outcome of pregnancy are well documented. A major consequence is low weight for gestational age. Reduced lean body mass, and relative placental hypertrophy have been reported. These effects may be the result of chronic fetal hypoxia from exposure to carbon monoxide or decreased uteroplacental blood flow from nicotine (Wigglesworth, 1966; Longo, 1976, 1977). Because tobacco smoke contains more than 4000 compounds, it is also possible that some other components such as cadmium contribute to growth retardation by interference with placental transfer of zinc and other metals (Fig. 4.12).

Fetal factors that tend to reduce size for gestational age are multiple pregnancies, sex (female infants are slightly smaller at any given gestational age), and insulin deficiency. Infants of small parents tend to be small, with maternal size having the greatest influence.

Injuries to the fetus early in gestation, such as the effects of chromosomal abnormalities or severe fetal infection as with rubella, interfere with cell growth and cause a reduction in cell number. They can produce profound disturbances in growth from which "catch up" never occurs. These insults are estimated to represent about 20% of growth retarded fetuses (type 1 fetal growth retardation). Other insults such as those secondary to maternal problems that occur later in pregnancy may also reduce cell number, and may or may not permit catch up growth postnatally (type 2 fetal growth retardation). Often conditions are overlapping, such as chronic malnutrition and cigarette smoking. In the best of hands, the cause of fetal growth retardation is not clear in about half the cases.

Diagnosis

The outstanding clinical features have been summarized and are shown in Table 4.13.

An estimate of gestational age can be made from examination of neuromuscular development, as illus-

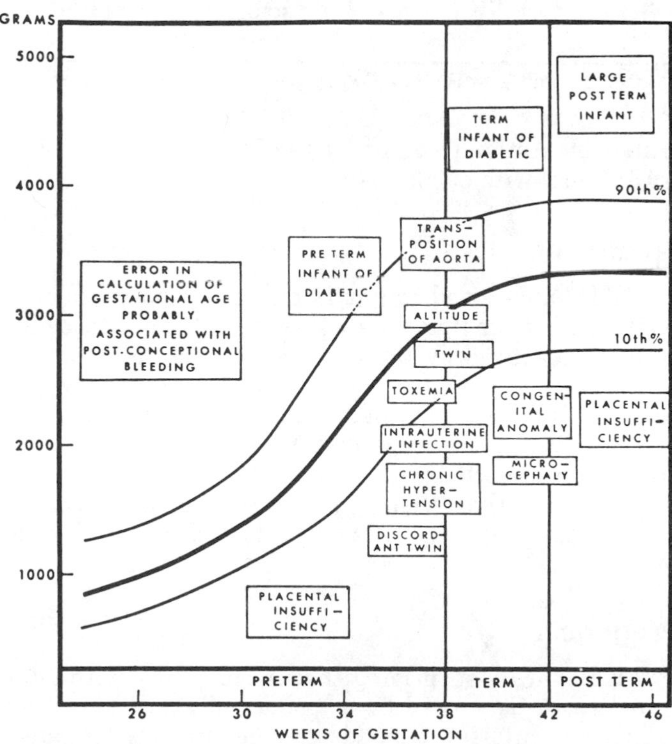

Figure 4.12. Graphic representation of conditions associated with deviations of intrauterine growth. The boxes symbolize the approximate birth weight and gestational age at which the condition is likely to occur. Lubchenco LD, et al: Factors influencing fetal growth. In Joxnis JHP, et al (eds): *Aspects of Praematurity and Dysmaturity*. Leiden, HG Stenfert Kroese, 1968.

Table 4.13
Clinical Criteria for Classification of Low Birth Weight Infants: Premature vs. Dysmature ("Small for Dates")[1]

Criteria	36 Weeks (Premature)	37–38 Weeks (Borderline Premature)	39 Weeks (Full-Term)
Creases on sole of foot	One or two transverse creases running anteriorly, smooth posterior ¾ of foot	More creases appear anteriorly, heel remains smooth	Creases extend throughout soles, prominent deep clefts
Size of breast nodule (large nodules, full term; but small ones may be found in premature or small for dates)	Not palpable before 33 weeks; rarely exceeds 3 mm by 36 weeks	Average is 4 mm	Average is 7 mm, sizable mass readily seen
Hair on head	Cotton wool quality, difficult to distinguish one strand from another	Same, with some progression toward 38 weeks characteristic	Silky texture because of thickening of hair; each strand of hair can be distinguished
Cartilaginous development of earlobe	Shapeless, pliable with little cartilaginous support		Rigid earlobe, stiffened with cartilage; folds of helix and anthelix prominent (distinct ridges)
Testicular descent and scrotal changes	Small scrotum with rugae on its inferior aspect limited to a small area; testes at junction of inguinal canal and superior aspect of scrotum not completely descended	Gradual descent with scrotal enlargement	Enlarged scrotum with fully descended testes, pendulous in appearance, inferior surface of scrotum completely covered with rugae

[1]Modified from Usher R, et al: *Pediatr Clin North Am* 13:835, 1966.

trated by Amiel-Tison or by the Dubowitz score (Fig. 4.13) (Dubowitz et al, 1970).

Treatment

The undersized infant is at risk of postnatal hypoglycemia from inadequate glycogen stores. Blood glucose is measured by the glucose oxidase method by 1 hour of age and frequently thereafter. Glucose and water in some form are provided no later than 1 hour after birth. Given their hypermetabolic state, the infants should be provided with about 10–15% more calories per kilogram than their appropriately grown counterparts. They may seem hungry and reach full oral feeds by 3 days.

Prognosis

It is hardly surprising that interference with fetal growth can be caused by a variety of conditions. The long-term outcome depends on the underlying cause rather than the degree of growth delay. In following these infants, Fitzhardinge and Steven (1972) identified two populations: those who remained undersized and those who "caught up." The best predictor of ultimate growth is the growth rate in the first year. Early failure of growth in utero can result in reduced growth at age 5 years; late onset impairment in fetal growth is associated with microcephaly (Sann et al, 1986). Neurological deficits are present in about 25% of growth-retarded infants. Poor performance in school and speech problems were found in one-half of the boys and more than one-third of the girls.

These observations were confirmed and extended to a group of VLBW infants (less than 1.5 kg) some of whom were appropriate for gestational age (AGA) and others small for gestational age (SGA), born during 1977–1978. Hack et al (1982) found by 8 months corrected age, 72% of AGA infants were within the normal weight range and 50% of SGA infants who remained undergrown, had lower developmental quotients on the Bayley examination. Allen (1984) found the majority of undersized infants caught up in both postnatal growth and development.

The persistent problems of all VLBW infants can be predicted from a neurologic evaluation at 1 year of age, according to Vohr and Garcia Coll (1985). They report that the need for special education at 7 years of age was predicted with considerable success in a study of 42 infants, 22 of whom were classified as normal, 12 suspect, and eight abnormal.

If hypoglycemia is untreated, the neurologic outlook is poor. If treated, the outlook is better (Haworth and McRae, 1965; Pildes et al, 1974).

Considerations Before Discharge of Low Birth Weight Infants

Throughout the nursery stay, the mother or other future caretaker should have the opportunity to ask questions, assist in the care of her infant, and become comfortable and confident in the new relationship. If the infant has been ill, a written discharge summary can be given to the mother to give to whomever will assume responsibility for the child in the future. This seems especially important in our mobile society where delays in access to information can be not only frustrating, but dangerous.

Questions for caregivers before the discharge of a premature infant

The following is a suggested check list for the pediatrician:

Is the infant gaining weight at an appropriate rate?

Are all medical conditions stabilized, and mother informed of future needs such as medications and follow-up visits?

Have hernias been repaired or will they be before discharge?

Has circumcision (pros and cons) been discussed?

If the infant is 2 months old the first immunization with diptheria-tetanus-pertussis (DTP) can be given, and plans made for a second at 3 months (regardless of gestational age).

Is the infant's hemoglobin at a satisfactory level (i.e., the infant is asymptomatic although pale)?

Has screening for congenital hypothyroidism, phenylketonuria (PKU), or maple syrup disease been done and recorded?

NEUROMUSCULAR MATURITY

NEUROMUSCULAR MATURITY SIGN	SCORE 0	1	2	3	4	5	RECORD SCORE HERE
POSTURE							
SQUARE WINDOW (WRIST)	90	60	45	30	0		
ARM RECOIL	180		100 -180	90 -100	90		
POPLITEAL ANGLE	180	160	130	110	90	90	
SCARF SIGN							
HEEL TO EAR							
						TOTAL NEUROMUSCULAR MATURITY SCORE	

SCORE

Neuromuscular _____

Physical _____

Total _____

MATURITY RATING

TOTAL MATURITY SCORE	GESTATIONAL AGE (WEEKS)
5	26
10	28
15	30
20	32
25	34
30	36
35	38
40	40
45	42
50	44

PHYSICAL MATURITY

PHYSICAL MATURITY SIGN	SCORE 0	1	2	3	4	5	RECORD SCORE HERE
SKIN	gelatinous red, trans-parent	smooth pink, vis-ible veins	superficial peeling, & or rash few veins	cracking pale area rare veins	parchment deep cracking no vessels	leathery cracked wrinkled	
LANUGO	none	abundant	thinning	bald areas	mostly bald		
PLANTAR CREASES	no crease	faint red marks	anterior transverse crease only	creases ant. 2 3	creases cover entire sole		
BREAST	barely percept.	flat areola no bud	stippled areola, 1-2mm bud	raised areola, 3-4mm bud	full areola 5-10mm bud		
EAR	pinna flat, stays folded	sl. curved pinna; soft with slow recoil	well-curv. pinna; soft but ready recoil	formed & firm with instant recoil	thick cartilage ear stiff		
GENITALS (Male)	scrotum empty no rugae		testes descend-ing, few rugae	testes down good rugae	testes pendulous deep rugae		
GENITALS (Female)	prominent clitoris & labia minora		majora & minora equally prominent	majora large, minora small	clitoris & minora completely covered		
						TOTAL PHYSICAL MATURITY SCORE	

Reference

Ballard JL, Novak KK, Driver M. A simplified score for assessment of fetal maturation of newly born infants. *J Pediatr* 95:769-774, 1979.
Reprinted by permission of Dr Ballard and *Journal of Pediatrics*.

GESTATIONAL AGE (weeks)

By dates _____

By ultrasound _____

By score _____

Figure 4.13. (*Upper panel*) Posture and passive tone at 26–44 weeks of gestation, indicating increasing muscle tone in upper and lower extremities, which develops with increasing age. *Lower panel* depicts scoring of physical signs. Devised by Ballard et al: *J Pediatr* 95:769, 1979.

CASE ILLUSTRATION

An infant was born to a 34-year-old mother with pre-eclampsia. This was her first pregnancy. She was admitted after a normal pregnancy at an estimated 29 weeks of gestation because of hypertension and mild edema. Maternal blood pressure was refractory to bedrest and an antihypertensive medication. Maternal urinary estriols dropped over the course of 4 days from 5.2 to 1.5 mg for 24 hours. Fetal ultrasonography revealed an infant without anomalies of approximately 700 g. Amniocentesis provided amniotic fluid with an L/S (lecithin/sphingomyelin) ratio of 1.5:1 and a saturated phosphatidylcholine of 215 g/dl, which suggested lung immaturity and surfactant deficiency. The mother was treated for 48 hours with dexamethasone phosphate (24 mg total) to accelerate fetal lung maturation and a girl was delivered by cesarean section. Apgar scores of 6 at 1 minute and 8 at 5 minutes and by Dubowitz examination gave an estimated age of 29 weeks' gestation. The birth weight was 720 g and the head circumference was 23.5 cm, both of which were under the 10th percentile for that stage of gestation.

The baby sustained good respirations in the first 2 hours after birth but, because $Paco_2$ rose from 35 to 50 torr, she was intubated and ventilated. Chest radiogram revealed a normal heart and reticulogranular densities consistent with mild hyaline membrane disease. The baby was ventilated for 6 days with low rates, pressures, and ambient oxygen. During that time several heart and head ultrasonographic examinations were normal. Thereafter, the hospital course was marked by apnea treated with theophylline; bilirubin that reached a total of 6 mg/dl that was treated with phototherapy; and several episodes of possible necrotizing enterocolitis and/or sepsis that were treated for 3 days with antibiotics. Blood cultures were negative. The infant was supported with parenteral alimentation until 3 weeks of age, when oral feeds of her mother's expressed breast milk were given. Evaluation such as cord blood IgM levels for other causes of fetal growth retardation was unremarkable and therefore poor growth was attributed to placental insufficiency associated with pre-eclampsia. The infant grew in parallel with predicted fetal growth curves with a weight of 900 g at 1 month of age, and 1500 g at an approximate age of 2½ months.

This case illustrates how the use of ultrasonography, measurement of maternal urinary estriol excretion, and amniocentesis as well as use of prenatal glucocorticoids permitted a successful outcome for this infant with intrauterine growth retardation.

COMMENT

Many issues common to infants of low birth weight for gestational age are illustrated by this pregnancy. Risk factors present here were first pregnancy, pre-eclampsia refractory to rest, and falling estriols. It would have been relevant to inquire whether the mother smoked or used alcohol or narcotics because all of these are associated with fetal growth retardation. Information on maternal height and weight is also useful because small mothers may have small infants.

The timing of delivery by section permitted use of dexamethasone (a synthetic glucocorticoid) to accelerate lung maturation. The mild nature of later respiratory distress is consistent with a beneficial effect from glucocorticoids.

The episodes of possible necrotizing enterocolitis were of concern but, in retrospect, may have been due to ileus. Blood cultures and abdominal radiographs were negative.

Hypoglycemia was not a problem in this infant because she (like all undersized infants) was given 5% glucose intravenously within the first hour of life. Larger, more vigorous infants would be offered the mother's breast, and supplements if needed.

Has a behavioral-developmental assessment been completed? Is early intervention appropriate and have parents been provided with information about location?

Has the infant had hearing and visual evaluation and have the parents been told the results?

Has social service been in touch with parents and are arrangements for the baby at home satisfactory?

Have the parents been instructed in cardiopulmonary resuscitation? Have they identified a doctor for the baby or an emergency center?

REFERENCES

Allen MC: Developmental outcome and followup of the small for gestational age infant. *Semin Perinatol* 8:123, 1984.

Battaglia FC, Lubchenco L: A practical classification of newborn infants by weight and gestational age. *J Pediatr* 71:159, 1967.

Campbell S, Thomas A: Ultrasound measurement of fetal head to abdomen circumference ratio in the assessment of growth retardation. *Br J Obstet Gynecol* 84:165, 1977.

Chessex P, Reithman B, Verellen G, et al: Metabolic consequences of intrauterine growth retardation in very low birthweight infants. *Pediatr Res* 18:709, 1984.

Dubowitz LM, Dubowitz V, Goldberg C: Clinical assessment of gestational age in the newborn infant. *J Pediatr* 77:1, 1970.

Fitzhardinge PM, Steven EM: The small-for-date infant. 1. Later growth patterns. *Pediatrics* 49:67, 1972.

Fitzhardinge PM: Early growth and development in low-birth-weight infants following treatment in an intensive care nursery. *Pediatrics* 56:162, 1975.

Gruenwald P, Minh HN: Evaluation of body and organ weights in perinatal pathology. *Am J Obstet Gynecol* 82:312, 1961.

Hack M, Merkatz I, Gordon D, et al: The prognostic significance of postnatal growth in very low-birth weight infants. *Am J Obstet Gynecol* 143:693, 1982.

Haworth JC, McRae TN: The neurological and developmental effects of neonatal hypoglycemia: A follow-up of 22 cases. *Can Med Assoc J* 92:861, 1965.

Pildes RS, Cornblath M, Warren I, et al: A prospective controlled study of neonatal hypoglycemia. *Pediatrics* 54:5, 1974.

Sann L, Darre E, Lasne Y: Effects of prematurity and dysmaturity on growth at age 5 years. *J Pediatr* 109:681, 1986.

Usher R, McLean F, Scott KE: Judgment of fetal age II. Clinical significance of gestational age and an objective method of its assessment. *Pediatr Clin North Am* 13:835, 1966.

Vohr BR, Garcia Coll CT: Neurodevelopmental and school performance of very-low birth weight infants: A seven year longitudinal study. *Pediatrics* 76:345, 1985.

Warshaw JB: Intrauterine growth retardation: Adaptation or pathology? *Pediatrics* 76:998, 1985.

Infants of Diabetic Mothers

6

Definition

Infants born to diabetic mothers are a special group that deserve extra care because of metabolic changes induced by maternal illness.

Epidemiology

The number of infants born of diabetic mothers in any given setting depends on local referral practices. Brigham and Women's Hospital serves the Joslin Clinic in Boston and delivers 60–80 infants of prediabetic and diabetic mothers per year.

Natural History

The infant of a diabetic mother is usually large for gestational age, if the mother has had significant hyperglycemia during pregnancy (Tables 4.14 and 4.15). Class A diabetics who may not know of their elevated sugars may have the largest infants. Diabetics with vascular disease may have a number of complications of pregnancy that can impair fetal growth, so that the birth weight of some of their infants will be low for gestational age.

Hypoglycemia

Nearly one-half of the infants of diabetic mothers will have blood glucose levels of less than 30 mg/dl during the first 2–6 hours of life. Rarely are they symptomatic. The mechanism of neonatal hypoglycemia in these infants is presumed to be excess insulin production by the fetus in response to maternal (hence fetal) hyperglycemia. Islet cell hypertrophy is evident histologically, and c-peptide levels are elevated. C-peptide, a by-product of the conversion of proinsulin to insulin, is secreted by B cells in equimolar amounts with insulin.

Fetal hyperinsulinemia is thought to be responsible for the macrosomia by enhancing protein synthesis, glycogen deposition, and lipogenesis. The weight discrepancy becomes apparent at about 1000 g, or 27–28 weeks' gestation.

Congenital Anomalies

The likelihood of serious anomalies is decreased when rigorous control of diabetes is established before and throughout pregnancy. Serial measurements of hemoglobin A_1c are useful to monitor degree of control. Among the anomalies over-represented in infants of diabetic mothers are the caudal regression syndrome, vertebral dysplasia, anencephaly, meningomyelocele, congenital heart disease, and small left colon syndrome. About 6–9% of infants will have a serious anomaly. The more severe the maternal diabetes, the greater the risk (Miller et al, 1981).

Respiratory Distress Syndrome

Infants of diabetic mothers have an average 5.6-fold relative risk of respiratory distress syndrome (RDS) when compared to infants of nondiabetic mothers of like gestational age, routes of delivery, and other maternal complications (Robert et al, 1976; Fig. 4.14). Although the lecithin-sphingomyelin ratio (L/S) in amniotic fluid may be normal, the infants may have classical and often severe RDS. (They are not likely to have RDS if L/S is > 3.) Apparently the phospholipids in the pulmonary lining layer are abnormal in other respects. The possibility of alterations in proteins associated with

Table 4.14
White's Classification of Maternal Diabetes[1]

Gestational diabetes (GD)	Glucose intolerance diagnosed during pregnancy
Class A:	Chemical diabetes; positive glucose tolerance tests prior to or during pregnancy
	Prediabetes; history of large babies more than 4 kg or unexplained stillbirths after 28 weeks
Class B:	Medication dependent; onset after 20 years of age; duration less than 10 years
Class C:	C_1: Onset at 10–19 years of age
	C_2: Duration 10–19 years
Class D:	D_1: Onset before 10 years of age
	D_2: Duration 20 years
	D_3: Calcification of vessels of the leg (macrovascular disease)
	D_4: Benign retinopathy (microvascular disease)
	D_5: Hypertension
Class E:	Same as D, but with calcification of pelvic vessels
Class F:	Nephropathy
Class R:	Malignant retinopathy
Class G:	Many reproductive failures
Class H:	Diabetic cardiomyopathy

[1]Sources: Kitzmiller, J.L., Cloherty, J.P. and Graham, C.A: Management of diabetes and pregnancy. In Kozak GP (ed): *Clinical Diabetes Mellitus*. Philadelphia, WB Saunders, 1982; Kitzmiller JL, et al: Diabetic pregnancy and perinatal mortality. *Am J Obstet Gynecol* 131:560, 1978; White P: Diabetes mellitus in pregnancy. *Clin Perinatol* 1:331, 1974.

Table 4.15
Frequency of Perinatal Complications in Insulin-Dependent Diabetic Women Compared with that in Women with Diabetic Nephropathy, 1975–1978, Brigham and Women's Hospital[1]

	White Classes B, C, D, R		White Class F	
	Number	Percent	Number	Percent
Number of pregnancies	232		26	
Polyhydramnios	62	26.7	7	26.9
Delivery (24 wk)	10	4.3	8	30.8
Fetal death	1	0.4	2	7.7
Intrauterine growth retardation	5	2.2	5	20.8
Macrosomia[2]	94	40.7	3	12,5
Major congenital anomalies	20	8.6	3	11.1
Neonatal [3]				
Respiratory distress syndrome	19	8.2	6	24.0
Hypoglycemia	113	48.7	11	44.0
Hypocalcemia	54	23.3	4	16.0
Jaundice, phototherapy	48	20.7	11	44.0
Death	6	2.6	1	4.0
Perinatal survival		97.0		88.9

[1]Data from Kitzmiller J, et al: *Am J Obstet Gynecol* 141: 741, 1981.
[2]One set of twins excluded from each column.
[3]Percentage of liveborn infants.

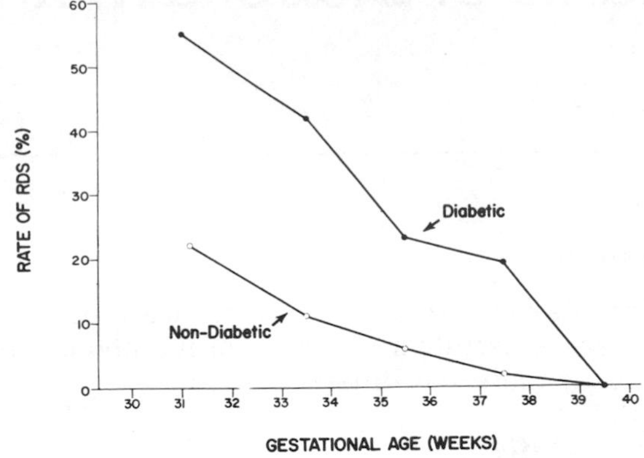

Figure 4.14. Rate of respiratory distress syndrome (RDS) versus gestational age. Each rate represents the rate for all the infants born in the week before and the week after gestational age designated. The high rate of respiratory distress in infants of diabetic mothers in the 1960s was related to the degree of prematurity. Elective cesarean section was carried out at 36–37 weeks' to avoid late fetal deaths. A change in management of mothers, to maintain close control of blood sugar levels and try to prolong pregnancy to term has resulted in a major reduction in respiratory distress and fetal and neonatal deaths. Obstetric management includes nonstress tests and ultrasonographs at intervals from 32 weeks. Amniocentesis to measure L/S ratio or saturated phosphatidylcholine at 36–37 weeks allows prediction of the risk of respiratory distress in a given infant. About 25% of diabetic mothers are delivered by section because of fetal distress.

surfactant is intriguing, and is supported by preliminary studies of Katyal et al (1984).

A possible mechanism of delayed lung maturation is the antagonism by insulin of cortisol action on lecithin synthesis (Smith et al, 1975). Carlson et al (1984) have shown in cell culture systems that insulin acts on the lung fibroblasts to inhibit glucocorticoid response. This explanation is compatible with the observation that after 38 weeks, the infant of the diabetic mother is not at increased risk of RDS since the effect of glucocorticoids as a timer of lung maturation is before 38 weeks.

Hypertrophic cardiomyopathy has been better defined in infants of diabetic mothers through the development of M-mode echocardiography. The cardinal feature in infants who have signs and symptoms of congestive failure shortly after birth is cardiac enlargement. They present with tachypnea, cyanosis, hepatomegaly, and signs of pulmonary venous congestion (Way et al, 1979). Electrocardiographic changes are variable, but may show acceleration of right ventricular hypertrophy. The echocardiographic changes include thickening of the anterior wall of the right ventricle and interventricular septum, and some left ventricular hypertrophy. Such changes are diagnostic and are reversible by about 1 month of age.

Other Problems

Hypocalcemia is sometimes present in infants of diabetic mothers. It resembles that of premature infants, with the nadir at about 24 hours. Total calcium may fall below 7 mg/dl, but ionized calcium does not fall proportionately. Although infants of diabetic mothers are jittery, no predictable relationship exists with either hypocalcemia or hypoglycemia.

An association between maternal diabetes and renal vein thrombosis is well known. Other thromboses and thromboembolic phenomena also occur in these infants, together with abnormalities of the microcirculation (Oppenheimer and Esterly, 1965). Among the possible explanations are polycythemia and fetal dehydration. Total body water content is relatively reduced as fat content is increased in the oversized infants (Osler and Pedersen, 1960).

An increase in conversion of arachidonic acid to a lipoxygenase metabolite in human endothelial cells and a decrease in prostacyclin production in umbilical arteries of infants of diabetic mothers have been reported, and may have a role in neovascularization that is seen in the microcirculation of diabetics (Setty and Stuart, 1986).

Prolonged elevation of unconjugated bilirubin (indirect) is present in about 20% of infants of diabetic mothers, presumably due to functional immaturity of hepatic enzymes.

OTHER EVIDENCE OF RELATIVE IMMATURITY

The normal switch from fetal to adult globin synthesis between 28 and 34 weeks' gestation is delayed in infants of diabetic mothers until after birth. These infants have elevated levels of glycosylated proteins including hemoglobin F (Perrine et al, 1985). Why this occurs and what its significance is await further study. Whether fetal oxygen delivery near term is compromised by the delay in switching is unknown.

Diagnosis

It is customary for the obstetrician to alert the pediatrician to the diabetic status of the mother. In the unusual event that this is not done, the diagnosis can be suspected from the Cushingoid appearance of the infant. Even though the weight is likely to be in the higher percentile range, the head may be in the lower percentile for height or age. The infants may be plethoric and prone to acrocyanosis. Most of them are jittery when stimulated, even when levels of blood sugar are normal. The significant depression in blood glucose that can occur is often without any evident change in symptoms. The behavior of the infants is reminiscent of babies delivered several weeks earlier, as if the infant of the diabetic mother has a relative delay in maturation, and thus paradoxically, is oversized but immature.

Treatment

MATERNAL ASPECTS

Throughout pregnancy, maternal blood sugars require strict regulation. During the last 2 months of pregnancy, hospitalization for control of blood glucose and blood pressure, and monitoring of c-peptide, as well as biweekly nonstress tests are often appropriate. Ultrasonic evaluations of the fetus are important to monitor growth.

INFANT ASPECTS

Blood glucose levels should be checked at 1, 2, 3, 6, 12, 24, 36, and 48 hours, and calcium levels at 1 and 24 hours. Most infants are placed in intensive care for observation, and kept under fluorescent lights for phototherapy to prevent the predictable rise in bilirubin. If the infant has respiratory distress, a chest film should be requested to evaluate cardiac size, pulmonary disease, and skeletal/vertebral anomalies.

Feedings of 10% dextrose (5 ml/kg) by bottle or gavage at 1 hour after birth, and hourly thereafter if the infant is over 2 kg, are recommended to lessen the reactive hypoglycemia. Smaller infants or those with respiratory distress are fed intravenously. Early nursing is desirable for both mother and infant. If blood glucose is found to be under 30 mg/dl, we give glucagon i.m. (300 µg/kg up to 1.0 mg). The effect is prompt and lasts 2–3 hours.

Prognosis

Individualization of treatment is the key to the greatly improved outlook for infants of diabetic mothers in recent years. The care of the mother, timing and route of delivery, and access to neonatal intensive care have increased perinatal survival from 82% in 1960 to 97% today (Jorge et al, 1981; Kitzmiller et al, 1978).

MACROSOMIA

Definition

Infants born above the 4.5-kg birth weight are arbitrarily considered to be macrosomic.

Epidemiology

In the United States, macrosomic infants are between 1.5% and 2.0% of all births.

Natural History

The most reliable predictor of excess fetal weight is excess maternal weight gain in pregnancy. Surprisingly, Klebanoff et al (1985) reported the next best predictor of macrosomia was the mother's own birth weight, which is a piece of historical information rarely collected. In a review of 33,545 births, Spellacy et al (1985) found 574 with birth weights of more than 4.5 kg, the largest of which was 5.9 kg. The most common cause of fetal macrosomia was maternal obesity. In general, the more obese the mother, the heavier the infant. The next most common association was postmaturity, followed by gestational diabetes, then insulin-treated diabetes. Of the macrosomic infants, 70% were males, for reasons we do not understand. Some association of large infants with maternal cystic fibrosis and maternal PKU has been noted.

Treatment

Obstetricians have the responsibility to monitor fetal growth and to be alert for possible problems with vaginal delivery of macrosomic infants. Pediatricians need to follow blood sugars in the first hours of life if hyperinsulinemia is suspected. The possibility of birth trauma, particularly to the clavicles, should be kept in mind.

Prognosis

The long-term prognosis of excessive fetal growth is not known. In general, large babies of large parents tend to remain in the upper percentiles of growth charts.

REFERENCES

Bourbon JR, Farrell PM: Fetal lung development in the diabetic pregnancy. *Pediatr Res* 19:253, 1985.

Carlson KS, Smith BT, Post M: Insulin acts on the fibroblast to inhibit glucocorticoid stimulation of lung maturation. *J Appl Physiol* 57:1577, 1984.

Cloherty JP, Epstein M: Maternal diabetes. In Cloherty JP, Stark A (eds): *Manual of Neonatal Care,* 2nd edition. Boston, Little, Brown & Co, 1985, p.3.

Jorge C, Artal R, Paul R, et al: Antepartum fetal surveillance in diabetic pregnant patients. *Am J Obstet Gynecol* 141:641, 1981.
Kitzmiller JL, Cloherty JP, Younger MD, et al: Diabetic pregnancy and perinatal morbidity. *Am J Gynecol* 131:560, 1978.
Klebanoff MA, Mills JL, Berendes HW: Mother's birth weight as a predictor of macrosomia. *Am J Obstet Gynecol* 153:253, 1985.
Miller E, Hare J, Cloherty J, et al: Elevated maternal HbAic in early pregnancy and major congenital anomalies in infants of diabetic mothers. *N Engl J Med* 304:1331, 1981.
Oppenheimer EH, Esterly JR: Thrombosis in the newborn; comparison between infants of diabetic and non-diabetic mothers. *J Pediatr* 67:549, 1965.
Osler M, Pederson J: The body composition of newborn infants of diabetic mothers. *Pediatrics* 26:985, 1960.
Papiernik E, Bouyer J, Dreyfus J, et al: Prevention of preterm births: A perinatal study in Itaguenu, France. *Pediatrics* 76:154, 1985.
Perrine SP, Greene MF, Faller DV: Delay in the fetal globin switch in infants of diabetic mothers. *N Engl J Med* 312:338, 1985.
Robert MG, Neff RK, Hubbell JP, et al: Association between maternal diabetes and respiratory distress syndrome in the newborn. *N Engl J Med* 294:357, 1976.
Setty BNY, Stuart MJ: 15-Hydroxy-5, 8, 11, 13-eicosatetraenoic acid inhibits human vascular cyclooxygenase. Potential role in diabetic vascular disease. *J Clin Invest* 77:202, 1986.
Smith BT, Giroud CJP, Robert M, et al: Insulin antagonism of cortisol action on lecithin synthesis by cultured fetal lung cells. *J Pediatr* 87:953, 1975.
Spellacy WN, Miller S, Winega A, et al: Macrosomia—maternal characteristics and infant complications. *Obstet Gynecol* 66:158, 1985.
Thorsson AV, Hintz RL: Insulin receptors in the newborn. *N Engl J Med* 297:908, 1977.
Way GL, Wolff RR, Eshaghpour E, et al: The natural history of hypertrophic cardiomyopathy in infants of diabetic mothers. *J Pediatr* 95:1020, 1979.

Respiration Around the Time of Birth 7

In the 1980s, methods of resuscitation of the newborn based on knowledge of ventilatory and circulatory needs of the infant should be well known. For the student of history, the reader is referred to the texts on the subject which brought us from the era of inversion and slapping or spanking at birth to the realization that aeration of the lungs and oxygenation of the infant are primary goals (Abramson, 1966).

ASPHYXIA

Definition

Asphyxia results from lack of ability to exchange oxygen and carbon dioxide. A patent airway is essential. In the absence of spontaneous breaths, air or oxygen-enriched air must be introduced within minutes of the time of occlusion of the umbilical cord to permit metabolism of the brain and myocardium and maintenance of life itself.

Epidemiology

Although, in a sense, every fetal death is due to asphyxia, neonatal deaths can be more definitively categorized. Improved obstetric monitoring, expanded criteria for delivery by section, and concerns of perinatologists for the immediate needs of the infant have resulted in a parallel decrease in fetal and early neonatal deaths from asphyxia in recent years, from approximately 20/1000 live births in 1950 to under 10/1000 (fetal deaths) and 10/1000 (neonatal deaths), all in the first 28 days in 1980 (National Center for Health Statistics, 1981). More precise figures are difficult to find because of differences in categorizing infants born with a heartbeat, but who never breathed. Technically, these are neonatal deaths. Actually they should be very rare because such infants should be resuscitated and ventilated mechanically.

Natural History

A first priority for a pregnant woman is that her obstetrician recognize the disorders that predispose to asphyxia of the infant at birth, and plan delivery in a setting where methods for resuscitation and continuing care of the infant will be optimal (Table 4.16; MacDonald et al, 1980).

Extensive clinical and experimental evidence documents the devastating effects of asphyxia at birth. From the first writings of Little (1861), the association of generalized spasticity with perinatal asphyxia was clear. Detailed clinical and pathologic studies by Banker (1962) stressed the vulnerability of the brain, especially in premature infants, to periventricular leukomalacia and more subtle changes in the gray matter. The pathology produced by asphyxia is related to the stage of vascularization in the developing brain.

Seen from another perspective, however, perinatal asphyxia is present in only about 20% of infants with cerebral palsy. Among 54,000 pregnancies studied be-

Table 4.16
Conditions Sometimes Associated with Asphyxia at Birth

I. Mechanical factors
 A. Cephalopelvic disproportion, shoulder dystocia
 B. Malposition of the infant
 C. Abnormal uterine contractions
 D. Prolapse of the umbilical cord or cord entanglement
 E. Multiple pregnancy
 F. Difficult forceps delivery
II. Maternal hemorrhage
 A. Abruptio placentae
 B. Placenta previa
 C. Other antepartum hemorrhage
III. Other maternal conditions
 A. Maternal age over 35 years
 B. Grand multiparity
 C. Toxemia of pregnancy
 D. Diabetes
 E. Cardiorespiratory disease
 F. Intrauterine infection
 G. Postmaturity
 H. Prolonged labor
IV. Iatrogenic factors
 A. Excessive maternal analgesia
 B. Excessive maternal anesthesia
 C. Antihypertensive agents
 D. Maternal hyperventilation
V. Fetal factors
 A. Erythroblastosis fetalis
 B. Passage of meconium
 C. Pneumonia
 D. Sepsis
 E. Malformations
 F. Fetal tachycardia (>160/min) and bradycardia (<100/min)

tween 1959 and 1966, with a 7-year follow-up, the conclusion was that maternal mental retardation, birth weight below 2001 g, and fetal malformation were the leading predictors of cerebral palsy. When all risk factors during pregnancy and throughout the nursery stay were considered, perinatal events (such as asphyxia) accounted for a portion of cerebral palsy only slightly higher than would have been predicted before the onset of labor (Nelson and Ellenberg, 1986).

Studies of cerebral blood flow with xenon-133 clearance show that, in asphyxiated hypotensive infants, the flow may be reduced to half the level observed in normal infants. Lack of autoregulation of cerebral blood flow under these circumstances predisposes to intraventricular hemorrhage, the incidence of which correlates with the degree of prematurity of the infant (Lou et al, 1979; Lazzara et al, 1980).

The sequelae of asphyxia are still being studied and documentation is necessary so that current methods of resuscitation and continuing care can be appropriately evaluated. The difficulties are multiple because the degree of asphyxia can be measured only by crude methods, such as by the Apgar Score (see pp. 156–157; Schachter and Apgar, 1959). In some instances, fetal scalp blood samples can be obtained to measure pH. Late adverse effects may be avoided if attention is paid to fluid status, acid-base balance, thermal environment, and the reasons for the initial asphyxial insult, such as infection or aspiration of meconium. If the evaluation is to be performed at 1, 3, or 7 years, intervening events may be more significant than the perinatal ones. Evaluation of gross motor deficits at 1 year is appropriate; 3 years permits assessment of language development and other higher intellectual capacities; 7 years permits evaluation of early school function and most accurately predicts later achievement. Furthermore, in the follow-up studies of premature infants, socioeconomic status of the parents is a strong predictor of outcome. This is both a sobering and also challenging observation (Drillien, 1964; Fisch et al, 1975).

Tolerance of the Newborn to Hypoxia

The observation that the newborn animal can survive longer than the adult animal in an oxygen-free environment, dates from Robert Boyle in 1670. Mott (1961) pointed out that during the period from midgestation to the early neonatal, the younger the animal, the longer the survival in anoxia. Anoxic animals that are more immature at term birth, such as rats and rabbits, survive longer than those that are more mature, such as lambs and monkeys.

The metabolic pathways that promote longer survival in an oxygen-free environment are not fully understood, but unquestionably, the major pathway is glycolysis, the activity of which must depend on cardiac glycogen stores (Stafford and Weatherall, 1960). The consequence of anaerobic metabolism is the accumulation of lactic acid.

Barbiturate narcosis also lowers metabolic needs, presumably by suppressing catecholamine production and depressing central medullary discharges (Miller and Miller, 1962). These and more recent observations have been applied clinically in the highly controlled settings of intensive care units to help in postoperative care of infants with diaphragmatic hernias. They have not, however, been applied to the care of infants in the delivery room. Early intubation and ventilation, and maintenance of a thermoneutral environment to reduce metabolic demands have proved so successful that it seems inappropriate even to evaluate the more drastic techniques of suppressing the normal biochemical mechanisms to delay postnatal adaptation because normal metabolism is ultimately needed for successful development.

New insight into the biochemical lesion in asphyxiated infants has been obtained from application of magnetic resonance imaging. Hope and colleagues (1984) identified spectral peaks that could be attributed to adenosine triphosphate, phosphocreatine, and other phosphorus-containing metabolites. They found that asphyxiated infants did not differ from normal ones on the first day, but from the second to ninth days there were major changes in the relationship of phosphocreatine to inorganic orthophosphate. The investigators propose that the changes in phosphorus metabolites represent interference with oxidative phosphorylation and some cellular injury. With further experience, it seems possible that the degree of injury and potential reversibility can be quantified by magnetic resonance imaging.

Circulatory Changes at Birth

Dramatic circulatory adjustments must occur within minutes (or seconds) of the initial inflation of the lungs with air or oxygen-enriched mixtures. The fetal circulation depends on the placenta as the gas exchanger. In the chronic fetal lamb preparation studied with labeled microspheres by Rudolph and Heymann (1970), 40–50% of the combined ventricular output was directed to the noninnervated placental vessels and only 3–7% goes to the lungs. During gestation, the intestine and the kidneys as well as the lung are relatively less well-perfused than after birth, presumably because the placenta also serves as the principal source of nutrition and excretion for the fetus.

With occlusion of the cord at birth and aeration of the lungs, increases in oxygen are accompanied by a major redirection of the circulation. The ductus arteriosus constricts, so that the site of right-to-left shunt in fetal life is reduced; a fall in pulmonary vascular resistance permits greater blood flow to the lungs through the pulmonary artery, and left-to-right shunt through the ductus unless it is totally occluded. Blood that returns to the right atrium is at relatively lower pressure than that in the left, so the foramen ovale (in fetal life, the site of right-to-left shunt) closes.

Response to β-adrenergic stimulation can be demonstrated in lambs early in gestation, although it is blunted in comparison to a mature response. Severe asphyxia is characterized by release of adrenaline and noradrenaline from the fetal adrenal medulla, and operates to maintain cardiac output, mostly by an increase in rate. Blood flow is increased in vital organs, and decreased in the periphery (Faxelius et al, 1984). Dopamine also can release noradrenaline stores in myocardium, but less well in the newborn compared with the adult.

A major determinant of pulmonary vascular tone is oxygen tension in the vessels, as has been extensively reviewed by Strang (1977). With the initiation of breathing, the key event is the fall in pulmonary vascular resistance and the increase in oxygenation from fetal levels of 25–30 cm H_2O to 40–60 cm H_2O. This is, in part, due to mechanical effects which result from the creation of an air-liquid interface, resorption of fetal lung liquid, and increased perfusion of pulmonary capillaries. In studies to quantify these events in the fetal lamb, Cassin et al (1964) found little effect on pulmonary blood flow with ventilation with 10% CO_2 in nitrogen, and a marked increase in blood flow after ventilation with air. In other words, the increase in oxygenation is the central factor in permitting increased flow. The effect is mediated by prostaglandin E (PGE). PGE has an important role in maintaining patency of the ductus in fetal life; an increase in oxygen saturation after birth decreases PGE availability and responsiveness (Coceani et al, 1978; Clyman et al, 1977).

Introduction of Air into Fetal Lung

Sufficient pressures must be generated by the muscles of respiration and laryngeal action to move air against the resistive opposing viscous flow and surface forces in the airways. Studies in animals and human infants show that, on average, pressures of 30–60 cm H_2O are applied with the first few breaths.

Lung expansion proceeds with serial aeration of terminal ventilatory units, with pathways of lowest resistance permitting initial aeration. Mechanical interdependence facilitates the application of pressure by inflated areas to uninflated ones to achieve full inflation. The time required for complete aeration varies, presumably as a function of the vigor of the infant, extent of crying, or adequacy of resuscitation if required. The persistence of rales for some hours after birth in some normal infants suggests that aeration may not be completed. Serial measurements of lung compliance and functional residual capacity document the wide variation in time required, which is usually about 30 minutes but may be as long as several days.

The fetal lung is distended to approximately the functional residual capacity with liquid secreted by the lung. Clearance of fetal lung liquid is accelerated by catecholamines released during the stress of delivery, and is more rapid during vaginal than cesarean delivery (Lagercrantz and Slotkin, 1986). The process begins before the onset of labor and is marked by a decrease in lung liquid secretion rate (Dickson et al, 1986).

Evaluation of the Infant at Birth

The most widely adopted system of evaluation at birth was proposed by Virginia Apgar[1] in 1953, and it has subsequently proved to be very useful (Table 4.17).

The equal weight given to signs of unequal importance and interdependence is a weakness, but is not so serious that it obviates the ability to distinguish severely depressed, moderately depressed, and vigorous infants. The 1-minute evaluation helps estimate the degree of asphyxia, but the 5-minute score correlates more closely with morbidity and mortality (Drage and Berendes, 1966).

The scores relate, in part, to the infant's level of maturity. Thus, most all infants less than 30 weeks' gestation have 1-minute scores of less than 6 and 5-minute scores of less than 8 in contrast to infants over 35 weeks of gestation who, on average, score higher. In a prospective evaluation of infants with normal cord blood gases, Catlin et al (1986) found no infants more than 31 weeks of gestation who required intubation, but more than half of those less than 30 weeks' did, on the basis of low scores that are descriptive of developmental difficulty with cardiorespiratory adaptations at birth.

[1]One of her favorite stories, a source of amusement, was to find her last name in lower case in the dictionary.

Table 4.17
Apgar Evaluation Method

Sign	0	1	2
Heart rate	Absent	<100/minute	>100/minute
Respiratory effort	Absent	Weak cry Hypoventilation	Good strong cry
Muscle tone	Limp	Some flexion of extremities	Well flexed
Reflex irritability (response to stimulation of skin of feet)	No response	Some motion	Cry
Color	Blue; pale	Body pink, extremities blue	Completely pink

Criteria and Methods for Resuscitation

Most perinatologists agree, in principle, on indications for resuscitation, although they differ on details and on the specificity with which they write their directions (Table 4.18).

Mechanical Ventilation

Adequate ventilation at the time of birth requires distention of both lungs and thorax over an appropriate volume range. Methods to accomplish this include:

1. Application of mask attached to inflating bag such as that used in anesthesia to deliver intermittent positive pressure (IPPB) or
2. Insertion of an endotracheal tube with attachment to a bag or ventilator.

Methods formerly advocated, but no longer considered safe or effective, include back pressure, arm lift, rocking, and mechanical stimuli, such as inversion and slapping.

Sustained ventilation is achieved by IPPB or intermittent mandatory ventilation (IMV). The latter, which is used to assist infants who make sporadic, but inadequate spontaneous breaths should be delivered at a lower rate than that shown by the patient.

Positive end-expiratory pressure (PEEP) is used with positive pressure in situations in which the infant cannot maintain a normal functional residual capacity, as in surfactant deficiency states or with a very compliant chest wall or flail chest. Alternatively, continuous positive airway pressure (CPAP) is applied throughout the respiratory cycle in a spontaneously breathing infant to maintain a normal functional residual capacity. This can be achieved with nasal prongs and avoids the necessity of endotracheal intubation (Wung et al, 1979).

Continuous negative airway pressure, (C Neg) applied by cuirass or similar device to the chest wall or trunk or whole body (cuirass ventilator, negative pressure incubator, or iron lung) has effects on distention of the lung similar to CPAP applied at the airway. (Cuirass ventilators have not been successfully adapted for infants.) Methods that apply subatmospheric pressure to the whole body share with positive pressure at the airway adverse effects on venous return to the heart and are contraindicated when the infant is in shock unless concurrent blood volume support is supplied.

However achieved, continuous distending airway pressure has been a major advance in successful ventilation of small infants. First evaluated by Gregory et al (1971), its efficacy has been widely affirmed. Early application of even a 5-cm H_2O continuous distending airway pressure aids restoration of blood gases toward normal levels so effectively that the need for sustained mechanical ventilation is reduced. Wung et al (1985) report the possibility of early weaning of infants given CPAP in the delivery room by nasal prongs. The reduced demands for high concentrations of inspired oxygen and high pressures for inspiration lessen the probability of injury to the trachea and airways.

Prolonged Ventilation

The most widely used ventilators are designed to permit changes in frequency, inspiratory-expiratory ratios, pressures, and gas flow rates. Initial settings are made on the basis of observation of chest wall movements and auscultation of breath sounds. If transcutaneous oxygen and carbon dioxide monitors are available (to measure P_s (skin) gases (P_sO_2 or P_sCO_2) an appropriate inspired oxygen concentration can be established. Initial indications for continued ventilation are frequent prolonged apneic spells, or a requirement of 70% oxygen to keep arterial levels at 50–70 torr, or a rising carbon dioxide tension (P_{CO_2} 60–70 torr). Initial settings of the ventilator may be 25 cm H_2O inspiratory pressure, 5 cm H_2O end-expiratory pressure, and a frequency of 25–30 breaths/minute, at whatever inspired oxygen concentration is needed to achieve arterial tensions of 50–70 torr. Inspiratory times are usually about 0.6 second (Avery et al, 1987).

CONTROVERSIES

Differences in settings of ventilators depend on the philosophy of the physician. If it is desired to keep P_{CO_2} between 35 and 45 torr to lessen vasodilatation of the cerebral vessels and promote pulmonary blood flow, relatively higher pressures and rates will be selected. If there is less concern about P_{CO_2} as long as pH is over 7.20, the focus will be on settings that produce optimal oxygenation (50–70 torr) regardless of P_{CO_2}.

Table 4.18
Indications for Resuscitation[1]

Apgar Score	Management
A. 8,9, or 10 = no asphyxia	Pink, active, responsive, crying baby with rapid heart rate: 1. Gentle suction airway, including nares, with bulb syringe. 2. Dry thoroughly, including head. 3. Maintain body temperature. 4. Perform brief physical examination. 5. Assign 5-minute Apgar score. 6. Unite baby with parents.
B. 5, 6, or 7 = mild asphyxia	Slightly cyanotic, moving with decreased muscle tone, breathing shallowly or periodically, heart rate >100: 1. Repeat steps 1, 2, 3 for management outlined in part A in rapid succession. 2. Stimulate to breathe more frequently by gentle but forceful slapping of soles of feet or rubbing of spine or sternum. 3. Provide enriched oxygen ambient atmosphere via anesthesia bag and mask held by baby's face. 4. If improving, complete steps 4, 5, 6 outlined in part A when Apgar score reaches 8. 5. If heart rate falls to <100, Apgar score is ≤4. 6. Administer naloxone 0.01 mg/kg intramuscularly if mother has received a narcotic analgesic during labor.
C. 3 or 4 = moderate asphyxia	Cyanotic, poor tone, weak respiratory efforts, slowing heart rate (<100): 1. Repeat steps 1, 2, 3 from part A and call for additional personnel to monitor heart rate continuously, manage airway, provide cardiac massage, etc. Resuscitation for the moderately to severely asphyxiated infant is a three-person job. 2. Provide brief trial of stimulation plus O_2 by mask. If there is no improvement by 1 minute, follow step 3. 3. Ventilate with bag and mask, using 100% oxygen and pressure adequate to move the chest. Continue bagging until heart rate >100, color is pink, and spontaneous respirations have begun. If the chest cannot be adequately moved with bag and mask ventilation, intubate. 4. If heart rate <60, intubate and begin cardiac massage at rate of 2 compressions/second, using fingers wrapped around back and thumbs over the sternum.
D. 0, 1, or 2 = severe asphyxia	Deeply cyanotic, no muscle tone, absent respiratory effort or periodic gasps, heart rate slow or absent: 1. Proceed directly to intubation and bag ventilation with 100% O_2 at 40–60 breaths/min at pressures great enough to move the upper chest wall. 2. Perform cardiac massage. 3. If heart rate is not >100 despite 2 minutes of adequate ventilation with 100% O_2 and cardiac massage, insert umbilical venous catheter and administer drugs. Insertion of the catheter is facilitated by cutting the cord at a point ≤1–2 cm from the abdominal wall. The catheter is most safely inserted only 2–3 cm to avoid administering hypertonic solutions directly into a small hepatic vein. All solutions must be flushed through the catheter to ensure their reaching the central circulation. Delivery room drug treatment is directed at improving myocardial contractility and rate by initally correcting metabolic acidosis (2–4 mEq $NaHCO_3$/kg body weight) and by providing carbohydrate substrate (equal volume of 50% dextrose). This combined $NaHCO_3$-dextrose solution can be infused over 3–5 minutes. Next, epinephrine (0.5–1.0 ml, 1:10,000) or atropine (0.1 ml/kg) can be injected to reverse bradycardia. Finally, a slow infusion of 1.0–2.0 ml/kg of calcium gluconate may provide for further enhancement of cardiac output. None of these drugs is effective unless adequate ventilation with oxygen has been achieved. If the heart rate >100 and adequate ventilation is achieved either spontaneously or via assisted ventilation, the use of drugs is not

Table 4.18
Indications for Resuscitation[1]

Apgar Score	Management
	necessary in the delivery room and the baby should be moved to the nursery. There, measurement of vital signs (including heart rate, respiratory rate, blood pressure, and temperature), arterial or capillary blood gases (Pa_{O_2}, Pa_{CO_2}, and pH), and a chest radiograph allow a rational basis for further care. The administration of hypertonic $NaHCO_3$, cardiotonic drugs, or volume expanders all carry risk. Their use should be withheld pending specific documentation of their need by the above studies if adequate ventilation and heart rate >100 can be achieved in the delivery room.

[1]Reproduced with permission from Epstein MF: In Avery ME, Taeusch HW (eds): *Diseases of the Newborns*, 5th edition. Philadelphia, WB Saunders, 1984.

Some physicians advocate a high inspiratory-expiratory ratio (I/E) to keep inspired air in the lung over a longer period. Although the effect of that maneuver is often to increase functional residual capacity by ending expiration early, prolonging inspiratory time may have an adverse effect by impeding venous return to the heart. The ratio should not exceed 1.5.

Of central importance is the need to individualize settings. Not all lungs are alike. Trial and error, with avoidance of extremes, and continuous monitoring of oxygenation remains reasonable advice (Ramsden and Reynolds, 1987).

High-Frequency (Hi-Fi) Ventilation

High frequency ventilators (up to 1500 breaths per minute) are under study to facilitate gas exchange by increasing turbulence in the airways. This approach has had promising results in interstitial emphysema and is being evaluated in comparison with conventional ventilation for early application in asphyxiated infants, and later (after 6 hours of age) in premature infants with surfactant deficiency (hyaline membrane disease). The theoretical advantages are improved distribution of ventilation at mean airway pressures similar to those with conventional ventilators, but without the elevated peak inspiratory pressures. Preliminary experience suggests that lower inspired oxygen concentrations may be sufficient (Frantz et al, 1980; 1983; Marchak et al, 1981; Vincent et al, 1984).

CONTROVERSY

Nasal Prongs, Masks, Oro- or Nasopharyngeal Tubes. Each of the above devices has advocates and critics. Wung et al (1979) have had success in delivering continuous distending airway pressure with prongs and face mask. Goldman et al (1979) found nasal prongs added significantly to the work of breathing and the mean Pa_{O_2} was lower by 8 torr. The possibility that bands that hold the mask can be too tight was raised by Pape et al (1976) who found intracerebellar hemorrhages in some infants.

Opponents of use of tubes in the trachea argue that they impair mucociliary clearance, may erode the tracheal wall, and increase the likehood of aspiration (Goodwin et al, 1985). Tube-induced tracheal stenosis is a recognized complication that may require laser therapy or plastic surgery (see Section 19).

Advocates of use of tubes claim that with careful insertion, loose-fitting tubes are safe for prolonged periods. They are not replaced unless the lumen is narrowed by inspissated secretions. Frequent suctioning can overcome the loss of mucociliary function. The conclusion is that more careful evaluation of the best way to connect an infant to a ventilator is required. In the absence of a perfect device, meticulous care must be taken in the use of existing methods.

The question of the oral versus the nasal route was considered by Donn and Blane (1985), who showed with radiographic studies that an orotracheal tube of constant 2.5 mm diameter moved less when the head was extended than did a nasotracheal tube. They suggest that tube motion is responsible for some instances of subglottic stenosis, and conclude the oropharyngeal route is preferable. We, on the other hand, prefer the nasotracheal route in small infants, and seldom see subglottic stenosis.

Muscle Relaxants

Muscle paralysis with agents such as Pavulon (pancuronium bromide, 0.1 mg/kg/dose) has been advocated in situations where inspired pressures of over 30 cm H_2O are required or when the infant "fights the machine," which occurs more often in term asphyxiated infants or those with persistent pulmonary hypertension. An improvement in oxygenation has been shown in some infants after paralysis. Reversal can be accomplished with atropine, 0.03 mg/kg, and prostigmine 0.06 mg/kg intravenously (Stark et al, 1979; Pollitzer et al, 1981; Crone and Favorito, 1980).

Other neonatologists manage to adjust the ventilator so that it is effective without use of relaxants (Wung et al, 1979). They fear depriving the infant of use of the muscles of respiration even for brief periods. The extensive edema that sometimes accumulates during paralysis is distressing and may negate the usefulness, if it involves the pulmonary circulation. The indications for and judicial use of muscle paralysis deserve further evaluation.

Extracorporeal Membrane Oxygenation (ECMO) for Respiratory Failure

Increasing experience with partial extracorporeal oxygenators has brought some success, particularly in term infants with persistent pulmonary hyptertension refractory to vasodilators. Among eight infants treated for a mean time of 164 hours, Kirkpatrick et al (1983) described six survivors. Central venous blood from internal jugular vein was oxygenated with a spiral coil membrane oxygenator and returned via the carotid artery to the ascending aorta (Subramanian et al, 1987). By 1987, approximately 20 centers in the United States are using ECMO. At Boston Children's Hospital, 30 infants have been treated for a variety of conditions that include diaphragmatic hernias and severe pneumonias. Some survivors of otherwise fatal disorders are normal. The ones that died may have died from their underlying condition. In a few instances, complications of ECMO and the necessary heparinization have proven lethal (Krummel et al, 1984).

No agreement exists on criteria for this therapy. Bedard et al (1985) reviewed the literature and found a 30% mortality rate among 47 treated infants. In untreated infants with an alveolar/arterial O_2 difference of over 600 for 12 hours, the mortality was 60% and morbidity among survivors was high. Krummell et al (1984) reported that six of nine were doing well 15–21 months later. Complications of the procedure, such as air embolism or intracranial hemorrhage, can lead to catastrophic outcomes.

Approach to an Infant with Continuing Respiratory Distress

One of the most alarming situations in the delivery room is an infant in respiratory distress after the initiation of breathing. Persistent or worsening labored breathing, nasal flaring, retractions, and poor air entry with or without visible cyanosis require immediate action such as increased inspired oxygen and a thermal neutral environment that can be achieved by a servo-controlled device to maintain skin temperature measured over the abdomen at 36.5°C. Intubation and mechanical ventilation may be required. As soon as the infant is stabilized, the reasons for the respiratory distress should be ascertained. The maternal history, gestational age, and observations on physical examination can provide useful clues.

It is important to look for upper airway obstruction such as choanal atresia. If the distress is overcome with intubation, some form of nasal, pharyngeal, or laryngeal obstruction is probable. If excess inspiratory effort persists, as seen by retractions and poor air entry, the problem is in the thorax and could be cardiac, pulmonary, or chest wall (including diaphragm) in origin. Examination of the heart for position of apical impulse, size and murmurs is mandatory, as is palpation of radial and femoral pulses. Careful attention to the thorax for size and asymmetry will indicate neuromuscular or skeletal defects, or the possibility of diaphragmatic hernia (especially likely if the abdomen is scaphoid). Palpation of the chest wall will help ascertain if air entry is bilateral. Transillumination will help identify a pneumothorax. Auscultation may be helpful in identifying wet lungs if rales are present, but is of less value in very small infants in whom sounds are so widely transmitted. The most important single diagnostic test is a radiograph that should include both chest and abdomen.

REFERENCES

Abramson H: *Resuscitation of the Newborn Infant.* 2nd edition. St. Louis, CV Mosby Co, 1966.

Apgar V: A proposal for a new method of evaluation of the newborn infant. *Anesth Analg* (Paris) 32:260, 1953.

Avery ME, Tooley WH, Keller JB, et al: Is chronic lung disease of prematurity preventable? A survey of eight centers. *Pediatrics* 79:26, 1987.

Banker BQ: Periventricular leukomalacia of infancy. *AMA Arch Neurol* 7:32, 1962.

Bedard MP, Splittgerber F, Bollinger RO, et al: Selection of infants with persistent fetal circulation (PFC) for extracorporeal membrane oxygenation. (ECMO). *Pediatr Res* 19:333A, 1985.

Cassin S, Dawes GS, Mott J et al: The vascular resistance of the foetal and newly ventilated lung of the lamb. *J Physiol* 171:61, 1964.

Catlin EA, Carpenter MW, Brann BS, et al: The Apgar score revisited: Influence of gestational age. *J Pediatr* 109:865, 1986.

Clyman RI, Heymann MA, Rudolph AM: Ductus arteriosus responses to prostaglandin E_1 at high and low oxygen concentrations. *Prostaglandins* 13:219, 1977.

Coceani F, Bishai I, White I, et al: Action of prostaglandins, endoperoxides, and thromboxanes on the lamb ductus arteriosus. *Am J Physiol* 234:117, 1978.

Crone RK, Favorito J: The effects of pancuronium bromide on infants with hyaline membrane disease. *J Pediatr* 97:991, 1980.

Dickson KA, Mahoney JE, Berger PJ: Decline in lung liquid volume before labor in fetal lambs. *J Appl Physiol* 61:2266, 1986.

Donn SM, Blane CE: Endotracheal tube movement in preterm infant: Oral versus nasal intubation. *Ann Otol Rhinol Laryngol* 94:18, 1985.

Drage J, Berendes H: Apgar scores and outcome of the newborn. *Pediatr Clin North Am* 13:635, 1966.

Drillien CM: *The Growth and Development of the Prematurily Born Infant.* Baltimore, Williams & Wilkins, 1964.

Faxelius G, Lagercrantz H, Yao A: Sympathoadrenal activity and peripheral blood flow after birth: Comparison in infants delivered vaginally and by cesarean section. *J Pediatr* 105:144, 1984.

Fisch, RO, Bilek MK, Miller LD, et al: Physical and mental status at 4 years of age of survivors of the respiratory distress syndrome. *J Pediatr* 86:497, 1975.

Frantz ID, Stark AR, Dorkin HL: Ventilation of infants at frequencies up to 1800/minute. *Pediatr Res* 14:642, 1980.

Frantz ID, Werthammer J, Stark AR: High frequency ventilation in premature infants with lung disease: Adequate gas exchange at low tracheal pressure. *Pediatrics* 71:483, 1983.

Goldman SL, Brady JP, Dumpit FM: Increased work of breathing associated with nasal prongs. *Pediatrics* 64:160, 1979.

Goodwin SR, Graven SA, Haberkern CM: Aspiration in intubated premature infants. *Pediatrics* 75:85, 1985.

Gregory GA, Kitterman JA, Phibbs RH, et al: Treatment of idiopathic respiratory distress syndrome with continous positive airway pressure. *N Engl J Med* 284:1333, 1971.

Hope PL, de L Costello AM, et al: Cerebral energy metabolism studied with phosphorus NMR spectroscopy in normal and birth-asphyxiated infants. *Lancet* 2:366, 1984.

Kirkpatrick BV, Krummel, TM, Mueller DG, et al: Use of extracorporeal membrane oxygenation for respiratory failure in term infants. *Pediatrics* 72:872, 1983.

Krummel TM, Greenfield L, Kirkpatrick BV, et al: The early evaluation of survivors after extracorporeal membrane oxygenation for neonatal pulmonary failure. *J Pediatr Surg* 19:585, 1984.

Lagercrantz H, Slotkin TA: The "stress" of being born. *Sci Am* 254:100, 1986.

Lazzara A, Ahmann P, Dykes F, et al: Clinical predictability of intraventricular hemorrhage in preterm infants. *Pediatrics* 65:30, 1980.

Lou HC, Lassen NA, Friis Hansen B: Impaired autoregulation of cerebral blood flow in the distressed newborn infant. *J Pediatr* 94:118, 1979.

MacDonald HM, Mulligan JC, Allen AC, et al: Neonatal asphyxia I. Relationship of obstetric and neonatal complications to neonatal mortality in 38,405 consecutive deliveries. *J Pediatr* 96:898, 1980.

Marchak BE, Thompson, WK, Duffty P, et al: Treatment of RDS by high frequency oscillatory ventilation: A preliminary report. *J Pediatr* 99:287, 1981.

Miller JA, Miller FS: Factors in neonatal resistance to asphyxia: III Potentiation by narcosis of the effects of hypothermia in the newborn guinea pig. *Am J Obstet Gynecol* 84:44, 1962.

Mott JC: The ability of young mammals to withstand total lack of oxygen. *Br Med Bull* 17:144, 1961.

Nelson KB, Ellenberg JH: Antecedents of cerebral palsy. Multivariate analysis of risk. *N Engl J Med* 325:81, 1986.

Pape KE, Armstrong DL, Fitzhardinge, PM: Central nervous system pathology associated with mask ventilation in the very low birth weight infant: A new etiology for intracerebellar hemorrhage. *Pediatrics* 58:473, 1976.

Pollitzer MJ, Reynolds, EOR, Shaw DG, et al: Pancuronium during mechanical ventilation speeds recovery of lungs of infants with hyaline membrane disease. *Lancet* 1:346, 1981.

Ramsden CA, Reynolds EOR: Ventilator settings for newborn infants. *Arch Dis Child* 62:529, 1987.

Rudolph AM, Heymann MA: Circulatory changes during growth in the fetal lamb. *Circ Res* 26:289, 1970.

Schachter FF, Apgar V: Perinatal asphyxia and psychologic signs of brain damage in childhood. *Pediatrics* 24:1006, 1959.

Stafford A, Weatherall JAC: The survival of young rats in nitrogen. *J Physiol* 153:457, 1960.

Stark AR, Bascom R, Frantz ID: Muscle relaxation in mechanically ventilated infants. *J Pediatr* 94:439, 1979.

Strang LB: *Neonatal Respiration: Physiological and Clinical Studies*. Oxford, UK, Blackwell Scientific Publications, 1977.

Subramanian KN, Keszler M, Hoy G: ECMO for severe neonatal respiratory failure. *Contemp Pediatr* 4:118, 1987.

Vincent RN, Stark AR, Lang P, et al: Hemodynamic response to high-frequency ventilation in infants following cardiac surgery. *Pediatrics* 73:426, 1984.

Wung J-F, James LS, Kilchevsky E, et al: Management of infants with severe respiratory failure and persistence of the fetal circulation without hyperventilation. *Pediatrics* 76:488, 1985.

Wung JT, Koons AN, Driscoll JM, et al: Changing incidence of bronchopulmonary dysplasia. *J Pediatr* 95:845, 1979.

Disorders of Respiration 8

We have elected to include in the section on neonatology a few disturbances of respiration that relate either to immaturity of the respiratory system or problems with postnatal cardiopulmonary adaptations. The many other respiratory problems that can occur in newborns or older children are discussed in Section 5, Pulmonology.

BREATHING RATES AND PATTERNS

Breathing rates and patterns are of major importance in revealing the degree of maturity and coordination of central and peripheral regulatory mechanisms. Fetal breathing movements, which are rapid and irregular, are present 10–90% of the time in late gestation (Dawes et al, 1972). Premature infants have respiratory irregularities characterized by brief recurrent pauses of 5–10 seconds (periodic breathing) or apneic intervals of longer duration associated with bradycardia (apneic spells). In general, respiratory patterns become more regular with increasing postnatal age; respiratory frequencies tend to decline from infancy to adolescence or with growth (Hathorn, 1975).

Fetal Breathing

The human fetus makes sporadic breathing movements from early gestation. Ultrasonography shows the fetus making sporadic gasps with long periods of quiescence, and as pregnancy advances, more frequent bursts of rapid, irregular diaphragmatic movements. Fetal breathing does not usually affect the flow of lung liquid in either direction because liquid viscosity is approximately 100 times that of air. It is remarkable that whereas these movements are present on average only half the time, with the advent of birth, a viable infant breathes continuously.

Fetal respiratory movements are inhibited by hypoxia, labor, general anesthesia, barbiturates, prostaglandin E_2, maternal smoking and alcohol ingestion. It is probable that the physiologic regulation of fetal breathing movements is by PGE_2.

The unusual intermittency of fetal breathing makes it an inappropriate short-term measure of fetal health. Evidence of diminished variability in fetal heart rate appears a more promising gauge of well-being, particularly in growth-retarded fetuses (Henson et al, 1985).

In summary, the central control mechanisms are present and responsive to chemical and neural influences by at least 24 weeks of gestation, and probably as early as 16 weeks (200 g weight). Quantitative studies are difficult to perform in the human fetus; studies in VLBW infants suggest diminished responses to changes in oxygen and carbon dioxide and more active responses to stimuli mediated via the vagus when compared to infants at term or adults.

Breathing Patterns in Immature Infants

The ontogeny of ventilatory control remains an active area of investigation, as new tools permit continuous recordings under normal and abnormal conditions, and quantification of responses to stimuli. No prognostic significance has been assigned to periodic breathing. Areas of agreement are summarized as follows:

1. Nearly all infants have some episodes of periodic breathing. The incidence of periodic patterns decreases with increasing gestational age. It is more common in infants at high altitudes, presumably from lower inspired oxygen tensions and in infants with deficient oxygenation from other causes;
2. periodic breathing persists until infants are about 36 weeks' gestational age, after which it usually becomes infrequent, at least at sea level;
3. the ventilatory responses to hypoxia in all infants are blunted in comparison to those of adults; transient hyperventilation follows depression;
4. the responses to an increase in carbon dioxide are usually brisk, but are a function in part of the rate of change of CO_2. A gradual decrease in alveolar ventilation with CO_2 accumulation is more likely to lead to further hypoventilation or even apnea than to sustained hyperventilation;
5. periodic breathing can be diminished by increased inspired oxygen;
6. brief ventilatory pauses are less common in the first 24 hours of life in preterm infants. Longer pauses—apneic spells—are often first observed on day 1;
7. periodic breathing is most commonly observed in REM sleep (Tables 4.19 and 4.20).

Table 4.19
Ventilation in Newborn During Sleep States[1]

Respiratory Variables	Active Sleep (REM)		Quiet Sleep (Non-REM)
Rate	↑ 22%	Above baseline	
Ventilation	↑ 18%	Above baseline	
O_2 consumption	↑ 16%	Above baseline	
Airway occlusion pressure (0.1 sec)	↑ 27%	Above baseline	
Periodic breathing	Common		Rare
Hering-Breuer reflex	Less active		
Head's reflex	Depressed		
Elastance of lung	No change		No change
CO_2 response	↓		↑
O_2 response	No change		No change
Arousal threshold to hypoxia	↑		No change
Paradoxical respiration (seesaw pattern)	Common		No change

[1]Reproduced with permission from Avery ME, Fletcher BD, Williams RG: *The Lung and its Disorders in the Newborn Infant*, 4th edition. Philadelphia, WB Saunders, 1981.

Maintenance of Lung Volume

Occasional deep breaths are triggered by deflation receptors. The consequence of such breaths is the recruitment of atelectatic regions of the lung which then contribute to the increase in functional residual capacity. This phenomenon can be seen in the smallest preterm infants. In term infants, it appears to be a second inspiration triggered at the end of a first. Designated an inspiratory augmentation reflex (or a breath upon a breath), it occurs more often in the first days of life than later. It is possible that all lung liquid is not cleared by the first few breaths, and the remaining alveolar and interstitial liquid stimulates irritant receptors to produce the inspiratory augmentation (Thach and Taeusch, 1976).

Expiration, normally passive in the adult, has an active component in infants. Toward the end of expiration, "braking" occurs to initiate a new inspiration. This can be seen from flow-volume tracings or even straight recordings of flow versus time (Fig. 4.15; Kosch and Stark, 1984). This phenomenon has an important role in preventing the volume of the lung being reduced to very low levels which would occur in infants by virtue of a nearly infinitely compliant chest wall. With advancing age, the greater stiffness of the chest wall operates to lessen the tendency to atelectasis.

The muscles of respiration respond to the central stimuli to maintain not only lung volume, but the patency of the upper airways as well. Brouillette and Thach (1980) demonstrated the role of the genioglossus as a muscle of respiration inasmuch as it undergoes phasic contractions; when relaxed, the upper airway is closed as after death.

The relationships between swallowing and apnea have led Menon et al (1984) to suggest that, in some infants, excessive secretions trigger both swallowing and apnea. They noted a temporal relationship between swallowing during apnea and recovery of the onset of breathing. Perhaps continued swallowing clears the secretions and terminates apnea.

Maturation of Central Control

The respiratory centers (Fig. 4.16) of the reticular formation of the medulla exhibit rhythmic discharges thought to be stimulated by at least two central oscillators. One theory of pathogenesis of recurrent apneic spells is that the central oscillators may be either un-

Table 4.20
Factors Known to Influence Respiration

Stimulants	Depressants
Chemical	
Arterial P_{CO_2} up to about 80 mm Hg	Arterial P_{CO_2} over 80 mm Hg
Arterial pH 7.0 to 7.4	Arterial pH <6.9 or >7.5
Arterial P_{O_2} < about 80 mm Hg (in adults)	
(Newborn infants with only mild hypoxemia are stimulated by inspired oxygen)	Profound hypoxia
Pharmacologic	
Epinephrine	Morphine
Lobeline	Barbiturates
Nicotine	Chloramphenicol
Salicylates	Neomycin, etc.
Picrotoxin	
Nikethamide	
Progesterone	
Methylxanthines	
Pulmonary Reflexes	
Deflation receptors (Hering-Breuer reflex)	Stretch receptors in lung
Stretch receptors (Head's reflex)	Stretch receptors in aortic arch and carotid sinus
Pressoreceptors	
Decrease in blood pressure	Increase in blood pressure
Bones and Joints	
Stretch receptors in muscles	
Tactile responses	
Thermal	
Fever	Hibernation
Sudden chilling	
Cortical	
Voluntary control of breathing is possible within limits.	

[1]Reproduced with permission from Avery ME, Fletcher BD, Williams RG: *The Lung and its Disorders in the Newborn Infant*, 4th edition. Philadelphia, WB Saunders, 1981.

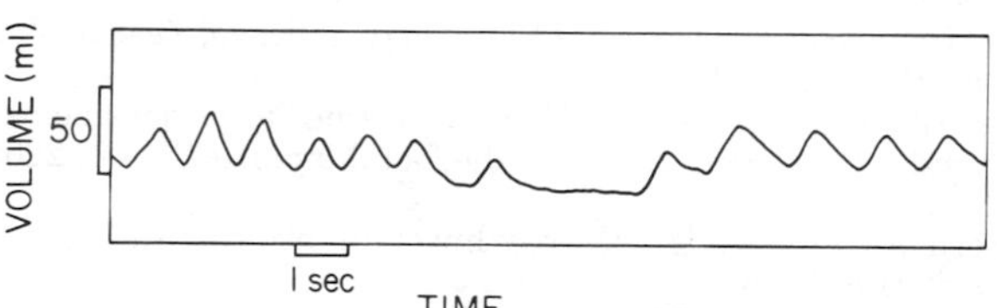

Figure 4.15. Recording of tidal volume in a healthy full-term newborn infant. Note that the dynamically maintained end-expiratory volume during breathing is higher than that during a brief unobstructed apnea. Mechanisms for active control of end-expiratory volume include timing reflexes and retardation of expiratory air-flow (braking) by upper airway muscles and diaphragm. Courtesy of Dr. Ann Stark.

derdamped or unstabilized in premature infants. Data of Waggener et al (1982) recorded from infants are consistent with this view. Immaturity of brainstem neural function as measured by auditory evoked responses has also been shown by Henderson-Smart et al (1983). The prolongation of brainstem conduction time is not sufficient to explain the spells because, in a given infant, the measurements may be the same on days on which many spells are recorded as on days with no spells.

Natural History

The natural history of apneic spells depends on recognition of precipitating or aggravating causes. Apneic spells with bradycardia can occur in most immature infants (40–50% of those less than 31 weeks' gestation, and 5–10% of those up to 35 weeks' gestation) on the basis of immaturity alone; that is, in the absence of demonstrable disease.

In some immature infants and in all other infants, such spells may herald underlying disease including intracranial pathology, RDS, pneumothorax, hypoxia from any reason, hypoglycemia, or hemorrhage with decrease in blood volume. They may be an early manifestation of sepsis, or occur in association with respi-

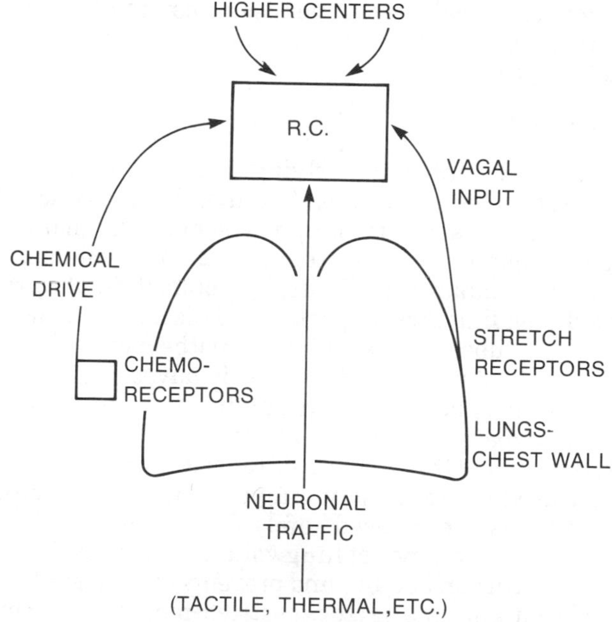

Figure 4.16. Schematic representation of central and peripheral modulators of breathing. Rhythmic discharges from the medullary respiratory centers can be modified voluntarily from higher centers, or regulated by a variety of chemical stimuli to maintain normal pH and oxygenation. Among the chemical stimuli are hydrogen ion, P_{O_2}, and P_{CO_2} operating at the carotid and aortic chemoreceptors and brain stem. Other stimuli include acetylcholine, amino acids, monoammines, adenosine, neuropeptides, and neurohormones. Progesterone and thyroid hormone influence breathing patterns and ventilation. Little is known of the site of action of these chemicals on the respiratory system.

ratory syncytial virus infection (Church et al, 1984). Episodes of apnea with bradycardia (<80/min) can result in a decrease in cerebral blood velocity as measured by the Doppler technique. Ischemic brain injury can result (Perlman and Volpe, 1985).

Fatigue can be a final common pathway to recurrent apnea, sometimes aggravated by malnutrition or deficient energy reserves. This can be decreased or prevented by assisted mechanical ventilation, attention to nutritional needs, or restoration of a thermoneutral environment to lessen oxygen consumption (see pp. 136).

Diagnosis

Consideration of possible underlying causes requires information on events surrounding delivery, previous stresses, or hypoxia that could promote intracranial bleeding, and evaluation of the current status with respect to oxygenation and nutrition.

In the event of extreme prematurity, the problem is most complex and requires judgment whether laboratory studies are required. Cranial ultrasonography is an important first step in evaluation. Blood counts and blood cultures are usually indicated as well as urinalysis, and possibly lumbar puncture. (Recall that when body weight is at its nadir, cerebrospinal fluid pressure is often subatmospheric and lumbar punctures are unrewarding.) Blood sugar and electrolytes with microchemical determinations can reveal aggravating biochemical imbalances. A persistent patent ductus with shunts in either direction can be associated with apnea and bradycardia.

Treatment

When treatable, underlying causes are eliminated, the question becomes what should be done to lessen the frequency and severity of apneic spells. The mainstay of treatment is the maintenance of lung volume, especially in immature infants, by application of continuous distending airway pressure. This can be achieved with nasal tubes because infants breathe mostly through the nose. The use of nasal tubes is advocated because the normal upper airway humidification mechanisms are not bypassed and the larynx and vocal cords are not irritated. Oro- and nasotracheal tubes are commonly used because suctioning is easier, and carefully placed tubes can be used safely for months.

The maintenance of lung volume improves the ventilation perfusion balance and prevents atelectasis. When muscle fatigue is a factor, assisted mechanical ventilation is indicated. The pressures required are relatively low, and increased inspired oxygen may or may not be needed. Usually, 24–26% oxygen is given to keep arterial tensions in the 60- to 70-torr range.

Stimulants such as methylxanthines are often used, and may be especially helpful during the period of weaning from the ventilator. Because infants differ markedly in their requirements, blood levels of theophylline should be maintained at 4–15 μg/L. The usual dose is 1–3 mg/kg/dose, one to three times daily, with the infant's response being the indication for change. Toxicity can be reflected in tachycardia; heart rate monitors are important in showing changes in heart rate.

Sometimes infants respond well to gentle rocking (as may be obtained with a rubber glove filled with water placed under the sheets on which the infant rests). A waterbed provides the degree of stimulus that may make respirations more regular. Once again, individual infants may be overstimulated by this maneuver and the best advice is trial and error to see what helps.

Outcome

With prompt intervention, apneic spells can be prevented, and many VLBW infants who received appropriate neonatal intensive care show normal outcome by all available measurements at 3 years of age.

A common question is what to do about a premature infant who is ready for discharge, but who has occasional apneic spells in spite of therapeutic blood levels of theophylline? Is a home cardiac or respiratory monitor indicated?

A prospective study of 1157 infants, many of whom had apneic spells showed that 11 infants died suddenly and unexpectedly (sudden infant death syndrome) but none of those infants had had apnea (Southall, 1983). Thus, pneumograms would not have predicted those at risk, and would identify children with apnea but not necessarily those in need of intervention. Bazzy et al (1983) studied respiratory patterns in infants who were found to be apneic and were resuscitated (near-miss SIDS) and compared them to age-matched controls. No differences in breathing patterns could be detected.

We do not think apneic spells alone are a sufficient indication for use of home monitors, although when parents request them, we prescribe them (see pp. 292).

REFERENCES

Avery ME, Taeusch HW Jr: *Diseases of the Newborn,* 5th ed. Philadelphia, WB Saunders Co, 1984.

Bazzy AR, Haddad GG, Chang SL, et al: Respiratory pauses during sleep in near-miss sudden infant death syndrome. *Am Rev Respir Dis* 128: 973, 1983.

Brouillette RT, Thach BT: Control of genioglossus muscle inspiratory activity. *J Appl Physiol* 49:801, 1980.

Church NR, Anas NG, Hall CB, et al: Respiratory syncytial virus-related apnea in infants: Demographics and outcome. *Am J Dis Child* 138:247, 1984.

Dawes GS: *Foetal and Neonatal Physiology.* Chicago, Year Book Medical Publishers, 1968.

Dawes GS, Fox HE, Leduc BM, et al: Respiratory movements and rapid eye movement sleep in the foetal lamb. *J Physiol* 220:119, 1972.

Hathorn MKS: Analysis of the rhythm of infantile breathing. *Br Med Bull* 31:8, 1975.

Henderson-Smart DJ: The effect of gestational age in the incidence and duration of recurrent apnoea in newborn babies. *Austr Paediatr J* 17:273, 1981.

Henderson-Smart DJ, Pettigrew AG, Campbell DJ: Clinical apnea and brain stem neural function in preterm infants. *N Engl J Med* 308:353, 1983

Henson G, Dawes GS, Redman WG: Characterization of the reduced heart rate variation in growth-retarded fetuses. *Obstet Gynecol Surv* 40:225, 1985.

Kosch PC, Stark AR: Dynamic maintenance of end-expiratory lung volume in full term infants. *J Appl Physiol* 57:1126, 1984.
Menon AP, Schefft GL, Thach BT: Frequency and significance of swallowing during prolonged apnea in infants. *Am Rev Respir Dis* 130:969, 1984.
Patrick J: Fetal breathing movements. *Clin Obstet Gynecol* 25:787, 1982.
Perlman JM, Volpe JJ: Episodes of apnea and bradycardia in the preterm newborn: Impact on cerebral circulation. *Pediatrics* 76:333, 1985.
Southall DP: Home monitoring and its role in sudden infant death syndrome. *Pediatrics* 72:133, 1983.
Thach BT, Taeusch HW Jr: Sighing in newborn human infants: Role of inflation augmenting reflex. *J Appl Physiol* 41:502, 1976.
Trippenbach T: Laryngeal, vagal and intercostal reflexes during the early postnatal period. *J Devel Physiol* 3:133, 1981.
Waggener TB, Frantz ID, Stark AR, et al: Oscillatory breathing patterns leading to apneic spells in infants. *J Appl Physiol* 52:1288, 1982.
Waggener TB, Stark AR, Cohlan BA, et al: Apnea duration is related to ventilatory oscillation characteristics in newborn infants. *J Appl Physiol* 57:536, 1984.

HYALINE MEMBRANE DISEASE OR RESPIRATORY DISTRESS SYNDROME

Definition

Hyaline membrane disease (HMD) is a pulmonary disorder of premature infants, first described by pathologists who noted widespread atelectasis and eosinophilic material lining the overdistended terminal bronchioles (hence the name). In deference to historic precedent we perpetuate the use of that name, although we recognize the appropriateness of indicating that during life the infants have respiratory distress syndrome (RDS; Fig. 4.17). Either designation is acceptable. The condition is a surfactant deficiency syndrome resulting from immaturity (Avery and Mead, 1959).

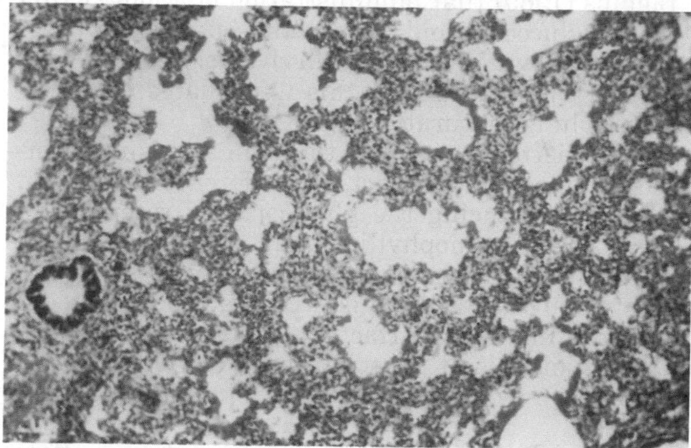

Figure 4.17. The histology of hyaline membrane disease shows the uneven (Swiss cheese) pattern of aeration, widespread atelectasis, and a pink-staining material that consists of fibrin and cellular debris in the overdistended airspaces. The eosinophilic hyaline membranes are resorbed after several days or weeks in infants who recover. Healing is characterized by a proliferation of type II cells and synthesis of pulmonary surfactant.

Epidemiology

This disorder remains one of the major respiratory problems of infancy and accounts for about 25% of all neonatal deaths in the United States (Farrell, 1983). The prevalence depends on the number of infants born prematurely, the number of very immature infants resuscitated in the delivery room, the reasons for early onset of labor, and use of tocolytics and glucocorticoids to delay labor and accelerate fetal lung maturation. The condition is about 1.7 times more common in males than in females, and more common in low birth weight whites than in nonwhite infants of like gestational age. Olowe showed precocious maturation of the L/S in amniotic fluid (an index of lung maturity) in pregnancies of black mothers in Nigeria compared to those of mixed groups (mostly white) in San Diego (Olowe and Akinkugbe, 1978).

Examination of death rates by race for low birth weight infants shows an excess in white/black deaths until approximately 1500 g. At term, mortality in black infants exceed that in white infants. For VLBW infants, the delay in lung maturation of the white infant imposes a risk. As term is approached, other factors are more significant in differential mortality.

Basic Science

HMD is the consequence of ventilation of lungs that have not achieved the capacity to synthesize the pulmonary surfactants. Differentiation of the type II alveolar cells, which are the sole site of surfactant synthesis, usually occurs at about 32 weeks' gestation. The time of differentiation is, in part, under genetic control, and is regulated by both endocrine and paracrine hormones. Thus, infants who have had intrauterine stress (such as those whose mothers are toxemic or who smoke and who are low birth weight for gestational age) have presumably been in a high glucocorticoid milieu before birth. They have less respiratory distress than expected. Conversely, infants of diabetic mothers, whose intrauterine environment was hyperinsulinemic, have a relative delay in lung maturation because of the antagonistic effect of insulin and cortisol on type II cell differentiation. Carlson et al (1984) have shown in tissue culture that this is manifested in the fibroblast, so that the peptide mediator of glucocorticoid function, fibroblast pnemonocyte factor (FPF) is inhibited.

The composition of the surfactants which line the alveoli and terminal airways has been defined as a complex mixture of mostly saturated phospholipids and lung-specific proteins. Essential to the requisite physical properties is a predominance of disaturated phosphatidylcholine (dipalmitoyl lecithin). The composition of human surfactant obtained by lung lavage is shown in Table 4.21.

The phospholipids are associated with proteins, which are presumed to facilitate movement of the newly synthesized phospholipids to the alveolar surface, or stabilize the lipid layer.

A group of glycoproteins has been identified in lung lavage that are not present in serum. Identification of

Table 4.21
Phospholipid Composition of Lamellar Bodies[1]

Phosphatidylcholine	71.1%
Saturated	48.3%
Unsaturated	22.9%
Phosphatidylserine	2.3%
Phosphatidylinositol	3.8%
Phosphatidylglycerol	9.9%
Phosphatidylethanolamine	7.7%
Sphingomyelin	2.2%
Lysophosphatidylcholine	2.9%

[1]Data of Post et al, 1982.

a 35,000 molecular weight species by cloning the DNA required for its synthesis has permitted precise definition of this protein. Its gene is on chromsome 10. Lower molecular weight hydrophobic proteins are also found associated with lung phospholipids and are under study (Jobe and Ikegami, 1987).

PHYSICAL PROPERTIES

Alveolar stability, or the prevention of atelectasis at end-expiration, requires that the alveolar lining layer be able to change surface tension with surface area. At large lung volumes, the expanded surface has a relatively high surface tension which augments elastic recoil of the lung. At low lung volumes, surface tension approaches zero so that alveoli become "stable bubbles" and resist collapse. These observations can be understood in the context of the LaPlace relationship for spherical surfaces. Pressure (P) across the surface is directly related to tension (T) in the surface and indirectly proportional to radius of curvature (r): $P = 2T/r$. As the radius decreases, tension must also decrease if pressure is to stay the same. Admittedly, alveoli are not necessarily spherical and may have different shapes dependent on adjacent supporting structures. They must have curved surfaces that operate to reduce volume or promote atelectasis unless the forces of surface tension are overcome by surface tension-lowering compounds (surfactants; Fig. 4.18).

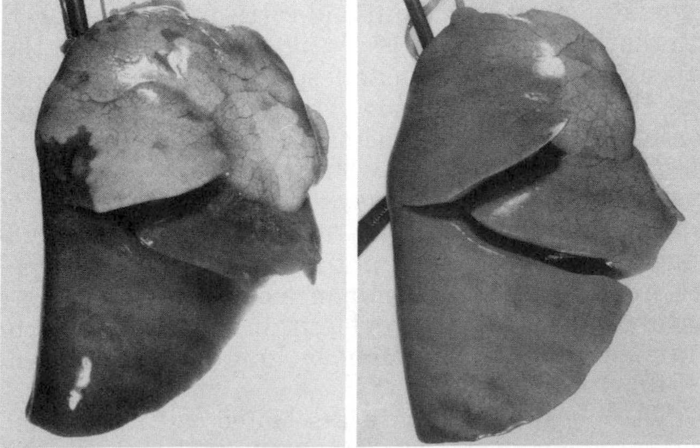

Figure 4.18. Fully inflated 130-gestation lamb lung (*right*) after deflation to atmospheric pressure (*left*). The upper lobe contains pulmonary surfactant, the lower lobes are less mature. From *J Clin Invest* 46:863, 1967.

SOURCE OF PULMONARY SURFACTANTS

The source of both phospholipid and glycoprotein components of human pulmonary surfactant is the alveolar type 2 cell, sometimes called the granular pneumonocyte or great alveolar cell. (The type 1 cell is an attenuated or squamous lining cell that is derived from the type 2 cell.) The type 2 cell has been identified as having storage granules for surfactants. They sometimes coalesce and can be secreted as vesicles, which then spread and line the alveolar surface. Release of osmiophilic inclusions can be stimulated by birth, large breaths, and both adrenergic and cholinergic agents (Wright and Clements, 1987).

Abundant evidence shows that the timing of lung maturation with respect to surfactant synthesis and secretion is under hormonal regulation. The best studied and clinically useful hormones are glucocorticoids, the physiologic example of which is cortisol. During gestation, serum cortisol levels are relatively low until about 34–36 weeks when a rapid increase parallels the increase in size of the adrenal cortex. This high level of cortisol affects the type 2 cell of the alveolus indirectly by way of the fibroblast pneumocyte factor from adjacent cells and directly through an increase in receptors in the cytosol and nucleus of the type 2 cell. Both in animals in vivo and in tissue culture, cortisol can accelerate the time of appearance of osmiophilic inclusions and the presence of surface-active phospholipids in lung lavage or in the medium of mixed cell cultures from the lung (Smith and Bogues, 1980).

These observations confirm the original findings of Liggins (1969) that administration of a long-acting synthetic glucocorticoid, betamethasone, to the pregnant ewe allows precocious survival of the newborn lamb and establishes that this is mediated by acceleration of lung maturation.

Other hormones such as thyroxin have similar effects in animals, but also act by a different mechanism, namely by enhancing the glucocorticoid receptors in the type 2 cell. Aminophylline and β-adrenergic agents presumably act in the same way. Ambroxol, a bromhexine metabolite, also causes proliferation of type 2 cells and stimulates surfactant synthesis. Estrogens enhance synthesis of phosphatidylcholine in rats and rabbits and may have a physiologic role in lung maturation.

Androgens inhibit the cortisol-stimulating effect and may delay lung maturation. Administration of an antiandrogen, flutamide, prevents delay in lung maturation in male fetal rabbits. Because androgens are present in male animals at higher concentrations, their action on the lung may be one reason for the relative delay in maturation of the male who is at nearly twice the risk of RDS as the female (Nielsen et al, 1982).

ONTOGENY

Lamellar bodies, or osmiophilic inclusions, the storage form of surfactant, have been seen in (20-week, 200-g) stillborn fetuses, but they are not normally found before about 5–6 months (900 g). Saturated phosphatidylcholine increases rapidly in association with appearance of increased numbers of lamellar bodies. Although less than half the amount of saturated phosphatidylcholine need be surfactant-related, the concentration increases about three-fold from 5 months' gestation to 7 months'. It is highest just before birth at term and decreases after the onset of air breathing.

SYNTHESIS

Most kinetic studies have focused on phosphatidylcholine on the premise that it is representative of the other phospholipids, although this may not be the case. The phospholipids are synthesized in endoplasmic reticulum and then migrate to the lamellar bodies. In the rabbit, Jacobs et al(1982) reported maximal specific activities of phosphatidylcholine at 4–6 hours in lamellar bodies and 12 hours in alveolar washes after administration of radiolabeled palmitate. The biologic half-life of saturated phosphatidylcholine in adult animals was about 17 hours. Recycling of surfactants is evident from the demonstration of uptake of aerosolized dipalmitoyl phosphatidylcholine by type 2 cells in the rat within 2 hours (Geiger et al, 1975). Labeled surfactant instilled in adult rabbit tracheas quickly became associated with tissue and only 8% of the injected dose was recovered in the alveolar wash at 6 hours (Hallman et al, 1981).

For a more complete discussion of the pulmonary surfactant, the reader is referred to Robertson et al, 1984; Rooney, 1985; Wright and Clements, 1987.

Natural History

The disorder almost always occurs after premature delivery, although it has been noted in infants born near term, at a frequency of about 1/6000 live births. Difficult deliveries and circumstances that produce asphyxia at birth predispose to later respiratory distress. Labored breathing begins at birth, but may worsen in the subsequent few hours. Tachypnea, retractions, and an expiratory grunt follow.

Gas exchange is impaired, with significant right-to-left shunts that are partly through the persistent patent ductus, foramen ovale, as well as perfusion of poorly ventilated regions of the lung. Hypercarbia may be present and a profound respiratory and metabolic acidosis occurs in the absence of ventilatory support and adequate oxygenation.

The chest radigraphs show a diffuse reticulogranular pattern, air bronchograms, and low lung volume from underinflation. The thymus may be prominent on the first day and less prominent after a few days of respiratory distress. Spontaneous pneumothoraces and interstitial emphysema can occur, although these instances of air leak are more common in association with mechanical ventilation (Figs. 4.19–4.21).

RDS usually persists for 3–7 days, but resolves by 7–10 days in infants over 1500 g. In smaller infants, the course may be prolonged. Requirements for increased inspired oxygen or mechanical ventilation lasting more than 7 days should alert the physician to other problems such as aspiration around an endotracheal tube, heart failure from left-to-right flow through an abnormally persistent patent ductus arteriosus, intercurrent infection, or bronchopulmonary dysplasia.

Infants who develop RDS have a number of markers of immaturity in addition to surfactant deficiency. In general, most of the reported measurements are similar to values seen at a lower gestational age in unaffected infants. These include, lower total serum proteins, α_1 antitrypsin, and fibrinolysins. Affected infants are at risk of intracranial hemorrhage, which may be aggravated by the disease, or represent relatively immature vascularization of regions of the brain. They also have more severe and prolonged physiologic jaundice which could reflect delay in maturation of the liver and its capacity to conjugate bilirubin. Alternatively, it could reflect increased uptake of bilirubin from the intestinal tract. Whereas early feeding stimulates motility of the gut, delayed feeding which is usual in infants with respiratory distress increases enterohepatic circulation of bilirubin.

Diagnosis

PRENATAL DIAGNOSIS

Basics. The prediction that a fetus if delivered preterm will be at risk of RDS is of great importance when the location and timing of delivery can be chosen

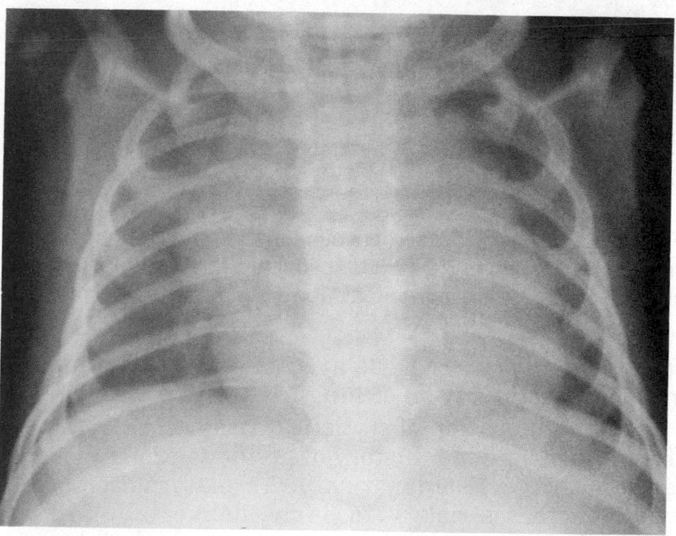

Figure 4.19. Normal inspiratory and expiratory films. The original AP radiograph obtained on this baby (Fig. 4.20) was an expiratory film. The novice can be misled by such a film thinking that mediastinal enlargement, cardiac enlargement, and pulmonary disease are all present.

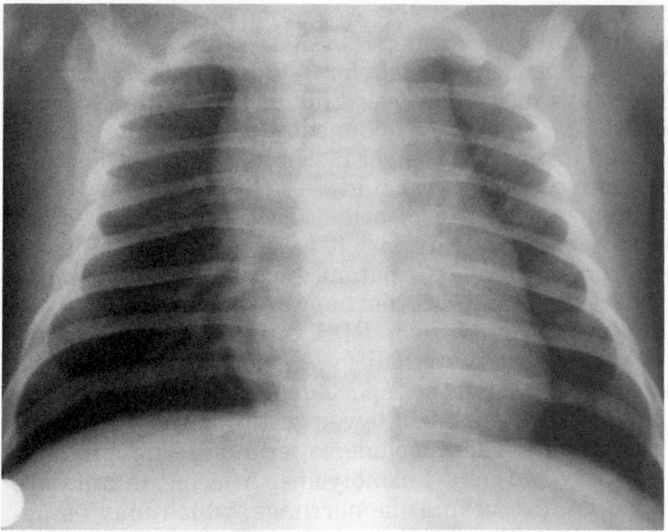

Figure 4.20. The inspiratory film shown for comparison shows a dramatic change in size of lungs. Notice also that the thymus has "shrunk" relative to the expiratory film and also that the cardiac silhouette is smaller relative to the size of the chest. This baby's chest is completely normal.

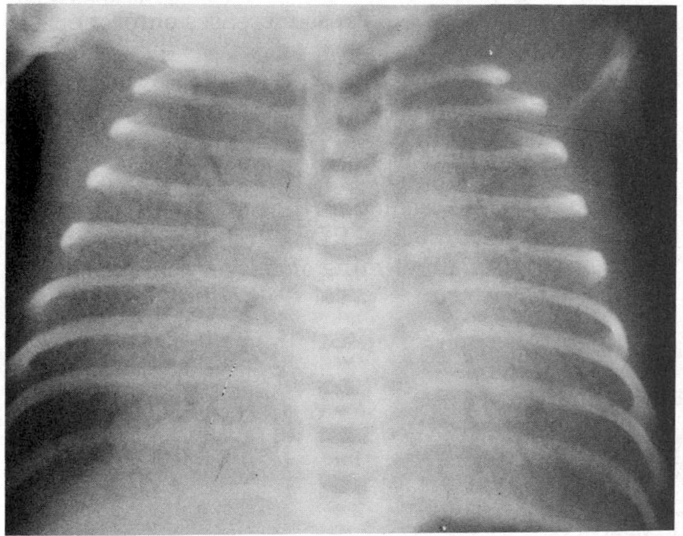

Figure 4.21. Radiograph of hyaline membrane disease on the first day of life. Note the diffuse reticulogranular pattern with an air bronchogram. An orotracheal tube can be seen in the trachea.

or when delivery can be delayed safely to permit pharmacologic acceleration of lung maturation.

Some indication of statistical risk can be obtained from knowledge of a history of previous premature infants with the disorder (risk 90%), maternal diabetes which increases risk 5- to 6-fold, delivery by section before the onset of labor, second born twin, and male sex.

Tests for lung maturity with respect to surfactant synthesis can be carried out on amniotic fluid. Because the lung is a source of amniotic fluid, tracheal effluent from fetal lung contains pulmonary surfactants. Gluck and Kulovich (1973) demonstrated an increase in lecithin with respect to sphingomyelin, an L/S ratio over 2 was predictive of normal postnatal lung function in most instances. Modifications of this test such as measurement of the amount of disaturated phosphatidylcholine (DSPC) or the stability of foam generated on shaking the fluid with carefully measured amounts of ethanol and saline (shake test) are also used to indicate lung maturity.

CONTROVERSY

No test of surfactant components in amniotic fluid is reliable in all circumstances. For example, all tests are unreliable in grossly contaminated specimens. DSPC is somewhat better than the L/S ratio with low levels of meconium or blood in the sample. The lung-specific protein may prove to be the best test, now that a radioimmunoassay is available, although much more clinical evaluation is needed. Errors can occur if the sample is taken from a portion of amniotic fluid containing mostly fetal urine. For reasons that are not clear, the L/S ratio may be normal (>2) in infants of diabetic mothers, even though they subsequently develop RDS. In that condition, the amounts of saturated phospholipids are not diminished. It seems possible, but not yet proven, that the protein components may be abnormal or decreased.

Treatment

BASICS

The treatment for HMD includes general supportive care as required by all low birth weight infants, such as optimal thermal environment (see pp. 136), nutritional support (pp. 139), protection from infection, and phototherapy in the face of a rising bilirubin. More specifically it is important to have access to arterial blood for blood gas determination. A catheter placed in an umbilical artery may be best in a very sick infant, or samples from a temporal or radial artery may be used. Infants seem to do best if arterial oxygen tensions are kept between 50 and 70 mm Hg. If they cannot be maintained by oxygen via hood, insertion of an endotracheal tube and application of continuous positive airway pressure is necessary. If the CO_2 rises above 60 mm Hg, mechanical ventilation should be considered.

CONTROVERSIES

Antibiotics. Because it is sometimes impossible to distinguish RDS from Group B streptococcal pneumonia clinically or radiographically, most infants are given intravenous antibiotics. Furthermore, during the course of treatment, exposure to infection is bound to occur which also mandates use of antibiotics. The choice of antibiotic depends on knowledge of the likely organisms and their sensitivities in a given nursery. A search for organisms by tracheal aspirate or gastric aspiration should be undertaken; if these are absent, broad spectrum coverage seems appropriate.

Muscle Relaxants. Pancuronium bromide to paralyze the infant is widely advocated by some, who find they can achieve more effective mechanical ventilation at lower pressures if the infant does not fight the respirator. Others believe suitable ventilatory adjustments can be made and relaxants should not be necessary. Paralyzed babies require diligent continuous nursing care and attention to fluid intake. The infants easily become edematous because of lack of muscle action.

Physical Therapy. The advocates of physical therapy believe that chest percussion and endotracheal suction facilitate removal of secretions. Others believe this added stimulation is not beneficial and may tire the infants and possibly predispose to intraventricular hemorrhage (Raval et al, 1987). For infants who show persistent atelectasis (often of the right upper lobe) during convalescence, gentle percussion, and changes of position may be useful. Continuous transcutaneous oxygen measurements allow an objective assessment of benefit from chest percussion.

Diuretics. If the baby's condition deteriorates after a few days of apparent improvement, it is possible that a left-to-right shunt through the ductus is causing pulmonary edema. Under these circumstances, furosemide, 1 mg/kg/dose has been found to be helpful. Prolonged use may cause hypercalciuria, hypocalcemia and nephrocalcinosis. Although limiting liquid intake has also been advocated, the benefit from decreasing fluid intake may be offset by the concomitant reduction in calories. Attempts to close the ductus with indomethacin (0.2 mg/kg intravenously) may be undertaken if renal function is adequate (see pp. 138). Indomethacin failure should prompt consideration of surgical ligation.

Surfactant Replacement. The discovery that RDS was the consequence of surfactant deficiency led to attempts to aerosolize purified components of the surfactant and deliver them via endotracheal tube. The first impressive result was obtained by Fujiwara et al (1980) who used an extract prepared from a minced cow lung with added surface-active phospholipids delivered as a liquid via endotracheal tube. Subsequent experience with that mixture (TA surfactant, Tokyo Tanabe Laboratories) has confirmed its efficacy. Long-term safety remains to be established but, to date, no adverse effects have been reported. Extensive studies in animals and humans are underway to evaluate such artificial surfactants, natural surfactants from lung lavage, and synthetic surfactants. From studies to date, it appears that one or two instillations may be adequate, and the earlier the first dose, the greater the benefit (Enhorning et al, 1985; Gitlin et al, 1987). Surfactant replacement before the first breath has been shown effective with both bovine and human preparations. Follow-up of treated infants is necessary before the experimental preparations are licensed (Enhorning et al, 1985; Merritt et al, 1986; Jobe and Ikegami, 1987).

Prevention

The prevention of premature birth would avoid nearly all cases of RDS. Because some infants undoubtedly always will be born early, attempts to accelerate lung maturation are worthwhile.

If delivery can be safely delayed for more than 24 hours, and preferably 48 hours, glucocorticoids such as dexamethasone or betamethasone have been shown to be effective. Their efficacy is greatest between 30 and 34 weeks of gestation, although they have been effective in earlier or later gestations when the L/S ratio indicates lung immaturity (Collaborative Group, 1981).

REFERENCES

Avery ME, Mead J: Surface properties in relation to atelectasis in hyaline membrane disease. *Am J Dis Child* 97:517, 1959.

Carlson KS, Smith BT, Post M: Insulin acts on the fibroblast to inhibit glucocorticoid stimulation of lung maturation. *J Appl Physiol* 57:1577, 1984.

Collaborative Group on Antenatal Steroid Therapy: *Am J Obstet Gynecol* 141:276, 1981.

Enhorning G, Shennan A, Possmayer F, et al: Prevention of neonatal repiratory distress syndrome by tracheal instillation of surfactant: A randomized clinical trial. *Pediatrics* 76:145, 1985.

Farrell PM: RDS today: Advances in treatment and prevention. *J Respir Dis* 4:80, 1983.

Farrell PM, Avery ME. Hyaline membrane disease. *Am Rev Respir Dis* 111:657, 1975.

Fujiwara T, Maeta H, Chida S, et al: Artificial surfactant therapy in hyaline membrane disease. *Lancet* 1:55, 1980.

Geiger K, Gallagher ML, Hedley-White J: Cellular distribution and clearance of aerosolized dipalmitoyl lecithin. *J Appl Physiol* 39:759, 1975.

Gitlin JD, Soll RF, Parad RB, et al: Randomized controlled trial of exogenous surfactant for the treatment of hyaline membrane disease. *Pediatrics* 79:31, 1987.

Gluck L, Kulovich MV: Lecithin/sphingomyelin ratios in amniotic fluid in normal and abnormal pregnancy. *Am J Obstet Gynecol* 115:539, 1973.

Hallman M, Epstein BL, Gluck L: Analysis of labeling and clearance of lung surfactant phospholipids in rabbit. *J Clin Invest* 68:742, 1981.

Jacobs H, Jobe A, Ikegami M, et al: Surfactant phosphotidylcholine source, fluxes and turnover time in 3-day-old, 10-day-old and adult rabbits. *J Biol Chem* 257:1805, 1982.

Jobe A, Ikegami M: State of art: Surfactant treatment for respiratory distress syndrome. *Am Rev Respir Dis* 136:1256, 1987.

Liggins GC: Premature delivery of foetal lambs infused with glucocorticoid. *J Endocrinol* 45:515, 1969.

Mendelson CR, Norwood N, Snyder JM, et al: CTP: choline phosphate cytidylyl transferase activity in developing fetal rabbit lung: Effect of cortisol. *Pediatr Res* 14:458, 1980.

Merritt TA, Hallman M, Bloom BT, et al: Prophylactic treatment of very premature infants with human surfactant. *N Engl J Med* 315:785, 1986.

Nielsen HC, Zinman HM, Torday JS: Dihydrotestosterone inhibits fetal rabbit pulmonary surfactant production. *J Clin Invest* 69:611, 1982.

Olowe SA, Akinkugbe A: Amniotic fluid lecithin-sphingomyelin ratio: Comparison between an African and a North American community. *Pediatrics* 62:38, 1978.

Post M, Batenburg JJ, VanGolde LMG, et al: The rate-limiting reaction in phosphatidylcholine synthesis by alveolar type II cells isolated from fetal rat lung. *Biochem Biophys Acta* 795:558, 1984.

Post M, Batenburg JJ, Schuurmause E, et al: Lamellar bodies isolated from human lung tissue. *Exp Lung Res* 3:17, 1982.

Ravel D, Yeh TF, Mova A, et al: Chest physiotherapy in preterm infants with RDS in the first 24 hours of life. *J Perinat* 7:301, 1987.

Robertson B, Van Golde L, Batenburg JJ (eds): *Pulmonary Surfactant.* New York, Elsevier Science Publishers, 1984.
Rooney SA: The surfactant system and lung phospholipid biochemistry. *Am Rev Respir Dis* 131:439, 1985.
Smith BT, Bogues WG: Effects of drugs and hormones on lung maturation in experimental animal and man. *Pharmacol Ther* 9:51, 1980.
Wright JR, Clements JA: State of art: Metabolism and turnover of lung surfactant. *Am Rev Respir Dis* 136:426, 1987.

BRONCHOPULMONARY DYSPLASIA OR CHRONIC LUNG DISEASE OF PREMATURITY

Definition

Bronchopulmonary dysplasia (BPD) is a chronic potentially reversible lung disease of prematurely born infants who have required mechanical ventilation and increased inspired oxygen concentrations in the first weeks of life. It was first described in 1967 when mechanical ventilation was beginning to prolong life in infants with severe HMD (Northway et al, 1967) and, most recently, extensively reviewed in 1985 (O'Brodovich and Mellins).

Basic Science

In the early stages, the lungs show atelectasis, edema, and hyaline membranes that are indistinguishable from HMD. Instead of resolution in 3–7 days, however, the lungs show persistent consolidation and by 10–20 days develop numerous cystic areas, which can be seen both radiographically and on gross inspection at autopsy (stage III disease). In the most advanced disease, stage IV, the lungs are hyperaerated with strand-like dense areas. Radiographic changes may vary depending on degree of airway plugging by secretions and intercurrent infections which are common. Pulmonary arteries have an abnormal extension of smooth muscle in their walls, as if in response to injury (Tomashefski et al, 1984).

Extensive squamous metaplasia involves trachea and bronchi. Cilia may be absent and mucus forms pools in the airways (Figs. 4.22–4.24). Examination of cilial ultrastructure from the nose of a severely affected infant showed few cilia with slow motion. Partial recovery was noted by 4 months and normal nasal epithelium and ciliary beat was present at 10 months, coincident with clinical recovery (Lee et al, 1984).

What insult (or insults) leads to bronchopulmonary dysplasia is uncertain. Initially, most, but not all infants have had severe HMD, nasotracheal or orotracheal intubation, need for increased inspired oxygen mixtures and mechanical ventilation. Because the underlying disease and/or aspects of therapy are all potentially injurious, it has not been possible to separate the results. Barotrauma and oxygen toxicity probably are most significant. An association with patent ductus arteriosus and fluid overload have suggested the possibility of chronic pulmonary edema as a contributing factor (Brown et al, 1978). Frequently, interstitial emphysema has been noted and hypothesized as an important precursor of cellular proliferation and compromise of air space (Stahlman et al, 1979). Chronic aspiration occurs in 80% of intubated infants, and may cause or aggravate chronic lung disease (Goodwin et al, 1985).

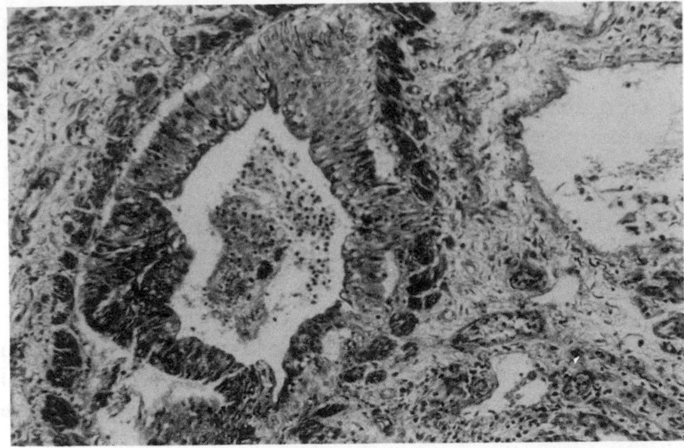

Figure 4.22. Section of small airway of an infant who died at 20 days of age after severe hyaline membrane disease and prolonged mechanical ventilation with over 90% oxygen. Note the loss of ciliated columnar epithelium, squamous metaplasia, and squamous debris in the airway.

Epidemiology

Difficulty in defining the disease, and finding the appropriate denominator have confounded efforts to ascribe an incidence. It is clear that the more premature the infant, the greater the likelihood of chronic lung disease. About half the infants who weigh under 1 kg at birth and survive for 28 days will have some continuing oxygen dependency, as will 10–20% of infants of 1- to 1.5-kg birth weight (Table 4.22). The incidence varies widely among centers, in part because of different populations of infants, and in part because of clinical practice inasmuch as the incidence may vary as much as five-fold among infants of comparable low birth weight in different centers (Avery et al, 1987). In most settings, the more premature the infant, the greater the risk. The condition is rarely, but sometimes, seen in infants weighing more than 2 kg at birth.

Diagnosis

A premature infant who had RDS and who requires oxygen because of chronic pulmonary changes for more than 28 days is assumed to have bronchopulmonary dysplasia. If death occurs, or oxygen is required for more than 3 months, the condition is defined as severe. Arbitrary as these definitions are, they are at least objective and allow comparison among institutions.

A clinical scoring system proposed by Toce et al (1984) is useful (Table 4.23). This system, coupled with a radiographic score is helpful in evaluating therapeutic interventions, and may be useful in multicenter comparisons (Table 4.24).

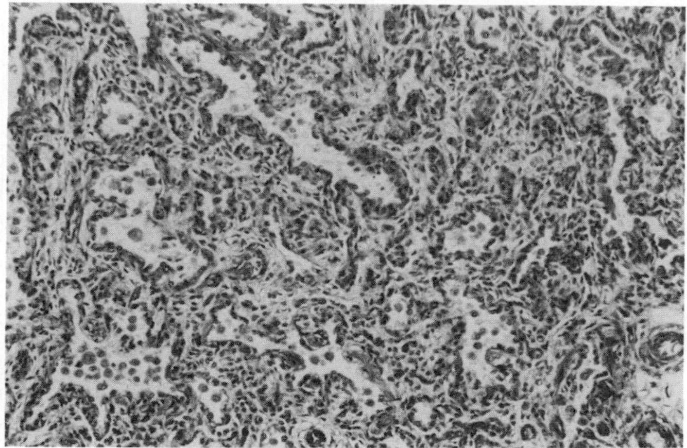

Figure 4.23. The lung parenchyma appears very cellular with loss of normal architecture. Alveolar lining cells have proliferated and sloughed into the airspaces.

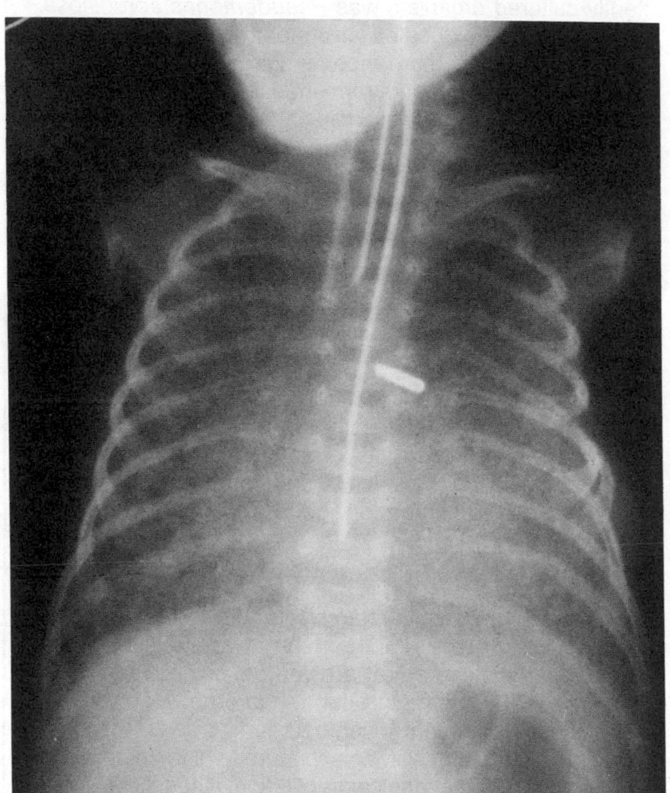

Figure 4.24. Chest radiograph of 800-g infant at 3 weeks of age who had hyaline membrane disease, and a patent ductus arteriosus that was symptomatic at 3 days of age and was closed with a metal clip. Note the distortion of the ribs at the operative site. An endotracheal tube and a feeding tube are both visible.

Treatment

In the absence of full understanding of the pathogenesis of the disorder, treatment must be supportive. All the interventions discussed elsewhere with respect to care of the premature infant apply here, such as optimal nutrition, a thermoneutral environment, maintenance of adequate oxygenation, and provision of appropriate periods of rest and stimulation.

Table 4.22
Survival Without Added Oxygen at 28 Days by Birth Weight[1]

Weight	Live Born	Without Oxygen No.	Without Oxygen %
701–800 g	142	34	23.9
801–900 g	202	63	31.2
901–1000 g	209	112	53.6
1001–1250 g	485	359	74.0
1251–1500 g	587	511	87.1
Total	1625	1079	66.4
Chi-square = 367.21	$p < 0.01$		

[1]These data are from eight centers in the United States who reported inborn infants born between January 1982 and December 31, 1984. Reproduced with permission from Avery et al: *Pediatrics*, 75:106, 1987.

Table 4.23
Bronchopulmonary Dysplasia Clinical Scoring Chart[1]

Variable	Score 0 (Normal)	1 (Mild)	2 (Moderate)	3 (Severe)
Respiratory rate (No./min)[2]	<40	40–60	61–80	>80
Dyspnea (retractions)	0	Mild	Moderate	Severe
F_{IO_2}[3] requirement (for Pa_{O_2} of 50–70 mm Hg), %	21	21–30	31–50	>50
P_{CO_2} (mm Hg)	<45	46–55	56–70	>70
Growth rate (g/day)	>25	15–24	5–14	<5

[1]Modified from the National Institutes of Health Workshop on Bronchopulmonary Dysplasia. Reproduced with permission from Farrell P: *Am J Dis Child* 13:582, 1984.
[2]Average per minute value over one nursing shift. If patient is receiving mechanical ventilation for respiratory failure, a total score of 15 points is assigned. Total score is the summation of values for the five categories, the maximum being 15 points.
[3]F_{IO_2} indicates fraction of inspiratory oxygen.

A specific concern for infants with impaired gas exchange is to provide enough oxygen for their needs, but not in excess, which would cause airway irritation. No agreement exists on optimal blood oxygen levels, but our bias is to try to keep arterial levels between 50 and 70 mm Hg. Sometimes this is best achieved by nasal catheter to avoid prolonged endotracheal intubation and to permit being maintained on oxygen at home. In the late stages of the disease, when the infants are home on oxygen, monitors of oxygen saturation are useful and 90–95% saturation is usually appropriate.

Intercurrent infections are common in any situation with impaired mucociliary function, and are particularly common in infants with BPD. Respiratory syncytial viruses are especially dangerous because they aggravate a preexisting tendency to bronchospasm. The severe airway obstruction that follows may require further hospitalization, intubation, and mechanical ventilation. When bacteria are obtained by tracheal aspirate, culture and sensitivities can direct optimal antibiotic regimens. As new drugs against viruses or vaccines become available they deserve a trial in these infants who are at great risk of fatal pneumonia in the first year of life.

During the acute stages of the disease, there should be concern about possible pulmonary edema. A left-to-right ductal shunt may aggravate the pulmonary dysfunction. Indomethacin or surgical ligation may be indicated. Fluid intake must be sufficient to provide basal calories at least, but should not be excessive. If weight gain is excessive and fluid retention is confirmed, diuretics such as furosemide are recommended (Kao et al, 1984). They are effective in the short term, but may lead to electrolyte and phosphorus depletion if used daily over weeks (Patel et al, 1985). During episodes of respiratory distress, antidiuretic hormone levels are elevated about five-fold which would promote hyponatremia and fluid retention (Rao et al, 1986).

Caloric requirements in the first week of life are usually met by the peripheral intravenous route and average 40–50 kcal/kg/day. As the infant improves, usually at 1–2 weeks of age, intravenous fat emulsions are added to increase calories to 65–85 kcal/kg/day.

VLBW infants have a reduced peripheral sensitivity to insulin and are at risk of hyperglycemia. The usual intravenous mixture in the first week is 10–12% glucose and 1.5% amino acids to give a caloric density of 0.46 kcal/ml. Higher concentrations of glucose are not well tolerated.

When the infant can tolerate oral feeds, 100–120 kcal/kg/day will permit weight gain in most infants. If not, the caloric intake is increased to 130–140 kcal/kg/day.

In infants with respiratory distress, it is particularly important to minimize energy expenditures by careful thermal control and reduction in the amount of handling or examining the infant.

CONTROVERSIES

Considering physical therapy as an aid in dislodging secretions in infants who cannot cough seems logical. Unfortunately, it is not always possible to move secretions by percussion if the mucociliary transport system is impaired. In the absence of consensus about the relative value of attempts to dislodge secretions versus concern for the stress of physical therapy for a fragile infant, it is appropriate to consider each case individually. Continuous transcutaneous oxygen monitoring or pulse oximetry provides an objective record of the efficacy of changes in any intervention.

Corticosteroids have been evaluated during the acute stages of HMD (Baden et al, 1972) without demonstrated benefit. In a prospective randomized study of infants weighing less than 1.5 kg between 2 and 6 weeks of age with chronic lung disease. Avery et al (1985) showed short-term improvement in lung function and more rapid weaning from ventilators in the infants who received the following regimen of dexamethasone sodium phosphate: 0.5 mg/kg/day intravenously in two divided doses for 72 hours, then 0.3 mg/kg/day for 72 hours, then decreased by 10% of the current dose every 3 days until 0.1 mg/kg/day was reached. The drug was

CASE ILLUSTRATION

A white male was born after 28 weeks' gestation and an otherwise unremarkable pregnancy. Birth weight was 1.2 kg and Apgar scores were 2 at 1 minute and 7 at 5 minutes. The infant developed severe HMD and was intubated and ventilated with 90% oxygen. An arterial line was placed in the right radial artery. By day 5, the infant required 60% oxygen to maintain an arterial level of 70 mm Hg and seemed better. Deterioration was evident on day 6, when rales were heard for the first time, and signs of a patent ductus were seen by ultrasonography. Fluid intake was controlled, diuretics were instituted, and indomethacin was started after confirmation of normal renal function.

Over the next 2 months, the infant had both inspiratory and expiratory air flow obstruction, and carbon dioxide retention (Pco_2 80 mm Hg). Copious mucoid secretions could be obtained by tracheal suction. The only consistently cultured organism was *Pseudomonas aeruginosa*. The infant was extubated at 5 months, but required 30–40% oxygen for 2 more months. His growth was among the third percentile and remained at this level until 10 months, at which time his clinical improvement was impressive.

Periodic annual evaluations showed a normal rate of growth (along the 10th percentile). The respiratory rate was elevated at rest to 25–35/minute, and mild expiratory prolongation was evident until about 2 years of age.

Upon physical examination, pulmonary function at 7 years of age was normal, but there was evidence of expiratory obstruction on flow-volume determinations. He had no exercise intolerance and no tendency to recurrent infections after 1 year of age. The residual volume/total lung capacity ratio was 0.34 compared to a normal of 0.20. Maximum midexpiratory flow rate was 60, in contrast to a predicted 98. The maximum inspiratory pressure was 87 cm H_20 (111 is average for age.)

COMMENT

Noteworthy in this example is that the infant was a white male. Severe HMD is nearly twice as common in males as females and, at a given gestational age, white infants have a less mature lung than do black ones.

The development of chronic lung disease occurred after premature birth, HMD, exposure to high percentages of oxygen, and mechanical ventilation. The infant had an asymptomatic patent ductus, and later developed chronic infection. The only known risk factor not present in this particular infant was interstitial emphysema.

Table 4.24
A System for Scoring Roentgenographic Severity of Bronchopulmonary Dysplasia[1]

Variable	Score 0	1	2
Cardiovascular abnormalities	None	Cardiomegaly	Gross cardiomegaly, *or* right ventricular hypertrophy, *or* enlarged main pulmonary artery
Hyperexpansion	Anterior plus posterior rib count of 14 or less[2]	Anterior plus posterior rib count of 14½ to 16	Anterior plus posterior rib count of 16½ or more, *or* hemidiaphragms flat or concave on lateral view
Emphysema	No focal areas seen	Scattered small abnormal lucencies	One or more large blebs or bullae
Fibrosis/interstitial abnormalities	None seen	Few streaks of abnormal density; interstitial prominence[3]	Many abnormal strands; dense fibrotic bands
Subjective[4]	Appears mildly diseased	Appears moderately diseased	Appears severely diseased

[1]Modified from Edwards, 1979. Reproduced with permission from Farrell P: *Am J Dis Child* 138:582, 1984.
[2]Rib counts of anterior and posterior ribs intersecting the level of the dome of the right hemidiaphragm. If the level of the right hemidiaphragm were at the sixth anterior rib and the eighth posterior intercostal space, the total rib count would be 14½.
[3]Enlarged lymphatics and areas of atelectasis cannot usually be distinguished from fibrosis.
[4]"Subjective" factor is based on overall roentgenographic judgment of the severity of disease.

then given on alternate days for 1 week and discontinued. If no benefit was observed in 6 days, the drug was discontinued (Avery et al, 1985). Toxicity from longer term administration is a concern.

Isoproterenol by inhalation has been used frequently for wheezing, especially in the presence of superinfection with respiratory syncytial virus. Kao et al, (1984) examined the responses of infants with BPD, born prematurely (at 30 weeks), and evaluated at 41 weeks. Isoproterenol 0.1% (Isuprel, Breon Laboratories, NY) was given by aerosol, and physiologic saline was given to a control group. Airway resistance was significantly reduced (by about 30%) for 1–2 hours after treatment with isoproterenol. No effect was seen with saline. Similar results were found by Motoyama et al even in the early stages of disease. Kao et al (1984) speculate that the abnormally muscular airways in infants with BPD are more responsive to β_2 sympathomimetic agents. Many infants will benefit from intermittent treatment with inhaled bronchodilators. Theophylline is helpful in some infants, but hazardous without monitoring blood levels (O'Brodovich and Mellins, 1985).

An association between low concentrations of retinol and retinol-building protein in the serum and risk of BPD was reported by Hustead et al (1984). The values are depressed for at least 3 weeks despite intake of recommended daily requirement of vitamin A. These findings have been confirmed by Shenai et al (1985) and suggest that more attention to the nutritional status of infants with respiratory distress would be worthwhile.

Vitamin E, an antioxidant, has been used to treat bronchopulmonary dysplasia with mixed results (Hansen et al, 1982).

Prognosis

The long-term morbidity after severe bronchopulmonary dysplasia is considerable. Sauve and Singhal (1985) report an 11.2% postdischarge mortality among 179 infants with BPD compared to a 0.9% mortality in controls. It is not certain that lung function ever returns to normal in severely affected infants. Coates et al (1978) found low air flow rates in children 8–10 years after their chronic neonatal pulmonary disease. Flow-volume curves were consistent with focal increases in compliance or resistance of terminal airways in a group of infants with Wilson-Mikity syndrome who had not been treated with added oxygen or by mechanical ventilation as infants. Nonetheless, most of these children showed normal growth and were not aware of their flow-volume abnormalities.

The possibility that infants who develop RDS have more reactive airways than those who do not was given support by the studies of Bertrand et al (1985). They found positive responses to a histamine challenge in children 7–12 years of age who survived RDS. The study was remarkable in that siblings also showed abnormal responses to histamine, as did two-thirds of their mothers. The authors speculate that a familial alteration in basic activity of uterine smooth muscle and bronchial smooth muscle could have a role in the onset of otherwise unexplained premature onset of labor and later airway hyperactivity.

Growth failure is common in infants with severe bronchopulmonary dysplasia. The reasons are probably multiple and include difficulty in providing sufficient calories for these infants whose resting oxygen consumption averages 25% higher than comparable infants with respiratory difficulties. The increase in oxygen consumption is presumably due to the overall increased respiratory effort (Weinstein and Oh, 1981). Too few long-term studies have been undertaken to permit a prediction about the ultimate height achieved by these infants.

REFERENCES

Avery GB, Fletcher AB, Kaplan M, et al: Controlled trial of dexamethasone in respirator dependent infants with bronchopulmonary dysplasia. *Pediatrics* 75:106, 1985.

Avery ME, Tooley W, Keller JB, et al: Is chronic lung disease in low birth weight infants preventable? A survey of eight centers. *Pediatrics* 79:26, 1987.

Baden M, Bauer CR, Colle E, et al: A controlled trial of hydroxycortisone therapy in infants with respiratory distress syndrome. *Pediatrics* 50:526, 1972.

Bertrand JM, Riley SP, Popkin J, et al: The long-term pulmonary sequelae of prematurity; the role of familial airway hyperreactivity and the respiratory distress syndrome. *N Engl J Med* 312:742, 1985.

Brown ER, Stark A, Sosenko I, et al: Bronchopulmonary dysplasia: Possible relationship to pulmonary edema. *J Pediatr* 92:982, 1978.

Coates AL, Bergsteinsson H, Desmond K, et al: Long term pulmonary sequelae of the Wilson-Mikity syndrome. *J Pediatr* 92:247, 1978.

Edwards DK, Colby TV, Northway WH Jr: Radiographic-pathologic correlation in bronchopulmonary dysplasia. *J Pediatr* 95 (part 2):834, 1979.

Goodwin SR, Graven SA, Haberkern CM: Aspiration in intubated premature infants. *Pediatrics* 75:85, 1985.

Hansen TN, Hazinshi TA, Bland RD: Vitamin E does not prevent oxygen-induced injury in newborn lambs. *Pediatr Res* 16:583, 1982.

Hustead VA, Gutcher GR, Anderson SA, et al: Relationship of vitamin A (retinol) status to lung disease in the preterm infant. *J Pediatr* 105:610, 1984.

Kao LC, Warburton D, Platzker ACG, et al: Effect of isoproterenol inhalation on airway resistance in chronic bronchopulmonary dysplasia. *Pediatrics* 73:509, 1984.

Lee RMK, Rossman CM: O'Brodovich H, et al: Ciliary defects associated with the development of bronchopulmonary dysplasia. *Am Rev Respir Dis* 129:190, 1984.

Motoyama EK, Fort MD, Klesh KW, et al: Early onset of airway reactivity in premature infants with bronchopulmonary dysplasia. *Am Rev Respir Dis* 136:50, 1987.

Northway WH, Rosan RC, Porter DY: Pulmonary disease following respiratory therapy of hyaline-membrane disease: Bronchopulmonary dysplasia. *N Engl J Med* 276:357, 1967.

O'Brodovich HM, Mellins RB: State of the Art. Bronchopulmonary dysplasia. *Am Rev Respir Dis* 132:694, 1985.

Patel H, Yeh TF, Jain R, et al: Pulmonary and renal responses to furosemide in infants with state III-IV bronchopulmonary dysplasia. *Am J Dis Child* 139:917, 1985.

Rao M, Eid N, Herod, et al: Anti-diuretic hormone response in children with broncho-pulmonary dysplasia during episodes of acute respiratory distress. *Am J Dis Child* 140:825, 1986.

Sauve RS, Singhal N: Long-term morbidity of infants with bronchopulmonary dysplasia. *Pediatrics* 76:725, 1985.

Shenai JP, Chytil F, Stahlman M: Vitamin A status of neonates with bronchopulmonary dysplasia. *Pediatr Res* 19:185, 1985.

Sickles EA, Gooding CA: Asymmetric lung involvement in bronchopulmonary dysplasia. *Radiology* 118:379, 1976.

Stahlman, Cheatham W, Gray ME: The role of air dissection in bronchopulmonary dysplasia. *J Pediatr* 95:878, 1979.

Toce SS, Farrell PM, Leavitt LA, et al: Clinical and roentgenographic scoring systems for assessing bronchopulmonary dysplasia. *Am J Dis Child* 138:581, 1984.

Tomashefski JF, Opperman HC, Vawter GF, et al: Bronchopulmonary dysplasia: A morphometric study with emphasis on the pulmonary vasculature. *Pediatr Pathol* 2:469, 1984.

Weinstein MR, Oh W: Oxygen consumption in infants with bronchopulmonary dysplasia. *J Pediatr* 99:958, 1981.

TRANSIENT TACHYPNEA OF THE NEWBORN (PLACENTAL TRANSFUSION)

Definition

Transient tachypnea of the newborn, sometimes called transient respiratory distress of the newborn or wet lung disease, is evident in the first hours of life in infants who are usually term or near term.

It is characterized by markedly elevated respiratory rates with minimal retractions or cyanosis and a tendency to recover over 24–48 hours (Avery et al, 1969).

Basic Science

It is assumed that infants with transient tachypnea are suffering from some degree of fluid overload which might result from a variety of reasons. For example, maternal fluid overload during labor can induce transplacental hyponatremia and increase the risk of tachypnea in the first days of life (Singhi and Chookang, 1984). Similarly, delayed clamping of the umbilical cord with a placental transfusion to the fetus induces radiographic findings that are similar to those found in transient tachypnea (Saigal et al, 1977). Elevated central venous pressure could delay clearance of lung liquid through the pulmonary lymphatics and the thoracic duct. Intrauterine aspiration of excessive amounts of amniotic fluid could overload the clearance system and lead to interstitial edema and an elevated respiratory rate. Delivery by section before the onset of labor prolongs clearance of lung liquid.

Natural History

This condition is diagnosed by exclusion of other causes of respiratory distress in the newborn infant. As such, it is poorly defined and there is no specific diagnostic test. This makes it difficult to define prevalence or indeed a classic natural history. In general, the infants appear only moderately ill, although some may be cyanotic and require increased inspired oxygen. Respirations are often very rapid, 100–120/minute and shallow. The infants do not show the extreme retractions characteristic of a surfactant deficiency state; instead, they appear to have some degree of overinflation of the lungs and vascular congestion. These findings characteristically begin to clear by the second or third day and the infant should be back to normal by 1 week. Most are normal by 2–3 days.

Diagnosis

The diagnosis is based on exclusion of other causes of respiratory distress and, thus, most of these infants should be treated with antibiotics. It is not possible to distinguish with certainty transient tachypnea from some forms of pneumonia, for which identification of the offending organism may require several days. If the infants have persistent pulmonary vascular engorgement and edema, it would be appropriate to consider using diuretics, although most infants recover so promptly that these are not required. Underlying cardiac disease, such as anomalous pulmonary veins, can present as tachypnea and vascular engorgement.

Treatment

Supportive care is usually all that is required in this self-limited disorder. If the infant is hypoxic, added oxygen is indicated. Rarely are ventilators required.

Prevention

Obviously, maintaining normal osmolality in the mother during labor and delivery promotes a more normal distribution of liquid in the baby. Likewise, the prevention of asphyxial episodes reduces the likelihood of the infant aspirating significant amounts of amniotic liquid. The position of delivery of the infant vis a vis the mother may be important, with milking of the umbilical cord tending to produce neonatal plethora and delay clearance of lung liquid. Delivering the infant at the same level as the mother with clamping of the cord promptly after the initiation of breathing is the best prevention of an excessive placental transfusion.

Prognosis

The process is self-limited and infants followed for as long as 1 year have not had recurrent tachypnea or other evidence of pulmonary dysfunction.

PERSISTENT PULMONARY HYPERTENSION (PERSISTENT FETAL CIRCULATION)

Definition

Elevated pulmonary vascular resistance sufficient to cause right-to-left shunting through the patent foramen ovale and ductus arteriosus is considered persistent fetal circulation (PFC) or persistent pulmonary hypertension.

Basic Science

The condition is most common in term or post-term infants, many of whom have aspirated meconium or other amniotic debris. Many affected infants have been asphyxiated in utero or around the time of birth. Thickening and extension of the smooth muscle in the small pulmonary arteries has been described in autopsy specimens (Murphy et al, 1981; Fig. 4.25).

Epidemiology and Natural History

Some patients have an underlying pulmonary disorder, and the prevalence of persistent pulmonary hypertension reflects that of the underlying condition. The most common association is with aspiration of meconium-stained amniotic fluid but it has also been seen with RDS, diaphragmatic hernia, and infectious (es-

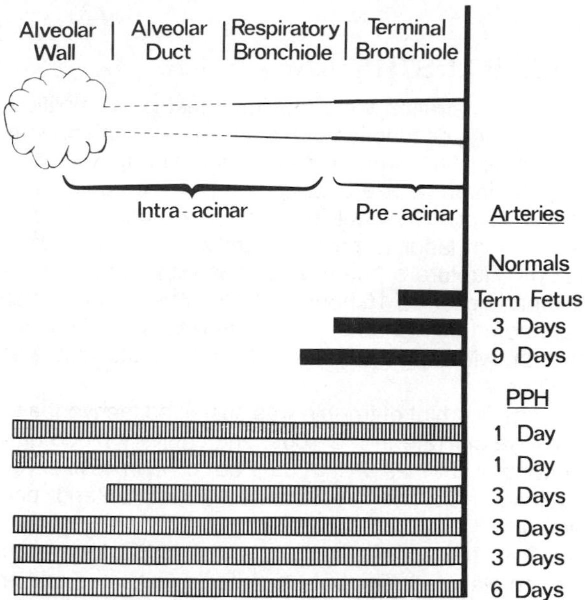

Figure 4.25. Diagrammatic location of muscle in the walls of the intracinar pulmonary arteries. All of the patients with persistent pulmonary hypertension (PPH) had an abnormal extension of smooth muscle into the small arteries. From Murphy JD, et al: *J Pediatr* 98:962, 1981.

pecially group B streptococcal) pneumonia. Sometimes congenital heart disease is present. In the University of Minnesota study, the condition was present in 1.5% of admissions to the newborn intensive care unit (Ferrara et al, 1984). We estimate the prevalence to be about 1.5/1000 births.

Diagnosis

The outstanding presenting finding is profound cyanosis resulting from right-to-left shunts through the foramen ovale or ductus arteriosus; pulmonary pathology is often present but not sufficient to explain the cyanosis or hyperventilation. Arterial carbon dioxide tensions are often normal or low in the early stages of the disorder. Chest radiographs are often clear, although some infiltrates may be present.

Treatment

The best results reported to date have employed a treatment regime that minimizes barotrauma. Peak inspiratory pressures were 25–45 cm H_2O and positive end-expiratory pressure was 5 cm H_2O. Arterial carbon dioxide tensions were in the 40–60 mm Hg range. Arterial oxygen tensions were 50–70 mm Hg. Neither hyperventilation nor muscle relaxants were used. Tolazoline was given to some infants, and dopamine to those who were oliguric (Wung et al, 1985).

Several groups have demonstrated improved oxygenation with deliberate hyperventilation and respiratory alkalosis (pH $>$ 7.55, $P_{CO_2} < 25$ torr). The rationale was to promote pulmonary vasodilation. However, results with this approach are not as good as

CASE ILLUSTRATION

The frustration we sometimes feel is exemplified in the following description of the course of an infant born in November 1984, who died at 41 hours of age.

The infant was a 3.12-kg boy delivered by cesarean section after a 39-week uneventful pregnancy, because of failure of labor to progress and cephalopelvic disproportion. Rupture of the membranes with release of clear fluid had occurred 16 hours before delivery. No problems were noted during labor. The infant was in good condition at birth, with Apgar scores of 8 at 1 minute and 9 at 5 minutes.

The first hint of trouble was sustained tachypnea with a respiratory rate in the 100s, and capillary blood gases showing pH of 7.29, Po_2 of 35, Pco_2 of 48 in 45% oxygen. Radiographs of the chest showed a small anterior pneumothorax.

Over the subsequent hours, the respiratory rate remained elevated. The baby vomited a few times and presumably aspirated. Arterial blood gases even in 100% oxygen failed to show improvement, and at 3 hours of age the pH was 7.16, Po_2 56, Pco_2 60 in 100% oxygen. A repeat chest film showed accentuation of the pneumothorax so that chest tubes were placed.

On physical examination, this term baby boy appeared to be well-developed, but was poorly perfused and dusky. No congenital malformations were evident. The only other abnormality on physical examination was a soft systolic murmur along the left sternal border. The liver and spleen were not abnormal.

Other laboratory data showed a hematocrit of 53, white count of 35,300 with 49 polys, 26 bands, 12 lympocytes, 13 monocytes. An electrocardiogram and ultrasonography of the heart were normal.

During the subsequent hours of life, vigorous attempts were made to promote pulmonary vasodilatation. Therapeutic trials of tolazoline, dopamine, isoproterenol, dobutamine, decadron, and continuous bicarbonate infusion were instituted. Each pharmacologic measure met with minimal or mixed response at best, and at no time did the Po_2 exceed 50 torr, even at 100% oxygen.

POSTMORTEM EXAMINATION

The most striking abnormalities on examination were the presence of polycystic disease of the kidneys, involving both cortex and medulla with "sponge-like" change. The kidneys were nearly four times expected weight. The lungs were hypoplastic, with poor aeration and marked edema. The heart was modestly enlarged and the patent ductus had a diameter equal to the preductal aorta. The pulmonary artery was enlarged. The foramen ovale was probe-patent, with a diameter of 1 cm. There was a mild preductal coarctation of the aorta (0.7 cm in diameter).

COMMENT

In retrospect, there was no clinical clue to the presence of polycystic kidneys, although whether on careful examination they would have been observed to be enlarged is not known. Certainly amniotic fluid was present as noted by the rupture of the membranes before delivery. This child must have had a form-fruste of Potter syndrome with involvement of both kidneys and lung. The profound hypoplasia of the lungs was suggested by the chest radiograph which showed decreased lung volume in a situation where hyperaeration would have been expected. Clearly these anatomic abnormalities made the heroic pharmacologic interventions futile.

QUESTIONS AND COMMENTS

Is persistent fetal circulation an appropriate name for this condition?

High pulmonary vascular resistance is present and appropriate in fetal life; with the onset of breathing, both mechanical events associated with an increase in oxygenation and with lung expansion operate to reduce pulmonary vascular resistance in normal newborns. A situation where this does not occur could be described as persistence of fetal pulmonary circulation. The name ignores the fact that when the cord is occluded, and placental circulation is eliminated, the circulation is no longer fetal.

Why are vasodilators unpredictable?

Vasodilators are shunted to the peripheral circulation through the foramen ovale and the ductus arteriosus and, thus, produce systemic shock, which may require use of vasopressors. The net effects are unpredictable, and require continuous close observation and adjustment of doses.

The early onset of pneumothorax in this infant in the absence of overdistended lungs was overlooked as a clue to the presence of pulmonary hypoplasia. Pulmonary hypoplasia is associated with pulmonary hypertension and was probably the primary lesion in this infant who was not asphyxiated in the perinatal period.

What might be complications of muscle relaxants and hyperventilation?

Complications of hyperventilation are possible injury to lung from barotrauma, and decreased cerebral blood flow. Use of muscle relaxants may be appropriate to dampen changes in cerebral blood flow velocity with muscle exertion by the infant.

What studies are advisable on parents and siblings of this infant?

The association of polycystic kidneys and pulmonary hypoplasia (Potter syndrome) is familial. Ultrasonographic studies of the urinary tract of relatives may reveal some correctable anomalies (Roodhooft and Holmes, 1981).

those of Wung et al who avoid hyperventilation and maintain a normal pH. Pulmonary vasodilatation is apparently more dependent on pH than on Pco_2, according to studies in lambs. Thus, maintenance of normal pH or moderate alkalosis could be achieved by bicarbonate administration. This approach needs to be studied (Schreiber et al, 1986). Vasodilators are often hazardous because they affect the systemic as well as pulmonary circulation. Systolic blood pressure can be maintained at >50 torr with dopamine, 5–20 μg/kg/

min i.v. In most centers, infants are treated with pancuronium to lessen their resistance to the ventilator. Although some infants respond well, others are not improved by alkalosis and hypocapnea, and some progress to bronchopulmonary dysplasia. Isoproterenol, dopamine, and tolazoline are sometimes used singly or in combination, with unpredictable results; occasionally they are life-saving.

CONTROVERSY

Every aspect of therapy of this serious condition is controversial. Extreme alkalosis may have deleterious effects on the cerebral circulation, although Ferrara et al (1984) found 16 survivors all had normal postnatal growth and development when observed at about 1 year of age. Mental development was normal but psychomotor indices were lower.

Hyperventilation reduces cerebral blood flow velocity in human infants, according to Peabody and Emery (1985), although the clinical significance of this observation awaits clarification.

Extracorporeal membrane oxygenation has been used in infants with diaphragmatic hernia and persistent pulmonary hypertension with some clear successes and some failures. It is too early to evaluate this approach.

Prognosis

The neonatal mortality associated with this condition is 20–30%. Few follow-up studies have been reported. Clearly some infants recover completely, and others have serious brain damage. Sell et al (1985) followed 40 survivors for 1–4 years and found that only 40% were normal. An important observation was that 20% had neurosensory hearing loss. Persistent EEG abnormalities are common, and cerebral infarction occurred in nearly one-half of the survivors in the series by Klesh et al (1987).

CHRONIC RESPIRATORY DISTRESS IN THE PRETERM INFANT (WILSON-MIKITY SYNDROME)

Definition

This disorder is characterized by diffuse cyst-like foci of hyperaeration in lungs of preterm infants who do not have severe respiratory illness in the days after birth, but show gradual onset of respiratory dysfunction in the first weeks of life.

Epidemiology

This condition is less common than chronic lung disease after RDS. The true incidence is not known because there is no pathognomonic test and overlap exists with other forms of chronic respiratory distress.

Natural History

This is a clinical-radiographic syndrome first described in 1960 (Wilson and Mikity, 1960). Some preterm infants have mild respiratory distress in the first days of life, which clears as shown clinically and by radiograph. Days, or even weeks later, respiratory distress recurs, and an unusual radiograph is observed, with multiple cyst-like foci throughout both lung fields. Mikity described two stages; the first between 1 and 6 weeks of age, with the cystic changes and diffuse interstitial infiltration. The second stage, at 1–6 months, shows coalescence of the cystic foci and overexpansion of the lower lobes in particular, consistent with air trapping. The changes resolve over the subsequent months (1983).

Pathologic studies suggest residual areas of immature lung with prominent interalveolar septa. The findings do not suggest a reaction to injury, which characterizes bronchopulmonary dysplasia. Rather there appears to be an arrest in alveolar proliferation in the lungs, which is potentially reversible.

Diagnosis

The diagnosis can be suspected from the radiograph and supported by a compatible clinical course. Laboratory studies to rule out pneumonia are important. No consistent changes in blood counts have been noted. Blood gases reflect the degree of respiratory compromise, with reduced compliance, evidence of intrapulmonary shunts, and increased resistance to expiratory flow.

Treatment

Maintenance of adequate caloric intake is important to ensure growth of these infants. They have less pulmonary hypertension if they are adequately oxygenated. Delivery of oxygen by nasal catheter is useful in the older infants who should experience life outside an oxygen tent.

Prognosis

With good supportive care, more than half will recover completely. Several of our early patients are now asymptomatic teenagers. Coates et al (1978), found lower airflow rates in children who had had the syndrome compared to preterm infants without respiratory distress.

PULMONARY HEMORRHAGE

Definition

Pulmonary hemorrhage can be predominately alveolar or interstitial and occurs mostly in low birth weight infants usually in association with other problems in the perinatal period.

Epidemiology

No current figures are available, but it appears to be rarer than in the 1960s when DeSa and MacLean (1970) found 0.21 cases per 1000 live births.

Natural History

This uncommon event can occur in isolation, or be massive and fatal. More commonly it is associated with profound asphyxia as with a nuchal cord, pulmonary edema, pneumonia, disseminated intravascular coagulation, hypothermia, and RDS. Occasionally, blood in the lung is aspirated maternal blood at the time of delivery.

Diagnosis

The only feature that distinguishes pulmonary hemorrhage from other causes of neonatal respiratory distress is coughing or regurgitating bloody material from nose, mouth, or tracheal suction. Adamson et al (1969) found the hematocrit of the fluid to be low, which led them to suggest the fluid was a filtrate from congested capillaries, hence a hemorrhagic pulmonary edema. The condition can be expected in an infant who suddenly goes into cardiovascular collapse. Radiographic changes can range from minimal streaking to massive consolidation.

Treatment

If the hematocrit has fallen, prompt restoration of blood volume with transfusions of fresh blood seems appropriate, although not always effective. A search for infection and appropriate treatment is indicated. Even if no infection is found, we would treat with intravenous antibiotics because of the association of infection and hemorrhage as reported by Landing (1957).

Prevention

The condition was more common when infants were allowed to be moderately hypothermic, before the era of prompt and vigorous resuscitation and maintainance of ventilation with respirators (Rowe and Avery, 1966). Careful attention to maintaining adequate circulatory and ventilatory support in the perinatal period would be the best approach to prevention.

REFERENCES

Adamson TM, Boyd RDH, Normand ICS, et al: Hemorrhagic pulmonary oedema in the newborn. *Lancet* 1:494, 1969.

Avery ME, Gatewood OB, Brumley G: Transient tachypnea of the newborn. *Am J Dis Child* 117:710, 1969.

Coates AL, Bergsteinsson H, Desmond K, et al: Long-term pulmonary sequelae of the Wilson-Mikity syndrome. *J Pediatr* 92:247, 1978.

Cole VA, Normand ICS, Reynolds EOR, et al: Pathogenesis of hemorrhagic pulmonary edema and massive pulmonary hemorrhage in the newborn. *Pediatrics* 51:175, 1973.

DeSa DJ, MacLean BS: An analysis of massive pulmonary hemorrhage in Oxford 1948–68. *J Obstet Gynaecol Br Commonw* 77:158, 1970.

Ferrara B, Johnson DE, Chang PN, et al: Efficacy and neurologic outcome of profound hypocapneic alkalosis for the treatment of persistent pulmonary hypertension in infancy. *J Pediatr* 105:457, 1984.

Klesh KW, Murphy TF, Scher MS, et al: Cerebral infarction in persistent pulmonary hypertension of the newborn. *Am J Dis Child* 141:852, 1987.

Landing BH: Pulmonary lesions of newborn infants: A statistical study. *Pediatrics* 19:217, 1957.

Mikity V: Chronic distress in the premature infant (Wilson-Mikity Syndrome). In Kendig E, Chernick V (eds): *Disorders of the Respiratory Tract in Children*. 4th edition. Philadelphia, WB Saunders, 1983, p. 243.

Murphy JD, Rabinowitz M, Goldstein JD, et al: The structural basis of persistent pulmonary hypertension of the newborn infant. *J Pediatr* 98:962, 1981.

Peabody J, Emery JR: Hyperventilation reduces cerebral blood flow velocity in newborns. *Pediatr Res* 19:356A, 1985.

Raval D, Yeh TF, Mora A, et al: Chest physiotherapy in preterm infants with RDS in the first 24 hours of life. *J Perinatol* 7:301, 1987.

Roodhooft AM, Holmes LB: Family studies: Potter's syndrome of renal agenesis and dysgenesis. *Am J Hum Genet* 33:91A, 1981.

Rowe S, Avery ME: Massive pulmonary hemorrhage in the newborn. II. Clinical considerations. *J Pediatr* 69:12, 1966.

Saigal S, Wilson R, Usher R: Radiological findings in symptomatic neonatal plethora resulting from placental transfusion. *Radiology* 125:185, 1977.

Schreiber MD, Heymann MA, Soifer SJ: Increased arterial pH, not decreased $PaCO_2$ attenuates hypoxia-induced pulmonary vasoconstriction in newborn lambs. *Pediatr Res* 20:113, 1986.

Sell EJ, Gaines JA, Gluckman C, et al: Persistent fetal circulation. Neurodevelopmental outcome. *Am J Dis Child* 139:25, 1985.

Singhi SC, Chookang E: Maternal fluid overload during labor; transplacental hyponatremia and risk of transient neonatal tachypnoea in term infants. *Arch Dis Child* 59:1155, 1984.

Wilson MG, Mikity VG: A new form of respiratory distress in premature infants. *Am J Dis Child* 99:489, 1960.

Wung JT, James LS, Kilchevsky E, et al: Management of infants with severe respiratory failure and persistence of the fetal circulation, without hyperventilation. *Pediatrics* 76:488, 1985.

Congenital Malformations

9

APPROACH TO A CHILD WITH CONGENITAL MALFORMATIONS

The pediatrician's first responsibility is a complete and careful evaluation of the nature of the presenting malformation, the documentation of any other malformations that may require radiographic or ultrasonographic studies, and, if necessary, consultation with geneticists and surgeons or others who may contribute to the subsequent care of the infant (Table 4.25).

These consultations and tests should be done promptly, but thoroughly, to avoid reaching conclusions with inadequate information. Parental reactions to a child with a congenital malformation appear to follow a reasonably predictable course (Fost, 1981). It is well to wait until the mother has recovered from anesthesia or sedation and until a careful examination of the infant has been done before introducing the parents to the problem. They will always express disbelief and sometimes great sadness or anger. This intense emotional reaction is followed by a period during which they ask many questions to which the pediatrician must give careful attention. The situation is always unique to a given couple but typical reactions are to turn their attention quickly to the other children, parents, neighbors, or to their own future economic status. They may jump from one question to another, and much of the time, even though immediate answers may be possible, they are not even necessary. The continuing presence of a pediatrician or individual who can respond to changes that may arise in the baby's condition is desirable. There may be a period of denial which may vary considerably in length but the mother's denial decreases as her attachment to her living, but damaged child increases. Once the parents take over the care of the child and they learn to cope comfortably, their sadness tends to abate.

It is desirable, if possible, to have the mother and the baby together for several days before interventions are undertaken. Even if immediate surgery is necessary, permitting the mother to relate to the infant is beneficial. It is encouraging to note that even where repair of a myelocele is necessary, there is usually no need for emergent surgical intervention. Several days can be taken to evaluate the infant and consider the most appropriate course (Charney et al, 1985).

Table 4.25
Approach to Child with Multiple Congenital Anomalies[1]

- History
  - Mother's previous reproductive history (spontaneous abortions, stillbirths)
  - Pregnancy
    - Infections
    - Drug exposure
    - Alcohol
    - Smoking
    - Maternal illness—diabetes, PKU, Marfan, etc.
  - Labor/delivery history
  - Family history
    - Relatives with neonatal deaths, children with birth defects, known chromosome abnormalities, multiple miscarriages
    - Consanguinity
    - Ethnic background
- Physical examination
  - Anthropometrics
    - Height
    - Weight
    - Head circumference
    - Inner and outer canthal distance
    - Chest circumference
    - Internipple distance
  - Dermatoglyphics
  - Facies
  - Presence of anomalies
- Laboratory evaluation
  - Radiographs
  - Chromosomes
  - Pathologic specimens (placenta)
- Additional studies
  - Examine parents/relatives

[1]Courtesy of Diana Bianchi, M.D.

Epidemiology

Among 10,000 consecutive births in a university hospital in Belgium, van Regemorter et al (1984) found major malformations in 2%. Seventy-eight percent of them were associated with a recurrence risk of over 1%; 9% had a recurrence risk of over 10%. In another survey in Wisconsin, Marden et al (1964) found minor abnormalities in nearly 15%.

ETIOLOGY OF CONGENITAL DEFECTS

The first question that occurs to physicians and parents of the newborn infant with a congenital defect is: how did it happen? The question is of great importance both with respect to directing therapy as well as counseling for subsequent pregnancies. Unfortunately, proof of the cause of disorders is often elusive (Table 4.26).

Among the known associations with certain groups of defects are chromosomal abnormalities, exposure to viruses or drugs at critical periods of development, prenatal irradiation, or oligohydramnios; another group

Table 4.26
Malformations by Apparent Etiology[1]

Apparent Etiology	Approximate % of All Malformations
Genetic Abnormalities	
Chromosome abnormalities	6–10%
Single gene abnormalities	3–8%
Familial, but pattern of inheritance uncertain	18%
Multifactorial Inheritance	20–30%
Environmental Factors	4–5%
Maternal conditions	3–4%
Teratogenic drugs	1–2%
Environmental exposures	
Unknown Cause	30–60%

[1]Courtesy of Diana Bianchi, M.D.

of abnormalities described by Smith (1982) as deformations rather than malformations result from an abnormal intrauterine environment which produces injury to the fetus through external mechanical forces. These abnormalities are characteristically asymmetric.

The physician caring for the infant should consult the appropriate specialists to establish the etiology and work out a plan of treatment. In many instances, the geneticist can be of special help, particularly through the use of laboratory diagnosis for chromosomal abnormalities. A genetics referral center should be consulted if a constellation of findings suggests a syndrome which may be unknown to the physician, but could be identified through computerized data retrieval. If a congenital infection is suspected, appropriate samples should be taken to identify the virus in the fetus or newborn, and to carry out appropriate serology on both mother and infant.

Viruses that Affect the Fetus and Newborn

Many viruses can produce illness in the fetus and, presumably, fetal death, but relatively few are teratogens. Of the latter, rubella is perhaps the best known, and when present in the first trimester of pregnancy can be associated with congenital heart defects, cataracts, and deafness in particular (see Infectious Diseases). Cytomegalovirus is known to be associated with low birth weight and microcephaly. Likewise, the herpes virus hominis has been known to produce chorioretinitis and microcephaly. Varicella zoster may be associated with hypoplasia of limbs and rudimentary digits (see pp. 1037).

Some fetuses infected with human immunodeficiency virus (HIV) show severe growth failure, microcephaly, relative hypertelorism, flat nasal bridge, and patulous lips (Marion et al, 1987). Experience is too recent to be certain the features are associated only with the virus because many AIDS mothers are exposed to narcotics, alcohol, cigarette smoking, and other risk factors.

CASE ILLUSTRATION

A 25-year-old mother of two healthy children gave birth by elective repeat cesarean section at 39 weeks to a grossly undersized infant weighing 1.86 kg. The Apgar scores were 4 and 6, respectively, and the baby was intubated.

It was immediately noted that the infant was dysmorphic with a prominent occiput, short sternum, low set ears, a small mouth, receding chin, and abnormalities of the digits of the hands and feet. Fingers were clenched. A grade 2 murmur was prominent in the right chest and a chest radiograph showed an elevated left hemidiaphragm and an enlarged heart consistent with dextrocardia. The clinical impression was that this was trisomy-18 syndrome and that was subsequently confirmed by chromosomal studies (47XX + 18).

A bone marrow aspirate can be a source of material for chromosome analysis. Results are available in 5–8 hours, but always confirmed with lymphocyte culture later. When information is urgent for therapeutic decisions, we request the shorter bone marrow examination.

The severe malformations and the bleak outlook for an infant with trisomy-18 could have dictated no intervention. The physicians caring for the infant elected, however, to intubate the baby, put her on ventilation, and treat with digitalis and diuretics. No surgery was contemplated. Throughout this period, the family was completely involved with the infant, given much counseling, and was fully aware of the grave prognosis. They participated with the staff in the decision to discontinue mechanical ventilation at 10 days of age.

COMMENT

This syndrome first recognized in 1960, is the second most common of the live births with chromosome abnormalities (prevalence, 0.3/1000 newborn babies). More than 130 different abnormalities have been described in patients with this syndrome, the natural history of which is now well documented. The infants characteristically are feeble at birth, have poor sucking ability, and require nasogastric feedings. Within the first month, 30% die, 50% die by 2 months, and of the 10% known to survive the first year most are severely mentally defective.

The great majority of these infants have trisomy-18 as a result of nondysjunction. When that occurs, it is presumed that the risk of recurrence is less than 1%. If the baby had a translocation it could have been de novo. If one of the parents was a carrier, then the risk would be higher.

The decision to support life with a ventilator for 10 days in this situation is somewhat unusual, but was done at the parents' request to allow time for full understanding of the nature of the problem. The decision should always be left with the individuals concerned with the care of each patient in full recognition of the parents' emotional needs.

Although no other viruses have been known to produce malformations, many can produce fetal or neonatal disease.

Maternal Drugs and Fetal Illness

Surprisingly few drugs are known teratogens and those that are depend on dose, route and timing of administration, and, presumably, the genotype of mother and infant for their teratogenicity (see also Genetics). They are important enough to warrant discussion. *Thalidomide* is the prototype of a drug that has a specific adverse effect on the fetus at a critical period. More than 90% of infants whose mothers received the drug between 34 and 50 days of gestation (postmenstrual) had major malformations, the most striking of which was phocomelia or profound disruption of limb development. Anomalies of eyes, ears, teeth, and intestine were also present in some infants.

Folic acid antagonists, such as aminopterin, have been associated with hydrocephalus, craniosynostosis, limb abnormalities, and mental deficiency.

Excess maternal *iodides* or propylthiouracil is associated with fetal goiter and hypothyroidism.

Warfarin, an anticoagulant, interferes with carboxylation of γ-carboxyglutamic acid (GLA) which is a component of cartilage. Infants may have hypoplasia of the nose, shortened digits, and stippled epiphyses.

Although the teratogenicity of most drugs is evident at birth, some may have their adverse effects many years later. The prototype of such an agent is *diethylstilbestrol* (DES). The initial association of maternal DES, prescribed to counteract threatened abortion, and the development of clear-cell adenocarcinoma of the vagina and cervix in the offspring many years later was made by Herbst in 1971. Subsequent follow-up of these children has confirmed the association, with the average age of detection at 19 years, and the oldest 33 years. Abnormalities of reproduction have also been noted in the daughters, with an 18% chance of poor outcome such as abortion or preterm delivery. A small increased rise of breast cancer has been described among 3033 women who had themselves taken DES between 1940 and 1960, with relative risk of 1.4 (Herbst, 1984).

At least two anticonvulsants are putative teratogens. *Valproic acid* during pregnancy is associated with a greater than expected incidence of neural tube defects, so that α-fetoprotein should be measured in serum or amniotic fluid in the event that the drug has been taken at the crucial stage (Lindhout and Menardi, 1984). Fetal hydantoin syndrome (Fig. 4.26) has been recognized in mothers on *diphenylhydantoin.* The most characteristic feature is hypoplastic nails, particularly the fifth. Rib, vertebral, and hip abnormalities have been noted. Hypertelorism and a flat facies, sometimes with cleft lip and cardiac defects, have also been noted (Meadow, 1968).

Organic mercury (Minimata disease) has been associated with greater than expected incidence of serious CNS toxicity, with microcephaly, mental deficiency, and spasticity.

Tetracycline in the last two trimesters can injure the tooth buds and result in enamel hypoplasia.

Strong presumptive evidence exists to incriminate large doses of *vitamin A* as teratogenic. From June, 1983 to April 1984, the United States Food and Drug Administration was notified of 10 infants with major malformations whose mother had taken *isotretinoin* for acne in the first trimester of pregnancy. Subsequently, other instances have been reported of infants with abnormal facies with hypoplasia of bones of midface and mandible, atretic auditory canal and malformed ears, hydrocephalus, and thymic dysplasia (Rosa, 1983; Hall, 1984). A higher proportion of spontaneous abortions has been noted. Many questions remain about this association, but the data are adequate to advise against excessive intake of vitamin A in pregnancy. The critical period for teratogenesis is probably in the first 8 weeks. It seems probable that the drug has a deleterious effect on cephalic neural crest activity (Lammer et al, 1985).

Androgenic hormones given very early in gestation can masculinize the female fetus and mimic the findings in congenital adrenal hyperplasia. Fusion of the labia and clitoral enlargement are the consequence. This association was first made by Lawson Wilkins and colleagues at Johns Hopkins in 1958. They identified 21 females born with partial masculinization of the external genitalia, female chromatin patterns, and low excretion of 17-ketosteroids. In 15 of the cases, the mothers had been treated for threatened abortion with an oral progestin that contained 17-ethinyltestosterone.

Phenylalanine. Mothers with untreated hyperphenylalaninemia have been reported to have infants with mental retardation, low birth weight, microcephaly, seizures, cerebral palsy, and congenital heart disease. In a summary of 293 births, 91% had mental retardation, and 84%, microcephaly when maternal blood levels were over 1.2 mMol/L. When maternal levels were < 0.65 mMol/L, 21% were retarded. The facies showed a long, underdeveloped philtrum, thin upper lip, flattened nasal bridge, and maxillary hypoplasia with micrognathia (Lipson et al, 1984).

Excess maternal *alcohol* intake was related to a recognizable syndrome by Jones and Smith in 1973.

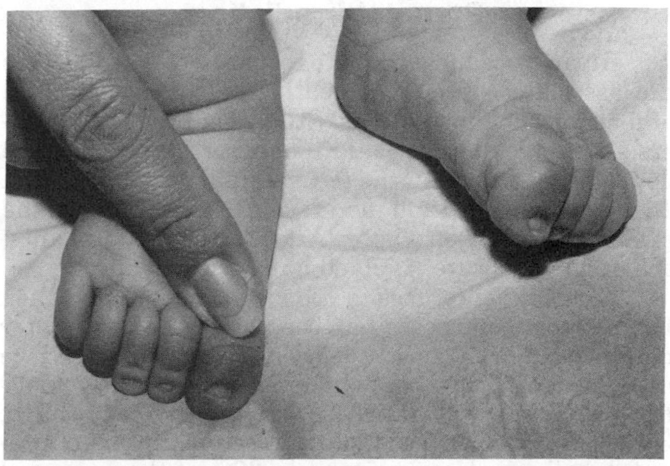

Figure 4.26. Fetal hydantoin syndrome: Note hypoplastic nails that are characteristic of this condition (courtesy of Dr. Lewis Holmes).

They noted growth retardation, narrow upper lip, small chin, and cardiac anomalies in up to 70% of infants whose mothers consumed substantial amounts of alcohol. Mental retardation is common, especially when mothers consume more than 60 ml of ethanol per day. Other features include postnatal growth deficiency, and irritability resulting from central nervous system dysfunction (Rosett and Weiner, 1984; Marbury et al, 1983).

There is little doubt that excess alcohol intake can damage the CNS. Studies on chick embryo show that ethanol alters certain metabolic processes in developing neurons (Dow and Riopelle, 1985), and interferes with their proliferation and migration in fetal rats (Miller, 1986). The evaluation of clinical and epidemiological studies in humans is difficult because mothers with high alcohol intake are likely to be smokers, and perhaps to be using other drugs as well. The most compelling human studies are those that document a dose-response relationship of maternal intake of ethanol and size at birth (Ouellette et al, 1977). Major malformations occur in a minority of infants (Smithells and Smith, 1984).

The prognosis for infants of severely alcoholic mothers is related to the severity of the craniofacial abnormalities. Microcephaly and short stature have been noted in follow-up studies of severely affected infants. Mothers who stopped drinking after the first month of pregnancy had normal infants whereas mothers who did not stop until the second trimester had affected infants. On follow-up, no affected infants had normal intellectual development and most were underweight for height. The influence of continuing maternal alcoholism may have contributed to some of the later adverse effects.

Deliberate sniffing of *leaded gasoline* during pregnancy has been associated with profound retardation, "chipmunk" facies, and spastic diplegia. Elevated blood lead levels found in the infants may have been teratogenic (DeSa et al, 1984).

Prenatal Irradiation

During organogenesis, exposures of 10–300 rads are associated with fetal death, skeletal defects, and other major malformations. Studies of pregnant mothers exposed to nuclear radiation in Hiroshima show the devastating effects on the fetus. Plummer (1952) found 11 women within 1200 meters of the hypocenter of the explosion, seven of whom had microcephalic infants; the other four were shielded by concrete walls.

Exposure of fetuses to prenatal radiographs taken for diagnostic purposes has been associated with later childhood cancer, mostly leukemia. In a retrospective case control study of twin pregnancies where radiographs were used to diagnose fetal position before birth, 31 cases of cancer were found. Documentation of prenatal radiographs was found in 39% of the cases and only 26% of age- and race-matched controls. Thus, the relative risk was 2.4; 95% confidence interval 1.0–5.9 (Harvey et al, 1985).

Most diagnostic studies involve <1 rad exposure to fetus (worst = barium enema 9–20 rads). We counsel people that teratogenicity is not usually seen if exposure is <25 rads after 8 weeks' gestation.

Amniotic Band Sequence

In this condition, amniotic bands are thought to be fibrous tissue formed aberrantly after rupture of the amnion and loss of amniotic fluid. When this happens early in gestation, the process could lead to compression of developing structures and result in a variety of malformations or deformations known as the amniotic band sequence. It is possible that this condition may be more common than reported because some anomalies may be attributed to other mechanisms. Regardless of mechanism, the incidence is about 1/1200 live births (Bieber et al, 1984).

The most common malformations attributed to constricting bands are congenital amputations. A portion of a limb may be missing at birth in an otherwise normal child whose family history lacks similar events.

However, some caution is warranted in genetic counseling. Etches et al (1982) described familial congenital amputations present in mother and son. In this situation, the similarity of the malformations makes it unlikely that these were caused by amniotic bands and lends support to Streeter's hypothesis of a focal degenerative process (Streeter, 1930). Some constricting strings of tissue could be remnants of dysplastic tissue and have nothing to do with fibrous adhesions resulting from rupture of the amnion.

Maternal Addiction and Infant Withdrawal

Drugs of Abuse

Most users of street drugs are addicted to multiple drugs, hence evaluation of the effect of a given drug becomes complex. Prematurity, low birth weight for gestational age, and perinatal asphyxia are more common among abusers of drugs, alcohol, and tobacco in combination than are congenital malformations. Adverse events in pregnancy, including spontaneous abortion, abruptio placenta, and stillbirth are associated with drug abuse.

Tobacco

The adverse effects of maternal cigarette smoking are well-documented and show a dose-response relationship. Overall perinatal mortality was 23.3/1000 births in nonsmokers, 28.0 in smokers of under 1 pack a day and 28.9 in smokers of over 1 pack a day (Meyer and Tonascia, 1977). Growth retardation and subsequent developmental delay have been found in excess in infants of cigarette-smoking mothers.

Cocaine

Use of cocaine by women in the child-bearing years has increased dramatically in the United States in the 1980s, yet the effects on the newborn are seldom described (Madden et al, 1986). When developmental assessments such as the Brazelton examination are carried out the infants are reported to be hypertonic, irritable and have depressed interactive behaviors (Chasnoff et al, 1985). Complications of pregnancy including abruptio placenta occur at a higher rate in cocaine abusers than in the general population, although cocaine abuse is not an isolated risk factor. The rate of congenital malformations is higher in cocaine abusers (Bingol, 1987).

CASE ILLUSTRATION (Courtesy of Dr. Paul Cotran)

A 2.9-kg boy was born to a 24-year-old white mother after 41 weeks' gestation. This was the first pregnancy for an unemployed middle-class mother with a history of polydrug abuse. She had been on intravenous heroin for about a year, including the first part of pregnancy. Six months before delivery she enrolled in a methadone clinic and began on 40 mg/day. She reported frequent use of intravenous and nasal cocaine throughout pregnancy, and oral Valium during the last 2 weeks.

Labor was precipitous. She received 11 mg methadone subcutaneously 20 minutes before vaginal delivery. No anesthesia was used.

At birth, the infant was covered with meconium. After intubation and suction of meconium from below the vocal cords, the infant was given 5 cm H_2O continuous positive airway pressure with oxygen. He was noted to be hypotonic and did not cry. He vomited thick green material on two occasions within the first hour and 30 minutes, but none thereafter. He did not require intubation or oxygen thereafter. On the second day of life he had episodic bradycardia to 80/minute and marked sinus arrhythmia which persisted over the next week.

Laboratory studies revealed positive results for both cocaine and opiates in the infant's urine on the first day. No methadone was present. Blood gases and blood chemistries, including calcium and glucose, were within the normal range on the second day of life.

The infant was started on diluted tincture of opium (0.05 ml/kg) every 4 hours. Although fretful and jittery, no seizures occurred. He was able to take formula well and gained weight at a normal rate during the 1 month of hospitalization. The tincture of opium was tapered daily and withdrawn at 1 month.

COMMENT

It seems probable that most of this infant's problems related to withdrawal from heroin. The unusual finding was bradycardia rather than the more common tachycardia. Experience with withdrawal from the combination of heroin and cocaine and methadone and Valium is too little to allow further comment about the relation of symptoms to drugs. Most of the concern about this infant was focused on the social scene. When both parents are on intravenous heroin and cocaine, who should assume responsibility for the infant? In this case, the maternal grandmother took over care of the infant.

Heroin

Maternal heroin injection is associated with evidence of fetal distress including low birth weight. Fetal pulmonary maturation is accelerated, presumably from endogenous release of glucocorticoids. The infants may have a severe withdrawal syndrome 24–72 hours after birth. They are hyperactive and, if severely affected, may have seizures. Tachycardia, vomiting, diarrhea, and fever may appear during the period of withdrawal. Irritability and jitteriness may persist for a month or longer.

Methadone

Methadone maintenance is prescribed for women dependent on heroin to lessen the likelihood of adverse effects on the fetus of uncontrolled maternal heroin withdrawal. The symptoms may be of later onset and more protracted than those seen in heroin-addicted infants. Some infants have had symptoms for more than a month.

Diagnosis

In the absence of a maternal history of drug ingestion, analysis of the first voided specimen of urine in the infant is diagnostic. After the first day, the newborn will probably have excreted most of the transplacentally absorbed drugs.

Treatment

Treatment of mothers can begin in the last trimester with very slow withdrawal of methadone. About half the infants of maternal narcotic addicts will not need any medication. Those who persist in hyperactivity or have gastrointestinal problems may be treated with phenobarbital, 5–8 mg/kg/day intramuscularly or by mouth in three divided doses and tapered over 2 weeks. For severely affected infants, tincture of opium, 10% solution diluted 25-fold with sterile water, two drops every 4 hours, tapered daily, is effective. Treatment duration is individualized, but may be 1–6 weeks. Side effects include constipation and sleepiness.

REFERENCES

Bieber FR, Mostoufi-Zadehm, Birnholz JC, et al: Amniotic band sequence associated with ectopia cordis in one twin. *J Pediatr* 105:817, 1984.

Bingol N, Fuchs M, Diaz V, et al: Teratogenicity of cocaine in humans. *J Pediatr* 110:93, 1987.

Brande MC, Szeto HH, Kuhn CM, et al: Perinatal effects of drug abuse. *Fed Proc* 46:2446, 1987.

Briggs GC, Freeman RK, Yaffe SJ: *Drugs in Pregnancy and Lactation: A Reference Guide to Fetal and Neonatal Risk.* Baltimore, Williams & Wilkins, 1986.

Charney EB, Weller SC, Sutton LN, et al: Myelomeningocele; time for a decision making process. *Pediatrics* 75:58, 1985.

Chasnoff IJ, Burns W, Schnoll SH, et al: Cocaine use in pregnancy. *N Engl J Med* 313:666, 1985.

DeSa DJ, Evans JA, Greenberg CR, et al: The fetal gasoline syndrome. *Pediatr Pathol* 2:492a, 1984.

Dow KE, Riopelle RJ: Ethanol neurotoxicity: Effects on neurite formation and neurotrophic factor production in vitro. *Science* 228:591, 1985.

Etches PC, Stewart AR, Ives EJ: Familial congenital amputations. *J Pediatr* 101:449, 1982.
Fost N: Counseling families who have a child with a severe congenital anomaly. *Pediatrics* 67:321, 1981.
Hall JG: Vitamin A: A newly recognized human teratogen. Harbinger of things to come? *J Pediatr* 105:538, 1984.
Harvey EB, Boice JD, Honeyman M: Prenatal x-ray exposure and childhood cancer in twins. *N Engl J Med* 312:541, 1985.
Herbst AL: Diethylstilbestrol Exposure-1984. Editorial. *N Engl J Med* 311:1433, 1984.
Jones K, Smith D: Recognition of the fetal alcohol syndrome in early infancy. *Lancet* 2:999, 1973.
Lammer EJ, Chen DT, Hoar RM, et al: Retinoic acid embyropathy. *N Engl J Med* 313:837, 1985.
Lindhout D, Menardi H: Spina bifida and in utero exposure to valproate. *Lancet* 2:396, 1984.
Lipson A, Beuhler B, Bartley J, et al: Maternal hyperphenylalaninemia fetal effects. *J Pediatr* 104:216, 1984.
Madden JD, Payne TF, Miller S: Maternal cocaine abuse and effect on the newborn. *Pediatrics* 77:209, 1986.
Marbury MC, Linn S, Monson R, et al: The association of alcohol consumption with outcome of pregnancy. *Am J Public Health* 73:1165, 1983.
Marden PM, Smith DW, McDonald MJ: Congenital anomalies in the newborn infant, including minor variations. *J Pediatr* 64:357, 1964.
Marion RW, Wiznia AA, et al: The AIDS fetopathy: A recognized pattern of craniofacial dysmorphism in children with AIDS. *Am J Dis Child* 141:429, 1987.
Meadow SR: Anticonvulsant drugs and congenital abnormalities. *Lancet* 2:1296, 1968.
Meyer MB, Tonascia JA: Maternal smoking, pregnancy complications and perinatal mortality. *Am J Obstet Gynecol* 128:494, 1977.
Miller MW: Effects of alcohol on the generation and migration of cerebral cortical neurons. *Science* 233:1308, 1986.
Ouellette EM, Rosett H, Rosman NP, et al: Adverse effects on offspring of maternal alcohol abuse during pregnancy. *N Engl J Med* 297:528, 1977.
Plummer G: Anomalies occurring in children exposed in utero to the atomic bomb in Hiroshima. *Pediatrics* 10:687, 1952.
Rosa FW: Teratogenicity of isotretinoin. *Lancet* 2:513, 1983.
Rosett HL, Weiner L: *Alcohol and the Fetus: A Clinical Perspective.* New York, Oxford University Press, 1984.
Rubin IL, Crocker A(eds): *Developmental Disabilities. Medical Care for Children and Adults.* Philadelphia, Lea & Febiger, 1987.
Smith DW: *Recognizable Patterns of Human Malformation,* 3rd edition. Philadelphia, WB Saunders, 1982.
Smithells RW, Smith IJ: Alcohol and the fetus. *Arch Dis Child* 59:113, 1984.
Solnit AJ, Stark MH: Mourning and the birth of a defective child. *Psychoanalyt Study Child* 16:523, 1961.
van Regemorter N, Dodion J, Druart C, et al: Congenital malformations in 10,000 consecutive births in a university hospital: Need for genetic counseling and prenatal diagnosis. *J Pediatr* 104:386, 1984.
Wilkins L, Jones HW, Holman GH, et al: Masculinization of the female fetus associated with administration of oral and intramuscular progestins during gestation: Non-adrenal femal pseudohermaphrodism. *J Clin Endocrinol Metabol* 18:559, 1958.

Multiple Pregnancies 10

In the United States about one of 80 pregnancies produces twins, about 1/1000 result in triplets and 2/10,000 results in quadruplets. Quintuplets and sextuplets are exceedingly rare. We know of only one instance of septuplets, reported in the news, May 21, 1985. Marked differences exist among races. For example, in the white population of the Western hemisphere twins occur at about one of 80 pregnancies. However, in Nigeria, in some tribes the occurrence may be as high as one in four. In Japan, on the other hand, the frequency of twins is only half that of the United States.

Twins can arise from a single ovum or from two ova. About one-third are from one ovum and, thus, are considered identical (1/200 births). Variations in twinning rate are almost all due to dizygotic twins.

It is probable that there is an hereditary predisposition to dizygotic (dissimilar) twins. The frequency of dizygotic twin births increases from 3/1000 when the mother is under age 20 years to 14/1000 at ages 35–40 years. There is also an increase with maternal parity independent of age.

Determination of twin zygosity is important but sometimes difficult, as discussed by Hrubec and Robinette (1984). Examination of the placentas is helpful only to establish monozygosity of monochorionic twins. For identification in other situations, immunologic typing of blood is necessary. Tissue typing is required when transplantation is contemplated. It is of interest that adult twins can classify themselves as identical or not within a 2–5% accuracy.

In most cases, it is thought that twinning is initiated after the blastocyst is established and, thus, the twins are enclosed in a single chorionic vesicle. In some instances, however, each embryo is surrounded by an individual amniotic sac contained in a common chorionic membrane. It is not always possible on examination of the placenta to be certain whether the twins were monovular or polyovular. Two embryos in a single sac are associated with a high mortality rate because of the likelihood of intertwining of the umbilical cords. It is also true that even single ovum twins may have very different malformations or one can be grossly abnormal and the other normal. Potter (1949) noted that although she has seen minor malformations of different varieties in both members of twins, she had never seen a severe abnormality present in both twins. Structural defects occur two to three times more often in monozygotic twins.

Triplet placentas may originate from one, two, or three ova. A single placenta and chorionic membrane is found in one-ovum triplets, but the fetuses may have separate amniotic sacs. More commonly, triplets are derived from two eggs.

Multiple pregnancies are at risk of abnormalities, such as limb deformations, that result from crowding in utero. Monochorionic twins are at risk of vascular interconnections in the placenta that may result in significant imbalance in the distribution of blood between the infants. Oligohydramnios is common. The anastomoses may be from artery to vein or artery to artery. The effect on the "giving" or arterial side of the anastomosis is to have some degree of malnutrition, significant anemia, hypovolemia, and even shock. The twin who receives more blood can be plethoric, polycythemic, hypervolemic, and in heart failure. This is designated the fetal-transfusion syndrome, in which an artery from one twin delivers blood which is drained through the vein of the other.

Studies on twins have been helpful in understanding the hereditary basis of disease. For example, if one twin has maturity-onset diabetes, the identical twin has a 90% risk of developing this disease, and is at nearly five times greater risk than a dissimilar twin would be (Tattersall et al, 1980). Twin concordances in juvenile-onset diabetes are lower, although this form is associated with specific HLA types.

CONJOINED TWINS

Frequency

Conjoined or siamese twins are fortunately very rare, (only 1% of monozygotic twins.) Symmetrical conjoined twins are almost never seen. The origin of such twins is probably the same as that of some normal separate monovular twins except that division occurs after day 13. If both twins are in the same amniotic sac, there may be incomplete separation and organs may be shared to various degrees. These can exist in a variety of ways from shared cranial contents to shared thoracic or abdominal contents. Occasionally, sacral areas are adjoined and genitalia are partially fused.

Management decisions depend on the extent of fusion and the possibility of surgical separation.

REFERENCES

Benirschke K, Kim CK: Multiple pregnancy. *N Engl J Med* 288:1276, 1329, 1973.

Hrubec Z, Robinette D. The study of human twins in medical research. *N Engl J Med* 310:435, 1984.

Potter EL: Multiple pregnancies at the Chicago Lying In Hospital 1941–1947. *Am J Obstet Gynecol* 58:139, 1949.

Potter EL: *Pathology of the Fetus and Infant.* Chicago, Year Book Medical Publishers, 1961.

Schinzel AA, Smith DW, Miller JR. Monozygotic twinning and structural defects. *J Pediatr* 95:921, 1979.

Strandskov HH, Edelou EW: Monozygotic and dizygotic twin birth frequencies in total white and colored US population. *Genetics* 31:438, 1946.

Tattersall R, Pyke D, Nerup J: Genetic patterns in diabetes mellitus. *Hum Pathol* 11:273, 1980.

Jaundice 11

Some forms of jaundice are most prominent, if not unique, in the first days of life. Their diagnosis and management are central to the care of the newborn infant, hence their inclusion in this section. A more detailed discussion of jaundice appears in Section 7.

PHYSIOLOGIC JAUNDICE

The normal newborn infant has some elevation in serum bilirubin detectable on the second day of life, which may persist for several days or even a week after birth. The bilirubin is unconjugated, or indirect reacting, and rarely exceeds 13 mg/dl in normal infants. The condition is considered "physiologic jaundice."

Basic Science

The elevation in bilirubin results in part from a destruction of red cells which were elevated in utero as an appropriate response to the needs of the fetus for a high oxygen-carrying capacity. The life span of fetal erythrocytes is 60–80 days which may contribute to the elevation in bilirubin (Pearson, 1967). With an increase in oxygen tension after birth, hemolysis occurs and the resulting bilirubin requires conjugation with glucuronide for excretion. Impaired conjugation by the liver results from deficient glucuronyltransferase activity. Jaundice is brought about by enterohepatic recirculation of bilirubin. Delay in passage of meconium for any reason exaggerates recirculation of unconjugated bilirubin. Inadequate production of ligandin, the hepatic cytoplasmic bilirubin-binding protein, also delays hepatic uptake.

Epidemiology and Natural History

Physiologic jaundice, defined as a peak bilirubin of over 10 mg/dl, in the absence of isoimmunization or prophylactic phototherapy, was studied in a review of 12,023 singleton deliveries by Linn et al (1985) in Boston. Perinatal events that were associated with jaundice were low birth weight, being Oriental, premature rupture of membranes, breast-feeding, neonatal infection, use of the pill at time of conception, bleeding in the first trimester, and male sex. These were all independently statistically significantly related to neonatal hyperbilirubinemia. Variables that were negatively related were mother smoking three or more cigarettes per day at delivery, and being black.

Diagnosis

Jaundice is most visible in the face and is less visible in the extremities. Light pressure applied to the tip of the nose blanches the skin and, on release, the yellow pigment is visible earlier than it is in well-perfused areas.

Factors that predispose to significant elevations in bilirubin can be obtained from history and physical examination. Delayed clamping of the umbilical cord with the baby in a dependent position with respect to the placenta leads to a "placental transfusion" which increases red cell mass. Reduced bowel motility in infants in whom initial feedings are delayed is associated with an increase in the enterohepatic recirculation of bilirubin. Glucuronidases in the bowel wall deconjugate bilirubin and allow reabsorption of the "indirect reacting" molecules. Delayed feeding with subsequent caloric deprivation may reduce levels of hepatic binding proteins. Bruising or cephalohematoma increases the load of bilirubin and may overwhelm the mechanisms of hepatic excretion. In some families, physiologic jaundice occurs in siblings who have higher bilirubin levels than expected, presumably on a genetic basis of delayed hepatic maturation. Hypothyroidism is associated with prolonged jaundice, probably for similar reasons.

CONTROVERSY

Breast-Milk Associated Jaundice. A long-standing clinical observation is an increase in indirect hyperbilirubinemia from the third to the seventh postnatal day in infants fed breast milk in contrast to those fed formula.

The explanation for this phenomenon is unclear, but several factors have been implicated. Pregnanediols in breast milk may interfere with conjugation of bilirubin in the liver through inhibition of glucuronyl transferase. Elevated lipoprotein lipase and nonesterified fatty acids have been found in milk from rats whose pups had elevated bilirubin levels. Delay in passage of meconium could also increase enterohepatic circulation of bilirubin. Breast-fed infants receive fewer calories in the first days of life than formula-fed infants, and the relative starvation could enhance enterohepatic circulation of bilirubin. For whatever reason, fecal excretion of bilirubin is lower in infants with hyperbilirubinemia in comparison to those with lower serum bilirubin levels.

Many opinions and little data exist to guide management of infants with rising indirect bilirubin on the third to fifth day of life. In general, when the serum bilirubin reaches 15–16 mg/dl, many physicians advise cessation of breast-feeding for 48 hours. If the bilirubin falls, breast-feeding can resume, with the expectation of a modest subsequent transient increase in bilirubin. The baby can be given formula for the 48 hours and mother should maintain lactation with a breast pump (Lascari, 1986). Other physicians take note of the absence of reports of kernicterus in otherwise healthy term infants with hyperbilirubinemia associated with breast feeding and urge it be continued. Keeping the infant undressed (but warm) near a window is an effective form of home phototherapy.

PHOTOTHERAPY

Visible light (daylight) therapy for neonatal jaundice may well have been used for centuries, but systematic evaluation of its efficacy awaited the observations of Cremer et al (1958) and Lucey et al (1968). Studies of the mechanism of action continue to the present. It is estimated that between 2% and 5% of all newborn infants are "put under the lights," naked, with eyes covered, for a few days to lower serum bilirubin.

Basic Science

EFFICACY

In 1974, a prospective controlled clinical evaluation of standardized approach to phototherapy was sponsored by the National Institute of Child Health and Human Development. For this study, 1339 infants from six centers were assigned to phototherapy at 24 ± 12 hours of age. The duration of therapy consisted of exposure for 96 hours to Westinghouse daylight fluorescent bulbs placed between 35 and 55 cm from the surface on which the infant lay. Phototherapy was effective in preventing hyperbilirubinemia in infants under 2 kg. It was also effective in infants of 2–2.5 kg when initiated after bilirubin was 10 mg/dl, and in infants weighing more than 2.5 kg when bilirubin was 13 mg/dl. Black and nonblack infants had similar responses. Phototherapy was not as effective in infants with ongoing hemolysis (Brown et al, 1985).

METABOLIC ASPECTS

Higher fluid and caloric intakes result in lower mean serum bilirubin levels in all infants. The effect is greater with oral than with intravenous calories. Phototherapy is most effective when infants receive at least 60 ml/kg/day of fluids. Presumably water-soluble bilirubin products are excreted in urine (Wu et al, 1985).

BILIRUBIN METABOLISM

Bilirubin is derived from degradation of heme. It is highly lipophilic and is usually rapidly cleared from the circulation after conjugation to a glucuronide in the liver. Neonatal hyperbilirubinemia in rats can be totally prevented by blocking the first step in the degradation of heme by a potent competitive inhibitor, tin protoporphyrin (Drummond and Kappas, 1981). The heme can be excreted in the bile. Studies in monkeys and humans are promising; further research is needed to assess its safety (Cornelius and Rodgers, 1984; Kappas et al, 1988).

The effect of phototherapy is to promote metabolism of bilirubin to byproducts that are more readily excreted than conjugated bilirubin, especially when conjugation is impaired as in physiologic jaundice (Ennever et al, 1985). The fastest reaction is a Z to E isomerization which, in infants, results in a bilirubin isomer (McDonagh et al, 1982). It is thought that up to 20% of total bilirubin can be converted to this isomer during phototherapy. The rate of elimination into bile is relatively slow, with a half life of 15 hours in preterm infants. Another minor isomer, lumirubin, has a shorter half-life and may make an important contribution to excretion.

CHARACTERISTICS OF LIGHT SOURCE

Optimal isomerization of bilirubin is highly correlated with the intensity of radiation within the bilirubin absorption spectrum and best results are achieved with a special blue lamp with narrow spectral output at 445 nm (McDonagh et al, 1980). Because the results are nearly as good with daylight sources, which are preferable for those taking care of the infants, we use fluorescent lights that have a daylight spectrum. In parts of the world where such light sources are unavailable, placing infants in warm environments near windows will reproduce the original observations of Cremer.

ISOIMMUNIZATION

Isoimmunization in a fetus or newborn is the result of the transplacental passage of maternal immunoglobulin G directed against red cells. During pregnancy, fetal cells that carry an antigen new to the mother induce in her an antibody response when they enter her circulation. The most common example of this process is in Rh hemolytic disease, or erythroblastosis fetalis. Other antigens on fetal red cells that can induce maternal antibodies are blood group A and B antigens, Kell, Duffy, Lutheran, and other very rare ones.

Epidemiology

Rh antigen is a protein with specific antigenic sites identified as C, c, D, E, e. The most common is D, and when present the blood is denoted as Rh positive; when absent it is designated "d" or Rh negative. Rh negativity is found in about 15% of caucasians, 5% of American blacks, and is negligible in Orientals.

A mother with type O blood with naturally occurring anti-A and anti-B antibodies and a type A or B fetus may have an infant with hemolytic disease. The set-up for ABO incompatibility is present in about 12% of pregnancies, but a positive direct Coombs test indicative of isoimmunization occurs in only 3%.

Natural History

Rh sensitization of the mother occurs in the first pregnancy, but does not usually become sufficient to affect the firstborn. Residual antibody may become a problem in the next pregnancy and increases in subsequent pregnancies.

In the 1% of instances in which the first Rh-positive infant is affected, maternal sensitization may have occurred through Rh-positive blood transfusions, presence of blood in older vaccines, tubal pregnancy, abortion, fetomaternal hemorrhage or amniocentesis without administration of immune globulin. The major sensitizing event in the absence of the above is the first delivery. Administration of high titer anti-D globulin at 28 weeks' gestation and again within 72 hours of delivery effectively reduces maternal sensitization to less than 1% (Freda et al, 1975).

ABO incompatibility is usually milder than Rh incompatibility, although severe hemolysis and hydrops have occurred. The firstborn may be affected; subsequent infants need not show more severe findings in contrast to Rh isoimmunization. The peripheral smear is characterized by spherocytosis, thought to be the result of reduced red cell surface area as antibody and membranes are removed by splenic macrophages. In some instances, the persistence of maternal antibody can lead to prolonged hemolysis and anemia progressing to 8–12 weeks of age more commonly after Rh isoimmunization.

Diagnosis

The blood group and antibody status of all pregnant women must be determined. In the event of Rh negativity, the mother should have serial determinations of IgG anti-D titers. If the titers rise, the status of the infant can be determined from measurements of optical density on amniotic fluid. In the presence, of bilirubin, absorption is increased at 450 nm. Currently, it is recommended that the first amniocentesis be performed at 22 weeks and repeated every 2 weeks. Serial examinations by ultrasonography will detect early stages of hydrops which may be followed with daily scans, or may require immediate delivery (Frigoletto et al, 1986).

After delivery, a hemoglobin, blood typing, and a Coombs test should be performed on cord blood. The direct Coombs test measures IgG anti-D in Rh-sensitized pregnancies.

In about 25% of affected infants, a significant hemolysis leads to hemoglobin values of less than 14 g/dl and cord blood bilirubin levels of over 4 mg/dl. Peripheral blood smears will show numerous nucleated red cells and, often, a decrease in platelets.

Treatment

PRENATAL

Severely affected infants less than 32 weeks' gestational age are candidates for intrauterine red cell transfusions (Liley, 1963). Red cells injected into the peritoneal cavity are absorbed by the lymphatic system and enter the circulating blood. The injected Rh negative cells replace fetal cells so that the infant at birth has a negative Coombs test and little or no fetal hemoglobin. Because the baby may continue to produce red cells, later hemolysis of the infant's cells may produce significant postnatal hyperbilirubinemia.

Less severely affected infants who are over 32 weeks of gestation may be candidates for planned preterm delivery. If the bilirubin in amniotic fluid rises above normal values, and the infant has a low L/S indicating inadequate pulmonary surfactants, dexamethasone given to the mother 48 hours before delivery will help postnatal pulmonary adaptations, and possible intestinal ones as well.

POSTNATAL

Anticipation of a rise in bilirubin is indication for phototherapy (pp. 186). If the levels exceed established guidelines (Fig. 4.27), exchange transfusion is required. In general, levels of 10–14 mg/dl in the first 24 hours, or 15–19 mg of bilirubin/dl by 48 hours are reasons for exchange.

Hydrops fetalis, or gross edema and anemia is the most severe manifestation of isoimmunization and should have been prevented by fetal transfusion or early delivery. If it occurs, an immediate transfusion followed

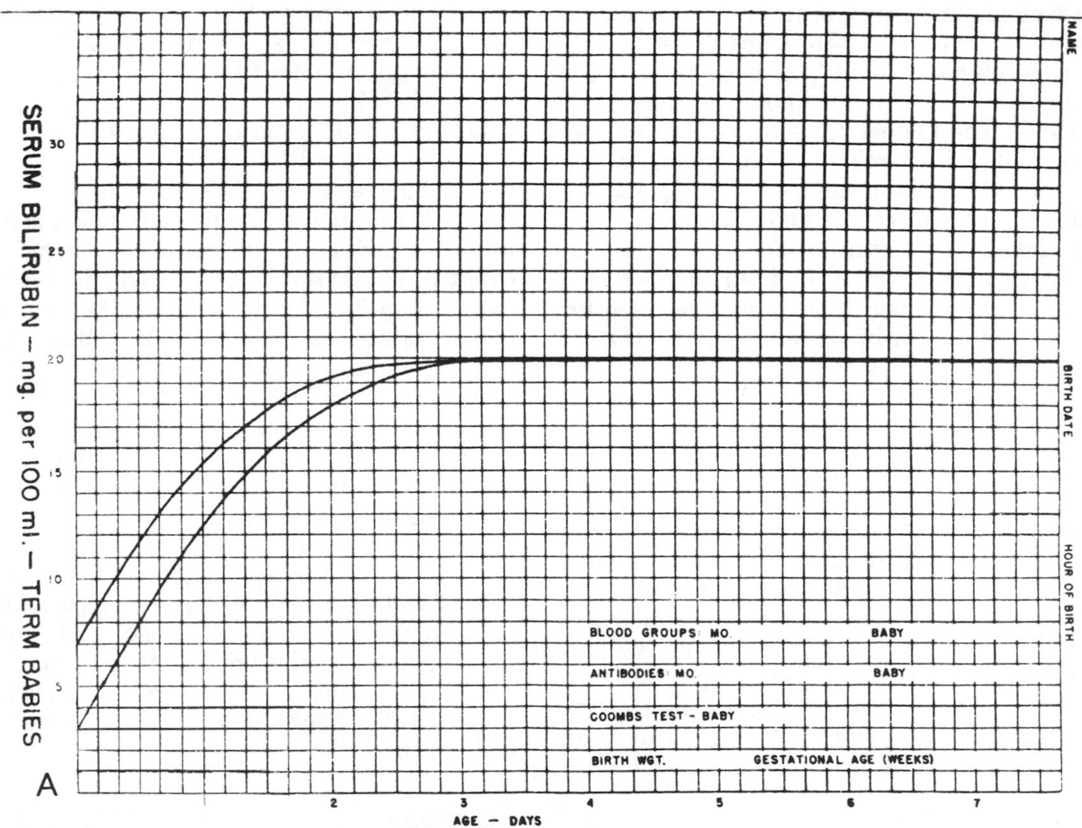

Figure 4.27A. Serum bilirubin levels are plotted against age in term infants with erythroblastosis. Levels that are above the top line at any time predict an ultimate level of 20 mg/dl or over, unless the infant is treated. Even though these diagrams were made before the era of phototherapy, they are a good reminder that the rate of rise of bilirubin is predictive. From Allen FH, Diamond LK: *Erythroblastis Fetalis: Including Exchange Transfusion Technique*. Boston, Little, Brown & Co, 1957.

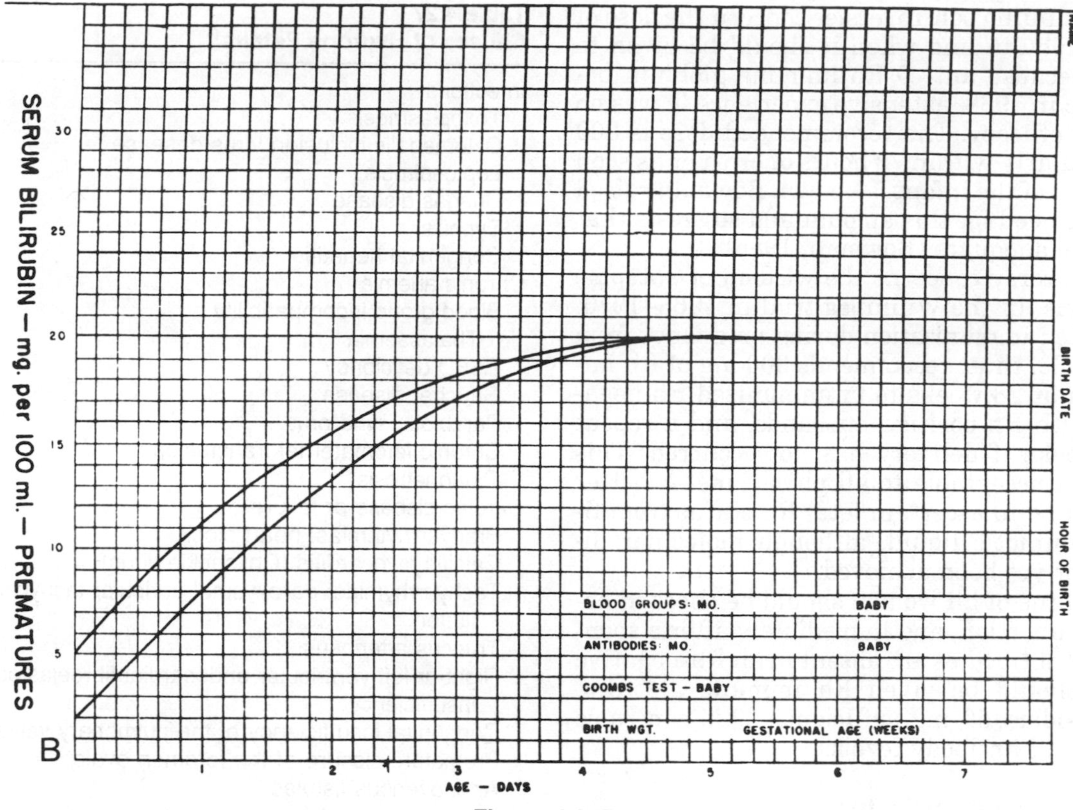

Figure 4.27B.

by partial exchange transfusion with fresh Rh negative blood relieves congestive failure and partially corrects the anemia. (If the anemia is severe, packed red cells (25 ml/kg) are preferred.) Other aspects of the management of hydrops are discussed on page 190.

Late complications: continued low grade hemolysis is to be expected, so that anemia several weeks after exchange is common. If the reticulocyte count is elevated and the infant is asymptomatic, no intervention is needed. If the infant has sustained tachycardia, or other symptoms of anemia, further transfusion is advised. Portal vein thrombosis may be a complication of exchange transfusion. No therapy has been proven effective once the condition is established.

CONTROVERSIES

Types of blood used for exchange transfusions are acid-citrate-dextrose (ACD) or citrate-phosphate-dextrose (CPD) with 65 ml of anticoagulant solution per 500 ml (CPD). Heparinized blood, by contrast, requires 25 mg/500 ml blood.

CPD blood is preferred over ACD because it has less than half the acid load and maintains a neutral pH after storage for 7 days.

Heparinized blood is probably the best, but has the disadvantage that it cannot be used after 24 hours. Its advantages are that it produces no change in ionized calcium, electrolytes, glucose, or acid-base status. It may, on the other hand, interfere with the infant's coagulation. For that reason, 2 mg of protamine for every 100 ml of blood exchanged is recommended.

For all transfusions in newborns, we recommend blood from donors known to be seronegative for cytomegalovirus (CMV). Yeager et al (1981) demonstrated reduced prevalence of excretion of CMV among hospitalized infants from 12.5% to 1.8% after institution of transfusion with seronegative blood. Other methods of prevention include use of filters, leukocyte-poor blood or frozen red cells, but none are more effective, and all are more expensive than careful selection of donors.

Screening blood for HIV is important in areas where AIDS positive donors have been identified. Deaths have occurred in premature infants within 7 months of receiving packed-cell transfusions from individuals who are seropositive for AIDS.

Frequent checks of the infant's blood glucose are advised in all erythroblastotic infants because islet hyperplasia occurs in erythroblastosis. In general, the more severe the hemolytic process, the more profound the hypoglycemia. Raivio and Hallman (1968) observed hypoglycemia before, during or after exchange transfusions in 18% of infants with cord hemoglobin < 10. Exchange transfusion with ACD blood produces a temporary hyperglycemia which then triggers a postexchange reactive hypoglycemia. If the infant's true blood glucose level is less than 40 mg, 5–10 ml of 5% dextrose can be given for every 100 ml of blood exchanged.

Other continuing controversies concern the dose of Rh immune globulin and when it should be given to the mother. Because anti-D Rh immune globulin became available in 1968, extensive experience leaves no question as to efficacy. The recommended dose is 300 mg intramuscularly within 72 hours of birth or as soon as the Rh status of the infant is known. Bowman raised the question of need for this amount and suggests that 100 mg may be adequate (Bowman, 1985).

One controversy concerns the wisdom of antepartum prophylaxis. In the Winnipeg trial in 1968–1976, Bowman reduced immunization during pregnancy from 1.8% to 0.1%. He, thus, recommends 300 mg of Rh immune globulin at 28 weeks to unimmunized Rh-negative women with Rh-positive husbands, and a repeat dose at 40 weeks if delivery has not occurred. This approach is not acceptable to all physicians. A better solution would be to ascertain fetal Rh status from fibroblasts in amniotic liquid, although molecular diagnosis has not yet been achieved.

The Rh status of all women should be checked before a planned abortion, and immediately after a spontaneous one. If antibodies are absent in an Rh-negative mother, she should be given Rh immune globulin. (Bowman considers 50 mg sufficient.) This can raise slightly maternal antibody levels.

Hydropic Infant

Definition

Edema, and anemia, with or without congestive failure constitute hydrops.

Epidemiology and Natural History

This complication of fetal life can be the final common expression of many underlying disorders that permit generalized edema. Its incidence depends on the occurrence of those disorders and the quality of prenatal care and ultrasonographic monitoring that could detect it early and prevent severe edema. The underlying conditions in which hydrops has been reported are listed in Table 4.27.

Diagnosis

Hydrops is obvious on inspection. The most difficult task is to pinpoint the cause and recognize the possibility that there may be several contributory causes in a given infant. For example, anemia contributes, as in hemolytic diseases of the newborn. The process is aggravated by the associated heart failure and decreased colloid osmotic pressure that results from fluid retention. Because the placenta is also edematous, the fetus has probably had some impairment in gas exchange before birth and may have suffered myocardial or cerebral hypoxia.

Treatment

Hydrops is lethal without appropriate intervention. Prompt resuscitation is required. If there is dif-

Table 4.27
Causes of Hydrops Fetalis[1]

Infections
- Toxoplasmosis
- Cytomegalic inclusion virus desease
- Leptospirosis
- Chagas disease
- Syphilis
- Congenital hepatitis

Chronic anemia
- Blood group incompatibility
- α-Thalassemia
- G6PD deficiency
- Gaucher disease
- Parabiotic syndrome
- Chronic fetomaternal transfusion
- Osteopetrosis

Cardiac disease or failure
- Bradyarrhythmias: heart block
- Calcific myocarditis (Coxsackie virus)
- Tachyarrhymias: paroxysmal auricular tachycardia, atrial flutter
- Truncus arteriosus
- Right or left ventricular endocardial fibroelastosis and mitral insufficiency
- Congenital insufficiency of the pulmonary valve
- Premature closure of the foramen ovale
- Arteriovenous fistulas
- Uhl anomaly, pulmonary atresia
- Cardiac neoplasm
- Twin pregnancy with "parasitic fetus"

Renal disease
- Congenital nephrosis
- Renal vein thrombosis

Malformations and congenital tumors
- Pulmonary hypoplasia
- Hemangioendothelioma
- Chorioangioma of the placenta
- Aneurysm of the umbilical artery
- Angiomyxoma of the umbilical cord
- Congenital neuroblastoma
- Cystic hygroma
- Cervical teratoma
- Pulmonary lymphangiectasia
- Cystic adenomatoid malformation of the lung
- Down syndrome
- Trisomy E
- Turner syndrome
- Sacrococcygeal teratoma

Miscellaneous
- Idiopathic arterial calcification
- Fetal retroperitoneal fibrosis
- Umbilical vein thrombosis
- Intrauterine intracranial hemorrhage
- Storage disease
- Small bowel volvulus
- Tuberous sclerosis

Maternal disorders
- Diabetes mellitus
- Toxemia of pregnancy
- Polyhydramnios

[1]Modified from Giacoia, 1980.

ficulty insufflating the lung, hydrothorax may be present and thoracentesis is indicated. Abdominal paracentesis is helpful if ascites limits diaphragmatic movement. Central arterial and venous pressures should be monitored. The need for packed red cells or whole blood, depending on the degree of anemia and edema, is urgent. If cardiac arrhythmia occurs, digitalization or cardioversion is necessary. If pulmonary edema persists, fluid restriction and diuretics are indicated.

Prognosis

Once regarded as uniformly fatal, hydropic infants can recover completely if given immediate and appropriate therapy.

Kernicterus

Definition

Yellow staining of the basal ganglia, globus pallidus, putamen, and caudate nuclei with cellular injury that leads to profound central nervous system dysfunction (cerebral palsy) is called kernicterus.

Basic Science

The degree of toxicity of bilirubin correlates with the severity of the hyperbilirubinemia. This stems from the clinical and histopathologic observations that have been made in the past, particularly in infants who have been Rh isoimmunized. Pathologic studies of late stages show neuronal loss and gliosis. More recently, clinical correlations have shown a number of potentiating factors especially in premature infants. Low levels of serum albumin reduce bilirubin binding and permit higher levels of diffusable bilirubin. Acidosis, sepsis, and meningitis appear to increase the likelihood of bilirubin encephalopathy. Competition for bilirubin-binding sites on albumin by drugs such as sulfonamides and salicylates and by nonesterified fatty acids, which are increased in cold stress and hypoglycemia, are associated with higher levels of diffusable bilirubin and increased nuclear staining. A number of different methods of assessing reserve albumin binding capacity have been developed over the years. However, there have been no appropriate clinical studies to correlate the findings of low reserve albumin-binding capacity with pathogenesis of the encephalopathy. The correlation between bilirubin levels and reversible damage to neural tissue was explored by Nakamura et al (1985). Abnormal values of brainstem auditory potentials were more closely related to unbound-bilirubin levels than total levels, and were reversed by exchange transfusion. The investigators concluded the auditory pathology in their infants was in the cochlea or auditory nerve, not the brainstem.

Hyperosmolarity can increase the permeability of the blood-brain barrier and, hence, the likelihood of kernicterus. Studies by Levine et al (1982) have demonstrated this very clearly in rats. They have suggested the possibility that bilirubin bound to albumin can diffuse into the brain through an opened blood-brain barrier if it has been so damaged. That bilirubin itself is toxic to the neural cell has been inferred from a number of studies on non-neural cells such as hepatocytes and fibroblasts. A number of different enzymatic processes have been impaired by bilirubin in these systems. However, what the target of bilirubin is in the neural cell has not been identified. Studies by Nagaoka et al (1978) have suggested the possibility that bilirubin is taken up by different phospholipids in the cell membrane. Brodersen and Bartels (1969) have also indicated that the bilirubin may be metabolized by bilirubin oxidase within the neural cell. Schiff et al (1985) have demonstrated that bilirubin can be taken up by neuroblastoma cell lines and that free bilirubin may have an effect on different aspects of these cells' function. They have suggested that the presence of albumin in the system may have a protective effect on bilirubin uptake by the neural cell. It may well be that the number of insults that the newborn experiences, i.e., hypoxemia, acidemia, hyperosmolarity, and infections may alter the function and integrity not only of the blood-brain barrier but the neural cell membrane as well, facilitating the entry of bilirubin into the cell.

CASE ILLUSTRATION

A 3.2-kg term male infant was born to a black mother, blood group O+, whose pregnancy had been uneventful. The infant was meconium-stained at birth, and was covered with petechiae. The liver was 4–5 cm enlarged and the spleen touched the pelvic brim. The hematocrit was 43, platelets 63,000, white blood count 22,000. Reticulocytes were 9%. The smear showed marked spherocytosis. The infant's blood group was B, Rh+, and the direct Coombs test was positive. The bilirubin rose to 8.0 indirect/5.4 direct at 8 hours, and 17 mg% indirect at 20 hours, when an exchange transfusion was performed. The infant improved immediately after the exchange and was discharged 4 days later, asymptomatic.

COMMENT

This unusually severe case of O-B incompatibility was not diagnosed until the blood smear was examined, and even then it was hard to believe all of the findings were on the basis of the usually mild O-B blood group incompatibility. Blood cultures and TORCH titers were negative. The prompt improvement after exchange transfusion established the diagnosis. Presumably the direct-reacting bilirubinemia was from prenatal liver damage and the thrombocytopenia from massive splenic enlargement. Extramedullary erythropoiesis was sufficient to prevent a severe anemia.

Epidemiology and Natural History

This preventable condition should not occur in this era. Before its pathogenesis was understood, or at least the relationship to hyperbilirubinemia and care in removing excess bilirubin by exchange transfusion was accomplished, the history of severe neonatal jaundice was commonly noted among children with athetoid cerebral palsy (Asher and Schonell, 1950).

The classic descriptions of the disease emphasize loss of suck, blunted Moro reflex, vomiting, and high-pitched cry. Muscle rigidity, paralysis of upward gaze, and periodic oculogyric crises and seizures occurred. Infants who survive the neonatal period have a characteristically high frequency of nerve deafness, dental enamel dysplasia, choreoathetosis, and mental retardation.

Diagnosis

No single test allows the definition of the potentially dangerous effect of bilirubin. Reserve albumin binding capacity, although widely used, has never been clinically tested to establish the exact safe level of free bilirubin. There is no question that with the greater awareness of the potential toxic effects of bilirubin, the closer monitoring of infants that has occurred, and the advent of phototherapy, the incidence of bilirubin encephalopathy has been significantly reduced. This has also been coupled by a significant reduction in the incidence of Rh isoimmunization, the single most common cause of bilirubin encephalopathy. Thus, it is recommended that the time-honored value of over 20 mg/100 ml as a danger level remains useful in a general way. The rate of rise of bilirubin is useful only in those situations before the initiation of exchange transfusion and/or the use of phototherapy. Once these modes of therapy are introduced this no longer becomes useful. Hence the following guidelines are recommended for initiation of either phototherapy and/or exchange transfusion (Schiff D, personal communication).

Indications for Phototherapy:	Weight	Level of Bilirubin
Infant of > 36 weeks' gestation	> 2500 g	12–14 mg/dl
Infant of < 36 weeks' gestation	> 1800 g	10 mg/dl
Infant of < 32 weeks' gestation	< 1800 g	8 mg/dl
Bilirubin Levels for Exchange Transfusion:		
Nonhemolytic jaundice if bilirubin exceeds term infant > 36 weeks' gestation	>2500 g	20 mg/dl
Premature infant of < 36 weeks' gestation	>1800 g	18 mg/dl
Infant of< 32 weeks' gestation	<1800 g	15 mg/dl

In the presence of hemolytic jaundice (i.e., Rh isoimmunization) when at birth a cord bilirubin of >4 mg/dl, hemoglobin of < 13 g/dl, and/or positive Coombs test occur, if two of these three situations exist, an immediate exchange transfusion should be carried out. In the absence of these indications, a rate of rise of bilirubin of >0.5 mg/dl/hour should indicate exchange transfusion within the first 24 hours of life.

Treatment

Once kernicterus is established, no definitive therapy is available. The care of the child is the same as that required for any neurologically disabled infant.

PERSISTENT UNCONJUGATED HYPERBILIRUBINEMIA

When levels of indirect reacting bilirubin remain elevated or fail to return to normal after about 9 weeks of age, a search for reasons other than "physiologic" is essential.

The most common condition is hemolytic anemia, either associated with infection or an inherited defect in red cell metabolism, such as congenital spherocytosis; also isoimmunization from blood group incompatibility can continue to produce low-grade hemolysis and anemia. These conditions are discussed in Section 8. A peripheral blood smear for determining red cell morphology, reticulocyte counts and Coombs tests are essential diagnostic tests.

Extravasation of blood in any location can result in continued elevation of bilirubin levels for some weeks after birth. Cephalohematomas are the most common sites of loculated blood.

Other conditions that require investigation are galactosemia, and hypothyroidism which should be observed on routine neonatal screening. Prolonged hyperbilirubinemia may be the first sign of these disorders.

Familial nonhemolytic jaundice, type 1, (Crigler-Najjar jaundice) is a much rarer condition. Bilirubin levels range from 14–50 mg/dl. Type 2, another glucuronide-conjugating defect differs from type 1 in being autosomal dominant, and by low levels of bilirubin in the range of 2–4 mg/dl. Jaundice may be exacerbated by infection or other illness. Kernicterus has been described in a few type 1 patients.

Gilbert disease is a more common disorder. Rarely diagnosed in children, it exists in 2–6% of the population. Bilirubin levels are usually under 5 mg/dl and the defect in conjugation is only partial. The condition is autosomal dominant. Treatment with phenobarbital corrects the hyperbilirubinemia, presumably by enhancing hepatic conjugation.

Some infants with prolonged and significant elevations of bilirubin have an inhibitor of conjugation in their sera, which eventually disappears from their circulation. The substance has not been identified, but is presumably a gestational hormone that can be detected in maternal as well as fetal serum (Lucey et al, 1960).

REFERENCES

Asher P, Schonell FE: Survey of 400 cases of cerebral palsy in childhood. *Arch Dis Child* 25:360, 1950.

Bowman JM: Controversies in Rh prophylaxis. *Am J Obstet Gynecol* 151:289, 1985.

Brodersen R, Friis-Hansen B, Stern L: Drug-induced displacement of bilirubin from albumin in the newborn. *Dev Pharmacol Ther* 6:217, 1983.

Brodersen R, Bartels P: Enzymatic oxidation of bilirubin. *Eur J Biochem* 10:468, 1969.

Brown AK, Kim MH, Wu PYK, et al: Efficacy of phototherapy in prevention and management of neonatal hyperbilirubinemia. *Pediatrics* 72 (Suppl) 393, 1985.

Cornelius CE, Rodgers PA: Prevention of neonatal hyperbilirubinemia in rhesus monkeys by tin-protoporphyrin. *Pediatr Res* 18:728, 1984.

Cremer RJ, Perryman PW, Richards DH: Influence of light on the hyperbilirubinaemia of infants. *Lancet* 1:1094, 1958.

DeVore G, Mayden K, Tortora M, et al: Dilation of the fetal umbilical vein in rhesus hemolytic anemia: A predictor of severe disease. *Am J Obstet Gynecol* 141:464, 1981.

Drummond GS, Kappas A: Prevention of neonatal hyperbilirubinemia by tin protoporphyrin IX, a potent competitive inhibitor of heme oxidation. *Proc Natl Acad Sci* 78:6466, 1981.

Ennever JF, Knox I, Denne SC, et al: Phototherapy for neonatal jaundice: In vivo clearance of bilirubin photoproducts. *Pediatr Res* 19:205, 1985.

Ennever JF, Sobel M, McDonagh, et al: Phototherapy for neonatal jaundice: In vitro comparison of light sources. *Pediatr Res* 18:667, 1984.

Freda VJ, Gorman JG, Pollack W, et al: Prevention of Rh hemolytic disease—10 years' clinical experience with Rh immune globulin. *N Engl J Med* 292:1014, 1975.

Frigoletto FD, Greene MF, Benacerraf BR, et al: Ultrasonographic fetal surveillance in the management of the isoimmunized pregnancy. *N Engl J Med* 315:430, 1986.

Giacoia GP: Hydrops fetalis (fetal edema). *Clin Pediatr* 19:334, 1980.

Hansen TWR, Bratlid D: Bilirubin and brain toxicity (review article). *Acta Pediatr Scand* 75:513, 1986.

Kappas A, Drummond GS, Manola T, et al: Sn-protoporphyrin use in the management of hyperbilirubinemia in term infants with direct Coombs-positive ABO incompatibility. *Pediatrics* 81:485, 1988.

Karp WB: Biochemical alteration in neonatal hyperbilirubinemia and bilirubin encephalopathy: A review. *Pediatrics* 64:362, 1979.

Levine RL, Fredericks WR, Rappaport SI: Entry of bilirubin into the brain due to opening of the blood-brain barrier. *Pediatrics* 69:255, 1982.

Liley AW: Intrauterine transfusion of foetus in hemolytic disease. *Br Med J* 2:1107, 1963.

Linn S, Schoenbaum SC, Monson R, et al: Epidemiology of neonatal hyperbilirubinemia. *Pediatrics* 75:770, 1985.

Lucey JF, Arias I, McKay R: Transient familial neonata; hyperbilirubinemia. *Am J Dis Child* 100:787, 1960.

Lucey J, Ferreiro M, Hewitt J: Prevention of hyperbilirubinemia of prematurity. *Pedatrics* 41:1047, 1968.

McDonagh AF, Palma LA, Lightner DA: Phototherapy for neonatal jaundice: Configurational isomers of bilirubin. *J Am Chem Soc* 104:6865, 1982.

McDonagh AF, Palma LA, Lightner DA: Blue light and bilirubin excretion. *Science* 208:145, 1980.

Nagaoka S, Cowger ML: Interaction of bilirubin with lipids studied by flourescence quenching method. *J Biol Chem* 253:2005, 1978.

Nakamura H, Takada S, Shimabuku R: Auditory nerve and brain stem responses in newborn infants with hyperbilirubinemia. *Pediatrics* 75:703, 1985.

Pearson, HA: The lifespan of the fetal red blood cell. *J Pediatr* 70:166, 1967.

Raivio KO, Hallman N: Neonatal hypoglycemia. I. Occurrence in patients with various neonatal disorders. *Acta Paediatr Scand* 57:517, 1968.

Schiff D, Chan G, Pozansky MJ: Bilirubin toxicity in neural cell lines N115 and NVR10A. *Pediatr Res* 19:908, 1985.

Wu PYK, Hodgman JE, Kirkpatrick BU, et al: Metabolic aspects of phototherapy. *Pediatrics* 72 (Suppl):427, 1985.

Yeager AS, Grumet FC, Hafleigh EB, et al: Prevention of transfusion-acquired cytomegalovirus infections in newborn infants. *J Pediatr* 98:281, 1981.

Neonatal Infections and Other Disorders 12

SEPSIS (IN THE NEWBORN)

Some considerations of infection are most pertinent to the care of newborn infants. We have selected topics of general interest to be included under neonatology. For a more complete discussion of specific infections, please refer to Section 17, Infectious Diseases.

Definition

Bacteremia is defined as a condition in which a microorganism is recovered from the blood stream. (Occasionally, in the presence of indwelling catheters, for example, blood aspirated through the catheter may contain bacteria that are not found when blood is sampled from a peripheral vein, which would not be considered bacteremia.) Infection implies that the body has mounted a response to the circulating microorganisms, a condition designated septicemia or sepsis. In many instances, no obvious focus of infection is found in infants.

Basic Science

In different regions organisms that most commonly cause septicemia change decade by decade (Freedman et al, 1981). In this country overall, for the past decade group B streptococci have been prominent. Group B streptococci together with other streptococci and species of *Escherichia coli,* contribute 85–95% of neonatal septicemia infections. *Staphylococcus epidermidis* is a relative newcomer as a pathogen, although it has long been recognized as a contaminant. Nontypeable *Haemophilus* species are encountered on occasion.

The most devastating organisms in the newborn are group B streptococci and *E. coli,* both of which invade the meninges. They also contribute to inhibition of phagocytosis, and neither activates the alternate complement pathway.

Epidemiology

Sepsis has become a more serious problem as more VLBW infants spend longer periods in intensive care nurseries. In the past, such infants did not live long enough to have recurrent bouts of sepsis. Infants born under 37 weeks' gestation are at 10 times the risk of sepsis, for complex reasons stemming from nosocomial exposure as well as their immature host defenses.

The rates of infection for each organism differ as a function of their virulence. With intrauterine exposure, the risk depends on the prevalence of maternal colonization. At Baylor, where careful documentation has been made, group B streptococcal sepsis occurs in 1.2–3.2/1000 live births (Baker C, personal communication).

In a prospective study of 182 sick infants (at home) under age 3 months who were febrile (over 38°C), a viral pathogen was isolated from 41%, bacterial pathogen in 27%, and no pathogen in the remainder. The final diagnoses were aseptic meningitis (often without pleocytosis) in 30%, urinary tract infection in 11%, otitis in 9%, gastroenteritis in 8%, and pneumonia in 5%. More than one-third of the infants had no specific diagnosis made (Krober et al, 1985).

Natural History

The fetus can be infected by transplacental passage of pathogens, by infection in the placenta and contamination of amniotic fluid, and retrograde extension from vaginal flora, which occurs most commonly with rupture of membranes.

Neonates can acquire infection from the environment by hand-to-infant transmission, or from contaminated formula, nipples, medical instruments, or other apparatus. Any break in the mucosal barrier can permit infection, as can indwelling catheters or other devices.

The signs of infections in the newborn can be very subtle and suspicion may be aroused only when several of them coexist. For example, temperature instability is one of the most common findings in infected infants, but this important sign may be masked by the environment of an incubator with servocontrolling devices. Nonetheless, the demand for more heat by the infant who is servocontrolling his own environment is an important sign of his own tendency to hypothermia. Alternatively, for other infants, any change in temperature in either direction should alert the physician to the possibility of a problem.

The degree of temperature elevation at the time that the problem is first recognized is important as described by Klein and colleagues in 1984. In their survey of infants 3 months of age or younger seen at The Boston City Hospital, the percentage with fevers under 100° F who had only mild illness was 79% and only 6% had severe illness. Conversely, if the temperature was over 100° F, mild illness accounted for 39% and severe illness was identified in 32%. The striking conclusion is that temperature elevation be taken seriously in infants under 3 months of age.

A change in any habit can be the signal of septicemia. Thus, a baby who has been taking an adequate amount of liquids, may suddenly want less or tire during feedings. An infant who has been vigorous with a lusty cry, suddenly is noted to be lethargic, less easily aroused, and to have apneic spells. Sometimes, apneic spells reflect the underlying more serious illness, but they can occur in infants less than about 35 weeks' in the absence of sepsis. Vomiting or diarrhea, or both, is not uncommon, and some of the systemic symptoms may well reflect underlying dehydration or acidemia. Persistent jaundice indicates underlying infection.

Infants unable to tolerate progressive oral feedings have a high rate of endotoxemia, as measured by a Limulus lysate test. Scheifele et al (1985) reported that 60% of infants tested during their stay in a tertiary care nursery had endotoxemia with evidence of infection. Bowel disease predisposed to endotoxemia; presumably as fecal flora develops, and the bowel wall remains permeable to macromolecules, endotoxins are absorbed (Beach et al, 1982).

The significance of these observations is not completely clear. They may explain, in part, the number of negative cultures obtained during work-ups to "rule out sepsis."

Diagnosis

The decision to subject an infant to a "sepsis work-up" depends on the severity of the situation as deduced both from the clinical signs and the possibility of exposure to infection. While the historical information is relevant, it is never sufficient. Laboratory studies can be helpful, by revealing an elevation or depression in the number of neutrophils, an increase in the number of bands, and an elevation in the sedimentation rate and/or the C-reactive protein. Initially, septic newborns usually show a polymorphonuclear response, but as the infection worsens the ability to respond is depressed and neutropenia occurs. Routine surveillance cultures from external ear, throat, or even Gram stain of gastric aspirate are not helpful in predicting whether there is need for a full septic work-up.

The components of the work-up on suspicion of infection include: one or more blood cultures of at least 1 ml from a peripheral vein (not from an indwelling catheter), a lumbar puncture, and collection of midstream urine or suprapubic aspiration for analysis and latex fixation. A chest film is appropriate.

Treatment

It is customary to initiate intravenous antibiotic therapy as soon as the cultures are obtained rather than to wait the day or two required for identification of the organism, or even the few hours to ascertain acute phase reactants. This approach is based on the rapidity and fulminant nature of some systemic infections in infants and requires the choice of antibiotics that will give broad coverage for the organisms most likely to be found in the given environment.

CONTROVERSY

The choice of antibiotic must depend on recent local experience. Penicillin is the best drug for streptococci, but ampicillin may be preferable if *Haemophilus* species have been identified locally. *S. epidermidis* is resistant to both penicillin and methicillin, and responds to vancomycin (10–15 mg/kg/dose, usually every 12 hours). Serum levels should be monitored since low birth weight infants may require less frequent doses. Ampicillin and gentamicin together give good broad spectrum coverage. Ampicillin and cefotaxime are especially effective if Gram-negative rods are present.

Prevention

The best method of prevention would be to reduce the number of premature births. Next best is to follow each mother carefully, and treat her infection vigor-

CASE ILLUSTRATION

A 3700-g infant was delivered to a 31-year-old mother who had a history of asthma but no problems during the pregnancy. She had had one bladder infection treated with antibiotics just before the onset of the current pregnancy, but had taken no medication during the pregnancy. After 41 weeks' gestation, there was spontaneous rupture of the membranes. Because of frank breech presentation, delivery was made by cesarean section 5 hours later. The male infant was vigorous at birth and had a normal physical examination. At 3 days of age, his rectal temperature was noted to be 101.4° F. It was later determined that the mother had had a slight temperature elevation on the 3 preceding days and was nursing her infant. No pathogens were recovered from her.

Because of the temperature elevation, sepsis was suspected and a white count was ascertained to be 18,300, with 26% neutrophils, 12% bands, 57% lymphocytes, and 5% eosinophils, and the hematocrit was 60. The infant's weight was 3320 g. Over the subsequent days, the only abnormality in examination was a reduction in intake from the breast and some lethargy. Chemical determinations showed mild dehydration with an elevation of the serum sodium to 152, potassium 4.6, chloride 118, CO_2 15, and BUN 31. With appropriate hydration, the electrolytes returned to normal levels and by 6 days of age, weight had increased to 3620 g. Cultures of blood, spinal fluid, and urine were negative at 1 week. The infant was treated first with ampicillin, 50 mg/kg/dose, and gentamicin, 2.5 mg/kg/dose, every 12 hours. Gentamicin levels in blood were maintained in the recommended range of 2–8 μg/ml. Throughout the first 5 days of therapy, the temperature instability was pronounced, with the baby requiring an incubator temperature as high as 91° to maintain body temperature of 97.4°. He was also noted to be unusually sleepy during that period and had several episodes of bradycardia. By the ninth day of life, he showed an increase in his desire to feed and maintained a normal body temperature. Antibiotics were continued for 15 days. The infant was then discharged home presumed to be well.

In retrospect, we have no evidence that this infant had sepsis, although the course was compatible with that possibility and recovery took place after antibiotic treatment. Alternatively, this illness could have been viral.

QUESTIONS AND COMMENTS

Why were a lumbar puncture and bladder aspirate undertaken?

Seeding of the meninges is very common in neonatal sepsis. Some physicians fear the possibility of the lumbar tap being the means of inoculating the spinal fluid. In our view, what is gained by knowledge of cells and cultures from spinal blood in a symptomatic infant outweighs the unproven risk of introduction of infection. Urine cultures are valuable inasmuch as congenital anomalies of the genitourinary tract may predispose the infant to infection. Also, organisms in the circulation may be concentrated in the urine.

Would you have requested one or two blood cultures in this infant?

Two blood cultures would have been preferable. *S. epidermidis* may be a contaminant or a pathogen. If present in both cultures, it would be presumed to be a pathogen.

How long should antibiotics be continued?

The answer must be individualized. Clearly coverage is required as long as symptoms persist, or blood or spinal fluid cultures remain positive. This can be as long as 6 weeks in some infants with meningitis, and longer in some instances of *Klebsiella* sepsis. When no organisms are recovered, as in our patient, we arbitrarily stop administering antimicrobials at 10 days to 2 weeks and observe the infant in hospital a few days to be certain that he remains asymptomatic. In an event with little likelihood of infection, we could discontinue antibiotics after 72 hours.

What is the best position for a spinal tap in a preterm infant?

Spinal taps in the lateral position with neck flexion are associated with hypoxemia. If the neck is not flexed, the lateral position is safer; alternately, the upright position can be used.

ously. Colonized mothers respond to intravenous ampicillin. Boyer et al (1983) showed that 2 g of ampicillin intravenously, followed by 1 g every 4 hours until delivery was effective in eliminating streptococcal disease in the infant. In their study, the infants were given four additional doses of ampicillin (50 mg/kg/intramuscularly) at 12-hour intervals. Some physicians would culture cord blood, and initiate penicillin therapy in the delivery room. It is possible that prompt administration of intravenous gamma-globulin will be useful, but it remains to be evaluated.

Granulocyte transfusions are probably not appropriate for neonatal sepsis, as there is no evidence of depletion of neutrophil pools in bone marrow. In contrast, there are definite risks from such transfusions, such as promotion of graft-versus-host disease, or transmission of some serious infections, such as AIDS or cytomegalovirus. If granulocytes or platelets are given, they must be irradiated first to lessen risks of infection and graft-versus-host disease.

NECROTIZING ENTEROCOLITIS

Definition

Necrotizing enterocolitis (NEC) is a serious intestinal disorder generally of preterm infants. It is characterized by abdominal distention, bloody stools, and air seen in the bowel wall on plain radiographs. It is thought to be the end-response of the immature intestinal tract to many insults to the mucosa, including infection. This condition was considered under many other names before the mid-1960s when the characteristic features were described by Misrahi et al (1965).

Epidemiology and Natural History

NEC tends to occur in clusters in tertiary care nurseries. Some institutions report it to be rare, whereas others find it sufficiently common to publish results of clinical trials to evaluate interventions. Overall, it occurs in about 10% of infants less than 1500 g birth weight (Davis et al, 1986).

Although it most often affects VLBW infants in the first week of life, it can occur in term infants. The mean age of onset of symptoms in Davis' series was 22.8 ± 4.7 days. The illness frequently occurs in sick infants who have umbilical artery lines in place, respiratory distress syndrome (RDS), patent ductus arteriosus, or sepsis.

No agreement exists on pathogenesis. In studies to evaluate the effects of breast versus cow's milk, no differences were detected between modified cow's milk and breast milk, although hyperosmolar formulas have been associated with increased gastrointestinal problems. No differences were noted among infants sustained by intravenous feeding in whom oral feedings were delayed for more than 14 days and no differences were noted when infants fed orally on the first day compared with 7 days of age (Ostertag et al, 1985).

Although many microorganisms have been associated with NEC, most of them are normal gut flora. No convincing evidence has been forthcoming about the association with rotavirus or corona virus, although the presence of both has been reported (Resta et al, 1985). No benefit has been reported from prophylaxis with gentamicin or oral antibiotics.

Diagnosis

Abdominal distention, bloody stools, ileus, and a pathognomonic radiographic picture of pneumatosis intestinalis confirm the diagnosis. In early stages, the

CASE ILLUSTRATION

A 1200-g infant was born at 30 weeks' gestation after a precipitous delivery to a 26-year-old mother in good health. The reason for preterm birth was unknown. The infant required resuscitation and mechanical ventilation for respiratory distress syndrome for 3 days, but then was weaned from the ventilator. An umbilical catheter was in place for 3 days to monitor blood gases. Gavage feedings with breast milk were started. By 9 days of age, the infant had apnea and bradycardia, pallor, and abdominal distention and absent peristalsis. Loose heme-positive stools were noted. Abdominal radiographs demonstrated pneumatosis. Intravenous alimentation was begun and the infant's condition improved. Oral feedings were resumed successfully after 10 days (age 19 days).

QUESTIONS AND COMMENTS

What would you do if the identical clinical picture was not associated with a positive radiograph?

We would probably culture the stool for bacteria and viruses, and repeat the film a day later. Intravenous alimentation would be required with or without pneumatosis. A nasogastric tube should be inserted to decompress the stomach and the infant would receive nothing by mouth until peristalsis returned.

What are the indications for antibiotics?

Although in most instances antibiotics have not been found of benefit, for these very sick infants who are prone to peritonitis and sepsis, we prescribe ampicillin and gentamicin. Blood levels of this antibiotic should be followed.

What are the indications for surgery?

Bowel perforation is a strong indication for surgery. If shock and disseminated intravascular coagulation cannot be managed medically, resection of necrotic bowel is indicated. Stricture formation late in the illness may require one or more operations.

What are the criteria for reintroduction of feedings?

We do not know of definitive studies to establish when oral intake should be reinstituted in infants recovering from NEC, nor what types of food should be given and how much. We reinstate feedings with small volumes of dilute elemental formula after the infant achieves thermal stability, normal peristalsis, good peripheral circulation, and the umbilical artery catheter is removed. Trial and error guide the rate of resumption of full feedings.

radiographs may simply show gaseous dilatation of small bowel and colon.

Laboratory findings may include a low granulocyte count, thrombocytopenia, and in the sickest infants, disseminated intravascular coagulation.

Treatment

We discontinue all oral feedings and initiate intravenous alimentation. A nasogastric tube should be used to prevent gastric distention. Consultation with a surgeon is imperative because bowel obstruction and perforation may require urgent intervention.

CONTROVERSIES

Prenatal glucocorticoids have been associated with less NEC in The Collaborative Trial (1981); however, no prospective study has been reported to confirm this association (Bauer et al, 1984).

Other interventions that have been recommended in these extremely ill infants are intravenous gammaglobulin, white cell transfusions, and exchange transfusions. None has been studied adequately to permit a recommendation.

Prognosis

In the first series described, the mortality rate was 75%. Early recognition and intravenous nutrition have improved the outcome, but about 10–20% of the infants die. Some have had such extensive bowel resection that although they survive, they have a short bowel and may need intravenous support for years. If the bowel was not significantly shortened, survivors evaluated at 1 year by Abassi et al (1984) had no adverse effects on growth or gastrointestinal function. Late onset (several months) intestinal obstruction has occurred from strictures.

NEONATAL MASTITIS

Definition

Breast inflammation with or without abscess formation in the first few months of life is termed neonatal mastitis.

Basic Science

Staphylococcus aureus is overwhelmingly the most common organism although infection with streptococci and Gram-negative organisms have been described. The condition occurs in term or post-term infants who have breast tissue from maternal estrogens absorbed in late fetal life. Pustules elsewhere on the skin are common and may be the source of infection by retrograde spread up the nipple.

Epidemiology

The condition has been described worldwide in 119 cases reviewed by Walsh and McIntosh (1986). They added 41 cases seen at The Children's Hospital, Boston in 1947–1983.

Natural History

Males and females are equally at risk for neonatal mastitis. The onset of inflammation is usually between the second and fifth week of life. The condition is most often unilateral but can be bilateral. In The Children's Hospital experience, 89% were fluctuant. In none were blood, urine, or spinal fluid cultures positive. The infant may have low-grade fever and leukocytosis.

Diagnosis

Needle aspiration and culture establish the etiology.

Treatment

Intravenous β-lactamase-resistant penicillin (oxacillin to start pending sensitivities) is appropriate initially if the infant is irritable, febrile, and likely to be a poor feeder or vomit. If the infant can tolerate oral intake, oral antibiotics for 10–14 days are usually effective.

If the lesion is fluctuant, surgical incision and drainage may be necessary.

NOSOCOMIAL INFECTION

Definition

Disease that is a consequence of medical care, in the sense that it was neither overt nor being incubated on admission to hospital,is considered to be a nosocomial infection. Infections in newborns that might have been acquired from the mother are not considered nosocomial.

Epidemiology

The incidence of nosocomial infection in a neonatal intensive care unit in a crowded antiquated nursery (1974–1978) and after relocation in a new, more spacious, better ventilated nursery (1977–1978) was evaluated in 1981 by Goldmann et al. In the crowded nursery, 5.2% of the infants had at least one major nosocomial infection. The risk was increased with low birth weight, patent ductus arteriosus, surgery, and requirement of multiple supportive measures. In the new, more spacious nursery in which the number of staff was increased, only 0.9% of the patients had a major nosocomial infection. One of the major differences in the environment was the presence of more sinks in convenient locations, which increased the opportunity for handwashing. Contaminated hands have been shown to be the major route of spread of nosocomial infection in nurseries (Hall et al, 1979).

Basic Science

The types of organisms identified at the intensive care nursery of The Children's Hospital, Boston, in 1974–

Table 4.28
Leading Etiologies of Major Nosocomial Infections
The Children's Hospital, Boston, MA, 1974–1978[1]

Bacteremia
Klebsiella pneumoniae
Staphylococcus epidermidis
S. aureus
Enterococcus species
Esherichia coli
Meningitis
K. pneumoniae
E. coli
Candida albicans
Pneumonia
Pseudomonas aeruginosa
P. cepacia
K. pneumoniae
E. coli

[1]Modified from Goldmann et al, 1981.

1978 were identified by Goldmann et al and are shown in Table 4.28.

Since then, coagulase-negative staphylococci, principally *S. epidermidis,* previously assumed to be nonpathogenic, have become the major pathogens of the blood stream. A wide variety of Gram-negative rods have been reported as causes of wound infections and blood stream infections related to indwelling intravascular catheters, especially in older children. *Serratia marcescens,* once thought to be nonpathogenic, has been cultured from the blood of infants with clinical illness (Smith et al, 1984). *Candida* remains a problem during intravenous alimentation. The fungus *Malassezia* has been associated with infection of the pulmonary vasculature in infants on intravenous lipids (Redline and Dahms, 1981).

Nosocomial viral infections have also been identified in careful studies by others. Hepatitis A has emerged as a major pathogen, and may be undetected until a staff member or parent develops jaundice. Respiratory syncytial virus has a high attack rate both among staff and infants, and has been shown to be spread to infants primarily by direct contact such as from the hand (Hall et al, 1979). Rotaviruses have been described as responsible for severe diarrhea in nursery epidemics (Steinhoff, 1980). Enteroviruses, once thought to be transmitted to the infant by the mother during vaginal delivery, can also be acquired by infants in a nursery. Modlin (1980) described an epidemic in Boston in which four infants died from echovirus II infection. In all instances, the infants had no detectable antibody in cord serum. When mothers had serum neutralizing antibody, cord sera were positive and the infants were not ill (Modlin et al, 1981).

Other enteroviruses that can be pathogenic include *Coxsackie* A and B, with B being more virulent. Myocarditis and aseptic meningitis are the most common infections. Infection presumably occurs in antibody-negative infants who acquire the organism from the maternal vagina.

Fungal infections may be introduced from contaminated skin by way of indwelling catheters. Organisms that rarely affect normal individuals may be pathogenic in preterm infants or immunocompromised older patients who are on intravenous alimentation with lipids. Infection with *Malassezia furfur* illustrates the point. The fungus is associated with tinea versicolor, a minor skin infection. It can induce fever or depression in temperature and thrombocytopenia in infants. The treatment is removal of the catheter (Dankner et al, 1987).

Diagnosis

The search for the source of infection may be a complicated and expensive undertaking, but must be done whenever an outbreak of illness occurs in a nursery. The most straightforward approach is a "case control" method, to ascertain what interventions the sick infants shared, and which personnel cared for all of them. Chronic carriers of *S. aureus* and group A streptococci should be identified by culture of nose and hands and suitably treated, or relocated. Phage typing is useful in identifying carriers.

Prevention

Recognition that sick newborn infants may harbor infection and that others, particularly those born before term, may be unusually susceptible to infection, has led to measures to control cross-infection. The level of concern and the extent of the protective measures have varied widely from decade to decade and nursery to nursery. Some nurseries continue to insist on use of caps, masks, gowns, and foot cover before any person may enter the area containing the babies. They also insist on hand-washing with an antiseptic soap between contact with babies. Some studies of the value of masks and gowns, in particular, have failed to show that such approaches are effective. In fact, sometimes the increased hand to mask contact when masks are worn for long periods actually enhances spread of infection by hand.

If an infant is found to have an infection he should be isolated from other infants insofar as possible. If the organism is resistant to most antibiotics, isolation of the infant in a separate room is desirable. A minimal requirement is that the infected infant and all other infants in the immediate area and in cohorts should be in incubators. The incubator should either be receiving outside air or in an environment where the climate control is sufficient to guarantee several air changes per hour. If the pathogen is airborne, a separate isolation room is essential. The use of gowns and disposable gloves by everyone in contact with the infant further reduces the spread of infection.

Our general nursery routines require handwashing by all persons before entry into the area containing the babies. We prefer the use of an organic iodine containing compounds (such as iodophor) or chlorhexidine gluconate. In addition, anyone who plans direct contact with an infant or equipment that will be in contact with the infant wears a sterile gown. Those who are visiting or viewing the nursery but who are not going to be in contact with the infants are not required to wear gowns. All individuals repeat handwashing before and after direct contact with the infant. Infants are bathed with sterile water and no antibiotics or antiseptics are applied. Specifically, we do not routinely bathe babies with hexachlorophene because it became clear that this and other substances can be absorbed through the skin in toxic amounts. If there is a problem with staphylococci, we insist that the caretakers use hexachlorophene soaps to try to reduce spread of infection.

The elimination of pools of water such as in incubator humidification trays lessens the likelihood of opportunistic organisms growing in this environment. Only sterile water should be used to provide humidity in incubators. Standards and recommendations for hospital care of newborns are regularly reviewed by the Committee on the Fetus and Newborn of the American Academy of Pediatrics. Reference to their latest handbook is advised by all who assume responsibility for nursery policies.

REFERENCES

Abassi SM, Pereira GR, Johnson L, et al: Long-term assessment of growth, nutritional status, and gastrointestinal function in survivors of necrotizing enterocolitis. *J Pediatr* 104:550, 1984.

Baker CT: Early onset group B streptococcal disease. *J Pediatr* 93:124, 1978.

Bauer CR, Morrison JC, Poole WK, et al: A decreased incidence of necrotizing enterocolitis after prenatal glucocorticoid therapy. *Pediatrics* 73:682, 1984.

Beach RC, Menzies IS, Clayden GS, et al: Gastrointestinal permeability changes in the preterm infant. *Arch Dis Child* 57:141, 1982.

Boyer KM, Gadzala CA, Kelly PD, et al: Selective intrapartum chemoprophylaxis of neonatal group B streptococcal disease III. Interruption of maternal-to-infant transmission. *J Infect Dis* 148:810, 1983.

Brown EG, Sweet AY(eds): *Neonatal Necrotizing Enterocolitis*. New York, Grune & Stratton, 1980.

Collaborative Group of Antenatal Steroid Therapy. Effect of antenatal dexamethasone administration on the prevention of respiratory distress syndrome. *Am J Obstet Gynecol* 141:276, 1981.

Dankner WM, Spector SA, Fierer J, et al: Malassezia fungemia in neonates and adults: Complication of hyperalimentation. *Rev Infect Dis* 9:743, 1987.

Davis JM, Abassi S, Spitzer AR, et al: Role of theophylline in pathogenesis of necrotizing enterocolitis. *J Pediatr* 109:344, 1986.

DeGamarra E, Helardot P, Moriette I, et al: Necrotizing enterocolitis in full-term newborns. *Biol Neonate* 44:185, 1983.

Freedman RM, Ingram DL, Gross I, et al: A half century of neonatal sepsis at Yale. *Am J Dis Child* 135:140, 1981.

Goldmann DA, Durbin WA Jr, Freeman J: Nosocomial infections in a neonatal intensive care unit. *J Infect Dis* 144:449, 1981.

Goldman DA, Leclair J, Macone A: Bacterial colonization of neonates admitted to a neonatal intensive care unit. *J Pediatr* 93:288, 1978.

Hall CB, Kopelman AE, Douglas RG Jr, et al: Neonatal respiratory syncytial virus infection. *N Engl J Med* 300:393, 1979.

Kleigman RM, Fanaroff AA: Neonatal necrotizing enterocolitis. *N Engl J Med* 310:1093, 1984.

Klein JO, Schlesinger PC, Karasic RB: Management of the febrile infant three months of age or younger. *Pediatr Infect Dis* 3:75, 1984.

Krober MS, Bass JW, Powell JM, et al: Bacterial and viral pathogens causing fever in infants less than 3 months old. *Am J Dis Child* 139:889, 1985.

McCracken GH Jr, Nelson JD, Kaplan SL, et al: Consensus report: Antimicrobial therapy for bacterial meningitis in infants and children. *Pediatr Infect Dis* 6:501, 1987.

Misrahi A, Barlow O, Berdon W, et al: Necrotizing enterocolitis in premature infants. *J Pediatr* 66:697, 1965.

Modlin JD, Polk BF, Horton P, et al: Perinatal echovirus infection: Risk of transmission during a community outreach. *N Engl J Med* 305:368, 1981.

Modlin JF: Fatal echovirus II disease in premature neonates. *Pediatrics* 66:775, 1980.

Murphy AM, Albrey MB, Crewe EB: Rotavirus infection in neonates. *Lancet* 2:1149, 1977.

Ostertag SC, LaGamma EF, Reisen CW: Early enteral feeding does not affect incidence of necrotizing enterocolitis. *Pediatr Res* 19:356A, 1985.

Redline RW, Dahms BB: Malassezia pulmonary vasculitis in an infant on long term intralipid therapy. *N Engl J Med* 305:1395, 1981.

Resta S, Luby JP, Rosenfeld CR, et al: Isolation and propagation of a human enteric coronavirus. *Science* 229:978, 1985.

Scheifele DW, Olsen E, Fussell S, et al: Spontaneous endotoxinemia in premature infants: correlations with oral feeding and bowel dysfunctions. *J Pediatr Gastro Nutr* 4:67, 1985.

Smith PJ, Brookfield DSK, et al: An outbreak of serratia marcescens infection in a neonatal unit. *Lancet* 1:151, 1984.

Steinhoff MC: Rotavirus: The first five years. *J Pediatr* 96:611, 1980.

Walsh M, McIntosh K: Neonatal mastitis. *Clin Pediatr* 25:395, 1986.

Yow MD, Mason ED, Leeds LJ, et al: Ampicillin prevents intrapartum transmission of group B streptococci. *JAMA* 241:1245, 1979.

Intestinal Disorders 13

INTESTINAL ATRESIA AND STENOSIS

Definition

Obstruction or narrowing of the lumen of the intestine can take place at any level and be isolated or multiple.

Basic Science

Duodenal atresia is most likely a congenital malformation because it occurs so commonly in association with other malformations. Trisomy 21, for example, is present in about 30% of babies with duodenal atresia. Congenital heart disease is found in approximately 20% of the babies, including some of those with trisomy 21. The obstruction can occur either proximal or distal to the ampulla of Vater. Sometimes the obstruction is a true atresia, other times it is partial caused by a diaphragm. An annular pancreas may cause narrowing of the duodenum and even complete obstruction.

Atresia and stenosis of the jejunum and ileum are most commonly the result of an ischemic insult in intrauterine life. The evidence in support of this is based on both clinical and experimental studies. Jejunoileal and colonic atresia have been produced in fetal pups by Louw and Barnard (1955) by devascularizing segments of the fetal intestine.

Epidemiology

Intestinal atresia was found to occur in 1/2710 live births in a nationwide survey by Ravitch and Barton (1974). It is, thus, the most common cause of congenital intestinal obstruction.

Atresia of the colon is relatively rare, accounting for only 10% of intestinal atresias or stenoses. The salient clinical and diagnostic features are similar to those with ileal obstruction. Other anomalies may be present, such as gastroschisis.

Natural History

Hydramnios occurs in about half of infants with duodenal or proximal jejunal atresia, but is uncommon in those with ileal or colonic obstruction. In the presence of hydramnios it is useful to examine the fetus by ultrasonography in search of associated lesions, which include diaphragmatic hernia or situs inversus.

Postnatally, the diagnosis should be considered in any infant who vomits green material, although intestinal obstruction will be found in only one-third of such infants. Infants with atresia usually begin to vomit shortly after birth, but the vomiting may be delayed for hours or even a few days. When the obstruction is distal to the duodenum, abdominal distention becomes evident and active peristalsis may be observed through the abdominal wall. Failure to pass meconium in the first 24 hours should raise a suspicion of intestinal obstruction but about a third of infants with duodenal atresia and about 20% of those with ileal atresia may evacuate a normal meconium stool. This observation, of course, substantiates the view that lower intestinal atresias are acquired in utero. Prolonged jaundice is also characteristic of intestinal obstruction through an increased enterohepatic recirculation of bilirubin.

Diagnosis

Once intestinal obstruction is considered a possibility, the most important next step in diagnosis is abdominal radiographic examination. Typically, air-filled intestinal loops become evident and air fluid levels are characteristic. Two air-filled structures containing fluid levels at the level of the duodenum are called the "double bubble" sign and are diagnostic of duodenal obstruction. A barium enema is indicated if the plain radiographs are not diagnostic or if lower intestinal or colonic obstruction is thought possible. The distinction from Hirschsprung disease may be made by barium enema, or, if equivocal, biopsy. Occasionally, the colon seems very small in the case of atresias or infants with meconium ileus. Infants of diabetic mothers have also been observed to have a microcolon. No therapy is indicated because the colon increases in diameter with oral feeding.

Treatment

The earlier the diagnosis, the earlier definitive surgical intervention can be undertaken. In the event of delayed diagnosis, it may be useful to reestablish normal acid base balance and adequate urine output before proceeding to operation. Preoperative decompression with a nasogastric tube is essential. The operation is usually a side-to-side duodenoduodenostomy or, occasionally, a duodenojejunostomy. Intravenous alimentation is required postoperatively in about half the patients (Rescorla and Grosfeld, 1985).

About 40% of all atresias occur in the jejunum and the ileum. The diagnosis is discussed previously. Treatment requires surgical intervention with an excellent chance of survival because other malformations are unusual.

Prognosis

Deaths from operation on duodenal atresia are unusual from the operation but occur in approximately 10–30% of infants in association with other major anomalies (Danismend et al, 1986). The outlook for infants with atresias depends on the amount of viable bowel that can be left in place.

Meconium Ileus

Definition

Abnormally viscous meconium may inspissate in the fetal gut. In some instances, perforation occurs causing meconium peritonitis.

Basic Science

Deficiency of pancreatic enzymes is probably the reason for the excessively viscous meconium in some infants who have cystic fibrosis (Shwachman and Antonowicz, 1981).

The reasons for gut perforation are not clear, but it is evident that healing can occur in utero. At birth, abdominal films may show flecks of calcium from previous peritonitis in otherwise asymptomatic infants.

Epidemiology

The condition occurs in individuals with cystic fibrosis and, thus, is most common in the caucasian population.

Natural History

If a family history is positive for cystic fibrosis, every new infant should be considered a candidate for meconium ileus. The first sign is abdominal distention by 12–24 hours, vomiting, and failure to pass meconium. Failure to recognize the condition increases the risk of perforation, peritonitis or volvulus, and death.

Diagnosis

No meconium is present in the rectal pouch. On palpation of the abdomen, dilated loops of bowel can often be felt and, occasionally, hard masses of meconium are palpable. Radiographs may show fluid levels and distention of small bowel. The distal bowel may show tiny bubbles of gas mixed with meconium.

The sweat chloride may be elevated at birth, or may not be outside the normal range for some weeks.

Treatment

Hyperosmolar enemas draw water into the intestinal tract and help dislodge the meconium. Care is required to provide fluids intravenously to prevent serum osmolarity from rising over 29 Osm/L (Noblett, 1969). Enemas are effective in about half the infants; in the remainder, surgery is required. Some surgeons create an ileostomy to permit irrigations with N-acetyl-cysteine for several weeks. In other respects, the infants are treated as if they had cystic fibrosis with oral pancreatic enzyme supplements (Caniano and Beaver, 1987).

Prognosis

The presence of meconium ileus is not a predictor of the severity of cystic fibrosis. Affected individuals may have episodes of fecal impaction in later life.

Annular Pancreas

Definition

Annular pancreas is a flat ring of pancreatic tissue that surrounds the duodenum distal to the ampulla of Vater. It may contain a duct which joins Wirsung duct but may empty by other orifices into the duodenum.

Epidemiology

This is an unusual condition. Between 1938 and 1977 at The Children's Hospital, Boston, 36 cases were seen. Frequently it was not discovered until adulthood.

Diagnosis

Inasmuch as annular pancreas may not constrict the duodenum at all, it may never be diagnosed. If it does constrict the duodenum, it can be hard to distinguish from duodenal stenosis or atresia.

Treatment

In order not to compromise the pancreatic ducts, the operation of choice is usually a bypass procedure, which is a side-to-side duodenojejunostomy.

Duplication of the Small Intestine

Duplication cysts may be attached to the duodenal wall or even imbedded in the pancreas. The majority of duplications are in the jejunum and ileum.

Diagnosis

Signs of intestinal obstruction may be present and, occasionally, a volvulus or intussusception results. Diagnosis is best made by radiographic examination or ultrasonography.

Treatment

Because all cysts and duplications may be pivotal sites for volvulus or even malignant change, surgical removal is advised once they are demonstrated. Complete excision of the cyst and attached bowel may be required.

Congenital Deformities of the Anus and Rectum (Imperforate Anus)

Congenital deformities of the anus and rectum can occur as (1) stenosis at the lower rectum or anus, (2) with a membranous obstruction of the anus, (3) with the rectum ending as a blind pouch at a variable distance from the perineum, and (4) the anal canal and lower rectum forming a blind rectal pouch. Approximately 55–82% of all reported cases have associated fistulas. In the female, they are usually rectovaginal or rarely rectoperineal. In the male, they are rectourinary usually terminating in the bladder or urethra. Other associated anomalies include upper urinary tract (25%), lower genital tract (27%), upper genital tract (35%), and other organ systems (50%) (Fleming et al, 1986).

Diagnosis

A standard part of the routine physical examination of the newborn infant is to examine the anus to see if it is of normal caliber, meaning for most infants, the ability to insert a little finger into the rectum. Occasionally, only a dimple is present or only a fine probe can be passed. A requirement that the initial temperature be measured per rectum ensures early diagnosis.

The membranous type of obstruction is very rare and can be overcome with the insertion of a probing finger.

Preoperative evaluation should include careful radiographic studies with barium injected vaginally as well as into the rectum to search for fistulas.

Treatment

Obstructive lesions with or without fistulas require surgical treatment. When the blind rectal pouch is at a considerable distance from the anus, a colostomy will be required to relieve the obstruction and definitive surgical repair awaits growth for 1–2 years.

NEONATAL ASCITES

Definition

Prominence of the abdomen with evidence of presence of fluid by clinical and radiographic examination establishes the diagnosis of ascites. This discussion will be limited to those infants in whom ascites is a dominant finding, although some may have a degree of peripheral edema or edema of the abdominal wall in association with fluid in the abdominal cavity. Infants with massive edema as in the case of erythroblastosis fetalis are considered on page 190.

Epidemiology and Natural History

The epidemiology and natural history are those of the underlying disorder (Table 4.29).

Diagnosis

Prominence of the abdomen should dictate examination to ascertain the presence of free fluid. Abdominal distention may be present at birth and, if so, may have been associated with hydramnios and dystocia. It may be difficult to measure amounts of peritoneal fluid by radiographs. Ultrasonography is better able to quantify the amount of fluid and provide information about possible etiologies (Newman and Teele, 1984).

Ascites may result from problems in the urinary gastrointestinal, cardiovascular, hepatic, or lymphatic systems and/or may be associated with an infectious etiology or ovarian cyst (Table 4.29). Thus, diagnostic studies starting with plain radiographs are important to determine the underlying cause for the accumulation of liquid. Cystography and intravenous urography are useful for pinpointing possible bladder perforation, neurogenic bladder, or posteriorly placed urethral valves. Chest radiographs may demonstrate cardiomegaly which most commonly results from paroxysmal supraventricular tachycardia. Even if tachycardia is not observed after birth, its occurrence in utero could have induced heart failure sufficient to result in ascites. If the problem is thought to be related to the gastrointestinal tract, a possibility highlighted by the association of maternal hydramnios and abdominal calcifications on the infant's radiographs, contrast studies with barium or water-soluble material would be useful. Ileal atresia with perforation has been associated with meconium and ascites at birth.

Although systemic infections are uncommon causes of isolated ascites, this condition has been the presenting symptom in hepatitis. Hepatosplenomegaly suggests the possibility of a systemic infection such as toxoplasmosis or cytomegalovirus infection.

Appendicitis can occur in newborn infants, although it accounts for only 2% of childhood appendicitis. Signs can be deceptive, from vomiting alone, to fever, abdominal distention or tenderness. The diagnosis is usually made at operation for suspected bowel rupture. Neonatal appendicitis can be associated with Hirschsprung disease.

Other anatomic malformations, such as mesenteric cysts, can mimic ascites or gross lymphatic abnormalities may be associated with the chylous ascites. Birth trauma can cause a tear in lymphatics with resultant leakage of chyle. Also, congenital lymphangiectasia can present as ascites. Exploratory laparotomy may be required if liquid reaccumulates after its removal.

Paracentesis is usually indicated to ascertain the nature of the liquid and to rule out the possibility of infection. If there is rupture of the bowel, grossly contaminated fluid may be present. Chylous fluid would turn milky after milk feedings, but would not be white before beginning oral nutrition. Protein concentrations can vary within the fluid and no patterns are associated with a particular etiology.

In seven of the 27 patients presenting with ascites in the first month of life reviewed by Griscom and colleagues (Griscom et al, 1977) no cause was demonstrated despite many diagnostic tests. Four of these infants survived, with gradual disappearance of their ascites.

Treatment

Inasmuch as the accumulation of fluid must be secondary to an underlying problem, the approach to

Table 4.29
Major Causes of Ascites in the Fetus and Neonate[1]

Etiology	Mechanism	Special Ultrasound Features
Genitourinary		
Obstruction of lower urinary tract most commonly posterior urethral values	Rupture of the fornix of a calyx with pyelosinus extravasation	May see hydronephrosis, hydroureters, distended thickened bladder, and sometimes dilated posterior urethra
Perforation of bladder usually secondary to birth trauma or occasionally bladder outlet obstruction	Urine enters the peritoneal cavity directly	
Congenital nephrosis	Proteinuria leads to hypoalbuminemia and decreased oncotic pressure	Kidneys may be unusually echogenic
Gastrointestinal		
Meconium peritonitis due to perforation of bowel secondary to atresia, stenosis, intussusception, volvulus, hernia, meconium ileus, or duplication	Direct Increased capillary fluid loss due to inflammation	Localized or widespread peritoneal calcifications Free and/or loculated fluid collections Obstructed loops of bowel
Fetal appendicitis with rupture		
Perforation of Meckel diverticulum		Obstructed fluid-filled loops
Imperforate anus		May be able to identify position of blind end of rectum
Portohepatic		
Congenital cirrhosis Biliary atresia Infections Glycogen storage disease Galactosemia Transplacental hepatitis Wilson disease Fibrocystic disease Cytomegalic inclusion disease	(i) Increased portal and intrahepatic hydrostatic pressure (ii) Hypoproteinemia and decreased oncotic pressure (iii) Sodium retention and impaired water excretion	Liver may be enlarged and unusual in its parenchymal pattern Spleen enlarges with increased portal pressure
Common duct perforation	Bile peritonitis	
Cardiac		
RH disease Severe anemia secondary to thalassemia, hemorrhage Major congenital heart disease Arrhythmia, e.g., supraventricular tachycardia	Ascites usually precedes hydrops fetalis (i) Major mechanism is probably congestive heart failure (ii) Hypoproteinemia (iii) Hepatic congestion and intrahepatic erythropoiesis may cause liver dysfunction	Enlarged, dilated, or malformed heart Pleural effusions When hydrops is present, may see scalp and body wall edema, hepatosplenomegaly, polyhydramnios, and placentomegaly Can pick up abnormal rhythm on real-time or Doppler study
Arteriovenous malformation		AVM in liver, head, or placenta
Miscellaneous		
Chylous ascites Lymphatic obstruction due to congenital malformation, e.g., cystic lymphangioma, lymphangiectasis, and neoplasm and inflammation Traumatic disruption of the thoracic duct	Lymphatic leak	Ascites may contain echogenic particles May see underlying mass or malformation

Table 4.29 *Continued*

Etiology	Mechanism	Special Ultrasound Features
Most cases are idiopathic infections Congenital syphilis, cytomegalovirus, and toxoplasmosis	(i) Peritonitis and increased capillary permeability (ii) Associated hepatic and cardiac pathology (iii) Hemorrhagic disorder	Hepatosplenomegaly

[1]Reproduced with permission from Newman B, Teele RL: *Sem Ultrasound CT, MR* 5:93, 1984.

management depends on the diagnosis of that problem. In all instances of meconium peritonitis, for example, a sweat test is required to identify those babies with cystic fibrosis. An abnormality of the urinary tract mandates appropriate surgical intervention. Systemic infections should be treated. Cardiovascular abnormalities require further definition by electrocardiography, ultrasonography, or catheterization.

Chylous ascites from whatever cause may require repeated paracenteses. A low fat diet with medium chain triglycerides is often helpful in lessening the formation of chyle. If chyle formation persists, intravenous alimentation allows the bowel to rest until recovery takes place spontaneously. Cautious reintroduction of elemental formulas can then occur. Most patients with lymphangectasia show eventual remission.

REFERENCES

Caniano DA, Beaver BL: Meconium ileus: A fifteen-year experience with forty-two neonates. *Surgery* 102:699, 1987.

Danismend EN, Brown S, Frank JD: Morbidity and mortality in duodenal atresia. *Z Kinderchir* 41:86, 1986.

Fleming SE, Hall R, Gysler M, et al: Imperforate anus in females: Frequency of genital tract involvement, incidence of associated anomalies and functional outcome. *J Pediatr Surg* 21:146, 1986.

Griscom NT, Colodny AH, Rosenberg WK, et al: Diagnostic aspects of neonatal ascites: report of 27 cases. *AJR* 128:961, 1977.

Louw JH, Barnard CN: Congenital and intestinal atresia: Observation on its origin. *Lancet* 2:1065, 1955.

Newman B, Teele RL: Ascites in the fetus, neonate and young child: Emphasis on ultrasonographic evaluation. *Sem Ultrasound CT MR* 5:85, 1984.

Noblett HR: Treatment of uncomplicated meconium ileus by gastrogroffin enema: A preliminary report. *J Pediatr Surg* 4:180, 1969.

Ravitch MM, Barton BA: The need for pediatric surgeons is determined by the volume of work and mode of delivery of surgical care. *Surgery* 76:754, 1974.

Rescorla FJ, Grosfeld JL: Intestinal atresia and stenosis: Analysis of survival in 120 cases. *Surgery* 98:668, 1985.

Shwachman H, Antonowicz I: Studies on meconium. In Lebenthal E (ed): *Textbook of Gastroenterology and Nutrition in Infancy*. New York, Raven Press, 1981.

Wedge JJ, Grosfeld JL, Smith JP: Abdominal masses in the newborn: 63 cases. *Am J Dis Child* 129:1096, 1975.

Intracranial Hemorrhage 14

As ever more low birth weight infants survive, the magnitude of the problem of intracranial bleeding will increase. This is one of the most important causes of neonatal morbidity, and sometimes death. In some instances, it occurs without any obvious explanation; in others, it is associated with respiratory distress and mechanical ventilation, and still others may be related to episodes of asphyxia, hyper- or hypovolemia, or hyperosmolarity. The following discussion reviews the state of knowledge in 1987, which we recognize is woefully inadequate.

Definition

Extravascular blood within the cranial cavity can vary from slight oozing to massive bleeding with extension to the subarachnoid space of the posterior fossa.

Basic Science

Pathologists have long agreed that hemorrhage in preterm infants most commonly originates from small vessels in the germinal layer of the brain in the periventricular areas. Babies up to 32 weeks' gestational age have a rich capillary bed in the subependymal region, particularly over the lower half of the head of the caudate nucleus. Small capillaries can be seen entering the major terminal vein branches, usually at right angles. All the small arteries, capillaries, and veins in the developing brain have a simple endothelial wall. After 32 weeks' gestational age, there is a diminution of the germinal layer and the capillary bed gradually merges with that of the rest of the corpus striatum. With the aid of injection studies and careful dissection, Hambleton and Wigglesworth (1976) confirmed the rich arterial supply to the germinal layer and found on injection that multiple leaks occur in the capillaries. They noted that during an apneic spell, infants often have sharp increases in arterial pressure by as much as 25 mm Hg and that these fluctuations in arterial pressure could well be transmitted to the germinal vessels and predispose them to hemorrhage.

Another possible explanation for intracranial bleeding after birth is the fluid shift that accompanies postnatal water loss. This is reflected in head shrinkage after birth; brain weights of infants with intraventricular hemorrhage are lower than those without (Williams et al, 1977; deCourten and Rabinowicz, 1981). Welch (1980) has reasoned that the decrease in spinal fluid pressure within the ventricular system exposes the vessels in the germinal matrix to increased transvascular pressure, which could promote rupture, particularly during episodes of hypertension or hypervolemia.

The fetus is exposed to the maternal hormonal milieu with its high levels of estrogen, progesterone, and prolactin levels. Fluid retention in pregnancy is shared by the fetus. After birth, intracellular water moves to the extracellular space and is lost through the kidney, skin, and lung. This postnatal shift results in weight loss, particularly from skin, but also from other organs, including the brain (Coulter, 1984). Coulter argues that a more gradual withdrawal from the intrauterine water-retaining hormones, particularly prolactin, could reduce the likelihood of postnatal intraventricular bleeding.

The possibility that fluctuations in cerebral blood-flow velocity could enhance the likelihood of intraventricular hemorrhage was examined by Perlman et al (1985). They eliminated the fluctuating velocities by muscle paralysis for the first 72 hours of life and found less hemorrhage in the treated infants. Other ways to reduce fluctuating cerebral blood flow velocity are to prevent respiratory distress syndrome (RDS) and the need for mechanical ventilation. The use of pancuronium or other muscle relaxants has its own hazards involving total dependence on mechanical ventilation and intubation.

Neonatal thrombocytopenia in infants under 1.5 kg birth weight is associated with severe intraventricular hemorrhage (Andrew et al, 1987).

An association between benzyl alcohol preservative used in solutions to flush intravascular catheters and subsequent intraventricular hemorrhage in small preterm infants was reported by Benda et al (1986). Discontinuation of the use of benzyl alcohol was followed by a significant reduction in intraventricular hemorrhage.

Epidemiology and Natural History

Intracranial hemorrhage, which is mostly intraventricular, or subependymal in preterm infants, is an increasing problem for infants with lower birth weight who are kept alive on mechanical ventilators for RDS.

In Children's and Brigham and Women's nurseries in 1975, intracranial hemorrhage was diagnosed in 19 infants, and in 1980, the number was 61. The only significant changes were survival of more VLBW infants and improvements in ultrasonographic diagnosis. Because almost half the infants were asymptomatic, the situation would not have been recognized without ultrasonography, which is now part of routine screening for VLBW infants.

The incidence of intracranial hemorrhage will depend, in part, on the population of infants in any given nursery and, thus, should be considered as a percentage of infants of given birth weight. With the use of CT and brain scans, Papile et al (1978) found hemorrhage in 20 of 46 infants weighing less than 1500 g who were admitted to a special care unit. Most observers report subependymal or intraventricular hemorrhages in 35–45% of infants born at less than 35 weeks' gestational age. The hemorrhages reach their maximum extent about 48 hours of age. Roughly one-third of them will bleed on the first day with the median age of onset about 16 hours. The optimal time for diagnosis by ultrasound is the end of the first week. Most infants who bleed will have some ventricular dilatation best seen by day 14, but often it resolves by 6 weeks (Szymonowicz et al, 1984).

Sixty-four infants between 580 and 1480 g at birth or 24–33 weeks' gestational age were studied sequentially with ultrasonography by Partridge et al in Cincinnati (1983). Hemorrhage in one or more sites was detected at some time in 55% of the patients. It was most common in the subependymal area, followed by ventricular hemorrhage with intraparenchymal bleeding in about 15%. Extension of the initial hemorrhage occurred in nearly half the infants by day 4 and maximum diagnostic efficiency was delivered on day 7. They agreed with others that the maximum efficiency for diagnosis of ventricular dilatation is on day 14.

Papile et al (1978) established grades for degrees of severity of intraventricular hemorrhage:

Grade I	Isolated subependymal hemorrhage
Grade II	Intraventricular hemorrhage without ventricular dilatation
Grade III	Intraventricular hemorrhage with ventricular dilatation
Grade IV	Intraventricular hemorrhage with parenchymal hemorrhage

Subarachnoid hemorrhage is more closely linked to birth trauma and asphyxia and occurs in infants of any gestational age. In an analysis of 104 infants in whom subarachnoid bleeds were found in the first week by CT scan, Adamkin et al (1985) reported mean birth weights of 3.11 kg and mean gestational age of 38.7 weeks. Twenty-two were delivered by emergency section for abnormal fetal heart tracings. The onset of symptoms of apnea, bradycardia seizures, cyanosis, and lethargy was usually within 24 hours. Rapid improvement and no long-term adverse effects are the rule.

Diagnosis

The most important and useful clinical signs of intracranial bleeding are falling hematocrit values and failure of the hematocrit to rise with transfusion. In about half the cases, the fontanelle will be full and frequently the infant will show changes in activity, such as unwillingness to suck, myoclonic movements, and even seizures. Decreased muscle tone is present in about half the infants in whom CT scan subsequently has shown bleeding (Lazzara et al, 1980; Fig. 4.28*A* and *B*).

Treatment

CONTROVERSIES

Central questions concern who should be treated and with what modality? If ventricular dilatation is progressive, and head growth accelerated, it is appropriate for neurosurgeons to establish a ventricular drainage either by ventriculostomy or by ventricular-peritoneal shunt. Kreusser et al (1985) advocate serial measurement of intracranial pressure indirectly with a fiberoptic sensor (Ladd intracranial pressure monitor). If it increases more than 20 mm of cerebrospinal fluid (CSF) in 1 week, they establish drainage.

The problem concerns the best approach to infants with progressive enlargement of the head but with lesser or no elevation in CSF pressure. Under these circumstances, daily serial lumbar punctures to remove as much fluid as will flow (often about 10–15 ml/kg) are useful. Acetazolamide and furosemide are sometimes effective. The results can be monitored by ultrasonography. In some infants, this intervention results in pressure returning to normal and ventricular size stabilizing. Others cannot be weaned from lumbar punctures and may progress to requiring a shunt, albeit at

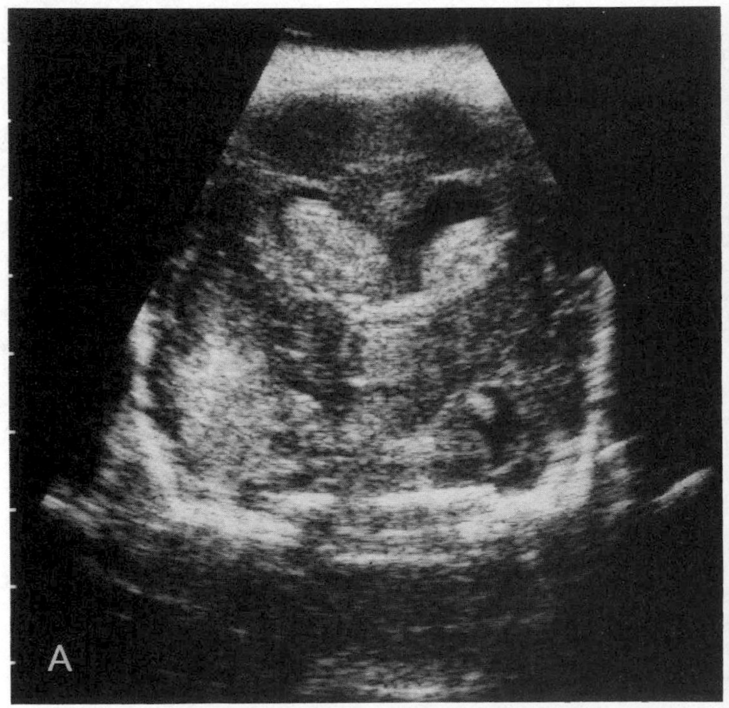

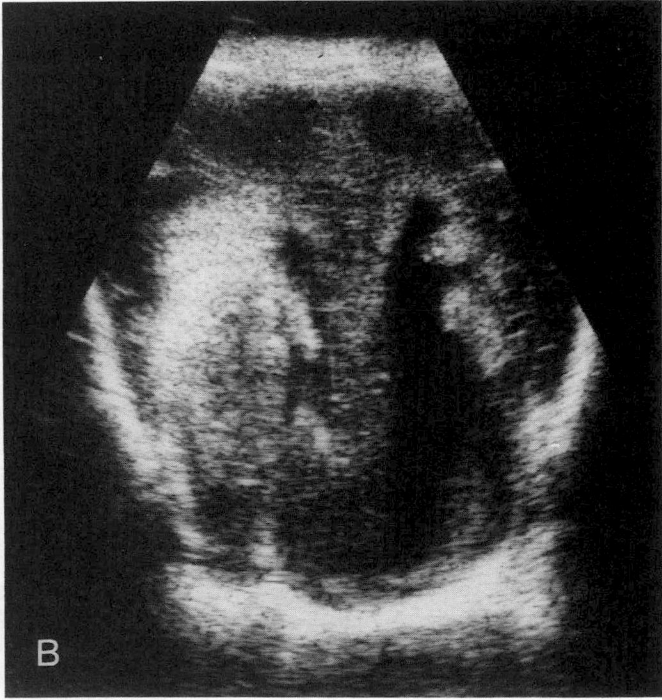

Figure 4.28. This baby was the 1-kg product of a 29-week gestation. He was delivered by cesarean section because of ruptured membranes and amnionitis. He had severe hyaline membrane disease and required mechanical ventilation for 42 days. On day 1, a cranial ultrasonogram was normal. On day 2, these coronal ultrasonograms demonstrate dilatation of lateral ventricles with blood filling the ventricles (**A**). There is an associated intraparenchymal hemorrhage on the right, involving parietal, occipital, and temporal lobes. This grade IV hemorrhage led to severe neurologic impairment. Serial ultrasonograms were done to follow resolution of blood clot, assess degree of ventricular dilatation, and determine the degree of parenchymal damage (**B**). The infant has bilateral ventricular-peritoneal shunts to relieve the obstructive hydrocephalus.

CASE ILLUSTRATION

A 790-g, 28-week gestational age male infant had respiratory distress, and was intubated and placed on mechanical ventilation from the first hour after birth. Oxygen requirements and ventilation pressures were stable until 18 hours, when the infant became ashen and the blood gases revealed a Pa_{O_2} of 40 on 80% oxygen, a deterioration from the earlier Pa_{O_2} of 60 at the same inspired oxygen concentration. A hematocrit at 18 hours was 38, a fall from an initial 43. The fontanelle was slightly tense. Cranial ultrasonography revealed a grade II intraventricular hemorrhage. Serial head circumference measurements and hematocrit levels did not change. No lumbar punctures were performed. The infant improved over the subsequent days with a decrease in ventilatory requirements as lung function improved and no increase in head circumference. Ultrasonographic examination at 2 weeks of age revealed minimal ventricular dilatation.

COMMENT

The benign course after intraventricular hemorrhage of modest degree provides a reminder that, in the past, this condition was probably not diagnosed on clinical grounds. Thus, the report of hemorrhage by ultrasonography should not be a signal to abandon hope.

a larger weight. According to Hill and Volpe (1981), about 40% will eventually undergo spontaneous arrest with partial or complete resolution of ventricular dilatation. The question of whether the lumbar punctures are beneficial remains moot.

Glycerol or head compression have had their advocates, but we are not among them.

Prevention

Prevention of prematurity would virtually eliminate intraventricular hemorrhage in the newborn. An increase in the section rate for premature infants has been associated with less subarachnoid or other traumatic bleeding. Discontinuation of benzyl alcohol as a

CASE ILLUSTRATION

A 600-g female infant born after an estimated 25-week gestation had a surprisingly uneventful first day of life. Apgar scores were 6 at 1 minute, and 8 at 5 minutes, with good air exchange. The chest film showed good bilateral aeration. On the second day of life, apneic spells with bradycardia were sufficient to require intubation and intermittent mandatory ventilation at peak pressures of 18, and end-expiratory pressure of 5. Over the next few days, the chest radiograph showed increasing opacification of both lungs. A ductus murmur was heard and echocardiography was consistent with a left-to-right ductal shunt. Oxygen requirements increased. Indomethacin was begun with a gradual improvement. The hematocrit fell from an initial 42 to 34 and the possibility of intraventricular hemorrhage was confirmed by ultrasonography, which showed a hemorrhage with dilatation of the ventricles.

Initial head circumference was 24.5 cm and, by 96 hours of age, had not changed. Serial measurements thereafter showed a greater than expected increase, so that by 10 days of age, it was 27 cm. Lumbar punctures were performed to remove spinal fluid and control intracranial pressure. After 5 weeks of continued taps, with no reduction in volume of fluid removed, and evidence of continued increase in ventricular size by ultrasonography examination, a ventriculoperitoneal shunt was inserted. The infant tolerated the procedure well, and showed normal weight gain and increase in head circumference in the following weeks.

Follow-up examination at 4 months after birth showed a nonfunctional shunt that was removed, without evidence of a return of hydrocephalus.

COMMENT

This infant posed the problem of how long to continue spinal taps to relieve pressure, when to insert a ventriculoperitoneal shunt, and what would be the ultimate prognosis. No precise answers were available. In general, we prefer to postpone shunts until the infant has been gaining weight and would presumably be in better condition to tolerate surgery. In this instance, the cardiopulmonary status was precarious when the bleeding was discovered, so serial lumbar taps were undertaken until the infant no longer required mechanical ventilation.

In some infants, as in case 1, observation alone is sufficient. In case 2, the relief of pressure required taps. (The infant had been on furosemide for the ductus, but had continuing increase in head size during that period.) When serial taps continue to be required, the decision of the timing of placement of a shunt remains a problem. This depends on the general condition of the infant, and the experience of neurosurgeons.

The outlook for infants who require shunts must be guarded but not hopeless. Some will have infections and require shunt revision. Others will have central nervous system damage, either cortical blindness or cerebral palsy. Even 2-kg preterm infants with early (median age 28 days) shunts may have a poor outcome. Boynton et al (1985) followed 28 preterm infants (mean birth weight 1338 g, gestational age 30 ± 2 weeks) with grade III or IV hemorrhages and found 17 required one or more shunt revisions; 10 had infections; three died; eight had profound visual loss and seven had hearing impairment; five had profound neurologic sequelae. Only five had normal developmental scores.

preservative in solutions used to flush intravascular catheters is essential (Benda et al, 1986) since it has been linked with an increase in incidence of intraventricular hemorrhage in small preterm infants.

The possibility of pharmacologic intervention in the first hours of life before bleeding is evident was raised by Donn et al in 1981. The rationale was to take advantage of the neuroprotective effects of barbiturates, which include decreased catecholamine release, decreased cerebral blood flow and metabolism, and possible enzyme induction. We do not advocate phenobarbital for prophylaxis because careful prospective controlled trials have not shown benefit (Bedard et al, 1984; Kuban et al, 1986).

Prognosis

The prognosis after intraventricular hemorrhage depends on the extent of bleeding, but also on the associated events during the neonatal and postneonatal course. For example, a small intraventricular hemorrhage (grade I and II) has a good likelihood of complete resolution, but the infant may have residual neuromotor dysfunction from other insults such as asphyxia or infection. More extensive hemorrhages which reach into the periventricular substance predictably have a worse prognosis. (Armstrong et al, 1987).

Of 129 preterm infants who were 27–34 weeks' gestational age followed prospectively by Dubowitz et al (1984), 29% had ultrasonographic evidence of periventricular hemorrhage in the newborn period; about one-third were normal at 1 year of age. The abnormalities were greater the larger the hemorrhage. Periventricular hemorrhage by itself was not as good a predictor of outcome as was the neurologic assessment at 40 weeks postmenstrual age (after mother's last menstrual period).

REFERENCES

Adamkin DH, Fleischaker JW, Cook LN, et al: The perinatal/neonatal profile of subarachnoid hemorrhage. *Pediatr Res* 19:330A, 1985.

Andrew M, Castle V, Saigal S, et al: Clinical impact of neonatal thrombocytopenia. *J Pediatr* 110:457, 1987.

Armstrong DL, Sauls CD, Goddard-Finegold J: Neuropathologic findings in short-term survivors of intraventricular hemorrhage. *Am J Dis Child* 141:617;, 1987.

Bedard MP, Shankarzn S, Slovis TL, et al: Effect of prophylactic phenobarbital on intraventricular hemorrhage in high-risk infants. *Pediatrics* 73:435, 1984.

Benda GI, Hiller JL, Reynolds JW: Benzyl alcohol toxicity: Impact on neurologic handicaps among surviving very low birth weight infants. *Pediatrics* 77:507, 1986.

Boynton CA, Boynton BR, Merritt TA, et al: Early ventriculo peritoneal shunts in infants weighing 2000 grams: Neurodevelopmental follow-up. *Pediatr Res* 19:387A, 1985.

Coulter DM: Differing effects of prolactin on the water content of individual tissues in the rabbit pup at 72 hours of age. *Biol Neonate* 46:131, 1984.

deCourten GM, Rabinowicz T: Analysis of 100 infant deaths and intraventricular hemorrhage: Brain weights and risk factors. *Dev Med Child Neurol* 23:287, 1981.

Donn SM, Roloff DW, Goldstein GW: Prevention of intraventricular hemorrhage in preterm infants by phenobarbital. *Lancet* 2:215, 1981.

Dubowitz LMS, Dubowitz V, Palmer PG, et al: Correlation of neurologic assessment in the preterm newborn infant with outcome at 1 year. *J Pediatr* 105:452, 1984.

Hambleton G, Wigglesworth JS: Origin of intraventricular haemorrhage in the preterm infant. *Arch Dis Child* 51:651, 1976.

Hill A, Volpe JJ: Normal pressure hydrocephalus in the newborn. *Pediatrics* 68:623, 1981.

Kreusser KL, Tarby TJ, Kovnar E, et al: Serial lumbar punctures for at least temporary amelioration of neonatal post hemorrhagic hydrocephalus. *Pediatrics* 75:719, 1985.

Kuban KC, Leviton A, Krishnamoorthy KS, et al. Neonatal intracranial hemorrhage and phenobarbital. *Pediatrics* 77:443, 1986.

Lazzara A, Ahmannn P, Dykes F: Clinical predictability of intraventricular hemorrhage in preterm infants. *Pediatrics* 65:30, 1980.

Papile LA, Burstein J, Burstein R, et al: Incidence and evolution of subependymal and intraventricular hemorrhage: A study of infants with weight less than 1,500 gm. *J Pediatr* 92:529, 1978.

Papile LA, et al: Cerebral intraventricular hemorrhage (CVH) in infants <1500 grams: Developmental follow-up at one year. *Pediatr Res* 15:528, 1979.

Partridge JC, Babcock DS, Steichen JJ, et al: Optimal timing for diagnostic cranial ultrasound in low birth weight infants; Detection of intracranial hemorrhage and ventricular dilatation. *Pediatrics* 102:281, 1983.

Perlman JM, Goodman S, Kreusser KL, et al: Reduction in intraventricular hemorrhage by elimination of fluctuating cerebral blood-flow velocity in preterm infants with respiratory distress syndrome. *N Engl J Med* 312:1353, 1985.

Szymonowicz W, Yu VYH, Wilson FE: Antecedents of periventricular haemorrhage in infants weighing 1250 g or less at birth. *Arch Dis Child* 59:13, 1984.

Welch K: The intracranial pressure in infants. *J Neurosurg* 52:693, 1980.

Williams J, Hirsch MJ, Corbet AJS, et al: Postnatal head shrinkage in small infants. *Pediatrics* 59:619, 1977.

Hematologic Disorders 15

Certain hematologic disorders are of significance only in the newborn period. One of them, isoimmunization from Rh or ABO incompatibility is so important a perinatal issue that it was discussed under jaundice in this section. Others that are discussed here include anemia of prematurity, neonatal polycythemia and thrombocytopenia. Other hematologic conditions that may affect infants and older children as well will be discussed in other sections (see Index).

ANEMIA OF PREMATURITY

Definition

A progressive decline in hemoglobin follows birth and is more pronounced in premature infants than those at term. The nadir is usually reached between 4 and 8 weeks. This phenomonen is so common, and the infants usually so asymptomatic, that the anemia of prematurity was, in the past, considered a normal neonatal adaptation. In infants who have had exchange transfusions or blood loss at the time of delivery, the anemia could be very severe and not respond to iron. These infants have required small transfusions.

The anemia of prematurity that reaches 7–9 g/dl in the absence of other causes such as blood loss and infection, has been thought to be related to vitamin E deficiency.

Basic Science

Oski and Barness (1967) demonstrated the beneficial effect of daily vitamin E by mouth (15 IU/day) and, at that dose, no demonstrable toxicity. Levels of linoleic acid comparable to those in human milk are important for the beneficial effect of vitamin E on hemoglobin levels.

Serum erythropoietin concentrations in preterm infants with anemia have been followed by several investigators. Evidence suggesting inadequate production of erythropoietin was reported by Shannon et al in 1987.

Treatment

Caution is advised in the use of vitamin E because, as in so many other situations, an excess can be harmful. In a clinical trial to evaluate the effect of vitamin E on the retinopathy of prematurity, Johnson and colleagues (1985) found that their vitamin E treated infants of less than 1500 g had a significant increase in neonatal sepsis and necrotizing enterocolitis. They had been given vitamin E in doses sufficient to maintain a serum level of 5 mg/dl. They believed the increased susceptibility to infection and late onset necrotizing enterocolitis was the result of excessive scavenging of oxygen radicals by the high levels of vitamin E. Their recommendation is, for optimal vitamin E nutrition, that the serum concentrations be kept between 1 and 3 mg/dl.

Glader's recommendations (1984) to prevent anemia of prematurity are (1) vitamin E (25 IU) daily until 8–10 weeks of age, (2) formulas should be similar to mother's milk with respect to linoleic acid content, (3) no iron supplements during the first 2 months, (4) supplement with iron to ensure 2 mg/kg/day to prevent the late anemia of prematurity when growth is rapid later in the first year of life.

CONTROVERSY

Although the relationship of low tocopherol levels and anemia have long been known, and vitamin E supplementation widely practiced, the causal relationship has been challenged. Multiple factors that contribute to late anemia include blood sampling, other illness, and rapid growth which had not always been considered by advocates of vitamin E supplementation.

Zipursky et al (1987) carried out a prospective randomized controlled trial of vitamin E supplementation in well infants weighing less than 1.5 kg. The treated group received 25 IU of *dl*-α-tocopherol by gavage for the first 6 weeks of life. No differences were found between treated and control infants in hemoglobin concentration, reticulocytes, platelet counts, or erythrocyte morphology. As the investigators commented, this study did not prove that vitamin E deficiency anemia does not occur, but it challenges the assumption that in well low birth weight infants, routine vitamin E supplementation is needed.

NEONATAL POLYCYTHEMIA

Definition

An increase in red cell mass to above-normal levels is polycythemia. The hematocrit may be elevated by increased numbers of red cells or by decreased plasma volume. A decrease in plasma volume is less common at birth than an increase in red cell mass. Hematocrits of over 65 are arbitrarily considered polycythemia in newborns.

Basic Science

The most common cause of an increase in blood volume is a "placental transfusion," meaning a shift of blood from the placental vascular bed to the fetus. Delay in clamping the cord, or positioning the infant below the level of the placenta can promote movement of as much as 100 ml of blood from placenta to infant. Twin-to-twin intrauterine transfusions can result in one polycythemic and one anemic twin. Sometimes an infant may be polycythemic from chronic placental insufficiency, perhaps from the hypoxic stimulus. Infants of diabetic mothers have increased red cell production and high fetal hemoglobin concentrations (Bard and Prosmanne, 1985).

Epidemiology

In several studies, the prevalence in appropriately grown term infants was 4% (Stevens and Wirth, 1980; Wirth et al, 1979). Although unusual, the condition occurs more frequently in infants of diabetic mothers, and in infants who are small for gestational age and in Down syndrome and Beckwith syndrome infants.

Natural History

Most infants with elevated hematocrit values remain asymptomatic, although in some the bilirubin-conjugation and excretion mechanisms may become overloaded so that the infants have significant "physiological" jaundice.

Some infants may have cardiorespiratory symptoms consistent with elevated venous pressures that delay clearance of lung liquid. Tachypnea, cyanosis, cardiomegaly, and even pulmonary edema have been described. An association between polycythemia and necrotizing enterocolitis has been noted. Some infants have seizures, and few have persistent neurological dysfunction, such as hemiparesis. Hypoglycemia has been associated with polycythemia even in the absence of a history of maternal diabetes.

Diagnosis

It is important to measure the hematocrit on central circulating blood, such as that obtained from an umbilical vein, or other major vein. Capillary blood hematocrits may be higher than values on central blood because of some peripheral stasis.

Treatment

In general, we treat the infant on the basis of anticipated problems. Because symptoms of cyanosis, priapism, persistent hypoglycemia, lethargy, and later jaundice are so likely at hematocrit values of over 65, we usually intervene. If the hematocrit is over 70, even in the absence of symptoms, we recommend partial plasma exchange to reduce the risk of thrombosis from viscous blood. No uniform approach to treatment has been accepted. Some physicians practice phlebotomy or phlebotomy with albumin or saline infusion sufficient to lower the hematocrit to 50%. An evaluation of partial plasma exchange and observation only, carried out by Black et al (1985), indicated no benefit in the neonatal period but, at 2 years, the group who received the exchange had fewer neurologic findings and abnormalities in fine motor function.

BLEEDING FROM PLATELET ABNORMALITIES

Platelet-related bleeding in the newborn is most commonly associated with thrombocytopenia, although abnormal platelet function can occur. When the platelets are low in number, the bleeding is characteristically superficial, petechial, and self-limited. This is in contrast to large hemorrhages seen in coagulopathies.

Isoimmune Thrombocytopenia

Definition

This condition is analogous to erythroblastosis fetalis, except that the sensitizing cells are infant's platelets entering the maternal circulation instead of infant's red cells producing maternal antibodies. The condition occurs most commonly when the mother is PL^{A1}-negative and the infant is PL^{A1}-positive (Shulman et al, 1964).

Epidemiology

Of all cases, 50% occur in the first pregnancy, and once this problem has occurred, there is a 70–85% probability of a repeat in later pregnancies.

Natural History

Infants with isoimmune thrombocytopenia usually have petechial, purpuric, and sometimes mucosal bleeding during the first 48 hours of life but, in other respects, they are usually entirely well. The platelet counts may be decreased to levels as low as 2000 and the platelets appear very large on the peripheral blood smear. Usually the mother has a normal platelet count.

Without treatment, the thrombocytopenia will resolve spontaneously over a period of 3–4 weeks as maternal antibodies decrease in the infant's circulation.

Diagnosis

The diagnosis can be suspected whenever a healthy infant has thrombocytopenia and the mother a normal platelet count. Definitive diagnosis depends on the detection of antiplatelet antibodies in the maternal circulation.

Treatment

Formerly, the mainstay of treatment was transfusion of maternal platelets that were washed and resuspended in AB-negative plasma (random donors were of little value because 97% of donors were platelet A1-positive). Treatment is generally advocated when platelet counts are less than 30,000, even in the absence of overt bleeding.

Hydrocortisone, 10 mg every 12 hours intravenously, or prednisolone are effective in gradually increasing the platelet count. Most infants achieve higher levels than in the absence of steroids, although the effect is not impressive until 10–15 days in children with idiopathic thrombocytopenic purpura. The time of the response in infants is not as well studied. Nonetheless, steroids are ineffective in stopping bleeding (Sartorius, 1984).

Of some promise is the use of intravenous immunoglobulin which stimulates a rise in platelets faster than adrenocorticosteroids in children with idiopathic thrombocytopenic purpura (Inbach et al, 1984). Derycke et al (1985) described a patient who was treated with an infusion of pH 4-treated immunoglobulin in 3% saline solution at a dose of 400 mg/kg/day on days 4–8 after birth. The infusions were given over a 3-hour period each day and were well tolerated. Correction of the thrombocytopenia was noted between day 8 and day 10.

Prevention

If a mother has had an affected child and is known to be PL^{A1}-negative, it is appropriate to measure platelet counts on the fetus. Traditionally, maternal PL^{A1}-negative platelets have been given to infants in utero. It is possible that intravenous gammaglobulin can be given as well, although that has not yet been evaluated.

A cesarean section is far better than a vaginal delivery to prevent obstetrical trauma to these infants since they are thrombocytopenic in utero.

Immune Thrombocytopenia Secondary to Maternal Disease

Definition

This is a condition in which a mother has evidence of active thrombocytopenia and a low platelet count, and her infant also has thrombocytopenia.

Basic Science

A mother with thrombocytopenia will have antibodies to her own platelets that can cross the placenta and cause immune thrombocytopenia in the infant.

Epidemiology

This rare condition occurs most commonly when mothers are thrombocytopenic near delivery. Steroid administration to the mother during the pregnancy can raise the infant's platelet counts and reduces the incidence of the disorder.

Natural History

There is no way to distinguish these babies from those born with isoimmune thrombocytopenia except by examination of their mothers. Occasionally, an infant of a mother with lupus erythematosus (LE) will have transient thrombocytopenia in association with LE cells in the peripheral blood.

Diagnosis

The diagnosis depends on ascertainment of a low platelet count; values of less than 100,000/ml^3 are characteristic of mothers who have infants with this disorder.

Treatment

The level of platelets at which one should treat the infant with hydrocortisone is debatable but, in general, values of less than 20,000 are indications for treatment (oral prednisone, 1 mg/kg/day). If there is severe hemorrhage, a transfusion of platelets or intravenous immunoglobulin should be given.

Other Causes of Neonatal Thrombocytopenia

Drug-Induced Maternal Thrombocytopenia

Some drugs, particularly quinine, sulfonamides and digitoxin, given to the mother can produce neonatal thrombocytopenia in both infant and mother. An antibody to the drug is produced by the mother, and the drug-antibody complex attaches to platelets and results in their removal. Significant bleeding in the infant is rare in this circumstance.

Thrombocytopenia with Infection

Most of the serious congenital infections, including cytomegalic inclusion disease, toxoplasmosis, rubella, and herpes simplex are associated with neonatal thrombocytopenia and often disseminated intravascular coagulation.

Thrombocytopenia with Giant Hemangiomas

Multiple hemangiomas are capable of trapping platelets and producing significant thrombocytopenia. The possibility of visceral hemangiomatosis should be considered whenever platelet levels are low in the absence of other known causes. When this condition is recognized, steroids (e.g., prednisone 20 mg/day for 2 weeks) may cause regression of hemangiomas, although they are not always successful.

Thrombocytopenia in Asssociation with Bone Marrow Hypoplasia

Decreased platelet production can take place in a variety of situations including Fanconi hypoplastic anemia, congenital leukemia, and a situation associated with bilateral absence of the radiae.

Hereditary thrombocytopenia (Wiskott-Aldrich syndrome) is characterized by thrombocytopenia thought to be related to an intrinsic platelet defect that leads to their decreased survival. The platelets in Wiskott-Aldrich syndrome are much smaller than normal, which distinguishes this disorder from many other thrombocytopenias (see pp. 535).

Platelet Dysfunction

Neonatal platelet aggregation may be abnormal and increase bleeding time. This possibility should be considered in infants who are bleeding and in whom coagulation studies are normal. The most usual cause for platelet dysfunction is maternal drug ingestion, with aspirin the worst offender. There have been reports wherein mothers have taken aspirin before delivery and their infants subsequently have large cephalohematomas and evidence of platelet dysfunction.

CONSIDERATIONS IN BLOOD TRANSFUSIONS

Frequent small transfusions have been widely used in nurseries for infants who have falling hematocrit values and who appeared lethargic or to be having apneic spells. No definitive criteria for transfusion have been formulated and no systematic evaluation of indications for transfusion has been made.

Transfusion-acquired cytomegalovirus (CMV) infections are recognized as a significant cause of morbidity in premature and newborn infants (Yeager et al, 1981). The rate of excretion of CMV by young infants who have not been transfused is 11–14%. Many of these infants remain asymptomatic. The rate of excretion of the virus among infants who have been transfused is twice as high, which clearly incriminates transfusion as a means of infecting a number of infants and producing significant illness in some. CMV can cause pneumonia, hepatitis, a hemolytic anemia, and thrombocytopenia in infants. Nursery epidemics can result when infants excrete virus and infect others.

Because transfusion-acquired CMV infections can cause fatal illness, it becomes imperative to break the chain of transmission of infection. The method currently advocated is the exclusive use of blood from CMV-negative donors, which is a very effective way in reducing infection in infants. Blood banks can identify a pool of CMV-negative individuals who can be screened periodically to ensure persistent CMV negativity; screening twice a year is advocated. Blood from these individuals is used for all transfusions in newborn infants.

Other potentially transfusion-related diseases include hepatitis B, and it should be routine for all blood banks to make sure that donors are hepatitis B-negative. Unfortunately, no screening is available for hepatitis non-A non-B infection.

Screening for HIV by several techniques is in current use in blood banks. Nevertheless, the presence of some false-negative tests, including individuals with active infection, means that even with screening there is a small chance of infecting infants (Ward et al, 1988).

Other situations in which infants have been infected included donors who were unaware, for example, of a past history of malaria. When their blood is donated and given to infants, full-blown malaria can result. With an increase in the number of individuals travelling to areas of the world in which malaria is endemic, we can expect to see more infected blood donors.

Another risk of transfusion in newborn infants is the production of graft-versus-host disease which can occur from the action of donor in a situation of congenital or acquired immune suppression. This is a particular problem after fetal transfusions unless the blood has been irradiated. Infants with severe combined immune deficiency disease should never be given blood transfusions unless white cells have been removed by appropriate filtration and irradiation.

Given these hazards, it is time to reexamine the iteria for administration of blood to newborn infants. It seems arbitrary to set a value for hemoglobin at which preterm infants should be transfused for the anemia of prematurity, for example. The nadir of their anemia is likely to be 5–6 weeks after birth and, if a reticulocyte count is elevated and the infants are asymptomatic, it seems quite unnecessary to transfuse because the hemoglobin or hematocrit are low. Breastfeeding, or use of formulas fortified with iron and vitamin E are appropriate (Zipursky et al, 1987).

REFERENCES

Bard H, Prosmanne J: Hemoglobin synthesis in cord blood of infants of insulin-dependent diabetic mothers. *Pediatrics* 75:1143, 1985.

Black VD, Lubchenco LO, Koops BL, et al: Neonatal hyperviscosity and randomized study of the effect of partial plasma exchange transfusion on long-term outcome. *Pediatrics* 75:1048, 1985.

Derycke M, Dreyfus M, Ropert JC, et al: Intravenous immunoglobulin for neonatal isoimmune thrombocytopenia. *Arch Dis Child* 60:667, 1985.

Glader BE: Erythrocyte disorders in infancy. In Avery ME, Taeusch HW (eds): *Diseases of the Newborn*. Philadelphia, WB Saunders, 1984.

Inbach B, Barandun S, et al: Intravenous immunoglobulin for idiopathic thrombocytopenic purpura (ITP) in childhood. *Am J Pediatr Hematol/Oncol* 6:171, 1984.

Johnson L, Bowen FW, Abassi S, et al: Relationship of prolonged pharmacologic serum levels of vitamin E to incidence of sepsis and necrotizing enterocolitis in infants with birth weight 1500 grams or less. *Pediatrics* 75:619, 1985.

Karpatkin M, Porges RF, Karpatkin S: Platelet counts in infants of women with autoimmune thrombocytopenia. *N Engl J Med* 305:936, 1981.

Oski FA, Barness LA: Vitamin E deficiency: A previously unrecognized cause of hemolytic anemia in the premature infant. *J Pediatr* 70:211, 1967.

Sartorius JA: Steroid treatment of idiopathic thrombocytopenic purpura in children. *Am J Pediatr Hematol/Oncol* 6:165, 1984.

Shannon KM, Naylor GS, Torkildson JC, et al: Circulatory erythroid progenitors in the anemia of prematurity *N Engl J Med* 317:728, 1987.

Shulman NR, Marder VJ, Hiller MC: Platelet and leukocyte isoantigens and their antibodies, serologic, physiologic, and clinical studies. *Prog Hematol* 4:222, 1964.

Stevens K, Wirth FH: Incidence of neonatal hyperviscosity at sea level. *J Pediatr* 97:118, 1980.

Ward JW, Holmberg SD, Allen Jr, et al: Transmission of human immunodeficiency virus (HIV) by blood transfusions screened as negative for HIV antibody. *N Engl J Med* 318:473, 1988.

Wirth FH, Goldberg KE, Lubchenco LO: Neonatal hyperviscosity: 1. Incidence. *Pediatrics* 63:833, 1979.

Yeager AS, Grumet FC, Hafleigh EB, et al: Prevention of transfusion acquired cytomegalovirus infections in newborn infants. *J Pediatr* 98:281, 1981.

Zipursky A, Brown EJ, Watts J, et al: Oral vitamin E supplementation for the prevention of anemia in premature infants: A controlled trial. *Pediatrics* 79:61, 1987.

Umbilicus 16

The umbilical cord is essential for intrauterine life, and interference with blood flow through it can be the cause of fetal death. If it has a velamentous attachment to the placenta, it can tear during delivery with resultant blood loss. Great variations in cord length have been documented. Purola (1968) found the range to be 22–135 cm, with the mean 59 ± 12 cm. The cord contains two arteries and a vein, embedded in a loose mucoid matrix called Wharton jelly. Stellate mesenchymal cells are normally present, but the cord is devoid of nerves, capillaries, or lymphatics.

ABNORMALITIES IN LENGTH

Apparently linear cord growth depends on intrauterine space and fetal movement. Miller et al (1981) noted short cords in conditions that restrict fetal movement, which include early amnion rupture, renal agenesis, and structural limb dysfunction, such as Werdnig-Hoffman disease of prenatal onset.

Data from 35,779 successful singleton pregnancies in the Collaborative Perinatal Study in the United States were analyzed by Naeye (1985). Short cords (less than 40 cm at 40–41 weeks' gestation) were associated with greater need for resuscitation, jitteriness, and later neurological abnormalities.

Unusually long umbilical cords are found in situations in which they have been wrapped around a fetal part, and probably subjected to abnormal stretch. Cord entanglements toward term are more probable with long cords.

The importance of measuring and recording cord length is to alert parents to possible problems that may not be detected until ages 4–7 years, and to point to a possible cause. There is no reason to expect a familial incidence of this condition unless the underlying condition is familial (as in renal agenesis). Naeye noted that when full-term same sex siblings had cord lengths that differed by more than 20 cm, those with shorter cords had lower IQ values and more neurologic abnormalities. He also noted that female infants have shorter cords on average.

ROUTINE CARE OF UMBILICAL CORD

The cord should be clamped or tied with sterile materials, and cut with sterile scissors. Colonization of the cord stump is inevitable from environmental sources. Most organisms produce minimal inflammation that remains localized. The question then is whether there is any purpose in the application of agents to prevent infection. A large literature describes attempts to prevent colonization with *Staphylococcus aureus,* which is the major cause of omphalitis (Cushing, 1985). Current practices favor use of dry-skin care, that is, no chemicals or moisture to avoid unnecessary treatment and emergence of resistant organisms. When the infant is bathed, care should be taken to keep the cord dry, or wipe with alcohol several times a day.

SINGLE UMBILICAL ARTERY

This abnormality occurs in 0.75% of infants. About 18% of those infants will show other malformations, according to Heinonen et al (1977), based on 45,192 infants in the Collaborative Perinatal Project. Cardiovascular and genitourinary tracts were most often affected. Examination of infants who died before 28 days of age, revealed twice the frequency of single umbilical artery compared with survivors.

About 1.5% of infants who died before 28 weeks had a single umbilical artery. Nearly one-half of those affected had chromosomal problems, and more than half had other serious malformations (Byrne and Blanc, 1985). Antenatal diagnosis by ultrasonography has been reported (Tortora et al, 1984).

SEPARATION

The normal time for separation of the cord is 5–8 days. Delay beyond 10 days requires investigation. Absence of bacteria, as in a germ-free environment, postpones separation time. The most serious concern is a lack of neutrophil motility. Hayward et al (1979) described six infants with that condition from two families in which cord separation did not occur until 3–6 weeks. Other instances of delayed separation occur in the absence of T-killer cell activity and deficient γ-interferon production (Davies et al, 1982).

GRANULOMA

After cord separation, the base usually epithelializes, but sometimes granulation tissue forms. The gray-red smooth appearance may be in the depth of the depression or project onto the abdominal wall. Differentiation from intestinal or gastric mucosa can be made by moistening the finger and noting if mucus is present. A granuloma feels like dry velvet with no mucus. Treatment is gentle application of desiccated silver nitrate from a stick. Care must be taken not to touch the surrounding skin.

ABERRANT MUCOSA

If gastric mucosa is present, acid secretions can be detected. Surgical removal is required.

OMPHALITIS

Definition and Epidemiology

Omphalitis is an infection of the tissues adjacent to the cord; it may extend into the blood stream.

Omphalitis occurs in about 2% of infants delivered in modern hospitals. Serious illness (sepsis) is less common.

Natural History

On the first day of life, almost all cords are sterile, but they gradually become colonized with *S. aureus, S. epidermidis,* or streptococci. Gram-negative rods are present in about one-third of cultures. In attempts to lower the incidence of staphylococci, hexachlorophene or triple dye solutions have been found effective. Nonetheless, some infants had cellulitis. Infants with surrounding tissue infection are most likely to have staphylococci as the offending organism.

Diagnosis

Because infection of the cord is necessary before sloughing, the presence of a positive culture does not denote disease. Only when there is an excess of purulent material, or erythema of the soft tissues, should treatment be considered. Sometimes aggressive treatment of a granuloma with silver nitrate can induce a chemical erythema at the cord base.

Significant erythema, swelling, tenderness, or even black discoloration or crepitus are found in severe infections.

Treatment

Serous, serosanguinous, or purulent secretions from the cord base after separation are common. If the surrounding skin is inflamed, or the secretions are frankly purulent, local application of bacitracin or neomycin ointments is indicated. Significant periumbilical infection or any evidence of systemic infection requires administration of systemic antibiotics, orally or intravenously. The antibiotic and route of delivery will depend on knowledge of likely organisms and sensitivities, and degree of illness. Erythromycin or cephalexin orally is useful in most mild cases. With severe infections, therapy against Gram-negative aerobic and anaerobic organisms, as well as staphylococci is indicated. Clindamycin and gentamicin would be appropriate (Cushing, 1985).

UMBILICAL HERNIA

Definition

A separation of the rectus muscles permits protrusion of abdominal viscera in the midline at the level of the umbilicus. Skin and subcutaneous tissue are intact. A hernia is considered present if abdominal contents protrude 0.5 cm or more and a palpable defect in fascia is at least 1 cm diameter.

Epidemiology

Umbilical hernias are present in about 30% of black infants and 4% of white infants under 6 weeks old. Seventy-five percent of infants weighing less than 1500 g have a defect which closes by 1 year, at which time the incidence of hernias in black infants is 12–13%, and in white infants about 2%. Half the hernias present in black children at ages 4–5 years close spontaneously by age 11 years.

Diagnosis and Treatment

Umbilical hernias range in size from barely perceptible to 10 cm or more in diameter, and reach maximal size at about 1–2 months.

Small hernias will close spontaneously within a few months to 3 years. The supine position is helpful in promoting spontaneous reduction. There is no evidence to indicate that taping is helpful. Incarceration is rare.

Hernias of 5-cm diameter or greater probably should be repaired early. Controversy, or at least uncertainty, exists about the management of hernias of 2–5 cm. Some advise taping, whereas others advise early surgery. Observation for several years seems appropriate. The rarity of umbilical hernias in older children even without earlier surgery provides reassurance that most all of them will resolve in time.

OMPHALOCELE AND GASTROSCHISIS

See also page 461, Section 7, Gastroenterology.

URACHUS

Urachus is the embryonic communication between bladder and umbilicus. It is usually a fibrous cord at the time of birth. A very rare event is patency of the urachus which permits discharge of urine through the umbilicus. Diagnosis depends on introduction of dye into the bladder, and observation of the colored urine on the abdominal wall. Excision is the treatment of choice to avoid infection.

REFERENCES

Byrne J, Blanc WA: Malformations and chromosome anomalies in spontaneously aborted fetuses with single umbilical artery. *Am J Obstet Gynecol* 151:340, 1985.
Cushing A: Omphalitis: A review. *Pediatr Infect Dis* 4:282, 1985.
Davies EG, Isaacs D, Levinsky RJ: A lethal syndrome of delayed umbilical cord separation, defection and neutrophil mobility and absent natural killer cell activity. Abstract. *Br Paediatr Assoc,* p 46, 1982.
Hayward AR, Leonard J, Wood CBS, et al: Delayed separation of the umbilical cord, widespread infections and defective neutrophil mobility. *Lancet* 1:1099, 1979.
Heinonen OP, Slone D, Shapiro S: *Birth Defects and Drugs during Pregnancy*. Little, MA, Publishing Sciences Group, 1977.
Hoyme HE, Higginbottom MC, Jones KL: The vascular pathogenesis of gastroschisis: Intrauterine interruption of the omphalomesenteric artery. *J Pediatr* 98:228, 1981.
Miller ME, Higginbottom M, Smith DW: Short umbilical cord: Its origin and relevance. *Pediatrics* 67:618, 1981.
Naeye RL: Umbilical cord length: Clinical significance. *J Pediatr* 107:278, 1985.
Purola E: The length and insertion of the umbilical cord. *Ann Chir Gynaecol* 27:621, 1968.
Tortora M, Chervenak FA, Mayden K, et al: Antenatal sonographic diagnosis of single umbilical artery. *Obstet Gynecol* 63:693, 1984.

GENERAL REFERENCES

Avery ME, Fletcher BD, Williams RG: *The Lung and its Disorders in the Newborn Infant*. Philadelphia, WB Saunders, 1981.
Avery ME, Taeusch HW Jr (eds): *Diseases of the Newborn*. Philadelphia, WB Saunders, 1984.
Cloherty JP, Stark AR: *Manual of Neonatal Care*. Boston, Little, Brown and Co., 1985.
Kendig EL, Chernick V (eds): *Disorders of the Respiratory Tract in Children*. 4th edition. Philadelphia, WB Saunders, 1983.
Purola E: The length and insertion of the umbilical cord. *Ann Chir Gynaecol* 27:621, 1968.
Roach MR: A biophysical look at the relationship of structure and function in the umbilical artery. In *Foetal and Neonatal Physiology*. Proceedings of the Sir Joseph Bancroft Centenary Symposium. Cambridge University Press, 1973, p. 141.
Roberts RS: *Drug Therapy in Infants. Pharmacologic Principles and Clinical Experience*. Philadelphia, WB Saunders, 1984.
Smith DW: *Recognizable Patterns of Human Malformation*. 3rd edition. Philadelphia, WB Saunders, 1982.
Volpe JJ: *Neurology of the Newborn*. Philadelphia, WB Saunders, 1981.

MARY ELLEN AVERY
HEIDELISE ALS

Consultants
Elizabeth Brown
Michael F. Epstein
Helen Liley
David Schiff
Janice Ware

Section 5

Pulmonology

Reference to the lung and its disorders occurs in many sections of this book, especially Neonatology (Section 4). The contents of this section were selected to provide some perspective on manifestations of pulmonary disease and approaches to diagnosis.

The grouping of disorders is designed to aid in differential diagnosis by predominant radiographic or clinical signs. Within obstructive diseases for example, asthma, bronchiolitis, and cystic fibrosis need to be distinguished from each other, as well as chronic aspiration.

When the etiology is known, a discussion of the given entity may appear under the name of the offending agent. For example, some pneumonias will be discussed under the organism responsible (Section 17). Some of the neuromuscular disorders will be clarified in Section 12.

Manifestations of Pulmonary Disease 1

PHYSICAL EXAMINATION

The classic methods of examination of the chest have much merit and deserve consideration in this section, even with awareness that roentgenographic and other imaging techniques have provided invaluable and indispensable aid in diagnosis.

Breathing Patterns

Tachypnea is the most common alteration in breathing and the most important clue to pulmonary dysfunction. Hypoxemia or infiltrative disease often require the patient to take frequent small tidal volumes to lessen the work of breathing and facilitate gas exchange. Conversely, obstructive lesions of the upper airway require prolonged inspiration and higher pressures that produce retractions or indrawing of soft tissues. Lower airway obstruction is associated with prolonged expiration and, frequently, an audible wheeze. Metabolic derangements that can be compensated by hyperventilation are accompanied by deep breathing, as in ketoacidosis; hypoventilation may be a response to metabolic alkalosis as in pyloric stenosis. Shallow irregular breathing or periodic breathing denotes cerebral dysfunction or drug intoxication.

Inspection of the chest wall will indicate the presence of increased transpulmonary pressure, as the soft tissues are drawn in with inspiration (called retractions). An abnormal configuration will indicate kyphoscoliosis, or guarding in the presence of pleural disease. Paradoxical movements of chest and abdomen may be the sign of diaphragmatic paralysis or chest wall muscular weakness. Hyperinflation is indicative of lower airway obstructive disease, or pneumothorax, and may be evident as an increase in the anteroposterior diameter of the chest.

A shift in the cardiac impulse can result from loss of volume in one lung, as in agenesis or atelectasis, or overdistention of the thorax caused by a space-occupying lesion such as an effusion, or adenomatoid malformation. Dextrocardia may occur in association with the immotile cilia syndrome.

Other clues to respiratory disease come from *examination of the extremities* for clubbing or edema. Clubbing is an enlargement of the terminal phalanges with loss of the normal angle at the base of the nailbed. It appears first in the thumb and index finger. It occurs most frequently in individuals with chronic hypoxemia as in congenital heart disease or cystic fibrosis, but can be seen in patients with cirrhosis or inflammatory bowel disease but is rarely, if ever, seen in asthma.

Observation of skin color is important, but a treacherous means of identifying cyanosis since it requires 5 g of unsaturated hemoglobin before cyanosis can be observed. Anemic individuals can be acyanotic with significant desaturation; polycythemic individuals can be dusky with adequate oxygenation.

Auscultation remains a useful way to assess distribution of ventilation, the presence of fluid that produces rales, and rubs that denote pleural or pericardial inflammation. Normal breath sounds are called vesicular. Sounds such as those heard over the normal trachea are accentuated and they are called bronchial when heard over the lung fields. They are prominent in areas of consolidation. Rales are sometimes coarse, and called rhonchi, or crackling, or fine crackling at end-inspiration. They are heard when edema fluid is present in the peripheral airways or in the presence of interstitial disease. A wheeze is a continuous, high-pitched musical expiratory sound and is usually associated with intrathoracic airway obstruction. Stridor, on the other hand, occurs during inspiration and is usually due to extrathoracic airway obstruction. Rubs are coarse, appear to be close to the end of the stethoscope, and vary with respiration. If coarse sounds or crackles are synchronous with the cardiac cycle they may be from mediastinal air.

Percussion is most useful to detect differences between regions of the lung. Flatness denotes consolidation; resonance comes from presence of air; and hyperresonance is characteristic of a pneumothorax, blebs, or poorly ventilated overdistended regions as in lobar emphysema.

In small infants, sounds are widely transmitted and percussion is difficult. *Palpation* may be the best approach to detect asymmetries or rales. Place both hands on the thorax, and observe excursion with ventilation and feel the effect of liquid in the airways as a vibration.

APPROACH TO CHILD WITH RECURRENT RESPIRATORY INFECTIONS

Definition

An acute inflammatory response to an inhaled pathogen is a respiratory infection.

Epidemiology

EPIDEMIOLOGY OF RESPIRATORY DISEASE

Nearly one-half of all ill children seen by practicing physicians present with acute respiratory complaints and most of these involve the upper respiratory tract. Children, on the average, experience six to eight acute respiratory illnesses each year, a large proportion of which have been ascribed to specific respiratory viruses and *Mycoplasma pneumoniae*.

The seasonal distribution has always been striking with a midwinter peak that often extends through late spring. Respiratory illnesses are infrequent during the summer but begin to increase again in the autumn. In this part of the world, the incidence of respiratory infection parallels the time when children are in school or other relatively closed environments.

In a classic longitudinal study in Chapel Hill, North Carolina from 1963–1971, Glezen and Denny documented the prevalence of lower respiratory tract illnesses. Seventy-five percent of the nonbacterial agents isolated from children with lower respiratory tract disease were from one of four groups: respiratory syncytial virus, parainfluenza virus types 1 and 3, and *M. pneumoniae*. They correlated the infections caused by viruses with distinct clinical features. Respiratory syncytial virus was the most important pathogen and was often associated with bronchiolitis in infants. Parainfluenza type 1 was the agent predominantly associated with croup. Parainfluenza type 3 was less predictable, but was associated with tracheobronchitis, especially in children over 2–3 years of age. *M. pneumoniae* infections were most frequently found in association with pneumonia. Clearly other viruses, such as epidemic strains of influenza, may alter these generalizations from time to time. Adenoviruses, particularly types 1, 2, and 5 can be associated with respiratory or even systemic illness but, in the North Carolina study, they were isolated from only 2% of the patients. They found rhinoviruses to be relatively uncommon in childhood respiratory infections.

The prevalence for boys under 6 years of age was 215/1000, substantially higher than that for girls, 145/1000. Boys were significantly over-represented among individuals with severe infections, such as croup or bronchiolitis, that required hospitalization. After age 6 years the rates were lower for both, and not too different, 66 and 68/1000, respectively.

The North Carolina group documented an experience which has certainly been generalizable. Respiratory syncytial virus produces yearly epidemics of lower respiratory disease characterized mostly by bronchiolitis and pneumonia in infants. In this part of the world, they are predictable in midwinter. On the other hand, croup tends to reach a peak in the autumn of even numbered years. The most susceptible group are boys between the ages of 8 and 30 months. Parainfluenza type 3 can occur at almost any age with no preference for one sex over the other. *M. pneumoniae* is the main cause of pneumonia in school-aged children of both sexes and infection is more likely to occur in the autumn and early winter than in any other season.

In a prospective study to identify all pathogens associated with acute lower respiratory tract infection in children, Paisley et al (1984) studied hospitalized children under 5 years of age from November 1978 through June 1979 in Denver. Figure 5.1 summarizes their findings by age. Note the overwhelming predominance of viral etiology. Table 5.1 lists the pathogens identified in 102 children and, once again, respiratory syncytial virus was found in 75% of the cases in the study. Unlike the Chapel Hill experience, rhinoviruses were more commonly isolated by the Denver group. This probably reflects differences in culture technique. This more recent review also highlights the importance of *Chlamydia trachomatis* infection as a frequent cause of afebrile pneumonia in infants.

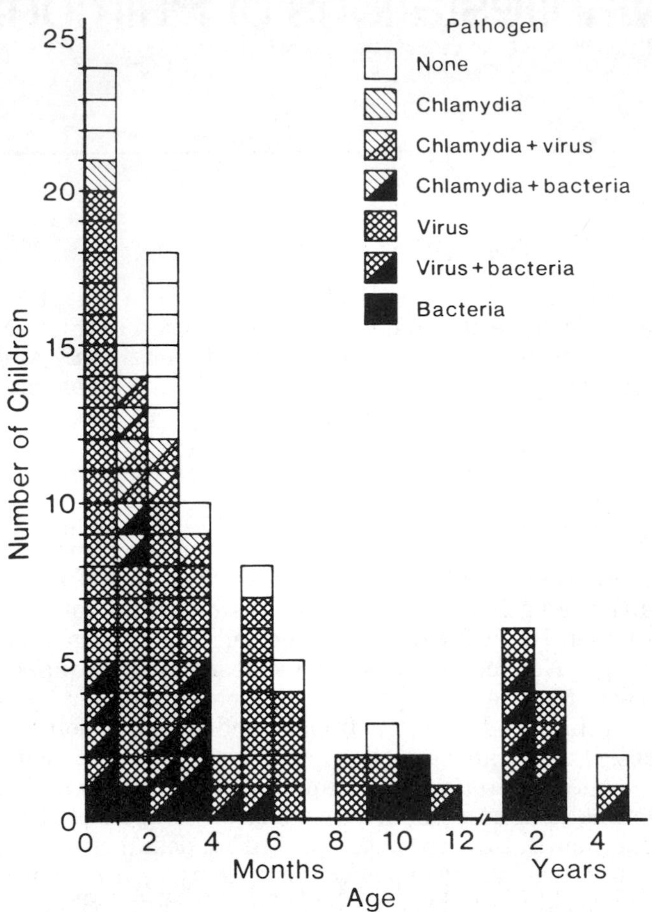

Figure 5.1. Distribution of age and pathogen of 102 children less than 5 years old hospitalized for acute lower respiratory infection. Reproduced with permission from Paisley JW, et al: *Pediatr Infect Dis* 2:14, 1984.

There are, of course, major differences in design of the Chapel Hill and the Denver Studies. In Chapel Hill, populations were seen longitudinally in physicians' offices and outpatient settings, whereas in Denver a study was made of organisms found in children hospitalized with either clinical or radiographic evidence of pneumonia. Nevertheless, several observations are shared by the two studies, namely, that respiratory syncytial virus is the most common cause of lower airway disease in infants and bacterial infections are much less common. Of the bacteria, however, the Denver group noted pneumococcus was the most common, followed by *Haemophilus influenzae*.

Natural History

A number of viruses and some bacteria are capable of causing upper and lower respiratory infections. Acute

Table 5.1
Pathogens Identified in 102 Children less than 5 Years Old Hospitalized with Acute Lower Respiratory Infection[1]

Pathogen(s)	No. of Children
Single (n = 54)	
Respiratory syncytial virus (RSV)	37
Rhinovirus	4
Parainfluenza virus	2
Cytomegalovirus (CMV)	2
Chlamydia trachomatis	1
Streptococcus pneumonia [2]	8
Multiple (n = 33)	
Rhinovirus + parainfluenza	2
RSV + parainfluenza	1
C. trachomatis + RSV	4
C. trachomatis + *S. pneumoniae*	2
C. trachomatis + CMV	2
C. trachomatis, RSV + rhinovirus	1
S. pneumoniae + RSV	10
Haemophilus influenzae + RSV [3]	4
S. pneumoniae + adenovirus	2
H. influenzae + influenza A_2[4]	1
Staphylococcus aureus + RSV	1
Klebsiella pneumoniae + RSV	1
Bordetella pertussis + RSV	1
B. pertussis, *S. pneumoniae* + RSV	1
No pathogen identified	15

[1]Data from Paisley JW, Lauer BA, McIntosh K, et al: Pathogens associated with acute lower respiratory tract infection in young children. *Pediatr Infect Dis* 3:14, 1984.
[2]Bacterial pathogens were detected by fluorescent antibody testing or culture for *B. pertussis*, blood culture, tracheal aspirate culture obtained by direct laryngoscopy or counterimmunoelectrophoresis of urine or nasopharyngeal secretions.
[3]Type b (3).
[4]Not type b.

inflammation of the pharynx is usually viral, but may be from Group A β-hemolytic streptococcus, pneumococcus, or coagulase-positive staphylococcus. Not uncommonly, the initial infection may be rhinitis or otitis, with extension to other mucous membranes including the bronchi. Illness of viral origin may be complicated by bacterial superinfection. (For discussion of a particular pathogen, see Section 17 on Infectious Diseases.)

The manifestations of recurrent infections will depend on whether they occur in an otherwise healthy infant or child, or are in a compromised host (Table 5.2).

Diagnosis

INFECTIONS

The majority of children in whom the complaint is "keeping a cold" or "always sick" are between ages 3 and 8 years. Presumably, contact with other children increases around age 3 years, and the normal child may be in an adverse environment. By age 8 years, tonsillar and adenoidal tissues are becoming less prominent, some immunity has been acquired and lower respiratory tract infection is less common (see also Section 17).

Some observations that are pertinent are the general health of the individual. Malnutrition, for example, impairs defense against infection. If pneumonia has recurred, a chest radiograph should be obtained during an asymptomatic period to rule out an underlying lesion such as sequestration.

Environmental factors may be significant. Children in households with adults who smoke have an increased risk of chest infection (Ware et al, 1984). In a longitudinal study of more than 10,000 Caucasian children in six different cities, maternal cigarette smoking was associated with increases of 20–35% in the rates of eight respiratory illnesses and symptoms investigated. The effect of paternal smoking was smaller. The strongest risk factor for respiratory illness in this study was parental respiratory illness, such as chronic bronchitis, asthma, and emphysema. After adjusting for the parental illness, the prevalence of respiratory disease in children of smokers remained increased.

When pulmonary infections are recurrent, a number of underlying conditions may be present. When to "rule them out" will depend on the severity of the illness and the general health and growth of the infant or child.

CASE ILLUSTRATION

A 6-year-old has a chronic cough, but no sputum, fever, or other signs of systemic illness. The cough is worse at night and after exercise. Treatment with antibiotics has been of no benefit.

Further questioning revealed that the mother smoked a pack of cigarettes a day and also had a chronic "smoker's cough." The father had had asthma as a child. The patient had had milk eczema on face and around skin creases as an infant.

COMMENT

At this point, the possibility of reactive airway disease, if not overt asthma comes into focus. The pulmonary function laboratory can be helpful in most children over 5–6 years of age who are cooperative. A 1-second forced expiratory volume may be prolonged, and a flow-volume curve may demonstrate a pattern consistent with airways obstruction. A provocative test with cold air, exercise, histamine, or methacholine may be appropriate if the other tests are normal. Demonstration of airway reactivity is an indication for oral theophylline at a dose that should be adjusted initially by monitoring serum levels. Usually children who have reactive airways will improve on this regimen in a few weeks. Inhaled bronchodilators may be useful in acute episodes or, in some instances, on a regular basis.

Advice to the mother on the adverse effects of smoking both to herself and her child is very much worthwhile, even if not always effective. Simple allergy precautions such as diminishing exposure to dust may be effective.

Table 5.2
Recurrent Pneumonia

Predisposing Factors	Pertinent History	Tests
Premature birth with mechanical ventilation	Neonatal events	Chest radiograph TORCH titers
Aspiration		
Swallowing incoordination	Cough with feeding, regurgitation	Barium (Ba) swallow for evidence of spillover into trachea
Gastroesophageal reflux	Cough or wheeze with feedings, or at night	Ba swallow, milk scan, pH probe, esophageal biopsy
Tracheoesophageal fistula	Symptoms with feeding	Ba studies of upper esophagus
Laryngotracheal cleft		Laryngoscopy
Foreign body	Toddlers, history of sudden onset	Inspiration-expiration Radiographs or chest fluoroscopy Bronchoscopy
Vomiting for any cause	Other illness	Fat-laden macrophages in lung lavage
Visceral larval migrans		Eosinophilia
Ascaris		Stool examination
Hereditary metabolic diseases	Affected sibling(s)	Screening for blood or urine metabolites
Cystic fibrosis	Affected sibling(s)	Sweat test
α_1 Antitrypsin deficiency	Family history Asthma or emphysema Onset usually in teens, may be earlier	P_i typing
Persistent lung infiltrates		
Cytomegalovirus	Maternal infection	Urine culture and cytology
Rubella	Maternal infection	Serology
Syphilis	Maternal infection	Serology
Pneumocystis carinii	Prematurity Immunocompromised	Lung aspirate or biopsy
Recurrent aspiration	See above	
Congenital lesions	See above	
Other		
Pulmonary embolism	Intravenous catheters Shunts Chest pain Hemoptyses	Serial ECG and chest radiographs Radionuclide scans
Infarction	Sickle cell disease	Hemoglobin electrophoresis
Compression of airways	Recurrent localized infection	Chest radiograph with obliques with barium
Vascular ring Anomalous bronchi Sequestered lung Congenital cysts Neoplasms		Ultrasound Possible angiography
Impairment host defenses		
Hyper IgE syndrome	Eczema, recurrent Staphylococcal abscesses	Defective neutrophil Chemotaxis IgE levels
DiGeorge syndrome	Recurrent fungal infections Thymic dysplasia Neonatal tetany	Chest radiograph Associated cardiac anomalies T-cell deficiency Serum Ca and P
Chronic granulomatous disease	Pneumonias Skin infections with catalase-producing organisms (*Staphylococci*, some Gram-negative organisms)	Chest radiograph Phagocytic function impaired

Table 5.2–*continued*

Predisposing Factors	Pertinent History	Tests
Cyclic neutropenia	Bacterial pneumonia	Neutrophil count low
Complement deficiency	Bacterial pneumonia Chronic otitis, sinusitis Recurrent *Neisseria* infections	C3, C6–C9
Graft-versus host disease	Transfusion in immunodeficient subject Bone marrow transplant	T-cell deficiency Opportunistic organism
Hypogammaglobulinemia	Bacterial pneumonias	Quantitative globulins
Selective IgA deficiency	Maternal rubella Family history Sinopulmonary infections Malabsorption, diarrhea	Serum IgA levels
Bronchiectasis	Recurrent bacterial pneumonia, often localized	Chest radiograph CT scan
Immotile cilia syndrome	Recurrent widespread pneumonias, sinusitis	Tracheal mucosal biopsy Sperm motility Radiographs for situs inversus
Severe combined immunodeficiencies	Early onset Severe pneumonias Opportunistic organisms Fungi	r-globulin Monilia skin test (T-cells deficient)
Wiscott-Aldrich syndrome	Family history (X-linked recessive) Eczema Purpura	IgE elevated Poor antibody production Thrombocytopenia Combined B- and T-cell deficiency
AIDS	Exposure to infected parent	AIDS antibodies
Congestive heart failure	Pulmonary edema	Full cardiac evaluation Cerebral aneurysms
Hypersensitivity states		
Asthma	Family history	RAST
Pulmonary hemosiderosis		Iron-laden macrophages
Milk allergy		Milk precipitins

CASE ILLUSTRATION

A 6-month-old infant boy had had a hoarse cry from birth and chronic cough especially with feedings. Occasionally, he regurgitated uncurdled formula and failed to take in an adequate amount. His weight was 4.8 kg at 6 months. Chest radiograph showed some localized hyperaeration, some atelectasis, and prominent perihilar markings, most suggestive of chronic aspiration.

COMMENT

The most direct approach to elucidate the possible cause of aspiration is to observe a barium swallow for coordination of swallowing, possible tracheal overflow, a midline laryngoesophageal cleft or tracheoesophageal fistula, gastroesophageal reflux, and gastric emptying time. A careful radiographic examination may reveal the answer. If a laryngeal fistula or cleft is suspected, direct laryngoscopy is helpful. In a severely malnourished infant, surgical repair may be deferred to allow restoration of good nutrition and growth via gastrostomy.

In the infant presented, laryngoscopy revealed a paralyzed vocal cord, but no evidence of a laryngeal-esophageal cleft. Pulmonary damage was extensive, with pulmonary artery pressures nearly equal to systemic pressures and arterial oxygen tensions between 50 and 60 on room air.

A gastrostomy was placed, but gastroesophageal reflux persisted despite medical management and gastric plication was carried out. Aspiration became less in time, and the pulmonary hypertension decreased over the subsequent year.

CASE ILLUSTRATION

A 12-year-old male was referred with the complaint of chronic sinusitis, productive purulent sputum, and clubbing. Examination revealed a youngster of normal height, who was underweight, and appeared chronically ill, although he was attending school regularly. He became short of breath with exercise and preferred watching television and reading to more active pursuits.

Chest examination revealed some increase in anteroposterior diameter, coarse rales throughout, and diminished air entry on the right. Chest radiograph showed hyperaeration with atelectasis of the right middle lobe (Fig. 5.2*A, B, and C*).

COMMENT

Possible diagnoses for this chronic illness are cystic fibrosis, chronic aspiration, immune defect, reaction to a foreign body, or immotile cilia syndrome. Differentiation is straightforward. The sweat test was negative, and mucosal biopsy from the trachea revealed abnormal cilia compatible with immotile cilia syndrome. In a large series of patients with immotile cilia syndrome, only half had situs inversus (Rossman et al, 1980).

Immune Deficiencies

In other instances of recurrent pneumonia, consideration of abnormal host defenses is appropriate. A history of recurrent pyogenic infections suggests an immunoglobulin deficiency, or rarely, a defect in complement. Quantitative measurement of immunoglobulins is essential (see Section 16). Infants with chronic pneumonias associated with combined immune deficiency should be on continuous chemoprophylaxis to prevent *P. carinii* pneumonia. Live virus vaccines are contraindicated in these infants. Similar considerations apply to infants with AIDS (acquired immune deficiency syndrome).

Anomalies

Recurrent infections can occur in anomalous lobes or other malformations. Pulmonary sequestration, cystic adenomatoid malformation, or other cysts are examples (see pp. 274).

Tracheal bronchus is a supernumerary or aberrant bronchus that arises from the right lateral wall of the trachea. It can be responsible for recurrent pneumonia in the right upper lobe. Tracheal bronchus was diagnosed at bronchoscopy in 18 patients from birth to 54 months over a 16-year period at The Children's Hospital, Boston (McLaughlin et al, 1985).

Tracheal bronchus occurs in association with malformations such as VATER syndrome, pectus excavation, abnormal ribs, omphalocoele, and others. The lesion must arise before 16 weeks of gestation when the tracheal-bronchial tree has all of its branches.

The diagnosis depends on findings at bronchoscopy, but the likelihood is greatest if right upper lobe pneumonia or atelectasis is present together with minor skeletal abnormalities or tracheoesophageal fistula.

Role of Bronchoscopy

A child with recurrent pneumonias in one area of the lung deserves either further imaging studies, such as a CT scan, or bronchoscopy to rule out a partial obstruction of a bronchus by foreign body or lesion.

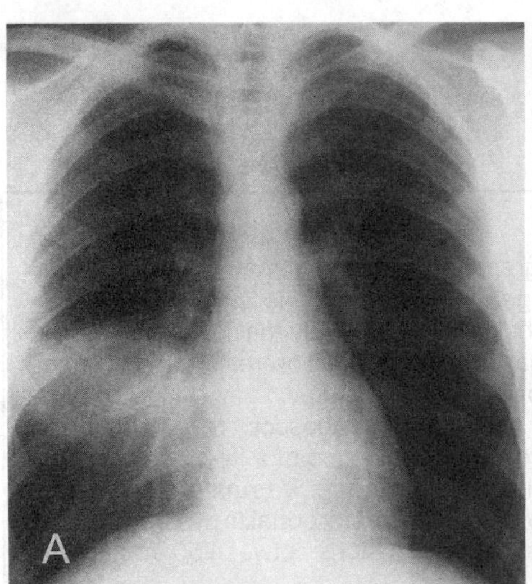

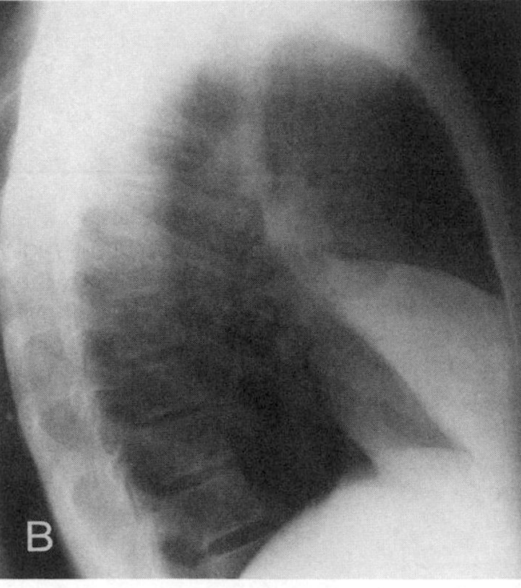

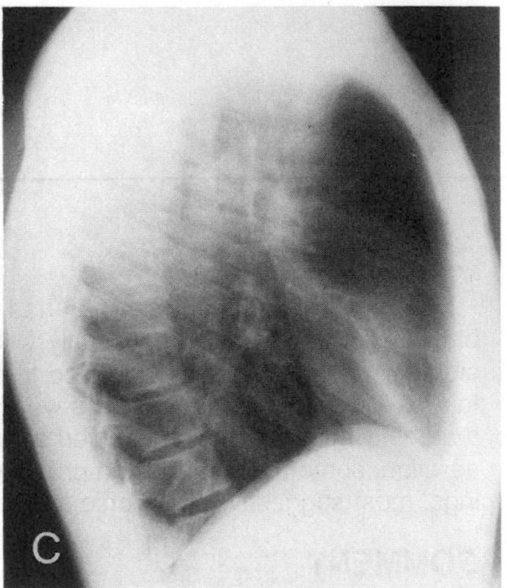

Figure 5.2.A, B, and **C.** An adolescent presented with high spiking fevers, right-sided pleuritic pain, and rales over the right anterior chest. His films show a typical right middle lobe pneumonia. **A** and **B.** Two months after the pneumonia, when he was clinically asymptomatic, there is still residual atelectasis. **C.** It is not unusual to see changes in the lung persisting some weeks after the acute infection. It is important to make sure that there is no underlying bronchial lesion, i.e., adenopathy, endobronchial foreign body, or mass.

Sometimes congenital deformities will be revealed that were not suspected on chest films. In a review of bronchoscopies at The Children's Hospital, Boston, over the years 1974–1980, 412 were performed in children under 5 years of age. Stridor was the indication in 47%, recurrent pneumonia in 25%, suspected foreign body in 20%, and miscellaneous reasons in 8%. Two percent of the children had a tracheal bronchus (McLaughlin et al, 1985).

Bronchoscopy with flexible fiberoptic instruments allows examination of upper airway function, collection of bronchial washings for culture, examination for fat-laden macrophages, and hemosiderin.

APPROACH TO CHILD WITH HEMOPTYSIS

Hemoptysis, the coughing of blood as a result of bleeding in the respiratory tract, is an unusual complaint in childhood.

Minor bleeding, or blood-streaked sputum is common, and not considered significant. In general, coughing up 5 ml of blood or a clot of blood would be considered abnormal in a child. Blood from the respiratory tract, including nose bleeds, may be vomited. Thus, a consideration of the likely site of bleeding is of first importance.

A systematic approach to differential diagnosis would be to "think anatomically" (see Table 5.3).

If bleeding is from the lung in older children and young adults, cystic fibrosis is an important cause. A number of other systemic disorders may present with hemoptysis and/or a glomerulopathy. Prominent among them is Goodpasture syndrome, notable for the triad of glomerulonephritis, pulmonary hemorrhage, and an antiglomerular-basement-membrane antibody.

Other systemic disorders that can be distinguished best by pulmonary or renal biopsy include periarteritis nodosa, hypersensitivity angiitis, and angiitis with granulomas as in Wegener granulomatosis, Churg-Strauss syndrome, and necrotizing sarcoid granulomatosis.

Collagen vascular disorders such as lupus and mixed cryoglobulinemia may involve lungs, kidneys, and other organs (see Section 22).

Table 5.3
Some Conditions that May Cause Hemoptysis

Larynx	Trauma from intubation
Trachea and bronchi	Bronchiogenic cyst Erosion by tuberculous node Erosion by tumor Telangiectasis
Small airways	Bronchiectasis Bronchopulmonary sequestration
Pulmonary parenchyma	Embolism, infarction Hypertrophied bronchial collateral circulation Fungal infection of cavities of any organ Hemosiderosis Granulomas Collagen vascular diseases
Clotting defects	Thrombocytopenia Diffuse intravascular coagulation Heparin therapy Fibrinolytic therapy
Cardiovascular	Mitral stenosis Congestive failure Pulmonary arteriovenous fistulas Aortic aneurysm

Localization of Bleeding

Sometimes the child can tell where the bleeding originates. Knowledge of underlying conditions such as heart disease or cystic fibrosis helps define the likely site of bleeding. A chest radiograph will define some of the obvious problems. A lung scan and angiography may clarify further the site of bleeding. Fiberoptic bronchoscopy is another approach to localization. When the reasons for bleeding are obscure and the bleeding is diffuse, examination of clotting factors is appropriate.

Treatment

Profuse pulmonary hemorrhage can be terrifying to the patient and physician alike. The principles of treatment are to prevent shock from exsanguination, prevent asphyxia from excess blood in the airways, attempt localization of hemorrhage and, if a site is determined, to try to occlude the bleeding vessel with catheterization and insertion of Gelfoam or selective intubation and inflation of balloon catheters, such as a Foley catheter, in the acute situation. Occasionally, surgical resection will be required.

Attention to clotting status, cardiac function, and possible infectious etiologies is required depending on the underlying condition.

To allay fear may be the most difficult challenge to physicians and nurses. Sedatives and narcotics are contraindicated. A prompt and systematic approach to diagnosis and therapy is the best reassurance.

PULMONARY HOST DEFENSE MECHANISMS

The lung, with an enormous surface area in contact with the environment, is protected from noxious agents by two principal types of defense: first, physical mechanisms, and second, cellular mechanisms.

The turbinates of the nose provide the first defense from inhalation of particles. Nearly all particles of more than 10 μ impact against the moist surfaces of the nose and nasopharynx. Smaller particles may impact at a lower level and may be moved up the mucociliary escalator. Particles of 2 μ and smaller can penetrate to peripheral airways: particles of 0.5 μ have sufficient aerodynamic stability to behave as a gas and may be exhaled.

Particles stimulate vagally mediated or trigeminal nerve-mediated reflexes that result in sneezing (from nasal stimulation) or coughing (from pharyngeal or tracheal stimulation). The rapid expulsions of expired air can accelerate the slower clearance by mucous flow.

The mucociliary escalator depends on adequate hydration and production of mucus by submucosal glands and goblet cells. Mucus is a complex mixture of lipids, carbohydrates, mucins, immunoglobulins, nucleic acids, electrolytes, and amino acids. Ciliary movement directs the flow up the tracheobronchial tree, and out of the nasal passages. Cilia beat at 1000–1500 cycles/minute and move almost all deposited material within 24 hours (clearance is faster for larger particles in trachea and large bronchi).

Among agents that slow mucociliary clearance are tobacco smoke, sulfur dioxide, and other air pollutants, alcohol, general anesthetics, and viral infections. Agents that can improve mucociliary clearance are adrenergic or cholinergic agents, and methylxanthines. Malformed cilia can be congenital (immotile cilia syndrome) or acquired and reversible as in some viral infections (Carson et al, 1985).

Cellular defense mechanisms are mediated, in part, by the alveolar macrophage. These remarkable cells can ingest foreign particles and microbes, and kill the microbes. During phagocytosis, oxygen radicals are formed that work with proteolytic enzyme to kill bacteria. They are largely responsible for clearance of *Staphylococcus aureus. Klebsiella pneumonia* and *Pseudomonas aeruginosa* require neutrophils for clearance, which are stimulated by chemotoxins secreted by the alveolar macrophage as well as other sources.

A complex series of interactions between alveolar macrophages and lymphocytes stimulates humoral and cell-mediated antibody production. The role of the macrophage appears to be to stimulate immune responses and regulate them as well (Harada and Repine, 1985). The secretory products of mononuclear phagocytes are shown in Table 5.4 (Fels and Cohn, 1986).

CASE ILLUSTRATION

A 17-year-old female presented with 1-day history of cough (with a few "clots of blood"). She had a similar episode 2 years previously diagnosed as "gastritis" with pregnancy (which the patient carried to completion). She had been on birth control pills since then and remained sexually active. She was found to be afebrile (although had been febrile by history) with a respiratory rate in the 30s at rest. She had a clear chest and diffuse abdominal tenderness. Pelvic examination confirmed cervical tenderness and discharge showing Gram-negative intracellular diplococci.

Despite the absence of respiratory difficulty or chest pain and normal blood gases on room air, the use of birth control pills and the diagnosis of pelvic inflammatory disease with possible pelvic thrombophlebitis raised the question of a pulmonary embolus. A lung scan was obtained and confirmed a perfusion defect in the left posterior lateral lung. Ultrasonography showed no evidence of clots in the inferior vena cava. The patient was treated with heparin and penicillin and recovered.

COMMENT

The only pulmonary symptom in this case of pulmonary embolism was hemoptysis. The coexistence of abdominal pain from pelvic inflammatory disease increased the possibility of embolism, as did the use of birth control pills.

Properties of Viruses that Promote Infection

Presumably, viruses enter the upper respiratory tract where they may or may not produce disease. They can enter the lower tract by aspiration or as inhaled droplet nuclei. The evidence for droplet nuclei as the source of infection is clearly established for tuberculosis and measles and inferred for other viruses (Riley and O'Grady, 1961). Once in the lower respiratory tract, viruses localize to certain regions and cell surfaces, presumably because of a match between virus and cell surface receptors, or cell proteases that can activate viruses. Local production of IgE and histamine through viral-host interaction, and immune complexes of virus and antibody stimulate the inflammatory responses.

The termination of viral infection depends primarily on cell-mediated immunity, since children with X-linked agammaglobulinemia do not have problems with viral infections, but those with severe combined immunodeficiency do.

Some viruses, particularly measles and types of influenza, suppress host defenses long after the acute infection has subsided. During either the acute symptomatic phase or in the more prolonged immunocompromised state, superinfection with other organisms can be serious.

Reinfection with the same viruses can occur if serotypes shift (as in influenza) or the immune response to the virus is poor (as in respiratory syncytial virus illness).

PNEUMONIA IN IMMUNOCOMPROMISED PATIENTS

Increasingly in referral centers that undertake bone marrow transplantation or have tumor therapy services, where many patients are immunocompromised by their therapy, diffuse interstitial pneumonia becomes a serious complication and, not infrequently, is the cause of death.

The etiologies of these pneumonias in a susceptible population are probably multiple. In some instances, dependence on high inspired oxygen concentrations sets

Table 5.4
Secretory Products of Mononuclear Phagocytes that Modulate the Inflammatory and Immune Response [1]

Complement components	Enzyme inhibitors	Chemotactic factors
C1	Plasmin inhibitors	For neutrophils
C4	α_2-Macroglobulin	For fibroblasts
C2		
C3	Binding proteins	Factors regulating synthesis of proteins by other
C5	Transferrin	Hepatocytes
Factor B	Transcobalamin II	Serum amyloid A
Factor D	Fibronectin	Haptoglobin
Properdin	Apolipoprotein E[2]	Synovial-lining cells
C3b inactivator		Collagenase
β1H	Oligopeptides	Prostaglandins
	Glutathione	Plasminogen activator
Coagulation factors		Adipocytes
X	Bioactive lipids	Lipoprotein lipase
IX	Arachidonate metabolites	
VII	Prostaglandin E_2	Growth-promoting factors
V	Prostaglandin $F_{2\alpha}$	Lymphocytes (T and B cells)
Thromboplastin	6-Ketoprostaglandin $F_{1\alpha}$ (from prostacyclin)	Myeloid precursors (colony-stimulating factors, factor inducing monocytopoiesis)
Prothrombin	Thromboxane A_2	Erythroid precursors
Prothrombinase	Leukotrienes B, C, D, E	Fibroblsts
	Monohydroxyeicosatraenoic acids (5-, 12-, 15-)	Capillaries (angiogenesis factor)
Other enzymes	Dihydroxyeicosatraenoic acids	
Lysozyme [2]	Platelet-activating factors	Factors inhibiting growth of
Neutral proteases		Lymphocytes
Plasminogen activator	Nucleosides and metabolites	Myeloid precursors
Collagenase	Thymidine	Tumor cells
Elastase	Uracil	Viruses (α- and β-interferons)
Angiotensin converting enzyme	Uric acid	
Acid hydrolases		Other hormone-like factors
Proteases	Reactive metabolites of O_2	Endogenous pyrogens (2 mol. wt. species)
Lipases	Superoxide anion	Insulin-like activity
Deoxyribonucleases	Hydrogen peroxide	Thymosin B_4
Phosphatases	Hydroxyl radical	
Glycosidases	Singlet oxygen (?)	
Sulfatases		
Arginase		
Lipoprotein lipase		

[1]The alveolar macrophage. From Fels AOS, Cohn ZA: *J Appl Physiol* 60: 353, 1986.
[2]Major bulk products.

the stage for pulmonary oxygen toxicity; in others, opportunistic infections with unusual organisms such as *Pneumocystis carinii, Candida,* or *Aspergillus* establish an interstitial pneumonic process which can be lethal.

The question then concerns how to establish a precise diagnosis in these patients or to establish an approach to therapy that covers the most likely etiologies. Although examination of sputum by culture and Gram stain appears to be an obvious starting point for diagnosis, these procedures have been shown to be of limited value in revealing the cause of pneumonia in immunocompromised patients. Generally, only 15–20% of the patients will show a predominant organism on Gram staining that clearly appears to be the offending agent.

Needle aspiration of the affected portions of lung has many advocates. The procedure is similar to that of a thoracentesis, in which an approximately 18-gauge needle is inserted quickly into pulmonary parenchyma while suction is maintained on a syringe which then allows prompt withdrawal of a small bit of tissue juice and a few drops of blood for Gram stain and culture.

Since the description by Klassen et al in 1949 of a procedure for open lung biopsy, this approach has been widely used and evaluated in several settings. McKenna et al (1984) described a 4-year experience at the M.D. Anderson Hospital in Houston. Their patients had an average age of 44 years (range, 7–72 years). All had been treated empirically with broad spectrum antibiotics, including agents that would be effective against *Legionella, Pneumocystis,* and fungi. When treatment failed, open lung biopsy was undertaken and found to be an accurate indicator of the underlying condition that was confirmed subsequently on follow-up or at autopsy. Very few false-positives or false-negatives were obtained. On the other hand, 66% of the patients were given the nonspecific diagnosis of granulomatus disease of unknown origin. An infectious etiology was identified in only 10% of that particular group of patients.

There is no reason to recommend the routine use of open lung biopsy in immunocompromised patients with acute interstitial pnemonitis who have failed to improve after treatment with broad spectrum antibiotics. We agree that the major indication for the procedure would be for patients who had had bone marrow transplantations or graft-versus-host reaction to their lungs. The reason to establish that diagnosis is that some of these patients will respond to steroids and it is important to know if infection is present, since steroids could aggravate existing infection. In general, it is clear that open lung biopsy has a role, but probably a modest likelihood of revealing important new findings that would be helpful to the patient.

APPROACH TO RECURRENT CHEST PAIN IN CHILDREN

Episodes of recurrent sharp pains or dull aches in the chest wall can be alarming, especially in young adults who may equate them with a heart attack. Although less common than headache or abdominal pain, it ranks high among complaints in adolescents (Coleman, 1984).

Basic Science

Sharp, superficial localized pain usually results from an irritation that sends a stimulus along an intercostal nerve. Deep, poorly localized visceral pain may arise from mediastinal structures and is most likely in the T1-T4 region of the thoracic spine. T5-T8 pain suggests diaphragmatic or upper abdominal peritoneal irritation. Pain of cardiac origin may be deep substernal, or referred to arm, shoulder, or neck.

Pain from pleural irritation or pneumothorax is exaggerated by deep inspiration and is phasic with respiration. It is usually well localized.

Natural History

Inflammation may cause localized pain as in the case of trauma to muscles and ligaments. Occasionally costochondritis can produce local tenderness. Shingles (herpes zoster infection), is a common cause of pain in adults but it is rare in children. Trauma from excessive coughing or overzealous physical therapy may also cause chest pain.

When breasts enlarge at puberty in both sexes (gynecomastia), they may have very tender nodules. In the male, they occur in 50% of individuals 11–18 years old, but then regress spontaneously if the testes and penis are of normal size at the time of gynecomastia.

Irritation of the parietal pleura from any cause can produce localized pain. Visceral pleura and pulmonary parenchyma have no sensory intervention.

Cardiovascular sources of pain are very few in children. Aberrant coronaries can produce angina and infarcts. Mitral valve prolapse has been associated with, but not proven to cause recurrent chest pain.

Myocarditis and pericarditis can be painful. Chronic recurrent pain from these conditions is seen in some viral conditions, such as coxsackie disease, or in systemic lupus erythematosus, and Kawasaki disease.

The most common abdominal source of chest pain is gastroesophageal reflux with esophagitis. The symptoms are the same as those in hiatal hernia, mainly postprandial discomfort.

Functional chest pain is most common in school-age children under stress. As with headache, its presence is probably real, but cannot be proven or disproven. Thus, it can become a reason for school absenteeism. The pain can be brought on by hyperventilation and relieved by calming the youngster.

For diagnosis and treatment, see the chapters on possible underlying conditions.

LUNG RESECTION

There are relatively few indications for lobectomy or pneumonectomy in childhood. Some of them require urgent intervention, such as an expanding emphysematous lobe in a newborn. Other times, lobectomy can be performed electively, as for benign cysts or pulmonary sequestration.

The question arises whether compensatory lung growth is more likely to occur in a younger individual at an age when new alveoli can be formed. Thurlbeck (1982) suggests that new alveoli continue to be formed until 2 years of age and Dunhill (1962) cited 8 years. Normal lung volumes were formed in children studied at ages 8–32 years after resection for congenital lobar emphysema in infancy (McBride et al, 1980). No effect of age on compensatory growth was found by Frenckner and Freyschuss (1982) in a group of children treated surgically at ages 12 hours to 11 years. Consequently, consideration of the nature of the lesion, its potential to be symptomatic, and the general condition of the child should take precedence over any evaluation of the stage of lung growth.

REFERENCES

Carson JL, Collier AM, Hu SS: Acquired ciliary defects in nasal epithelium of children with acute viral upper respiratory infections. *N Engl J Med* 312:463, 1985.

Coleman WL: Recurrent chest pain in children. *Pediatr Clin North Am* 31:1007, 1984.

Denny FW, Clyde WA: Acute lower respiratory tract infections in nonhospitalized children. *J Pediatr* 108:635, 1986.

Dunhill MS: Postnatal growth of the lung. *Thorax* 17:329, 1962.

Fels AOS, Cohn ZA: The alveolar macrophage. *J Appl Physiol* 60:353, 1986.

Frenckner B, Freyschuss U: Pulmonary function after lobectomy for congenital lobar emphysema and congenital cystic adenomatoid malformation. *Scand J Thorac Cardiovasc Surg* 16:293, 1982.

Glezen WP, Denny FW: Epidemiology of acute lower respiratory disease in children. *N Engl J Med* 288:498, 1973.

Harada RN, Repine JE: Pulmonary host defense mechanisms. *Chest* 87:247, 1985.

Hunninghake GW, Gallin JI, Fauci AS: Immunologic reactivity of the lung. *Am Rev Respir Dis* 117:15, 1978.

Kaufman R, Fields BN: Pathogenesis of viral infections. In Fields et al (eds): *Virology*. New York, Raven Press, 1985.

Klaussen KP, Anlyan AJ, Curtis GM: Biopsy of diffuse pulmonary lesions. *Arch Surg* 59:694, 1949.

Landing BH, Dixon LG: Congenital malformations and genetic disorders of the respiratory tract. *Am Rev Respir Dis* 120:151, 1979.

McBride JT, Wohl MEB, Strieder DJ, et al: Lung growth and airway function of the lobectomy in infancy for congenital lobar emphysema. *J Clin Invest* 66:962, 1980.

McKenna RJ, Mountain CF, McMurtrey MJ: Open lung biopsy in immunocompromised patients. *Chest* 86:671, 1984.

McLaughlin FJ, Strieder DJ, Harris GBC, et al: Tracheal bronchus: Association with respiratory morbidity in childhood. *J Pediatr* 106:751, 1985.

Paisley JW, Lauer BA, McIntosh K, et al: Pathogens associated with acute lower respiratory tract infection in young children. *Pediatr Infect Dis* 3:14, 1984.

Pennline KJ, Herscowitz HB: Dual role for alveolar macrophages in humoral and cell-mediated immune responses: Evidence for suppressor and enhancing functions. *J Reticuloendothel Soc* 30:205, 1981.

Riley RL, O'Grady F: *Airborne Infection Transmission and Control*. New York, MacMillan Co, 1961.

Rossman CM, Forrest JB, Rubbin RE: Immotile cilia syndrome in persons with and without Kartagener's syndrome. *Am Rev Respir Dis* 121:1011, 1980.

Rubin BK: The evaluation of the child with recurrent chest infections. *Pediatr Infect Dis* 4:88, 1985.

Thurlbeck WM: Pneumonectomy compensatory lung growth. *Am Rev Respir Dis* 128:965, 1983.

Wanner A: Clinical aspects of mucociliary transport. *Am Rev Respir Dis* 116:73, 1977.

Ware JH, Dockery DW, Spiro A, et al: Passive smoking, gas cooking and respiratory health of children living in six cities. *Am Rev Respir Dis* 129:366, 1984.

Diagnostic Methods 2

PULMONARY FUNCTION TESTS

The respiratory system depends on a CNS mechanism that involves conscious (cortical) control, and unconscious (automatic) functions in the brain stem. The central oscillators dictate respiratory frequency which is communicated to the lungs via the vagus nerves. Modulation of this system depends on the integrity of different signals from chemoreceptors (carotid and aortic bodies) that detect changes in blood gases, from stretch receptors in lungs and airways and irritant receptors in the lungs (mediated via the vagus) as well as chest wall reflexes. The firing of the inspiratory and expiratory neurons in the reticular substance of the medulla is enhanced by nonspecific afferent information from peripheral nerves stimulated by position and exercise, as well as by pain and changes in blood gases.

The output of the respiratory system depends on the integrity of the central neural mechanisms, the distensibility of the lung parenchyma and airways, and the ability to move air by contraction and relaxation of the muscles of respiration.

Abnormalities at any level of this complex system can result in impaired gas exchange and respiratory failure. Pulmonary function tests are designed to localize, measure and define an abnormality and its effect on the system as a whole. Each test has specific limitations and some may only quantify the overall deficit. In other circumstances, they define the functional problem and direct the physician to appropriate therapeutic interventions. They are most useful in evaluating responses to therapy.

In this section, we offer a critique of currently available tests to elucidate pulmonary dysfunction in infants and children.

Arterial Blood Gases (Pa_{O_2}, Pa_{CO_2})

Since the primary function of breathing is to maintain arterial blood gases within a narrow range, it is not surprising that the most useful measures of overall lung function are the P_{O_2} and P_{CO_2}, pH, and bicarbonate (HCO_3) values. The level of ventilation is defined in terms of Pa_{CO_2}. Elevation indicates hypoventilation;

depression indicates hyperventilation, regardless of cause. Adequate perfusion and a balance between ventilation and perfusion dictate the Pa_{O_2} value.

Methods

Arterial punctures can be performed on individuals of any age, irrespective of their state of health. Capillary samples provide values that are close enough to arterial values if the extremity is well perfused and warmed to arterialize the capillary blood. In newborn infants, a catheter inserted into the umbilical artery allows access for repeated determinations with minimal trauma. Prolonged use of this route is unwise because of risk of infection or clotting. The blood should be collected in a heparinized tube. If the catheter is to remain patent, constant perfusion with dilute heparin in physiologic saline is helpful (1 unit/ml at 3–5 ml/hour).

Noninvasive methods are available for continuous measurement of O_2 and CO_2 tensions by transcutaneous recordings. The oxygen measurements are more reliable since the electrodes are relatively stable and do not require calibration as frequently as do CO_2 electrodes. They are not adequate for single measurements, but do show trends. End-tidal CO_2 can be measured continuously, and corresponds to arterial values unless there is very uneven distribution of ventilation. The usual nomenclature is $T_cP_{O_2}$ but P_sO_2 (for skin) is preferable. Changes in oxygenation can be followed reliably by ear or finger oximetry which measures oxygen saturation.

Interpretation

Arterial oxygen tensions range 50–80 torr on the first days of life and should be over 80 torr by about a week of age. In general, oxygenation improves with age, with the normal range of 75–100 torr at sea level. Continuous monitors show that wide variations occur with crying, eating, and even change of position. The average values are about 15 torr higher in the prone compared with those in the supine position (Martin et al, 1979).

The Pa_{CO_2} values are 30–45 torr, and intervention is not usually required unless they rise above 50–60 torr. pH is usually 7.30–7.38 during the first days of life and 7.37–7.40 thereafter. Knowledge of HCO_3 concentrations is essential to distinguish respiratory from metabolic compensation in accord with the Henderson-Hasselbalch relationship.

$$pH = pK + \log [(HCO_3)/0.03\ P_{CO_2}]$$

It is useful to consider HCO_3 as being under renal regulation, and Pa_{CO_2} as controlled by the lung. Thus, pH ~ kidneys/lungs. The lung is a kind of tonometer that brings inspired air rapidly into equilibrium with blood. Renal compensation is slower, since it requires adjustments in HCO_3, but may take place within an hour or so. Thus, HCO_3 levels reflect the duration of a ventilatory abnormality.

Normal blood gases depend on the integrity of all parts of the respiratory system and, thus, are the best overall indicators of its functions.

Spirometry

Simple spirometry is the mainstay of evaluation of lung function. A number of inexpensive electronic devices are now available which can measure and record vital capacity (VC), 1-second forced expiratory volume (FEV_1), maximal midexpiratory flow rate (MMEF), and peak expiratory flow (PEF). VC, which is an index of lung size, is reduced if restrictive lung disease is present, airways are obstructed, or muscles are weak. Prolongation of expiration or reduced peak flow occurs with partial airway obstruction, as in asthma. Spirometry is a very simple and useful method for evaluating function in individuals who can cooperate (usually those over 6 years of age). Normal values with age, race, and sex are shown in Table 5.5 and Figure 5.3.

Lung Volumes

Functional residual capacity (FRC), the volume of air in the lungs at resting end-expiration, is a useful measure of lung size and airway integrity. In the older child, it is determined by the balance between elastic lung recoil (the tendency of the lung to become smaller), and the outward recoil of the chest wall. Residual volume is the air remaining after a forced expiration. FRC plus inspiratory capacity is total lung capacity. It is reduced in restrictive diseases, in the presence of space-occupying lesions, and with deformities of the chest wall.

Methods

FRC is measured either by gas dilution techniques, such as helium or nitrogen washout, or by body plethysmography.

Body plethysmographs are useful in cooperative children who can be coaxed to breathe through a mouthpiece with a pneumotachograph screen to permit measurement of airway resistance as well. Measurements of FRC in the first year of life were accomplished with a helium dilution method by Tepper et al (1986).

Airway obstruction is commonly assessed by *peak flow rate.* This simple test measures effort as well as airway patency, but is most useful in the emergency room to assess the response to bronchodilators in children with asthma.

The MMEF is less dependent on effort than peak flows. It is measured as the slope of the line between 25 and 75% of the vital capacity on the spirogram. *Flow-volume relationships* describe a loop the shape of which suggests the nature of the problem. Volume is reduced in restrictive disease; flow is reduced in obstructive disease. In a fixed obstructive lesion, located in the central airway (i.e., tracheal stenosis) inspiratory and expiratory flows may be about equal and constant, producing a flow-volume relationship resembling

Table 5.5
Summary of Normal Data [1]

Index	Group	Predictive Equation	% Mean Predicted Value That is equal to 1 Standard Deviation (SD)
Peak flow [2] (L/second)	Female		
	MA[3]	$9.23 \times 10^3 \times H^{2.12}$	15
	White	$4.63 \times 10^2 \times H^{2.00}$	14
	Black	$4.59 \times 10^3 \times H^{2.25}$	16
	Male		
	MA	$8.21 \times 10^3 \times H^{2.15}$	15
	White	$3.15 \times 10^3 \times H^{2.33}$	14
	Black	$2.26 \times 10^3 \times H^{2.39}$	19
Forced vital capacity [2] (L/second)	Female		
	MA	$1.25 \times 10^3 \times H^{2.92}$	14
	White	$2.57 \times 10^3 \times H^{2.78}$	14
	Black	$8.34 \times 10^4 \times H^{2.98}$	15
	Male		
	MA	$1.06 \times 10^3 \times H^{2.97}$	13
	White	$3.58 \times 10^4 \times H^{3.18}$	13
	Black	$1.07 \times 10^3 \times H^{2.98}$	17
Forced expiratory volume [2] (L)	Female		
	MA	$1.61 \times 10^3 \times H^{2.85}$	14
	White	$3.79 \times 10^3 \times H^{2.68}$	14
	Black	$1.14 \times 10^3 \times H^{2.89}$	15
	Male		
	MA	$1.73 \times 10^3 \times H^{2.85}$	13
	White	$7.74 \times 10^4 \times H^{3.00}$	13
	Black	$1.03 \times 10^3 \times H^{2.92}$	17
Forced expiratory flow $_{25-75\%}$ [2] (L/second)	Female		
	MA	$1.20 \times 10^3 \times H^{2.40}$	24
	White	$3.79 \times 10^3 \times H^{2.16}$	28
	Black	$1.45 \times 10^3 \times H^{2.34}$	30
	Male		
	MA	$9.13 \times 10^4 \times H^{2.45}$	25
	White	$7.98 \times 10^4 \times H^{2.46}$	26
	Black	$3.61 \times 10^4 \times H^{2.60}$	36
Flow-volume curve[4] $Vmax_{50\%}$ VC − (L/second)	Male	(0.113 × inches) − 3.653	13
	Female	(0.109 × inches) − 3.336	15
$Vmax_{25\%}$ VC − (L/second)	Male	(0.040 × inches) − 1.167	13
	Female	(0.057 × inches) − 1.960	16

[1] From Lemen RJ: In Kendig E, Chernick V (eds): *Disorders of the Respiratory Tract in Children*, 4th edition. Philadelphia, WB Saunders, 1983.
[2] Normal data with height in centimeters from Hsu et al: *J Pediatr* 95:192, 1979. Values for sitting height can be found in Hsi et al: *J Pediatr* 102:861, 1983.
[3] Mexican American.
[4] Normal data with height in inches from Taussig (unpublished data). Values for sitting height can be found in Hsi et al: *J Pediatr* 102:861, 1983.

a rectangle. A fixed obstruction in one bronchus will appear as a fast and slow component during expiration.

Comparison of the flow-volume relationship can be made with a patient breathing air and then a less dense gas, such as helium (He) and oxygen. The 80% He mixture reduces turbulence and, normally, the maximum expiratory flow increases by about 1.4–1.7 times. With disease of the small airways, flow is less affected by turbulence and there is little change with He-O_2 mixtures. For serial values, spirometry is acceptable; for more accurate determinations, volume should be measured with a body plethysmograph (Fig. 5.4).

Airways reactivity can be measured with particular challenges such as cold air, histamine, exercise, or reversal of airflow limitation with bronchodilators. In general, a change in airway resistance, measured by a change in the 1-second FEV of over 10% from baseline is evidence of increased bronchial lability. The risk of

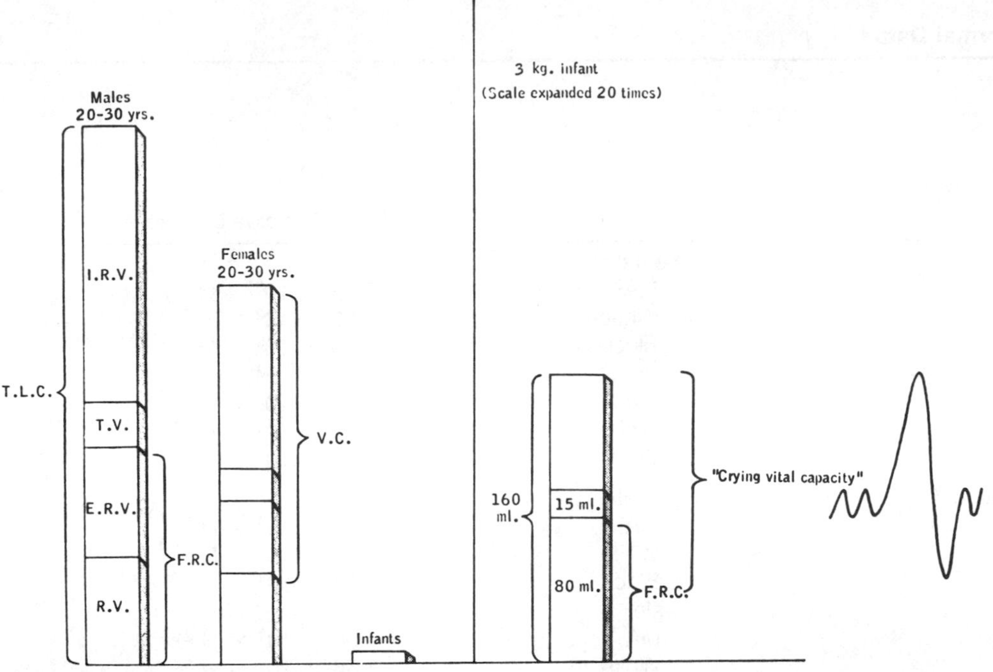

Figure 5.3. The lung volumes. A volume is a single subdivision; a capacity is more than one subdivision. Abbreviations: *T.L.C.*, total lung capacity (6 liters in an average male, 4.2 liters in an average female); *I.R.V.*, inspiratory reserve volume; *T.V.*, tidal volume; *E.R.V.*, expiratory reserve volume; *R.V.*, residual volume; *F.R.C.*, functional residual capacity; *V.C.*, vital capacity. The spirogram shown on the right is a tracing from a revolving drum attached to a water-filled spirometer. *T.V., I.R.V., E.R.V.*, and Chernick V (eds): can be measured from such a tracing. Reproduced with permission from Chernick V, Avery ME: In Kendig EVC (ed): *Disorders of Respiratory Tract in Children.* Philadelphia, WB Saunders, 1977.

producing severe bronchospasm in susceptible individuals requires caution with these tests.

Lung compliance or change in volume with changes in pressure is another measure of lung function. A balloon catheter in the esophagus allows measurement of transpulmonary pressures at different volumes from which compliance can be calculated. The compliance of lung and thorax together can be measured by pressure

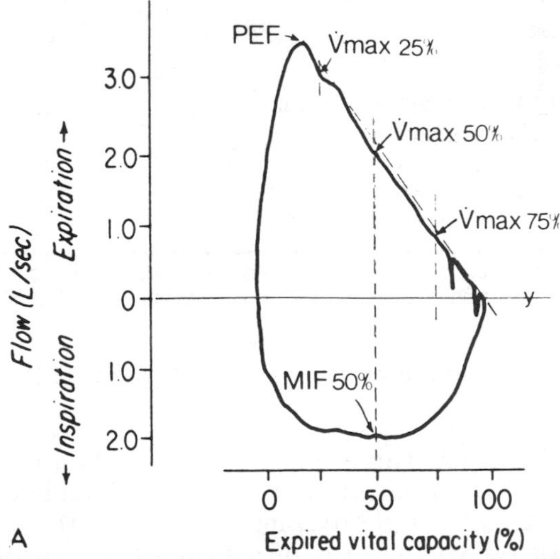

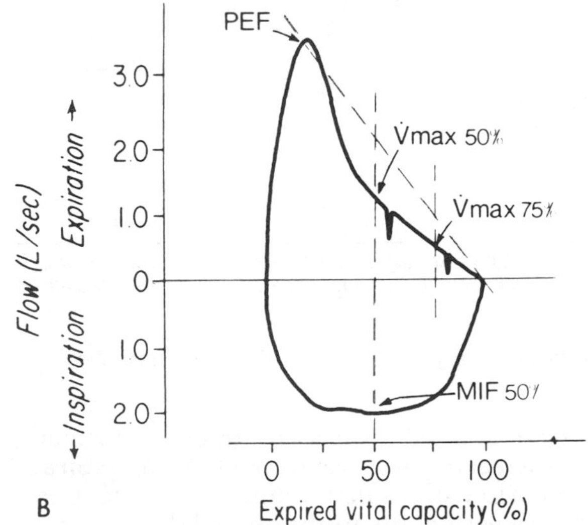

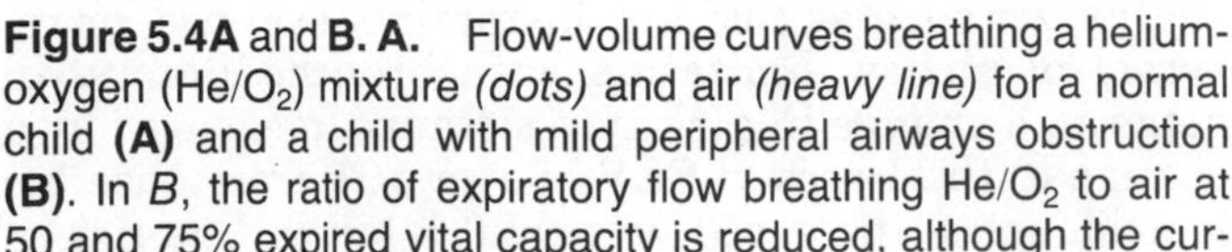

Figure 5.4A and **B. A.** Flow-volume curves breathing a helium-oxygen (He/O_2) mixture *(dots)* and air *(heavy line)* for a normal child **(A)** and a child with mild peripheral airways obstruction **(B)**. In *B*, the ratio of expiratory flow breathing He/O_2 to air at 50 and 75% expired vital capacity is reduced, although the curvilinearity score in air is near normal. Reproduced with permission, from Lemen RJ: In Kending EL, Chernick V (eds): *Disorders of The Respiratory Tract in Children*, 4th edition. Philadelphia, WB Saunders, 1983.

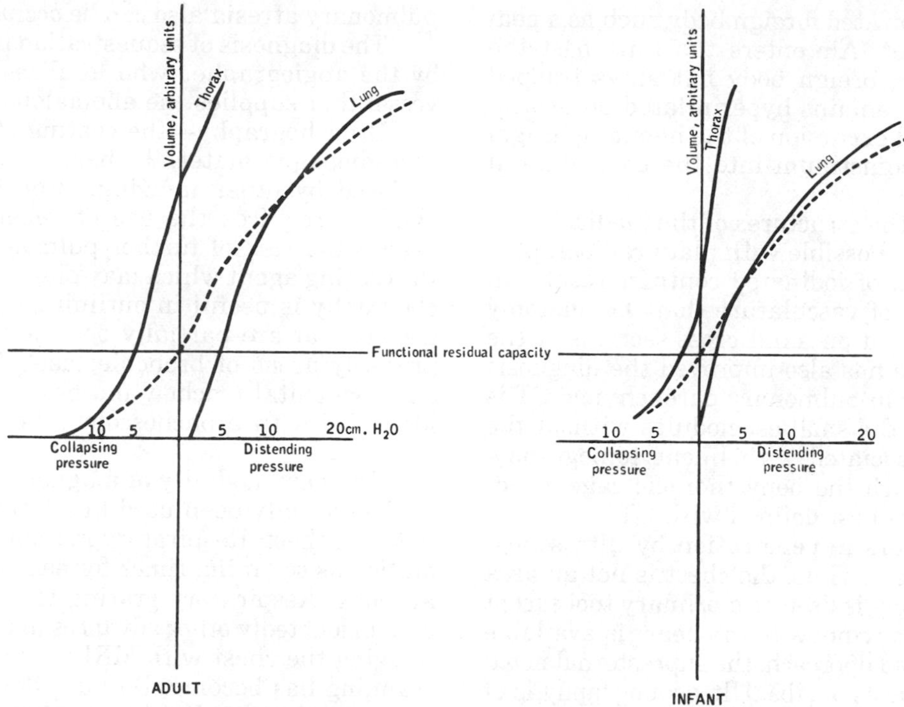

Figure 5.5. Pressure-volume relations of lungs and thorax in an adult on the left, in an infant on the right. The *dashed line* represents the characteristic of lungs and thorax together. Transpulmonary pressure at the resting portion (functional residual capacity) is less in the infant, and thoracic compliance is greater in the infant. Reproduced with permission from Chernick V, Avery ME: In Kendig E, Chernick V (eds): *Disorders of the Respiratory Tract in Children*. Philadelphia, WB Saunders, 1977.

changes at the mouthpiece or in the airway if the individual is on a ventilator. Since the compliance of the chest wall in infancy is nearly infinite, the total compliance depends mainly on the elasticity of the lung in the range of tidal volume (Fig. 5.5).

Respiratory muscle strength can be measured by recording maximal inspiratory and expiratory pressures at residual volume and total lung capacity, respectively, or with a simple aneroid manometer with a fast response time and minimal overshoot. These measurements are affected adversely by malnutrition, fatigue, and lack of cooperation. Their interpretation depends on knowledge of the general status of the individual; most cooperative individuals produce both inspiratory and expiratory pressures greater than 80 cm H_2O.

Regional distribution of ventilation and perfusion can be ascertained with radionuclide scans in individuals of any age. Inhalation of xenon, krypton, or nitrogen 15 will allow assessment of distribution of ventilation. Regional perfusion can be seen with labeled macroaggregated albumin or xenon injected into the circulation. The tests are best interpreted in a stable patient, since regional mismatching can occur in asthma or pneumonia. They have been of the greatest value in suspected pulmonary embolism.

PULMONARY IMAGING

No area of clinical practice is more dependent on radiology than is pulmonology. Some of the earliest medical investigations using the magical X-rays that had been discovered by Roentgen in 1895, were of the chest. Thomas Morgan Rotch, professor of pediatrics at Harvard and The Children's Hospital in the early part of this century, was able to compile, in 1910, the first textbook of pediatric radiology. He drew on a file of 2300 cases that had been collected in the previous year. Examples of pneumonia, miliary tuberculosis, hydropneumothorax, pericardial effusion, and aspirated foreign body (a china doll's arm) are among the illustrations.

Many years later, we still rely on the routine posteroanterior and lateral radiographs to give anatomic information regarding large airways, pulmonary parenchyma, mediastinum, heart, pulmonary vasculature, and pleural spaces. Other techniques that refine diagnosis have been added over the years. Fluoroscopy of the upper airway is useful when a suspected mass—inflammatory or neoplastic—impinges on the pharynx or trachea. Motion of vocal cords can be studied. Barium swallow can be added in the evaluation of swallowing disorders and suspected aspiration. The esophagus, outlined with barium, acts as a flexible probe through the mediastinum, a probe that is pushed or pulled by vascular structures—normal or anomalous—and mediastinal masses—inflammatory, developmental, or neoplastic.

Fluoroscopy of the mediastinum can differentiate a large thymus from a pathologic anterior mediastinal mass. Mediastinal swing associated with limited unilateral diaphragmatic motion—especially on expiration—is diagnostic of obstruction of a large bronchus, typically from an aspirated foreign body such as a peanut or piece of carrot. Air enters the lung past the partially obstructing foreign body but stays trapped behind it. That lobe remains hyperinflated on expiration, limiting upward excursion of the hemidiaphragm and pushing the mediastinum into the contralateral hemithorax.

CT has exposed the structures of the mediastinum in a way that was not possible with plain radiography. Intravenous injection of iodinated contrast results in enough opacification of vasculature that the anatomy is beautifully displayed on axial cross-sections of the chest. This technique has also improved the diagnosis of metastatic disease in pulmonary parenchyma. CT is now able to identify the smallest nodules without the streaky artifacts associated with linear tomography. Masses associated with the bony thoracic cage or adjacent soft tissues are best defined with CT.

The major barriers to penetration by ultrasonography are bone and air. Thus, the chest is not an area where ultrasonography is used as a primary tool except in cardiology where a window to the heart is available through the subxiphoid approach, the suprasternal notch and anterior interspaces of ribs. Ultrasonography is of use in establishing a peripheral pulmonary mass as cystic or solid, in characterizing and localizing pleural fluid for thoracentesis, and in evaluating the opaque hemithorax to determine whether the parenchyma, pleura, or both, are the source of the findings on plain radiographs. Because ultrasonography is generally used in the real-time mode, diaphragmatic motion can be monitored although it is easiest to do this in babies where both hemidiaphragms are visible simultaneously while liver provides an acoustic window.

Radionuclide imaging contributes substantially to the diagnosis of pulmonary embolization. The ventilation-perfusion mismatch—lack of perfusion shown by an absence of radionuclide in a segment of lung associated with normal ventilation of that segment—is the classic appearance of pulmonary embolus. Pulmonary scanning is also useful in providing physiologic information in children who have chronic lung disease. This is especially true in patients with cystic fibrosis whose radionuclide scans may indicate significant abnormality in areas that on plain radiographs appear unremarkable. Radionuclide angiography in the determination of both central and peripheral shunts has been developed in the past 15 years. Its use is best discussed in Section 6, Cardiology.

Angiography is no longer simply a diagnostic procedure. The angiographers have exchanged their diagnostic catheters for those that carry therapeutic drugs, balloons, and coils. The patient with chronic lung disease, typically cystic fibrosis, develops thin-walled bronchial collateral arteries in areas of intense chronic inflammation. These vessels may bleed, resulting in life-threatening hemoptysis. The angiographer can identify the site of bleeding by injection of contrast material through the bronchial circulation, then occlude the offending vessel with pieces of Gelfoam, balloon, or coil. Systemic collateral arteries associated with pulmonary atresia also can be occluded in this fashion.

The diagnosis of sequestration is usually confirmed by the angiographer who localizes the aortic feeding vessel that supplies the anomalous pulmonary tissue.

Bronchography—the coating of bronchial mucosa by radiopaque material—has, to a large degree, been replaced by other imaging. Bronchography in small children requires the use of general anesthesia and carries the risk of further pulmonary compromise by the coating agent which may plug small airways. Bronchography is useful in outlining small intrabronchial lesions that are partially obstructing and in defining precisely areas of bronchiectasis. Anomalous bronchi and congenital trachea and bronchial stenosis can be identified with bronchoscopy followed by bronchography.

The new modality of magnetic resonance imaging (MRI) has only been used in a limited fashion to evaluate the chest. Respiratory motion interferes with resolution as scanning times for each cross-sectional area are long. Respiratory grating is now being attempted and undoubtedly other advances in technology will make imaging the chest with MRI as straightforward as CT scanning has become. Because flowing blood does not return a signal, MRI has applications in cardiology. Radiographs of patients who have chronic pulmonary disease often show areas of opacity that may be either vascular or result from parenchymal consolidation. MRI can differentiate these. Further characterization of tissue is anticipated in the future (Smith, 1983).

ENDOSCOPY

Direct examination of larynx, trachea, and bronchi is sometimes the only way to ascertain the nature of a lesion. Hoarseness that persists is reason to inspect the vocal cords. Inspiratory stridor may require direct visualization, although radiographs of the upper airway should precede direct inspection. Clearly, any suggestion of obstruction of a bronchus by a foreign body requires a therapeutic bronchoscopy. Persistent atelectasis may be the consequence of a lesion in a bronchus which could be biopsied through a bronchoscope.

Flexible fiberoptic bronchoscopes have facilitated diagnosis by providing greater safety and less morbidity than rigid instruments. Older children and adults tolerate the procedure with orotracheal topical anesthetics such as xylocaine. Patients receive supplemental oxygen and cardiac monitoring. Young children usually require anesthesia (Wood and Postma, 1988).

Cultures obtained through the suction channel of the bronchoscope are usually contaminated with upper airway pathogens. A specimen brush contained within a double catheter can be used to sample cells and microorganisms in the airways. Cuffing of the scope makes it possible to wedge it in a lobar bronchus and lavage a portion of the lung. (The external diameter of available scopes range from 3–6 mm.)

ALVEOLAR WASH

Bronchoalveolar lavage is considered to be the most reliable method of evaluation of inflammatory and immune processes in the lung (Keough and Crystal, 1982).

The procedure can be carried out on an anesthetized child during bronchoscopy. Aliquots of 5–25 ml of sterile saline solution at 37° C are introduced through a wedged fiberoptic bronchoscope, and removed with immediate gentle suction. In adults a minimum of 100 ml total delivered in aliquots is recommended (Summary Report, 1985). The aspirated material is kept cold and filtered through sterile gauze. The cells can be separated by low-speed centrifugation and resuspended in Hank solution for total cell count and differential. Identification of lymphocytes by surface markers with use of monoclonal antibodies allows measurement of the proportion of helper and suppressor cells.

Insufficient experience with this diagnostic approach in children precludes generalizations about its role in diagnosis. The significance of lipid-containing alveolar macrophages, once thought to indicate aspiration, remains uncertain in light of finding them in a variety of parenchymal diseases (Corwin and Irwin, 1985). The possibility of lavage to remove inspissated sputum in cystic fibrosis deserves evaluation in selected patients, but is rarely undertaken.

NEEDLE ASPIRATION

Although noninvasive imaging has advanced our ability to localize infection, and endoscopy, lung wash, and culture are sometimes sufficient to establish etiologic diagnosis, lung aspirate or biopsy is sometimes required to establish the cause of disease.

Lung aspiration, like a thoracentesis, requires sterile preparation, and is most useful in a cooperative patient who can hold his breath throughout the procedure. For this, a syringe containing a few milliliters of saline (without antibacterial additives) attached to a no. 18 or no. 20 gauge needle is inserted quickly along the top of a rib (to avoid blood vessels) about a centimeter through the chest wall into the lung. Gentle suction is applied and the needle is withdrawn. The saline is flushed through the needle, and needle itself is inserted into the culture medium. Sometimes enough serosanguinous material is available for Gram stain as well as culture. If the needle has penetrated an area of disease, offending bacteria or viruses usually can be cultured.

OPEN LUNG BIOPSY

When other diagnostic methods have been unrevealing, and the disease is progressive, open biopsy of the involved area may be required.

In a review of 36 consecutive patients who underwent lung biopsy at Columbus Children's Hospital, about one-third had an infectious agent identified (Early et al, 1985). *Pneumocystis carinii* was most common in this group of patients, 22 of whom had preoperative diagnoses of compromise of the immune system. The noninfectious diagnoses were eosinophilic pneumonia, radiation pneumonitis, interstitial fibrosis, and desquamative interstitial pneumonia. The diagnosis led to a change in therapy in 15 patients (43%). Nevertheless, five of these very sick children died after their biopsies, although not as a direct result of the procedure. Delayed healing, late bleeding from the wound, and pneumothorax were ascribed to the procedure.

Our results are similar, and lead us to view open lung biopsy as a procedure to be used only when the course of disease is progressive and the patient has not responded to therapy.

REFERENCES

Avery ME, Fletcher BD, Williams RG: *The Lung and its Disorders in the Newborn Infant.* 4th ed. Philadelphia, WB Saunders, 1981.

Coleman DL, Dodek PM, Luce JM, et al: Diagnostic utility of fiberoptic bronchoscopy in patients with *Pneumocystis carinii* pneumonia and the acquired immune deficiency syndrome. *Am Rev Respir Dis* 128:795, 1983.

Corwin RW, Irwin RS: The lipid-laden alveolar macrophage as a marker of aspiration in parenchymal lung disease. *Am Rev Respir Dis* 132:576, 1985.

Crystal RG, Reynolds HY, Kalica AR: Bronchoalveolar lavage. The report of an international conference. *Chest* 90:122, 1986.

Doershuk CF, Downs TD, Matthews LW, et al: A method for ventilatory measurements in subjects 1 month to 5 years of age: Normal results and observations in disease. *Pediatr Res* 4:165, 1970.

Doershuk CF, Fisher BJ, Matthews LW: Specific airway resistance from the perinatal period into adulthood. *Am Rev Respir Dis* 109:452, 1974.

Early GI, Williams TE, Kilman JW: Open lung biopsy: Its effect on therapy in the pediatric patient. *Chest* 87:467, 1985.

Fox WW, Bureau M, Taussig LM, et al: Helium flow-volume curves with detection of early small airway disease. *Pediatrics* 54:293, 1974.

Fulkerson WJ: Fiberoptic bronchoscopy. *N Engl J Med* 311:511, 1985.

Haller JO, Schneider M, Kassner EG, et al: Sonographic evaluation of the chest in infants and children. *AJR* 134:1019, 1980.

Keough BA, Crystal RG: Alveolitis: The key to the interstitial lung disorders. *Thorax* 37:1, 1982.

Kilman JW, Clatworthy HW, Hering J, et al: Open pulmonary biopsy compared with needle biopsy in infants and children. *J Pediatr Surg* 9:347, 1974.

Kirks DR, Korobkin M: Computed tomography of the chest in infants and children: Techniques and mediastinal evaluation. *Radiol Clin North Am* 19:409, 1981.

Klein JO: Diagnostic lung puncture in the pneumonias of infants and children. *Pediatrics* 44:456, 1969.

Mansell AL, Bryan AC, Levison H: Relationship of lung recoil to lung volume and maximum expiratory flow in normal children. *J Appl Physiol* 42:817, 1977.

Martin RJ, Okken A, Rubin D: Arterial oxygen tension during active and quiet sleep in the normal neonate. *J Pediatr* 94:271, 1979.

McBride JJ, Wohl MEB: Pulmonary function tests. *Pediatr Clin North Am* 26:537, 1979.

Polgar G, Promodhat V: *Pulmonary Function Testing in Children: Techniques and Standards.* Philadelphia, WB Saunders, 1971.

Polgar G, Weng TR: The functional development of the respiratory system. *AM Rev Respir Dis* 129:625, 1979.

Rotch TM: *The Roentgen Ray in Pediatrics.* Philadelphia and London, JB Lippincott, 1910.

Smith FW: The value of NMR imaging in pediatric practice: A preliminary report. *Pediatr Radiol* 13:141, 1983.

Summary and Recommendations of a Workshop on the investigative use of fiberoptic bronchoscopy and bronchoalveolar lavage in asthmatics. *Am Rev Respir Dis* 132:180, 1985.

Taussig LM, Chernick V, Wood R, et al: Standardization of lung function testing in children. *J Pediatr* 97:668, 1980.

Taussig LM, Cota K, Kattenborn W: Different mechanical properties of the lung in boys and girls. *Am Rev Respir Dis* 123:640, 1981.
Tepper RS, Morgan WJ, Cota K, et al: Physiologic growth and development of the lung during the first year of life. *Am Rev Respir Dis* 134:513, 1986.
Wagener JS, Hibbert WE, Landau LI: Maximal respiratory pressures in children. *Am Rev Respir Dis* 129:873, 1984.
Wallaert B, Colombel JD, Tonnel AB, et al: Evidence of lymphocyte alveolitis in Crohn's disease. *Chest* 87:363, 1985.
Weiss ST, Tager IB, Weiss JW, et al: Airway responsiveness in a population sample of adults and children. *Am Rev Respir Dis* 129:898, 1984.
Wimberley NW, Bass JB, Boyd BW, et al: Use of a bronchoscopic protected catheter brush for the diagnosis of pulmonary infections. *Chest* 81:556, 1982.
Wood RE, Postma D: Endoscopy of the airway in infants and children. *J Pediatr* 112:1, 1988.
Yahav J, Mindorff C, Levison H: The validity of transcutaneous oxygen tension method in children with cardiorespiratory problems. *Am Rev Respir Dis* 124:586, 1981.

Obstructive Disease 3

Upper airway obstruction can occur in the presence of anomalies of the oropharynx (e.g., Pierre Robin syndrome), with masses in the nasal or oropharynx (e.g., adenoids and tonsils), or obstructions from atresias, tumors, or chronic inflammation at any level of the extrathoracic airway.

The pathophysiology is a narrowing of the airway during inspiration with heightened inspiratory effort, stridor, and prolongation of inspiratory time.

Lower airway obstructive disease is found in asthma, cystic fibrosis, α-1 antitrypsin deficiency and bronchopulmonary dysplasia, as well as in other forms of chronic infection as seen with ciliary dyskinesis or chronic sinusitis and bronchitis.

The pathophysiology involves narrowing of the intrathoracic airways during forced expiration with prolongation of expiration and wheeze. An increase in functional residual capacity (FRC) occurs to compensate for airway narrowing.

Methods of Evaluation of Chronic Obstructive Disease

Measurement of blood gases with samples taken with the subject at rest are essential. Continuous transcutaneous recordings are of help in assessing changes during sleep. Oximetry may be used on outpatient visits to monitor serial changes in a given child (Monaco et al, 1983; Yahave et al, 1981).

Meaurements of FRC, airway resistance, and flow rates will reflect mechanical derangements, and are valuable for following the course of disease and measuring the effects of therapy.

Changes During Sleep

Children with chronic obstructive disease of either upper or lower airways are more likely to have impaired gas exchange when asleep. Gaultier et al (1985) reported blood gas values on a group of 17 children ages 3–20 years, with obstructive disease. When awake, mean Pa_{O_2} values were 72 torr and Pa_{CO_2} values were 38 torr. During sleep, Pa_{O_2} values were about 14 torr lower (range 8–29), and Pa_{CO_2} values were 9 torr higher (range 6–13). Some periodic breathing was observed, as were paradoxical inward rib cage motions. Severe hypoventilation in sleep occurs with central respiratory failure (Ondine curse; see pp. 290).

Individuals with chronic hypoxemia during sleep are at increased risk of altered vascular development. For example, Ryland and Reid (1975) found a decrease in the number of arteries per unit area of lung section in children with cystic fibrosis and correlated these changes with right ventricular hypertrophy. They suggest that vascular hypoplasia and remodeling of the pulmonary circulation contribute to cor pulmonale.

BRONCHIOLITIS

Definition

Bronchiolitis, an inflammation of the bronchioles and neighboring air passages is an acute (often severe) respiratory illness in children who are mostly under 2 years of age.

Epidemiology

Epidemics occur between October and April with alternating 7- to 12-month or 13- to 16-month intervals between epidemic peaks (Glezen and Denny, 1973). In general, the most susceptible group are infants between 1 month and 1 year of age. Infection can occur at any age but bronchiolitis is unusual before 1 month and unusual after 2 years.

The attack rate is very high in a day care setting; a value of 98% of previously uninfected infants has been reported (Henderson et al, 1979). We have noted that, for an infant hospitalized on an open ward with other infants, the attack rate is high and the risk of cross-infection very great. Although about half the hospital personnel working with infants acquire infection during an epidemic, their symptoms are not those of bronchiolitis. Adults have nasal congestion, cough, and sometimes severe bronchitis (Hall et al, 1975).

Basic Science

See Section on Epidemiology of Acute Lower Respiratory Disease.

Natural History

The disease is usually caused by the respiratory syncytial virus, although a similar response can be found with parainfluenza and some adenoviruses. The latter viruses are more commonly associated with upper respiratory tract disease. The virus continues to be shed from the respiratory tract for an average of 9 days even with clinical improvement. Infants with immunodeficiency syndromes may shed virus for months after infection (Fishaut et al, 1980).

An unusual response of the immune system may indeed be responsible for most of the manifestations of respiratory syncytial virus infections in infants. This was brought into focus by the work of Chanock et al, 1970, who gave infants a killed respiratory syncytial virus vaccine and found that when they were exposed subsequently to the infection their disease was more severe than it had been in control infants. More recent studies with purified RSV glycoprotein are promising but not tested in infants as of 1987. Thus, it is possible that the presence of antibody contributes to the production of disease.

Diagnosis

The diagnosis is straightforward if it is known that there is an epidemic of respiratory syncytial virus in the community and a previously well infant acquires asthma-like symptoms; low grade fever may be present and the chest radiographs are nonspecific (Fig. 5.6*A* and *B*). Peribronchial thickening and patchy atelectasis may be evident in some but, in others, only hyperinflation is seen. The infant is likely to be symptomatic for 4 or 5 days and symptoms may not clear completely for 10 days to 2 weeks. The white blood count averages 5000–24,000 cells/mm^3 with a preponderance of polys.

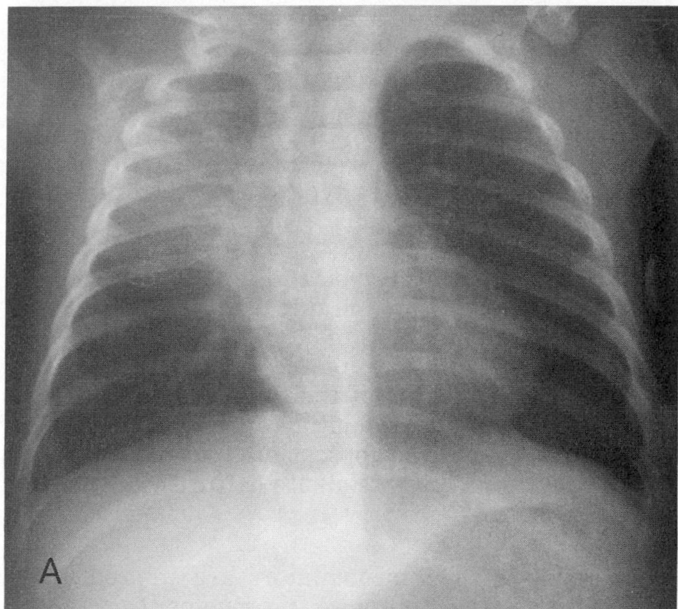

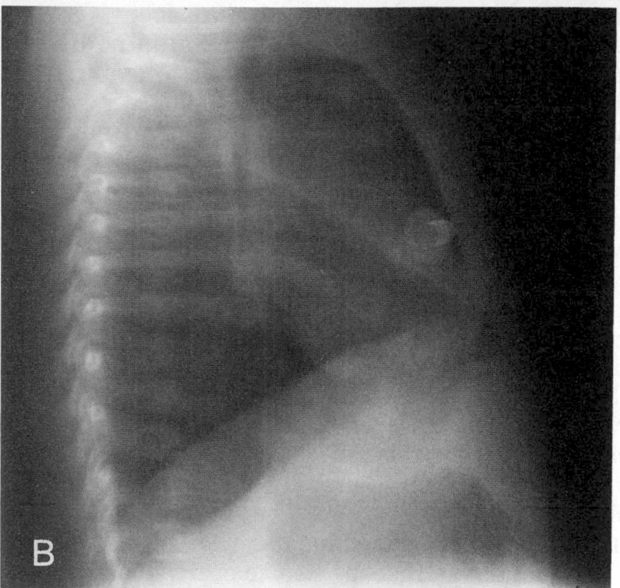

Figure 5.6.A and **B**. Radiographs of the chest (**A** and **B**) in this 2-month-old baby with broncholitis from respiratory syncytial virus show volume loss of the right upper lobe and hyperinflation of other lobes. These children have alternating areas of hyperinflation and atelectasis but quite often, the atelectasis involves right upper lobe.

Laboratory diagnosis depends on isolation of the virus or the use of immunofluorescent techniques applied to nasal aspirates. The latter is useful since it can be accomplished within 24 hours. Respiratory syncytial virus-specific IgE in nasopharyngeal secretions after infection points to the possibility that immune responses may be triggered by this particular virus (Welliver et al, 1980).

Treatment

Infants with severe bronchiolitis are indeed very sick and often profoundly hypoxemic. Therefore, a mainstay of treatment is to increase the inspired oxygen mixture. Occasionally, an infant who has previously been restless, with tachypnea and tachycardia will have his first good rest once inside an oxygen tent. It is important not to have a high density of mist in the tent since mist can exacerbate bronchospasm in these infants: rather, the oxygen should be humidified but water droplets should be evaporated before the infant breathes them.

If the infant has been sick for a few days, he may show some dehydration and intravenous fluids should be administered slowly to make up for deficits.

It is unlikely that antibiotics will be beneficial for these infants. However, if the diagnosis is uncertain and there is lobar consolidation with a very elevated white count, it would be appropriate then to administer antibiotics after taking requisite cultures.

CONTROVERSY

Responses to bronchodilators are unpredictable. Some infants have a prompt improvement on inhalation with Bronkosol or some similar agent. Others apparently resist such treatment and gain no benefit. A number of prospective control trials to evaluate corticosteroids in the treatment of bronchiolitis have been inconclusive. Whereas some infants show slight benefit, it has not been demonstrated in the major systematic studies.

Ribavirin aerosol treatment has been evaluated by several groups with mixed results. It acts by limiting viral replication with cells. In a small series, Taber et al (1983) found neither benefit nor toxicity. In a larger trial, Hall et al (1983) reported modest success when the drug was given in a tent 12–18 hours a day. Since ribavirin is effective in vitro, other means for delivering the drug deserve exploration. Its ultimate role may be to prevent shedding of virus in infants who are in hospital or even to provide some prophylaxis to infants at risk. Further work is needed in this area. It is currently recommended for use in high-risk patients.

Chest physiotherapy has no positive benefit on the course of the disease (Webb et al, 1985).

Prognosis

Most infants appear to recover fully from an attack of bronchiolitis. Some long-term studies of hospitalized infants are sobering, however, since some of the infants will show persistent evidence of lower airway obstruction (Rooney and Williams, 1971; Kattan et al, 1977). It is not clear whether the infants who had severe bronchiolitis had reactive airways that made them prone to severe infections, or whether the infection caused a persisting abnormality in the airways.

Prevention

There is no means of immunizing against respiratory syncytial virus infection and, indeed, it seems unlikely that one will be developed. Repeated infections are the rule and immunity is short-lasting.

One effective approach to prevention is to recognize that the virus is spread by hand or contact with infected objects. Thus, strict hand-washing and cohorting of infants in institutions is very important. Routine use of gloves and gowns diminishes nosocomial spread of the virus.

BRONCHIOLITIS OBLITERANS

Definition

Progressive inflammation and occlusion of the bronchioles is called bronchiolitis obliterans.

Epidemiology

The disease is most common in young adults, but may follow some infections (such as adenovirus) in children. It has been noted in half the survivors of heart-lung transplantation (Burke et al, 1986) and occurs after bone marrow transplantation as a manifestation of graft-versus-host disease (Ostrow et al, 1985).

Natural History

The onset may be acute or insidious with dyspnea, cough, and chest pain for 1–2 weeks. Chest radiographs may show diffuse interstitial infiltrates. After the acute onset, the symptoms may subside for a few months when gradual dyspnea and cyanosis are noted. The course is variable. Some patients die within weeks, others develop the unilateral hyperlucent lung syndrome.

Diagnosis

Given the severity of the disease, confirmation of the diagnosis by biopsy is appropriate.

Treatment

Corticosteroids deserve a trial and are of benefit in a few instances.

CHRONIC BRONCHITIS

Definition

Chronic bronchitis is arbitrarily defined as a chronic productive cough for at least 3 months a year for 2 consecutive years in children with no obvious underlying disease.

Epidemiology

The true "incidence" is unknown since the condition is not reported to any center and individuals may seek several different physicians in search of relief. Surely it is more common than recognized by references to it in the current pediatric literature (Taussig et al, 1981).

Natural History

Most children with chronic coughs are considered to be reactive to some inhalant, such as cigarette smoke, pollens, or pollutants. Many such children have some bronchospasm and find relief from bronchodilators.

Diagnosis

The diagnosis is unsatisfactory since it depends chiefly on exclusion of sinusitis, cystic fibrosis, immune deficiency disorders and, when radiographs demonstrate localized abnormalities, bronchoscopy and CT scans. Clearly not all these conditions need to be excluded in every youngster with a chronic cough. The severity of the cough, evidence of systemic illness (fever, weight loss, etc) would be reasons for a more extended work-up. The designation of "allergic cough" is a problem because it is not provable except by a therapeutic trial of bronchodilators and expectorants. The possibility of cough-variant asthma deserves consideration in any child with a seasonal cough or a cough induced by cold air or exercise. Bronchial provocation testing can suggest if a trial of bronchodilator therapy is warranted.

Treatment

Given the vagueness of the diagnosis and the lack of long-term follow-up of children with chronic bronchitis, there is little wonder that no agreement exists on treatment. Cloutier and Loughlin (1981) reported 15 children whose chronic cough was an isolated symptom of airway hyperreactivity. They found a good clinical response to theophylline, and a recurrence when it was discontinued.

When signs of infection are present, courses of antibiotics seem warranted; if response is inappropriate, investigation for immunodeficiencies and ciliary function is in order.

BRONCHIECTASIS

Definition

Bronchiectasis refers to dilatation and distortion of the architecture of the bronchi, usually accompanied by inflammation and the accumulation of purulent material in the airway.

Basic Science

Congenital deficiency of bronchial cartilage is a rare form of generalized bronchiectasis. More commonly, bronchiectasis evolves in the wake of infection, most commonly in the first 3 years of life. It can occur at any age as a postinfectious event. Aspiration of a foreign body is currently the most likely cause of bronchiectasis if the foreign body is not removed completely by bronchoscopy or vigorous coughing.

Epidemiology

Once a common and serious consequence of measles, pertussis, and tuberculosis, childhood bronchiectasis is rarely seen in the absence of a generalized disease such as cystic fibrosis or ciliary dyskinesis. Congenital cartilage deficiency is very rare. Over a 20-year period (1940–1960), Avery et al (1961) found records of only 66 children less than 14 years of age with documented bronchiectasis at Johns Hopkins Hospital. The numbers have declined subsequently; most of the children currently under our care for postpneumonic bronchiectasis in Boston are immunodeficient (1986).

Natural History

The course of bronchiectasis depends on the cause. If it is in association with ciliary dysfunction or cystic fibrosis, it is progressive. If it follows pneumonia, it may resolve completely with extended antibiotic therapy. If it is the consequence of a foreign object, even extensive saccular changes can reverse, after removal of obstruction. No evidence supports the argument that an area of purulent bronchiectasis will seed normal lung with infection. Instances of multilobe involvement have had underlying disease as the basic problem.

Diagnosis

When rales persist in one region, with or without symptoms, it is important to ascertain the integrity of the bronchus, particularly to rule out foreign body. Bronchoscopy is appropriate to localize sites of inflammation, bronchial compression, or strictures.

Plain chest films will often show dilated bronchi; but may not delineate the extent of involvement. CT scans are most helpful in diagnosis, and have made bronchography (instillation of radiopaque material) outmoded (Fig. 5.7*A*, *B*, and *C*).

Persistent bronchiectasis may be the sequel to repeated infection on the basis of impaired immune responses, cystic fibrosis, endobronchial tuberculosis, or immotile cilia. Appropriate studies should be undertaken to rule out these conditions.

Treatment

Culture, appropriate early use of antibiotics for prolonged periods, and postural drainage are the mainstays of treatment. Segmental resection should be considered only for localized disease that fails medical management.

Prevention

Childhood immunization with DPT, measles, and polio vaccines all serve to reduce the likelihood of severe pneumonias and subsequent bronchiectasis. In the areas of the world where tuberculosis is prevalent, BCG at birth is recommended.

Prompt removal of aspirated foreign bodies by an experienced otolaryngologist is the best prevention of injury to the bronchus.

DISORDERS OF CILIA

Cilia can have two functions: When attached to free-swimming organisms, such as spermatozoa, cilia or flagella propel the organisms; when attached to a fixed cell, as in respiratory epithelium, cilia permit movement of a liquid over the surface. Ciliary function is integrally related to structure, which is remarkably similar in a wide variety of organisms. Mobility is conferred by bending motions of the shaft that result from

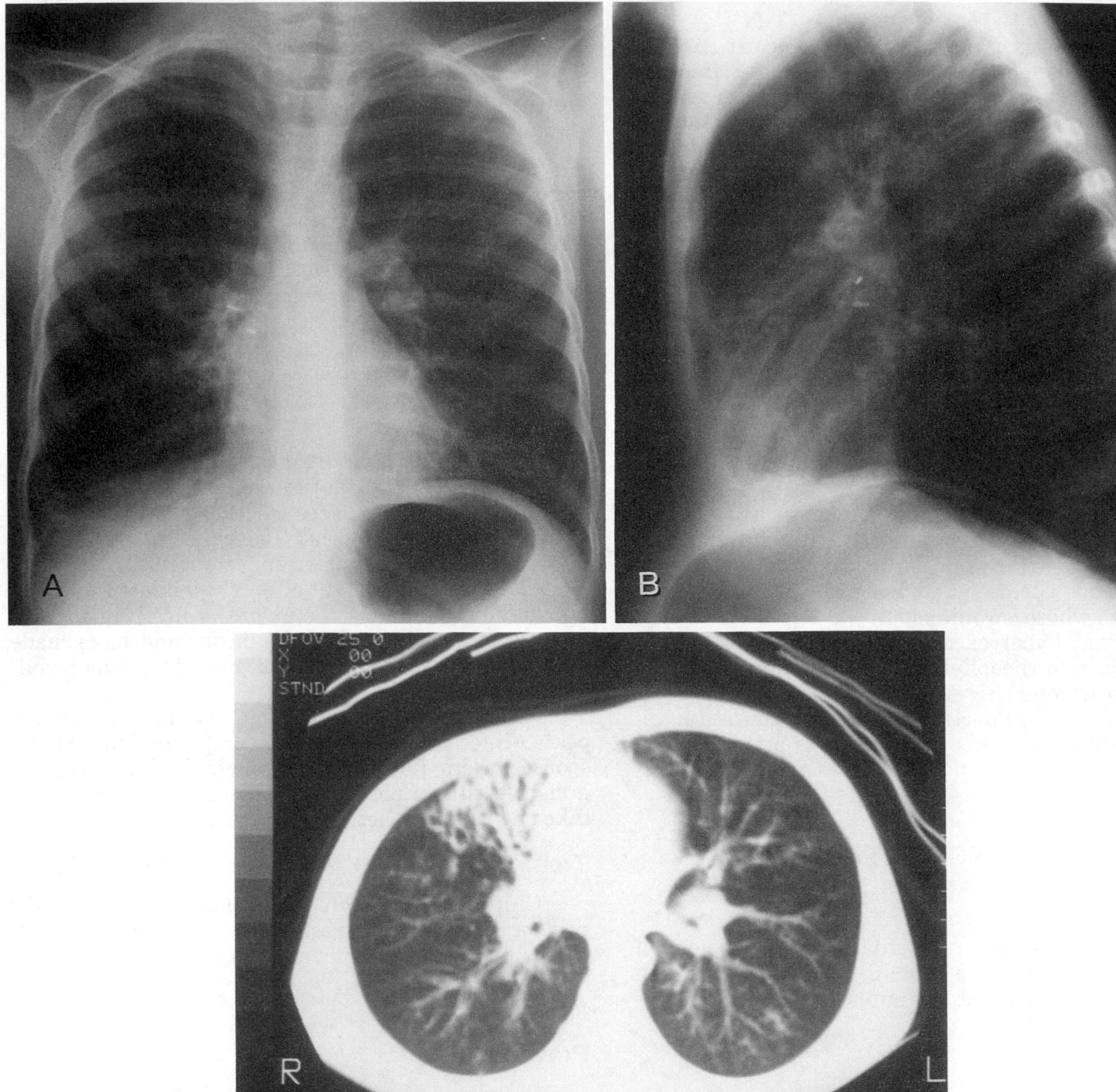

Figure 5.7. This 8-year-old boy has had T-cell deficiency associated with chronic infections all his life. He has had partial resection of right lung in part for chronic infection. His chest radiographs (**A** and **B**) show streaky interstitial markings with more irregular densities in the right middle lobe seen best on lateral (**B**). The CT scan (**C**) demonstrates thick-walled bronchi with mucous plugs, typical of bronchiectasis. CT has, in most cases, replaced bronchography in the diagnostic evaluation of this disease.

sliding of peripheral pairs of microtubules. Alignment of central ciliary microtubules is essential for maintenance of beat synchrony (Eliasson et al, 1977).

Definition

Immotile cilia syndrome is a congenital ciliary abnormality associated with chronic airway infection and male sterility.

Basic Science

The absence of dynein arms from the tails of spermatozoa results in normal appearing, but immotile sperm. Individuals with this condition also have chronic sinusitis and bronchitis. Brushings of their nasal epithelia show almost absent dynein arms. Some individuals have abnormalities in the ciliary spoke. Measurements of mucociliary clearance show essentially nonfunctional cilia and a high retention of inhaled particles. This association of defective cilia in sperm and in respiratory epithelium was first described by Afzelius in 1976 in three men without situs inversus, and in three men and one woman with situs inversus. Confirmation of the association has come from many centers (Sleigh et al, 1988)

A group of related disorders has been described as ciliary morphology as has been examined more frequently. Many different types of structural abnormalities have been described and all result in some degree of diminished function. The immotile ciliary syndrome is distinguished from primary ciliary dyskinesia, in which the proportion of cilia with ultrastructural abnormalities is significantly greater than normal. Beat frequency is reduced and mucociliary clearance is absent. Kartagener syndrome can be considered a subgroup of primary ciliary dyskinesia. A necessary component of the syndrome is situs inversus. Visceral heterotoxy with polysplenia and extrahepatic biliary atresia is also associated with abnormal cilia (Teichberg et al, 1982).

In healthy subjects, about 5% of cilia have either extra or missing peripheral microtubules or altered central microtubules. In individuals with poor ciliary function, as measured by beat frequency or mucociliary clearance, as many as 95% of cilia may be abnormal. Perhaps surprisingly, the proportion of atypical cilia is not increased in cystic fibrosis (Rossman et al, 1984).

Acquired ciliary defects have been associated with acute viral respiratory infections in children. Influenza A and B, adenoviruses types 1 and 5, parainfluenza, and respiratory syncytial viruses have all been associated with an increase in central microtubular defects. The increase is about sixfold, from 2% abnormal in controls and 11.7% in the first week of illness, with return to normal by 10 weeks (Carson et al, 1985).

Epidemiology

The syndrome is probably under-recognized, but is reported to occur in 1/12,500 live births. It is considered an autosomal recessive disorder.

Natural History

The common triad in all patients with immotile cilia are sinusitis, otitis, and a productive cough. In the series of Turner et al (1981), about half of the patients had situs inversus (Kartegener syndrome). Nasal polyps and anosmia have been reported.

The earliest presenting clinical problem may be persistent otitis media. Sometime in early childhood, these children may come to medical attention because of a chronic cough that is often productive of yellow or green sputum. Chest films may show air trapping and multiple infiltrates.

Pulmonary function studies confirm gas trapping and often show an increase in lower airway resistance. A ventilation-perfusion imbalance can lead to hypoxemia.

Although symptoms are usually present from early childhood, they may be delayed as long as 20 years. Height tends to be normal, although many of the affected individuals are underweight.

Diagnosis

In the presence of chronic or recurrent sinusitis, otitis, and bronchitis, ciliary dyskinesia should be considered. The diagnosis can be made by electron microscopy of cells brushed from the nasal turbinates with a cytologic brush. The sample should be fixed immediately for best results. Turner et al (1981) reported better results with bronchial biopsy.

CONTROVERSY

The congenital disorders appear to be clearly related to ciliary dysfunction. Acquired defects are subject to confirmation. The mechanisms involved are speculative. Carson et al (1985) show a viral particle adjacent to ciliated nasal epithelial cells and suggest that it may interfere with cilioneogenesis. This possibility is consistent with the fact that recovery occurred in a finite period.

Treatment

No means of improving defective ciliary motility are known. Daily use of an antihistamine decongestant and a bronchodilator may be helpful. Treatment must be directed toward control of infection and excessive secretion. Immunization with pneumococcal vaccine and influenza viral vaccines is appropriate. The dangers of smoking and exposure to smoke should be emphasized.

Prognosis

Experience is too recent to be sure of the long-term prognosis.

REFERENCES

Afzelius BA: A human syndrome caused by immotile cilia. *Science* 193:317, 1976.

Avery ME, Riley MC, Weiss A: The course of bronchiectasis in childhood, *Bull Johns Hopkins Hosp* 109:20, 1961.

Burke CM, et al: Twenty-eight cases of human heart-lung transplantation. *Lancet* 1:517, 1986.

Carson JL, Collier AM, Hu SS: Acquired ciliary defects in nasal epithelium of children with acute viral upper respiratory infections. *N Engl J Med* 312:463, 1985.

Chanock RM, Kapikian AZ, Mills J, et al: Influence of immunilogical factions in respiratory syncytial virus disease of the lower respiratory tract. *Arch Environ Health* 21:347, 1970.

Cloutier MM, Loughlin GM: Chronic cough in children: A manifestation of airway hyperreactivity. *Pediatrics* 67:6, 1981.

Eliasson R, Mossberg B, Camner P, et al: The immotile-cilia syndrome. *N Engl J Med* 294:1, 1977.

Ellis DA, Thornley PE, Wightman AJ, et al: Present outlook in bronchiectasis: Clinical and social study and review of factors influencing prognosis. *Thorax* 36:659, 1981.

Epler GR, Colby TV: The spectrum of bronchiolitis obliterans. *Chest* 83:161, 1983.

Fishaut M, Tubergin D, McIntosh K: Cellular response to respiratory viruses with particular reference to children with disorders of cell-mediated immunity. *J Pediatr* 96:179, 1980.

Gaultier C, Praud JP, Clement A, et al: Respiration during sleep in children with COPD. *Chest* 87:168, 1985.

Glezen WP, Denny FW: Epidemiology of acute lower respiratory disease in children. *N Engl J Med* 288:498, 1973.

Gosink BB, Friedman PJ, Liebow AA: Bronchiolitis obliterans: Roentgenographic-pathologic correlations. *AJR* 117:816, 1973.
Hall CB, Douglas RG, Geiman JM, et al: Nosocomial respiratory syncytial virus infections. *N Eng J Med* 293:1343, 1975.
Hall CB, McBride JT, Walsh, EE, et al: Aerosolized ribavirin treatment of infants with respiratory syncytial virus infection. *N Engl J Med* 308, 1443, 1983.
Henderson FW, Collier AM, Clide WA Jr, et al: Respiratory syncytial virus infections, reinfections, and immunity. *N Engl J Med* 300:530, 1979.
Kattan M, Keens TG, Lapierre J, et al: Pulmonary function abnormalities in symptom-free children after bronchiolitis. *Pediatrics* 59:683, 1977.
Monaco F, McQuitty JC, Nickerson BG: Calibration of a heated transcutaneous carbon dioxide electrode to reflect arterial carbon dioxide. *Am Rev Respir Dis* 127:322, 1983.
Muller NL, Francis PW, Gurwitz D, et al: Mechanism of hemoglobin desaturation during rapid eye-movement sleep in normal subjects and in patients with cystic fibrosis. *Am Rev Respir Dis* 121:463, 1980.
Ostrow D, Buskard N, Hill RS, et al: Bronchiolitis obliterans complicating bone marrow transplantation. *Chest* 87:829, 1985.
Rooklin AR, McGready SJ, Mikaelian DO, et al: The immotile cilia syndrome: A cause of recurrent pulmonary disease in children. *Pediatrics* 66:526, 1980.
Rooney JC, Williams HE: The relationship between proved viral bronchiolitis and subsequent wheezing. *J Pediatr* 79:744, 1971.
Rossman C, Lee RMK, Forrest JB, et al: Nasal ciliary ultrastructure and function in patients with primary ciliary dyskinesia compared with that in normal subjects with various respiratory diseases. *Am Rev Respir Dis* 129:161, 1984.
Ryland D, Reid L: The pulmonary circulation in cystic fibrosis. *Thorax* 30:285, 1975.
Sleigh MA, Blake JR, Liron N: The propulsion of mucus by cilia. *Am Rev Respir Dis* 137:726, 1988.
Stokes DS, McBride, JT, Wall MA, et al: Sleep hypoxemia in young adults with cystic fibrosis. *Am J Dis Child* 134:741, 1980.
Taber LH, Knight V. Gilbert BE, et al: Ribavirin aerosol treatment of bronchiolitis associated with respiratory syncytial infection in infants. *Pediatrics* 72:613, 1983.
Taussig LM, Smith SM, Blumenfeld R. Chronic bronchitis in childhood: What is it? *Pediatrics* 67:1, 1981.
Teichberg S, Markowitz J, Silverberg M, et al: Abnormal cilia in a child with the polysplenia syndrome and extrahepatic biliary atresia. *J Pediatr* 100:399, 1982.
Turner JAP, Corkey CWB, Lee JYC, et al: Clinical expressions of immotile cilia syndrome. *Pediatrics* 67:805, 1981.
Webb MSC, Martin JA, Cartlidge PH, et al: Chest physiotherapy in acute bronchitis. *Arch Dis Child* 60:1078, 1985.
Welliver RC, Kaul TN, Ogra PL: The appearance of cell-bound IgE in respiratory tract epithelium after respiratory syncytial virus infection. *N Engl J Med* 303:1198, 1980.
Welliver RC, Rinaldo D, et al: The effect of viral lower respiratory tract infection in infancy on pulmonary function in childhood: A prospective study. *Pediatr Res* 19:210A, 1985.
Wohl ME: Bronchiolitis. *Pediatr Ann* 15:307, 1986.
Wohl ME, Chernick V: Bronchiolitis. *Am Rev Respir Dis* 118:759, 1978.
Yahav J, Mindorff C, Levison H: The validity of transcutaneous oxygen tension method in children with cardiorespiratory problems. *Am Rev Respir Dis* 124:586, 1981.

ASTHMA

Definition

The definition of asthma has been attempted by a number of people, with no agreement that helps to classify patients. Our definition is "asthma is reactive lower airway disease, characterized by recurrent episodes of bronchospasm and mucosal edema." Scadding has defined it "asthma is a disease characterized by wide variations over short periods of time in resistance to flow in intrapulmonary airways." Godfrey suggests "asthma in childhood is a disease characterized by wide variations over short periods of time in resistance to flow in intrapulmonary airways and manifest by recurrent attacks of cough or wheeze separated by symptom-free intervals. The airflow obstruction and clinical symptoms are largely or completely reversed by treatment with bronchodilator drugs or steroids" (Godfrey, 1985).

Epidemiology

The prevalence of asthma in infancy is thought to be between 5 and 10%, although regional differences exist (Gergen et al, 1988). Asthma affects 2.4 million children in the United States under age 17 years. The urban poor are most at risk for a variety of reasons, including, in particular, increased exposure to respiratory infections and air pollution. Asthma has a genetic basis, but inheritance must be multifactorial. Monozygotic twins have a 19% concordance for asthma; but dizygotic twins have a 5% concordance.

A striking increase in rates of hospitalization for asthma in the 0- to 14-year age group have been reported in many countries. The reasons are not understood, but the observation underscores the importance of asthma as a health problem (Fig. 5.8; Mitchell, 1985).

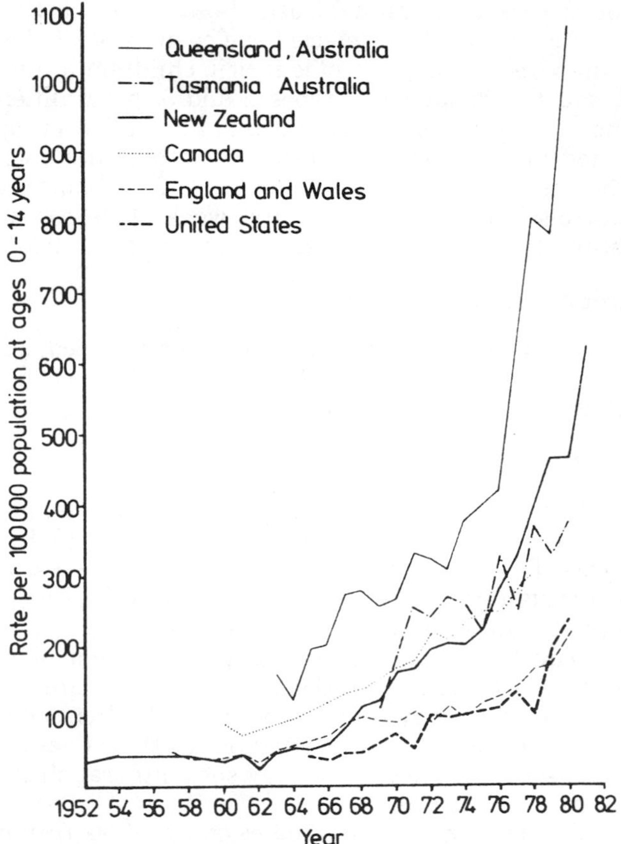

Figure 5.8. Hospital admission rates for asthma in the 0- to 14-year age group for New Zealand, England and Wales, the United States, Canada, and Queensland and Tasmania (Australia.) Reproduced with permission from Mitchell EA: *Arch Dis Child* 60:376, 1985.

Before puberty, asthma is twice as common in boys; after puberty, it is equally distributed between sexes.

Onset can be at any age, but 75% of childhood asthmatics have their first attack between ages 4 and 5 years. No clear relationship between age of onset and prognosis has been defined. Longitudinal studies show that about half of all asthmatic children will be symptom-free by adulthood. The relationship of childhood asthma to airway reactivity and emphysema in adults has not been documented (McNicol and Williams, 1973; Cropp, 1985).

An infant with eczema in addition to wheezing during the first 2 years has a much greater chance of having asthma after age 10 years. More than 90% of such infants continue to wheeze, compared to only about 25% of those without eczema.

Basic Science

During an attack of asthma the patient is most acutely aware that breathing is work. The physician who observes the action of the accessory muscles of respiration (neck, back, and abdominal muscles) is also aware that the patient is doing heavy physical labor, sometimes to the point of exhaustion.

The functional lesion is a prolonged, tetanic contraction of the smooth muscle of the bronchial tree. In addition, there is excessive secretion of mucus from the mucous glands, further obstructing the airway. Because of the increased resistance to airflow, passive expiration is no longer possible in the time allotted, the functional residual capacity increases and the tidal volume is now at a different absolute lung volume. This midpositional shift tends to increase the diameter of the airway and to stretch the expiratory muscles, thus, permitting greater force and assisting expiration.

GAS EXCHANGE

In severe asthma, arterial oxygen saturation falls, probably due to venous admixture that is the result of well-perfused, but poorly ventilated lung units. The arterial P_{CO_2}, which is almost exactly the same as alveolar P_{CO_2} is usually maintained at the normal level by appropriate alveolar ventilation. When respiratory work increases very greatly, the increase in CO_2 produced by the respiratory muscles may not be compensated for by the increase in alveolar ventilation, and CO_2 retention (respiratory acidosis) results.

The problem of therapy in the case of the asthmatic who is hypoxic and has hypercapnea is complicated by the need to give oxygen, but the fear that in so doing the hypoxic stimulus to ventilation may be depressed. In the event of severe CO_2 retention, the respiratory center is no longer sensitive to small changes in P_{CO_2} and the hypoxic drive is essential. On the other hand, hypoxia itself can be fatal. Clearly an "appropriate" amount of oxygen is required. "Appropriate" in this case means an amount which relieves the hypoxia but does not depress respiration. In an asthmatic, a major ventilatory drive also results from obstruction. An asthmatic given O_2 so that the P_{O_2} is > 100 can still have dyspnea.

Assessment of blood gases is essential in evaluating individuals with severe airway obstruction. If an elevated P_{CO_2} increases still further after oxygen therapy, ventilation has been depressed. If it decreases, ventilation has improved.

The interaction of potential bronchoconstrictors was demonstrated by Strauss et al (1977) in a study of the separate and combined effects of cold air challenge in exercise-induced asthma. Noting that individuals whose bronchospasm was evoked during exercise often commented that the problem was worse in cold air, Strauss et al conducted careful pulmonary function studies on eight asymptomatic adults with such a history. They found that cold-air breathing magnified the response to exercise, while at rest, little effect was noted. Isocapnic hyperventilation with cold air can provoke bronchoconstriction.

How the exercise response is mediated is not known with certainty, although humoral mediators of immediate hypersensitivity appear to be the most likely candidates. The response to cold air, on the other hand, is not inhibited by prior administration of atropine, which rules out upper airway reflexes as important in the response. During exercise, incompletely warmed and humidified air may enter thoracic airways. Deal et al (1979) suggested that mucosal cooling may release humoral mediators since cromolyn sodium blunts the response and is useful in treatment of cold-induced bronchospasm. Respiratory tract infections, which sensitize the airways to histamine (and other agents such as cigarette smoke), also act as stimuli in the production of bronchospasm (Strauss et al, 1977).

It is partly because the triggers to bronchospasm may be multiple and operate through different mechanisms, that it is often difficult to ascertain which stimulus precipitated a given attack. Although patterns of responses may emerge in a given individual, such as seasonal attacks, irritation from pollens, smoke, or infections, bronchospasm may develop from different combinations of trigger events. Knowledge of the more common ones, with avoidance when possible, is the only reasonable approach. Sometimes avoidance is increased by air-conditioning, and air-filtering, humidification if dry air is especially irritating to upper airways, move to a more compatible environment if cold air challenge elicits a response, avoidance of exposure to smoke and reduction in exposure to respiratory viruses especially for young children.

Recent advances in the chemistry of the chemical mediation of bronchospasm have shown that certain metabolites of arachidonic acid, especially prostaglandins and leukotrienes, have potent effects on vascular permeability and bronchomotor tone. Moreover, sensitive biologic assays now permit detection of these compounds in pathologic processes. Leukotrienes C_4, D_4 and E_4 are smooth muscle constrictors and account for the biologic activity of "slow-reacting-substance" or SRS-A. Studies on airway smooth muscle have documented their effect in vitro. Antigen challenge leads to release of the leukotrienes, which also mediate mucus production, mucociliary clearance, eosinophil accumulation, and vascular permeability. Leukotrienes are thought to be the major mediators of smooth muscle contraction in asthma.

In some patients, pollens and dust induce IgE formation. This form of extrinsic asthma has given rise to the concept that asthma is an allergic disorder, which is true in only a very limited sense. For example, most children who wheeze in association with viral infections do not have excess IgE, but presumably have a lowered threshold for vagal stimulation of the cholinergic system. Clearly bronchospasm is a response to a variety of stimuli, only some of which could be categorized as "allergic."

Pathology

Knowledge of the structural derangements in asthma is based mostly on the study of lungs of patients who have died during status asthmaticus. In those patients, there is increased vascular permeability and the plasma proteins can be demonstrated in the mucus plugs in the airway. There is an inflammatory reaction with eosinophils prominent in the tissue. Hypersecretion of mucus results in excessive plugging of the airways. The airways obstruction is partly from edema and partly from smooth muscle contraction. Presumably the inflammatory reaction is the underlying process which induces hypersecretion and bronchoconstriction.

Diagnosis

The first episode of wheezing in an infant may represent a single illness in response to respiratory syncytial virus, parainfluenza virus, or rhinoviruses and is usually designated bronchiolitis, especially if the infant is under 8 months old. Recurrent attacks carry a different prognosis, and deserve careful consideration and appropriate diagnostic tests. Among possible causes are aspiration, bronchiolitis obliterans, bronchopulmonary dysplasia, cystic fibrosis, gastroesophageal reflux, heart disease, laryngeal polyps, mediastinal masses, tracheobronchial tree anomalies, and vascular rings. When specific etiologies are ruled out and wheezing recurs, we then ascribe it to asthma.

Digital clubbing would necessitate a sweat test to rule out cystic fibrosis as it is rarely, if ever, associated with asthma.

The major physical findings are tachypnea, with prolonged expiration and some hyperinflation of the chest. In more severe attacks, intercostal retractions are prominent, and accessory muscles of respiration are recruited to assist expiration. Difficulty feeding, dehydration, vomiting, and irritability are common. Excessive irritability may indicate hypoxemia before cyanosis is visible. In older children, digital clubbing may occur in severe chronic asthma.

A chest radiograph is essential if wheezing persists, especially in the first episode since it can provide evidence of a foreign body or a mediastinal mass, or cardiac enlargement. Overdistention and small areas of atelectasis are commonly seen. A barium swallow can be helpful in chronic or recurrent cases if an underlying congenital anomaly or gastroesophageal reflux is suspected.

Eosinophilia is common, but not necessary for the diagnosis. A very high or very low leukocyte count should stimulate pursuit of an infectious agent.

OTHER TESTS

Pulmonary Function Tests. The main value of pulmonary function tests is to establish reversibility of bronchospasm during an asymptomatic interval and to provide an objective measure of response to therapy (such as before and after administration of salbutamol or other β-sympathomimetic agents).

The most commonly used test is the forced expiratory volume delivered in 1 second as expressed as percent of total expired volume. For young children who are not able to sustain an expiratory effort, the peak flow is readily measured. Usually serial measurements made with much encouragement give reproducible values. A wide variety of instruments are commercially available to make these measurements, some complete with computer screen depicting candles to be blown out. Forced oscillation to measure total respiratory resistance can be obtained during normal tidal breathing in young children. This method can be used to elicit responses as bronchial provocation (Lebeque et al, 1987).

More formal tests with flow-volume curves measured before and after airway challenge (cold air, histamine) are discussed under pulmonary function tests.

Total IgE. Elevated levels of total serum IgE support the diagnosis of atopic disease. It should be emphasized that values of IgE for normal and atopic individuals overlap, and that a normal IgE for age does not rule out allergic disease. Elevated levels of IgE are often seen in children with atopic dermatitis as well as in children with allergic respiratory diseases.

Test for Allergen-Specific IgE. These tests are useful for evaluation of specific allergens as a cause for asthma. The results for such tests must be correlated with the history and physical findings in each patient.

Immediate-Type Skin Tests. For these tests, a small quantity of suspected allergen is introduced by prick or scratch or intradermally; 15–20 minutes later, a wheal and flare indicates a positive reaction. Both histamine control to establish reactivity of the skin and a saline or diluent control to rule out nonspecific reactions should be included.

RAST. The radioallergosorbent test (RAST) is an in vitro assay for allergen-specific IgE. Since it can be performed in vitro it is advantageous in infants for whom skin tests may be contraindicated, in patients in whom skin reactivity is modified by disease or drugs, or in patients whose history suggests exquisite sensitivity to antigens where the risk of anaphylaxis is great. The disadvantages of RAST testing include decreased sensitivity compared with skin testing, lack of immediate results, and increased relative cost compared with skin testing.

Treatment

ACUTE ATTACK (TO CONTROL SYMPTOMS)

Sympathomimetic bronchodilators are the first line drugs to alleviate bronchospasm. In mild attacks, aerosols such as isoetharine (Bronkosol) 0.25–0.5 ml diluted in 2 ml of physiologic saline can be administered by nebulized inhalation. Increasingly, metered dose inhalers are used to deliver β-agonists for relief of acute bronchospasm. Administration by intermittent positive pressure is no longer appropriate due to the increased incidence of pneumothorax.

If there is an inadequate response, epinephrine subcutaneously can be given; 0.01 mg/kg (1:1000 dilution) with a maximum of 0.3- to 0.4-mg dose is recommended. It can be repeated two to three times at 20-minute intervals. A positive response is followed with a dose of long acting epinephine (Sus-Phrine 0.005 ml/kg, maximum 0.15 ml).

SEVERE ATTACK

If these measures fail, intravenous aminophylline is the main agent used for severe or prolonged attacks. A bolus of 5–8 mg/kg in 30–50 ml saline is given over 20 minutes and administration can be repeated in 4–6 hours. In patients already on theophylline, the loading dose should be 2.5 mg/kg or 5 mg/kg if it has been more than 4 hours since the last dose if the patient is on rapid release or 8 hours on slow-release preparation. Serum levels should be maintained at 10–20 μg/ml for the best results. Maintenance requires 12–30 mg/kg/day in most instances, but since the drug is metabolized at different rates in certain individuals, serum levels must be monitored. Theophylline can be given by continuous intravenous infusion to maintain desired blood level. Tachycardia and vomiting are early signs of toxicity and signal the need for lowering the dose. Rectal suppositories are not advisable because of variable rates of absorption. Intravenous steroids should be started early (Littenberg and Gluck, 1986).

CHRONIC ASTHMA

In patients with chronic asthma, the goals of treatment are directed at controlling symptoms so that normal activities are possible with the minimum number of medications. A major modality in the treatment regimen includes education regarding the disease and instruction in avoiding precipitating or aggravating factors, and in early and aggressive use of medication to reduce symptoms once they occur.

Cromolyn sodium is the primary drug in long-term management of asthma. In children over age 5 years, 2 mg, four times a day by metered-dose inhaler reduces the number and severity of attacks (Eigen et al, 1987). The action of the drug is to stabilize mast cells and inhibit activation of inflammatory cells.

Oral methylxanthines, such as sustained release theophylline preparations, with or without adrenergic drugs by aerosol are useful in management of chronic asthma. The dose has to be individualized to avoid gastrointestinal and CNS toxicity.

Glucocorticoids are the most effective agents in treatment of chronic asthma, but their side effects mandate consideration of their use. Glucocorticoids in clinical use are all analogs of cortisol and bind selectively to glucocorticoid receptors. They affect nuclear DNA to make new RNA for synthesis of new proteins. Since protein synthesis is necessary, a time lag of hours to days may be needed before the full effect is seen. Glucocorticoid action affects many target tissues other than lung. For that reason inhalants such as beclomethasone dipropionate have an advantage in maximizing tissue concentration in the airways.

The pulmonary effects of glucocorticoids include suppression of acute and chronic inflammation by lessening recruitment of leukocytes and suppression of binding of complement components and IgE and IgG to leukocytes. They also block synthesis of some lymphokines and release of histamine from mast cells. Synthesis of prostaglandins (PGE_2 and prostacyclin) is blocked. Glucocorticoids also potentiate pulmonary response to β-agonists, presumably by externalizing receptors to the surface of the cell membrane. Later, an increase in β-agonist receptors is seen after glucocorticoid administration.

The effect of glucocorticoids on breathing in status asthmaticus is seen after 6 hours, and may not be impressive for 24 hours. Thus, other agents such as theophylline are needed to initiate therapy.

Hazards of prolonged steroid therapy include development of Cushing disease and possible lowered resistance to infection.

Prednisone or methyl prednisolone, 1–2 mg/kg/day in divided doses for 7–10 days, may be required. Some severely affected children will need long-term therapy with corticosteroids on an every other day basis. Children over age 6 years may respond to flunisolide by aerosol twice each day and require a lower dose of oral prednisone and consequently fewer side effects.

Treatment

CONTROVERSIES

Asthma can be such a severely debilitating disease that there is little wonder that many interventions have been tried, with much controversy as to their efficacy.

A careful history may point to a component of the diet that initiates an attack. If so, the effect of eliminating that food should be tested. Usually, however, no such history is forthcoming, and batteries of skin tests with subsequent dietary changes are of little benefit. For all asthmatic children, the reduction of dusts or pollutants such as tobacco smoke is appropriate. Tests for specific allergens that require methods of measurement of IgE (i.e., RAST) have their advocates. Few data exist to show benefit except in isolated instances. Nonetheless, they may point to a useful specific intervention.

Physical therapy may be helpful in a superinfection or in the presence of a productive cough to help move sticky mucus, but routine physical therapy has little to recommend it.

Severely disabled youngsters may be more comfortable sleeping in 25–30% humidified oxygen. Mist tents are potentially harmful, however, since water inhaled as droplets can induce bronchospasm.

Psychiatric support is indicated in circumstances where the history documents attacks induced by stress or in response to a given individual, such as a parent or other caretaker. Sometimes the illness itself serves as a strain on family relations. When to intervene with psychiatric or social service supports is a matter for individual interpretation.

Infants with wheezing have a less predictable response to *bronchodilators* than older children with asthma. Despite much speculation, no convincing reasons for this effect have been proposed. Some infants have a prompt and clearly beneficial response (Lenney and Milner, 1978); whereas, others have none. In the absence of an ability to predict, a therapeutic trial with inhaled Bronkosol or subcutaneous epinephrine seems appropriate (Table 5.6).

Oxygen is a mainstay of treatment of an acute attack. Only enough should be given to bring the arterial oxygen to comfortable levels of 70–80 torr. The oxygen should be appropriately humidified, but not supersaturated with a water fog. A large mist tent with water vaporized as a humidifier is satisfactory. A smaller "croupette" with a dense fog may trigger further bronchospasm.

Much debate has centered on the role of *exercise,* particularly since the recognition that exercise can induce attacks in some individuals. Swimming has been advocated for asthma and cystic fibrosis patients, since most of the accessory muscles of respiration are used. Since muscle fatigue is a liability during an acute exacerbation, training for fitness seems sensible. Nickerson and colleagues (1983) have tested the effect of vigorous exercise in 15 children taking theophylline and beclomethasone for their asthma. After a 6-week program in running, overall fitness improved and no deterioration in pulmonary function was evident.

Sinusitis and asthma are so often associated that it seems appropriate to consider the possibility that treatment of the upper airspace infection will lessen

Table 5.6
Drugs Used to Treat Infants with Asthma

Drug	Nebulized solution	Oral preparation	Parenteral solution
Albuterol Ventolin Proventil	0.5% solution, 0.01–0.03, ml/kg diluted to 2 ml, up to four times daily	2 mg/5 ml/syrup, 0.1–0.15 mg/kg/dose every 6 hours	Not available
Cromolyn Intal	1% solution, 2 ml/dose initially four times daily, then two times daily	Not available	Not available
Epinephrine	Not available	Not available	1:1,000, 0.01 ml/kg subcutaneously, 2 doses every 20 minutes × 3
Hydrocortisone sodium succinate	Not available	Not available	4 mg/kg/hour to start, then 1 mg/kg/hour
Isoetharine Bronkosol	1% solution, 0.25 ml diluted to 2 ml, up to four times daily	Not available	Not available
Isoproterenol Isuprel	0.5% solution, 0.03 ml/kg diluted to 2 ml, up to four times daily	Not available	0.1 μg/kg/minute intravenously; may be increased to 0.8 μg/kg/minute
Prednisone	Not available	2 mg/kg/day; wean to minimum within 5 days	Not available
Theophylline	Not available	Multiply age in weeks by 0.3, add 8 mg/kg/day, up to 24 mg/kg; regular release, every 6 hours; sustained release, every 8–12 hours	6 mg/kg to start, then 1 mg/kg/hour

[1]Reproduced with permission from Robertson C, Ronchetti R, Levison H: *J Respir Dis*, March, 1984.

the lower airway reactivity. The question is whether sinus films or otolaryngologic consultation are required to make the diagnosis. Alternatively a 10-day course of a broad spectrum antibiotic could be a diagnostic-therapeutic trial. The answer must be individualized, on the basis of the presence of physical signs such as sinus tenderness, purulent nasal discharge or chronic cough from postnasal drips. Also, sinus films may be misleading, and should not be repeated often because of radiation hazards.

Some gastroenterologists have put forward the idea that gastroesophageal reflux may trigger bronchospasm by a reflex mechanism or aspiration. They advocate pH probes in the lower esophagus, technetium scans, barium swallows, and, if positive, esophagoscopy and bronchoscopy with alveolar lavage as means of diagnosing aspiration in individuals whose chest radiographs are consistent with it. As of this writing (1987), no prospective controlled clinical trials support the likelihood of gastroesophageal reflux as important in producing recurrent wheezing nor have we seen therapeutic success from medical or surgical interventions. More systematic experience is needed before we can decide who might profit from a full-scale work-up. If reflux is evident clinically, our first intervention is to reduce the dose of theophylline, which is known to promote vomiting and lower gastroesophageal sphincter tone. We doubt if many asthmatics would profit from further evaluation.

CASE ILLUSTRATION

An 8-year-old schoolboy was in excellent general health and had no respiratory symptoms until a month before being brought to the pediatrician. When he was competing in sports contests after school, he began to cough for periods as long as 20–30 minutes. The problem was worse on cool days. The diagnosis of exercise-induced asthma was considered despite a normal physical examination. Referral for pulmonary function evaluation showed that his peak expiratory flow rate fell from 250 L/minute before exercise to 100 L/minute after 5 minutes of exercise. Over the subsequent hour, there was a gradual return to baseline.

When he was scheduled to participate in competitive sports, he inhaled a β-adrenergic agonist about 15 minutes before starting exercise. This measure brought significant relief.

COMMENT

It is important to inform the child of the nature of the problem and to allow him to select sports that are tolerated. Swimming is one of the best. It is essential not to let exercise-induced bronchospasm be an excuse for not participating in sports. Some top athletes have had exercise-induced asthma and have overcome the problem by warm-up before competing and proper use of bronchodilators.

Prognosis

The majority of asthmatic children have fewer attacks after puberty and about 30% never have recurrences. Infection-induced asthma in early life is said to have a better prognosis than asthma triggered by allergens.

Deaths from asthma continue to occur, although rarely. In several long-term studies, death occurred in about 1% of children whose asthma began under age 12 years and were followed for more than 20 years (Blair, 1977). However, only one death occurred in the last 5 years among 8000 asthmatics followed at The Children's Hospital, Boston. The causes of death include asphyxia from severe bronchospasm, inappropriate sedation, pneumothorax (especially with intermittent positive-pressure breathing), adverse reactions to β-blockers, and hypersensitivity to drugs.

Deaths are more common at night or in the early morning. Among the possible reasons are sleep-related hypoxemia and diurnal variation in bronchial reactivity (Benatar, 1986).

Prevention

Many of the 2–3 million asthmatic children less than 17 years old in the United States lead unnecessarily restricted lives. Several pediatric asthma self-management programs have taught parents and children to recognize and respond to symptoms. They aim to help the child achieve independence and, by so doing, to relieve stresses within the family. When these programs have been evaluated, school attendance has improved and the number of attacks decreased.

AIR POLLUTION

The possibility that agents that incite bronchospasm in susceptible individuals may act synergistically when in combination has long been suspected from epidemiologic evidence.

For example, temperature inversions that have concentrated air pollutants over urban areas and produced epidemic illness and excess deaths have had the worst effect on individuals with preexisting reactive airway disease. In Donora, Pennsylvania in 1948, a 4-day fog with zinc sulfate and sulfur dioxide among the pollutants made nearly half the population of 14,000 ill and 20 died. In London in 1952, from December 5 to December 8, during a particularly severe "smog," 4000 deaths were recorded in excess of those expected at that time of the year. These extreme illustrations are convincing evidence that air pollution can kill. More subtle levels of pollution unquestionably increase the frequency of "asthmatic" attacks, as is often observed by correlating the increased numbers of emergency room visits during high levels of air pollution.

REFERENCES

Benatar SR: Fatal asthma. *N Engl J Med* 314:423, 1986.
Blair H: Natural history of childhood asthma: 20 year follow-up. *Arch Dis Child* 52:613, 1977.

Cheng TO, Godfrey MD, Shepard RH: Pulmonary resistance with state of inflation of lungs in normal subjects and in patients with airway obstruction. *J Appl Physiol* 14:727, 1959.
Cropp GJA: Special features of asthma in children. *Chest* 87:57S, 1985.
Dahlen S, Hansson G, Hedquist P, et al: Allergen challenge of lung tissue from asthmatics elicits bronchial contraction that correlates with the release of leukotrienes C_4, D_4, and E_4. *Proc Natl Acad Sci* 80:1712, 1983.
Deal EC, McFadden ER, Ingram RH, et al: Hyperpnea and heat flux: Initial reaction sequence in exercise-induced asthma. *J Appl Physiol* 46:476, 1979.
Eigen H, Ried JJ, Dahl R, et al: Evaluation of the addition of cromolyn sodium to bronchodilator maintenance therapy in the long term management of asthma. *J Allergy Clin Immunol* 80:612, 1987.
Ford-Hutchinson AW: Leukotrienes: Their formation and role as inflammatory mediators. *Fed Proc* 44:25, 1985.
Gergen PJ, Mullally DI, Evans R: National Survey of prevalence of asthma among children in the United States, 1976 to 1980. *Pediatrics* 81:1, 1988.
Godfrey S: What is asthma? *Arch Dis Child* 60:997, 1985.
Godfrey S, Konig P: Inhibition of exercise-induced asthma by different pharmacological pathways. *Thorax* 31:137, 1976.
Hogg JC: The pathology of asthma. *Chest* 87:152S, 1985.
Lebecque P, Spier S, Lapierre J, et al: Histamine challenge test in children using forced oscillation to measure total respiratory resistance. *Chest* 92:318, 1987.
Lenney W. Milner AD: Alpha and beta adrenergic stimulants in bronchiolitis and wheezy bronchitis in children under 18 months of age. *Arch Dis Child* 53:707, 1978.
Littenberg B, Gluck EH: A controlled trial of methylprednisolone in the emergency treatment of acute asthma. *N Engl J Med* 314:150, 1986.
McNicol KN, Williams HB: Spectrum of asthma in children. I. Clinical and physiological components. *Br Med J* 4:7, 1973.
Mitchell EA: International trends in hospital admission rates for asthma. *Arch Dis Child* 60:636, 1985.
Morris HG: Mechanisms of glucocorticoid action in pulmonary disease. *Chest* 88:1335, 1985.
Nickerson BG, Bautista DB, Namey MA, et al: Distance running improves fitness in asthmatic children wihout pulmonary complications or changes in exercise induced bronchospasm. *Pediatrics* 71:147, 1983.
Otis AB: The work of breathing. *Physiol Rev* 34:449, 1959.
Riley RL: The work of breathing and its relation to respiratory acidosis. *Ann Intern Med* 41:172, 1954.
Robertson C, Ronchetti R, Levison H: When infants wheeze is it asthma? *J Respir Dis* Vol. 5, March, 1984.
Samuelsson B: Leukotrienes; mediators of immediate hypersensitivity reactions and inflammation. *Science* 220:568, 1983.
Strauss RH, McFadden ER, Ingram RH, et al: Enhancement of exercise-induced asthma by cold air. *N Engl J Med* 297:743, 1977.
Wells RE, Mechanics of respiration in bronchial asthma. *Am J Med* 26:384, 1959.

CYSTIC FIBROSIS

Definition

Cystic fibrosis (CF) is a disorder of the exocrine system that produces abnormalities in secretions in many glands. The onset of symptoms referable to pancreatic and/or pulmonary dysfunction usually dates from early childhood, but the symptoms may be mild or unrecognized until young adult life. The condition is so strongly associated with elevated concentrations of chloride in sweat that a positive "sweat test" is at the current time the sine qua non of diagnosis.

Basic Science

The Mendelian recessive mode of inheritance makes it probable that the protean manifestations of CF result from a single abnormal or missing gene with very major adverse effects on the eccrine gland system. No identifiable abnormal gene product has to date been found. The many studies on etiology have provided an enormous amount of descriptive data on epiphenomena. Since the basic defect is unknown, it is impossible to distinguish the carrier state with a high probability of success; carriers do not have any recognizable clinical or biochemical markers.

Progress in localizing the gene moved rapidly in the mid-1980s with identification of markers that can be linked to the gene within certain families. At least the common form of CF is related to a gene on the long arm of chromosome 7 near the centromere (Knowlton et al, 1985; Tsui et al, 1985).

Among the candidates for the basic defect is deficiency of the enzyme that cleaves the arginine-aspartine peptide bond in cholecystokinin to produce octapeptide CCK-8. This product normally stimulates exocrine secretion in pancreas, gall bladder, and intestine (Gosden and Gosden, 1984). The observations were based on examination of fetuses with CF identified by abnormal structural features in pancreas (disorganized acini and long-distorted tight junctions between epithelial cells.)

Interest has been focused on the regulation of airway epithelial cell chloride channels (Welsh, 1986). One provocative observation is that the regulation of chloride channel activity normally stimulated by β-adrenergic agents is deficient in airway epithelial cells from patients with CF studied in culture (Frizzell et al, 1986). Similarly secretory coils isolated from sweat glands do not respond to β-adrenergic (isoproterenol) stimulation. The relation of these observations to the basic biochemical defect in CF remains to be demonstrated.

The major demonstrable metabolic abnormality that is present from birth is an elevation of the sodium and chloride content in sweat, but not predictably in tears or saliva. The increases in sodium and chloride concentration in sweat result from a decrease in sodium reabsorption in the sweat duct. The pancreatic lesion is characterized by impaired secretion of water, electrolytes, and bicarbonate with resultant protein hyperconcentration (Kopelman et al, 1985). Mucous secretions in the lungs are viscid (hence, an earlier name of the disorder, mucoviscidosis). Whether the abnormality in mucus is primary or secondary to chronic infection is not established. It is probable that the water content is low in all mucus, including intestinal, which gives rise to an abnormally viscid meconium in the fetus and newborn. Despite many studies, no consistent abnormalities of other components of sweat or mucous glands have been described. As of 1988, no satisfactory unifying hypothesis to explain this disease has been forthcoming.

The pulmonary lesion may be evident at birth, but usually infants with meconium ileus and elevated sweat chloride have normal lungs. The earliest lesion is hypertrophy of the bronchial glands followed shortly by plugging of small peripheral airways. Obstruction produces chronic infection, bronchiectasis, loss of pulmonary function, cyanosis, pulmonary hypertension, and cor pulmonale. Collateral circulation through bronchial arteries can be very pronounced, and bleeding from these vessels is a serious and often fatal event, especially in young adults.

The initial colonization and occasional serious attack of pneumonia is caused by *Staphylococcus aureus*, but may result from a number of pathogens. Very quickly after initial infection mucoid strains of *Pseudomonas aeruginosa* enter the lung and aggravate the chronic pneumonia. It is very difficult, if not impossible, to eradicate *Pseudomonas*, which is known to be the principal pathogen in CF. The reason for this symbiosis between *Pseudomonas* and the lung in CF is unknown. Immune complexes to *Pseudomonas* antigens may have deleterious effects on the lung (Pier, 1985). Recently, multiply-resistant species, among them, *P. cepacia*, have been found in increasing frequency. *P. cepacia* seems especially harmful in females who have been doing reasonably well before becoming infected. Males are less likely to have an adverse reaction (Thomassen et al, 1985; Tablan et al, 1985; Goldmann and Klinger, 1986).

Clinical severity sometimes correlates with the number of bacteria in the sputum; treatment with suitable antibiotics can alleviate symptoms even though total eradication of *Pseudomonas* does not occur. Some investigators believe clinical deterioration represents an overexuberant immune response; and therapy with corticosteroid on an alternate day basis has been associated with a reduction in pulmonary deterioration (Matthews et al, 1980; Auerbach et al, 1985). A clear association between the frequency of viral respiratory infections and pulmonary deterioration was shown in a prospective study by Wang et al (1984).

Epidemiology

The prevalence of CF varies among and within the races. It is most common in the white population in the United States, where it occurs in about 1/1,600–1/2,000 births. The estimated prevalence in the United States black population is 1/17,000, and the disease seems less severe among blacks. It is rarest among Asian peoples, but has been reported in Asians living in Hawaii at a rate of 1/90,000. Approximately 1200 cases are newly diagnosed each year in the United States. The male to female ratio is 1.3:1 (Table 5.7).

Natural History

The disease may present in the neonatal period with meconium ileus (approximately 10% of cases) or prolonged jaundice. Failure to gain weight in infancy is another common finding. Protein deficiencies may ensue, with edema as an early manifestation. Fat malabsorption can lead to bulky stools, abdominal protuberance, and reduced subcutaneous tissue. Rectal prolapse is common.

Table 5.7
Risks of Producing a Child with Cystic Fibrosis [1]

One Parent	Other Parent	Risk of CF in Each Pregnancy
With no CF history	With no CF history	1/1600
With no CF history	With first cousin having CF	1/320
With no CF history	With aunt or uncle having CF	1/240
With no CF history	With sibling having CF	1/120
With no CF history	With CF child by previous marriage	1/80
With no CF history	With parent having CF	1/80
With no CF history	Has CF	1/40
With sibling having CF	With sibling having CF	1/9
With CF child	With CF child	1/4

[1] From Shwachman H: Cystic fibrosis. In *Current Problems in Pediatrics*. Vol VIII. Chicago, Year Book Medical Publishers, 1978, p. 7.

Recurrent pneumonias or persisting pulmonary infiltrates with or without wheezing at any age should raise suspicion of CF, as should the recovery of mucoid *P. aeruginosa* from sputum. Pulmonary symptoms of chronic hacking (or later productive) cough with episodic wheezing are characteristic. The initial pulmonary lesion results in increased lower airway resistance, with significant hyperinflation. Later, lesions produce tissue destruction and widespread bronchiectasis. Although sometimes more prominent in one lobe or another, eventually all portions of the lung are involved (Fig. 5.9). When the lung disease is associated with hypoxemia, clubbing of the fingers and toes becomes prominent, usually toward the end of the first decade.

Eighty-five percent of patients with CF have severe pancreatic disease. The lesion is demonstrable in utero, at 32–38 weeks after conception, with a deficiency in acinar tissue. The resulting deficiency in trypsin and lipolytic enzymes results in malabsorption, steatorrhea, and a celiac-like syndrome. Some infants have low levels of serum proteins and may even present with edema.

Hypogammaglobulinemia has been noted in about one-quarter of the children less than 10-years-old. Matthews et al (1980) noted a milder disease in those with low levels of γ-globulin. Older patients were found to have elevated γ-globulin coincident with progression of disease, indicating that a hyperimmune response and complement activation indicate a poor prognosis (Moss et al, 1986).

In an older age group, cirrhosis with portal hypertension may be the only manifestation of CF (except for the elevated sweat electrolytes) which are the sine qua non of the diagnosis (Fig. 5.10*A* and *B*). Nasal polyps are found in some CF patients in association with multiple allergies. Pansinusitis is almost always present. Aspermia is a uniform finding in affected males

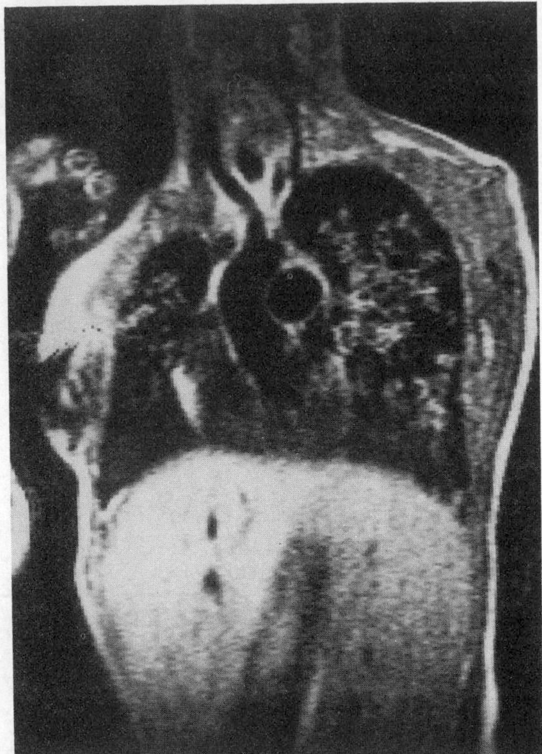

Figure 5.9. MRI—CF. T1-weighted coronal image from magnetic resonance imaging (MRI) unit, 0.6 Tesla, with 45-cm body coil, is of a patient with cystic fibrosis. Because flowing blood gives no signal, pulmonary disease (*areas of white*) can be differentiated from patent pulmonary vessels. Gated MRI also has applications in the diagnosis of cardiac disease. Note how well the ascending aorta and its branches are displayed. Case is courtesy of David Kushner, M.D., MGH, Boston.

from obliteration of the vas deferens. This lesion can be identified in affected fetuses.

About 1% of patients with CF may develop an adult-type diabetes mellitus. It is estimated that by age 18 years 15% of patients will have diabetes, and about 50% will have a diabetic-type glucose tolerance test. Ketoacidosis and vascular complications are rare in these patients, although those who live into the third decade may develop proliferative diabetic retinopathy (Dolan, 1986) and diabetic renal disease.

Osteoarthropathy with bone pain and joint effusion is also a recognized complication which can flare during respiratory exacerbations. (Braude et al, 1984).

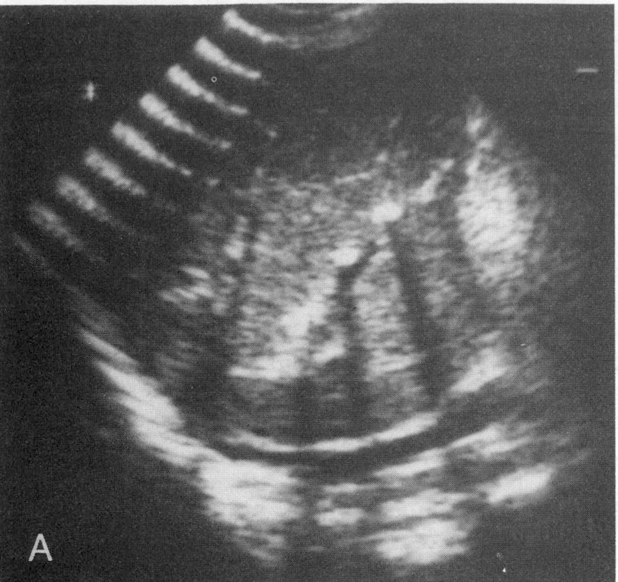

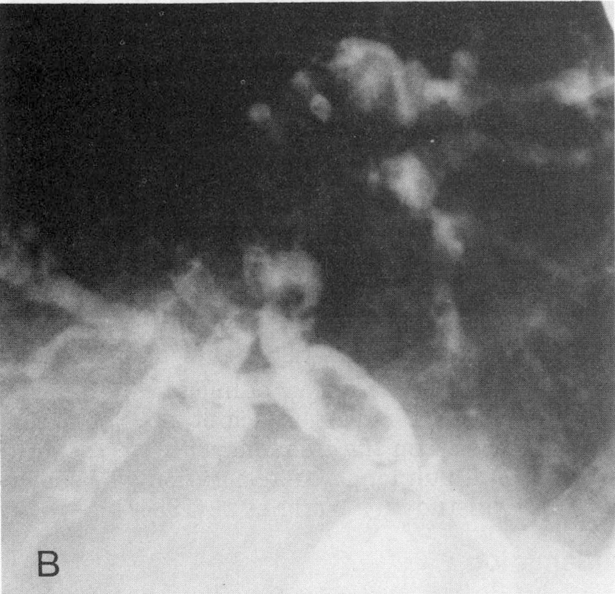

Figure 5.10.A and **B.** This patient with cystic fibrosis presented with painless jaundice as a young man. Ultrasonogram of the upper abdomen **(A)** shows multiple echogenic foci within the liver which are casting shadows. These are intrahepatic calculi and are confirmed on the ERCP **(B)** as multiple filling defects within dilated biliary radicals. This is a very difficult condition to treat. Sphincteroplasty and choleretics were used in this patient. Intrahepatic calculi are rare in childhood. When seen, they are typically associated with cystic fibrosis.

Diagnosis

SWEAT TEST

A standard approach to collection and measurement of sweat chloride is essential to obtain accurate results. Short cuts in which sweat from palms is used or extremities are heated are to be avoided, mainly because the concentration of chloride in sweat varies with the rate of sweating.

WHEN TO DO A SWEAT TEST

1. Infants who pass their initial meconium late, i.e., after approximately 30 minutes of age
2. Intestinal obstruction in the newborn
3. Failure to thrive in infancy or childhood
4. All siblings of patients with CF, including the newborn
5. All patients suspected of having CF or celiac disease

6. Infants and children with steatorrhea or chronic diarrhea
7. Infants with rapid respirations and retraction with chronic cough
8. Infants with diagnosis of asthma, especially if digits are clubbed
9. Infants with hypoproteinemia, especially when on soybean formula
10. Infants who show hyperaeration on chest radiographs or have atelectasis
11. Infants with hypoprothrombinemia, excluding major hematologic disease
12. Infants and children with rectal prolapse
13. All patients suspected of having disaccharidase intolerance or diagnosed as having celiac disease
14. Infants and children who "taste salty"
15. Patients with recurrent pneumonia, chronic atelectasis, chronic pulmonary disease, bronchiectasis, or chronic cough or staphylococcal pneumonia
16. Children and adults with nasal polyposis even though they may be allergic
17. Children and young patients (nonalcoholics) with cirrhosis of the liver and portal hypertension
18. Infants of a CF parent; the obligate heterozygote
19. Infant with unexplained hyponatremia
20. Finally, in response to parents who request a sweat test on their child

Modified from Shwachman H: Cystic fibrosis. In *Current Problems in Pediatrics.* Vol VIII. Chicago, Year book Medical Publishers, 1978, p. 11.

The most widely used test involves iontophoresis of pilocarpine into the skin of the volar surface of forearm (Gibson and Cooke, 1959). A 3-ma electric current carries pilocarpine into the skin to stimulate sweating locally. Sweat is collected from filter paper that is kept covered to prevent evaporation. After 30-60 minutes, the paper is removed, weighed, eluted with distilled water, and chloride concentration is measured. The amount of sweat measured should be reported, since errors can occur with too little sweat production, especially in the first 2 weeks of life.

In general, normal values, although very variable, are usually under 40 mEq/L. A level of more than 60 mEq/L is considered diagnostic. For intermediate, values other criteria for diagnosis should be carefully considered. All questionable or elevated tests should be repeated to lessen risk of misapplication of this essential information.

A few conditions may show elevation of sweat chlorides, but are clearly distinguishable from CF. These are: adrenal insufficiency, hypothyroidism, severe malnutrition, ectodermal dysplasia, nephrogenic diabetes insipidus, and some mucopolysaccharidoses.

Tests for Pancreatic Function

Qualitative examination of stool fat is useful. Often the stools are described as bulky, foul-smelling, greasy, and floating. A 3-day collection with controlled fat intake is needed to document steatorrhea. Quantitative assay of trypsin and chymotrypsin in a fresh specimen is helpful. Duodenal intubation, formerly the main diagnostic test, is not used routinely, although in borderline cases, it may be useful.

Vitamin E levels may be low even if pancreatic enzyme replacement has been inadequate; reversible neurological dysfunction has been described in severe vitamin E deficiency (Bye et al, 1985).

Presenting Problems

Presenting problems may relate to the gastrointestinal tract, the lung, the upper airways, or the liver. In infancy, meconium ileus heralds CF in an otherwise normal infant (Table 5.8). Hypoproteinemia, with associated edema, also may be the presenting finding. Later, malabsorption, especially of protein and fat from deficient pancreatic enzyme secretion leads to poor weight gain, diminished subcutaneous fat, and occasionally a distended abdomen, as is also observed in celiac disease. Rectal prolapse may complicate the picture. The pulmonary dysfunction may present as recurrent or persistent infiltrates with some degree of hyperinflation. Not infrequently, infants are diagnosed

Table 5.8
Conditions to Consider in the Differential Diagnosis of Cystic Fibrosis [1]

Pulmonary	Disaccharidase deficiency
Aspiration pneumonia	Jaundice
Foreign body	Diarrhea
Asthma	Steatorrhea
Recurrent viral or bacterial respiratory infection	Hypoproteinemia and anemia
Bronchitis and bronchiolitis	Protein-losing enteropathy
Pneumonia: viral, mycoplasma, or bacterial	Failure to gain weight (pancreatic infantilism, short stature)
Bronchiectasis	
Staphylococcal empyema	Shwachman syndrome
Pertussis and parapertussis	Recurrent abdominal pain
	Recurrent acute pancreatis
Pulmonary tuberculosis	Cirrhosis of liver
Histoplasmosis	Hypersplenism
Ascariasis	Portal hypertension
Pulmonary aspergillosis	Intussusception (over 3 years of age)
α_1-Antitrypsin deficiency	
Emphysema	Fecal impaction
Kartagener's syndrome	Regional enteritis
Pneumothorax	Sweat gland defect
Pulmonary hemorrhage	"Rusters"
	Heat stroke and circulatory collapse
Gastrointestinal	Other conditions
Meconium ileus, simple	Agammaglobulinemia
Meconium ileus complicated by atresia, volvulus, or peritonitis	Familial dysautonomia
	Aspermia
	Amenhorrhea
Hirschsprung disease	Inguinal hernia
Meconium plug syndrome	Gum hypertrophy

[1] From Shwachman H: Cystic fibrosis. In *Current Problems in Pediatrics*. Vol VIII, Chicago, Year Book Medical Publishers, 1978, p. 11.

as having bronchiolitis and asthma before a sweat test distinguishes those conditions from CF. In addition, chronic sinusitis and especially nasal polyps should signal the possibility of cystic fibrosis (Stern et al, 1982b).

In older children, the insidious onset of adult type diabetes may be a complication of severe pancreatic dysfunction that eventually compromises islet secretions. Recurrent acute pancreatitis occurs in this age group.

Focal biliary cirrhosis, secondary to bile-containing mucous plugs, may occur in 2–3% of youngsters with CF, and may, although rarely, be the only manifestation. Advanced cirrhosis is complicated by portal hypertension, esophageal varices, and hypersplenism.

Chronic salt depletion may occur, especially in the summer because of salt loss through sweating, or during episodes of gastroenteritis when they may develop a hypochloremic alkalosis. Parents sometimes report that their children "taste salty" when they kiss them.

Delayed sexual maturation is a problem in teenagers; reassurance is helpful. Counseling about sterility in males and cervicitis in females is appropriate (Stern et al, 1982a).

General Approach to Therapy

It is essential to confirm the diagnosis by ensuring that the child has a sweat test carefully performed in an experienced laboratory. Often hospitalization is appropriate to document the extent of pulmonary and pancreatic dysfunction, to plan a nutritional regimen with replacement of pancreatic enzymes, vitamin supplements, and to initiate appropriate chest physical therapy. Cultures of sputum should dictate the choice of antibiotics. The prevalence of mucoid strains of *Pseudomonas* resistant to most antibiotics poses the greatest challenge. Some of the wide-spectrum cephalosporins, such as ceftazidime, seem promising (Moellering, 1985). Any acute pulmonary exacerbation is an indication for intensive antibiotic therapy, usually intravenous, for an arbitrary period of 10 days to 2 weeks. Formerly this required hospitalization, but now some older children can be managed by a home care team. Immunization against influenza is warranted.

With greater awareness of the disease that has prompted early diagnosis and treatment, the prognosis for CF patients has improved in recent years. Some individuals are aided by administration of isoproterenol or terbutaline; others may be made worse by these interventions. Pulmonary function evaluation before and after bronchodilators is important to permit individualization of optimal treatment. Mucolytic aerosols are probably ineffective, although an occasional patient reports improvement. Growth can be promoted with nutritional supplements aiming at 130% of requirement to meet extra metabolic costs of breathing and coughing (Parsons et al, 1985) (Table 5.9).

In a preliminary report, Auerbach et al, (1985) showed a delay in the progression of pulmonary disease in patients given 2 mg/kg of prednisone every other day for 4 years to suppress the inflammatory response.

Table 5.9
Daily Nutrient Guidelines for Patients with Cystic Fibrosis[1]

Age	kcal/kg	Protein (g/kg)	Fat (g/kg)	
0–1 year	150–200	4	Normal intake	>6.0
			Moderate intake	4.5–6.0
			Low intake	<4.5
1–9 years	130–180	3	Normal intake	3.0
			Moderate intake	2.0–3.0
			Low intake	1.0–2.0
9–18 years (males)	80–130	2.5–3.0		
9–18 years (females)	80–110	2.5–3.0		

Vitamins and Minerals
- Routine Supplementation
- Multivitamins
  - 0–1 year: 0.6 ml bid water miscible
  - 1–18 years: 0.6 ml water miscible or chewable tablet bid
- Vitamin E
  - Asymptomatic patients: 5–10 mg/kg up to 300 mg/day
  - Symptomatic patients with severe muscle cramps: 5–10 mg/kg bid until remission
- Vitamin K
  - Infants to 1 year with prolonged prothrombin time, active bleeding, liver cirrhosis: 5 mg 1–5 times per week
- Vitamin A
  - Patients with below normal levels
  - Children weighing 20 kg or less: 1250 IU per day Aquasol A
  - Children weighing more than 20 kg: 2500 IU per day Aquasol A
- Sodium chloride
  - Varies depending on amount of sweat, exercise, temperature increases: 0.5–2.0 g tid NaCl given in addition to salt in the diet.

Additional Supplementation
- Zinc
  - 15 mg/day elemental zinc or 75 mg/day zinc sulfate
- Iron
  - Infants: 1–2 mg/kg/day
  - Children: 10–18 mg/day elemental iron or 50–100 mg/day ferrous sulfate
- Selenium
  - 0.05–0.2 mg/day elemental selenium or 0.5 mg/day sodium selenium sulfate
- Vitamin B_{12}
  - 0.1 μg/day or larger amounts with deficiency states
- Folic acid as recommended for age.
- Linoleic acid
  - Essential fatty acid intake should make up 3–5% of caloric intake

[1]Reproduced with permission from Howard RB, Winter HS (eds): *Nutrition and Feeding of Infants and Toddlers*. Boston, Little, Brown & Co., 1984.

No adverse side effects were noted. This observation will undoubtedly stimulate a search for the best anti-inflammatory drugs to use in this condition and to identify the individuals most likely to benefit.

Enzyme replacement therapy can be achieved by use of tablets, capsules, or microspheres. The highest lipase activity is in Ilozyme, followed by Cotazym and Pancrease. Viokase has somewhat less. Enzyme replacement can be monitored by measurements of fecal fat and patient tolerance. Antacids with meals sometimes improve tolerance.

Late Complications

As the life-span of individuals with CF has increased, late complications have become a greater problem. In particular, massive hemoptysis may occur as the result of chronic enlargement of bronchial collateral arteries.

Hemoptysis occurs mostly in teenagers or in those in their 20s. Bleeding may be precipitated by cough, but can occur during sleep. Although the initial episode is sometimes fatal, the condition is more likely to subside, only to recur later. Hemoptysis is most likely to occur during a pulmonary exacerbation. Occasionally the patient may feel an unusual sensation near the site of bleeding and can even suggest which lobe is involved. A bubbling or gurgling sensation with localized warmth may precede the event (Fig. 5.11*A* and *B*). It must be differentiated from bleeding from esophageal varices.

Management requires immediate replacement of lost blood, correction of any clotting defect, and angiography to identify the site of hemorrhage. Insertion of pledgets can arrest bleeding. In a series of 25 patients seen over 9 years at The Children's Hospital in Boston, bleeding stopped after bronchial artery embolization. However, half the patients had a recurrence within 32 months (Sweezey and Fellows, 1986).

Pneumothorax. As individuals with CF survive longer they become more prone to pneumothorax. During the period January 1969–1981 in The Children's Hospital, Boston, among 3,340 admissions of patients with CF, 150 were for management of pneumothorax. In the study of McLaughlin et al, 67 patients experienced 170 pneumothoraces during that period. No consensus exists on the management of these painful (and sometimes fatal) episodes. Recurrence rates are high after needle aspiration, trochar thoracotomy and sclerosis with tetracycline or silver nitrate. The best results were with quinacrine sclerosis, and if that failed, partial pleurectomy. No recurrences were reported after partial pleurectomy (McLaughlin et al, 1982).

The frequency of meconium-ileus equivalent increases in the older patient population. Dietary man-

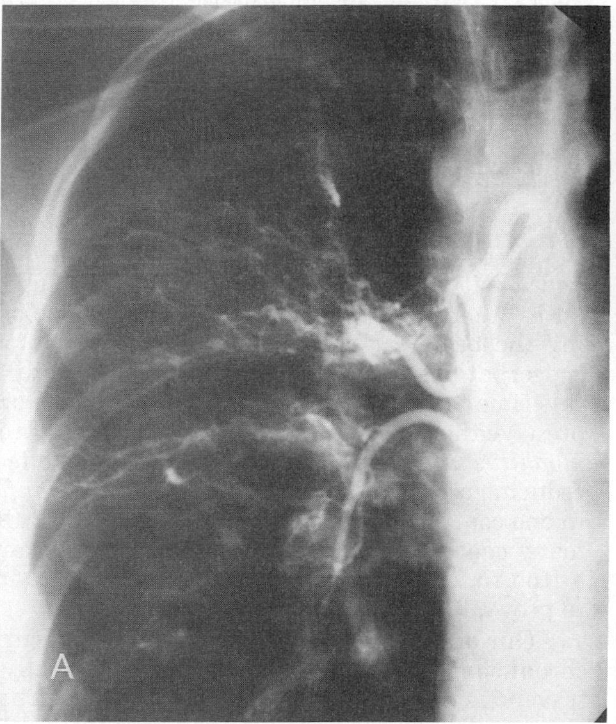

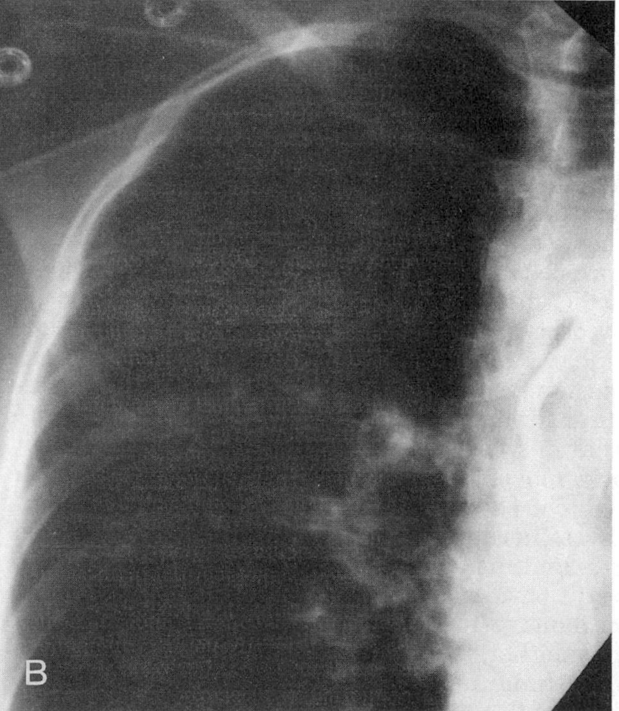

Figure 5.11.A. Selective bronchial arteriograph in this patient with cystic fibrosis and hemoptysis shows hypertrophy of the vessels supplying right upper lung. These vessels were embolized with particles of Gelfoam and the patient's hemoptysis stopped. **B.** Chronic inflammation in the lungs appears to stimulate development of bronchial, intercostal, and pleural collaterals. These thin-walled vessels may bleed with quite dramatic hemoptysis ensuing. Often, patients are able to localize their bleeding to right or left hemithorax; plain radiographs of the chest are rarely helpful in localizing the site of bleeding. Films courtesy of K. Fellows, M.D.

agement, mucolytic agents orally and ultimately enemas and lavage may be required (Cleghorn et al, 1986).

Cor pulmonale is seen with increasing frequency as the patients live longer. When right-sided heart failure ensues, the prognosis is poor. The question of treatment is difficult. Digitalis is not beneficial and vasodilators do not reduce pulmonary hypertension. The only known effective therapeutic intervention is to increase inspired oxygen to 30–50% (Geggel et al, 1985). However early use of oxygen in patients with significant hypoxemia does not appear to affect mortality or rate of progression of disease (Zinman et al, 1987).

Amyloidosis is a severe complication, reported in a total of nine patients, mostly in their 20s. Proteinuria, edema, hepatosplenomegaly, and renal failure after some months of presentation were most common (Castile et al, 1985).

Acute deterioration in pulmonary function has been associated with the development of allergic bronchopulmonary aspergillosis.

CONTROVERSY

Mist therapy, once the mainstay of pulmonary therapy, is no longer advocated because of failure to show benefit in prospective controlled trials, and the possibility that water droplets may promote bronchospasm. Contamination of equipment with opportunistic organisms is a persistent concern. When children require oxygen, it is usually delivered by nasal cannula. The generation of mist, especially by ultrasound, is contraindicated.

The adverse effects of inhalation of ultrasonically nebulized distilled water ("fog") on normal lungs has been documented by Borland et al (1985). An aerosol of water labeled with techneticum 99 was generated by ultrasound and clearance of the isotope was measured with scintillation counters. Distilled water fogs delayed clearance by a mean value of 38%; whereas no change in clearance was found after inhalation of physiologic saline (Fig. 5.12). Thus, if medications are to be delivered by aerosol, it may be preferable to use saline as the vehicle.

Chest physiotherapy to promote clearance of infected mucus has long been advocated. During acute exacerbations, especially among debilitated patients, it promotes movement of sputum and benefit has been documented. The question arises as to the merit of routine physiotherapy at home. One widely used regimen requires 2 minutes of percussion and vibration in each of 11 positions. An evaluation of sputum expectorated and pulmonary function was undertaken before and after physiotherapy and before and after 10 minutes of deep breathing and vigorous coughing. There was no clear benefit from physiotherapy over cough alone. For these reasons, it seems wise to individualize use of physiotherapy, and consider the alternative of vigorous coughing (de Boeck et al, 1984).

Antibiotic prophylaxis. If an infant is identified as having CF in the absence of any pulmonary symptoms, we do not routinely recommend antibiotic prophylaxis. However, most children are diagnosed be-

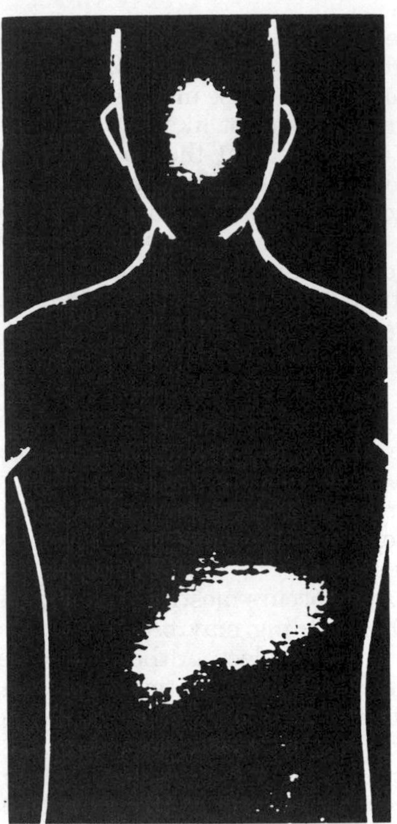

Figure 5.12. Scan of patient with cystic fibrosis after 1 hour of breathing a radioaerosol from a mist tent. Patients who are nose breathers accumulate aerosal in the nares and nasopharynx and then swallow it. Very little enters the lungs. Evidence such as this led to the abandonment of routine nightly mist tent therapy for cystic fibrosis. Data of Bau et al: *Pediatrics* 48:605, 1971.

symptoms, we do not routinely recommend antibiotic prophylaxis. However, most children are diagnosed be-
cause of pulmonary infection and most physicians treat the current infection on the basis of sputum culture and sensitivity tests. The use of continued suppressive antibiotic therapy is undertaken in the hope of reducing the bacterial burden and the frequency of acute exacerbations. Since no oral antibiotics available at this time are effective against *Pseudomonas*, oral suppressive therapy is directed against *S. aureus* and *Haemophilus influenzae*. Cephalexin was found effective in reducing colonization with *S. aureus* and *H. influenzae* in one controlled trial (Loening-Baucke et al, 1979). In many centers oral antibiotics are used intermittently at the time of respiratory tract infections in an effort to prevent colonization with *S. aureus*.

Our practice is to admit patients with recurrent or chronic pneumonias to the hospital periodically for intravenous therapy with anti-*Pseudomonas* drugs such as ticarcillin and tobramycin, and with intensive physical therapy. If the organisms are resistant to those drugs, ceftazidime or imipenem are sometimes effective (in Boston in 1987). These admissions, termed "clean outs", are undertaken empirically to try to reduce the degree of chronic infection. When acute exacerbations occur, intravenous treatment is undertaken based on drug sensitivities, for 14 days or until pulmonary function returns to baseline. A number of cephalosporin derivatives and oral quinolones are available in the event of ticarcillin and tobramycin resistance to *Pseudomonas* (currently found in 23% of our patients).

We are concerned about increasing drug resistance, toxicity, and cost of these unproven approaches to management. Admittedly, many times the patients feel better after hospitalization (or more recently after home intravenous therapy) (Donati et al, 1987). It is distressing that sputum concentrations of bacteria return to pretreatment levels on an average of 4 weeks after discharge (Table 5.10).

Prognosis

Overall, the outlook for survival is related to the severity of the pulmonary lesion. Severely affected patients may die in the first year of life. When the response to treatment is good, more than 90% of these patients can expect to live at least 18 years. Overall, cumulative survival is about 78% at 20 years of age. The mean survival was over 4 years in 1950 and 19 years in 1976. At least one CF patient is over 60 years in 1988. Heart-lung transplants have been successful for at least 2 years in a few patients.

Prevention

SCREENING

Screening for evidence of the disease in the newborn period is advocated by some, but not all pediatricians. Since the basic defect is unknown, screening depends on detection of manifest disease, such as excess albumin in meconium or elevated serum trypsin levels (Wilcken et al, 1983). Both false-positive and false-negative findings are sufficiently common to discourage wide use of these tests. The controversy surrounds the value of early detection of the disease. Proponents argue that optimal nutrition and early treatment of infection may lessen lung damage and improve the quality of life. We do not screen all infants for CF, but screen all siblings of affected individuals with a sweat test. In some countries routine screening for elevated immunoreactive trypsin in dried blood spots is routine.

Prenatal diagnosis by detection of gene markers is now possible as well as by analysis of intestinal enzymes in the amniotic fluid at 16–18 weeks' gestation. If blood is available from both parents and from the patient, siblings may be studied to determine whether or not they carry the gene.

REFERENCES

Auerbach H, Williams M, Kirkpatrick JA, et al: Alternate-day prednisone reduces morbidity and improves pulmonary function in cystic fibrosis. *Lancet* 2:686, 1985.

Borland C, Chamberlain A, Barber B, et al: Pulmonary epithelial permeability after inhaling saline, distilled water "fog" and cold air. *Chest* 87:373, 1985.

Braude, S, Kennedy H, Hodson M, et al: Hypertrophic osteoarthropathy in cystic fibrosis. *Br Med J* 288:822, 1984.

Bye AME, Muller DPR, Wilson J, et al: Symptomatic vitamin E deficiency in cystic fibrosis. *Arch Dis Child* 60:162, 1985.

Castile R, Schwachman H, Travis W, et al: Amyloidosis as a complication of cystic fibrosis. *Am J Dis Child* 139:728, 1985.

Chang N, Levison H, Cunningham K, et al: An evaluation of nightly mist therapy for patients with cystic fibrosis. *Am Rev Respir Dis* 107:672, 1973.

Cleghorn GI, Stringer DA, Forstner GG, et al: Treatment of distal intestinal obstruction syndrome in cystic fibrosis with a balanced intestinal lavage solution. *Lancet* 1:8, 1986.

de Boeck C, Zinman R: Cough versus chest physiotherapy: A comparison of acute effects on pulmonary function in patients with cystic fibrosis. *Am Rev Respir Dis* 129:182, 1984.

Di Sant'Agnese, PA, David PB: Research in cystic fibrosis. *N Engl J Med* 295:481, 534, 597, 1976.

Dolan TF Jr: Microangiopathy in a young adult with cystic fibrosis and diabetes mellitus. Letter. *N Engl J Med* 314:991, 1986.

Table 5.10
Antibiotic Regimens for Cystic Fibrosis

Chronic Suppressive Antibiotic Therapy

Aim: To reduce pulmonary bacterial burden, retard pulmonary damage, and to decrease the frequency of acute pulmonary exacerbations requiring hospitalization. Therapy directed primarily against *S. aureus* and *H. influenzae*.

Trimethoprim, 10–20 mg/kg/day and sulfamethoxazole, 50–100 mg/kg/day orally in 2–3 divided doses
and Cephalexin, 25–50 mg/kg/day orally in 3–4 divided doses
or Dicloxacillin, 25–50 mg/kg/day orally in 3–4 divided doses

Acute Pulmonary Exacerbation

Aim: Relief of the symptoms of acute pulmonary exacerbation. Treatment is directed against the predominant pathogens isolated from sputum, usually *Pseudomonas aeruginosa* although *S. aureus* and *Enterobacteriaceae* can also be found. Standard therapy employs the combination of an aminoglycoside and an anti-pseudomonal β-lactam selected on the basis of antibiotic susceptibility testing. The pharmacokinetics of aminoglycosides and most β-lactam antibiotics are altered in patients with cystic fibrosis requiring higher dosages to achieve therapeutic serum levels.

Tobramycin, 240 mg/m^2/day intravenously in 4 divided doses *with* Mezlocillin, 500 mg/kg/day intravenously in 6 divided doses
or Azlocillin, 450 mg/kg/day intravenously in 6 divided doses
or Ticarcillin, 500 mg/kg/day intravenously in 6 divided doses
or Ceftazidime, 150 mg/kg/day intravenously in 3 divided doses
or Cefoperazone, 150 mg/kg/day intravenously in 3 divided doses
or Timentin, 500 mg/kg/day (based upon ticarcillin content) intravenously in 6 divided doses if *S. aureus* and *P. aeruginosa* are isolated. Otherwise, Oxacillin, 250 mg/kg/day intravenously in 6 divided doses in addition to above.

[1]Courtesy of Dr. William Gerson.

Donati MA, Guenette G, Auerbach H: Prospective controlled study of home therapy of cystic fibrosis pulmonary disease. *J Pediatr* 111:28, 1987.
Frizzell RA, Rechkemmer G, Shoemaker RL: Altered regulation of airway epithelial cell chloride channels in cystic fibrosis. *Science* 233:558, 1986.
Geggel RL, Dozor AJ, Fyler DC, et al: Effect of vasodilators at rest and during exercise in young adults with cystic fibrosis and chronic cor pulmonale. *Am Rev Respir Dis* 131:531, 1985.
Gibson LE, Cooke RE: A test for concentration of electrolytes in sweat in cystic fibrosis of the pancreas utilizing pilocarpine iontophoresis. *Pediatrics* 23:545, 1959.
Goldmann D, Klinger JD: *Pseudomonas cepacia:* Biology, mechanisms of virulence, epidemiology. *J Pediatr* 108(2):806, 1986.
Gosden C, Gosden JR: Fetal abnormalities in cystic fibrosis suggest a deficiency in proteolysis of cholecystokinin. *Lancet* 2:541, 1984.
Holsclaw DS, Grand RJ, Shwachman H: Massive hemoptysis in cystic fibrosis. *J Pediatr* 76:829, 1970.
Knowlton RG, Cohen-Haguenauer O, et al: A polymorphic DNA marker linked to cystic fibrosis is located on chromosome 7. *Nature* 318:380, 1985.
Kolata G: A new approach to cystic fibrosis. *Science* 228:167, 1985.
Kopelman H, Durie P, Gaskin K, et al: Pancreatic fluid secretion and protein hyperconcentration in cystic fibrosis. *N Engl J Med* 312:329, 1985.
Landon C, Rosenfeld RG: Short stature and pubertal delay in male adolescents with cystic fibrosis. *Am J Dis Child* 138:388, 1984.
Loening-Baucke VA, Mischler E, Myers MG: A placebo controlled trial of cephalexin therapy in the ambulatory management of patients with cystic fibrosis. *J Pediatr* 95:630, 1979.
MacLusky I, McLaughlin FJ, Levison H: Cystic Fibrosis Part I. *Curr Probl Pediatr* 15:4, 1985.
Matthews WJ, Williams M, Oliphint B, et al: Hypogammaglobulinemia in patients with cystic fibrosis. *N Engl J Med* 302:245, 1980.
McLaughlin FJ: Clinical and bacteriological responses to three antibiotic regimens for acute exacerbations of cystic fibrosis: Ticarcillin-tobramycin, azlocillin-tobramycin and azlocillin-placebo. *J Infect Dis* 147:559, 1983.
McLaughlin FJ, Matthews WJ, Strieder DG, et al: Pneumothorax in cystic fibrosis. Management and outcome. *J Pediatr* 100:863, 1982.
Mearns MB, et al: Bacterial flora of the respiratory tract in patients with cystic fibrosis 1950–71. *Arch Dis Child* 47:902, 1971.
Moellering RC: Ceftazidime: A new broad spectrum cephalosporin. *Pediatr Infect Dis* 4:390, 1985.
Moss RB, Hsu YP, Lewiston NJ, et al: Association of systemic immune complexes complement activation and antibodies to *Pseudomonas aeroginosa* lipopolysaccharide and exotoxin A with mortality in cystic fibrosis. *Am Rev Respir Dis* 133:648, 1986.
Motoyama EK, Gibson LE, Zigas CJ: Evaluation of mist tent therapy in cystic fibrosis using maximum expiratory flow volume curve. *Pediatrics* 50:299, 1972.
Parsons HG, Beaudry P, Pencharz PB: The effect of nutritional rehabilitation on whole body protein metabolism of children with cystic fibrosis. *Pediatr Res* 19:189, 1985.
Piedra P, Ogra PL: Immunologic aspects of surface infections in the lung. *J Pediatr* 108:817, 1986.
Pier GB: Pulmonary disease associated with *Pseudomonas aeruginosa* in cystic fibrosis: Current status of host-bacterium interaction. *J Infect Dis* 151:575, 1985.
Roy CC (ed): The pancreas in cystic fibrosis. *J Pediatr Gastroenterol Nutr* 3:Suppl 1, 1984.
Shwachman H: Cystic fibrosis. In *Current Problems in Pediatrics.* Vol VIII. Chicago. Year Book Medical Publishers, 1978.
Stern RC, Boat TF, Doershuk CF: Obstructive azoospermia as a diagnostic criterion for the cystic fibrosis syndrome. *Lancet* 1:1401, 1982a.
Stern RC, Boat TE, Wood RE, et al: Treatment and prognosis of nasal polyps in cystic fibrosis. *Am J Dis Chil* 136:1067, 1982b.
Sweezey NB, Fellows KE: Embolization of bronchial arteries for severe hemoptysis in cystic fibrosis. *Am Rev Respir Dir* 133:A248, 1986.
Tablan OC, Chorba TL, Schidlow DV, et al: *Pseudomonas cepacia* colonization in patients with cystic fibrosis. *J Pediatr* 107:382, 1985.
Taussig LM (ed): *Cystic Fibrosis.* New York, Thieme-Stratton Inc, 1984.
Thomassen MJ, Demko CA, Klinger JD, et a: *Pseudomonas cepacia* colonization among patients with cystic fibrosis. A new opportunist. *Am Rev Respir Dis* 131:791, 1985.
Tsui LC, Buchwald M, et al: Cystic fibrosis locus defined by a genetically linked polymorphic DNA marker. *Science* 230: 1054, 1985.
Wang, EEL, Prober CG, Manson B, et al: Association of respiratory viral infections with pulmonary deterioration in patients with cystic fibrosis. *N Engl J Med* 311:1653, 1984.
Wilcken B, Brown ARD, Urwin R, et al: Cystic fibrosis screening by dried blood spot trypsin assay: Results in 75,000 newborn infants. *J Pediatr* 102:383, 1983.
Welsh MJ: An apical-membrane chloride channel in human tracheal epithelium. *Science* 232:1648, 1986.
Wood RE, Boat TF, Doershuk CF: State of the art cystic fibrosis. *Am Rev Respir Dis* 113:833, 1976.
Zinman R, Corey M, Coates AL, et al: Noctornal oxygen therapy in the treatment of cystic fibrosis. *Am Rev Respir Dis* 135:A287, 1987.

OVERDISTENTION (RESPIRATORY AIRSPACE ENLARGEMENT AND EMPHYSEMA)

The National Heart, Lung, Blood Institute, Division of Lung Diseases suggested the following definitions (*Am Rev Respir Dis* 132:182, 1985):

"Respiratory airspace enlargement is defined as an increase in airspace size as compared with the airspace of normal lungs. The term applies to all varieties of airspace enlargement distal to the terminal bronchioles whether occurring with or without fibrosis or destruction."

"Emphysema is defined as a condition of the lung characterized by abnormal permanent enlargement of airspaces distal to the terminal bronchioles, accompanied by the destruction of their walls, and without obvious fibrosis."

Three anatomic subtypes of emphysema are recognized, mainly in adults; these are: centriacinar emphysema, panacinar emphysema, and distal acinar emphysema. Centriacinar type is mostly associated with cigarette smoking, panacinar can occur in smokers, but also in homozygous α-1-protease inhibitor deficiency; distal acinar emphysema may be regional and is associated with bullae and spontaneous pneumothorax in young adults.

Congenital Lobar Emphysema

Congenital lobar emphysema is rare, but the incidence is not known. About 10% of affected infants have heart disease or other malformations.

Natural History

One lobe, usually an upper one, but occasionally the right middle lobe, is overdistended. In some infants, the overdistention can progress from the initiation of air-breathing at birth, and if not recognized as a cause of severe respiratory distress, can be fatal. In other instances, overdistention is not progressive, and may be unrecognized until a chest radiograph is obtained for other reasons at a later age.

Sometimes lesions are identified at operation or autopsy that account for the overdistention. They include redundant bronchial mucosa, deficient bronchial cartilage, bronchiogenic cysts, or even mucous plugs. Extrabronchial compression by aberrant vessels or the ductus arteriosus can partially obstruct a bronchus.

Diagnosis

Clinical signs are decreased air exchange over the distended lobe and, occasionally, an expiratory wheeze. Mediastinal shift depends on the degree of overdistention.

Care must be taken to ascertain whether the overdistention is primary, or secondary to atelectasis elsewhere. If it is compensatory, breath sounds will be accentuated over the distended lobe; if primary, they will be decreased.

Radiographs are invaluable in defining the location and progression or diminution in the lesion, and respiratory—expiratory films can elucidate whether the affected region deflates. Air trapping would favor a primary process (Fig. 5.13*A* and *B*).

Treatment

If respiratory distress is severe, endoscopy with preparation for immediate surgical resection is urgent, and may be lifesaving. If the infant is asymptomatic, it is possible to observe him for some weeks, and even years, inasmuch as overdistended lobes have been found to return to normal volume (Roghair, 1972; Eigen et al, 1976).

Prognosis

In general, the infants do well after resection. DeMuth and Sloan (1966) found residual symptoms in two of six children studied 5–14 years after resection. These findings suggest the disease is not always restricted to the overdistended lobe (Fig. 5.14). Lobar resection in infants under age 3 years was followed by compensation of volume loss by ages 8–30 years in the study of McBride et al (1980). Our second forced expiratory volumes were reduced below 85% of total in 14 out of 15 patients.

Lobar Overdistention

Bronchial Agenesis

When a lobar or segmental bronchus is atretic, the distal lung may be ventilated by collateral pathways. Air exit may be impeded and lobar emphysema results. This rare lesion has a characteristic radiograph, with the atretic bronchus opaque from an occluding mucous plug. The left upper lobe is most often affected (Fig. 5.15*A* and *B*).

The lesions are usually asymptomatic, and may not be found until a routine chest radiograph is obtained later in life (Fig. 5.16*A* and *B*). Cystic changes and recurrent pneumonias occur in some individuals.

In a review of 56 cases, Jederlinic et al (1987) report the lesion has been seen in stillborn infants, and in a 44-year-old female. Seventy-two percent of the patients had surgery for a variety of indications, but rarely for recurrent pneumonia.

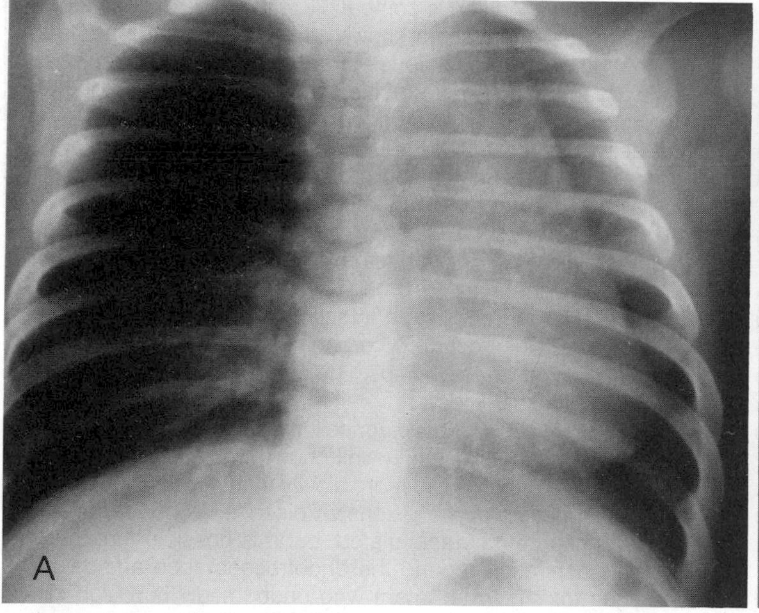

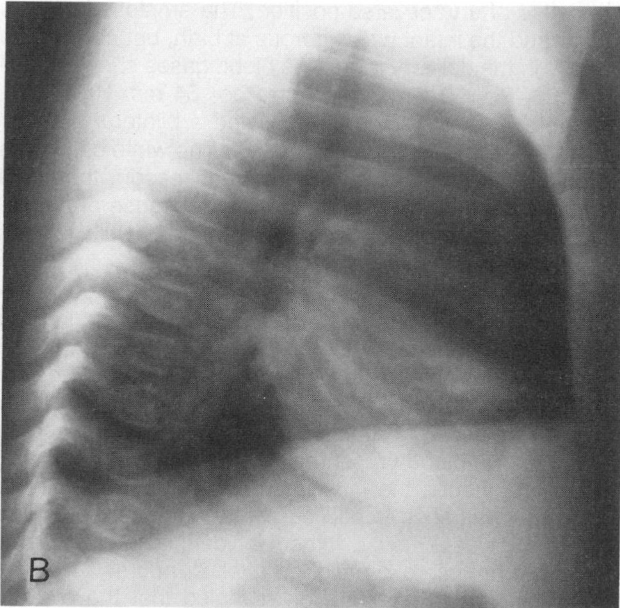

Figure 5.13.A and **B.** A 3-month-old boy had a 3-week history of progressively worsening cough and wheezing which failed to respond to bronchodilators. The chest films **(A** and **B)** show a hyperlucent right upper lobe which is acting as a mass, depressing the minor fissure, and causing atelectasis in the lower lung. There is shift of mediastinum to left and herniation of right upper lobe across midline. These findings are typical of congenital lobar emphysema which presents at this age and commonly affects upper lobes as opposed to lower lobes. Right upper lobe lobectomy was performed on this patient. The excised lobe in this child was of the overinflation type. Some cases of congenital lobar emphysema have a polyalveolar pattern, i.e., more alveoli than normal. Some cases of congenital lobar emphysema are caused by obstructing bronchogenic cysts or other masses.

TYPES OF CHILDHOOD EMPHYSEMA

	Airway number	Alveoli number	Alveoli size
Overinflation			
Compensatory	N	N	↑
Check valve	N	N *	↑
Hypoplasia	↓	↓	↑
Atresia of Bronchus	N	N *	↑
Polyalveolar Lobe	N	↑ *	N or ↑

N = normal ↑ = increased ↓ = decreased

* Alveoli do not multiply normally, so number becomes low for age.

Figure 5.14. Types of childhood emphysema. Courtesy of Dr. Lynne Reid.

Generalized Overdistention

Definition

Overdistention of all portions of the lung with or without alveolar wall destruction is considered generalized overdistention.

Epidemiology

This condition occurs as a complication of CF, acute bronchiolitis, some forms of pneumonia, and chronic asthma. It can also occur in association with congenital heart disease.

Diagnosis

The chest appears enlarged in anteroposterior diameter on radiograph. The diaphragms are flat and pushed down by overinflated lung. The auscultatory finding is a prolongation of expiration, with or without a wheeze. Air exchange appears to be reduced.

Pulmonary function tests show a delay in 1-second forced expiratory volume, a characteristic flow-volume curve, and an increase in functional residual capacity.

CASE ILLUSTRATION

A 3.2-kg white male was born after 37 weeks to a 19-year-old mother, whose pregnancy had been complicated in the second and third trimesters with urinary tract infection. The infant was delivered by elective cesarean section because of a transverse position. The amniotic fluid was clear and the infant was vigorous at birth, but noted to be dusky in the delivery room. His blood gases showed a pH of 7.23, Po_2 59 mm Hg, and a Pco_2 64 mm Hg in 40% oxygen. A chest radiograph showed a bilateral granular pattern which was hazier on the left. The white count was 35,000 with 48% polys, and, for that reason, the infant was given ampicillin and gentamicin. Because of a deteriorating Po_2 the infant was maintained in 100% oxygen throughout the subsequent course.

The major abnormalities were best delineated by serial chest radiographs which showed gradual clearing and eventual hyperlucency of the left upper lobe, with increased density in the left lower lobe and some evidence of loss of volume on the right. The infant remained critically ill and required ventilatory support and use of pressors to maintain the blood pressure.

At 48 hours, the infant had a left upper lobectomy. The lobe was seen to pop out through the incision in the chest and was removed without incident. The infant, however, did not improve and died after 72 hours.

Postmortem examination revealed that the excised lobe weighed twice as much as expected. The bronchi were patent and no obstructive lesion was evident. On section, it appeared as if there were an immense number of very small air spaces and the pulmonary arteries leading to them were more muscular than usual. The infant had necrotizing bronchitis and some hemorrhage and hyaline membrane formation in the remaining lung. No other lesions of note were found at autopsy.

COMMENT

This condition is compatible with the form of congenital lobar emphysema known as a polyalveolar lobe. It is not unusual for such lobes to appear fluid-filled or at least hazy in the first hours of life; with gradual clearing of that lung liquid an overdistended aerated lobe becomes evident. The downward course of this infant probably was related to the increasing size of that lobe through which air could enter but could exit only with difficulty.

The puzzling situation was why the infant was not improved after the lobectomy. The autopsy findings revealed a necrotizing bronchitis of considerable severity and although coexisting infection was suggested by the elevated white count, no organisms were cultured during life or postmortem. Thus, the cause of the necrotizing bronchitis is unclear.

In retrospect, this diagnosis might have been obtained earlier inasmuch as it is well known that the polyalveolar lobes clear their liquid more slowly than normal lobes. The pathogenesis of the extensive disease in the rest of the lung can only be speculated, but it is possible that there was aspiration around the endotracheal tube and/or oxygen toxicity in an infant who undoubtedly had high circulating epinephrine and cortisol levels at some stage, both of which increase pulmonary oxygen toxicity in animals (Clark and Lambertsen, 1971).

Localized airspace enlargement can occur whenever partial obstruction of an airway allows air entry but impedes air egress.

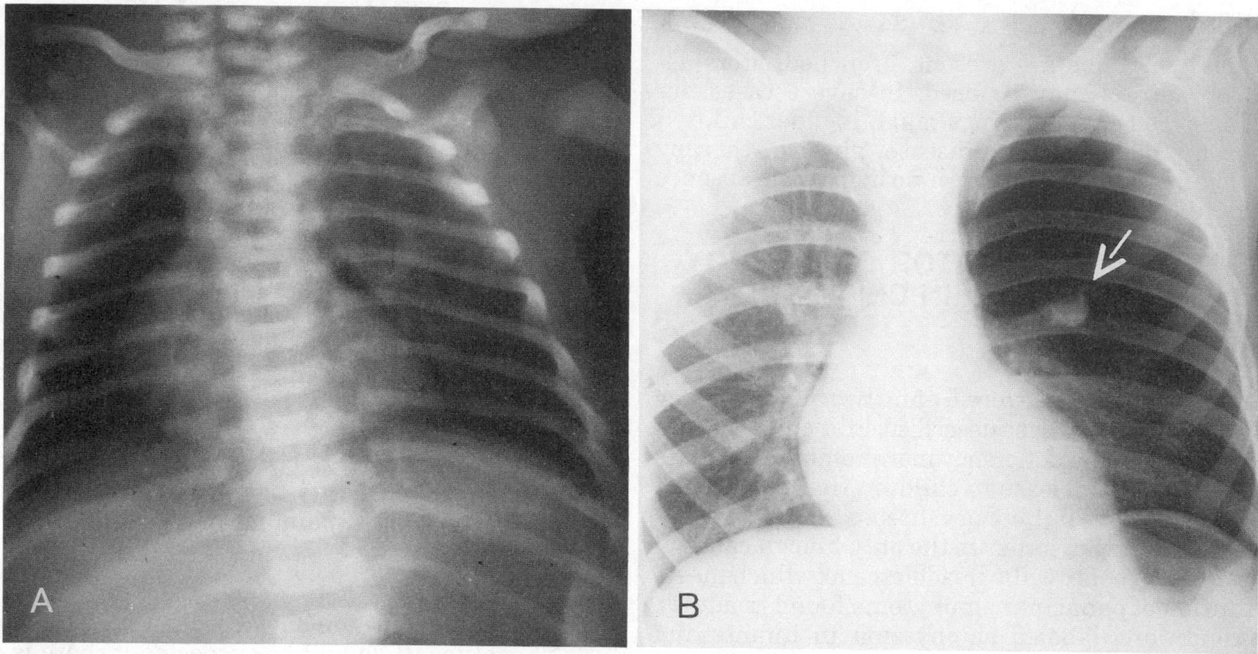

Figure 5.15.A. Atresia of the apical-posterior bronchus of the left upper lobe in a newborn presenting as haziness, presumably from delayed clearance of fetal lung liquid. **B**. 19 months later, the mucus-filled bronchus plug in the proximal part of an atretic bronchus is indicated by the *arrow*. The upper lobe is hyperinflated air entry through collateral pathways. Reproduced with permission from Avery et al: *The Lung and Its Disorders in the Newborn Infant,* 1981, p. 150.

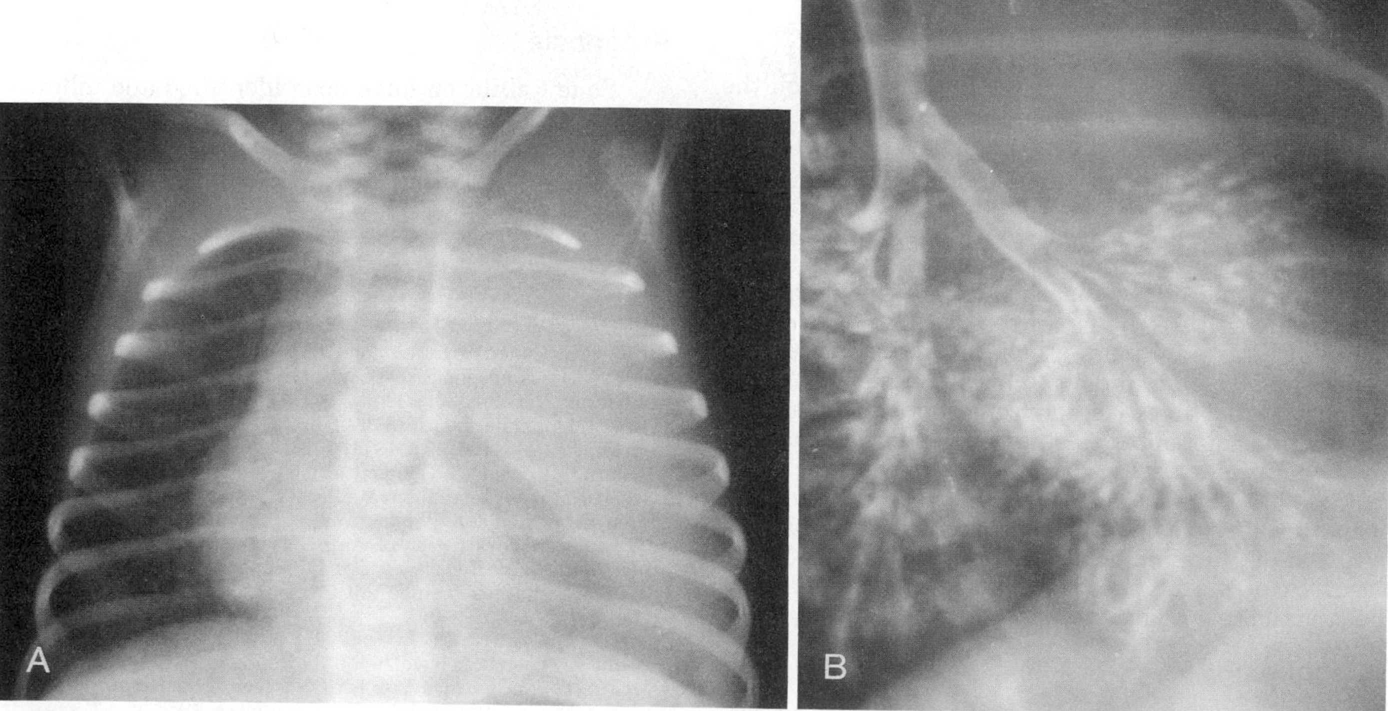

Figure 5.16.A. This radiograph is of a patient who has retained fetal lung fluid beyond a bronchial obstruction in the left upper lobe. Because the bronchus is obstructed, normal removal of fetal lung fluid is prevented. **B.** Bronchogram showed no communication of upper lobe to bronchial tree. Thoracotomy in this patient revealed an airless accessory upper lobe connected to the hilum by a pedicle which contained artery and vein but no bronchus.

Treatment

When symptoms are present, bronchodilators delivered by aerosol may be used. In severe cases, increased inspired oxygen brings relief. In older children with chronic purulent lung disease, physical therapy is beneficial, but it is of limited or no help in the absence of debris in the airway.

α-1-PROTEASE INHIBITOR DEFICIENCY (A1-P_i α_1-ANTITRYPSIN DEFICIENCY)

Definition

The association of severe α_1-antitrypsin deficiency and emphysema was first described in a child by Talamo et al (1971). The deficiency more commonly causes a progressive liver disease in children that can coexist with the obstructive pulmonary disease. Strictly speaking this hereditary disorder is the only known cause of disruption of alveolar walls in adolescence which meets the definition of panacinar emphysema found in adults. Other conditions labeled emphysema in infants and children are much more likely to be overdistention, which implies reversibility with removal of obstruction.

Basic Science

α_1-Antitrypsin is one of several well-characterized protease inhibitors in human serum. Their major function is to inhibit tissue enzymes such as elastases that are normally released from polymorphonuclear leukocytes.

α_1-Antitrypsin is synthesized in the liver and secreted into the circulation where it has a half-life of 4–6 days. It has been found in the cytoplasm and on the surface of pulminary alveolar macrophages, platelet granules and along the airway lining at the level of the terminal bronchiole. It is an acute phase reactant whose concentration may double or triple with acute inflammatory processes. Synthesis by human mononuclear cells and macrophages has been shown by Perlmutter et al (1985) and allows identification of the phenotype from tissue culture.

α-1-Protease inhibitor is believed to protect the lung from proteolytic breakdown, chiefly by elastase. P_iZZ patients with severe emphysema have measurable amounts of neutrophil elastase in their bronchoalveolar lavage fluid.

The biochemical basis for A1-P_i deficiency in P_iZZ phenotypes is a point mutation resulting in the substitution of glutamic acid for lysine at position 342 in the DNA of the Z gene. How this substitution affects the function of the mutant A1-P_i is not known.

Epidemiology

Although very rare, the condition is often unsuspected and probably under-reported. It is inherited through an autosomal recessive trait. The system of nomenclature is P_i (for protease inhibitor) and normal individuals are P_iMM phenotype; those with severe deficiency are P_iZZ. Heterozygotes P_iMZ have intermediate levels of α_1-antitrypsin, but are not at risk of lung disease (Bruce et al, 1984).

In the Caucasian population, 90% are P_iMM, 2–3% P_iMZ. The incidence of P_iZZ is 1/3000–6000 live births. Of individuals with severe functional deficiency, 90% will eventually develop emphysema.

Natural History

Most individuals are asymptomatic until the end of the third decade, when the gradual increase in dyspnea is noted. Chest radiographs may show hyperaeration especially at the lung bases, which eventually become underperfused. The course is progressive and complicated by infection, bronchiectasis, and emphysema. Digital clubbing occurs in severe cases.

Screening of infants has demonstrated an association with prolonged jaundice (Sveger, 1976).

Diagnosis

Diagnosis depends on laboratory identification of the phenotype. It should be suspected if there is a positive family history of emphysema in any child with respiratory symptoms where another diagnosis is not established, or when liver disease of unknown origin is present.

Treatment

Infusions of α_1-antitrypsin can reverse the biochemical abnormalities. The long-term benefit awaits further evaluation (Wewers et al, 1987).

Prognosis

So few children have been identified and followed that no generalizations about the course of the disease would be useful. Clearly homozygous individuals should avoid smoking and air pollution, which could precipitate lung disease.

REFERENCES

Bruce RM, Cohen BH, Diamond EL, et al: Collaborative study to assess risk of lung disease in P_iMZ phenotype subjects. *Am Rev Respir Dis* 130:386, 1984.

Clark JM, Lambertsen CJ: Pulmonary oxygen toxicity: A review. Pharmacol Rev 23:37, 1971.

DeMuth GR, Sloan H: Congenital lobar emphysema: Long-term effects and sequelae in treated cases. *Surgery* 59:601, 1966.

Eigen H, Lemen RJ, Waring WW: Congenital lobar emphysema: Long-term evaluation of surgically and conservatively treated children. *Am Rev Respir Dis* 113:823, 1976.

Eriksson S: Studies in alpha$_1$antitrypsin deficiency. *Acta Med Scand* 117:432, 1965.

Griscom TN, Harris GBC, Wohl ME, et al: Fluid filled lung due to airway obstruction in the newborn. *Pediatrics* 43:383, 1969.

Kendig EL Jr, Chernick V (eds): *Disorders of the Respiratory Tract in Children.* Philadelphia, WB Saunders, 1983.

McBride JT, Wohl MEB, Strieder DJ, et al: Lung growth and airway function after lobectomy in infancy for congenital lobar emphysema. *J Clin Invest* 66:962, 1980.

Morse JO: Alpha-1-antitrypsin deficiency. *N Engl J Med* 299:1049, 1978.

Perlmutter DH, Cole FS, Killbridge P, et al: Expression of the $\alpha_1$proteinase inhibitor gene in human monocytes and macrophages. *Proc Natl Acad Sci* 82:795, 1985.
Roghair GD: Non-operative management of lobar emphysema: Long-term followup. *Radiology* 107:125, 1972.
Schuster SR, Harris GBC, Williams AJ, et al: Bronchial atresia: A recognizable entity in the pediatric age group. *J Pediatr Surg* 13:682, 1978.
Sveger, T: Liver disease in alpha$_1$antitrypsin deficiency detected by screening 200,000 infants. *N Engl J Med* 294:1316, 1976.
Talamo RC, Levison H, Lynch MJ, et al: Symptomatic pulmonary emphysema in childhood associated with hereditary alpha-1-antitrypsin and elastase inhibitor deficiency. *J Pediatr* 79:20, 1971.
Wewers MD, Casolaro A, Sellers SE, et al: Replacement therapy for alpha$_1$-antitrypsin deficiency associated with emphysema. *N Engl J Med* 316:1055, 1987.

Infiltrative Disorders 4

Fibrosing Alveolitis (Honeycomb Lung, Hamman-Rich Syndrome)

Definition

One response of the lung to injury of various sorts is a fibrosing alveolitis, which is usually progressive and may terminate in respiratory failure. This heterogeneous group of disorders can result from more than 100 agents, although in two-thirds of the cases, no cause is identified (Crystal et al, 1984).

Nomenclature is confusing, because the same symptom complex has been designated Hamman-Rich syndrome since their description of four patients with acute progressive dyspnea died within 6 months (1944). Subsequently, older patients with chronic interstitial fibrosis have lived longer; the disorder is not always progressive or fatal. It has been called chronic interstitial pneumonia, idiopathic pulmonary fibrosis, fibrosing alveolitis, and cryptogenic fibrosing alveolitis (Scadding, 1978).

Basic Science

The initial lesion in interstitial pulmonary disease is an alveolitis with an accumulation of inflammatory cells. The associated disorder, when known, is characterized by distinct types of infiltrate. For example, sarcoidosis is distinguished by activated lymphocytes, with a marked increase in the ratio of helper to suppressor T cells. This mononuclear inflammatory response precedes granuloma formation and suggests that pulmonary manifestations may be the result of an overactive immune system. In histiocytosis X, the cells are mostly mononuclear phagocytes, thought to be closely related to Langerhans' cells in normal skin. The reaction to these cells in the lung is alveolitis, bronchiolitis, and obliteration of capillaries. Idiopathic pulmonary fibrosis is characterized in its initial stages by the presence of neutrophils and macrophages. The macrophages release fibronectin, which is chemotactic for fibroblasts. Fibroblasts proliferate and make type I collagen, which produces the increase in interstitium.

Epidemiology

The prevalence of chronic interstitial pneumonia depends on the underlying disease. In general, all forms of progressive alveolitis are rare. Those of unknown etiology occur in 5–10 cases/100,000 population. The disorders with which alveolitis is associated include environmental causes such as radiation, and some chemotherapeutic agents to treat cancer. Some forms of interstitial pneumonia show deposition of immunoglobulin in the lung and circulating immune complexes, as in rheumatoid arthritis, and systemic lupus erythematosus. Interstitial pneumonia occasionally complicates sarcoidosis and neurofibromatosis. In about 5% of patients it appears in an autosomal dominant form, which can present in infancy. It can complicate some cases of histiocytosis X and Weber-Christian disease.

Natural History

The onset may be as early as 4 months, but most commonly is in late adolescence or young adults. Anorexia, dyspnea, fatigue, and pleuritic pain may have an insidious onset, and any one can be the presenting symptom. Hemoptysis and spontaneous pneumothorax may also be the first indication of trouble. The course is variable, like most of the associated underlying conditions.

Diagnosis

Physical examination may be normal or may disclose rapid shallow breathing and end-inspiratory rales. Later, hypoxemia and clubbing occur. Classically, chest radiographs show a diffuse reticulonodular infiltrate, and later, small cystic lesions appear (Walters et al, 1986). There are no definitive laboratory studies. Elevated sedimentation rates and hypergammaglobulinemia may be present. Pulmonary function studies show a reduction in all lung volumes, diminished compliance, and reduced diffusing capacity. Blood gases show a low Po_2 and low Pco_2 until late in the disease. Open lung biopsy is the best approach to diagnosis.

Another important diagnostic tool to distinguish persistent infiltrative disorders is bronchoalveolar lavage, introduced by Reynolds and Newball (1974). Examination of the cells in the lavage provides some guides to etiology and therapy.

Treatment

No definitive treatment is known, but high doses of prednisone, monitored by serial pulmonary function tests is worth a trial. All other approaches to therapy, such as penicillamine await confirmation of efficacy by randomized trials.

Prognosis

The course is unpredictable, but usually is slowly progressive.

Desquamative Histiocytic Interstitial Pneumonia (DIP)

Definition

This form of interstitial pneumonia has pathognomonic histologic features and, in contrast to fibrosing alveolitis, is potentially reversible.

Epidemiology

Although this is a very rare disorder, it has been detected as early as 2½ weeks of age. It is also seen in adults, but occurs only about 25% as often as fibrosing alveolitis.

Natural History

The cause is unknown. The onset often follows an acute respiratory infection and may have a viral etiology. The clinical features are the same as those in fibrosing alveolis. A mild fever may occur. Radiographs may be normal or show haziness radiating from the hila, described as a ground-glass appearance. DIP has been reported in children with inflammatory bowel disease on long-term sulfasalazine therapy (Teague et al, 1985).

Diagnosis

Open lung biopsy is preferred by pathologists who report a proliferation of type II cells that line the alveoli and give a glandular appearance to the lung. The cells may lie free in the air spaces with macrophages. A mild interstitial infiltrate with lymphocytes, plasma cells, and eosinophils is common. The alveolar walls are fibrotic.

No other laboratory tests are helpful, except pulmonary function studies to follow the course of disease and response to therapy. Some patients have a mild eosinophilia.

Treatment

Corticosteroids may be of great benefit or have no effect at all. As many as 20% of patients improve without treatment; nearly 60% improve with it (Carrington et al, 1978).

Lymphoid Interstitial Pneumonia

Definition

Lymphoid interstitial pneumonia (LIP) is one of the rare chronic interstitial pneumonias of unknown etiology that may be familial. It is found in children

CASE ILLUSTRATION

An infant of Moroccan origin presented at age 1 month with cough and cyanosis. He had a respiratory rate of 45/min with nasal flaring. In other respects he seemed well. All laboratory studies were normal except for a Po_2 of 50 torr in room air, and a chest radiograph which revealed interstitial pneumonia. Treatment with ampicillin was started. No pathogens were isolated from deep tracheal aspirates. An open lung biopsy showed desquamative interstitial pneumonia. Despite treatment with prednisolone, antibiotics, and cyclophosphamide the infant died at 11 weeks of age.

COMMENT

This patient and two siblings were described by Tal et al (1984). No response to therapy was noted in these siblings. The authors cite positive experience with chloroquine, which is worthy of a trial in situations as desperate as this one.

Another instance of familial lung disease in infancy characterized by proliferation and desquamation of type II pneumocytes was described by Farrell et al (1986). Their patient had the insidious onset of interstitial pulmonary disease and poor weight gain at 4 months of age. Two siblings of the father had died at 7 and 8 months of age with a similar illness. She did not respond to prednisone, but did respond to oral chloroquine phosphate at 10 mg/kg/day. She was better after 2 weeks of therapy, which was continued. At 4 years of age, she was reported doing well, although with tachypnea and slight intercostal retractions.

Whether the child described above had DIP, or another process is hard to decide. The rarity of inflammatory cells seen on biopsy led Farrell et al to distinguish their patient from others with DIP. It seems probable that an inflammatory reaction could be present at one stage of the process and not another. At any rate, chloroquine is surely worth a trial in treatment of these rare disorders.

with acquired immune deficiency syndrome (AIDS) often in association with Epstein Barr (EB) virus infection.

Basic Science

The possibility that malfunction of the immune system is involved in the pathogenesis of this disorder was proposed on the basis of its association with autoimmune diseases such as hemolytic anemia, chronic thyroiditis, and myasthenia gravis. Positive tests for rheumatoid factor have been reported. Histologic similarity to lung lesions in Waldenström macroglobulinemia and Hashimoto thyroiditis have been noted. Yoshizawa et al (1984) reported the case of an adult with enhanced humoral immunity, as demonstrated by increased circulating immunoglobulins, and depressed cellular immunity. As the condition improved so did cellular immunity, although the patient was still hypergammaglobulinemic.

In biopsy specimens, Andiman et al (1985) recovered EB virus in 8 of 10 specimens with LIP.

Epidemiology

As of 1980, only seven cases were known to have been reported in children, two of which were siblings (O'Brodovich et al, 1980). Since then a number of cases have been reported (Church, 1985). The disorder may become more common as the number of infants with AIDS increases.

Natural History

It is difficult to generalize about a disease this rare. One of the siblings described by O'Brodovich had onset of clubbing at 3 years and died at 12 years of progressive pulmonary insufficiency unresponsive to prednisone. The other child had rapid breathing noted at 1 year, but was 13 years old at the time of the report and had few symptoms other than fatigue. The clinical symptoms in patients reported by Rubinstein et al (1986) are in Table 5.11.

Table 5.11
Clinical Symptoms During Episodes of *Pneumocystis Carinii* Pneumonia or Pulmonary Lymphoid Hyperplasia [1]

	P. carinii pneumonia	Pulmonary lymphoid hyperplasia
Cough	3/8	11/11
Tachypnea with retractions	8/8	1/11
Fever	8/8	1/11
Auscultatory findings		
Diminished breath sounds	8/8	1/11
Wheezes	4/8	0/11
Rhonchi	5/8	0/11
Digital clubbing	0/8	11/11
Salivary gland enlargement	0/8	11/11
Generalized lymphadenopathy (nodes >2 cm)	0/8	11/11
Nodular roentgenographic lung pattern	0/8	11/11

[1] Data of Rubinstein A, Morecki R, Silverman B, et al: Pulmonary disease in children with acquired immune deficiency syndrome and AIDS-related complex. *J Pediatr* 108:498, 1986.

Diagnosis

Lung biopsy is essential to establish this diagnosis. As first described by pathologists in 1966, there is massive perivascular accumulation of small mature lymphocytes and plasma cells. Extreme metaplasia of alveolar type II cells is evident, with some airways full of phagocytic cells. The pulmonary vasculature is intact. Pulmonary function studies show restrictive lung disease with low compliance and hypoxemia on exercise.

Treatment

The treatment is supportive only.

Prognosis

The prognosis is variable. The classification of chronic interstitial pneumonias is based on morphology only. Until more biochemical and immunochemical studies are done, we cannot be certain the entities described are really different. Perhaps in some instances genetic differences promote different responses to common insults. The outlook for infants or children with AIDS associated LIP is bleak. None are known to have recovered as of 1988.

REFERENCES

Andiman WA, Eastman R, Martin K, et al: Opportunistic lymphoproliferation disease associated with Epstein-Barr viral DNA in infants and children with AIDS. *Lancet* 2:8469, 1985.

Carrington CB, Gaensler EA, Contu RE, et al: Natural history and treated course of usual and desquamative interstitial pneumonia. *N Engl J Med* 298:801, 1978.

Church JA: Lymphoid interstitial pneumonia and rheumatoid arthritis. Letter to editor. *J Pediatr* 107:485, 1985.

Crystal RG, Gadek JE, Ferrans VJ, et al: Interstitial lung disease: Current concepts of pathogenesis, staging and therapy. *Am J Med* 70:542, 1981.

Crystal RG, Bitterman PB, Rennard SI, et al: Interstitial lung diseases of unknown cause. *N Engl J Med* 310:154, 1984.

Farrell PM, Gilbert EF, Zimmerman JJ, et al: Familial lung disease associated with proliferation and desquamation of Type II pneumoncytes. *Am J Dis Child* 140:262, 1986.

O'Brodovich H, M oser MM, Lu L; Familial lymphoid interstitial pneumonia: A long-term follow-up. *Pediatrics* 65:523, 1980.

Reynolds HY, Newball HH: Analysis of proteins and respiratory cells obtained from human lung by bronchial lavage. *J Lab Clin Med* 84:559, 1974.

Rubinstein A, Morecki R, Silverman B, et al: Pulmonary disease in children with acquired immune deficiency syndrome and AIDS-related complex. *J Pediatr* 108:498, 1986.

Scadding JG: Talking clearly about diseases of the pulmonary acini. *Br J Dis Chest* 72:1, 1978.

Tal A, Maor E, Bar-Ziv J, et al: Fatal desquamative interstitial pneumonia in three infant siblings. *J Pediatr* 104:873, 1984.

Teague WG, Sutphen JL, Fechner RE: Desquamative interstitial pneumonia complicating inflammatory bowel disease of childhood. *J Pediatr Gastroenterol Nutr* 4:663, 1985.

Walters LC, Talmadge EK, Schwarz MI, et al: A clinical, radiographic, and physiologic scoring system for the longitudinal assessment of patients with idiopathic pulmonary fibrosis. *Am Rev Respir Dis* 133:97, 1986.

Yoshizawa Y, Ohdoma S, Ikeda A, et al: Lymphoid interstitial pneumonia associated with depressed cellular immunity and polyclonal gammopathy. *Am Rev Respir Dis* 130:507, 1984.

PULMONARY HEMOSIDEROSIS

Definition

Pulmonary hemosiderosis is the accumulation of iron in the form of hemosiderin in the lung as a consequence of diffuse alveolar hemorrhage.

Epidemiology

Isolated or primary pulmonary hemosiderosis is very rare. Chronic low grade pulmonary hemorrhage with similar manifestations can accompany milk allergy, which is also rare. Other forms of hemosiderosis can be associated with glomerulonephritis (Goodpasture syndrome) or with collagen vascular diseases, all of which occur uncommonly in childhood. Systemic granulomatoses such as Wegener have been reported in children in whom hemoptyses have been the major finding (Grupe et al, 1986; Levy and Wilmott, 1986).

Natural History

Recurrent episodes of bleeding may be asymptomatic, or associated with fever, tachycardia, cough, hemoptysis, and be undistinguishable from infectious pneumonia. The chronicity of the bleeding may result in an iron-deficiency anemia, since red cells in the lung are sequestered and iron is not readily available for new blood formation, although eventually some utilization is possible.

The course is unpredictable. Some individuals have long remissions, or even cures, while others may have a fulminant and fatal course.

Diagnosis

Chest radiographs may be normal or show minimal transient infiltrates or even massive ones. The radiographs may be similar to those for pulmonary edema or interstitial fibrosis (Fig. 5.17).

Because blood from the lung may be swallowed, tests for blood in the stools are pertinent. Gastric aspirate or lung lavage may reveal iron-laden macrophages, sometimes called siderophages, which are diagnostic.

Lung biopsy may be appropriate to permit immunofluorescent studies, and electron microscopy. Focal rupture of the basement membrane with collagen deposition is characteristic of primary pulmonary hemosiderosis. Linear deposition of immunoglobulin and complement along the alveolar basement membrane is consistent with an underlying allergic component.

Tests for antibodies to milk in the serum are important. Although their presence does not prove that milk allergy is an underlying cause, clearly elimination of milk from the diet is indicated.

Pulmonary function studies do not clarify the diagnosis, but serial studies are of value in documenting

CASE ILLUSTRATION (Courtesy Dr. Mary Ellen Wohl)

S.F. was in excellent health with normal growth and development and no family history of renal or lung disease until age 6 years when she developed anemia associated with fluffy infiltrates on chest radiographs. The diagnosis of idiopathic pulmonary hemorrhage was made based on the absence of abnormalities in urinary sediment, normal serum creatinine, presence of hemosiderin-laden macrophages in bronchial washings, a normal tracheobronchial tree, and a lung biopsy when she was relatively well which showed evidence of interstitial fibrosis and failed to bind antiglomerular basement membrane antibody (GBM). Multiple RAST tests to milk proteins and tests for serum anti-GBM antibody were negative. She was initially treated with a trial of milk-free diet and courses of prednisone were administered for each acute attack. However, frequent pulmonary exacerbations and apparent clinical response to steroids led her clinicians to institute alternate day prednisone therapy. She continued to have two or three exacerbations per year which typically were associated with a prodrome of epistaxis followed by dyspnea, occasionally hemoptysis, a decline in hematocrit of about 5% and the development of new, bilateral infiltrates on chest radiographs. She complained of occasional arthritis in both knees which was not temporally associated with pulmonary exacerbations.

Rheumatoid factor, antinuclear antibody, and anti-GBM antibody were repeatedly negative and she had no evidence of renal disease or of a systemic vasculitis, even on muscle biopsy. She developed evidence of a progressive restrictive defect on pulmonary function testing. During her 12th year, she developed several episodes of microscopic hematuria without hypertension or creatinine elevation.

About 6 months after the appearance of the episodes of microscopic hematuria, she developed dark urine, hypertension, and peripheral edema. Several days later, she developed massive pulmonary hemorrhage. Treatment included intubation and ventilation, prednisone, plasmapheresis, and cyclophosphamide. Renal biopsy revealed advanced focal glomerulosclerosis. The biopsy was not consistent with Goodpasture disease or vasculitis. Following recovery from this episode, she has stabilized with no further hemoptysis and a glomerular filtration rate of 30% normal.

COMMENT

This patient illustrates a number of the dilemmas in idiopathic pulmonary hemorrhage or pulmonary hemosiderosis. A number of patients with pulmonary hemosiderosis develop renal involvement which may or may not be typical Goodpasture syndrome. When to biopsy the kidney is a critical issue. Whether or not to immunosuppress this patient was an important issue, as was the use of repeated plasmapheresis. The prognosis of both the pulmonary restriction and the renal disease and whether the therapy instituted has actually altered the course is unknown.

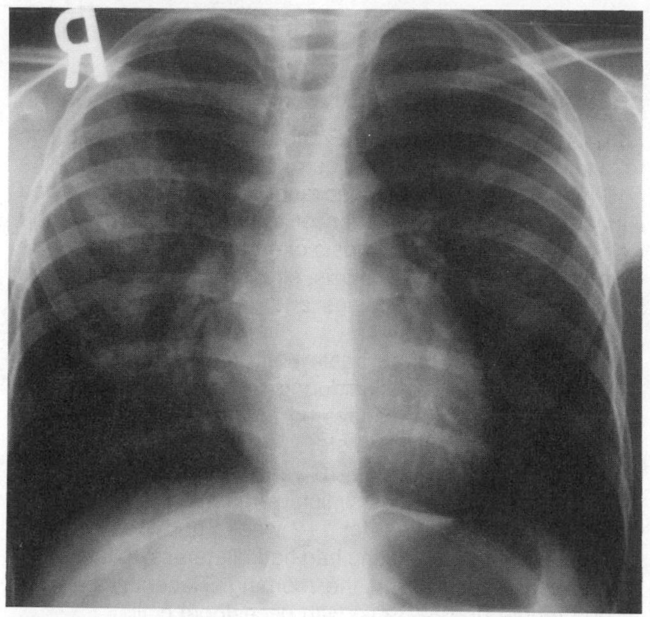

Figure 5.17. Pulmonary hemosiderosis. This patient had had malaise and unexplained iron deficiency anemia at age 6 years. A year later, she developed hemoptysis. Radiographs of the chest taken over the next several years showed changing location of pulmonary infiltrates. Idiopathic pulmonary hemosiderosis, the diagnosis in this case, is a rare abnormality which typically is associated with hemoptysis, cough, fever and dyspnea, changing infilatrates on chest radiographs, and chronic iron deficiency anemia. Hemosiderin in the sputum is diagnostic. Patients are treated with supplemental iron and steroids. Cause is still unknown.

the course of disease. Electrocardiograms are also important to assess possible strain on the right side of the heart.

Treatment

When an underlying disorder, such as collagen vascular disease is present, treatment should be directed toward it. Prednisone, 1–2 mg/kg/day orally is sometimes helpful. The anemia should be treated with iron, or transfusions if onset is sudden and severe.

In severe cases, other immunosuppressant drugs, such as azathioprine or cyclophosphamide have been tried. No systematic experience is reported, hence these drugs should be monitored in terms of individual responses.

Prevention

None is known.

SARCOIDOSIS

Definition

Sarcoidosis is a chronic granulomatous disorder of unknown cause that generally affects lymph nodes, lung, liver, skin, and eye.

Epidemiology

The disease is rare in children, and has its peak incidence in young adults of 20–40 years. The youngest reported patient was 2 months old. In the United States, the disease is 10–20 times more common in blacks. The disorder has been reported worldwide (with Sweden having the highest reported incidence, about 40/100,000 population).

Natural History

Sarcoidosis appears to be an unusual host response to an unidentified exogenous agent. The portal of entry of the agent is also unknown, but resemblances to tuberculosis make an airborne route likely. Erythema nodosum is common and suggests an allergic response.

Affected individuals have a defect in cell immunity characterized by anergy to delayed hypersensitivity antigens.

Diagnosis

The most common symptom is weight loss. Fever is present intermittently in about half the children. Respiratory symptoms may be a dry cough, with mild or moderate dyspnea. On radiograph, bilateral hilar adenopathy is often prominent, with pulmonary infiltrations of fine or coarse nodules, some of which may be cotton-wool in type. Late in the illness, fibrosis and bullae may be seen.

Involvement of the lung occurs in 80–90% of adults, but only 55% of children, according to Jasper and Denny (1968).

Ocular lesions include uveitis and iritis, but also keratitis, retinitis, glaucoma, and involvement of lacrimal glands.

Uveoparotid fever consists of uveitis, parotitis, and sometimes facial nerve palsy. It occurs in 10–20% of children with sarcoidosis.

Osseous lesions occur in adults and may be punched-out areas in metacarpals or distal phalanges. Bone lesions are very unusual in childhood sarcoid.

Liver enlargement may be present and may be documented by needle biopsy.

A rare but important manifestation is diabetes insipidus, sometimes associated with panhypopituitarism (Nora et al, 1959; Fig. 5.18).

LABORATORY STUDIES

Classically, hypergammaglobulinemia, eosinophilia (>6%), leukopenia, hypercalcemia, and elevated alkaline phosphatase may be found. None of these findings need be present. Angiotensin-converting enzyme may be elevated, but need not be. The sedimentation rate is a good indicator of disease activity. Analysis of cells obtained by lung lavage has proved useful in the diagnosis of pulmonary sarcoidosis, (Hance et al, 1985). Ia^+ lung cells were exclusively of the $ORT4^+$ helper phenotype in patients studied by Costabel et al (1985). Gallium scans of lacrimal glands are useful if positive,

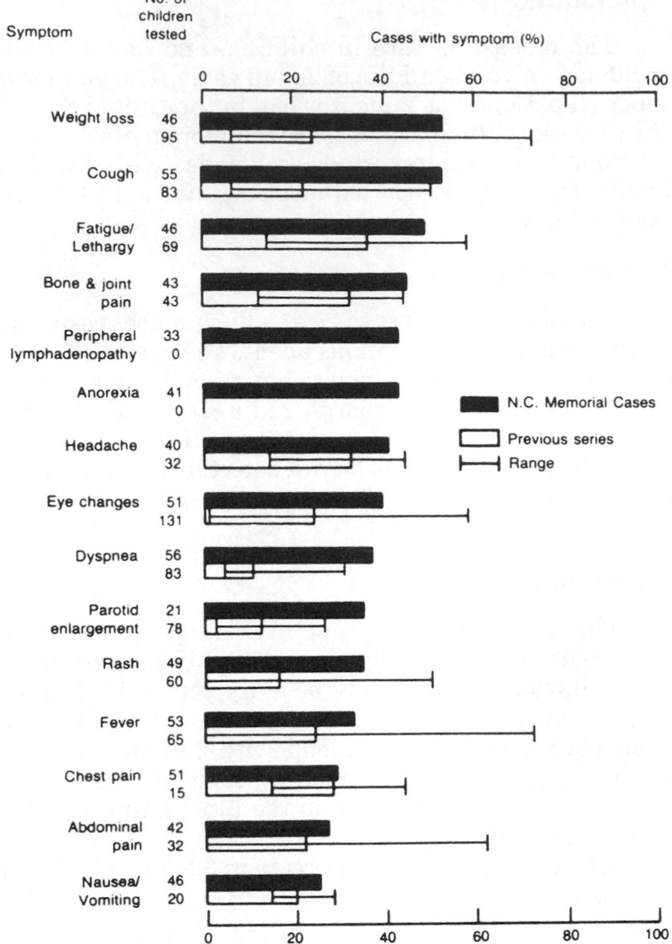

Figure 5.18. Proportion of sarcoid patients with symptoms compared to the mean and range of the previous series. The number represents the total in whom symptoms were documented and was used to calculate the proportions in the corresponding row. Peripheral lymphadenopathy and parotid enlargement were included as symptoms when they were presenting complaints. Reproduced with permission from Pattishall et al: *J Pediatr* 108:169, 1986.

but should be followed with biopsy to confirm the diagnosis.

CONTROVERSY

Angiotensin-converting enzyme has two roles, one to convert angiotensin I to angiotensin II, and the degradation of bradykinin into an inactive form. For reasons that are unclear, the enzyme is elevated in a number of conditions that have little relationship to each other, including Gaucher disease and sarcoidosis. The test for angiotensin-converting enzyme produces significant numbers of false-positive and false-negative values and, in our view, little confidence should be placed in it.

The Kveim skin test has been less than satisfactory, and scarcity of test materials makes it unavailable in most centers.

CASE ILLUSTRATION

A white female from Boston was first seen at The Children's Hospital at the age of 16 months because of a 10-month history of a purpuric rash. The skin biopsy showed focal perivascular infiltration of the subcutaneous tissue compatible with the diagnosis of erythema nodosum. She was evaluated for tuberculosis, streptococcal infection, and lupus with negative findings and her bone marrow was normal.

She was not seen again until age 8 years. Loss of visual acuity was identified during a screening examination at school. She was discovered to have uveitis and was treated intermittently with steroid optic drops.

The follow-up at age 13 years revealed raised purpuric lesions on the legs, which were tender and erythematous. They would last for 1–2 weeks and then resolve. She also reported that she had had bilateral swollen, painful knees, especially in the morning. Recently she had been febrile (to 38–39°C) with occasional chills.

The only abnormalities on physical examination were the persistent uveitis and a liver palpable 5 cm below the right costal margin and the spleen down 4 cm. The multiple raised, round, nontender lesions were now brown. Blood count showed a hematocrit of 40%, white count of 4000/mm^3 with a normal differential, and normal platelets. The sedimentation rate was 26 mm/hour. Electrolytes, liver function tests, and serum protein profiles were all within the normal limits. She had a normal chest radiograph. However, a Gallium scan showed uptake in both lacrimal glands and the right parotid gland consistent with sarcoidosis. The serum angiotensin converting enzyme activity was at the upper range of adult normal, 31 nm/ml, but well within normal for children. A biopsy of the lacrimal gland showed chronic inflammation and biopsy of the liver revealed a noncaseating granuloma compatible with sarcoidosis.

She began therapy with prednisone, 1 mg/kg/day, and continued optic steroids. The symptoms resolved and she remains on therapy.

COMMENT

Although in retrospect this youngster had a number of findings compatible with sarcoidosis, the diagnosis was not made immediately, because of the unequivocally normal chest radiograph and the absence of lymphadenopathy. The most important clue was the persistent uveitis, which is uncommon in children and should suggest the possibility of tuberculosis or sarcoidosis. Tuberculosis was unlikely in this situation, despite the chronic course, and a positive tuberculin test was not obtained. The youngster was well-developed and well-nourished. The evidence of anergy as indicated by a negative Monilia skin test was consistent with sarcoidosis.

Ocular involvement occurs in nearly all younger patients with keratitic precipitates, iris nodules, and posterior synechiae. Chorioretinitis occurs in approximately 25%.

Treatment

No specific treatment exists for this disorder of unknown cause. The symptoms can be suppressed with corticosteroids, which are advocated only during acute or dangerous episodes. The initial dose is prednisone, 1 mg/kg/day, with gradual reduction as symptoms disappear. The disease is characterized by relapses and remissions, and therapy needs to be adjusted for the individual.

REFERENCES

Costabel U, Bross KF, Ruhle KH, et al: Ia-like antigens on T cells and the subpopulations in pulmonary sarcoidosis and in hypertensitivity pneumonitis. *Am Rev Respir Dis* 131:337, 1985.

Hance AJ, Douches S, Winchester RJ, et al: Characterization of mononuclear phagocyte subpopulations in the human lung by using monoclonal antibodies: Changes in alveolar macrophage phenotype associated with pulmonary sarcoidosis. *J Immunol* 134:284, 1985.

Jasper PL, Denny FW: Sarcoidosis in children. *J Pediatr* 73:499, 1968.

Kendig EL, Peacock RL, Ryburn S: Sarcoidosis: Report of three cases in siblings under 15 years of age. *N Engl J Med* 260:962, 1959.

Kendig EL, Jr: The clinical picture of sarcoidosis in children. *Pediatrics* 54:289, 1974.

Kendig EL: In Kendig EL, Chernick V (eds): *Disorders of the Respiratory Tract in Children*, 4th edition. Philadelphia, WB Saunders, 1984.

Nora JR, Levitsky, JM, Zimmerman HJ: Sarcoidosis with panhypopituitarism and diabetes insipidus. *Ann Intern Med* 51:1400, 1959.

Pattishall EN, Strope GL, Spinola SM, et al: Childhood sarcoidosis. *J Pediatr* 108:169, 1986.

Rodriguez GE, Shin BC, Abernathy RS, et al: Serum angiotensin converting enzyme activity in normal children and in those with sarcoidosis. *J Pediatr* 99:68, 1981.

Low Lung Volume 5

ATELECTASIS

Definition

Atelectasis refers to closure or collapse of previously expanded regions of lungs. It can be diffuse from inadequacy of pulmonary surfactants, as in respiratory distress syndrome (RDS) or hyaline membrane disease (HMD) (pp. 165–69). Collapse (or more precisely airway closure) can be lobular or lobar or involve a whole lung as a consequence of obstruction or disease. Regions of loss of aeration can be identified by physical examination if they are extensive, but more commonly are brought to attention by a chest radiograph with consolidation of a region associated with diminution in size in comparison to the aerated state.

Basic Science

Widespread atelectasis is usually the result of immaturity with respect to surfactant synthesis or secretion, or a consequence of lung injury, as in phosgene or mercury vapor inhalation, oxygen toxicity, smoke inhalation, or adult RDS. The pathophysiology is a decrease in compliance in association with loss of volume, decreased oxygenation from venous admixture, and hypoventilation in severe cases. Patchy atelectasis is the hallmark of most infectious pneumonias in toddlers.

The degree of pulmonary shunt of blood through atelectatic regions has been well-studied in dogs and, clearly, similar events occur in humans (Lopez-Majano et al, 1966). When an airway was occluded in an animal breathing pure oxygen, the lung distal to occlusion became completely atelectatic (liver-like in appearance). When ventilation was maintained in the unoccluded lung with intrapleural pressure swings of -3 to -12 cm H_2O, blood flow through the atelectatic lung was reduced from 45% to 22.% of pulmonary flow. With larger distending pressures (from -7.5 to -24 cm H_2O) blood flow increased to the airless lung probably because of partial tamponade of the vessels in the overdistended lung (Finley, 1963).

On a microscopic level, the capillary network can be compressed by overdistention of surrounding airspaces. Probably intrapulmonary shunting is an advantage from the point of view of shifting blood from poorly ventilated to better ventilated regions. However, overdistended regions can become unperfused. These considerations are all important if mechanical ventilation is undertaken in the presence of significant atelectasis.

When lobar collapse occurs in association with infection in infants, the right upper lobe is most commonly involved. In children, the order of preference for pneumonia is left lower lobe, right middle lobe, right lower, right upper, lingula, and left upper. The likelihood of persistent collapse is greatest in right middle, lingula, and to a much lesser degree, the lower and upper lobes. Persistent collapse (over 2 years) occurs in less than 5% of children with atelectasis (James et al, 1956).

Epidemiology

Small areas of atelectasis are probably always present in normal individuals particularly after breathing quietly without periodic deep breaths or sighs. Pathologic atelectasis is arbitrarily considered what the radiologist can see on chest radiographs. Often, even significant collapse, such as an entire right upper lobe in infants, may be without symptoms or abnormalities in blood gases. Only significant mediastinal shift toward the side of reduced lung volume is likely to produce discomfort in an older child.

Since atelectasis is a component of most pneumonias, and is also frequently seen in postoperative patients, it is of course very common. No "incidence" as such can be stated.

Natural History

The most common cause of radiographically demonstrable atelectasis is lower respiratory tract disease. So-called postpneumonic atelectasis usually clears in a few weeks, but can persist for months. Atelectasis in association with asthma usually clears as the bronchospasm resolves. Aspiration of any foreign material, from upper respiratory tract mucus to peanuts can produce an obstruction that results in resorption atelectasis. A third mechanism is lung compression from enlargement of other intrathoracic structures, such as massive pericardial effusions, pleural effusions, or herniated abdominal viscera. Lower lobe atelectasis is seen in patients with neuromuscular disease in which each is significantly impaired. In this setting it is usually a poor prognostic mediator.

Diagnosis

The cardinal physical findings are loss of aeration and dullness to percussion. If extensive, mediastinal shift will be evident. The radiologist usually denotes areas of opacification with loss of volume as atelectasis. The pathologist considers airless lung as atelectatic, although often cannot differentiate the degree of expansion during life from postmortem changes. Experimentally, pressure-volume studies on excised lobes or lungs will delineate these regions with inability to expand or with premature closure after inflation. The latter condition reflects deficiency or alteration in pulmonary surfactants.

Treatment

Identification of the underlying reason for atelectasis is the first step toward therapy. The condition almost always disappears with treatment of infection or removal of a foreign body or space-occupying masses.

Postoperative atelectasis can be prevented or treated by periodic deep breaths, which recruit airless alveoli. No gain is achieved by breathing against a resistance. For individuals on ventilators, judicious use of continuous distending airway pressure of 4–6 cm H_2O will help overcome a predisposition to atelectasis from increased surface forces as in RDS, some pneumonias and pulmonary edema.

Prognosis

Recurrent collapse is most common in children with sinobronchitis of any cause (including cystic fibrosis) and asthma. The duration is usually less than 3 months, but re-expansion is still possible after an interval of several years (James et al, 1956). Persistent collapse and symptoms suggest bronchiectasis, but it is now a rare event.

HYPOPLASIA

Definition

Pulmonary hypoplasia can occur in many degrees of severity, but the term has usually been restricted to instances with gross diminution in lung mass, incompatible with life. The early literature was contributed almost exclusively by pathologists who were able to weigh lungs and compare them to an expected weight or express a lung weight/body weight ratio. Infants with congenital disorders of the chest wall, such as in asphyxiating thoracic dystrophy, have small lungs, presumably the consequence of a small thoracic volume. Small thoracic volume can occur from paralysis of the diaphragm as in the case of an infant born with congenital absence of both phrenic nerves and a profoundly hypoplastic lung (see Case Illustration). Diaphragmatic hernias are often associated with lung hypoplasia. Patients with oligohydramnios, if associated with renal agenesis, have hypoplastic lungs and it is now recognized that milder degrees of oligohydramnios from any cause can be associated with a reduction in lung size, at least in the experimental animal. A clinical definition of the lower limit of normal lung size has not been established, hence, the diagnosis of pulmonary hypoplasia is usually restricted to the more severe forms.

Basic Science

Some forms of pulmonary hypoplasia are clearly influenced by genetic factors. The observation that relatives of infants with Potter syndrome are known to have more than the expected renal abnormalities makes it clear that there is a familial predisposition to that malformation. It is not known whether the relatives of such infants have any pulmonary hypoplasia. Further evidence for a genetic basis of some forms of pulmonary hypoplasia comes from the observations of Cooney and Thurlbeck (1982) who noted a diminished number of alveoli in relation to alveolar ducts in seven patients of various ages who had Down syndrome. Five of the seven had associated congenital heart disease, most commonly an atrioventricular canal. Demonstration of unusual adhesiveness of fibroblasts from heart and lung tissue of abortuses with Down syndrome has lead to the suggestion that the extra genetic material on chromosome 21 is expressing itself through surface markers on these fibroblasts (Wright et al, 1984).

Any condition that limits space for the lung to develop in fetal life will be associated with hypoplasia. For example, with a diaphramatic hernia and abdominal viscera occupying some of the thorax, the lung on the ipsilateral side will be hypoplastic. If the abdominal contents shift to the mediastinum, then both lungs can be hypoplastic, although the greatest diminution in growth will be on the side of the hernia. deLorimier et al (1967) have reproduced this phenomenon in fetal lambs in whom diaphragmatic hernias were created.

The relationship between oligohydramnios and pulmonary hypoplasia is thoroughly established from a number of clinical and experimental observations. For example, one of a pair of monoamniotic monochorionic twins with renal agenesis had normal lungs, probably because the other twin was capable of urine production and, thus, amniotic fluid formation (Mauer et al, 1974).

The role of lung liquid in determining lung size was evaluated experimentally by Alcorn et al in 1977 in fetal lambs. They altered fetal lung volume in lambs by tracheal ligation at 105–110 days and by tracheal drainage into the amniotic sac at the same time in other fetuses. The lungs were studied 3–4 weeks later. Those in the ligated group were large, but relatively immature with respect to type 2 cells. The drained lungs were only half the expected size and had thick alveolar walls with abundant type 2 cells. The question of whether prolonged leakage of amniotic fluid in the human can affect lung size remains controversial. Perlman et al (1976) found a reduced number of alveolae after leakage.

From studies in rats, it is probable that as lung tissue becomes stretched, somatomedins are released and these can accelerate lung growth. This is thought to be the basis of the hyperplasia after pneumonectomy in infancy. However, similar studies have not been undertaken in the evaluation of fetal lung growth.

Other observations on rats suggest that maternal smoking during pregnancy can impair fetal lung growth. Collins et al (1985) described fewer and larger saccules and reduced lung weight and surface area available for gas exchange. They suggest a diminution in the length of elastic tissue as the underlying defect. These provocative findings await further study to ascertain their relevance in humans.

Diagnosis

The diagnosis of pulmonary hypoplasia may be evident on physical examination. When profound, obviously ventilation is clearly impossible. With modest degrees of hypoplasia, the infant assumes a higher respiratory frequency to achieve adequate ventilation with a reduced tidal volume. If lung compliance is low, higher pressures are required, as is often the case with infants with diaphragmatic hernia. In fact, pneumothoraces can occur bilaterally after diaphragmatic hernia presumably because of the high pressures applied across relatively poorly distensible lung tissue. A straightforward way to assess pulmonary hypoplasia is to measure chest circumference at the nipple line and compare it to maximal head circumference. In most infants, these numbers are similar. A significant reduction in chest circumference usually is associated with descent of the diaphragm and protruberance of the abdominal wall. Most infants with asphyxiating thoracic dystrophy have poorly distensible thoraces, depressed diaphragms, and significant prominence of the abdomen.

The presence of hypoplastic lungs should raise questions as to whether there are malformations in other organs such as heart or kidneys, and whether there is a familial predisposition. Possibility of amniotic fluid leak should be entertained.

CASE ILLUSTRATION

A 3.6-kg male infant was delivered after an uneventful pregnancy of 42 weeks. The 22-year-old mother had had a normal infant, and this was her second pregnancy. No fetal distress was observed during labor, but the Apgar scores were 1 and 2 at 1 and 5 minutes, respectively. No spontaneous breaths were noted. After intubation and mechanical ventilation with 100% oxygen, his arterial Po_2 was 70 mm Hg. A chest film (Fig. 5.19) showed elevation of both diaphragms and evidence of gastric distention with air. At autopsy, the diaphragms were fibrous sheaths with no muscle, and phrenic nerves were absent (from Goldstein JD, Reid LM: *J Pediatr* 97:282, 1980).

COMMENT

This is the only instance of absence of both phrenic nerves we have observed. Experimental production of pulmonary hypoplasia is possible by cutting the phrenic nerves in the first trimester. The failure of muscle development in the diaphragm made fetal breathing impossible, and presumably led to pulmonary hypoplasia by compromise of thoracic volume.

The profound neonatal depression and no spontaneous respiratory movements in the absence of fetal distress, in retrospect were suggestive of hypoplastic lungs and absent phrenic nerves.

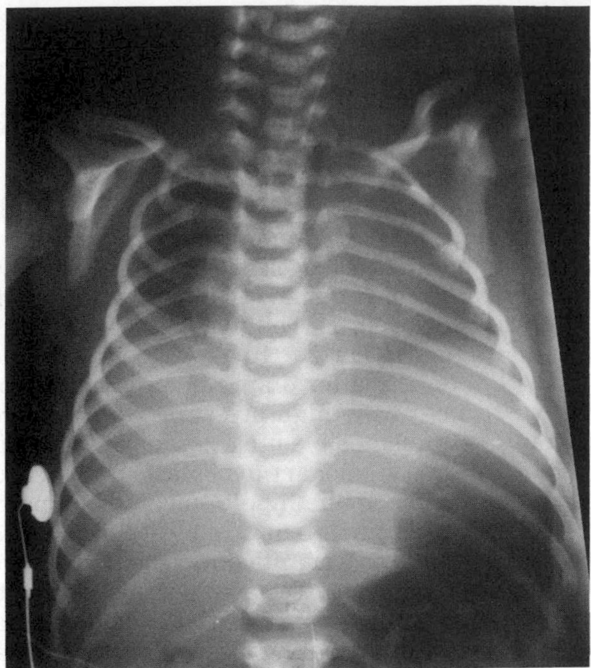

Figure 5.19. This infant had profound pulmonary hypoplasia in association with absence of birth phrenic nerves. The diaphragm was a fibrous sheath devoid of muscle. Reproduced with permission from Goldstein JD, Reid, LM: *J Pediatr* 97:282, 1980.

Treatment

Mechanical ventilation with appropriate end-expiratory pressure offers the only known support for these infants. Clearly, if the underlying effect of lung hypoplasia can be remedied, as in diaphragmatic hernia, some further growth can occur. The numbers of alveoli will increase, although the total may never reach normal. Lung volume is restored by overdistention of existing air spaces (Thurlbeck et al, 1979). Wohl et al (1977) demonstrated a reduction in blood flow to the ipsilateral lung in nine patients who had hernia repair before age 1 year, and studied at ages 6–18 years. These findings are consistent with a reduction in the number of branches of pulmonary arteries.

AGENESIS OF THE LUNG

Definition

Agenesis of the lung is a developmental defect with complete absence or profound hypoplasia of one or both lungs.

Epidemiology

The incidence of this lethal condition is not known. When it occurs on only one side and is found later in life, it remains unusual with one report of four patients among 114,569 admissions (Borja et al, 1970).

Natural History

The majority of reported cases of unilateral or bilateral agenesis of the lung have had significant associated congenital anomalies involving the heart, skeleton, or gastrointestinal tract. In a group of four patients reported from Riyadh, Saudi Arabia, an additional malformation was ipsilateral abnormalities of the thumbs (Mardini and Nyhan, 1985).

It is thought that the malformations must result from an interference with embryologic development at about the fourth week of fetal life, when the primitive lung buds are forming.

There are a number of variations of anomalies that have been reported with pulmonary agenesis. Sometimes the entire lung and its pulmonary artery are absent, with or without a rudimentary bronchus from the trachea. In another, the lung is hypoplastic but there is a fully formed bronchus. Apparently, embryonic pulmonary tissue is important for the growth and vascularization of the pulmonary artery.

Diagnosis

Patients with absence of one lung and the pulmonary artery may be asymptomatic, and the diagnosis may not be made until a chest film is taken for some reason in later life. Most of the time however, the diagnosis is made in childhood because many of the patients have respiratory difficulties, persistent cyanosis, and a significant mediastinal shift. Some of the children have pulmonary hypertension and congestive heart failure may result in association with intercurrent in-

CASE ILLUSTRATION

A 2-week-old female from Saudi Arabia was delivered by cesarean section for fetal distress. Parental consanguinity was present. The infant had frequent attacks of respiratory infection and wheezing during the first few weeks, and at 2 weeks of age was noted to be cyanotic with crying. The chest was slightly asymmetric with decreased motion on the right. Bilateral inspiratory and expiratory wheezes were heard and a short systolic murmur with a split-second sound was present. A chest film demonstrated agenesis of the right upper and right middle lobes, with atrial septal defect and an absent pulmonary artery.

This infant had malformation of the right thumb, with only three phalanges and a hypoplastic middle phylanx. She also had fused ribs and subluxation of the hips. Simian lines were present bilaterally.

It was thought that there was no specific therapy indicated, and gradually over the subsequent years, the respiratory symptoms became fewer, and by 6 years of age, she was asymptomatic (patient of Mardini and Nyhan, 1985).

fections. Tracheal compression has been noted in association with a normal but deviated aorta in the presence of a right-sided pulmonary agenesis (McCormick and Kuhns, 1979).

If the patient is symptomatic and it is thought that a hypoplastic lung may be the site of a right-to-left shunt and the source of recurrent infections, consideration of surgical resection is appropriate. Bronchoscopy may be indicated to be certain of the anatomy. Cardiac catheterization and angiography will help evaluate the nature of associated congenital heart disease. The indication for resection should be a hypoplastic lung that is sequestered with a systemic blood supply.

Inasmuch as no two instances are exactly alike, careful radiographic and cardiovascular studies are necessary.

REFERENCES

Alcorn D, Adamson TM, Lambert TF, et al: Morphologic effects of traceal ligation and drainage in fetal lamb lung. *J Anat* 123:649, 1977.

Borja AR, Ransdell HT, Villa S: Congenital developmental arrest of the lung. *Ann Thorac Sug* 10:317, 1970.

Collins MH, Moessinger AC, Kleinerman J, et al: Fetal lung hypoplasia associated with maternal smoking: A morphometric analysis. *Pediatr Res* 19:408, 1985.

Cooney TT, Thrulbeck WM: Pulmonary hypoplasia in Down's syndrome. *N Engl J Med* 307:1170, 1982.

Dolan CJ, Strodes CH, Duffey FD: Idiopthic pulmonary hemosiderosis: Electron microscopic, immunofluorescent and iron kinetic studies. *Chest* 68:577, 1975.

deLorimier AA, Tierney DF, Parker HR: Hypoplastic lungs in fetal lambs with surgically produced congenital diaphragmatic hernia. *Surgery* 62:12, 1967.

Finley TN, Hill TR, Bonica JJ: Effect of intrapleural pressure on pulmonary shunt through atelectatic dog lung. *J Appl Physiol* 205:1187, 1963.

Grupe WE, Colvin RB, Mark EJ: A 15-year-old boy with hemoptysis and occult blood in the urine. Case Records of the Massachusetts General Hospital. *N Engl J Med* 314:834, 1986.

Heiner DC: Pulmonary hemosiderosis. In Kending E, Chernick V (eds): *Disorders of the Respiratory Tract in Children,* 4th edition. Philadelphia, WB Saunders, 1983, p. 430.

James U, Brimblecombe FSW, Wells JW: The natural history of pulmonary collapse in childhood. *Quart J Med* XXV 97:121, 1956.

Jederlinic PJ, Sicilian LS, Bagelman W, et al: Congenital bronchial atresia. A report of 4 cases and a review of the literature. *Medicine* 66:73, 1987.

Levy J, Wilmott RW: Pulmonary Hemosiderosis. *Pediatr Pulmonol* 2:384, 1986.

Lopez-Majano V, Wagner HN, Twining RH, et al: Effect of regional hypoxia on the distribution of pulmonary blood flow in man. *Circ Res* 1966.

Mardini MK, Nyhan WL: Agenesis of the lung: Report of four patients with unusual anomalies. *Chest* 87:522, 1985.

Mauer SM, Dobrin RS, Vernier RL: Unilateral and bilateral renal agenesis in monoamniotic twins. *J Pediatr* 84:236, 1974.

McCormick TL, Kuhns LR: Tracheal compression by a normal aorta associated with right lung agenesis. *Pediatr Radiol* 130:659, 1979.

Moessinger A, Bassi CA, Ballantyne G, et al: Experimental production of pulmonary hypoplasia following amniocentesis and oligohydramnios. *Early Human Devel* 8:343, 1983.

Perlman M, Williams J, Hirsch M: Neonatal pulmonary hypoplasia after prolonged leakage of amniotic fluid. *Arch Dis Child* 51:349, 1976.

Ross A, Naeye RL: Racial and environmental influences on fetal lung maturation. *Pediatrics* 68:790, 1981.

Thurlbeck WM, Kida K, Langston C, et al: Postnatal lung growth after repair of diaphragmatic hernia. *Thorax* 34:338-1979.

Wohl MEB, Griscom NT, Strieder DJ, et al: The lung following repair of congenital diaphragmatic hernia. *J Pediatr* 90:405, 1977.

Wright TC, Orkin RW, Destremps M, et al: Increased adhesiveness of Down syndrome fetal fibroblasts. *Proc Nat Acad Sci USA* 81:2426, 1984.

Space-Occupying Lesions

6

PNEUMOTHORAX AND OTHER AIR LEAKS

Definition

The abnormal presence of air in any tissue space constitutes pneumothorax-pneumomediastinum or pneumopericardium, interstitial, or subcutaneous emphysema.

Epidemiology

Pneumothorax may occur spontaneously at any age, but is most common in the first days of life, in adolescents and in young women during delivery. It may also be a complication of injury by mechanical ventilation, in which case the incidence depends on the number of individuals who receive mechanical ventilation. Among infants with HMD (Fig. 5.20), air leak of some degree occurs in 10–40% of those ventilated (Madansky et al, 1979). Chest catheters and catheters passed too far through the endotracheal tube also have been incriminated in lung rupture. Children with Marfan syndrome have a 4–5% incidence of pneumothorax in association with apical blebs (Hall et al, 1984).

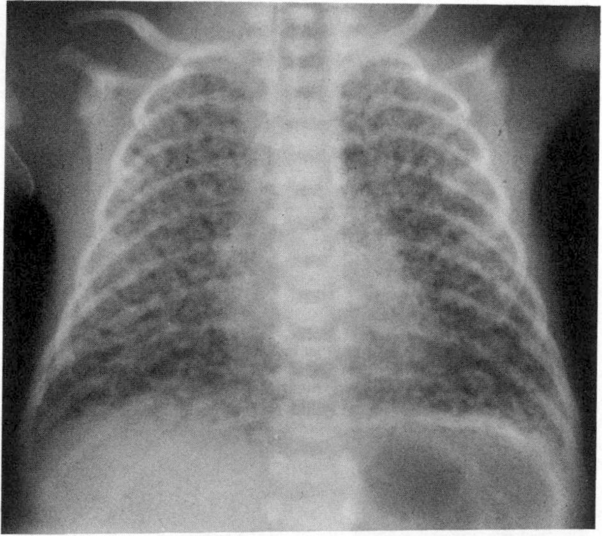

Figure 5.20. This infant had been ventilated at high pressures for hyaline membrane disease (HMD) when his condition suddenly deteriorated. Extensive dissection of air into the interstitial spaces throughout both lungs is evident on the radiograph.

Natural History

Lung rupture allows air to dissect along vascular sheaths to the lung root. Mediastinal walls rupture and air enters the pleural space as well as mediastinum. Usually some predisposing condition increases the possibility of rupture. For example, a vigorous infant who has aspirated meconium may have plugged some bronchi. The mechanical advantage of the elevated diaphragm, when it contracts, will allow a higher than normal transpulmonary pressure across aerated sections of the lung.

In older children, pneumothorax can occur in association with infection or from rupture of a pleural bleb. The genesis of blebs or bullae is not clear, but presumably they occur mainly after infection. Patients with Marfan syndrome are at risk of pneumothorax (Hall et al, 1984).

Diagnosis

The possibility of spontaneous pneumothorax should be considered in vigorous infants, mostly at term or postmature, who may have aspirated meconium or squamous debris. Air leak in association with mechanical ventilation should be considered whenever there is an otherwise unexplained deterioration in the infant's course. In the older child pneumothorax may be associated with asthma, histiocytosis, dermatomyositis, and cystic fibrosis.

Treatment

Transillumination is a useful clinical tool in an emergency. If the infant has signs of severe respiratory distress, with mediastinal shift, needle aspiration of pleural air is lifesaving. Later, a catheter can be inserted and attached to continuous suction.

If the pneumothorax is discovered incidentally on a chest radiograph, no immediate treatment is needed. The infant requires careful following to ascertain if the loculated air is increasing or decreasing. The absorption of the air can be accelerated if the infant breathes 100% oxygen, but oxygen breathing will not help clear nonloculated air.

Interstitial emphysema of the lung is more serious because the air can cause gross enlargement of one or all lobes. The air may compress vessels and lead to hypoperfusion and, eventually, to fibrosis. There is some urgency, therefore, to treat this condition. The most effective treatment is high frequency ventilation, as used in this condition by Frantz et al (1983). If that is not available, a lobe may be decompressed by temporary occlusion of its bronchus to allow the loculated gas to be resorbed (Brooks et al, 1977).

Pneumopericardium can cause cardiac tamponade and death. Thus, any evidence of circulatory embarrassment is an indication for needle aspiration via the subxiphoid route and possibly catheter drainage if air reappears.

Recurring pneumothorax in children and adolescents is usually associated with an underlying disease such as cystic fibrosis. No consensus exists on management, but in general quinacrine sclerosis has been successful in some children, and if it fails partial pleurectomy is advised (McLaughlin et al, 1982)

Prognosis

Spontaneous pneumothorax in the newborn is usually an isolated event related to the stresses on lung parenchyma in the transition from fetal to neonatal life. Pneumothorax that occurs during mechanical ventilation in newborns is also an isolated event. Survivors of neonatal respiratory illnesses are not prone to recurrent pneumothorax in childhood.

Children with lung cysts, or underlying disease such as cystic fibrosis are prone to recurrent pneumothoraces. If they recur, or are bilateral, the prognosis is guarded. Pleurectomy is indicated.

PLEURAL EFFUSION AND EMPYEMA

Definition

Pleural effusions are an abnormal accumulation of fluid in the pleural space. Empyema denotes a purulent exudate, often with bacteria present.

Basic Science

The initial stage of inflammation results in accumulation of fibrinous liquid with a few polymorphonuclear cells. When permeability of pleural capillaries increases, high protein fluid enters the pleural space and favors transfer of liquid by colloid osmotic effects. Bacterial invasion and loculation of the liquid follow. If the liquid is not drained, fibroblasts enter from both pleural surfaces and form an inelastic membrane.

Epidemiology

Small pleural effusions can occur in a number of situations and their prevalence reflects that of the underlying condition. About half of patients with acute bacterial pneumonia have some parapneumonic effusion. Its prevalence has decreased since the development of antimicrobial agents but empyema occurs several times a year in our hospital, mostly in youngsters whose initial pneumonia was untreated, or those who have impairment of host defenses. About 70% of cases of childhood empyema occur in the first 2 years of life (Nelson, 1985).

Natural History

Liquid can accumulate in the pleural space from a wide variety of organisms. Bacterial infections associated with empyema include tuberculosis, *Staphylococcus aureus, Haemophilus influenzae, Streptococcus pyogenes, Diplococcus pneumoniae, Mycoplasma* (about 20% of patients), and others. Anerobic bacteria also may be involved, most commonly microaerophilic streptococcus from periodontal infections (Fine et al, 1970; Fig. 5.21), and the organisms in the neurologically impaired child with recurrent aspiration.

Although some viral pneumonias, particularly adenovirus, can be associated with massive pleural effusions, most viruses do not cause effusions.

Diagnosis

The diagnosis can be suspected on the basis of physical findings of decreased air entry, dullness to percussion, and occasionally mediastinal shift to the opposite side. Pleuritic pain may or may not be present. In severe cases, dyspnea and severe chest pain are prominent. Persistent fever, vomiting, anorexia, and prostration may be present. A paralytic ileus can induce abdominal distention. Muffling of heart sounds and a pericardial rub suggest extension to the pericardial sac.

The chest radiograph is the most useful aid. The earliest sign of liquid is obliteration of the costophrenic angle. Ultrasonography helps to distinguish loculated liquid from a mass.

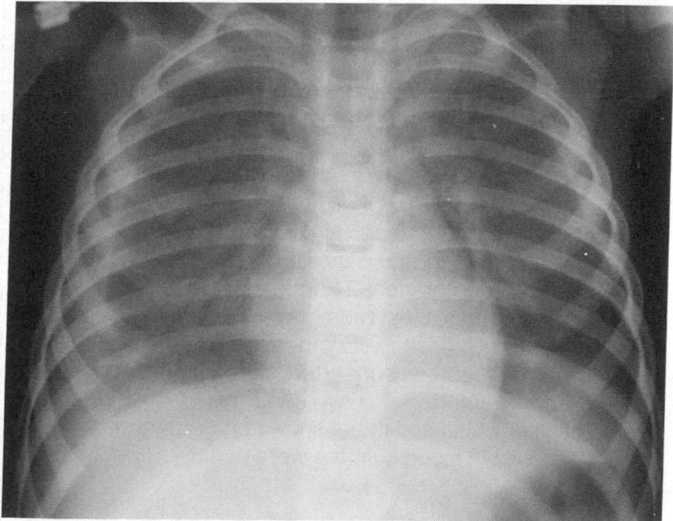

Figure 5.21. This patient had hemolytic uremic syndrome and presented in respiratory distress. The radiograph shows bilateral pleural effusions as well as pulmonary edema. The heart is not enlarged. When pleural effusion is identified clinically or radiographically, it is usually associated with underlying inflammatory disease, failure, or, less likely, tumor.

The essential test is examination of the pleural fluid after thoracentesis. The needle should be inserted into the area of maximal density as determined by chest radiograph. Usually the seventh posterolateral intercostal space, just above the rib, is the best site for obtaining nonloculated fluid. The aspirated material should be submitted for Gram stain, culture, cell count, and cell block. Blood cultures can enhance the likelihood of identifying the pathogen. Determination of protein, lactic dehydrogenase, and amylase are useful. Countercurrent immunoelectrophoresis can help identify the pathogen. If the diagnosis remains uncertain, pleural biopsy is indicated, either by needle, or open thoracotomy. Complicated effusions that require a chest tube for drainage usually have a pleural fluid pH below 7.00, glucose below 40 mg/dl and LDH over 100 IU/L. Conversely, effusions having a pleural fluid pH above 7.20 and glucose over 40 mg/dl, and a negative Gram stain usually respond to antibiotics without drainage. (Light, 1985). Interpretation of values in pleural fluid depends on knowledge of simultaneous blood values.

Treatment

Appropriate antibiotic therapy is indicated in pneumonia with effusions. The question arises when thoracentesis is required. In general, with small effusions that simply blunt the costophrenic angle on radiograph, we do not tap. If the effusion is increasing, the patient is short of breath, or there is mediastinal shift, removal of fluid for both diagnostic and therapeutic reasons is indicated.

If the fluid is thick and purulent or if fever persists, closed chest drainage is important. Areas of loculated fluid can often be localized with ultrasonography. Chest tubes are usually required for about 10 days.

CASE ILLUSTRATION

A 5-year-old boy, previously well, developed a barking cough, followed by complaint of right upper quadrant abdominal pain. Five days later he was first seen by a physician who found a temperature of 38°C, but nothing to explain the persistent cough. A few hours after returning home, his temperature rose to 41°C, and he was in acute respiratory distress. He arrived at the hospital emergency room cyanotic and acutely ill. A white blood count of 19,000 mm^3 had 35% polymorphonuclear cells. A chest radiograph showed right upper and lower lobe infiltrates. He was given ampicillin and oxacillin for presumed bacterial pneumonia. Over the next 24 hours, his respiratory status deteriorated, and a chest radiograph showed opacification on the right. A thoracentesis produced 600 ml of purulent liquid. A chest tube was inserted, penicillin was administered, and he improved slowly over the next week. Cultures of pleural fluid and throat showed group A β-hemolytic streptococci, but blood cultures were negative (Fig. 5.22*A*-*C*).

COMMENT

Streptococcal pneumonia is rare, but when it occurs it is accompanied by empyema. We assume that this child had had an untreated throat infection for about a week, with sudden extension to the lungs and pleura. In the prepenicillin era, we expect this boy would have died.

Prognosis

In a follow-up study of children 1–15 years of age who had had empyema that was surgically drained, McLaughlin et al (1984) found most were asymptomatic, with pulmonary function studies in the normal range.

CONGENITAL CYSTS

Definition

Congenital cysts result from abnormal development of airways and are usually confined to one lobe.

Epidemiology

Congenital cysts are rare, and outnumbered by those acquired in infancy. A peculiarly high incidence was reported among individuals in Yemen and Iraq, but it is not certain they were congenital (Baum et al, 1966).

Natural History

The usual type is in the lung periphery and probably represents disordered bronchial growth at a late stage in fetal life. They can be simple or multiple and may expand after the onset of air breathing. Recurrent infections are a hazard.

Diagnosis

In the first days of life, fetal lung liquid may not be cleared from the cavity because of abnormal bronchial connections. Thus, the presentation is that of an area of increased parenchymal density on chest radiographs. With further air breathing, their cystic nature becomes evident. Careful radiographic studies may be required to distinguish multiple cysts from herniated bowel or lobar emphysema.

An unusual variant is cystic adenomatoid malformation, which is a type of pulmonary hamartoma with cystic structures. Maternal hydramnios and fetal hydrops may be present. This lesion can be immense and cause symptoms by crowding normal lung and producing mediastinal shift. Associated malformations are present in about 20% of affected infants (Stocker et al, 1978). Prenatal diagnosis by ultrasonography can allow plans for resection immediately after delivery in compromised infants (Adzick et al, 1985).

Treatment

Small, sharply circumscribed cysts may resolve in time. The larger cystic adenomatoid malformation or

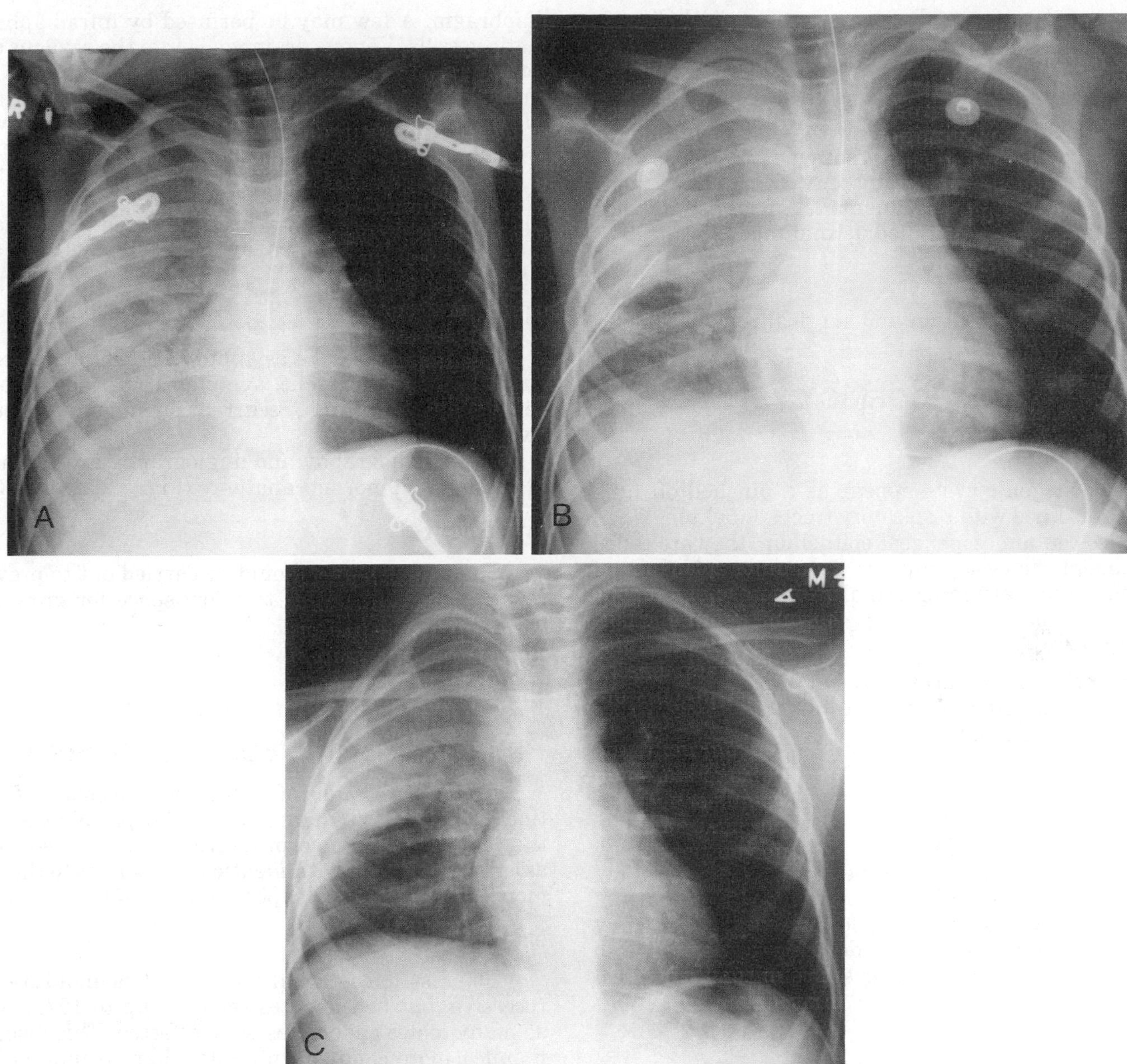

Figure 5.22.A, B, and C. This 5-year-old with right-sided pneumonia and pleural effusion proved to have β-streptococcal pneumia. Other common bacterial agents producing such a radiographic picture include *Pneumococcus* and *Staphylococcus*. If pleural fluid is loculated, it can be localized and drained under ultrasonic guidance. It is not unusual for the pleural reaction to take weeks or months to resolve.

multiloculated cysts may require urgent resection to avoid further compression of normal lung.

ENTERIC CYSTS: GASTROENTERIC, GASTRIC, OR ESOPHAGEAL DUPLICATION

Enteric cysts represent a congenital malformation often associated with abnormalities in the dorsal spinal column as the result of a fistula between the neural canal and the primitive foregut. They are usually in the posterior mediastinum, and represent one form of alimentary-tract duplication.

Epidemiology

The lesion is rare. Among mediastinal cysts and tumors in children, it accounted for 11–20% in one study (Whittaker and Lynn, 1973), but was less common in Pokorny's series (1980).

Natural History

Enteric cysts may present in infancy if they are large enough to compress adjacent bronchopulmonary structures, or if not, they may be undetected for years. About half of them contain gastric mucosa which can ulcerate and perforate. Respiratory tract epithelium is present in a small percentage.

Diagnosis

Dyspnea and tachypnea, with some degree of cyanosis is usually present in symptomatic lesions. Swallowing difficulty and vomiting may occur. Radiographs typically show vertebral anomalies in upper thoracic spine associated with a mediastinal mass.

Treatment

Proper identification and surgical removal should result in a cure.

BRONCHOGENIC CYSTS

Definition

Bronchogenic cysts appear as a pinched off lung bud that is lined with respiratory tract epithelium. When they also contain esophageal epithelium, they are called bronchoenteric cysts, and are part of the spectrum of bronchopulmonary foregut malformations.

Epidemiology

Bronchogenic cysts are rare but appear to be slightly more common than other enteric cysts based on most series (Eraklis et al, 1969).

Diagnosis

Bronchogenic cysts are usually close to the carina, and may compress a bronchus partially or completely. Thus the presentation could be lobar or unilateral overdistention, or atelectasis. Radiographs with barium are helpful in outlining the lesion. Ultrasonography can be used if an acoustic window is available. CT also displays the relationship of cyst to normal structures.

Treatment

Surgical excision should produce a cure.

PULMONARY SEQUESTRATION

Definition

Pulmonary sequestration represents a disturbance in embryogenesis that results in a cystic mass of nonfunctioning lung tissue that may have gastrointestinal communications and abnormal vascular connections.

Epidemiology

Exact figures are not available, although Carter (1969) reported sequestration in 1.1–1.8% of all pulmonary resections, about a third of which were in children younger than 10 years of age.

Natural History

Between 85 and 90% of sequestered tissue is perfused by anomalous arteries that originate above the diaphragm. A few may be perfused by infradiaphragmatic vessels. Venous drainage is into the azygous system or portal vein. The majority of sequestrations are on the left. In a series of 12 intralobular sequestrations, Alivizatos et al (1985) identified five in whom all venous blood from the right lung drained into the inferior vena cava. This draining vessel produced the "scimitar" shadow on chest radiograph. Associated cardiac malformations occur in nearly half these children. A familial incidence was noted by Neill et al (1960) and Tomsick et al (1976).

Diagnosis

Individuals may be asymptomatic. If foregut communications are present, symptoms are more prominent and include cough, recurrent pneumonia, sputum, fever, or hemoptysis.

Chest radiography and angiography are essential to define the abnormal anatomy (Fig. 5.23*A* and *B*).

Treatment

Surgical excision should be carried out to prevent recurrent infection, and to allow space for growth of normal lung.

Prognosis

Postoperative results are excellent.

PULMONARY ALVEOLAR PROTEINOSIS

A very rare cause of widespread alveolar infiltration in infancy is pulmonary alveolar proteinosis. It is the consequence of overproduction or decreased clearance of lipoprotein with identical properties to the pulmonary surfactant (Claypool et al, 1984).

Natural History

The disorder is usually inherited as an autosomal recessive, but in the cases reported up to 1971, twice as many males as females were affected. This disorder is much more common in adults than in infants, but has been singled out as an uncommon cause of chronic neonatal respiratory distress (Avery et al, 1984).

Diagnosis

The findings may be present at birth when significant respiratory distress is noted. Chest radiographs may show widespread infiltrates that are often confused with neonatal pneumonia. The condition is distinguished from pneumonia by its failure to respond to antibiotics.

Treatment

Experience with this disorder has been so sporadic that there has been no systematic evaluation of its treatment in the newborn. Trials of steroids have been without effect as has administration of acetylcysteine by inhalation. The treatment of choice in adults is pulmonary lavage; it has been successful in at least one infant as young as 18 months.

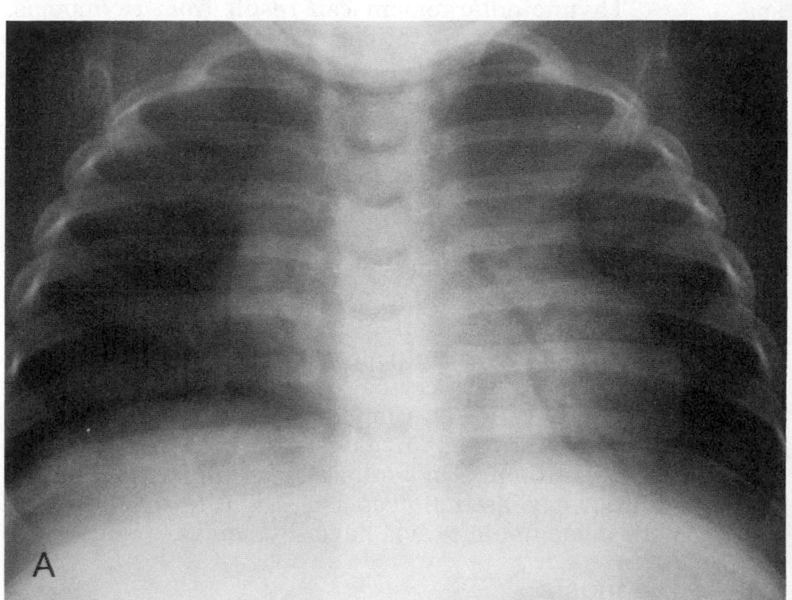

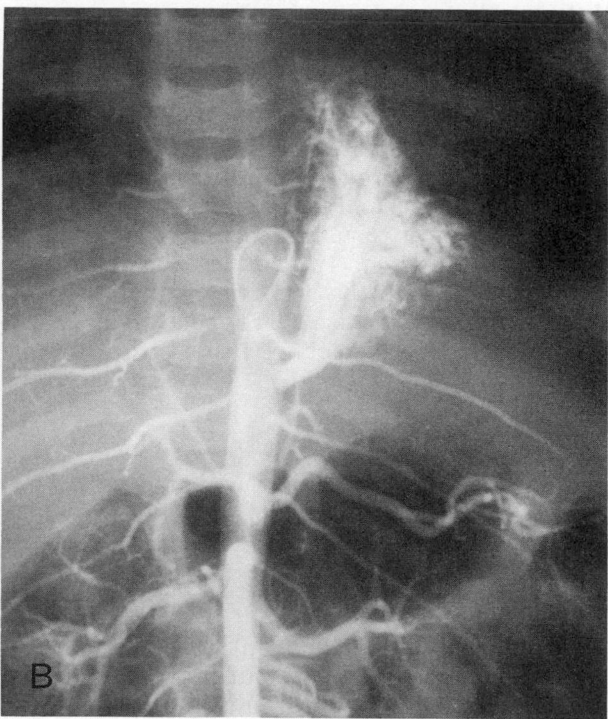

Figure 5.23.A and **B.** Pulmonary sequestration. This baby had been a premature infant and had had multiple chest films in the newborn period. **A.** At that time, both lungs had been diffusely abnormal from HMD and the left lower lobe density, which is appreciated on this film taken at 1 year of age, had not been evident. She was evaluated further with angiography. **B.** This radiograph shows a mass being supplied by a systemic artery arising from the aorta below the diaphragm. At surgery, sequestered lung was removed. Typically, sequestration involves left lower lobe and presents as an asymptomatic mass or as a source of respiratory infection. Films courtesy of K. Fellows, M.D.

LUNG ABSCESS

Definition

Lung abscess is a circumscribed, thick-walled cavity that contains purulent material from necrosis of lung tissue.

Epidemiology

Formerly a common complication of pneumonia, lung abscesses are now rare unless the child has incompetence of some component of the immune system. Asher et al (1982) reported the prevalence to be 1.3/10,000 hospital admissions at the Montreal Children's Hospital.

CASE ILLUSTRATION

A 3.36-kg infant born at term was noted to have moderate respiratory distress after birth. A chest radiograph was interpreted as showing bilateral bronchopneumonia. Antibiotics and oxygen were administered without response.

The mother's history is relevant in that three boys who had breathing problems that started on the day of birth died early in the neonatal period. No diagnosis was ever made. This same couple had two girls who were well. The mother and father were distant cousins.

The respiratory distress worsened over the subsequent weeks of life with flaring, grunting, retractions, and cyanosis even on 100% oxygen. Hemogram was normal. A tracheal aspirate at 1 week of age grew *Klebsiella*. There was no improvement on amikacin, although the infection apparently was controlled.

Open lung biopsy at 14 days of age revealed alveoli that were dilated with a granular material and many desquamated alveolar cells. On electron microscopy, it was evident that numerous lamellated structures derived from osmiophilic bodies of type 2 pneumonocytes filled the air spaces. The material in the alveoli was strongly PAS-positive and stains for *Chlamydia* or other organisms were negative. Squamous metaplasia was not present. Viral cultures were negative. The diagnosis was alveolar proteinosis.

The infant had a progressively downhill course and died at 6 weeks of age (Avery et al, 1984).

Natural History

Lung abscesses can occur at any age, more often in males than females (1.6:1). The organisms associated with abscess are overwhelmingly staphylococcal species, often resistant to penicillin. Many other organisms, including streptococci, *Haemophilus*, and even anaerobes have been recovered.

Symptoms are usually those of pneumonia, but persistent. A putrid odor to the breath may be present. Blood cultures may be positive if lung abscess is secondary to infection elsewhere, such as osteomyelitis, but they are rarely positive with a postpneumonic abscess (Fig. 5.24*A*, *B*, and *C*).

Diagnosis

The white count may be elevated with a predominance of polymorphonuclear cells. If sputum is available, it should be examined by smear and culture.

CONTROVERSY

It may be difficult to identify the offending organism, particularly because sputum production by children is unusual. If sputum contains mixed organisms, they are likely to be anaerobic organisms from the mouth. Needle aspirate is tempting, but may be dangerous and may even seed the pleural space with organisms.

Wire brushing through a fiberoptic bronchoscope has been tried, but with both false-positive and false-negative results.

Treatment

A trial of antibiotics that will cover resistant *Staphylococci, Streptococci,* and *Haemophilus* is appropriate, and has been found successful (Asher et al, 1982). Surgical drainage or resection are rarely indicated. Physical therapy has not been found helpful.

Usually fever resolves in 1–3 weeks after starting antibiotics. Complete resolution of the cavity may require months, during which time antibiotics should be continued.

Prognosis

The outcome is excellent when the patient responds to antibiotics, as is usual in an immunocompetent host.

SPACE-OCCUPYING TUMORS

A number of tumors can present in the thorax in infancy and childhood (Fig. 5.25). These include neurogenic tumors in the posterior mediastinum or metastatic tumors from other locations. Teratomas account for more than 30% of primary mediastinal cysts and neoplasms (Ellis, 1955). Cystic hygromas or lymphangiomas are more commonly found in the neck or axilla but may be located entirely in the mediastinum. (For a more extended discussion of tumors, see Section 9.)

THYMIC TUMORS

Definition

Thymic enlargement can result from thymomas, which are cystic dilatations of embryonic remnants.

Epidemiology

All thymic tumors are rare in children.

Natural History

Inflammatory cysts are rare, but have been a complication of congenital syphilis or tuberculosis. The congenital cyst may be large, and present as an anterior mediastinal mass that can extend into the posterior mediastinum. An outpouching of the midline of the sternal notch with crying may represent a position of thymus that did not complete migration to the usual substernal location. Thymomas are exceedingly rare in children although in adults they are the most common anterior mediastinal neoplasm. Eight to 15% of adults with myasthenia gravis have thymomas.

Diagnosis

Thymic lesions are usually asymptomatic and diagnosed incidentally on chest radiographs.

Treatment

Resection of cysts or tumors is advisable.

PULMONARY ARTERIOVENOUS MALFORMATIONS

Definition

Direct connections between branches of the pulmonary artery and pulmonary vein are variously called malformations, fistulae, angiomas, or hematomas. They are congenital benign lesions, whose size and number determine whether symptoms occur (Kafka et al, 1961).

Epidemiology

Several hundred cases have been reported in the literature, about one-third of whom have Osler-Weber-Rendu disease (hereditary hemorrhagic telangiectasia) (Burke et al, 1986). Lesions may be single or multiple, aneurysmal or microscopic. Fistulous vascular connections between pulmonary artery and vein are unusual.

Natural History

The condition is rarely diagnosed in infancy or childhood. The onset of symptoms is most common in the second decade. Progressive enlargement occurs with age, with eventual necrosis of the vascular wall. Thus, either a right-to-left shunt or rupture of the malformation may be responsible for the onset of cyanosis or hemoptysis, respectively. Dyspnea, cough, and chest

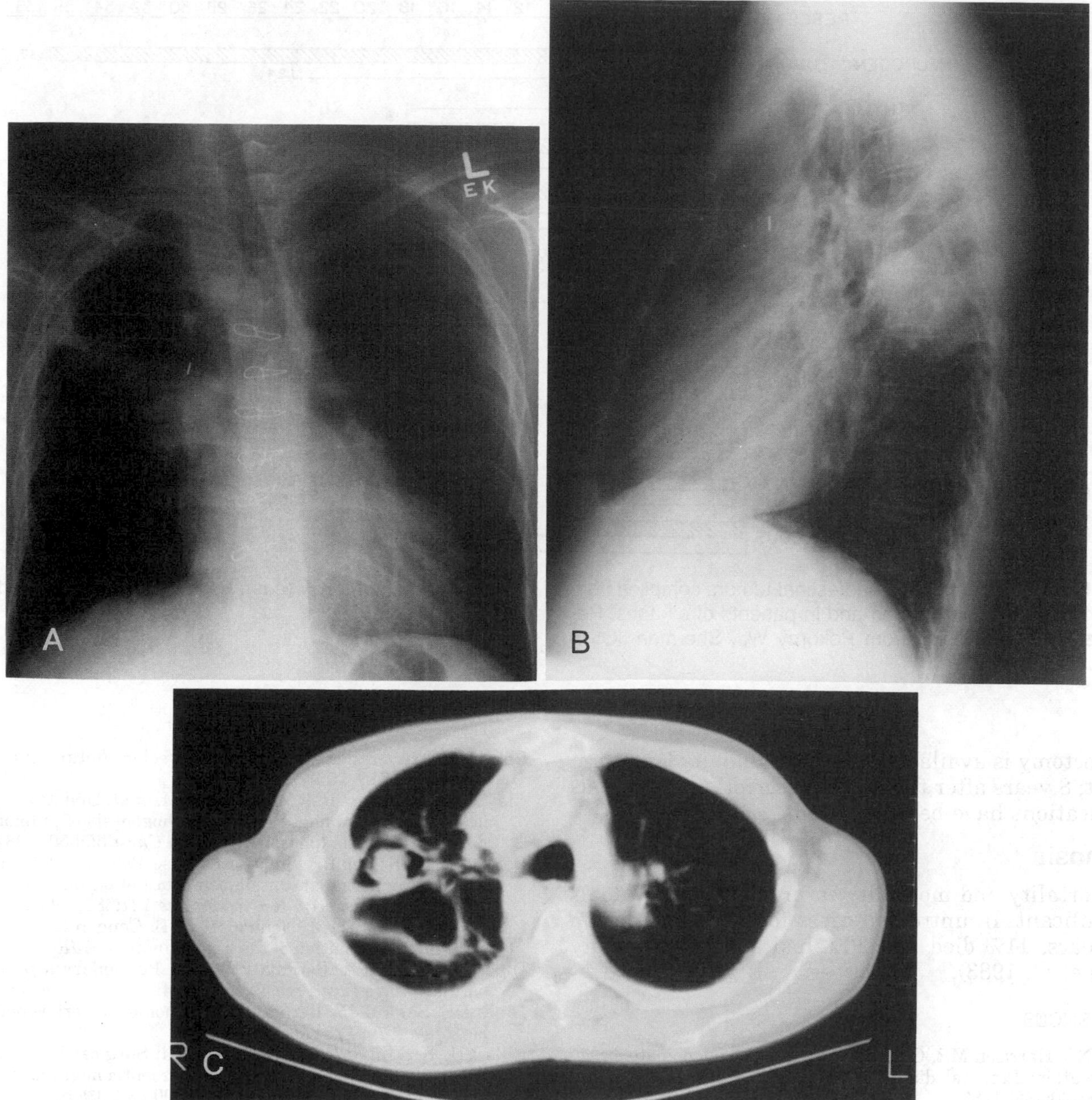

Figure 5.24.A, B, and **C.** This teenage boy with severe complex cyanotic congenital heart disease developed cavitary lesions in the right lung **(A** and **B)** which were evaluated with CT scan **(C)**. The cross-sectional image shows, to good advantage, one of the cavitations with a solid mass—a fungus ball—within. Fungal infections can also complicate the course of children who are immunosuppressed.

pain may prompt investigation and diagnosis. Hemoptysis is rare.

Arterial desaturation can result in polycythemia and clubbing. The condition can be distinguished from congenital cyanotic heart disease by normal electrocardiograms and hemodynamic studies.

Diagnosis

Soft systolic or continuous murmurs may be heard over the site of the fistula. Chest radiographs reveal a peripheral circumscribed lesion that is not calcified, but has vascular connections to the hilus of the lung. CT scans and radionuclide angiography are useful in confirming the diagnosis. Angiography is mandatory before definitive treatment.

Treatment

Embolotherapy is useful for some lesions, either by insertion of a coil or a balloon. In some instances, excision is appropriate. Insufficient experience with

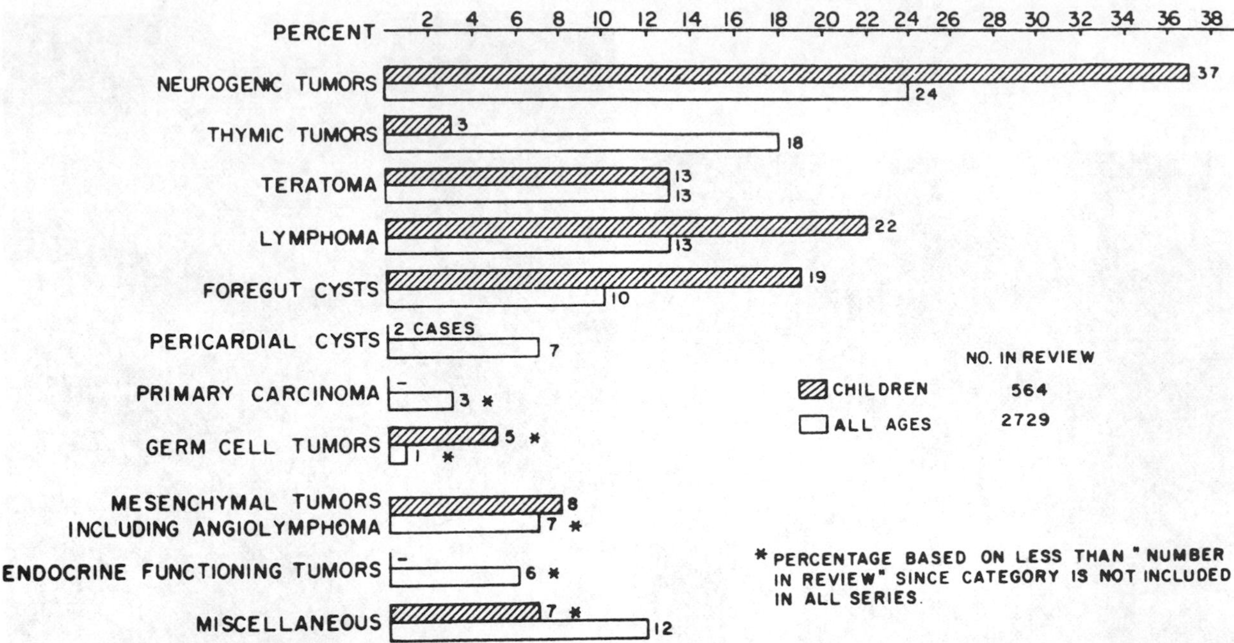

Figure 5.25. Percentage of mediastinal tumors compiled from several large series in children and in patients of all ages. Reproduced with permission from Pokorny WJ, Sherman JO: In Holder TM, Ashcraft KW (eds): *Pediatric Surgery*. Philadelphia, WB Saunders, 1980.

embolectomy is available to be certain of its long-term benefit; 8 years after the initial description, no serious complications have been reported.

Prognosis

Mortality and morbidity in untreated individuals is significant. In untreated cases followed for a mean of 6 years, 11% died and 26% had serious morbidity (Dines et al, 1983).

REFERENCES

Adzick NS, Harrison MR, Glick PC: Fetal cystic adenomatoid malformation: Prenatal diagnosis and natural history. *J Pediatr Surg* 20:483, 1985.

Alivizatos P, Cheatle T, deLeval M, Stark J: Pulmonary sequestration complicated by anomalies of pulmonary venous return. *J Pediatr Surg* 20:76, 1985.

Asher MI, Spier S, Beland M, et al: Primary lung abscess in childhood. The long-term outcome of conservative management. *Am J Dis Child* 136:491, 1982.

Avery ME, Fletcher BD, Williams RG: *The Lung and its Disorders in the Newborn Infant*, 4th edition. Philadelphia, WB Saunders, 1981.

Avery ME, Ohlsson A, Cummings W, et al: Clinical Pathologic Conference. The King Faisal Medical Specialist Hospital Medical Journal, 4:33, 1984.

Baum GL, Racz I, Bubis JJ, et al: Cystic disease of the lung. *Am J Med* 40:578, 1966.

Brooks JG, Bustamante SA, Koops BL, et al: Selective bronchial intubation for the treatment of severe localized pulmonary interstitial emphysema in newborn infants. *J Pediatr* 91:648, 1977.

Burke CM, Safai C, Nelson DP, et al: Pulmonary arteriovenous malformations: A critical update. *Am Rev Respir Dis* 134:334, 1986.

Carter R: Pulmonary sequestration. *Ann Thorac Surg* 7:68, 1969.

Case Records of Massachusetts General Hospital. *N Engl J Med* 310:36, 1984.

Chernick V, Avery ME: Spontaneous alveolar rupture at birth. *Pediatrics* 32:816, 1963.

Claypool WD, Rogers RM, Matuschak GM, et al: Update on the clinical diagnosis, management and pathogenesis of pulmonary alveolar proteinosis (phospholipidosis). *Chest* 85:550, 1984.

Coleman M, Dehner LP, Sibley RK: Case Reports; Pulmonary alveolar proteinosis; an uncommon cause of chronic neonatal respiratory distress. *Am Rev Respir Dis* 121:583, 1980.

Craig JM, Kirkpatrick J, Neuhauser EBD: Congenital cystic adenomatoid malformation of the lung of infants. *AJR* 76:516, 1956.

Dines DE, Arms RA, Bernatz PE, et al: Pulmonary arteriovenous fistulas. *Mayo Clin Proc* 49:460, 1974.

Dines DE, Seward JB, Bernatz PE: Pulmonary arteriovenous fistulas. *Mayo Clin Proc* 58:176, 1983.

Ellis FH, Kirklin JW, Hodgson JR, et al: Surgical implications of the mediastinal shadow in thoracic roentgenograms of infants and children. *Surg Gynecol Obstet* 100:532, 1955.

Eraklis AJ, Griscom NT, McGovern JB: Bronchogenic cysts of the mediastinum in infancy. *N Engl J Med* 281:1150, 1969.

Fine NH, Smith LR, Sheedy PF: Frequency of pleural effusions in mycoplasma and viral pneumonias. *N Engl J Med* 288:790, 1970.

Fox LS, Buntain WL, Brasfield D, et al: Pulmonary arteriovenous malformations in children. *J Pediatr Surg* 14:53, 1979.

Frantz ID, Werthammer J, Stark AR: High-frequency ventilation in premature infants with lung disease: adequate gas exchange at low tracheal pressure. *Pediatrics* 71:483, 1983.

Gerle RD, Jaretzki A, Ashley CA, et al: Congenital bronchopulmonary foregut malformation. *N Engl J Med* 278:1413, 1968.

Griz A, Giammona ST: Pneumonitis with pleural effusion in children due to *Mycoplasma pneumoniae*. *Am Rev Respir Dis* 109:665, 1974.

Hall JR, Pyeritz RE, Dudgeon DL, et al: Pneumothorax in the Marfan syndrome: Prevalence and therapy. *Ann Thorac Surg* 37:500, 1984.

Kafka V, Padorcova H, Kabelka M et al: A congenital arteriovenous pulmonary aneurysm in a two and one half year old boy. *J Cardiovasc Surg* 2:396, 1961.

Kevy S: Streptococcal pneumonia and empyema in childhood. *N Engl J Med* 264:738, 1963.

Krech WG, Storey CF, Umiker WC: Thymic cysts: A review of the literature and report of two cases. *J Thorac Surg* 27:477, 1954.

Landing BH: Congenital malformations and genetic disorders of the respiratory tract. (Larynx, trachea, bronchi and lungs.) *Am Rev Respir Dis* 120:151, 1979.

Laurence KN: Congenital pulmonary cystic lymphangiectasis. *J Pathol* 70:325, 1955.

Light RW: Parapneumonic effusions and empyema. *Clin Chest Med* 6:55, 1985.

Madansky DL, Lawson EE, Chernick V, et al: Pneumothorax and other forms of pulmonary air leak in newborns. *Am Rev Respir Dis* 120:729, 1979.

Massaro D, Katz, S, et al: Von Recklinghansen's neurofibromatosis associated with cystic lung disease. *Am J Med* 38:233, 1965.

McLaughlin FJ, Goldman DA, Rosenbaum DM, et al: Empyema in children: Clinical course and long-term follow-up. *Pediatrics* 73:587, 1984.

McLaughlin FJ, Matthews WJ, Strieder DJ, et al: Pneumothorax in cystic fibrosis: Management and outcome. *J Pediatr* 100:863, 1982.

Neill CA, Ferencz C, Sabiston D, et al: The familial occurrence of hypoplastic right lung with systemic arterial supply and venous drainage "scimitar syndrome." *Bull Johns Hopkins Hosp* 107:1, 1960.

Nelson JP: Pleural empyema. *Pediatr Infect Dis* 4:531, 1985.

Noonan JA, Walters LR, Reeves JT: Congenital pulmonary lymphangiectasis. *Am J Dis Child* 120:314, 1970.

Pokorny WJ, Sherman JO: Mediastinal tumors. In Holder TM, Ashcraft KW (eds): *Pediatric Surgery*. Philadelphia, WB Saunders, 1980.

Stocker JT, Drake RM, Maxwell JE: Cystic and congenital lung disease in the newborn. *Perspect Pediatr Pathol* 4:93, 1978.

Teja K, Cooper PH, Squires JE, et al: Pulmonary alveolar proteinosis in four siblings. *N Engl J Med* 305:1390, 1981.

Thompson RE, Lowe WG: Persistent cervical thymoma apparent with crying. *Am J dis Child* 124:761, 1972.

Tomsick TA, Niesber SE, Smith WL: The congenital pulmonary venolobar syndrome in three successive generations. *J Can Assoc Radiol* 27:196, 1976.

Tucker TT, Smith WC, Smith JA: Fluid-filled cystic adenomatoid malformation. *AJR* 129:323, 1977.

Whittaker LD, Lynn HB: Mediastinal tumors and cysts in the pediatric patient. *Surg Clin North Am* 53:893, 1973.

Lymphatics 7

LYMPHANGIECTASIS

Definition

Abnormal dilatation of pulmonary lymphatics from a congenital defect is called pulmonary lymphangiectasis.

Epidemiology

This disorder is very rare. It has been reported twice as commonly in males, and has been seen in families (Scott-Emuakpor et al, 1981).

Natural History

In its severe diffuse form, this disorder is associated with parenchymal hypoplasia or congestion and may be lethal in infancy. In other individuals with a milder expression, it may be detected by an incidental chest radiograph. It may be isolated or coexist with generalized lymphatic disorders. Hyperaeration is regularly noted and helps to distinguish the condition from HMD with which it may sometimes be confused.

In the majority of infants, respiratory distress is noted at birth and cyanosis is marked and persistent. The duration of life in most symptomatic infants ranges from 30 minutes to 30 days. Very rarely, symptoms abate and survivals up to 4 years are known in infants who are symptomatic in infancy.

Children who are asymptomatic in infancy may have associated malformations of the lymphatic system such as lymphangiomas of the extremities or the intestine. In such instances, the pulmonary lesion may first have been recognized only after a routine chest radiograph, the classic appearance of which is a diffuse reticular pattern with prominent fissures.

Diagnosis

Pulmonary lymphangiectasis is usually associated with lymphedema elsewhere, as in Noonan syndrome. It can also be present in severe pulmonic stenosis. The radiologist is often the first to suggest the diagnosis on the basis of dilated lymphatics and sometimes pleural fluid on the chest radiograph. The diagnosis is more difficult when the infant or child has had no symptoms or has a late onset chylous effusion.

Removal and examination of the pleural fluid is essential. Mononuclear cells, elevated protein to about 4%, and chyle (if the patient has had milk or other sources of lipid) are diagnostic in the presence of a compatible radiograph and the absence of fever or other signs of systemic illness.

Lung biopsy is not indicated and can be hazardous. Once distended lymphatic channels are severed, they can leak fluid for weeks. Only if the possibility of malignancy is considered, or if the patient is not improved with repeated thoracenteses should open lung biopsy be considered and then undertaken with great care.

Treatment

Treatment is supportive only.

CONTROVERSY

The postmortem diagnosis of lymphangiectasis may be straightforward if dilated lymphatics are visible grossly. In other circumstances, it is less clear. Some infants have extensive pulmonary interstitial emphysema that may persist for weeks. In these conditions when lobectomy has been carried out to permit expansion of more normal lung, the lymphatics in the excised lobe may be dilated. Interstitial spaces may also appear to have lining cells, and their appearance is strikingly similar to some reported cases of pulmonary lymphangiectasis.

It could be argued that lobes in which interstitial air persists are abnormal, and a form of lobar lymphangiectasis could be hypothesized. Further careful examination of infants with lymphatic abnormalities as well as a study of animal models may clarify the picture.

CHYLOTHORAX

Definition

Accumulation of chylous fluid in the pleural space is known as chylothorax.

Epidemiology

Congenital chylothorax is rare. Only 12 cases were diagnosed over a 22-year period at the Hospital for Sick Children in Toronto. Acquired chylous effusions are more common, especially in centers in which cardiac surgery is performed or after prolonged intravenous alimentation with obstruction of superior vena cava.

Natural History

Pleural effusion in the absence of infection may present at any time within the first weeks of life. Tachypnea, retractions and mediastinal shift with decreased air entry on the affected side should alert the physician to the diagnosis. Spontaneous effusions are most common on the right, but may be bilateral, and rarely only on the left.

The cause of spontaneous chylothorax is not clear. Some cases can be related to birth trauma, and rupture of the thoracic duct has been repaired surgically. Most instances are not related to trauma, and a congenital defect is assumed. Clearly, because most infants recover, new growth of lymphatics must occur.

Spontaneous chylothorax has been associated with fetal hydrops, hydramnios, and Down, Noonan, and Turner syndromes.

Diagnosis

Thoracentesis before oral feeding will produce a clear fluid with several thousand white cells, over 90% of which are mononuclear. After milk feeding, the liquid becomes white or chylous. It contains, on average, 4% protein.

Treatment

Thoracentesis, repeated as long as liquid reaccumulates, eventually leads to cure. A serious complication of prolonged removal of liquid is malnutrition from protein depletion and decreased immunocompetence from lymphocyte depletion. Substitution of an elemental formula with medium-chain triglycerides helps to reduce chyle formation.

Prognosis

Most forms of chylothorax are self-limited. Rarely, when it occurs as a postoperative complication, exploration for the site of blockage may be indicated.

CONTROVERSY

How long should liquid continue to be removed before surgical exploration? We are willing to be patient for several months; but continuous drainage should be avoided since it operates as a siphon. If a chest tube is inserted, it should be clamped except for active drainage once or twice a day.

REFERENCES

Noonan JA, Walters LR, Reeves JT: Congenital pulmonary lymphangiectasis. *Am J Dis Child* 120:314, 1970.

Scott-Emuakpor AB, Warren ST, Kapur S, et al: Familial occurrence of congenital pulmonary lymphangiectasis. Genetic implications. *Am J Dis Child* 135:532, 1981.

VanAerde J, Campbell AN, Smythe JA, et al: Spontaneous chylothorax in newborns. *Am J Dis Child* 138:961, 1984.

Diaphragm and Chest Wall

8

MUSCLES OF RESPIRATION

The diaphragm is the principal muscle of respiration, but only one of many muscles that can operate to expand or contract the thoracic cage. The contraction of the diaphragm causes descent of its dome and aids in elevation of the lower ribs. The costal part of the diaphragm innervated by C5 is crucial in this inspiratory activity. Among the numerous other muscle groups that are important are the intercostal, abdominal, scalene, and sternocleidomastoid muscles. In disease states, these muscles may be very visibly at work as is evident to any individual in respiratory distress.

While it is important to realize that the weakness of respiratory failure can be due to failure of respiratory muscles as in neuromuscular diseases, whether respiratory muscle fatigue can ever limit performance remains uncertain.

Very few studies of this sort have been undertaken in children (Gaultier et al, 1985), but there has been some important information obtained from studies on adults. We know, for example, from histochemical studies that there are three types of muscle fibers in the diaphragm, and from physiologic investigations they can be classified as those which are slow-twitch fatigue-resistant, those which are fast-twitch fatigue-resistant, and the third type being the fast-twitch fatigable group. The fatigue-resistant groups have a high oxidative capacity which apparently increases with training. The oxidative capacity is relatively decreased in preterm infants.

The assessment of respiratory muscle activity is an important part of the physical examination. The diaphragm can be seen by observing movements of the lower rib cage and abdominal wall. In inspiration, the lower rib cage operates to expand the abdominal cavity to permit the diaphragm to descend. With diaphragmatic fatigue, the lower rib cage is drawn in with inspiration.

Diaphragmatic function can be studied with ultrasonography or with magnetometers to assess movement. The pressures exerted by the diaphragm can be measured by occluding the airway during normal breathing and measuring the maximal pressure that can be generated with an inspiratory effort in the airway. A normal value is about 100 cm H_2O (Gaultier and Zinman, 1983).

The nutritional status of the individual is important in determining the inspiratory muscle strength. In a group of malnourished adults who were receiving total parenteral nutrition, the reduction in body cell mass was correlated positively with the reduction in the maximal inspiratory pressure these individuals could generate. When their nutritional status improved so did their inspiratory muscle strength.

CASE ILLUSTRATION

The patient was a 14-year-old boy who had been evaluated 6 months before because of an 8-year history of clamp-like tightening and difficulty in relaxing limb muscles. On several occasions, he had fallen to the ground in a rigid position. The symptoms were notably reduced by preliminary warm-up. Electromyography of several limb muscles showed typical changes seen in myotonia congenita.

Although he had no respiratory symptoms at rest, he described an uncomfortable sensation of chest-tightening and dyspnea on exertion. These sensations were most prominent at the beginning of effort, but improved thereafter.

A detailed investigation of respiratory muscle function was undertaken. Routine pulmonary function tests, including static respiratory pressures, had been found to be within normal limits. The respiratory muscles showed increased excitability, impaired relaxation, and transient weakness similar to the findings in skeletal muscle. The authors remark that without the evaluation of respiratory muscles, in particular, the respiratory sensations experienced by the patient at the beginning of exercise would have been unexplained.

COMMENT

It becomes obvious that we have much to learn about the normal maturation of respiratory muscle strength and coordination, particularly in the newborn infant, and about the effects of long-term use of mechanical ventilation or muscle relaxants on developing muscle strength. Although the data are not available, it seems probable that the need for ventilatory assistance may be prolonged in many instances by not allowing the respiratory muscles to operate during periods of illness and the situation may well be compounded by some degree of malnutrition in the individuals who are chronically ill.

One mechanism by which chronic malnutrition could have an adverse affect on diaphragmatic function is through hypophosphaturia, which could limit available ATP. Thus, maintaining normal serum inorganic phosphate is important in the care of individuals with respiratory failure (Aubier et al, 1985).

The value of an assessment of respiratory muscle function in neuromuscular disease was highlighted by a report from Belgium (Estenne et al, 1984).

CONGENITAL DIAPHRAGMATIC HERNIA

Definition

A defect in the diaphragm that permits herniation of abdominal viscera into the thoracic cavity is a congenital diaphragmatic hernia.

Epidemiology

The reported prevalence of diaphragmatic hernias is between 1/2500 live births (Collaborative Perinatal Project 1959–1966), and 1/5000 live births (Hansen et al, 1984).

Basic Science

The diaphragm consists of two muscles: one derived from myoblasts in the lateral body wall forms the costal part; the other from the dorsal mesentery of the esophagus forms the crural part (DeTroyer et al, 1981). In dogs and probably in humans, the costal diaphragm is in series with intercostal muscles, and the crural diaphragm is in parallel. Contraction of the costal part expands the rib cage. In instances when the muscles do not join in development, the resulting defect may be the site of herniation of abdominal viscera. The most common defect is situated in the posterolateral aspect of the diaphragm and it occurs about 5 times as often on the left (foramen of Bochdalek). Less common are herniations through the substernal sinus of Morgagni. A thoracic stomach with short esophagus is discussed in Section 7.

Natural History

Small defects may never be recognized during life. Others may have intermittent herniation and the condition may not be recognized for some days or even months or years (Hight et al, 1982). The most severe, as in congenital absence of a leaf of the diaphragm, may have allowed the bowel to be in a hemithorax from early fetal life with hypoplasia of the ipsilateral lung. Hydramnios is present in 75% of infants with diaphragmatic hernia.

Between 60 and 80% of these infants die within the first 24 hours. Nearly all who survive that period will withstand operative repair and will recover.

Diagnosis

The infant born with bowel or other viscera in one side of the thorax is in no trouble until after birth. Very soon severe respiratory distress and cyanosis become marked. Initially the abdomen may be scaphoid. With resuscitative efforts, overdistention of the stomach can occur unless relieved by a nasogastric tube.

Auscultation may reveal bowel sounds in the chest, and absence of gas exchange on one side. The heart may be displaced to the side opposite the hernia. Given these findings, radiographs are essential. Contrast studies are indicated only if the diagnosis is in doubt (Fig. 5.26*A* and *B*).

In the older child these may be vague intermittent gastrointestinal symptoms or the finding may be incidental.

Treatment

It is urgent to prevent gastric distention that would further compromise space for pulmonary expansion. An indwelling feeding tube with continuous suction is essential. Inspired oxygen should be increased, but care should be taken to ensure that mechanical ventilation does not cause rupture of hypoplastic lungs. Consultation with a pediatric surgeon is urgent.

Many problems may occur, including a tendency to bilateral pneumothorax, persistent pulmonary hypertension, and hypoplastic lungs. The outlook for survival depends on the severity of these problems.

CONTROVERSY

Heroic measures may be rewarding for some of these infants; some respond to intravenous vasodilators such as tolazoline with support of the systemic circulation with dopamine. Others have responded to extracorporeal membrane oxygenation for a few days. These interventions require heparinization, and are not advised in premature infants. More experience is needed to assess their ultimate role (see pp. 160) (Towne et al, 1985; Bartlett et al, 1986; Langham et al, 1987).

Intrauterine diagnosis is possible. In situations where early delivery has been undertaken with pediatric surgeons alerted to operate as soon as the infant is delivered, the outcome is bleak if profound pulmonary hypoplasia is present. In a review of 94 infants in whom prenatal diagnosis was made with ultrasonography, 80% died in the neonatal period despite prompt surgical intervention (Adzick et al, 1985).

Prognosis

Infants with posterolateral hernias operated on in the first 24 hours have only about a 50% chance of survival. Those who can survive longer have hernias of lesser degree and fare better.

The prognosis depends on the degree of pulmonary hypoplasia and other malformations, such as hydrocephaly and Arnold-Chiari malformations, and cardiac and renal malformations.

Evaluation of survivors in later childhood shows reduced pulmonary blood flow persisting on the side of the hernia.

DIAPHRAGMATIC PARALYSIS

Bilateral diaphragmatic paralysis can be devastating at any age and is lethal in infancy. One reason for bilateral diaphragmatic paralysis includes congen-

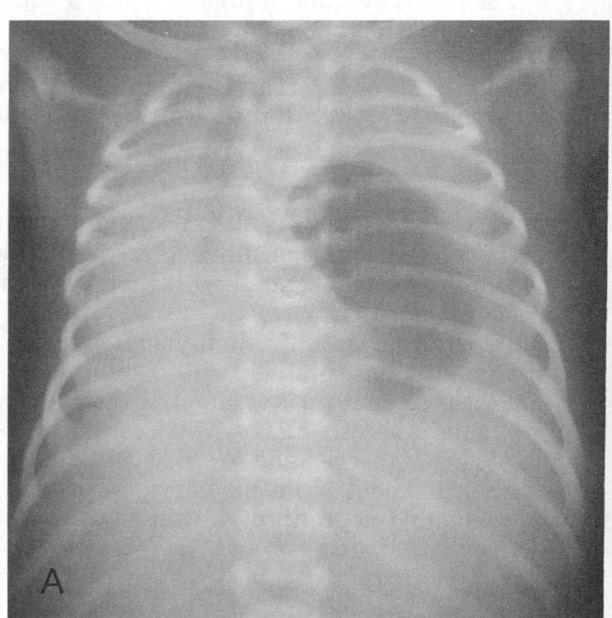

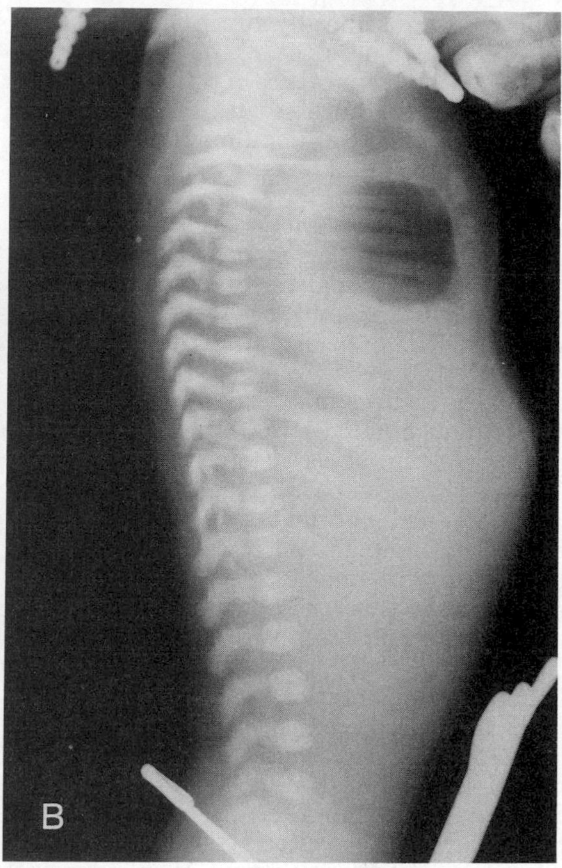

Figure 5.26.A and **B.** Patient was referred at 24 hours of age after clinical examination revealed cyanosis and respiratory distress. Anteroposterior and lateral views of chest and abdomen show an air-filled stomach in the left hemithorax. There is shift of mediastinum to the right. Both lungs are opacified. The lateral view of the abdomen shows a scaphoid appearance with no air containing loops of bowel. This baby, who was born 30 years ago, died 4 hours after admission. Now, diagnosis of diaphragmatic hernia is frequently made in utero on prenatal scans. The baby is delivered, a nasogastric tube is placed immediately, the hernia is repaired, and respiratory function is carefully monitored and supported with rapid progression to extracorporeal membrane oxygenation (ECMO) in selected cases if it is necessary.

ital absence of the phrenic nerve, and when this has been reported it has been associated with extremely hypoplastic lungs and has been fatal.

When one or both hemidiaphragms are paralyzed later in life, or during the course of delivery, lung size may be normal and some recovery is possible.

Basic Science

In infants, diaphragmatic muscles contain relatively few fatigue-resistant type 1 fibers, which is clearly one of the reasons for such infants being prone to apneic spells. When they spend much of their time lying supine and there is diaphragmatic weakness, lung function is further compromised.

Diagnosis

Because paralysis of one diaphragm is most commonly associated with Erb palsy, it is essential to determine if there were any complications during delivery of the infant; weakness of the arm would point toward a traumatic injury to the nerve routes of C3–5. Under these circumstances, respiration is obviously exceedingly difficult and retractions of the chest wall are seen during inspiration. The diagnosis can be established readily by fluoroscopy; during inspiration, both hemidiaphragms move upward with bilateral paralysis.

Treatment

The indications for diaphragmatic plication are controversial. Some surgeons recommend plication when a diaphragm has been paralyzed for longer than 2–6 weeks. Plication does not always improve the function of the diaphragm but it may help prevent atelectasis and significant mediastinal shift.

Bilateral plication is of dubious value, according to Aldrich et al (1980). In the literature reviewed to 1980, which included five bilateral plications, only one patient was alive 10 months later.

SCOLIOSIS

One of the most common reasons for deformity of the chest wall is scoliosis, which is usually detected for the first time during adolescence. In some instances where there is neuromuscular dysfunction or vertebral anomalies, scoliosis can occur at a much earlier age.

The extent to which curvature of the spine impairs lung function is of importance as surgical correction is possible and knowledge of cardiopulmonary status has some role in the timing of intervention. (For discussion of scoliosis, see Section 23.)

Abnormalities in lung function show a reduction in total lung capacity as well as in maximal inspiratory airway pressure at functional residual capacity. Both static and dynamic lung compliance can be reduced. In an evaluation of patients before and after surgery for scoliosis, Cooper et al (1984), reported that both maximal inspiratory pressures and peak expiratory flows increased in patients studied 1 year after the Harrington procedure (insertion of a rod to correct the curvature). The investigators compared lung volumes in these patients with expected normal values by using arm span instead of linear height inasmuch as height was shortened in those with more severe scoliosis. Even though the patients in this study had mild to moderate scoliosis, they were free of respiratory symptoms both at rest and during exercise. Others have found, however, that there can be deterioration in lung function in adults with untreated scoliosis characterized by elevation of functional residual capacity and a fall in arterial oxygen saturation (Kafer, 1976).

The decision on when to intervene depends on the rate of progression of the scoliosis as well as the deterioration in lung function (see pp. 1283). Surgical correction is usually performed in adolescents with curves of 40 to 50°. This degree of curvature is not associated with a reduction in total lung capacity. Nonetheless, a measurement of lung function is of value because of the possibility of an additional neuromuscular problem.

ASPHYXIATING THORACIC DYSTROPHY

Many of the generalized chondrodystrophies can involve the rib cage. One of these is asphyxiating thoracic dystrophy of Jeune, or thoracic-pelvic-phalangeal dystrophy. The small thorax, with hypoplastic lungs, impairs ventilation from birth. The diaphragm is flattened, and liver and spleen are pushed down and readily palpable. Renal dysplasia may be present. Almost all infants reported in the literature have died in the first year of life, although one gradually improved and was short but otherwise normal at age 15 years (Oberklaid et al, 1977). The disorder is familial and is inherited as autosomal recessive (Fig. 5.27*A* and *B*). Attempts at operative correction have not been successful. Prenatal diagnosis with ultrasonography is possible (Lipson et al, 1984).

OTHER DISORDERS

Osteopenia from any cause may involve the ribs and impair their ability to augment normal resting lung volume. The most common cause of osteopenia in infancy is rickets, which in its severe form can result in a flail chest.

Multiple rib fractures, as in osteogenesis imperfecta, hypophosphatasia, or copper deficiency in preterm infants, can impair normal chest wall function.

Pectus Excavatum and Carinatum

Definition

Pectus excavatum, funnel chest, is a depression of the lower portion of the sternum from an overgrowth of anterior costal cartilage that fixes the sternum in a posterior position. Pectus carinatum (pigeon breast) causes the lower sternum to protrude anteriorly.

Epidemiology

Pectus excavatum is the most common chest wall deformity; pectus carinatum is rarely seen. Pectus excavatum may be associated with Pierre Robin or Marfan syndrome. Family members are affected in more than a third of patients. It is about four times more common in males than females (Table 5.12).

Pectus carinatum is symmetric in about two-thirds of patients. A family history was present in 26% in the series of Shamberger and Welch (1987). Associated anomalies includes scoliosis, Morquio disease, Poland syndrome, and neurofibromatosis.

Natural History

Pectus excavatum is rarely present at birth, but becomes more prominent in the first years of life. Occasionally, with growth, the deformity becomes less apparent.

A pseudopectus deformity is frequently seen in premature infants who have had chronic lung disease, and usually becomes less prominent with recovery.

In severe cases, anterior compression of the heart against the vertebral column is thought to be the cause of mitral valve prolapse in nearly half of patients (Shamberger, et al 1987).

Diagnosis

A 2-cm depression is considered significant. Serial photographs provide the best documentation of changes with time. When severe, the heart is shifted to the left. Evaluation of cardiopulmonary function is appropriate. Progression of the defect, or impairment in pulmonary function are indications for operative repair.

Treatment

In pectus excavatum, many surgeons recommend removal of abnormal cartilage at 5–6 years of age, when normal growth and development of the chest wall can ensue. The operation is a major one and results in considerable discomfort, and a midline scar. In pectus carinatum, operative repair is deferred until midteens, after the growth spurt to reduce risk of recurrence. The effect of repair on function is of questionable benefit. In most situations this is done for cosmetic purposes (Shamberger and Welch, 1987).

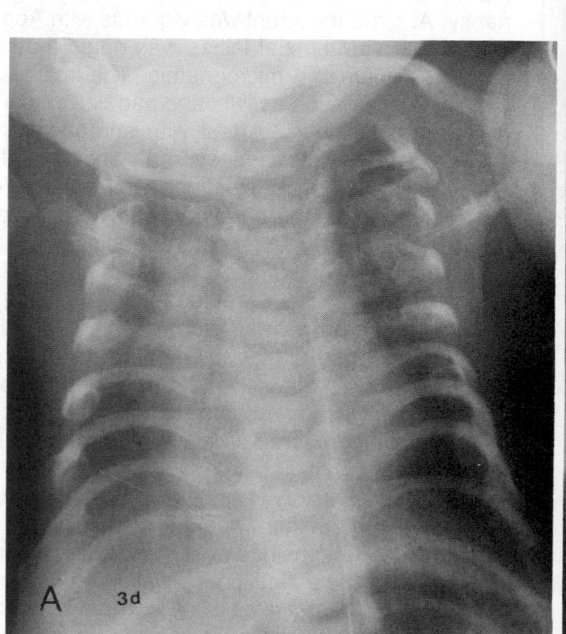

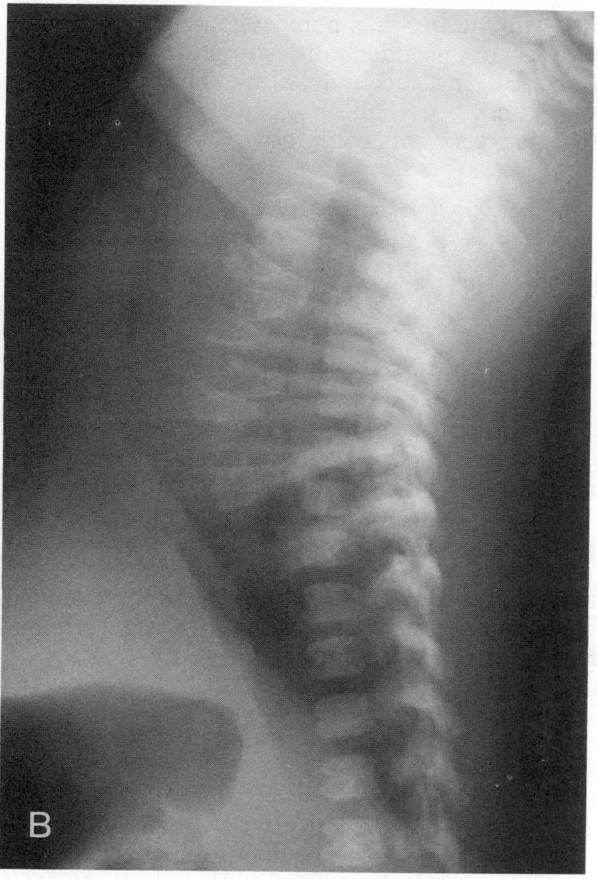

Figure 5.27.A and **B.** Asphyxiating thoracic dystrophy (Jeune disease). This baby had mild respiratory distress at birth. Radiographs, taken at that time, show her abnormally small thorax. She died at 5 months of chronic respiratory failure. The appearance of the chest is typical of Jeune thoracic dystrophy with rather horizontal short ribs, narrow shallow thorax, and low, flat hemidiaphragms. It is interesting that on postmortem examination, lungs were normal in weight for the child's age and there were the normal number of airways and alveoli. Gross and microscopic features of one rib showed a severely disordered endochondreal ossification at both costovertebral and costochondral junctions. Jeune syndrome is an autosomal recessive disease which typically leads to death in early life. Interstitial nephritis is an associated abnormality.

Table 5.12
Surgical Correction of Anterior Chest Wall Deformities in Patients at Children's Hospital, Boston 1952–1982 [1]

Type of Deformity	No. of Patients
Pectus excavatum	970
	M 775
	F 195
Pectus carinatum	138
	M 95
	F 43
Recurrent pectus excavatum	14
Poland's syndrome	12
Vertebral and rib anomalies	7
Lower sternal cleft	7
Upper sternal cleft	5
Ectopia cordis	3
Total	1156

[1]Courtesy of Dr. Kenneth Welch.

Prognosis

Results are considered excellent in 90% of patients with pectus excavatum repaired before the adolescent growth spurt. Recurrences are rare.

NEUROMUSCULAR DISORDERS

Myopathies

The diaphragm and chest wall muscles may be weak from any one of a number of congenital myopathies (see also Section 12) (reviewed in detail by Dubowitz, 1978). Usually the disorders involve all striated muscle.

Intrauterine or acquired poliomyelitis can result in asymmetric muscle paralysis and involve the muscles of respiration.

Transient muscle weakness has been described from transplacental passage of succinylcholine (Hoefnagel et al, 1979). The mother was homozygous for the atypical allele for serum pseudocholinesterase, and became apneic after receiving succinylcholine. The infant, delivered by section, breathed once, and was apneic for 20 minutes. Recovery was complete.

Myasthenia Gravis

Infants of mothers with myasthenia gravis (see also pp. 736, Neurology) can have transient neonatal myasthenia which reverses after a few weeks.

Basic Science

Antibodies to maternal acetylcholine receptors can cross the placenta and adversely affect neurotransmission in the infant.

Epidemiology

About 12% of infants of symptomatic mothers have the condition, but it is much more rare among asymptomatic mothers who have had thymectomy.

Natural History

The infants may be born with a weak cry and symmetrical hypotonia. They may have difficulty sucking and some of them have difficulty with clearing secretions. In the neonatal form, their eyes are usually open and extraocular muscles work well. Facial weakness is, however, very evident. The condition is usually present within a few days of birth and may last for several weeks. Recovery may be quite sudden so that there is a danger of overdose of neostigmine.

Diagnosis

Diagnosis should be expected in any "floppy" infant with a weak Moro reflex but normal knee jerks. The differential diagnosis is extensive but transient myasthenia should be suspected if the mother has myasthenia. Rarely a congenital persistent form of the disease may occur and present in the newborn period. This is not caused by receptor antibodies and may respond poorly to therapy. Presumably, it results from a genetic abnormality of the acetylcholine receptor protein. The differential diagnosis includes infant botulism and other congenital myopathies.

The diagnosis of the transient form is made with a test dose of neostigmine 0.02 mg/kg subcutaneously, usually given with atropine 0.01 mg/kg subcutaneously. After about 10 minutes, the infant should be manifestly stronger. It is possible to measure serum acetycholine receptor antibodies to confirm the diagnosis.

Treatment

The infants should continue to receive neostigmine methylsulfate in doses of 0.1–0.2 mg/kg subcutaneously as long as muscle strength is impaired.

CASE ILLUSTRATION

A 3.5-kg baby girl was born at term to a 31-year-old mother who had had a thymectomy for myasthenia gravis. She was on alternate-day low-dose prednisone therapy during the pregnancy. Her acetylcholine receptor antibodies were markedly elevated before and during the pregnancy. At birth, the infant was vigorous with Apgar scores of 7 and 9. An unusual facies was noted, however, with epicanthal folds and micrognathia. The infant was hypotonic with decreased activity and had flexion contractures of hands and fingers. A test with edrophonium chloride (Tensilon), was not diagnostic but, because of the suspected diagnosis of transient neonatal myasthenia gravis, the infant was started on pyridostigmine bromide (Mestinon), 5 mg every 4 hours, before feedings. The response to therapy was equivocal. At 6 days of age the infant had a mild cholinergic crisis that led to discontinuing the medication. The infant slowly improved and was discharged on the eighth day of life, still moderately hypotonic. She gained strength progressively over the next 3 months. The infant's acetylcholine receptor antibody titer in cord blood was 50 units compared with a normal value of less than 5.

The family history is significant in that the mother had experienced intermittent weakness and diplopia since age 15 and the symptoms had worsened with each pregnancy. Her firstborn male had poor swallowing, cyanosis, and apnea for the first 2 weeks of life and, at that time, no cause was found. The second male infant was normal, but the third male infant had multiple contractures, hypoplastic lungs, and unusual facies and died despite ventilator therapy. The diagnosis was trisomy 18. During genetic counseling of the mother, the pediatrician made the diagnosis of maternal myasthenia gravis on the basis of the fact that the mother could not keep her eyelids open. In retrospect, it seems possible that both the first- and third-born infants had some degree of neonatal myasthenia.

Prognosis

The prognosis for infants with the congenital persistent form is poor because, often, the diagnosis is not considered and not all infants respond to medication. The outlook for those with the transient form is excellent because the maternal history makes the diagnosis almost certain and careful care in the neonatal period with judicious use of neostigmine should produce permanent recovery.

The possibility that maternal myasthenia gravis can be associated with contractures in a newborn infant (arthrogryposis multiplex congenita) was raised by observations of Holmes et al (1980).

REFERENCES

Adzick NS, Harrison MR, Glick PL, et al: Diaphragmatic hernia in the fetus: Prenatal diagnosis and outcome in 94 cases. *J. Pediatr Surg* 20:357, 1985.

Aldrich TK, Herman JH, Rochester DF: Bilateral diaphragmatic paralysis in the new born infant. *J. Pediatr* 97:988, 1980.

Aubier M, Muirciano D, Lecocguic Y, et al: Effect of hypophosphatemia on diaphragmatic contractility in patients with acute respiratory failure. *N. Engl J Med* 313:420, 1985.
Avery ME, Fletcher BD, Williams RG: *The Lung and its Disorders in the Newborn Infant*, 4th edition. Philadelphia, WB Saunders, 1981.
Bartlett RH, Gazzaniga AB, Toomasian J, et al: Extracorporeal membrane oxygenation (ECMO) in neonatal respiratory failure in 100 cases. *Ann Surg* 204:236, 1986.
Castile RG, Staats BA, Westbrook PR: Symptomatic pectus deformities of the chest. *Am Respir Dis* 126:564, 1982.
Cooper DM, Rojas JV, Mellins RB, et al: Respiratory mechanics in adolesents with idopathic scoliosis. *Am Rev Respir Dis* 130:16, 1984.
DeTroyer A, Sampson M, Sigrist S, et al: The diaphragm: Two muscles. *Science* 213:237, 1981.
Drachman DB: Present and future treatment of myasthenia gravis. *N Engl J Med* 316:743, 1987.
Dubowitz V: *Muscle Disorders in Childhood.* Philadelphia, WB Saunders, 1978.
Estenne M, Borenstein S, DeTroyer A: Respiratory muscle dysfunction in myotonia congenita. *Am Rev Respir Dis* 130:681, 1984.
Fenichel GM: Clinical syndroms of myasthenia in infancy and childhood. *Arch Neurol* 35:97, 1978.
Gaultier C, Boule M, Tournier G, et al: Inspiratory force reserve of the respiratory muscles in children with chronic obstructive pulmonary disease. *Am Rev Respir Dis* 131:811, 1985.
Gaultier C, Zinman R: Maximal static pressures in healthy children. *Respir Physiol* 51:45, 1983.
Hansen J, James S, Burrington J, et al: The decreasing incidence of pneumothorax and improving survival with congenital diaphragmatic hernia. *J Pediatr Surg* 19:385, 1984.
Hight DW, Hixson SD, Reed JO: Intermittent diaphragmatic hernia of Bochdalek report of a case and literature review. *Pediatrics* 69:601, 1982.
Hoefnagel D, Harris NG, Kim TN: Transient respiratory depression of the newborn. Its occurrence after succinylcholine administration to the mother. *Am J Dis Child* 133:825, 1979.
Holmes LB, Driscoll SG, Bradley WG: Contractures in a newborn infant of a mother with myasthenia gravis. *J Pediatr* 96:1067, 1980.
Kafer E: Idiopathic scoliosis, gas exchange and the age-dependence of arterial blood gases. *J Clin Invest* 58:825, 1976.
Langham MR Jr, Krummel TM, Greenfield LJ, et al: Extracorporeal membrane oxygenation following repair of congenital diaphragmatic hernias. *Ann Thorac Surg* 44:247, 1987.
Lipson M, Waskey J, Rice J, et al: Prenatal diagnosis of asphyxiating thoracic dystropy. *Am J Med Genet* 18:273, 1984.
McLean WT, Mickone RC: Congenital myasthenia gravis in twins. *Arch Neurol* 35:97, 1978.
Moxham J, Edwards RHT, Aubier M, et al: Changes in EMG power spectrum (high-to-low ratio) with force fatigue in humans. *J Appl Physiol* 53:1094, 1982.
Muller NL, Bryan AC: Chest wall mechanics and respiratory muscles in infants. *Pediatr Clin North Am* 26:503, 1979.
Oberklaid F, Danks DM, Mayne V, et al: Asphyxiating thoracic dysplasia: Clinical, radiological and pathological information on 10 patients. *Arch Dis Child* 52:758, 1977.
Roussos C: Function and fatigue of respiratory muscles. *Chest* 88:1245, 1985.
Roussos CS, Macklem PT: Diaphragmatic fatigue in man. *J Appl Physiol* 43:189, 1977.
Shamberger RC, Welch KJ: Surgical correction of pectus carinatum. *J Pediatr Surg* 22:48, 1987.
Shamberger RC, Welch KJ, Sanders SP: Mitral valve prolapse associated with pectus excavatum. *J Pediatr* 111:404, 1987.
Towne BH, Lott IT, Hicks DA, et al: Long-term follow-up of infants and children treated with extracorporeal membrane oxygenation (ECMO): A preliminary report. *J Pediatr Surg* 20:410, 1985.
Welch KJ: Chest wall deformities. In Holder TM, Ashcraft KW (eds): *Pediatric Surgery*. Philadelphia, WB Saunders, 1980, p. 162.
Wohl MEB, Griscom NT, Strieder DJ, et al: The lung following repair on congenital diaphragmatic hernia. *J Pediatr* 90:405, 1977.

Respiratory Failure 9

DISORDERS OF VENTILATORY CONTROL (see also pp. 161, Neonatology, Section 4)

Fatigue

Respiratory failure depends on either failure of the neuromuscular system that constitutes the ventilatory pump or a problem with the lungs, which must have adequate ventilation, perfusion and surface area for gas exchange. Failure of the pump is shown by hypercapnia; failure of gas exchange is initially shown by hypoxemia. Some problems with the muscles and skeleton were discussed in Chapter 8. In this chapter, we will focus on disorders of central control mechanisms which, in turn, are the engine, for the respiratory pump.

Central Alveolar Hypoventilation

Definition

Alveolar hypoventilation is defined in terms of a persistently elevated P_{CO_2} with a reciprocally reduced P_{O_2}. Usually the respiratory acidosis is compensated so that the bicarbonate level is elevated.

Epidemiology

There are relatively few causes of alveolar hypoventilation from respiratory center dysfunction. Nocturnal hypoventilation can result from upper airway obstructive disease as with significantly hypertrophied tonsils and adenoids. In some of these children, severe pulmonary hypertension can result, which is reversed when the upper airway obstruction is removed. This has been associated with Arnold-Chiari malformation and syringomyelia.

An even more unusual form of alveolar hypoventilation is that due to a disturbance in the respiratory center called Ondine curse.

Basic Science

Infants with alveolar hypoventilation have a depressed ventilatory response to CO_2, but have a normal hypoxic response during quiet sleep. Fleming et al (1980) report that behavioral inputs in the awake state and during REM sleep increased ventilation, but not to the expected normal levels.

It should be noted that breathing is the only autonomic function controlled entirely by skeletal muscle. It serves both metabolism and behavior. Awake states allow voluntary alteration of breathing depth and patterns. Thus, individuals with disorders of metabolic control may be symptomatic during quiet sleep, but be able to override the problem when awake.

Pathologic studies of the brain stem in children with congenital alveolar hypoventilation have failed to reveal structural lesions thought to be severe enough to explain the clinical findings (Liu et al, 1978).

Natural History

The severely affected infants (Ondine curse) usually present on the first day of life with cyanosis and slow or shallow respirations, particularly during sleep. Hypotonia and hyporeflexia are also described.

Abnormalities in brain stem auditory evoked responses have included a delay in wave III latency from the area of the superior olives, which is anatomically near the medullary chemoreceptors.

Central hypoventilation has been seen in infants with pyruvate dehydrogenase complex deficiency (Johnston et al, 1984).

Treatment

When the condition is profound, the only treatment is mechanical ventilation. Trials of theophylline and methylphenidate have not been found helpful. Many of these children can function quite well when awake, but need to be returned to a ventilator during sleep (Oren et al, 1987).

Prognosis

The ultimate prognosis is unclear. The disorder is apparently not familial.

SUDDEN INFANT DEATH SYNDROME

Definition

Sudden Infant Death Syndrome (SIDS), otherwise known as sudden unexpected death or cot death is defined as sudden death unexpected by history in which a postmortem examination fails to demonstrate an adequate cause of death. Despite enormous efforts to unravel the epidemiology of this condition and a search for etiology from many postmortem examinations, the reason or reasons for sudden infant death remains obscure.

Epidemiology

In the United States, SIDS is the leading cause of death of infants between the ages 28 days and before the first birthday. In 1980, more than 5500 deaths were ascribed to SIDS in the United States alone.

There is some racial predilection for SIDS; the National Center for Health Statistics in the United States (1980) reported 1.5 deaths per 1000 live births overall; black infants have a rate of 2.8/1000; 0.5/1000 for Asian infants; and 5.93/1000 for American Indians. (Subsequently the SIDS rate in Oklahoma Indians was found to be 2.32/1000 live births, still higher than the 1.8/1000 among white infants in the same area.) Males have had consistently higher rates of SIDS, regardless of race. Infants with bronchopulmonary dysplasia and others with achondroplasia are at increased risk of SIDS.

Although formerly thought to be uncommon in Japan, recent reports are 3.6/1000 live births (Kubota, 1986).

Diagnosis

The diagnosis of sudden infant death depends on the suddenness and unexpectedness of a usually silent death, most often in an infant between 2 and 8 months of age, and a thorough postmortem examination that fails to reveal another cause of death. It can occur at any age, but is rare in infants over 18 months. A home visit to examine the setting in which the infant was found dead may reveal contributing factors, such as a very soft mattress or pillow that could allow smothering (Bass et al, 1986).

Pathology

Pathologists have variously described abnormalities in pulmonary vessels with peripheral extension of smooth muscle, gliosis of the brain stem, and a decrease in myelinated fibers in the vagus nerve. Many of these findings are consistent with chronic or recurrent hypoxia, which raises the question of central respiratory failure as a basis for the sudden death.

CONTROVERSIES

The major controversy has been whether infants who have episodes of apnea and cyanosis, but are successfully resuscitated are "near miss" sudden deaths,

CASE ILLUSTRATION

A 1690-g male infant of a 33-week gestation was born to a 22-year-old gravida 4 para 3 white female. Past history indicated a healthy 2-year-old sibling. The first child was given up for adoption, the third was born at 33 weeks of gestation and subsequently died at 2½ months, apparently of SIDS. In this pregnancy, a repeat cesarean section was performed after premature onset of labor followed by rupture of membranes. Apgar scores were 8 and 5. Grunting, flaring, and retraction were noted in the delivery room and chest radiograph revealed a ground-glass pattern with air bronchogram consistent with HMD. The infant was intubated and remained on the ventilator for 6 days. The highest FIO_2 was 0.95 on day 2 and 0.45 on day 5. A pneumomediastinum developed on day 2 and interstitial emphysema developed on day 3, both resolving by day 6. On day 5, several episodes of bradycardia without apnea occurred for which low-dose aminophylline was administered for 4 days. On day 7, a grade 2 intraventricular hemorrhage was documented by ultrasonography which had resolved by day 9. He did not exhibit any neurologic complications and was transferred to the referring hospital on day 11.

At 3 weeks of age, while the infant was not receiving theophylline, a pneumogram revealed frequent bradycardia with heart rates of less than 70/minute for greater than 10 seconds at least once per hour. One episode lasted 50 seconds. Therefore, theophylline was reinstituted with a plasma level of 11 μg/ml. A repeat pneumogram was within normal limits, and the infant was discharged from the hospital.

Another pneumogram, done at 6 weeks of age while the infant was still receiving theophylline, was within normal limits. At 2 months of age and a weight of 4.2 kg, the infant had a bilateral inguinal herniorrhaphy after which he had multiple prolonged apneic spells requiring intubation and mechanical ventilation. Supplementary history from the mother indicated that in the preceding weeks, she had observed several periods during which the infant looked grey, but regained pink color after shaking. The infant had another apneic episode at 3 months and 1 week of age and another pneumogram showed a very rare short apnea to 5 seconds, a resting pulse of 140–150, and one episode of brief bradycardia to 75. An upper gastrointestinal series did not reveal reflux. The infant was placed on a monitor at this time.

One week before death at 6 months of age, he was admitted to the hospital after an episode of choking and change of color on feeding. There was a questionable infiltrate on chest radiography and amoxicillin was instituted. Weight was 5.2 kg, length 24 inches, and head circumference 41 cm. The theophylline dosage was 20 mg qid and blood level was 11.5 μg/ml. The pneumogram was repeated and interpreted as showing improvement. The baby was discharged and was active and playful during the same day. He was placed in a playpen at 8:30 p.m. with the monitor not connected and at 9:00 p.m. he was found not to be breathing. Resuscitation attempts were unsuccessful.

No lesion was found at postmortem to explain death. (Case taken from The Children's Hospital, Boston Clinico-Pathologic Conference Wednesday, November 21, 1984).

COMMENT

Extensive epidemiologic surveys have identified some of the risk factors, many of which are apparent in the illustrative case history. The mother was relatively *young* with *short intergestational intervals.* She was *multiparous* and a *cigarette smoker.* The infant, a *male* was born *prematurely* and graduated from the neonatal intensive care unit in the *winter months.* A *sibling had previously died* of SIDS. The risk is increased about four-fold in subsequent siblings, and reaches 4% in a surviving twin. Each one of these observations constitutes a risk factor and when they occur together such an infant was indeed at extraordinary risk. This was undoubtedly the reason for frequent evaluations by pneumogram and the use of theophylline as a respiratory stimulant. Although there is no evidence that apneic intervals demonstrated on a pneumogram are predictive of SIDS, current practice is based on the assumption that they may be related, particularly in an infant of high risk. When the apneic episodes were identified, the infant was investigated further for the possibility of gastroesophageal reflux but it was not present. The infant was on a monitor, but monitoring is not used continuously and it is not unusual for such an infant to be placed in a playpen without a monitor connected. The tragedy in this instance is that ½ hour after that happened, the previously active and playful infant was found not breathing. In this situation, death is typically quiet, without evidence of struggle and is more likely to occur in the evening than in the daytime.

or whether there is no relationship between these infants and those who are actually found dead. (The phrase "near miss" is widely used, although some experts prefer "apparent life threatening event" (ALTE). Because it seems possible that episodic apnea may precede the fatal apneic episode, intensive study of cohorts of infants who are labeled "near miss" have been undertaken with comparable controls. The most extensive study was made prospectively by 24-hour recordings of respiratory wave form and ECG on low birth weight infants within 1 week of discharge from neonatal intensive care units. This study conducted by Southall et al (1982) included 1157 infants, 11 of whom died. Five were victims of SIDS and others had associated problems. None of the six infants who died suddenly and unexpectedly had had apnea of greater than 20 seconds or bradycardia of less than 50 beats per minute or cardiac arrhythmias on their 24-hour recordings. A number of infants had episodes of apnea and bradycardia, but these were not the ones who died suddenly and unexpectedly. Similar results have been reported from France (Monod et al, 1986). Despite the overwhelming evidence provided by this study that pneumograms are not predictive, there continues to be a dependence on this form of testing in the absence of something better.

When an infant has had respiratory irregularities, it has become the custom to treat with theophylline, but as in the case illustrated, it provides no guarantee of effectiveness.

A major question confronting pediatricians is, what is an appropriate work-up for an infant who has respiratory irregularities or an apneic episode from which it was successfully resuscitated. The differential diagnosis is extensive. Among the possibilities are seizure disorders, reflex abnormalities of the upper airways, failure of automatic ventilation (Ondine curse), congenital heart disease, cardiac arrhythmias, hyponatremia, hypocalcemia, hypoglycemia, sepsis and meningitis, respiratory infections, anemia, or CNS tumors or compression of the spinal cord. Given this wide differential diagnosis, the pediatrician is obliged to obtain a careful history as to the frequency of spells and other abnormal movements that might be suggestive of a seizure. Commonly, a normal EEG is found to be reassuring.

The diagnosis of upper airway problems may be difficult to prove, but it is clear that some young animals can go into fatal breath-holding episodes from reflex stimulation of laryngeal chemoreceptors. Apneic spells in association with swallowing might suggest this mechanism. Since gastric reflux can produce laryngospasm, many believe that serious apneic episodes should be evaluated with a barium swallow, a technetium-labeled milk scan, or a pH probe in the esophagus to evaluate gastroesophageal reflux. Here individual discretion is indicated. There is no evidence that fatal SIDS has been associated with gastroesophagheal reflux.

Many studies of ventilatory responses to hypercarbia or hypoxia have provided contradictory results in siblings of victims and in the near miss group. The most reliable test is the arousal response to 17% inspired oxygen which is not present in some siblings of victims. Further evaluation of this test is warranted to detect infants at risk (Brady and McCann, 1985).

Even though sepsis, meningitis, and metabolic disorders should have manifestations in addition to apnea, they should be considered when apneic spells are recurrent or prolonged. Furthermore, respiratory syncytial virus infection and pertussis are clearly associated with increased numbers of apneic episodes in infants.

Treatment

Obviously, any underlying condition deserves specific treatment. If apneic episodes continue in the absence of an underlying problem, methylxanthines are used. The compounds should be used cautiously at first, with a low starting dose of 2–2.5 mg/kg every 8–12 hours after a single loading dose of 5 mg/kg. If the heart rate is elevated above baseline, it is advisable to defer the next dose. Serum theophylline concentrations of 3–11 μg/ml provide sufficient respiratory stimulus in the apnea of prematurity, but whether such doses would be appropriate for older infants at risk of SIDS is not known.

If an infant has symptoms suggesting gastroesophageal reflux, elevation of the head of the bed is appropriate and the infant should be kept upright for 30–60 minutes after feeding. Careful attention should be paid to adequate burping and possibly thickening of the infant formula may be helpful.

The most controversial of all interventions is home cardiorespiratory monitoring (Southall, 1983; Kelly et al, 1978). Only anecdotal evidence suggests that it is effective. Nonetheless, it is one of the few actions that can alleviate anxiety of parents whose infant previously required resuscitation.

Home monitoring is usually dependent on the infant's heart rate and chest wall movement. The most common monitor uses three electrodes attached to the chest, with a device that permits adjustable alarms. Individuals who are experienced with home monitors underscore the need for preparation of parents in cardiopulmonary resuscitation, availability of reliable instrumentation and maintenance, and appropriate psychosocial support (Kelly et al, 1978). The question of how and when to discontinue monitoring has to be individualized. On average, most parents continue until the infant is 9 months old, when the likelihood of sudden unexpected death is very low (Consensus statement, 1987).

REFERENCES

Bass M, Kravath RE, Glass L: Death-scene investigation in sudden infant death. *N Engl J Med* 315:100, 1966.

Beckwith JB: The sudden infant death syndrome. *Curr Probl Pediatr* 3:1, 1973.

Brady JP, McCann EM: Control of ventilation in subsequent siblings of victims of sudden infant death syndrome. *J. Pediatr* 106:212, 1985.

Consensus statement: NIH Consensus Development conference on infantile apnea and heart monitorings. Sept 29 to Oct 1, 1986. *Pediatrics* 79:292, 1987.

Fleming PJ, Cade D, Bryan MH: Congenital central hypoventilation and sleep state. *Pediatrics* 66:425, 1980.

Ingress LM, Skjaerven R, Peterson DR: Prospective assessment of recurrence risk in sudden infant death siblings. *J Pediatr* 104:349, 1984.

Johnston K, Newth CJ, Sheu K-F, et al: Central hypoventilation syndrome in pyruvate dehydrogenase complex deficiency. *Pediatrics* 74:1034, 1984.

Kaplan DW, Bauman AE, Kraus HF: Epidemiology of sudden infant death syndrome in American Indians. *Pediatrics* 74:1041, 1984.

Kelly DH, Shannon DC, O'Conner K: Care of infants with near miss sudden infant death syndrome. *Pediatrics* 61:511, 1978.

Kubota Y in *Bull Int Pediatr Assoc* 7:310, 1986.

Liu HM, Lowe JM, Hunt CE: Congenital central hypoventilation syndrome: A pathologic study of neuromuscular system. *Neurology* 28:1013, 1978.

Mellins RB, Balfour HH, Turino GM, et al: Failure of automatic control of ventilation (Ondine's curse). *Medicine* 49:487, 1970.

Monod N, Plouin P, Sternberg B: Respiratory patterns for detecting infants at risk for SIDS (abstr.) *Early Human Devel* 14:152, 1986.

Oren J. Kelly DH, Shannon DC: Long Term follow-up of children with congenital hypoventilation syndrome. *Pediatrics* 80:375, 1987.

Pauli RM, Scott CI, Wassman ER, et al: Apnea and sudden unexpected death in infants with achondroplasia. *J Pediatr* 104:342, 1984.

Peterson DR, Sabotta MA, Daling JR: Infant mortality among subsequent siblings of infants who died of sudden infant death syndrome. *J Pediatr* 108:911, 1986.

Southall DP: Home monitoring and its role in the sudden infant death syndrome. *Pediatrics* 72:133, 1983.

Southall DP, Richards JM, Rhoden KJ, et al: Prolonged apnea and cardiac arrhythmias in infants discharged from neonatal intensive care units: Failure to predict an increased risk for sudden infant death syndrome. *Pediatrics* 70:844, 1982.

Stevens V, Wilson AJ, Southall DP, et al: Analysis of the heart rate and breathing patterns of infants destined to suffer sudden infant death syndrome: Probability density function analysis. *Pediatr Res* 19:1327, 1985.

Lung Injury from Aspiration 10

ASPIRATION OF INJURIOUS SUBSTANCES

Aspiration remains a common and potentially serious form of injury to the lung. Aspirated materials can be those that are ingested by mouth, or secretions from the mouth or upper airways, or regurgitated gastric contents.

The association of upper respiratory tract infection including sinusitis, chronic bronchitis, and bronchiectasis, has long been observed and has been explained as reactive respiratory mucosa (unusually responsive to infection) in all areas, or the combined infections represent spread from sinus and upper airways to lower ones (the leaky roof-wet cellar theory). Indirect evidence suggests that aspiration of secretions from the upper airway may be a major factor in some bacterial pneumonias. Normal subjects, particularly in deep sleep, have been observed to aspirate small quantities of pharyngeal contents throughout the night. This has been confirmed many times by instillation of small amounts of traceable materials into the nose or mouth of sleeping subjects and recovering the material later from the lung. Clearly, patients with abnormal swallowing mechanisms are at special risk of aspiration. Sick or debilitated infants appear to be at increased risk and those with intratracheal tubes in place for long periods may indeed aspirate around the tube, as was demonstrated by Goodwin et al (1985). One mechanism that the infant frequently uses to prevent aspiration is the so-called nonfeeding swallow. Episodes of swallowing increase in frequency during brief respiratory pauses.

Regurgitation immediately after feeding is very common in both normal and sick infants. Frequent spitting is as regular an event as drooling. Actual vomiting is rarer, but it is not infrequently observed in infants who consume their formula rapidly and swallow some air, and have not had satisfactory burping. Apnea itself has been observed to be associated with milk visible in the posterior pharynx. Some regurgitation can result from incompetence of the gastroesophogeal sphincter (see Section 7). Usually during regurgitation, upper airway closure and swallowing occur in close temporal sequence and appear to be the major mechanisms for protection of the airway.

Once foreign material is in the lung, a number of irritant receptors appear to respond. If the stimulus is severe, there may be periods of breath-holding interspersed with gasps, coughs, and bronchoconstriction. The afferent pathways for these reflex effects are mainly through the vagus nerve, and rise from stretch receptors in the conducting airways from the trachea to the smaller bronchi.

Newborn infants are handicapped with respect to some of the defenses against aspiration. Not only can there be pharyngeal incoordination, but there is a less easily provoked cough in most infants. Less than half of newborns cough spontaneously, even on direct laryngeal stimulation. Clearly any infant with an endotracheal tube cannot clear secretions distal to the tube very efficiently. Such infants are also unable to cough.

In the months after birth, maturation of the neurologic control mechanisms increase musculoskeletal coordination. Growth and decrease of compliance of the chest wall is all important in enhancing the efficiency of the cough. Documentation of the changes in the first year of life has now been undertaken (Leith, 1985).

ASPIRATION IN FETUS AND NEWBORN

The stressed fetus can aspirate whatever is in amniotic liquid, including squamous cells, bacteria, or meconium.

Epidemiology

No accurate figures are available. In general, significant aspiration is becoming less common as labor is monitored and infants are delivered at the first signs of distress. Prompt suction of the infant's airway through a laryngoscope can remove much of the aspirated material before it enters deep airways (Gregory et al, 1974). Thus, in centers that practice optimal obstetrics and resuscitation severe meconium aspiration is rarely seen.

Natural History

The risk of meconium aspiration increases with gestational age. In preterm infants, it is rare; at term, it may accompany severe intrauterine hypoxia; postterm, it becomes increasingly common, presumably as peristalsis begins. Meconium stained infants may present with tachypnea only, and then become indistinguishable from those with persistent fetal circulation (see pp. 175). Infection may accompany aspiration or cause it. Sometimes the differential diagnosis between intrauterine pneumonia and meconium aspiration is difficult. Experimentally, intratracheal instillation of meconium in animals enhances infection with *E. coli* (Bryan, 1967).

Diagnosis

Inspection of the larynx with visualization of aspirated meconium establishes the diagnosis. In severe cases radiographs will show widespread infiltrates. Hyperinflation alternating with atelectasis is the rule. Occasionally loculated air can produce pneumatoceles. Death may occur a few minutes after birth or at any time within the first days of life, usually as a consequence of severe pulmonary hypertension and heart failure. Infants who recover may have a prolonged course of weeks of tachypnea.

Treatment

Prevention is the answer. Only supportive treatment, including oxygen, mechanical ventilation, and antibiotics are available. If pneumothorax is present, chest drainage may be required.

CASE ILLUSTRATION

A 4-kg male infant was delivered vaginally after an uncomplicated 42-week gestation. Meconium staining of the skin was evident at birth and the perineum was covered with thick meconium. Catheter suction of the oropharynx did not remove much material. Apgar scores were 5 at 1 minute and 8 at 5 minutes, although the infant was reported to be gasping. A chest radiograph at 1 hour showed a small right pneumothorax, but no significant infiltrates. Treatment with ampicillin and gentamicin was started and 30% oxygen was administered.

Over the subsequent hours, respiratory distress worsened, oxygen requirements increased, and the infant was intubated and ventilated. Pancuronium was given as a muscle relaxant. Echocardiogram and ECG were normal.

Laboratory studies showed the initial hematocrit was 56% and later rose to 70%. Platelets fell to 43,000 mm^3 and,at 14 hours,the infant was given a platelet transfusion, followed by a partial exchange with 5% albumin. Blood cultures were negative. Blood gases showed progressive deterioration despite 90% oxygen and mechanical ventilation.

COMMENT

The tragedy of this case is the unanticipated demise of a normally developed term infant associated with aspiration. It seems clear that the initial suctioning was inadequate. Laryngoscopy and deep tracheal suction would have been more appropriate. Even so, the relatively normal appearance of the chest radiograph suggests the major lesion was in the pulmonary arterioles. This patient might well have been viewed as illustrative of persistent fetal circulation since echocardiography showed right-to-left shunting at the atrial level. Too little is understood about the pathophysiology of disturbances in postnatal adaptation illustrated here.

QUESTION AND COMMENT

What is the effect of meconium on the lung?

The viscous material may obstruct the airway and promote resorption atelectasis or produce a check-valve effect and permit air-trapping. Alternately, the principal fatty acids in meconium (palmitic, stearic, and oleic) are capable of inactivating the pulmonary surfactants and producing atelectasis and edema (Terasaka et al, 1986).

ASPIRATION IN OLDER INFANTS AND CHILDREN

Definition

Ingestion of hydrocarbons, such as lighter fluid, cleaning fluid, mineral seal oil, and kerosene represent a major threat to the toddler who may vomit and aspirate the materials.

Epidemiology

Health education on the hazards of ingestion, as well as the establishment of poison-control systems have had a favorable impact in the reduction of deaths. The prevalence is not documented.

Natural History

Hydrocarbons can cause gastric irritation, vomiting, and aspiration. Experimental studies in animals show the gastrointestinal problems to be the major hazard. Pneumonia may not be evident for several hours after ingestion and aspiration after which it may become fulminant. Air-trapping, areas of atelectasis, and pneumatoceles may progress for about 72 hours before slow resolution. The asymptomatic child should be observed for 6–8 hours.

Most deaths from hydrocarbon ingestion are the consequence of aspiration, particularly of the low viscosity fuels (30–60 ssu). Systemic absorption may produce central nervous system depression, and renal damage, but these are self-limited. More viscous products (150–250 ssu), such as mineral oil, and motor oil are less commonly ingested but, if aspirated, produce a lipoid pneumonia.

Diagnosis

If aspiration has occurred, retractions, bronchospasm, cough, and fever become prominent. With severe injury, hemoptysis and pulmonary edema can develop rapidly. Blood gases reveal hypoxemia before hypercarbia, suggesting ventilation perfusion abnormalities.

Treatment

Gastric lavage or induced emesis should be avoided to lessen the likelihood of aspiration. If a toxic compound has been ingested at the same time, cautious lavage may be necessary. The most useful intervention is to increase delivery of humidified oxygen. Bacterial infections are rare, and antibiotics are not indicated unless other infections are present. No benefit has been shown for treatment with corticosteroids in humans or in animal models.

Prognosis

Survivors can show persistent abnormalities in pulmonary function even though asymptomatic. Gurwitz et al (1978) found small airway obstruction in 14 of 17 patients tested 14 years after an episode of aspiration.

ADULT RESPIRATORY DISTRESS SYNDROME

Definition

Adult respiratory distress syndrome (ARDS), sometimes called shock lung, is a diffuse injury to the alveolar capillary membrane that results in acute onset of respiratory failure from an increase in microvascular permeability. It can occur in children of any age (Royall and Levin, 1988.)

Epidemiology

This condition is well-known to individuals involved in respiratory intensive care. It most commonly follows multiple trauma, but can be associated with septic shock from bacteremia, or any severe infection in which hypovolemia can occur (Table 5.13). The incidence of this disorder will be a function of the number of individuals with overwhelming infection and trauma. The condition was recognized as a major cause of death in soldiers injured during the Viet Nam war. It is of much less importance in a civilian population.

Table 5.13
Conditions That May Be Associated with ARDS

Injury via inhalation
Gas inhalation
Smoke inhalation
Oxygen toxicity
Injury from aspiration
Gastric contents
Near drowning
Injury to pulmonary capillaries via blood stream
Sepsis
Fat embolism
Radiation pneumonitis
Paraquat poisoning
Drug-induced pulmonary edema

Natural History and Diagnosis

The phrase adult respiratory distress syndrome (ARDS) was applied to distinguish this form from that which occurs in the first days of life in preterm infants. It is probable that they share surfactant deficiency.

ARDS can occur in children or young adults as well as individuals of advanced age. Characteristically there is a lag period of some hours between injury and onset of respiratory difficulty. However, the onset of the respiratory difficulty is typically precipitous and is associated with profound hypoxemia that is usually not very responsive to administered oxygen. Thus, the individuals are often treated with positive end-expiratory pressure in an effort to prevent atelectasis and lessen the extent of intrapulmonary venous mixture.

Granulocytes in thc peripheral blood have been shown to be metabolically active. Zimmerman et al (1983) found that granulocytes from patients with ARDS generate increased quantities of active oxygen metabolites and that this effect was not reduced by glucocorticoid. The superoxide anion that is released can be a mediator of endothelial cell injury, which is thought to be one of the primary lesions in this condition.

Despite very many studies, it is not clear what factors specifically mediate the increase in permeability of the microvascular epithelium. Pulmonary edema is one of the early lesions in this condition followed by injury to interstitial elements and alveolar lining cells as well. Aggregates of polymorphonuclear cells have been found in the capillaries of the lung and have been found in increased numbers during bronchoalveolar lavage in patients with ARDS. Surfactant inactivation may result from increased capillary permeability (Seeger et al, 1985).

Treatment

Massive doses of glucocorticoids have been tried but there is no convincing evidence that they alter the course of the disease. Treatment consists of developing positive end-expiratory pressure with only enough increased inspired oxygen to maintain arterial concentrations at 50–60 mm Hg because presumably, oxygen therapy can aggravate the injury. Full recovery is possible over a matter of weeks with appropriate respiratory and general supportive care. Surfactant replacement may have a role in some circumstances.

Prognosis

The disorder carries approximately a 50% mortality. Survivors usually recover completely.

LUNG DISEASES CAUSED BY CHEMOTHERAPEUTIC AGENTS

A number of agents used to treat childhood cancer are responsible for a diffuse interstitial pneumonitis and fibrosis, or bronchiolitis obliterans.

Epidemiology

As ever more potent antitumor drugs are used, more serious side effects are expected. The major offender in childhood is bleomycin, which is variably reported to produce pneumonitis in 3–40% of individuals treated. Bulsulfan injures lung in 2–11% of patients, and a number of other agents have been incriminated in individual case reports.

Natural History

The pulmonary lesions may be evident as pulmonary edema or pleural effusions during treatment, but others such as those produced by cyclophosphamide have a delayed onset and appear weeks or even years after treatment. The mechanism of toxicity is not usually known. Bleomycin is an inhibitor of DNA synthesis and probably facilitates production of superoxide anions. Supplemental oxygen may increase the severity of the lung injury. Risk of development of the disease depends largely on the total dose of drug administered (Cooper et al, 1986).

Diagnosis

Patients with pulmonary involvement develop cough, shortness of breath, fatigue, and weight loss. They may or may not be febrile. Pulmonary function tests indicate a restrictive lung disease, not unlike that found in interstitial pulmonary fibrosis from alveolitis.

The treatment of these unfortunate complications is, of course, to withdraw the chemotherapeutic agent. On the other hand, if it is the one that is responsible for suppression of the malignancy, the clinical decision can be very difficult.

Prevention

Not enough is known of the long-term effects of some of the newer chemotherapeutic agents. It is incumbent on all those using these agents to record the complications and assess what kinds of drugs are likely to have similar side effects and which can be used as alternative therapy.

THERMAL INJURY TO THE LUNG

The chief cause of early death after burns is injury to the respiratory tract from inhalation of gases or particulate matter that reach the airways. In some instances, death presumably follows upper airway obstruction from laryngeal edema or spasm. In other instances, there is a lag period of 4–6 hours, after which a fulminant pulmonary edema appears. Injury to the respiratory tract may occur in the absence of any demonstrable facial burns. Highly irritating fumes contain large quantities of sulfur and nitrogenous materials which can be very toxic.

If patients survive the early fulminant edema and receive appropriate ventilatory support, they may proceed to extensive bronchopneumonia, usually from *Staphylococci*, and are at risk for coliform organisms or *Pseudomonas*. The impaired mucosa allows stasis of organisms in the absence of ciliary action.

Treatment

If there is severe upper airway obstruction, emergency tracheostomy may be necessary. Mechanical ventilation with end-expiratory pressure of about 5 cm H_2O reduces the likelihood of atelectasis. Inhalation of cold air is desirable, if possible, and it should be humidified, although water droplets are not useful.

CONTROVERSY

There is some suggestion that 4 mg/kg/day of methylprednisolone may reduce bronchial edema. This has not been confirmed, however, and the suppression of inflammatory response could be a disadvantage.

REFERENCES

Batist G, Andrews JL: Pulmonary toxicity of antineoplastic drugs. *JAMA* 246:1449, 1982.

Bryan CS: Enhancement of bacterial infection by meconium. *Johns Hopkins Med J* 121:9, 1967.

Coleridge JCG, Coleridge HM: Lower respiratory tract afferance stimulated by inhaled irritants. *Am Rev Respir Dis* 131:S51, 1985.

Cooper JAD, White DA, Matthay RA: Drug-induced pulmonary disease. *Am Rev Respir Dis* 133:321, 1986.

Cope O: Management of the Coconut Grove burns at the Massachusetts General Hospital. *Ann Surg* 117:801, 1943.

Eade NR, Taussig LM, Marks MI: Hydrocarbon pneumonitis. *Pediatrics* 54:351, 1974.

Gregory GA, Gooding CA, Phibbs RH, Tooley WH: Meconium aspiration in infants—a prospective study. *J Pediatr* 85:848, 1974.

Goodwin SR, Graves SA, Haberkern CM: Aspiration in intubated premature infants. *Pediatrics* 75:85, 1985.

Gurwitz D, Kattan M, Levinson H, et al: Pulmonary function abnormalities in asymptomatic children after hydrocarbon pneumonitis. *Pediatrics* 62:789, 1978.

Leith DE: The development of cough. *Am Rev Respir Dis* 131:S39, 1985.

Lloyd EL, MacRae WR: Respiratory tract damage in burns. *Br J Anaesth* 43:365, 1971.

McGuire WW, Spragg RG, Cohen AB, et al: Studies on the pathogenesis of the adult respiratory distress syndrome. *J Clin Invest* 69:543, 1982.

Mellins RB, Park S: Respiratory complications of smoke inhalation in victims of fires. *J Pediatr* 87:1, 1975.
Moseley PL, Shasby M, Brady M, et al: Lung parenchymal injury induced by bleomycin. *Am Rev Respir Dis* 130:1082, 1984.
Petty TL: Adult respiratory distress syndrome: Historical prospective and definition. *Sem Respir Med* 2:99, 1981.
Rinaldo JE: Mediation of ARDS by leukocytes: Clinical evidence and implications for therapy. *Chest* 89:590, 1986.
Royall JA, Levin DL: Adult respiratory distress syndrome in pediatric patients. 1. Clinical aspects, pathophysiology and mechanisms of lung injury. *J Pediatr* 112:169, 1988.
Seeger W, Stöhr G, Wolf HRD, et al: Alteration of surfactant function due to protein leakage: Special interaction with fibrin monomer. *J Appl Physiol* 58:326, 1985.
Terasaka D, Clark DA, Singh BN, et al: The free fatty acids of meconium. *Biol Neonate* 50:16, 1986.
Thack BT, Menonb A: Pulmonary protective mechanisms in human infants. *Am Rev Respir Dis* 131:S55, 1985.
Wall MA, Wohl ME, Jaffe N, et al: Lung function in adolescents receiving high dose methotrexate. *Pediatrics* 63:741, 1979.
Zapol WM, Snider MT: Pulmonary hypertension in severe acute respiratory failure. *N Engl J Med* 296:476, 1977.
Zimmerman GA, Renzetti AD, Hill HR: Functional and metabolic activity of granulocytes from patients with adult respiratory distress syndrome. *Am Rev Respir Dis* 127:290, 1983.

INHALATION OF PARTICLES

Inhaled particles of 10-μ or less can penetrate the peripheral airways, particularly during mouth or endotracheal tube breathing.

The risks to children's lungs of exposure to air pollutants is of increasing concern in our industrialized societies. Considerations that dictate airway deposition include particle size and density in inspired air, airway size and branching, rate and depth of ventilation, patterns of airflow, and minute ventilation.

The findings of Phelan et al (1985) using measurements of airway casts from individuals 11 days to 21 years of age (and assumed values for other variables) show 5-μ particles have six times the deposition in the mouth-breathing resting newborn compared to that of the adult. In general, deposition is greatest in the smallest lungs in whom respiratory rates are higher and minute ventilation proportionally greater than in larger lungs. Pulmonary retention of particles tends to decrease with age, with most of the decrease occurring in the first 2 years.

Nose breathing is the best protection against lung injury from particles. About 90% of labeled water droplets from jet or ultrasonic nebulizers were found in the upper respiratory tract.

OXYGEN TOXICITY

Pulmonary oxygen toxicity is underappreciated as a problem despite extensive studies in experimental animals and clinical observations. Pure oxygen is eventually lethal to all mammals studied (Kafer, 1971). The level at which it produces irreversible injury is a function of host factors and duration of exposure.

In general, agents that increase metabolism increase susceptibility to pulmonary oxygen toxicity. These include glucocorticoids, epinephrine, amphetamines, thyroid hormones and hyperthermia. Tolerance to high oxygen can be shown experimentally when metabolism is lowered. Age is another factor in susceptibility, with newborn animals tolerating high oxygen longer than their nursing mothers. Quantitative data on the human infant is not possible to obtain; human infants do show pulmonary lesions after prolonged high oxygen exposure, although usually they are also on ventilators and barotrauma could aggravate the injury. Newborn lambs breathing pure oxygen died from pulmonary edema after 40–60 hours of exposure (deLemos et al, 1969).

Basic Science

Oxygen-free radicals evolve during normal tissue metabolism and form a perhydroxy radical (HO_2) that can penetrate cell membranes and is highly toxic. In hyperoxic states, excess amounts of free radicals can overwhelm the systems for neutralization of the radicals, mainly the metalloproteins superoxide dismutases. The reaction product is hydrogen peroxide which, in the presence of catalase and glutathione peroxidase is degraded to water. In addition to antioxidant enzymes, most cells contain other antioxidants such as ascorbic acid, α-tocopherol, and ceruloplasmin. Activity of superoxide dismutase, catalase and glutathione peroxidase is low before 26–28 weeks' gestation, and increases several-fold by term (Frank and Sosenko, 1987). There is also an increase in production of oxygen-free radicals during reoxygenation of hypoxic tissues. The mechanism relates to the accumulation of hypoxanthine during hypoxia which is washed out of tissues during reoxygenation and metabolized via the xanthine oxidase system to produce free radicals (Saugstad, 1985).

Pathological changes, studied mostly in animals exposed to 40–100% oxygen, show swelling of capillary endothelium, edema, and injury to alveolar type 1 cells. Fibrin thrombi were found in capillaries and hyaline membranes in overexpanded airspaces. Later, alveolar type 2 cells proliferate as do alveolar septal cells. These changes have been described as an early exudative phase and a later proliferative phase, and eventual fibrosis.

Similar pathologic findings are seen in some patients with ARDS even in the absence of high inspired oxygen. Thus, the findings are nonspecific.

Lung injury may partially resolve on weaning from high oxygen. Monkeys exposed to pure oxygen for 8 or 13 days recovered after about 3 months (Kaplan et al, 1969). Residual scarring persisted, but function was normal.

Natural History

In awake subjects who have been studied as volunteers in high oxygen environments, the earliest symptoms are substernal distress described as aching, and some pleuritic pain after 12–14 hours. Later, cough and dyspnea appear, usually after 30–74 hours.

The earliest measurable changes are a reduction in tracheal mucociliary transport, which can be seen after only 3 hours in 90–95% oxygen (Jackson, 1985).

Chronic oxygen toxicity can develop in animals exposed to 60–80% oxygen. They may become cyanotic whenever the inspired levels are reduced, and thus exhibit oxygen dependency. Although it is difficult to prove, it seems probable that some infants with bronchopulmonary dysplasia who are oxygen dependent have had as part of their problem, pulmonary oxygen toxicity.

Treatment

No pharmacologic agents have been found helpful. Avoidance of those drugs that increase metabolism would seem reasonable when there are other compelling indications for their use. Further evaluation of antioxidants as therapeutic agents would seem worthwhile. Preliminary observations on administration of bovine superoxide dismutase to preterm infants are promising (Rosenfeld et al, 1984).

Prevention

Careful monitoring of oxygen needs is now possible with transcutaneous measurements in infants and periodic blood gas or oximetry measurements in other individuals. No benefit accrues to the patient from blood oxygen tensions over 90–100 torr and most are comfortable at 70–80 torr. Weaning from high inspired mixtures should be undertaken as soon as possible. No symptoms or other evidence of pulmonary toxicity have been noted at inspired levels below 40%, and rarely (if ever) below 50%.

REFERENCES

Clark JM, Lambertsen CJ: Pulmonary oxygen toxicity: A review. *Pharmacol Rev* 23:37, 1971.

deLemos R, Wolfsdorf J, Nachman R, et al: Lung injury from oxygen in lambs. *Anesthesiology* 30:609, 1969.

Frank L, Sosenko IRS: Development of lung antioxidant enzyme system in late gestation: Possible implications for the prematurely born infant. *J. Pediatr* 110:9, 1987.

Jackson RM: Pulmonary oxygen toxicity. *Chest* 88:900, 1985.

Kafer ER: Pulmonary oxygen toxicity: A review of the evidence for acute and chronic oxygen toxicity in man. *Br J Anaesth* 43:687, 1971.

Kapanci Y, Weibel ER, et al: Pathogenesis and reversibility of the pulmonary lesions of oxygen toxicity in workshops. II. Ultrastructural and morphometric studies. *Lab Invest* 20:101, 1969.

Kaplan H, Robinson F, Kapanci Y, et al: Pathogenesis and reversibility of pulmonary lesions of oxygen toxicity in monkeys. I. Clinical and light microscopic studies. *Lab Invest* 20:94, 1969.

Phelan RF, Oldham MJ, Beaucage CB, et al: Postnatal enlargement of human tracheobronchial airways and implications for particle deposition. *Anat Rec* 212:368, 1985.

Rosenfeld W, Evans H, Concepcion L, et al: Prevention of bronchopulmonary dysplasia by administration of bovine superoxide dismutase in preterm infants with respiratory distress syndrome. *J Pediatr* 105:781, 1984.

Saugstad OD: Oxygen radicals and pulmonary damage. *Pediatr Pulmonol* 1:167, 1985.

Smaldone GC, Messina MS: Enhancement of particle deposition by flow-limiting segments in humans. *J Appl Physiol* 59:509, 1985.

Wolfsdorf J, Swift, DL, Avery ME: Mist therapy reconsidered: an evaluation of the respiratory deposition of labelled water aerosols produced by jet and ultrasonic nebulizers. *Pediatrics* 43:799, 1969.

MARY ELLEN AVERY

Consultants
Raif Geha
Mary Ellen B. Wohl
Raezelle Zinman

Section 6

Cardiology

Diagnostic Tools

1

History

Cardiac evaluation of a child includes a review of the child's physical capabilities, growth, and developmental progress. In early infancy, consistent tachypnea suggests congestive heart failure, whereas poor growth or delayed development may be the result of serious cardiac impairment. At the end of the interview, the physician should have a sense of the daily life of the child and his physical capabilities.

Physical Examination

Physical examination begins with an estimation of growth. Generally, cardiac disease dating from birth will affect the weight before the height, resulting in a scrawny infant. Those with severe problems will show delays in both height and weight. In general, obstructive lesions such as coarctation, aortic stenosis, or pulmonary stenosis, without congestive failure, are associated with normal growth. Patients with cyanotic lesions such as tetralogy of Fallot may show generalized growth retardation, while those having lesions associated with congestive heart failure such as left-to-right shunts (septal defects) show poorer weight than height growth. Complete cessation of growth, even weight loss, is seen in patients with severe congestive heart failure. Growth charts are a vital and indispensible tool in the assessment of infants with congenital heart disease.

SCOLIOSIS

Scoliosis is common among adolescent children with cyanotic congenital heart disease, the severity being roughly proportional to the severity of the arterial unsaturation. Examination of the spine with this possibility in mind is a required part of the examination of cyanotic girls (Roth et al, 1973).

EXTRACARDIAC ANOMALIES

The overall incidence of extracardiac anomalies among children with congenital heart disease is about 20% of all patients (Greenwood et al, 1975). There is considerable variation: with some cardiac defects (e.g., truncus arteriosus), there is an incidence of extracardiac anomalies as high as 50%, whereas in others the incidence of associated anomalies seems lower than in the general population (e.g., transposition of the great arteries). Some extracardiac anomalies tend to be associated with a particular cardiac disease (e.g., Down syndrome with atrioventricularis communis (Table 6.1) (Fyler, 1985).

CHEST DEFORMITY

Left chest deformity is a feature of congenital heart disease. This is believed to result largely from increased cardiac size and activity during the time that the chest wall is being formed. It is commonly seen in patients with large left-to-right shunts.

RESPIRATION

The respiratory rate and possible subcostal retractions should be observed with the patient quiet, and the infant's response to his respiratory problems should be noted. Rapid, shallow respiration in excess of 50–60 breaths per minute in an otherwise happy newborn infant is abnormal and implies elevated pulmonary venous pressure until proven otherwise. This pattern is particularly common in infants with excessive pulmonary blood flow. The anxious infant with rapid deep respirations associated with retractions may have severe congestive heart failure or, more likely, pneumonia.

PULSES

Observation of the radial, carotid, and femoral pulses should be a routine matter. Specific simultaneous comparison of the strength and timing of femoral and right radial pulses is mandatory to evaluate the possibility of coarctation of the aorta. Bounding peripheral pulsations suggest systemic hypertension or lesions associated with an aortic run-off (e.g., aortic regurgitation or patent ductus arteriosus). Prominent carotid pulsations may be seen in patients with hypertrophic subaortic stenosis.

BLOOD PRESSURE

It is difficult to obtain satisfactory blood pressures in an infant or toddler. Nevertheless, many pediatricians do much better than others, the conclusion being that a lot depends on how the child is approached. In the most difficult situations (e.g., an apprehensive infant with the suspicion of coarctation), we prefer to use a Doppler sensing device as the best tolerated approach. Small children are examined on the mother's lap. It may be necessary to resort to blood pressure measurements under sedation, often in association with sedation for other frightening tests such as echocardiography.

Normal systemic blood pressure gradually rises over the lifetime of children.

For a detailed discussion of hypertension in childhood, the reader is referred to the excellent monograph by Ingelfinger (1987).

Table 6.1
Types of Extracardiac Anomalies Listed by Diagnostic Categories[1,2]

Cardiac Diagnosis	No. of Infants	% Noncardiac Anomalies	Skeletal	Respiratory	CNS	GI	Urinary	Genital	Down Syndrome	Other Syndrome	Chromosomes
Endocardial cushion	119	63	***	*	*	***	**	*	****	*	*
Truncus arteriosus	33	48	****	*	**	**	***			**	**
Atrial defect	70	43	****	*	*	*	**	*	*	*	*
Patent ductus	146	40	***	***	***	***	***	*	*	***	*
Ventricular defect	374	33	***	**	**	**	**	*	*	*	**
Heterotaxias	95	32	**	**	**	***	***	*		*	*
Tetralogy of Fallot	212	31	**	*	**	**	**	*	*	*	*
Myocardiopathy	61	31	**	*	**	**	*	*		*	
Coarctation	179	26	***	**	*	*	***	*		*	*
Tricuspid atresia	61	20	**	*	*	**	*	*	*		*
Double-outlet right ventricle	35	20	***	*		*	**		**		*
Pulmonary stenosis	79	19	**	*	**	*	*			*	
Single ventricle	58	17	***	**	*		*		*		*
Hypoplastic left ventricle	177	12	**	*	*	*	**	*		*	*
Total anomalous pulmonary veins	63	11	*	*	*	*	*			*	*
D-transposition	236	9	**	*	*	*	*			*	*
Aortic stenosis	45	7	**	*	*	*	**				
Pulmonary atresia	75	4	*	*	*	*	*				
Other	133	29									

[1]One infant may be shown several times because of multiple anomalies.
[2]Key: **** = more than 20% of diagnostic category; *** = 10–20% of diagnostic category; ** = 5–10% of diagnostic category; * = any percent less than 5% of diagnostic category if only one anomaly, or if the total number of cases was small (10) and the number of anomalies was one or two; NS = intact ventricular septum; CNS = central nervous system; GI = gastrointestinal; RV = right ventricle; LV = left ventricle.

NECK VEINS

Distended or pulsating neck veins are normal in a recumbent child but should not be seen in a 10-year-old child of normal size in the sitting position. This observation is valuable and easily accomplished in a cooperative child. Distended or pulsating neck veins require explanation.

HEPATOMEGALY

Another evidence of elevated central venous pressure is the presence of hepatomegaly. A liver edge of more than 3 cm below the right costal margin as a sign of congestive heart failure has been overemphasized in the past. Tachypnea is a more important and reliable indicator of congestive failure. Apparent hepatomegaly often results from respiratory distress and thereby a lower diaphragm. Furthermore, most normal infants have a palpable liver. Generally, if there is abnormal hepatomegaly in an older child, the neck veins will also be visible in the sitting position.

CARDIAC IMPULSE

Any diagnosis that is being entertained should be reconciled with the observation and palpation of the cardiac impulse. It is hard to imagine a patient suffering from severe mitral regurgitation without having a prominent cardiac impulse. Similarly the diagnosis of a small patent ductus arteriosus associated with a grossly hyperactive cardiac impulse is suspicious.

AUSCULTATION

The most cost-effective tool for cardiac diagnosis is the stethoscope. Systematic evaluation of heart sounds and murmurs is inexpensive, often diagnostic, readily repeated, and can be learned by most everyone. For some cardiac lesions (e.g., aortic regurgitation), it is the most sensitive diagnostic tool. It is an efficient means of discovering new cases and accounts for most of the new patients encountered by a cardiology unit each year. This is the one cardiac diagnostic tool remaining to the pediatrician. The "experts" have expropriated most of the other tools and charge handsomely for them.

First Heart Sound. The first heart (Fig. 6.1) (Leatham, 1975) sound is produced by a combination of mitral and tricuspid valve closures at the beginning of systole. The fourth heart sound may add to the intensity of the first heart sound if the P-R interval is short. The first heart sound tends to be of decreased intensity if the P-R interval is long. Early systolic clicks may be easily confused with the first sound. Generally, fourth sounds are dull, low frequency, distinct, soft thuds, audible with a bell, whereas a click is a short snappy, higher frequency, clicking noise best heard with a diaphragm. First sounds are louder in patients with mitral stenosis or those with atrial septal defects.

Second Heart Sound. In most instances, the second heart sound (Fig. 6.3) is audibly split (at least 0.03 sec) into two components, originating from the aortic and the pulmonary valves. Because of the differences in spread of electrical activation of the ventricles

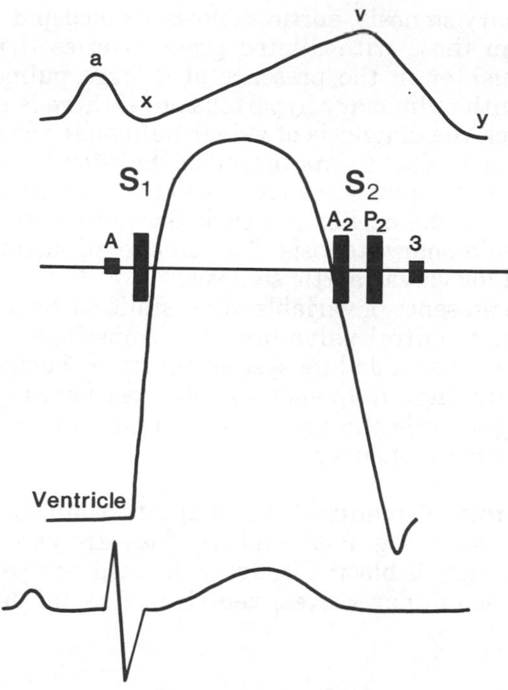

Figure 6.1. Schema of the relations of the jugular venous pulse (showing the *a wave, v wave, x descent,* and *y descent*) heart sounds showing the fourth sound *(A),* the first sound, the second sound, aortic closure *(A_2)*, pulmonary valve closure *(P_2)*, and (the third heart sound), the ventricular pressure tracing, and the electrocardiogram.

and differences between pressure in the aorta and pulmonary artery, pulmonary valve closure normally is heard later than is aortic valve closure. Respiration produces differential effects on the pulmonary and systemic circulations, inspiration being associated with greater inflow of systemic venous blood into the thorax. The result is variation in splitting of the second heart sound depending on whether the right ventricle has received more or less blood because of the coincident phase of respiration. The degree of splitting increases with inspiration and decreases, usually to the point of no audible split, on expiration (Fig. 6.2). If no split is observed on inspiration, an explanation is needed. Is there perhaps only one semilunar valve (e.g., pulmonary valve atresia)? Is there pulmonary artery hypertension at systemic levels, or do the ventricles eject simultaneously because of a large ventricular septal defect? With open communication between the atria via an atrial septal defect, the effect of respiration on the splitting of the second heart sound is diminished. Further, the atrial left-to-right shunt greatly increases the right ventricular stroke volume, accentuating the split. Thus, a widely split second heart sound which does not vary with respiration is almost diagnostic of an atrial septal defect.

Children less than 5 years old can rarely control respiration on demand, hence observing the effects of inspiration and expiration in young children requires some other approach. A useful technique is to listen

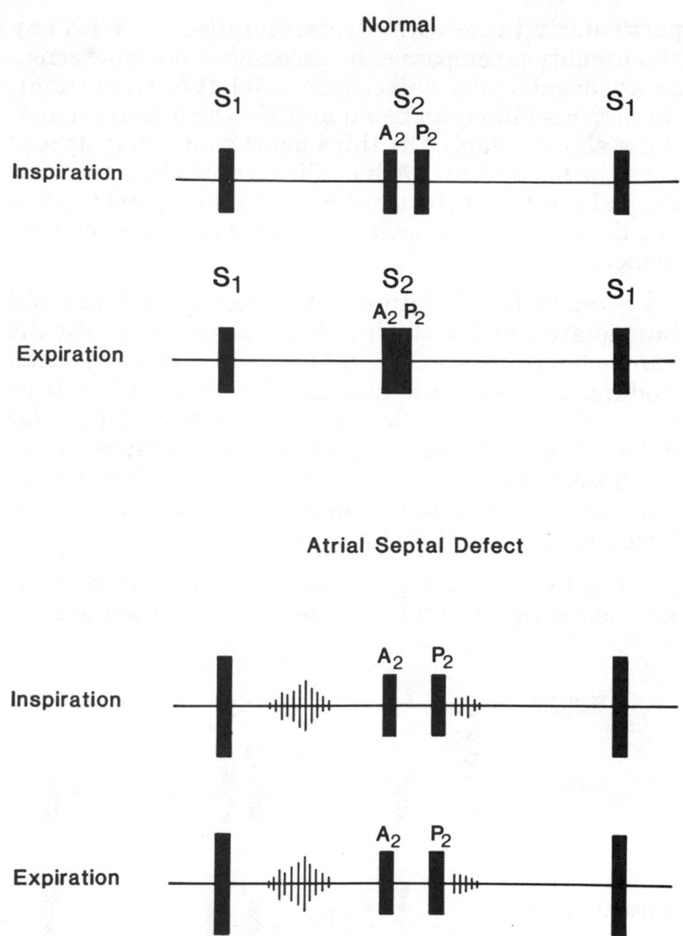

Figure 6.2. Heart sounds diagram comparing the splitting of the second heart sound in a normal child with the second sound in a child who has an atrial septal defect. *S_1*, first heart sound; *S_2*, second heart sound; *A_2*, aortic valve closure; *P_2*, pulmonary valve closure. Note the variation in splitting of the second heart sound in a normal child and the lack of variation in splitting in the child with an atrial septal defect.

while the child is lying down and, while continuing to listen, to sit the child upright. The first several beats while sitting will show variation in splitting; if not, the split may be fixed.

While the intensities of the aortic and pulmonary closure sounds are dependent on the aortic and pulmonary arterial pressure, they are also dependent on the distance of the valve from the chest wall. Consequently, systemic or pulmonary hypertension only rarely may be diagnosed confidently by auscultation.

Third Heart Sound. The third heart sound (Fig. 6.1) is heard during the first period of rapid inflow into the ventricle. In adults, a third sound is almost invariably pathologic. By contrast, many normal, thin children have a readily audible third heart sound. The sound, being of low frequency, is best heard with the bell of the stethoscope. A third sound heard in the presence of tachycardia is called a gallop rhythm. Third heart sounds, particularly in the context of a gallop, are heard in patients with congestive heart failure, particularly those with myocardial disease. With any abnormality accompanied by excessive blood flow across an atrioventricular valve, such as a left-to-right shunt, there is also likely to be an audible third heart sound. If the shunt is large the third heart sound may appear to be the beginning of a diastolic rumble. As a practical clinical matter, if the third heart sound seems to have any duration, an associated diastolic rumble should be suspected.

Fourth Heart Sound. A remote, brief thud heard immediately before the first heart sound is usually the fourth heart sound (Fig. 6.1) and is rarely a normal finding. This sound is associated with atrial contraction, with excessive flow across the atrioventricular valves and with atrial hypertension. Because fourth heart sounds result from atrial contraction,they are not audible in rhythm abnormalities such as atrial fibrillation or junctional tachycardia.

Clicks. Brief, high-frequency, early systolic clicks are heard in patients with semilunar valvar lesions (pulmonary stenosis, aortic stenosis, or bicuspid aortic valve), in those with dilated great arteries (truncus arteriosus), or in the presence of a large pulmonary artery with pulmonary hypertension. If there is no audible click the diagnosis of valvar pulmonary or aortic stenosis is in doubt. The timing of the click in pulmonary stenosis gives some clue as to the severity of the obstruction; the earlier the click the more severe the valvar pulmonary stenosis. The same relationship does not hold for valvar aortic stenosis.

The presence of variable midsystolic clicks is characteristic of mitral valve prolapse, sometimes associated with a variable late systolic murmur. Such clicks are usually high frequency sounds, best heard with a diaphragm while the patient is standing up or doing the Valsalva maneuver.

Systolic Murmurs. The majority of murmurs occur in systole (Fig. 6.3*A* and *B*). They are associated with passage of blood through a limited orifice (e.g., stenotic semilunar valves, ventricular septal defects,

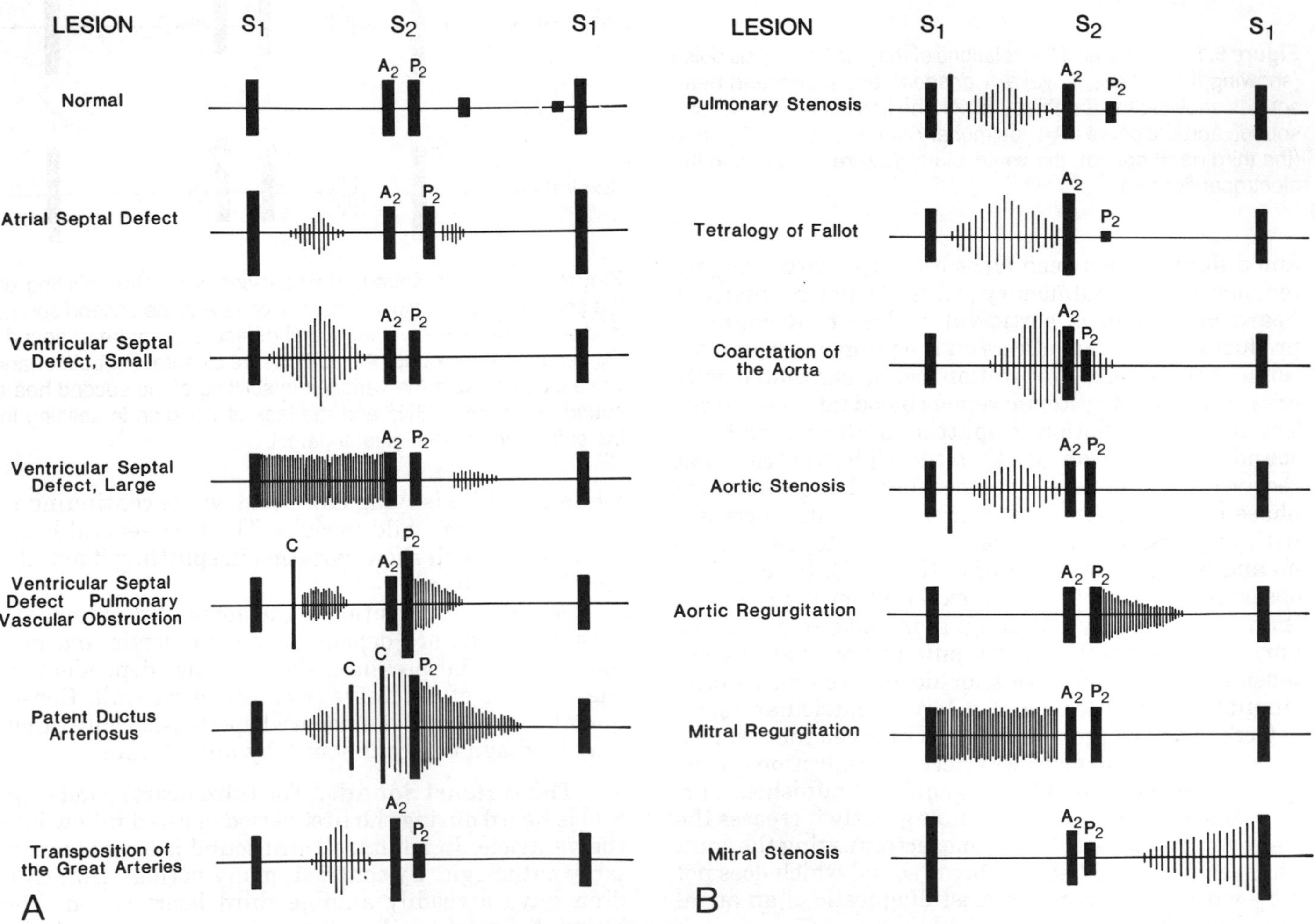

Figure 6.3 A and B. Schema of auscultatory findings in selected circumstances. S_1, first heart sound; S_2, second heart sound with its components; A_2, aortic valve closure; P_2, pulmonary valve closure shown separately; *C*, systolic click. Murmurs between S_1 and S_2 are systolic murmurs and between S_2 and S_1 are diastolic murmurs. The relation of intensity and frequency of murmurs is schematically shown.

atrioventricular valve regurgitation, or mild obstructions within the pulmonary arteries or the aorta, as in coarctation of the aorta). In general, the intensity of the murmur is proportional to the pressure loss across the orifice or to the amount of blood involved.

A very loud murmur may produce palpable vibrations of the chest wall. The lower the frequency of the murmur the more likely a thrill will be palpable; the higher the frequency, the less likely. For these reasons the murmur of aortic stenosis is often associated with a thrill, while the murmur of mitral regurgitation rarely is.

Much has been made of the characteristics of systolic murmurs. Murmurs with maximal intensity in midsystole are described as ejection murmurs (diamond-shaped) and those with the same intensity throughout systole are regurgitant murmurs (plateau type). In general, diamond-shaped murmurs are associated with larger pressure gradients (as in aortic stenosis) and plateau murmurs with little or no pressure gradient (as in mitral regurgitation). While these descriptions are correct, their practical value is limited, particularly for small children.

The location of maximal intensity of a systolic murmur may be of diagnostic help. A murmur localized to the left infrascapular area suggests coarctation of the aorta: a murmur at the right lower sternum, increasing with inspiration, indicates tricuspid valve incompetence, and an apical murmur radiating toward the axilla indicates mitral regurgitation.

Diastolic Murmurs. The early diastolic murmur of aortic regurgitation has a high-frequency, blowing quality (Fig. 6.3*A* and *B*). Because of the logarithmic nature of human hearing, the murmur of minimal aortic regurgitation is detectible almost before aortic regurgitation can be discerned by any other means. The murmur is best heard along the left sternal border, with the patient in the sitting position, in expiration, and leaning forward; the diaphragm is used to exclude lower frequency sounds. The murmur of pulmonary regurgitation in patients with low pulmonary artery pressure is of low frequency and is heard best in the pulmonary area or the lower left sternal border. Confusion between the two may arise in patients with high pulmonary artery pressure where the long, loud, early diastolic murmur may sound just like aortic regurgitation. Pulmonary regurgitation is most often heard after pulmonary valvotomy, whereas aortic regurgitation is usually a natural phenomenon. Furthermore, a wide pulse pressure may help identify the presence of aortic regurgitation.

While diastolic blowing murmurs have the highest frequencies encountered in auscultation, mid and late diastolic rumbles have the lowest—so low as to be occasionally palpable but inaudible. Rumbles are mostly heard at the lower sternal border and apex, and occur at either of the two points of maximal diastolic inflow into the ventricles. These murmurs are best heard with the bell held lightly against the chest. Excess inflow through a normal atrioventricular valve, as in left-to-right shunts, or pathologic narrowing of the inflow orifice can result in a diastolic rumble. The timing of diastolic rumbles in children is almost invariably at the first period of rapid inflow, immediately after the third heart sound. A severely obstructed mitral valve may produce a rumble audible in presystole. Presystolic accentuation of the diastolic rumble occurs at the second period of rapid inflow during atrial contraction.

Continuous Murmurs. A murmur extending from systole into diastole, through the second heart sound and sometimes even throughout the entire cardiac cycle, is described as continuous (Fig 6.3*A* and *B*), and generally results from communication between two structures with a continuous, though possibly variable, pressure difference. Connections between arteries and veins, between the systemic arterial and pulmonary circulation, or between systemic arteries and cardiac chambers can result in continuous murmurs. The classic example is a patent ductus arteriosus, heard best at the second left interspace. Other common causes include: excessive bronchial collateral circulation (often over the back), coronary arteriovenous fistula (often at the third or fourth interspace), and systemic arteriovenous fistula (anywhere over the body). The intensity of the murmurs is an indication of the pressure difference between the two structures as well as of the amount of blood being shunted. Consequently, some murmurs are loudest during systole and diminish over the course of diastole, as the pressure differences become smaller. In children with patent ductus arteriosus and pulmonary hypertension, the differences in pressure during diastole may be sufficiently small that the murmur becomes inaudible in early or mid-diastole. It follows that the point of maximal intensity of the murmur is at about the second heart sound giving a crescendo-decrescendo quality. This is useful in recognizing patients who have systolic murmurs by reason of valvar stenosis or ventricular defects associated with pulmonary or aortic regurgitation. In this case (to-and-fro murmur) the systolic component may appear to extend into diastole but careful auscultation will reveal that the peak intensity of the systolic murmur is before the second heart sound. Because maximal flow occurs during diastole in a coronary arterial fistula, this variety of continuous murmur has its peak intensity in diastole.

Innocent Murmurs (Functional, Insignificant, Physiologic, Benign, No Significant Heart Disease). As many as 50% of school-age children have an audible, but faint, systolic murmur that often varies in intensity with time, position, and activity level. In the absence of other evidence of heart disease, these murmurs have been labeled "innocent" or "functional."

For some years now, in the cardiac department of The Children's Hospital in Boston the term "no signficant heart disease" has been used for conditions judged by the cardiologist to carry an excellent prognosis. In other words, the condition, to the best of the cardiologist's knowledge, will never cause disability or require treatment, medical or surgical. Such situations are almost always associated with a murmur but have no symptoms or signs such as an abnormality of the second heart sound, or abnormal film or electrocardiogram. It is helpful for classification of the following conditions to designate them as representing no significant heart disease: trivial ventricular septal defect, mild pulmonary stenosis, trivial mitral regurgitation, or physiologic ejection murmur or Still murmur. The murmur may not be "innocent," but the condition and its prognosis are of no significance to the patient.

Commonly encountered innocent murmurs include the mildest variations of well-known lesions such as tiny ventricular defects, minimal mitral regurgitation, mild peripheral pulmonary stenosis, and trivial valvar pulmonary stenosis. The presence of a click might point toward mitral valve prolapse or a bicuspid aortic valve. A low hemoglobin count, excitement, or fever may explain a murmur which might otherwise not be present.

An innocent murmur varies with position becoming less loud when the patient is in the supine position. Clearly, any murmur that disappears from one day to the next, with position, or with variations in respiration, is likely to be innocent. An example is the right infraclavicular continuous murmur (venous hum) often heard clearly when the patient is sitting, but which disappears when the patient lies down or turns the head. A vibratory ("plucking string") murmur of the lower left sternal border (musical murmur) is commonly encountered and has been designated as Still murmur (Still, 1915).

It should be remembered also that the presence of an innocent murmur does not exclude heart disease.

Minor Laboratory Tests

HEMATOCRIT

In following any patient with congenital heart disease, it is important to observe the hematocrit. Among those who are cyanotic the hematocrit is largely reflective of the prevailing arterial oxygen content in the blood during the course of the day. The hemoglobin level may serve the same purpose. Cyanotic children with low hematocrit may be in particular difficulty. They may exhibit hypoxic spells more readily than if the oxygen-carrying capacity is normal. Whereas it is important that such children receive iron therapy, it is equally important that the course of response to iron therapy be monitored carefully, inasmuch as the hematocrit may be driven quickly to undesirably high levels, causing high blood viscosity.

BLOOD OXYGEN

In following children with cyanosis, it is useful to have some measurement of arterial oxygen saturation. We have used the measurement of transcutaneous Po_2 but have found this sufficiently unstable to be of some concern. Perhaps more reliable, although not perfect, is the measurement of fingertip oxygen saturation. Often observations of indirect oxygen saturation at rest and on exercise are useful. In some situations, particularly in cyanotic newborns, measurements of blood gases may be especially useful. The discovery of acidosis or retained carbon dioxide requires an explanation.

Comparison of right arm or right temporal arterial blood gases with those obtained from the umbilical artery is a useful test. If there is notable difference in the partial pressure of oxygen in these two areas it can be concluded that there is right-to-left shunting through a patent ductus arteriosus.

Having the patient breathe 100% oxygen while measuring arterial Po_2 can be revealing. Any cyanotic child who can raise his Po_2 to levels higher than 200 torr probably has a primary pulmonary problem (including pulmonary edema) which accounts for the low arterial oxygen saturation. Individuals who cannot raise their Po_2 higher than 100 torr while breathing 100% oxygen for 10 minutes probably have congenital heart disease with a right-to-left shunt, particularly if there is no obvious lung disease on a chest film.

Electrocardiography

The electrocardiogram is the specific test for any rate or rhythm disturbance and, for all children with heart disease, gives an inexpensive, easily obtained, reasonably accurate estimate of ventricular hypertrophy. The nomenclature of electrocardiographic deflections and intervals is shown in Figure 6.4 (Burch and Windsor, 1945).

RHYTHM DISTURBANCES

A long strip (10 inches) of electrocardiographic tracing (usually lead II), showing P waves, is desirable for rhythm evaluation. Occasionally, atypical leads, such

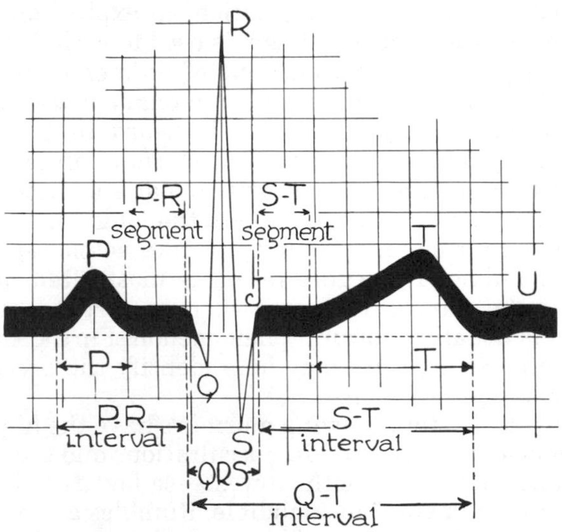

Figure 6.4. Nomenclature of electrocardiographic deflections and intervals. Reproduced with permission from Burch GE, Windsor T: *A Primer of Electrocardiography.* Philadelphia, Lea & Febiger, 1945.

as an esophageal lead, are needed to get the most helpful recording. For more detailed discussions of rhythm disturbances, see the monographs by Roberts and Gelband (1983) and Gillette and Garson (1981).

Sinus Arrhythmia. Variation in the heart rate with respiration is a normal finding beyond infancy and, at slower heart rates may be especially noticeable. A variation in cycle length of as much as 10% is known as sinus arrhythmia (Fig. 6.5).

Sinus Tachycardia. Sinus tachycardia is rapid heart rate, with a normally shaped P wave and a P-R interval of appropriate length, without any other abnormality in the sequence of conduction. This may be caused by exercise, fever, anxiety, and other manifestations of increased sympathetic tone or by congestive heart failure. In small infants with rates around 200, the differentiation between paroxysmal tachycardia and sinus tachycardia may be difficult. Sinus tachycardia with rates greater then 180 beats/min is rare.

Sinus Bradycardia. A slow heart rate with no abnormalities in the sequence of conduction is designated as sinus bradycardia (Fig. 6.5). The slowest of possible heart rates, still within "normal" limits, has been steadily redefined in recent years. The use of 24-hour tape-recording techniques has demonstrated that

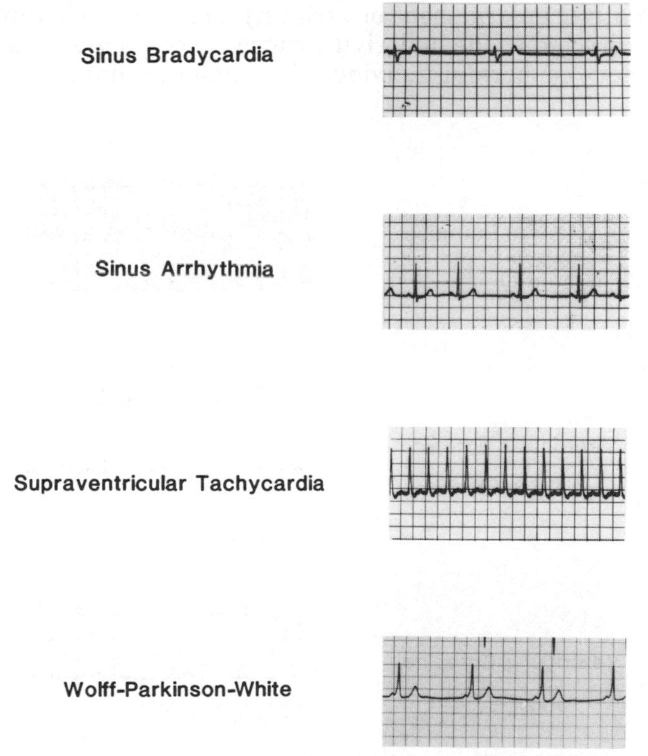

Figure 6.5. Sinus bradycardia. Rate of less than 40 beats/min. *Sinus arrhythmia.* Note variation in cycle length, R wave to R wave, in an otherwise normal tracing. *Supraventicular tachycardia.* Heart rate of 200. *Wolff-Parkinson-White syndrome.* Note short P-R interval and slurred initial portion of the QRS complex (delta wave).

in many normal individuals, the pulse rate drops to the 50s and even the 40s during sleep. The acceptable limits of sinus bradycardia in newborns is in the range of 80 beats/min; in older infants, 60 beats/min, in small children 50–60 beats/min, whereas in young athletic adults rates in the 40s and 50s may be usual provided they are of sinus origin. Rates below these arbitrary limits should raise the suspicion of complete heart block, and a 12-lead electrocardiogram should be recorded.

Supraventricular Tachycardia. Supraventricular tachycardia (Fig. 6.5) is characterized by a sudden onset of rates greater than 180 beats/min, as fast as 300 beats/min (in small infants), with sudden reversion to sinus rhythm. The rate is rigidly fixed without any appreciable variations. Often, the P waves are not readily seen. When the tachycardia arises from the atrioventricular node, the P-R interval may be very short and the P waves may be absent, or even follow the QRS (junctional tachycardia). The QRS complex is almost invariably normal (less than 0.10 sec); rarely, the conduction distal to the atrioventricular node may be aberrant, with a wide QRS complex resembling ventricular tachycardia. Differentiation between supraventricular tachycardia with a wide QRS complex and ventricular tachycardia can be extremely difficult, and is best determined by experts (see Wide QRS Complex Tachycardia).

The mechanism of supraventricular tachycardia is thought to be either a *re-entry* phenomenon or *automaticity*, with an arrhythmogenic focus outside the sinus node.

Re-entry. Re-entry occurs when dual atrioventricular nodal pathways or an accessory pathway allows return of the impulse conducted from the atrium to the ventricle through the bundle of His, back to the atrium from the ventricle. A repetitive, circular movement down the bundle of His and up the accessory pathway restimulates the atrium, resulting in a fast regular heart rate. This "circus" movement continues until the relative conductivity of the pathways is changed.

The Wolff-Parkinson-White syndrome (WPW), an ECG phenomenon, is the first recognized example of an accessory pathway (bundle of Kent) which allows "circus" movement to develop. The ECG of WPW is characterized by a short P-R interval (less than 0.1 sec), a slurred initial QRS deflection (delta wave) and a widened, bizarre QRS complex with an inverted T. This pattern is readily recognized but may be only intermittently present (Fig. 6.6). The Lown-Ganong-Levine syndrome is a variation on the WPW phenomenon and is characterized by a short P-R interval without the other features of WPW. It is associated less frequently with supraventricular tachycardia (Gillette et al, 1979).

Many patients with supraventricular tachycardia based on re-entry have "concealed" accessory pathways recognizable only at intracardiac electrode catheter study. Still, the majority of classical episodes of supraventricular tachycardia have re-entry as the underlying electrophysiologic mechanism.

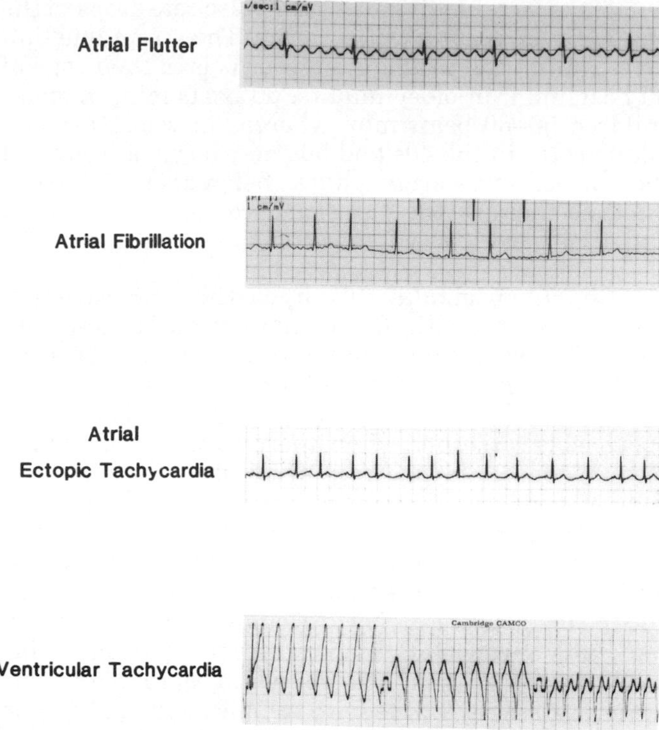

Figure 6.6. *Atrial flutter* with an atrial rate of more than 250 and a ventricular rate of about 50 beats/min. The saw-tooth pattern of P waves is characteristic. *Atrial fibrillation.* Note the completely irregular QRS cycle length and the evidence of chaotic atrial activity. *Atrial ectopic tachycardia.* Note the atrial activity (P waves) at a rate of 150 and a ventricular rate (QRS complexes) of 110. Sometimes the atrial activity stimulates the QRS complex and sometimes it does not. This rare form of supraventricular tachycardia is particularly resistant to therapy. *Ventricular tachycardia.* This tracing is three leads reported consecutively, each showing a bizarre widened QRS complex at a rate of more than 200 beats/min.

Automaticity. An automatic focus, producing impulses at a faster rate than the sinus node may be located anywhere within the atria or the atrioventricular node. An automatic focus tachycardia usually shows some variation in the heart rate, with P waves of abnormal morphology, introduced by warm-up and terminated by a cooling off period, but without of electrophysiological study it is usually indistinguishable from re-entry tachycardia.

Atrial Flutter. Atrial flutter (Fig. 6.6) is characterized by regular atrial rates around 300 beats/min. The saw-toothed atrial deflections are best seen in lead II, AVF and the right precordial leads. Fortunately, the atrioventricular conduction system usually is unable to respond to this rapid rate and the ventricles beat at fractions of the atrial rate. Thus, atrial flutter with 2:l or 3:l atrioventricular block results in ventricular rates of 150 or 100 (fractions of 300).

Atrial Fibrillation. Atrial fibrillation (Fig. 6.6) implies a completely chaotic, usually very rapid, atrial rate with irregular rapid stimulation of the ventricles. Fibrillatory waves are often barely discernible in the electrocardiogram.

Ventricular Tachycardia. In ventricular tachycardia (Fig. 6.6), at a rate between 150 and 250 beats, there are wide QRS complexes with no relation to the P waves. It may be difficult to distinguish this from supraventricular tachycardia with aberrant conduction, but all cases of wide QRS complex tachycardia should be considered to be ventricular tachycardia until proven otherwise because this rhythm is potentially lethal.

Ectopy. Ectopic beats (beats which are not part of the usual rhythm) should be recorded on an electrocardiogram, and the plan of management should be based on the specific diagnosis. Fetal ectopy is best documented by two-dimensional echocardiography (Kleinman et al, 1981).

Atrial Ectopy (Fig. 6.7). A premature atrial beat has a P wave unlike others in that lead, and is usually followed by a normal QRS complex. There is invariably a fixed relationship to the preceding abnormal P wave, irrespective of the morphology of the QRS. If the abnormal P wave immediately precedes the QRS, is buried in the QRS, or immediately follows the ventricular complex at a fixed interval, the term "junctional ectopy" is used. Barring the presence of cardiotoxic drugs or electrolyte imbalance, atrial ectopy is often related to atrial enlargement or atrial hypertension. Therapy is directed at the underlying cause. Atrial ectopy in an otherwise normal individual is a benign condition.

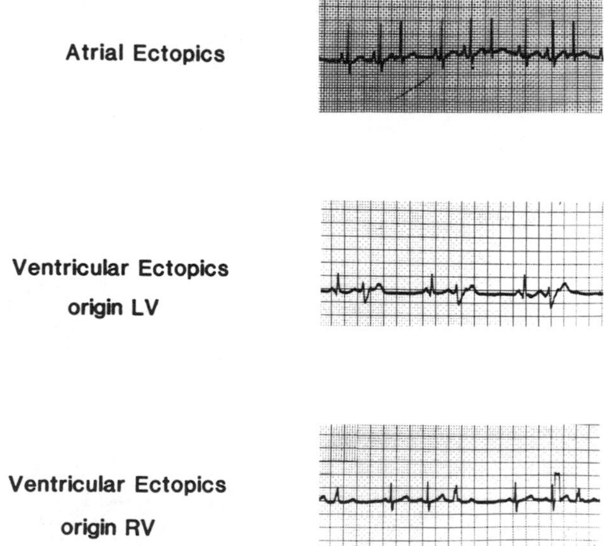

Figure 6.7. *Atrial ectopics* are recognized by a premature beat of normal QRS duration and morphology, which is preceded by a P wave of different origin than the fundamental rhythm. *Ventricular ectopics* are characterized by a premature beat of widened and often bizarre QRS morphology. Whether the ectopic beat originates from the right or left ventricle can be estimated by calculating the QRS axis of the ectopic beats.

Ventricular Ectopy (Fig. 6.7). Ventricular premature beats are characterized by a widened, bizarre QRS complex, occurring without consistent relationship to P waves. Alternating normal and ectopic beats are called "bigeminy." Two ectopic beats in sequence are couplets; three consecutive beats are triplets, and six or more ventricular beats in sequence are described as "a run of ventricular tachycardia." Ventricular premature beats with different QRS morphology are described as multifocal. While isolated ventricular premature beats may be benign, the potential for development of ventricular tachycardia (a dangerous rhythm) requires at least minimal documentation. For practical purposes, all individuals with known heart disease who have any form of ventricular ectopy must undergo complete examination beginning with a 24-hour tape-recorded electrocardiogram and exercise testing. Some estimation of the frequency of ectopic beats and the response to exercise should be recorded. Children with only occasional ventricular beats on a 24-hour monitoring tape require no further study.

Heart Block. First degree heart block is characterized by prolongation of the P-R interval.

Second degree heart block (Fig. 6.8) is characterized by variable atrioventricular conduction, including blocked beats. The Wenckebach phenomenon (1903) with progressively lengthening P-R intervals until the QRS complex drops out is an example of this.

Third degree heart block (complete heart block) (Fig. 6.8) is characterized by totally unrelated atrial and ventricular complexes. The rates of the atrial contractions and ventricular contractions are different, the ventricular rate being slower. Complete heart block can be suspected when the pulse rate is consistently less than 80 in a small infant and consistently less than 60 in a child or adult. An electrocardiogram clearly shows the unrelated P waves and QRS complexes at different rates.

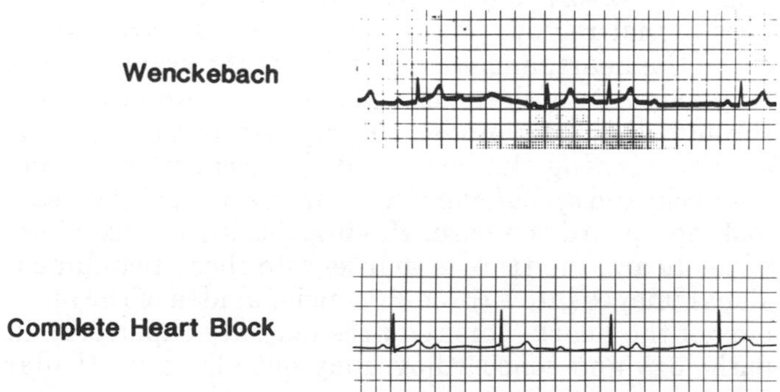

Figure 6.8. The Wenckebach phenomenon is characterized by an increasingly prolonged P-R interval until a P wave occurs without a following QRS complex. At that point, a beat following a normal P-R interval restarts the phenomenon. *Complete heart block* is characterized by independent unrelated P waves and QRS complexes. In the example presented, the ventricular (QRS) rate is 40/min, while the atrial rate varies from 75–85.

HYPERTROPHY

The relative thickness of the right versus the left ventricle is reflected in the electrocardiogram, which normally shifts from right ventricular dominance to left ventricular dominance by 2 years of age. Because of the variation with growth, reference to standards of normal evolution are helpful in assessing evidence of hypertrophy (Davignon et al, 1980).

Right ventricular hypertrophy is characterized by: (*a*) a positive TV4R-V5, (Fig. 6.9) (*b*) a dominant RV4R and RV1, (*c*) an axis greater than +120, (*d*) dominant SV5 and SV6, (*e*) voltage criteria for RV4R and RV1 which exceed age standards, (*f*) voltage criteria for SV5 and SV6 which exceed age standards, and (*g*) rSR1 in which R1 is greater than 10 millivolts. All of these criteria are seen in normal newborns through the first week of life.

Left ventricular hypertrophy is characterized by: (*a*) SV4R and SV1 which exceed voltage criteria for age, (*b*) RV5 and RV6 which exceed voltage criteria for age, (*c*) ST depression or T wave inversion in V5 and V6, and (*d*) a leftward superior axis. Practice provides confidence in recognizing abnormal patterns of ventricular voltages. It will be recognized that estimation of ventricular hypertrophy is a statistical conclusion and should be thought of as such in arriving at a diagnosis. A small percentage of normal children, by definition, will fall outside the limits of the standard

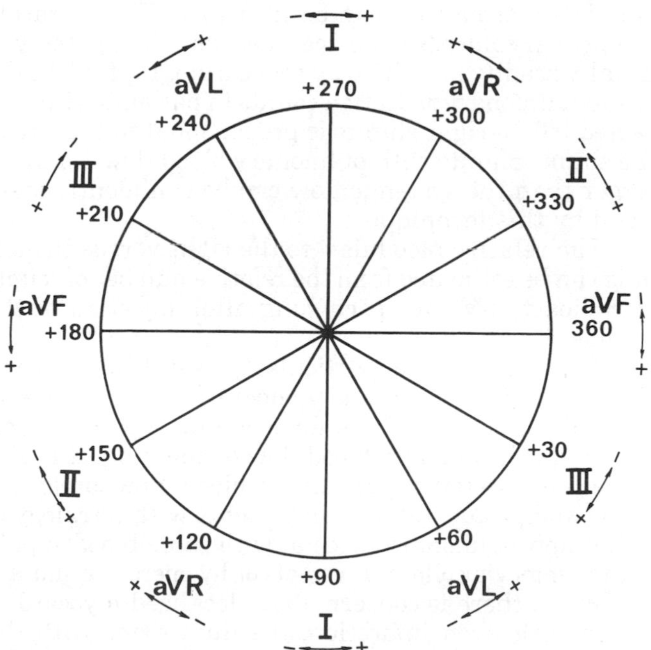

Figure 6.9. Diagram for estimation of the QRS axis: The positive and negative signs indicate the dominant direction of the QRS complex in that lead. Thus, if the dominant QRS direction in lead aVF is negative and the dominant QRS direction in lead aVR is also negative, the axis must lie between +300° (−60)° and 360 (0)°. Reference to the QRS direction in lead II will add further precision. If lead II is equiphasic, i.e., equal positive and negative QRS deflection, the axis is +330 (−30).

deviation. At the same time, serial evaluations showing changing patterns of ventricular hypertrophy over time can be particularly valuable in understanding the course of the patient's disease.

Radiography

CHEST FILM

A chest radiograph provides an estimation of the overall cardiac size and an estimation of the pulmonary blood flow. If it were for these features alone, echocardiograms would be more revealing without the necessity for exposure to X-radiation. The major value of the chest film is as a screen for ancillary observations such as: abnormal vessels, right aortic arch, scimitar syndrome, aberrant pulmonary vessels, vascular rings, associated pulmonary abnormalities, pneumonia, atelectasis, or emphysema.

RADIOISOTOPE SCANS

Radioisotopes provide information not otherwise readily available in some children with heart disease. The techniques vary. Either the initial bolus of radioisotopes is followed through the intrathoracic circulation (first pass) or the patient is observed after the radioisotope has been distributed throughout the circulation (equilibrium).

A first-pass scan is a crude angiogram; gross anatomic abnormalities can be identified. This is rarely the primary purpose of a scan because the anatomy is usually readily identified by echocardiography. The decay in pulmonary radiation counts in patients with suspected left-to-right shunts is proportional to the size of the shunt. Shunts with pulmonary blood flow 1.5 times larger than the systemic flow can be confidently identified by this technique.

The relative blood flow to the right versus the left lung can be estimated from the relative number of counts of radioactivity over each lung after injection of the isotope.

This technique is particularly useful in assessing the possibility of success preoperatively for patients who might be candidates for a Fontan operation but who might have major blood flow to one lung. It is also useful in assessing pulmonary blood flow preoperatively and postoperatively in patients with tetralogy of Fallot and pulmonary atresia, with some blood supply to the lungs via collateral vessels or by operative shunts.

When there is concern about localized myocardial ischemia or even infarction, thallium scans with the patient at rest and during exercise may help to demarcate the area and therefore the extent of injury. With increasing interest in arterial switching operations for transposition of the great arteries and the consequent necessity to manipulate coronaries, thallium scans have become a useful tool in determining success.

Echo-Doppler Study

Echocardiography is the prime method for evaluating cardiac anatomy in children with heart disease. As a diagnostic tool it has several important advantages. Modern echo equipment provides real-time imaging at 30 frames per second, with resolution to 1 mm. Because the ultrasonic beam is relatively harmless studies can be as prolonged as needed for optimal understanding and may be repeated as often as necessary. The equipment is reasonably mobile, although sometimes cumbersome and always expensive. Because structures at short distances are easier to image, pediatric patients with small chests are particularly favorable subjects for this technique.

With the advent of pulsed Doppler technology, further information became available through evaluation of the direction and velocity of blood flow. The discovery of a jet of blood into the right ventricle may signify a ventricular defect not visualized by inspection of the septum. The velocity of flow through a narrowed orifice, as in aortic stenosis, can be measured by a continuous-wave Doppler study and indicates the severity of the stenosis. Doppler measurements of flow velocity coupled with echo estimation of great vessel diameter in the pulmonary artery and aorta allow estimations of relative pulmonary and aortic blood flow.

Two-dimensional echocardiography is so valuable and used so often that some understanding of the technical details is desirable. Complete discussions are available in the echo texts (Williams et al, 1986).

METHODOLOGY

Echocardiography is a sonar technique. Thousands of pings of high frequency sound are directed toward the organ of interest. Tissues of different acoustic density reflect varying echos from the target, which, when corrected for transit time, can be processed to produce a faithful image. The more pings, the better the resulting image.

There are four usual views (windows) of observation (Fig. 6.10*A* and *B*): *parasternal*, viewing the left parasternal region, producing a short-axis transverse cut of the heart, and with rotation of the transducer, a long-axis view of the heart; *subcostal*, viewing the heart through the liver, under the xiphoid process; *suprasternal*, viewing the heart and the great vessels from the neck; and *apical*, viewing from the apex of the heart looking toward the base. Having obtained these views of the heart, the trick is to integrate these two-dimensional images into a three-dimensional idea of the anatomy of the heart. This requires not only experience in pathology and echocardiography but also a particular talent for spatial relations.

USES

Doppler studies are based on measuring the variations in frequency of reflected sounds. The difference between the transmitted and the reflected frequency of

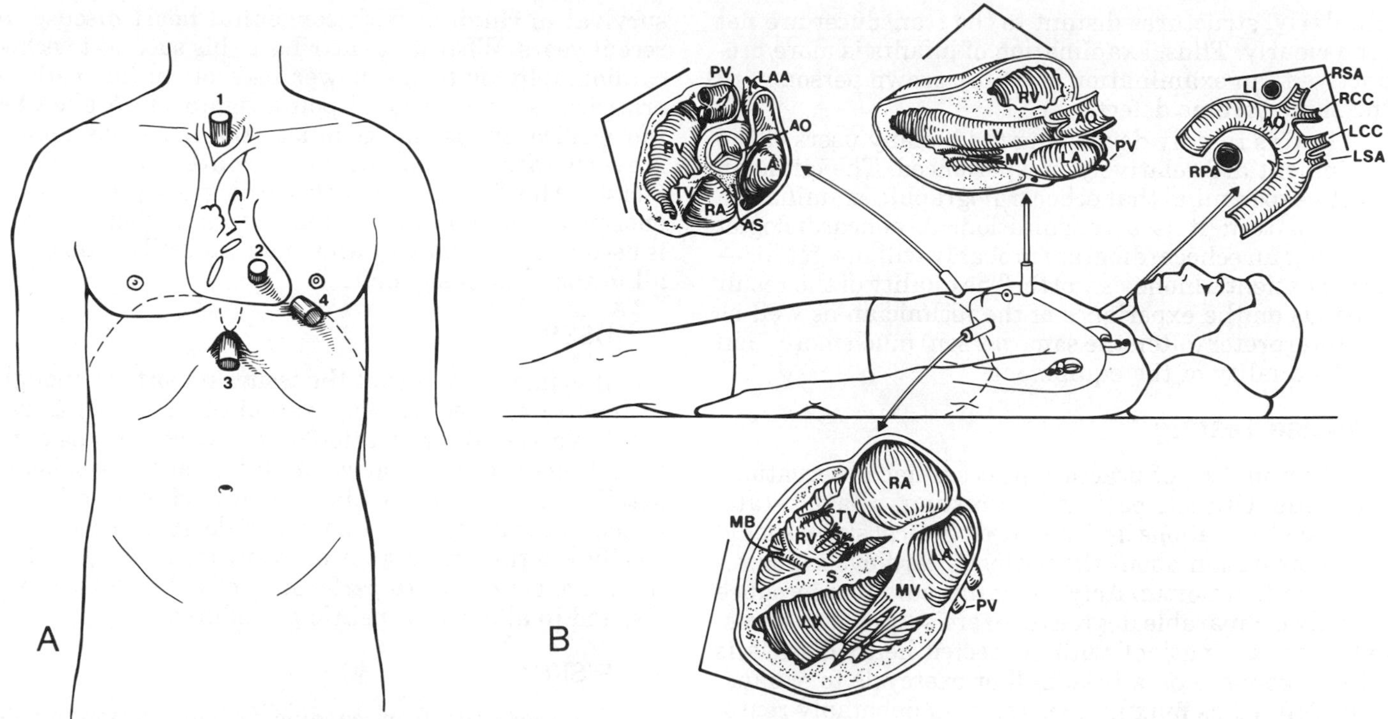

Figure 6.10 A. Routine echocardiographic views: *(1)* suprasternal, *(2)* parasternal, *(3)* subxyphoid, and *(4)* apical. **B.** Routine echocardiographic views. *LI,* left innominate vein; *RSA,* right subclavian artery; *RCC,* right common carotid; *LCC,* left common carotid; *LSA,* left subclavian artery; *PV,* pulmonary veins; *RA,* right atrium; *LA,* left atrium; *RV,* right ventricle; *LV,* left ventricle; *AO,* aorta; *MV,* mitral valve; *LAA,* left atrial appendages; *AS,* atrial septum; *TV,* tricuspid valve; *S,* ventricular septum; *MB,* moderate band.

sound is proportional to the velocity of pulsing blood flow. Thus, it is possible to measure the velocity of blood flow at selected points in the circulation (Goldberg et al, 1985).

Many foreign objects in the circulation reflect the ultrasonic signals. Monitoring lines in the intensive care unit and cardiac catheters may be observed; indeed, cardiac catheterization may be carried out under echocardiographic control. Induced microbubbles after an injection of saline or other fluid may provide a kind of angiocardiogram, allowing detection of right-to-left shunting.

If the ultrasonography is confined to a single narrow beam (M-mode), improved resolution in estimating the axial distance between two reflecting surfaces is obtained. Thus, precise measurements of the distance between the inner walls of the cardiac chambers at various times during contraction are possible. By choosing a standardized point of reference, the size of the chamber in systole and diastole, as well as the rate at which the size changes during contraction (a useful measure of myocardial function), can be estimated.

The main value of two-dimensional echocardiography is in delineating anatomy; Doppler cardiography provides complimentary physiologic information. The ability to recognize confidently virtually all cardiac abnormalities has dramatically changed pediatric cardiology. Nowadays, the anatomic diagnosis is known within hours of admission of a critically ill newborn.

Of potential value are estimations of ventricular function, particularly in documenting myocardial changes over time, as in healing myocarditis or worsening aortic regurgitation.

LIMITATIONS

Any structural detail, as small as 1 mm, can be discovered by ultrasonography, but to examine the heart millimeter by millimeter is impractical. The echocardiographer, to avoid unduly prolonged examination, must rely on the clinician's diagnostic acumen. It cannot be emphasized too strongly that echocardiograms are most useful when the time used is focused on particular questions raised, rather than on an uninformed search of the heart for possible abnormality. The echocardiographer should know in advance whether there is (*a*) a murmur; (*b*) cyanosis; (*c*) congestive heart failure; (*d*) concern about bacterial endocarditis; (*e*) concern about the severity of a known defect; or (*f*) concern about function of the heart when the anatomy has already been established.

It will be remembered that structures behind the air-filled lung and behind opaque bone are difficult, if not impossible, to visualize on the echocardiogram.

Similarly, structures distant to the transducer are not seen clearly. Thus, examination of infants is more productive than examination of a fully grown person with the same cardiac defect.

In this rapidly developing field, many users of the equipment are relatively inexperienced. The clinician must keep in mind that echocardiographic examination is not a test; it is a consultation. A noncardiologist ordering an echocardiogram probably will not get his—or his patient's money's worth. The quality of the result depends on the experience of the technician as well as the interpreter (often the same person) much more than on the quality of the equipment.

Exercise Testing

As a matter of practice most cardiac observations are made with the patient in a resting, relaxed state. Further observations under graded physical stress should add information about the patient's cardiovascular reserve, but, unfortunately, it is difficult to reproduce reliably comparable degrees of exercise. So, at the present time, the patient with suspected heart disease is either exercised on a treadmill or exercycle to exhaustion (defined as maximal exercise—a debatably reproducible point) or until some distinctly abnormal observation occurs (e.g., arrhythmia, abnormalities in the ST segments and T waves, or a drop in blood pressure). On a first visit, for a child with possible heart disease, one can simply ask the child to run down the hall or upstairs and note the rate and rhythm changes that occur.

Maximal exercise testing is most useful for serial observations of a patient's progress, particularly to monitor effects of pharmacologic interventions.

Children with aortic stenosis in whom changes occur in the ST and T waves during exercise are considered candidates for surgery, regardless of other abnormalities.

In many children arrhythmias develop during exercise, but in some, arrhythmias are suppressed with increased heart rate on effort. It is our belief that children with frequent ventricular ectopy should undergo exercise testing. Sometimes otherwise well children develop ventricular tachycardia under stress (Coelho et al, 1986).

Children who seem physically unable to perform up to expectation are often helped by maximal exercise testing. That the child can perform adequately often clears the air for a more realistic approach to life. Alternatively, the discovery of an abnormality leads to further study.

Cardiac Catheterization

In the 1980s echocardiography became the prime method for delineating cardiac anatomy in pediatric patients. Armed with information obtained at echocardiography the issues to be clarified by cardiac catheterization (Keane and Freed, 1980; Freed and Keane, 1980) have been extended. The increased information thus provided has clearly contributed to the improved survival in children with congenital heart disease in recent years. Whether to attribute this success to echocardiography or to the newer uses of cardiac catheterization is an emotional point vigorously argued by the medical-industrial complex (the more passionate "reverberators" and the more contentious "catheteers"). The fact is that echocardiography makes an enormous contribution and that cardiac catheterization is used more extensively and more fruitfully than ever, all to the patient's benefit.

USES

It is fair to state that the issues important enough to require cardiac catheterization are still being defined. We use catheterization to resolve conflicting clinical observations, to show anatomic and physiologic details not otherwise available, to provide data relative to the natural history of poorly understood lesions, to clarify life-threatening situations that develop in the intensive care unit, to perform electrophyiologic studies, and to allow therapeutic procedures.

RISKS

The mortality from cardiac catheterization is less than 0.1% for individuals older than 4 months of age. At less than 4 months of age, the risk is higher (about 1%), largely because the lesions that require study in the first days of life are particularly lethal (Cohn et al, 1985). The sickest patients find their way into the cardiac catheterization laboratory, often for emergency studies in the middle of the night. Many have life-threatening problems. It is inevitable that some will die.

Other risks include: blood loss at the point of insertion of the catheter; thrombosis of the artery used for entry of the catheter; thrombosis of the veins used for entry; rhythm disturbances with catheter manipulation; rarely, perforation of the heart; occasionally, provocation of a cyanotic spell; and, very rarely, cerebral vascular accidents in patients with intracardiac left-to-right shnting (Terplan, 1973).

Blood Loss. Often, a hematoma will develop at the site of percutaneous catheter entry. In small infants, blood loss at the wound site and in sampling requires transfusion. Potential for passage of the catheter outside of the circulation exists, and occasionally this occurs.

TECHNIQUE OF CARDIAC CATHETERIZATION

The child or infant is sedated, restrained on a fluoroscopy table, and given additional sedation as needed. A mixture of meperidene, promethazine, and chlorpromazine has sufficed for children beyond their first birthday. Chloral hydrate or Valium are often added. Using a sterile technique, a needle is inserted into the right femoral vein (umbilical vein in a newborn). A guidewire is passed into the vessel and the needle is removed. A sheath is inserted over the guidewire. The wire is then removed and an appropriate catheter is passed through the sheath into the circulation. This technique allows the use of a variety of catheters because changing the catheter is relatively easy.

In general, duplicate measurements of pressure and oxygen saturation, under conditions as near basal as can be obtained, are observed. Estimation of cardiac output is made by means of measured oxygen consumption and the Fick principle or by using injections of cold saline and thermodilution catheters. Occasionally, the responses to inhalation of 100% oxygen and to 15% oxygen are useful. Angiographic demonstration of the desired anatomy is undertaken. The patient is positioned to provide the best view of the anatomy. The angled views fundamental to successful angiography are shown in Figure 6.11 *A, B,* and *C* (Kelly et al, 1982). Biplane studies reduce the amount of contrast agent needed and the duration of the procedure. Digital subtraction may be useful in further reducing the dose of contrast (Bogren and Bursch, 1984; Capp and Oritt, 1984; Chung and Hesselink, 1984).

Electrophysiologic Studies. Placement of several, multiple-electrode catheters in various parts of the heart allows for timing of the passage of the impulse through the various parts of the heart under varying conditions. Precise definition of the electrophysiologic abnormality is possible. Stimulation to produce various rhythm problems and to convert them with medications may be a part of this procedure (Gillette and Garson, 1981).

AMBULATORY CATHETERIZATION

Many catheterization studies can be handled as outpatient procedures. Routine studies are accomplished the day before on an outpatient basis; the next morning the child is given no breakfast and is taken directly to the catheterization laboratory. At the conclusion of the study the patient is observed until completely awake and, barring complications, is discharged that evening. The prime impetus for this approach is to allay the child's and the parents' fears about separation. The misconception that this approach somehow really reduces the cost is unwarranted. Savings are minimal.

THERAPEUTIC CATHETERIZATION

Occasionally, therapeutic catheterizations are undertaken immediately after a diagnostic study, but of-

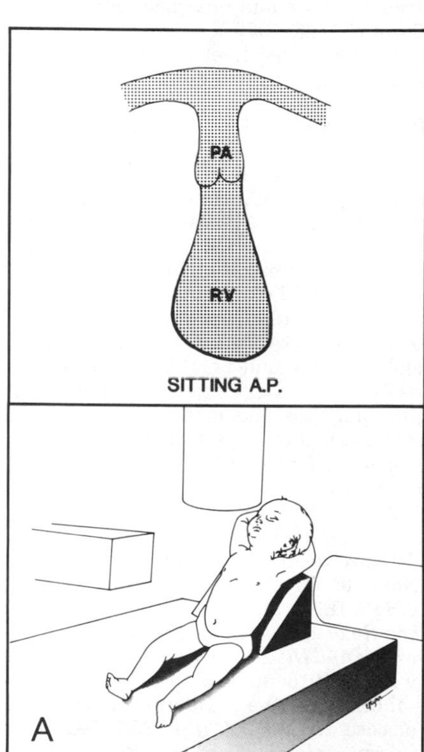

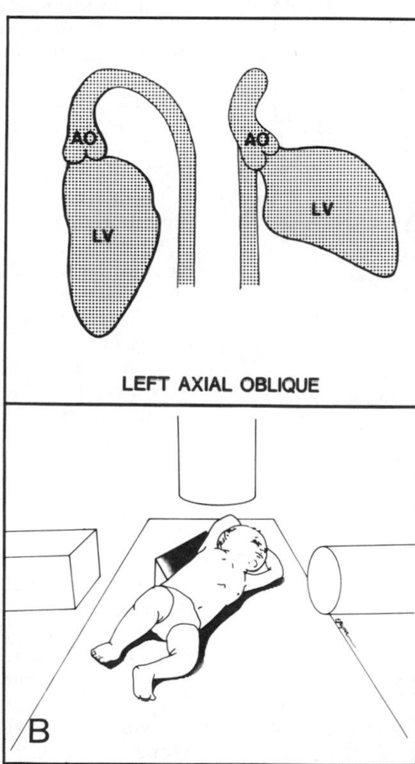

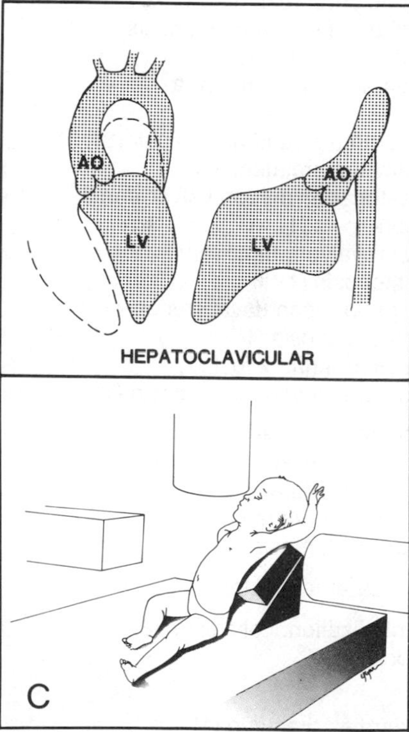

Figure 6.11 A. In the sitting up view, the right ventricular outflow tract, the main pulmonary artery and the right and left main pulmonary arteries are elongated. An angiogram with injection into the right ventricle in this position allows better recognition of obstructive abnormalities in these areas. This is a standard view for all patients with tetralogy of Fallot. **B.** In the left axial oblique view, the ventricular septum is seen at its greatest length and the outflow region for the left ventricle is seen to advantage. With contrast injection into the left ventricle this view allows discovery of several types of ventricular septal defects and shows left ventricular outflow obstructions. **C.** The hepatoclavicular (four-chamber) position allows a view of both the ventricular and atrial septa. Both ventricles and both atria are seen. Injection of contrast material into the left ventricle shows no ventricular septal defect. The location of the right ventricle and the left atrium are shown as dotted lines. The effect of changing the position of the child can also be achieved by changing the position of the radiographic tubes.

ten they are planned as separate procedures. Special balloons designed to stretch or rip open a stenotic valve and to dilate an acquired or postoperative stenosis of a vessel, such as peripheral pulmonary stenosis or coarctation of the aorta, are remarkably successful. Coils may be deposited in collateral vessels to promote clotting. Myocardial biopsy is possible and is particularly useful for patients with cardiac transplants. Placement of various devices to occlude patent ductus arteriosus, atrial defects, and other structures has been successful but must be considered as experimental (Table 6.2; Hoffer et al, 1985; Park et al, 1978).

Table 6.2
Interventional Catheterizations at Boston Children's Hospital, 1985[1]

Procedure	Number	Success
Balloon dilation		
Valvar pulmonary stenosis	24	23
Obstructed porcine valve	3	2
Peripheral pulmonary stenosis	42	18
Valvar aortic stenosis	17	14
Recoarctation of the aorta	13	13
Other	13	8
After interrupted arch repair (3),		
Native coarctation (4)		
Postoperative supravalvar aortic stenosis (1)		
Supravalvar pulmonary stenosis (1)		
Superior vena caval stenosis (1)		
Mitral stenosis (1)		
Dilation atrial defect (1)		
Pulmonary venous stenosis (1)		
Double umbrella device closure	13	8
Patent ductus arteriosus (9)		
Glenn procedure		
Left superior vena cava		
Potts anastomosis		
Park blade atrial septostomy	4	4
Coil embolization, collaterals (8), Blalock (2)	10	9
Other	4	4
Pericardiac drainage (1), Foreign body removal (3)		

[1]Reproduced with permission of Dr. James Lock.

REFERENCES

Bogren HG, Bursch JH: Digital angiography in the diagnosis of congenital heart disease. *Cardiovasc Intervent Radiol* 7:180-188, 1984.

Burch GE, Windsor T: *A Primer of Electrocardiography*. Philadelphia, Lea & Febiger, 1945.

Capp MP, Ovitt TW: Digital angiography in the diagnosis of congenital heart disease: An alternative viewpoint. *Cardiovasc Intervent Radiol* 7:190-191, 1984.

Chung KJ, Hesselink JR: Review of digital subtraction angiography in the diagnosis of congenital heart disease. *Cardiovasc Intervent Radiol* 7:188-189, 1984.

Coelho A, Palileo E, Ashley W, et al: Tachyarrhythmias in young athletes. *J Am Coll Cardiol* 7:237-243, 1986.

Cohn HE, Freed MD, Hellenbrand WF, et al: Complications and mortality associated with cardiac catheterization in infants under 1 year. A prospective study and review of 12 years' experience in the New England Regional Infant Cardiac Program. *Pediatr Cardiol* 6:123-132, 1985.

Davignon A, Rautaharju P, Boissele E, et al: Normal ECG standards for infants and children. *Pediatr Cardiol* 1:123-131, 1980.

Freed MD, Keane JF: Profiles in congenital heart disease. In: Grossman W (ed): *Cardiac Catherization and Angiography*. Philadelphia, Lea & Febiger, 1980, pp. 377-400.

Fyler DC, Buckley LP, Hellenbrand WE, et al: Report of the New England Regional Infant Cardiac Program. *Pediatrics*. 65 Suppl: 376-460, 1980.

Gillette PC, Garson A: *Pediatric Cardiac Dysrhythmias*. New York, Grune & Stratton, 1981.

Gillette PC, Garson A, Kugler JD: Wolff-Parkinson-White syndrome in children: Electrophysiologic and pharmacologic characteristics. *Circulation* 60:1487-1495, 1979.

Greenwood RD, Rosenthal LA, Parisi L, et al: Extracardiac abnormalities in infants with congenital heart disease. *Pediatrics* 55:485-492, 1975.

Goldberg SJ, Allen HD, Marx GR, et al: *Doppler Echocardiography*. Philadelphia, Lea & Febiger, Philadelphia, 1985.

Hoffer FA, Fellows KE, Wyly JB, et al: Therapeutic catheter procedures in pediatrics. *Pediatr Clin North Am* 32:1461-1476, 1985.

Ingelfinger JR: *Pediatric Hypertension*. Philadelphia, WB Saunders, 1982, pp. 296.

Keane JF, Freed MD: Cardiac catheterization in infants and children. In Grossman W (ed): *Cardiac Catheterization and Angiography*. Philadelphia, Lea & Febiger, 1980, pp. 70-77.

Kelley MJ, Jaffe CC, Kleinman CS: *Cardiac Imaging in Infants and Children*. Philadelphia, WB Saunders, 1982, pp. 441.

Kleinman CS, Hobbins JC, Lynch DC, et al: The use of fetal echocardiography in the diagnosis and management of antenatal arrhythmias. Abstract. *Am J Cardiol* 47:457, 1981.

Leatham A: *Auscultation of the Heart and Phonocardiography*. New York, Churchill Livingstone, 1975.

Park SC, Neches WH, Zuberbuhler JR, et al: Clinical use of blade atrial septostomy. *Circulation* 58:600–606, 1978.

Roberts NK, Gelband H: *Cardiac Arrhythmias in the Neonate, Infant and Child*, ed 2. Norwalk, CT, Appleton-Century-Crofts, 1983.

Roth A, Rosenthal A, Hall JE, et al: Scoliosis in congenital heart disease. *Clin Orthop Related Res* 93:95–102, 1973.

Still GF: *Common Disorders and Diseases of Childhood*, ed 3. London, Oxford University Press, 1915, pp. 495-496.

Terplan KL: Patterns of brain damage in infants and children with congenital heart disease. *Am J Dis Child* 125:175–185, 1973.

Wenckebach KF: *Die Arhythmie als Ausdruck Bestimmter Funktionsstorungren des Herzens*. Leipzig, W. Engelmann, 1903.

Williams RG, Bierman FZ, Sanders SP: *Echocardiographic Diagnosis of Cardiac Malformations*. Boston, Little, Brown, 1986.

Therapeutic Tools

2

Increased use of conduits, pacemakers and prosthetic valves prompted preparation of this chapter. More than 500 children who have been seen at The Children's Hospital in Boston now survive because of one or the other of these devices.

Conduits

Woven plastic conduits, valved or nonvalved, and aortic homografts are a necessary part of modern surgery for congenital heart disease. Conduits are used to bridge a gap between the right ventricle and the pulmonary artery in patients with tetralogy of Fallot, or as part of a Rastelli repair for transposition of the great arteries with ventricular defect and pulmonary stenosis. Conduits are used in the repair of truncus arteriosus, double-outlet right ventricle and corrected transposition of the great arteries with ventricular defect and pulmonary stenosis. Modified Fontan repairs, using conduits from the right atrium to the right ventricle or pulmonary artery, are less common nowadays.

Although conduits cannot grow, the disproportion in size because of growth has not been a major problem except in very small infants. Rather, the development of neointima causes obstruction for virtually all patients, particularly those in whom the conduit was inserted in childhood. Peeling of the neointima has been observed but is thought to be uncommon with the use of more modern conduits (Jonas et al, 1985; Schaff et al, 1984). Aortic homografts, with or without valves, have been used extensively in other countries with good results and may be the method of choice at the present time.

Replacement of obstructed conduits has proved to be less of a problem than the initial surgery. Balloon dilatation for internal obstruction of conduits and obstructions at the ends of conduits may be the answer to this problem.

Pacemakers

There are 150 surviving children who have had pacemakers inserted at The Children's Hospital in Boston. Fortunately, pacemakers today are highly reliable over long periods of time. The battery life averages 10 years. Other mechanical failures, including problems with fixed-length leads in a growing child have been resolved. Most of these pacemakers have been inserted either because of heart block (surgical or congenital) or because of the adminstration of powerful antiarrhythmic agents which might cause cardiac arrest (i.e., sick sinus syndrome) (Frye, 1984; Gillette et al, 1983; Parsonnet and Bernstein, 1983).

Pacemakers should be checked at least yearly and more frequently near the projected decay time. Some checks can be made by telephone, others require the use of external magnets to alter rates and determine function. Some pacemakers even record arrhythmogenic experience. The power supply is usually inserted in the upper chest or axilla, although in small infants the abdominal wall may be used. Sepsis at the implant site is a serious and difficult problem. The pacemakers are attached to electrode-tipped catheters which are inserted transvenously and impinge on the apical portion of the right ventricle. For children with interventricular or great vessel right-to-left shunting, pacemaker leads are placed epicardially. Recent experience indicates that the electrode can be inserted safely and effectively inserted into an anatomic left ventricle (L-transposition of the great arteries).

Prosthetic Values

Insertion of a prosthetic valve in a growing child is not desirable unless it is unavoidable. Although the need to change these devices regularly with growth is much less than was originally expected, nevertheless, changes are frequently required because of malfunction. The growth of pannus (an exuberant fibrinoid reaction) around the valve has led to severe malfunction over a period as short as 1 or 2 years. Deformity of the valve structure itself does not constitute a problem. Acute malfunction is a dramatic episode requiring immediate attention.

A surprisingly large valve can be inserted in a small child who has mitral regurgitation inasmuch as the condition dilates the valve ring. Insertion of an artificial valve because of mitral stenosis is another matter and may not be possible in a small child. Occasionally, insertion above the valve ring is possible. Anticoagulation is mandatory. Coumadin is used most often; prothrombin time checks should be made at least once a month. Problems with bleeding are not common if there are regular checks and the prothrombin time is kept at twice control. Occasionally, children have problems with control and treatment is changed to Persantine or aspirin. It is important to remember that in the rare cyanotic patient who has a high hematocrit, routine prothrombin times are not reliable unless there is compensation for the abnormal hematocrit.

The half-life of plastic prosthetic valves is about 5 years in children (Schaff et al, 1984). The half-life of porcine valves in a growing child is shorter and, for this reason, this type of valve has been abandoned (Sanders et al, 1980). We are hopeful that aortic homografts will provide a longer lasting solution.

REFERENCES

Gillette PC, Shannon C, Blair H, et al: Transvenous pacing in pediatric patients. *Am Heart J* 105843–847, 1983.

Frye RL (chairman): A Report of the Joint American College of Cardiology/American Heart Association Task Force on Assessment of Cardiovascular Procedures. Guidelines for permanent cardiac pacemaker implantation, May 1984. *J Am Coll Cardiol* 4:434-442, 1984.

Jonas RA, Freed MD, Mayer JE, et al: Long term followup of patients with synthetic right heart conduits. *Circulation* 72 Suppl II: 77–83, 1985.

Parsonnet V, Bernstein AD: Cardiac pacing in the 1980s: Treatment and techniques in transition. *J Am Coll Cardiol* 1:339-354, 1983.

Sanders SP, Levy RJ, Freed MD, et al: Use of Hancock porcine xenografts in children and adolescents. *Am J Cardiol* 46:429–438, 1980.

Schaff HV, Danielson GK, DiDonato RM, et al: Late results after Starr-Edwards valve replacement in children. *J Thorac Cardiovasc Surg* 88:583-589, 1984.

Schaff HV, DiDonato RM, Danielson GK, et al: Reoperation for obstructed pulmonary ventricle-pulmonary artery conduits. *J Thorac Cardiovasc Surg* 88:334–343, 1984.

Congenital Heart Disease 3

Epidemiology

About 1% of newborns have congenital heart disease. Excluding bicuspid aortic valve and mitral valve prolapse, conditions that are almost never recognized in the newborn period, the figure is closer to 750/100,000 live births (Mitchell et al, 1971; Carlgren, 1969). One-third of these will require hospitalization in the first year of life because of symptoms (Fyler et al, 1980; Ferenz et al, 1984); one-third will require attention later in life, and in one-third, there is little functional consequence. Of those hospitalized in the first year, one-half will require cardiac surgery before their first birthday.

When patients are listed in diagnostic categories (Table 6.3), ventricular septal defect is the lesion most commonly encountered in the clinic and in the cardiac catheterization laboratory. Tetralogy of Fallot is the leading reason for cardiac surgery; hypoplastic left heart syndrome is the number one cause of death. Mitral valve prolapse accounts for the significant group of patients with mitral valve disease seen in the clinics.

Ventricular septal defect is the most common anomaly in all age groups, even among adults (Table 6.4). Hypoplastic left heart syndrome and transposition of the great arteries are problems of infancy. Mitral valve prolapse is common in childhood. Aortic stenosis rises from the tenth place (3% of patients) in infancy to third place (14%) in the second decade. Coarctation of the aorta and endocardial cushion defects each constitute 5% of patients in all age groups.

The median age of patients at clinic visits at The Children's Hospital is about 10 years, with 15% of patients being older than 20 years (Table 6.5). The median age at cardiac catheterization is about 5 years and at cardiac surgery is between 1 and 5 years. Almost half (43%) of the deaths occur in the first month of life; almost three-quarters (70%) occur in the first year of life.

At The Children's Hospital in Boston about 70% of patients of all ages who have congenital heart disease require an operation. Because many are referred to this hospital specifically for surgery this is not a representative figure. Dickinson (et al (1981a) estimates 53% of all patients with congenital heart disease will require surgery. One-third never require major investigation or surgery and 1–2/1000 live births will undergo nonsurgical cures. These will occur largely in babies with low birth weight who have patent ductus arteriosus and in larger infants with ventricular septal defects and, to a lesser extent, atrial septal defects. The total mortality of patients from all congenital heart disease is about 10%, of whom three-quarters will have died before the first birthday.

Survival among children with congenital heart disease has improved considerably in the past quarter of a century. Much of this is due to improved surgery.

Table 6.3
Patient Experience: Percentage and Rank (in Parentheses)[1,2]

Diagnosis	NERICP, 1968–1981 At birth	The Children's Hospital, Boston, 1973–1985 All Ages Clinic	Catheterization	Surgery	Death
VSD	15.7(1)	26.1(1)	15.7(1)	13.3(2)	8.4(4)
TGA	9.9(2)	3.0(10)	7.4(5)	8.8(4)	10.4(2)
TF	8.9(3)	8.7(4)	15.0(2)	13.9(1)	8.6(3)
Coarc	7.5(4)	4.2(7)	5.6(7)	8.0(6)	4.3(10)
HLV	7.4(5)	0.4	2.6	2.2	15.6(1)
PDA	6.1(6)	3.7(8)	1.9	9.8(3)	3.5
ECD	5.0(7)	3.6(9)	6.5(6)	7.7(7)	6.9(5)
Hetero	4.0(8)	1.0	1.1	1.1	4.3
PS	3.3(9)	13.8(2)	8.8(4)	5.2(8)	0
PA & IVS	3.1(10)	0.2	1.2	1.8	0.9
ASD2	2.9	6.4(5)	4.3(8)	8.6(5)	5.2(6)
TAPVR	2.6	0.5	1.5	1.6	1.4
Myocard	2.6	2.1	1.5	0.2	3.2
TA	2.6	0.8	1.9	1.7	2.0
SV	2.4	1.3	3.3(9)	2.6	2.9
Aortic val	1.9	9.9(3)	8.9(3)	4.9(9)	4.9(7)
Mitral val	0	6.2(6)	2.6	1.1	1.2
DORV	1.5	0.9	3.2(10)	3.2(10)	4.9(9)
Trunc	1.4	0.4	1.3	1.3	4.9(8)
LTGA	0.7	1.0	1.0	0.9	0.6
Others	10.5	5.8	4.7	2.1	5.9

[1]Infants in the New England Regional Infant Cardiac Program (NERICP) (Fyler et al, 1980a) were hospitalized in the first year of life and underwent cardiac catheterization, cardiac surgery, or died in their first year. The diagnosis at birth is listed. Among patients at The Children's Hospital in Boston, the diagnosis listed is that at death, at last surgery, last cardiac catheterization, or last clinic visit. Children with no heart disease have been excluded; those with mitral valve prolapse are included. The percentages presented are based on the number of patient encounters with a given diagnosis. Hence, diagnoses that might require more frequent clinic visits, multiple catheterizations, or repeat surgery are overemphasized.

[2]Abbreviations used in Table 6.3: NERICP, New England Regional Infant Cardiac Program; Cath, catheterization; VSD, ventricular septal defect; TGA, transposition of the great arteries; TF, tetralogy of Fallot; Coarc, coarctation of the aorta; HLV, hypoplastic left ventricle; PDA, patent ductus arteriosus; ECD, endocardial cushion defects; Hetero, Heterotaxic malposition or splenic abnormality; PS, pulmonary stenosis; PA & VS, pulmonary atresia with intact ventricular system; ASD2, atrial septal defect secundum; TAPVR, total anomalous pulmonary venous return; Myocard, myocardial disease; TA, tricuspid atresia; SV, single ventricle; Aortic val, aortic valve disease; Mitral val, mitral valve disease; DORV, double-outlet right ventricle; Trunc, truncus arterious communis; LTGA, corrected (L) transposition of the great arteries.

Surgical results have improved not only because of newer operative procedures, but because, for some reason, older operations are being performed better. It is our impression that this results from earlier and improved diagnosis and improved postoperative care.

The congenital heart lesions will be discussed in order of their rank in prevalence among infants seen in the New England Regional Infant Cardiac Program (Fyler et al, 1980a). Added emphasis will be given to those seen in increased numbers in childhood and later. Mitral valve prolapse (±5% of population, Table 6.3) (Jeresaty, 1979) and bicuspid aortic valve (±1% of population) (Keith et al, 1979) are considered variants of normal, producing no physiological problems, and will not be mentioned further except as they relate to specific cardiac lesions.

DEVELOPMENT OF CIRCULATION

Fetal Circulation

Before birth, the two ventricles share in providing roughly equal amounts of blood to the placenta and to the body (Fig. 6.12). The ventricles, however, do not pump precisely equal shares; the volume of blood handled by the right ventricle is greater than that in the left (as much as 50%) varying somewhat from individual to individual. The inferior vena caval blood, carrying the newly oxygenated blood from the placenta, tends to go through the patent foramen ovale into the left atrium, left ventricle and out the ascending aorta toward the head (perhaps a fortunate arrangement), while the less oxygenated blood, coming from the superior vena cava and coronary sinus, passes through the right ventricle into the pulmonary artery. From here most of the blood goes through the ductus arteriosus, down the descending aorta, and only a small percentage (less than 10%) goes through the lungs into the left atrium. Because of the potential for mixing in the right atrium where the two caval flows meet, the actual difference between the blood oxygen saturation in the ascending and descending aorta is not great.

During fetal life, the right and left sides of the heart work as parallel circuits, jointly pumping the systemic circulation. For a more detailed discussion of fetal hemodynamics see Barcroft (1947), Lind et al (1964), Dawes (1969), and Rudolph (1974).

Table 6.4
Rank and Frequency of Cardiac Diagnoses among Different Age Groups between 1973 and 1985 at the Boston Children's Hospital[1,2]

	Age in Years							
	0–1		1–10*		10–20		20+	
Rank	Dx	%	Dx	%	Dx	%	Dx	%
1	VSD	30	VSD	23	VSD	18	VSD	17
2	PDA	11	PS	12	PS	14	TF	17
3	TGA	8	TF	10	AS	14	AS	15
4	TF	8	ASD	10	MV	10	PS	11
5	PS	6	AS	8	TF	9	ASD	5
6	Coarc	5	ECD	5	ASD	6	ECD	5
7	ECD	5	Coarc	5	Coarc	5	MV	5
8	HLV	4	PDA	5	ECD	4	Coarc	5
9	ASD	4	TGA	4	Hyper	3	PH	2
10	AS	3	MV	3	Myocard	2	TGA	2
	Other 16		Other 15		Other 15		Other 16	

[1]Each patient seen between 1973 and 1985 has been assigned a single categorical diagnosis based on the last surgical or catheterization encounter or on findings at autopsy or, if no other data, on the first clinic encounter. Each appears only once. Patients with no heart disease have been excluded. Table 6.4 is based on experience with 11,105 patients.
[2]Abbreviations as in Table 6.3; other abbreviations: Dx, diagnosis; %, percent; AS, aortic stenosis; MV, mital valve; Hyper, hypertension; PH, pulmonary hypertension.

Fetal Heart Disease

Because the two ventricles pump blood in parallel before birth, most congenital cardiac lesions are well tolerated by the fetus. Given a cardiac lesion which that limits entry or exit of blood from a ventricle, the other ventricle simply assumes the work. It is an accepted principle of embryologic growth that vascular structures assume the size needed to accommodate the blood flow that is presented. Thus, with pulmonary valve atresia, the left ventricle assumes the entire pumping responsibility and with aortic atresia the right ventricle becomes the sole pump. It is easy to see why problems occur at birth.

Table 6.5
Percent of Patients with Congenital Heart Disease by Age and Events, 1973–1985[1]

Age	Clinic	Catheterization	Surgery	Death
1–6 days	0.4	6.9	4.0	24.5
7–30 days	2.3	3.8	8.5	18.2
31–365 days	11.7	17.3	24.0	27.4
1–4 years	17.7	25.8	25.5	13.8
5–9 years	16.6	15.0	16.4	4.6
10–14 years	17.3	11.9	9.3	2.9
15–19 years	16.1	9.8	6.5	3.2
20–24 years	8.1	5.0	2.8	1.2
25–80 years	7.1	4.4	2.9	3.2

[1]The patient experience at The Children's Hospital in Boston listed by age at the time of clinic visits, cardiac catheterization, cardiac surgery, or death.

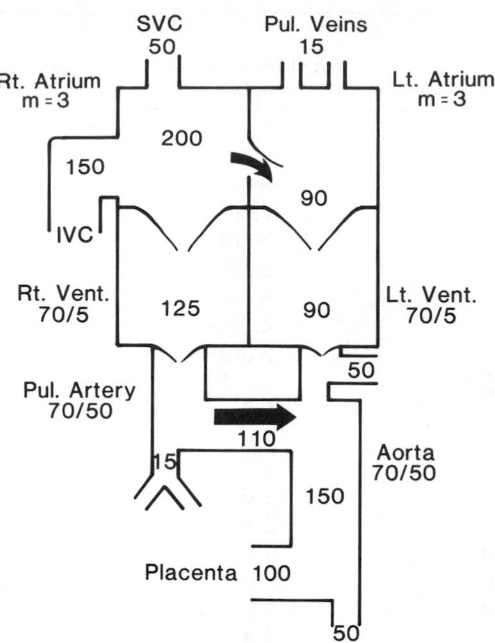

Figure 6.12. The numbers within each chamber represent the relative contributions to volume flow. The numbers outside represent the fetal pressures. Note that the placental blood flow is approximately equal to systemic blood flow and that the right and left ventricles carry approximately equal amounts of blood. It can be appreciated that during fetal life the relative amount of blood carried by each ventricle could vary widely while still providing adequate output to the patient and placenta.

Although most cardiac anomalies are not associated with congestive heart failure before birth, intrauterine heart failure can occur and may be documented by two-dimensional echocardiogram (Gillette et al, 1979). The manifestations of congestive heart failure are hepatomegaly, edema, and anasarca. The underlying cause may be anemia or prolonged supraventricular tachycardia (Griscom et al, 1977; Hutchinson et al, 1982). Atrial flutter may also occur but it is usually blocked to a 2:1, or lower, response and, therefore, does not usually produce intrauterine failure.

Large systemic arteriovenous fistulae can cause congestive heart failure before birth and presumably the largest ones cause intrauterine death. Lesser arteriovenous malformations allow normal intrauterine growth and survival with normal birth weights. Immediately after birth, however, with the requirement for pumping the systemic circulation through the heart twice, a systemic arteriovenous fistula (cerebral or hepatic) results in an intolerable load to the heart within days (Holden et al, 1972).

Myocardial disease, viral or hypoxic, before birth can also be the cause of intrauterine congestive failure (Griscom et al, 1977; Hutchinson et al, 1982), which may be expected to worsen with birth. The New England Regional Infant Cardiac Program found that the number of newborns with myocardial difficulties is higher in the first days of life than at any time thereafter (Fyler et al, 1980a).

Valvar regurgitation may also contribute an added load to both intrauterine and extrauterine circulations and, thus, is a potential cause for intrauterine congestive heart failure. The fetus with Ebstein disease, undefended tricuspid orifice, or absence of the pulmonary valve may be born with gross cardiac enlargement, clearly having had this for some time before birth.

Events at Birth

After birth, each ventricle pumps the cardiac output in sequence; first the right ventricle to the lungs, then the left ventricle to the body, the amount of blood pumped to the body having gone through the heart twice (serial circulation; Fig. 6.13). Despite this rough approximation of the amount of blood pumped by the heart before and after birth, there is, nonetheless, substantial added cardiac work after birth. With removal of the low-resistance placenta and equalization of the blood volume between the left and right ventricles, the added effort falls mainly on the left ventricle, which must supply an increased blood flow at higher pressure. In contrast, the right ventricle with involution of the pulmonary arteriolar bed, experiences decreased pressure work and is no longer required to supply the descending aorta through the ductus arteriosus with a large part of the cardiac output. Along with the requirement to provide temperature regulation, a prenatal surge of thyroid hormone adds to the work of the heart (Breall et al, 1984). Oxygen consumption increases. The suspicion that the left ventricle is working at maximum capacity at birth has been confirmed by studies showing minimal cardiac reserve in the first days and weeks of life (Rudolph, 1970). Within weeks the circulation gradually stabilizes to adult status.

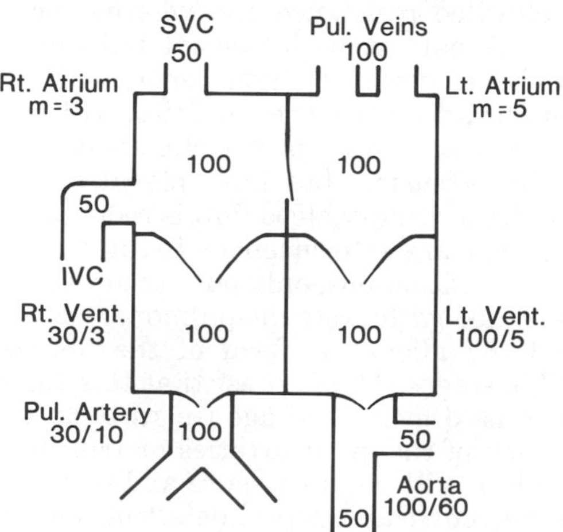

Figure 6.13. At birth, the amount of blood pumped by the heart is approximately the same as before birth, but it must pass through the two ventricles in sequence. The pressures are largely achieved within days of birth.

At birth, the *ductus arteriosus* may briefly contribute to shunting right to left or left to right for some hours or days, depending on the level of pulmonary resistance. Within a few days, often as long as a week in premature infants, regardless of whether the pulmonary resistance remains high or regresses normally, the ductus follows its programmed course of closure.

Pulmonary arterial pressure falls in proportion to the drop in *pulmonary arteriolar resistance*. The initial decrease is steep (in the order of 50% with the first few breaths), the subsequent fall being more gradual. Within 2 weeks, 90% of the change has occurred and, after 3–4 months, residual abnormality of pulmonary resistance can be detected only with refined methods.

Timing of the closure of the *ductus venosus* is less well documented but it occurs within a few days after birth, often to the dismay of the cardiac catheterization team who may try to use the umbilical vein as an entry site to the heart.

The *foramen ovale* is functionally closed by the flap of septum primum within minutes or hours of birth because of the rise in left atrial pressure needed to fill an overworking left ventricle. Nonetheless, a newborn infant with straining or grunting can occasionally create enough right-to-left shunt to cause visible cyanosis. Anatomic closure of the foramen ovale depends on the relative right and left atrial pressures; closure is earlier in patients with elevated left atrial pressure (e.g., ventricular septal defect, patent ductus arteriosus) and later in patients with somewhat higher right atrial pressures (e.g., valvar pulmonary stenosis). In 5% of people without heart disease the foramen ovale may remain probe-patent for life.

Mature Circulation

A schema of the mature circulation is presented in (Fig. 6.13). Reflex control of the circulation is largely in place within weeks of birth. The systemic blood pressure gradually rises as a child grows.

Handicaps Resulting from Congenital Heart Disease

Pulmonary Hypertension

Anatomy

Pulmonary arterial hypertension is a consequence of arteriolar obstruction to pulmonary blood flow. The obstruction may occur because of reduction in the average arteriolar cross- section (anatomic and/or vasoconstrictive), because of insufficient numbers of arteries, or because of stenoses of peripheral pulmonary arteries proximal to the arterioles. The latter is not common and can be readily recognized by angiography. An inadequate number of vessels is encountered when the lungs are hypoplastic (diaphragmatic hernia) or when there is limited available lung (repaired tetralogy of Fallot with absence of the left pulmonary artery). For practical purposes, the bulk of clinical pulmonary hypertension results from pulmonary arteriolar narrowing, and in late stages of the disease, from a reduced number of arterioles as well.

Heath and Edwards (1958) graded the microscopic findings of pulmonary vascular abnormalities associated with pulmonary hypertension. After the first months of life, normal pulmonary arterioles are thin-walled, without visible medial muscle, and are indistinguishable from veins. The earliest appearance of abnormality in the pulmonary arterioles is increased medial muscle (grade 1) compromising the arteriolar lumen. Later, there is patchy, intimal hyperplasia (grade 2), and ultimately occlusion of the lumen by excessive, concentric layers of intimal collagen (grade 3). At this stage larger vessels are also compromised. There may be angiomata (probably a recanalization phenomenon) (grade 4) and, ultimately, arteriolar necrosis with intimal and medial fibrosis (grades 5 and 6). Reid and associates (Hislop and Reed, 1973; Haworth et al, 1977; Rabinovitch et al, 1982), using morphometric techniques, showed that in the initial stages of pulmonary vascular obstructive disease arteriolar muscle is present more peripherally than normal when exposed to higher flow (grade A). If accompanied by increased thickness of the wall (medial muscle) (grade B), pulmonary hypertension is present. Finally, the number of arterioles is diminished (grade C).

Heath's and Edwards' (1958) grade 3 and Hislop's and Reid's (1973) grade B may be largely reversible, but beyond these, the pathologic changes of pulmonary vascular disease are probably irreversible. It is obviously of considerable interest that only a few vessels in any biopsy specimen of lung tissue may show advanced changes and that biopsies from different areas of the lungs may not be representative. Perfusion of lobes, or whole lungs, provide pathological demonstrations but some means of examining the lungs in toto during life are needed. Rabinovitch et al (1984) tried to do this using multiple wedge angiograms with some success. For the immediate future, it seems that the best way to demonstrate pulmonary arteriolar disease is to measure physiologically, in the catheterization laboratory, the pulmonary artery pressure and the pulmonary flow under various circumstances such as rest, exercise, inhalation of 100% oxygen, or during the use of vasodilators (e.g., tolazaline). These observations give the best functional estimate of the total pulmonary vascular bed—the observation most valuable to the clinician.

Physiology

Normally, the pulmonary arterioles can accommodate at least a 3- to 4-fold increase in pulmonary arterial blood flow without a rise in pressure. A healthy individual, exercising moderately, scarcely raises pulmonary artery pressure. However, given limitation in the number or average internal diameter of the pulmonary arterioles, vigorous exercise causes pulmonary arterial pressure to rise (Maron et al, 1973). When there is increased pulmonary blood flow because of a secundum atrial septal defect, the pulmonary arterial pressure is not elevated unless there is pulmonary arteriolar abnormality. However, a newborn with a large interventricular or great vessel communication (single ventricle or patent ductus arteriosus) will have pulmonary hypertension because the fetal arteriolar musculature has not had an opportunity to resolve and, indeed, cannot resolve if the patient is to survive. Otherwise he would bleed into his lungs.

These relationships between pressure, blood flow and pulmonary arteriolar resistance can be crudely, but usefully, shown by the equation:

$$\frac{\text{mean Ppa} - \text{mean Ppv}}{\text{Qp/min/m}^2} = \text{pR (Wood unit)}$$

where Ppa = pulmonary arterial pressure; Ppv = pulmonary venous pressure; pR = pulmonary resistance; Qp = pulmonary blood flow; min = minutes; and m^2 = square meter of body surface area. Normally, the pulmonary resistance is three units/m^2 or less, about one-tenth of the systemic resistance. Any higher number is abnormal and must be explained. Whether the estimated resistance will readily resolve in time with correction of the underlying problem, or is an irreversible phenomenon, cannot be predicted with certainty through simple resistance calculations. A variety of other items act as risk factors for persistent elevation of pulmonary resistence: the age of the child, the duration of increased resistance, the cause of the elevated resistance, and inducible variation in pulmonary arterial pressure through a variety of maneuvers (Hoffman et al, 1981).

The relation between physiologic and pathologic findings should not be oversimplified. A patient with high pulmonary resistance can have irreversible arteriolar disease (large ventricular defect in a child), but not necessarily (high altitude, mitral stenosis). The combination of a large systemic-pulmonary opening and hypoventilation (Down syndrome and atrioventricular canal) often causes confusion about which one is causing the elevated resistance and whether or not it is reversible. A patient with normal pulmonary resistance can have pulmonary hypertension and abnormal pulmonary arterioles (ventricular defect with high flow). Another patient with no pathologic abnormality may have no hypertension, but have elevated pulmonary resistance if pulmonary blood flow is reduced (bypassed lung in pulmonary arteriovenous fistula).

With few exceptions, only pulmonary vascular disease associated with systemic-pulmonary communications and the idiopathic form of the disease reach irreversible stages. The earliest that this can occur is thought to be 6 months of age (in rare patients with transposition of the great arteries or truncus arteriosus). Children with high pressure and flow from birth and a large ventricular septal defect or patent ductus arteriosus begin to get permanent changes at about 2 years of age, although some patients having irreversible pulmonary vascular obstructive disease have been seen as early as 1 year of age. Untreated, all surviving patients with truncus arteriosus and transposition of great arteries will have irreversible pulmonary vascular obstructive disease at a young age. In many with a large ventricular septal defect, large patent ductus arteriosus or atrioventricular canal defect, permanent changes will occur, albeit somewhat later. In only about 10% of those with secundum atrial septal defect (high flow, low pressure) will irreversible changes occur, and then only after two to three decades of exposure to high pulmonary blood flow.

The reversibility of pulmonary vascular abnormality is thought to be a function of duration. Thus, major elevation of pulmonary vascular resistance that has occurred in the past 6 months is more likely to be reversible than that which has lasted for 20 years. This is a difficult point to prove but seems empirically correct.

Testing the lability of pulmonary vascular resistance by using vasoactive agents, such as oxygen, may be helpful. Significant changes in pulmonary artery pressure or flow upon administration of 100% oxygen suggest that the vascular abnormality is labile vasoconstriction. On the other hand, a complete lack of response does not necessarily mean that there will be no regression after correction of the underlying cardiac defect. If the patient is a young infant, there may still be a reasonable chance of regression of pulmonary vascular disease, albeit not complete.

Elevated pulmonary resistance is produced by a variety of physiologic states, but the reaction of pulmonary arterioles to a variety of stimuli is not thought to be genetically predetermined, although variation in degree of response may be. Given sufficient stimulation, over a long enough period of time, elevated pulmonary resistance and pulmonary hypertension would develop in all patients. There are many stimuli known to produce elevated pulmonary vascular resistance and pulmonary hypertension:

1. Systemic-pulmonary communications: Patent ductus arteriosus, ventricular septal defect, atrial septal defect, truncus arteriosus
2. Pulmonary venous hypertension: Mitral stenosis, pulmonary venous stenosis, coarctation of the aorta, left ventricular failure, cor triatriatum
3. Reduced pulmonary alveolar oxygen: High altitude, hypoventilation, obstructed ventilation, pulmonary parenchymal disease, cystic fibrosis, Down syndrome
4. Idiopathic pulmonary vascular disease
5. Persistent pulmonary hypertension of the newborn
6. Pulmonary hypoplasia
7. Drugs: Aminorex, rape seed oil, bleomycin, estrogen contraceptives
8. Metabolic syndromes: Nonketotic hyperglycinemia
9. Thromboembolic disease
10. Collagen vascular disease: Lupus erythematosus

SYSTEMIC-PULMONARY COMMUNICATIONS

Patients having pulmonary hypertension associated with systemic-pulmonary communications, by far the most common group seen by pediatric cardiologists, can be subdivided into those having lesions where survival is not possible without increased pulmonary arteriolar muscle (truncus arteriosus) and those in whom this is not a necessity (atrial septal defect secundum).

With the normal fall in pulmonary resistance at birth, newborns with a large ventricular septal defect or a single ventricle face the possibility that blood will be preferentially recycled to the lungs. In fact, this does not occur. The regression of the fetal pulmonary resistance is delayed and incomplete, resulting in pulmonary blood that is greater than in normal individuals, and is accomplished at systemic pressure levels but does not cause demise in the first days of life. The mechanism for this persistence of fetal arteriolar musculature is not understood, but it must be related to the ever increasing pulmonary blood flow as the pulmonary resistance begins to fall. Continued high flow and high pressure with persistent arteriolar constriction results, after a year or two, in irreversible pulmonary vascular disease (Eisenmenger syndrome).

Although in most patients pulmonary vascular disease progressively limits pulmonary blood flow, the progression slows down as the pulmonary flow approaches the systemic cardiac output. If pulmonary vascular obstruction were inexorably progressive, steadily decreasing blood flow and increasing cyanosis would be expected. This usually does not occur. Once the Eisenmenger reaction is well established, the patient continues with the same degree of cyanosis and pulmonary hemodynamics for years, often decades. High-flow situations which do not require pulmonary hypertension to survive—such as atrial septal defect of the secundum type—are a different matter. In these individuals, pulmonary flow is gradually increased in infancy and early childhood as the fetal resistance resolves. They may then experience 20–30 years of increased pulmonary blood flow at low pressure before progressive pulmonary vascular changes occur. Unlike the usual Eisenmenger reaction, in these patients, once vascular disease has developed, long survival is rare.

PULMONARY VENOUS HYPERTENSION

Pulmonary venous hypertension from any cause may trigger elevated pulmonary arteriolar resistance. The classic example is mitral stenosis, but any reason for elevation of left atrial pressure (cor triatriatum, pulmonary venous stenosis, elevated left ventricular end diastolic pressure) may be associated with this phenomenon. As with any other acute stimulus causing development of pulmonary hypertension the initial response is minimal and only later will gross elevation of pulmonary arterial pressure take place. Thus, sudden acquired mitral regurgitation, as with rupture of a chorda tendinea, results initially in pulmonary edema and, with survival, in late development of pulmonary arteriolar vasculature. With gradual development of left atrial hypertension, the changes in the pulmonary arterioles may occur gradually and pulmonary edema may never be experienced. With pre-established medial muscular hypertrophy, the response to pulmonary venous hypertension in the newborn is immediate. This is why severe pulmonary hypertension results from left ventricular failure in infants with critical aortic stenosis or coarctation of the aorta.

For unknown reasons, pulmonary vascular pathology associated with pulmonary venous hypertension does not progress to irreversible stages. In practical terms, pulmonary arterial hypertension secondary to pulmonary venous hypertension is rapidly and completely reversible, given surgical alleviation of the cause (mitral stenosis, cor triatriatum) almost irrespective of the duration.

REDUCED PULMONARY ALVEOLAR OXYGEN

Exposure of a normal person to low ambient oxygen may induce pulmonary arteriolar constriction and a few millimeters of rise in pulmonary arterial pressure. With prolonged exposure, the arteriolar musculature increases and the obstruction becomes greater, leading to greater calculated pulmonary resistance and higher pulmonary artery pressure. Individuals living at high altitude, usually over 10,000 feet, may have elevated pulmonary artery pressures, at least on exercise. This is not a direct relationship, the degree of hypertension varying greatly among individuals. Hypoxic pulmonary hypertension may be completely reversible within days after descent to sea level. It is clear that the hypoxic effect is not mediated through low systemic arterial oxygen because many cyanotic patients do not have pulmonary hypertension. Indeed, the initiating mechanism must reside within the alveoli or immediately adjacent structures.

Examples of hypoxic pulmonary hypertension include obstruction of the airway by unusually large tonsils (Johnson and Todd, 1980), hypoventilation (Glenn et al, 1973), sleep apnea (Cherniak, 1981), and a wide variety of pulmonary parenchymal diseases that may limit oxygenation (e.g., cystic fibrosis) (Geggel et al, 1985; Noonan, 1971).

!DIOPATHIC PULMONARY VASCULAR DISEASE

Rarely, pulmonary vascular disease will develop in a child without a ready explanation. As such patients have been studied over the years, reasonable explanations for the pulmonary hypertension have been found for many. These include a closing ventricular septal defect, pulmonary venous stenosis, pulmonary venoocclusive disease, the effects of bleomycin therapy, or cor triatriatum.

The remaining, truly "idiopathic" pulmonary vascular disease, a disease of young, adult women (rare in childhood), is almost uniformly fatal within 2–5 years. The pathologic changes are indistinguishable from those seen in the Eisenmenger syndrome.

PERSISTENT PULMONARY HYPERTENSION OF THE NEWBORN

This syndrome is characterized by pulmonary hypertension which, when severe, results in right-to-left shunting through the still patent ductus arteriosus and foramen ovale. For this reason, the term *persistent fetal circulation* (PFC; Gersony et al, 1969) has been applied to this condition. Sometimes the cause may be obvious (i.e., pulmonary hemmorhage, atelectasis, aspiration, or pneumonia) but often it is unknown. It has been proposed that prenatal events are responsible for the unexplained cases (Murphy et al, 1984) and, of these unexplained cases the majority survive without permanent injury. Depending on the criteria used to define persistent fetal circulation, the mortality may be as high as 50%. The role of inflammation in chronic pulmonary hypertension is reviewed by Meyrick et al, 1987.

Diagnosis

When there are intact atrial and ventricular septums and no ductus arteriosus, children with systemic levels of pulmonary hypertension may be symptomatic. This occurs primarily among those with idiopathic pulmonary hypertension, among otherwise normal newborns with pulmonary hypertension (PFC), and among those who have had a pulmonary systemic communication surgically closed (ventricular septal defect, patent ductus arteriosus) and the associated pulmonary hypertension did not regress. Such patients have difficulty in providing systemic cardiac output with exercise. Right ventricular pressure may rise to suprasystemic levels but, even so, cardiac output may still be inadequate. Syncope and sudden death may occur; angina-like pain, probably originating in the distended main pulmonary artery, has been described.

In contrast, in the more commonly encountered patients with communication between the systemic and pulmonary circuits, whether the vascular abnormality is reversible or not, symptoms are less marked for comparable levels and duration of pulmonary hypertension and sudden death occurs only in advanced stages. As long as there is a communication between the right and left heart—particularly at the ventricular level—cardiac output, albeit with low systemic arterial oxygen saturation, can be maintained through right-to-left shunting as needed.

Patients with systemic-pulmonary shunts and irreversible pulmonary vascular disease seldom have significant symptoms until cyanosis develops. At that point, the most common complaint is limitation of exercise capacity and, in the later stages, beginning at the end of the third decade, anginal pain, hemoptysis, syncope, and, rarely, congestive heart failure.

On physical examination, whether or not there is cyanosis, the pulmonary component of the second heart sound is accentuated and the degree of splitting of the second heart sound is diminished. There may be an early diastolic regurgitant murmur (pulmonary regurgitation). The murmur, in contrast to pulmonary regurgitation with pulmonary stenosis, resembles that of aortic regurgitation, but does not produce a wide pulse pressure.

MINOR LABORATORY TESTS

The arterial oxygen level may be reduced, especially on exercise, and the hematocrit is high, sometimes more than 70%.

ELECTROCARDIOGRAPHY

The electrocardiogram shows right ventricular hypertrophy and evidence of right atrial hypertension.

RADIOGRAPHY

On chest films, the main pulmonary artery and the right and left main pulmonary arteries are larger than normal. This provides an overall impression of increased pulmonary vasculature with particularly large central vessels.

CARDIAC CATHETERIZATION

Given the clinical suspicion of pulmonary hypertension (cyanosis, narrow S2, loud P2, right ventricular hypertrophy, a large main pulmonary artery, compatible echocardiography) any time after the first few weeks of life, cardiac catheterization is mandatory. The confusion produced by noninvasive estimation of pulmonary hemodynamics is unacceptable given the importance of the condition. Even patients with idiopathic pulmonary hypertension, in whom there is more than 10% mortality associated with cardiac catheterization (Keane et al, 1978) should undergo study. Because idiopathic pulmonary hypertension is an almost uniformly fatal disease, attempted discovery of an identifiable cause (i.e., lupus erythematosus, unsuspected ventricular septal defect, pulmonary venous stenosis, cor triatriatum, mitral stenosis) is well worth the risk. Well-documented pulmonary capillary wedge pressures are essential observations in these patients, because some of the causes of pulmonary venous hypertension are completely curable. Cardiac catheterization carries little or no added mortality for other patients with pulmonary hypertension, irrespective of the degree of pulmonary vascular change.

Management

Treatment should be directed at the underlying cause; otherwise there is no specific treatment for pulmonary hypertensive vascular disease today. Vasoactive drugs to reduce pulmonary vasoconstriction in the advanced stages are not effective. Nighttime administration of oxygen may provide some comfort. Steps to prevent infective endocarditis are desirable; anesthetic agents should be used with caution. Sexually active females should avoid pregnancy and delivery because mortality among recently delivered patients with advanced pulmonary vascular disease is high (>50%; Pitts et al, 1977). Estrogen-containing contraceptive pills should be avoided and tubal ligation should be seriously considered. Usually it is not necessary to limit activity because the patient does this herself. Living at a high altitude would be foolhardy for such a patient. Regular checks of the hematocrit are needed inasmuch as some symptoms due to poor oxygen delivery (fatigue, headache, lassitude, breathlessness) are partly the result of polycythemia and may be helped by red cell pheresis.

Course and Prognosis

When there are no advanced and irreversible changes of pulmonary vascular disease, there are no late problems specific to pulmonary hypertension. When irreversible arteriolar pathology is present, the impression that the patient is doomed has been overemphasized in recent years. In fact, the majority are cyanotic and have a limited exercise tolerance, but the main symptoms are psychologic, stemming in part from the physician's overt and covert suggestions of doom. Most can work and support themselves, some for three to four or more decades. While it is difficult to remove empathy from clinical assessment, the adjustment which many of these patients achieve is remarkable.

Infective endocarditis and brain abscess are always a threat. Late in the disease hemoptysis may be a problem, sometimes fatal. Congestive heart failure is not a common problem until the end stages of the disease. The appearance of syncope is an ominous sign. Sudden death, presumed to result from ventricular tachycardia, is a common mode of exitus.

Hypoxemia

Hypoxemia is defined as lower than normal arterial oxygen concentration (oxygen saturation less than 93%, partial pressure of oxygen less than 100 torr at sea level). The precise figure below which hypoxemia is considered to be present varies somewhat with age and altitude, normally being lower both in early infancy and at higher altitudes. Clinical cyanosis is hardly visible until the arterial oxygen saturation is around 85% and then only if the hematocrit is high (5.0 g of reduced hemoglobin are required before cyanosis can be seen). In a small infant, arterial saturation as low as 70% may be overlooked if the hematocrit is low. It is important to distinguish between hypoxemia resulting from intracardiac right-to-left shunting and hypoxemia based on pulmonary problems. When the pulmonary venous blood has reduced oxygen concentration, the pulmonary resistance and pulmonary pressure may be secondarily elevated to a degree comparable to the effects observed in patients exposed to low ambient oxygen (e.g., high altitude). Since atelectasis, pneumonia and pulmonary edema are common concomitants of heart disease, especially in infancy, confusion resulting from hypoxemia of pulmonary origin must be kept in mind. As a principle, all measurements of pulmonary pressure and resistance should be made both in room air and after the adminstration of 100% oxygen to ensure that these effects have been compensated for, particularly in sick infants.

Acute Effects

Acutely, hypoxemia reduces peripheral resistance without affecting the pulmonary resistance (unless the hypoxemia has a pulmonary origin). Reduction in peripheral resistance because of right-to-left shunting promotes more right-to-left shunting. This phenomenon is the fundamental basis for cyanotic spells. As the patient becomes more hypoxemic, he becomes breathless (Guntheroth et al, 1965) and frightened, cries, and is agitated; this further reduces his peripheral resistance and peripheral arterial oxygenation, until he ultimately lapses into unconsciousness. This phenomenon is damped in patients who have chronic hypoxemia and is most dramatic in those who become acutely cyanotic. It is particularly accentuated in patients with tetralogy of Fallot where muscular infundibular pulmonary stenosis may spasmodically promote right-to-left shunting by increasing the obstruction to pulmonary blood flow while simultaneously reducing systemic resistance.

Chronic Effects

Chronic hypoxemia is associated with the limitation of exercise ability because of the inability to increase delivery of oxygen to the exercising tissues. The patient tires sooner and becomes short of breath and increasingly cyanotic. Chronically cyanotic children have depressed intelligence quotients (presumably more depressed with greater degrees of cyanosis; Newburger et al, 1984), and have delayed neuromuscular development (Newburger et al, 1983) and poor growth.

Chronic hypoxemia results in polycythemia which is mediated through erythropoitin produced by the kidneys. Consequently, patients with differential upper and lower body cyanosis have somewhat different responses to hypoxemia. The level of polycythemia increases with age, the hematocrit of the teenager and adult patient with cyanotic congenital heart disease often reaching levels in the range of 65–75%. As the hematocrit rises the blood viscosity rises, with the result that circulation times are reduced, and the turbulence produced by cardiac anomalies is less. Murmurs may become less intense, even disappear, and symptoms that can be related to reduced cardiac output may be encountered. These symptoms disappear with red cell pheresis.

Generally, red cell pheresis is considered for anyone whose hematocrit (accurately measured—equipment measuring hematocrit through optical density is unreliable in the higher ranges) is in excess of 70%. Some patients get relief of symptoms with red cell pheresis when the hematocrit is 65–70%. How often this needs to be repeated varies considerably from patient to patient and from time to time in the same patient. Red cell pheresis is most elegantly accomplished by continuous centrifugation of the blood from one arm with return of the lower hematocrit blood to the other. Equally satisfactory is the removal of blood and the return of equal amounts of plasma or albumin. Simply to remove blood and expect the patient to compensate is an unacceptable procedure and dangerous because of systemic hypotension (Rosenthal et al, 1971).

The turnover of red cells is increased in patients with cyanosis; the excess of bile pigments may result in *gallstones* in these patients. This diagnosis should be considered when seeing a cyanotic teenager with abdominal pain.

Cyanotic patients tend to *bleed*; this may be related to platelet abnormalities (Paul et al, 1961).

There is a tendency toward *cerebral vascular accidents* among children with hypoxemia. This is more common in infants who are anemic or relatively anemic, but it is also reported among young adults with polycythemia. In the older patients it is presumed to result from clotting or stasis, though this is not well documented among our patients with congenital heart disease.

Pregnancy in the cyanotic patient carries increased maternal mortality depending somewhat on the cardiac defect and the degree of cyanosis. The more cyanotic the mother the less likely is the infant to survive. Infants of mothers with congenital heart disease have a greater chance of having a cardiac abnormality.

Brain abscess in the pediatric age group is almost entirely encountered in cyanotic patients and, while rare, is potentially such a devastating event that the appearance of severe headache, convulsions, and new symptoms suggesting neurologic disorder in a cyanotic child should suggest this possibility. Computerized axial tomography (CAT scan) usually clarifies this question.

Scoliosis in a cyanotic female patient is surprisely common, occurring in proportion to the arterial oxygen saturation. The reasons for this are not clear. Examination of the spine of a teenage patient with cyanosis is part of the routine pediatric cardiology examination. Nevertheless, most patients with this problem are discovered through routine cardiac chest radiology.

Clubbing of the fingers and toes and, in extreme situations the ends of the larger bones, is characteristic of chronic cyanosis. This abnormality disappears with surgical correction of the congenital heart disease.

Congestive Heart Failure

Definition

When the heart cannot supply the blood flow demanded by the tissues, a clinical syndrome of symptoms and signs largely resulting from elevated atrial pressures can be recognized as congestive heart failure (Artman and Graham, 1982; Artman et al, 1984; Beekman et al, 1982; Berman et al, 1983).

Basic Science

PHYSIOLOGY

The principal function of the heart may be summarized briefly as follows:

The atria receive blood at low pressure and pass it on to the ventricles, from where it is propelled at a higher pressure into the great arteries. The right ventricle fills the pulmonary arteries under relatively low pressure (<20 mm Hg, mean), whereas the left ventricle generates higher aortic pressure (>60 mm Hg, mean). The pulmonary flow has to be sufficient to allow for an adequate supply of oxyhemoglobin to meet the metabolic needs of the body.

The heart may fail if it is confronted with (a) an abnormally high afterload (coarctation, aortic stenosis), (b) an excessive preload (left-to-right shunts beyond the atrial level, mitral regurgitation), (c) impaired myocardial contractility (myopathy), or (d) inadequate diastolic filling (constrictive pericarditis, chronic tachyarrhythmias).

Diagnosis

The above principles are equally valid for adults, children, and infants. The types of heart failure and their clinical manifestations, however, have age specificity. In terms of *FORWARD/BACKWARD* failure, an artifical distinction, most pediatric patients suffer from backward failure, meaning that although the cardiac output may be in the low range of normal, the ventricular end-diastolic pressures are elevated. In terms of *RIGHT/LEFT-SIDED* failure, most infants and children suffer from left-sided failure, and manifestations of right-sided failure, if any, are only secondary to this. In terms of *HIGH/LOW CARDIAC OUTPUT* failure, most of our patients suffer from low output states, although it has to be emphasized that in the great majority the cardiac index is higher than 2.0 L/min/m^2, meaning the lower range of normal.

It follows, from the physiologic considerations above, that the *clinical picture* in pediatrics is dominated by low output, left-sided, backward failure.

The paragraphs that follow will relate principally to congestive heart failure in infants; manifestations in children and adolescents are virtually indistinguishable from those observed in adults and, thus, are well described in texts on Cardiology.

The most common clinical sign is *rapid and labored respirations*. This, of course, has to be distinguished at the bedside from the tachypnea of pneumonia, a common occurrence in babies. A good clinical sign in differential diagnosis is that the babies in left-sided failure seem relatively undisturbed by their rapid respirations, whereas those with pneumonia are clearly having pain (? of pleuritis) on breathing. Low-output failure is manifested by *pallor* (? tinged with cyanosis) and *feeble pulses*. *Cyanosis* is due to pulmonary edema, secondary to increased left ventricular end-diastolic pressure with increased pulmonary venous pressure, and is improved by the administration of 100% oxygen for 10 minutes. Evidence of *systemic congestion* (edema), so common in adults, is *relatively rare* in children and even more so in infants. Distended jugular venous pulses may well be seen, although they are hard to observe in infants with short necks; hepatomegaly is rare and fluid retention (edema, ascites, anasarca) is seldom visible except in babies with coarctation of the aorta (decreased renal perfusion). Chronic congestive heart failure sometimes may manifest itself only by *failure to thrive*. On a growth chart, it becomes obvious that in most instances the infant's position on the height chart is appreciably higher than on the weight curve. More important, height growth continues, while the weight curve levels off.

MINOR LABORATORY TESTS

Mild elevations of the *white blood count* may be noted without obvious infection. *Anemia* may precipitate congestive failure in a patient with borderline compensation. *Low urinary output* with high specific gravity and albuminuria are characteristic of congestive failure. Increased urinary output with a decrease in specific gravity may be a sign of improved compensation after adequate treatment. *Hypoglycemia* and *hypocalcemia* may occur in infants with heart failure: spectacular improvements have been noted after correction of these metabolic derangements. Low serum sodium in a patient with heart failure and obvious fluid retention is often due to dilution, with an actual increase in total body sodium. This is of poor prognostic significance and management can be quite tricky.

Severe volume overloading (ventricular septal defect, patent ductus arteriosis) is characterized by mild respiratory acidosis. In total anomalous venous return with obstruction, respiratory acidosis tends to be more severe and hypoxia is usually, though not invariably, marked. In the hypoplastic left heart syndrome, metabolic acidosis dominates the picture, whereas transposition of the great arteries (with intact ventricular septum) is accompanied by severe hypoxia with a large systemic flow and only modest acidosis.

ELECTROCARDIOGRAPHY

The electrocardiogram is almost totally useless in diagnosing heart failure, although by demonstrating chronic tachyarrhythmia it may explain the etiology of heart failure diagnosed by other means.

RADIOGRAPHY

The chest x-ray is not nearly as sensitive as the echocardiogram in assessing heart failure. On the other hand, for the average cardiologist, this is a more obvious manifestation; a normal-sized or only slightly enlarged heart is generally incompatible with congestive failure. The most common exceptions to this rule are patients with total anomalous venous return and older children with constrictive pericarditis.

ECHO-DOPPLER STUDY

Echocardiograms with decreased ejection fraction and low circumferential fiber shortening are direct evidence of heart failure. Response to treatment may be monitored accurately by these noninvasive means.

CARDIAC CATHETERIZATION

Cardiac catheterization with good angiograms is an excellent, although not totally innocuous, way of documenting heart failure. The most sensitive hemodynamic index is the presence of "cardiac inflation," a left ventricular end-diastolic pressure higher than needed in normal individuals to produce any given cardiac work (flow × pressure).

It should be noted, that right atrial hypertension in infants is not nearly as common as in adults, a finding giving physiologic explanation for the relative rarity of evidence of systemic congestion. On the other hand, left atrial pressures are elevated more nearly to the level expected from the degree of heart failure. This pressure difference between the atria may result in a left-to-right shunt due to a stretched foramen ovale, further aggravating a bad situation. Wide arteriovenous oxygen differences reflect the low cardiac output. The angiograms show poor contractility.

AGE OF ONSET

Congestive heart failure in the first hours of life may be caused by a large systemic arteriovenous fistula (vein of Galen), intrauterine supraventricular tachycardia, profound fetal anemia, fetal myocardial disease, severe atrioventricular valve incompetence (Ebstein disease), and an unguarded tricuspid orifice.

In the first week of life, congestive heart failure is associated with the hypoplastic left heart syndrome, interrupted aortic arch, and large left-to-right shunts (patent ductus arteriosus, truncus arteriosus, total anomalous pulmonary veins, single ventricle).

Infants first admitted in the second week of life with congestive heart failure most often have coarctation of the aorta, large left-to-right shunts (ventricular septal defects, patent ductus arteriosus, common atrioventricular canal) or aortic stenosis.

Ventricular septal defects and the other left-to-right shunts are the leading causes of congestive heart failure in patients admitted after the second week of life.

Management

It is almost axiomatic that all patients with congestive heart failure due to congenital heart disease will need corrective surgery. The timing of surgery is one of the most crucial decisions the pediatric cardiologist has to make. It may be advantageous to procrastinate judiciously and treat medically for days, weeks or even months for one of two reasons only: (a) to allow the patient to reach the operating room in better hemodynamic and metabolic states or (b) to give an opportunity for spontaneous improvement of the defect. For practical purposes, this fortunate course of events occurs (among those with congenital heart disease) in only two conditions: patent ductus arteriosus in premature infants and ventricular defect within the first 6 months of life. In all other situations, our policy is to operate as soon as possible.

MEDICAL MANAGEMENT

As a rule, infants first seen in congestive failure should not be treated on an outpatient basis. Given an exceptionally good home situation and no significant respiratory distress, one might try the cautious administration of diuretics or digoxin (probably not both, initially) at home. A return office appointment within a week at the latest is mandatory. Obviously, this policy holds only for first encounters; infants with known and clearly understood heart failure can, and probably should, be managed as outpatients as long as some kind of equilibrium and clear understanding has been achieved through previous hospitalization.

The virtually mandatory hospitalization of all infants with newly discovered heart failure is recommended for many reasons:

1. Congestive heart failure is life-threatening in infants.
2. The administration of therapeutic agents in this age group is far from routine; the selection of drugs and determination of appropriate dosages might best be done in an inpatient setting. Of course, later adjustments may be made on an outpatient basis.
3. A complete anatomic and physiologic understanding should be accomplished as soon as possible after the baby has stabilized, to help decide whether and when cardiac surgery should be performed.

Once the patient is admitted to the floor, most conveniently on the way to the ward, a chest film and an electrocardiogram should be taken and blood for blood counts, gases and chemistries should be obtained. On the ward, after a careful history and physical examination, a working diagnosis should be proposed and treatment started. The reader should note that we, prejudiced old-timers, do not include two-dimensional echocardiography as part of the initial diagnostic approach. There are two rationalizations for this proposal: first, it is an attempt at forcing pediatricians, house staff, and fellows to arrive at their own working hypotheses; and second, careful two-dimensional echo-Doppler study is an exhaustive procedure and to achieve first class results the baby, if possible, should be in relatively stable condition. Clearly, all of this is predicated on the assumption that the infant is not at death's door. If the patient is desperately ill, two-dimensional echocardiography may be the very first thing that should be done, simultaneously with starting an intravenous line, delivery of oxygen by mask, and inotropic agents.

Once a working diagnosis is proposed and judgment is made that no emergency surgery is indicated, most doctors today would probably start intravenous diuretics, provided that the serum potassium is normal. Furosemide is used to improve ventricular function through preload reduction, as long as the ECG does not indicate that the cause of heart failure is tachyarrhythmia. In the latter instance, an antiarrhythmic is the first drug of choice. Simultaneously, if there is considerable respiratory distress, the baby is given oxygen, with or without intubation, and is sedated (morphine sulphate, meperidine) if restless. Desperately ill infants may be given parenteral inotropics (digoxin, dopamine) simultaneously with the intravenous furosemide.

In the second 24 hours, assuming that the patient has had a good diuresis and the respiratory distress has lessened, oral digoxin is started and the diuretics are switched to the oral route (two to three times a day).

Assuming that the baby has improved sufficiently, this is the time to do a careful, deliberate two-dimensional echo-Doppler study.

If inotropics and preload reducers do not produce the desired effect, afterload reducers (captopril) should be considered. Treatment of infections is a very important part of management, as is the correction of low hematocrit (less than 30%). The latter may best be accomplished by very careful, slow, small red cell transfusions without increasing the blood volume (Lister et al, 1982).

When the baby has improved enough to tolerate room air and has developed an appetite sufficient to weight gain, it must be decided whether and when cardiac catheterization should be performed. Because, in most instances, although not invariably, surgical treatment will be necessary for any congenital cardiac malformation causing heart failure, probably most of these babies should be catheterized, depending on the preference of the local surgeons and cardiologists. A case may be made for catheterization during the initial hospitalization, everything else being equal. This does not necessarily mean that surgery should follow immediately; if good echo studies are made virtually simultaneously with the catheterization, the patient's progress can be followed adequately with echocardiography, and a decision can be made whether and when surgery should follow.

Assuming that the initial hospitalization alleviated most of the respiratory distress and the baby has started feeding and does not need any more oxygen, after hospitalization for at least 1 week, discharge may be in order. Medications should be given orally and frequent office visits (i.e., once a week to once a month) are essential. Perhaps the most sensitive index of the baby's condition is the weight gain. Without appropriate weight increments, it cannot be assumed that heart failure has been alleviated. In judging weight gain, the "false" weight gain due to water retention must be taken into account; a baby with a poor appetite and striking increase in weight is particularly suspect in this regard. Suffice it to say that a baby who maintains a satisfactory weight curve at home on appropriate medications is probably not in chronic congestive failure; thus, timing and even the necessity for surgery can be determined with some deliberation. In contrast, a baby who does not follow his developmental curve, particularly if the curve flattens out, should be considered urgently for cardiac surgery.

A final word about the rare, happy event when the baby seems to thrive to the extent where consideration may be given to omitting medications and questioning the necessity of surgery. As stated before, this happens only in patients with large left-to-right shunts (at atrial, ventricular, or great artery levels) whose communications have become smaller. An alternative and quite malignant cause for "improvement" in congestive failure is the development of right ventricular outflow obstruction, either at the infundibular or pulmonary arteriolar level. An electrocardiogram showing increasing right ventricular hypertrophy is the easiest way to identify this situation, which should serve as a clear indication for immediate surgical consideration.

Two general therapeutic principles to be applied both in the hospital and at home should be touched upon briefly:

1. Salt restriction should not interfere with the baby's eating. Our authors' philosophy is to make sure that the infants eat enough of the appropriate foods to gain and grow; if salt restriction interferes with appetite, forget it. Give more diuretics! A high calorie-low sodium formula may help the infant gain weight, particularly if administered through a nasogastric tube, or through gastrostomy in very chronic situations.
2. Obviously, restriction of physical activity in infants is a not an issue. Even for toddlers physical restrictions may be counterproductive; they consume more oxygen fighting their constraints than they would by doing what they wanted to do in the first place.

SURGICAL MANAGEMENT

As indicated in the introductory paragraphs, most, if not all, infants whose congenital cardiac lesions lead to heart failure will have to be treated surgically.

Details of surgical management will be discussed under the individual lesions. A few general principles may be mentioned here briefly.

1. Once it has been decided by the cardiologists and cardiovascular surgeons that an operation is indicated, it should be performed at the youngest age that the intervention can be performed as safely as it ever will be. There is much to be gained by allowing the infant to grow normally as soon as possible. In skillful surgical hands, age probably is not a significant risk factor for operative mortality.
2. Although every possible effort should be exerted to have the baby in as good a metabolic state as possible when it is taken to the operating room, some derangements (acidosis, pulmonary edema) will not be corrected until after successful operative intervention.
3. At The Children's Hospital in Boston, corrective surgery, whenever possible, is preferable to palliation (pulmonary artery banding, shunt procedures).
4. An unsatisfactory postoperative state often is the result of an inadequate operation. No diagnostic effort should be spared, including emergency postoperative catheterization, if the baby does poorly in the intensive care unit.

VENTRICULAR SEPTAL DEFECTS

Definition

An opening in the ventricular septum which allows communication between the right and left ventricles is called a ventricular septal defect. By convention, at The Children's Hospital in Boston, ventricular septal defects include isolated lesions with or without associated atrial defects, ductus arteriosus, or mild pulmonary stenosis. The more complicated anatomies are considered elsewhere.

Basic Science

ANATOMY

A ventricular septal defect is a delay in closure of the ventricular septum beyond 5–6 weeks of embryological life. The defects are of variable size and may be located in any part of the ventricular septum as single or multiple lesions (Goor et al, 1970; Lincoln et al, 1977; Edwards, 1960; Soto et al, 1980; Hagler, 1985; Capelli et al, 1983). Classifications of ventricular septal defects vary but all are based on the anatomical location of the defect (Fig. 6.14). Defects in the lower trabecular septum are described here as muscular and can be further specified as apical, midmuscular, anterior, or posterior defects. A large apical muscular defect may be partially covered by right ventricular trabeculations and appear to be many small ventricular defects when viewed from the right ventricle (Swiss cheese defect), but appear as a single defect when viewed from the left ventricle. Defects in the right ventricular outflow (in the infundibular septum) are referred to here as subpulmonary defects. Viewed from the left ventricle, these defects are located just below the aortic valve. Those largely involving the subaortic region of the membranous septum, when viewed from either ventricle, are described as membranous or perimembranous defects. Because ventricular defects often involve, but are not confined to, the membranous septum, the term perimembranous often has been used in recent years. Defects associated with overriding of the aorta are called malalignment defects. Defects in the inflow of the right ventricle are called atrioventricular canal defects but are not always associated with other stigmata of endocardial cushion abnormalities (e.g., cleft mitral valve). Combinations of defects and extension of a defect from one area into another are common (Fig. 6.15).

The distribution of the various types of ventricular septal defects, except for the muscular ones, is not age-dependent. In early infancy, the incidence of muscular defects is highest, gradually decreasing over the years. Otherwise the relative frequency of the types of defect does not vary even into third decade.

PHYSIOLOGY

A ventricular septal opening allows shunting of left ventricular blood into the right ventricle. The amount of shunting depends on the size of the defect and the relative pulmonary and systemic resistances. The amount of blood shunted can exceed the cardiac output by 3- to 4-fold and, at that level, often causes more work than the left ventricle can manage, resulting in congestive failure. A large left-to-right shunt is associated with increased water in the lung (Vincent et al, 1985), perhaps accounting for the symptom of tachypnea. The largest shunts produce elevated left atrial and pulmonary venous pressure as well, the picture being readily recognized as pulmonary edema. Increased left ventricular pressure, as with coarctation of the aorta or aortic stenosis, is associated with a larger shunt, while an increasing degree of pulmonary stenosis or pulmonary vascular obstructive disease is associated with a decreasing size of left-to-right shunt, and even a right-to-left shunt. Large defects (more than 50% of aortic diameter) allow equalization of pressure between the right and left ventricles. The size and direction of the shunt through a large defect is decided by the relative pulmonary and systemic resistance. When there is a large ventricular defect combined with a large duc-

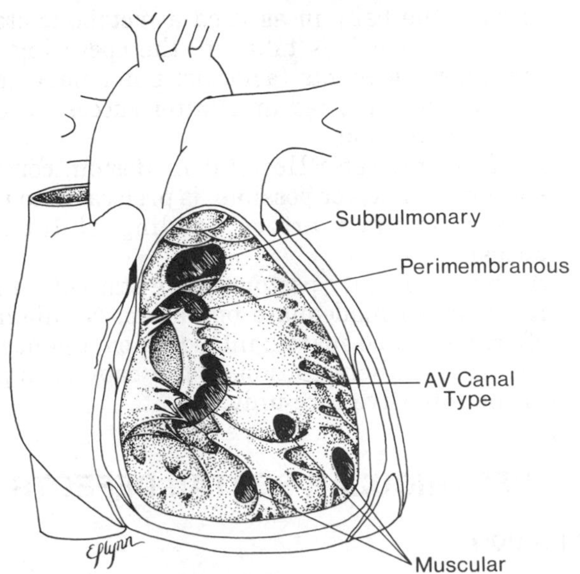

Figure 6.14. Location of ventricular septal defects.

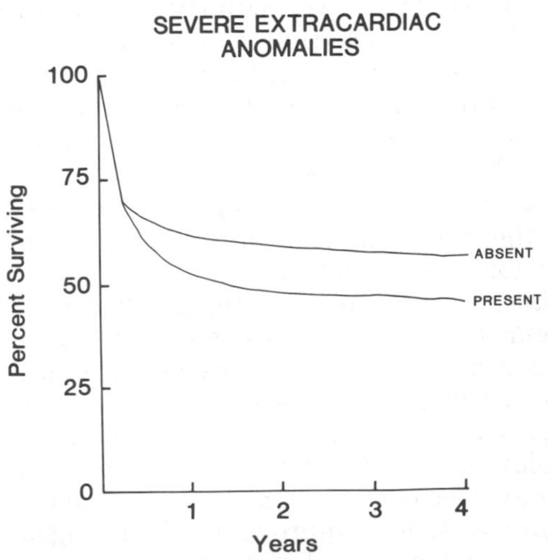

Figure 6.15. Comparative life-table analysis of survival of infants with critical congenital heart disease with and without other congenital anomalies.

tus arteriosus, division of the ductus might be expected to cut down the size of the shunt. In fact, if the residual ventricular septal defect is large, the determinants of shunting (i.e., the pulmonary and systemic vascular resistances) remain the same and division of the ductus has little effect.

Epidemiology

Isolated ventricular defects are the most common congenital cardiac anomalies and the most common defects occurring after the newborn period and through the third decade. They are encountered in 100–200/100,000 live births (Mitchell et al, 1971), 15% of critically ill infants with heart disease (Fyler et al, 1980a) (see Table 6.3). About one-third are sufficiently large to cause symptoms or are complicated by major extracardiac anomalies requiring hospitalization in infancy. Ventricular septal defects are the most common form of congenital heart disease in all age groups after the first weeks of life and through the third decade (see Table 6.4) If all ventricular septal defects that are associated with other cardiac lesions (such as transposition of the great arteries, tetralogy of Fallot, tricuspid atresia, truncus arteriosus, etc) are included, well over 50% of children with congenital heart disease have a ventricular septal opening.

Diagnosis

A ventricular septal defect is most often detected by the discovery of a murmur on routine examination (Fig. 6.3*A*). The murmur is not usually heard at birth, but appears later, in the first week of life, as pulmonary resistance resolves after discharge from the hospital. The absence of a murmur at birth, and its appearance a few days later, is characteristic of ventricular septal defects. By contrast, the murmur of infundibular pulmonary stenosis (which is virtually identical on auscultation) is heard at birth.

Often, discovery of a ventricular defect occurs because of extracardiac anomalies (e.g., tracheoesophageal fistula) which prompt a search for other malformations, including the heart. Less commonly, ventricular defects are discovered because of the appearance of congestive heart failure which, in its mildest form, consists of tachypnea (more than 60 breaths per min), not accompanied by sternal or costal retractions. Often the infants seem relatively well in other respects.

The readily audible murmur leads to cardiac evaluation and establishment of the diagnosis. It is our practice to investigate all infants thought to have a significant cardiac problem without delay, even in the absence of symptoms. Nowadays, there is little excuse to be surprised by the unexpected occurrence of cardiovascular collapse, cyanosis, or gross congestive heart failure in an infant known to have a significant heart murmur, who in the newborn period seemed well. Examination, including chest films, electrocardiograms, and consultation with an echocardiographer usually provides a precise diagnosis.

The clinical problems that are direct consequences of ventricular septal defect occur in the first 6 months of life or not at all. The appearance of symptoms suggesting congestive heart failure after the age of 6 months requires some other explanation, for example, associated acquired myocardial disease. The larger the defect, the earlier the symptoms appear. Tachypnea is the most common symptom, often remembered to be present from birth. The tachypnea may interfere with feedings and result in poor weight gain. While a normal infant can vigorously consume the bulk of his usual bottle within minutes before dawdling, the infant with tachypnea often takes much longer, 30 minutes to an hour, with resting between nursing. Frequent feeding is required to maintain an adequate intake. Breast-fed babies are substantially more difficult to evaluate; plotting growth may be the only secure source of useful data.

Sternal or costal retractions imply either a very large shunt or, more commonly, superimposed pneumonia, atelectasis, or aspiration.

These infants are often irritable and difficult, although occasionally, especially if the birth weight is low, they are lethargic while simultaneously tachypneic.

There is a high incidence of low birth weight. In 27% of symptomatic babies with ventricular defect, the birth weight was found to be less than 2.5 kg and 16% were born before the 36th week of gestation (Fyler et al, 1980a). When estimations of gestational age and appropriate weight are made, these infants do not appear to have suffered from intrauterine growth retardation, but rather to have been born earlier than expected.

In New England, as many as 9% of babies symptomatic with ventricular septal defect are first admitted to cardiac units by the 2nd day of life, with a total of 16% being hospitalized by the age of 1 week. Nevertheless, more than 50% are not sufficiently sick to be hospitalized before the age of 2 months (Fyler et al, 1980a).

Growth among infants with larger ventricular septal defects tends to be poor (Yeager et al, 1984; Levy et al, 1978) and is the prime reason for hospitalization. Any infant with a ventricular defect who is below the fifth percentile for height and weight or whose growth does not seem appropriate for his potential should be studied as a possible surgical candidate.

PHYSICAL EXAMINATION

An infant with a small ventricular septal defect and no other cardiac problems appears normal. There is a loud murmur, usually loudest at the lower left sternal border (Fig. 6.3*A*). Trivial defects may produce a slight murmur of debatable significance.

By contrast, the infant with a large ventricular defect is often scrawny, with discordant height and weight, although both measures may be below the fifth percentile. Tachypnea as high as 100 breaths/min is common. The peripheral pulses are small. Femoral pulses should be examined with care since association with coarctation of aorta is common; this is a particularly dangerous combination, which can lead to episodes of sudden collapse. The liver is often enlarged. The cardiac impulse is visibly and palpably hyperactive because of the large excess of blood recirculated through the lungs and heart. Indeed, in a small infant, the diagnosis of a large ventricular septal defect without a hyperactive cardiac impulse should be viewed with suspicion.

On auscultation there is a pansystolic murmur, loudest at the lower left sternal border (Fig. 6.3*A*). This murmur may not be as loud as that of smaller ventricular defects and may not cause a palpable thrill. Without treatment, the heart rate is fast and a gallop rhythm (S3) may be present at the apex. The gallop sound in diastole at a fast heart rate may become a mid-diastolic rumble as the heart slows with digoxin therapy. Both first and second heart sounds are loud. There is a single or narrowly split second heart sound. Pulmonary rhonchi and rales are common.

ELECTROCARDIOGRAPHY

In the patient with a small ventricular septal defect, the electrocardiogram is normal. With increasingly larger defects there is, first, left ventricular hypertrophy, and then, with the largest defects, both left and right ventricular hypertrophy. Right ventricular hypertrophy without evidence of left ventricular hypertrophy in an infant thought to have a ventricular septal defect is unusual and is reason to question the diagnosis. Is there associated pulmonary stenosis, mitral stenosis or some other problem that causes increased right ventricular work?

RADIOGRAPHY

Both the heart size and the pulmonary vasculature are normal in infants with small ventricular defects. With larger defects, the heart is proportionally large, with increased pulmonary vascularity. The left atrial shadow may be large. Pneumonitis, atelectasis, or aspiration may be evident. The diagnosis of a large ventricular septal defect with a large left-to-right shunt, associated with normal pulmonary vascularity on the chest x-ray, certainly is suspect.

ECHO-DOPPLER STUDY

Larger defects are readily recognized and accurately localized by two-dimensional echocardiography (Hagler, 1985). With smaller defects, not seen directly on two-dimensional echo, Doppler evidence of a left-to-right shunt into the right ventricular chamber can be discovered.

A Doppler search for additional associated ventricular septal defects should be made in all cases. Differences between right ventricular and left ventricular pressures are recorded and possible pressure gradients between the right ventricle and the pulmonary artery are estimated. Search should made for an associated patent ductus arteriosus or atrial septal defect. The enlargement of chambers resulting from a left-to-right shunt through a ventricular septal defect (left ventricle, right ventricle, pulmonary arteries, left atrium) should be noted and recorded.

CARDIAC CATHETERIZATION

With a reliable echo diagnosis, the infant with an isolated ventricular septal defect is managed without cardiac catheterization until surgery is contemplated. Continued congestive heart failure, difficulty in feeding, poor growth, recurrent pulmonary complications, and associated extracardiac anomalies suggest the need for cardiac surgery. With surgery under consideration, cardiac catheterization is carried out. The useful information to be obtained includes demonstration of the level of pulmonary hypertension, the level of atrial and end-diastolic ventricular pressures, the confirmation of the size and location of the defect or defects, confirmation of the size of the left-to-right shunt and, most of all, confirmation of the overall clinical impression. Based on this information a decision to proceed to cardiac surgery is on firm ground.

The spectrum of physiologic observations obtained at cardiac catheterization in patients with ventricular septal defect is shown in Table 6.6.

Management

SMALL VENTRICULAR DEFECT

The majority of patients with ventricular septal defect are and remain asymptomatic because the defects are small. Only 15% of all patients with ventricular septal defect require surgical intervention; even among the symptomatic infants only 30% come to surgery (Fyler et al, 1980a; Yeager et al, 1984; Weidman et al, 1977; Corone et al, 1977; Dickinson et al, 1981b).

The management of small defects requires only observation to detect the development of aortic regurgitation (see Ventricular Septal Defect and Aortic Regurgitation) and the use of prophylactic antibiotics to prevent bacterial endocarditis.

LARGE VENTRICULAR DEFECT

With large defects, the most common problems are congestive heart failure and failure to thrive. Congestive heart failure is managed initially with digoxin and diuretics, but only rarely is there more than minimal relief of symptoms. Berman et al (1983), using sophisticated techniques, has shown that digoxin has a measurable effect on up to 50% of patients; the remainder must depend on ancillary therapeutic measures for benefit (Beekman et al, 1982; Lister et al, 1982).

Efforts to provide adequate calories at the lowest cost (e.g., nasogastric feedings) are tried but are usually inadequate to reverse growth failure. The malnourished infant with increased lung water or outright pulmonary edema is a candidate for secondary pulmonary difficulties. Because ventricular septal defects commonly become smaller in the first months of life, a

Table 6.6
Comparison of Physiologic Data for Various Types of Ventricular Septal Defect

Chamber	Small Ventricular Septal Defect		Large Ventricular Septal Defect		VSD with Pulmonary Stenosis		VSD with Pulmonary Vascular Obstruction	
	Oxygen sat %	Pressure mm Hg	Oxygen sat %	Pressure mm Hg	Oxygen sat %	Pressure mm Hg	Oxygen sat %	Pressure mm Hg
Superior vena cava	70		70		70		60	
Right atrium	71	M=3	71	M=3	71	M=3	60	M=8
Right ventricle	80	35/2	88	90/5	80	90/5	65	90/8
Pulmonary artery	81	35/15	88	90/60	81	20/10	65	90/60
Pulmonary capillary		m=8		m=15		m=4		m=8
Left atrium	100	7	100	14	100	m=3	95	m=7
Left ventricle	100	90/7	100	90/14	100	90/3	92	90/7
Aorta	100	90/70	10	90/70	100	90/70	88	90/70

waiting plan, gambling on the natural diminution in the size of the defect, may be justifiable, provided there is a possibility, based on the anatomy, that the particular defect will get smaller. However, even with a defect known to be in a favorable location (muscular, perimembranous), the decision to resort to surgery may be inescapable after vigorous medical management has failed to produce improvement in congestive heart failure or weight gain. Continued conservative management is possible if there is a significant pressure gradient in the right ventricular outflow (see Table 6.6). The absence of pulmonary hypertension and the presence of normal atrial pressures are favorable observations. Equal pulmonary and systemic pressures and elevated atrial pressures are unfavorable. When making the decision to recommend surgery, the physician should keep in mind that although there is a somewhat higher mortality with a lower age at surgery (Yeager et al, 1984), it is entirely possible that this is not an independent variable, but rather is a direct function of the size of the defect itself.

SURGERY

For the past 12 years, surgeons at The Children's Hospital in Boston have patched ventricular defects through the tricuspid valve. Rarely, a right ventricular incision is needed: even more rarely, a left ventricular apical incision is used to close a large apical muscular defect. In a few instances it is not possible to close multiple defects and a band is put on the pulmonary artery.

Even with a selected group of severely ill infants, all below the third percentile for height and weight, the mortality at The Children's Hospital in Boston is 12%. With successful surgical repair of the ventricular septal defect the infant almost invariably begins to gain weight (Yeager et al, 1984). About 10% of them have a small residual shunt and even smaller numbers require late reoperation to close a residual opening, often an unrecognized second defect.

PULMONARY HYPERTENSION

In the management of children with ventricular septal defect and pulmonary vascular obstructive disease, the first hurdle is to decide whether the child can possibly undergo cardiac surgery for the ventricular septal defect. Given minimal elevation of the pulmonary vascular resistance, as estimated at a stable catheterization, we favor closing the ventricular septal defect. Given pulmonary vascular resistance of eight Woods units or higher, we tend, in general, to avoid surgical repair except in the very young. Since this disease is acquired and is progressive, it is reasonable to assume that in small infants, the disease was only recently acquired and, thus, is likely to be reversible. Consequently, the discovery of ventricular septal defect with severe pulmonary vascular obstructive disease in a small infant is likely to lead to surgery whereas the same findings in a child more than 2 years old will indicate an inoperable situation.

Course and Prognosis

The noncardiac factors which unfavorably influence the outcome of a patient with ventricular septal defect include associated extracardiac anomalies and low birth weight (Fyler et al, 1980a; 1980b). Extracardiac anomalies occur in 33% of infants with significant ventricular septal defects. Twenty-five percent of these are of major importance, often require surgery (tracheoesophageal fistulae), and clearly influence the survival of these infants. Fifteen percent of all patients with large ventricular septal defects have major extracardiac defects that cannot be corrected (e.g., chromosomal abnormalities; Fyler et al, 1980a). Twenty percent of infants who underwent cardiac catheterization in the first year of life for ventricular septal defect had major extracardiac anomalies or low birth weight. The first year mortality in this group was 35%, while in those without these additional problems there was a mortality of only 10% (Fyler et al, 1980a). The important effects of other anomalies or low birth weight on survival of infants with congenital heart disease are readily demonstrated through life table analysis (Figs. 6.15 and 6.16). Depending on birth weight, the size of the ventricular defect, and the presence of extracardiac anomalies, growth may be very poor (Levy et al, 1978). Fifty percent of the infants who were not treated or who received palliative treatment were below the third

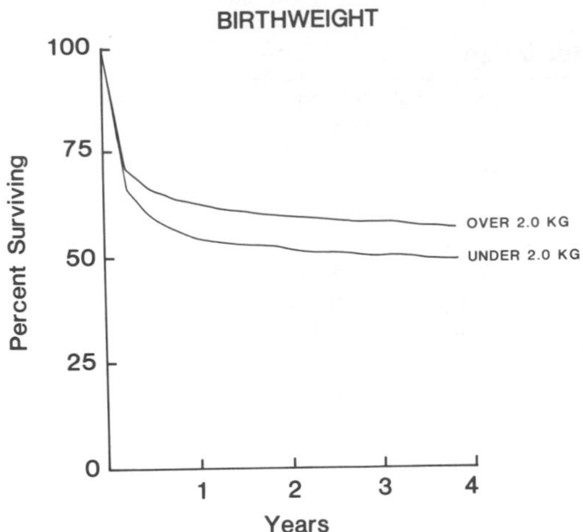

Figure 6.16. Comparative life-table analysis of survival of infants with critical congenital heart disease with birthweights of more or less than 2.0 kg.

percentile for height or weight at 1 year of age and 25% of the survivors were still below the fifth percentile at 5 years of age despite surgical management for some (Levy et al, 1978). Growth failure was the major reason for recommending surgical repair; Yeager et al (1984) reported that virtually all infants undergoing surgical repair were below the third percentile at the time of operation. In contrast, infants deemed sick enough to undergo cardiac catheterization but whose defects later spontaneously closed had normal growth.

The physiologic abnormalities encountered in patients with ventricular septal defects are not necessarily static. Defects may become smaller (never larger) and many close entirely. Pulmonary stenosis or excessive right ventricular muscle bundles may become gradually more obstructive, thereby temporarily improving the patient's status. About 5% of patients develop some aortic valve abnormality.

The natural history of ventricular septal defect emphasizes, more than that of other congenital heart defects, the dynamic nature of congenital cardiac anomalies. Changes over time are more likely to occur than not. The delusion that once a patient is categorized his classification is forever solved should be recognized for what it is.

SPONTANEOUS CLOSURE

The disappearance of a murmur typical of ventricular septal defect during the first months of life is a common phenomemon. As many as 30% of ventricular septal defects have been documented to close completely with no treatment (Hoffman and Rudolph, 1965). It is generally believed that the smaller defects are more likely to close (Hoffman and Rudolph, 1965; Alpert et al, 1979); however, up to 12% of larger defects have also been documented to close (Fyler et al, 1980a). The available data suggest that muscular defects are most likely to undergo spontaneous closure. Decrease in size of a ventricular septal defect is common and occurs in up to 50% of all patients (Hoffman and Rudolph, 1965). A decrease in size of membranous ventricular septal defects is well documented, but in our experience complete closure of a membranous defect is not common. Five to 11% of very small membranous defects are reported to close spontanously (Beerman et al, 1985, Ramaciotti et al, 1986). The aneurysm (Freedman et al, 1974; Anderson et al, 1983b), or "windsock" that partially occludes the membranous ventricular opening is primarily a distortion of the septal tricuspid valve leaflets. Indeed, some minor deformity of the tricuspid valve is usual with membranous defects (Anderson et al, 1983b). There has been no suggestion that subpulmonary, malalignment or atrioventricular canal defects ever close or get smaller, even though some must either have extension into other areas of the septum or be associated with other defects, allowing for diminution in the size of the total ventricular opening and a clinical picture suggesting decreasing size.

PULMONARY VASCULAR DISEASE

The tendency for pulmonary vascular obstructive disease to develop in patients with ventricular septal defect is well known (Nadas et al, 1977). Permanent pulmonary vascular obstructive disease rarely develops before the age of 2 years and where, formerly, this problem developed in as many as 20% of surviving patients, it is now rare. The New England Regional Infant Cardiac Program found no case of pulmonary vascular obstructive disease in more than 800 children with ventricular septal defect seen over a 13-year period.

Patients diagnosed as having ventricular defect and pulmonary vascular obstructive disease should undergo cardiac catheterization, primarily to exclude other forms of pulmonary hypertension and to confirm unequivocally a diagnosis with a relatively poor outcome. Causes of elevated pulmonary resistance which are reversible (such as cor triatriatum, mitral stenosis, hypoventilation) should be diligently excluded.

Ventricular Septal Defect And Patent Ductus Arteriosus

About 15% of infants with a ventricular defect also have a persistently open ductus arteriosus after the age of 10 days (Fyler et al, 1980a). Any combination of small-to-large ductus arteriosus and small-to-large ventricular defects may occur. In practical terms, the two lesions are additive in their physiologic consequences, because both produce left-to-right shunts and, if large, are associated with pulmonary hypertension.

There is a higher percentage of extracardiac anomalies (48%) among these patients than among those who have only a ventricular defect (Fyler et al, 1980a). The increased tendency to find this combination in females is understandable (see Patent Ductus Arteriosus).

The clinical findings are those of the dominant defect (Fyler et al, 1968). With a large patent ductus arteriosus and a small ventricular septal defect there is a crescendic systolic murmur and a wide pulse pressure, while a dominant ventricular defect presents the clinical picture of a ventricular septal defect. The film and electrocardiogram are not helpful in this distinction. A two-dimensional echocardiogram may discover the second defect, as may cardiac catheterization.

The mortality associated with this combination of defects is higher than that for isolated ventricular defect (Fyler et al, 1980a). Associated extracardiac anomalies may contribute to this difference, but are not the sole explanation.

Most patients with ventricular septal defect and patent ductus arteriosus require early surgical intervention since the total shunt is large and anticongestive medications are relatively ineffective. Alhough the possibility of simply dividing the patent ductus arteriosus is present if the ventricular septal defect is known to be small, more often both defects are closed through a single operative procedure.

Ventricular Septal Defect And Atrial Septal Defect

Ten percent of infants with ventricular defect have an additional atrial shunt (Fyler et al, 1980a). Usually it is not possible to be certain whether the atrial opening is no more than a dilated, incompetent foramen ovale or a true secundum defect. The tendency to female dominance, the increased numbers of extracardiac anomalies (44%), and a poor survival rate compared to that for ventricular septal defect alone, suggest that a majority have a disease different from an isolated ventricular septal defect and a patent foramen ovale.

Clinical recognition of the associated atrial defect is difficult and depends on echocardiographic evaluation and cardiac catheterization.

Children with ventricular septal defect and atrial septal defect almost invaribly require surgical intervention, inasmuch as there is a tendency toward rather large shunts.

Ventricular Septal Defect And Pulmonary Stenosis

In infants with ventricular septal defect, a small pressure gradient across the right ventricular outflow is often the result of excessive blood flow (flow gradient) because of the left-to- right shunt. In some infants, the pressure gradient results from a mild anatomic obstruction of the type seen in tetralogy of Fallot, or is caused by excessive right ventricular muscle bundles (moderator bands, double-chambered right ventricle) or by valvar pulmonary stenosis. The tetralogy type is associated with a malalignment ventricular septal defect; double-chambered right ventricle and valvar pulmonary stenosis are usually associated with a membranous ventricular septal defect. Each of the three types of pulmonary stenosis may be progressive. As outflow obstruction increases, the amount of left-to-right shunting through the ventricular defect decreases. For this reason, these infants may have congestive failure early, later improve, and finally, weeks to decades later, become cyanotic (Gasul et al, 1957). This is particularly evident in those with tetralogy of Fallot. Right ventricular outflow obstruction from valvar pulmonary stenosis or from abnormal right ventricular muscle bundles is more likely to be associated with a progressively smaller ventricular defect. Increasing right ventricular outflow obstruction with an increasingly restrictive (smaller) ventricular defect may result in suprasystemic right ventricular pressure. In any case, these infants tend to have less congestive failure and, in the absence of cyanosis, to grow well. Whereas the murmurs of ventricular defect and pulmonary stenosis are blended at first, later the murmur of pulmonary stenosis is dominant. The electrocardiogram initially may show left ventricular hypertrophy, later combined ventricular hypertrophy and finally pure right ventricular hypertrophy. On a chest film, the heart size initially may be large with increased pulmonary vasculature; it becomes smaller over time and ultimately is associated with decreased pulmonary vascularity. Two-dimensional echocardiography generally demonstrates the anatomy, although confusion over minor degrees of obstruction early in the course is to be expected.

Survival during the first year is improved by the presence of pulmonary stenosis as shown by comparison of survival rates for other patients with ventricular septal defects. There is no escape from surgery with this combination of defects, however, unless the "pulmonary stenosis" is a flow gradient and not based on an anatomic abnormality.

Ventricular Septal Defect And Aortic Regurgitation

Aortic regurgitation and infundibular pulmonary stenosis (most often with a small left-to-right shunt) develop in about 5% of patients with ventricular septal defects, particularly the subpulmonary variety, who have not undergone surgery (Keane et al, 1977; Momma et al, 1984; Van Praagh and McNamara, 1968). How often this is caused by anomalies in the aortic valve leaflets and how often it is a consequence of leaflet abnormalities caused by the jet of shunted blood is a matter of debate. The aortic leaflets immediately adjacent to the ventricular defect are defective, sometimes prolapsing through the ventricular defect into the right ventricle, further reducing the size of the left-to-right shunt. In any case, progressive aortic regurgitation may develop after the age of 18 months and before the age of 20 years. Pulmonary hypertension is almost unknown in this group of patients; mild to moderate pulmonary stenosis, sometimes caused by the prolapsing aortic cusp, is common. Initially, a diastolic blowing murmur (see Diastolic Murmurs) is discovered in a patient thought to have only a small ventricular defect. Progressively severe aortic regurgitation may ensue, ultimately leading to left ventricular hypertrophy and gross cardiomegaly.

Children with aortic regurgitation from any cause are particularly prone to bacterial endocarditis.

The management of patients with ventricular septal defect and aortic regurgitation depends on the location of the ventricular defect. All patients with subpulmonary ventricular septal defect probably ought to undergo surgery at some convenient time after the discovery since that defect is often large, has not been shown to become smaller with time, and is known to lead to development of aortic regurgitation. It seems reasonable, although not proved in our experience, to assume that closing the subpulmonary ventricular defect will influence the later development of aortic regurgitation.

On the other hand, the value of closure of subaortic defects to prevent aortic regurgitation is debatable. The incidence of aortic regurgitation with membranous ventricular defects is small and the defect is likely to become smaller with time. For these reasons, we do not favor closing the smaller membranous defects for the purpose of preventing aortic regurgitation.

Whether to recommend immediate cardiac surgery on discovery of aortic regurgitation, whatever the location of the ventricular defect, is a different and more difficult question. Improvement of aortic valve function through valvoplasty is desirable but there is a possibility that aortic valve replacement will be required. It is our impression that the older the patient the less likely will valvoplasty be successful, and the more likely will aortic valve replacement be needed. The decision, whether to follow the patient without surgery or to recommend surgery must be reviewed regularly. We recommend surgery when the aortic regurgitation is mild in a young child, particularly if the ventricular defect is subpulmonary. In older patients with membranous ventricular defects we require documented progression.

The lesson of this disease is that clinically small ventricular septal defects cannot be ignored. Some systematic scheme for monitoring the appearance of aortic regurgitation is needed for those with subaortic or subpulmonary ventricular defects.

Ventricular Septal Defect And Subaortic Stenosis

The appearance of subaortic stenosis in an infant with ventricular septal defect has been noted increasingly in recent years (Lauer et al, 1960; Freed et al, 1973; Vogel et al, 1983). Sometimes this is a variation of the syndrome of coarctation, ventricular defect and aortic stenosis (see Coarctation of the Aorta). Occasionally, it is a feature of the group of patients who have double-chambered right ventricle. Sometimes it may be associated with pulmonary artery banding, or it may simply represent the natural history of otherwise uncomplicated ventricular septal defect.

Subaortic stenosis as an isolated lesion is rare in infancy and is not seen at birth. There are, however, 2–3% of infants with ventricular septal defect in whom subaortic stenosis will develop. Characteristically, it produces progressive obstruction.

Subaortic stenosis should be thought of when the clinical picture of ventricular defect includes excessive left ventricular hypertrophy, when the murmur tends to be louder toward the base of the heart, and when the patient is responding poorly to treatment. Sometimes, poor recovery after surgical repair of ventricular septal defects leads to the observation that the ventricular defect is closed and that there is no pulmonary stenosis. In this case, the explanation for the loud murmur may be subaortic stenosis. Because the lesion is progressive, it is possible that subaortic stenosis will appear to have been excluded by cardiac catheterization in early infancy, only to be discovered later.

Children with ventricular septal defect and subaortic stenosis almost always come to cardiac surgery for the subaortic stenosis at some point, since the stenosis is progressive. The criteria for attempting surgical correction of the subaortic stenosis are those described under the section on Subaortic Stenosis.

TRANSPOSITION OF THE GREAT ARTERIES

Definition

D (dextrorotary)-transposition of the great arteries is present when the aorta arises from an anterior anatomic right ventricle receiving systemic venous blood and the pulmonary artery arises from a posterior anatomic left ventricle receiving pulmonary venous blood.

Basic Science

ANATOMY

D-transposition of the great arteries refers to patients whose ventricles have the normal D relationship, with the right ventricle rightward and anterior and the left ventricle leftward and posterior (Fig. 6.17). The

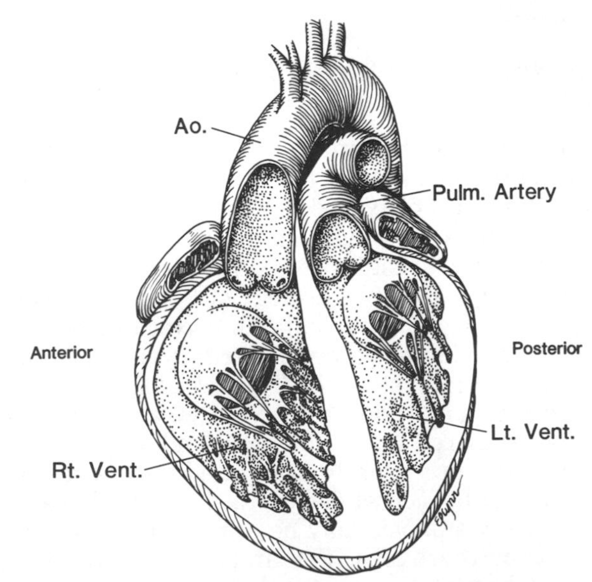

Figure 6.17. Anatomy of transposition of the great arteries as viewed from the left chest.

CASE ILLUSTRATION

At hospital discharge at 3 days of age, this 3-week-old, first born, male infant appeared well but was noted to have a systolic murmur. Because his grandmother thought he was breathing too fast he was brought to his pediatrician for early follow-up examination at 3 weeks. He had regained his birth weight but feeding had been slow requiring up to 30 minutes to take 2–3 oz. He vomited occasionally.

Physical examination showed a scrawny infant with a respiratory rate of 80, without retractions. The peripheral pulses were present and equal. The liver was palpable 3.0 cm below the right costal margin. The heart rate was 150 beats/min and regular. There was a grade 4 systolic murmur maximal at the lower left sternal border; a gallop was audible at the apex. A chest film showed the heart to be moderately enlarged with an area of possible atelectasis or pneumonia in the right upper lobe. The pulmonary vasculature was engorged. The electrocardiogram had an axis of +120° with sinus rhythm. There was right and left ventricular hypertrophy. A two-dimensional echocardiographic examination showed a membranous ventricular septal defect, with an additional smaller defect in the muscular septum detected by Doppler examination. Administration of digoxin and furosemide resulted in slowing of the heart rate to 120/min and a decrease in respiratory rate. A diastolic rumble became audible at the apex.

After obtaining cultures, antibiotic treatment was begun because of the area of density in the right upper lobe, and was continued for 1 week. The infant tolerated feedings of formula strengthened to 26 calories per ounce given every 3 hours. A decision was made to discharge the infant and observe him at home inasmuch as the family situation was favorable. At 2 months the baby had grown but was below the third percentile for both weight and height. The electrocardiogram was unchanged. The chest film continued to show a large heart with increased pulmonary vascular markings. The density in the right upper lobe had cleared. Because of poor growth and, therefore, the probability that surgery would be indicated, cardiac catheterization was carried out. This showed systemic pressure in the pulmonary arteries. There was a large left-to-right shunt. Left ventricular angiography showed a large membranous ventricular defect and several small, apical, muscular defects. Further increase in the caloric content of the formula resulted in vomiting. Cardiac surgery was carried out at 10 weeks of age. The large membranous ventricular defect was patched through the tricuspid valve and attempts were made to close the muscular defects. During the postoperative period, a loud murmur of ventricular septal defect persisted. Two-dimensional echocardiography with a Doppler examination identified the opening to be in the muscular septum.

Over the next year the infant improved in growth and had satisfactory developmental milestones. At 1 year of age, a cardiac catheterization showed a small residual ventricular septal defect at the edge of the patched membranous defect. The muscular defects had closed. Pulmonary arterial pressure was normal.

QUESTIONS AND COMMENTS

Are prophylactic antibiotics during dental surgery to prevent bacterial endocarditis needed after corrective surgery?

If there is a residual systolic murmur prophylactic antibiotics should be used. If there is no murmur in the postoperative period and there is positive evidence that the ventricular defect is closed, prophylactic antibiotics are used for the first few months after surgery at which time it can be assumed that the patching material used for closing the ventricular septal defect has become endothelialized.

Should a small subpulmonary ventricular septal defect be closed?

Yes! Commonly, the subpulmonary ventricular defects seem small but, in fact, are large openings partly occluded by a prolapse of the aortic valve into the defect.

If advanced prolapse of the aortic valve without aortic regurgitation is encountered in association with a ventricular septal defect, should aortic valve surgery be undertaken?

This is a difficult question. Valvoplasty may result in residual aortic regurgitation. We favor closure of the ventricular septal defect and valvoplasty.

Should vasodilator therapy be used for people with ventricular septal defect and pulmonary hypertension?

Vasodilator therapy (afterload reduction) helps patients with ventricular defect and congestive heart failure but there is no evidence that vasodilator therapy has any beneficial effect on the pulmonary hypertension associated with ventricular defects.

Given a loud murmur following surgery for ventricular septal defect, is there reason for concern?

If the patient appears well, there is clearly no reason for immediate concern. On the other hand, if the postoperative course is proceeding poorly, cardiac catheterization should be carried out to discover the reason for the murmur. It is possible that an unexpected lesion will be uncovered and the situation salvaged through better information. In general, the systolic murmurs audible after cardiac surgery result from an incompletely closed ventricular defect, from a second unrecognized ventricular defect, from subaortic stenosis, from pulmonary stenosis, or from tricuspid regurgitation.

One cardiologist says that the child has a double-outlet right ventricle with ventricular septal defect and, on second opinion, another cardiologist says that there is only a ventricular septal defect. What is the explanation of these differences?

There is a spectrum of patients ranging from those with simple uncomplicated ventricular septal defect through those with obvious double-outlet right ventricle and ventricular septal defect. In the area of overlap it is expected that two experienced people reviewing the same data may decide on different labels for the same lesion.

pulmonary artery is connected to the left ventricle and almost invariably lies in a posterior position behind the aorta. The aorta is anterior and is connected to the right ventricle. The coronary circulation arises from the root of the aorta, although the pattern of the coronary arterial circulation varies considerably from normal. Except for these abnormalities, the ventricles, the valves, and the great vessels are usually normal. However, many other congenital cardiac anomalies may be associated with transposition of the great arteries. By convention, at The Children's Hospital in Boston, infants with transposition and atresia of an atrioventricular valve, with single ventricle, and most with heterotaxy are characterized separately whereas transposition of the great arteries with any other defect is considered under the rubric, D-transposition. Some patients with transposition physiology have variations of double-outlet right ventricle (see Double-Outlet Right Ventricle).

Among newborns with transposition of the great arteries, two-thirds have no additional cardiac defects except for a patent foramen ovale and a ductus arteriosus. The remainder have an associated ventricular septal defect. All varieties of ventricular septal defects are known to occur in patients with transposition of the great arteries (Penkoske et al, 1983).

PHYSIOLOGY

Normal cardiopulmonary circulation is a serial circulation; blood passes from one area of the heart along to the next without re-entering that heart chamber again until it is passed through systemic capillaries. The patient with transposition of the great arteries has two parallel circulations; blood may recirculate repeatedly through the same chamber before returning to either the systemic or pulmonary capillaries. The unoxygenated systemic venous return passes through the right ventricle to the aorta and back to the systemic capillaries. The oxygenated pulmonary venous return passes through the left ventricle and returns to the lungs. It is obvious that the transposed circulation is incompatible with life unless there is communication between the two circuits. It is also obvious that the amount of blood passing from the systemic to the pulmonary circulation must equal exactly that which returns from the pulmonary to the systemic. Furthermore, the equilibration of blood flowing toward and away from the pulmonary circulation must be maintained on virtually a beat to beat basis. If this were not true, one parallel circulation could empty into the other in a very short time. The subtle mechanisms that control homeostasis in patients with transposition of the great arteries are not well understood. Empirically, the measured pulmonary blood flow is greater than the systemic blood flow. The mechanisms that determine why one patient settles at a particular pulmonary blood flow while the next patient with apparently the same anatomy selects a much larger or smaller pulmonary flow are not known. An atrial or a ventricular septal defect allows equal shunting in opposite directions through a single orifice. By contrast, patients cannot survive with a patent ductus arteriosus alone; blood passes through the ductus arteriosus toward the lungs but, of necessity, there must be another means of returning oxygenated blood to the systemic circulation. The combination of a patent ductus arteriosus and a dilated patent foramen ovale is common in newborns with transposition of the great arteries and intact ventricular septum. Such patients rapidly deteriorate as the ductus arteriosus follows its programmed course of closure. The greater the movement of blood into and out of the pulmonary circulation (mixing), the less cyanotic is the patient. With large pulmonary blood flow, congestive heart failure is common.

The most common problem for infants with transposition and intact ventricular septum is low-arterial blood oxygen, due to inadequate mixing. For the majority this is not a subtle problem. The newborn is severely cyanotic; there may be hypoxia, tachypnea and even death within hours of birth. In those with excessive mixing through a ventricular defect or a large patent ductus arteriosus, cyanosis is minimal and can be overlooked. The pinker the infant, the more likelihood of congestive heart failure. Additional defects, such as pulmonary stenosis, coarctation of the aorta, and various types of septal openings influence the physiologic state of the patient and result in varying degrees of pulmonary blood flow and arterial oxygenation, producing a spectrum of clinical pictures from deep hypoxia with a small heart, to no visible cyanosis, a large heart, and congestive heart failure.

Epidemiology

Among individuals with congenital malformations of the heart, transposition of the great arteries is the most common reason for admission to a cardiac hospital in the first week of life; it is the second most common defect encountered in the first year of life, (Fyler et al, 1980a) and is among the top five cardiac lesions requiring cardiac catheterization or cardiac surgery in all age groups (Table 6.3). The number of infants born with transposition of the great arteries is remarkably constant, 21/100,000 live births (Fyler et al, 1980a). Over the past 15 years, the prognosis for infants with transposition of the great arteries has improved from an almost universally fatal outlook to a 90% chance of survival and long-term well-being. Since systematic salvage of these infants has become a reality only in the past 15 years, long-term survivors with transposition of the great arteries can be expected to receive increasing attention from physicians in the coming decade.

Diagnosis

For clinical purposes the patients are divided into those with an intact ventricular septum and those with ventricular septal defects. Although pulmonary stenosis does occur in patients with intact ventricular septum, it is not often severe. By contrast, among those with moderate-to-large ventricular septal defects, pulmonary stenosis of varying severity, up to pulmonary atresia, is encountered.

Infants with transposition of the great arteries are most often discovered in the newborn nursery because they are cyanotic, in congestive failure, or because there is an audible murmur. More than 50% have been referred to a cardiac unit by the age of 2 days. The majority arriving at a cardiac unit after the age of 2 weeks has a ventricular septal defect (Fyler et al, 1980a).

SYMPTOMS

The usual presenting symptom is severe cyanosis, varying somewhat with crying but not influenced by adminstration of high concentrations of oxygen. The deeply cyanotic newborn may also have tachypnea.

Infants with greater mixing are less cyanotic, and with large amounts of mixing may be so pink that oxygen unsaturation may be overlooked. However, such a baby, will have tachypnea, with or without subcostal retractions, because of excessive pulmonary blood flow and congestive heart failure.

PHYSICAL EXAMINATION

These newborns are predominantly male (64%) and seem large to pediatric cardiologists dealing primarily with infants who are malnourished. In the New England Regional Infant Cardiac Program, babies with transposition of the great arteries had the highest birth weights; only 6% had birth weights of less than 2.5 kg and 1% less than 2.0 kg. Nevertheless, when comparisons are made to a suitable normal control group, these infants are not unexpectedly large.

Associated extracardiac anomalies are not common, occurring in about 9% of infants, and are only rarely of major importance.

Obvious cyanosis and mild tachypnea may be the only recognizable physical abnormalities in a newborn male of normal or large size. Auscultation may be completely unrevealing. A systolic murmur along the left sternal border suggests the presence of a ventricular defect or of pulmonary stenosis (Fig. 6.4*A*). Evidence of gross congestive failure without a systolic murmur suggests a diagnostic error.

MINOR LABORATORY TESTS

A test of the response of blood gases to 100% ambient oxygen may be helpful. Measurement of of the patient's arterial oxygen before and after 5 minutes of breathing 100% oxygen (delivered by a hood) may show little change because of the limited opportunity for mixture of oxygenated and unoxygenated blood.

Arterial oxygen saturations as low as 30–40% (Po_2, 20 torr) are regularly encountered and emphasize the precarious situation of the patient.

ELECTROCARDIOGRAPHY

At birth, the electrocardiogram shows normal right ventricular hypertrophy, reflecting the prior 9 months. Later, the fact that the right ventricle acts as the systemic ventricle is reflected in persistent marked right ventricular hypertrophy.

RADIOGRAPHY

At birth the chest film is often normal. Later, the heart may be variably enlarged with increased pulmonary vascularity.

ECHO-DOPPLER STUDY

The transposed nature of the great arteries can be readily identified with two-dimensional echocardiography. The patency of the ductus may be demonstrable and the characteristics of an atrial defect can be defined. Is there an incompetent patent foramen ovale or true atrial defect? Are there other defects?

CARDIAC CATHETERIZATION

Cardiac catheterization should be carried out as soon as possible after the diagnosis has been established by echocardiography. The purposes of cardiac catheterization are: (a) therapeutic (i.e., balloon septostomy), (b) to establish the number and the location of ventricular septal defects, and (c) to learn other details necessary for the proposed surgery.

Therapeutic Maneuvers. Balloon atrial septostomy, introduced by Rashkind et al in 1966, rapidly became the standard management aimed at increasing mixing at the atrial level, supplanting surgical atrial septostomy (Blalock-Hanlon operation). A balloon mounted on the tip of the catheter is placed through the foramen ovale into the left atrium, inflated with contrast material to about the size of the left atrium and forcibly pulled back through the septum. This maneuver produces a tear in the atrial septum that heals to a sizeable atrial defect.

Anatomic and Physiologic Data. The size and location of ventricular septal defects are vital data. Will surgery for the defect be required? Will the defects be likely to close spontaneously? Will the defect be accessible to the surgeon through the tricuspid valve as opposed to a left ventricular incision? Is the location of the ventricular septal defect more favorable for an atrial or an arterial switching operation? Is the pulmonary artery pressure favorable for an arterial switching operation?

If there is no ventricular defect, and if atrial switching correction is planned, little additional information is required from cardiac catheterization. If an arterial switching operation is planned, the ability of the left ventricle to manage the systemic circulation must be estimated. The coronary anatomy and the relative size of the great arteries may be useful information in planning an arterial switching procedure. The degree of pulmonary stenosis and the size and location of the ventricular septal defect may prompt the use of a Rastelli type of operation (Rastelli et al, 1969)

Management

A deeply cyanotic newborn almost invariably does better on prostaglandins therapy because prostaglandins dilate the ductus arteriosus, allowing greater entry of blood into the lungs. The return of oxygenated blood takes place through the foramen ovale from the left atrium to the right. This phenomenon requires a progressively incompetent foramen, which is believed to be produced by ever-increasing left atrial size and pressure caused by excessive blood entering the lungs via the ductus arteriosus. The circulation stabilizes for days, often with good arterial saturation, although elevation of left atrial pressure and secondary pulmonary edema may be encountered. Prostaglandins often tide the baby over until cardiac catheterization can be arranged. Because prostaglandins sometimes cause apnea, this therapy should not be used without equipment and capability for intubation and ventilation immediately at hand. Prostaglandins improve the possibility of successful transport to a distant center.

Balloon atrial septostomy is routinely carried out in all patients except those who undergo immediate arterial switching. The naturally occurring large atrial septal defect is sufficiently rare to be effectively discounted in deciding whether to carry out balloon septostomy or not. Having stabilized the patient with balloon septostomy, attention turns to the surgical options.

ATRIAL SWITCHING

Mustard's (1964) operation, a variation on the theme for correction introduced by Senning (1959), revolutionized the care of infants with transposition of the great arteries (Marx et al, 1983). Conceptually, the circulation is converted from two parallel circuits to "normal" serial circulation by redirecting the systemic venous blood, with a baffle, into the left ventricle and thence to the pulmonary artery. The pulmonary venous blood cascades around the baffle to the right ventricle. The right and left ventricles, therefore, have reversed roles, the left ventricle pumping the pulmonary circulation under low pressure and the right ventricle pumping the systemic circulation at systemic pressures. At the same time, the right atrial blood is directed to the pulmonary artery and left atrial blood to the aorta in the normal fashion.

This arrangement can also be accomplished through a modified Senning approach that uses largely native structures to baffle the blood. There seems to be little difference in the results of the two operations. How the baffle is placed influences the possibility of pulmonary venous or systemic venous obstruction, perhaps the most common complications of this kind of surgery.

ARTERIAL SWITCHING

This operation was first done successfully in significant numbers by Jatene et al (1976). Through this technique, serial circulation is established by surgically transposing the pulmonary artery to the native aortic valve and the right ventricle. The aorta is transposed to the native pulmonary valve and the left ventricle. The trick is to move the coronary arteries with the aorta without compromising the coronary circulation. A variety of techniques are used to accomplish this purpose. Obviously, the left ventricle must be sufficiently muscular to maintain the systemic circulation. Within 1–2 weeks after birth, the left ventricle may no longer be able to adapt suddenly to pumping at systemic pressure. Hence, these newborns require an arterial switching operation within the first 10 days of life (de Leon et al, 1984). Alternatively, Yacoub and Radley-Smith (1984) have banded the pulmonary artery in this situation so that the left ventricle remains accustomed to pumping at higher pressures. Later within months, the band is removed and the arterial switching procedure is carried out.

Among patients with ventricular septal defects the small defects are ignored (virtually intact septum). Larger defects may be closed through the tricuspid valve if an atrial switching operation is being carried out. Clearly, a right ventricular incision to close a ventricular defect in a patient who will need his right ventricle to pump his systemic circuit is risky. By the same token, closure of apical muscular defects through a left ventricular incision may be better tolerated in a patient undergoing an atrial switching procedure.

Ideally, transposition of the great arteries associated with a ventricular septal defect is repaired by using an arterial switching approach, the ventricular defect being closed through the tricuspid valve or even possibly through a right ventricular incision. This approach is desirable if the ventricular defect is large and particularly if it is inaccessible through the tricuspid valve. Anatomic pulmonary stenosis prohibits this surgical procedure.

RASTELLI PROCEDURE

Children with D-transposition, ventricular septal defect, and severe pulmonary stenosis are not candidates for arterial switching, since artificial conduits are usually required for repair in such patients and since these conduits are prone to early malfunction if the small diameters required for infants are used. Because small infants are not candidates for conduit repair a palliative central shunt or modified Blalock shunt is carried out. Repair is scheduled 4–5 years later by means of a Rastelli procedure (Rastelli et al, 1969). With a large ventricular septal defect appropriately located, the left ventricular outflow is directed into the aorta by use of a patch. A conduit is then placed between the right ventricle and the main pulmonary artery, which has been disconnected from the left ventricle.

PALLIATIVE ATRIAL SWITCHING

Pulmonary vascular obstructive disease has almost invariably developed in individuals appearing at an older age who have survived without corrective surgery; almost without exception a large ventricular septal defect is present. In these patients atrial switching procedures have been carried out to reduce the cyanosis, improve symptoms, and prolong life to a limited extent, without closing the ventricular septal defect (Lindesmith et al, 1975).

Course and Prognosis

The natural history of D-transposition of the great arteries is early demise; untreated, 51% of infants with this diagnosis are dead within the first month and 90% within the first year. Those with an intact ventricular septum are more at risk for early death, there being one to two infants each year in New England who die the first day of life before reaching an appropriate hospital. Survival beyond the first birthday implies a ventricular defect with pulmonary stenosis or possible pulmonary vascular obstructive disease.

In the New England Regional Infant Cardiac Program, the incidence of CNS injury associated with D-transposition of the great arteries was high (20%). Some of this represents surgical accidents, but much occurs naturally. The later corrective surgery is carried out, the lower is the ultimate intelligence quotient and the more delay there is in motor development (Newberger et al, 1983; 1984). The conclusion that injuries of the CNS relate to the duration (and probably the degree) of cyanosis is inescapable. Growth is directly proportional to the child's age and to the success of the corrective surgery. The earlier surgery is carried out, the

CASE ILLUSTRATION

A male infant, with birth weight of 3.3 kg, was noted to be cyanotic at 6 hours of age in a hospital in New Hampshire. The infant had a respiratory rate of 50, but otherwise seemed normal; there were no abnormalities on auscultation.

On chest film the heart size was at the upper limits of normal with normal pulmonary vascular markings (Fig. 6.18). An electrocardiogram showed normal right ventricular dominance. Right radial arterial Po_2 was reported as 33 torr rising to 35 torr when 100% oxygen was administered by hood.

Because a long trip to the nearest cardiac center was required, prostaglandins therapy was started and, as a safety measure, the infant was intubated before the transport. On arrival at the cardiac unit an echocardiogram showed D-transposition of the great arteries, a moderate-sized patent ductus arteriosus and a dilated patent foramen ovale. Cardiac catheterization was carried out and confirmed the echocardiographic observations. Before balloon septostomy in the arterial oxygen saturation was 60%; after the procedure it rose to 80%.

The infant was safely weaned from the ventilator over the next day, but with each attempt to discontinue prostaglandins, he became more cyanotic with arterial oxygen saturations falling to 30%.

By the age of 8 days, it seemed unlikely that prostaglandins could be safely discontinued. In deciding among surgical options, and after discussion with the family, the option of arterial switching was chosen.

This was accomplished. Recovery was uneventful. On discharge, the infant had a grade II systolic murmur but otherwise seemed well.

At recatheterization, 6 months later a pressure gradient of 30 mm Hg in the main pulmonary artery was discovered at the suture site. The infant had gained to 9.0 kg and was sitting up and creeping.

QUESTIONS AND COMMENTS

Are there circumstances where transposition of the great arteries is not an emergency problem?

Yes, if there is good mixing, as in transposition with a large ventricular defect, transposition with single ventricle, transposition with a straddling tricuspid valve, or in some variants of double-outlet right ventricle. Unfortunately, those defects that allow a longer life without surgery are the very defects that are most difficult to repair.

Why is a pacemaker needed for the sick sinus syndrome?

The sick sinus syndrome occurs after extensive intra-atrial surgery and is characterized by episodes of very slow heart rate, often associated with episodes of supraventricular tachycardia. Medications needed to control the supraventricular tachycardia may further depress the rate when the heart is slow. Hence, it is commonly necessary to use a pacemaker in conjunction with antiarrhythmic medications (Flinn et al, 1984).

What are the late complications of chronic cyanosis?

These include a depressed intelligence quotient (Newburger et al, 1984), poor growth, poor motor function (Newburger et al, 1983), and CNS injuries (Terplan, 1973).

How long can surgery be delayed in a reasonably growing and developing child with transposition of the great arteries and a ventricular septal defect?

Good arterial oxygen saturation is implied by the question; hence, the only real concern is the development of pulmonary vascular disease. This occurs as early as the second half of the first year. Consequently, surgery of some sort is required between the ages of 6 and, at the latest, 12 months. If pulmonary arterial pressure is normal because of pulmonary stenosis or a pulmonary artery band, surgery can be safely delayed.

Is balloon septostomy needed if arterial switching is contemplated?

No. The defect caused by balloon atrial septostomy requires surgical closure during the repair. Balloon atrial septostomy does improve arterial oxygen saturation and does provide protection before surgery if any delay is expected.

If the diagnosis of transposition of the great arteries is discovered by fetal ultrasonography, does this affect the management?

It does not affect the management except that the mother should be delivered in a hospital near a cardiac center.

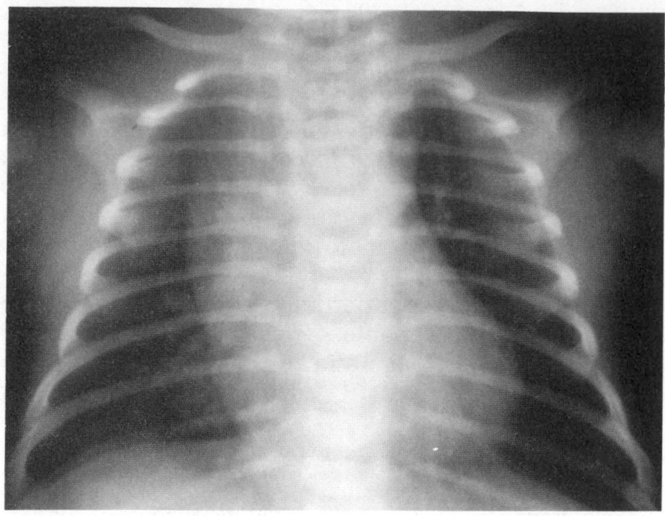

Figure 6.18. Chest film from patient with D-transposition of the great arteries. Note the virtually normal appearance.

more likely will the child be within normal growth percentiles at a later period.

These considerations lead to the recommendation that corrective surgery be carried out as early as is compatible with acceptable surgical mortality.

ATRIAL SWITCHING

There is a high incidence of atrial arrhythmias after atrial switching procedures, whether Mustard or Senning techniques are utilized. The number of patients with junctional rhythm or "sick sinus syndrome" and other atrial rhythm problems appears to increase with increasing years of follow-up, possibly occurring in 90% of patients after 5 years (Hayes and Gersony, 1986; Flinn et al, 1984). Late sudden deaths are a matter of concern, reaching 3% in the follow-up period after the Mustard operation (introduced in 1966), although initially many of these patients do not have detectable rhythm disturbances. Pacemakers are used in as many as 3% of patients.

The number of patients with late myocardial dysfunction has been debated (Hurwitz et al, 1985; Trowitzsch et al, 1985a, 1985b; Borow et al, 1984, 1984, 1981; Parrish et al, 1983). Patients with repaired ventricular septal defect have more right ventricular failure (systemic ventricular failure) than do those without ventricular septal defect. Impaired myocardial function is more often seen when corrective surgery is carried out at an older age. Tricuspid valve insufficiency is encountered in approximately 3% of the patients with repaired ventricular septal defects; tricuspid valve replacement is an unpleasant complication. Whether this is the result of surgery (unlikely) or, as is more likely, the result of an associated anomaly of the tricuspid valve is yet to be proven (Deal et al, 1985; Huhta et al, 1982).

ARTERIAL SWITCHING

The late problems following arterial switching procedures include obstruction at the site of the anastomosis of either the aorta or the main pulmonary artery. There are problems in transposing the coronaries as well. The minimal follow-up that has been available thus far suggests that there may be fewer arrhythmias and less myocardial dysfunction in the systemic ventricle in these patients than in comparable patients who have had atrial switching procedures.

It remains to be seen whether arterial switching procedures, performed of necessity in the first week of life, will have a lower long-term mortality and fewer complications than Senning or Mustard procedures performed later.

RASTELLI PROCEDURE

After successful Rastelli operations, concerns center around patency of the conduit from the right ventricle to the pulmonary artery. Dacron conduits usually become sufficiently obstructed with pannus to require replacement within 5 years (McGoon et al, 1982). The use of homografts may reduce the frequency of replacement. Patch closure of the ventricular septal defect is more of a baffle connecting the left ventricle to the aorta than a patch closure of a ventricular septal defect in the usual sense. Nevertheless, problems with the inappropriately placed or leaking patch are minimal.

Regardless of the surgical procedure many questions remain about patient survival. Systematic monitoring for rhythm difficulties, myocardial dysfunction, tricuspid valve function and obstructive suture lines will be needed for some years.

TETRALOGY OF FALLOT

Definition

The tetralogy of Fallot may be defined in a number of ways. Historically, Stensen (Goldstein, 1948), in the late 1600s, described an anatomic abnormality of the heart consisting of a ventricular defect, pulmonic stenosis and a dextroposed aorta. In the late 1800s, Fallot (1888) described the entity, adding the fourth component, right ventricular hypertrophy, as underlying the clinical syndrome of "cyanose cardiac." At present, Monsieur Fallot's name is attached to the malformation, though those familiar with the condition, refer to it often simply as tetralogy (tet or tetrad).

Basic Science

For the clinical physiologist, the abnormality consists of a large ventricular defect leading to systemic pressure in the right ventricle, with pulmonary stenosis resulting in a right-to-left shunt through the ventricular septum. From the surgical point of view, there is always infundibular stenosis (or atresia) with or without associated valvar stenosis. The large ventricular defect is always subaortic (when viewed from the left ventricle), malaligned (as seen from the right ventricle) and somewhat more anterior than the usual solitary ventricular defect. Note that the surgical definition, like the pathologic one, does not include cyanosis, but insists on the appropriate morphology of the ventricular defect and the pulmonary stenosis. Clinical cardiologists, on the other hand, may (perhaps incorrectly) refer to patients with pulmonary stenosis, ventricular defect and a right-to-left shunt (Fig. 6.19) irrespective of the anatomic minutiae, as "tets."

Epidemiology

Nine percent of infants born with critical congenital heart disease have tetralogy of Fallot, making this the third most common lesion among the patients in the New England Regional Infant Cardiac Program (Fyler et al, 1980a). Certainly, it is the most common cyanotic lesion among children surviving without operation beyond the first birthday. The overall incidence among all children with congenital heart disease is thought to be between 10% and 15% (see Table 6.3). It is axiomatic that a cyanotic patient, surviving beyond infancy, in all likelihood has tetralogy of Fallot or one of its variants.

Diagnosis

HISTORY

There is no single clinical profile of patients with tetralogy of Fallot; the manifestations, given the constancy of ventricular defect morphology, depend on the severity of the pulmonary stenosis, almost invariably a progressive lesion. Newborns (often) and children (less commonly) may be admitted with evidence of left-sided failure, indistinguishable from that seen in patients with large ventricular defect (see Ventricular Septal Defects). These patients have only mild pulmonary stenosis at this time. Older children and adults with tetralogy of Fallot who have not undergone surgical repair almost never show evidence of congestive heart failure unless there are complicating factors (bacterial endocarditis, anemia, aortic regurgitation). They have cyanosis and exercise intolerance of varying degrees; they have moderate or severe pulmonary stenosis. They are cyanotic and have clubbing of the fingers and toes; after running, even walking, they may assume a squatting position. Hypercyanotic spells occur mostly in infants; these consist of uncontrollable crying (? "teething") with increasing cyanosis, tachycardia, and tachypnea, leading occasionally to unconsciousness, and sometimes even to a cerebral vascular accident. The frightening part of these "spells" is that they may occur in otherwise healthy looking, pink infants. The conventional explanation, based on less than unassailable evidence, is that the attacks are due to infundibular spasm. Others (Guntheroth et al, 1965) suggest that hyperpnea, leading to an increase in right-to-left shunt, elevation of P_{CO_2} and a drop in P_{O_2} and pH, is the primary cause. Usually, these attacks occur in the morning and last from several minutes to an hour or more.

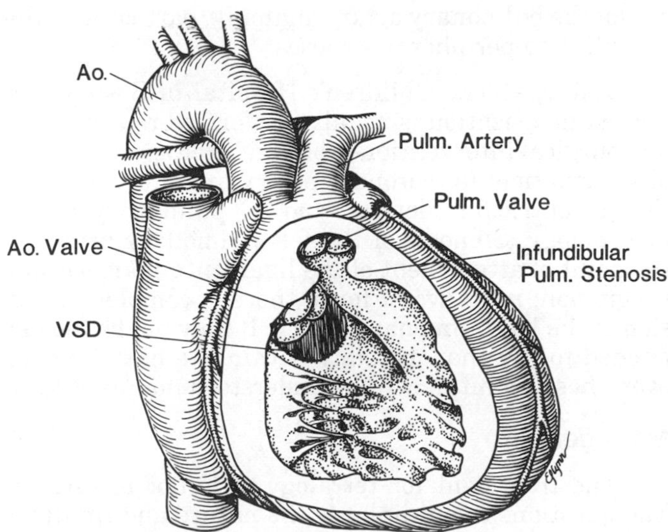

Figure 6.19. Anatomy of tetralogy of Fallot. Note relatively small size of the pulmonary arteries, the right aortic arch, and the relation of the aortic valve to the ventricular defect (overriding aorta).

PHYSICAL EXAMINATION

Results of the physical examination of patients having tetralogy with mild pulmonary stenosis are virtually indistinguishable from those for patients with large ventricular defects. In patients with moderate-to-severe pulmonary stenosis, cyanosis and clubbing dominate the picture. A systolic thrill is palpable at the left sternal border, transmitting to the suprasternal notch, but usually not to the carotids. This distinguishes it from aortic stenosis. On auscultation, there is usually an apical click (large aorta), a single loud second sound (A_2), and a grade IV-VI systolic murmur at the lower left sternal border transmitting well to the suprasternal notch; no diastolic murmur is heard (Fig. 6.3*B*). There are a number of variations on this theme. In those who have maximal pulmonary stenosis (pulmonary atresia), a systolic murmur may result from tricuspid incompetence. The dominant murmur in these patients may be a continuous one due to aortopulmonary collaterals, audible diffusely over the front and the back, or to a large patent ductus arteriosus, noted at the second left interspace. It should be emphasized here that a clearly audible systolic ejection murmur in an infant without cyanosis may disappear transiently owing to obliteration of the left-to-right shunt and virtual disappearance of the pulmonary flow during a hypercyanotic spell.

MINOR LABORATORY TESTS

Increased hematocrit (50–75%) is characteristic of cyanotic heart disease in children and adults. Infants, particularly during the first year of life, during the period of the developmental anemia of the newborn, may be "relatively anemic," i.e., having hematocrit normal for age but insufficient for a patient with a low blood oxygen content. Severe polycythemia (hematocrit higher than 65%), unusual in infancy, may increase the viscosity of the blood to a level that would impede oxygen delivery to tissues; the usual manifestations of this are symptoms of the CNS (dizziness, headaches, blackouts).

There are abnormalities of clotting factors and decreases in platelets that cannot be explained completely (Paul et al, 1961).

ELECTROCARDIOGRAPHY

The electrocardiogram always shows right ventricular hypertrophy with upright T waves in the right chest leads, often associated with peaked P waves (P pulmonale). The QRS axis is between 90 and 150°; occasionally a patient with an endocardial cushion-type of ventricular defect may have a superior frontal plane axis at −30 to −90°.

RADIOGRAPHY

The film in a patient with a right-to-left shunt shows a normal-sized heart with right ventricular contour ("boot-shaped," like a Dutch wooden shoe), a large aorta (right aortic arch in 20%), and normal or decreased pulmonary vasculature. The main pulmonary artery segment on the left border of the heart is diminished, and may even be concave (Fig. 6.20).

ECHO-DOPPLER STUDY

The echo-Doppler study demonstrates the subaortic malaligned ventricular defect and the infundibular stenosis, which establishes the morphologic diagnosis of tetralogy of Fallot.

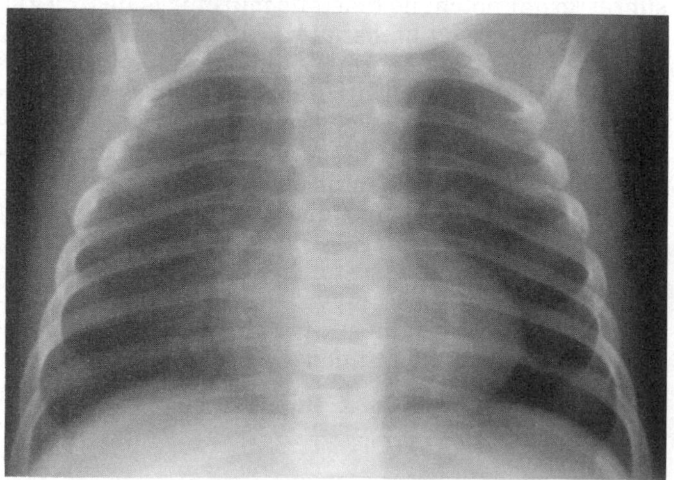

Figure 6.20. Chest film of baby with tetralogy of Fallot. Note the absence of a pulmonary artery segment and the small heart. The pulmonary vascular markings are diminished.

CARDIAC CATHETERIZATION

Cardiac catheterization with angiography provides the morphological and physiological details necessary for intelligent surgical handling of the problem.

1. Oxygen studies indicate only trivial, if any, left-to-right shunt at the ventricular level. If there is an additional patent ductus or large collaterals are present, an increase in oxygen saturation is noted at the pulmonary arterial level. The systemic artery is unsaturated to varying degrees. Steep drops in arterial saturation may be noted during a catheter study because of infundibular spasm or systemic vasodilation.
2. The pressure tracings are characterized by virtual identity of right ventricular and left ventricular pressure pulses. The pulmonary arterial pressure is low (less than 12 mm Hg, mean) and looks damped. There may be a slight increase in the A wave in the right atrium.
3. Systemic flow is normal; pulmonary flow is low (1–3 L/m^2 of body surface area).
4. Angiocardiograms, in angled position, show anatomic details characteristic of the abnormality. One issue that the angiocardiogram can solve with certainty is the course of the coronary arteries, visualized through a supravalvar aortic injection. The important point is to exclude the presence of a so-called "conus coronary," that is, the anterior descending coronary artery originating from the right coronary artery (5% of patients) that courses through the area of the usual surgical incision to correct the ventricular defect and the infundibular pulmonary stenosis. Failure to recognize this and transecting the artery may result in myocardial infarction. Angiographers should also spend an appreciable amount of time in outlining the details of the pulmonary artery anatomy, particularly relative to peripheral stenoses.

Today, at The Children's Hospital in Boston, cardiac catheterization is usually performed routinely before surgical intervention to obtain three specific points of information: (a) coronary artery anatomy, (b) additional ventricular defects, and (c) pulmonary artery morphology. Stenosis of the left pulmonary artery at the point of attachment of the ligamentum arteriosum is common; in its worst form, there is complete occlusion of the left pulmonary artery. It may not be too far-fetched to say that, possibly within the next 5 years, even these minutiae will be understood noninvasively.

Management

The treatment for tetralogy of Fallot is surgery. The questions remaining are the nature and timing of the operation. We emphasize that the approach to surgical management outlined in these pages reflects the experience at The Children's Hospital in Boston. Other institutions and other physicians and surgeons may approach the problem differently, reflecting, appropriately, the local skills and preferences.

INDICATIONS FOR SURGICAL CORRECTION

Everything else being equal, all patients with tetralogy of Fallot should electively undergo surgery before 2 years of age. Clearly, this is a totally arbitrary statement based on the recognition that the average toddler is becoming increasingly active at that age and, as pediatricians, we ought to strive to give the child adequate tools for locomotion. Another psychologic issue is the increasing trend to socialize, to play with other children. It is hard to be "one of the kids" if you have to squat every few minutes. From the surgical point of view, our colleagues tell us that opening up the infundibulum is easier in a young patient where the intima is not yet sclerosed and the muscle bundles have not hypertrophied.

Earlier correction can be performed with equal or almost equal safety at any time from the neonatal period on, if indicated (Castaneda et al, 1977). The principal indications are hypercyanotic spells (often not identified by intelligent parents of first children when pediatricians are not tuned in), noticeable limitations of effort (including sucking), frequent squatting and severe polycythemia (hematocrit greater than 55% in an infant).

Hospital mortality among infants at The Children's Hospital in Boston is less than 10%, when all patients are considered. Probably those without complicating anatomic factors, with good pulmonary arteries, classical ventricular defects and good clinical condition face half this risk. There is an impression that infants less than 3 months of age face higher risks; so far this has not been proved to everybody's satisfaction. The results of corrective operations are very good immediately and have stood the test of time for more than 25 years. Postoperative complications are increasingly rare; they include (a) heart block, (b) ventricular ectopic activity, (c) pulmonary regurgitation, and (d) aortic regurgitation.

SURGICAL PALLIATION

More than 40 years ago, Drs. Helen Taussig and Alfred Blalock (1945) performed the first aortopulmonary shunt by anastomosing the subclavian artery, contralateral to the aortic arch, to the pulmonary artery. This historic tour-de-force probably alleviated as much suffering as any subsequent undertaking in pediatric cardiac surgery. The drama was exciting. Surgery was performed on desperately ill, deformed, acutely suffering children; not prophylactically, to prevent something that might or might not happen in the future. The only other surgical triumph that we can compare with this is the relief of tight stenosis of the mitral valve in women with severe intractable dyspnea and hemoptysis.

Recognizing the enormous significance of this palliative operation should not stop us from looking at it realistically in the 1980s. The fact that it is palliative indicates that it is only a first stage; the second shoe will drop. The mortality rate of the Blalock-Taussig palliative operation should be judged in combination with the mortality rate of the subsequent corrective surgery. Only if the addition of the two risks equals or is less than the risk of one-stage correction should it be considered as an option. Even under these circumstances, the disadvantage to the parents of waiting with apprehension for definitive surgery should be taken into consideration, as well as the complications inherent in palliative operations (cerebrovascular accident, bacterial endocarditis, brain abscess).

Nevertheless, there are distinct indications even today for Blalock-Taussig shunts in the treatment of tetralogy of Fallot: (a) pulmonary atresia with ventricular defect and small pulmonary arteries in infants, (b) conus coronary artery, and (c) as an emergency measure for severe hypoxic spells, not manageable by medical means. The hospital mortality of the Blalock-Taussig operation depending on the age of the patients and the skill of the surgeons is 1–3%. The results in the survivors are very good. Cyanosis and clubbing decrease markedly and rarely is there congestive heart failure secondary to left ventricular volume overload. Although the development of pulmonary vascular obstructive disease is rare after the Blalock-Taussig operation, most pediatric cardiologists and cardiac surgeons prefer to follow it with definitive correction, electively, within a year or two (Lamberti et al, 1984; Rittenhouse et al, 1985; Karpawich et al, 1985; Kirklin et al, 1983).

Course and Prognosis

It is unrealistic to spend much time on the course of patients who do not undergo surgery for tetralogy of Fallot. In the developed countries, and most of the underdeveloped ones as well, almost all patients undergo surgery, palliative or corrective, at some time. With increasing surgical skills, effective correction of the malformation may be achieved at younger and younger ages.

Clearly, uncorrected pulmonary stenosis is a progressive condition and malalignment ventricular septal defects seldom change through the years. It follows from these facts that although infants may behave initially like those with ventricular defects in left-sided failure, eventually, through months or years, they become increasingly cyanotic and severely limited. Despite this, before the days of surgical repair, patients were reported to lead very restricted but, nevertheless, reasonably satisfactory lives into the fourth and fifth decades and even longer.

A word should be said here about patients who have severe tetralogy of Fallot with pulmonary atresia and large aortopulmonary collaterals; they have their own particular natural history (Fig. 6.21). Rarely, in infants, heart failure may occur because of the large collaterals. With growth, increasing pulmonary resistance, and anticongestive measures, most survive this period of stress. For many years and even decades they do well, only to develop complications again in the third or fourth decade. There may be a recurrence of congestive heart failure as occurs with any other large left-

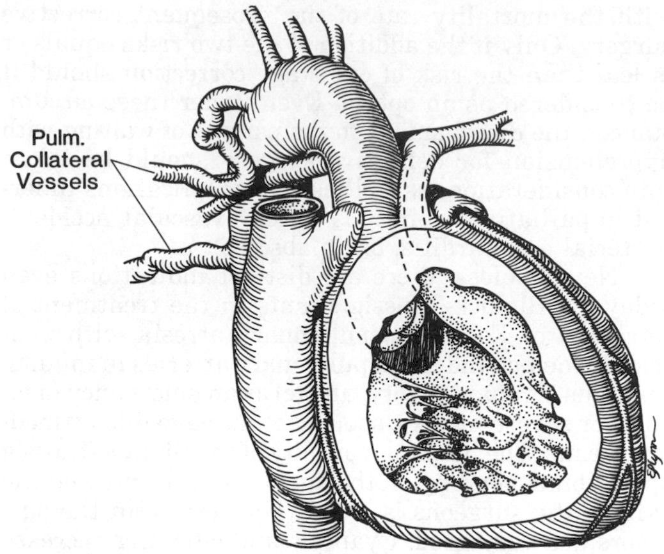

Figure 6.21. Anatomy of tetralogy of Fallot with pulmonary atresia. Note the diminutive size of the pulmonary artery and the presence of bizarre, primitive collateral vessels supplying the lung. Similar collaterals arising from the descending aorta supply the right and the left lung.

to-right shunt. In others, pulmonary vascular obstruction develops, the shunt through the collaterals decreases, and the patients become severely limited and deeply cyanotic. Still others may succumb to severe hemoptysis from an erosion of the large collaterals into the bronchi.

Children with tetralogy of Fallot and absent pulmonary valve have a unique syndrome recognizable by a very large main pulmonary artery and a loud systolic-diastolic murmur (Rabinovitch et al, 1982). Cyanosis is minimal. Fatal pulmonary complications, probably resulting from inherent pulmonary anomalies, occur in some of these infants. Others survive to undergo surgical correction at a later date (McCaughan et al, 1985).

COMPLICATIONS

Most complications are, or should be, of only historical interest in the 1980s and 1990s. Early surgery has decreased their incidence markedly.

Brain Abscess. Evidence of an acquired, localized lesion of the CNS beyond early infancy, in a cyanotic patient, should suggest the presence of brain abscess unless proven otherwise. Immediate CT scan and neurosurgical consultation are mandatory. Interestingly, brain abscess is almost never associated with infective endocarditis.

Cerebral Vascular Accident. This is the principal differential diagnostic issue when considering brain abscess. Inasmuch as nothing dramatic can be done for cerebral vascular accidents and because surgical drainage, after intravenous antibiotic treatments, brain abscess can be cured, the policy at The Children's Hospital in Boston is first to ascertain the presence or absence of brain abscess. Often, the circumstances under which cerebral vascular accidents occur clarify the diagnosis. Hemiplegia after a hypoxic spell or occurring during or immediately after cardiac catheterization or surgery is clearly not brain abscess. The anatomy and physiology of cerebral vascular accident, not caused by brain abscess, is not clear; hypoxia leading to encephalomalacia, embolic phenomena, or associated cerebral vascular anomalies have all been blamed for these episodes by respectable pathologists, without adequate proof. One item to be stressed here is that polycythemia, a relatively common cause of cerebral vascular accident in adults, almost never is the underlying cause in infants and young children with smooth intimal surfaces. By contrast, relative anemia (hematocrits within normal

CASE ILLUSTRATION

A 2-month-old boy was brought to the cardiac clinic at The Children's Hospital in Boston in October, 1985. He was born in West Germany where his father was serving in the U.S. army. His birth weight was 4.77 kg. This was the first baby of this young couple.

When the child was 3 days old, a murmur was discovered at the U.S. Army Hospital. According to the parents, an echocardiogram showed a small ventricular septal defect. This was not thought to be of major importance; the baby was discharged and the parents were told to bring him back to the hospital in 2 months. At home he gained weight and acted like a normal baby to the inexperienced parents. At 7 weeks, his weight was 11 lbs, 12 oz. The cardiologist who saw him on the return visit thought that he might be cyanotic. In retrospect, the grandmother thought that she had noticed tachypnea from the first day of life. The cardiologist in Germany diagnosed a large ventricular defect with pulmonary hypertension and suggested catheterization. The parents wanted to have the baby taken care of closer to home and brought him back to the United States. The local cardiologist diagnosed tetralogy of Fallot clinically and had it confirmed by two-dimensional echocardiogram.

At the first office visit in Boston, at 2 months, he seemed like a well-developed, well-nourished infant. He was slightly, but definitely, blue and tachypneic. His heart rate was 126; the respiratory rate, 50. The parents maintained that he was doing fine, although they were somewhat concerned about his color. He had a lot of "gas pains" and maybe a couple of times a week he had episodes of uncontrollable crying lasting between 30 and 60 minutes.

At auscultation, both the first and second heart sounds were single and the second sound was loud at the lower left sternal border. There was a constant ejection click at the apex. A grade III systolic ejection murmur was noted at the lower left sternal border, transmitting up the left sternal border. There were no diastolic murmurs. The electrocardiogram showed a mean frontal plane axis of +110° with right ventricular hypertrophy, probably abnormal for that age. The chest film revealed a small heart with right ventricular contour and ischemic lung fields (Fig. 6.20). The hematocrit was 45%. Two-dimensional echocardiogram confirmed the diagnosis of tetralogy of Fallot, with good-sized pulmonary arteries, normal coronary arteries, and a left aortic arch.

The parents brought the baby to Boston originally for a second opinion. They wanted to know whether, indeed, the diagnosis was correct and, if so, what we thought of the management plans suggested by the local cardiologist. The plan, as outlined to them locally, was that because the baby was "doing well" he should be watched for a few weeks or months and then have a Blalock-Taussig shunt, with repair to follow in a year or two.

The parents were told that, indeed, the diagnosis was as stated. There was some doubt that he was really "doing well," however, and some concern about the crying episodes, of which he produced a good example in the office. It was thought also that a hematocrit of 45% was on the high side for a 2-month-old infant and might indicate a relatively low "prevailing" arterial saturation. They were told that the management plan as outlined by the local cardiologist was perfectly acceptable in many institutions, but would not be the one preferred here. It was a difficult situation, inasmuch as the family came to Boston only for a consultation and had no idea that the baby might be kept in the hospital. The doctors certainly did not want to appear to pressure them. Nevertheless, the parents went along with their suggestion.

He was admitted and a skin Po_2 electrode was placed on his abdomen. When the baby was resting during the ensuing hours in the ward, readings averaging 50 torr were obtained, but suddenly, on two or three occasions, it dropped to 10 torr during the night in the hospital. The next morning he was sent to the catheterization laboratory where the echo diagnosis was confirmed and the anatomy was deemed to be favorable. Surgery was planned in 2 or 3 days, on a Monday, but because of several more episodes of spontaneous hypoxia during the second 24 hours, the surgeons operated on him on a Saturday morning, 2 days after admission. Under deep hypothermic cardiac arrest, his large malaligned ventricular defect was closed with Dacron, the tight infundibular obstruction and the pulmonary valve annulus were incised, and a transannular pericardial patch was placed. He was discharged 10 days postoperatively. He returned for a postoperative check-up 2 weeks later and was doing fine. He has had no more crying spells, he seemed happy, and had a good appetite. On physical examination, he did not appear to be cyanotic, the second sound was split, and the P_2 moved appropriately with respirations. He had a grade III ejection murmur without a diastolic component. His chest film was unchanged, but his right ventricular hypertrophy may have diminished slightly on the electrocardiogram. His hematocrit was 40%. He will be recatheterized 1 year postoperatively.

QUESTIONS AND COMMENTS

What are the indications for surgery in infants with tetralogy of Fallot in the newborn period?

Deep cyanosis and cyanotic spells are the usual reasons for requesting cardiac surgery in newborns with tetralogy of Fallot.

What is the role of β-blockers in the management of babies with tetralogy of Fallot?

There is no reason to use β-blockers in infants with tetralogy of Fallot. If the infant has had a convincing cyanotic spell then surgery, either primary repair or palliation and secondary repair, is needed.

Are there factors other than infundibular spasm which contribute to cyanotic spells?

Anemia, excitement, physical activity, dyspnea, systemic vasodilators, or cardiac catheterization tend to promote cyanotic spells.

A 15-year-old-boy with tetralogy of Fallot, surviving because of an arterial shunt develops increasing cyanosis and congestive heart failure with persistence of a systolic and diastolic murmur. How is this possible?

An increasing shunt would tend to make the patient pinker and might cause congestive failure. Given evidence for congestive heart failure and increasing cyanosis, an enlarging shunt (a rare phenomenon) cannot be the cause of the failure. Rather, some other cause for the congestion must be sought. A reasonable explanation would be the development of aortic regurgitation. The aortic valve ring is dilated in all patients with tetralogy of Fallot, particularly those with pulmonary atresia. In addition, infective endocarditis on the aortic valve may have caused the aortic regurgitation.

What are the possible mechanisms for the development of congestive heart failure in patients with tetralogy of Fallot in addition to aortic regurgitation?

As a matter of clinical experience, cyanotic patients with tetralogy of Fallot do not have congestive heart failure in childhood; if congestive failure is evident, some other explanation should be sought. Congestive heart failure is occasionally seen in infants with tetralogy of Fallot, pulmonary atresia and large collaterals, where there is excessive pulmonary flow. It may be seen after shunt surgery when the shunt is too large. The infant with tetralogy of Fallot and an absent pulmonary valve often appears to have congestive heart failure when the problem is primarily pulmonary.

Why is it necessary for patients with tetralogy of Fallot to have cardiac catheterization when the diagnosis can be established by echocardiography?

Cardiac catheterization is undertaken to clarify three anatomic problems that may complicate surgery. A conus coronary is a particular problem. Rarely, a patient will have additional ventricular septal defects and often there is stenosis at the junction of the main and left main pulmonary arteries. All of these problems require special attention at the time of surgery.

range for children with full arterial saturation, but inadequate for cyanotic patients) is fairly commonly associated with cerebral vascular accidents. The conventional explanation is the inadequate oxygen content of the blood delivered to the central nervous system.

Infective Endocarditis (see pp. 390). Patients who have uncorrected tetralogy of Fallot, even those with adequate oxygen saturation because of well-functioning arterial shunts, are prone to the development of endocarditis. It may not be too far-fetched to suggest that aortic regurgitation, a not uncommon complication of tetralogy of Fallot, might make the aortic valve a site for infective endocarditis. No data are available on the vulnerability of patients to infective endocarditis after "complete repair." It does make sense, and experience supports the thesis, that the incidence is much lower than in patients who have not undergone surgical treatment. Remembering the complexity of the anatomy, however, we continue to insist on meticulous dental hygiene as well as penicillin prophylaxis even after first-class repair.

Hemorrhagic Disorders. Hemoptysis may occur rarely in older patients with large collaterals and may be due to erosion into the pulmonary artery of these large systemic vessels. Bed rest with moderate sedation is the usual treatment. Aggressive radiologists and cardiologists are contemplating obliteration of these collaterals at catheterization (see Therapeutic Catheterization). No large scale experience is available at present. Bleeding and clotting problems, referred to earlier, are not uncommon in older patients with severe polycythemia.

COARCTATION OF THE AORTA

Definition

Coarctation of the aorta is a narrowing or constriction of the aortic isthmus. It is a common, potentially fatal congenital cardiac malformation, clearly progressive through the years. In a minority of instances, the defect is solitary; more often it is combined with other serious malformations.

Basic Science

ANATOMY

The localized, constricted segment of the aortic isthmus is almost invariably juxtaductal (Fig. 6.22), with some progression from preductal to postductal as the child grows older (Gitterberger-deGroot and Elzinga, 1983). It may be caused by ductal fibers surrounding—"almost lassoing"—the aortic wall. If not corrected, the narrowing eventually becomes more severe through the progressive intimal proliferation. This is the anatomy of discrete uncomplicated coarctation, representing probably no more than 20% of the total identified in infancy.

Complex coarctations, associated with other cardiac malformations also have this discrete juxtaductal component but, in addition, there is often tubular hypoplasia of the aortic arch. A ventricular defect is found in at least half of the complex coarctations; mitral regurgitation, mitral stenosis, aortic stenosis, and great vessel anomalies are also frequently present.

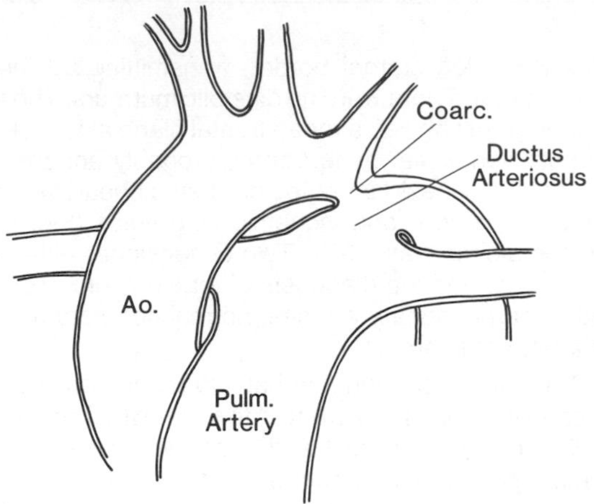

Figure 6.22. Diagram of coarctation of the aorta and a patent ductus arteriosus.

PHYSIOLOGY

The physiology of coarctation of the aorta may best be discussed first in terms of constriction of the isthmus. During the fetal circulation (see Fetal Circulation), the isthmus is bypassed by the ductus arteriosus carrying 90% of the right ventricular output down the descending aorta. After birth, under normal circumstances, the duct constricts and the right ventricular output enters the left heart through the pulmonary capillaries. At the same time, the placental circulation is eliminated. Under normal circumstances, this causes a sizeable increase in both flow and pressure work on the left ventricle. If, in addition to this physiologic left ventricular stress, the aortic isthmus is also constricted because of the ductal fibers surrounding it, it is not surprising that the left ventricle fails, with increased end-diastolic and pulmonary capillary pressure, pulmonary edema, a low output state and often sudden circulatory collapse. Sudden circulatory collapse is associated with closure of the ductus arteriosus and usually occurs in the second week of life, although it may happen in the first days and weeks.

In complex coarctation with tubular hypoplasia and a ventricular defect, with or without other defects, all of the above difficulties are compounded. A catastrophe may occur earlier and may lead to death sooner, because of a huge left-to-right shunt resulting in pulmonary hypertension.

Beyond the newborn period, two other elements are added to the physiologic picture. First, collaterals allow a run-off from the ascending to descending aorta, resulting in a decrease in ascending aortic pressure and a bypass of the systemic output into the descending aorta. The second factor is the hypertrophy, and even hyperplasia, of the left ventricular myocardium, enabling the left ventricle to cope with the increased work load.

Epidemiology

Coarctation of the aorta, as a solitary lesion or associated with patent ductus arteriosus, ventricular septal defect, or mitral or aortic valve lesions was found to be the fourth most common defect among infants in the New England Regional Infant Cardiac Program. It occurred in 7.5% of a total of 2251 babies born with congenital cardiac malformation (Table 6.3), or about 15 patients per 100,000 live births (Fyler et al, 1980a).

Diagnosis

At least two-thirds of the patients with coarctation in the New England Regional Infant Cardiac Program were admitted to a cardiac center within the first 2 months of life (Fyler et al, 1980a).

The history is often that of a baby (56% males) with normal birth and development doing well during the first days of life. He may even be discharged from the hospital at a usual time, only to develop tachypnea, tachycardia, or pallor tinged with cyanosis at 1–3 weeks of age.

PHYSICAL EXAMINATION

Physical examination, in addition to the above, reveals a hyperactive large left ventricle with decreased and delayed femoral pulses. On auscultation, the second sound is narrowly split, if at all, with a loud pulmonary component. There is a third sound at the apex, possibly prolonging into a diastolic rumble. Murmurs are not striking and may even be absent. An apical systolic blow, resulting from mitral incompetence may be heard. More characteristic is a loud stenotic murmur over the spine due to the coarctation itself, or at the second right interspace or suprasternal notch, caused by associated aortic valve disease (Fig. 6.3*B*). A diastolic rumble is present in 25% of patients. The liver may be enlarged and sometimes, though rarely in infants, there may be edema. In patients with complex coarctation, a ventricular defect murmur predominates and, because of the tubular hypoplasia, the left radial pulse may also be diminished, contrasting markedly with the hyperactive apex.

ELECTROCARDIOGRAPHY

Irrespective of the complexity of the lesion, the electrocardiogram in newborns with congestive failure shows right ventricular hypertrophy. In those with unrepaired solitary coarctation left ventricular hypertrophy gradually develops through months and years. Even in older children with isolated coarctation, a left ventricular strain pattern is seldom seen. If such is noted, associated anomalies, particularly aortic stenosis, should be suspected.

RADIOGRAPHY

Chest films in infants with isolated coarctation and heart failure show a large heart with passive congestion of the pulmonary vasculature. Those with complex coarctation may have huge hearts with both active and passive vascular congestion. Children and adolescents who have not undergone surgery and who have well-developed collaterals and hypertrophied, compensated left ventricles, may have normal-sized hearts with normal pulmonary vasculature. In the barium-filled esophagus, there is an indentation at the narrow coarcted segment of the aorta, with dilated segments before and after the coarctation.

ECHO-DOPPLER STUDY

A two-dimensional echocardiogram usually demonstrates the coarcted segment as well as any other associated anomalies, including a patent ductus arteriosus.

CARDIAC CATHETERIZATION

For practical purposes, at The Children's Hospital in Boston, cardiac catheterization with angiography is performed in infants only when there is congestive failure, for the purpose of clearly identifying the associated anomalies. It is rare that a child or adolescent with isolated coarctation is catheterized preoperatively.

Catheterization reveals the following:

1. Oxygen saturation studies show a left-to-right or right-to-left shunt if there is an open ductus. With a right-to-left shunt the saturation in the descending aorta is lower than in the right brachial artery, unless there is associated transposition in complex coarctations. Ventricular shunts are noted and the pulmonary veins may have reduced oxygen saturation if there is pulmonary edema. In uncomplicated coarctations without failure, the systemic arterial saturation is normal.
2. Pressure data indicate hypertension in the left ventricle and in the precoarcted segment of the ascending aorta. With heart failure, left ventricular end-diastolic pressures and left atrial pressures are elevated. In critical coarctations, there is pulmonary hypertension at the systemic level and, occasionally, an aortic valve gradient may be demonstrated resulting from a bicuspid aortic valve.
3. The cardiac output is normal except in critically ill infants, who have a low output.
4. Angiocardiograms are probably the most important part of the study. They outline the anatomy of the arch, the site and number of the ventricular defects, and the status of the mitral valve, as well as the size of the two ventricles.

Management

The treatment of coarctation is surgical. The rationale for this dogmatic statement for the complex lesion is clearcut; patients with tubular hypoplasia and a ventricular defect do not survive without surgery. For patients with isolated coarctation, the issues are a bit more cloudy. Neonates with discrete coarctation and heart failure should be managed first medically with prostaglandins, diuretics, and digitalis (in this order). This may bring them out of their precarious state within days. The dilemma then is: Should surgery be performed right away, within weeks, or should it be postponed for months, even a couple of years, to ensure better, long-term results? This issue has not been completely settled; our personal opinion is that surgery should be performed sooner rather than later, for the following reasons: (a) patients who responded well to medical management may still relapse into a critical state at home after discharge, (b) after 3 months of age, the operative results do not improve further with age, and (c) there is some evidence that long-term results on blood pressure may be better if patients are operated on early.

Whether, and when, patients with isolated coarctation without heart failure or other symptoms should be operated on at any age is still another problem. The conventional wisdom that all these patients need surgery is based on poor control data from the 1940s (Reifenstein et al, 1947). Nevertheless, these are the only data in the literature and conform with individual observations of experienced clinicians. Rarely do we encounter asymptomatic patients with coarctation beyond the fourth and fifth decades. Whereas this may occur, it cannot be counted upon. Given the safety of surgical intervention and the total impossibility and probably unethical nature of setting up a randomized study to-

CASE ILLUSTRATION

A 10-day-old male infant was reported to have had an increased respiratory rate from birth. The baby nursed well but grunted and wheezed.

On physical examination, the respiratory rate was 100, the pulse was 140, and blood pressure in the right arm was 87/57 and in the right leg 80/50. There were audible wheezes. There was a grade II systolic murmur, equally loud in the back, with a gallop sound at the apex. The liver was palpable 2 cm below the right costal margin. The pulses in the upper extremities were more readily palpable than were those in the lower, where the pulse was delayed.

The arterial blood gases showed a pH of 7.4 and the Po_2 was 44 with an oxygen saturation of 88%. The electrocardiogram showed right ventricular hypertrophy. The chest film showed a large heart with increased pulmonary vascularity and evidence of pulmonary edema (Fig. 6.23). A two-dimensional echocardiogram showed a large midmuscular ventricular septal defect and a coarctation of the aorta.

The baby was treated with digoxin, furosemide, and spironolactone. Two days later, cardiac catheterization showed severe coarctation of the aorta with a large left-to-right shunt through a midmuscular ventricular septal defect. There was pulmonary hypertension (75/28 mean = 50). At 2 weeks of age, the coarctation was resected and an end-to-end anastomosis accomplished. The baby improved slowly and was discharged 2 weeks later at 1 month of age with a respiratory rate varying between 60 and 70, a heart rate of 130 and blood pressure in the arm of 90/50. He had a grade IV harsh systolic murmur and a grade II mid-diastolic rumble. He was receiving digoxin, furosemide, and spironolactone.

At age 6 months, the infant is growing well and at the 75th percentile for height and weight. His heart rate is 120, his respiratory rate is 36, and blood pressure is 110/70 in the right arm and 90/- in the right leg. The baby appears well. He has a grade II systolic murmur with no diastolic murmur. The electrocardiogram is normal and, on the chest film, his heart size is within normal limits, with normal pulmonary vascularity.

QUESTIONS AND COMMENTS

Can and should a baby with coarctation of the aorta and congestive heart failure be managed medically?

Newborns and babies with any suggestion of complicating cardiac defects usually cannot. Infants with isolated coarctation of the aorta in whom congestive failure develops after the first month of life often can be safely managed medically. Whether or not medical management should be used depends on the circumstances. Is the family reliable? Do they live near by? How well did the infant respond initially to treatment? It should be clearly understood that the advantage of medical management is perhaps to avoid reoperation for recoarctation when coarctation repair is carried out in early infancy.

How does the treatment of interrupted aortic arch differ from that of coarctation?

In principle, the plan is to establish a connection between the proximal and distal sections of the aorta and to manage the other defects. In practice, the problem is more complicated because these infants are very ill, often require a conduit to establish a connection and consistently have other defects, often including subaortic stenosis.

What are the chances that a ventricular septal defect associated with a coarctation of the aorta will spontaneously close up?

Ventricular defects close up at the same rate whether they are associated with coarctation of the aorta or not (±30%). Consequently, when evaluating a patient with complex coarctation, a moderate-sized membranous defect might kept under observation while a similar-sized subpulmonary defect would be scheduled for surgery.

A baby in the newborn nursery was carefully examined and found to have good femoral pulses. Two weeks later the infant was admitted to a hospital in profound congestive heart failure because of coarctation of the aorta. Where was the error?

There was no error! This is not an unusal observation. Femoral pulses may be good at birth because the blood supply is via a ductus arteriosus that later closed or because the coarctation was not present at birth and appeared later because of ductal fibers constricting the aorta.

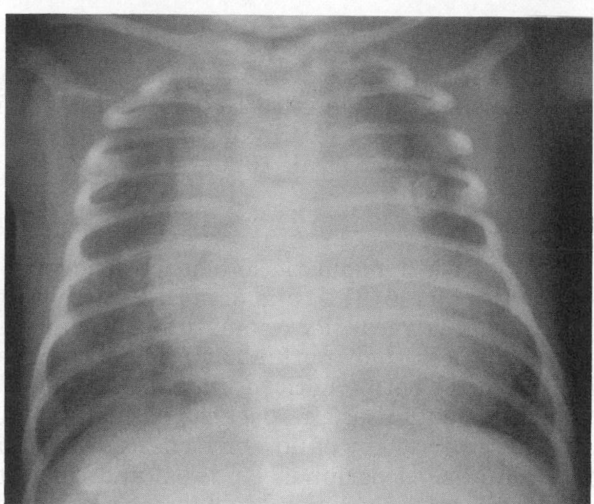

Figure 6.23. Chest film of baby with coarctation of the aorta. Note the large heart with increased pulmonary vascular markings and pulmonary congestion.

day, the dictum remains, based on a number of reasons, that all should be treated surgically. Given the information alluded to earlier, to the effect that control of systemic hypertension is more reliable the earlier surgery is performed, we arbitrarily recommend elective relief of coarctation in asymptomatic children under school age even if there is normal or only slightly elevated right arm blood pressure.

The operative technique has not yet been definitely settled. In the original publications of Gross (1950), the coarctation was resected and an end-to-end anastomosis was established. If the coarcted segment was long, it was bridged with a homograft or Dacron prosthesis. Waldhausen and Nahrwold (1966) suggested a subclavian flap aortoplasty, using the left subclavian artery as a "roof" over the narrowed segment. The enthusiasm for this procedure has abated somewhat (Zeimer et al, 1986), but it is still a useful surgical tool.

The lesions associated with complex coarctation have to be dealt with individually by the experienced surgeon. The technical details are beyond the scope of this volume. The ventricular defect in infants with tubular hypoplasia may be left open after the coarctation is dealt with, hoping that it may close spontaneously, as it does in about 20% of the cases. The practicality of this depends in part on the location of the defect and the clinical postoperative course. Some babies in the intensive care unit just do not tolerate the ventricular defect. Some of these may have to undergo banding; in others, the ventricular defect should be closed.

Surgical mortality after the subclavian flap technique is cited as 3% by Waldhausen and Nahrwold (1966). The majority of the babies had associated lesions.

Course and Prognosis

The matter of postoperative "recurrences" is a serious problem; the possibility remains that, for one reason or another, the obstruction was inadequately relieved at surgery. At any rate, it cannot be automatically assumed that the operation is curative; these patients should be followed carefully with blood pressure measurements at rest and on the treadmill. Most of the residual hypertension is probably due to a persistent gradient; small pressure differences between the right arm and leg at rest may become significant on strenuous effort (Freed et al, 1979). Incidence figures for residual hypertension are hard to obtain, but our personal estimate is that it occurs in at least 25% 5 years postoperatively. Persistent postoperative hypertension in both upper and lower extremities is another worry; this is less common than is the residual gradient and may be related to the age at operation. These are all worrisome questions, with no precise, unbiased answers. Therefore, we stress that surgery for coarctation may just be a palliative procedure in a not inconsequential percentage of patients.

A recent approach to the management of "recoarctation" is balloon angioplasty, introduced in 1983 by Lock et al (Table 6.2). Although the procedure is not eminently successful on virginal lesions, it is a reasonable alternative for re-operation.

COMPLICATIONS

Infective endocarditis is a relatively common complication of coarctation. Whether the site of infection is in the aorta itself or on the bicuspid aortic valve is hard to determine. For this reason, however, endocarditis prophylaxis is mandatory even after apparently successful relief of the obstruction.

Vascular complications—cerebral vascular accidents, ruptured aorta, or cerebral thrombosis—are rare in pediatric practice. Systemic hypertension, even occasionally with readings of close to 200 mm Hg in the right arm, seldom should be regarded as a prime indication for surgery. With the development of collaterals, the pressure usually drops.

Aortic regurgitation and *aortic stenosis* are often associated with the bicuspid aortic valve and should be judged and managed on their own merits. The problem of which lesion, the coarctation or the aortic valve, should be operated on first, depends on the respective severities.

HYPOPLASTIC LEFT VENTRICLE

Definition

Hypoplastic left ventricle is a general term Noonan and Nadas (1959) used clinically to describe a variety of cardiac anomalies associated with a diminutive left ventricle so small as to prohibit normal function. The majority of patients with these anomalies have aortic atresia, mitral atresia, or a combination of severe mitral and aortic stenosis associated with hypoplasia of the aorta.

Basic Science

It is presumed that the hypoplasia of the left ventricular structures is related to diminished left-sided blood flow during fetal development. This hypothesis is supported by demonstration of a small, or even prematurely closed, foramen ovale in some of these patients. The left ventricle may be minuscule and the ascending aorta is so small that it carries only coronary blood flow (Fig. 6.24). The mitral and aortic valve rings are small and the mitral and aortic valves are either severely stenotic or atretic. The left atrium is small.

Little or no blood passes through the left atrium to the left ventricle and to the aorta pre- or postnatally. Fetal circulation (essentially a right-sided circulation) is thought to be adequate, inasmuch as birth weights in these babies are normal. At birth, the problems presented are formidable. The small left atrium must accommodate a greater than normal pulmonary blood flow. Exit from the left atrium is usually entirely left to right through the foramen ovale. To survive, it is required that there be an atrial defect or an incompetent foramen ovale. The right ventricle provides both the systemic and pulmonary blood and, therefore, is large and hypertrophied. The ductus arteriosus supplies the entire cardiac output relatively satisfactorily at first. In the vast majority of patients, however, the ductus closes, as programmed, suddenly causing signs of low output in the first days of life. The effects of hypoxia and reduced peripheral perfusion result in acidosis and transient relaxation of the ductal spasm. The patient recovers, only to go through the cycle again, ultimately, without medical intervention, succumbing to low output in the first week of life.

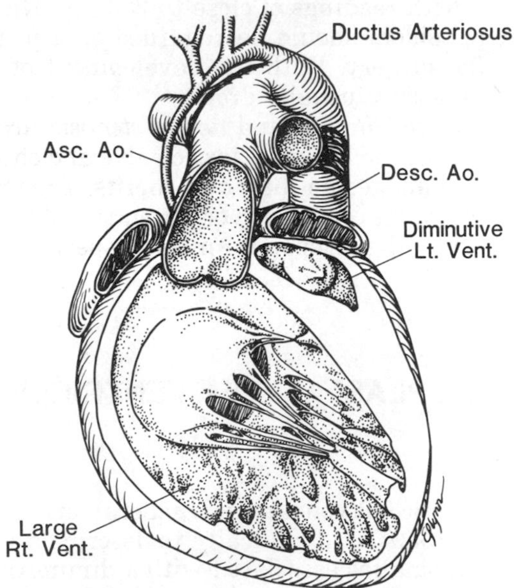

Figure 6.24. Anatomy of aortic atresia. Note the tiny ascending aorta which carries blood retrograde to the coronary arteries. Note the large ductus arteriosus which carries the entire cardiac output.

Epidemiology

Using the definition presented, the prevalence of hypoplastic left ventricle is 16/10,000 live births (fifth most common cardiac defect among critically ill infants; Table 6.3; Fyler et al, 1980a).

Diagnosis

Infants with hypoplastic left heart syndrome are predominantly male (67%) and of normal birth weight; only 10% have extracardiac anomalies. Although these infants have less than normal arterial oxygen saturation, this may not be noticed until an episode of reduced cardiac output occurs because of ductal closure. This is characterized by pallor (often described as "poor color"), diminished peripheral pulses, and congestive heart failure (tachycardia and tachypnea). With recovery, these observations regress; indeed, the infant may recover sufficiently that the pediatrician arriving at the nurse's request may question the validity of the observations, only to have the infant repeat the same sequence within minutes or hours. There may be a minimal systolic murmur.

MINOR LABORATORY TESTS

There is a reduced level of umbilical arterial oxygen saturation which, even with exposure to 100% ambient oxygen, rises to levels less than normal (Po_2, 150 torr). Comparison of oxygen levels in the right radial artery and the descending aorta shows no significant difference.

ELECTROCARDIOGRAPHY

The electrocardiogram shows a dominant right ventricle, often with absence of left ventricular forces.

RADIOGRAPHY

The heart is enlarged and there is increased pulmonary vascularity.

ECHO-DOPPLER STUDY

Two-dimensional echocardiographic examination of the heart reveals the diminutive left heart structures and establishes the diagnosis.

CARDIAC CATHETERIZATION

There is little value in cardiac catheterization unless some surgical procedure is being considered.

Management

Prostaglandins are life-saving for these babies. With the first episode of low cardiac output, prostaglandins help to resuscitate the infant and permit continued survival until the diagnosis is established and a plan of management can be formulated. There is no universally accepted surgical management for infants with hypoplastic left ventricle. Two methods are being tested. More than 50% of patients survive initial palliation

CASE ILLUSTRATION

A male, full-term infant, weighing 3.5 kg, appeared normal at birth but twelve hours later had a transient episode of "poor color." On the second day of life a more profound episode of pallor and tachypnea was noted. An echocardiogram demonstrated the hypoplastic left heart syndrome.

The patient was transferred to The Children's Hospital in Boston while receiving intravenous prostaglandins and oxygen (Fig. 6.25). The diagnosis was confirmed by a second echocardiogram and cardiac catheterization was carried out to document the status of the aorta before to surgery. No coarctation was seen, but typical aortic hypoplasia associated with aortic atresia was noted. The mitral valve was atretic.

On the fourth day of life, the baby underwent palliative cardiac surgery in which the pulmonary artery was divided and attached entirely to the arch of the aorta; the pulmonary blood flow was supplied through a Blalock operation to the pulmonary artery distal to the division. An atrial septal defect was created. There appeared to be some evidence for coarctation at the time of surgery. The ductus was ligated.

The infant had a somewhat stormy postoperative course but was discharged at 3 weeks of age.

By 2 months, it was clear that there was coarctation of the aorta. Angiograms demonstrated severe coarctation at the usual site. This responded to balloon dilatation.

At 11 months of age cardiac catheterization demonstrated a mean pulmonary artery pressure of 13 mm Hg, with right and left pulmonary arteries of normal size and shape and without obstruction. The right ventricular end-diastolic pressure was 8. The arterial oxygen saturation was 75%.

QUESTIONS AND COMMENTS

Should all patients with hypoplastic left heart syndrome undergo palliative surgery?

Attempts to salvage these babies by transplantation or by palliative surgery, such as described in this case, are being made. The mortality is high, the risk of complication is high and the long range results are not clear. This surgery should not be considered as standard practice.

Is it not unusual to see coarctation of the aorta associated with the hypoplastic left heart syndrome?

When children began to survive after palliative surgery for hypoplastic left heart syndrome, it was learned that coarctation of the aorta is a common concomitant. When studied at birth coarctation is relatively rare but among the surviving children coarctation is relatively common some weeks later.

How many survivors are there who have had successful Fontan procedures or transplantation?

As of August 1986, there are three with Fontan procedures and one with transplantation.

consisting of (a) connecting the main pulmonary artery to the aorta, (b) dividing the ductus arteriosus, and (c) providing for pulmonary blood flow through a systemic pulmonary shunt distal to ligation of the main pulmonary artery. Methods of converting the main pulmonary artery into an ascending aorta vary: a number

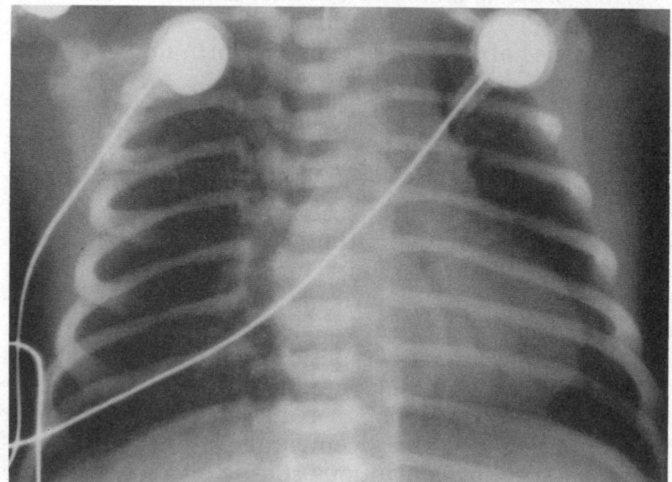

Figure 6.25. Chest film of infant with a hypoplastic left ventricle. Note cardiac enlargement and pulmonary vascular engorgement.

of them have been successful. These maneuvers allow the patient to grow up to become a candidate for a modified Fontan operation at a later date (Norwood et al, 1983). While more than 50% survive this first stage palliation, the numbers of patients surviving after a second stage Fontan operation are too few to be sure what the future holds.

Another approach has been cardiac transplantation (Bailey et al, 1986). Perhaps the kindest, and in many instances the wisest, decision is to accept the inevitable.

Course And Prognosis

Without surgery these infants die within days or weeks of birth.

PATENT DUCTUS ARTERIOSUS

Definition

A patent ductus arteriosus (PDA) is the persistent patency of the normal fetal structure beyond the expected time of closure, usually within the first hours or days of life. Within the past several years, as physiologists and pediatric cardiologists have been concentrating on the ductus arteriosus of premature infants, a distinction has been made between a "persistent ductus arteriosus" (delayed closures in small prematures) and "patent ductus arteriosus" which stays open permanently unless closed by surgical means.

Basic Science

ANATOMY

The ductus arteriosus is the remnant of the left sixth aortic arch, connecting the distal portion of the main pulmonary artery, near the bifurcation, to the aorta, just beyond the left subclavian artery (Fig. 6.26). During early fetal life, the lumen is large—as large as the aorta; in the course of normal development, the lumen narrows through constriction and thickening of the intima with endocardial "mounds." Under pathologic conditions (i.e., intrauterine German measles or infection) the normal ontogenetic process is interfered with and the ductus arterious remains open until it is medically or surgically closed. It is the prevailing opinion that the basic developmental process is not disturbed in the ductus of premature infants. The process goes on, only the baby is born too soon. Both administration of corticosteroids to the mother during pregnancy and indomethacin treatment for the baby hasten the process of closing.

PHYSIOLOGY

In its pure form, the ductus arteriosus represents a left-sided volume overload. The left ventricle has to pump a larger volume of blood to allow for the runoff, through the ductus, into the low-resistance pulmonary artery and still furnish the systemic circulation with an adequate cardiac output under adequate pressures; this demands increased volume work from the left ventricle. The large pulmonary flow, sometimes four to six times normal, representing the combined right ventricular and ductal output, is returned to the left atrium, which must dilate to accommodate it. Under these circumstances the right atrium and right ventricle are relatively unaffected. This theoretical situation, produced by a laboratory model of the circulation, rarely exists in real life. A patent ductus arteriosus of any size will be associated with some degree of pulmonary hypertension owing to arteriolar obstruction, which then will impose a pressure load on the right ventricle.

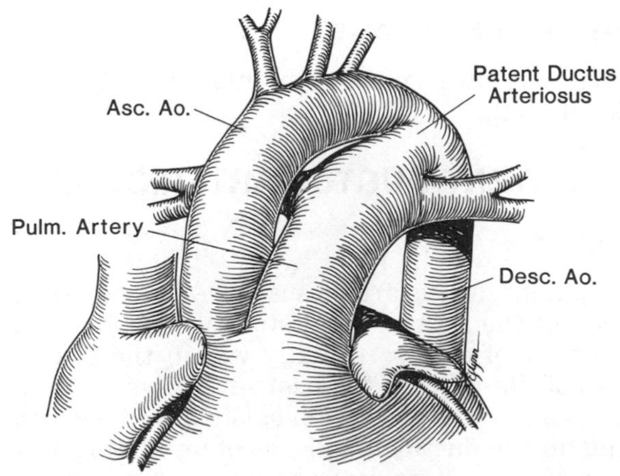

Figure 6.26. Anatomy of patent ductus arteriosus.

Epidemiology

Among the critically ill infants studied by the New England Regional Infant Cardiac Program, patent ductus arteriosus was sixth in ranking order, with a prevalence of less than 7% (Table 6.3; Fyler et al, 1980a). In two large pediatric cardiology units with active surgical services (The Children's Hospital of Boston and The Hospital for Sick Children in Toronto) (Nadas and Fyler, 1972; Keith et al, 1979) patent ductus arteriosus was second in ranking order (15% and 12% prevalence, respectively) among a pediatric population representing the entire age spectrum. It is assumed that these figures represent real "PDAs" and not the "persistency" of premature babies.

Diagnosis

Patent ductus arteriosus (the condition not associated with prematurity) may be familial in nature, may occur in babies born at high altitudes, may be the consequence of a rubella pregnancy, or, as in most instances, have an unknown etiology. The largest may manifest themselves in early infancy (although not usually in the newborn period) through congestive failure. An unusual group of patients has been described with large ductus arteriosus in whom heart failure never develops; they may, indeed, have persistence of the fetal arteriolar pattern and follow the course of progressive pulmonary vascular obstructive disease (Eisenmenger syndrome, see Pulmonary Arterial Hypertension). This group is ill-defined, occurrence is rare, and descriptions are mostly anecdotal; the patients are discovered later in childhood with evidence of cyanosis, without ever having gone through the congestive heart failure phase.

Moderate-to-small patent ductus arteriosus is usually discovered by the pediatrician on routine checkups, because of the characteristic continuous murmur.

PHYSICAL EXAMINATION

The physical examination is dominated by the continuous systolic and diastolic murmur, not necessarily occupying the entirety of both systole and diastole, but certainly going through the second sound in a crescendo-decrescendo fashion. This is the typical Gibson murmur (Fig. 6.3*A*), heard best at the second left interspace; the transmission varies with intensity. Often the murmur assumes a stenotic character at the second right interspace, corresponding to that of relative or absolute aortic stenosis. If a ductus is very large or very small it is often accompanied by atypical murmurs, lacking the continuous character, and it may be entirely systolic in nature. The first heart sound is usually not remarkable; the second sound is well split with a loud pulmonary component, moving appropriately with respirations.

The patients, usually female (2:1), are slender with left chest deformity, a hyperkinetic apex and pulsatile carotids. The pulse pressure is wide and peripheral pulses are bounding. There is no cyanosis except late in the disease with pulmonary vascular obstruction or in the very young with severe heart failure and pulmonary venous unsaturation. As mentioned earlier, the largest ductus in the youngest patients are accompanied by evidence of left-sided failure.

MINOR LABORATORY TESTS

Routine laboratory tests are unremarkable.

ELECTROCARDIOLOGY

The cardiogram in the patient with classical patent ductus arteriosus shows a normal inferior mean frontal plane axis (between 30° and 90°) and left ventricular hypertrophy in the chest leads with P mitrale. Pure right ventricular hypertrophy, even combined ventricular hypertrophy, should serve as a warning sign of pulmonary hypertension or even a different diagnosis (truncus arteriosus, aortopulmonary window, etc).

RADIOGRAPHY

The chest films show a large aorta and an equally large pulmonary artery with left ventricular and left atrial enlargement and pulmonary vascular engorgement.

ECHO-DOPPLER STUDY

Two-dimensional echocardiography shows a nonspecific left ventricular overload with an increased left atrial-aortic ratio and it identifies the presence and morphology of the patent ductus. Doppler estimates of the volume and direction of the flow are relatively accurate. Two-dimensional echocardiography is the best tool for differential diagnosis against common truncus as well as aortopulmonary window. It is not unreasonable to suggest that all patients with an "atypical" ductus should have expert echocardiographic evaluation.

CARDIAC CATHETERIZATION

There is no need for routine catheterization of patients with classical patent ductus arteriosus. The experienced cardiologist or cardiac surgeon needs only a stethoscope to make the diagnosis. Chest films, ECGs and, in rare instances, echocardiograms should confirm the clinical impression in the vast majority. Catheterization should be reserved for patients with less than classical profiles and for those who are suspected of having pulmonary vascular disease. More recently, aggressive interventionist cardiologists have suggested cardiac catheterization not for diagnosis but for therapy.

At catheterization, typically, the following information is collected:

1. There is a left-to-right shunt with pulmonary systemic flow ratios varying from 1.5:1 to 4:1. The oxygen step-up occurs at the pulmonary artery, particularly at the left pulmonary artery level. Systemic arterial saturation is normal unless there is pulmonary venous unsaturation due to pulmonary edema. At times, it may be confusing to find a sizable atrial left-to-right shunt as well, because of a stretched foramen ovale caused by left atrial dilatation. The systemic cardiac output is normal.
2. Left atrial pressure may be elevated. The systemic artery shows a wide pulse pressure. In the classical, moderate-sized patent ductus arteriosus, pulmonary arterial pressure is normal; in infants and children with a large ductus there is hyperkinetic pulmonary hypertension of varying degrees. Adults who have not had surgical repair and the rare child with a very large ductus may have pulmonary vascular obstructive disease with increased resistance and marginally increased pulmonary flow.
3. Angiography with retrograde injection into the aortic arch clearly shows the ductus arteriosus, although passing of the catheter through its proper course from pulmonary artery to aorta provides equally good proof.

Management

All patent ductus should be closed, with few exceptions. Until the last few years, closure was exclusively surgical, with a mortality of less than 1% and with no significant incidence of complications or recanalization as long as the structure was divided, not ligated. Within the last year or two, aggressive "catheterizers" have been working, lately with some success, on creating umbrella-like devices to be introduced into the pulmonary artery, through the ductus, from the aorta, and obliterating the flow in that way. Today, some degree of success has been obtained, but the procedure is still viewed as an experimental one. Within the next 5 years, it will be decided whether a proven, virtually no risk, and 100% effective surgical procedure should be abandoned for a catheter approach, essentially for economic and cosmetic reasons.

In our view, the exceptions to closing the patent ductus are patients with pulmonary vascular disease resulting in a net right-to-left shunt. In experienced surgical hands, closure of bidirectional shunts may be attempted if the patient is young (less than 10 years old) and temporary closure on the catheter table with a balloon is well tolerated. This difficult proposition, however, should be handled by a very experienced cardiologist and cardiovascular surgeon. The other issue is whether a ductus with a trivial shunt (a pulmonary-systemic flow ratio of less than 1.5:1) is worth closing. In 1986, considering the risks of infective endocarditis, the unlikely possibility of the development of pulmonary vascular disease and the "nuisance value" of insurance hassles, we would be inclined to suggest closure even for a "mini ductus" in a young person, given competent surgical support.

The timing of surgery is not important; surgical division may be done at any time, at the convenience of the family and the surgeon. The operative risk, even in the smallest infant, is negligible. As an elective procedure, we suggest surgery at about 1 year of age.

Course and Prognosis

The clinical course of patients successfully operated upon for patent ductus without pulmonary obstructive disease is indistinguishable from that of patients born with normal hearts. For all practical purposes there are no complications and there is no recanalization. If the patient has pulmonary hypertension before surgery, the course will depend on the age at surgery as well as the level of pulmonary resistance. These issues have been discussed already in the section on Pulmonary Hypertension.

We shall not waste too much time in discussing unrepaired patent ductus; this does not occur today in the United States or any of the developed countries. Those who have been in the field for a long time remember adults with patent ductus arteriosus and pulmonary vascular disease, with the classic Eisenmenger syndrome. The course in these patients is similar to that of patients with Eisenmenger syndrome as a whole, only they may live somewhat longer (five to six decades) and may have better functional capacity than do those with ventricular defect. These are unsubstantiated impressions, however, unlikely to be validated in the future.

Persistent Ductus Arteriosus (Premie Ductus)

Definition

Persistent ductus arteriosus represents delayed closure in small prematures, commensurate with the immaturity of the baby. It has been well-documented for more than a decade that the left-to-right shunt through the ductus contributes significantly to the morbidity and mortality from the respiratory distress syndrome (Jones and Pickering, 1977). Interruption of the ductus arteriosus was undertaken first by surgical (Kitterman et al, 1972), then by medical means (Gersony et al, 1983). Because of the success of these procedures in the 1980s in the United States, in most situations, "delayed" closure cannot be documented. The definition

CASE ILLUSTRATION

A boy lives in a distant city at an elevation of 8600 feet. Three weeks after birth a murmur was heard. From birth he was bothered by a cough and vomiting associated with feeding; nonetheless his growth and development were excellent.

On examination in Boston at 6 months of age, a day after the plane trip from Bogota, the baby appeared well with a grade III systolic murmur. His chest film showed a normal-sized heart and his electrocardiogram showed combined ventricular hypertrophy. On two-dimensional echocardiography, no specific abnormality was seen, although the left atrium was large. He was studied for gastric reflux.

On return to Boston 3 years later, this time having been in the United States for 6 weeks, he was re-examined and found to have a roaring continuous murmur. His electrocardiogram showed right ventricular hypertrophy. He derwent cardiac catheterization because the combination of right ventricular hypertrophy and a continuous murmur cannot be readily explained. A small ductus arteriosus with normal pulmonary artery pressure was discovered and was closed during the procedure, using an umbrella occluding device. When examined 6 months later he was well.

QUESTIONS AND COMMENTS

Why was there no continuous murmur at the age of 6 months and a typical one at the age of 3 years?

Ordinarily, a patent ductus arteriosus produces a continuous murmur by the age of 6 months. This child had been at sea level for only 24 hours when examined at 6 months and is presumed to have had high altitude pulmonary hypertension. The murmur of patent ductus arteriosus is not typical, more often just systolic, when there is pulmonary hypertension. The second time he was seen, his high altitude pulmonary hypertension had had 6 weeks to resolve.

Is it not customary to close a patent ductus arteriosus based on typical clinical findings alone?

Yes, but although this boy had a typical murmur he also had right ventricular hypertrophy, not a feature of patent ductus arteriosus—particularly in the presence of a continuous murmur. Because this was an atypical combination, he underwent cardiac catheterization to rule out some unexpected problem. The right ventricular hypertrophy was not due to the patent ductus arteriosus but to the high altitude.

Why was the ductus closed with an experimental device?

The ductus was small and the pulmonary hypertension was documented to have resolved. The idea of closing the ductus with a transcatheter device as opposed to surgery was discussed with the family and they agreed. Whether this method of ductal closure will become standard practice is not clear. Clearly, there are significant details to be learned about this method before its general use.

Why didn't the right ventricular hypertrophy on the electrocardiogram not resolve as the pulmonary hypertension disappeared with the patient at sea level?

While high altitude pulmonary hypertension can resolve completely in a matter of days, the muscle in the right ventricle takes somewhat longer to regress.

then becomes simply "the ductus arteriosus occurring in a small premature baby, the natural history of which is assumed, not proven." That this distinction between premie ductus (persistent ductus) and "regular" patent ductus arteriosus is probably valid is supported by the lack of female dominance among premature infants with ductus arteriosus as well as by the histology of the structure itself (Ross Conference, 1977).

Basic Science

The histology of the persistent ductus "capable of constricting in time with or without indomethacin administration" is indistinguishable from the permanently patent ductus (Gitterberger-deGroot et al, 1980).

The hemodynamics are similar to those described for a large ductus. The confounding feature here is the presence of the respiratory distress syndrome owing to surfactant deficiency. The ductus arteriosus probably does not *cause* the respiratory distress syndrome but it certainly exaggerates the severity of hyaline membrane disease through the interplay of increased pulmonary capillary pressure and hypoxia, secondary to pulmonary edema. There is undoubtedly pulmonary hypertension.

Epidemiology

Among the approximately 1700 premature babies weighing less than 1750 g studied within the framework of a national collaborative randomized study (Gersony et al, 1983), 20.5% were diagnosed as having a hemodynamically significant patent ductus. The incidences ranged from 42% among those weighing less than a 1000 g to only 7% among those who weighed more than 1500 g (Ellison et al, 1983).

Diagnosis

The typical patient with a persistent ductus arteriosus is a small premature in whom the respiratory distress syndrome develops and does not improve under conventional medical management, including respiratory support for 48 hours. Alternatively, the baby improves for a day or two, only to require increased ventilatory support again to maintain adequate blood gases.

On physical examination, respiratory distress usually dominates the picture. A typical continuous murmur is seldom heard; the murmur, if any, is systolic, often with a crescendo quality at the second left interspace. The pulses are bounding and the pulse pressure is wide. The heart sounds are often difficult to analyze, because of the noisy respirations, but the second sound is usually single and loud at the second left interspace. The liver is usually palpable; how much of this is due to actual enlargement and how much to downward displacement due to hyperinflation is hard to judge.

The electrocardiogram shows sinus tachycardia with moderate right axis deviation and right ventricular hypertrophy, and sometimes combined ventricular hypertrophy.

The chest film, like the physical examination, is dominated by the respiratory distress syndrome. The degree of cardiac enlargement is hard to appreciate because of the hyperinflated lungs and the infiltrates.

Echo-Doppler is the diagnostic tool of choice. There is an increased left atrial-aortic ratio. The two-dimensional echo outlines the ductus and Doppler estimates the flow with reasonable accuracy.

Cardiac catheterization is seldom performed on these fragile, tiny babies; the history, physical, and echocardiogram almost invariably establishes the diagnosis without serious doubts. A retrograde aortogram nicely outlines the ductus, but in the 1980s its use is limited.

Management

The National Collaborative Study on Patent Ductus Arteriosus in Prematures (Gersony et al, 1983) recommended the following treatment regimen for babies with hemodynamically significant patent ductus (diagnosed by clinical means and confirmed by echocardiography):

1. There should be 48 hours of conventional management (respiratory assistance and anticongestants).
2. If no closure occurs, indomethacin (0.2 mg/kg, first dose) is administered intravenously, to be followed by two doses at 12-hour intervals. For babies less than 48 hours old, on account of their poor renal function, the subsequent second and third doses should be 0.1 mg/kg. Those older than 48 hours receive 0.2 mg/kg twice.

With this management schema, about 80% of the ductus will close or become hemodynamically insignificant and remain so. For babies in whom this plan is ineffective, surgery (with a risk of less than 3%) is recommended (Wagner et al, 1984).

Course and Prognosis

The overall mortality rate at 1 year in the National Collaborative Study was around 20%, principally due to pulmonary insufficiency, intracranial hemorrhage, necrotizing enterocolitis, and sepsis. It is unlikely that the ductus played a major role in the ultimate outcome of these babies; severe untoward events and death were mostly due to prematurity and the respiratory distress syndrome. At 1 year, 65–70% of the original group were alive without major handicaps.

Aortopulmonary Window

Definition

The communication between the aorta and pulmonary artery right above the valve rings, considerably proximal to the huge ductal site, having no length, is referred to as an aortopulmonary window. Its significance lies in its hemodynamic resemblance to a large patent ductus.

Basic Science

The defect varies in diameter between 5 and 30 mm. The ventricular septum is usually, but not invariably, intact (as distinguished from common truncus arteriosus).

The physiology is indistinguishable from that of a large patent ductus arteriosus.

Diagnosis

The clinical picture is virtually identical to that seen in patients with a large ductus. Distinguishing features include early congestive failure, a very loud continuous murmur lower down at the left sternal border, marked left ventricular hypertrophy or combined ventricular hypertrophy, and a very large heart with markedly increased pulmonary vasculature.

Two-dimensional echocardiography, in expert hands, establishes the diagnosis. It is strongly recommended that any patient with a large patent ductus arteriosus and an atypical clinical profile should undergo echocardiography.

The passage of the catheter through the window is pathognomonic and before the advent of two-dimensional echocardiography was the gold standard of diagnosis (Fig. 6.27).

Management

Surgery is mandatory on diagnosis if the window is large. Operation with cardiopulmonary bypass, with or without deep hypothermia, is much trickier than a simple division of a ductus.

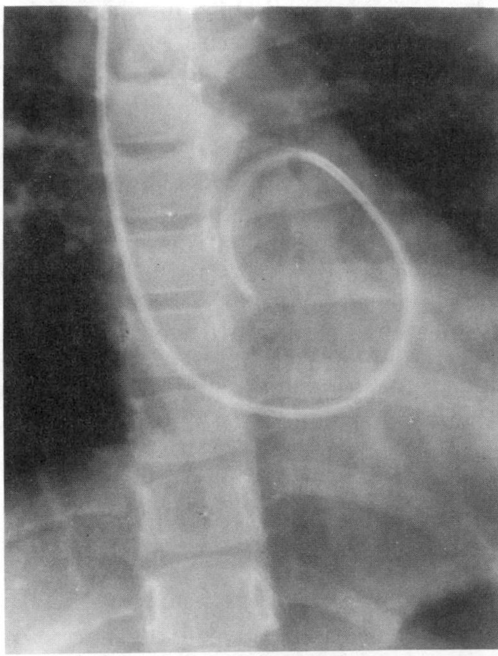

Figure 6.27. Passage of the catheter through the superior vena cava, right atrium, right ventricle, main pulmonary artery and through an aortopulmonary window into the ascending aorta. The tip of the catheter lies just above the aortic valve.

Course and Prognosis

Successful early surgery should yield results comparable to those achieved for a patent ductus.

ENDOCARDIAL CUSHION DEFECTS

Definition

The four endocardial cushions are embryologic structures that contribute to the development of the atrial and ventricular septa at the point of junction with the atrioventricular valves and to the development of adjacent septal leaflets of both the mitral and tricuspid valves. Cardiac defects involving the above structures derived from the endocardial cushions are so labeled.

Basic Science

ANATOMY

Only a limited area of the atrial and ventricular septa is truly derived from the endocardial cushions. By convention, septal defects that extend into other areas of the ventricular and atrial septa are described as cushion defects:

1. If both atrial and ventricular septa are involved, together with both atrioventricular valves, the lesion is designated as atrioventricularis communis (Fig. 6.28).
2. If, principally, the atrial septum is involved with only a small ventricular defect, with or without clefts in the medial leaflets of the atrioventricular valves, an ostium primum defect is present.
3. If there is a ventricular defect alone in the specific location, it is referred to as a ventricular defect of the endocardial cushion type.
4. Complete absence of the atrial septum is called a common atrium.

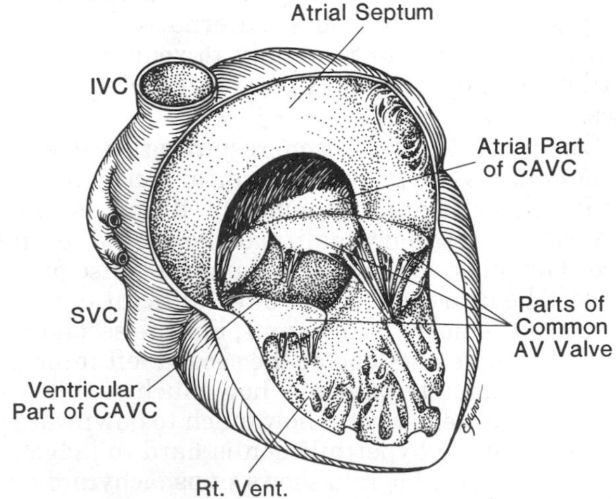

Figure 6.28. Anatomy of common atrioventricular canal as viewed from opened right ventricle.

5. Complete absence of the ventricular septum in the context of endocardial cushion defects, is called a single ventricle of the atrioventricular canal type (Feldt, 1976).

The septal leaflets of the atrioventricular valves are abnormal to a greater or lesser degree in all these varieties. They are joined in a single common atrioventricular valve in atrioventricularis communis lesions. Sometimes the abnormal atrioventricular valves misdirect blood flow so that one or the other ventricle receives less than the usual amount of blood, resulting in a disproportionately small ventricular cavity.

PHYSIOLOGY

The physiologic abnormalities include left-to-right shunting at the atrial or ventricular level or both, with systemic levels of pulmonary artery pressure if the ventricular septal opening is large enough. There may be mitral regurgitation if the mitral valve has short chordae tendinae; but often the mitral cleft or even the common atrioventricular valve is quite competent. Pulmonary vascular disease is common after a few years of survival with an atrioventricularis communis; pulmonary artery hypertension is much less common among the children who have only an ostium primum defect. Infants with Down syndrome and hypoventilation confuse the issue by having, simultaneously, two causes for pulmonary hypertension (hypoxia and left-to-right shunting) which must be sorted out before intelligent assessment of operability can be made. Severe pulmonary stenosis in a patient with atrioventricularis communis or endocardial cushion ventricular defect results in a tetralogy of Fallot type of clinical profile.

Epidemiology

Endocardial cushion defects are the seventh most common form of critical congenital heart disease in infants (11–14/100,000 live births; Table 6.3; Fyler et al, 1980a). Of these, 45% have Down syndrome. Of those with Down syndrome and congenital heart disease, nearly 80% have atrioventricularis communis (complete atrioventricular valve canal defect; Table 6.7).

Diagnosis

The discovery of heart disease is dependent on the appearance of congestive heart failure, finding a murmur on routine examination or, most commonly, on recognition of an extracardiac anomaly (i.e., Down syndrome), which directs attention to the possibility of congenital heart disease.

On physical examination, other than the possibility of seeing extracardiac anomalies, there may be no specific abnormality. If there is no pulmonary stenosis, congestive heart failure dominates the picture. In infants with severe hypoventilation, there may be only limited left-to-right shunting and no atrioventricular valve regurgitation. In an infant with a major abnormality of the heart, there may be only a trivial murmur and no congestive heart failure. In the majority, however, there is a murmur of ventricular defect, of mitral regurgitation or of pulmonary stenosis; the diastolic rumble of excessive shunting is often encountered.

Table 6.7
Diagnostic Distribution of Congenital Heart Defects among Patients with Down Syndrome

Diagnosis	No. with Down Syndrome	No. without Down Syndrome
Endocardial cushion defect	54	65
Atrioventricular canal	43	28
Atrial septal defect 1	2	19
Other	9	18
Ventricular septal defect	14	360
Tetralogy of Fallot	7	205
Patent ductus arteriosus	3	143
Double-outlet right ventricle	2	33
Tricuspid atresia	1	60
Atrial septal defect 2	1	69
Single ventricle	1	57
Other	1	116
Remainder	0	1059[1]
Total	84	2167

[1] Includes: truncus arteriosus, coarctation of aorta, myocarditis, pulmonary stenosis, hypoplastic left heart syndrome, total anomalous pulmonary veins, transposition of great arteries, aortic stenosis, and pulmonary atresia with intact ventricular septum (Fyler, 1980).

ELECTROCARDIOLOGY

The electrocardiogram is almost pathognomonic showing a leftward superior axis with a counterclockwise loop. The axis is deviated to the extreme northwest sector in those with atrioventricularis communis and toward the northeast sector with ostium primum defects. The presence and degree of ventricular hypertrophy depends on the amount of left-to-right shunting and on the balance of atrioventricular valve regurgitation, pulmonary stenosis, and pulmonary hypertension.

RADIOGRAPHY

Depending on the size of the shunt and the amount of atrioventricular valve regurgitation, the heart may be large. The amount of pulmonary vascularity depends on the amount of left-to-right shunting and the degree of pulmonary stenosis.

ECHO-DOPPLER STUDY

The various forms of endocardial cushion defect are particularly well delineated anatomically as well as physiologically by two-dimensional echocardiography with color-Doppler.

CARDIAC CATHETERZATION

All infants with the clinical diagnosis of endocardial cushion defect probably should undergo cardiac catheterization before surgery at the present time. In patients with atrioventricularis communis there may be additional muscular ventricular septal defects, which can be particularly troublesome to manage. Often the child with Down syndrome and atroventricularis communis has less than normal pulmonary venous oxygen saturation (hypoventilation) and secondary pulmonary hypertension, which limits the size of the left-to-right shunt and would suggest an inoperable defect. Efforts to clarify this question (administration of 100% oxygen or vasoactive drugs) are undertaken during cardiac catheterization. Generally, the degree of left-to-right shunting increases substantially during oxygen administration. This phenomenon can be detected using nuclear scanning techniques to compare pulmonary blood while breathing air and while breathing oxygen (Fujii et al, 1982).

Management

ATRIOVENTRICULAR CANAL

The infant in congestive heart failure with a common atrioventricular canal, a common atrioventricular valve and pulmonary hypertension is managed with anticongestive medications at first. For those who respond and grow, corrective surgery is delayed until the second half of the first year of life (but no later because of the danger of pulmonary vascular obstructive disease), at which time elective repair of the anomaly is undertaken. Those who cannot be encouraged to grow and who remain in congestive heart failure are referred to the surgeon as soon as this fact is clearly established, usually at 4–6 weeks of age. In our experience, hospital surgical mortality is below 15% and is about the same in patients with Down syndrome (Table 6.8); not all agree (Bull et al, 1985). Within the past decade our surgeons have abandoned palliative pulmonary artery banding for management of these patients (Chin et al, 1982; Mavroudis et al, 1982).

OSTIUM PRIMUM DEFECTS

Children with ostium primum defects all suffer left-to-right shunting through the atrial defect with or without mitral regurgitation of varying severity. Sur-

Table 6.8
Atrioventricular Canal Repair 1980–1985 at The Children's Hospital, 30-Day Mortality

	With Down Syndrome		Without Down Syndrome	
Age	No. of Patients	% Mortality	No. of Patients	% Mortality
Less than 1 year	70	13	21	14
More than 1 year	41	2	15	7

CASE ILLUSTRATION

A 5-month-old female infant was admitted for elective cardiac catheterization. The baby was thought to be normal until the age of 2 months when, during a regular checkup, a murmur was heard. Retrospectively, the mother reported episodes of poor color associated with grunting respiration. An echocardiogram showed an atrioventricular canal with severe atrioventricular valve regurgitation. Treatment with furosemide and digoxin was begun. She continued relatively well.

On physical examination her length was 61 cm (25%), weight 5 kg (3%), pulse rate 132, and respiratory rate 36. This was a somewhat thin child who was in no distress. There was a grade IV harsh systolic murmur at the lower left sternal border. The liver was palpable 2 cm below the costal margin.

The ECG showed a leftward superior axis. On a chest film, the heart size was large, with increased pulmonary vascularity (Fig. 6.29). Echo-Doppler study showed a common atrioventricular canal, a patent foramen ovale, and atrioventricular regurgitation.

At cardiac catheterization, it was possible to demonstrate the presence of an atrioventricular canal. There was mild atrioventricular valve regurgitation with systemic pressure in the pulmonary artery and a huge left-to-right shunt was demonstrated. The arterial oxygen saturation was 92%. There were no additional ventricular defects.

The child was discharged having been scheduled for surgical repair in 2 months. This was accomplished without complication.

QUESTIONS AND COMMENTS

Is there any difference in survival with repair of atrioventricular canal in patients with Down syndrome as compared to those who do not have Down syndrome?

There is no demonstrable difference. Surgical mortalities seem to be identical.

Wouldn't salvage be greater if the patient first had a pulmonary artery band and then had a band takedown and repair of the arterioventricular canal when the child was larger?

Our experience indicates no advantage in the two-stage approach, either in terms of survival or the quality of repair.

How often must the mitral valve be replaced in atrioventricular canal defects?

An attempt is made to provide a mitral valve that is reasonably functional at the first operation, but later it is sometimes discovered that there is important mitral regurgitation. Replacement, formerly common, is now relatively unusual and is required in less than 5% of patients.

How early does pulmonary vascular obstructive disease occur in children with an atrioventricular canal defect?

Pulmonary vascular obstructive disease occasionally is encountered in the first year of life but is not common before the age of 2 years. Elective surgical repair is carried out between 6 and 12 months of age to avoid this possiblity.

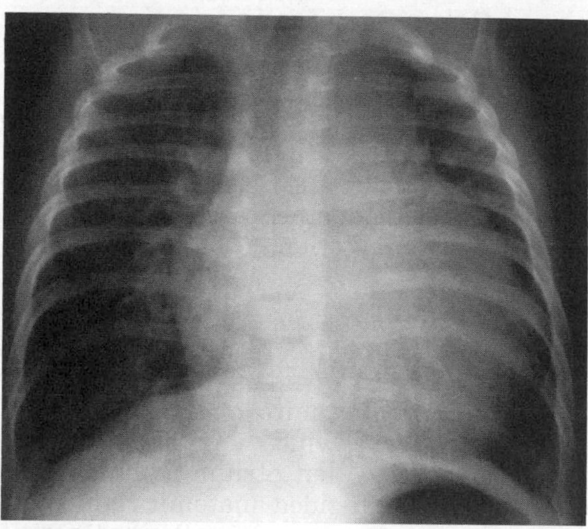

Figure 6.29. Chest film showing a common atrioventricular canal. Note the large heart with increased pulmonary vascular marking.

gery for mitral regurgitation is rarely needed in infancy, although the condition tends to become progressively more severe with age. Those patients without significant mitral regurgitation may undergo surgery for repair in the first 2–4 years of life. Those with huge left-to-right shunts or severe mitral regurgitation may require repair earlier. The atrial defect is closed and the mitral valve is repaired with surprisingly good results. Most patients have some residual abnormality of the mitral valve. Occasionally a patient will need replacement of the mitral valve. It should be stressed that in patients with severe mitral regurgitation and an atrial defect, closure of the atrial defect without complete amelioration of the mitral regurgitation will result in elevated left atrial pressure and pulmonary edema (Portman et al, 1985).

Course and Prognosis

Children who have survived corrective surgery with endocardial cushion defects have chronic atrioventricular valve problems of various degrees and require prophylactic antibiotics to prevent bacterial endocarditis for the rest of their lives. The amount of residual difficulty is usually well tolerated although, occasionally, a child will require replacement of the mitral valve some years later. Infants with repaired common atrioventricular canal have had an extensive surgical procedure and occasionally, the reconstructed mitral valve which has been sewn to the artifically implanted septum will tear loose. The sudden appearance of gross mitral regurgitation is a particularly dramatic event manifested by a very fast pulse, cardiovascular collapse, high fever, a grossly elevated white count, and all of the features of overwhelming sepsis. Such a patient can only survive if the valve is restored to competency. Delay to sort out the question of sepsis can be fatal. We have seen this phenomenon in the immediate postoperative period and as late as several months after surgery.

ABNORMALITIES OF CARDIAC POSITION AND ABNORMAL SEGMENTAL RELATIONSHIPS

Definition

In this section, abnormalities of the position of the heart itself and of its segments (atria, ventricles, or great arteries) will be discussed.

Basic Science

The heart may be abnormally located in the right chest where it is described as dextrocardia or mesocardia depending on how far into the right chest it is positioned. Dextrocardia may be caused by the push or pull of external forces (hypoplastic right lung, diaphragmatic hernia), or by abnormal development of the heart itself. In dextrocardia, the relationship of the segments of the heart may be normal and without other congenital anomalies (24%; Van Praagh et al, 1983) or there may be segmental abnormalities with or without other cardiac anomalies, such as septal defects, valvar abnormalities, or transposition.

The relative positions of the atria, ventricles and great arteries can be normal or inverse, independent of the location of the heart in the chest. Any form of congenital heart disease can be superimposed. The permutations and combinations of possible abnormalities are numerous.

Many authors have sought to simplify this complexity. The segmental approach suggested by Van Praagh et al (1983) solves the problem of position of the heart in the chest by ignoring it, focusing instead, on the structure and position of the chambers. According to this method the visceral situs (position of the spleen, liver, bronchi) may be solitus (S), inversus (I), or ambiguous (A). The discovery of situs solitus effectively locates the systemic venous atrium. Clinically, it is necessary to establish the position of the liver or the initial branching pattern of the bronchi to indicate which side the systemic venous "right" atrium is located. Since the inferior vena cava almost invariably connects to the right atrium, inversion of abdominal contents signifies a left-sided inferior vena cava connecting to a systemic venous "right" atrium on the left side.

The ventricles may also be normal or inverted (reversed in their right-to-left position). Identification of the ventricles is possible at autopsy, echo-Doppler examination, or by angiography since the anatomic "right ventricle" is grossly trabeculated, U-shaped, and has the tricuspid valve, whereas the anatomic "left ventricle" has the mitral valve, is oval-shaped, and smooth-walled. Ventricles are described as D (dextrorotatory) if normally related (right ventricle on right side) and L (levorotatory) if inversely related (right ventricle on left side).

The great arteries may also arise normally or in an inverse position. The great arteries may not only be inverse, opposite to normal, as in situs inversus universalis (mirror image dextrocardia) but are often also transposed with the aorta related to the anatomic right ventricle and the pulmonary artery to the anatomic left ventricle (usually with the aorta anterior and the pulmonary artery posterior). This situation is reversed with "corrected" transposition (the aorta is still anterior and the pulmonary artery posterior, with the aorta related to the anatomic right ventricle, but it carries pulmonary venous blood from the left atrium).

The location of the liver or stomach or bronchi may be ambiguous. Additionally, sometimes the liver or the stomach may seem to move from one side to the other. The bronchial branching pattern may resemble that for two right lungs or two left lungs. Indeed, it has been proposed that these patients may be divided into those with bilateral left-sidedness (polysplenia) or bilateral right-sidedness (asplenia).

The problem of ambiguous visceral sidedness is largely confined to patients with splenic dysgenesis (asplenia, polysplenia, accessory spleen). Patients with the heart in the left side of the chest who have abdominal heterotaxy almost invariably have some intracardiac abnormality, often involving splenic dysgenesis.

The interrelationships of cardiac position (dextrocardia, isolated levocardia), situs (solitus, inversus, ambiguous), splenic dysgenesis (asplenia, polysplenia, accessory spleen) and looping (D, L) are presented in Tables 6.9–6.11. For a more detailed discussion, the reader is referred to the papers of Van Praagh et al (1983), Van Mierop et al (1972), Ivemark (1955), and Peoples et al (1983).

Epidemiology

Abnormal segmental interrelationship (heterotaxia) comprised the eighth most common category of critically ill infants found by the New England Infant Cardiac Program (Fyler et al, 1980a) and represented 10 infants per 100,000 thousand live births (Table 6.3). This figure nearly doubles if infants with abnormal segmental relationships, in the context of single ventricle, double-outlet right ventricle, and L-transposition of the great arteries are included.

Corrected Transposition

Definition

Corrected transposition (L-transposition of the great arteries) denotes a heart with normally positioned atria, inverse ventricles and transposition of the great arteries (SLL), which, without other cardiac anomalies, would provide a normal circulation.

Basic Science

The cardiac segments are oriented SLL in situs solitus or IDD in situs inversus (p). The right atrium conveys blood through a mitral valve to a right-sided anatomic left ventricle, which empties into a posterior pulmonary artery. The left atrium pumps pulmonary venous blood into a left-sided anatomic right ventricle, which empties into an anterior left-sided aorta. The systemic atrioventricular valve is tricuspid and is sometimes incompetent, when it may appear to have an Ebstein-like deformity.

Inherent in this segmental arrangement is the tendency to atrioventricular block. Some of these children are born with complete heart block, some acquire it at cardiac catheterization, some with cardiac surgery, but in most, presumably all, complete heart block will develop sometime during their life. The conduction system distal to the atrioventricular node is inverted and perhaps this anatomy accounts for the tendency to atrioventricular block.

Only a rare patient has no other cardiac anomalies. Indeed, the most common variety of the SLL segmental arrangement includes a single left ventricle. Ventricular defects and combinations of ventricular defect and subvalvar pulmonary stenosis are common.

Epidemiology

L-transposition without single ventricle comprised 1–2 infants per 100,000 thousand live births in the New England Regional Cardiac Program. With single ventricle, it was substantially more common (Table 6.3).

Table 6.9
Viscero Atrial Situs

	Solitus		Inversus		Ambiguous Asplenia		Ambiguous Polysplenia	
	D Loop	L Loop	D Loop	L Loop	D Loop	L Loop	D Loop	L Loop
Dextrocardia[1]								
Normally related great vessels	24	2	1	7		2	2	10
Transposition of great arteries	4	28	4	8	4	8		6
Double-outlet right ventricle	1				2			
Other	1	4		4	1	8		
Levocardia								
Normally related great vessels					3	2	8	
Transposition of great arteries			7		5	1	1	
Double-outlet right ventricle			2		17	1	4	
Other						1		

[1]Modified from Van Praagh et al, 1983.

Table 6.10
Cardiac Anatomy in Dextrocardia and Isolated Levocardia[1]

Cardiac Anatomy	Dextrocardia Situs Solitus		Dextrocardia Situs Inversus		Levocardia Situs Inversus
	D Loop n=30	L Loop n=35	D Loop n=5	L Loop n=19	D Loop n=9
Normal	7			2	
Ventricular septal defect	11	19	2	3	1
Pulmonary stenosis or pulmonary atresia	2	26	3	7	8
Transposition of the great arteries	4	28	4	8	7
Double-outlet right ventricle	1	4		4	2
Atrial septal defect 2	6			4	
Coarctation of the aorta	4				
Single ventricle		5			3
Common atrioventricular canal	2	6	1	1	6
Pulmonary vein anomaly	3				4
Atrioventricular valve atresia	1	4	1		

[1]Modified from Van Praagh et al, 1983.

Table 6.11
Cardiac Anatomy in Asplenia and Polysplenia[1]

Cardiac Anatomy	Asplenia		Polysplenia	
	Dextrocardia n=27	Levocardia n=33	Dextrocardia n=18	Levocardia n=13
Common atrioventricular canal	24	27	5	5
Common atrium	13	17	4	1
Total pulmonary vein abnormality	19	23	2	3
Pulmonary stenosis or atresia	23	27	5	5
Single ventricle	5	11	1	2
Interrupted inferior vena cava			8	5
Bilateral superior vena cava	13		7	

[1]Modified from Van Praagh et al, 1983.

Diagnosis

The history and physical examination depend on the associated cardiac anomalies.

ELECTROCARDIOGRAPHY

The inverse conduction system has led many observers to suggest that corrected transposition could be recognized by observing the presence of right-sided Q waves in the chest leads and the absence of Q waves in the left chest leads. This is probably true on a statistical basis but is scarcely useful in making the diagnosis in an individual case. The presence of atrioventricular block has been discussed.

RADIOGRAPHY

The leftward anterior aorta presents a relatively characteristic shadow in the posteroanterior radiograph. The size of the heart and amount of pulmonary vasculature depend on the underlying defects.

ECHO-DOPPLER STUDY

Transposition of the great arteries with inverse ventricles can be recognized by two-dimensional echocardiography.

Management

Management is directed toward the associated lesions. All patients should have pacemaker wires inserted when cardiac surgery is undertaken since complete heart block may occur regardless of the operative procedure performed. Symptomatic patients with complete heart block who have not had surgery also require pacemakers (Estes et al, 1983). Conduits from the anatomical left ventricle to the pulmonary artery are often required in patients with pulmonary stenosis and ventricular defect to relieve the outflow obstruction. As a consequence, these patients will be subjects for repeated surgery during their lifetime (Hwang et al, 1982).

Course and Prognosis

Inasmuch as all such patients are expected to acquire complete heart block, any episode of sudden collapse or fainting requires consideration of a Stokes-Adams episode. Nevertheless, with skillful medical and surgical management, patients may lead normal lives, at least into the fourth and fifth decades (Graham et al, 1983).

PULMONARY STENOSIS WITH INTACT VENTRICULAR SEPTUM

Definition

This anomaly has been variously described as "pure" pulmonary stenosis, "valvar" pulmonary stenosis, or "pulmonary stenosis with a normal aortic root." Our definition is a physiological one, allowing for the development of suprasystemic right ventricular pressure even in the face of a tiny, restrictive opening in the ventricular septum; thus, the entity to be discussed includes those with a "virtually intact" septum as well. However, this diagnosis does not include patients with pulmonary atresia and intact ventricular septum, which is a different clinical entity with a very different surgical implication.

Basic Science

ANATOMY

As indicated previously, there is no significant opening in the ventricular septum. In contrast, often an opening is present in the atrial septum, either in the area where secundum atrial defects would occur or through a foramen ovale.

Pulmonary stenosis is almost invariably (more than 90%) valvar, with fused and thickened commissures (Fig. 6.30). The main and branch pulmonary arteries are well developed, even "poststenotically" dilated, particularly the left main pulmonary artery. The degree of poststenotic dilatation is *not* proportionate to the severity of stenosis. Additional infundibular obstruction, probably secondary to ventricular hypertrophy, may be seen in 25% of the patients and is rarely of any surgical significance. Isolated infundibular stenosis is rare and is often regarded as part of a ventricular defect with muscle bundles (double-chambered right ventricle), where the ventricular defect closed spontaneously. Pulmonary stenosis is the most common congenital cardiac lesion in patients with Noonan syndrome; the valve is "dysplastic" or in these patients thickened, without commissural fusion, but often has a small annulus.

PHYSIOLOGY

The level of right ventricular systolic pressure is determined by the severity of the obstruction; the pressure rises to the level necessary to achieve sufficient pressure and flow in the pulmonary artery to fill the left atrium and the left ventricle in diastole. Given normal left heart structures, the mean pulmonary arterial pressure is approximately 10 mm Hg (enough to fill the left atrium with an average pressure of 8 mm Hg). On exercise, with an increased cardiac output, right ventricular systolic pressure often rises well above systemic levels. Given an adequate myocardium, right ventricular end-diastolic pressure is normal. As the ventricle thickens, and later becomes fibrotic, right ventricular end-diastolic pressure rises, causing the right atrial pressure to be elevated also. There has been some suggestion within recent years that myocardial disease involving both ventricles may be an intrinsic part of the syndrome (Becu et al, 1976). Once the right atrial pressure rises secondary to elevation of the right ventricular end-diastolic pressure, the foramen ovale is forced open, equalizing pressures between the left and right atria and causing an atrial right-to-left shunt and cyanosis. With few exceptions systemic arterial unsaturation in these patients is indicative of at least moderately severe obstruction.

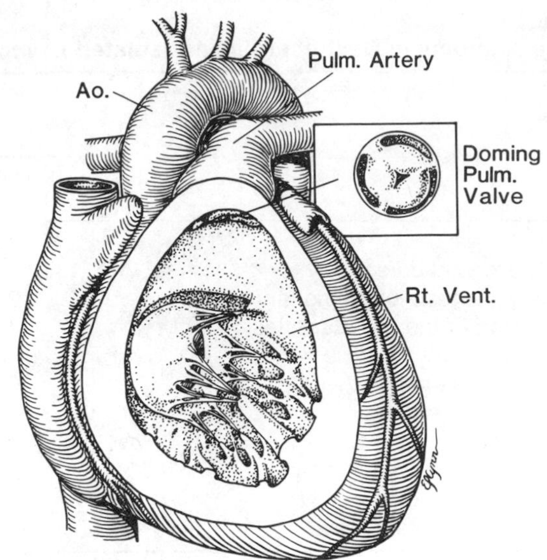

Figure 6.30. Anatomy of pulmonary stenosis. In the inset, the pulmonary valve is maximally open showing a diminutive orifice. The main pulmonary artery is dilated. Often the left main pulmonary artery is dilated as well.

Epidemiology

Among infants with critical congenital heart disease, pulmonary stenosis with intact ventricular septum is the ninth most common lesion (3.3%, 7/100,000 live births; Table 6.3; Flyer et al, 1980a). In a mixed hospital population, including infants and children, the prevalence is close to 12.5%, ranking second.

Diagnosis

HISTORY

Symptomatology depends primarily on the severity of the obstruction and secondarily on the age of the patient. Mild stenosis, arbitrarily defined as resting right ventricular systolic pressure that is less than half of systemic arterial pressure, rarely causes symptoms. Pressures beyond this level, often suprasystemic even at rest, are accompanied by exercise intolerance of varying degrees, ranging from inability to suck in infancy to limitations in athletics for school-age children. Occasionally, there is chest pain and even syncope. As noted earlier, severe obstruction is almost invariably associated with cyanosis and consequent dyspnea. Newborns with critical pulmonary stenosis may be desperately ill, with poor cardiac output, right-sided failure and severe hypoxia, requiring emergency intervention (Awariefe et al, 1983; Daskalopoulos et al, 1982).

PHYSICAL EXAMINATION

On physical examination, the patients, at whatever age, are relatively well developed; their faces are usually round (moon-faced) and they tend to be hyperteloric. Those with severe obstruction are blue; the cyanosis is partly central, due to the atrial right-to-left shunts, and partly peripheral, with a reddish tinge due to low cardiac output. With severe obstruction, a prominent A wave is visible on the jugular venous pulse. There is a thrill at the second left interspace and the suprasternal notch. The xiphoid impulse is heaving. Significant hepatomegaly is rare and peripheral edema is almost never seen. At auscultation, a variable ejection click is noted at the pulmonary area followed by a loud ejection murmur (Fig. 6.4*B*). The splitting of the second sound and the intensity of pulmonary closure are roughly proportionate to the severity of the stenosis. Respiratory variations of the second sound may be noted. This is important in the differential diagnosis of a secundum atrial defect where, with a pulmonary ejection murmur, the split second sound is almost invariably fixed. A low-frequency early diastolic blow is the hallmark of trivial stenosis. A loud right ventricular fourth sound indicates critical pulmonary stenosis.

MINOR LABORATORY TESTS

Routine laboratory findings are unremarkable, except for elevated hematocrit in patients with hypoxia.

ELECTROCARDIOGRAPHY

The electrocardiogram, reflecting right ventricular and right atrial hypertrophy, is a good clinical index of the severity of pulmonary stenosis. Severe right ventricular hypertrophy with strain and P pulmonale indicate right ventricular pressure at or above the systemic level. There is an occasional newborn with critical pulmonary stenosis resembling pulmonary atresia whose right ventricle is so small and contains so little blood that there is no right ventricular hypertrophy although there still is a murmur of pulmonary stenosis (Freed et al, 1973).

RADIOGRAPHY

A chest film shows normal or decreased pulmonary flow and a normal or severely dilated cardiac silhouette, depending on the severity of the disease. Poststenotic dilatation of the main and left main pulmonary artery is clearly visible in children unless the heart is very large. Some of the severe cardiac enlargement, particularly in infants with congestive failure, may be due to pericardial effusion. The dilated right atrium may be visible at the right lower border.

ECHO-DOPPLER STUDY

The echocardiogram clearly demonstrates the anatomy of the obstruction and gives a good estimate of the pressure gradient.

CARDIAC CATHETERIZATION

With the excellent qualitative and quantitative assessment of valvar pulmonary stenosis, there is some question whether cardiac catheterization is necessary in these patients. As a matter of fact, for a number years at least one-third of the children with valvar pulmonary stenosis at The Children's Hospital in Boston underwent surgery without preoperative physiologic study, even before the introduction of echocardiography. The diagnosis in these cases was based on the classic profile at physical examination and the chest film, with the electrocardiogram furnishing quantitative data. As indicated earlier, two-dimensional echo-Doppler studies have improved appreciably our already good diagnostic abilities. Today, however, almost all patients (infants and children) with pulmonary stenosis and intact ventricular septum are catheterized, not primarily for diagnosis, but for balloon angioplasty. This procedure, first proposed (Kan et al, 1982) in 1982, is now almost routine in many cardiac centers. Its effectiveness will be discussed under Management.

Physiologic data reveal: (a) right ventricular and right atrial hypertension with a gradient across the right ventricular outflow tract, (b) arterial unsaturation, in those with severe obstruction, due to atrial right-to-left shunt, (c) normal or low normal cardiac output, and (d) at angiography, a restrictive pulmonary valve orifice, doming in systole. Often there is secondary, functional, infundibular obstruction.

Management

Until a few years ago, the treatment of pulmonary stenosis with intact ventricular septum, was exclusively surgical; the only question was who should be operated on and when. In the National Collaborative Study of the Natural History of Congenital Heart Disease (Nadas et al, 1977), it was arbitrarily decided that patients with systolic gradients of 75 mm Hg or more across the right ventricular outflow tract should undergo surgery. The results of this policy were highly satisfactory: in the 1970s in six United States centers, the mortality was 3% and deaths were restricted to newborns with critical disease. The physiologic outcome was excellent and, during an 8-year follow-up, no reoperation was necessary. Pulmonary incompetence postoperatively was common, but during the 8-year period this seemed to cause no problems. In view of the excellent clinical results obtained, physiologic indications for surgery at The Children's Hospital in Boston have been extended to resting pressure gradients between the right ventricle and the pulmonary artery at or above 50 mm Hg.

In 1986, at The Children's Hospital in Boston, in spite of the excellent results of cardiac surgery, balloon angioplasty is the procedure of choice on account of the simplicity of the procedure, the absence of a need for thoracotomy, and last but not least, the economy. The experience compared to that of surgery is limited, but it seems to work. Among patients with gradients ranging 40–120 mm Hg, there was no mortality or severe morbidity. The average gradient was reduced from 75 to 25 mm Hg and no restenosis has been observed so far (Radtke et al, 1986). Clearly, the obstruction has to be valvar. Dysplastic valves are better handled on the operating table. Secondary infundibular obstruction seems to resolve after the valvar stenosis has been relieved. Patients with primary infundibular stenosis (moderator bands, double-chambered right ventricle) are candidates for surgery as well (Byrum et al, 1982; Restivo et al, 1984). Minimal physiologic indications for balloon angioplasty may be set at resting gradients of perhaps 40 mm Hg. This number is clearly arbitrary; results of long-term follow-up will have to serve as criteria for final judgment of the procedure.

Course and Prognosis

As indicated, the clinical course of successfully treated patients having pulmonary stenosis with intact

CASE ILLUSTRATION

A 3.9-kg male infant was noted to be cyanotic at birth. A loud systolic murmur was present. The electrocardiogram showed no ventricular hypertrophy. The chest film showed a large heart. On two-dimensional echocardiography there was valvar pulmonary stenosis.

On the third day of life, cardiac catheterization showed the right ventricular systolic pressure to exceed left ventricular pressure by 20 mm Hg (right ventricle, 107/7 mm Hg versus left ventricle, 80/5). The arterial saturation was 83% because of a right-to-left shunt through the foramen ovale.

On the fourth day of life, under inflow occlusion, a pulmonary valvotomy was accomplished. Postoperatively the baby remained cyanotic. The arterial saturation gradually improved to 88% on discharge at 10 days of age.

Now 3 years later he continues to do well.

QUESTIONS AND COMMENTS

What is the difference between pulmonary atresia with an intact ventricular septum and isolated pulmonary valvar stenosis?

There is an opening, sometimes miniscule, in the pulmonary valve of patients with pulmonary stenosis and, consequently, some blood passes through the right ventricle. In patients with pulmonary atresia no blood passes out of the right ventricle except by abnormal sinusoids or tricuspid regurgitation. The chest film, the electrocardiogram, and even the echocardiogram, may be similar in both conditions. There is no murmur of pulmonary stenosis in patients with pulmonary atresia but there can be a systolic murmur of tricuspid regurgitation. The key reason for believing the two conditions are different is the fact that there is much better survival with pulmonary stenosis than with pulmonary atresia.

What are the similarities between Ebstein disease and isolated pulmonary stenosis?

In both cases there is diminished blood flow out of the right ventricle; the needed extra amount to make up the cardiac output is provided by right-to-left shunting through the foramen ovale. Both are cyanotic; the heart is large in Ebstein disease and may be large with pulmonary stenosis. Both may be discovered at birth. The systolic murmur of critical pulmonary stenosis may be minimal as it is in patients with Ebstein disease.

What are the indications for interventional relief of valvar pulmonary stenosis?

The indications are: (a) cyanosis, (b) right-sided congestive heart failure, (c) cardiomegaly, (d) severe right ventricular hypertrophy on the electrocardiogram and (e) a pressure measurement in the right ventricle greater than 50% of systemic pressure with normal pulmonary artery pressures.

What is the significance of postoperative pulmonary regurgitation?

If the pulmonary artery pressure is normal, when a murmur of pulmonary regurgitation implies a good surgical result. If the pulmonary artery pressure is high, the resulting excessive pulmonary regurgitation may be a crippling volume load on the right ventricle.

What is the difference between the murmur of aortic regurgitation and the murmur of pulmonary regurgitation?

The murmur of pulmonary regurgitation is of lower freqency than is the murmur of aortic regurgitation, except when the pulmonary artery pressure is high (Eisenmenger syndrome).

Is an aortopulmonary arterial shunt ever needed to relieve cyanosis in patients with valvar pulmonary stenosis?

Rarely, there is severe cyanosis after pulmonary valvotomy which is so slow to regress that an arterial shunt is used to improve the infant's arterial oxygen saturation. By comparison with infants who have pulmonary valvar atresia with intact septum, however, the need for arterial shunts is much less.

ventricular septum is excellent. We have watched these patients for at least three decades postoperatively and they seem to do beautifully, leading normal, active lives, working full-time, having babies, and acting like people without heart disease. We have not even insisted on dental prophylaxis in view of the extreme rarity of bacterial endocarditis in these patients, with the possible exception of intravenous drug addicts. Whether the outcome of balloon angioplasty will be equally favorable remains to be seen, but there is no reason to assume otherwise.

The course of patients with trivial (less than 25 mm Hg) and mild stenosis (less than 50 mm Hg) seems equally favorable. There is no evidence so far that the obstruction becomes more severe after infancy if the gradient is small. Nevertheless, it would not be surprising if the minimal indications for balloon angioplasty were dropped further at some future date, once the benign nature and effectiveness of the procedure is further proven.

Variations

Congenital absence of the pulmonary valve or its minor variant, *idiopathic dilatation of the pulmonary artery*, should be mentioned here briefly. The latter is characterized by a large main pulmonary artery observed in the chest film coupled with a low-frequency to-and-fro murmur in the pulmonary area (sawing wood). The right ventricular pressure is normal, the gradient is trivial, and the electrocardiogram shows only right intraventricular conduction disturbance. If the pulmonary valve is totally absent, the radiographic appearance, with the huge main pulmonary artery segment, is similar, and the to-and-fro murmur is also noted, but is much louder. The difference is that the cardiac silhouette, reflecting the major abnormality of the valve, is large. These babies may be quite sick in infancy owing to congestive failure or bronchial obstruction, sometimes caused by the huge pulmonary artery, but often the result of diffuse pulmonary, bronchial, and vascular congenital abnormalities. Surgery in these infants is difficult and dangerous. Approaches include lifting the pulmonary artery off the compressed bronchus with or without replacing the pulmonary valve.

PULMONARY ATRESIA WITH INTACT VENTRICULAR SEPTUM

Definition

In this condition, there is *complete obstruction* to normal outflow from the right ventricle and no ventricular septal defect. While in many ways similar, patients who have *nearly atretic* right ventricular outflow (critical pulmonary stenosis) have better survival and, therefore, are considered elsewhere (see Pulmonary Stenosis with Intact Ventricular Septum).

Basic Science

The right ventricle and the tricuspid valve are variably and proportionally small, ranging from near normal size to a chamber only a few millimeters across (Patel et al, 1980; Bull et al, 1982). Pulmonary atresia with intact ventricular septum, in contrast to pulmonary atresia within the framework of tetralogy of Fallot, is usually valvar with a good-sized main pulmonary artery.

With isometric ventricular contraction, the pressure in the right ventricle may rise above systemic levels, particularly if the tricuspid valve is competent. Rarely, with a grossly incompetent tricuspid valve, the ventricular pressure is lower, even in the normal range, and the size of the ventricle is larger than normal.

With no outlet from the right ventricle, the entire cardiac output passes through the foramen ovale, with some egress through myocardial sinusoids of the right ventricle to the coronary circulation (O'Connor et al, 1982). Pulmonary circulation is maintained by the ductus arteriosus, which, however, usually closes on schedule. Survival after the first week of life requires a patent ductus arteriosus or, extremely rarely, excessive pulmonary collateral circulation.

Epidemiology

Pulmonary atresia with intact ventricular septum is the 10th most common cardiac defect requiring hospitalization in the first weeks of life (7/100,000 live births) (Fyler et al, 1980a). However, because of poor survival, it constitutes less than 1% of overall congenital cardiac experience (Table 6.3).

To include, by definition, patients with similar anatomy and physiology whose pulmonary valve is not atretic is misleading since infants with maximal pulmonary stenosis are more likely to survive (de Leval et al, 1982; see Case Illustration under Pulmonary Stenosis).

Diagnosis

Within 24–48 hours of birth, cyanosis is noted, and for this reason the infant is referred to a cardiologist. Eighty-seven percent of these babies have already undergone cardiac examination by the end of the first week of life (Fyler et al, 1980a).

Extracardiac anomalies and low birth weight are not common. Other than cyanosis, the physical findings are not characteristic. There may be a murmur of tricuspid regurgitation and in some infants, the open ductus arteriosus is recognizable because of the continuous murmur.

The electrocardiogram usually has a normal QRS axis (+30 to +75) without the normal degree of right ventricular dominance for age. This feature distinguishes these patients from those with tricuspid atresia where the absence of right ventricular hypertrophy is associated with a superior axis and those with critical pulmonary stenoses who normally have severe right ventricular hypertrophy. The chest film shows a heart that may vary from normal to being considerably enlarged. The pulmonary vasculature is also variable. On two-dimensional echocardiographic examination, the small right ventricle and tricuspid valve can usually be recognized, although confusion with tricuspid atresia is obviously possible.

The factors that determine outcome are still unclear. For this reason, precise data available from cardiac catheterization are being collected. The right ventricle can usually be entered through the tricuspid valve if a determined effort is made. Occasionally, however, the right ventricle is overlooked and an erroneous diagnosis of tricuspid atresia is made at catheterization. Often there is great excessive right ventricular pressure, and angiography shows a very small ventricle often barely accommodating the catheter.

Management

As soon as can be arranged, pulmonary valvotomy should be undertaken (Cobanoglu et al, 1985). If the right ventricle is more than half its normal size, as determined by angiography, valvotomy may be sufficient. Otherwise, a systemic-pulmonary arterial shunt, nowadays a modified Blalock procedure, should be established simultaneously (deLeval et al, 1982; Cobanoglu et al, 1985). If a shunting procedure is required, the right ventricular outflow is patched open some weeks to months later and the shunt is occluded. For those infants in whom the right ventricle is extremely small, the shunt is removed and a Fontan procedure is attempted at a later date. We believe that decompression of the right ventricle is desirable in any case, to prevent future potentially fatal arrhythmias.

Course and Prognosis

Without surgery, the immediate outlook for these patients is death. With surgery, the initial mortality is high and late deaths are common. It is interesting that patients with pulmonary atresia and intact septums do poorly, whereas patients with tricuspid atresia do better, even though the circulations are comparable in the two. The obvious difference is the obstructed, isometrically contracting, high-pressure, tiny right ventricle in patients with pulmonary atresia and intact septum. Comparable ventricular pressures are not encountered in patients with tricuspid atresia.

Pulmonary valvotomy alone (a satisfactory operation in no more than 10% of the patients) has provided the best results in our series. The number of long-term survivors is small, but the result is a near normal individual. Those who have undergone outflow reconstruction, and later removal of the systemic arterial shunt, generally have limitations and require medication. Those who have survived the Fontan procedure seem to do well, but one wonders what the long-term effect of the residual, tiny high-pressure right ventricle will be.

SECUNDUM ATRIAL SEPTAL DEFECT

Definition

A secundum atrial defect is a hole in the septum primum (at the site of the foramen secundum) not covered by the septum secundum.

Basic Science

ANATOMY

The defect is high in the atrial septum, and may vary from dime size to virtual absence of the atrial septum. In contrast to the ostium primum defect, there is seldom an associated ventricular defect or atrioventricular valve cleft; the most common associated lesions are partial anomalous venous return and pulmonary stenosis. Openings at the top of the atrial septum, being straddled by the superior vena cava, are referred to as sinus venosus defects and are almost invariably associated with anomalous drainage of the right upper pulmonary vein into the superior vena cava (Fig. 6.31).

PHYSIOLOGY

In the vast majority of instances, the shunt across the defect is from the left to the right atrium in diastole. The two atria act as a single filling chamber with identical pressures if the hole is at least 1 cm in diameter; in this instance, the flow in diastole is toward the ventricular chamber which is thinner walled and more

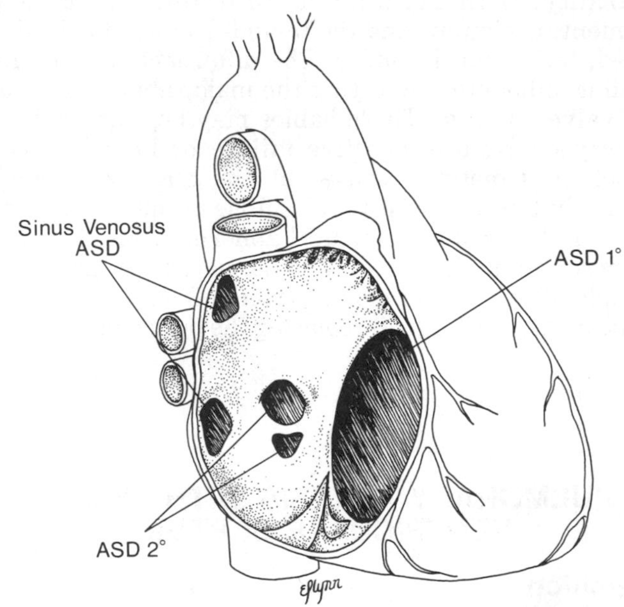

Figure 6.31. Anatomy of atrial septal defects. Sinus venosus defects are often associated with partial anomalous pulmonary veins entering the superior vena cava. Ostium primum defects (ASD 1°) are usually associated with mitral valve defects. ASD 2° may be single or multiple. All of these defects can be of variable size, although sinus venosus defects tend to be smaller.

compliant, i.e., the right ventricle. This concept explains why there is no significant left-to-right shunt, and there may even be a right-to-left shunt in early infancy, and why there is an increasing left-to-right shunt through the years as the left ventricle becomes thicker with increased left ventricular end diastolic pressure. At low pressure the flow through the defect is a cascading phenomenon, phasically bidirectional, net left-to-right, with a large pulmonary blood flow calculated at catheterization from oxygen data. The pulmonary arterial pressure is normal in spite of the huge flow, owing to the distensibility of the normal pulmonary arterioles. Pulmonary vascular obstructive disease, a common early consequence of intraventricular communications as well as patent ductus arteriosus, is relatively rare in patients with atrial septal defect (less than 10% overall) and seldom occurs before the third decade. The extra work of the heart is carried almost exclusively by the right ventricle and in uncomplicated defects consists of increased volume work only. Increased pressure work is a late phenomenon if arteriolar obstruction appears, at which time the shunt becomes bidirectional or even net right-to-left (see Pulmonary Hypertension: Physiology).

Epidemiology

Among infants with critical congenital heart disease who were included in the New England Regional Infant Cardiac Program, secundum atrial defect was relatively rare, 4% (70 babies of 2251 with heart disease), about 11th in ranking order (Table 6.3; Fyler et al, 1980a). In a mixed age pediatric hospital population, underrepresenting the critically ill infants who died young, the ranking order of secundum atrial defect is eighth (4.5%). It may be the most common congenital cardiac lesion first discovered in adolescence or adulthood in the United States today (Hamilton et al, 1985).

Diagnosis

With few exceptions, patients with secundum atrial defect do not become symptomatic until childhood or adolescence, if at all; almost one-half of our patients were asymptomatic at the time of surgery. This phenomenon may explain the late discovery of the malformation. The symptoms, when they occur, consist principally of failure to thrive, dyspnea, and palpitations.

PHYSICAL EXAMINATION

The typical patient with a secundum atrial defect is usually a tall, thin girl (almost 2:1). Cyanosis is rare and almost invariably indicates right ventricular outflow tract obstruction (pulmonary stenosis or pulmonary vascular obstructive disease). The jugular veins are strongly pulsatile with a tall V wave preceded by a systolic collapse. There is left chest prominence with a hyperkinetic xiphoid (right ventricular) impulse. At auscultation, the first sound tends to be loud; the almost pathognomonic feature is a widely split second sound (more than 5 msec) with a pulmonary closure of normal intensity, barely moving with respirations (fixed split) (Fig. 6.3). There is a soft ejection murmur at the second left interspace (louder if there is associated pulmonary stenosis) and a low-frequency early diastolic rumble at the lower left sternal border (Fig. 6.3*A*). The sounds, the murmurs, and the palpable impulse with left chest prominence all indicate a hyperkinetic circulation.

MINOR LABORATORY TESTS

Routine laboratory tests are not remarkable.

ELECTROCARDIOGRAPHY

The electrocardiogram typically shows a frontal QRS axis of approximately +120° with right intraventricular conduction delay. Severe right ventricular hypertrophy indicates obstruction of the right ventricular outflow tract.

RADIOGRAPHY

The chest film shows mild-to-moderate right ventricular and right atrial enlargement with pulmonary vascular engorgement and a prominent main pulmonary artery segment. The sinus venosus defect is characterized by the absence of the right superior vena cava shadow and entrance of the horizontal pulmonary vein into the right upper cardiac shadow.

ECHO-DOPPLER STUDY

Two-dimensional echocardiography in expert hands identifies the size and location of the defect in young, nonobese people. Additional nonspecific evidence of right ventricular overload with "paradoxical" septal motion is needed to confirm left-to-right shunting. The Doppler echocardiogram, particularly in color, gives a good estimate of the size and direction of the shunt. A warning note should be sounded here lest a patient be referred for surgery on the basis of a false-positive echocardiogram without supporting data from the physical examination, chest film, and electrocardiograph.

CARDIAC CATHETERIZATION

At The Children's Hospital in Boston, in 1986, patients with a classic picture of secundum atrial septal defect are not catheterized. Only those with features that do not conform to the expected profile undergo cardiac catheterization. These situations include discrepancies between the physical examination and the echocardiogram, the presence of cyanosis, early symptomatology, etc. With the rapid strides being made in interventional catheterization, we would not be surprised if, within the next decade, catheter closure of secundum atrial defects might become the preferred approach; today this is not the case.

CASE ILLUSTRATION

A female born in 1947 was found to have a murmur at the age of 4 years. The pediatrician obtained a chest film, which was read as normal, and an ECG which showed questionable right ventricular hypertrophy. She was totally asymptomatic. Thus, the issue was not pursued any further at that time. The clinical impression was "mild pulmonary stenosis."

At 8 years, a cardiologist saw her and found the murmur, the film, and the ECG to be unchanged. At 12 years, with identical clinical findings, and still without symptoms and with good growth and development, she underwent a two-step exercise test which showed a "normal response."

At 16 years, another cardiologist saw the patient in the same city and suggested cardiac catheterization because of persistent, although mild, evidence of right ventricular hypertrophy in the ECG with a mean frontal plane axis of 110° and a 5 mm S wave in V_5 (R/S = 2/1). Catheterization at the University Hospital showed a small oxygen step-up at the right atrial level, confirmed by dye curves. The pressure in the right ventricle was 32/0 and in the pulmonary artery 20/7. The catheteer, a young cardiologist, suggested that the atrial defect be closed "as a precaution against any future difficulties, particularly when the problem of pregnancy arises." This was in 1963. The parents, apparently intelligent, well-to-do people, sought a second opinion in another metropolitan area from a very good, somewhat older and thus, presumably wiser, cardiologist who had seen the girl 7 or 8 years before. He was more conservative than the younger man who had carried out the catheterization and said, "It has been our policy for some time not to recommend surgery for minimal atrial defect or pulmonary stenosis of such mild degree."

Having obtained the desired favorable opinion, the patient, now having entered adulthood, started taking charge of her own destiny and stopped going to the doctors. She was fully active, feeling fine, presumably "on the Pill" until around the age of 30, when she started experiencing tightness in the chest (usually in the morning) and very mild dyspnea on exertion.

Her local cardiologist at that time (1972) sent this young woman to Boston for a second opinion. At this time, she was slightly, but definitely, cyanotic, without any significant murmur. There was a narrowly split second sound with a loud pulmonary component and without significant respiratory variations. Her chest films showed no significant cardiac enlargement, but a prominent main pulmonary artery and increased pulmonary vasculature. Her ECG still showed a mean frontal plane axis of +110° with more right ventricular hypertrophy than before, with a dominant R wave in V_1 and a deep S wave in V_5 (R/S = 1/2). Recatheterization was then performed in Boston. This showed a trivial, bidirectional shunt at the atrial level; the pulmonary arterial pressure was two-thirds of the femoral arterial pressure and the pulmonary resistance was three-fourths of the systemic resistance. The resting systemic arterial saturation was 92%.

On the basis of these findings, specifically the pulmonary artery pressures and resistances within systemic range and the equal bidirectional shunt, it was decided not to recommend surgery.

She continued to lead a slowly declining, but reasonably satisfactory existence until 1982, age 35 years. At that time she began to have severe left-sided headaches and fever; later there was confusion and aphasia. On admission to The Children's Hospital, a CT scan revealed a 3-cm diameter abscess in the left temporoparietal region. After 4 days of medical management with steroids and antibiotics, the abscess was surgically evacuated through a burr hole. The ensuing weeks in the hospital were characterized by steady improvement; however, on the 28th hospital day, she was found dead in her bed.

Postmortem examination revealed (a) left frontotemporal brain abscess with postsurgical drainage, (b) a very large atrial defect of the secundum type with a virtually absent septum primum, (c) markedly dilated main and branch pulmonary arteries, and (d) pulmonary vascular obstructive changes (Heath Edwards grade 5).

COMMENT

There are many conclusions to be drawn from this tragic case of death in a 35-year-old female with pulmonary vascular obstructive disease and a secundum atrial septal defect.

The first and most important lesson is that, for practical purposes, all atrial defects diagnosable clinically should be closed surgically in childhood. Had this young woman been so managed, irrespective of flow calculations, and in spite of a normal pulmonary arterial pressure and resistance, the catastrophe of pulmonary vascular obstructive disease and brain abscess *might* not have happened. In all honesty, it is not possible to be certain of this, since the pulmonary vascular changes might have been due to contraceptive pills or even to so-called "idiopathic pulmonary artery hypertension." Nevertheless, given the real safety and effectiveness of surgical closure of atrial defects, we continue to believe that closing *all* left-to-right shunt atrial defects is a rational policy.

What should be done with a patient who already has a right-to-left shunt? Would surgery not be recommended in 1986 as was the case in 1972? Probably, because she had the lethal combination of arterial unsaturation (92%) with increased pressure and resistance in the pulmonary circuits. Eliminating the safety valve of right-to-left shunt across the atrial septum may actually result in early demise because of the difficulty in maintaining the systemic output. The prevailing opinions however, have been changing to some extent within the past few years; adults with borderline, bidirectional shunts and pulmonary artery hypertension have been helped by surgical closure. As a rule, at The Children's Hospital in Boston, surgery still is *not* recommended for these patients. Perhaps when noninvasive approaches to atrial defect closure become available, this policy might change, but that is not yet a reality.

A few words regarding follow-up may be warranted here. If for some reason (parental or patient reluctance, geography, philospohy, or whatever) a patient with a definite secundum atrial defect is not going to be operated on, how closely should he or she be followed? Surely, more often than the 10-year span that was the case in this patient. Visits are strongly recommended yearly or at least every 2 years, including careful clinical evaluation with radiography, ECG, and echocardiography. Any change should prompt reassessment of previous decisions for procrastination.

All of the above comments relate to secundum-type atrial defects. Primum atrial defects, so-called endocardial cushion defects, are a completely different matter with more complex anatomy and physiology. Surgery in these patients is also indicated, but the operation is not quite as simple and the results are not as uniformly good as for the secundum variety. With today's knowledge of the worrisome clinical course of these patients, however, and the very good surgical results obtained by experienced cardiovascular surgeons, there is no doubt that operation, even in patients with ostium primum defect, is indicated, electively, in childhood and for symptomatic patients in infancy.

The final item to be considered is that of brain abscess. In any cyanotic patient, beyond infancy, localizing neurological signs (cerebrovascular accident) should lead to prompt investigation of the possibility of brain abscess, through CT scans and neurosurgical consultation. In contrast to embolic or hypoxic phenomena, this is a highly treatable condition. The patient generally should be treated with intravenous antibiotics for a few days to allow localization of the abscess; this is followed by drainage of the abscess through burr holes.

Findings at cardiac catheterization include: (a) The pulmonary systemic flow ratios are at or above 2:1 with the step-up occurring principally, although not exclusively, at the mid-right atrial level. The systemic cardiac output is normal to low-normal and the systemic arterial saturation is normal. (b) The right atrial and left atrial pressures are virtually identical, with prominent V waves and a mean pressure of well under 10 mm Hg. The pulmonary arterial pressure is normal as is the pulmonary capillary wedge pressure. The systemic pulse pressure may be slightly narrow. (c) Angiography with injection into the main pulmonary artery clearly outlines the atrial septal defect and may demonstrate anomalous pulmonary venous return.

Management

It has been the policy at The Children's Hospital in Boston for decades to close surgically all secundum atrial defects any time on diagnosis. The possibility that closure may be accomplished through catheter techniques in the not too distant future has already been alluded to. The question that arises frequently, is how small a defect is worth closing. Our answer has been, and still is, that all defects that can be diagnosed clinically probably should be closed. With the increased sensitivity of two-dimensional echocardiograms, this has become a problem; as of now, however, we still demand clinical criteria for surgical referral unless the diagnosis is confirmed at catheterization. In many institutions, surgeons demand precise delineation of the anomalous venous return before operation; hence the demand for preoperative catheterization. In our hands, two-dimensional echocardiography is quite sensitive in this regard; also, our surgical colleagues have proven repeatedly that they can cope with unexpected partial anomalous venous returns. Surgical mortality is less than 1%, postoperative complications, with the exception of postpericardial syndrome, are virtually nil, and the vast majority of defects are closed completely and stay that way.

Patients who have secundum atrial defect and cyanosis associated with systemic right ventricular hypertension probably should not be operated on. There is a small, but very important, group of patients with arterial unsaturation but normal right ventricular pressure, probably caused by the inferior vena cava draining directly into the left atrium through the foramen ovale (as in the fetus). In this situation, after precise catheter and angiographic delineation, surgery is mandatory to avoid all the complications of an intracardiac right-to-left shunt.

Course and Prognosis

It has been demonstrated repeatedly by older clinicians that persons with unrepaired secundum atrial defects may live normal lives for six to seven decades. However, it is our assumption (probably a correct one, although not proven for obvious reasons by a prospective randomized study) that the likelihood of a normal life is much greater if the defect is closed in childhood, even in asymptomatic patients. Patients with secundum atrial defect may remain asymptomatic through childhood and early adulthood. Often they become symptomatic in the fourth or fifth decade. Symptoms include supraventricular arrhythmias (atrial flutter and fibrillation), congestive failure, pulmonary vascular obstructive disease, and associated complications of cyanosis (cerebral vascular accidents, brain abscess, etc). At the present time, inasmuch as one cannot predict which patients will live a normal life and which will become invalids in their 40s (the size of the defect is surely not a good indicator), given the fact that surgery is safe and effective, it seems far wiser to operate on everybody.

Patients operated on in childhood and early adulthood may look forward to normal lives. In many instances, in patients without residual murmur, not even dental prophylaxis is mandatory. Two caveats should be mentioned. The first is that after the age of 20 years the later surgery is performed the less likely is the future to be symptom-free, particularly if the pulmonary arterial pressure is elevated at the time of operation. The second point is that arrhythmias in the fourth and fifth decade may occur even when faultless surgery has been performed at an appropriately young age; it seems almost as though the arrhythmia may have a "life of its own" over and beyond hemodynamics. All in all, however, as shown by a 40-year clinical postoperative follow-up on these patients, the vast majority seem to live a full normal existence.

TOTAL ANOMALOUS PULMONARY VENOUS RETURN

Definition

Total anomalous pulmonary venous return is described as absence of a normal connection of the pulmonary veins to the left atrium and entry of all the pulmonary veins into the systemic venous circulation. Entry of less than all pulmonary veins into the systemic circulation (partial anomalous pulmonary veins) causes circulatory abnormalities that resemble secundum atrial septal defects and will be discussed under that heading.

Basic Science

ANATOMY

Usually, but not invariably, the pulmonary veins collect into a single common pulmonary venous structure, which then enters an anomalous vertical vein to the innominate vein, directly to the superior vena cava, the portal vein, the right atrium, or the coronary sinus. In 46%, the site of entry is supracardiac, with the pulmonary veins entering directly into the superior vena cava or the left vertical vein; in 24%, it is cardiac, with entry directly into the right atrium or coronary sinus; in 22%, it is infracardiac (portal vein); and in 8%, the site is mixed. For the most part, the common collecting vein lies immediately behind the left atrium. Less commonly, individual veins or pairs of veins may enter the systemic venous circulation separately (Fig. 6.32).

Rarely is the left heart is abnormally small in volume but is usually dwarfed by a grossly enlarged right side, carrying the huge pulmonary blood flow. Thirty percent of patients may have total anomalous pulmonary veins associated with heterotaxy and other complex cardiac and noncardiac anomalies, as discussed under the asplenia-polysplenia syndromes. In 70% there are no other cardiac anomalies and in these extracardiac anomalies are rare.

PHYSIOLOGY

These patients present a spectrum of problems varying from greatly excessive pulmonary blood flow, which gradually appears as fetal pulmonary vasculature resistance, drops after birth, to the opposite extreme: individuals who have congenital obstruction of the pulmonary venous channels producing pulmonary venous hypertension, secondary pulmonary arterial hypertension (sometimes at suprasystemic levels), pulmonary edema, and right-to-left shunting through a ductus if it is patent. Without pulmonary venous ob-

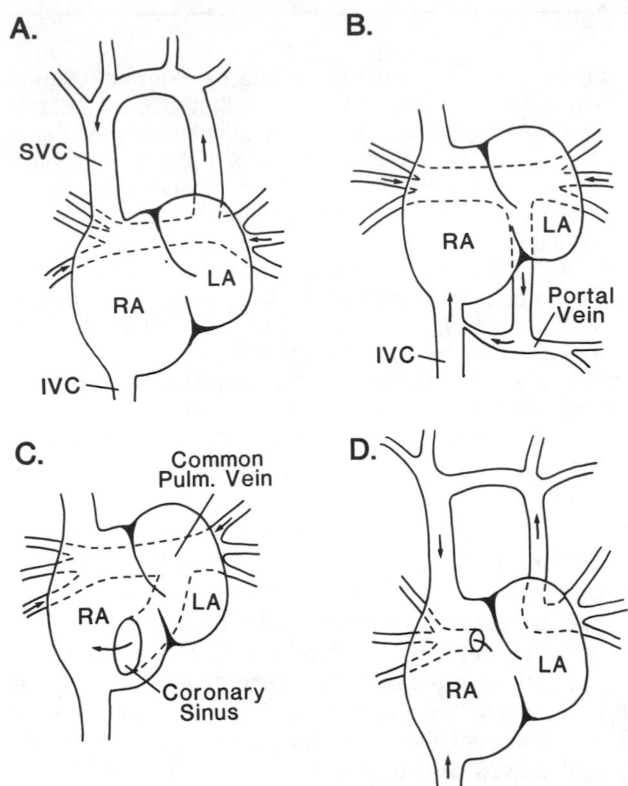

Figure 6.32. Schema of total anomalous pulmonary venous return. **A.** Supracardiac: pulmonary venous blood returns to a common pulmonary vein, then through a left vertical vein to the innominate vein, to the right atrium. **B.** Infracardiac: pulmonary venous blood returns to a common pulmonary vein, from which it passes inferiorly to the portal system. Exit from the portal system is obstructed by the requirement to pass through an obstructed ductus venosus or the liver. **C.** Cardiac: after passing through the common pulmonary venous channel, blood enters the right atrium via the coronary sinus. **D.** Mixed: the diagram depicts entry of the left veins to a left vertical vein, the innominate, and the superior vena cava. The right veins enter the right atrium directly.

struction, the large pulmonary blood flow, when mixed with the systemic venous return, results in relatively normal systemic arterial oxygen content. By contrast, with severely obstructed pulmonary veins, there is a much smaller pulmonary blood flow and, after it mixes with the systemic venous return, there may be a very low arterial oxygen saturation. All types of pulmonary venous anomalies may be obstructive, but those entering the portal system are invariably obstructed, commonly at the point of passage through the diaphragm and perhaps even more often by the spontaneous closure of the ductus venosus.

Obstruction is most common below the diaphragm and least common among those with entry into the coronary sinus. In either case the entire systemic blood flow (the cardiac output) passes through the foramen ovale, the only point of entry into the left heart. In our experience, the foramen is rarely small enough to limit cardiac output significantly.

Epidemiology

Among infants requiring hospitalization for cardiac problems, those with total anomalous pulmonary drainage constitute 2.6% of critically ill infants (Table 6.3). It is the 12th most common problem—7–9/100,000 live births (Fyler et al, 1980a).

Diagnosis

Infants with severely obstructed total anomalous pulmonary veins become cyanotic within a few hours or days of birth. Sometimes there are episodes of paroxysmal dyspnea. In contrast, infants without pulmonary venous obstruction may be discovered weeks or months after birth because of a murmur, tachypnea, cardiac hyperactivity, or poor growth.

On examination, a child with obstructive total pulmonary venous anomaly is typically deeply cyanotic and may have findings suggesting pulmonary edema. Often no murmur is audible, the second heart sound is loud and single, and confusion with persistent fetal circulation is possible. Infants with unobstructed pulmonary venous anomaly are minimally cyanotic and present a picture similar to that in patients with a large secundum atrial septal defect (e.g., a hyperactive heart, a well-split second heart sound without respiratory variation, a systolic ejection murmur, and a tricuspid diastolic rumble).

MINOR LABORATORY TESTS

If obstructed, the arterial Po_2 may be low, with a significant response after administration of 100% oxygen by hood. Among unobstructed patients, the arterial Po_2 is higher and occasionally may rise to more than 150 torr in the hyperoxia test because of greatly excessive pulmonary blood flow.

CASE ILLUSTRATION

This infant was born in 1986 of an uncomplicated pregnancy and delivery with a birth weight of 2.8 kg. Within hours of birth he was noted to have increased respiratory rate and looked pale. He was transferred to the newborn intensive care unit, evaluated for sepsis and treated with ampicillin and gentamicin. He seemed much improved by 1 week of age but the respiratory rate was noted to be 100. An echocardiogram was obtained and was interpreted as showing a normal heart.

Over the next week, the respiratory rate varied between 60 and 70 and by the age of 2 weeks, this was thought to be caused by pulmonary edema. The infant was transferred to a hospital with a pediatric cardiac unit where he was found to have tachypnea (80–100/min) and tachycardia (160/min). He was not cyanotic and there was no murmur. His electrocardiogram showed right ventricular hypertrophy, and on the chest film there was generalized haziness compatible with pulmonary edema. He was thought to have total anomalous pulmonary venous return. All arterial oxygen saturations were lower than 70% and some were as low as 40%. An echocardiogram showed a large right atrium, a large right ventricle, a small left atrium, a small left ventricle and entry of the pulmonary veins into the left atrium.

With no explanation for the low arterial oxygen saturation, cardiac catheterization was carried out and showed total anomalous veins below the diaphragm without any other significant abnormality. There was suprasystemic pulmonary artery pressure, the ductus was closed, and the pulmonary artery wedge pressure was 20.

The patient was transferred to Boston for surgery and, within 24 hours of arrival, underwent successful repair. The postoperative course was uncomplicated except for transient complete heart block which resolved in 4–5 days.

QUESTIONS AND COMMENTS

Management appears delayed and confused. Why was the diagnosis not made sooner?

In the best of hands, management which in retrospect seems confused occurs in many infants with total anomalous pulmonary venous return. The reasons for this are (a) it is a rare disease and (b) the obstructive (more common) variety mimics lung disease. The echocardiogram supports the diagnosis of lung disease by readily establishing that the heart has a normal number of chambers and valves. Nonetheless, a wary and experienced echocardiographer should not miss this diagnosis, providing he can obtain a good quality view.

Why was this diagnosis missed by two echocardiographers?

Experience is essential for reliable echocardiography.

Is it reasonable to worry about the left atrial-common pulmonary vein anastomosis which may be adequate at first but later, with growth, could become obstructive?

The late appearance of obstruction has not been observed. Either an obstructed anastomosis is discovered within weeks or months of surgery or else it will not occur.

Why did this patient's arterial saturations vary so much?

In patients with obtructed total anomalous pulmonary venous return, the amount of pulmonary edema varies depending on treatment with drugs and oxygen. When pulmonary edema is largely under control, the patient is relatively pink but when there is widespread pulmonary edema, the patient may be quite cyanotic.

How can there be complete heart block after an operation that involves only the atrial wall? Is this surgery not a long way away from the atrioventricular node and the conduction?

The actual surgery in this situation is away from the atrioventricular node and ordinarily is not associated with complete heart block. It is proposed that the trauma of vigorously pulling or stretching the atrium caused the block. Transient complete heart block (rarely permanent) is known to occur with surgery confined to the atria.

ELECTROCARDIOGRAPHY

The electrocardiogram shows severe right ventricular hypertrophy.

RADIOGRAPHY

Obstruction of all pulmonary veins causes minimal, if any, cardiac enlargement, and is often associated with evidence of pulmonary edema. Unobstructed pulmonary venous anomaly produces considerable cardiomegaly and pulmonary vascular engorgement.

ECHO-DOPPLER STUDY

Two-dimensional echocardiography readily identifies the absence of entry of pulmonary veins into the left atrium and establishes the mode of drainage of the pulmonary veins.

CARDIAC CATHETERIZATION

Cardiac catheterization is not a routine procedure for these patients; however, if there is diagnostic confusion, or poor delineation of the anatomic drainage of pulmonary veins by echo, catheterization may be needed. All children suspected of having mixed total anomalous pulmonary venous return should undergo cardiac catheterization, since detailed anatomy is required for successful surgery in this difficult group.

Management

The treatment for total anomalous pulmonary venous return is surgical correction immediately after diagnosis. In the mid 1980s, the mortality is about 10% regardless of the age at operation. At surgery, the common pulmonary vein is anastomosed to the back of the left atrium. Surgery for those with entry into the coronary sinus involves opening the coronary sinus into the left atrium and closing the coronary sinus orifice into the right atrium. For those with mixed entry of pulmonary veins, a baffle is tailored to direct the pulmonary venous flow into the left atrium (Norwood et al, 1980; Hawkins et al, 1983; Reardon et al, 1985).

Course and Prognosis

The majority of survivors are asymptomatic healthy children and have normal physiologic findings when evaluated. Pulmonary venous obstruction develops in a small number. When this involves only the point of connection between the common pulmonary vein and the left atrium, successful reoperation is possible. When individual pulmonary veins are involved in these obstructions, the outcome can be grim.

TRICUSPID ATRESIA

Definition

There are two current definitions of tricuspid atresia. One requires absence of the right-sided atrioventricular valve, whatever its morphology, whereas the other demands atresia of the morphologic tricuspid valve wherever it is located. In this section, right-sided atresia of the tricuspid valve will be discussed. According to present understanding the tricuspid valve is not really atretic; rather it never existed.

Basic Science

Caval blood flow returns normally to the right atrium, but there being no other egress, it is directed through the foramen ovale to the left atrium and left ventricle. Usually the great arteries are not transposed. Pulmonary blood flow is solely through a patent ductus arteriosus (type 1A) or through a small ventricular defect (type 1B). If the ventricular defect is large and there is no pulmonary stenosis, pulmonary blood flow is large, often large enough to cause congestive heart failure (type 1C). Less commonly (25% of the total), the great arteries are transposed (type 2), the amount of pulmonary blood flow being determined by the presence and degree of pulmonary stenosis.

In either case, the ventricular defect is likely to become smaller with time. With normally related great arteries, this will result in progressive limitation of pulmonary blood flow, decreasing evidence of congestive failure, and increasing cyanosis. With transposed great arteries, progressively higher ventricular pressures are required to produce an adequate flow through the subaortic obstruction. With rising ventricular pressure, increasing pulmonary blood flow makes a pulmonary artery banding procedure mandatory (Dick et al, 1975).

Epidemiology

Tricuspid atresia is the 14th or 15th most common cardiac defect in infants, comprising 2.6% of critically ill infants (4–6/100,000 live births; Table 6.3; Fyler et al, 1980a).

Diagnosis

Infants with tricupsid atresia are discovered early in infancy, more than 50% being admitted to a cardiac hospital during the first week of life.

PHYSICAL EXAMINATION

On physical examination, there is cyanosis of variable degree and often a murmur produced by the ventricular defect or a stenotic pulmonary outflow.

RADIOGRAPHY

A chest film usually shows a small heart if the pulmonary blood flow is low (type 1a + 1b). Occasionally (type 1c + 2) there is a large heart, sometimes with increased pulmonary blood flow, when the predominant symptom is congestive heart failure.

ELECTROCARDIOGRAPHY

The electrocardiogram is almost pathognomonic in a cyanotic baby showing a leftward superior axis and left ventricular dominance. Without this finding, the diagnosis is suspect.

ECHO-DOPPLER STUDIES

The diagnosis is confirmed by recognizing the anatomy on two-dimensional echocardiography.

CARDIAC CATHETERIZATION

Cardiac catheterization is usually carried out to confirm the diagnosis. The pulmonary arterial anatomy and the size and location of the ventricular defect may present problems in planning surgery.

Management

The goal is for the infant to reach a suitable size and age with undistorted pulmonary arteries and pulmonary pressures acceptable for a Fontan operation (Fontan and Baudet, 1971; Fontan et al, 1983; Laks et al, 1984). Rarely, particularly in those with a large ventricular defect or with transposition, a pulmonary arterial banding procedure may be required (5% of infants). Fortunately, the majority of large ventricular defects get smaller during the first months of life, obviating the need for a banding procedure. Because of this, a conservative approach toward pulmonary artery banding is recommended unless there is transposition, in which case pulmonary vascular disease is a risk. Others with decreased pulmonary flow require a systemic-pulmonary arterial shunt in early infancy to pro-

CASE ILLUSTRATION

At 1 month of age, this infant was admitted because of a loud murmur found on routine examination. There was a grade IV stenotic systolic murmur over the base of the heart. The baby seemed mildly cyanotic. The electrocardiogram showed left ventricular hypertrophy with a QRS axis of 0°. Chest film showed the heart to be moderately enlarged with increased pulmonary vascularity.

Cardiac catheterization revealed tricuspid atresia with transposition of the great arteries and a large ventricular defect. Because the baby was doing well and the arterial saturation was acceptable he was followed over the course of the next 2 years. He grew at the 50th percentile but became increasingly cyanotic. At 2 years of age, a Blalock operation was performed because of irritability and increased cyanosis. The child did well and at 5 years of age underwent cardiac catheterization which showed a mean pulmonary artery pressure of 8 mm Hg, arterial oxygen saturation of 82%, mean left ventricular end-diastolic pressure of 10, good sized pulmonary arteries without distortion, and a bulboventricular foramen which was not obstructive.

At the age of 7 years, a Fontan operation was carried out. The main pulmonary artery was ligated and the right atrial appendage was attached to the pulmonary artery. The Blalock procedure was taken down. The postoperative course was benign except for the development of junctional rhythm which has continued ever since.

At cardiac catheterization 1 year later, the cardiac output was normal and arterial saturation was 95%. The boy continues in junctional rhythm.

Since the Fontan operation he has done well in school. He rides a bike, swims, and plays football. There is no residual murmur. The neck veins are not visibly distended and the liver is not enlarged. On the chest film, his heart size is normal with normal pulmonary vascularity.

QUESTIONS AND COMMENTS

Is it true that patients who have had a Fontan operation can accomplish less exercise than normal individuals?

Although many patients can perform apparently normal activity after the Fontan procedure, it is true that their measured exercise tolerance as well as the increase in cardiac output on effort is usually less than normal for their age.

How long can a Fontan procedure be expected to function satisfactorily?

This operation was first performed in 1972. Those patients continue to do well and unexpected late problems have not been reported. Those requiring conduits as part of their Fontan operation are expected to have the late problems of conduits (see Conduits) and those in whom arrhythmias develop will also have well-recognized problems. Late unexpected difficulties resulting from the Fontan procedure are otherwise not common. The operation has been performed successfully in age groups through age 35 years.

Can the Fontan procedure be performed in infancy?

Technically the procedure can be done in infancy but survival is poor. Whether this is because the younger children proposed for Fontan procedures are sicker (unable to wait for late surgery) or because of other problems is not clear. In the first months of life, the naturally high pulmonary resistance argues against this operation being attempted.

What supplies the energy to move blood through the pulmonary circuit?

It was thought that a muscular atrium was required to pump the pulmonary circulation. In fact, right atrial pumping contributes little to the propulsion of blood; the residual energy from the left ventricular contraction provides the propelling forces. Contrary to early opinion, artificial valves are not required.

Is persistent pleural effusion common after Fontan surgery?

The Fontan operation, despite its rewarding features, has some drawbacks. Some patients, after surgery, are plagued by persistent pleural effusions for weeks or months. With continued thoracic drainage, the effusions eventually will dry up but the experience is difficult, not only for the patient but for all concerned.

vide enough pulmonary blood flow to allow survival with adequate arterial oxygen saturation and good growth; the shunt must be small if a later Fontan operation is to be possible. In a few patients, no surgery is needed in infancy (10%), inasmuch as the physiology will allow survival with good growth. Over the years, it has been recommended that balloon septostomy be carried out routinely in children with tricuspid atresia. The foramen ovale is viewed as a limitation to cardiac output. This has not been our experience and it has not been our practice to use balloon septostomy unless a pressure gradient of greater than 4 mm Hg has been demonstrated.

Course and Prognosis

Survivors with undistorted pulmonary arteries and pulmonary arterial mean pressures of less than 15 mm Hg are candidates for elective Fontan procedures at an acceptable mortality (less than 10%). Cardiac catheterization must be carried out before the Fontan operation to establish these features. If the pulmonary arteries are distorted, it may be useful to attempt reconstruction of these vessels as a primary procedure before the Fontan operation is attempted. Infants with transposition and obstruction at the level of the ventricular septal defect present a particularly difficult problem which, at least theoretically, can be approached by creating an aortopulmonary window, ligating the pulmonary artery, and providing an aortopulmonary shunt. Later, a Fontan operation may be possible.

The number of children who are born with tricuspid atresia and who will be brought through to successful Fontan procedures is not yet known (deBrux et al, 1983). Considering the relative well-being of the survivors, maintaining suitable Fontan physiology and anatomy can be a rewarding goal.

After the Fontan operation, the survivors show limited exercise tolerance when tested on a treadmill, but still are often able to engage in sports and to function without obvious problems. Their cardiac outputs measure lower than normal and do not increase normally with exercise. What will happen as the years go by is a matter of great interest.

SINGLE VENTRICLE

Definition

In recent years there has been considerable, less than productive, debate between those who use the term *single ventricle* to describe a single ventricle with two atrioventricular valves and those who use the term *univentricular* heart to describe a single ventricle with one or two atrioventricular valves (Van Praagh et al, 1979, 1982; Anderson et al, 1979, 1983c). We prefer to divide all functionally single ventricles into (a) *single ventricle* with two atrioventricular valves, (b) *tricuspid atresia*, (c) *mitral atresia*, and (d) *atrioventricular canal* with a common atrioventricular valve. If there is doubt about the anatomy of the atrioventricular valves, the terms right- or left-sided atrioventricular valve atresia are accurate and useful.

Often there is a rudimentary second ventricle serving as an outflow chamber to one of the great arteries. Roughly half of the patients have anatomic transposition of the great arteries and half have pulmonary stenosis or atresia, with or without transposition. A complex of single left ventricle, rudimentary right ventricle supplying a transposed aorta, and atrioventricular valves that are transposed comprises three-quarters of all cases diagnosed as single ventricles. The remaining 25% have a variety of other cardiac anomalies.

Basic Science

Since both pulmonary and systemic blood returns to the same ventricular chamber, there is a "common mixing chamber" with the result that the aorta and pulmonary artery contain the same amount of oxygen. The level of oxygen saturation is determined by the amount of pulmonary blood flow and by the proportion of pulmonary-to-systemic venous blood entering the common ventricle. Without pulmonary stenosis there is excessive pulmonary flow, higher systemic arterial oxygen saturation, and higher pulmonary pressure. With pulmonary stenosis the pulmonary blood flow is less, the pulmonary artery pressure is lower and the patient is more cyanotic. The communication between the common ventricle and the rudimentary outflow chamber is embryologically a ventricular septal defect (bulboventricular foramen) (Freedom et al, 1986). It is not surprising that in many of these patients, if they survive, there is spontaneous reduction in the size of the ventricular defect resulting in outflow obstruction equivalent to subaortic stenosis. Since 75% of the patients have L-malposition, heart block and left atrioventricular valve malfunction may be encountered (see Abnormalities of Cardiac Position: Corrected Transposition).

Epidemiology

Among infants transferred for cardiac examination in the first year of life, single ventricle is the 15th most common lesion (5–10/100,000 live births; Table 6.3; Fyler et al, 1980a).

Diagnosis

Depending on the amount of pulmonary blood flow relative to the systemic venous return, these babies are discovered to have heart disease in the first days of life because of cyanosis or congestive heart failure. Generally, in the 1980s, diagnostic studies are completed and a surgical plan is formulated in the newborn period before there is time for significant growth retardation.

PHYSICAL EXAMINATION

On physical examination there is cyanosis, varying in degree, depending on the severity of pulmonary stenosis.

RADIOGRAPHY

A chest film gives some idea of the relative pulmonary blood flow: the more flow, the larger the heart and the more pronounced the pulmonary vascularity.

ELECTROCARDIOGRAPHY

The electrocardiogram is rarely helpful, but often indicates that all is not normal. Often a large posterior ventricle is suggested by deeply negative QRS complexes across the chest. Attempts to decide which ventricle is which by the electrocardiogram are misleading.

ECHO-DOPPLER STUDY

Echocardiography is usually anatomically diagnostic but may be misleading or, at least, imprecise in physiological interpretation. Estimations of amounts of regurgitation, stenosis, and flow should be taken for what they are—attempts at estimates rather than definitive values.

CARDIAC CATHETERIZATION

Cardiac catheterization and angiography are routinely carried out to confirm the echocardiographers anatomic and physiological impressions.

Management

The plan of management in infancy is to provide sufficient arterial oxygen saturation, to allow growth, control congestive heart failure, prevent the development of pulmonary vascular disease and preserve the integrity of the pulmonary arteries so that a Fontan operation can be carried out later. In the 1980s, we believe that careful use of prostaglandins, pulmonary artery banding, systemic pulmonary arterial shunting procedures, and anticongestive medications will enable a child to reach a suitable size and age for a Fontan operation (Fontan and Baudet, 1971) or, less likely, ventricular septation (McKay et al, 1982).

Course and Prognosis

With the best of management, mortality in early infancy is high (25–50%; Gale et al, 1979). Many of those who survive with natural pulmonary stenosis are able to have successful modified Fontan operations; there is a reasonable operative mortality (10%). Those who have had a pulmonary artery banding procedure are less fortunate. In some there is major distortion of the pulmonary artery from a migratory band, which prohibits a Fontan operation at acceptable risk. Others have inadequate bands resulting in pulmonary vascular obstructive disease. In still others, progressive obstruction of the embryologic ventricular defect (bulboventricular foramen) develops; this is the functional equivalent of subaortic stenosis (Freedom et al, 1983). Attempts to get around this obstruction by making a proximal aortopulmonary window, distally ligating the pulmonary artery and providing a systemic-pulmonary arterial shunt, are sometimes successful. Overall, those requiring banding procedures do not do nearly as well as those who have native pulmonary stenosis with or without a shunting procedure.

Children with single ventricle who have survived a modified Fontan procedure are remarkably well. Although there is abundant information indicating limited cardiac output and exercise tolerance, thus far survivors of Fontan operations live nearly normal lives.

AORTIC STENOSIS

Definition

Obstruction of the outflow of the left ventricle may occur, most commonly, at the aortic valve level or, less frequently, below or above the valve.

Basic Science

ANATOMY

All degrees of *aortic valve* obstruction, including atresia, may be present at birth. In the neonate these valves often seem uncorrectably abnormal, appearing jelly-like and lumpy (Messina et al, 1984). With survival, this embryonic tissue continues to develop in extrauterine life and becomes more typical of a diseased aortic valve. The valve may be bicuspid (bicommissural) or, occasionally unicuspid; for practical purposes, it remains abnormal, although the degree of obstruction is likely to worsen with time. By the third decade, the abnormal valve tissue begins to calcify.

Membranous *subvalvar* aortic stenosis is an acquired problem, virtually never diagnosed at birth, consisting of a progressively obstructive membrane beneath the aortic valve. Occasionally it takes the form of fibrous tissue, obstructing over some length, and involving the insertion of the mitral valve at the point of aortic-mitral continuity. In contrast to valvar aortic stenosis, this type of left ventricular outflow obstruction is often associated with other congenital cardiac defects, such as ventricular septal defect, interrupted aortic arch and coarctation of the aorta. There may be additional muscular obstruction, actually becoming more obstructive with cardiac contraction. This feature will be discussed under the heading of obstructive cardiomyopathy (see Myocardial Disease). The subvalvar obstruction produces a jet of blood which, with time, damages the aortic valve itself, producing aortic insufficiency.

Supravalvar aortic stenosis can be described as a supravalvar coarctation. There is sometimes discrete, at other times a tunnel-like, narrowing beginning right above the valve, sometimes extending as far as the first branches of the brachiocephalic vessels. There may also be associated obstruction at the takeoff of the branches, or even typical coarctation at the usual site; finally, there may be stenosis of the renal or pulmonary arteries. Many of these patients have Williams syndrome (Williams et al, 1961), some of whom have been shown to have a problem with calcium and vitamin D metabolism in infancy (Black and Bonham-Carter, 1963).

PHYSIOLOGY

The more obstruction there is, the greater is the left ventricular pressure needed to provide the required systemic output at adequate systemic pressure (mean 40–60 mm Hg needed for renal perfusion). In a normal individual the systemic pressure rises with exercise, often reaching as high as 200 mm Hg. Given the fact that even moderate aortic stenosis may result in a resting left ventricular pressure of 180 mm Hg having to provide a systolic pressure of 120 mm Hg at rest, the problem for the left ventricle during exercise is apparent. To produce the needed pressures the left ventricle must hypertrophy, and with severe aortic stenosis the degree of ventricular hypertrophy may be massive.

Epidemiology

Valvar aortic stenosis seldom causes problems in early infancy (4/100,000 live births and the 16th most common defect—1.9% of total; Table 6.3; Fyler et al, 1980a), but it is the second most common congenital cardiac defect in young adults (only ventricular septal defect occurs more frequently). There are more than 1300 cases of aortic stenosis in the files of The Children's Hospital, Boston. Subaortic obstruction was documented about 250 times and supravalvar aortic stenosis is mentioned less than 100 times.

Diagnosis

Since aortic stenosis of any type produces a stenotic murmur, the diagnosis is commonly made on routine examination with the discovery of a loud systolic murmur with wide transmission to the suprasternal notch and carotids. Children with supravalvar aortic stenosis may have the features of Williams syndrome, with a decreased left radial pulse because of stenosis at the take-off of the left subclavian. Those with other lesions, interrupted aortic arch or coarctation of the aorta, may, as neonates, have symptoms of congestive failure resulting from the associated defects, only to have subaortic stenosis discovered later.

Children with isolated obstruction are rarely symptomatic, although a few with severe obstruction may have anginal pain on exercise and, occasionally, syncope. Sudden death, as the first symptom, accounts for some unfortunate events associated with vigorous sports. Rarely does this occur without symptoms of left ventricular strain. Infants with valvar aortic stenosis, by contrast, are critically ill, with congestive heart failure and a cardiac output so low that a murmur is noted only after adequate anticongestive treatment.

On physical examination beyond infancy, the intensity of the systolic ejection murmur is proportionate with the severity of the obstruction (Fig. 6.3*B*). It is generally true that patients with severe aortic stenosis beyond infancy have a thrill at the second right interspace and the suprasternal notch. There is a constant ejection click at the apex. With subaortic stenosis, the murmur may be maximal along the left sternal border and there is no ejection click. The presence of an early diastolic murmur indicates aortic incompetence; it may be present in both valvar and subvalvar lesions. With valvar lesions, it suggests a bicuspid valve. Usually the murmur of supravalvar aortic stenosis is maximal over the base of the heart and may be noted as among the loudest murmurs of the whole group.

ELECTROCARDIOGRAPHY

There is left ventricular hypertrophy proportionate with the amount of obstruction. ST and T wave changes ("strain pattern") suggest critical stenosis.

RADIOGRAPHY

The heart size is usually normal with left ventricular contour despite massive hypertrophy.

ECHO-DOPPLER STUDY

The anatomic defects can be well-documented by two-dimensional echocardiography. Doppler estimation of pressure gradients across obstructions is reasonably accurate but usually catheter gradients are overestimated.

CARDIAC CATHETERIZATION

All patients with aortic stenosis suspected of needing surgery should undergo cardiac catheterization. Those with valvar stenosis may be candidates for aortic balloon valvuloplasty although, in 1986, this is still an experimental procedure. In those with subaortic or supravalvar stenoses a search should be made for associated lesions.

Management

VALVAR STENOSIS

The routine management of valvar aortic stenosis in 1986 is surgical valvotomy. This procedure has stood the test of many years. Patients with moderate or severe aortic regurgitation need aortic valve replacement. Arbitrarily, patients with gradients of 75 mm Hg or more should have a valvotomy. Those with lesser gradients, with strain, also should be operated on as should those who are symptomatic. Critically ill infants may require prostaglandins to provide an output sufficient for survival (Jonas et al, 1985).

Balloon valvuloplasty has been developed in the past 2 years and may become the treatment of choice for the future. Some details related to this plan remain to clarified. It is not clear whether it is useful for individuals of all ages. Certainly it seems effective for very old adults and very young children. A stiff balloon is inflated in the aortic valve and the valve is torn open. The result is approximately comparable to that of open surgical relief, and there is the advantage that repeated dilatation is possible; if surgery is still needed it is available (see Table 6.2). Valvuloplasty is undertaken when the pressure gradient is greater than 40–50 mm Hg. Patients who have ST and T changes with an even lesser gradient are also candidates for valvuloplasty,

CASE ILLUSTRATION

A 6-year-old asymptomatic male was discovered to have a grade III stenotic systolic murmur, loudest at the second right intercostal space, during evaluation before tonsillectomy. The chest film and electrocardiogram were normal. The diagnosis of aortic stenosis was made.

At the age of 11 years the boy continued to be asymptomatic, but the murmur was louder. The electrocardiogram showed left ventricular hypertrophy without "strain." Cardiac catheterization was carried out and a gradient of 40 mm Hg of systolic pressure between the left ventricle and the ascending aorta was documented.

At age 13 years, because of the appearance of ST and T wave changes on the electrocardiogram, a valvotomy was carried out. Postoperatively, the electrocardiogram was unchanged and a grade III diastolic murmur of aortic regurgitation was noted.

At the present time this young man is 18 years old. The heart is enlarged on the chest film (Fig. 6.33). His electrocardiogram shows left ventricular hypertrophy with ST and T changes. He continues to be asymptomatic. His echocardiogram shows normal left ventricular function. There is a grade III stenotic systolic murmur maximal at the second right intercostal space and a grade II blowing diastolic murmur of medium duration at the third left intercostal space. His blood pressure is 120/60. This boy is an unusually talented athlete. He has limited his competitive sports to varsity baseball during school.

QUESTIONS AND COMMENTS

Is the systolic gradient of only 40 mm Hg between the left ventricle and aorta sufficient to recommend surgery?

In the face of ST and T changes ("left ventricular strain"), it was concluded that a valvotomy should be carried out.

Is the degree of aortic regurgitation a high price to pay for the reduction of a systolic gradient in an asymptomatic patient?

Possibly. The goal of surgery for aortic stenosis is to minimize the possibility of sudden death and to preserve myocardial function. Management is designed to provide reasonable function for decades. In attempting to reach these goals some risks are involved. How many decades this young man will be asymptomatic remains to be seen.

How is it possible to miss the murmur of congenital aortic stenosis until the age of 6 years?

Because of the dangers of sudden death during varsity sports, high school athletes are screened for heart murmurs. A surprising number of individuals are discovered to have aortic stenosis who have no prior history of a heart murmur. This and catheterization documentation of increasing severity of aortic stenosis over the years has led to the conclusion that it is a progressive disease. Presumably this young man's aortic stenosis was milder and did not produce a particularly noticeable murmur before the age of 6 years.

If there is danger associated with varsity sports, why was this boy allowed to play varsity baseball?

While no vigorous competitive sports are desirable for these patients, the passionate involvement with sports among some teenage boys requires a compromise between the risk of death and the satisfaction of participation. In this case, pitching baseball was chosen as the least violent exercise, over the boy's favorite activities (basketball, hockey, track, and swimming).

open or closed, since they are prone to sudden unexpected death.

SUBAORTIC STENOSIS

Because of the tendency of the left ventricular jet to damage the aortic valve, the indications for relief of subaortic stenosis are more liberal. Unfortunately, this lesion is particularly progressive, but fortunately, surgery is particularly effective. Any patient having a gradient of 25–30 mm Hg with a clearly demonstrable membranous obstruction is referred for surgical resection. The results are particularly gratifying (Wright et al, 1983).

SUPRAVALVAR AORTIC STENOSIS

Supravalvar aortic stenosis must be evaluated in relation to the other vascular problems present. A gradient of 50–60 mm Hg can be relieved, but surgical relief of coarctation may be a priority. Discrete supravalvar stenosis can be handled effectively, but success of surgery for long tunnel-like obstruction is dubious (Keane et al, 1976).

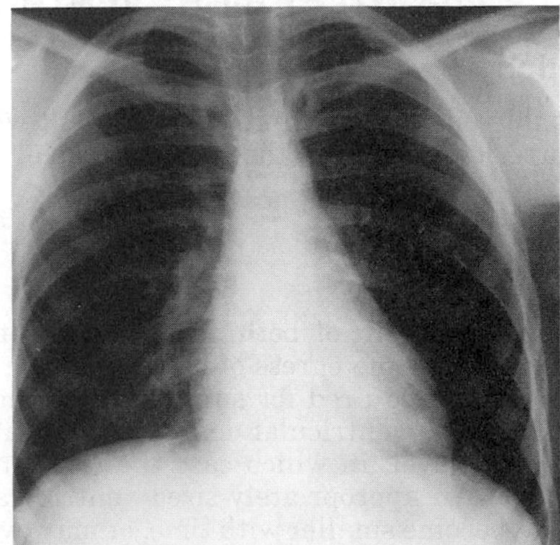

Figure 6.33. Chest film of patient with aortic stenosis. It shows no abnormality.

Course and Prognosis

Valvar aortic stenosis requires continuing attention at least yearly throughout the patient's life. The tendency toward progression is well-documented. Calcification of the valve by the third decade is common. Valve replacement and re-replacement may ultimately be the final steps. At all times, the goals of management are prevention of sudden death and preservation of the myocardium. Often the patient looks and acts well, despite repeated hospitalizations, operations, and chronic therapy. With as much manipulation as is required, however, it is not surprising that there is, over the years, a steady loss of life.

Infectious endocarditis is perhaps more common among people with this congenital anomaly than with any other disorder.

Resection of a subvalvar membrane may be curative. Nevertheless, such patients should also be regularly observed indefinitely for evidence of recurrence. When an attempt has been made to open up fibrous subaortic stenosis of some length, the result is rarely completely satisfactory. Sometimes there is mitral valve damage and rarely is the subaortic obstruction relieved completely. Infectious endocarditis is common.

Patients having supravalvar obstructions should be observed indefinitely, because the vascular obstructions seem to be progressive in some and relief of the supravalvar obstruction is rarely complete.

Most of these patients are males and many are "jocks." The question of how much athletics these patients should be allowed is a real problem. Our policy is to prohibit *competitive* sports in all, whether or not our patients have undergone surgery. Recreational sports are to be encouraged; the level of activity may be evaluated by periodic stress testing. The whole issue is a very tricky one; it needs a great deal of understanding on everybody's part and tact and wisdom from the cardiologist.

DOUBLE-OUTLET RIGHT VENTRICLE

Definition

Double-outlet right ventricle is present when both great arteries arise from the right ventricle.

Basic Science

ANATOMY

With the origin of both great arteries from the right ventricle, some egress of blood from the left side of the heart is required for survival. This most often occurs through a ventricular defect, but may also occur at the atrial level, in which case the left ventricle is diminutive. An appropriately-sized ventricular septal defect can become smaller with time, or may even close, and result in a fatal outcome for these patients. When a ventricular septal defect is positioned immediately below the great arteries, it is not always obvious that both great arteries arise from the right ventricle (Anderson et al, 1983a). Arbitrarily, if no more than one-half of a great vessel appears to arise from the left ventricle the patient is considered to have a double-outlet right ventricle. The great arteries and the underlying conal tissue may assume a variety of relative positions. Often the two semilunar valves lie side by side when viewed anteroposteriorly.

There is potential confusion between double-outlet right ventricle and (a) ventricular defect, (b) tetralogy of Fallot and (c) transposition of the great arteries, with or without pulmonary stenosis. There is a spectrum of patients ranging from those classified as having typical ventricular septal defect to those with double-outlet right ventricle with the *aorta committed to the left ventricle*. All positions of the aorta ranging from being directly over the left ventricle to being unequivocally committed to the right ventricle are seen. A similar range of anomalies is encountered when the pulmonary artery relates to the left ventricle. Thus, there is another spectrum ranging from patients with typical D-transposition of the great arteries with a ventricular septal defect to those having double-outlet right ventricle with ventricular septal defect, with the *pulmonary artery committed to the left ventricle*. Finally, there are patients with *uncommitted great arteries* whose great vessels are not clearly committed to either of the ventricles.

Double-outlet right ventricle is often associated with abnormal segmental relationships and with dextrocardia, mesocardia, and splenic agenesis. Mitral valve anomalies are common as is coarctation of the aorta.

Whichever great artery relates more closely to the left ventricle generally determines the physiology. If the aorta receives most of its blood from the left ventricle, the physiology is that of a ventricular septal defect. If the pulmonary artery relates best to the left ventricle, the physiology is that of transposition of the great arteries.

Epidemiology

The prevalence of double-outlet right ventricle depends on what criteria are used to decide whether the great vessels lie dominantly over the right or left ventricle. Since this is a subjective observation, prevalence varies considerably. The New England Regional Infant Cardiac Program placed a conservative 1.5% of the critically ill infants in the double-outlet right ventricle category (3/100,000 live births; Table 6.3; Fyler et al, 1980a).

Diagnosis

The clinical picture depends on the anatomic and physiologic situation. Those who have the aorta committed to the left ventricle may appear to have ventricular septal defect, or, if there is pulmonary stenosis, a variant of tetralogy of Fallot. Patients with the pulmonary artery committed to the left ventricle may be admitted as infants with transposition of the great arteries. Those patients with double-outlet right ventricle whose great arteries are committed to neither ventricle may have a wide range of symptoms and physical findings.

ELECTROCARDIOGRAPHY

The electrocardiogram is variable, often showing right ventricular hypertrophy but, on occasion, showing combined or left ventricular hypertrophy. A leftward superior QRS axis is often encountered.

RADIOGRAPHY

The degree of pulmonary stenosis determines the pulmonary flow, the size of the heart, the amount of shunting, and the degree of congestive failure.

ECHO-DOPPLER STUDY

The echocardiographer will generally recognize the internal anatomy in detail and will look specifically for mitral valve problems and for coarctation of the aorta.

CARDIAC CATHETERIZATION

Cardiac catheterization is used preoperatively to confirm the detailed anatomy. Occasionally, data concerning physiologic streaming from the left ventricle to either great artery is helpful in defining probable commitment of a great artery to the ventricle.

Management

Because of the wide variability in the anatomic and physiologic abnormalities, surgery for these patients is also variable (Luber et al, 1983; Piccoli et al, 1983). Corrective procedures range from those typically used for ventricular septal defect or tetralogy of Fallot to those used for transposition of the great arteries with ventricular septal defect. Surgery is tailored to the case. The outcome of surgery depends on the anatomy and the operative procedure used.

Course and Prognosis

The course of patients with double-outlet right ventricle varies widely because a large variety of physiologic problems are presented.

TRUNCUS ARTERIOSUS

Definition

Truncus arteriosus is characterized by the origin of a single great artery from the heart which gives rise to the pulmonary arteries and the aorta. There is almost invariably an associated ventricular septal defect.

Basic Science

The single arterial trunk may give off a single main pulmonary artery (type I) or separate right and left pulmonary arteries (type II) just above the semilunar valves. There may be stenosis at the origin of the right and left pulmonary arteries and occasionally patients have only a single right pulmonary artery. The semilunar valve is usually abnormal, often having misshapen cusps with up to five leaflets. The ventricular defect is subaortic and occasionally the aortic arch is interrupted (Hernanz-Schulman and Fellows, 1985). The thymus is often absent and variations of the DiGeorge syndrome (pp. 845) are common (Raatikka et al, 1981). As many as half of the patients with truncus arteriosus have some additional noncardiac anomaly (Fyler et al, 1980a).

All left and right ventricular blood passes through the single semilunar valve which, therefore, is large and often incompetent, sometimes to a severe degree. Pulmonary flow is usually large and, therefore, the arterial oxygen saturation is 80–90%. Pulmonary arterial pressure is systemic. Congestive failure is common.

Epidemiology

Truncus arteriosus is a rare lesion occurring in 3–4 infants/100,000 live births, the 18th most common cardiac defect among sick infants (Table 6.3; Fyler et al, 1980a).

Diagnosis

These infants become ill over the course of the first days and weeks of life with symptoms of congestive failure. Cyanosis is often overlooked. There is evidence of congestive failure with a hyperactive cardiac impulse, an enlarged liver, and tachypnea. Usually there are murmurs, sometimes loud to-and-fro murmurs.

ELECTROCARDIOGRAPHY

The electrocardiogram usually shows left ventricular hypertrophy, but may show right or combined ventricular hypertrophy; it is never normal. In contrast, in patients with pulmonary atresia and ventricular septal defect the electrocardiogram almost invariably shows right ventricular hypertrophy.

RADIOGRAPHY

The heart size is large, with increased pulmonary vascularity. The pulmonary artery segment is diminished or absent.

ECHO-DOPPLER STUDY

The echocardiographer rapidly discovers the typical anatomy.

CARDIAC CATHETERIZATION

Cardiac catheterization is usually carried out as soon as the defect is discovered, because surgery is imminent. The critical questions relate to the anatomy and function of the semilunar valve. The degree of truncal regurgitation is assessed, the location of the coronaries and the origin of the pulmonary arteries are noted. Additional anomalies are evaluated (i.e., second ventricular defects, interrupted aortic arch, peripheral pulmonary stenosis).

Management

Once associated extracardiac anomalies are evaluated and controlled as well as possible and congestive failure is treated, an attempt to gain growth is made. It is usually apparent within days or weeks whether this is likely to succeed or that surgical options offer the most benefit for the least risk. While successful banding of both the right and left pulmonary arteries has been accomplished, it is difficult to provide ideal pulmonary flow under these circumstances. Consequently, surgical repair is required for virtually all such infants relatively early in life (Ebert et al, 1984). Enthusiasm for surgery is greatly dampened by the presence of more than minimal truncal regurgitation. Depending on how cases are selected, survival varies widely.

Course and Prognosis

The natural course is rapidly downhill, the average age at death being a matter of weeks. Successful repair includes closure of the ventricular defect and connection of the right ventricle to the pulmonary artery by an artifical conduit. It is to be hoped that there will be no need for an artifical semilunar valve. The conduit will need replacement with growth; however, the surviving child may be surprisingly well.

OTHER CONGENITAL HEART DISEASES

Mitral Stenosis and Related Problems

Congenital mitral stenosis (Ruckman and Van Praagh, 1978; Collins-Nakai et al, 1977), parachute mitral valve (Shone et al, 1963), cor triatriatum (Marin-Garcia et al, 1975; Richardson et al, 1981; Oglietti et al, 1983), supravalvar mitral ring (Richardson et al, 1981; Oglietti et al, 1983; Sullivan et al, 1986), and pulmonary venous stenosis (Pacifico et al, 1985; Bini et al, 1984) are all very rare defects (Fyler et al, 1980a).

Basic Science

ANATOMY

Obstructive deformity of the mitral leaflets is rare and often is associated with chordal fusion (*mitral arcade*; Castaneda et al, 1969). Attachment of the two mitral leaflets to a single papillary muscle results in what is usually described as *parachute mitral valve*. An obstructive ring of tissue immediately above the mitral valve and downstream from the atrial appendage is called *supravalvar mitral stenosis*. This defect and parachute mitral valve are often associated with coarctation of the aorta and subaortic stenosis (Shone syndrome; Shone et al, 1963). *Cor triatriatum* consists of an obstructive membrane upstream from the atrial appendage. Finally, the individual pulmonary veins may acquire progressive obstruction at their orifices.

CASE ILLUSTRATION

A infant is a fraternal twin who did well until the age of 7 weeks, when he developed tachypnea, tachycardia, and radiographic signs of interstitial pneumonia. There was no fever. He was hospitalized and treated for pneumonia for 7 days without significant response. Because of the course which could be explained by congestive failure, a cardiac consultation was obtained. There was a grade I systolic murmur, but no diastolic murmur. There was tachypnea at 80 beats/min and tachycardia at 130 beats/min. The chest film suggested pulmonary edema (Fig. 6.34). The electrocardiogram showed right ventricular hypertrophy. A two-dimensional echocardiogram revealed a membrane bisecting the left atrium and obstructing blood flow out of the lungs.

The diagnosis of cor triatriatum was confirmed at cardiac catheterization. There was severe pulmonary hypertension and a pulmonary arterial wedge pressure was recorded as 26 mm Hg. Anomalous entry of the right upper pulmonary vein into the right atrium was found. The next day a left atrial membrane was excised, and the anomalous right pulmonary vein was anastomosed to the left atrium. The child has been well since.

COMMENT

The reason for including a case report on this rare disease is self-evident. If recognized, the patient can be cured.

PHYSIOLOGY

All of these lesions produce pulmonary venous hypertension in proportion to the severity of obstruction. When the obstruction is severe there is pulmonary edema and pulmonary arterial hypertension.

Except for mitral valve stenosis (Fig. 6.3*B*), there usually is no diastolic murmur despite a diastolic pres-

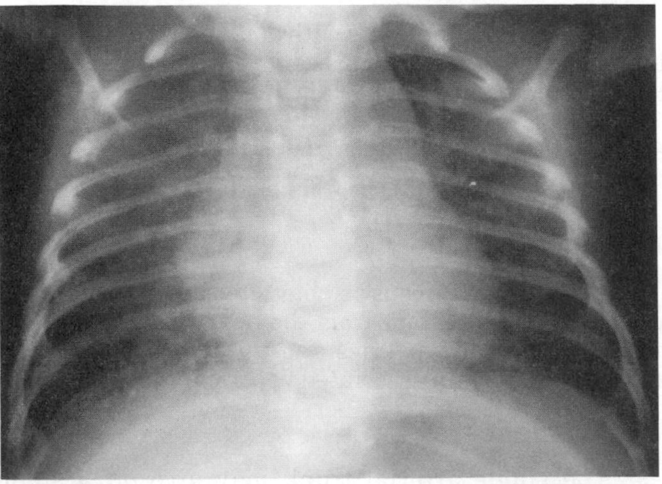

Figure 6.34. Chest film of infant with cor triatriatum shows a normal-sized heart with evidence of pulmonary edema initially interpreted as interstitial pneumonia.

sure gradient from the pulmonary veins to the left ventricle. Diagnostic confusion centers around the distinction between intraparenchymal pulmonary disease and pulmonary edema. Signs suggesting cor pulmonale are the rule. Lack of fever, lack of response to antibiotics, and possible presence of other cardiac defects (coarctation, ventricular defects, subaortic stenosis) lead to the correct diagnosis.

The electrocardiogram shows right ventricular hypertrophy. The chest film may show pulmonary vascular congestion, even pulmonary edema. Two-dimensional echocardiography confirms the diagnosis. At cardiac catheterization the severity of the defect can be measured and the surgical anatomy confirmed.

Supravalvar mitral rings and cor triatratum respond readily to surgery. Naturally occurring pulmonary venous obstruction rarely responds to any form of intervention (Bini et al, 1984) and is almost invariably fatal. Obstructive mitral arcade, obstructive mitral parachute valve, and congenital mitral stenosis are treated conservatively as long as possible before surgery is attempted since the outcome is less than satisfactory and mitral valve replacement may be required.

As indicated, the pulmonary arterial hypertension secondary to pulmonary venous hypertension is reversible; hence early elective surgery is not necessary except to relieve symptoms (see Pulmonary Venous Hypertension). If valve replacement is a possibility, there is good reason to procrastinate with surgery, if possible, to avoid or at least diminish multiple valve replacements in a lifetime.

Ebstein Anomaly

Ebstein anomaly consists of variable degrees of downward displacement of the tricuspid valve with "atrialization" of the inflow portion of the right ventricle and a small, thin-walled "true" right ventricular cavity.

Basic Science

The septal leaflet and, less frequently, the posterior leaflet of the tricuspid valve are displaced downward and are redundant. The right atrium is large, including the "atrialized" portion of the right ventricle. Ebstein disease accounts for some of the largest cardiac silhouettes seen in childhood (Fig. 6.35). The physiologic abnormality is under debate. There is tricuspid regurgitation in most patients, but why tricuspid regurgitation produces such profound changes in this disease as compared to other forms of tricuspid regurgitation is not clear. There is limitation of passage of blood through the right ventricle and consequently, some may pass right to left through the patent foramen ovale, producing cyanosis.

Epidemiology

This anomaly was found in 13 of 2251 consecutive infants with heart disease (Fyler et al, 1980a) or approximately 1/100,000 live births. It seems probable that, since the disease is quite variable and may be so mild that recognition is delayed for decades, this prevalence number may be low (Watson, 1974).

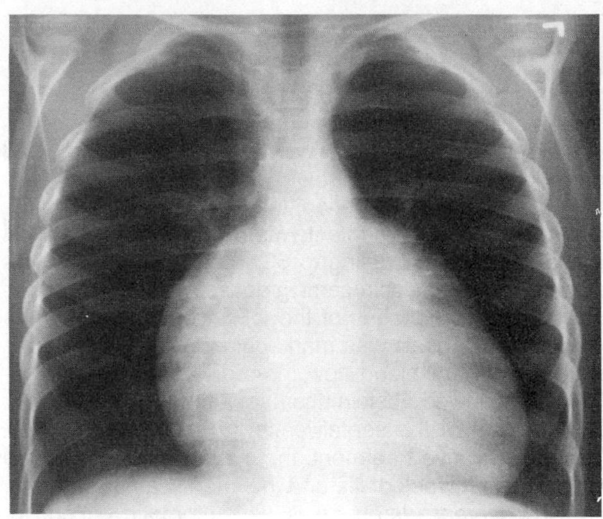

Figure 6.35. Chest film of child with Ebstein disease. Note the large heart with large, dilated, right-sided (right atrial) structures.

Diagnosis

Cyanosis may be present at birth, may be profound in infancy, and is associated with a high mortality. Mild forms of the disease are not associated with cyanosis and cause relatively few symptoms. Most patients are discovered because of cyanosis or are accidentally found because of cardiac enlargement on a chest film taken for some other purpose.

On auscultation, there is usually a loud third or fourth heart sound with a widely split second sound, giving rise to a quadruple rhythm at the apex. Classically, the electrocardiogram has wide QRS complexes and large bizarre P waves; occasionally the Wolff-Parkinson-White syndrome is present. In contrast to critical valve pulmonary stenosis, there rarely is severe right ventricular hypertrophy. The chest film shows a large, occasionally huge, heart with decreased pulmonary vasculature. Two-dimensional echocardiography is diagnostic. Cardiac catheterization is rarely needed unless there is evidence to suggest an associated cardiac abnormality. Electrophysiologic studies may be needed to sort out supraventricular arrhythmias and are used to establish electroventricular dissociation.

Management

Treatment is usually expectant even in newborns with severe cyanosis. Arrhythmias are treated as they develop. Congestive heart failure or severe cyanosis may serve as an indication for tricuspid valvuloplasty (Oh et al, 1985) or replacement of the tricuspid valve and closure of the foramen ovale in adults (less than 10% of the patients in the first 20 years of life).

CASE ILLUSTRATION

A newborn was noted to have dusky color during his first bath at 8 hours of age. A murmur was discovered and on the chest film, the heart was noted to be very large.

On physical examination, there was a loud gallop audible at the apex. The infant was cyanotic. The umbilical arterial Po_2 was 52, rising to 63 when 80% oxygen was administered. The electrocardiogram showed large P waves and decreased voltages of the QRS complexes. On the chest film, the heart was markedly enlarged, with diminished pulmonary blood flow. Two-dimensional echocardiography showed Ebstein anomaly with the classic inferior displacement of the septal leaflet of the tricuspid valve. With conservative treatment, the cyanosis cleared by the end of the first week of life and the infant was discharged.

Now 6 years later, he is asymptomatic except for some minimal limitation in exercise tolerance. He is going to school and is well. In a single episode, supraventricular tachycardia was converted and he is taking propranolol. At cardiac catheterization with electrophysiologic studies, no bypass tract could be identified.

COMMENT

The reason for including a case report of this rare disease is that despite the combination of cyanosis, a gallop rhythm, and a huge heart on the chest film, survival in the first months of life may indicate many good years ahead.

Course and Prognosis

With the involution of neonatal pulmonary hypertension, a cyanotic baby may become pink within the first weeks of life. Most of those who survive infancy live active, vigorous lives for many years, even decades. Rhythm abnormalities are common in adults. Congestive heart failure is rare in children. It is important to note that the heart size has little relationship to the prognosis.

Coronary Artery Fistulas

Fistulas between a coronary artery and a cardiac chamber (the right ventricle, the right atrium or, rarely, pulmonary artery) result in a loud systolic-diastolic murmur, usually not at the location of a ductus arteriosus. The atypical location of the continuous murmur thereby suggests this diagnosis. An unusual bulge in the cardiac silhouette may be seen and excess pulmonary blood flow may be demonstrable on the chest film. These anomalies can be identified readily by echocardiography and delineated in detail at cardiac catheterization before surgical closure of the fistula, which generally completely abolishes the shunt (Lowe et al, 1981).

Kawasaki disease is discussed in Section 17, page 1108.

REFERENCES

Alpert BS, Cook DH, Varghese PJ, et al: Spontaneous closure of small ventricular septal defects: Ten year follow-up. *Pediatrics* 63:204-206, 1979.

Anderson RH, Becker AE, Freedom RM, et al: Problems in the nomenclature of the univentricular heart. *Herz* 4:97-106, 1979.

Anderson RH, Becker AE, Wilcox BR, et al: Surgical anatomy of double outlet right ventricle—A reappraisal. *Am J Cardiol* 52:555-559, 1983a.

Anderson RH, Lenox CC, Zuberbuhler JR: Mechanisms of closure of perimembranous ventricular septal defect. *Am J Cardiol* 52:341-345, 1983b.

Anderson RH, Macartney FJ, Tynan M, et al: Univentricular atrioventricular connection: The single ventricle trap unsprung. *Pediatr Cardiol* 4:273-280, 1983c.

Artman M, Graham TP Jr: Congestive heart failure in infancy: Recognition and management. *Am Heart J* 103:1040-1055, 1982.

Artman M, Parrish MD, Boerth RC, et al: Short-term hemodynamic effects of hydralazine in infants with complete atrioventricular canal defects. *Circulation* 69:949-954, 1984.

Awariefe SO, Clarke DR, Pappas G: Surgical approach to critical pulmonary valve stenosis in infants less than six months of age. *J Thorac Cardiovasc Surg* 85:375-387, 1983.

Bailey L, Concepcion W, Shattuck H, et al: Method of heart transplantation for treatment of hypoplastic left heart syndrome. *J Thorac Cardiovasc Surg* 92:1-5, 1986.

Barcroft J: *Researches of Prenatal Life*, Springfield, IL, Charles C Thomas, 1947, 287 pp.

Becu L, Somerville J, Gallo A: "Isolated" pulmonary valve stenosis as part of more widespread cardiovascular disease. *Br Heart J* 38:472-482, 1976.

Beekman RH, Rocchini AP, Rosenthal A: Hemodynamic effects of hydralazine in infants with a large ventricular septal defect. *Circulation* 65:523-528, 1982.

Beerman LB, Park SC, Fischer DR, et al: Ventricular septal defect associated with aneursym of the membranous septum. *J Am Coll Cardiol* 5:118-123, 1985.

Berman W, Yabek SM, Dillon T, et al: Effects of digoxin in infants with a congested circulatory state due to a ventricular septal defect. *N Engl J Med* 308:363-366, 1983.

Bini RM, Cleveland D, Cebailos R, et al: Congenital pulmonary venous stenosis. *Am J Cardiol* 54:369-375, 1984.

Black JA, Bonham-Carter RE: Association between aortic stenosis and facies of severe infantile hypercalcemia. *Lancet* 2:745-748, 1963.

Blalock A, Taussig H: The surgical treatment of malformation of the heart. *JAMA* 128:189, 1945.

Borow KM, Arensman FW, Webb C, et al: Assessment of left ventricular contractile state after anatomic correction of transposition of the great arteries. *Circulation* 69:106-112, 1984.

Borow KM, Keane JF, Castaneda AR, et al: Systemic ventricular function in patients with tetralogy of Fallot, ventricular defect and transposition of the great arteries repaired in infancy. *Circulation* 64:878-885, 1981.

Breall JA, Rudolph AM, Heymann MA: Role of thyroid hormone in postnatal circulatory and metabolic adjustments. *J Clin Invest* 73:1418-1424, 1984.

Bull C, de Leval MR, Mercanti C, et al: Pulmonary atresia and intact ventricular septum: A revised classification. *Circulation* 66:266-280, 1982.

Bull C, Rigby ML, Shinebourne EA: Should management of complete atrioventricular canal defect be influenced by coexistant Down syndrome. *Lancet* 1:1147-1149, 1985.

Byrum CJ, Dick M, Behrendt DM, et al: Excitation of the double chamber right ventricle: Electrophysiologic and anatomic correlation. *Am J Cardiol* 49:1254-1258, 1982.

Capelli H, Andrade JL, Somerville J: Classification of the site of ventricular septal defect by 2-dimensional echocardiography. *Am J Cardiol* 51:1474-1480, 1983.

Carlgren LE: The incidence of congenital heart disease in Gothenburg. *Proc Assoc Eur Paediatr Cardiol* 5:2-8, 1969.

Castaneda AR, Anderson RG, Edwards JE: Congenital mitral stenosis resulting from anomalous arcade and obstructing papillary muscles. *Am J Cardiol* 24:237-240, 1969.

Castaneda AR, Freed MD, Williams RG, et al: Repair of tetralogy of Fallot in infancy. Early and late results. *J Thorac Cardiovasc Surg* 74:372-382, 1977.

Cherniack NS: Respiratory dysrrhythmias during sleep. *N Engl J Med* 305:325-330, 1981.

Chin AJ, Keane JF, Norwood WI, Castaneda AR: Repair of complete common atrioventricular canal in infancy. *J Thorac Cardiovasc Surg* 84:437-445 1982.

Cobanoglu A, Metzdorff MT, Pinson CW, et al: Valvotomy for pulmonary atresia with intact ventricular septum. *J Thorac Cardiovasc Surg* 89:482-490, 1985.

Collins-Nakai RL, Rosenthal A, Castaneda AR, et al: Congenital mitral stenosis: A review of 20 years experience. *Circulation* 56:1039-1047, 1977.

Corone P, Doyon F, Gaudeau S, et al: Natural history of ventricular septal defect; A study involving 790 cases. *Circulation* 55:908-915, 1977.

Daskalopoulos DA, Pieroni DR, Gingell RL, et al: Closed transventricular pulmonary valvotomy in infants. *J Thorac Cardiovasc Surg* 84:187-191, 1982.

Dawes GS: *Foetal and Neonatal Physiology: A Comparative Study of the Changes at Birth.* Chicago, Year Book Medical Publishers, 1969, pp 91-101; 160-187.

Deal BJ, Chin AJ, Sanders SP, et al: Subxiphoid two-dimensional echocardiographic identification of tricuspid valve abnormalities in transposition of the great arteries with ventricular septal defect. *Am J Cardiol* 55:1146-1151, 1985.

deBrux JL, Zannini L, Binet JP, et al: Tricuspid atresia: Results of treatment in 115 children. *J Thorac Cardiovasc Surg* 85:440-446, 1983.

deLeon VH, Hougen TJ, Norwood WI, et al: Results of the Senning operation for transposition of the great arteries with intact ventricular septum in neonates. *Circulation* 70:121-125, 1984.

de Leval MR, Bull C, Stark J, et al: Pulmonary atresia and intact ventricular septum: Surgical management based on a revised classification. *Circulation* 66:272-280, 1982.

Dick M, Fyler DC, Nadas AS: Tricuspid atresia: The clinical course in 101 patients. *Am J Cardiol* 36:327-337, 1975.

Dickinson DF, Arnold R, Wilkinson JL: Congenital heart disease among 160,480 live born children in Liverpool 1960 to 1969. *Br Heart J* 46:55-62, 1981a.

Dickinson DF, Arnold R, Wilkinson JL: Ventricular septal defect in children born in Liverpool 1960 to 1969. *Br Heart J* 46:47-54, 1981b.

Ebert PA, Turley K, Stanger P, et al: Surgical treatment of truncus arteriosus in the first six months of life. *Ann Surg* 200:451-456, 1984.

Edwards JE: Congenital malformations of the heart and great vessels. In Gould SE (ed): *Pathology of the Heart.* Springfield, IL, Charles C Thomas, 1968, pp. 280–311.

Ellison RC, Peckham GJ, Lang P, et al: Evaluation of the preterm infant for patent ductus arteriosus. *Pediatrics* 71:364-372, 1983.

Estes NAM, Salem DN, Isner JM, et al: Permanent pacemaker therapy in corrected transposition of the great arteries: Analysis of site of lead placement in 40 patients. *Am J Cardiol* 52:1091-1097, 1983.

Fallot A: Contribution a l'anatomie pathologique de la maladie bleue (cyanose cardiaque) *Marseille Med* 25:77, 138, 207, 270, 341, 403, 1888.

Feldt RH: *Atrioventricular Canal Defects.* Philadelphia, WB Saunders, 1976, 145 pp.

Ferencz C, Rubin JD, McCarter RJ, et al: Congenital heart disease: Prevalence at live birth; the Baltimore-Washington infant study. *Am J Epidemiol* 121:31-36, 1984.

Flinn CJ, Wolff GS, Dick M, et al: Cardiac rhythm after the Mustard operation for complete transposition of the great arteries. *N Engl J Med* 310:1635-1638, 1984.

Fontan F, Baudet E: Surgical repair of tricuspid atresia. *Thorax* 26:240, 1971.

Fontan F, Deville C, Quaegebeur J, et al: Repair of tricuspid atresia in 100 patients. *J Thorac Cardiovasc Surg* 85:647-660, 1983.

Freed MD, Rocchini A, Rosenthal A, et al: Exercise induced hypertension after surgical repair of coarctation of the aorta. *Am J Cardiol* 43:253-258, 1979.

Freed MD, Rosenthal A, Bernhard WF, et al: Critical pulmonary stenosis with diminutive right ventricle in neonates. *Circulation* 48:875-881, 1973.

Freed MD, Rosenthal A, Plauth WH, et al: Development of subaortic stenosis after pulmonary artery banding. *Circulation* 47(suppl III):7-10, 1973.

Freedom RM, Benson LN, Smallhorn JF, et al: Subaortic stenosis, the univentricular heart, and banding of the pulmonary artery: An analysis of the courses of 43 patients with univentricular heart palliated by pulmonary artery banding. *Circulation* 73:758-764, 1986.

Freedom RM, White RD, Pieroni DR, et al: The natural history of the so-called aneurysm of the membranous ventricular septum in childhood. *Circulation* 49:375-384, 1974.

Fujii AM, Rabinovitch M, Keane JF, et al: Radionuclide angiocardiographic assessment of pulmonary vascular reactivity in patients with left-to-right shunt and pulmonary hypertension. *Am J Cardiol* 49:356-360, 1982.

Fyler DC, Buckley LP, Hellenbrand WE, et al: Report of the New England Regional Infant Cardiac Program. *Pediatrics* 65 (Suppl): 376-460, 1980a.

Fyler DC, Gallaher ME, Nadas AS: Auscultation in the evaluation of children with heart disease. *Prog Cardiovasc Dis* 10:363-384, 1968.

Fyler DC, Rothman KJ, Buckley LP, et al: The determinants of five year survival of infants with critical congenital heart disease. In Brest AN, Engle MA (eds): *Pediatric Cardiovascular Disease, Cardiovasc Clinic.* Philadelphia, FA Davis, 1980b, pp. 393-405.

Gale AW, Danielson GK, McGoon DC, et al: Modified Fontan operation for univentricular heart and complicated congenital lesions. *J Thorac Cardiovasc Surg* 78:831-838, 1979.

Gasul BM, Dillon RF, Vrla V, et al: Ventricular septal defects, their natural transformation into those with infundibular stenosis or into the cyanotic or noncyanotic type of tetralogy of Fallot. *JAMA* 164:847-853, 1957.

Geggel RL, Dozor AJ, Fyler DC, et al: Effect of vasodilators at rest and during exercise in young adults with cystic fibrosis and chronic cor pulmonale. *Am Rev Respir Dis* 131:531-536, 1985.

Gersony WM, Duc GV, Sinclair JC: "PFC" (persistence of the fetal circulation) *Circulation* 40:III, 1969.

Gersony WM, Peckham GJ, Ellison RC, et al: Effects of indomethacin in premature infants with patent ductus arteriosus: Results of a national collaborative study. *J Pediatr* 102:895-906, 1983.

Gillette PC, Garson A, Knight JD: Wolff-Parkinson-White syndrome in children: Electrophysiologic and pharmacologic characteristics. *Circulation* 60:1487-1495, 1979.

Gitterberger-deGroot AC, Elzinga NJ: Localised coarctation of the aorta; an age dependent spectrum. *Br Heart J* 49:317-323, 1983.

Gitterberger-deGroot AC, van Ertbruggen I, Moulaert AJMG: The ductus arteriosus in the preterm infant: Histologic and clinical observations. *J Pediatr* 96:88-93, 1980.

Glenn WWL, Holcomb WC, Hogan J, et al: Diaphragmatic pacing by radio frequency transmission in the treatment of chronic ventilatory insufficiency: Present status. *J Thorac Cardiovasc Surg* 66:505-520, 1973.

Goor DA, Lillehei CW, Rees R, et al: Isolated ventricular septal defect. Developmental basis for various types and presentation of classification. *Chest* 58:468-482, 1970.

Graham TP, Parrish MD, Boucek RJ, et al: Assessment of ventricular size and function in congenitally corrected transposition of the great arteries. *Am J Cardiol* 51:244-251, 1983.

Griscom NT, Colodny AH, Rosenberg HK, et al: Diagnostic aspects of neonatal ascites. Report of 27 cases. *AJR* 128:961-969, 1977.

Gross RE: Coarctation of the aorta. Surgical treatment of one hundred cases. *Circulation* 1:41-55, 1950.

Guntheroth WG, Morgan BC, Mullins GL: Physiologic studies of paroxysmal hyperpnea in cyanotic congenital heart disease. *Circulation* 31:70-76, 1965.

Hagler DJ: Standardized nomenclature of the ventricular septum and ventricular septal defects, with applications for two-dimensional echocardiography. *Mayo Clin Proc* 60:741-752, 1985.

Hamilton WT, Haffajie CI, Salem JE, et al: Atrial septal defect secundum: Clinical profile with physiologic correlates in children and adults. In Roberts WC (ed): *Congenital Heart Disease in Children*, Philadelphia, LA Davis Co, 1985, pp 267-277.

Hawkins JA, Clark EB, Doty DB: Total anomalous pulmonary venous connection. *Ann Thorac Surg* 36:548-560, 1983.

Haworth SG, Sauer U, Buhlmeyer K, et al: Development of the pulmonary circulation in ventricular septal defect: A quantitative structural study. *Am J Cardiol* 40:781-788, 1977.

Hayes CJ, Gersony WM: Arrhythmias after the Mustard operation for transposition of the great arteries: A long-term study. *J Am Coll Cardiol* 7:133-137, 1986.

Heath D, Edwards JE: The pathology of hypertensive pulmonary vascular disease. *Circulation* 18:533-547, 1958.

Hernanz-Schulman M, Fellows KE: Persistent truncus arteriosus: Pathologic, diagnostic and the therapeutic considerations. *Semin Roentgenol* 20:121-129, 1985.

Hislop A, Reid L: Pulmonary arterial development during childhood: Branching pattern and structure. *Thorax* 28:129-135, 1973.

Hoffman JIE, Rudolph AM: The natural history of ventricular septal defects in infancy. *Am J Cardiol* 16:634-653, 1965.

Hoffman JIE, Rudolph AM, Heymann MA: Pulmonary vascular disease with congenital heart lesions: Pathologic features and causes. *Circulation* 64:873-877. 1981.

Holden AM, Fyler DC, Shillito J, et al: Congestive heart failure from intracranial arteriovenous fistula in infancy. *Pediatrics* 49: 30-39, 1972.

Huhta JC, Edwards WD, Danielson GK, et al: Abnormalities of the tricuspid valve in complete transposition of the great arteries with ventricular septal defect. *J Thorac Cardiovasc Surg* 83:569-576, 1982.

Hurwitz RA, Caldwell RL, Girod DA, et al: Ventricular function in transposition of the great arteries: evaluation by radionuclide angiocardiography. *Am Heart J* 110:600-605, 1985.

Hutchinson AA, Drew JH, Yu VYH, et al: Nonimmunologic hydrops fetalis: A review of 61 cases: *Obstet Gynecol* 59:347-352, 1982.

Hwang B, Bowman F, Malm J, et al: Surgical repair of congenitally corrected transposition of the great arteries: Results and follow-up. *Am J Cardiol* 50:781-785, 1982.

Ivemark B: Implications of agenesis of the spleen on the pathogenesis of conotruncus anomalies in childhood. *Acta Paediatr Scand* 44(Suppl 104):7-84, 1955.

Jatene AD, Fontes VF, Paulista PP, et al: Anatomic correction of transposition of the great vessels. *J Thorac Cardiovasc Surg* 72:364-370, 1976.

Jeresaty RM: *Mitral Valve Prolapse*. New York, Raven Press, 1979, 251 pp.

Johnson GM, Todd DW: Cor pulmonale in severe Pierre Robin syndrome. *Pediatrics* 65:152-154, 1980.

Jonas RA, Lang P, Mayer JE, et al: Importance of prostaglandin E1 in resuscitation of the neonate with critical aortic stenosis. *J Thorac Cardiovasc Surg* 89:314-315, 1985.

Jones RWA, Pickering D: Persistent ductus arteriosus complicating the respiratory distress syndrome. *Arch Dis Child* 52:274-281, 1977.

Kan JS, White RF, Mitchell SE, et al: Percutaneous balloon valvuloplasty: A new method for treating congenital pulmonary valve stenosis. *N Engl J Med* 307:540-542, 1982.

Karpawich PP, Bush CP, Antillon JR, et al: Modified Blalock-Taussig shunt in infants and young children. *J Thorac Cardiovasc Surg* 89:275-279, 1985.

Keane JF, Fellows KE, LaFarge CG, et al: The surgical management of discrete and diffuse supravalvar aortic stenosis. *Circulation* 54:112-117, 1976.

Keane JF, Fyler DC, Nadas AS: Hazards of cardiac catheterization in children with primary pulmonary vascular obstruction. *Am Heart J* 96:556-558, 1978.

Keane JF, Plauth WH, Nadas AS: Ventricular septal defect and aortic regurgitation. *Circulation* 56(Suppl):I72-I77, 1977.

Keith JD, Rowe RD, Vlad P: Bicuspid aortic valve. In *Heart Disease in Infancy and Childhood*, ed 3. New York, Macmillan, 1979, pp. 3–13, 728-735.

Kirklin JW, Blackstone EH, Kirklin JK, et al: Surgical results and protocols in the spectrum of tetralogy of Fallot. *Ann Surg* 198:251-265, 1983.

Kitterman JA, Esmunds H, Gregory GA, et al: Patent ductus arteriosus in premature infants. Incidence, relation to pulmonary disease and management. *N Engl J Med* 287:473-477, 1972.

Laks H, Milliken JC, Perloff JK, et al: Experience with the Fontan procedure. *J Thorac Cardiovasc Surg* 88:939-951, 1984.

Lamberti JJ, Carlisle J, Waldman JD, et al: Systemic-pulmonary shunts in infants and children. *J Thorac Cardiovasc Surg* 88:76-81, 1984.

Lauer RM, DuShane JW, Edwards JE: Obstruction of left ventricular outlet in association with ventricular septal defect. *Circulation* 22:110-125, 1960.

Levy RJ, Rosenthal A, Miettinen OS, et al: Determinants of growth in patients with ventricular septal defect. *Circulation* 57:793-797, 1978.

Lincoln C, Jamieson S, Joseph M, et al: Transatrial repair of ventricular septal defects with reference to their anatomic classification. *J Thorac Cardiovasc Surg* 74:183-190, 1977.

Lind J, Stern L, Wegelius C: *Human Foetal Neonatal Circulation*. Springfield, IL, Charles C Thomas, 1964, 153 pp.

Lindesmith GG, Stanton RE, Lurie PR, et al: An assessment of Mustard's operation as a palliative procedure for transposition of the great arteries. *Ann Thorac Surg* 19:514-520, 1975.

Lister G, Hellenbrand WE, Kleinman CS, et al: Physiologic effects of increasing hemoglobin concentration in left-to-right shunting in infants with ventricular septal defects. *N Engl J Med* 306:502-506, 1982.

Lock JE, Bass JL, Amplatz K, et al: Balloon dilation angioplasty of coarctaion in infants and children. *Circulation* 68:109-116 1983.

Lowe JE, Oldham HN, Sabiston DC: Surgical management of congenital coronary artery fistulas. *Ann Surg* 194:373-380, 1981.

Luber JM, Castaneda AR, Lang P, et al: Repair of double- outlet right ventricle: Early and late results. *Circulation* 68(Suppl II):144-147, 1983.

Marin-Garcia J, Tandon R, Lucas RV, et al: Cor triatriatum: A study of 20 cases. *Am J Cardiol* 35:59-66, 1975.

Maron BJ, Redwood DR, Hirshfeld JW, et al: Postoperative assessment of patients with ventricular septal defect and pulmonary hypertension; response to intense upright exercise. *Circulation* 48:864-874, 1973.

Marx GR, Hougen TJ, Norwood WI, et al: Transposition of the great arteries with intact ventricular septum: results of Mustard and Senning operations in 123 consecutive patients. *J Am Coll Cardiol* 1:476-483, 1983.

Mavroudis C, Weinstein G, Turley K, et al: Surgical management of complete atrioventricular canal. *J Thorac Cardiovasc Surg* 83:670-679, 1982.

McCaughan BC, Danielson GK, Driscoll DJ, et al: Tetralogy of Fallot with absent pulmonary valve. *J Thorac Cardiovasc Surg* 89:280-287, 1985.

McGoon DC, Danielson GK, Puga FJ, et al: Results after extracardiac conduit repair for congenital cardiac defects. *Am J Cardiol* 49:1741-1749, 1982.

McKay R, Pacifico AD, Blackstone EH, et al: Septation of the univentricular heart with left anterior subaortic outlet chamber. *J Thorac Cardiovasc Surg* 84:77-87, 1982.

Messina LM, Turley K, Stanger P, et al: Successful aortic valvotomy for severe congenital valvular aortic stenosis in the newborn infant. *J Thorac Cardiovasc Surg* 88:92-96, 1984.

Meyrick B, Perkett EA, Brigham KL: Inflammation and models of chronic pulmonary hypertension. *Am Rev Respir Dis* 136:765, 1987.

Mitchell SC, Korones SB, Berendes HW: Congenital heart disease in 56,109 births. *Circulation* 43:323-332, 1971.

Momma K, Toyama K, Takao A, et al: Natural history of subarterial infundibular ventricular septal defect. *Am Heart J* 108:1312-1317, 1984.

Murphy J, Vawter GF, Reid LM: Pulmonary vascular disease in fatal meconium inspiration. *J Pediatr* 104:758-762, 1984.

Mustard WT: Successful two stage correction of transposition of the great vessels. *Surgery* 55:469-472, 1964.

Nadas AS, Ellison RC, Weidman WH: Pulmonary stenosis, aortic stenosis, ventricular septal defect: Clinical course and indirect assessment. *Circulation* 56:I1-I87, 1977.

Nadas AS, Fyler DC: *Pediatric Cardiology*. Philadelphia, WB Saunders, 1972, pp. 293-294.

Newburger JW, Silbert AR, Buckley LP, et al: Cognitive function and duration of hypoxemia in children with transposition of the great arteries. *N Engl J Med* 310:1495-1499, 1984.

Newburger JW, Tucker AD, Silbert AR, Fyler DC: Motor function and timing of surgery in transposition of the great arteries, intact ventricular septum. (Abstract). *Pediatr Cardiol* 4:317, 1983.

Noonan JA: Pulmonary heart disease. *Pediatr Clin North Am* 18:1255-1272, 1971.

Noonan JA, Nadas AS: The hypoplastic left heart syndrome: An analysis of 101 cases. *Pediatr Clin North Am* 5:1029-1056, 1959.

Norwood W, Hougen TJ, Castaneda AR: Total anomalous pulmonary venous connection; surgical consideration. *Pediatr Cardiovasc Dis* 11:353-363, 1980.

Norwood WI, Lang P, Hansen DD: Physiologic repair of aortic atresia—hypoplastic left heart syndrome. *N Engl J Med* 308:23-26, 1983.

O'Connor WN, Cottrill CM, Johnson GL, et al: Pulmonary atresia with intact ventricular septum and ventriculocoronary communications: Surgical significance. *Circulation* 65:805-809, 1982.

Oglietti J, Cooley DA, Izquierdo JP, et al: Cor triatriatum: Operative results in 25 patients. *Ann Thorac Surg* 35:415-420, 1983.

Oh JK, Holmes DR, Hayes DL, et al: Cardiac arrhythmia in patients with surgical repair of Ebstein's anomaly. *J Am Coll Cardiol* 6:1351-1357, 1985.

Pacifico AP, Mandke NV, McGrath LB, et al: Repair of congenital pulmonary venous stenosis with living autologous atrial tissue. *J Thorac Cardiovasc Surg* 89:604-609, 1985..RF

Parrish MD, Graham TP, Bender HW, et al: Radionuclide angiographic evaluation of right and left ventricular function during exercise after repair of transposition of the great arteries. Comparison with normal subjects and patients with congenitally corrected transposition. *Circulation* 67:178-183, 1983.

Patel RG, Freedom RM, Moes CAF, et al: Right ventricular volume determinations in 18 patients with pulmonary atresia and intact ventricular septum. Analysis of factors influencing right ventricular growth. *Circulation* 61:428-440, 1980.

Paul MH, Currmibhoy Z, Mieler RA, et al: Thrombocytopenia in cyanotic congenital heart disease. (Abstract) *Circulation* 24: 1013, 1961.

Penkoske PA, Westerman GR, Marx GR, et al: Transposition of the great arteries and ventricular septal defect: Results with the Senning operation and closure of the ventricular septal defect in infants. *Ann Thorac Surg* 36:281-288, 1983.

Peoples WM, Moller JH, Edwards JE: Polysplenia: A review of 146 cases. *Pediatr Cardiol* 4:129-137, 1983.

Piccoli G, Pacifico AD, Kirklin JW, et al: Changing results and concepts in the surgical treatment of double-outlet right ventricle: analysis of 137 operations in 126 patients. *Am J Cardiol* 53:549-554, 1983.

Pitts JA, Crosby WM, Basta LL: Eisenmenger's syndrome in pregnancy. *Am Heart J* 93:321-326, 1977.

Portman MA, Beder SD, Ankeney JL, et al: A twenty year review of ostium primum defect repair in children. *Am Heart J* 110:1054-1058, 1985.

Raatikka M, Rapola J, Tuuteri L, et al: Familial third and fourth pharyngeal pouch syndrome with truncus arteriosus. *Pediatrics* 67:173-175, 1981.

Rabinovitch M, Grady S, David I, et al: Compression of intrapulmonary bronchi by abnormally branching pulmonary arteries associated with absent pulmonary valves. *Am J Cardiol* 50:804-813, 1982.

Rabinovitch M, Haworth SG, Castaneda AR, et al: Lung biopsy in congenital heart disease: Morphometric approach to pulmonary vascular disease. *Circulation* 58:1107-1122, 1978.

Rabinovitch M, Keane JF, Norwood WI, et al: Pulmonary hypertension before and after repair of congenital heart defects. *Congenital Heart Disease* 1(1):65, 1984.

Radtke W, Keane JF, Fellows KE, et al: Percutaneous balloon valvotomy of congenital pulmonary stenosis. *J Am Coll Cardiol* 8:909-915, 1986.

Ramaciotti C, Keren A, Silverman NH: Importance of (perimembranous) ventricular septal aneurysm in the natural history of isolated perimembranous ventricular septal defect. *Am J Cardiol* 57:268-272, 1986.

Rudolph AM: *Congenital Diseases of the Heart.* Chicago, Year Book Publishers 1974.

Rudolph AM: The changes in the circulation after birth: Their importance in congenital heart disease. *Circulation* 41:343-359, 1970.

Rashkind WJ, Miller WW: Creation of an atrial septal defect without thoracotomy. A palliative approach to complete transposition of the great arteries. *JAMA* 196:991-992, 1966.

Rastelli GC, Wallace RB, Ongley PA: Complete repair of transposition of the great arteries with pulmonary stenosis. A review and report of a case corrected by using a new surgical technique. *Circulation* 39:83-95, 1969.

Reardon MJ, Cooley DA, Kubrusly L, et al: Total anomalous pulmonary venous return: Report of 201 patients treated surgically. *Texas Heart Inst J* 12:131-141, 1985.

Reifenstein GH, Levine SA, Gross RE: Coarctation of the aorta; a review of 104 autopsied cases of the "adult type" 2 years of age or older. *Am Heart J* 33:146-168, 1947.

Restivo A, Cameron AH, Anderson RH, et al: Divided right ventricular: A review of its anatomical varieties. *Pediatr Cardiol* 5:197-204, 1984.

Richardson JV, Doty DB, Sievers RD, et al: Cor triatriatum: (subdivided left atrium). *J Thorac Cardiovasc Surg* 81:232-238, 1981.

Rittenhouse EA, Mansfield PB, Hall DG, et al: Tetralogy of Fallot: Selective staged management. *J Thorac Cardiovasc Surg* 89:772-779, 1985.

Rosenthal A, Button LN, Nathan DG, et al: Blood volume changes in cyanotic congenital heart disease. *Am J Cardiol* 27:162-167, 1971.

Ross Conference on Pediatric Research: The Ductus Arteriosus. Proceeding of the Seventy-fifth conference on Pediatric Research. Palm Beach, Florida, 1977.

Ruckman RN, Van Praagh R: Anatomic types of congenital mitral stenosis: Report of 49 autopsy cases with diagnostic and surgical implications. *Am J Cardiol* 42:592-601, 1978.

Senning A: Surgical correction of transposition of the great vessels. *Surgery* 45:966-980, 1959.

Shone JD, Sellers RD, Anderson RC, et al: The developmental complex of "parachute mitral valve," supravalvar ring of the left atrium, subaortic stenosis and coarctation of the aorta. *Am J Cardiol* 11:714-725, 1963.

Soto B, Becker AE, Moulaert AJ, et al: Classification of ventricular septal defects. *Br Heart J* 43:332-343, 1980.

Stenson N: Quoted by Goldstein HI: *Bull Hist Med* 29:526, 1948.

Sullivan ID, Robinson PJ, de Leval M, et al: Membranous supravalvular mitral stenosis: A treatable form of congenital heart disease. *J Am Coll Cardiol* 8:159–164, 1986.

Terplan KL: Patterns of brain damage in infants and children with congenital heart disease. *Am J Dis Child* 125:175-195, 1973.

Trowitzsch E, Colan SD, Sanders SP: Global and regional right ventricular function in normal infants and infants with transposition of the great arteries after Senning operation. *Circulation* 72:1008-1014, 1985a.

Trowitzsch E, Colan SD, Sanders SP: Two-dimensional echocardiographic estimation of right ventricular area change and ejection fraction in infants with systemic right ventricle (transposition of the great arteries or hypoplastic left heart syndrome). *Am J Cardiol* 55:1153-1157, 1985b.

Van Mierop LHS, Gessner IH, Schiebler GI: Asplenia and polysplenia syndromes. *Birth Defects* 8:36, 1972.

Van Praagh R, David I, Van Praagh S: What is a ventricle? The single ventricle trap. *Pediatr Cardiol* 2:79-84, 1982.

Van Praagh R, McNamara JJ: Anatomic types of ventricular septal defect with aortic insufficiency: Diagnostic and surgical considerations. *Am Heart J* 75:604-619, 1968.

Van Praagh R, Plett JA, Van Praagh S: Single ventricule. Pathology, embryology, terminology and classification. *Herz* 4:113-150, 1979.

Van Praagh R, Weinberg PM, Matsuoka R, et al: Malpositions of the heart. In Adams FH, Emmanoulides GC (eds): *Heart Disease in Infants, Children and Adolescents.* Baltimore, Williams & Wilkins, 1983, pp. 422-458.

Vincent RN, Lang P, Elixson EM, et al: Extravascular lung water in children after operative closure of either isolated atrial septal defect or ventricular septal defect. *Am J Cardiol* 56:536-539, 1985.

Vogel M, Freedom RM, Brand A, et al: Ventricular septal defect and subaortic stenosis; an analysis of 41 patients. *Am J Cardiol* 52:1258-1263, 1983.

Wagner HR, Ellison RC, Zierler S, et al: Surgical closure of patent ductus arteriosus in 268 preterm infants. *J Thorac Cardiovasc Surg* 87:870-875, 1984.

Waldhausen JA, Nahrwold DL: Repair of coarctation of the aorta with a subclavian flap. *J Thorac Cardiovasc Surg* 51:532-533, 1966.

Watson H: Natural history of Ebstein's anomaly of the tricuspid valve in childhood and adolesence: an international co-operative study of 505 cases. *Br Heart J* 36:417-427, 1974.

Weidman WH, Blount SG, DuShane JW, et al: Clinical course in ventricular septal defect. *Circulation* 56(Suppl I):I56-I71, 1977.

Williams JCP, Barrett-Boyes BG, Lowe JB: Supravalvar aortic stenosis. *Circulation* 24:1311-1318, 1961.

Wright GB, Keane JF, Nadas AS, et al: Fixed subaortic stenosis in the young: medical and surgical course in 83 patients. *Am J Cardiol* 52:830-835, 1983.

Yacoub MH, Radley-Smith R: Anatomic correction of the Taussig-Bing anomaly. *J Thorac Cardiovasc Surg* 88:380-388, 1984.

Yeager SB, Freed MD, Keane JF, et al: Primary surgical closure of ventricular septal defect in the first year of life: Results in 128 infants. *J Am Coll Card* 3:1269-1276, 1984.

Zeimer G, Jonas RA, Perry SB, et al: Surgery for coarctation in the neonate. *Circulation* 74(Suppl 1): I25-I31, 1986.

Rheumatic Fever

4

Rheumatic fever is a social disease, rampant in economically depressed societies, and is probably the most common cause of heart disease in children in the world. In sharp contrast, it is now an insignificant public health problem in industrialized nations, i.e. the United States, Europe, U.S.S.R., Canada, Japan, and The Peoples Republic of China, where only sporadic cases are seen.

Definition

Rheumatic fever is an abnormal, delayed, often recurrent, probably autoimmune reaction to group A β-hemolytic streptococcal pharyngitis, involving the joints, skin, brain, serous surfaces and, most important, the heart valves. Were it not for the valve damage, the disease would have little practical consequence.

Basic Science

The pathogenesis of rheumatic fever is not clear. Whatever theory is proposed, the following observations must be accounted for. Rheumatic fever is predominantly, although not exclusively, a disease of socially and economically disadvantaged people. It is the sequela of a group A β-hemolytic streptococcal pharyngitis and occurs in 3% of infected individuals. It does not follow nonpharyngeal streptococcal infections. It is rare in small children and virtually unknown in infants before the second birthday. There is a familial tendency. Recently, an antigen was identified on the β-cells in 90% of patients who have had rheumatic fever, whereas this antigen is detectable in only 20% of the general population (Zabriskie, 1985).

Evidence has accumulated to suggest strongly that rheumatic fever is an immunologic aberration. Sera of patients with rheumatic fever react with cardiac muscle (Kaplan et al, 1964) and sera of patients with chorea are reported to react with tissue from the caudate nucleus. The level of circulating streptococcal antibodies is greater in patients with rheumatic fever than in patients with streptococcal infections who do not have rheumatic fever. There is cross-reactivity of several antigens from the streptococcus with antigens obtained from heart muscle. The disease is suppressed, although not eradicated, through the use of cortisone. The antistreptolysin titer is higher than with ordinary streptococcal infections.

An excellent summary of the present status of the basic science of rheumatic fever has been provided by Zabriskie (1985; see also pp. 1089).

PATHOLOGY

The pathology of rheumatic fever includes inflammatory and exudative lesions in the heart, blood vessels, brain, and serous surfaces of the joints pleura pericardium. Active disease is characterized by a distinctive and pathognomonic granuloma consisting of a perivascular aggregation of cells and fibrinoid protoplasma (Aschoff nodules). Aschoff nodules are found in all patients with clinical rheumatic activity and in many with chronic rheumatic valvar abnormalities as well, suggesting that in many patients the disease is subclinically active and smoldering for years. This view corresponds with years of clinical observation of gradually progressive valvar abnormalities. The mitral valve is most commonly involved and in the late stages is thickened, verrucous, nodular and, first incompetent, later stenotic. Less commonly, similar changes occur in the aortic valve, producing incompetence but almost never producing stenosis. Aortic regurgitation is rare as a solitary lesion (<10%) but it occurs in combination with mitral regurgitation in about half of the patients with rheumatic heart disease. Mitral regurgitation alone or associated with aortic regurgitation is by far the most common lesion (>95%). The diagnosis of rheumatic heart disease without mitral disease is suspect.

Epidemiology

There are no reliable data on the incidence of rheumatic fever. Where the disease is reportable, the data are flawed by imprecise diagnosis and among populations where the disease is known to be common, reporting seems least reliable. Nonetheless, in the United States, most reports suggest a decreasing incidence of first attacks of acute rheumatic fever, decreasing recurrences, and, most important, decreasing prevalence of rheumatic heart disease. Not all agree, however. Tolaymat, in 1984, reported 128 patients with rheumatic fever in 1 year in a population of 600,000.

Diagnosis

Careful questioning elicits a history of pharyngitis within 2 weeks of the onset in about half of the patients with rheumatic symptoms. An acute attack is characteristically associated with low grade fever and sometimes not much else. Polyarthritis and polyarthralgia are common. Erythema marginatum is rare. Subcutaneous nodules are seen only in chronic, recurring severe disease. Chorea is often an isolated phenomenon but may be seen with other evidence of active disease. If heart disease is to be a problem, a murmur is usually present in the first 2 weeks of the illness, although appearance of a murmur weeks or months later may be observed.

Since there is no laboratory test for rheumatic fever, the diagnosis is made on clinical grounds. Using Jones' criteria (1944, 1965) in addition to evidence of a preceding group A β-hemolytic streptococcal infection, two major manifestations or one major manifestation plus two minor manifestations strongly indicate the presence of acute rheumatic fever. Jones listed the major manifestations as: (a) polyarthritis, (b) carditis, (c) erythema marginatum, (d) subcutaneous nodules, and (e) Sydenham's chorea. He listed minor manifestations as: (a) fever, (b) arthralgia, (c) previous rheumatic fever or rheumatic heart disease, (d) an elevated sedimentation rate or positive C-reactive protein, and (e) a prolonged P-R interval.

POLYARTHRITIS

Multiple joint involvement is the most common major manifestation of rheumatic fever. There may be vague migratory joint pain (arthralgia) or full-blown arthritis with swelling, redness, and even exquisite tenderness of the larger joints. In contrast to rheumatoid arthritis, the fingers and toes are rarely involved. Joint symptoms are usually migratory, rarely involving a single joint for more than 48 hours, and are usually self-limited within a few days, but persistence of untreated arthritis (nowadays rarely observed) has been reported for as long as 2 months.

CARDITIS

Carditis is manifested most commonly by a new murmur of mitral regurgitation (Fig. 6.3*B*) and, occasionally, by myocarditis and pericarditis, with or without pericardial effusion. Most patients who ultimately will have significant valve damage from the first attack will have a mitral murmur in the first 2 weeks of the illness (more than 80%; Massell et al, 1958). Late appearance of valvar abnormality is well documented. The abnormality may appear as long as 15–22 years after the initial attack, particularly in patients with pure chorea, often without intervening episodes of obvious acute rheumatic fever. Pericarditis, manifested by friction rub, documents the presence of carditis. Pericardial effusion is occasionally large but rarely sufficient to require more than observation; even when large it rarely accumulates rapidly enough to require drainage. Pericarditis or myocarditis is never rheumatic in origin without associated evidence of valvar involvement. Myocarditis is suspected when there is cardiomegaly and congestive failure early in the disease. Months and years later cardiomegaly is almost invariably the result of valve dysfunction unless there is strong evidence to suspect recurrent rheumatic activity.

ERYTHEMA MARGINATUM

This distinctive exanthem is not a common feature of rheumatic fever but is virtually diagnostic of active disease when present. The irregular, circinate, evanescent, red, marginate patterns over the torso are accentuated by a hot bath and do not itch.

SUBCUTANEOUS NODULES

Nontender subcutaneous nodules over the bony surfaces of the wrists, elbows, knees, ankles, vertebrae, and skull are found in patients with recurrent active rheumatic fever and well established rheumatic heart disease. These nodules are best detected under side lighting when the skin is slowly moved over bony surfaces such as the elbows or the knees. When nodules are present, rheumatic activity is almost invariably present.

SYDENHAM CHOREA

There is virtually no other disease that resembles Sydenhams chorea. The purposeless, choreiform movements, aggravated by emotional stress in an emotionally labile child (usually teenage female) characterize this disease. In its worst form, the child may be unable to use a spoon to eat and may bruise her extremities. Chorea may be associated with other manifestations of rheumatic fever (never arthritis) and is often seen as an isolated phenomenon even without evidence of a preceding group A streptococcal infection ("pure chorea"). However, mitral stenosis develops in 30% of children with pure chorea 15–20 years later.

MINOR MANIFESTATIONS

Migratory arthralgia involving the larger joints, with or without objective signs of arthritis, is perhaps the most common feature of acute rheumatic fever. Fever is rarely higher than 103°F and in the untreated patient may persist for several weeks, gradually decreasing. An elevated sedimentation rate or a C-reactive protein is characteristic of acute active rheumatic fever. Except for pure chorea, the diagnosis of rheumatic activity without elevation of the sedimentation rate is suspect. Evidence of a prior streptococcal infection is required whether in the form of a positive throat culture or a rising antistreptolysin titer. A prolonged P-R interval, reversible with atropine, is commonly observed. Oddly, this cardiac abnormality has no relation to subsequent valvar disease (Roy et al, 1957).

Management

PRIMARY PREVENTION

Rheumatic fever can be prevented if treatment of group A β-hemolytic streptococcal pharyngitis is begun within 9 days of onset and is continued for 10 days (Rammelkamp et al, 1961). This fact, more than any other, may account for the remarkable reduction in cases of rheumatic fever and rheumatic heart disease in the United States (Zabriskie, 1985). A single injection of benzathine pencillin (0.06 million units to 1.2 million units), oral pencillin G (200,000 units three to four times a day for 10 days), or the antibiotic equivalent in allergic patients eradicates β-hemolytic streptococci in 95% of patients. It is worth stressing that group A β-hemolytic streptococci in contrast to α-streptococci do not become resistant to penicillin.

ACUTE ATTACK

When the diagnosis of acute rheumatic fever is seriously considered, a throat culture is taken and pencillin therapy to eradicate β-hemolytic streptococci is begun. Simultaneously, for the milder forms of acute rheumatic fever without evidence of carditis, suppression of rheumatic activity is begun by using high doses of salicylates until salicylate levels of 20–25 mg/100 ml are attained (Table 6.12). Weeks later, after suppression is documented by absence of symptoms and a normal sedimentation rate, the dosage is reduced. For patients with carditis, practically those with a murmur, suppression with prednisone for the first 2–4 weeks, with conversion to salicylates later, is recommended. For patients with pancarditis (congestive heart failure, pericarditis, valvulitis), the use of steroids is mandatory and is life-saving. Treatment is continued for 8–16 weeks depending on evidence of carditis and evidence of rheumatic activity. In the final days of treatment, as antirheumatic medication is withdrawn, the patient may experience a return of symptoms and laboratory evidence of active rheumatic fever. Often this is mild and requires no more than observation for a few days. Sometimes, however, antirheumatic drugs must be restarted.

Table 6.12
Recommended Anti-Inflammatory Agents for Acute Rheumatic Fever

Arthritis	Definite Carditis, No Cardiomegaly	Severe Carditis, Cardiomegaly, or Congestive Failure
Salicylates, 100 mg/kg/day In 1 week, reduce dose to 65 mg/kg/day Continue for 3–4 weeks	Salicylates, 100 mg/kg/day In 1 or 2 weeks, reduce dose to 65 mg/kg/day Continue for 6–8 weeks Change to prednisone if cardiomegaly develops	Prednisone, 2 mg/kg/day 2–4 weeks, then taper Begin salicylates in final week of prednisone and continue for 6–12 weeks

There is no certain evidence that pharmacologic suppression of acute rheumatic fever prevents valve damage, even though it may be lifesaving in fulminating cases (Markowitz and Hordis, 1972).

SECONDARY PREVENTION

Oral pencillin (125 mg) is taken twice daily (200,000 units of pencillin G twice daily) and is continued "indefinitely" if there is evidence of valvar damage. Alternatively, 1.2 million units of benzathine pencillin administered intramuscularly is given monthly. If there is no valvar damage oral prevention is continued for 5 years.

Patients with rheumatic fever, with or without carditis, should be systematically observed over their lifetime for evidence of late valvar disease and possible recurrence of rheumatic fever.

Chorea without other evidence of rheumatic activity is managed with sedation, tranquilizers or, more recently, Haldol. Prophylactic pencillin to prevent secondary rheumatic activity is recommended even though the initial documentation of β-hemolytic streptococcal infection may be lacking. Long range follow-up is desirable since late mitral stenosis develops in as many as 30% of these individuals.

Course and Prognosis

An episode of active rheumatic fever usually lasts 8–16 weeks. Rarely, patients continue to show evidence of chronic activity with intermittent low grade fever,

CASE ILLUSTRATION

A 14-year-old black male had a sore throat in May, 1985. It was not treated with antibiotics. Over the next few weeks he became chronically fatigued, lost 5 lbs, had vague aches and pains, and was intermittently febrile. Two months after the episode of pharyngitis an apical systolic murmur and a blowing diastolic murmur at the left sternal border were discovered (Fig. 6.3*B*). His antistreptolysin O titer was 2000 units; his sedimentation rate was elevated. There was cardiomegaly on the chest film. Treatment with prednisone resulted in control of fever and reduction in the sedimentation rate.

After a 10-week course of prednisone, he was given aspirin. His rheumatic activity rebounded and the prednisone was reinstated. Five months later, he was still showing evidence of rheumatic activity each time the prednisone dosage was decreased. Nonetheless, it was decided that it should be discontinued and 10 days later he became short of breath, had limited exercise tolerance and, over the course of 3–4 weeks, became seriously ill, being admitted to his local hospital with florid pulmonary edema. After being stabilized, he was transferred to The Children's Hospital in Boston.

On physical examination, there was evidence of gross congestive heart failure with hepatomegaly,orthopnea, neck vein distention, and pulmonary rales. There were murmurs of mitral regurgitation and aortic regurgitation. His blood pressure was 110/40. On the chest film, his heart was grossly enlarged (Fig. 6.36). At cardiac catheterization, he was shown to have markedly elevated left atrial pressure, severe mitral regurgitation, and moderately severe aortic incompetence.

The next day, at surgery (February, 1986), he was found to have deformed aortic and mitral valves with ruptured mitral chordae tendinae. He underwent mitral and aortic valve replacement. He returned from the operating room looking better than when he went in and was discharged from the hospital to his local institution several days later with his sedimentation rate still elevated. Arrangements were made for him to resume his antirheumatic therapy.

The excised valve tissue showed Aschoff nodules. Some weeks later, his chest film was considerably improved (Fig 6.37).

QUESTIONS AND COMMENTS

Is this an extreme case?

Yes, but it is important to note that we are not completely rid of this disease even in 1986.

Was this a native of some other country?

No, this was a native-born black American male.

Is this a rather protracted course?

It is definitely protracted. We wonder if complete suppression had been maintained and continued for a period of time, whether the course would have continued this long.

How do you know that this was this boy's first attack of rheumatic fever? Is it possible that this was a recurrent episode?

That is possible and could account for some of the features of his course. Prolonged activity, "chronic rheumatic fever," is more common in recurrent attacks. However, this boy was not known to have had a murmur and had been examined by his physician before the initial episode of pharyngitis.

How do you decide whether the congestive heart failure is the result of myocardial or valvar disease?

Early in the course, in the first 6 months of illness, the dominant cause of congestive heart failure is myocardial. It is extremely rare for congestive heart failure to develop from valvar disease in the first 6 months of an acute attack in the United States, although it is described in other countries. After 6 months the contribution to congestive failure becomes dominantly valvar.

What will happen to these artificial valves?

It is unrealistic to believe that they will last more than 5–10 years. Regular echocardiographic checks of valve function will be needed for the rest of his life, and the valves will be replaced at about 10-year intervals.

The aortic and mitral valves having been replaced, is there any point in trying to prevent further rheumatic fever?

Admittedly, the major lesions caused by rheumatic fever are mitral and aortic valve disease. Nevertheless, it seems worthwhile to prevent further rheumatic myocarditis, and right-sided valvar disease has been well documented in patients with chronic rheumatic fever in the past.

Do you believe that, had the initial pharyngitis been treated with pencillin in the usual dosage for 10 days, this whole episode could have been prevented?

There is a 95% chance that that is correct.

elevation of sedimentation rate, and progression of valvar damage. In any patient with a history of acute rheumatic fever, a late β-hemolytic streptococcal infection, either as a breakthrough of pencillin prophylaxis or because of poor compliance, may result in a further episode of acute rheumatic fever and further valve damage.

REFERENCES

Jones TD: Criteria for guidance in diagnosis of rheumatic fever (revised). *Circulation* 32:664-668, 1965.

Jones TD: The diagnosis of rheumatic fever. *JAMA* 126:481-484, 1944.

Kaplan EL: Acute rheumatic fever. Symposium on Pediatric Cardiology. *Pediatr Clin North Amer* 25.4:817-829, 1978.

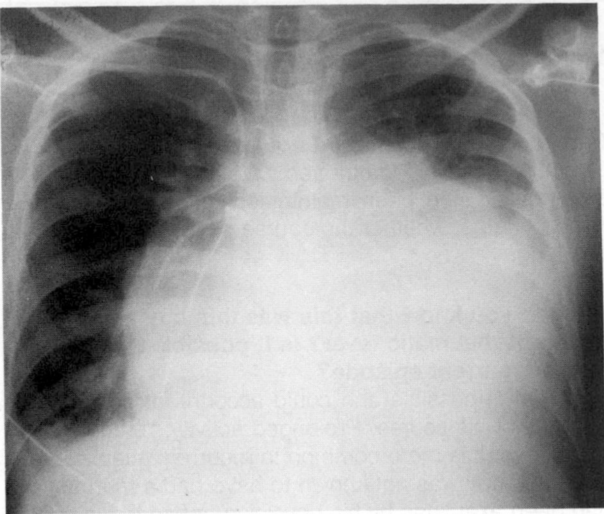

Figure 6.36. Preoperative chest film of child with acute rheumatic fever. Note grossly enlarged heart. There was minimal pericardial effusion.

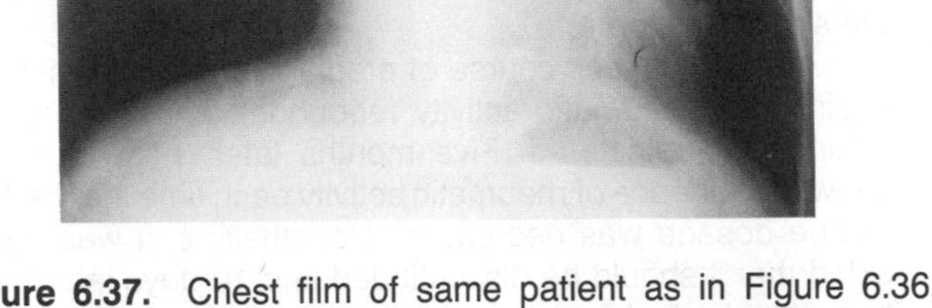

Figure 6.37. Chest film of same patient as in Figure 6.36, several weeks after replacement of the aortic and mitral valves.

Kaplan MH, Bolande R, Rakita L, Blair J: Presence of bound immunoglobulins and complement in the myocardium in acute rheumatic fever. *N Engl J Med* 271:637-645, 1964.

Markowitz M, Gordis L: *Rheumatic Fever*, ed 2. Philadelphia, WB Saunders, 1972.

Massell BF, Fyler DC, Roy SB: The clinical picture of rheumatic fever. Diagnosis, immediate prognosis, course and therapeutic implications. *Am J Cardiol* 1:436-449, 1958.

Rammelkamp CH Jr, Stolzer BL: The latent period before the onset of acute rheumatic fever. *Yale J Biol Med* 34:386-398, 1961.

Roy SB, Fyler DC, Massell BF: Prolongation of PR interval in prognosis of rheumatic fever. *Proc N Engl Cardiovasc Soc* 15:31, 1957.

Tolaymat A, Goudarzi T, Soler GP, et al: Acute rheumatic fever in north Florida. *South Med J* 77:819-823, 1984.

Wannamaker LW, Kaplan EL: Rheumatic fever. In Adams FH, Emmanouilides GG (eds): *Heart Disease in Infants, Children and Adolescents*. ed 3. Baltimore, Williams & Wilkins, pp. 534-552.

Zabriskie JB: Rheumatic fever: The interplay between host, genetics, and microbe. *Circulation* 71:1077-1086, 1985.

Infective Endocarditis 5

Definition

Bacterial endocarditis may develop in any patient with a valvar abnormality, septal defect, or vascular lesion, i.e., coarctation of the aorta. For practical purposes a pre-existing murmur is always present, albeit very faint, except for endocarditis as part of generalized sepsis, where infection may develop on a normal valve. Bacterial endocarditis may develop in any patient with a bicuspid aortic valve, even if the associated aortic regurgitation is trivial. In general, regurgitation is more often associated with endocarditis than are other types of physiologic dysfunction. Thus, although aortic stenosis is relatively common in children and aortic regurgitation is less common, bacterial endocarditis is more common when aortic regurgitation is present. Endocarditis often develops on prosthetic materials that are not endothelialized. In the past, the term "subacute" bacterial endocarditis (SBE) implied, an indolent course (endocarditis lenta), sometime extending over months, even years. Nowadays, a child who has been ill for more than a week or so is the exception. Thus, the term subacute is probably inappropriate in 1986. Most people today prefer to drop the terms acute or subacute, as having no useful meaning and refer to the condition as infective endocarditis.

Basic Science

Vegetations appear at a point of turbulent flow (e.g., at the place of impact of a high velocity jet of blood through a ventricular defect on the right ventricular wall, on the back wall of the left atrium in mitral regurgitation or on the regurgitant aortic valve leaflets themselves). Low velocity flows (atrial septal defect secundum) do not predispose to the condition. Kaplan (1986) examined the distribution of cardiac lesions associated with endocarditis among 266 children (Fig. 6.38). The development of blood clots is not a predisposing factor since clots regularly form in huge atria (giant left atria) without endocarditis developing. Rather, the original focus may be an area of erosion due to flow dynamics, followed by bacterial invasion of the damaged endothelial surface. Among the bacteria cultured from the blood of children with endocarditis (Fig. 6.39), mouth organisms are common enough to implicate poor oral hygiene more than oral surgical manipulations. The prevalence of such manipulation by dentists in over 1000 cases of bacterial endocarditis was less than 5% (Guntheroth, 1984). The vegetation that develops encloses live bacteria, not readily accessible to circulating antibiotics, hence the requirement for prolonged, intensive bactericidal therapy. Occasionally especially virulent bacteria invade adjacent tissues as well, specifically the ventricular septum, producing a septal abcess.

We believe that mechanical factors and infective agents may not be the only issues, in addition to the edentulous state, explaining the virtual absence of the disease in infancy and the increasing incidence with age. Immunologic factors, in addition to dental decay, may play a role.

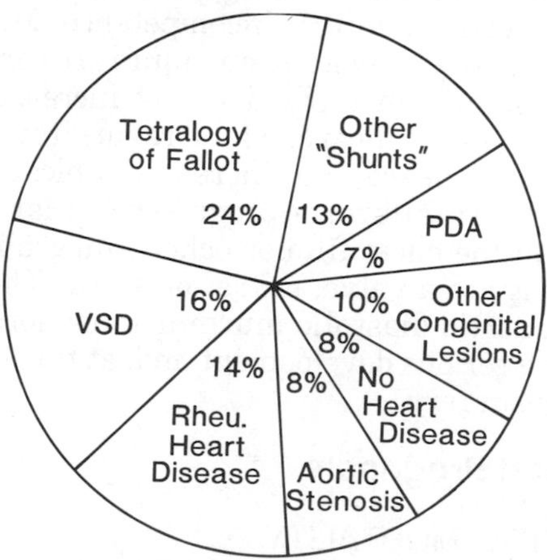

Figure 6.38. Frequency distribution of cardiac lesions in children with infective endocarditis. Reproduced with permission from Kaplan EL: Infective endocarditis: Aspects unique to children and of special interest to pediatric cardiologists. In Doyle EF, Engle MA, Gersony WM, Rashkind WJ, et al (eds): *Pediatric Cardiology*. New York, Springer-Verlag, 1986, p. 1031.

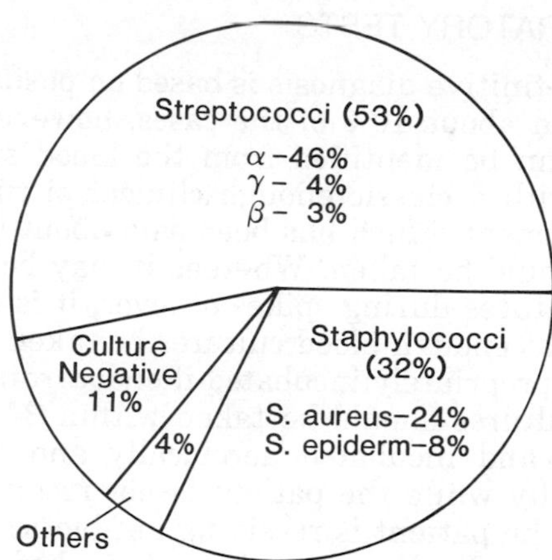

Figure 6.39. Frequency distribution of bacteria cultured from patients with infective endocarditis. Reproduced with permission from Kaplan EL: Infective endocarditis: Aspects unique to children and of special interest to pediatric cardiologists. In Doyle EF, Engle MA, Gersony WM, et al (eds): *Pediatric Cardiology*. New York, Springer-Verlag, 1986, p.1033.

Epidemiology

The prevalence of infective endocarditis in children is difficult to establish, but it is the impression of most pediatric cardiologists that the incidence may be increasing. The incidence among children per pediatric hospital admission in the 1980s seems to be around 1/1000. How this relates to actual incidence is unknown.

Diagnosis

Any patient with a known cardiac lesion, particularly if there is a murmur, who has unexplained fever, may have infective endocarditis. The clinical picture may be explosive with sudden chills and high fever or there may be a gradual realization that fever has been present for many days or weeks. Some systemic features of bacterial infection are usually present; lassitude, night sweats, and malaise are common. Major embolic phenomena may be seen but, fortunately, are not common. A cerebral vascular accident in a young person, an embolus to an extremity, or a shower of petechiae should raise the question of bacterial endocarditis even in the absence of known heart disease. Sore fingertips (Janeway spots), retinal conjunctival petechiae, appearance of a palpable spleen, discovery of microscopic hematuria, or the appearance of a new murmur or exaggeration of a known one should raise the question of endocarditis. In this country today, the disease rarely goes unrecognized long enough to produce anemia, weight loss, or clubbing, as reported in the older literature.

LABORATORY TESTS

The definitive diagnosis is based on positive blood cultures. In about 10% of the cases, however, no organisms can be identified from the blood stream in patients with a classic enough clinical picture to require treatment. Much has been said about when the culture should be taken. Whereas it may be of value to take cultures during spikes of fever, it is more important that enough blood cultures be taken and that they be appropriately incubated if endocarditis is suspected. Cultures should be taken within 24 hours of admission and incubated aerobically and unaerobically, ideally while the patient is not receiving antibiotics. If the patient is receiving antibiotics, waiting for a day or so for clearance of antibiotics before taking culture is a sensible approach if the patient is not critically ill, inasmuch as identification of the organism will allow the most effective therapy.

Virtually any bacterium can cause endocarditis, even organisms otherwise viewed as contaminants, particularly in individuals with cardiac prostheses. Repeated blood cultures of even a saprophytic organism, for example diphtheroids, should be considered seriously. By far the most common organism is the *alpha streptococcus*, the green alpha-strep, which is also the organism implicated in tooth decay. The staphylococcus is a close second (Fig. 6.39; Kaplan et al, 1986).

The white blood count is usually elevated, sometimes greatly so, with a shift to the left, but rarely it may be normal. The sedimentation rate is usually but not invariably elevated. Two-dimensional echocardiograms should be taken to search for vegetations even though the chance of discovering vegetations early is small.

Rarely, the electrocardigram shows the appearance of complete bundle branch block or an unequivocally prolonged P-R interval (longer than 20 msec) which was not present earlier. These observations in a child who has symptoms suggestive of endocarditis, or appearing in the course of treatment of bacterial endocarditis, suggest the presence of a septal abscess that may require drainage.

Management

When an organism has been recovered from the blood stream, sensitivities to a variety of antibiotics are tested and, based on these observations, the appropriate antibiotic is selected. Bacteriostatic agents or levels are inadequate; bactericidal effects are mandatory. Without exception, hospitalization with bed rest and intravenous antibiotic treatment, in our view, is the management of choice; this is too serious a disease to be managed on an outpatient basis. We cannot think of any good reason for a child with this serious illness not to be managed, at least initially, in the hospital. The duration of intravenous antibiotic treatment depends on the organism. *Staphylococcus aureus*, in our view, requires 6 weeks of treatment without exception. Endocarditis in patients with prostheses or with negative blood cultures also requires 6 weeks at least. Other bacteria, particularly the α *streptococcus*, may be treated intravenously for 2–4 weeks to be followed by oral administration of the drug, producing bactericidal levels, to complete 6 weeks of treatment, assuming a satisfactory clinical response.

If the suspicion of infective endocarditis is strong, particularly in patients with an artificial valve, visible vegetations on echocardiogram, or a cerebral vascular accident, six blood cultures should be taken over a matter of hours and the administration of broad-spectrum antibiotics in high dosage should be started. A specific antibiotic regimen can be initiated after the organism has been identified.

Large vegetations should raise the possibility of surgical excision, particularly if they are a source of embolism to the systemic circulation (Lutas et al, 1986). Bacterial endocarditis in patients with prosthetic materials, if not responding to antibiotics promptly, may also have to be treated surgically through removal of the infected material. Obviously this is not a decision to be taken lightly.

We have had sufficient accumulated experience with endocarditis to be leary of abbreviated, poorly controlled therapy. The disaster of recurrent endocarditis requiring a second full course of therapy is indelibly imprinted on those patients and physicians unfortunate enough to have gone through it. Consequently, the use of oral therapy and the management of patients at home is to be undertaken very cautiously if at all.

COMPLICATIONS

Major embolic phenomena may occur before or during the course of treatment. Each is treated accordingly. It should be emphasized that emboli may occur after the blood stream has been sterilized. Valvar damage should be suspected if a new murmur appears or there is evidence of increasing congestive heart failure. Of particular interest is the appearance of evidence of significant aortic or mitral incompetence. Minor variations in intensity of systolic murmurs are common but have little significance. Evidence of increased valvar regurgitation in the form of a loud regurgitant murmur not previously heard, an increased apical impulse, congestive heart failure, or progressive enlargement of the heart on the chest film or echocardiogram suggest major damage to a valve, mitral or aortic. The appearance of an aortic diastolic murmur (new aortic regurgitation) is a serious development and, at times, requires emergency surgery.

Course and Prognosis

HOSPITAL MORTALITY

Overall, hospital mortality is still about 20%. Younger patients, those with *S. aureus* infection, and postoperative patients carry a relatively higher risk, while children infected with the green streptococcus have a lower mortality rate.

INCOMPLETE TREATMENT

In this era of wide use of antibiotics, the number of patients with endocarditis who are incompletely treated (given antibiotics for some other reason) has risen, possibly to the benefit of the patient even though the resulting diagnostic confusion has obvious dangers. At the same time, the numbers of patients who are treated for infective endocarditis without positive blood cultures has also risen (10%), again probably to the benefit of all concerned.

Recurrence

It is an obvious conundrum. Is the patient who has had endocarditis somehow more prone to a second episode? Without good evidence we are prepared, on intuitive grounds, to believe that this is true. The significance of this is that any patient who has had bacterial endocarditis should have any cardiac defect repaired, if possible, especially if he has had endocarditis twice almost irrespective of the physiologic severity of the defect.

Table 6.13[1]
Summary of Recommended Antibiotic Regimens for Dental/Respiratory Tract Procedures

Standard Regimen	
For dental procedures that cause gingival bleeding, and oral/respiratory tract surgery	Penicillin V 2.0 g orally 1 hour before, then 1.0 g 6 hours later; for patients unable to take oral medications, 2 million units of aqueous penicillin G iv or im 30–60 minutes before a procedure and 1 million units 6 hours later may be substituted
Special Regimens	
Parenteral regimen for use when maximal protection desired; e.g., for patients with prosthetic valves	Ampicillin 1.0–2.0 g im or iv plus gentamicin 1.5 mg/kg im or iv, ½ hour before procedure, followed by 1.0 g oral pencillin V 6 hours later; alternatively, the parenteral regimen may be repeated once 8 hours later
Oral regimen for penicillin-allergic patients	Erythromycin 1.0 g orally 1 hour before, then 500 mg 6 hours later
Parenteral regimen for pencillin-allergic patients	Vancomycin 1.0 g iv slowly over 1 hour, starting 1 hour before; no repeat dose is necessary

[1]From Shulman et al, 1984.

Table 6.14[1]
Summary of Recommended Regimens for Gastrointestinal/Genitourinary Procedures

Standard Regimen	
For genitourinary/gastrointestinal tract procedures listed in the text	Ampicillin 2.0 g im or iv plus gentamicin 1.5 mg/kg im or iv, given ½–1 hour before procedure; one follow-up dose may be given 8 hours later
Special Regimens	
Oral regimen for minor or repetitive procedures in low risk patients	Amoxicillin 3.0 g orally 1 hour before procedure and 1.5 g 6 hours later
Penicillin-allergic patients	Vancomycin 1.0 g iv slowly over 1 hour, plus gentamicin 1.5 mg/kg im or iv given 1 hour before procedure; may be repeated once 8–12 hours later

[1]From Shulman et al, 1984.

Prevention

The use of antibiotics during oral surgical procedures to prevent bacterial endocarditis is based on the fact that an oral source for the bacteria is suspected in most cases. Whether rational or not, the conventional medical wisdom in 1986 is to require the use of antibiotics (penicillin or erythromycin) before major oral manipulations (those that cause bleeding) if a known cardiac lesion is present. Recommendations for specific prophylaxis are standardized at intervals by the American Heart Association (Table 6.13 and 6.14; Shulman et al, 1984). Almost more important, in our view is the maintenance of meticulous oral hygiene in patients with heart disease, particularly those with cardiac prostheses.

REFERENCES

Guntheroth WG: How important are dental procedures as a cause of infective endocarditis. *Am J Cardiol* 54:797–801, 1984.

Johnson DH, Rosenthal A, Nadas AS: A forty year review of bacterial endocarditis in infancy and childhood. *Circulation* 51:581-588, 1975.

Kaplan EL: Infective endocarditis: aspects unique to children and of special interest to pediatric cardiologists. In Doyle EF, Engle MA, Gersony WM, et al (eds): *Pediatric Cardiology*. Springer-Verlag, New York, 1986, pp. 1030-1037.

Lutas EM, Roberts RB, Devereux RB, et al: Relation between the presence of echocardiographic vegetation and the complication rate in infective endocarditis. *Am Heart J* 112:107-113, 1986.

Shulman ST, Amren DP, Bisno AL, et al: Prevention of bacterial endocarditis. A statement for health professionals by the committee on rheumatic fever and infective endocarditis of the council on cardiovascular disease in the young. *Circulation* 70:1123a-1127a, 1984.

Van Hare GF, Ben-Shachar G, Liebman J, et al: Infective endocarditis in infants and children during the past 10 years. A decade of change. *Am Heart J* 107:1235-1240, 1984.

Primary Myocardial Disease

6

Definition

This discussion is concerned with any condition that primarily affects the myocardium.

Basic Science

In the course of infectious illness, myocardial involvement is suggested by electrocardiographic ST and T changes. This observation is relatively common and reported with many diseases. Congestive heart failure associated with an infectious illness is much less common. Biopsy of the myocardium at catheterization shows evidence of inflammation in less than 10% of reported cases, although most biopsies may be obtained too late in the illness to be diagnostic (Lewis, 1985). The pathogenesis of myocardial involvement is unclear and may include direct invasion, immune reactions, toxins, or an inherited predisposition to cardiomyopathy, possibly triggered by infection. Cardiomyopathy is a deliberately vague term, only marginally clarified by the terms "dilated" (dilated heart with congestive heart failure), "hypertrophic" (excessive thickness of ventricular muscle, with or without obstruction), "restrictive" or "obliterative" (small, noncompliant ventricular cavity). From an etiologic point of view, a cardiomyopathy may result from a prior infectious episode (coxsackie, diphtheria, *Rickettsia*), nutritional problems (Kwashiorkor, beriberi), metabolic abnormalities (Pompe disease, carnitine deficiency, infants of diabetic mothers), collagen diseases (dermatomyositis, lupus erythematosus, scleroderma), neuromuscular diseases (muscular dystrophy, Friedreich ataxia), parasitic diseases (Chagas disease), immunologic diseases (rheumatic fever), syndromes (Noonan syndrome), mucopolysaccharidoses (Hurler disease), endocardial fibroelastosis, an anomalous left coronary arising from the pulmonary artery, drugs (adriamycin toxicity), X-radiation, or postsurgical trauma. In many, if not most, the etiology is not identified. Familial cardiomyopathy, however, is often recognized (Gutgesel et al, 1980; Lewis et al, 1981; Marin-Garcia et al, 1981; Tripp et al, 1981; Wynne and Braunwald, 1980). The manifestations of myocardial disease range from muscle sufficiently diseased to interfere with ejection of blood to a thickened stiff myocardium that prevents adequate filling. In the hypertrophic form there may be muscular obstruction of the left ventricular outflow, which is accentuated during myocardial contraction (idiopathic hypertrophic subaortic stenosis). Arrhythmias are common in all varieties of myocardial disease, and are probably the cause of the sudden, unexpected deaths, particularly common in hypertrophic varieties. Coronary artery disease (Kawasaki syndrome and congenital abnormalities of the coronaries) may produce myocardial dysfunction, even myocardial infarction (anomalous origin of the left coronary from the pulmonary artery).

Epidemiology

Primary myocardial disease requiring hospitalization in childhood is rare, less than 1% of the patient experience at the Boston Children's Hospital Cardiology Department. The New England Regional Infant Cardiac Program found 2.6% of acutely ill infants to have primary myocardial problems (Table 6.3). This incidence is perhaps accentuated by the left ventricular stress that occurs naturally immediately after birth (see Events at Birth, pp. 319).

Diagnosis

In many acute viral illnesses evanescent ST and T changes on the electrocardiogram may be the only evidence of myocardial involvement. More extensive myocardial damage can result in left-sided failure, the inflamed myocardium being incapable of supplying an adequate cardiac output. The child exhibits progressive exercise intolerance, and later, shortness of breath, loss of appetite, and often vomiting. Either the congestive symptoms (sometimes acute, even catastrophic) or the onset of arrhythmia brings the patient to the attention of physicians.

Myocardial problems are discovered because of symptoms of congestive heart failure or as part of an examination for some disease or syndrome known to have an associated myocardial problem (e.g., Friedreich ataxia).

Hypertrophic cardiomyopathy is often familial and asymmetric septal hypertrophy may be discovered through systematic echocardiographic examination of relatives. These surveys of relatives produce more patients with this problem than does any other mechanism of discovery. Occasionally patients who have obstructive hypertrophic myopathy will have murmurs of mitral regurgitation or aortic stenosis that bring them to the physician's attention. Some have arrhythmias.

ELECTROCARDIOGRAPHY

With viral myocarditis, there may be acute changes in the ST and T waves, and even Q waves, sometimes so pronounced as to suggest myocardial infarction. Often in the cardiomyopathies, particularly the hypertrophic varieties, there are prominent Q waves, changes in the ST and T waves, promiment P waves, and occasionally a widened QRS. Rhythm problems, including ventricular ectopy and atrial fibrillation, are not uncommon.

RADIOGRAPHY

On chest films, the heart is visibly enlarged. There may be pulmonary congestion and Kerley B lines.

ECHO-DOPPLER STUDY

The patients with asymmetric septal hypertrophy can be readily identified by echocardiography. The presence of associated pericardial effusion, the size of the chambers, the thickness of the ventricular muscle, and estimations of ventricular function can be recorded. The presence and degree of mitral regurgitation can be documented. Determination of left ventricular size and function are useful in following the course of the disease.

CARDIAC CATHETERIZATION

If the child is known to have formerly had a normal heart, there is little value in cardiac catheterization. If not, it is possible that a coronary anomaly accounts for the myocardial problem. In this case cardiac catheterization may be particularly rewarding. Cardiac catheterization or Swan-Ganz monitoring of pulmonary blood flow, pulmonary artery pressure, and pulmonary wedge pressures provides useful management information and should be used in desperate situations. There are not sufficient data to recommend routine myocardial biopsies (Sekiguchi et al, 1985); the risk is small but, so far, the benefit is small also.

Management

ACUTE MYOCARDIAL DECOMPENSATION

These patients are a prime test of the physician's skill in managing congestive heart failure. Since the myocardial abnormality is sometimes reversible, it is possible that with the most sophisticated medical management (an approach similar to that practical for acute myocardial infarction in the adult), the patient will survive and become well. There are several pitfalls. With an inflamed myocardium the tendency to arrhythmia may be accentuated by digoxin. For this rea-

CASE ILLUSTRATION

A 18-month-old girl was well until 3 weeks before to admission when she developed a cough, worse at night, with vomiting and loss of appetite. Her physician discovered gross congestive failure and transferred her to The Children's Hospital in Boston.

On physical examination she was pale, tachypneic (50/min), and her liver was enlarged 4 cm below the right costal margin. The cardiac impulse was quiet. The heart rate was 140; there was a loud gallop sound, and a minimal apical systolic murmur. The electrocardiogram showed generalized low voltage, ST and T changes and an axis of $+150°$. The echocardiogram showed no pericardial effusion, an enlarged left ventricle and an enlarged left atrium (Fig. 6.40). On the chest film, there was moderate cardiomegaly and evidence of pulmonary edema.

Treatment with digoxin, furosemide, spironolactone and mechanical ventilation improved the situation somewhat, but the child was stabilized on mechanical ventilation in chronic congestive failure. Cardiac catheterization was undertaken to determine her response to afterload reduction. At the outset of this procedure, the pH was 7.28. During catheterization, the right atrial pressure was: V wave, 23 mm Hg; A wave, 28 mm Hg; the mean pressure was 18 mm Hg. The mean pulmonary arterial wedge pressure was 24. There was no evidence for intracardiac shunting. The pulmonary artery pressure was 60/40 with a mean of 45 mm Hg, while the aortic pressure was 80/50 with a mean of 63 mm Hg. Systemic cardiac output was 2.8 L/m^2 while systemic resistance was 21 units. With nitroprusside infusion the resistance gradually fell while cardiac output improved (Table 6.15).

Over the course of the next several days, with administration of hydralazine, she steadily improved and 2 weeks after admission she was discharged with instructions to continue treatment with digoxin, hydralazine, Diuril, and Aldactone. Some months later, her medications were discontinued with no return of congestive heart failure. Her heart size was normal and her electrocardiogram became normal.

QUESTIONS AND COMMENTS

The heart was not grossly enlarged. Isn't it more likely that the heart will be very large with this degree of congestive heart failure?

It is currently thought that an acute onset of myocardial disease may not result in immediate gross dilatation of the heart. Only with prolonged myocardial abnormality does the heart dilate to a giant size. This child had a relatively recent onset of congestive heart failure.

Is the response to afterload reduction particularly dramatic?

It was in this child, yet most patients with myocardial disease make a similar initial response. In some, the chronic effect is less noticeable.

Is complete recovery from myocarditis unusual?

At least 20–30% of patients recover completely even with some have congestive failure as difficult to control as was this patient's. Every effort to control congestive failure is worthwhile since, if given some time, the disease may resolve, if not completely, at least leaving the patient in a survivable state.

Is it necessary to carry out cardiac catheterization before starting afterload reduction?

This is not customary at the present time. This child was admitted during a period when we were collecting physiologic information about the effects of afterload reduction.

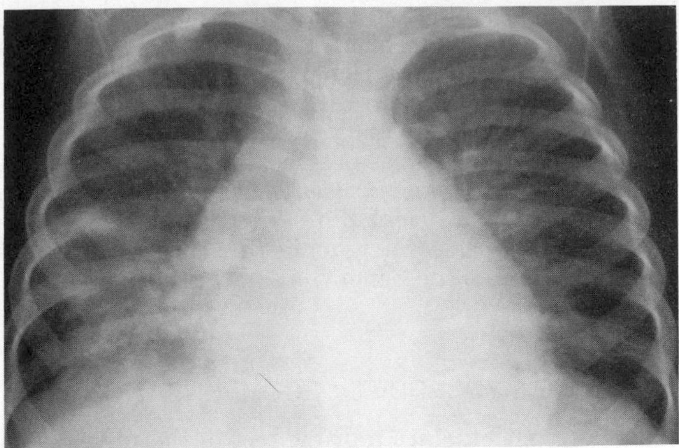

Figure 6.40. Chest film of patient with myocarditis showing a grossly enlarged heart and evidence of congestive heart failure. This child recovered completely and is now reported to have a normal-sized heart.

Table 6.15
Effects of Nitroprusside Infusion in this Patient During Cardiac Catheterization

Nitroprusside infusion (μg/kg/min)	Cardiac Output, (L/m^2/min)	Systemic Vascular Resistance (Wood units)	Right Atrial Pressure (Mean)	Pulmonary Arterial Wedge Pressure (Mean)
Baseline	2.8	21	14	33
1.0	3.4	15	13	24
2.0	3.6	15	11	22
3.0	4.1	12	12	18

son, careful monitoring is required as the dose is increased and as serum potassium levels fluctuate with the coincident use of diuretics. The sudden appearance of arrhythmia may be fatal with a damaged myocardium, hence the requirement for electrocardiographic monitoring in the acute stages. Limitation of salt and fluid intake may be helpful. Vigorous use of diuretics may be the most effective measure used may be even with digitalis. On occasion, afterload reduction is lifesaving. Increased ambient oxygen, even assisted ventilation, may be required. In the worst situations Swan-Ganz catheters may provide useful management information. With chronic congestive heart failure bed rest, limitation of exercise and use of home teachers may be advisable.

Finally, cardiac transplantation can be considered in intractable situations.

HYPERTROPHIC CARDIOMYOPATHY

With obstructive hypertrophic cardiomyopathies, digoxin is contraindicated since increased strength of myocardial contraction may limit diastolic filling and increase outflow obstruction. Patients with this problem may do well if such agents as propanolol or verapamil are administered; these effectively reduce the strength of myocardial contraction, allow better filling, and reduce outflow obstruction. Arrhythmias are common and may be the cause of sudden death. For this reason, strict attention to pharmacological control of rhythm is required.

Patients with obstructive cardiomyopathy who have treatment-resistant angina may benefit symptomatically from surgical resection of the obstructing outflow muscle without changing the ultimate prognosis.

ANOMALOUS ORIGIN OF THE LEFT CORONARY ARTERY

Anomalous origin of the left coronary artery from the pulmonary artery should be considered in any infant 3–4 months old with a large heart and an electrocardiogram showing a pattern suggesting myocardial infarction (inverted T_1, T_2, TAVL, and T in left chest leads, Q_1, QAVL, and Q in midprecordial leads, ST elevation in the precordial leads, and left ventricular hypertrophy). If the anomalous coronary is large it may be recognized at echocardiography but any suspicion of this diagnosis should lead to cardiac catheterization.

In the past 5 years it has been our policy to implant the origin of the anomalous coronary into the aorta in these patients on diagnosis. Even when this is done some years after birth, the improvement in the electrocardiographic abnormalities and the echocardiographic evidence of myocardial function is sometimes quite gratifying.

REFERENCES

Gutgesell HP, Speer ME, Rosenberg HS: Characterization of the cardiomyopathy in infants of diabetic mothers. *Circulation* 61:441-450, 1980.

Lewis AB: Findings on endomyocardial biopsy in infants and children with dilated cardiomyopathy. *Am J Cardiol* 55:143-145, 1985.

Lewis AB, Crouse VL, Evans W, et al: Recovery of left ventricular function following discrimination of anthracycline chemotherapy in children. *Pediatrics* 68:67-72, 1981.

Marin-Garcia J, Gooch WM, Coury DL: Cardiac manifestations of Rocky Mountain Spotted Fever. *Pediatrics* 67:358-361, 1981.

Sekiguchi M, Olsen EGJ, Goodwin JF: Myocarditis and Related Disorders: Proceedings of the International Symposium Cardiomyopathy and Myocarditis. Tokoyo, Springer-Verlag, 1985.

Tripp ME, Katcher ML, Peters HA, et al: Systemic carnitine deficiency presenting as familial endocardial fibroelastosis. *N Engl J Med* 305:385-390, 1981.

Wynne J, Braunwald E: The cardiomyopathies and myocardities. In Braunwald E (ed): *Heart Disease: A Textbook of Cardiomuscular Medicine*. Philadelphia, WB Saunders, 1980, pp. 1437-1498.

Pericardial Disease

7

Definition

Acute pericardial disease in pediatric patients may be caused by viruses (coxsackie), bacteria (Feldman, 1979; Morgan et al, 1983) (*Staphylococcus, tuberculosis*), collagen disease, postpericardiotomy syndrome (Engle et al, 1980), hemorrhage, primary pericardial tumors (teratoma), and metatastic neoplastic disease. Constrictive pericarditis is a distinct clinical entity, the etiology of which is seldom obvious. Tuberculous pericarditis used to be blamed for the majority of constrictive cases. In 1986, in the United States, this is not necessarily true.

Basic Science

When serous membranes of the pericardium are diseased, sufficient fluid may accumulate to interfere with cardiac filling. The effusion could be serous, serosanguinous or purulent. With appreciable fluid accumulation—tamponade—the pericardium becomes increasingly tense, limiting diastolic filling, and thereby reducing cardiac output. This occurs rapidly as the pericardial fluid accumulates. If the accumulation is slow, allowing for stretching of the pericardium over time, the fluid collection may be very large without dangerously limiting inflow. If the fluid accumulation is rapid, the obstruction to inflow and the drop in cardiac output may occur in a matter of hours—rarely minutes. Whenever an inflammatory process is occurring in the pericardium, the subepicardial layers of the myocardium are involved as well.

Epidemiology

Pericardial disease occurring as an isolated entity is rare, whereas pericardial problems occurring in patients postoperatively (hemorrhage, tamponade, postpericardiotomy syndrome) are common.

Diagnosis

The clinical picture is dominated by symptoms and signs of inflammation of the pericardium and limitation of cardiac inflow. An inflamed pericardium may produce dull, aching pericardial pain, associated with nausea, or sometimes sharp, stabbing pain referred to the shoulder or epigastrium. Sitting up and leaning forward sometimes relieves the pain; it is often associated with a dry cough.

Because the limitation of inflow into the heart results in reduced cardiac output, there is also limitation of exercise, fatigue, and weakness. The symptoms may become overpowering as tamponade—a life-threatening event—develops, the patient becoming anxious, leaning forward for relief, and racked by cough. Tachycardia is invariably noted; tachypnea and dyspnea occur but are rarely predominant unless the limitation of inflow into the systemic circulation is different from that into the pulmonary circulation (an unusual occurrence). If the disease involves infection the symptoms associated with empyema, such as fever or evidence of pneumonia, may be present.

PHYSICAL EXAMINATION

The patient with severe disease is pale, anxious, leaning forward on a pillow, and sitting up in bed. When there is no limitation of inflow, there are usually no specific signs of pericardial disease except in those who have a friction rub. The movement of the inflamed parietal and visceral pericardial surfaces against each other may produce a characteristic scraping, scratching sound, which varies in quality and intensity in systole and diastole, varies with position, and is not limited to either cardiac cycle. A friction rub often sounds close to the ear with the danger that it may be discounted as an adventitious noise. The presence of a friction rub is pathognomonic for pericardial inflammation and may be the only physical sign of a problem. The larger the effusion, the less obvious the friction rub.

Evidences of limited cardiac inflow, and therefore limited output, include a small pulse, small arterial pulse pressure, and low systolic blood pressure. There may be excessive respiratory variation in the systolic pressure. This is normally only a few mm Hg (±10), but in pericardial disease it may be as high as 20–30 mm Hg (paradoxical pulse). The liver may be enlarged but is not pulsating. The neck veins may be distended well above the clavicle when the patient is sitting. With constriction, sharp X and Y descents in the jugular venous pulse may be noted. The cardiac impulse is quiet, never hyperactive, and there may be a friction rub.

MINOR LABORATORY TESTS

With purulent pericarditis there is usually leukocytosis with a high polymorphonuclear count. The sedimentation rate and other phase reactants are elevated. The serum protein may be abnormal with the hypersensitivity type of pericarditis. If there is any suggestion of constrictive disease, a tuberculin skin test might be warranted.

ELECTROCARDIOGRAPHY

The ECG may show characteristic elevation of the ST segments, sometimes with changes in the T wave and rarely with small QRS complexes in all the chest leads. There is a characteristic evolution from an elevated ST segment to inverted T waves and back to normal. The ECG often returns to normal while the inflammatory process, including a friction rub, is still present.

RADIOGRAPHY

The heart size depends on the size of the effusion. The heart may be huge with minimal clinical evidence of tamponade if fluid has accumulated over weeks, or the heart may be mildly enlarged with severe symptoms if the fluid has accumulated in a short time.

ECHO-DOPPLER STUDY

The echocardiographer can recognize the presence and volume of the pericardial fluid and give some impression of the degree of tamponade (Weitzman et al, 1984).

CARDIAC CATHETERIZATION

Cardiac catheterization is not needed for the diagnosis of pericarditis or effusion. It may be essential, however, in the differential diagnosis of constrictive pericardial versus myocardial disease. In constrictive pericarditis, characteristically, although not invariably, the diastolic pressures in the two ventricles are virtually identical and closely approximate atrial pressures and pulmonary arterial diastolic pressures. By contrast, in the cardiomyopathies, the abnormalities are more marked and may be largely limited to the left-sided chamber. A sharp dip in the ventricular pressure pulse at the onset of ventricular diastole is characteristic of constrictive pericarditis.

Management

When tamponade has not occurred, treatment is directed at the underlying cause. Often a sample of pericardial fluid, obtained through pericardiocentesis while the patient is being monitored by electrocardiography, is desirable for diagnostic purposes. A small collection of pericardial fluid is likely to result in a bloody and unhelpful pericardial tap. If there is a strong possibility of bacterial pericarditis, a diagnostic tap and arrangements for chronic drainage are mandatory.

With tamponade, a pericardial tap is performed for relief of symptoms and even as a lifesaving measure. When it has been demonstrated that tamponade is developing (low blood pressure, paradoxical pulse, pulsatile jugular veins, ascites), a pericardial tap is performed as soon as it can be arranged. The services of an experienced cardiologist or surgeon should be sought. If none is available, insertion of a needle at the xiphoid, directed toward the left shoulder may solve the problem. Removal of a small amount of fluid (10–50 ml depending on the size of the child) will relieve pericardial tension, pain, cough, and the threat of imminent death. Initial removal of small amounts of fluid is important, particularly if the fluid is bloody, since a decision whether the fluid comes from a cardiac chamber or the pericardium must be made. A drop of bloody fluid on a towel will give an immediate clue which can be confirmed by later centrifugation. Blood which has been in the pericardium for more than a few hours has a much lower hematocrit than the patient's blood does. Once the diagnosis of constrictive pericarditis has been made with reasonable certainty, exploration through a small window of the pericardial space may be indicated. If indeed constrictive disease is found, stripping of the pericardium is highly effective in alleviating, even curing, the process (McCaughan et al, 1985).

Medical management of pericardial disease depends on the course. For patients with postpericardiotomy syndrome, unless they are critically ill, treatment usually is started with salicylates. If these are not effective within a few days, a shift should be made to indomethacin; only if this fails to control the effusion and the symptoms should one resort to prednisone, which is almost invariably effective. The pericardial fluid should be cultured and examined for cell counts, protein, and tumor cells. The amount of fluid to be removed is always a matter of debate. There is little reason for excessive drainage since it is possible to remove more fluid later. If the cardiologist or surgeon can be found who has the appropriate equipment, a catheter can be inserted over a guide wire and left in the pericardium as a safety measure against future difficulty.

Course and Prognosis

The course of pericardial disease depends on the underlying cause. Pericardial teratoma is managed with surgical removal of the teratoma. Bacterial sepsis is treated with specific bactericidal antibiotics if an organism can be identified. Otherwise, treatment is with broad spectrum coverage. Collagen diseases respond to anti-inflammatory agents such as steroids but only rarely is treatment for the pericardial effusion needed as specific therapy. Acute hemorrhage into the pericardium requires pericardial drainage and even autotransfusion. The postpericardiotomy syndrome usually responds to therapy with aspirin or indomethacin.

REFERENCES

Engle MA, Zabriskie JB, Senterfit LB, et al: Viral illness and the postpericardiotomy syndrome; A prospective study in children. *Circulation* 62:1151-1158, 1980.

Feldman WE: Bacterial etiology and mortality of purulent pericarditis in pediatric patients: Review of 162 cases. *Am J Dis Child* 133:641-644, 1979.

McCaughan BC, Schaff HV, Piehler JM, et al: Early and late results of pericardiectomy for constrictive pericarditis. *J Thorac Cardiovasc Surg* 89:340-350, 1985.

Morgan RJ, Stephenson LW, Woolf PK, et al: Surgical treatment of purulent pericarditis in children. *J Thorac Cardiovasc Surg* 85:527-531, 1983.

Weitzman LB, Tinker WP, Kronzon I, et al: The incidence and natural history of pericardial effusion after cardiac surgery—an echocardiographic study. *Circulation* 69:506-511, 1984.

Arrhythmias

8

BRADYCARDIA

Sinus Bradycardia

A slow heart rate does not cause concern unless the rate is slower than 50–60 beats/min in an otherwise well child or adolescent. After intra-atrial surgery, as in a Senning procedure or atrial septal defect repair, episodes of supraventricular tachycardia and long pauses, at rates in the range of 20 beats/min, are described as *sick sinus syndrome*. These children often require medication to control the tachycardia which has the side effect of further increasing the length of the pauses. Consequently, this combination of problems sometimes requires a demand pacemaker to take over at extremely slow rates, making it possible to continue tachycardia-supressing medication without danger of cardiac arrest.

Complete Heart Block

Complete heart block is suspected when the heart rate is found to be unexpectedly slow; less than 80 in the fetus and newborn, less than 60 in a child and less than 50 in an awake adolescent. The diagnosis in the fetus is best established by two-dimensional echocardiography demonstrating discordant atrial and ventricular beats.

In some individuals with complete heart block, a sudden loss of consciousness occurs due to cardiac arrest or ventricular fibrillation (Stokes-Adams attacks). The diagnosis of Stokes-Adams attacks should be considered as the most likely possibility in any patient with complete heart block and syncope. Although a patient with a Stokes-Adams attack, particularly the first one, usually recovers, death may occur in subsequent episodes. For reasons that are not clear, Stokes-Adams attacks are more common after surgically induced block and less common in children with naturally occurring complete heart block, with or without associated heart disease. Electrophysiologists attribute the difference in severity between natural and surgical third degree block to the site of the interruption in the bundle of His. A single Stokes-Adams episode, or reasonable facsimile, requires that a pacemaker be inserted (Karpawich et al, 1981).

Complete Heart Block without Congenital Heart Disease

Rarely, an otherwise normal infant is found to have complete heart block (Gochberg, 1964; Michaelsson and Engle, 1972; Nakamura and Nadas, 1964; Pinsky et al, 1982) in the perinatal period. The possibility that the mother has lupus erythematosus should be explored since association between maternal lupus erythematosus and complete heart block in infants has been reported (Chameides et al, 1977; Scott et al, 1983). If there are no cardiac defects, the treatment is expectant. If there is no suggestion of Stokes-Adams attacks, the infant is allowed to grow and behave normally. With a single episode of syncope or other suggestion of Stokes-Adams phenomenon (lightheadness, near syncope) insertion of a pacemaker is mandatory.

Complete Heart Block with Congenital Heart Disease

Although the association of complete heart block with inverted ventricles (corrected transposition) is well established (Huhta et al, 1983) it has been seen in association with a variety of other cardiac defects, notably atrial septal defects.

With increasing numbers of individuals surviving with inverted ventricles, the appearance of complete heart block as the individuals grow older (fourth to fifth decade) is likely (Esscher, 1981). Given sufficient survival time perhaps complete heart block will occur in all of these patients. Its development during cardiac catheterization has been observed.

Surgical Heart Block

Surgical complete heart block is seen less often now that the anatomic location of the atrioventricular node and the bundle of His in most varieties of congenital heart disease has been established. Complete heart block after ventricular septal defect surgery, after tetralogy of Fallot repair, and after surgery for other defects is now relatively rare (less than 1%). Patients in whom complete heart block develops with cardiac surgery should have pacing wires inserted and should be observed closely. If the complete block is transitory the patient can be safely observed without a pacemaker. If the block persists more than a few days, insertion of a pacemaker should be seriously considered (Karpawich et al, 1981; see Pacemakers).

ECTOPY

Ectopic beats originating outside the prevailing pacemaker and appearing prematurely should be recorded on an electrocardiogram if they are frequent, cause symptoms or are associated with heart disease. Management should be based on the specific diagnosis.

Fetal ectopy is best documented by two-dimensional echocardiography.

Supraventricular Ectopy

Barring the presence of alcohol, tobacco, cardiotoxic drugs, electrolyte imbalance, or hyperthyroidism, supraventricular ectopy may be related to atrial enlargement or atrial hypertension. Supraventricular ectopy in an individual with a normal heart is a benign condition, requiring no specific therapy. Treatment, if any, is directed at the underlying cause.

Ventricular Ectopy

Although rare ventricular premature beats may be benign, the potential for a dangerous rhythm to develop, particularly if the beats are frequent, associated with effort, or multifocal, is real and requires at least minimal documentation. For practical purposes, all individuals with known heart disease who have more than occasional ventricular ectopy must be studied beginning with a 24-hour tape-recorded electrocardiogram (Holter monitoring) and exercise testing. Asymptomatic young people who do not have congenital heart disease and have only an occasional ventricular beat during a 24-hour monitoring particularly if they disappear in exercise, require no further study. By contrast, children who produce couplets or runs of ventricular beats on exercise should receive appropriate medication to suppress the ectopy. Some children with no cardiac abnormality, who have asymptomatic ventricular ectopy, including bursts of ventricular tachycardia, do well without any medication (Bricker et al, 1986). This rare and worrisome phenomenon is under study at the present time in a number of centers. Patients of this type should be referred to a pediatric cardiologist since the principles of management are in flux.

A chaotic rhythm, with multifocal ventricular premature beats, couplets or runs of ventricular tachycardia, is sufficiently dangerous to require hospitalization, monitoring and treatment. In the more stable patient a baseline 24-hour tape-recording is made, the response to exercise is recorded, an appropriate medication is chosen and treatment is started. After a suitable interval the exercise and tape-recorded electrocardiogram are repeated to evaluate the result of treatment. Unfortunately, individual responses to any given medication are sufficiently varied that often a series of tests is required before suppression is achieved. Suppression has occurred with phenytoin, propranolol, procainamide, quinidine, disopyramide and amiodarone (Table 6.16). If there are problems with control, an intracardiac electrophysiologic study, with drugs administered during the procedure, may be desirable (Gillette and Gearson, 1981).

In general, attempts to control runs of ventricular tachycardia, couplets, and even bigeminy are probably best left to the expert pediatric cardiologist since these problems are often intractable and carry significant risk.

TACHYCARDIA

Narrow QRS Complex Tachycardias

A practical division of patients into those with narrow QRS complexes and those with wide QRS tachycardia has stood the test of time and is a safe basis for management. The principle behind this grouping is that a wide QRS complex tachycardia usually, although not invariably, arises from below the atrioventricular node. These ventricular tachycardias are more dangerous and require a specific form of treatment. Confusingly, some forms of supraventricular tachycardias are also associated with a wide QRS complex and are clinically indistinguishable from ventricular tachycardia. In the absence of sophisticated pediatric electrophysiologic opinion, all wide QRS tachycardias (QRS longer than 0.11 sec) should be managed as ventricular tachycardia (see Wide QRS Complex Tachycardia).

Sinus Tachycardia

In response to fever, some drugs, and toxins, a sinus heart rate of more than 160 is common; rarely in very small children, particularly premature babies, it may exceed 200 beats/min. A gradual increase or decrease in the rate, as well as well-defined P waves in the ECG, suggest the underlying mechanism to the clinician. Treatment is directed to the underlying cause.

Supraventricular Tachycardia

Definition

Supraventricular tachycardia is defined as a very rapid heart rate (≥200/min) with narrow QRS complexes.

Basic Science

The mechanism is thought to be either a *re-entry* phenomenon or *automaticity*, an arrhythmogenic focus outside the sinus node (see Diagnostic Tools: Supraventricular Tachycardia).

Supraventricular tachycardia which lasts for many hours or days results in congestive heart failure in infancy, even when the heart is structurally normal, since the time for diastolic filling of the ventricles and the coronaries can be too short to produce a normal cardiac output. Clearly, if the patient has congenital heart disease the critical period may be much shorter. This life-threatening feature is a practical consideration in early infancy where paroxysmal heart rates of 300 beats/min are observed. Small infants with rates higher than 300 are known to succumb to congestive heart failure within 48 hours of onset. The rare death from supraventricular tachycardia in the pediatric age group occurs within the first year of life whether there is underlying congenital heart disease or not (Garson et al, 1981).

Epidemiology

Supraventricular tachycardia is the most common arrhythmia in childhood. Approximately one new patient with this problem is seen each month at The Chil-

Table 6.16
Dosage of Common Cardiovascular Drugs

Drug	Usual dose and interval	Route
Antiarrhythmics		
Lidocaine	Bolus: 1 mg/kg every 20–60 min	IV
	Infusion: 10–50 μg/kg/min	IV
Propranolol	10–20 μg/kg over 10 min q 6–8 h	IV
	1–8 mg/kg/day given q 6 h	PO
Quinidine sulfate	15–60 mg/kg/day given q 6 h in 4 doses	PO
Procainamide	15–60 mg/kg/day given q 4–6 h in 4–6 doses	PO
Phenytoin	3–5 mg/kg over 5 min	IV
	3–8 mg/kg/day in 2–3 divided doses	PO
Verapamil	0–1 year: 0.1 mg/kg over 2 min May repeat dose 0.1–0.2 mg/kg in 30 min	IV
	1–15 years: 0.1–0.3 mg/kg (maximum 5 mg) over 2 min, may repeat dose (maximum 10 mg) in 30 min	IV
Disopyramide	0–1 years: 10–30 mg/kg/day 1–4 years: 10–20 mg/kg/day 4–12 years: 10–15 mg/kg/day 12–18 years: 6–15 mg/kg/day PO in 4 equal doses, q 6 h	PO
Diuretics:		
Furosemide (Lasix)	1.0 mg/kg/dose over 1–2 min	IV
	2–3 mg/kg/day	PO
Chlorothiazide (Diuril)	20–30 mg/kg/day in 2 doses	PO
Hydrochlorothiazide (Hydro-Diuril)	2–3 mg/kg/day in 2 doses	PO
Spironolactone (Aldactone)	1–3 mg/kg/day in 1–2 doses	PO
Positive Inotropes		
Digoxin		
Initial digitalizing dose	Initially ½ total dose, then ¼ of digitalizing dose every 6 hours for 2 days	
Premature:	0.035 mg/kg/24 hr	PO
Newborn:	0.05 mg/kg/24 hr	PO
2 years:	0.05–0.07 mg/kg/24 hr	PO
>2 years:	0.03–0.05 mg/kg/24 hr	PO
Daily maintenance dose	¼ of digitalizing dose/24 hr in 2 doses	PO
Dopamine	2–10 μg/kg/min	IV
Isoproterenol	0.1 μg/kg/min	IV
Dobutamine	1–2 μg/kg/min	IV
Systemic Vasodilators:		
Nitroprusside	3 μg/kg/min	IV
Hydralazine	1 mg/kg/day 3–4 doses	PO
Captopril	0.1 mg/kg/day 3–4 doses	PO

dren's Hospital in Boston. Except for episodes induced during cardiac catheterization, or as a result of cardiac surgery, this arrhythmia usually occurs in children with otherwise normal hearts. It is most common in male infants less than 4 months old and is occasionally detected in utero.

Diagnosis

Supraventricular tachycardia is documented by electrocardiography (see Diagnostic Tools). Although the diagnosis may be clinically suspected because of the absolutely regular, very fast heart rate (>200 beats/

min), with a sudden onset and sudden termination, an electrocardiogram is mandatory for precise diagnosis. Although the generic diagnosis of supraventricular tachycardia can be readily recognized, the precise diagnosis of the various types often requires an experienced electrocardiographer and even an electrophysiologic study.

Management

Supraventricular tachycardias with a narrow QRS complex, particularly in infants, have been treated successfully with digoxin for many years. Generally, in the small infant, treatment is begun with parenteral digoxin (to prevent vomiting) and the full digitalizing dose is given over a matter of 12 hours. The majority respond within hours. Over the years, a variety of other proposals for the treatment of critical supraventricular tachycardia have been put forward. At the present time a favorite is the intravenous administration of verapamil for children, not for infants. The attractiveness of an intravenous drug that stops supraventricular tachycardia within minutes is obvious. Whether this turns out to be as safe as digoxin remains to be seen.

Intractable supraventricular tachycardia, or frequent recurrences despite full digitalization, occasionally requires the addition of β-blockers. For older children and adults with demonstrated Wolff-Parkinson-White syndrome and supraventricular tachycardia, beta blockers are the drugs of choice, with the addition of quinidine for the resistant ones. Theoretical considerations, based on unfavorable differential conduction in the two limbs of the re-entrant pathways with digoxin, argue against the use of glycosides.

Direct current countershock invariably stops supraventricular tachycardia and has the favorable feature that no potentially toxic agent has been introduced, irretrievably, into the patient. The argument, still occasionally heard, that direct current countershock may cause ventricular tachycardia is specious since a second shock will stop ventricular tachycardia.

Fetal supraventricular tachycardia has been successfully controlled (Dumensic et al, 1982) with material digitalis administration.

Course and Prognosis

Most individuals who have had an attack of supraventricular tachycardia are subject to recurrences, but a male infant without a demonstrable accessory pathway is likely to stop having recurrent attacks around the age of six months. Individuals with demonstrable accessory pathways allowing re-entry (such as are present in Wolff-Parkinson-White syndrome) continue to be subject to recurrent attacks for many years, as are most individuals whose first episode occurred beyond infancy. The frequency and duration of recurrent attacks are unpredictable except that many individuals follow a pattern that becomes recognizable over time. In some individuals episodes of paroxysmal tachycardia clearly develop in association with stressful situations, physical or emotional (Lundberg, 1982).

Prevention of Recurrence

All patients prone to have recurrences of supraventricular tachycardia, whether a re-entry tract is identified or not, are candidates for chronic preventive treatment if the attacks are prolonged or frequent enough to interfere with a comfortable lifestyle. In those whose attacks are short and infrequent, a cost/benefit decision must be made between tolerating an occasional and predictable "spell" and taking daily medication.

Digoxin, as a prophylactic, should be tried first and will almost invariably reduce or eliminate the number of attacks. Occasionally, propanolol is required and, rarely, other drugs such as quinidine or procainamide are useful. All infants should be kept on digoxin for at least 6–12 months after an initial episode; at that time an attempt to discontinue the drug can be made. If there is a recurrence, the drug should be restarted and continued for an additional 1–2 years.

Refractory tachycardias should be viewed with some suspicion and an electrophysiologic study considered. This allows for sharper definition of the nature of the rhythm, more precise use of specific antiarrhythmic agents and the location of possible re-entry tracts. Rarely, a child may require surgical division of the re-entry pathway to control recurrences of the arrhythmia.

Atrial Flutter

Atrial flutter is defined as atrial rates around 300 beats/min, with variable ventricular conduction of 1:1 or with atrioventricular block of 2:1 or 3:1. For this reason, a tachycardia with a fixed ventricular rate of 150 should raise the possibility of atrial flutter with 2:1 block. In lead II, the ECG shows the characteristic "sawtooth" flutter waves. Aside from being associated with cardiac diseases that cause very large atria, naturally occurring atrial flutter is seen largely in the newborn. The risk to the patient is directly related to the ventricular rate and to the possibility, even in older patients, that a 1:1 mechanism may suddenly take over and produce an extremely dangerous situation. Treatment for atrial flutter begins with digitalization if the patient is not in critical condition to produce atrioventricular block. Direct current countershock is highly effective for conversion and is the method of choice for critical and resistant flutter.

Atrial Fibrillation

Structural heart disease that causes an atrium to become large may cause atrial fibrillation characterized by an irregular rhythm at varying rates, referred to as irregular irregularity. Rhythms shifting from characteristic atrial flutter to atrial fibrillation (flutter-fibrillation) are encountered. Atrial fibrillation, without structural heart disease, is seen at birth and occasionally among adolescents. Digoxin will control the ventricular rate and direct current countershock will terminate the rhythm. Occasionally, prevention of recurrent episodes is best managed with quinidine.

Chronic Atrial Ectopic Tachycardia

A particularly resistant, fortunately rare, form of atrial tachycardia, which is repetitive, variable in rate and characterized by ectopic P waves is referred to as chronic ectopic tachycardia or repetitive tachycardia. Children with this chronic type may have tachycardia for days, months, or years. Sometimes, with medication, the rhythm breaks to 2:1 or 3:1 atrioventricular block, providing a more physiologic ventricular rate. Treatment is best left to the experts.

Wide QRS Complex Tachycardia

Ventricular Tachycardia

Any tachycardia that on electrocardiographic documentation is found to have wide QRS complexes (longer than 0.10 msec) should be managed as ventricular tachycardia until proven otherwise. Ventricular tachycardia is rare in childhood. It is often associated with major structural disease, although rarely it may be encountered in otherwise normal children (Deal et al, 1986) (see Diagnostic tools). Often treatment must be begun before the diagnosis is confirmed; until proven otherwise, a wide QRS complex tachycardia must be considered to be ventricular in origin. The patient often, although not invariably, may show signs of low cardiac output (pallor, sweating, and hypotension) and have generally slower rates (160–180 beats/min) than occur with supraventricular tachycardia.

Treatment requires an electrocardiographic monitor, an intravenous line and handy apparatus for direct current countershock. A bolus of lidocaine is often successful in terminating ventricular tachycardia. With worsening clinical condition, countershock is used. Prevention of recurrence includes continued intravenous administration of lidocaine until pharmacologic control, with other drugs such as quinidine, disopyramide, and propranolol, is established.

CASE ILLUSTRATION

This previously well, 1-month-old male infant became irritable and restless and fed poorly over the preceding 24 hours. With the onset of vomiting, he was brought to the hospital.

On examination, there was tachypnea (60/min) without retractions. The liver was enlarged 3.0 cm below the right costal margin. The heart rate was more than 200 beats/min. An ECG showed a heart rate of 280 beats/min (Fig. 6.5) without visible P waves and with clock-like regularity. The QRS duration was 0.08 sec. The chest film showed a moderately enlarged heart.

An electrocardiographic monitor was set up and an intravenous line was established. Digitalization was begun. Six hours later, after the second intravenous dose of digoxin, the rhythm suddenly converted to a normal sinus mechanism.

Two days later the child was discharged on maintenance digoxin therapy and arrangements were made for follow-up.

At 6 months of age, there having been no further episodes, digoxin was discontinued.

QUESTIONS AND COMMENTS

Is 6 months of preventive treatment sufficient?

The majority of male infants with narrow QRS complex tachycardia do not experience recurrence after the age of 6 months. Female infants and infants with known Wolff-Parkinson-White syndrome are more likely to suffer recurrences and are kept on preventive medication through the age of 2 years.

How will a mother know there is a recurrence?

Generally the mother has little difficulty in recognizing a recurrent attack; there is return of symptoms. The onset of tachycardia is often associated with sudden pallor; later, other symptoms such as irritability, tachypnea and vomiting call attention to the problem.

Should the parents have a stethoscope to monitor the infant?

No! It is obvious that the mother could be taught to use a stethoscope and to count the heart rate. Similarly, an ECG monitor could be rented, but, in our view, this should be avoided. Early detection and early treatment is unneccessary since a recurrent attack is well tolerated for 12–24 hours and longer. The spectre of the parents checking the child every hour, day after day, is appalling.

Why not use direct current countershock for all patients?

Although direct current countershock almost invariably results in conversion to sinus rhythm, without preventive medicine a return to supraventricular tachycardia is likely. Hence, treatment is begun with digoxin and only if symptoms require emergency intervention, is direct current countershock used.

Does a child with Wolff-Parkinson-White syndrome require preventive therapy forever?

With no recurrent attacks, the preventive medication is discontinued perhaps every 2 years to see how the child does. Since the problem can be readily recognized by the patient there should be no fear of unrecognized attacks.

Can a child who has been free of recurrent attacks for 10 years be considered unlikely ever to have attacks again?

No one who has ever had supraventricular tachycardia (including male infants) is free from possible subsequent attacks up to many years later.

Who should have electrophysiologic study?

If, despite preventive therapy, a child has recurrent tachycardias that interfere with his lifestyle, electrophysiologic study will locate the re-entry circuit. It may be possible to identify the most effective drug to use and it may be possible to suggest surgical division of the reentry circuit in extreme cases.

The differential diagnosis between supraventricular tachycardia with aberrant conduction (a less dangerous rhythm) and ventricular tachycardia may require intracardiac electrophysiologic study, with controlled induction of the tachycardia and demonstration of the relationship, or lack of it, between the P waves and the QRS complexes.

REFERENCES

Bricker JT, Traweek MS, Smith RT, et al: Exercise-related ventricular tachycardia in children. *Am Heart J* 112:186-188, 1986.

Chameides L, Truex RC, Vetter V, et al: The association of maternal systemic lupus erythematosis and congenital complete heart block. *N Engl J Med* 297:1204-1207, 1977.

Deal BJ, Miller SM, Scagliotti D, et al: Ventricular tachycardia in a young population without heart disease. *Circulation* 73:1111-1118, 1986.

Dumensic DA, Silverman NH, Tobias S, et al: Transplacental cardioversion of fetal tachycardia with procainamide. *N Engl J Med* 307:1128-1131, 1982.

Esscher EB: Congenital complete heart block in adolescence and adult life: A followup study. *Eur Heart J* 2:281-288, 1981.

Garson A, Gillette PC, McNamara DG: Supraventricular tachycardia in children: Clinical features, response to treatment, and long term followup of 217 patients. *J Pediatr* 98:875-882, 1981.

Gillette PC, Garson A: *Pediatric Cardiac Dysrhythmias*. New York, Grune & Stratton, 1981.

Gochberg SH: Congenital heart block. *Am J Obstet Gynecol* 88:238-241, 1964.

Huhta JC, Maloney JD, Ritter DG, et al: Complete atrioventricular block in patients with atrioventricular disorder. *Circulation* 67:1374-1377, 1983.

Karpawich PP, Gillette PC, Garson A, et al: Congenital complete atrioventricular block: Clinical and electrophysiologic predictors of need for pacemaker insertion. *Am J Cardiol* 48:1098-1102, 1981.

Lundberg A: Paroxysmal atrial tachycardia in infancy: Long term followup study of 49 subjects. *Pediatrics* 70:638-642, 1982.

Michaelsson M, Engle MA: Congenital heart block: An international study of natural history. In Brest AN, Engle MA (eds): *Cardiovascular Clinics*. Philadelphia, FA Davis, 1972, p 85-101.

Nakamura FF, Nadas AS: Complete heart block in infants and children. *N Engl J Med* 270:1261-1268, 1964.

Pinsky WW, Gillette PC, Garson A, et al: Diagnosis, management and long-term results in patients with congenital complete heart block. *Pediatrics* 69:728-733, 1982.

Scott JS, Maddison PJ, Taylor PV, et al: Connective tissue disease, antibodies to ribonucleoprotein and heart block. *N Engl J Med* 309:209-212, 1983.

DONALD C. FYLER
ALEXANDER A. NADAS

Section 7

Gastroenterology

Upper Gastointestinal Tract Diseases: Approaches by Symptom

1

APPROACH TO DYSPHAGIA

Definition

Dysphagia is any difficulty in swallowing. It can arise from structural or inflammatory abnormalities of the oral pharynx, esophagus, or thorax, or from neurologic or neuromuscular disorders. Both structural and neurologic etiologies may be either congenital or acquired.

Basic Science and Natural History

Pathophysiologic descriptions of specific entities and their natural histories are included in the appropriate sections elsewhere in this book.

Diagnosis

Even before the baby is born it may be possible to suspect dysphagia. For example, polyhydramnios may herald esophageal atresia, along with other upper GI anomalies. Myasthenia gravis in the mother could also result in temporary dysphagia in a newborn owing to passage of maternal antibodies. If an infant is comfortable at birth but becomes dyspneic with the first feed, a structural abnormality such as Pierre-Robin syndrome, macroglossia, or esophageal atresia should also be suspected. Failure to suck is a common finding in premature infants who have been intubated for prolonged periods.

A few anatomic lesions can present after the neonatal period. If the infant chokes on solid foods, has frequent upper respiratory infections and pneumonia, and intermittent episodes of wheezing, anatomic lesions such as vascular compression of the esophagus or an esophageal duplication should be considered. In addition, if a child fails to grow and has a history of persistent vomiting, and dysphagia, esophageal stenosis resulting from esophagitis is a possibility.

In an older child, dysphagia may serve as a signal for other more systemic diseases such as dermatomyositis or scleroderma. It even can be a component of inflammatory bowel disease. Other possible causes when dysphagia occurs for the first time in an older child are obstructive lesions such as mediastinal masses, foreign bodies, thyroiditis, progression of lesions in Stevens Johnson syndrome into the esophagus, achalasia, epidermolysis bullosa, or even globus hystericus. Neurologic disorders at this stage could include brain tumors and demyelinating diseases.

Physical examination may reveal an obstructive abnormality of the nasal or oral pharynx, which can be ruled out by successfully passing a catheter through each nostril into the stomach. This eliminates choanal atresia, obstructing pharyngeal masses and esophageal atresia. Watching the infant feed and noting the strength and coordination of sucking, swallowing, and breathing are useful to assess the neurologic problems in an infant. Radiographic procedures include fluoroscopic evaluation of lateral neck, airway and diaphragm, in association with a barium swallow to reveal structural and physiologic abnormalities of pharynx and esophagus. If dysphagia occurs later in childhood, endoscopy and laryngoscopy may be indicated as well as motility and manometric studies.

Treatment

See specific section for an approach to treatment once the underlying cause has been ascertained.

APPROACH TO RUMINATION

Definition

Rumination constitutes a syndrome in which food is regurgitated, then partially or completely rechewed, reswallowed, or expelled. Because it frequently occurs when an infant is alone, it is often difficult to diagnose. Nevertheless, rumination can result in weight loss, poor weight gain, electrolyte imbalance, dehydration, and possibly death.

Basic Science

There is some controversy as to the etiology of rumination with possibilities ranging from organic and anatomic to psychodynamic and behavioral. The leading organic theory is that rumination is a sequela of gastroesophageal reflux and that oral movements are attempts to empty the esophagus of refluxed gastric contents. When reflux cannot be demonstrated, however, psychodynamic theories are considered. For example, rumination has been proposed as a somatic symptom reflecting an unsatisfactory mother-infant relationship or as a way for the infant to "recoil from the environment and the people in it" (Lourie, 1954). Endorphin stimulation by rumination has been considered by Herman and Panksepp (1978).

Natural History

Rumination is most commonly seen in infants, but has been described in children and adults. Age of onset is typically between 3 weeks and 12 months in infants who demonstrate no known neurologic disorder. In children with a neurologic dysfunction, rumination may not occur until they are several years of age.

Diagnosis

A history of a preceding illness associated with vomiting such as otitis media or an anatomic problem such as hiatal hernia may often precede the onset of the syndrome. Once an infant learns to initiate the vomiting, rumination can become part of a self-regulation process. The relationship between vomiting and an infant's feeding schedule should be determined; vomiting after and between feedings suggests the possibility of rumination.

If rumination is expected, the basic examination should include observation of the interaction between the infant and its parent during feeding and play. Such observations can provide valuable information as to whether the rumination is used to relieve tension or as a way of self-stimulation if parent-child interaction is inadequate.

CONTROVERSY

Whether an extensive work-up should be performed to elicit gastroesophageal reflux remains controversial. A barium swallow can demonstrate anatomic abnormalities, but should not be used to evaluate reflux since reflux of barium may be seen in healthy infants as well as in ruminators. If the patient fails to gain weight or has recurrent episodes of pneumonia, evaluation of reflux is appropriate (see pp. 417).

Treatment

If gastroesophageal reflux has been documented as a cause of rumination, appropriate treatment should follow. If, however, rumination is seen as a somatic symptom that becomes a learned habit, a psychodynamic and behavioral approach to therapy is in order, which would be geared toward helping parents understand the meaning of the symptom and helping the child and parents modify their interactions and their response to stress. One approach to therapy is a combination of social punishment after verbal punishment. In other words, parents scold the child who is ruminating, place the child down and leave the room for several minutes. If the infant is not ruminating on return, the child is picked up, cleaned, and played with.

APPROACH TO VOMITING

Definition

Vomiting represents the forceful ejection of stomach contents. Nausea is a conscious recognition of impending vomiting, thought to be stimulated by irritated nerve impulses coming either from the GI tract or the brain itself.

Basic Science

Vomiting represents a response to afferent stimuli that are mediated by a vomiting center thought to be located in the lateral reticular formation in the medulla. These afferent stimuli arise from the pharynx, intestines, pleura, heart, urogenital and biliary tracts in response to such mechanisms as obstruction or infection of a viscus. Moreover, the vestibular apparatus, metabolic factors (such as electrolyte imbalances), azotemia, and certain drugs (particularly morphine derivatives and cardiac glycosides), have all been reported to stimulate the vomiting center, acting either directly or indirectly through another medullary area—the chemoreceptor trigger zone.

The act of vomiting itself is usually precipitated by responses from the vomiting center that include (1) a deep breath, (2) raising of the hyoid bone in the larynx to pull the cricoesophageal sphincter open, (3) closing the glottis, and (4) lifting of the soft palate to close the posterior nares. These responses result in contraction of the gastric outlet and duodenum, with subsequent contraction of abdominal muscles and diaphragm. When the cardia of the stomach and esophagus relax, gastric contents are forced upward with reverse antral peristalsis. It is thought that impulses can be submitted either by vagal or sympathetic afferents to the vomiting center (Borison et al, 1984).

Epidemiology

The prevalence of vomiting depends on the age of the child and the nature of the stimulus that triggered the vomiting mechanism.

Although studies suggest that over 50% of infants experience spitting, vomiting, or rumination as an isolated complaint, only 5% have significant underlying disease. The remaining episodes reflect either improper feeding techniques, psychosocial disturbances between parent and infant, or simply physiologic immaturity of the gastroesophageal junction.

Diagnosis

Because various causes of vomiting in infants or children depend on age and sex, these factors should be taken into account in evaluating the disorder. A history should focus on an accurate description of the vomiting, e.g., whether it involves forceful ejection or just spitting or ruminating. The nature of the emesis is also important in making a diagnosis. The presence or absence of bile, blood, or undigested food will help direct the focus of further diagnostic investigation. The timing of vomiting with regard to feeding can also be important, as can the quality, quantity, and frequency of feeding itself, particularly in the infant and young child. If a child is not acutely ill, psychosocial problems contributing to poor feeding techniques may be responsible for the symptom. The inability to gain weight in the setting of vomiting may suggest a more chronic process. Vomiting in the setting of an intercurrent illness may simply be an acute episode that will resolve with appropriate treatment of that intercurrent illness.

In the newborn period, vomiting with the first feed or with abdominal distention can represent anatomic obstruction that should be investigated further with appropriate radiologic studies and use of contrast. If vomiting is bilious, it should be considered a surgical

CASE ILLUSTRATION

A 15-year-old white female presented to our emergency room for evaluation of sporadic vomiting over the past several months. She was previously well except for a history of "weak" stomach pains over the past 2 years, and intermittent, nonbilious vomiting that had increased in frequency, prompting the visit. Past medical history and family history were entirely benign. She was a high school junior who was described as being "nervous but studious" in her quest to go to college and eventually medical school. Initial physical examination was notable for a depressed, anxious female in no acute distress, afebrile with stable vital signs. Examination was entirely benign except for a large 10 × 10 cm hard mass extending from below the right costal margin across the midline above the umbilicus. The mass was nontender and did not vary much with respirations. Bowel sounds were present. There was no splenomegaly. Liver function tests were normal.

QUESTION AND COMMENT

What is the differential diagnosis and how is this diagnosis best obtained?

Since the liver remains a leading possibility in the differential diagnosis of a right upper quadrant abdominal mass, ultrasonography is probably the most useful test to assess whether the liver is distinguishable from the unknown mass. In this patient, ultrasonography revealed a normal sized liver alongside a large calcified mass. A plain radiograph of the abdomen and an upper GI series then showed a large gastric bezoar. In retrospect, the patient had a history of trichophagia but not enough to cause alopecia.

Trichobezoars, composed of firmly matted together hairs, are more common in older children, although they have also been noted in children as young as 15 months. Trichobezoars should be differentiated from phytobezoars (usually composed of vegetable matter), which can occur in patients taking anticholinergic medications that hamper gastric emptying or in patients without teeth. Occasionally, they may manifest as complete gastric obstructions; trichobezoars have been reported to cause small intestinal obstruction as well. The association of eating hair in the setting of iron deficiency anemia has been suggested, although anemia was not noted in our patient.

Since medical management is not helpful with trichobezoars, the patient subsequently underwent a gastrostomy for removal of the bezoar (which revealed brown hair matted with mucus occupying almost the entire gastric space). Postoperatively, behavioral "antistress" therapy was started to prevent recurrence of the gastric mass. We report this case as a reminder that right upper quadrant mass in a child who has progressive anorexia and vomiting need not always involve the hepatobiliary tree.

emergency until proven otherwise. In early infancy, however, vomiting can also be due to sepsis, intracranial diseases, such as bleeding or subdural effusions, narcotic withdrawal, peptic ulcer disease, and the adrenogenital syndrome. Inborn errors of metabolism may initially present with vomiting.

In the postneonatal period, spitting and regurgitation are most likely to be secondary to a feeding disorder. Nonetheless these can be equally responsible for an inability to gain weight and occasionally lead to dehydration. Hypertrophic pyloric stenosis is common during this period. Vomiting accompanied by a history of diarrhea and abdominal pain is most often attributable to gastritis, gastroenteritis, or other infectious disorders, and is usually an acute problem. Urinary tract infection and peptic ulcer disease may also present with vomiting. Vomiting and fever in the absence of diarrhea should prompt a chest radiograph to rule out pneumonia and/or reactive airway disease.

In older children, persistent vomiting usually is associated with abdominal pain and may represent mechanical obstruction and/or inflammation of an abdominal viscus such as the appendix. Vomiting may herald an upper respiratory infection, varicella exposure, usage of aspirin, hepatitis, or even Reye syndrome. Particularly in adolescent females, vomiting and weight loss may signify bulimia.

Treatment

Treatment for vomiting depends on the specific entity associated with the symptom, and is discussed under that condition.

APPROACH TO UPPER GASTROINTESTINAL BLEEDS

Definition

Upper gastrointestinal (UGI) bleeding refers to hemorrhage proximal to the ligament of Treitz that may present as hematemesis, melena, abdominal pain, or as a combination of these features.

Epidemiology and Natural History

UGI bleeding accounts for the majority of all episodes of GI bleeding in children (excluding anal fissures). Although UGI bleeding (secondary to ulcers or gastritis) can occur at any age, some conditions appear more prominent at certain ages. For example, neonates are likely to present with hematemesis as a result of swallowed maternal blood, hemorrhagic gastritis, or hemorrhagic disease of the newborn. UGI bleeding due to complications of a gastric volvulus or foreign body ingestion are most commonly seen in infants and toddlers. Mallory-Weiss gastric tears that cause UGI bleeding are most frequent from preschool age to adolescence.

Diagnosis

Particular emphasis should be placed on a careful drug history, especially for salicylates and ethyl alcohol. A family history is important not only for GI diseases but also for bleeding disorders. Previous episodes of chronic cough, hemoptysis, or even epistaxis should be considered to ensure that the blood being vomited is not just swallowed blood from other non-GI locations. A history of stress or a stressful event may also be useful in deciding whether to search further for possible mucosal erosions as a source of bleeding. Did vomiting precede the appearance of the blood (e.g., consistent with a Mallory-Weiss tear)? Constitutional symptoms and usage of gastric irritants (e.g., aspirin or alcohol) or other drugs (e.g., chemotherapy) may provide some information and should also be elicited. A description of the blood, vomitus, or abdominal pain may be useful for localizing a lesion, but is never pathognomonic. Quantitation of blood loss may be very helpful in assessing how quickly to intervene, both diagnostically and therapeutically.

A history of neonatal hepatitis from exchange transfusions, omphalitis, use of umbilical vein catheters, cystic fibrosis, or radiation therapy may antedate the appearance of varices secondary to portal venous obstruction. In older children, painless hematemesis is most likely to be due to variceal bleeding.

In newborns, a maternal history of a difficult labor or prolonged rupture of membranes has been associated with stress gastric ulcers or hemorrhagic gastritis. Medications administered to the infant during the perinatal period should be reviewed to ensure that vitamin K has been given to prevent a bleeding diathesis.

Abnormal vital signs are the best indicators of the need for emergency intervention. Postural changes, sweating, mental confusion, or simply hypotension and tachycardia while the patient is lying down indicate an unstable blood volume. Skin pallor can also be a useful sign of blood volume instability. Examination of the skin may also provide information on possible etiologies for the bleed. For example, the presence of telangiectasias may suggest a vascular malformation syndrome such as Osler-Weber-Rendu. The presence of petechiae, purpura, or ecchymoses might suggest a bleeding dyscrasia. Hemangiomas on the skin may suggest an arteriovenous malformation. Mucosal pigmentation may signify Peutz-Jeghers disease and evidence of polyps. Physical signs of liver disease should also be looked for including hepatomegaly, icterus, spider nevi, or ascites. Splenomegaly may suggest portal hypertension. Nasal passages should be examined to ensure that epistaxis has not caused the hematemesis. The presence of rectal bleeding should also be ascertained.

The vomitus or a nasogastric aspirate should be examined for diagnostic characteristics. For example, bright red blood or coffee-ground material usually suggests that there is a lesion proximal to the ligament of Treitz. Bright red blood that pours out of the oral pharynx often arises from varices.

Baseline laboratory studies should include a complete blood count with differential, platelet count, reticulocyte count, peripheral smear, coagulation studies, liver function tests, and urinalysis. A clot should be sent to the blood bank for typing and cross-matching. The initial hemoglobin value may not represent the true severity of an acute bleeding episode because of the delay in hemodilution that occurs after acute blood loss. While a low white blood count and platelet count may suggest hypersplenism from portal hypertension, these may also indicate sepsis and a subsequent stress gastritis or ulceration. In a newborn, a test for fetal hemoglobin should be performed to determine whether the blood is actually from the mother (e.g., a cracked nipple that bleeds during breast feeding) or whether it represents bleeding derived from the newborn.

It is essential to pass a nasogastric tube to detect the presence of blood in a gastric aspirate, although traumatic passage itself can cause bleeding. If blood is present, a bleeding site proximal to the ligament of Treitz is strongly suggested. If the test is negative, however, bleeding may not have stopped but may be distal to the pylorus. Further steps in a diagnostic work-up, including when to use barium, endoscopy, angiography, or radionucleotide studies are somewhat controversial and are discussed below.

CONTROVERSIES

Diagnostic Studies. There has been much debate over which procedure is most effective for diagnosing UGI bleeding. The advantages and disadvantages of each procedure are examined in Table 7.1.

What conclusions can be drawn from Table 7.1? If the nasogastric aspirate is positive and there is evidence of active ongoing bleeding, endoscopy is the procedure most likely to provide an accurate diagnosis, although it will not decrease the duration of hospital stay or mortality, nor will it improve outcome unless it can be used to cauterize an ongoing site of bleeding. Certain subgroups of patients as mentioned above will benefit from having this procedure done early in the hospitalization, particularly those with liver disease, or recurrent bleeding. The diagnostic information from endoscopy 12–24 hours after admission is as good as when the procedure is performed immediately on admission (Eastwood, 1977).

If the nasogastric aspirate is negative for blood or there is no evidence for active bleeding, a site distal to the ligament of Treitz should be investigated (see discussion of lower GI bleeding). If the barium study is normal and bleeding recurs, endoscopy should be carried out to aid in the diagnosis of an ulcer, gastritis, varix, or Mallory-Weiss tear that the UGI series failed to show.

Angiography is rarely the first choice for diagnostic study since a tagged red cell scan may identify the same rate of bleeding and is less invasive. Angiography is useful, however, in the setting of brisk bleeding where an exact site must be identified for therapeutic intervention (e.g., vasopressin infusion or embolization). It is also useful for identifying varices.

Treatment

ACUTE STABILIZATION

On the basis of the diagnostic work-up, therapy is directed not only at stopping bleeding at the source,

Table 7.1
Diagnostic Procedures for Upper Gastrointestinal Bleeding

Advantages	Disadvantages
UGI Barium Contrast	
1. Noninvasive and easy to do 2. Able to detect site of UGI bleed with with 50–66% accuracy in pediatric studies particularly if double air contrast is used (Cox and Ament, 1979)	1. Sensitivity limited for superficial mucosal lesions (20%) (Cox and Ament, 1979) 2. May visualize an innocent varix and miss more active variceal bleeding site, i.e., unable to distinguish active from inactive site if more than one are seen 3. Clotted blood obscures mucosal detail 4. Barium may interfere with other tests (e.g., radionucleotide studies)
Endoscopy	
1. Most sensitive test to detect bleeding source (90%; Cox and Ament, 1979) 2. Provides most rapid diagnosis 3. Allows direct visualization, biopsy, and potential therapeutic intervention (e.g., cauterization) 4. Beneficial to certain subgroups e.g., those with liver disease, recurrent, or persistent bleeding	1. Invasive 2. No change in mortality rate, number of transfusions, need for surgery, duration of hospitalization despite accurate diagnosis with the procedure (Peterson et al, 1981) 3. No benefit to patients whose bleeding stops in the hospital (Peterson et al, 1981), although cauterization may alter morbidity
Angiography	
1. Allows a selective visualization of a bleeding source 2. Very specific 3. Useful for selective infusion of vasopressin or embolization	1. Invasive 2. Detects only brisk hemorrhage (>0.5 cc/min)
Radioisotope Scans (labeled RBC and/or TC-99m pertechnetate)	
1. Noninvasive with minimal radiation 2. Useful if Meckel diverticulum is suspected 3. Useful for vascular tumors and lower intestinal lesions	1. False-positives include inflammatory lesions, intussusception, and vascular malformations 2. Barium in gut may obscure the scan results and result in a false-negative study 3. Detects only brisk bleeding (at least 1 cc/min)

but also at maintaining blood volume. This is done in the following manner.

The patient should be placed in a semisitting position (with legs elevated) in a calm environment. Vitamin K (5 mg iv) should be given as soon as blood has been drawn for clotting studies. If hypotension or orthostasis is evident, volume should be expanded with the use of a plasma expander (saline, Ringer lactate, or 5% albumin) until blood products are available. The solution should be given at a rate of 20 cc/kg/hour until intravascular volume has been restored as evidenced by improved perfusion and/or blood pressure. At this point, the rate of perfusion should be adjusted to keep up with rate of blood loss since too large a volume may exacerbate bleeding varices.

Once a gastric aspirate has been obtained and is positive for blood, gastric lavage should be started with use of a saline solution until a clear or only blood-tinged aspirate is obtained. This procedure may stop most UGI bleeding and is not contraindicated in suspected variceal bleeding. In the acute situation, antacids or cimetidine have no effect unless the bleeding is secondary to ulcer disease. In this case, iv cimetidine at a dose of 10 mg/kg every 6 hours has been shown to stop bleeding faster than gastric lavage alone.

Failure to control the bleeding after 30–60 minutes of lavage requires endoscopy with the hope of localizing the lesion. If angiography is performed to isolate a specific bleeding site, intra-arterial or intravenous vasopressin should be used before embolization with a gelatin preparation is considered, although the latter has been found more effective in the treatment of a bleeding pyloroduodenal ulcer.

Once bleeding has stopped, antacids or cimetidine may prevent the recurrence of UGI hemorrhage, especially in the treatment of ulcer disease (more effective for gastric than for duodenal ulcer). Antacids are usually administered 1 hour and 3 hours after meals, while cimetidine is given four times a day or just nightly if antacids are used as well. These agents have also been advocated as prophylactics against initial bleeding in the presence of ulcer disease as discussed in the section on ulcer diseases.

CONTROVERSY

Whether gastric lavage actually controls UGI bleeding has not been clearly documented. While lavage at cold temperatures has been shown to reduce gastric blood flow, such temperatures also impair platelet function and promote temperature instability in small infants. Several studies on dogs suggest that lavage with saline at room temperature is as effective as lavage with iced saline (Ponsky, 1980). Until these studies have been performed in humans, iced lavage remains the treatment of choice. Moreover, some recent case reports discuss the addition of norepinephrine to the saline solution as a means of promoting vasoconstriction but no subsequent studies have been done to date (Boyle, 1983); nor is there evidence that the addition of pitressin or antacids to the lavage is useful.

CASE ILLUSTRATION

A 2½-year-old white male presented with hematemesis. The patient was well until the day of admission when he began suddenly vomiting bright red blood. Two days before admission he ingested two aspirin. There was no prior history of GI disturbance or bleeding problems. Past medical history was notable for bilateral ureteral obstruction noted prenatally, requiring ureteric reimplantation and associated with an episode of *Klebsiella* sepsis in the postoperative period. Since then the patient had had two urinary tract infections and was receiving Bactrim prophylaxis.

Physical examination revealed an afebrile male who was vomiting bright red blood with clots, with vital signs of heart rate 200, blood pressure 140 by palpation, and a respiratory rate of 20 breaths/min. The abdomen was soft and nontender with a liver edge just palpable at the right costal margin, and the spleen, enlarged 2 cm below the left costal margin, was firm in texture. Initial laboratory values were notable for hematocrit of 27.7%, a white blood count of 13,500/mm^3 with 65% neutrophils, 2% bands, 32% lymphs, and 1% mono. Platelets of 314,000/mm^3, clotting studies that were slightly prolonged, a blood sugar of 104 mg/dl, a BUN of 35 mg/dl, and normal liver function tests, albumin, and a serum aspirin level of 6 mg/dl. Creatinine was 0.2 mg/dl.

QUESTION AND COMMENT

What are the possible diagnoses for this patient's hematemesis and splenomegaly?

Once the hematemesis has been documented to be of an UGI nature following passage of a nasogastric tube, the causes of splenomegaly should be sought, including those that relate to proliferation of the reticuloendothelial system, immune stimulation, infiltration of abnormal cells and/or protein in the spleen, its congestion with fluid, or expansion via extramedullary hematopoiesis. For this patient, the combination of UGI bleeding and splenomegaly suggests a congestive process due to portal hypertension, which is normally classified as either being pre-, intra-, or posthepatic in nature. Since the liver was of normal size in this patient, posthepatic causes, including hepatic vein thrombosis, inferior venacaval abnormalities, and constrictive pericarditis, were less likely. The normal size of the liver also argued against liver disease unless the liver was already cirrhotic, which seemed unlikely since the liver function tests, clotting studies, and albumin were normal. Thus, a prehepatic cause of portal hypertension was most likely, with the UGI bleeding being due to varices.

Therefore, after the child was stabilized, endoscopy was performed and showed large esophageal varices and distal esophagitis, with stomach and duodenum normal. Among causes for extrahepatic portal venous obstruction are infection (sepsis, intra-abdominal or umbilical), umbilical vein catheterization, abdominal trauma, coagulopathy, and congenital defects of the portal vein. Twenty percent of congenital defects of the portal vein have been associated with cardiovascular, urinary or biliary congenital malformations, and the time from neonatal event to the first hemorrhage is variable, with a mean age at first bleed of about 4 years (Alvarez et al, 1983). In our patient, an ultrasonographic examination revealed cavernous transformation of the portal vein. The first bleed is rarely fatal and, for this reason, therapy, such as sclerotherapy or portosystemic shunt, which carries significant risks of complication, has been withheld pending a recurrence of the hematemesis which, to date, has not occurred.

Other agents currently under investigation for stopping bleeding include somatostatin, glucagon, and prostaglandins, although none has been clinically proven to be effective to date. Among the new H_2-receptor antagonists, ranitidine has been found to be effective in preventing recurrence of bleeding from mucosal ulceration, but clinical prospective studies in children have not yet been reported (Zeldis et al, 1983).

APPROACH TO ABDOMINAL PAIN—ACUTE

Definition

Abdominal pain is a subjective sensation of discomfort that may originate from abdominal structures or be referred from extra-abdominal sites.

Basic Science

Any pain-sensitive structure that can refer pain to the abdomen represents a potential cause for an acute episode. The specific diseases that can result in abdominal pain are discussed in their respective sections.

Three neural pathways are responsible for symptomatic abdominal pain—(1) visceral, (2) somatic, and (3) referred. Visceral pain results from distention of a viscus that stimulates nerves locally, initiating an afferent nerve impulse that leads to efferent innervation in the midabdominal, upper gastric, or lower abdominal region. Since nerve fibers in this area overlap to different organs, visceral pain may often be nonspecific and bilateral. Somatic pain is transmitted by somatic nerves located in the muscle, skin, or parietal peritoneum, where the afferent track leads it to the spinal cord level from T6-L1 unilaterally before it is transmitted efferently to a well-localized area of the abdomen that has been initially stimulated. Referred pain is perceived distant from the organ from which the nerve fibers are initially emanating, because different organs or tissues may share common afferent nerve pathways centrally.

Diagnosis

Eight questions should be asked of the child or parents whenever an episode of acute abdominal pain occurs.

1. When did the pain start?
2. Where is the pain, and where does it radiate to?
3. How long does the pain last?
4. What does the pain feel like?

5. What makes the pain better?
6. What makes the pain worse?
7. Is the pain intermittent or constant?
8. Is the pain associated with any other symptoms, for example, fever, difficulty with breathing, particular foods, nausea, vomiting, bloating, or diarrhea?

A newborn or infant may simply cry during an exacerbation of acute abdominal pain. While intermittent episodes of crying accompanied by flexion of the legs or distended or tight abdomen relieved by passage of flatus, is usually attributed to "colic," or overfeeding, colicky behavior requires careful attention if it becomes more constant. Possible causes include a medical illness, such as milk protein allergy, or, if episodes are severe, mixed with brief pain-free periods or even lethargy, the possibility that the child has an intussusception must be considered. An intussusception may be suspected even before bile-stained vomitus or the classic "currant jelly" (burgundy red, clot-like) stools appear.

In the preschool child, abdominal pain is rarely of psychogenic origin and an organic source should be carefully sought. Again, associated symptoms such as fever, vomiting, or diarrhea may be helpful in determining whether there is a surgical or medical problem. For example, in acute appendicitis, periumbilical pain often occurs before the onset of vomiting, whereas in gastroenteritis, vomiting usually precedes the onset of the crampy abdominal pain. In addition, in these children it is important to keep in mind that abdominal pain may be a manifestation of an extra-abdominal problem. For example, pneumonia or genitourinary disease may first present as periumbilical abdominal pain.

In older children, appendicitis looms as the number one surgical possibility, yet most patients actually have gastroenteritis or pain that is psychogenic in origin. In addition, adolescent females may experience abdominal pain as mittelschmerz related to their menstrual cycle. Even when it is suspected that a child's recurrent abdominal pain does not require surgical intervention, each acute exacerbation requires careful physical examination in case a surgical abdomen has developed.

Radiography is particularly useful in the diagnosis of an acute episode of abdominal pain to provide evidence of obstruction or perforation. Occasionally, an appendicolith or opaque renal stones can be visualized on a plain film. Radiographs also can visualize pneumonia mimicking an acute abdomen, abnormal gas patterns in inflammatory bowel disease, soft tissue masses, organomegaly, and stool content. Further diagnostic work-up for possible causes for abdominal pain is discussed under the individual sections for specific disease entities.

APPROACH TO ABDOMINAL PAIN—CHRONIC

Definition

Recurrent abdominal pain (RAP) is arbitrarily defined as the presence of at least three discrete episodes of debilitating pain occurring over at least a 3-month period during the year preceding clinical examination (Apley, 1975).

The pain can be considered "organic," "dysfunctional," or "psychogenic." The addition of dysfunctional pain is used to characterize pain that is thought to be the result of normal physiologic functions that are more sensitive or more reactive, perhaps secondary to an autonomic abnormality.

RAP is believed by some to be the product of multiple predisposing factors that converge to produce the pain and to regulate its severity and impact. These factors include (1) a somatic predisposition, dysfunction, or disorder; (2) a patient's lifestyle and habits; (3) the influence of critical events in a child's life; and (4) temperament and learned response patterns to stress, with diagnosis based upon weighting the importance of each of these four factors in producing the pain (Levine and Rappaport, 1984).

Epidemiology

Fourteen percent of school children will complain of RAP (Apley and Nash, 1958). In far fewer will an organic cause be found. Preschool children are much less apt to experience RAP. When they do, their episodes are much briefer than are those of the school-aged child. RAP is more common in girls than boys, and becomes particularly noticeable in early adolescence (Barbero, 1982; Wald et al, 1982).

Diagnosis

RAP of organic origin is a consistent and localized pain, that is related to daily events, and is apt to interrupt sleep and may penetrate into the back. There are usually fewer nonintestinal symptoms, such as the headache, dizziness, visual symptoms, or fatigue that often accompany a more dysfunctional or psychogenic presentation.

Colonic distention secondary to constipation can be a trigger for intermittent crampy abdominal pain, and chronic constipation requires treatment to relieve the disorder.

Certain foods may precipitate an episode in a child who has some degree of malabsorption, perhaps secondary to lactose or sucrose intolerance, pancreatic insufficiency, or celiac disease. A food allergy, or excessive usage of some ingredients, such as caffeine or carbonated beverages may predispose to pain. Other conditions to consider are shown in Table 7.2.

Eliciting a history of the child's lifestyle and habits including his or her daily agenda may pinpoint stress issues that exacerbate the pain stimulus, and, more importantly, reveal a reason for erratic bowel habits leading to constipation with resultant abdominal pain. Although, no study has proved conclusively that environmental stress or setbacks directly cause RAP, it is clear that an association exists between stressful life events and RAP. The home environment, the child's interactions with neighborhood friends, and behavior and performance in school should all be scrutinized.

Table 7.2
Conditions Associated with Recurrent Abdominal Pain

Gastrointestinal
Congenital anomalies (e.g., malrotation volvulus)
Inflammatory (ulcer disease, Crohn, ulcerative colitis)
Infectious (*Yersinia*, *Giardia*, ascaris, viral hepatitis)
Neoplastic (e.g., lymphosarcoma)
Obstructive (hernias, intussusception, foreign body, bezoar, chronic constipation)
Metabolic (lactose intolerance, celiac disease, hyperlipidemia, cystic fibrosis)
Peri-Gastrointestinal
Renal (pyelo, hydronephrosis, stones, ureteropelvic junction obstruction)
Gynecologic disorders
Pneumonia
Systemic disorders
Lead
Diabetes
Asthma
Sickle cell anemia
Familial Mediterranean fever

A detailed family history may reveal numerous relatives with a history of strong functional conditions, such as irritable colon, spastic colitis, anxiety attacks, and mental illness. Positive family history for migraines is also common in these patients. Indeed, 50% of children with functional disorders have a parent with a history of irritable bowel or another functional complaint.

The child with more functional RAP tends to have a characteristic personality profile that fits into one of two categories. Either they are superachievers who tolerate failure very poorly and are obsessive-compulsive in their mannerisms, or they are children who are average in intelligence but immature in speech and behavior, and are frequently being compared to siblings who set higher standards. This latter group can develop anxiety reactions converted into RAP when they feel they cannot fulfill their parents' expectations.

It is recommended that the physician elicit a history initially with the parents alone. This is followed by an interview with the child alone, during which time further aspects of the history as well as a physical examination can be performed. If this is done without the parents in the room, additional information may be uncovered.

Signs suggestive of functional RAP include height and weight unaffected by the duration of symptoms, or heightened anxiety, characterized by cold extremities, mottled skin, nail biting, trichotillomania, or dilated pupils. Although examination of the abdomen if a nonorganic etiology is suspected usually results in verbal response of pain to deep palpation there is seldom guarding and, if present, it is usually voluntary. The child's verbal reponse to palpation may outweigh the degree of discomfort that the physician is attempting to elicit. Loops of hard stool in the descending colon and sigmoid can be palpated in 20–30% of children with functional RAP. A gynecologic examination is mandatory in any adolescent female.

The initial visit should consist of some baseline laboratory studies (complete blood count, a sedimentation rate, urinalysis, and guaiac of stool). If these are normal and the history points to a nonorganic complaint, no further laboratory work-up should be done. If an organic etiology still cannot be ruled out, however, a lactose hydrogen breath test, liver function tests, amylase, total protein and albumin, and stool cultures for bacteria and parasitic organisms should be obtained. A plain abdominal radiograph, though relatively easy to obtain, is rarely helpful in these patients. On the basis of these results, further work-up becomes much more selective and should include a repeat of the first studies during a pain attack, a lead level, lipoprotein and porphyria screens. An upper GI radiographic series and barium enema are rarely indicated. An EEG, neurologic, psychiatric, or surgical consultation may be required. Endoscopy is rarely useful, but a chest radiograph to detect asthma with atelectasis as the source of recurrent abdominal pain may be helpful.

A characteristic feature of nonorganic RAP is a failure to obtain any relief from antacids or anticholinergic medications. This may be frustrating to both child and family since inability to obtain relief may exacerbate their feeling that pain episodes are serious. Moreover, if recurrent abdominal pain has a dysfunctional or psychogenic cause, specific dietary elimination will rarely produce a useful response.

Treatment

Clearly a somatic predisposition should be treated (e.g., treatment of constipation or repair of a linea alba hernia). Since these problems are dealt with in other chapters, the remainder of this section is concerned with the treatment of patients with functional RAP.

After the initial visit, the most helpful treatment is simple reassurance that no serious organic abnormality has been detected; at this point, psychosocial problems may resurface and be discussed with parents and child. When the parents realize the importance of the psychosocial situation, they can work with the child and the pain will subsequently subside. Whatever the outcome, a follow-up visit is usually suggested as a supportive measure, to reassure the family that the pediatrician is still available should the pains recur, and indeed to examine the child in the setting of an acute episode.

If the pain persists, a repeat physical examination is appropriate. Pressure by a child's family for medication may result in prescription of an anticholinergic antispasmodic agent, but studies suggest that these are usually of minimal value. If the pain is severe enough that it is preventing a child from attending school or normal daily activities, further investigation is needed. Some physicians recommend hospitalization for observation of the patient and frequently discover that the pain diminishes or actually disappears during the time of the inpatient hospitalization. During hospitalization, psychosocial experiences can be explored in greater depth, and psychiatric and social service consultants can be involved in teaching the family how to cope with such stresses.

Prognosis

Children who are given an adequate explanation for their pain have a 2:1 chance of recovering, but retain an increased susceptibility of having nervous disorders in adult life (Barbero, 1982). Follow-up studies suggest that prognosis is worse for children whose pain episodes begin before 5 years of age, and for males than females. If the history indicates that other family members have other functional disorders, a first attempt at treatment for these episodes is less likely to be helpful. In addition, prognosis is likewise pessimistic if symptoms have been continuing for over 6 months. The most important factor in prognosis for the child is that the pediatrician be available to continue to investigate and intervene with therapy for the child and family when abdominal pain presents. No prospective studies of outcome based on any treatment have been reported.

REFERENCES

Alvarez F, Bernard O, Brunelle F, et al: Portal obstruction in children. I. Clinical investigation and hemorrhage risk. *J Pediatr* 103:696, 1983.

Apley J: *The Child With Abdominal Pains.* Oxford, Blackwell Scientific Publications, 1975.

Apley J, Nash N: Recurrent abdominal pains: A field survey of 1000 school children *Am J Dis Child* 33:165, 1958.

Athanasoulis CA: I. Severe upper gastrointestinal bleeding II. X-ray diagnosis and therapy. *Clin Gastroenterol* 10:26, 1981.

Barbero GJ: Recurrent abdominal pain in childhood. *Pediatr Rev* 4:29, 1982.

Borison HL, Borison R, McCarthy LE: Role of the area postrema in vomiting and related functions. *Fed Proc* 43:2955, 1984.

Castell DO, et al: Dysphagia. *Gastroenterology* 76:1015, 1979.

Chatoor I, Dickson L, Einhorn A: Rumination: Etiology and treatment. *Pediatr Ann* 13:924, 1984.

Chojkier M, Conn HO: Esophageal tamponade in the treatment of bleeding varices; a decadal progress report. *Dig Dis Sci* 25:267, 1980.

Christie DL, Ament ME: Upper gastrointestinal fiberoptic endoscopy—pediatric patients. *Gastroenterology* 72:1244, 1977.

Conn H: To scope or not to scope. *N Engl J Med* 306:967, 1981.

Cox K, Ament ME: Upper gastrointestinal bleeding in children and adolescents. *Pediatrics* 63:408, 1979.

Eastwood GL: Does early endoscopy benefit the patient with active upper gastrointestinal bleeding. *Gastroenterology* 72:737, 1977.

Farrell MK: Abdominal pain. *Pediatrics* 74:955 (Suppl), 1984.

Folkman J: Appendicitis. In Ravitch MM (ed): *Pediatric Surgery,* 3rd edition. Vol 2. Chicago, Year Book Medical Publishers, 1979, pp. 1004.

Galler JR, Neustein S, Walker WA: Clinical aspects of recurrent abdominal pain in children. *Adv Pediatr* 37:31, 1980.

Gryboski J, Walker WA: *Gastrointestinal Problems in the Infant.* Philadelphia, WB Saunders, 1983, p. 243.

Guyton AC: *Textbook of Medical Physiology,* 2nd edition. Philadelphia, WB Saunders, 1961.

Herman BH, Panksepp J: Effects of morphine and naloxone on separation, distress, and approach attachment: Evidence for opiate medication, mediation of social affect. *Pharmacol Biochem Behav* 9:213, 1978.

Hyams JS, Leichtner AK, Schwartz AN: Recent advances in diagnosis and treatment of gastrointestinal hemorrhage in infants and children. *J Pediatr* 106:1, 1985.

Larson P, Farnell M: Upper gastrointestinal hemorrhage. *Mayo Clin Proc* 58:371, 1983.

Lebenthal E: Recurrent abdominal pain in childhood. *Am J Dis Child* 134:347, 1980.

Levine MD, Rappaport LA: Recurrent abdominal pain in school children: The loneliness of the long-distance physician. *Pediatr Clin North Am* 31:969, 1984.

Liebman WM: Recurrent abdominal pain in children. *Clin Pediatr* 17:149, 1978.

Lourie RS: Experience with the therapy of psychosomatic problems in infants. In Hoch PH, Zubin J (eds): *Psychopathology of Children.* New York, Grune & Stratton, 1954.

McGehee FT, Buchanan GR: Trichophagia and trichobezoar: Etiologic role of iron deficiency. *J Pediatr* 97:946, 1980.

Olson A: Recurrent abdominal pain: An approach to diagnosis and management. *Pediatr Ann* 16:834, 1987.

Peterson WL, Barnett CC, Smith HJ, et al: Routine early endoscopy in upper gastrointestinal tract bleeding; a randomized, controlled trial. *N Engl J Med* 304:925, 1981.

Ponsky JL: Saline irrigation in gastric hemorrhage; effect of temperature. *J Surg Res* 28:204, 1980.

Priebe HJ, Skillman JJ, Bushnell LS, et al: Antacid versus cimetidine in preventing acute gastrointestinal bleeding. *N Engl J Med* 302:426, 1980.

Riff EJ, Hayden PW, Stevenson JK: The detection of acute gastrointestinal bleeding by in vivo technetium 99m pertechnetate-labeled erythrocytes. *J Pediatr* 97:956, 1980.

Roy CC, Morin CL, Weber AM: Gastrointestinal emergency problems in pediatric practice. *Clin Gastroenterol* 10:225, 1981.

Ruddy R: Abdominal pain. In Fleischer G, Ludwig S (eds): *Textbook of Pediatric Emergency Medicine.* Baltimore, Williams & Wilkins, 1983.

Silverman A, Roy CC (eds): Symptoms. In *Pediatric Clinical Gastroneurology,* 3rd edition, St. Louis, CV Mosby, 1983, p. 3.

Silverman A, Roy CC (eds): Psychophysiologic recurrent abdominal pain. In *Pediatric Clinical Gastroenterology,* 3rd edition. St. Louis, CV Mosby, 1983, p. 418.

Stickler GB, Murphy DB: Recurrent abdominal pain. *Am J Dis Child* 133:486, 1979.

Thoeni RF, Cello JP: A critical look at the accuracy of endoscopy and double contrast radiography of the upper gastrointestinal tract in patients with substantial UGI hemorrhage. *Radiology* 135:305, 1980.

Wald A, Chandra R, Fisher SE, et al: Lactose malabsorption in recurrent abdominal pain of childhood. *J Pediatr* 100:65, 1982.

Zeldis JB, et al: Ranitidine: A new H2-receptor antagonist. *N Engl J Med* 309:1368, 1983.

Diagnosis and Therapy of Specific Diseases of the Upper Gastrointestinal Tract

2

INFLAMMATORY DISORDERS

Gastroesophageal Reflux

Definition

Gastroesophageal reflux (GER) represents the retrograde flow of gastric contents into the esophagus. Chalasia refers to GER without a hiatal hernia or other anatomic defects. Hiatal hernia is an anatomic and pathologic term signifying the transposition of a portion of the stomach into the lower mediastinum. The presence of a hiatal hernia does not automatically lead to GER. Moreover, symptoms are not usually related to the hernia unless it is very large, but to the reflux of the acidic gastric contents into the esophagus.

Basic Science

Various gastric factors have been implicated in causing GER. For example, delayed gastric emptying has been associated with chronic reflux which increases the potential for postprandial reflux (Hillemeier et al, 1981). A vicious cycle ensues in which gastric contents enter the esophagus, irritate the mucosa, and result in esophagitis. Esophagitis can decrease the ability to maintain adequate sphincter pressure, resulting in even more reflux activity. This sequence is supported by studies in animals with normal sphincter pressures; the introduction of acid into the midesophagus has been shown to result in significant decreases in pressure in the lower esophageal sphincter (Richter and Castell, 1982).

Pathologic findings are often normal, but gross erythema, edema, friability of the mucosa, and/or discrete ulcerations may be observed. The earliest histologic finding is an increase in the basal layer of the stratified squamous epithelium that lines the esophagus, in association with an increase in the height of the dermal pegs and the presence of eosinophils. This represents proliferation of esophageal cells in response to inflammatory insult (Biller et al, 1983).

Under normal circumstances, a functional lower esophageal sphincter (LES), partly from musculature at the gastroesophageal junction and partly from the crural portion of the diaphragm, operates to prevent reflux of gastric contents. Episodes of reflux are related to transient complete relaxation rather than persistent low resting pressures across the sphincter (Dodds et al, 1982). Such transient relaxation can occur during normal activities such as defecation or crying (Helm et al, 1984).

Epidemiology

All children (especially those less than age 1 year) will at one time or another have reflux of their acidic gastric content into the esophagus, particularly in the postprandial period. Only in 1 of 300–1000 children is reflux pathologic or abnormal and causes excessive problems including vomiting, aspiration, and recurrent pneumonia, with failure to gain weight. About 95% of children with reflux present to their physicians by 6 weeks of age. GER is especially common in children with chronic debilitating disorders of the CNS (e.g., mental retardation and cerebral palsy). In addition, it appears to be present in over half the patients who have had a tracheal esophageal fistula (Herbst, 1981).

Natural History

GER that goes untreated can result in failure to gain weight, poor growth, aspiration or recurrent pneumonias, hematemesis, postprandial cyanosis, and Sandifer syndrome. This syndrome is characterized by an odd, head-tilted movement associated with wild thrashing, almost athetoid motions, in combination with severe reflux esophagitis and subsequent chronic blood loss and iron deficiency anemia.

It is possible (but not established) that reactive airway disease may result from aspiration, reflux bronchospasm, or lowered sphincter pressure from secondary theophylline medication. Rumination, although often believed to result from psychosocial behavioral abnormalities, can also be exacerbated with abnormal esophageal function.

Diagnosis

The most useful initial study is the UGI series with barium and fluoroscopy, less for the ability to diagnose reflux than to rule out anatomic lesions that can mimic or be responsible for the reflux, such as pyloric stenosis or a bowel obstruction (Fig. 7.1). If the UGI series is normal and reflux is suspected, a trial of frequent small feedings and placing the infant in the prone position with a 30% angle, may be helpful.

An ever-growing list of tests is being used to document reflux; these tests are indicated only in the presence of failure to gain weight from excessive vomiting, recurrent pulmonary illness thought to be related to

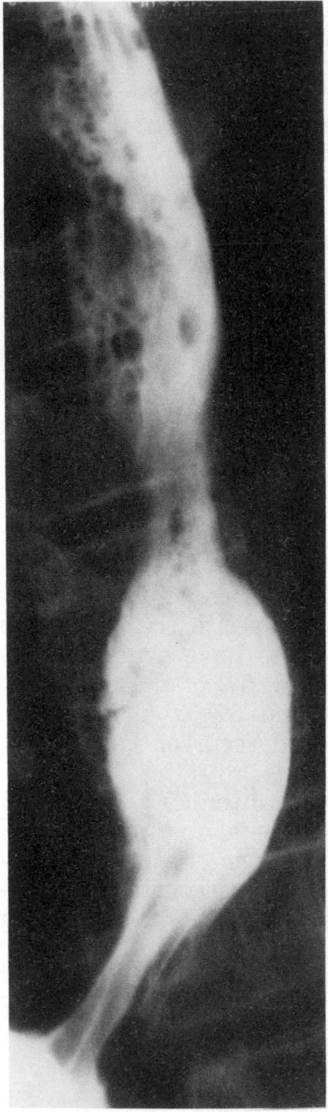
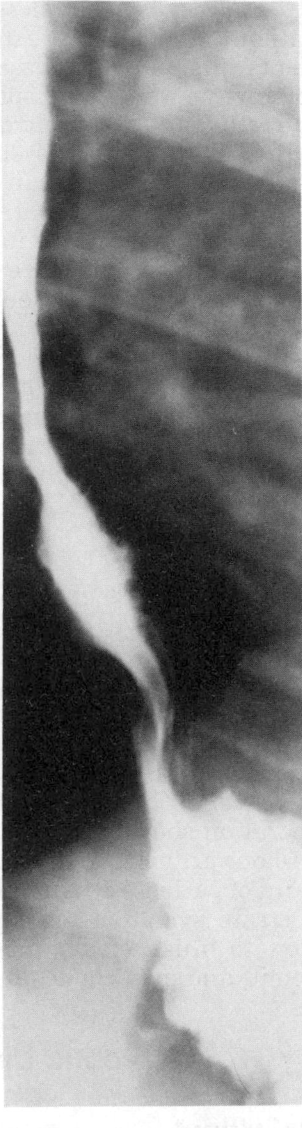

Figure 7.1. These two views of the esophagus show irregularity of the esophageal wall and segmental narrowing of the lumen from the esophagus. This boy had Down syndrome and duodenal stenosis which resulted in gastroesophageal reflux and peptic esophagitis.

Table 7.3
Tests to Document Reflux

Test	Interpretation
Chest radiograph	Evaluate aspiration
Abdominal radiograph	Dilated stomach or small bowel would be consistent with obstruction
Fluoroscopy with barium	Reflux may exist in the absence of vomiting; if vomiting is present, a barium study is helpful in establishing presence or absence of obstruction of gastric outlet
Radionuclide studies	Technetium^{99m} sulfur colloid in milk is given to the child; scintillation scanning of esophagus and stomach over a few hours may show intermittent reflux that would be missed on fluoroscopy; also evaluates gastric emptying
Esophageal manometry	Lower esophageal pressures of less than 12 mm Hg may indicate a poor response to medical management
Intraesophageal pH monitoring for 8, 12, or even 24 hours	Episodic drop in pH documents reflux
Endoscopy and biopsy	Specimens taken 3 cm above the sphincter may show an inflammatory response consistent with acid reflux (Euler and Ament, 1977)

aspiration or a fistula, or chronic blood loss (Table 7.3). The most useful of these tests is intraesophageal pH monitoring. If the pH of the distal esophagus is less than 4.0 for more than 5.2% of monitored time, the child is thought to have reflux (Sondheimer, 1980).

Evidence of aspiration may appear on a chest radiograph.

Treatment

There has been a paucity of well-controlled therapeutic trials testing the efficacy of various treatments for GER. Nevertheless, the major modalities include feeding modification, positional therapy, medications, and surgery, the selection of which depends upon the severity of the disease.

The feeding schedule is altered to provide small volumes more frequently rather than larger volumes with fewer feeds. Frequent "burping," as well as the thickening of feeds with rice cereal are often used in infants to reduce the amount of vomiting and regurgitating.

"Positioning" refers to a simple therapeutic maneuver by which the child is placed in a prone position on a 30° plane after meals. The prone rather than the supine position keeps the esophagogastric junction at the most superior part of the stomach, making it more difficult for stomach contents to be projected upward (Herbst, 1982). Unfortunately, positioning is not as useful in older infants who are too active and resist being confined in the proper position.

If physiologic interventions are not successful, antacids will neutralize gastric contents. Antacids may be more successful in patients with heartburn, consistent with esophagitis, than in those who are vomiting without other symptoms. Cimetidine, a histamine antagonist, reduces gastric acid secretion, but does not affect lower esophageal sphincter pressure. The side effects of cimetidine in children, including behavioral difficulties, confusion, bone marrow depression, and hemorrhage may overshadow the benefits of using this drug as a treatment for reflux.

Metoclopramide, a dopamine antagonist, has also been found to be effective in patients with reflux. This agent increases intestinal tract motility and, thus, speeds up gastric emptying. Because this drug can cross the blood-brain barrier, it may cause oculogyric crises and, hence, is not recommended in infants less than 6 months of age. Metoclopramide can also cause anxiety, tremors, and gynecomastia in children. It should not be given at the same time as cimetidine, since major alterations in mood and behavior are noted when the two agents are being used concurrently (Jewett and Siegel, 1984).

Bethanechol is an alternative to metoclopramide and has been found to be useful in decreasing the frequency of vomiting and increasing weight gain in reflux patients with poor growth (Strickland and Chang, 1983). This agent increases peristaltic activity in the UGI tract and, hence, increases lower esophageal sphincter pressure.

If a pharmacologic agent is used, the first clinical response may be a gain in weight rather than a decrease in the frequency of vomiting. If symptoms have been controlled for 4–6 weeks, however, it is reasonable to begin to decrease the intensity of therapy.

In the rare event that the diagnostic work-up reveals an esophageal stricture, or the child presents with a history of multiple life-threatening choking and apneic episodes or severe symptoms persist after 6 weeks of medical management, surgical procedure should be considered. About 5–10% of patients with symptomatic GER reflux fail to respond to the medical therapy proposed above, and have been treated surgically (Richter and Castell, 1982). The only absolute indication for surgery is esophageal stricture secondary to esophagitis. Nevertheless, other children who fail to gain weight, have persistent vomiting, chronic respiratory symptoms, near-miss sudden death, or esophagitis, and who do not respond to medical management after 1–2 months of therapy, become candidates for a surgical operation.

CONTROVERSY

The most common procedure for surgical repair of esophageal reflux is a Nissen fundoplication, in which the gastric fundus is wrapped around the distal esophagus. It is believed that fixation of the lower esophageal sphincter below the diaphragm, creating a longer narrowing of the distal esophagus, may improve the competence of the lower esophageal sphincter. If the lower esophageal sphincter is found to be normal, and the reflux is solely due to delayed gastric emptying, surgery should consist of a long myotomy with extension over the antrum of the stomach. This may relieve obstruction in some children and result in resolution of vomiting and reflux.

Surgery is said to lessen vomiting in about 95% of patients who are so treated. Nevertheless, 15% of patients who receive a Nissen fundoplication do not have improvement in their respiratory symptoms even though the reflux has been controlled (Herbst, 1983). The mortality rate for the Nissen fundoplication ranges 0.2–1.6%. Complications can include esophageal perforation, vascular injury, paraesophageal hernia, dumping syndrome, vagal nerve injury, as well as the inability to burp or vomit, slower eating, and the presence of gas bloating (the latter seen in one-third of patients) (Harnsberger et al, 1983).

Unfortunately, few clinical trials have compared the long-term effects of medical versus surgical therapy for chronic reflux utilizing current pharmacologic agents. Given the gravity of the complications of surgery, we rarely recommend it.

Prognosis

At least 60% of patients will be symptom-free by 18 months of age (even without specific treatment); no more than 30% will continue to have symptoms requiring treatment. If untreated, 5% of these will develop esophageal strictures and 5% eventually die, usually from malnutrition and recurrent aspiration pneumonia (Herbst, 1983).

Over 50% of patients 6 years after a fundoplication operation show no reflux symptoms, and have normal 24-hour pH monitoring (Harnsberger et al, 1983). One-third of patients 5 years after surgery continue to demonstrate symptoms of gas-bloating, as well as being slow to finish meals and 25% are unable to burp or vomit, and may choke on some solids.

Peptic Ulcer Disease

Definition

Peptic ulcers are localized areas of inflammation that occur anywhere in the GI tract where acid and pepsin come in contact with mucosa.

Basic Science

Understanding how ulcers develop requires knowledge of the basic physiology of gastric secretion. The process of secreting acid occurs in three phases. The first phase is mediated by the vagus nerve, which directly stimulates the parietal cells of the stomach for production of acid and the gastrin-producing cells in the antrum of the stomach and duodenum. The latter cells are responsible for the release of the hormone gastrin into the blood stream from which it reaches receptor sites on the parietal cells and further promotes the release of acid. Histamine release from mast cells may be a final common pathway in parietal cell stimulation. The second phase of acid secretion occurs where the stomach is distended by food or liquids and again causes the release of gastrin and increases acid secretion. In the third phase, digested protein reaches the duodenal mucosa causing the release of secretin and other intestinal hormones. These hormones then act both competitively and noncompetitively on the parietal cell to inhibit both acid secretion and the release of pepsin from chief and mucous-neck cells in the stomach. In addition, dietary fatty acids in the proximal part of the duodenum release gastric inhibitory peptide, which can inhibit gastrin release and hence inhibit acid secretion. Finally, acid itself can inhibit further release of gastrin if the intragastric pH decreases to 2.5 . Therefore, a duodenal ulcer can result when the hormonal balance is altered and there is either an increased capacity to secrete acid, an increased responsiveness to stimuli for acid secretion, or defective inhibition of acid secretion.

Most gastric ulcers in children occur in the antral mucosa which is adjacent to acid-secreting fundic mucosa. This gastric mucosa can maintain a large concentration gradient of hydrogen between the gastric lumen and plasma of over 1,000,000 to 1. In the presence of agents such as aspirin, bile salt, or ethanol, however, this barrier breaks down and there is back diffusion of hydrogen ion into the gastric mucosa leading to edema, hemorrhage, mucosal erosions, and hence, ulceration.

Nonsteroidal anti-inflammatory agents such as indomethacin and ibuprofen can also cause gastric damage, although changes are less pronounced and occur with much higher doses than with aspirin. These agents inhibit prostaglandin synthesis and since prostaglandin inhibits gastric acid secretion, the mucosa is no longer protected against injury from increased acid and pepsin production. The association with corticosteroids is weak, although some studies have suggested that there is a close association between ulcers and steroid usage.

Stress or secondary ulcers usually occur in the corpus of the stomach. These lesions are usually multiple and superficial and appear within hours of the insult.

Duodenal ulcers are associated with the following abnormalities: (1) an increased responsiveness to gastrin and pentagastrin, (2) an increased capacity to secrete gastrin and pepsin, with the mass of the parietal cell and the amount of acid secretion being twice normal, (3) a defective inhibition of gastrin release by hydrochloric acid that has been secreted, and (4) rapid emptying of the stomach and, therefore, inability to provide complete buffering of an acid load before it moves on to the duodenum.

Campylobacter pylori has been identified in the mucosa of some patients with peptic ulcer disease (Drumm et al, 1987). It is not clear whether the organism is the cause of the ulcer.

Epidemiology

Peptic ulcer disease in children is relatively uncommon, with an estimated incidence of 3.4–4.4/10,000 inpatient admissions (Tolia and Dubois, 1983). Gastric ulcers occur with the same frequency as duodenal ulcers in children, but duodenal ulcers occur four times as frequently in males as females, while gastric ulcers occur with equal frequency in both sexes. Most gastric ulcers in children are found in association with aspirin usage and/or stress.

Although peptic ulcers have been observed as early as the neonatal period, they are found most frequently in children between the ages of 12 and 18 years, with boys being affected twice as often as girls, particularly among teenagers. A positive family history is found in 20–63% of children with ulcers (Nord et al, 1981).

Diagnosis

In the neonatal period, peptic ulcers can present as GI hemorrhage or as perforation. They almost always are associated with stress. Associated signs and symptoms can include abdominal distention, vomiting, and lethargy.

During infancy, stress is also responsible for the majority of ulcers. Again, vomiting or abdominal fullness in association with GI bleeding can aid the diagnosis. Severe respiratory tract infection, increased intracranial pressure, or ingestion of aspirin can predispose an infant to development of an ulcer.

As the child becomes older, secondary stress ulceration becomes less common relative to primary ulcer formation—i.e., ulcer in the absence of any underlying cause. Older children usually present with hematemesis, melena, and/or recurrent vomiting. Abdominal pain can be present but is poorly localized, usually in the midepigastric or periumbilical area, especially before eating. One-third of patients may be awakened in the middle of the night by pain. Painful attacks can be sporadic, occurring weeks or even months apart. Usually children who present with hematemesis or melena rarely complain of any pain before the onset of hemorrhage. The family history of ulcer disease can be useful, particularly in the older child. A primary cause for the ulcer should be sought if the child is less than 6 years of age. In an older child, a therapeutic trial of antacids might be instituted before pursuing further invasive diagnostic studies.

If a patient presents solely with melena, a nasogastric tube should be inserted to assess whether there is fresh blood in the gastric aspirate, which would localize the lesion to the UGI tract. A UGI series is the diagnostic radiologic test of choice in a stable child, although barium studies detect only half of duodenal and gastric ulcers in children (Silverman and Roy, 1983a). The diagnosis of duodenal ulcer should not depend on a barium study unless a persistent crater is demonstrated. A deformed duodenal bulb without evidence of a crater could signify a previous ulcer with subsequent scar formation rather than an active ulcer. If symptoms are prominent, however, endoscopy possibly with biopsy, should follow.

A fasting and a 60-minute postprandial gastrin level should be obtained in children with recurrent peptic disease to rule out the presence of a gastrinoma (see section on Zollinger-Ellison syndrome).

Treatment

Fifty percent of ulcers will heal spontaneously. Nonetheless, objectives of treatment are: (1) to relieve ulcer pain, (2) to hasten healing, and (3) to prevent recurrences and complications. No diets have been proven to be advantageous over regular diets for ulcer patients. Nonetheless, it is still widely held that alcoholic beverages, coffee, or caffeine-containing soft drinks should not be given to individuals who have peptic ulcer disease.

Antacids are the most effective drugs (Fordtran et al, 1973). When given 1 hour after meals, they last about 2–3 hours; whereas, if given before meals, they last for less than 30 minutes. While antacid tablets may be more convenient for older children, they are less well-tolerated, and less effectively chewed by younger children for whom liquid antacids are more potent buffers. The most common side-effect is diarrhea secondary to the magnesium contained in many antacids. If a patient has renal insufficiency, the magnesium level should be monitored. Overusage of aluminum hydroxide antacid can result in phosphate depletion, osteomalacia, and osteoporosis. Therefore, the normal procedure is to alternate magnesium hydroxide with aluminum hydroxide antacids to minimize diarrhea and to prevent phosphate depletion. Calcium-containing antacids can result in acid rebound and further release of gastrin. Sodium-containing antacids can result in salt and water retention.

Cimetidine, an antihistamine which acts as an H_2 blocker effectively inhibits all phases of acid secretion. It is only required four times a day in doses of 20–40 mg/kg/day for 6–12 weeks. Side effects of cimetidine include gynecomastia (in less than 5%), an occasional rash, or behavioral abnormality, as well as reports of decreases in sperm counts and thrombocytopenia. Rebound hypersecretion of hydrochloric acid has been described after discontinuation of the drug. Another H_2 receptor blocker, ranitidine, has recently been found to be as potent and is longer acting than is cimetidine, thus allowing twice a day dosage to inhibit acid secretion.

The usual surgical procedure includes ligation of the bleeding artery, oversewing of the ulcer, vagotomy, or pyloroplasty. For intractable peptic gastric ulcer disease, the most common surgical procedure is a bilateral truncal vagotomy with antrectomy followed by a gastrojejunostomy or gastroenterostomy (Mohammed and Mackay, 1982).

Prognosis

Fifty percent of children and adolescents with peptic disease have a recurrence within a year and 70% will have repeated relapses afterwards (Silverman and Roy, 1983a).

Zollinger-Ellison Syndrome

Definition

Zollinger-Ellison syndrome is a condition in which there are high levels of circulating gastrin that originate from a gastrinoma, usually in the pancreas but occasionally found in the duodenum or stomach. This condition leads to peptic ulcers and to functional and morphologic abnormalities of the small intestine including duodenitis and stunting of villi.

Basic Science

Gastrin release from a gastrinoma is not influenced substantially by the chemical compositions of the contents in the gastric lumen or by neuropathways. On the other hand it is not completely autonomous in that secretin and increased serum calcium levels have both been shown to cause substantial increases in serum gastrin in patients with a gastrinoma, but do not do so in patients without the tumor (Jenson et al, 1983).

Epidemiology

This syndrome is rare in children. More than 25 cases have been reported in the literature, however, with the youngest patient being a 5-year-old female (Drake et al, 1980). It occurs in boys four times as frequently as in girls (Silverman and Roy, 1983b). The syndrome is associated with other islet cell tumors of the endocrine organs, especially those involving the adrenal and parathyroid as well as the pituitary and thyroid. Fifty percent of the other islet cell tumors in children are malignant.

Diagnosis

Clinical features that warrant investigation for Zollinger-Ellison syndrome include: peptic ulcerations associated with diarrhea; recurrent postoperative peptic ulceration; peptic ulceration of the distal duodenum or jejunum; peptic ulceration associated with hypercalcemia or other manifestations of a multiple endocrinopathy. The most common symptom is abdominal pain usually accompanied by vomiting, passage of tarry stools, and occasionally diarrhea. Most suggestive is massive hemetemesis, severe anemia, multiple ulcer and/or perforation.

Over the past decade, the availability of a serum gastrin radioimmunoassay has permitted diagnosis early in the disease.

Treatment

Localizing the tumors by CT scan or ultrasonography is rare and, often, surgical exploration fails as well. Moreover, there is no definitive evidence that primary resection of the gastrinoma without a chemical or surgical total gastrectomy is useful. The treatment of choice in children is cimetidine. Vagotomy, pyloroplasty, or total gastrectomy should be reserved for only those with severe symptoms or with complications of pharmacologic therapy. Even after complete excision of gross tumor these patients may continue to show elevated gastrin levels and require lifetime cimetidine therapy.

Prognosis

In cases where no tumor has been seen, the survival rate is 100%. If gross tumor is removed, there is about a 75% 5-year survival versus 20% when all gross tumor is not removed (Silverman and Roy, 1983b).

OBSTRUCTIVE DISORDERS

Tracheoesophageal Fistulas and Esophageal Atresia

Definition

Tracheoesophageal fistulas with or without esophageal atresia are congenital malformations that are associated 30% of the time with other major malformations.

Basic Science

The trachea develops as an outpouch from the portion of the foregut that is destined to be esophagus. A complex series of events before the eighth week of gestation permits differentiation into the two primitive tubes. Incomplete separation or canalization of the tubes can result in a spectrum of abnormalities depicted in Figure 7.2.

The most frequently associated malformations are cardiovascular abnormalities, other GI malformations, and renal dysgenesis. One constellation of findings includes vertebral, anal, tracheoesophageal, radial and renal abnormalities, named VATER syndrome by Quan and Smith (1973).

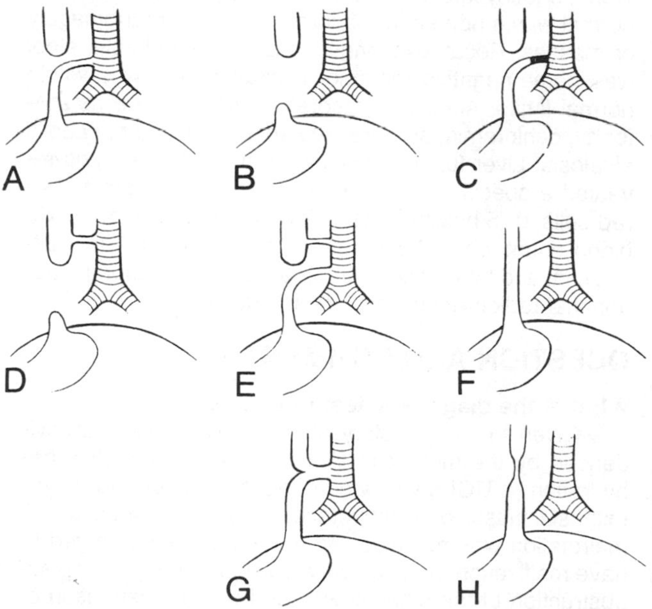

Figure 7.2. Types of tracheoesophageal fistulas. The type labeled *A* is overwhelmingly the most common, accounting for over 85% of esophageal malformations. *B* is the next most common and can be distinguished from *A* by the absence of air in the intestinal tract on roentgenogram. All other types have been noted sporadically. Reproduced with permission from Avery ME, et al: *The Lung and its Disorders in the Newborn Infant*, 4th edition. Philadelphia, WB Saunders, 1984.

Epidemiology

In the United States in 1959–1966, tracheoesophageal fistulas were found in 1/10,000 live births enrolled in a national collaborative survey. Other studies have reported the incidence as high as 1/2500 live births. Several reports of occurrence in siblings and of vertical transmission suggest a genetic predisposition to these lesions (Ericksen et al, 1981).

Natural History

About one-third of infants with esophageal atresia weigh less than 2.5 kg and are mostly low birth weight for gestational age, but may be premature as well. When esophageal atresia is present, and swallowing of amniotic fluid is prevented, hydramnios results, and is the first sign of possible atresia at some level in the UGI tract.

Most infants with tracheoesophageal fistulas with or without atresia have no problems with the initiation of breathing at birth. After a few minutes (or hours), excess mucus may accumulate in the pharynx and respiratory difficulties may be evident. Attempted feedings may exacerbate respiratory distress or be associated with choking and regurgitation.

If no gas is present in the abdomen, it is unlikely there is a fistulous connection between the trachea and lower esophageal pouch. More commonly, the abdomen rapidly distends with air that flows from the lung through the fistula into the lower esophagus.

Diagnosis

Gentle insertion of a soft catheter into the upper esophagus is the first step in investigation. If there is doubt about a possible obstruction, examination under fluoroscopy will clarify the situation. Fistulas without atresia require careful fluoroscopic examination with radiopaque material injected at different levels in the esophagus.

Treatment

Initially, continuous suction should be applied to the upper esophageal pouch to lessen the likelihood of aspiration. The semiupright position may reduce regurgitation of stomach contents into lung. Surgical intervention should be undertaken as soon as the infant's condition permits. If the infant is very premature, or the atretic segment is long, the initial operation may be a gastrostomy for feeding until the infant is ready for a major corrective procedure. (Care must be taken to reduce the likelihood of regurgitation and aspiration.) An upper pouch cervical salivary fistula reduces aspiration.

The operation of choice for atresia is end-to-end anastomosis of the esophagus as a primary repair in every infant. If that is not possible, some kind of neoesophagus is created at 12–18 months of age. The interposition of a segment of colon to act as the missing esophagus is one approach, although ischemic complications can occur.

Some infants require prolonged parenteral alimentation, especially if their stomachs are small.

Prognosis

The earlier the creation of a gastrostomy, or total repair of the atresia and fistula, the better the outlook. The survival rate for infants over 2.5 kg without pneumonia or associated anomalies should be 95% (Rickham, 1981). Occasionally, strictures develop at the site of anastomosis and require dilatation either using bouginage or balloon dilatation. Disordered esophageal motility is usually present and may require the patient to have frequent feedings and the upright position after feeds. If gastric emptying is delayed, a clinical trial of metoclopramide hydrochloride is indicated.

Malrotation

Definition

Malrotation predisposes to obstruction between the pylorus and the ligament of Treitz. It occurs secondary to the abnormal movement of the intestine around the superior mesenteric artery during embryologic development. Obstruction can result from midgut volvulus or inappropriate positioning of peritoneal bands which, if present, will usually obstruct the distal portion of the third part of the duodenum.

Epidemiology

Malrotation is thought to occur in about 1/6000 live births (Stewart et al, 1976).

Natural History

The majority of children who are born with a malrotation will show evidence of an obstruction within the first 2 weeks of life. These infants usually are able to retain feeds for the first 24–48 hours and then will begin to experience bilious vomiting, upper quadrant abdominal distention, prominent peristalsis, and pain. Twenty-five percent of malrotations are associated with other congenital anomalies including an annular pancreas, duodenal atresia, or stenosis. Malrotation occurs in association with omphaloceles, with gastroschisis and diaphragmatic hernias. If the common bile duct is twisted, jaundice may occur as well, although this is rare. Twenty percent of children develop symptoms after the first month of life or may not present until later childhood or, occasionally, even adulthood. Frequently, in older children vomiting is uncommon, but intermittent crampy abdominal pain and diarrhea occur.

The wide spectrum of clinical presentation in malrotation results from the lack of fixation of the small bowel mesentery, which may involve the duodenojejunal segment, the cecal-colic segment, or both, becoming twisted around themselves (a volvulus). Twisting of the bowel around the superior mesenteric artery can lead to major complications, including lymphatic obstruction with diarrhea and protein loss or vascular obstruction leading to ischemia, necrosis, sequestration of blood into the bowel, and hypotension.

Diagnosis

If a child has patency of the GI tract, demonstrated either by radiograph or by rectal passage of gas or stools, subsequent obstruction cannot be considered a congenital atresia, and a malrotation or volvulus remain likely. Some distention of the stomach and duodenum may be present, with gas scattered distally. A UGI series will demonstrate obstruction often with a twisted contour near the duodenal-jejeunal junction, and with little or no contrast passing distal to that junction (Fig. 7.3). If obstruction is demonstrated, an operation is urgently

CASE ILLUSTRATION

An 18-year-old male presented with episodes of vomiting since early childhood. These episodes have occurred every 1–2 months since 2 months of age. Episodes begin with a sense of heaviness in the epigastrium followed 1 day later with the onset of vomiting, which lasted for 3–5 days. Occasionally, the vomitus was reported to have a greenish hue, but never blood. After the 3–5 days of vomiting, the patient would have several watery stools and then feel fine. On the day of admission, the patient reported the vomiting having begun 7 days earlier.

Past medical history revealed that at 5 years of age because of the vomiting he had had an EEG which showed abnormal β activity on the right temporal region. He was diagnosed as having abdominal migraines, and was treated with dilantin and mysoline. However, since vomiting episodes continued to occur, these drugs were discontinued.

His initial examination revealed a young man who was afebrile, tachycardic, and orthostatic. Bowel sounds were normal with a nontender abdomen without organomegaly or masses. Rectal examination was unremarkable, stool was heme-negative, neurologic examination was within normal limits. Admission laboratory values were notable for hypochloremia, an increased anion gap, and metabolic alkalosis. Liver function tests were normal, urinalysis revealed a specific gravity of 1.029, with 2+ protein, 1–2 red cells, 3–5 hyaline, and 1–2 granular casts/hpf. White blood count was 13,000/mm^3 with an unremarkable differential and hematocrit was 55%. Supine and upright abdominal radiographs were unremarkable.

QUESTION AND COMMENT

What is the diagnostic test of choice?

Given the long history of recurrent vomiting as evidenced by the metabolic alkalosis and presumptive dehydration, a UGI series was performed to look for ulcer, extrinsic mass, or a malrotation causing obstruction. A malrotation was revealed. At operation, he was noted to have malfixation of the colon, a volvulus without complete obstruction of the small bowel, and partial obstruction of the duodenum from colonic bands extending to the right gut. A modified Ladd procedure was done and his postoperative course was unremarkable. This case is notable because of the late age at which the patient presented, although it appears he had had many warning signals ever since he was 2 months old.

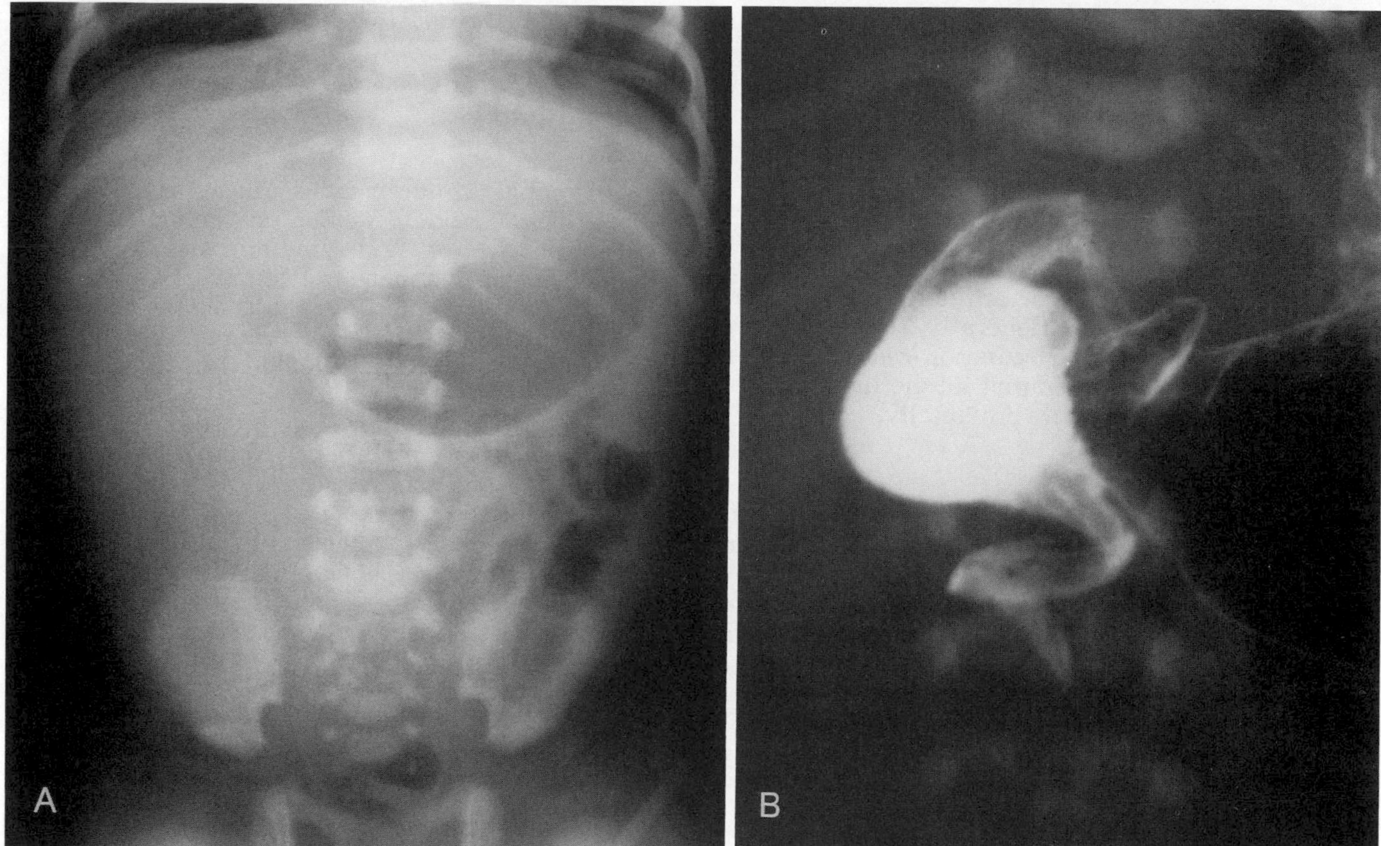

Figure 7.3. Plain radiograph **(A)** shows little gas distal to stomach and duodenum. UGIs **(B)** followed in this baby who presented with bilious vomiting and shows the "corkscrew" appearance of malrotation with midgut volvulus.

needed. Only with a UGI series showing an unequivocally normal c-loop of the duodenum and a left-sided, duodenojejunal junction can malrotation be ruled out as a possible cause for the obstruction. A barium enema may demonstrate a high medial cecum but it does not substitute for the benefits of the UGI series and, if negative, does not rule out a more proximal malrotation or volvulus.

The presence of bands will cause partial intestinal obstruction. If a barium enema shows an incompletely descended cecum, this may not be of any clinical significance and, in fact, a "high riding" cecum is quite common in the newborn infant. Occasionally, a volvulus may occur without malrotation due to twisting of bowel around the Meckel diverticulum, a small bowel duplication, the presence of a mesenteric cyst, or adhesions from prior surgery.

Treatment

Treatment of a symptomatic malrotation or midgut volvulus is surgical, in which case the volvulus is first reduced by twisting the bowel in a counter-clockwise direction and then dividing the peritoneal bands. The intestine may be viewed via a "second look" operation 36–48 hours after the initial procedure. This "second look" procedure, although relatively uncommon, may be able to save bowel that would otherwise have been resected, and supportive therapy including antibiotics can be administered between operations. Intestinal fixation to decrease the possibility of recurrence of intestinal obstruction has not been shown to be of benefit (Stauffer and Hermann, 1980).

Prognosis

Mortality from volvulus of the mid gut is about 35%. Ten percent of children will have recurrence of intestinal obstruction after surgery, usually due to adhesions. In the newborn period, the mortality rate is 15% with malrotation often complicated by intestinal necrosis, gangrene, perforation with peritonitis (Stewart et al, 1976). Other associated congenital anomalies can also be present and lead to death. If bowel resection is necessary, often a significant amount of small intestine is removed, leading to a short bowel syndrome and malabsorption.

Intussusception

Definition

Intussusception is a condition that occurs when a portion of the intestine invaginates into itself. In most cases, the intussusception begins at a point proximal to the ileocecal valve, although ileo, ileal and colocolic invaginations can also occur.

Basic Science

Only 6% of intussusceptions have a known cause; for the majority, the etiology is obscure (Ravitch, 1986). Once the invagination begins, venous return becomes compromised and an intense localized edema results because of compromised blood supply. This process leads to progressive swelling of tissues and even more venous compression. The engorged intestine can begin to ooze blood, which mixes with mucous secretion from the bowel to form the characteristic "currant jelly" stools or burgundy-red, clot-like stools. Generally, tissue pressure exceeds arterial pressure, circulation ceases, and necrosis ensues, usually beginning at the distal end of the invagination and moving proximally.

Epidemiology

Intussusception remains one of the most frequent causes of intestinal obstruction in infants. More than 50% of cases occur within the first year of life, usually between the fifth and ninth month. A strong male predominance has been noted and the condition occurs in children of all races. There is no known seasonal incidence.

Natural History

Several diseases are associated with intussusception. In younger children, intussusception has been associated with Meckel diverticulum, polyps, large and discrete patches of ileal lymphoid tissue, Henoch-Schönlein purpura, appendiceal stumps, hemangiomas, parasites, and foreign bodies. Cystic fibrosis is also associated with intussusception, perhaps secondary to inspissated fecal material in the distal ileum, appendix, or colon.

Classically, the first symptom that develops in intussusception is abdominal pain. Nonetheless, it is usually vomiting and the passage of a bloody stool that prompts the seeking of medical attention. The pain is colicky, with the infant becoming progressively apathetic between episodes of pain. If diagnosis is delayed, the presence of currant jelly stools is frequently noted. In 50% of cases, a sausage-shaped mass may be pal-

CASE ILLUSTRATION

A 6-month-old Hispanic male presented with difficulty breathing after 1 week of upper respiratory symptoms. He was described as being restless, irritable, somewhat indifferent to feeding, and very congested. He was found on examination to be afebrile, with bilateral otitis, but he had no other obvious focus for infection. His hematocrit was 31%, white count 19,300/mm^3, with 58% polys, 10% bands, and a normal urinalysis, chest radiograph, and spinal fluid findings. He was discharged home receiving amoxicillin.

Six hours after discharge, the patient developed fever and vomiting with generalized apathy progressing to lethargy, prompting a return to hospital where he arrived with a temperature of 38.8°C, heart rate 140/min, respiratory rate 30/min, blood pressure 120/80. Examination was unchanged except for a 200-g weight loss and mild dehydration, a slightly protuberant abdomen with some tenderness to palpation in the right lower quadrant, without frank peritoneal signs, and stool that was trace guaiac-positive. Laboratory findings were essentially unchanged. Because his lethargy far outweighed his degree of dehydration, it was decided to admit this child for further evaluation. Just before leaving the emergency room on his way to the ward, a repeat rectal examination elicited a large currant jelly stool. A radiograph of the abdomen subsequently showed large dilated loops of bowel without evidence of free air, and a water-soluble contrast enema was unable to pass a mass in the hepatic flexure confirming the diagnosis of an intussusception.

QUESTION AND COMMENT

Could this diagnosis have been made earlier, i.e., during the patient's first visit?

We mention this case because of the unusual way in which this patient presented with intussusception. While the location and age are appropriate for this type of obstruction, the classic triad of vomiting, paroxysmal abdominal pain, and bloody stools were not at all apparent in the setting of this patient's upper respiratory symptoms and otitis. Yet, in reviewing the literature, viral infections have been found to be associated with intussusception. For example, a series of patients from Johns Hopkins had a 21% incidence of upper respiratory infections or otitis media at the time of their diagnosis (Silverman and Roy, 1983b). In addition, numerous case reports discuss the findings of adenovirus or rotavirus at the time of surgical repair.

In retrospect, perhaps the most notable clue to the diagnosis was the parents' history of "indifference" or apathy to his environment, almost mimicking an encephalitic picture. In fact, a number of reports in the past few years have focused on this altered consciousness as not only a late but also an early indicator of abdominal intussusception (Singer, 1979). The cause of this neurologic manifestation is unknown. Although it is hypothesized that a toxic substance may be released from ischemic bowel, this is not sufficient to explain the degree of CNS change noted early in the disease before abdominal symptoms consistent with the ischemia manifest themselves (as in our patient). Therefore, intussusception should be considered in the differential diagnosis of the lethargic infant.

Our patient subsequently underwent laparotomy where a reduction of an ileocolic intussusception was performed and the bowel was preserved. The child continued to do well postoperatively.

pated in the upper abdomen, with the right lower quadrant feeling empty.

Diagnosis

The classic triad of intermittent abdominal pain, vomiting, and blood in stools should suggest the diagnosis. A radiographic contrast study should follow. Less than one-third of patients will show evidence of intestinal obstruction on a plain radiograph without having a barium study. For those patients, the use of barium becomes a therapeutic rather than a diagnostic maneuver.

Treatment

More than half the intussusceptions in children can be reduced by hydrostatic pressure resulting from the insertion of barium that is being used to make the diagnosis. In those patients showing peritoneal signs, however, a barium hydrostatic reduction should not be attempted. Indeed, some studies suggest that if the radiograph shows intestinal obstruction, a hydrostatic reduction should usually not be attempted, since the involved bowel may be incarcerated and gangrenous. Reduction using rectal insufflation of air or oxygen has also been successful and perhaps safer than barium if a perforation is feared (Jinzhe et al, 1986).

Follow-up and Prognosis

Any recurrence of the intussusception usually occurs within the first 36 hours after the reduction. Overall, recurrence rates of 4–6% of primary cases of intussusception have been reported (Ravitch, 1986). If reduction is not accomplished radiographically or surgically, an intussusception is fatal, although overall mortality stands at 1–2%.

Pyloric Stenosis

Definition

Hypertrophic pyloric stenosis represents an increase in the size of the circular muscle of the pylorus, resulting in an inability of the pylorus to open, thus, creating an anatomic and functional obstruction.

Basic Science

The reason for the increase in the size of the circular muscles surrounding the pylorus remains unknown. Hypergastrinemia has been suggested but has yet to be confirmed, particularly since patients with Zollinger-Ellison syndrome show hypergastrinemia but do not have hypertrophic pyloric stenosis. An increased association with renal anomalies, inguinal hernias, cryptorchidism, and hypospadias is apparent, but many cases occur independent of these anomalies.

Epidemiology

The disease occurs in 1 of every 500 births with males being four to five times more often affected than females. It has been found to occur in members of the same families and in twins and triplets, with higher rates of concordance in both monozygotic and dizygotic twins. Sons of affected parents have a 5–20% chance of stenosis, whereas daughters of affected parents have a 3–7% chance. No seasonal incidence has been observed (Benson, 1979).

Natural History

The disease is usually heralded by bile-free vomitus that becomes projectile, usually occurring in infants who are 2–3 weeks old, with peak obstruction by 4–6 weeks of age, although cases have been observed from 3 days to 5 months. Of interest is a study of 1000 infants who received UGI barium studies at birth for a variety of reasons, but none of whom showed evidence of pyloric stenosis (Benson, 1979). One month later, however, 5% did develop radiographic and clinical evidence for the disorder. It is more likely to occur in a full-term than in a premature infant. Usually the vomiting may be diminished somewhat by oral rehydration, but this is usually temporary. These infants usually are extremely hungry and yet fail to gain weight or even lose weight from their persistent vomiting.

Diagnosis

Physical examination is usually notable for some degree of dehydration. The hypertrophic pylorus can be felt as an olive or small mass in more than half the patients, particularly if the stomach is aspirated before attempts at palpation. The olive can be best felt with the left hand approaching from the patient's left side. A lubricant on the abdomen facilitates palpation of the mass. Gastric peristaltic waves are often seen. Laboratory studies are most notable for a hypochloremic metabolic alkalosis as well as severe potassium depletion. Hyperbilirubinemia may be protracted in infants with pyloric stenosis, the mechanism for which remains unclear. Radiographic and ultrasonographic studies can be extremely useful in confirming the diagnosis. A plain abdominal radiograph may show a dilated air-filled stomach and a paucity of gas in the abdomen. UGI will reveal fixed elongation and narrowing of the antrum and pylorus. Ultrasonography can demonstrate the thickened pyloric muscle; if ultrasonography is normal, UGI series may be needed to search for other etiologies for vomiting (Fig. 7.4*A* and *B*).

Treatment

Once the pylorus is known to be narrowed and the vomiting is persistent, the infant should be placed on nasogastric suction to decompress the stomach, and hydrated intravenously to correct the hypochloremic metabolic alkalosis. Once hydrated, a pyloromyotomy is the procedure of choice. The muscle is split without entering the bowel lumen. It is essential to split all fibers

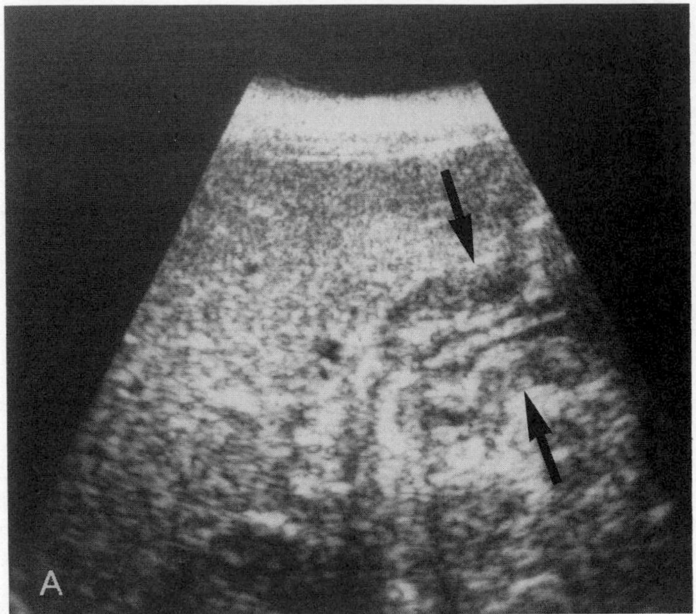

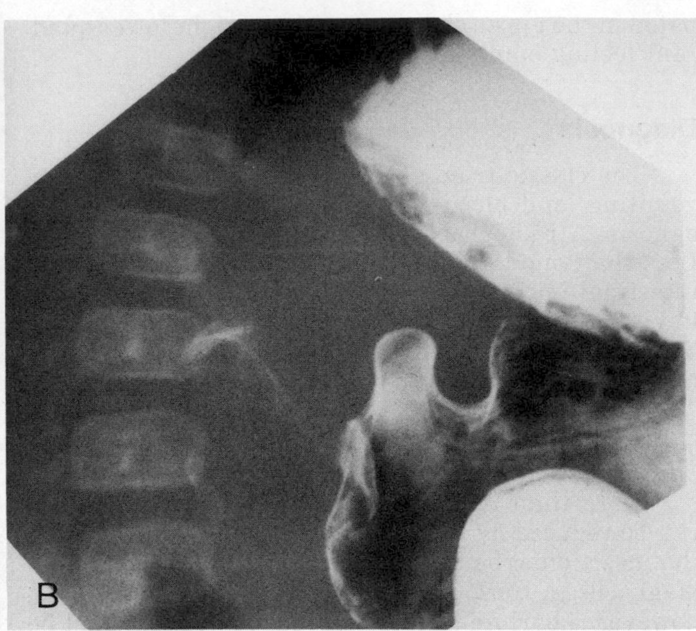

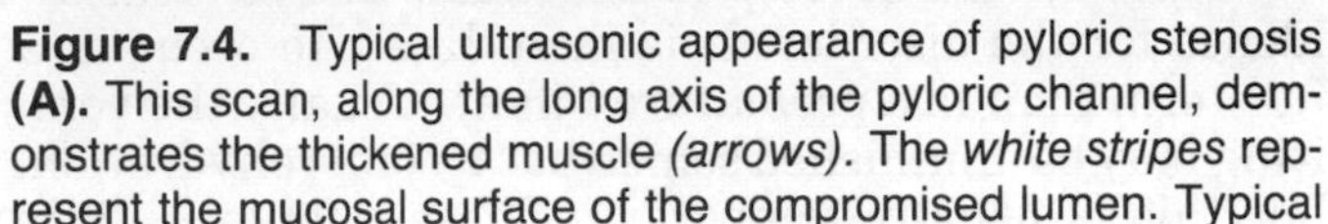

Figure 7.4. Typical ultrasonic appearance of pyloric stenosis **(A).** This scan, along the long axis of the pyloric channel, demonstrates the thickened muscle *(arrows)*. The *white stripes* represent the mucosal surface of the compromised lumen. Typical radiographic appearance of pyloric stenosis **(B).** Elongation of the pylorus and narrowed lumen result from the muscular hypertrophy.

down to the mucosa, however, and if the lumen is entered it can be readily repaired. Following the pyloromyotomy, most patients can usually be restarted on feedings within 24 hours, with the average hospital stay being 2–3 days.

Prognosis

Postoperative vomiting is common, with many infants exhibiting some vomiting during the initial 24–48 hours following the surgery. If vomiting persists for more than 4–5 days, reoperation may be necessary; this occurs in about 0.3% of patients. Recurrence later is very rare (Vilmann et al, 1986).

Motility Disorders

Motility represents the whole spectrum of motor function that enables nutrients to be ingested and moved along the intestinal tract and allows residual material to be removed from the body as feces at the appropriate time. While motility disorders can occur at any point along the entire digestive tract, most information is known about disorders in the most proximal and distal areas of the tract.

A fetus is able to swallow by the end of the 11th gestational week, and is able to produce meconium in utero beginning in the third trimester (Herbst, 1981). While a normal full-term infant demonstrates sucking and swallowing on the first day of life, a premature infant may require a period of weeks before achieving this milestone.

Sucking is normally coordinated with swallowing and as such is considered "nutritive." When an infant sucks in bursts of high frequency (about 120/min) the sucking is considered "non-nutritive," but has an important role in enhancing maturation of nutritive sucking ability, which is usually achieved by 33–34 weeks' gestation. Bernbaum et al (1983) underscore the importance of use of a pacifier for non-nutritive sucking in preterm infants who may be fed intravenously or by gavage. Weight gain was better in the infants with pacifiers than in those without, even with the same caloric intake. Presumably sublingual lipase and pancreatic secretions were stimulated by non-nutritive sucking.

Multiple mechanical factors can interfere with sucking and swallowing, causing dysmotility disorder; these are shown in Table 7.4.

In older children, dermatomyositis can also involve striated muscles of the proximal esophagus, causing

Table 7.4
Possible Factors in Swallowing Dysfunction in Infancy

Macroglossia
Cleft palate
Micrognathia
Hemangioma of tongue
Esophageal atresia or stenosis
Vascular rings
Neuromuscular disorders
  Werdnig-Hoffman
  Myasthenia gravis
Metabolic disorders
  Hypoglycemia
  Hyperbilirubinemia
Infection
Chromosomal disorders
Familial dysautonomia

problems with motility. The most common causes of neuromuscular motility disorders in older children include the infectious diseases, diphtheria, tetanus, and botulism. Achalasia is a motility disorder in which it is difficult for the food to be transported past the lower esophageal sphincter into the stomach—i.e., there is a lack of propulsive peristaltic waves in the smooth muscle of the distal esophagus. In this case, the resting pressure of the lower esophageal sphincter is elevated and does not decrease with swallowing.

In the distal bowel, motor disorders can be functional or due to obstruction. If mechanical, possibilities include atresia, obstructing bands, volvulus, intussusception, postoperative adhesions, or a strangulated hernia. Occasionally, tumor masses may cause obstruction. From a functional standpoint, systemic diseases that affect motor function of skeletal muscles will also affect colonic motility. These include, for example, hypothyroidism with associated constipation, dermatomyositis, or scleroderma. The most common motor disorders of the colon are aganglionosis of the colon (Hirschsprung disease) and functional constipation (see appropriate sections).

Diagnosis

A history of dysphagia or a history of coughing or choking in association with the swallowing mechanism is a clue that a motor disorder may be present.

Physical examination can be useful for excluding anatomical changes that can lead to a suspected neuromuscular disorder. The most helpful diagnostic tool for an oral, pharyngeal, or esophageal motility disorder is to watch the child eat and drink.

If a proximal motility disorder is suspected, a barium swallow can define anatomical abnormalities and a radionucleotide scan can detect reflux and delayed gastric emptying. Rectal monometry is the diagnostic test of choice for suspected Hirschsprung disease. If a systemic disease is suspected, standard electromyography of the skeletal muscles may aid diagnosis of a systemic disorder that affects the intestinal muscle as well.

Achalasia

Definition

Achalasia is a motility disorder of the esophagus that is characterized by the absence of peristaltic waves in the body of the esophagus and by failure of the lower esophageal sphincter to relax. As a result, it is difficult for food to pass from esophagus to stomach during the process of swallowing.

Epidemiology and Basic Science

The cause of esophageal achalasia is unknown and even the site of the primary lesion remains controversial.

CASE ILLUSTRATION

A 6-year-old male with growth retardation, being followed for growth hormone deficiency, presented for evaluation of dysphagia. Symptoms began at 18 months of age when the child was first noted to have intermittent difficulty swallowing food. One year later, he began regurgitating at night in bed, often with nocturnal coughing and sputtering, progressing to regurgitation during meals. He learned to "force" food down but took 45 minutes to finish an average meal. He gained weight poorly despite provision of adequate calories. He had a history of wheezing since 1 year of age. On physical examination, the height and weight were below the third percentile, but head circumference was at the 50th percentile. Breath sounds were occasionally coarse bilaterally, but otherwise the physical examination was unremarkable.

QUESTION AND COMMENT

What are some diagnostic possibilities for this child's symptoms and inability to gain weight? What further diagnostic work-up is indicated?

In light of the poor weight gain, regurgitation, pulmonary symptoms, and dysphagia, the esophagus is implicated as the likely source of pathology. In a young child, difficulty must be inferred from observations such as slow eating, a preference for liquids over solids, consumption of large amounts of liquids while eating, repeated swallowing maneuvers to pass food, vomiting (often self-induced) of undigested food, with small amounts of vomitus on the pillow in the morning, and obvious signs of substernal pain with eating.

The differential diagnosis of the esophageal pathology in the case described could include congenital and intrinsic anatomic abnormalities such as stenosis, webs, duplications, rings, or diverticulae; acquired intrinsic abnormalities such as strictures due to ulcers, esophagitis, perforations, or burns; extrinsic sources of obstruction such as vascular rings or mediastinal masses; an esophageal dysfunction such as collagen vascular diseases including scleroderma or dermatomyositis achalasia, Chagas disease, Riley-Day syndrome. The most direct way to distinguish among these possibilities is the barium swallow under fluoroscopy. In this child, a barium swallow showed normal deglutition, an absence of anatomic malformations, but most notably, a massively dilated esophageal body and a very narrow distal esophagus, which are classical signs of achalasia.

This case is unusual in that less than 100 reported cases of achalasia in children exist. Moreover, fewer than 5% of all affected patients with achalasia present in childhood or early adolescence (Azizkhan et al, 1980). Usually these cases are associated with disturbances in growth and development and severe pulmonary symptoms. This patient was treated successfully with pneumatic dilatation. Myotomy is more commonly recommended in younger children less than 9 years of age who are at risk of perforation from the dilatation.

Natural History

The mean age of diagnosis of achalasia in childhood is 9½ years, with a range of 1–15 years. The interval between onset and diagnosis averages 21 months. Reports of familial cases have been infrequent, although occasional case reports have suggested transmission of the disease in autosomal recessive fashion (Westerley, 1975).

For patients 1 year or older, a history of having difficulty swallowing solid food should suggest achalasia. Symptoms of achalasia are very slowly progressive and, in the most long-standing cases, are often associated with failure to gain weight. A history of dysphagia is present in 80% of patients, impairment of growth in 70%, and substernal pain or respiratory symptoms in less than half of children with this disorder (Azizkhan et al, 1980).

Diagnosis

A history of difficulty swallowing food for a period of months is suggestive. The child may experience retrosternal pain and frequent episodes of feeling that food is stuck in the throat or upper chest. Relief of dysphagia by repeated swallowing movements or by regurgitation is often reported.

The vomitus will not show evidence of significant digestion. A plain radiograph of the chest may reveal evidence of bronchopneumonia caused by aspiration, or may show a dilated esophagus full of food due to distal obstruction or poor propulsion. Rarely is air in the stomach visualized. A barium swallow shows a dilated esophagus with narrowing at the gastroesophageal junction and fluoroscopic examination reveals absence of normal peristalsis and failure of relaxation of the lower esophageal sphincter. Manometry should confirm that the lower esophageal sphincter pressure at rest is twice normal and that it is not reduced to the level of gastric pressure during swallowing.

Treatment

Pharmacologic therapy, although often unsuccessful, is the first line of therapy in children. If this fails, partial destruction of the lower esophageal sphincter is the treatment of choice and can be achieved by pneumatic dilation of the sphincter with a dilating balloon and with surgery if this fails.

Prognosis

If disease is suspected and treated at an early stage when proximal motility is less disturbed, return of the esophagus to normal caliber after surgical myotomy is good. Poorer results, however, can be expected if forceful dilatation and eventually surgery are carried out in long-standing cases.

REFERENCES

Azizkhan RG, Tapper D, Eraklis A: Achalasia in childhood: A 20 year experience. *J Pediatr Surg* 15:452, 1980.

Benson CD: Infantile hypertrophic pyloric stenosis. In Ravitch MM, Welch KJ, Benson CD, et al (eds): *Pediatric Surgery*, 3rd edition. Chicago, Year Book Medical Publishers, 1979.

Bernbaum JC, Pereira GR, Watkins J: Nonnutritive sucking during gavage feeding enhances growth and maturation in premature neonates. *Pediatrics* 71:41, 1983.

Berquist WE: Gastroesophageal reflux in children: Clinical review. *Pediatr Ann* 11:135, 1982.

Berquist WE, Byrne WJ, Ament ME, et al: Achalasia: Diagnosis, management and clinical course in 16 children. *Pediatrics* 71:798, 1983.

Biller JA, Winter MD, Grand RJ, et al: Are endoscopic changes predictive of histologic esophagitis in children? *J Pediatr* 103:215, 1983.

Boyle JT, Cohen S, Watkins JB, et al: Successful treatment of achalasia in childhood by pneumatic dilatation. *J Pediatr* 99:35, 1981.

Breaux CW, Georgeson MD, Royal SA, et al: Changing patterns in the diagnosis of hypertrophic pyloric stenosis. *Pediatrics* 81:213, 1988.

Carre IJ: Clinical significance of gastroesophageal reflux. *Arch Dis Child* 59:911, 1984.

Christie DL, Ament ME: Gastric acid hypersecretion in children with duodenal ulcer. *Gastroenterology* 71:242, 1976.

Dodds WJ, Dent J, Hogan WJ, et al: Mechanisms of gastroesophageal reflux in patients with reflux esophagitis. *N Engl J Med* 307:1547, 1982.

Drake DP, Maciver AG, Atwell JD: Zollinger-Ellison syndrome in a child: Medical treatment with cimetidine. *Arch Dis Child* 55:226, 1980.

Drumm B, Sherman P, Cutz E, et al: Association of *Campylobacter pylori* on the gastric mucosa with antral gastritis in children. *N Engl J Med* 316:1557, 1987.

Ericksen C, Hauge M, Madsen CM, et al: Two generation transmission of oesophageal atresia with tracheo-oesophageal fistula. *Acta Pediatr Scand* 70:253, 1981.

Fordtran JS, Morawski SG, Richardson CT: In vivo and in vitro evaluation of liquid antacids. *N Engl J Med* 288:923, 1973.

Harnsberger JK, Corey JJ, Johnson DG, et al: Long-term follow-up surgery for gastroesophageal reflux in infants and in children. *J Pediatr* 102:505, 1983.

Helm JF, Dodds WF, Pele LR, et al: Effect of esophageal emptying and saliva on clearance of acid from the esophagus. *N Engl J Med* 30:284, 1984.

Herbst JJ: Diagnosis and treatment of gastroesophageal reflux in children. *Pediatr Rev* 5:75, 1983.

Herbst JJ: Gastroesophageal reflux. *J Pediatr* 98:859, 1981.

Herbst JJ: Motility disorders of the intestine. *Pediatr Gastroenterol* 6:19, 1982.

Hillemeier AC, Lange R, McCallum R, et al: Delayed gastric emptying in infants with gastroesophageal reflux during infancy. *Gastroenterology* 84:741, 1983.

Jaffe BM: Surgical treatment of peptic ulcer disease: Parietal cell vagotomy. *Drug Ther* p. 89, 1983.

Jenson RT, Gardner JD, Raufman J-P, et al: Zollinger-Ellison syndrome: Current concepts in management. *Ann Intern Med* 98:59, 1983.

Jewett TC, Siegel M: Hiatal hernia in gastroesophageal reflux. *J Pediatr Gastroenterol Nutr* 3:340, 1984.

Jinzhe Z, Yenxia W, Linchi W: Rectal inflation reduction of intussusception in infants. *J Pediatr Surg* 21:30, 1986.

Khamapirad T, Athey PA: Ultrasound diagnosis of hypertrophic pyloric stenosis. *J Pediatr* 102:23, 1983.

Konno T, Suzuki H, Kutsuzawa T, et al: Human rotavirus in intussusception. *N Engl J Med* 297, 945, 1977.

Liu KW, MacCarthy J, Guiney EJ, et al: Intussusception—current trends in management. *Arch Dis Child* 61:75, 1986.

McGuigan J, Trudeau W: Differences in rates of gastrin release in normal persons and patients with duodenal ulcer disease. *N Engl J Med* 288:64, 1973.

Muhammed R, Mackay C: Peptic ulceration in adolescence. *Br J Surg* 69:525, 1982.

Nord KS, Rossi TM, Lebenthal E: Peptic ulcer disease in children. *Am J Gastroenterol* 75:153, 1981.

Orenstein SR, Whitington PF: Positioning for prevention in infant gastroesophageal reflux. *J Pediatr* 103:534, 1983.

Petersen H, Schrumpf E, Myrin J: Fasting serum gastrin in basic gastric acid secretion. *Scand J Gastroenterol* 10:721, 1975.

Quan L, Smith DW: The VATER association: Vertebral defects, anal atresia, T-E fistula with esophageal atresia, radial and renal dysplasia. A spectrum of associated defects. *J Pediatr* 104:7, 1973.

Rachmel A, Rosenbach Y, Amir J, et al: Apathy as an early manifestation of intussusception. *Am J Dis Child* 137:702, 1983.

Ravitch MM: Intussusception. In Welch KJ, Randolph JG, Ravitch MM, et al (eds): *Pediatric Surgery,* 4th edition, vol 2. Chicago, Year Book Medical Publishers, 1986.

Richter JE, Castell DO: Gastroesophageal reflux: Pathogenesis, diagnosis and therapy. *Ann Intern Med* 97:93, 1982.

Rickham PP: Infants with esophageal atresia weighing under 3 pounds. *J Pediatr Surg* 16:595, 1981.

Rudd TG, Christie DL: Demonstration of esophageal reflux in children by radionuclide gastroesophagography. *Radiology* 131:483, 1979.

Silverman A, Roy C: Peptic disease. In: *Pediatric Clinical Gastroenterology*. St. Louis, CV Mosby, p, 165, 1983a.

Silverman A, Roy CC: Malrotation with or without volvulus of the mid gut. In: *Pediatric Clinical Gastroenterology,* 3rd edition. St. Louis, CV Mosby, 1983b, p. 61.

Singer J: Altered consciousness as an early manifestation of intussusception. *Pediatrics* 64:93, 1979.

Sondheimer JM: Continuous monitoring of distal esophageal pH: A diagnostic test for gastrointestinal reflux in infants. *J Pediatr* 96:804, 1980.

Sondheimer JM: Gastroesophageal reflux: Update on pathogenesis and diagnosis. *Pediatr Clin North Am* 35:103, 1988.

Stauffer UG, Hermann P: Comparison of late results in patients with corrected intestinal malrotation with and without fixation demesentary. *J Pediatr Surg* 15:9, 1980.

Stevenson RJ: Nonneonatal intestinal obstruction in children. *Surg Clin North Am* p. 1223, 1985.

Stewart DR, Clodney AL, Daggett WC: Malrotation of the bowel in infants and children: A 15 year review. *Surgery* 79:716, 1976.

Strickland AD, Chang JH: Results of treatment of gastroesophageal reflux with bethanechol. *J Pediatr* 103:311, 1983.

Teele RL, Smith EH: Ultrasound in the diagnosis of idiopathic hyperthrophic pyloric stenosis *N Engl J Med* 296:1149, 1975.

Thomas GG, Zachary RB: Intussusception in twins. *Pediatrics* 58:754, 1976.

Vilmann P, Hjortrup A, Altmann P, et al: A long-term gastrointestinal follow-up in patients operated on for congenital hypertrophic pyloric stenosis. *Acta Pediatr Scand* 75:156, 1986.

Westerley CR, Herbst J, Goldman S, et al: Inheritance of infantile achalasia. *J Pediatr* 87:243, 1975.

Wilson SD, Schulte WJ, Meade RC: Longevity studies following total gastrectomy in children with the Zollinger-Ellison syndrome. *Arch Surg* 103:108, 1971.

Winter HS, Mandara JL, Stratford RJ, et al: Delayed acid clearance and esophagitis after repair of esophageal atresia. *J Gastroenterol* 80:1317, 1981.

Winter HS, Kleinman RE: Stretching strictures. *J Pediatr Gastroenterol Nutr* 5:171, 1986.

Zeldis JB, Friedman LS, Isselbacher KJ, et al: Ranitidine: A new H_2 receptor antagonist. *N Engl J Med* 309:1368, 1983.

Lower Gastrointestinal Tract Diseases: Approaches by Symptom 3

APPROACH TO ACUTE DIARRHEA

Diarrhea is an increase in frequency and a change in character of stool. When untreated, acute diarrhea can result in rapid dehydration, progressive acidosis, significant morbidity, and in areas of poverty and poor sanitation, significant mortality. While the differential diagnosis for a child who experiences a change in the character and frequency of stools is a large one, an organized approach to this symptom can be useful in determining its cause.

Diarrhea results when there is a decrease in the net movement of water from the intestinal lumen to plasma, and the volume of liquid that is subsequently delivered to the colon surpasses its reabsorptive ability. One of the primary mechanisms for acute diarrhea is an osmotic overload into the gut because of ingestion of poorly absorbable solutes, resulting in a more hypertonic environment in the lumen and increased water and electrolyte excretion on a solute load basis.

A second mechanism involves increased secretion. This can occur either passively from elevated hydrostatic pressure or actively by ion secretion by the mucosa. A third mechanism involves a decrease in the normal active ion absorption owing to a decrease in anatomic or functional surface area. Finally, acute diarrhea may result from motility disturbances that may be secondary to an underlying disease or previous surgery. In this situation, a mixed disorder involves the osmotic effect of increased solute load as well as an increased rate of secretion from the rapid transit and decreased absorption time.

Cyclic adenosine monophosphate (AMP) has been found to increase secretion and inhibit absorption of sodium chloride. Stimulators of cyclic AMP include vasoactive intestinal peptide, prostaglandins, deconjugated bile acids, and hydroxy fatty acids. In addition, mechanisms not involving cyclic AMP have been found to mediate secretion. These are through other GI hormones such as gastrin, cholecystokinin, glucagon, secretin, calcitonin, and serotonin. Intake of food can also increase secretion and lead to increased diarrhea.

If an infectious etiology is suspected, the diarrhea should be classified as inflammatory or noninflammatory. Inflammatory diarrhea results from infection localized to the distal small intestine and colon and is characterized by stools containing mucus, blood, and/or pus (fecal leukocytes). Noninflammatory organisms localize toward the proximal small bowel and produce a more watery, voluminous stool, but without the blood and pus. Organisms responsible for these two mechanisms are listed in Table 7.5.

Epidemiology

About 1 billion episodes of acute diarrhea occur each year among third world children, leading to a mortality of 5 million (Snyder and Merson, 1982). At the turn of the century diarrheal disease was a major cause of infant and early childhood mortality in the United States (McCormick, 1982). Improvements in sanitation and nutrition, however, have resulted in virtual eradication of deaths due to diarrheal disease in this country.

From a standpoint of morbidity, acute diarrhea accounts for 7–8% of all inpatient hospitalizations in children under age 15 in the United States (McCormick, 1982). It has been the third most frequent reason for hospitalization of children, following respiratory illness and injuries. Most hospitalizations are for children under age 1 year and again represent the third most frequent cause of hospitalization in children in this age bracket, following congenital anomalies and respiratory illness (McCormick, 1982). With increasing use of oral rehydration, hospitalization for rehydration is declining.

Acute diarrheal complaints account for 7% of all visits to pediatricians for children 15 years of age or younger (McCormick, 1982). Males and females are equally affected, although diarrhea is more likely to occur in infants than in older children. In developing countries, increased incidence is linked to poor sanitation and hygiene, which can lead to increased exposure to pathogenic organisms. In addition, malnutrition results in decreased caloric intake reducing the gut's resistance and predisposing it to increased risk of infection. Breast-feeding has been associated with a decrease in morbidity due to diarrheal disease, perhaps as a result of reduced exposure to organisms and of the immunoprotection provided in breast milk (Larsen and Homer, 1978). Increased prevalence can be seen in the United States in settings where a number of children are cared for in close proximity. In developed countries diarrhea is a cold weather disease, primarily reflecting the viral origin of diarrhea in these countries. In the less developed countries, summer outbreaks are largely due to bacterial agents. A child who travels especially to tropical or subtropical areas, may also show increased risk for acute diarrheal disease, usually within the first 2 weeks of arrival (see pp. 55–56).

Table 7.5
Some Organisms Associated with Diarrhea

Inflammatory	Noninflammatory
Salmonella	Rotavirus
Shigella	*Giardia lamblia*
Campylobacter jejuni	Toxigenic *E. Coli*
Yersinia enterocolitica	Cryptosporidium
Clostridium difficile	Norwalk virus

Diagnosis

Since the diagnosis of acute diarrhea depends on a sudden change in a patient's bowel habits, the history should focus on possible reasons for such a change. For example, new foods or contaminated foods may be a possible cause for acute diarrhea. The bowel status of other family members should be elicited, especially in regard to dietary change. The presence of other associated symptoms such as fever, vomiting, or abdominal pain may also be useful in characterizing the acuity of the diarrhea and may be able to classify it as part of a larger symptom complex.

A complete physical examination including a rectal examination should be performed. The physical examination should include weight and height. Hydration status should also be assessed as well as other associated symptoms of the disease.

Stools should be inspected and described, and tested for heme, fecal leukocytes, pH, and reducing substance, the latter to assess carbohydrate intolerance. If stools contain evidence for white or red blood cells, stool cultures should also be obtained. If a malabsorption is being considered and a chronic etiology cannot be ruled out, the stools should also be examined by sudan stain to seek increases in neutral fat. Urinalysis for specific gravity, and BUN and electrolytes to assess the hydration status of the child, are also useful.

Treatment

In general, antibiotics should not be started empirically unless the diarrhea is likely to be bacterial. Even then many bacterial enteritides resolve spontaneously without antibiotics. Antispasmodic and nonspecific antidiarrheal agents have not been found to be effective in children and are rarely recommended. Therefore, the mainstay of treatment is assurance of adequate hydration status by maintaining good fluid and electrolyte balance and an appropriate osmotic load. Usually this can be done with the appropriate oral rehydrating solution (see pp. 601).

Prevention

Proper sanitary conditions including handwashing, refrigeration, and adequate cooking are standard health measures that have resulted in significant reduction in the incidence of diarrhea. Although immunological approaches are being tested in high-risk areas, it is doubtful that an overall immunological solution will be found because of the multiplicity of etiologies responsible for acute diarrhea.

APPROACH TO CHRONIC DIARRHEA

Chronic diarrhea is usually defined as passage of formless stools for 14 or more days. It may be persistent or intermittent, with weeks of diarrhea alternating with weeks of normal stool.

Basic Science

Chronic diarrhea usually begins with a transient insult similar to that in an acute diarrheal episode, followed by secondary intestinal mechanisms that prolong the process. Transient insults may include an infectious enteritis, a dietary manipulation, or use of antibiotics or other medications. Secondary mechanisms that can prolong or result in a second osmotic or secretory process include mucosal damage resulting in disaccharide imbalance; increased motility from food ingestion; dietary imbalance, for example, with a low-fat, high-carbohydrate intake; starvation; or increased mucous secretion. The overall mechanisms responsible for the diarrhea, i.e., osmotic, secretory, decreased absorption, or motility disturbances are similar to those discussed in the section on acute diarrhea.

Natural History

The natural history of the specific disorders varies with the specific etiology and the reader is referred to the appropriate section for further discussion. Despite the wide range of causes, 95% of cases of chronic diarrhea can be attributed to fewer than a half dozen disease entities (Silverman and Roy, 1983).

Diagnosis

Diagnosis of chronic diarrhea is based on a careful history, since many patients will have few if any positive physical findings. Nonetheless, the physical examination as described below can also be useful.

Historical ascertainment of growth measurements as well as a thorough dietary record are essential in the evaluation. Alterations in diet should be correlated with changes in stool frequency and character. It is useful to separate the diet into its metabolic components, including protein, carbohydrate, and fat contents of foods and formulas. Poor growth may result from either malabsorption or persistent feedings of dilute, hypocaloric formulas or clear liquids that were begun in an effort to reduce acute diarrheal symptoms. Knowledge of the sequence of introduction of all food products into the diet of an infant and its temporal relationship to the diarrhea is crucial. For example, a child who develops chronic diarrhea while breast-fed may be demonstrating congenital lactase deficiency or glucose-galactose malabsorption. On the other hand, a breast-fed infant who gets diarrhea only after introduction of solid foods may have sucrase or isomaltase deficiency. A switch to a soy-based formula will usually successfully treat cow's milk protein allergy as well as lactose intolerance, although 30% of milk protein allergic children will also be soy allergic. A soy and milk protein-free formula might then be considered.

Oral medications, particularly antibiotics, used within 6 weeks of onset of diarrhea could be primarily responsible for the symptoms. Cystic fibrosis, celiac disease, protein intolerance, disaccharidase deficiencies, or inflammatory bowel disease could also be revealing.

Characterization of the stool is also important, for it may be helpful in determining the cause of the chronicity of the disease. For example, foul-smelling stools may represent a bacterial infection or steatorrhea.

Physical examination should include current anthropometric measurements. Most important is weight-for-height, since this is the best single index for growth failure secondary to malnutrition. Weight for age and height for age are also useful measurements. While physical findings are often rare in chronic diarrhea, they should nonetheless be looked for. Vitamin deficiencies can signal a malabsorptive process. For example, cheilosis or a smooth red tongue suggests vitamin B deficiency and dry, scaly skin indicates either fatty acid or vitamin A deficiency. An enlarged liver or spleen with hair thinning suggests protein malnutrition, and severe protein deficiency may be heralded by peripheral edema and depigmentation. Cystic fibrosis may be suspected if nasal polyps, rectal prolapse, or abnormal pulmonary findings are noted. The presence of iritis, arthritis, or erythema nodosum suggests inflammatory bowel disease.

Abnormal constituents of stools that can be identified easily include reducing sugars (use of Clinitest tablets), sucrose (Clinitest tablets after hydrolysis with 1 N hydrochloric acid and heating), occult blood (heme-occult paper), leukocytes (methylene blue staining of a stool specimen on a glass slide), bacteria (Gram stain), and neutral fat globules (sudan stain). These simple tests can suggest potential causes of chronic diarrhea. Significant carbohydrate malabsorption may reflect small intestinal mucosal injury, a disaccharidase deficiency, or a monosaccharide transport defect. Fecal leukocytes can signify infection, enteritis, or colitis, effect of drugs, intolerance to formula in infants, or inflammatory bowel disease. The more common microorganisms are *Salmonella, Shigella, Campylobacter jejuni, Yersinia enterocolitica, Clostridium difficile, Vibrio parahemolyticus,* invasive *Escherichia coli,* and *Entamoeba histolytica* and *Giardia*. Fat globules may suggest steatorrhea, but their absence does not exclude the diagnosis since fat ingestion may have been limited at or before the time of the examination. Stool electrolytes should also be assayed to determine whether an osmotic or secretory process is occurring.

A number of other studies are possible to evaluate metabolic deficiencies (folate, B_{12}, iron levels, etc) or malabsorption (d-xylose test and a lactose breath test).

In some instances, UGI series with small bowel follow through or barium enemas are appropriate, particularly if inflammatory bowel disease is a consideration.

In the unusual situation of a chronic secretory diarrhea, serum hormone levels to detect gastrin or vasoactive peptides, and urinary collections to measure catecholamine levels can be useful.

Treatment

Treatment will depend on the cause of the chronic diarrhea. A more aggressive approach to treatment, particularly if a child is having difficulty gaining weight, requires hospitalization and intravenous therapy. For most patients with chronic diarrhea, however, oral alimentation and dietary manipulations successfully abate the symptoms. Medications that affect or slow down motility have no place in the treatment of the child with chronic diarrhea.

MALABSORPTION

Definition

Malabsorption represents conditions in which dietary nutrients cannot be properly absorbed and/or transported across the intestinal mucosa.

Epidemiology

The major malabsorptive abnormalities in children are those involving carbohydrate absorption, gluten-induced enteropathy, and cystic fibrosis, a triad that accounts for over 90% of all malabsorption.

Diagnosis

Loose and bulky stools, poor weight gain, and abdominal distention characterize malabsorption. A complete and accurate dietary history is essential. A review of extraintestinal systems can also be useful to detect other associated disorders.

For example, various mineral and vitamin deficiencies can cause malabsorption and also present with a bleeding or bruising tendency, cheilosis, glossitis, or a peripheral neuritis. Edema, muscle cramping, tetany, bone pain, and anemia can also be manifestations of a protein or mineral disorder. A history of respiratory dysfunction in conjunction with chronic diarrhea may signify the presence of cystic fibrosis. Hepatomegaly and edema associated with diarrhea might point to liver disease or a protein-losing enteropathy as a possible cause for malabsorption. Pancreatic insufficiency and neutropenia are suggestive of Shwachman-Diamond syndrome.

Linear growth is markedly hampered in chronic diseases such as cystic fibrosis, celiac disease, and chronic inflammatory bowel diseases, such as ulcerative colitis and regional enteritis (Crohn disease). Patients with cystic fibrosis may have growth failure in early infancy, whereas those with gluten-induced enteropathy can grow normally for up to 2 years of age before a change is noted.

Physical examination can also document recent weight loss by observation of thickness of subcutaneous tissue and by examination of elasticity of the skin. Muscle-wasting can best be detected in the buttocks, thighs, and arms. Peripheral edema should also be sought since it can accompany a protein-losing enteropathy or severe malnutrition. Clubbing of fingers may point to cystic fibrosis or chronic liver or bowel disease in association with malabsorption. The abdominal examination may show enlargement, distention, or generalized discomfort secondary to a localized painful area or a mass. Examination of the skin may identify a vitamin deficiency. For example, an acute dermatitis may result from zinc deficiency whereas skin bruising may signify vitamin K deficiency and associated liver disease. Neurologic examination will reveal muscle weakness and cramping associated with the tetany seen in celiac disease. Patients with malabsorption are often irritable, uncooperative, and difficult to approach, or may be lethargic.

Table 7.6
Tests or Procedures Suggested to Aid Diagnosis of Malabsorption

Potential Abnormality	Test or Procedure
Fat malabsorption	72-hour fecal fat excretion
Carbohydrate malabsorption	d-Xylose or lactose breath test
B_{12} or folic acid	Shilling test Serum levels of B_{12} or folate (bone marrow)
Iron	Serum ferritin or iron levels
Bacteria present	Duodenal aspirate
Giardia	
Inflammation or obstruction or anatomical abnormality	Upper GI series
Pancreatic exocrine function	Stool trypsin or chymotrypsin levels;
Carbohydrate digestive enzymes	Laboratory analysis; small bowel biopsy

A careful history and physical examination may signal the need for further laboratory tests. A baseline work-up should include a complete blood count, urinalysis and urine culture, stool cultures for bacteria and parasites, a chemical profile, and a sweat test. In addition, stool should be examined for the presence of neutral fat, blood, and reducing substance, and, if any of these is detected, a more quantified stool collection might be useful. (Malabsorption of non-neutral fats, however, will not be identified by sudan stain.) The presence of edema, or a suspected protein-loosing enteropathy, or recurrent infections requires a serum protein analysis with immunoglobulin electrophoresis. If the linear rate of growth appears to have decreased, assessment of bone age is useful. The presence of pulmonary symptoms mandates a chest radiograph to detect infection and possible cystic fibrosis (see Table 7.6).

Lactase Deficiency

Definition

Lactase deficiency may be congenital and acquired. Congenital lactase deficiency is very rare, whereas the late-onset acquired lactase deficiency represents the most common disaccharide intolerance. Lactase deficiency manifests when the disaccharide lactose cannot be hydrolyzed to galactose and glucose for absorption.

Basic Science

It is believed that congenital lactase deficiency represents a reduction in the production of the enzyme rather than its absence, suggesting a defect in a regulatory protein, rather than in the gene (Freiburghaus et al, 1976).

Secondary or late-onset lactase deficiency is transmitted as an autosomal recessive disorder, and also is believed to represent a regulatory abnormality in that a low level of lactase activity is detectable. It is not clear why the deficiency does not present itself until 3–6 years after birth.

Both primary and acquired lactase deficiency should be distinguished from a transient lactose intolerance noted in both term and premature newborns. This early malabsorptive condition, in which a decreased amount of available lactase activity is observed that increases after 2 months of age, is rare. In addition, since lactase is superficially located on the brush-border, it may also be transiently reduced after damage to villus architecture, such as occurs following acute gastroenteritis. This type of secondary lactase deficiency is reversible with regeneration of normal villi.

Epidemiology

Inherited delayed-onset lactase deficiency has a prevalence related to ethnic background. Black children have been reported to have a higher percentage of milk intolerance than white children, with one study suggesting that 33% of black children and 10% of white children demonstrate abnormal lactose absorption. (Angelides and Davidson, 1985).

Natural History

Congenital lactase deficiency often presents as diarrhea with the onset of the first feeding of a lactose-containing formula or breast milk. Vomiting, colicky pain, and abdominal distention are common. In an older child who first presents with the genetic deficiency, diarrhea, flatulence, and crampy abdominal pain occur within 8 hours of the ingestion of lactose (from 2 to a maximum of 50 g/kg). Because of its high prevalence, it has also been evoked as a possible cause for children who present with recurrent abdominal pain, although these studies were not prospective.

Diagnosis

Suspected lactase deficiency may be confirmed by certain diagnostic tests. Stools should be acidic and the pH can be less than 4. The stools usually contain reducing substances. In infants, amino aciduria, proteinuria, and an elevated blood urea nitrogen have been described. Because this condition is so rare in infants, it is important to make sure that it is not secondary to mucosal damage, and a small bowel biopsy to assess the lactase level directly is recommended. A normal brush border may not rule out the presence of a lactase deficiency, since activity does not return for periods of up to 6 months.

Breath test analysis (by measuring the end-products of digestive metabolism [carbon dioxide and hydrogen] that represent gases that are transported by the blood stream and eliminated by the lungs) can aid diagnosis. Any increased tendency toward malabsorption will result in delivery of a larger amount of carbohydrate to the colon where, after bacterial fermentation, an increasing amount of carbohydrate and hydrogen is excreted by the lungs. If the disaccharide is radioactively labeled, the amount of hydrogen excreted by the lungs correlates directly with the amount of disaccharide reaching the colon, with larger amounts being excreted by the lungs in the presence of malabsorption. In normal children, less than 20 ppm of hydrogen is expired compared with more than 800 ppm in malabsorbers (Barr et al, 1979).

False-positives can occur if there is bacterial overgrowth (and consequently increased fermentation in the small bowel), small bowel obstruction, or in older children with regional enteritis. False-negatives can be caused by delayed gastric emptying or with rapid intestinal transit time and increased colonic evacuation that prevents sufficient fermentation to occur. Moreover, it has been reported that certain individuals may lack hydrogen-producing colonic bacteria. Nonetheless, the overall reliability of the test and its noninvasiveness make it the diagnostic choice in children suspected of having disaccharide malabsorption.

The definitive diagnosis of the specific enzyme deficiency can only be made by doing a mucosal enzyme assay via a jejunal biopsy. For patients with only mild symptoms or those who can manage a relatively normal diet, a small bowel biopsy is not necessary. If severe dietary restriction is required, a biopsy may be indicated to clarify the appropriate diet.

Treatment

In the rare case of infants with lactase deficiency, a lactose-free formula should be started as soon as the diagnosis is suspected. Most older children and adults with low lactase levels tolerate a certain amount of lactose, most successfully in its fermented form, such as in cheese or yogurt. Usually a child is started on cheese (with 2% lactase), followed by yogurt (33% lactase), and finally milk. They should also limit the amount of milk consumed. In younger children who consume large amounts of milk, a yeast lactase enzyme preparation can be added to milk to cleave the disaccharide and allow adequate absorption.

Celiac Disease or Gluten-Sensitive Enteropathy

Definition

Celiac disease is a condition in which small bowel mucosa is damaged when gluten-containing foods are introduced. It may also occur after an infectious insult to the small bowel.

Basic Science

Gluten, a grain protein extract, is believed to be responsible for the mucosal injury. More specifically, it is the gliadin fraction of the gluten that has been shown to be toxic to the small bowel. It is possible that susceptible patients lack an intestinal enzyme that can detoxify the gluten. On the other hand, such an enzyme deficiency might be a secondary rather than a primary cause of the disease. Another theory holds that the disorder results from an immunologic dysfunction of the intestinal mucosa with the gluten fraction eliciting an antigenic response that subsequently results in injury to the small bowel mucosa. Both antigen-antibody-mediated and cell-mediated responses have been explored as possible mechanisms for the disorder, but thus far, no definitive mechanism for the gluten-induced injury has been described.

The introduction of gluten results in a flattening of the intestinal mucosal brush border, with decreased disaccharidase enzyme levels and subsequently secondary lactose and sucrose intolerance and osmotic diarrhea. Proteins and fats may also be malabsorbed. Serum levels of secretin and cholecystokinin are decreased because of injury to the small intestine, from which these enzymes originate, and result in restricted exocrine pancreatic and biliary secretions. The enterohepatic circulation of bile acids may be diminished resulting in further fat malabsorption. All of these symptoms will abate with the institution of a gluten-free diet.

Epidemiology

Celiac disease is one of the most common causes of malabsorption in infants and children. The incidence is believed to be between 1:300 and 1:6500 and is highest in the western part of Ireland. There are no data on the incidence of celiac disease in the United States. It is possible, however, that reported prevalence is less than the true prevalence since many asymptomatic individuals with mucosal injury may exist among family members of patients with celiac disease. The disease occurs more frequently in families of patients with celiac disease than in those without—with a 5–10% increase in frequency in first degree relatives (Lebenthal and Branski, 1981).

Natural History

The characteristic child usually presents at about 18 months of age with a history of diarrhea beginning between 6 and 12 months of age. Both height and weight are diminished, the abdomen is often distended, and the child is described as being irritable and/or anorexic. While between 8 and 24 months is the usual time of onset, cases also have been reported in teenagers. The mode of onset tends to be more acute in the younger child. Muscle-wasting and hypotonia are particularly common in younger children, whereas in older children, retarded growth and delayed sexual development along with diarrhea are more characteristic. Symptomatic improvement may occur during adolescence with recurrence of symptoms in early adulthood.

The diarrhea in celiac disease is usually foul-smelling, bulky, pale, oily, and characteristic of fat malabsorption. Of importance, 10–25% of children will not present with diarrhea, although these tend to be the older children. The abdominal distention that occurs is caused by poor abdominal musculature, hypertonia, decreased intestinal motility, and accumulation of fluid and gases in the intestinal lumen secondary to bacterial action on undigested foods.

In adults, an association between recurrent aphthous stomatitis and celiac disease has been noted. Other associated abnormalities include a hypochromic microcytic anemia secondary to iron deficiency. Deficiencies in the fat-soluble vitamins are also common. Rare metabolic abnormalities include calcium malabsorption owing to defective calcium transport via the small intestine, with accompanying bone pain, tetany, and osteomalacia being more common than rickets in these patients. Exacerbations follow intercurrent infections and, in young children, may be so severe as to be called a celiac crisis. Celiac crisis is a medical emergency and requires treatment with intravenous fluids and electrolyte replacement and, occasionally, steroids.

Diagnosis

The definitive diagnosis of celiac disease is made by obtaining an initial biopsy while the patient is receiving a gluten diet that will show the characteristic flat villous lesion; a second biopsy obtained after the patient is placed on a gluten-free diet for 6 months; and a third biopsy after a repeat gluten challenge to show a return of the disease.

Since a biopsy is invasive, we usually proceed initially with a laboratory evaluation in a patient who has suspected celiac disease. This entails an analysis of fecal fat excretion, including sudan staining of stool for excessive neutral fats and a 3-day stool collection, which is analyzed for percentage of fat intake excreted. A concomitant dietary diary is needed to assess total fat intake over this time. While steatorrhea is often seen in gluten-sensitive enteropathy, up to one-third of patients may not have this symptom since steatorrhea depends more on the extent of involvement rather than the severity of the lesion itself. Analysis of fecal fat requires that the patient has had a diet containing at least 40% fat. Some caution in interpretation is necessary since collecting stool for 3 days is usually difficult for a young child and family and incomplete collection or an inadequate prior fat intake may occur. The d-xylose absorption test, while considered the best screening test for celiac disease for an overall estimate of large numbers of individuals, can produce false positive and false negative results. Absorption of xylose can be influenced by intestinal transit time, bacterial overgrowth, medications, and an abnormal liver metabolism. Therefore, it does not circumvent the need for small bowel biopsy.

A sweat test is indicated once the diagnosis of steatorrhea is obtained, not only to eliminate the diagnosis of cystic fibrosis, but also because of the increased frequency with which cystic fibrosis and celiac disease are found to be associated.

Radiographic evaluation is not pathognomonic of celiac disease but the presence on barium studies of bowel dilatation, edema, segmentation, fragmentation, and hypersecretion has been associated with the diagnosis (Fig. 7.5). The use of barium, however, is not required unless an anatomic lesion such as malrotation, an inflammatory lesion such as Crohn disease, or lymphoma, are considered possibilities. Moreover, a normal radiographic study does not rule out the diagnosis. Bone radiographs may show diffuse demineralization and a decrease in cortical thickness. Osteoporosis and osteomalacia are also frequently seen. Rickets, however, is much rarer in celiac disease, presumably because patients are not growing.

Treatment

Removal of gluten-containing foods usually results in improvement in the child's behavior and weight gain within 2 weeks of changing the diet. A complete list of gluten-free products can be obtained from the Celiac Society of the USA (45 Glifford Avenue, Jersey City, NJ 07304). Sucrose and lactose should be restricted until the enzyme levels in the small bowel increase as the villi regrow. Iron, folate, and rarely B_{12} also may be needed if significant areas of the distal small bowel have been damaged. After 6–12 months on a gluten-free diet, the patient should be rechallenged with a gluten-containing product and then monitored for occurrence of mucosal relapse, usually within 6 months to 1 year after reintroduction of gluten. A mucosal relapse after a gluten rechallenge reinforces the need to maintain a gluten-free diet.

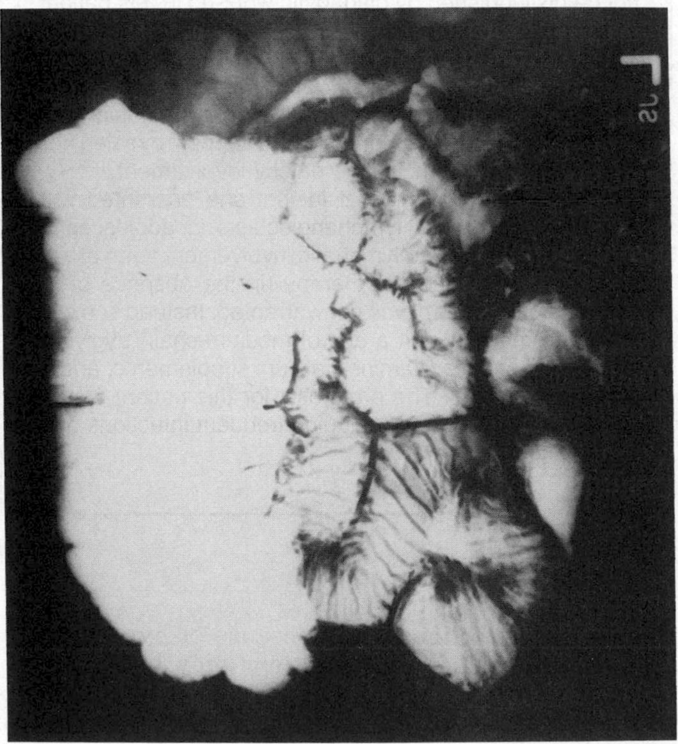

Figure 7.5. Celiac disease is one of the disorders of small bowel that is associated with increased diameter of the lumen. Note the prominent valvulae conniventes that result from the dilation.

NEW DEVELOPMENTS

Measurement of serum ferritin levels has been found to distinguish between a patient with nontreated celiac disease and other GI disorders. An initially low ferritin level will show improvement when a patient is put on a gluten-free diet and will subsequently decrease when gluten is reintroduced, hence obviating the need for repeat biopsy. Another serologic method is a direct and indirect leukocyte migration inhibition factor assay in which cells sensitized to alpha-gliadin are found circulating in the peripheral blood of patients with celiac disease (Bertell et al, 1985).

Follow-up

Children with celiac disease may be predisposed as adults to developing malignancies including small intestinal carcinoma and lymphomas, carcinoma of the esophagus, and less frequently of the stomach and colon. There are no data that suggest that a properly managed celiac disease patient will have a shortened life expectancy, nor is there evidence in adults that a gluten-free diet will provide protection from an increased risk of malignancy. Complete restoration of normal small bowel morphology usually takes at least 1–2 years. If a gluten rechallenge results in recurrence of symptoms, a life-long gluten-free diet is required. A relapse rate of 75% has been reported in patients who do not adhere to the diet.

Lymphangiectasia

Definition

Lymphangiectasia is a disorder of the intestinal lymphatic system that results in bulk loss of lymph into the bowel lumen and a subsequent protein-losing enteropathy. The lymphatic dysfunction may be primary or secondary to an obstructive lesion.

Basic Science

The primary form of intestinal-lymphangiectasia is congenital and is frequently associated with other lymphatic aberrations (e.g., in the extremities). It may be seen in patients with Turner or Noonan syndrome. The secondary form is the result of obstruction to lymph flow, either from anatomic malformations such as a malrotation, or from inflammatory infiltrative disorders affecting the intestine and its mesentery, such as regional enteritis, scleroderma, retroperitoneal tumors, or lymphomas. In both forms, massive protein leakage into the lumen of the bowel exceeds the ability of the liver to synthesize amino acids at the rate that they are being lost, culminating in hypoalbuminemia and edema. Malabsorption of fat is also associated with this disorder. Furthermore, the large volume of lymph that leaks into the bowel leads to humoral and cellular immunologic abnormalities including hypogammaglobulinemia, lymphocytopenia, anergic responses to cutaneous stimulation, and an increased frequency of neoplasia.

Natural History

A child with intestinal lymphangiectasis will most commonly present with peripheral edema. In addition, diarrhea, abdominal distention, lymphadematous extremities, failure to gain weight with repeated infections, are often common presentations. Secondary pleural, ascitic, and pericardial effusions may occur due either to hypoalbuminemia or to secretion of lymph fluid in these areas stemming from a congenital lymphatic anomaly. While other etiologies for protein-losing enteropathy should be considered in a patient who is hypoalbuminemic, the absence of liver, heart, or kidney disease will often point to intestinal lymphangiectasia. Moreover, ascites, pleural effusion, or lymphadematous limbs are concurrent with the abdominal symptoms most often found in congenital intestinal lymphangiectasia.

Diagnosis

Laboratory findings are notable for hypoalbuminemia, hypogammaglobulinemia, and lymphopenia. (Renal, hepatic, and nutritional causes for those findings must also be eliminated.) Serum calcium may also be depressed, whereas stool fat content can be elevated. Examination of stool may reveal large numbers of lymphocytes. Radiographic evaluation may reveal a normal small bowel pattern. Abnormalities, however, can include nodular thickening of the bowel wall and dilution of the barium as it flows distally and mixes with the lymph secretions. A small bowel biopsy is recommended and will confirm the diagnosis of lymphangiectasia by revealing dilated lymphatic lacteals in the villi. If the lymphangiectasia involves only the submucosa, then the mucosal biopsy may be normal. Although a lymphangiogram is difficult to perform in a child, it can reveal stasis and reflux of lymphatics into the abdominal and mesenteric lymphatic system with subsequent extravasation of contrast into the proximal small intestine. A lymphangiogram will more commonly show diffuse hypoplasia of peripheral lymphatics, periaortic lymph nodes and often total absence of the thoracic duct.

Treatment

Medical therapy is directed toward reducing intestinal lymphatic pressure via elimination of long chain fats from the diet. The use of medium-chain triglycerides is, therefore, recommended for these patients, but is largely effective only where the lymphangiectasia is limited to the lamina propria. Water-soluble vitamins and calcium supplements are also necessary. If frequent infections occur because of hypogammaglobulinemia, γ-globulin injections may be necessary, with appropriate use of antibiotics for a specific infection. The use of albumin with a diuretic will provide only short-term symptomatic relief.

In rare cases if the lesion is localized to only a small area of the bowel, surgery can be performed. Surgery is also indicated if the pleura and pericardium are involved.

CASE ILLUSTRATION

A 17-year-old white female presented with intermittent abdominal pain, vomiting, and ankle edema for 1 month. Her examination was unremarkable but initial laboratory values were notable for a hematocrit of 41%, a white blood count of 8100/mm^3, with 91% polys, 6% lymphs, a sedimentation rate of 3 mm/hr, a total protein of 3.3 mg/dl, and an albumin of 2 mg/dl. Urinalysis, electrolytes, liver function tests, and amylase were all normal. An IgG, however, was 80 mg/dl.

QUESTION AND COMMENT

What are the diagnostic possibilities and what further work-up is needed?

The lymphopenia, hypogammaglobulinemia, and hypoalbuminemia are consistent with lymphatic dysfunction and a protein-losing enteropathy, suggestive of lymphangiectasis, although a primary (congenital) versus a secondary (acquired obstructive) form could not be initially differentiated. Therefore, an upper GI series was performed and revealed a wide duodenal loop consistent with a mass effect, although no discrete mass could be identified on CT or ultrasonography. A CT scan did, however, show an ill-defined mass that appeared to blend in with the head of the pancreas although a subsequent endoscopic retrograde cholangiopancreatogram showed a normal unobstructed pancreatic duct.

Since primary and secondary lymphangiectasis could not be distinguished by diagnostic work-up in this patient, an exploratory laparotomy was performed. Operative findings revealed distended lymphatic channels in small bowel mesentery, retroperitoneum, and peripancreatic areas consistent with primary congenital lymphangiectasia of the mesenteric lymphatics. A small bowel biopsy revealed normal lamina propria indicating patchy involvement.

This patient is unusual in that she presented with presumed congenital lymphangiectasis in adolescence. Because of the diffuse lymphatic involvement seen at laparotomy, further surgical therapy (in the absence of localizable obstruction) was not warranted. Instead she was managed medically on a diet of medium-chain tryglycerides, water-soluble vitamins, calcium supplements, and γ-globulin injections. The prognosis for this patient is variable with complications including frequent infections and/or episodes of tetany.

Prognosis

Despite medical and surgical manipulations, a total remission is rare and exacerbations continue to occur throughout the patient's lifetime.

Short Bowel Syndrome

Definition

The short bowel syndrome encompasses a spectrum of GI problems that can result after an extensive small bowel resection. These problems can include alterations in digestion, motility, absorption, and secretion.

Basic Science

The degree of GI difficulty that a child experiences after small bowel resection depends on the extent of resection, the area of small bowel involved, the function of bowel that remains, the preservation of the ileocecal valve, and the ability of the shortened intestine to readapt after the surgery. GI motility may be increased owing to a decrease in the surface area available for absorption, increased bacterial overgrowth, gastric hypersecretion, and increased secretion of deconjugated and dehydroxylated bile acids which can serve as potent cathartics. Digestion is impaired secondary to impaired pancreatic function. Gastric hypersecretion and a decreased transit time diminish the transformation of zymogens into active proteolytic enzymes and also decrease the hydrolysis of fat by lipase. In addition, lack of conjugated bile acids also leads to poor micelle formation and inhibits lipid digestion. Disaccharides and polypeptides are also poorly digested owing to accelerated transit time and changes in the brush border stemming from bacterial contamination. The loss of the jejunum will also impair absorption of disaccharides and peptides. Maintaining the ileocecal valve at the time of surgery is always advantageous in terms of preventing massive malabsorption of water, electrolytes, fat, protein, carbohydrates, and vitamins, since it prevents further bacterial overgrowth and helps to slow transit time. Gastric hypersecretion is thought to be due to the removal of an inhibiting intestinal factor. The hypersecretion can predispose to peptic ulcer disease as well as malabsorption via destruction by acid of the mucosal surface.

Natural History

A resection of up to 40% of the total length of the small bowel is usually well-tolerated, assuming the duodenum, jejunum, distal half of the ileum (for B_{12}, folate, and bile acid absorption), and the ileocecal valve remain in contact. Otherwise, serious functional problems including diarrhea and malabsorption will result. Resections of over 70% of the small bowel can be life-threatening. In neonates, most resections are performed to correct congenital malformations such as intestinal malrotation, ileal or jejunal atresia, meconium ilius, volvulus, and duplications. Necrotizing enterocolitis may require extensive bowel resection. In older children, regional ileitis (Crohn disease) and intussusceptions are the most common causes of intestinal resection. The hypersecretion that results postoperatively is often self-limited and does not require immediate vagotomy or pyloroplasty since a decreased emptying time following surgery may, in fact, worsen steatorrhea.

The most common clinical finding in a patient with the short bowel syndrome is diarrhea. Vomiting after surgery should suggest a stricture at the anastomotic site or the presence of a stagnant loop. Often the diarrhea will improve as the absorptive surface increases in diameter and thickness, with the villi showing increased arborization. A decrease in the gastric hypersecretion and in the motility of the stomach and small bowel effectively increases the functional absorptive capacity for fat, proteins, and carbohydrates. This is more often seen when the ileum is left after a proximal resection than when the jejunum remains after a distal resection. The body habitus shows a rapid weight loss with diminished body fat and increased muscle wasting. Some patients become rapidly dehydrated and need increased salt. Anemia and hypoproteinemia may accompany the syndrome.

Bacterial overgrowth, the introduction of colonic bacteria into the small intestine, may complicate short bowel syndrome, as well as other chronic intestinal conditions. It is characterized by steatorrhea, weight loss, and anemia.

Diagnosis

Clinical manifestations of short bowel are diarrhea and rapid weight loss, anemia and hypoproteinemia. Evidence of vitamin D deficiency and low serum calcium levels secondary to malabsorption of calcium are common. Low magnesium will parallel hypocalcemia. Iron deficiency anemia is more likely if the upper small bowel has been resected, whereas B_{12} deficiency can result from removal of the lower small bowel. A patient who presents with bleeding and/or purpura may have coagulation difficulties from malabsorption of the fat-soluble vitamin K. Diagnostic work-up for a child with suspected short bowel syndrome should include documentation of intestinal transit time by use of nonabsorbable marker such as carmine red. Radiographic studies can also be used to estimate the length of remaining bowel and to ensure that there is normal caliber without stenosis or stricture throughout. If dilatation is observed proximal to the anastomosis, cultures of small bowel contents should be obtained to assess bacterial overgrowth and institute appropriate treatment.

Diagnostic tests are useful for evaluating the status of the appropriate absorptive mechanisms for carbohydrates (d-xylose and lactose absorption tests), fat and proteins (stool collections to document fat and nitrogen balance and with measurement of serum, protein, and albumin), and for bile acids, vitamins, and iron absorption.

Treatment

There are three mainstays of conventional treatment: (1) use of antimotility agents; (2) treatment of small bowel bacterial overgrowth with antibiotics; and (3) cholestyramine to bind bile acids. Dietary needs deserve close attention to avoid problems with malnutrition. Usually parenteral alimentation is needed to supplement the oral calories, which are often insufficient. Even when a few calories are obtained by mouth, this route of administration should be kept "active" as tolerated to stimulate intestinal development. A low osmolar solution consisting of protein hydrolysates and monosaccharides in a solution containing medium-chain versus long-chain triglycerides is likely to be tolerated. If the stool is positive for reducing substance or increased in amount, the limit of the ability of the bowel to tolerate the formula has been reached and a formula of lower caloric density should be tried after a 1- to 2-day fasting period.

Continuous enteral feeding has an advantage over boluses given every 3 or 4 hours, in that low osmolality is maintained while the number of calories is increased. Elemental diets have also been used to aid in the induction of adaptive changes in the bowel that remains. Once a hypo-osmolar formula has been tolerated, it may be increased to an isosmolar formula containing glucose polymers and eventually to a complex formula with disaccharides and even lactose as a source of carbohydrate. During this period, frequent small meals are better than a few large ones. The use of medium-chain trigylcerides should be maintained as a source of fat. Appropriate iron, trace elements, and vitamins should be administered.

The use of antacids or cimetidine to combat the initial gastric hypersecretion has been found to be of more benefit in adults than in children. Cholestyramine has not been found to be any more effective than the institution of a low-fat diet with medium-chain triglycerides to prevent the voluminous watery diarrhea that can be associated with losses of bile acids. If bacterial overgrowth is detected, antibiotics should be used unless such overgrowth is due to presence of a stagnant loop, in which case surgery to remove the site in the small bowel is the treatment of choice. If bacterial overgrowth is found on biopsy, courses of antibiotics that are active against anaerobic as well as aerobic bacteria are useful.

Prevention and Prognosis

A study of 50 infants who had extensive small bowel resections before age 2 months revealed that those who had at least 38 cm of small bowel remaining had a mortality rate of less than 5%. If 15–38 cm of small bowel were left the mortality rate increased to 50%. Survival, however, correlated significantly with the presence of the ileocecal valve. All 11 patients who had less than 40 cm of small bowel and who had lost their ileocecal valve died (Bohane et al, 1979). Of note, this study was performed before the addition of parenteral hyperalimentation and more recent clinical studies have suggested improved mortality with this therapeutic modality. In addition, it is not clear what role intestinal transplantation (if it becomes possible) will play in improving the prognosis of these patients, nor what complications will result in those children who remain hyperalimentation dependent throughout life (Caniano and Kanoti, 1988). If children survive the first year after surgery, they will usually be able to resume a normal diet except for some moderate reduction of fat. Moreover, they demonstrate good catch-up growth.

Approach to Rectal Bleeding

Definition

Hemorrhage occurring in any region of the GI tract can present as rectal bleeding in childhood.

Basic Science

The pathophysiology of rectal bleeding depends upon the anatomic site from which the bleeding originates. If bleeding is believed to originate from the UGI tract, the stool is usually melanotic, although occasionally it may be bright red if transit through the GI system is rapid. UGI tract bleeding presenting per rectum is most likely to occur secondary to ulcer disease. Esophageal varices can also present with rectal bleeding, although rarely within the first year of life.

Lower GI tract bleeding (that is, bleeding distal to the ligament of Treitz) can originate from a multiplicity of sites and for a variety of reasons, many of which are age dependent. For example, in the first year of life, anal fissures are the most common etiology while colitis secondary to infection or milk protein or soy intolerance is the second most frequent diagnosis (see specific disease entity for pathophysiologic mechanism).

Diagnosis

It is essential in ascertaining the cause of rectal bleeding to be aware of the child's age and the conditions that are age-specific. Other important points in the history are the quantity of blood per rectum, the color of the blood, although this is not necessarily pathognomonic in that esophageal varices may present as hematochezia, while a bleeding polyp may present as melena or black tarry stools. It is also important to ascertain by the history that the child is actually producing blood since ingested food coloring, beets, and some gelatins can resemble rectal bleeding.

Physical examination should focus on the condition of the patient which may warrant volume resuscitation for significant blood loss. A rectal examination is mandatory to ascertain the presence of anal fissures, polyp, stricture, or stenosis. The presence or absence of abdominal pain, pallor, diarrhea, fever, or vomiting can help pinpoint a diagnosis.

The most helpful initial diagnostic test is the use of a nasogastric tube to determine whether a gastric aspirate is heme-positive. A positive nasogastric aspirate identifies UGI bleeding (i.e., proximal to the ligament of Treitz) in a large percentage of patients (Hillemeir, 1983). If the nasogastric aspirate is negative, stools should be cultured, and rectosigmoidoscopy should be performed since the latter can distinguish inflamed mucosa from simply blood-covered mucosa, in that the inflamed or active colitis areas will appear erythematous, friable, granular, or ulcerated. Detection of a pseudomembrane may indicate the presence of *Clostridium difficile* toxin although other infectious organisms can be identified only from stool cultures. A history of delayed growth, weight loss, fevers, and/or abdominal pain, should suggest a more chronic process and raise the suspicion of an inflammatory bowel disease such as ulcerative colitis or regional enteritis (Crohn disease).

A fecal smear for Gram or Wright stain should be performed to document colitis and possible infection. Barium enema, radionucleotide scanning, or colonoscopy might also be considered. The precise order by which these studies should be performed remains somewhat controversial. In one clinical series, examination of the anal region and rectosigmoidoscopy with stool cultures were able to disclose the source of bleeding in 75% of children who presented with problems in the lower GI tract (Cucchiara et al, 1983). Yet while rectosigmoidoscopy enables stool to be obtained for culture and microscopic examination thus permitting a histologic diagnosis of colitis, it will not demonstrate colitis in other anatomic areas of the colon that can be seen by radiography with air contrast with barium. Radionuclide scintiscanning is also useful in diagnosis. The use of 99-TC sodium pertechnetate utilized by parietal cells in the gastric mucosa also permits visualization of ectopic gastric mucosa, such as that in a Meckel diverticulum. The precise sequence of procedure that should follow rectosigmoidoscopy depends on the leading clinical suspicion as no proven algorithm accounts for all diagnostic possibilities. For example, if intestinal obstruction is suspected, barium may be slowly inserted rectally although this will hamper subsequent colonoscopy. On the other hand, if the bleeding persists with a negative sigmoidoscopy and no evidence of obstruction, a Meckel scan might precede the use of barium. If the bleeding is life-threatening, angiography is in order to try to identify the vessel.

Treatment

If the rectal bleeding is profuse and associated with vascular instability, volume resuscitation is the most important priority in therapy. Once volume has been re-expanded through the use of crystalloid or, if necessary, emergency blood replacement, therapeutic efforts should be directed toward blocking the site of hemorrhage. If volume replacement is not adequate and bleeding is life-threatening, a surgical diagnostic and therapeutic approach may be used to tamponade the bleeding, although this is rarely useful in the setting of severe inflammatory bowel disease or in localizing an arteriovenous malformation. Selective angiography has allowed the injection of vasoconstrictive drugs or embolization materials into specific sites of vascular leakage.

Approach to Constipation

Definition

Constipation refers to the passage of a hard or firm stool. The definition is not dependent upon the frequency by which stools are passed since this can vary greatly during childhood and is influenced to a large extent by dietary and social patterns. However, if the intervals between passage of hard stools are extremely prolonged, the condition is referred to as obstipation. If constipation persists on a chronic basis such that there is also fecal soiling, the condition is known as encopresis (see pp. 39–41).

Basic Science

Rectal continence is a function of both voluntary and involuntary muscle activities. The internal sphincter represents a smooth muscle that relaxes upon distention by gas or fecal material. With relaxation of the internal sphincter, pressure increases on the external sphincter (under voluntary control) which can relax to allow defecation by utilizing the abdominal muscles, diaphragm, and the levator ani muscle complex. Rectal continence is usually achieved between the second and third year of life. Simple constipation occurs when mechanisms exist that increase the rate of water and electrolyte absorption in the colon and, hence, cause hardening of the stools. This increased absorption may be a result of inappropriate diet (e.g., excess intake of cow's milk or lack of bulk), excess use of certain medications that will delay colonic motility, anatomical defects of the GI tract, an obstruct passage of normal fecal material, and neuromuscular diseases. In addition, psychosocial factors have been associated with the development and course of acute episodes of constipation.

The development of fecal incontinence is believed to result from the build-up of a large fecal mass in the rectosigmoid area such that the sleeve and sling of the levator ani become relaxed, allow shortening of the anal canal (so that there is essentially no distance between the internal and external sphincter), and hence produce constant leakage. Moreover, recent studies show that patients with chronic constipation have associated disorders, e.g., some form of outlet obstruction, such as a painful anal fissure or polyp and/or abnormal manometric studies indicating that a higher than normal intrarectal pressure is required to relax the internal sphincter, an increased anal resting pressure, or a blunted subjective perception of the urge to defecate.

Epidemiology

Constipation accounts for 3% of all medical referrals and 3–6% of psychiatric referrals (Levine, 1981). A study of 186 children suggested that over 50% of the patients had a familial incidence of constipation, suggesting an underlying genetic predisposition to this disorder (Abrahamian and Lloyd-Still, 1984). Encopresis by definition is rare before age 3 years, and affects males more than females.

Natural History

Constipation noted during the newborn period is never functional and intestinal obstruction must be ruled out. The inability to pass meconium during the first 24 hours of life may signify obstruction. Newborns will often show abdominal distention, bilious vomitus, and respiratory distress when failure to pass meconium is due to bowel obstruction. During infancy, constipation usually is secondary to dietary manipulations, most commonly, the introduction of solid foods. In addition, excess intake of cow's milk or change from breast to bottle can result in the passage of decreased numbers of firm hard stools.

In older infants, environmental or dietary changes or an intercurrent illness are largely responsible for the onset of an episode of acute constipation. In addition, anal fissures continue to play an important role in the young child and the pediatrician should ask about blood-streaking around stools. As the child is taught toilet training, the interplay of familial and psychosocial factors contribute to the onset of constipation. It may not be until the child is past the age of toilet training when fecal soiling begins, that constipation first arises. In the school-age child if the urge to defecate arrives at inopportune times, the suppression or the withholding of defecation may lead to chronic constipation. Toilet training that can never be completed may also be a clue to the presence of localized neurologic lesion affecting sphincter competence, such as a myelomeningocele or a tumor of the cauda equina. Failure to gain weight is very uncommon in the setting of constipation. Studies on encopretic patients show that 40% were never toilet trained, and enuresis is an associated problem in 30%, with the likelihood of urinary tract infections also being increased (Levine, 1981).

Diagnosis

The diagnostic evaluation should begin with a careful bowel history that focuses on frequency, descriptive characteristics, and any therapeutic interventions previously tried. Associated symptoms such as abdominal pain, distention, vomiting, or growth problems, that can point to an organic cause require further diagnostic work-up. The use of any medications should also be ascertained since anticholinergic agents, antacids, some anticonvulsants, diuretics, and iron preparations can lead to constipation. Before doing a rectal examination, however, the perineal area and most important, the anus, the perirectal tissues, and lower spine should be inspected. If the anus is anteriorly displaced, a posterior shelf on the back lip of the anus can be palpated, which can become obstructive and be the source for constipation. If constipation has been chronic, the child may be withdrawn and depressed and unwilling to discuss his condition. A rectal examination in the chronically constipated child may show a much shortened anal canal with minimal sphincter tone. In addition, the rectal ampulla is usually large and filled with fecal material. In this situation, further diagnostic tests may be needed to rule out short segment Hirschsprung disease. In chronic constipation, a radiograph of the abdomen shows a colon completely dilated with stool. A plain radiograph usually does not distinguish between chronic constipation and Hirschsprung disease. A barium enema, on the other hand, will show a completely dilated colon extending to the anus, whereas aganglionic megacolon will have a narrow segment in the area that is devoid of ganglia. The barium enema, however, is not useful in making this diagnosis in infancy before a "transition zone" between the ganglia and aganglionic region has developed.

Treatment

A brief episode of constipation usually requires alterations in diet and the use of a stool softener. Dietary changes should include an increase in fluid intake and in fiber that can prevent stool hardening. Many infants have been found to produce softer stools when excess carbohydrate and prune juice are added to the diet. Stool softeners increase water and electrolyte secretion into bowel contents, hence, softening the stool. However, these softeners and laxatives can result in significant abdominal discomfort and cramping. If retention of stool is on a voluntary basis, however, laxatives and stool softeners will not be successful. Cathartics can lead to some degree of dependence, in addition to causing cramping and abdominal pain. The only laxative in the short-term constipated child that has been found to be of some use has been mineral oil, although the child should be old enough to swallow the substance without increased risk of aspiration. On a long-term basis, mineral oil is subject to poor compliance.

A much more aggressive and organized approach is required for treatment of a child with chronic constipation, particularly if there is fecal impaction. Impaction can be treated first by the administration of a hypertonic phosphate enema at a dose of 3 ml/kg, but this approach carries the possibility of hypertonic dehydration, hypocalcemic tetany, and hyperphosphatemia. Isotonic saline enemas may be used 1–2 hours after the administration of a hypertonic phosphate enema that has been unsuccessful, although shock has been reported after instillation of even small amounts of a saline solution. Tap water enemas are not recommended in children because of the possibility of water intoxication. Digital disimpaction is rarely necessary.

Concurrent with the initial catharsis is an initial counseling period at which time the child is educated not to feel embarrassed about the urge to defecate and to understand the mechanisms involved in causing the bowels to lose their muscular tone. Once the impaction has been remedied, the institution of a maintenance program involving dietary adjustment, mineral oil, and an oral laxative is helpful. During this time, required toilet-sitting periods should be inserted into the child's day so that regular bowel habits are developed. If an anteriorly displaced anus with a posterior shelf has been detected, an anoplasty may be necessary. Behavior modification techniques and biofeedback maneuvers are beginning to be used with increased effectiveness. Treatment for chronic constipation usually requires at least 6 months of maintenance therapy because partially treated conditions result in recurrence of symptoms. Parental guilt over the problem must be recognized. In those instances where therapeutic efforts may fail because of serious family psychopathology, psychiatric referral may be needed, but medical management must continue as well.

Prevention and Follow-up

About 20–40% of all patients with chronic constipation show relapse over a 5-year follow-up period (Abrahamian and Lloyd-Still, 1984). The only predictor of poor outcome is persistent soiling. Roughly one-third of patients will have resolved their symptoms within the first 6 months of treatment and over 90% of those cured after the initial episode will have recovered completely after 24 months of treatment. Usually treatment (especially diet) should be continued for at least 1 year and, in some cases, 3 years or more. One of the major reasons for recurrence is patient noncompliance owing to the long duration and poor tolerance of the agents used for therapy. Some studies suggest that the parents, rather than the children, are responsible for noncompliance, by failure to insist that their children follow the recommended treatment regimen (Abrahamian and Lloyd-Still, 1984).

REFERENCES

Abrahamian FP, Lloyd-Still JD: Chronic constipation in childhood: A longitudinal study of 186 patients. *J Pediatr Gastroenterol Nutr* 3:460, 1984.

Ament ME, Barclay GM: Chronic diarrhea. *Pediatr Ann* 11:124, 1982.

Anderson CM: Malabsorption in children. *Clin Gastroenterol* 6:355, 1977.

Angelides AG, Davidson M: Lactase intolerance and diarrhea: Are they related? *Pediatr Ann* 14:62, 1985.

Auricchio S, Greco L, Troncone R: Gluten-sensitive enteropathy in childhood. *Pediatr Clin North Am* 35:157, 1988.

Banarll JG: Pathophysiology of diarrhea. In Gorbavk JL (ed): *Infectious Diarrhea*. Boston, Blackwell, 1986, p. 1.

Barr RG, Levine MD, Watkins JB: Lactase intolerance in recurrent abdominal pain in childhood. *N Engl J Med* 300:1449, 1979.

Berg NO, Borulf S, Jakobsson I, et al: How to approach the child suspected of malabsorption. *Acta Pediatr Scand* 67:403, 1978.

Bertele RM, Burgin-Wolff A, Berger R, et al: The fluorescent immunosorbent test for IgG gliadin antibodies and the leucocyte migration inhibition test in coeliac disease; comparison of diagnostic value. *Eur J Pediatr* 144:58, 1985.

Bishop WP, Ulshen MH: Bacteral gastroenteritis. *Pediatr Clin North Am* 35:69, 1988.

Blacklow NR: CPC. *N Engl J Med* 313:805, 1985.

Bohane TD, Haka-Ikse K, Biggar WD, et al: The clinical study of young infants after small intestinal resection. *J Pediatr* 94:552, 1979.

Caniano DA, Kanoti GA: Newborns with massive intestinal loss: Difficult choices. *N Engl J Med* 318:703, 1988.

Clayden GS, Lawson JON: Investigation and management of long standing chronic constipation in childhood. *Arch Dis Child* 51:918, 1976.

Committee on Nutrition of AAP: The practical significance of lactase intolerance in children. *Pediatrics* 62:240, 1978.

Cucchiara S, Guandalini S, Staiano A, et al: Sigmoidoscopy: Colonoscopy, and radiology in the evaluation of children with rectal bleeding. *Pediatr Gastroenterol Nutr* 2:667, 1983.

Freiburghaus AU, Schmitz J, Schindler M, et al: Protein patterns of brush-border fragments in congenital lactase malabsorption and in specific hypolactasia of the adult. *N Engl J Med* 294:1030, 1976.

Hendren WH: Constipation caused by anterior location of the anus and its surgical correction. *J Pediatr Surg* 13:505, 1978.

Hillemeier C: Rectal bleeding in childhood. *Pediatr Rev* 5:35, 1983.

Kerzner V: Pathogenesis of diarrhea. From *Diagnosis and Management of Acute Diarrhea*. Ross Roundtable, p. 39, Aug 1982.

Larsen SA, Homer DR: Relation of breast versus bottle feeding to hospitalization for gastroenteritis in a middle-class U.S. population. *J Pediatr* 92:417, 1978.

Lebenthal E, Branski D: Childhood celiac disease: A reappraisal. *J Pediatr* 98:681, 1981.

Levine MD: The school child with encopresis. *Pediatr Rev* 2:285, 1981.

Lifshitz F: Acute and chronic diarrhea in childhood. *Pract Gastroenterol Ent* 6:8, 1982.

Lifshitz F: Childhood diarrhea. In Silverberg M (ed): *Pediatric Gastroenterology*. New Hyde Park, NY, Medical Examination, 1983, p. 286.

Lifshitz F, Fagundes-Neto U: The malabsorption syndrome. In Silverberg M (ed): *Pediatric Gastroenterology*. New Hyde Park, New York, Medical Examination, 1983, p. 313.

Lo CW, Walker WA: Chronic protracted diarrhea of infancy: A nutritional disease. *Pediatrics* 72:786, 1983.

MacLean WC, Fink BB: Lactase malabsorption by premature infants: Magnitude and clinical significance. *J Pediatr* 97:383, 1980.

McCormick MC: Epidemiology of diarrhea in the United States. From *Diagnosis and Management of Acute Diarrhea,* 13th Ross Roundtable, 1982, p 1.

Merritt RJ, Shah PH, et al: Treatment of protractive diarrhea of infancy. *Am J Dis Child* 138:770, 1984.

Olness K, McFarland FA, Piper J: Biofeedback: A new modality in the management of children with fecal soiling. *J Pediatr* 96:505, 1980.

Savilahti E, Launiala K, Kuitunen P: Congenital lactase deficiency. *Arch Dis Child* 58:246, 1983.

Schussheim A: Gastrointestinal bleeding. In Silverberg M (ed): *Pediatric Gastroenterology*. New Hyde Park, New York, Medical Examination, Chapter 11, 1983, p. 255.

Schuster MM: Chronic constipation in children: The need for hard data about normal stools. *J Pediatr Gastroenterol Nutr* 3:336, 1984.

Shah PC, Lebenthal E: Gluten-sensitive enteropathy: A practical approach. *Pediatr Basic* 34:4, 1983.

Silverberg M (ed): Celiac disease: Gluten-sensitive enteropathy. In: *Pediatric Gastroenterology*. New Hyde Park, New York, Medical Examination, 1983, p. 315.

Silverberg M (ed): Chapter 10—Constipation. In: *Pediatric Gastroenterology*. New Hyde Park, New York, Medical Examination, 1983, p. 247.

Silverman A, Roy CC: *Pediatric Clinical Gastroenterology*. St. Louis, CV Mosby, 1983, pp. 25, 249, 308.

Snyder JD, Merson MH: The magnitude of the global problem of acute diarrheal disease; a review of active surveillance data. *Bull WHO* 60:605, 1982.

Sunshine P: What pediatricians should know about malabsorption but are afraid to ask. *Current Concepts,* Spring, 1974.

Williams CB, et al: Total colonoscopy in children. *Arch Dis Child* 57:49, 1982.

Wilmore DW: Factors correlating with the successful outcome following extensive intestinal resection in newborn infants. *J Pediatr* 80:88, 1972.

Diagnosis and Therapy of Specific Diseases of the Lower Gastrointestinal Tract

4

INFLAMMATORY DISORDERS

Appendicitis

Definition

Appendicitis is an acute inflammation of the appendix.

Basic Science

The pathophysiologic origin for the pain in appendicitis begins with obstruction of the appendix, often secondary to impacted fecal material. This causes a closed viscus to swell secondary to the obstruction. Stretch receptors located in the small blood vessels of the swollen appendix will send nerve impulses along mesenteric fibers that refer pain to the dermatome innervated by the 10th thoracic nerve at the level of the umbilicus; hence, the initial origin of periumbilical pain in this disorder.

As the localized swelling continues, small amounts of exudative inflammatory fluid leak through the walls of the appendix into the parietal peritoneum. The purulent fluid and not the appendix itself, upon contact with the parietal peritoneum, causes a localized and more intense pain than that which is being referred to the periumbilical area and overshadows this earlier referred pain. It is the localized area of the peritoneum with which the inflammatory fluid comes into contact that determines where the patient perceives the localized pain. For example, in a retrocecal appendicitis, the right lower quadrant parietal peritoneum never receives the fluid and, hence, periumbilical pain may persist for a much longer time. If a perforation occurs, a child may momentarily feel better because of relief of intraluminal pressure; however, the increased seepage of inflammatory fluid and contents will soon intensify the localized and eventually generalized abdominal pain, and peritonitis results.

Epidemiology

Appendicitis is one of the most common causes of a surgical abdomen. Perforation rate at time of diagnosis varies from 17–40%, with the higher frequency occurring in younger age groups. The mean age of presentation is 10 years of age, although cases have been reported in newborn infants. The mortality rate for a child with appendicitis ranges from 0.1–1% (Hatch, 1985).

Natural History

The importance of understanding the natural history of a developing appendicitis is to be able to make a diagnosis before perforation. In children, the appendix commonly perforates at about 36 hours after pain begins. By 24 hours after onset of pain (which can often be documented as the time of the child's last good meal), 20% of children will already have perforated and, by 48 hours, 80% will have suffered a perforated appendix with peritonitis (Brender et al, 1985). The first symptom is usually periumbilical pain, which is often associated with nausea and vomiting. After a few hours, the pain will shift to wherever the inflammatory fluid makes contact with parietal peritoneum, most often in the right lower quadrant in older children and adults.

The diarrhea of appendicitis is low volume and contains mucus, secondary to localized irritation of the colon or rectosigmoid area by inflammatory fluid. High volume frequent watery diarrhea is more often associated with a viral gastroenteritis.

Once the appendix has perforated, the child will often lie still with legs drawn up. There may be increased tachypnea with inspirations being stopped short secondary to abdominal pain. Vomiting is more frequent following perforation and vomitus may contain small bowel contents because of a paralytic ileus. The child will often develop a temperature over 38.5°C and complain of pain and muscle spasms over the entire abdominal wall, rather than just in the right lower quadrant. In older children, the inflamed area around the perforation may be walled off to form an appendeceal abscess. It is only when this abscess ruptures that the child will begin to show signs of extreme toxicity and sepsis, often over a week after the initial perforation.

Diagnosis

From a historical standpoint, the onset of pain relative to when the last meal was eaten should be documented. A description of the pain and whether it has changed over a period of time is useful, together with information on what makes the pain better or worse; what other symptoms are associated with that pain; and whether anyone else in the family has a concurrent illness. Inquiring about the ride to the hospital or whether the child desires his favorite food often aids in ascertaining the severity of pain. With peritoneal irritation any movement will make the pain worse and the child will want to curl up and splint to bring temporary relief. The differential diagnosis of the acute abdomen includes gastroenteritis, urinary tract infection, constipation, pelvic inflammatory disease (in an older child), a bacterial enteritis (e.g., especially *Yersinia),* and occasionally a right or left lobe pneumonia that will also refer pain to the regions innervated by the 10th and 11th thoracic nerves.

The physical examination can become the basis for surgical intervention. Much can be gleaned from observation of the child and his position and whether he can be consoled when held by a parent. Asking the child to point to the area of most irritation or allowing your hand to guide the child's hand over to the area of most irritation can be a helpful way to elicit tenderness, guarding, spasm, and rebound. Guarding represents voluntary stiffening of the rectus muscle, whereas spasm is involuntary rigidity of this muscle secondary to localized peritoneal irritation. Rebound tenderness reflects the rate of stretch of the parietal peritoneum. Other conditions that are nonsurgical can also result in rebound tenderness, including severe gastroenteritis, pneumonia, lead poisoning, and Henoch-Schönlein purpura.

If the anterior abdominal wall is involved, with peritoneal irritation, the maximum point of tenderness will be an area two-thirds of the way between the umbilicus and the anterior iliac spine, referred to as McBurney point because of the physician who first identified that area.

Guarding, spasm, and rebound tenderness are signs that occur on the anterior abdominal wall. The abdomen, however, is a six-sided cavity and if the inflammatory fluid has not involved the anterior abdominal wall, these physical findings may be absent. The subdiaphragmatic peritoneum, pelvic peritoneum, and the posterior and lateral aspects of the abdomen will also be important areas from which to attempt to elicit pain. Hence, a child may only have costovertebral angle tenderness, shoulder pain, or pain solely on rectal examination, if other areas of the peritoneal wall are involved. The rectal examination will help determine whether pain persists in other areas of the peritoneum. Asking the child to try and have a bowel movement at the time of doing a digital rectal examination will make the examination less stressful on the child and provide a much more accurate assessment of the degree of pain being elicited. Fever usually will not be elevated more than 1°C in a child unless the appendix has perforated, in which case the temperature may be higher.

In a child with an unperforated appendix the white count will usually be between 5000 and 20,000/mm^3 and may go higher if perforation occurs. Urinalysis can aid differentiation between a urinary tract infection, pyelonephritis, renal stone, and acute appendicitis. A child with acute appendicitis will have no more than 5–10 white cells per high power field and a few red cells. Often the urine specific gravity will be elevated with acute appendicitis.

A chest radiograph is appropriate to see if pneumonia is present. A radiograph of the abdomen can have several signs that are not pathognomonic but are suggestive of acute appendicitis, including a concave curvature of the spine to the right due to spasm of abdominal musculature, loss of peritoneal fat planes, disturbance of gas pattern in small and large bowel, a calcified fecalith, a paucity of bowel gas in the right lower quadrant, an increase in the thickness of the lateral abdominal wall owing to soft tissue edema, or evidence of free peritoneal fluid or air as confirmed by an upright film, although it is rare to see air as this is a closed space perforation (Fig. 7.6*A* and *B*). Fifty percent of children with fecaliths are likely to have a perforated appendix particularly if they are infants and toddlers (Brender et al, 1985). Although a barium enema may be helpful in difficult diagnoses, it should not be the sole basis for performing surgery since a high num-

CASE ILLUSTRATION

A 6-year-old male presented with a 2-day history of periumbilical pain. About 12 hours before admission, he became nauseated and started vomiting. Pain became acutely worse and was accompanied by more severe nausea and vomiting. The patient walked into the emergency room slowly and cautiously as if protecting his abdomen. When asked about the automobile ride to the hospital he described it as "very bumpy." On examination, he was alert but in some distress. He lay in a fetal position on the examining table, flushed and grunting with pain. Temperature was 40.2°C, respiration 20/min, pulse 124/min, blood pressure 104/72. Mucous membranes were slightly dry and abdominal examination was notable for rigid and board-like abdomen, with tenderness, both to direct palpation and on rebound. Bowel sounds were absent. On rectal examination, there was tenderness toward the right lower quadrant with guaiac-negative stool present in the ampulla. The blood count was 27,000/mm^3, with 61% polys, 17% bands. Electrolytes were within normal limits and urinalysis was unremarkable.

QUESTION AND COMMENT

Should this patient have an operation or should further work-up be performed?

Because of this patient's clinical presentation, the diagnosis of acute appendicitis with perforation was made, antibiotics were given, and the child was whisked to the operating room without a single additional test being performed. However, while waiting to be wheeled into the operating room, for inexplicable reasons, the patient's symptoms suddenly disappeared. On re-examination, his condition appeared entirely benign. As the discomfort subsided a productive cough developed. A portable chest radiograph was obtained outside the operating room and revealed a prominent right lower lobe pneumonia. The child was then admitted and treated with intravenous antibiotics, and observation, defeversed over the next 48 hours and was discharged to continue his course of antibiotic therapy as an outpatient. We present this case as a reminder that a right lower lobe pneumonia can masquerade as appendicitis.

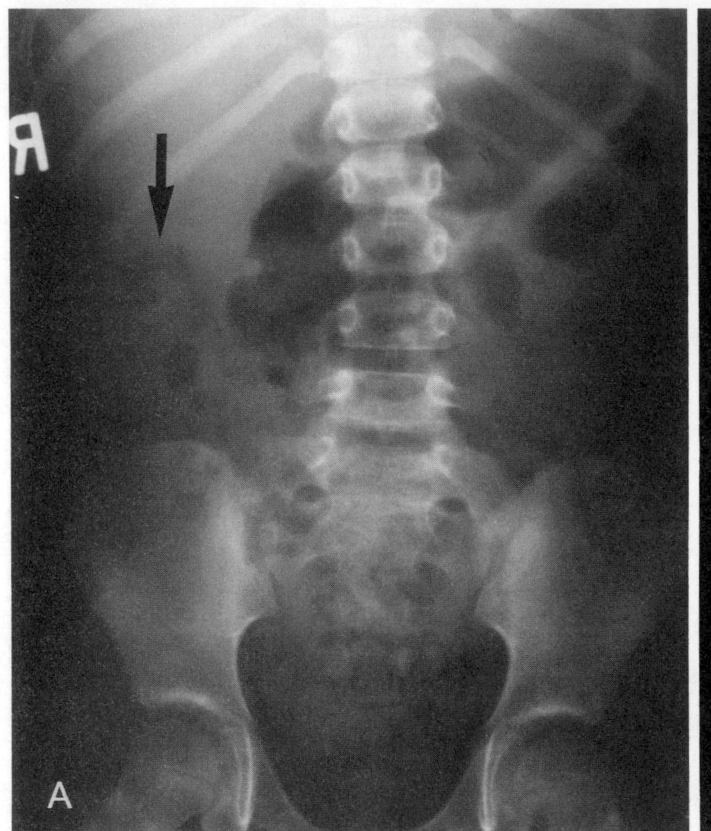

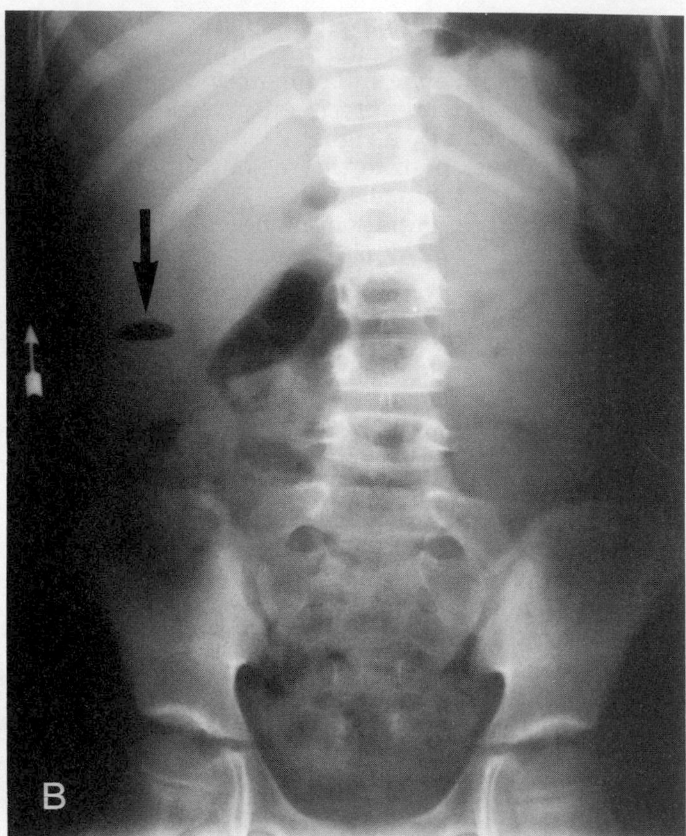

Figure 7.6. Supine **(A)** and upright **(B)** radiographs in this child show a gas-containing appendiceal abscess in the right hemiabdomen lateral to colonic gas *(arrows)*. The spine is curved, because the child is splinting her right side. A radiopaque appendicolith is not present.

ber of false-positives and false-negatives occur. Ultrasonography has been used in diagnosis of patients with appendiceal abscesses but to date has been of little value in diagnosing the child with early acute appendicitis.

Treatment

Appendectomy is the treatment of choice once the diagnosis is suspected. Antibiotics should be started as soon as the diagnosis is made, and should include either a broad spectrum cephalosporin or the combination of ampicillin, gentamicin, and clindamycin. A nasogastric tube is inserted to decompress the stomach and a right lower quadrant transverse incision is usually made to gain access to the peritoneal cavity. The appendix is removed and the appendiceal stump is ligated, rather than inverted (Malt, 1986). If no perforation is noted, the child should begin ambulation and activity early (on the second or third day following surgery) and be advanced quickly thereafter onto a normal diet with the return of peristaltic activity. If perforation has occurred, adequate drainage is needed for several days postoperatively.

If a right lower quadrant mass is present on presentation, intensive antibiotic therapy should be initiated, and the mass may resolve. If not, simple evacuation of pus may be needed. The appendix need not be removed unless signs and symptoms persist (Malt, 1986).

Prognosis

Complications of operation, which have included infertility from obstruction of Fallopian tubes and intestinal obstruction, chronic abdominal pain, and recurrent infections, occur at a frequency of less than 5% (Hatch, 1985).

Pseudomembranous Colitis

Definition

Pseudomembranous colitis (see also pp. 1063) represents a form of inflammatory bowel disease in which plaque-like lesions composed of fibrin, sloughed epithelial cells, mucin, and inflammatory cells are found throughout the intestines. At the beginning of this century, it was associated with patients who had had intestinal surgery, intestinal obstruction, colonic carcinoma, heavy metal poisoning, or ischemic cardiovascular disease. Over the past 20 years, however, it has become highly associated with use of antibiotics and, indeed, has also been referred to as antibiotic-associated pseudomembranous colitis.

Basic Science

Recently it has been discovered that toxins produced by the organism *Clostridium difficile* cause antibiotic-associated pseudomembranous colitis. One toxin designated a "cytotoxin" is potent in tissue culture assays and is a sensitive and specific marker for *C. difficile*-induced disease. The other toxin, referred to as toxin A, is much more potent in biologic assays of enterotoxins in animal models and is believed to be more important in causing the clinical gastrointestinal complications (Wald et al, 1980).

Epidemiology

The prevalence of antibiotic-associated pseudomembranous colitis appears to rise with increasing age and has been documented more often in adults than in children. Nevertheless, pediatric cases have been reported, often associated with antimicrobial usage. Amoxicillin and ampicillin are the most common offenders followed by clindamycin, lincomycin, and penicillin. Only with some aminoglycosides and vancomycin has the disease not been reported (Gebhard, 1985).

Natural History

There is a wide spectrum of clinical severity in pseudomembranous colitis. Diarrhea is the presenting symptom in almost all cases. In 50% of patients, diarrhea will occur while antibiotics are being administered. In the remainder, it will not develop until 4–6 weeks after antibiotic therapy has stopped. Antibiotic-associated diarrhea is often defined as 2–5 semisolid or liquid stools a day that represents a change in a patient's usual bowel pattern, with the change occurring within the time frame of antibiotic use described above. The diarrhea progresses to frank colitis in a minority of cases. Usually it will only last for 8–10 days after the antibiotic has been discontinued, but it has been reported to last for periods of 1–2 months. If colitis occurs in addition to diarrhea, the patient will have abdominal cramping and pain, fever, vomiting, tenesmus, abdominal distention, and dehydration. Late complications include electrolyte imbalance, hypoalbuminemia, anasarca, and toxic megacolon with perforation.

Diagnosis

The patient who meets diagnostic criteria on the basis of history of antibiotic use and physical examination should have the diagnosis confirmed by detection of *C. difficile* toxin, in tissue culture facilities that allow measurement of toxin titers or by simply detecting the toxin with an enzyme-linked immunoabsorbent assay (ELISA) or by counterimmunoelectrophoresis (CIE). The anatomic diagnosis can be made by sigmoidoscopy since the distal colon is usually involved, but if involvement is restricted to right colon or small bowel, colonoscopy may be needed. Endoscopic findings in patients with antibiotic-associated diarrhea range from a normal mucosa to a spectrum of changes including erythema and edema, friability, ulceration, and hemorrhage as well as the plaque-like lesions representing pseudomembranes. Sigmoidoscopy will show raised yellowish white plaques. A barium enema is contraindicated since the risk of perforation is high. Laboratory values will usually show hypoproteinemia, and a leukocytosis ranging from 10,000–20,000, although cases with white counts greater than 40,000 have been reported. Fever over 100°F is also common.

Treatment

Immediate therapy includes stopping administration of the antibiotic and rehydration that focuses on electrolyte replacement and correction of the hypoproteinemia with albumin. If symptoms of severe diarrhea persist after cessation of antibiotics, an alternative antibiotic, vancomycin, should be administered; usually within 2–3 days clinical improvement is noted. Therapy with vancomycin should be continued for at least a week. Use of vancomycin does have disadvantages, however: (1) it has a 20% relapse rate; (2) it is expensive; and (3) it has an unpleasant taste. If relapse does occur, vancomycin can be reused, although subsequent recurrences are equally possible with 20% frequency. Metronidazole and cholestyramine have also been used with some success.

Prognosis

With the use of vancomycin and appropriate rehydration, mortality in children with antibiotic-induced pseudomembranous colitis is virtually nil. However, the frequency of relapse ranges from 15–20% and multiple courses of vancomycin may be necessary (Bartlett et al, 1980).

Henoch-Schönlein Purpura

Definition

Henoch-Schönlein purpura (HSP) is a disease of unknown origin characterized by colicky abdominal pain, purpuric rash, and arthritis. Renal involvement characterized by hematuria, proteinuria, and/or hypertension is also commonly associated with the disease.

Basic Science

The pathophysiology of the disease is believed to be a vasculitis of unknown cause. Although cause and effect cannot be proven, strong associations exist between possible food and drug allergies or exposure to bacterial and viral infections (in particular, *Streptococcus, Mycoplasma pneumoniae,* and *Varicella),* in patients who subsequently develop HSP. The renal lesion shows diffuse mesangial proliferation with some focal variation. An excess IgA deposition can be demonstrated in the glomerular mesangium and, occasionally, along the basement membrane in severe cases. Whether IgA deposition in other organs, including the skin, plays a role in the disease has yet to be determined. IgA rheumatoid factor is elevated in about half the patients during the acute phase (Saulsbury, 1986).

Biopsy of the skin lesions reveals perivascular infiltration and thrombi in smaller vessels.

Epidemiology

HSP can affect any age group, but is most frequently found in patients between the ages of 6 months and 7 years. It is more common in males than females. Renal involvement has been reported to vary between 20% and 100%, with the disease being responsible for 15% of children who require dialysis for end-stage renal failure (Koskimies et al, 1981). There appears to be a seasonal incidence, with more cases in the spring and fall months (Silber, 1972).

Natural History

In most cases of HSP, an upper respiratory infection antedates the onset of the syndrome by 1–3 weeks. The skin rash is essential for the diagnosis, but need not occur before the abdominal pain or joint symptoms, although this is more common. The rash is usually urticarial initially, fading to a red macular or, occasionally, a red papular lesion which becomes purpuric, blotchy, and confluent. These lesions most often occur on the extensor surfaces of the lower extremities and on the buttocks and hands. The rash may persist for several weeks or may occur transiently over a period of months or even years. Recurrences of the rash may not be associated with other symptoms, despite multiple system involvement during the primary episode. In younger children, edema of scalp, face, upper and lower extremities may develop, which is thought to be due to a protein-losing enteropathy secondary to intestinal involvement. Two-thirds of patients will have joint findings which usually involve the ankles and knees, and less commonly the wrists and fingers. Usually only arthralgia is observed, with pain due to periarticular involvement rather than to bleeding or effusion into the joint. Joint symptoms may be recurrent as well but usually resolve completely with no permanent sequelae.

Abdominal symptoms consist of colicky abdominal pain which can mimic an acute abdomen and can cause a diagnostic problem if the rash is absent. Eighty percent of cases demonstrating abdominal symptoms will develop GI hemorrhage as characterized by melena, or occult blood in the stools and, more rarely, hematemesis. The mechanism appears to be submucosal hemorrhage, which may lead to localized ulceration of the mucosa associated with diffuse arterial inflammation and fibrinoid necrosis. Ileoileal or ileocecal intussusception has been described in 2–3% of patients with HSP (Meadow, 1979).

All affected children tend to have hematuria, and even those children who have normal urinalyses have been found to have an abnormal histologic picture on renal biopsy (Greifer et al, 1966). About 50% demonstrate albuminuria and microscopic hematuria and 20% show macroscopic hematuria. Those patients who have microscopic hematuria are likely to be completely normal subsequently, whereas 20% of the group with asymptomatic gross hematuria and proteinuria will develop permanent renal damage. Half of those few children who have acute nephritis with nephrosis will develop renal insufficiency. Less common features of the disease are CNS findings including headache, convulsions, hemiparesis, and coma often attributed to hypertensive encephalopathy, although intracerebral hemorrhages have also been reported. Testicular pain and scrotal swelling have also been noted (Byrn, 1976).

Diagnosis

The purpuric rash is essential for the diagnosis, with joint, renal, and GI symptoms being manifest either before, during or after the appearance of the skin rash. No laboratory studies are diagnostic of the disease, although stool should be tested for occult blood and a urinalysis is required in those presenting with a purpuric rash. Platelet counts are either normal or, in some cases, elevated and coagulation studies are normal also. The erythrocyte sedimentation rate has been reported to be both elevated and normal. Eosinophilia is rare, in contrast to periarteritis nodosa where peripheral eosinophilia is observed. IgA levels have been reported to be both elevated and normal within 3 months of onset of the skin rash and, thus, are of little diagnostic value. A serum complement level can distinguish poststreptococcal glomerular nephritis, in which the C3 level is low, from nephritis secondary to HSP, in which the level is normal. Radiographic studies with barium will show thumb printing of the barium column in small bowel from submucosal hemorrhage and, occasionally, an intussusception—typically ileoileal.

Treatment

Treatment remains strictly supportive, with no known therapeutic modality yet established. Although the rash appears urticarial, antihistaminic agents do not appear to ameliorate the course of the disease. Anti-inflammatory agents and salicylates have not been found to be effective for reducing joint symptoms, and they carry an increased risk for GI hemorrhage.

CONTROVERSIES

The question of steroid therapy in the treatment of HSP continues to be debated (Rosenblum and Winter, 1987). At present, it is commonly agreed that such therapy has no role in the treatment or prevention of the renal disease. It continues to be used for abdominal pain, but no adequate double-blind controlled study has evaluated the efficacy of steroids in influencing the course of the disease. The nephritic picture either will resolve spontaneously or progress to require dialysis for end-stage renal failure. Immunosuppressive agents other than steroids have not been found effective for the renal problems in this disorder.

CASE ILLUSTRATION

An 11-year-old male presented with a 10-day history of intermittent fever and abdominal pain, a 2- to 3-day history of an enlarged left testis and scrotum, and a 1-day onset of a rash in the lower extremities. His physical examination was notable for rash in the proximal thighs that was described as purpuric with central crusting, sparing the buttocks, and diffuse abdominal tenderness without rebound or guarding. Stool was guaiac-positive. His left scrotum was enlarged, tender, and indurated, with a swollen left testicle and epididymis. Laboratory values were notable for hematocrit of 32%, white count 9000/mm^3 with a normal differential and platelet count, and an ESR of 55 mm/hpf. Urinalysis showed 5–7 red cells but was otherwise normal. Ultrasonography and nuclear medicine scan ruled out a testicular torsion, evidence of testicular mass, or epididymitis and the patient's clinical status was considered to be most consistent with the vasculitic picture seen in HSP.

QUESTION AND COMMENT

How consistent is this case with HSP? How should this child be treated?

This case is unusual in that the abdominal pain preceded the rash by more than a week, whereas the opposite is more common. Testicular involvement has been noted in 2–38% of males with HSP. It is believed that the swelling represents edema in congestion of the cord, epididymis, and testes, along with inflammatory infiltrate and necrosis of blood vessels.

The abdominal symptoms were not considered severe enough to merit use of steroids which remains a controversial treatment for HSP. There is no report of steroids as treatment for the scrotal swelling and, in fact, with just heat and elevation the patient's testicular symptoms improved dramatically.

Prognosis

Mortality is estimated at 2%, solely due to renal involvement. Morbidity can result from the pain and severity of symptoms and/or the need for surgical intervention, for example, if an intussusception occurs. The overall prognosis in children, however, continues to be a good one.

Crohn Disease

Definition

Crohn disease or regional enteritis represents a chronic inflammatory disorder that can affect any part of the GI tract, from mouth to anus.

Basic Science

The etiology of Crohn disease remains unknown despite many hypotheses involving genetic predisposition, infectious agents, or autoimmune mechanisms. The possibility that genetic factors may be involved is supported by the higher incidence in family members, a greater than expected occurrence in Jewish population, and an increased association of Crohn disease in patients with Turner syndrome who demonstrate serum IgA deficiency. From an immunologic standpoint, a variety of abnormalities in immunoregulatory mechanisms and circulating lymphocytes has been noted but no consistent pattern has emerged. Recent immunologic studies have shown increased amounts of IgA, IgM, and IgG in the lamina propria of the intestinal mucosa. The possibility has been raised that some agent damages the colonic epithelial cells such that the body no longer recognizes its own cells and reacts against them, and the resultant inflammatory reaction to gut protein results in the inflammatory bowel disease. Although many infectious agents have been investigated, no one agent has been implicated.

Regardless of etiology, once Crohn disease has occurred in a child, growth failure is likely because of decreased nutrient intake, increased nutritional requirements and protein catabolism, and increased nutrient losses. The decreased nutrient intake may be a result of postprandial pain, anorexia, and a specific nutrient deficiency. Increased nutritional requirements and protein catabolism result from the inflammation, fever, and administration of steroids during treatment. Increased nutrient losses stem from mucosal inflammation leading to a protein-losing enteropathy and blood loss. In addition, diarrhea, use of steroids, and malabsorption will also lead to deficiencies in mineral and protein content.

The pathologic features of Crohn disease are limited to the terminal ileum in half the patients. They are focal inflammation, ulceration consisting of deep fissuring, and edema that narrows the lumen. Microscopically, the inflammatory changes are transmural and are most notable for the presence of noncaseating granulomas, lymphatic dilatation, and lymphoid aggregation.

Epidemiology

The prevalence of Crohn disease has increased over the past 20 years, involving 4.8–8.3/100,000 population per year (Calkins et al, 1984). There is a predilection for urban areas and it has not been seen in underdeveloped countries, suggesting an environmental influence as well. About 35% of patients with Crohn disease have a sibling, parent, or relative with the same diagnosis. The incidence among males and females is equal.

Natural History

There is usually a 1-year lag between onset of symptoms and diagnosis. During that time, patients may be thought to have infectious colitis, appendicitis, collagen vascular diseases, rheumatoid arthritis, and fever of unknown origin before the correct diagnosis is made. In children, extensive proximal small bowel involvement is far more common than the pure colonic form, which is more frequent in adults and older adolescents. Diffuse disease involving stomach, jejunum, ileum, and often colon occurs in fewer than 5% of patients.

The classic symptom triad of Crohn disease is abdominal pain, weight loss, and diarrhea (in about 50% of patients). The pain of Crohn disease can be diffuse, periumbilical, epigastric, or most often localized to the lower quadrants. It is cramping and intermittent, usually follows meals, and is relieved by defecation. Rectal bleeding is observed in more than two-thirds of children afflicted with colonic disease. Weight loss may be the first manifestation of growth failure and is a result of either anorexia or fear that abdominal pain will be induced by eating.

The disease may also present as arthritis and if so, usually it is HLA-B27-associated spondylitis rather than peripheral joint involvement. Over half of children with Crohn disease will have ileal and colonic involvement at the time of presentation. Moreover, most children with colonic involvement will have some anal-rectal abnormality, most likely anal fissure or fistulae at some time during the course of their disease.

The diarrhea consists of loose frequent stools if the colon is involved. If the disease is confined to the small bowel, the diarrhea can be less frequent and often is not an associated symptom. A variety of extraintestinal manifestations can occur, including stomatitis, arthritis, erythema nodosum, pyoderma gangrenosum, conjunctivitis, and uveitis, although the most frequent extraintestinal manifestation is growth retardation. Fever is usually intermittent and will rarely exceed 39°C, in the absence of complications such as perforation.

Crohn disease rarely presents with acute fulminating episodes, but rather pursues a more chronic and remitting course. Complications are related to the transmural inflammation which can result in intestinal obstruction, a stagnant loop syndrome, internal fistulization, and abscess formation. Although rarer than ulcerative colitis, toxic megacolon may occur as well. The ureter and bladder may occasionally be involved with the inflammatory process, resulting in hydronephrosis secondary to compression of ureters. Renal stone formation particularly of the oxalic and uric acid type has also been associated with the disease. In addition to calorie and protein malnutrition, deficiencies of vitamins A, D, C, folic acid, and B_{12} and the minerals calcium, magnesium, zinc, and copper may occur. These mineral deficiencies contribute to the already existing growth retardation, anorexia, hypogonadism, and skin lesions.

Diagnosis

On physical examination, most children with Crohn disease appear thin and pale, although a minority will appear entirely normal. Ten to 20% will demonstrate extraintestinal manifestations such as arthritis, erythema nodosa, or apthous ulcerations of the anal mucosa (Greenstein et al, 1976). Ten to 20% of children display digital clubbing consistent with the chronicity of the disease. Malnutrition is often associated with the disease and children show muscle-wasting and peripheral edema. Examination of the abdomen is notable for localized areas of tenderness over the areas of diseased bowel, mild guarding, and abnormally high- or low-pitched bowel sounds. Anal fissuring, ulceration, abscess, fistulae, or skin tags, may precede other abdominal symptoms.

Laboratory studies are not diagnostic, but are often helpful. Stool cultures should be obtained for bacteria and parasites. The anemia of Crohn disease is a hypochromic and microcytic anemia, secondary to chronic blood loss. If a macrocytic anemia is detected, a malabsorptive problem is also involved, usually suggestive of a B_{12} deficiency. Leukocytosis may occur but, in the presence of severe protein loss, neutropenia and lymphopenia may result. The sedimentation rate is usually elevated and correlates with disease severity. Hypoalbuminemia is also a good indicator of severity, although γ-globulin levels may be either elevated or decreased. Lactose intolerance is seen in 50% of children with diffuse small bowel disease, but not in those with only terminal ileum or colonic disease. Impaired d-xylose absorption is seen in 35% and impaired fat absorption in 25–40%. Hypocalcemia, hypozinc, and hypomagnesemia are all believed to be secondary to steatorrhea.

Radiographic studies should include a plain radiograph of the abdomen to show an abnormal gas pattern in colon and small bowel and any displacement of bowel loops to suggest an abscess. However, the UGI study with small bowel follow-through is the most useful study (Fig. 7.7). If the colon lacks stool, is air-filled, or if there is brisk bleeding, the barium enema should be withheld, nor should preparatory laxative "cleanouts" be used since they could lead to perforation. If a barium study is performed, colonic findings will include segmental areas of colonic edema, narrowing, and cobblestoning, generally with sparing of the rectum. Transmural ulcerations appear as "rose thorn" or "collar stud" ulcerations. If the disease is confined to the colon and includes the presence of pseudo polyps, the radiograph may resemble that seen in ulcerative colitis. Small bowel findings include thickening of the valvulae conniventes, cobblestoning from transverse and longitudinal ulceration, and thickening of the ileocecal valve. In later disease, the mucosal pattern is lost and the small bowel appears rigid, with generalized thickening of bowel loops. Sinus and fistulous tracts are also common. Duodenal and jejunal disease will be characterized radiographically by the presence of stenotic segments and strictures with dilatation of proximal loops.

Rectosigmoidoscopy is mandatory in any child suspected of having Crohn disease. While in over 50% of cases a normal rectum will be visualized, erythema, edema, increased friability, and aphthous ulcerations will occur in 10% or less, as well as pathognomonic noncaseating granulomas (Gryboski, 1981). A rectal

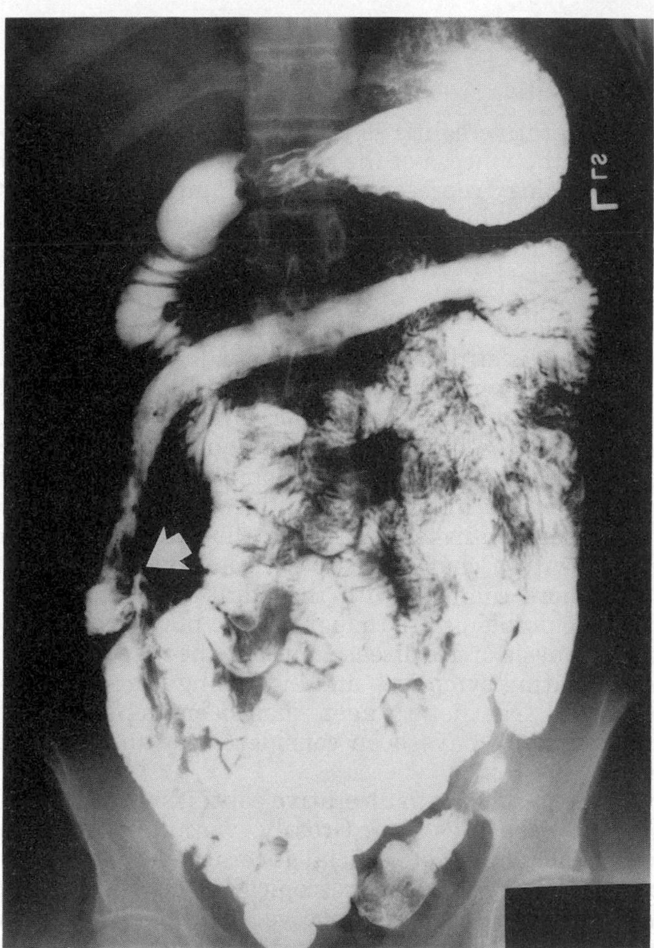

Figure 7.7. This adolescent girl had terminal ileal and colonic Crohn disease. This radiograph was taken at the end of the small bowel follow-through and shows the ileal disease, the abnormal ileocecal valve *(arrow)*, and the right colonic disease.

biopsy will often be nonspecific and show focal or diffuse inflammatory changes with mucosal ulceration and lymphoid hyperplasia, rather than the noncaseating granulomas. However, if the barium studies in combination with the rectosigmoidoscopy suggest the diagnosis, surgical specimens need not be obtained. Colonoscopy is useful if the rectosigmoidoscopy demonstrates normal tissue and if a barium enema cannot rule out colonic disease. It is also useful preoperatively to determine the extent of colonic involvement. Occasionally, UGI endoscopy is also indicated in patients who have an abnormal upper small bowel series.

Treatment

Crohn disease cannot be cured, but requires management by medical and surgical means. The goal of therapy is to achieve remission of clinical symptoms and resumption of normal growth and near normal activity. No single medication, treatment regimen, or surgical procedure can be recommended for all patients with Crohn disease. Treatment must be tailored to an individual's condition and ability to tolerate the disease. In the absence of an acute relapse or flare-up, management focuses on appropriate dietary care and reduction of inflammation. The diet is designed to provide high protein and abundant calories with supplemental vitamins and minerals. Only if the disease flares up should fiber be restricted in the diet. Often, small frequent meals rather than a few large ones will reduce the postprandial abdominal pain that discourages patients from eating. High caloric formulas may also provide a source of extra calories and nutrients for ambulatory patients who dislike large meals. No conclusive studies suggest the value of complete bowel rest, although this has been in more frequent practice for patients with acute abdominal symptoms. Continuous enteral alimentation with an elemental diet is being used with some success for a period of up to 6 weeks, in association with anti-inflammatory agents. These elemental diets may be of some use also for treatment of complications such as fistulas and perianal disease.

In the most severely ill patients with Crohn disease and in those in whom enteral alimentation has failed, total parenteral nutrition is necessary. Home intravenous alimentation is possible under some circumstances. Initially, such therapy should focus on achieving an increase in calories and protein 40% above the amounts normally required for a patient's height and age.

Steroids are the most useful anti-inflammatory agents available for the treatment of Crohn disease, particularly hydrocortisone or methylprednisolone given intravenously or prednisone given orally. In controlled studies, prednisone has been shown to be effective in the acute stage of the disease but has not yet proved to be effective in preventing relapses (Malchow et al, 1984). The recommended dose is 1–2 mg/kg/day up to a maximum dose of 40 mg/day for 4–6 weeks, with a gradual tapering over the subsequent month. Most patients are steroid-dependent, remaining on alternate-day therapy or a small daily dose. Notably, a smaller steroidal dosage will provide the same resolution of symptoms if an enteral alimentation regimen is also concurrently prescribed. There has been no evidence that topical steroids are effective in the treatment of Crohn disease.

Sulfasalazine is useful for treatment of Crohn colitis with bacterial overgrowth and colonic involvement. The drug has not been found to have a synergistic effect when used in combination with steroids in small bowel disease, nor has it been found effective once a remission has been obtained (Malchow et al, 1984). Fifteen percent of children experience side effects of the drug, including headache, increased abdominal pain, and rash. Hemolysis and folic acid deficiency have also been noted with chronic usage.

Immunosuppressive agents such as imuran or azathioprine allow reduction of corticosteroid dosage, but their complications tend to outweigh the benefits. More recently, 6-mercaptopurine has been found to be effective when used over a period of 3–6 months, particularly in patients with ileocolitis rather than those with disease limited to the small bowel (Present et al, 1980).

Its main indication is for patients who cannot be weaned from steroids and are beginning to show complications from that agent.

Surgery is utilized only when all dietary and pharmacologic treatments fail. It is indicated in the presence of abdominal obstruction, hemorrhage, toxic megacolon, and/or abscess, as well as for unrelenting disease requiring steroids for a period greater than 2 years. Nonetheless, resection of diseased bowel is only 20–50% effective and is found to be most successful between the ages of 12 and 16 years (Wesson and Schandling, 1981). Total colectomy and proctectomy are recommended in those with total colonic disease since the rectum has been shown to be a site of recurrence. Growth failure and intractability of the disease remain the number one indication for performing elective surgery in Crohn disease.

Prognosis

Although a small percentage of patients will go into permanent remission with either medical or surgical management, most will continue to have a smoldering disease that will occasionally demonstrate acute exacerbations, despite strict adherence to diet. Ileocolic involvement carries the highest frequency of recurrence and relapse, with the median relapse time of 16 months after medical therapy and 4 years after surgery. Twenty percent will have only a few symptoms and describe themselves as perfectly healthy, whereas 20% will have a severe disabling disease leading to growth failure and endocrinologic problems. The most favorable prognosis is for children in whom the disease is limited to the small intestine, with the occasional obstructive symptoms constituting the only complication. One clinical series in adults suggested that over 70% would require surgery 15 years after diagnosis (Farmer et al, 1985). Moreover, those with ileocolic disease most frequently undergo surgery versus those with simply ileal, colonic, or anal-rectal disease (Sales and Kirsner, 1983). In addition, patients who initially have fistulas, tend to have early recurrences often with recurrent fistulas. The presence or absence of demonstrable disease at the margins of surgical resection granulomas in the resected specimen has not been found to correlate with recurrence rates.

Although there is an increased incidence of carcinoma, particularly in the distal ileum of patients with Crohn disease who have had the disease over 10 years, it appears to be much lower than that experienced in patients who have ulcerative colitis.

The overall mortality rate from Crohn disease is highest during the first 5 years of the disease, but the relative risk of death decreases as the duration of the disease increases (Farmer et al, 1985). The site of involvement has little importance in survival. Overall, however, despite its chronic course and recurrence rate, most patients, particularly those with localized disease (e.g. terminal ileum), do enjoy a surprisingly good quality of life.

Ulcerative Colitis

Definition

Ulcerative colitis is an inflammatory disease involving the mucosa of the colon and rectum. Although the pathology represents acute inflammation, the disease runs a chronic course with multiple remissions and exacerbations.

Basic Science

There is still no known etiology for ulcerative colitis, although many hypotheses point to a combination of genetic susceptibility and/or environmental influences. The possibility that an autoimmune phenomenon causes the acute inflammation is evoked frequently, but as yet, no humoral or cell-mediated mechanisms have been confirmed. Although the disease has been linked with a characteristic personality, this appears to be more common with the adult-onset form. Psychologic problems are thought not to play a role in the pathogenesis of the disease, but may be responsible for accentuating symptoms and increasing the severity of a relapse. No dietary agent has been implicated although many have been considered on an anecdotal basis.

The pathology in ulcerative colitis is a diffuse nonspecific tissue reaction. Grossly, vascular congestion and hemorrhage, superficial ulcerations, and pseudo polyps are observed. Microscopically, only the mucosa and mucosal layers are involved. Although the presence of crypt abscesses is characteristic, such abscesses are not pathognomonic for the disease as they can be seen also in acute bacterial colitis and occasionally in Crohn disease. Occasionally, the submucosa may be so inflamed that further layers of bowel may also become involved. Nonetheless, the involvement of mucosa and submucosa can aid distinction of ulcerative colitis from Crohn disease. The area of inflammation in ulcerative colitis usually extends proximally into the colon, beginning often with rectal involvement.

Epidemiology

The incidence of ulcerative colitis varies between 3 and 15/100,000 per year (Calkins et al, 1984). Both sexes are equally affected. An increased incidence has been observed in patients of Jewish descent living in Europe and North America. Urban populations are at higher risk than are rural ones.

Natural History

The mean age of presentation is 11 years. The time from onset of symptoms to time of diagnosis is usually in the range of 3–6 months. The predominant symptom is bloody diarrhea, often in combination with abdominal pain, tenesmus, and less often with nausea, vomiting, and anorexia. In older children and adolescents, extraintestinal clinical features may precede by months, and even years, the initial presentation of the intestinal symptoms. Although less prominent than in Crohn disease, growth retardation and delayed puberty have been reported in up to 20% of cases. In addition, these children may present with fevers of unknown origin and for evaluation of muscular skeletal and/or ocular involvement, including episodes of arthralgia, arthritis, conjunctivitis, and uveitis. Erythema multiforme or erythema nodosum may also herald the onset of the disease as well as fatty infiltration of the liver and/or chronic active hepatitis. Liver function should be assessed in all patients for whom the diagnosis is being considered.

Ulcerative colitis shows considerable variability in severity, clinical course, and outcome. An exacerbation may be abrupt in onset or gradually progressive in severity. Neither the presence nor absence of a particular symptom complex nor the severity of an initial attack carries any prognostic value. Nonetheless, two patterns of the disease have been characterized in children: one is a remitting colitis, with multiple remissions and exacerbations during the first few years of the disease, followed by a permanent remission; the second pattern is a chronic continuous colitis in which patients do not have an initial exacerbation, but are never completely well and a complete remission is never documented. This type of colitis is characterized by chronic malnutrition and anemia with mild diarrhea and mild rectal bleeding. Children with this type of chronic continuous colitis are believed to respond poorly to conventional medical therapy.

Ulcerative colitis is also associated with a variety of local and systemic complications that occur as the disease becomes chronic. These can include hemorrhoids, anal fissures, perforations in fistulas, particularly in patients with toxic megacolon, strictures of the intestine, particularly in the rectosigmoid area, and pseudopolyps (representing islands of inflamed mucosa surrounded by damaged atrophic mucosa eventually appearing polypoid in nature). More systemic complications include ankylosing spondylitis, nephrolithiasis, hepatic lesions including chronic active hepatitis, and thrombophlebitis. Finally, increased susceptibility to carcinoma of the colon in patients with ulcerative colitis is apparent, particularly in those affected for 10 years or longer. Patients who have total colonic involvement are most at risk; those least at risk have only left-sided colitis or proctitis.

Diagnosis

An abnormal sigmoidoscopic examination showing diffusely friable rectal mucosa is necessary to make the diagnosis since 99% of cases will initially involve the rectum. Large discrete ulcerations with surrounding normal mucosa are more consistent with Crohn disease or amebiasis. Rectal biopsy is of limited diagnostic value, although it can confirm the diagnosis of amoebic granulomatous or pseudomembranous colitis. Rectal biopsy findings in ulcerative colitis are usually nonspecific and include chronic inflammation, crypt abscesses, and decreased presence of goblet cells.

A barium enema done early in the course of the disease may be normal. Air contrast is better at showing subtle ulceration. As the disease progresses, haustra become thicker and ulcerations are more obvious. At time of diagnosis, 25% of children will show involvement of their entire colon (Kelts and Grand, 1980). In long-standing chronic ulcerative colitis, when the disease has extended to the submucosa, a uniform reduction in the caliber of the colon occurs often referred to as "lead pipe colon." Segmental stricturing may occur similar in appearance to that in colonic carcinoma.

Laboratory findings, while not diagnostic, will help characterize some of the complications of the colitis. For example, hypochromic anemia occurs in many patients secondary to chronic blood loss. In addition, most patients show an elevated erythrocyte sedimentation rate and hypoalbuminemia, both indicators of an exacerbation consistent with a protein-losing enteropathy.

If the patient presents with abdominal distention, tenderness, tacycardia, hypotension, anemia, dehydration, and leukocytosis, toxic megacolon should be considered and surgery contemplated. Barium enema is contraindicated in a child with these signs and symptoms. Plain films show air and fluid in a colon that has lost the normal haustral pattern. Pseudopolyps appear as soft tissue masses within the air column. Perforation is evident if free air is present.

Treatment

Treatment goals in ulcerative colitis include decreasing the inflammation, minimizing side-effects of medications, and monitoring secondary complications. While dietary changes including a high protein, high carbohydrate, normal fat, high vitamin diet are often recommended, there is no evidence that such dietary management is effective. In severe exacerbations, hospitalization is necessary and parenteral alimentation is required for maintainance of adequate body nutrient stores. Neither opiates nor anticholinergic agents have been found to be effective. Patients with milder limited disease have benefitted from steroidal enemas or suppositories in combination with sulfasalazine. Sulfasalazine consists of two pharmacologic agents—5-aminosalicylic acid, the active component decreasing inflammation, and sulfapyridine, which acts as a carrier allowing the 5-aminosalicylic acid to reach the colon, where it is cleaved by colonic flora, releasing an active component. For children with active disease, the dose is 50–75 mg/kg/day. If remission occurs, a low dose of 50 mg/kg/day should be maintained since recurrence has been found to be four times higher in patients who stopped taking the drugs. Complications of this medication include reversible oligospermia, infertility, and inhibition of folate absorption. It is safe, however, in pregnancy. Since the efficacy of sulfasalazine depends on its being cleaved by bacteria in the colon, antibiotics should not be used concomitantly when the drug is given by mouth. Usually, sulfasalazine and steroidal enemas are effective if the disease is limited to the rectum or rectosigmoid junction.

If, however, the disease is believed to be more severe or the colonic involvement more extensive, oral steroids should be administered as well. Intravenous ACTH is the more effective for patients not previously treated with corticosteroids, while intravenous hydrocortisone 10 mg/kg/day is preferable for those patients already taking steroids (Meyers et al, 1983).

Azathioprine may play a role in maintenance treatment of the disease, and allow reduction in the frequency and dependency on steroid use. Azathioprine is usually given 2 mg/kg/24 hours and relapses can occur upon withdrawal of the immunosuppressive therapy. Cyclosporin A may also be a useful therapeutic agent (Kirschner, 1988).

If the disease becomes chronic and unresponsive to steroid therapy or the patient has complications of steroidal therapy, resection should be considered. Surgery normally consists of complete colectomy with removal of the rectum and creation of an ileostomy as a curative procedure. It is also performed for toxic megacolon with potential perforation, bleeding that is uncontrolled, or malignancy. At least 25% of patients with ulcerative colitis have indications for operation. Since the creation of an abdominal stoma may be disturbing to many young patients, recently some sphincter-saving operations have been performed, involving colonic resection and creation of an ileoanal anastomosis. Cumulative colectomy rates range from 4–9% after 1 year of disease, 6–27% after 5 years, and 14–50% after 10 years (Sales and Kirsner, 1983).

Prognosis

The extent of initial disease and severity of the first attack may be useful prognostic indicators. In younger patients who present with anemia, hypoalbuminemia, and severe abdominal pain, the response to medical management may be satisfactory initially, but these patients usually require resection within a few years. Exacerbations in children may follow respiratory infections, emotional stresses, or even the administration of a barium enema. In children, the chances of a complete and permanent remission after the first bout are less than 10%. From 25–50% of patients with the chronic continuous form will require curative surgery within 5 years (Michener et al, 1979). Because children who respond to medical therapy still have an increased risk of developing colonic carcinoma, a surveillance program consisting of frequent endoscopy and biopsy procedures is instituted to detect mucosal dysplasia. Moreover, carcinoma has been reported in disease limited to the rectum and in the rectal stump after colectomy and ileorectal anastomosis. Overall mortality from ulcerative colitis itself ranges from 1–12%, being higher in adults than in children, although with the improvement in medical management and the introduction of better surgical techniques, mortality continues to decrease across all age groups.

OBSTRUCTIVE DISORDERS

Meckel Diverticulum

Definition

Meckel diverticulum is a remnant of the fetal omphalomesenteric duct. It is usually composed of heterotopic tissue, including gastric, jejunal and colonic mucosa, and pancreatic tissue. It is located at the distal ileum within 100 cm of the ileocecal valve. It has a wide base with a lumen that is usually narrower than that of the ileum. Occasionally, its apex is connected to the umbilicus by a fibrous band or cord.

Basic Science

Complications caused by a Meckel diverticulum can be related to its anatomic location, as well as to the heterotopic mucosa that composes it. For example, hemorrhage may result from peptic ulceration occurring in eroded gastric mucosa making up the diverticulum. The diverticulum can also serve as a lead point for an intussusception, volvulus, torsion, or a herniation of a loop of bowel. Moreover, acute inflammation or diverticulitis from suppuration and subsequent perforation can mimic the pain and presentation of acute appendicitis.

Epidemiology

Meckel diverticulum is the most frequent malformation of the GI tract and occurs in 1.5% of the population, although only 2% of patients with this malformation are symptomatic, with males being three to five times more frequently symptomatic than females.

Natural History

Bleeding is usually painless and slight, although over a long period of time it may produce iron deficiency anemia. In severe circumstances, ulceration has resulted in perforation or significant bleeding, and surgery may be required to remove the diverticulum. Less common complications include an ileocolic intussusception characterized by vomiting and intestinal infarction, usually not reduced by barium enema. Most symptomatic cases will appear within the first 2 years of life.

Diagnosis

An infant or child who presents with massive, painless, bright red, or dark red rectal bleeding must be considered as having a Meckel diverticulum until proven otherwise. Diagnostic work-up should include a rectosigmoidoscopy, stool cultures, and plain radiographs of the abdomen to eliminate other diagnostic possibilities. In addition, a nasogastric tube can be useful to rule out UGI bleeding proximal to the ligament of Treitz. A technetium-99M radionucleotide scan is helpful since with pentagastrin stimulation it allows detection of sites of ectopic gastric mucosa and thus demonstrates a Meckel diverticulum (Fig. 7.8). While a radionucleotide scan can be 80–90% accurate, prior use of barium, or inflammation that destroys ectopic gastric mucosa may give a false-negative result. On the other hand, hemangiomas, abdominal aneurysms, hydronephrosis, lymphoma, peptic ulcerations of the small intestines, Peutz-Jegher syndrome, and an additional small bowel intussusception can all result in false-positive results with the scan and lead to unnecessary surgery. Therefore, the scan should supplement clinical suspicion and should not replace it. Hence, if a child continues to have major rectal bleeding and a negative scan, further work-up will be required, including an arteriogram if bleeding is active, or a colonoscopy if it is not.

Treatment

Treatment is surgical, with attention directed to correction of hypovolemic shock and blood replacement if hemorrhage has been significant. In addition, antibiotics should be used if inflammation and/or perforation are observed.

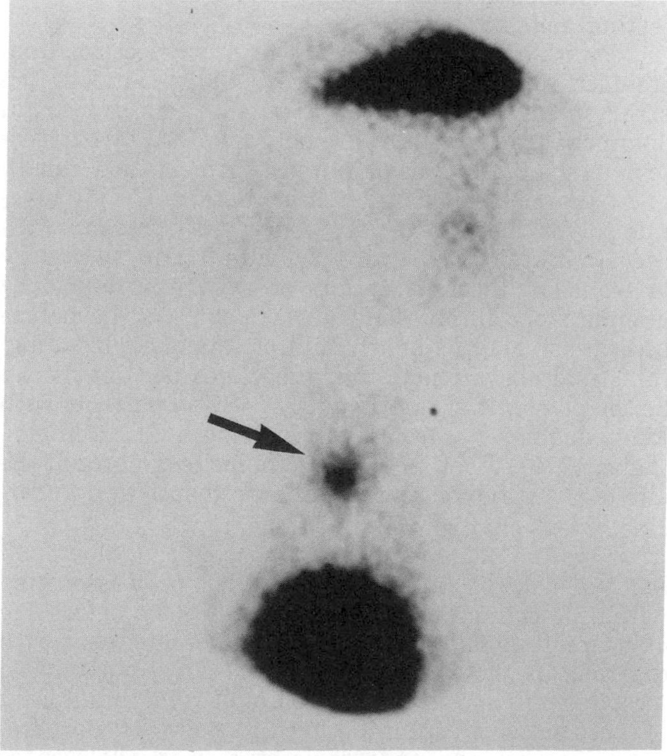

Figure 7.8. This is a technetium-99m pertechnetate scan of a boy who presented with painless rectal bleeding. The ectopic gastric mucosa in his Meckel diverticulum takes up radionuclide *(arrow)* as does gastric mucosa. Lower activity is from excretion into bladder.

Anal-Rectal Malformations

Definition

Anal-rectal anomalies include anal stenosis, an imperforate anal membrane, anal-rectal agenesis, and atresia. They result from embryologic events that occur sometime between the fourth embryonic week and the sixth month of gestation.

Basic Science

There are about 30 subtypes of anal-rectal anomalies, comprising two major categories—the supralevator and the translevator types, with classification based upon location of the anomaly, either above or below the puborectalis sling. In each category, a rectal pouch may be noncommunicating or communicate via a fistula with a neighboring viscus or the perineal surface. Usually fistulas are more common in patients with supralevator anomalies and involve the genitourinary tract.

Epidemiology

Anal-rectal anomalies occur 1 in every 3000–5000 live births and are more common in males. Familial incidence is rare and supported by only anecdotal reports. Of importance, however, is that 50% of patients will have other concomitant congenital malformations, particularly esophageal atresia. Twenty-five percent of cases are detected in low birth weight infants.

The other most common associated anomalies are vertebral column defects (28%), GI tract complications (9%), cardiac problems (9%), and CNS (18%) defects (Kieswetter et al, 1976).

Natural History

Low-lying anomalies tend to have fewer complications than do higher lying anomalies in which fistulae are more abundant and can cause difficulties in control of feces, flatus, and urine. If a stenotic lesion is present, most of these diagnoses can be detected at birth or shortly thereafter. Inability to pass meconium or difficulty with defecation are consistent with the diagnosis. Rectal agenesis and anal agenesis together account for over three-quarters of anal-rectal anomalies. The "higher" the anomaly, the more difficult the surgical procedure required to correct it.

Diagnosis

Radiologic work-up should consist of plain radiographs an ultrasonogram for renal anomalies, and a retrograde urethrogram in the male, to demonstrate the presence of a fistula. In addition, a cathether should be passed into the stomach to rule out associated esophageal atresia. Physical examination may give clues as to the level of the anomaly. A dimpled area will suggest a low-lying problem, with the dimple usually lying anterior to the normal position of the anus. A detailed neurologic examination should also be performed since sacral roots that can supply the levator ani muscles also innervate vesical sphincters and perineal dermatomes and abnormalities can, therefore, be detected before operation. For example, the presence of an atonic bladder or perineal anesthesia will be associated with a weak levator ani muscle and would mandate a permanent colostomy since there would be no point in constructing a functioning anus if the mechanism for defecation were abnormal. The level of the rectal pouch determines the definitive treatment, i.e., whether a simple sacral perineal repair will suffice, or whether a more complex abdominal sacral perineal approach is required.

Treatment

If a low pouch has been noted by radiographic studies, a primary anoplasty should be performed. If bowel appears to be more than 2 cm from the skin, a colostomy is required but investigation should also be carried out to rule out a fistula involving colon distal to the colostomy. A simple anoplasty can be performed shortly after birth, whereas definitive surgical procedures are carried out between 6 and 10 months of age. A pull-through procedure is required for the high-lying anomalies with their associated rectal vaginal fistulae. Several different operations for this corrective surgery have been devised and a pediatric surgeon should be consulted. Regardless of the surgical procedure, however, significant fecal incontinence is often a complication.

Prognosis

Often it is the associated anomalies and low birth weight that influence the prognosis far more than the type of anal rectal anomaly and/or the presence of a fistula. Overall mortality with this anomaly is 20%, however, and it can be as high as 50% in very low birth weight premature infants. In normal birth weight full-term infants, mortality is less than 5% and few if any associated anomalies have been detected.

Polyps

Definition

Polyps are the most common tumors of the GI tract. They appear as visible protrusions from a mucosal surface and can be found in any location from the stomach to colon. The four major types of polyps are (1) juvenile polyps (hamartomatous epithelial retentions), (2) Peutz-Jeghers polyps (hamartomatous), (3) hyperplastic polyps (hyperplasias), and (4) adenomatous polyps (neoplasias). While most polyps in children are benign, some carry an increased risk of carcinoma.

Epidemiology

Juvenile polyps are rare before the age of 1 year, although their incidence increases rapidly thereafter and reaches a maximum between 4 and 5 years of age, to become rare after 15 years of age. Peutz-Jeghers polyps are most often seen in adolescents in early adulthood. Adults tend to have hyperplastic polyps and in late adulthood adenomatous polyps. If an adenoma is found in an individual under the age of 30 years, familial polyposis should be considered.

Natural History

Bright red blood in the stools is often the presenting symptom in juvenile polyps. Occasionally occult bleeding can occur and lead to anemia. At other times, juvenile polyps may have a long stalk and predispose to a colocolic intussusception, although more commonly they are associated with rectal prolapse. More than three-quarters of these polyps are within reach of a sigmoidoscope, usually within the first 10 cm from the anus. Juvenile polyps are painless and bleeding can sometimes be confused with that from a Meckel diverticulum, although the latter usually results in greater blood loss and affects younger children. Juvenile polyps are associated with three syndromes: juvenile polyposis coli, generalized juvenile polyposis, and the Cronkhite-Canada syndrome (juvenile polyposis and ectodermal lesions).

In generalized GI juvenile polyposis, the polyps can form anywhere from the stomach through the small intestine sometimes into the colon, making removal almost impossible. Occasionally, these polyps may have adenomatous features, again predisposing them to intestinal malignancy.

Peutz-Jeghers polyps can occur in any location from stomach to anus, but they are usually found in the small intestine. They are inherited as an autosomal dominant trait, and also are characterized by extraintestinal manifestations of mucosal pigmentation (mouth and anus) noted during birth or infancy. Unlike juvenile polyps, this type of polyposis usually presents with recurrent attacks of severe abdominal pain, secondary to transient intussusception, or with iron deficiency anemia from chronic GI loss of blood. As the polyps ulcerate and subsequently infarct, vomiting, bleeding, intestinal obstruction, and sometimes peritonitis can be the presenting sign. Roughly 2–3% of patients with Peutz-Jeghers syndrome will develop a GI carcinoma (Erbe, 1976). Whether this carcinoma originates at the site of the polyp or represents a predisposition to carcinomatous change remains unclear.

Familial adenomatous polyposis of the colon is an autosomal dominant condition that is highly associated with development of carcinoma of the colon before age 40 years. It usually presents during the late teens with diarrhea as the first symptom and subsequent blood loss, anemia, and abdominal pain. Careful monitoring of these patients beginning in childhood with more frequent barium and endoscopic studies in adolescence and adulthood decreases the early mortality associated with this syndrome. Adenomatous polyps also occur in two polyposis syndromes—Gardner and Turcot syndromes. In Gardner syndrome, polyps are associated with soft tissue tumors, lipomas, fibromas, and bone tumors, usually osteomas involving the mandible, other facial bones, and the skull and occasionally long bones. Patients with Gardner syndrome have the same risk of developing colorectal carcinoma as do patients with the familial adenomatous polyposis of the colon. The triad of bone tumor, soft tissue tumor, and polyp rarely occurs in the first two decades of life. Turcot syndrome consists of adenomatous polyposis in conjunction with the malignant tumor of the CNS, usually a medulloblastoma or a glioblastoma. It is believed to be transmitted in autosomal recessive genes, although some authors have suggested that it is a variant of Gardner syndrome.

Finally, lymphoid polyposis or nodular lymphoid hyperplasia of the colon and rectum can present with rectal bleeding and nonspecific abdominal pain, in conjunction with diarrhea. These polyps may represent a temporary response to infection or an immune response. They have occurred following a necrotizing enterocolitis, in Hirschsprung disease complicated by colitis, and in chronic and inflammatory bowel disease. They do not have any increased risk of malignancy. Peak incidence is from 1–3 years, although they may occur at any time between 6 months and puberty.

NEW DEVELOPMENTS

A mixed hyperplastic-adenomatous polyp has been described, in which a transition appears to be occurring from hyperplasia to an adenomatous state. The hyperplastic areas continue to remain free of carcinoma whereas the adenomatous dysplastic component of the polyp is thought to be the precursor of cancer (Fenoglio-Preiser and Hutter, 1985).

Diagnosis

The most common polyps in children, juvenile polyps, are usually detected on rectal examination, followed by rectosigmoidoscopy. If this examination is negative, then a barium enema with air contrast should be performed (Fig. 7.9). If that study is negative and rectal bleeding persists, a Meckel scan should be performed before colonoscopy. Physical examination should also focus on extraintestinal manifestations of some of the polyposis syndromes. Any polyp localized on rectosigmoidoscopy should be excised for biopsy. If a juvenile polyp is detected, no further therapy is indicated. If barium enema detects polyps not accessible to a sigmoidoscope, colonoscopy should be performed for biopsy and eventual diagnosis.

Treatment

The treatment for juvenile polyps is conservative, unless pain or profuse bleeding are present. Nonetheless, barium studies should be repeated every 3–5 years in patients with more than one polyp, since recent reports have indicated the presence of dysplastic polyps in patients with juvenile polyps (Grotsky et al, 1982). For Peutz-Jeghers polyps, segmental resections can be successful in alleviating symptoms if the polyps are well-localized to a short segment of intestine. Patients with familial polyposis require frequent monitoring: in the first decade of life no more than every 3 years, but more frequently in adolescence so as to detect possible dysplastic change before it becomes malignant. Proctocolectomy with ileostomy or colectomy with an ileoendorectal pull-through is the treatment of choice, since any patient who has familial polyposis left untreated will eventually develop carcinoma of the colon. Genetic counseling is also useful in these patients because of its autosomal dominant inheritance pattern. Lymphoid polyposis only requires treatment if symptomatic as it is not associated with an increased risk of malignancy.

Prognosis

Predictive factors that indicate the likelihood of carcinoma developing arising from adenoma include

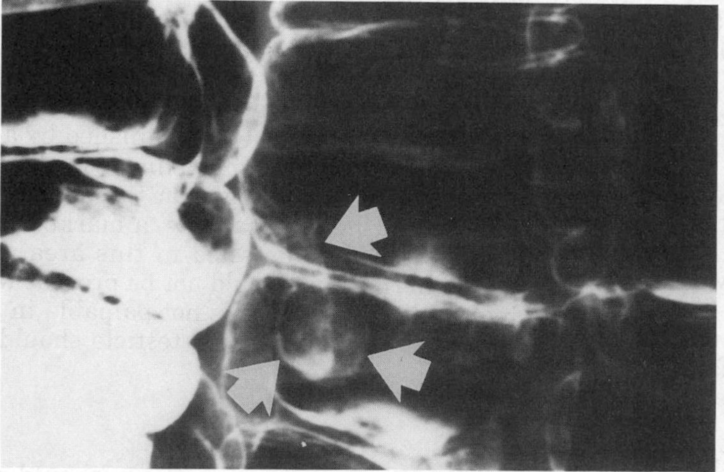

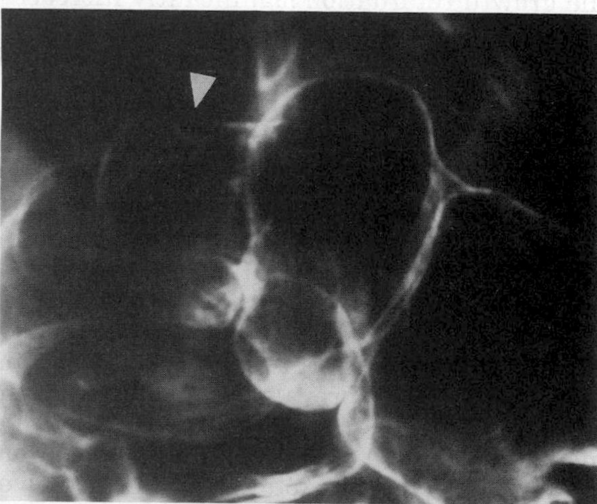

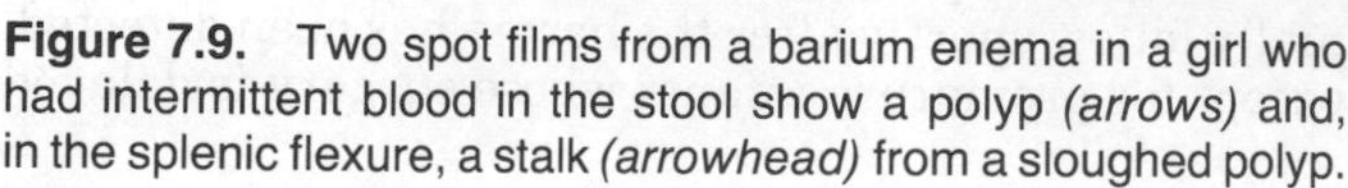

Figure 7.9. Two spot films from a barium enema in a girl who had intermittent blood in the stool show a polyp *(arrows)* and, in the splenic flexure, a stalk *(arrowhead)* from a sloughed polyp. By colonoscopy and histologic examination, she had juvenile polyps.

the size of the polyp, the growth pattern (pedunculated being more benign than the semisessile or sessile), the degree of differentiation, the proportion of carcinoma to adenoma within the polyp, the depth of invasion, the presence or absence of lymphatic vascular invasion, and the patient's age. If cancer is detected in a poorly differentiated polyp, with tumor at the margin of excision, and the patient is younger than age 40 years, this patient is at increased risk for metastases (Fenoglio-Preiser and Hutter, 1985).

Inguinal Hernia

Definition

Inguinal hernias occur when abdominal contents are pushed into the processus vaginalis, a peritoneal sac that should normally atrophy at birth. If the small intestine cannot recede from the sac, the hernia is said to be incarc erated. An *indirect* inguinal hernia exits the abdomen through the deep inguinal ring and passes down obliquely through the inguinal canal, lateral to the inferior epigastric artery. A *direct* inguinal hernia or internal hernia is rare in children and represents the protrusion of bowel emerging between the inferior epigastric artery and the edge of the rectus muscle.

Basic Science

The reasons for predisposition to hernias are unknown but some evidence suggests that events leading to increased intra-abdominal pressure both in utero and after birth will hasten the appearance of indirect inguinal hernias. For example, patients with a ventriculoperitoneal shunt who show increased pressure and fluid within the peritoneal cavity have been shown to have an increased incidence of inguinal hernias. If fluid rather than bowel enters the processus vaginalis, the condition is referred to as a hydrocele.

In infants of 32 weeks' gestation or less, intrauterine growth retardation significantly increases the risk of development of inguinal hernias, although the mechanism for this is unknown (Peevy et al, 1986).

Epidemiology

Inguinal hernia is the most common cause of intestinal obstruction in infants from the first week of life to age 4 months, when it becomes second to intussusception.

While hernias may be present at birth, 40% will become apparent before the age of 6 months, and the majority of patients with this diagnosis present in the first year of life. The prevalence in a general infant population is believed to range from 1–5%, with a ratio of nine males to one female. About 60% appear on the right side, 25% on the left, and 15% bilaterally. Overall, premature infants have a 5% higher frequency of inguinal hernias; among infants weighing less than 1000 g, about 30% have hernias (Harper et al, 1976).

Natural History

A nonincarcerated hernia is usually painless and appears to increase in size when a child strains or coughs and decreases when a child is sleeping. It is often initially noted on a routine physical examination shortly after birth. Normally, mild external pressure will bring about reduction of the herniated bowel into the abdominal cavity. When the sac contents cannot be reduced, the hernia becomes incarcerated and the bowel may undergo ischemic and even necrotic change secondary to the obstruction to blood flow. An incarcerated hernia will present with tenderness and pain and if obstruction has occurred, nausea, vomiting, and abdominal distention. Incarcerated hernias occur most often during the first 6 months of life.

Diagnosis

A bulge in the groin may be from a hernia, a hydrocele, an undescended testes, or torsion of the cord. Normally, inguinal hernia in a child is located along the inguinal canal and the bulge is easily reducible. If the bulge is below the inguinal canal, a femoral hernia should be considered. Increased thickness of the inguinal canal, ascertained by palpation of the structure between the index finger and the pubic tubercle, is also consistent with the diagnosis of inguinal hernia. If a hernia is suspected and cannot be palpated on physical examination, inguinal herniography may be used, although this procedure is being done less and less frequently. A radiopaque material is injected into the peritoneal cavity, after which a radiograph of the abdomen and inguinal canal is obtained. If the processus vaginalis remains patent, dye will be present in the extension of the peritoneal cavity and scrotum. Herniography is most useful in a patient in whom the presence or absence of an inguinal canal on the contralateral side cannot be definitively determined by physical examination.

If a child presents with a groin mass that appeared acutely and with pain, an incarceration should be suspected. Again, lack of mobility of the groin mass as well as increased thickness extending from the mass up to and including the internal ring of the inguinal canal are consistent with an incarcerated hernia. This increased thickness may also be distinguished by a bimanual examination: with the index finger in the rectum and the opposite index finger on the abdominal wall over and under the internal ring, a markedly increased thickening can be detected in this area with an incarcerated hernia that would not be present with an acute hydrocele. If a testicle is not palpable in the scrotum, torsion of an undescended testicle should be considered.

Treatment

Surgical repair of an inguinal hernia should normally follow shortly after the hernia has been detected, except for premature infants whose surgery is delayed until 4–6 months of age. If the hernia is incarcerated, manual reduction can be attempted. Using adequate sedation and elevation of the lower torso and limbs, firm pressure in the direction of the inguinal canal is usually effective. A complete surgical repair should be carried out about 48 hours after the reduction.

Complications of surgery include hematomas in the scrotum, testicular atrophy secondary to an excessively tight internal or external ring, poor placement of a suture, or excessive manipulation of the vascular supply of the testicle. The vas deferens may also be damaged by an incorrectly placed hemostat or by crushing with forceps. Inaccurate placement of the testicle on the scrotum can result in a malpositioned testicle. An unrecognized tear in the neck of the hernia may result in recurrence of symptoms after repair. Occasionally, a femoral or direct inguinal hernia may develop after an indirect inguinal hernia repair.

CONTROVERSIES

Controversy exists over the question of whether to operate on the contralateral side. Currently, it is believed that 50% of children 6 months of age or younger have a patent processus vaginalis on the opposite side, with this incidence decreasing as the child gets older, such that after 1 year of age it is unlikely that the opposite side sac remains open. On the other hand, the risk of dissecting an asymptomatic opposite side may well outweigh the benefits of performing a surgical repair for a potential hernia. Lowering the age of automatic exploration from 1–2 years to 6 months does not increase the rate of positive findings on the asymptomatic side (McGregor et al, 1980).

Hirschsprung Disease

Definition

Hirschsprung disease or congenital aganglionic megacolon is a congenital anomaly that occurs between the fifth and twelfth week of gestation. It is characterized by partial or complete obstruction of the intestine due to the absence of ganglion cells in the myenteric plexus of Auerbach and the submucosal plexus of Meissner, in the rectum or rectosigmoid area of the bowel.

Basic Science

The defect in Hirschsprung disease is the result of defective migration of ganglion cell precursors of the neurocrest. Many studies focus on the pathophysiology for the obstruction. The current hypothesis suggests that neurons of a nonadrenergic inhibitory system are located in the myenteric plexus, and when these inhibitory nerves cannot form synapses in ganglion cells (which are absent), a state of constant contraction takes place. There have been descriptions of patients who have ganglion cells present, but who still have symptoms consistent with hypo- or aganglionosis, suggesting that these neurons are defective.

Epidemiology

Hirschsprung disease occurs in about 1/5000 live births. The male to female ratio is 4:1, although when the aganglianosis extends beyond the sigmoid colon (long segment disease), the ratio drops to 3:1. Long segment disease may appear in siblings. Some patients also have Down syndrome, and 5% show associated

CASE ILLUSTRATION

A 3-month-old male with birth weight of 1.2 kg (29 weeks' gestation) was admitted for elective bilateral hernia repair. The patient had had a benign perinatal course except for some episodes of apnea and bradycardia, requiring brief intubation during the first week of life, without residual lung disease. He was discharged home at 9 weeks of life to be readmitted at this time (3 months) for elective hernia repair. The patient received general anesthesia by mask (nitrous oxide and halothane), and began to display shallow respirations and bradycardia that progressed to a respiratory arrest complicated by hemorrhagic pulmonary edema. Subsequently, the patient had a stormy course complicated by pneumothoraces and pneumoperitoneum, from which he slowly recovered.

COMMENT

We present this case because elective herniorraphy is not often complicated. In fact, early repair of congenital hernias (at 4–6 months of postnatal age) is usually recommended to prevent incarceration since most occur within the first year of life. Unfortunately, the risks of this operation on a very small infant may outweigh the benefits. Complications include testicular atrophy, secondary to spermatic vessel injury, division of the vas deferens, unnecessary bladder entry and iatrogenic cryptorchidism. In a premature infant with a low hematocrit (this patient's was 30), the risk of transfusion should be weighed against the risk of incarceration, or waiting for an acceptable blood count. Premature infants show increased frequency of aspiration pneumonia, atelectasis, and postextubation stridor (Steward, 1982). The mechanism for the apnea has not been elucidated, but it may represent the effects of halothane as a respiratory depressant on intercostal muscle activity and/or easy fatigability of the preterm newborn's ventilatory muscles.

Postnatal age, size, and general condition warrant consideration in choice of time for elective repair of the hernia. We refrain from outpatient elective surgery when possible for at least 4 months, and prefer an inpatient facility staffed by pediatric surgeons and anesthesiologists who are experienced in managing intubation for those less than 4 months. Occasionally, repair may be done under local anesthesia.

neurologic abnormalities such as cerebral palsy, mental retardation, or developmental delay (Martin and Torres, 1985). It is rare in low birth weight infants and there is no racial predilection. Hirschsprung disease is responsible for approximately 25% of the cases of neonatal intestinal obstruction.

Natural History

Hirschsprung disease is rarely detected during the first month of life, but two-thirds are diagnosed by age 3 months. Only a rare case will be diagnosed after age 5 years, although it has been diagnosed in adults with a history of lifelong constipation. The presenting signs and symptoms most frequently associated with Hirschsprung disease in the newborn are illustrated in Table 7.7.

If not diagnosed early in infancy, within several months an infant will usually present with abdominal distention, vomiting, and failure to grow. Often, severe diarrhea may result after a prolonged period of constipation and is usually indicative of enterocolitis and is associated with a high mortality. Enterocolitis is rarely seen after 2 years of age, but can occur in over one-third of cases presenting by 3 months of age. Perforation and sepsis in this setting are common.

If the disease is not diagnosed in infancy, it can present in early childhood as chronic constipation with abdominal distention. If limited to an ultrashort segment (less than 5 cm), the disease may mimic encopresis. Severity of symptoms is not related to the length of the segment.

In addition to enterocolitis, patients with Hirschsprung disease may occasionally also present with intestinal perforation, chronic malnutrition, anemia, and a protein-losing enteropathy. Use of multiple tap water enemas as treatment for the disorder, may result in water intoxication.

Diagnosis

Hirschsprung disease must be distinguished from a functional stool retention problem. Both will affect males predominantly; functional problems are rare in newborns. Patients with a functional problem will have trouble with toilet training, whereas patients with Hirschsprung disease will not. Patients with Hirschsprung disease will often report no stools for the first 24–48 hours of life. Stools in patients with Hirschsprung disease are often thin, whereas in patients with functional bowel disease, they appear large and bulky. Abdominal pain is rare in patients with Hirschsprung disease unless there is obstruction, whereas it is more common in patients with functional bowel problems. Unlike patients with Hirschsprung disease, patients with encopresis usually do not show growth failure. Stool in the ampulla is diminished on rectal examination in Hirschsprung disease, but present in a functional stool retention situation. Patients with Hirschsprung disease will also have tight anal sphincter tone.

A radiograph of the abdomen may show a narrow rectum in Hirschsprung disease whereas there will be a dilated distended rectum in a functional bowel problem. A barium enema can confirm localized constriction with proximal dilatation, whereas with functional stool retention, a diffuse megacolon is found. The tip of the barium enema catheter should be inserted only just beyond the anal sphincter so that a clear-cut zone of transition between the aganglionic narrow distal segment and the dilated proximal segment with normal ganglion cells can be noted. This clear-cut zone is often not present at birth or early infancy, thus making a barium study less specific at this age. Contrast introduced into the colon of a baby should be expelled by 24 hours. Retention of barium is a good supporting sign for diagnosis of Hirschsprung disease (Fig. 7.10*A-C*).

If the barium study is inconclusive, rectal manometry should be considered. Patients with Hirschsprung disease will not show internal sphincter relaxation in response to transient rectal distention by the manometric balloon. Unfortunately, this test also carries false-negative results in patients who have had chronic constipation with or without encopresis.

Rectal biopsy provides the most reliable diagnosis and if radiographic or manometric studies are suggestive, biopsy should be performed to confirm the diagnosis. Initially, a suction biopsy should be done. If ganglion cells are found, Hirschsprung disease can be ruled out. In addition, acetylcholinesterase, which can be assessed by staining of a suction biopsy specimen is elevated in a patient with Hirschsprung disease (Huntley et al, 1982). If this enzyme is detected in the mucosa, it is unnecessary to do a full-thickness biopsy. Suction biopsy specimens should be obtained 1, 3, and 5 cm from the anal margin.

Table 7.7
Presenting Signs in Hirschsprung Disease in the Newborn[1]

Abdominal distention	54%
Failure to pass meconium in the first 48 hours	46%
Constipation	34%
Intestinal perforation	6%
Enterocolitis	60%
Associated malformations	26%

[1] Data of Polley and Coran: *Pediatr Surg Int* 1:80, 1986.

Treatment

Treatment consists of a colostomy in the neonatal period and definitive corrective surgery when the child is bigger, usually about 1 year of age. The best repair procedure remains controversial but includes an abdomino-anal pull-through (Swenson procedure), or a one-half aganglionic anastomosis excluding the rectum (Duhamel procedure), or a seromuscular cylinder (Soave procedure). Regardless of the procedure, goals of surgery are to permit normal defecation and to ensure continence. Before surgery, daily rectal irrigations may be needed to provide decompression.

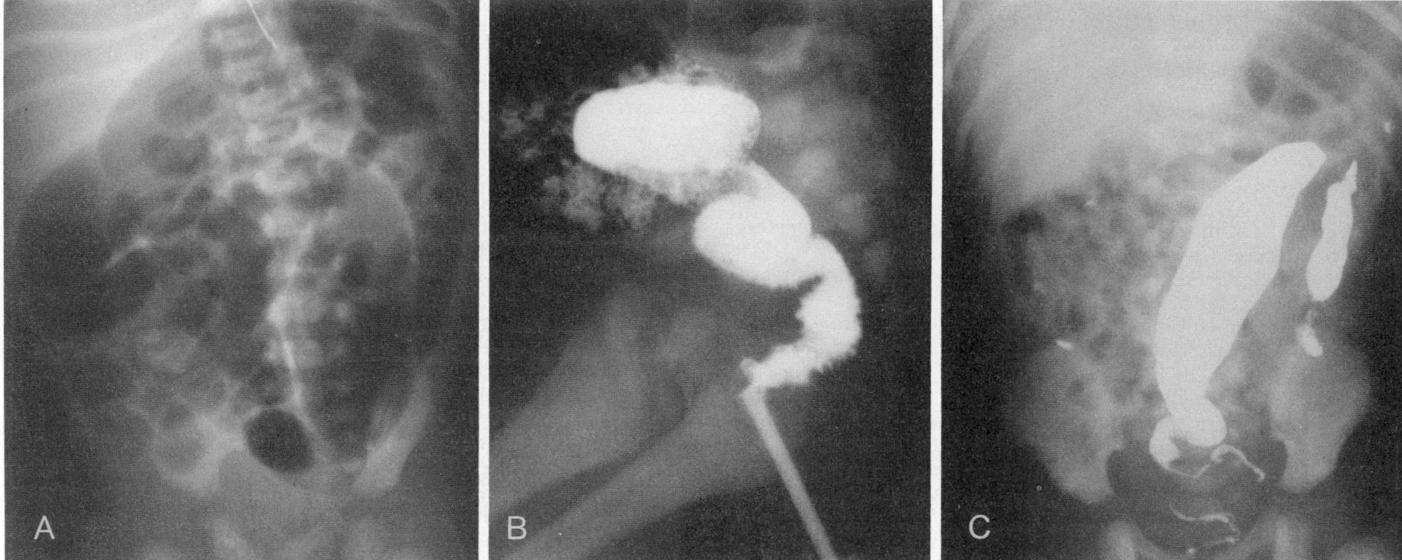

Figure 7.10. This baby had failed to pass meconium. Plain radiograph **(A)** shows distended loops of bowel; site of obstruction is indeterminate. Enema with barium demonstrates irregular narrowing of rectum **(B)**, and 24 hours later, **(C)** persisting contrast with a more obvious transition between dilated sigmoid colon and narrowed rectum. Biopsy of rectum confirmed aganglionosis.

Prognosis

Whatever surgical procedure is used, complications have been reported with an incidence as high as 45–60%. Postoperatively, complications include enterocolitis, incontinence, anal stenosis, recurrent obstruction, fecal fistula, and disruption of the anastomosis. In addition, Hirschsprung disease has been reported to occur postoperatively as well, perhaps secondary to vascular impairment or due to chronic inflammatory changes leading to recurrent stenosis. Mortality is as high as 25% if surgery is performed in the neonatal

CASE ILLUSTRATION

A 7-month-old white male had a history of vomiting, low grade fever, and constipation for 5 days. The vomiting was described as being bilious with brown flecked material and was associated with abdominal cramping. In the first days of life, he had abdominal distention with vomiting. Studies at that time included a barium enema and rectal manometry on the second day of life with a negative evaluation for Hirschsprung disease. The episode was ascribed to constipation and, subsequently, the infant began passing stools, feeding well, and gaining weight. However, at age 4–5 months, he began to have repeated episodes of constipation with radiographs demonstrating abundant stool throughout the colon, but otherwise a nonspecific bowel gas pattern with no evidence of perforation or obstruction. He had a low-grade fever of 38.5°C and appeared pale, tired, uncomfortable, and dehydrated, with a distended firm abdomen, hypoactive bowel sounds, and an empty rectal vault on digital examination. The white blood count was 6500/mm^3 with 12% polys, 10% bands. Urinalysis was notable for a specific gravity of 1.035 with large amounts of ketones. A radiograph of the abdomen revealed an airless large bowel with an enormous amount of stool in the colon and several air-fluid levels in the small bowel.

QUESTION AND COMMENT

What disease process is responsible for this patient's symptoms?

At the time of presentation, it was unclear whether there was a new intra-abdominal catastrophe such as an intussusception or volvulus or whether this was related to the patient's chronic history of constipation despite what was reported to be a negative work-up for Hirschsprung disease. Unfortunately, the definitive test for Hirschsprung disease, i.e., the rectal biopsy, had never been performed in this child. In the full-term infant, a barium enema can be difficult to interpret during the first 6 days of life because there is often a normal transition zone where a characteristic narrowing segment is simply not seen. Although manometric studies provide an excellent diagnostic tool, false-positives and -negatives are observed in early infancy. This patient underwent a water-soluble contrast enema shortly after arrival and displayed the classic transition zone in the sigmoid colon, with a massively distended proximal zone most consistent with Hirschsprung disease. He subsequently underwent a transverse colostomy to decompress the colon and allow the enterocolitis to resolve. Biopsy performed at surgery confirmed the diagnosis of Hirschsprung disease.

period (Martin and Torres, 1985). Otherwise, enterocolitis is the major cause of death in these patients either before or after surgery.

REFERENCES

Balistreri WF: Minimizing the effects of idiopathic inflammatory bowel disease. *Contemp Pediatr* 2:24, 1985.

Bartlett JG: *Clostridium difficile* in inflammatory bowel disease. *Gastroenterology* 80:863, 1981.

Bartlett JG, Moon N, Chang TW, et al: Role of *Clostridium difficile* in antibiotic associated pseudo membranous colitis. *Gastroenterology* 75:778, 1978.

Bartlett JG, Tedesco FJ, Shull S, et al: Symptomatic relapse after oral vancomycin therapy of antibiotic-associated pseudomembranous colitis. *Gastroenterology* 78:431, 1980.

Benson CD: Surgical complications of Meckel's diverticulum. In Ravitt MM, Welch KJ, Benson CD, et al (eds): *Pediatric Surgery*, 3rd edition. Chicago, Year Book Medical Publishers, 1973.

Bishop HC, Schnaufer L: Abdominal emergencies. Chapter 59. In Fleisher G, Ludwig S (eds): *Textbook of Pediatric Emergency Medicine*. Baltimore, Williams & Wilkins, 1983, p.837.

Brender JD, Marcuse EK, Koepsell TD, et al: Childhood appendicitis: Factors associated with perforation. *Pediatrics* 76:301, 1985.

Byrn JR, Fitzgerald JF, Northway JD, et al: Unusual manifestations of Henoch-Schönlein syndrome. *Am J Dis Child* 130:1335, 1976.

Calkins BM, Lilienfeld AM, Garland CF, et al: Trends in incidence rates of ulcerative colitis and Crohn's disease. *Dig Dis Sci* 29:913, 1984.

Cope Z: *Cope's Early Diagnosis of the Acute Abdomen,* 16th edition. Revised by William Silen. New York, Oxford University Press, 1983.

Cox JA: Inguinal hernia of childhood. *Surg Clin North Am* 65:1331, 1985.

Douglas JR, Campbell CA, Salisbury DM, et al: Colonoscopic polypectomy in children. *Br Med J* 281:1386, 1980.

Erbe RW: Inherited gastrointestinal-polyposis syndromes. *N Engl J Med* 294:1101, 1976.

Farmer RG, Whelan G, Fazio VW: Long-term follow up of patients with Crohn's disease. *Gastroenterology* 88:1818, 1985.

Fenoglio-Preiser CM, Hutter RVP: Colorectal polyps, pathologic diagnosis and clinical significance. *CA-A Cancer J Clin* 35:322, 1985.

Folkman J: In Ravitch MM, et al (eds): *Pediatric Surgery*, 3rd edition. Chicago, Year Book Medical Publishers, 1978.

Gebhard RL: Clinical and endoscopic findings in patients early in the course of *Clostridium difficile* associated pseudo membranous colitis. *Am J Med* 78:45, 1985.

Greenstein AJ, Janowitz HD, Sacher DB: The extra-intestinal complications of Crohn's disease and ulcerative colitis: A study of 700 patients. *Medicine* 55:401, 1976.

Greenstein AJ, Sacher DB: Pucillo A, et al: Cancer in universal and left-sided ulcerative colitis. *Mt Sinai J Med* 46:25, 1979.

Greifer I, Bernstein J, Kikkawa Y, et al: Histologic evidence of nephritis in patients with Henoch-Schönlein syndrome without clinical evidence of renal disease. In the Proceedings of the American Society of Nephrology (1966).

Grosfeld JL, Cooney DR: Inguinal hernia after ventriculo-peritoneal shunt for hydrocephalus. *J Pediatr Surg* 19:311, 1974.

Grotsky HW, Rickert RR, Smith WD, et al: Familial juvenile polyposis coli. *Gastroenterology* 82:494, 1982.

Gryboski J: Crohn's disease in children. *Pediatr Rev* 2:244, 1981.

Hamilton JR, Bruce GA, Abdourhaman M, et al: Inflammatory bowel disease in children and adolescents. *Adv Pediatr* 26:311, 1979.

Harper RG, Garcia A, Sia C: Inguinal hernia a common problem of premature infants weighing 1000 grams or less at birth. *Pediatrics* 56:112, 1975.

Hatch EI: The acute abdomen in children. *Pediatr Clin North Am* 32:1151, 1985.

Huntley CC, et al: Histochemical diagnosis of Hirschsprung's disease. *Pediatrics* 69:755, 1982.

Kelts D, Grand R: Inflammatory bowel disease in children and adolescents. *Curr Probl Pediatr* 10:1, 1980.

Kieswetter WB, Bill AH, Nixon HH, et al: Imperforate anus. *Arch Surg* 111:518, 1976.

Kieswetter WB, Chang JHT: Imperforate anus: A 5-30 year followup perspective. *Prog Pediatr Surg* 10:81, 1977.

Kirschner, BS; Inflammatory bowel disease in children. *Pediatr Clin North Am*, 35:189, 1988.

Koskimies O, et al: Henoch-Schönlein nephritis: Long-term prognosis of unselected patients. *Arch Dis Child* 56:482, 1981.

Malchow H, Ewe K, Brandes JW, et al: European cooperative Crohn's disease study: Results of drug treatment. *Gastroenterology* 86:249, 1984.

Malt RA: The perforated appendix. *N Engl J Med* 315:1546, 1986.

Martin GI, Kutner FR, Moser L: Diagnosis of Meckel's diverticulum by radioisotope scanning. *Pediatrics* 57:11, 1976.

Martin LW, Torres AM: Hirschsprung's disease. *Surg Clin North Am* 65:1171, 1985.

McGregor DB, Halverson K, McVay CB: The unilateral pediatric inguinal hernia: Should the contralateral side be explored? *J Pediatr Surg* 15:313, 1980

Meadow R: Schönlein-Henoch syndrome. *Arch Dis Child* 54:822, 1979.

Medical Staff Conference University of California, San Francisco: Crohn's disease newer aspects of etiology, prognosis and therapy. *West J Med* 128:419, 1978.

Meyers S, Sachar DB, Goldberg JD, et al: Corticotropin versus hydrocortisone in the intravenous treatment of ulcerative colitis. *Gastroenterology* 85:351, 1983.

Michener WM, Farmer RG, Mortimer EA: Long-term prognosis of ulcerative colitis with onset in childhood or adolescence. *J Clin Gastroenterol* 1:301, 1979.

Peevy KJ, Speed FA, Hoff CJ: Epidemiology of surgical hernias in preterm neonates. *Pediatrics* 77:246, 1986.

Polly TZ, Coran AG: Hirschsprung's disease in the newborn. *Pediatr Surg Int* 1:80, 1986.

Present DH, Korelitz BI, Wisch N, et al: Treatment of Crohn's disease with 6-mercaptopurine. *N Engl J Med* 302:981, 1980.

Ravitch MA: Appendicitis. *Pediatrics* 70:414, 1982.

Rosenblum ND, Winter HS: Steroid effects on the course of abdominal pain in children with Henoch-Schönlein purpura. *Pediatrics* 79:1018, 1987.

Sales DJ, Kirsner JB: The prognosis of inflammatory bowel disease. *Arch Intern Med* 143:294, 1983.

Saulsbury FT: IgA rheumatoid factor in Henoch-Schönlein purpura. *J Pediatr* 108:71, 1986.

Silber DL: Henoch-Schönlein syndrome. *Pediatr Clin North Am* 19:1061, 1972.

Silverberg M: Imperforate anus. In: *Pediatric Gastroenterology*. New York, Medical Examination, 1983, p. 125.

Silverman A, Roy CC: Ulcerative Colitis. In: *Pediatric Clinical Gastroenterology*. St. Louis, CV Mosby, 1983, p. 353.

Silverman A, Roy CC: *Pediatric Clinical Gastroenterology*. St. Louis, CV Mosby, 1983, p. 455.

Smith CD: Complications of pediatric surgery—prevention and management. In Welsh KJ: *The Abdominal Parietes*. Philadelphia, WB Saunders, 1982, p. 211.

Steward DJ: Preterm infants are more prone to complications following minor surgery than are term infants. *Anesthesiology* 56:304, 1982.

Tauscher JW, Bryant DR, Gruenther RC: False positive scan for Meckel's diverticulum. *J Pediatr* 92:1022, 1978.

Thomas DFM, Fernie DS, Malone M, et al: Association between *Clostridium difficile* and enterocolitis in Hirschsprung's disease. *Lancet* 1:78, 1982.

Viidik T, Marshall DG: Direct inguinal hernias in infancy and early childhood. *J Pediatr Surg* 15:646, 1980.

Wald A, Mendelow H, Bartlett JG: Nonantibiotic associated pseudo membranous colitis due to toxin produced *Clostridia*. *Ann Intern Med* 92:798, 1980.

Weber TR, Grosfeld JL, Bergstein J, Fitzgerald J, et al: Massive gastric hemorrhage: An unusual complication of Henoch-Schönlein purpura. *J Pediatr Surg* 18:576, 1983.

Wesson DE, Schandling, B: Results of bowel resection for Crohn's disease in the young. *J Pediatr Surg* 16:449, 1981.

Approaches to Other Conditions

5

OMPHALOCELE AND GASTROSCHISIS

Definition

Omphalocele and gastroschisis represent the two major abdominal wall developmental defects. Gastroschisis is a herniation without a covering sac of small intestine through a full-thickness complete abdominal wall defect, usually to the right of the normal umbilicus. An omphalocele is a congenital hernia that contains the intestine covered by an avascular sac composed of fused layers of amnion and peritoneum. An omphalocele that ruptures in utero will be indistinguishable from gastroschisis. An omphalocele may contain other organs of the abdominal cavity, whereas this is rarely observed in a gastroschisis, except that occasionally the liver is involved.

Basic Science

The pathogenesis of gastroschisis has yet to be definitively described. Hypotheses range from a congenital failure of formation of one of the lateral plates of the abdominal wall to an antenatal or perinatal tear or rupture through the membrane of a hernia of the umbilical cord, with a visceration subsequently through the less well-supported and more vulnerable side of an umbilical hernia sac. Omphalocele results from failure of the intestine to return to the abdominal cavity before birth, or a failure of closure of the umbilical ring, sealing abdominal contents back into the abdomen. No familial tendency has been confirmed for omphalocele, although congenital anomalies are reported in 40% of cases in first degree relatives suggesting that omphalocele is more likely to be a result of a genetic insult, whereas gastroschisis results from environmental (e.g., drugs and pollutants) influences (Moore and Nor, 1986).

Epidemiology

The incidence of these abdominal defects is estimated to be in 1/6000 births (Martin and Torres, 1985). Gastroschisis is associated with prematurity in 60% of patients, but rarely is associated with other malformations. Omphaloceles, on the other hand, are not associated with prematurity but often occur (60% of patients) with other anomalies, including intestinal obstruction, extrophy of the bladder, renal anomalies, and cardiovascular defects. In addition, omphalocele has been found in infants with Beckwith-Wiedemann syndrome in which macroglossia, microcephaly, macrosomia, renal hyperplasia, and severe hypoglycemia are associated with the defect.

Natural History

Most gastroschisis occurs to the right of the umbilical cord and usually varies from 2–15 cm in size. Gastroschisis appears as an edematous, viscerated mass of small bowel loops, usually of dark color, and encased in a thick gelatinous matrix of greenish fibrinous material. There is no peristalsis and the mesentery appears thick and edematous. Often jejeunoileal atresias or stenoses are evident as a result of autoamputation due to small strangulating defects that are caused by intrauterine volvulus of a viscerated intestine. The exposure of intestine to amniotic fluid will produce an intense peritonitis. The longer the intestine is exposed to amniotic fluid, the longer the time it will take for normal intestinal function to return. An omphalocele usually presents with the umbilical cord inserted into the sac and umbilical vessels running radially within its wall. There is usually no fixation of the midgut with resultant incomplete rotation. If the sac is ruptured earlier, similar to gastroschisis, the intestines may appear edematous and matted together by the fibrinous material characteristic of gastroschisis.

Diagnosis

Diagnosis is made at birth upon observation of the abdomen.

Treatment

A nasogastric tube should be placed shortly after birth to prevent further GI distention secondary to swallowing air, which will hinder closure of the defect. If no sac is present to contain the abdominal contents, the child will probably have increased fluid and heat losses.

Gastroschisis should be treated surgically as soon as possible to minimize the possibility of bacterial infection. Most patients with gastroschisis require staged surgical procedures to introduce the extra-abdominal contents back into the peritoneal cavity. About 10% of patients will be able to receive the abdominal contents in a one-stage procedure. During staged procedures, parenteral nutrition is essential until the defect can be closed. Paralytic ileus may persist in these patients for weeks, and sometimes months, and mechanical obstruction, wound infection, volvulus, constricting bands, bowel necrosis, and fistulae are common.

The initial management of an omphalocele is to cover the sac with moist gauze sponges and to wrap the abdomen without any pressure being applied to the sac. If the defect is less than 5 cm in diameter, a one-stage repair can be done. If the omphalocele is too large for primary repair and there is too little skin to cover the sac for repair when the child is older, the sac is covered with prosthetic material such as Silastic. Occasionally, if the omphalocele sac is intact, painting the sac with alcohol or tincture of merthiolate to promote skin growth will suffice for initial management. Later, the eventual hernia can be repaired once the abdominal cavity has grown sufficiently to accommodate the viscera that have been extruded. Complications of omphalocele surgery include prolonged ileus, duodenal obstruction or midgut volvulus, gastroesophageal reflux, and obstruction due to adhesions.

Prognosis

There is a 30% mortality in patients with gastroschisis, usually due to infection, prematurity, gangrenous small bowel, or paralytic ileus noted at birth, and, less commonly, due to complications of the surgical repair. Over the past several years, the use of parenteral alimentation has dramatically reduced surgical complications and mortality from this disease. Omphalocele mortality is also 30%, but is usually attributable to associated malformations rather than to the defect itself or the postoperative problems (Martin and Torres, 1985). Long-term follow-up studies in patients who survive to age 1 year have not been reported.

ASCITES

Definition

Ascites is defined as a transudate—that is, a fluid of low specific gravity (less than 1.015), and low protein concentration (less than 3 g/dl), containing only a few lymphocytes (less than 10–15)—that has passed through a membrane or been extruded from a tissue into the abdominal cavity.

Basic Science

Mesenteric attachments and peritoneal reflections are responsible for the natural pathways for and barriers to the spread of free abdominal fluid, with the transverse colon and the mesentery of the small bowel being the two most important anatomic barriers. There are two types of ascitic fluid: (1) simple ascites, the clear transudate produced as a result of a metabolic neoplastic or inflammatory disturbance; and (2) complex ascites, an exudate that is usually more viscid containing proteinaceous material. Inflammatory, neoplastic chylous, or hemorrhagic ascites are examples of the more complex type, which has a greater tendency to loculate.

The changes in the homeostasis existing between capillary hydrostatic pressure, colloid oncotic pressure, and capillary permeability promote a net tendency for fluid to move to the extravascular, extracellular space and, hence, produce ascites and/or edema.

Epidemiology

See specific disease entity for a discussion of epidemiology.

Natural History

The causes of ascites in childhood are multiple (Table 7.8).

Diagnosis

Abdominal distention is the hallmark of ascites. This may be associated with abdominal pain and/or dyspnea. Physical examination is notable for bulging flanks and a fluid wave. Although shifting dullness to percussion may be a sensitive indicator for identifying ascites, it is nonspecific. Ultrasonography is most useful and can detect as little as 100 ml of fluid in adults and even smaller amounts in infants. Ascites can also be diagnosed in utero through ultrasonography, permitting appropriate plans for the delivery of such a high-risk infant.

Once identified, ascitic fluid must be obtained for further diagnostic evaluation. Aspiration under ultrasonographic guidance is the most effective procedure, particularly for small amounts of fluid. The gross appearance of ascitic fluid is of limited value, since over one-third of adult patients with uninfected ascites have hazy or turbid fluid because of the presence of lipids or small amounts of blood. Moreover, in patients who have spontaneous bacterial peritonitis clear fluid has been found to contain over 10,000 white cells/mm^3. Cloudy fluid usually requires over 40,000 cells/mm^3. The specific gravity or protein concentration is not helpful except for aiding diagnosis of pancreatitis. The glucose concentration is less useful as an indicator than it is in cerebral or synovial fluids since it will rarely be less than half the serum level in a peritonitis episode. In pancreatitis the fluid amylase will often, but not always, be higher than the serum amylase. The number and type of leukocytes can be of critical diagnostic importance. The normal range is 0–500 white blood cells/mm^3. In spontaneous bacterial peritonitis the white

Table 7.8
Conditions Associated with Ascites

Decrease in venous return to heart
- Constrictive pericarditis
- Heart failure (cardiac arrhythmias in utero)

Generalized edema
- Hypoproteinemia
- Renal failure (posterior urethral valves in infants)

Portal vein obstruction
- Cirrhosis
- Enlarged lymph nodes
- Thrombosis

Chronic peritonitis
- Pancreatitis
- Tuberculosis
- Other bacteria

Ovarian tumors

count is usually greater than 2000 and three-quarters of the cells are polys. Gram stain aids bacterial identification in only one-fourth of infected patients, so that culture is mandatory. Since over 20 different organisms have been identified in ascitic fluid, broad spectrum coverage is useful in treatment.

Treatment

Before treatment, a Gram stain and culture should be obtained, but any patient suspected of having an infectious peritonitis should be treated, regardless of the number of white cells noted in the ascitic fluid. Any patient with more than 1000 white cells should be treated with broad spectrum antibiotics, even in the absence of symptoms, unless a predisposing malignancy or a pancreatitis that could contribute to the leukocytosis in the ascitic fluid has been identified. Ascites secondary to cirrhosis can be treated with sodium restriction and diuretics. Diuresis in such patients should be limited to achieve a weight loss of 200–300 g/day, which can be increased if peripheral edema is also present. Spironalactone is the agent of choice, followed by or combined with furosemide. An infusion of albumin, 30–60 minutes before the intravenous administration of furosemide is also useful in refractory cases of ascites. The patient should be monitored for hyponatremia and hypokalemia during treatment with the diuretic.

For symptomatic abdominal pain or respiratory distress, the child may undergo paracentesis although the volume removed should be limited to less than 1–2 L/24 hours, depending on the child's size, to prevent acute reaccumulation and worsening of symptoms. Paracentesis is often combined with the use of diuretics. Another approach is a peritoneojugular venous shunt which serves as an artificial lymphatic system between the abdominal cavity and the blood stream. While this procedure acts as a one-way valve to channel fluid from the peritoneum, it is more commonly used in adults and its complications have included disseminated intravascular coagulation, fever, shunt oclusion, embolisms, and infection. Moreover, it does not reverse the hepatorenal syndrome. In intractible ascites, portal systemic shunting can be attempted, although this procedure carries a high operative mortality (greater than 40% in children), and significant morbidity as well (Wyllie et al, 1980).

PERITONITIS

Definition

Peritonitis is acute inflammation of the peritoneal cavity. It may either be primary or secondary in etiology: primary represents inflammation when a perforation of an abdominal viscus cannot be demonstrated; secondary peritonitis represents inflammation due to bacteria, bile, or pancreatic enzymes released because of rupture or perforation of an intra-abdominal viscus.

Basic Science

Peritonitis usually occurs following bacterial infection introduced into the peritoneal cavity. The most common organisms are *Escherichia coli,* with group A streptococcus and pneumococcus now reported less frequently. In girls aged 5–10 years, a Gram-negative infection causing primary peritonitis is usually due to entry via the vagina. This occurs when the cervix is open, but the vaginal fluid is not yet acidic enough to hinder the ascent of infection. Most cases of secondary peritonitis occur early in life usually due to necrotizing enterocolitis or spontaneous perforation of the stomach. In childhood, a ruptured appendix is the most likely cause of secondary peritonitis, although any other abdominal viscus that ruptures may be responsible, including peptic ulcer, volvulus, intussusception, strangulated hernia, trauma, or chronic ulcerative colitis. The flora in secondary peritonitis depend on those found in the perforated organ. In these patients, multiple aerobic and anerobic organisms can be grown. The most frequently found are *E. coli, Klebsiella, Proteus,* and *Enterobacter,* with *Bacteroides* the most likely anerobic organism. In older children the infection may localize, whereas in younger children it tends to spill diffusely into the peritoneal cavity, perhaps due to infants having a shorter omentum providing less protection.

Some degree of immunologic incompetence may play a role in primary peritonitis and the disease is found in patients who are often immunologically compromised, including those with nephrotic syndrome or chronic liver disease.

Epidemiology

Primary peritonitis accounts for less than 1% of acute abdomens in children. A 10-year survey in Cleveland reported 26 cases, in which only six cases of primary peritonitis presented in the first 2 months of life, with the remaining 20 cases presenting at an average age of 8.5 years (McDougal et al, 1975).

Natural History

The signs and symptoms of peritonitis may closely mimic those of a perforated appendix, including abdominal pain preceding vomiting, presence of small loose stools, and fever. There is usually abdominal distention with diffuse tenderness and rigidity.

Diagnosis

A patient with nephrosis, chronic liver disease, or status postsplenectomy, for example, should raise the possibility of primary peritonitis rather than a perforated appendix. The white blood count is usually greater than 15,000/mm^3, with a left shift. Diagnosis rests on paracentesis, which can be safely performed in patients in whom primary peritonitis is suspected. Normal ascitic fluid contains less than 300 white cells/mm^3 with 75% polys. Gram stain of the peritoneal fluid should reveal a suspected organism, which can be identified by culture.

Plain radiographs of the abdomen may be useful to localize an intra-abdominal abscess responsible for a secondary peritonitis; as can ultrasonography or CT. A blood culture should also be obtained, as it can be positive in up to 30% of cases of secondary peritonitis. Acute pyelonephritis can mimic peritonitis.

Treatment

In primary peritonitis, treatment is conservative and consists of broad spectrum antibiotics until an organism has been identified by culture. Useful antibiotic coverage would be a combination of ampicillin, clindamycin, and gentamicin or an appropriate cephalosporin.

If secondary peritonitis is diagnosed, surgical correction is the treatment of choice. In preparation for surgery, the patient should be adequately rehydrated, and receive gastric suction to prevent further abdominal distention. Antibiotic treatment is still mandatory and should be broad spectrum until either the peritoneal, blood, or urine cultures reveal the organism.

Prognosis

Prognosis for both primary and secondary peritonitis is good, with less than 10% mortality in childhood.

PANCREATITIS

Definition

Pancreatitis is inflammation of the pancreas, which can result from a number of causes and can be either acute or chronic. If the attacks become recurrent, the condition is defined as chronic pancreatitis. Chronic relapsing pancreatitis is most often a familial, autosomal dominant disease.

Basic Science

While alcoholism and biliary tract disease are responsible for most cases of pancreatitis in adults, childhood cases of pancreatitis have other causes including drug toxicity, trauma, infection (e.g., viral infections and mycoplasma), genetic, or idiopathic. Pancreatitis has been associated with some systemic diseases such as lupus, inflammatory bowel disease, cystic fibrosis, and diabetes. Biliary tract disease including choledocal cysts, gallstones, as well as direct injury to the pancreas can result in acute inflammation. Metabolic disease such as α-1-antitrypsin deficiency and hyperlipidemia types 1 and 5 are also associated with pancreatitis.

Regardless of etiology, the exact mechanism by which the inflammatory process is triggered remains unknown. Currently it is believed that a sequence of events occurs leading to the release of a variety of proteolytic proenzymes that begin to autodigest the gland. Among these enzymes are trypsin, elastase, phospholipase, and ribonuclease. Amylase released from destroyed acinar tissue enters the blood and provides a useful laboratory diagnostic test.

Drugs that have been associated with pancreatitis include azathioprine, thiazide diuretics, furosemide, estrogens, and sulfonamides and L-asparaginase.

Epidemiology

Pancreatitis rarely occurs in children under 5 years of age. Of reported cases, 25% have the acute hemorrhagic form and the remainder an interstitial form of the disease. About half the cases appear secondary to trauma or infectious etiology, most notably mumps virus (Jordan and Ament, 1977).

Natural History

Abdominal pain, nausea, and vomiting are the three most common symptoms and occur in over three-quarters of children who present with pancreatitis. Children experience pain in the upper quadrants and periumbilical region of the abdomen, whereas in adults, pain usually is localized to the midepigastric area and then radiates to the back. Regardless of age, the pain is constant and is usually worsened by eating and relieved when a child is placed in a knee-chest position. Vomiting is usually worsened by eating or drinking and does not bring relief for the pain. An average attack lasts 24–72 hours and is considered severe if there is a bluish discoloration around the umbilicus (Cullen sign) or in the flanks (Grey-Turner sign); cardiovascular instability (shock or arrythmias); renal insufficiency (oliguria); pulmonary involvement (dyspnea or rales secondary to hemorrhagic pleural effusions); metabolic disturbances (fever, irritability, fluid retention, confusion); and/or protracted ileus with a tense abdomen. While hypovolemia and hemoconcentration may be common early in an episode of acute pancreatitis, several days after onset of symptoms, hypervolemia and congestive heart failure may occur because of sudden absorption of fluids from the peritoneal and pleural cavities back into the circulation. In addition, 15% of patients with acute disease develop an inflammatory mass, usually a pancreatic pseudocyst or pancreatic abscess (Winship et al, 1977).

Diagnosis

Physical examination will disclose minimal to moderate guarding, with maximal tenderness in the midepigastric region. Rebound tenderness also can be localized to the upper quadrants. Bowel sounds will vary from hyper- to hypoactive to absent depending on the degree of peritoneal inflammation. Fever, which can be as high as 39.5°C, will last for 3–5 days, and on rare occasions for weeks. Laboratory tests required for diagnosis are an elevated serum and urine amylase, and a raised serum lipase level. Rarely are these three tests all negative (Moosa, 1984).

The serum amylase may be normal for the first 24 hours, only to become abnormal and reach a peak within 48–72 hours from onset of the episode. The serum lipase remains elevated for several days after the serum amylase has returned to normal. The advantage of obtaining a serum lipase is that the pancreas is the only major source of the enzyme. Lipase is not detectable in urine. The severity of the pancreatic episode does not correspond to the degree of serum amylase or lipase elevation. If the serum amylase has not diminished in 2 weeks, a pancreatic pseudocyst should be suspected and abdominal CT scan obtained.

Other useful laboratory values are determination of hypocalcemia and hyperglycemia, which suggest more widespread destruction of the gland. Supportive evidence can also be obtained from plain radiographs of the abdomen which, while not diagnostic for pancreatitis, may help to rule out other entities in the differential diagnosis, including pneumoperitoneum, small bowel obstruction or aortic aneurysm. Air-fluid levels suggest small bowel obstruction rather than acute pancreatitis. A plain radiograph may also show a localized ileus, pancreatic calcification, or gallstones. Hypoalbuminemia, glycosuria, hypolipidemia, and an elevated ESR, white blood count, bilirubin, and liver function tests have been associated with pancreatitis.

In the acute situation, CT scan is considered to be more useful than ultrasonography since an associated paralytic ileus will hinder thorough examination of the gland by ultrasonography. CT will demonstrate the pancreas as a focal mass with irregular borders. It is most helpful to identify complications such as a pseudocyst and can help to determine whether the cyst contains blood and/or pus, or if gas bubbles are seen, it would suggest a pancreatic abscess. If GI bleeding has occurred, angiography may be useful to pinpoint and aid treatment of hemorrhagic complications. Chronic pancreatitis is best evaluated using endoscopic retrograde cholangiopancreatography (ERCP).

Treatment

Objectives of treatment are to reduce pancreatic exocrine secretion, relieve pain, and treat any contributing shock and electrolyte abnormalities. Normally the patient should receive nothing by mouth and be treated with maintenance fluid and electrolytes via parenteral therapy. A nasogastric tube is placed if nausea and vomiting or an ileus occur. Feeding can be restarted with carbohydrate-containing solutions when abdominal tenderness has disappeared, the ileus has resolved, and the amylase clearance is normal. Later, low-fat, low-protein diets are appropriate. If bowel rest continues for more than 5 days, parenteral hyperalimentation should be started.

Antibiotics are not recommended since the inflammatory reaction is apparently not provoked by bacterial infections and studies show that the rate of improvement is not increased in patients given antibiotics.

Pain is treated with meperidine, given intravenously every 3–4 hours. Morphine and codeine will produce a greater degree of spasm of the duodenum and sphincter of Oddi and are, therefore, not recommended.

Surgery is indicated only when the diagnosis is unclear. Surgical resection of the pancreas is usually reserved for cases of fulminant hemorrhagic pancreatitis, which represent less than 3% of all cases. Surgery is sometimes used for debridement of necrotic tissue or for drainage of an abscess, at which time the lesser peritoneal sac and gutters are also drained.

CONTROVERSIES

The use of anticholinergic drugs is controversial in that the side effects may offset the benefits of decreased pancreatic secretion.

Prognosis

No correlation has been observed between elevation of serum amylase and the severity of the pancreatic inflammation. Mortality for acute interstitial pancreatitis in childhood is about 17%, whereas for acute hemorrhagic pancreatitis, it is over 85% (Jordan and Ament, 1977). Death is believed to be due to the extreme fluid losses that occur in acute hemorrhagic pancreatitis. If recurrent episodes and relapse occur, surgery may eventually be necessary. If there is underlying renal or hepatic disease, the prognosis also remains poor. If severe recurrent pain continues, other complications may be narcotic addiction, depression, and suicide in adolescence, although again these events are rare and recurrence in general is rare in children.

PANCREATIC PSEUDOCYST

Definition

Pancreatic pseudocyst is a cystic structure usually located in the lesser sac of the omentum. Its walls are composed of granulation tissue and its lining is devoid of epithelium. The boundaries of the pseudocyst are determined by the organs that outline the lesser peritoneal cavity. It may or may not communicate with the pancreatic duct system. It is usually unilocular and volumes in excess of a liter have been encountered.

Basic Science

Pancreatic pseudocysts develop in or from the head, body, or tail of the pancreas and consist of collections of blood, pancreatic enzymes, tissue fluid and debris from the pancreas that progresses over a period of days to weeks after an attack of acute pancreatitis. In children, trauma is the predominant cause, with the remaining cases being either idiopathic or secondary to hereditary pancreatitis, cholelithiasis, or mumps virus.

Epidemiology

Twenty percent of cases of traumatic pancreatitis in children will result in a pancreatic pseudocyst. If the pseudocyst is due to pancreatitis, it is more apt to occur in children under 5 years than in older children, whereas if it is due to trauma it may occur in any age group (Winship et al, 1977).

Natural History

With the use of ultrasonography it now appears that up to 85% of pseudocysts resolve spontaneously and usually do so within a 2-week period. The majority of cases are uncomplicated, despite their persistence. In one-third of cases, pain occurs owing to expansion of the lesion with pressure on other organs. A pseudocyst is palpable in at least one-third of patients and will displace some portion of the upper GI tract radiographically in three-quarters of patients. If the common bile duct is compressed, jaundice and pain may result. If the stomach is encroached, a sense of fullness or nausea and vomiting may occur. Rupture, particularly into the peritoneal cavity, carries significant morbidity and mortality. The highest mortality results if there is hemorrhage into the pseudocyst, since in roughly half of such cases, bleeding into the cyst arises from a major artery, thus creating a pseudoaneurysm. Occasionally, the pseudocyst may be converted to an abscess, usually during the second week to the sixth month after an attack of pancreatitis. Frequently, these abscesses follow inadequate surgical drainage or needling of the pseudocyst.

Diagnosis

Elevated serum amylase or lipase values occur in less than half the patients, although an elevated urinary excretion of amylase relative to creatinine clearance sometimes occurs.

Treatment

No specific therapy is available. Serial observations should include frequent physical examinations, serum creatinine to amylase clearance ratio determinations, and serial ultrasonography. Indications for surgery are continuous growth of the cyst or persistent symptoms. Fever, leukocytosis, and ileus may suggest an abscess and require immediate surgical intervention. The child with contraindications to anesthesia and/or surgery is a candidate for percutaneous drainage of the cyst.

If surgery can be postponed for 6 weeks, the cyst wall is thicker and the outlook is better. Complications can include hemorrhage from the pseudocyst or from the anastomosis, or from the viscus into which the pseudocyst has drained, or recurrent pancreatitis, and death. Often, definitive treatment can be postponed while an initial operation to drain the pseudocyst is performed. If an abscess is present, without surgical drainage, death is inevitable. Even with the appropriate use of antibiotics, mortality with drainage approaches 50% (Winship et al, 1977).

JAUNDICE

Definition

Jaundice is a term to describe a condition in which bile production or flow is impaired. (see also pp. 200–208) When there is a problem in biliary flow, the condition is referred to as cholestasis. The obstruction can be at the intra- or extrahepatic level, and if it is intrahepatic, it can involve bile formation, secretion, or transport because of hepatocellular dysfunction or disruption of the continuity of smaller intrahepatic bile ducts. Extrahepatic obstruction can occur in any location along the bile duct from the hilum of the liver to the duodenum.

Basic Science

Heme is the ultimate source of bilirubin. It comes from a variety of sources in the body, including heme-containing enzymes in the liver (e.g., cytochrome P-450, catalases and peroxidases), which can be degraded into bilirubin in a matter of a few hours to a few days. Bilirubin is also derived from degradation of red cells, which have a half-life of about 120 days in adults and 80 days in newborns. Heme oxygenase, which is present in many different types of cells but has highest activity in organs responsible for the sequestration of cells, such as spleen and liver, converts heme to bi-

CASE ILUSTRATION 1

A 7-year-old male presented to the hospital for evaluation of obstructive jaundice. He had been treated with phototherapy at birth for hyperbilirubinemia which resolved, only to develop recurrent jaundice with elevation in liver function tests at 2 months of age. Liver biopsy at that time showed "giant cell" neonatal hepatitis and a repeat biopsy at 10 months (with jaundice no longer clinically evident, but persistently elevated liver function tests) revealed a resolving hepatitis without evidence of cholestasis. The patient was well for the next 6 years, until 2 months before admission when jaundice and acholic stools developed and were treated with cholestyramine. Initial physical examination was notable for marked icterus with a slightly enlarged liver span. Laboratory values included a bilirubin 14.4 mg/dl total with a 14.0 mg/dl direct, an alkaline phosphatase of 612 U/L and a normal SGOT and SGPT. Clotting studies were slightly prolonged, but easily correctable with vitamin K. Ultrasonography and CT scan were normal and a Bida scan revealed no excretion after 4 hours. An ophthalmologic examination was negative for Kaiser-Fleischer rings.

QUESTION AND COMMENT

What further work-up is indicated and what are the diagnostic possibilities?

In this patient, liver biopsy was performed and showed a paucity of intrahepatic ducts, consistent with a cholestatic picture most often seen with intrahepatic ductal hypoplasia. This entity has been described in infants with neonatal hepatitis who subsequently developed cholestasis over a period of 5 months to 22 years. The histologic changes apparently represent a continuum that begin with the hepatitis, regress to the ductal hypoplasia and then may go on to portal fibrosis and cirrhosis. Complete biliary atresia, however, has not been noted in these patients despite 20 years of follow-up. Symptomatic improvement has been obtained with cholestyramine and with phenobarbital, both of which were instituted in this patient before discharge.

liverdin by cleaving heme at the the α-carbon bridge. The biliverdin is then further degraded to bilirubin by biliverdin reductase, which is present in the cytosol. (Of interest is the recent discovery that tin protoporphyrin is a potent inhibitor of heme oxygenase and prevents the degradation of heme so that it is excreted as free heme in bile. This discovery may be useful in the future for treatment of neonatal hyperbilirubinemia (Kappas et al, 1988).

Once formed, bilirubin is referred to as unconjugated bilirubin and is transported to the liver bound to serum albumin. Upon reaching the liver, albumin becomes detached and returns to the circulation and the bilirubin gets transported at an as yet unidentified binding site on the hepatocyte across the plasma membrane surface. This transport of bilirubin appears to be carrier-mediated and exhibits saturation and competitive inhibition kinetics.

Once bilirubin has crossed the hepatocyte plasma membrane, it binds to cytoplasmic hydrophobic proteins, principally glutathione S-transferase B, also known as ligandin. This protein is the major transport protein for bilirubin. Once bound to ligandin, the bilirubin is then acted upon by UDP-glucuronyltransferase, a microsomal enzyme that polarizes the bilirubin by adding a polar sugar to the proprionic acid groups so that it can be excreted into the bile. The addition of these sugars, either mono- or diglucuronides, is known as conjugation. The absence of one form of glucuronyltransferase can create a genetic predisposition for jaundice, known as the Crigler-Najjar syndrome. In infants, bile acids are mainly conjugated with taurine; in adults, glycine predominates. The bilirubin conjugated is transported from the cytoplasm of the hepatocyte across the canalicular membrane and into the bile. This is believed to be the rate-limiting step in the overall transport of bilirubin from blood to bile, and to be responsible for hyperbilirubinemia associated with hepatocellular and hepatocanalicular disorders.

Three mechanisms of bile production have been identified: (1) A bile salt-dependent flow in which osmotically active bile salts create an osmotic force which promotes water flow into canaliculi; (2) a bile salt-independent flow linked to an active sodium transport mediated by sodium/potassium-ATPase activity; and (3) ductular bile flow in which an inorganic electrolyte solution consisting of sodium chloride and sodium bicarbonate further modifies bile composition. Moreover,

CASE ILLUSTRATION 2

A 2-month-old white male infant presented to the hospital for evaluation of cholestatic jaundice. He was the 3.4-kg product of a full-term unremarkable pregnancy, labor, and delivery, with Apgar scores of 9 at both 1 min and 5 min. He was discharged home on day 3 of life, and at 6 weeks of age, jaundice was noted by his parents, resolving after several days, but subsequently followed by vomiting and poor weight gain. The patient had been breast-fed but nursing was discontinued and replaced by feeding on elemental formula and the vomiting resolved. Three days before his admission, the vomiting recurred along with dark urine and jaundice. He had a hematocrit of 34%, a white count of 16,500/mm^3 with 24% polys and 54% lymphs, 16% atypical lymphs, and 6% monos, normal platelets and a bilirubin of 3.4 mg/dl total over 2.9 mg/dl direct. An abdominal ultrasonographic examination was reported as showing a choledochal cyst, prompting his admission to the hospital.

Initial physical examination revealed a mildly jaundiced male infant whose height, length, and head circumference were in the 60th percentile. There was slight scleral icterus and the liver was palpable 1 cm below the right costal margin. There was no splenomegaly. Laboratory evaluation revealed a bilirubin of 1.1 mg/dl total over 0.7 mg/dl direct, an SGOT of 20 U/L, SGPT of 65 U/L, LDH of 136 U/L, amylase of 17 U/L, and albumin of 3.8 mg/dl.

QUESTION AND COMMENT

What further diagnostic and therapeutic work-up is indicated?

The presentation appeared to be compatible with the diagnosis of a choledochal cyst. A nuclear medicine scan may be useful to rule out the presence of accompanying proximal ductular atresia and to show excretion into gut. If anatomy is not clear, a transhepatic cholangiogram may be able to define the anatomy before surgery, although the procedure is difficult to perform and may be unrevealing in infants.

In this patient, a repeat ultrasonographic examination was done before the transhepatic cholangiogram. The cyst seen on a previous ultrasonography was not present, but there was intra- and extrahepatic ductular dilatation. On that day, the baby also developed a fever and a diffusely tender abdomen and was treated with ampicillin and gentamycin for a possible cholangitis. A blood culture subsequently grew *E. coli* and the BIDA scan showed delayed but eventual passage of the radionucleotide into the bowel. Gallbladder was visualized, and the findings at that time pointed to obstruction at the level of the distal common bile duct.

What are some possible causes for this obstruction?

Causes could include a stone, bile sludge or a stricture, an intramural choledochocele in the duodenum or extrinsic compression from a duodenum duplication, or a tumor such as a rhabdomyosarcoma. An upper GI study revealed a round smooth impression on the medial aspects of the duodenal loop. Definitive diagnosis resulted from the transhepatic cholangiogram, which showed almost complete obstruction of the biliary tree by a 1-cm mass in the distal common bile duct. A laparotomy was done once the infection had been brought under control and a common bile duct stone was demonstrated at the ampulla of vater. There was no other abnormality. The stone was removed and the infant recovered. Possibly the prior diagnosis of choledochal cyst had been based on visualizing an enlarged gallbladder and mistaking it for an enlarged choledochus.

Table 7.9
Some Causes of Prolonged Hyperbilirubinemia in Infants

Conjugated	Predominantly Unconjugated
Hepatic cell injury	Hemolysis
Infection	Isoimmunization
Bacteria	Defects in red cell metabolism
Syphilis	Infection
Listeriosis	Increased enterohepatic circulation
Viral	Intestinal obstruction
Rubella	Meconium ileus
Cytomegalovirus	Pyloric stenosis
Herpes	Paralytic ileus
Hepatitis	Hypothyroidism
Parasites	Hypopituitarism
Toxoplasmosis	Gilbert disease
Toxic	Familial nonhemolytic jaundice
Sepsis	Extravasation of blood
Intravenous alimentation	Cephalohematomas
Drugs	Bruises
Inborn errors	Swallowed blood
Galactosemia	Chronic bilirubin overload
Tyrosinemia	Erythroblastosis
α-1-Antitrypsin deficiency	G6PD deficiency
Obstruction to bile flow	Congenital hemolytic anemias
Biliary atresia	
Choledochal cyst	
Cystic fibrosis	
Tumors	

bile flow is modulated by various endogenous compounds. Thyroxine and cortisone increase bile salt-independent flow, while ethinyl estradiol decreases this flow. Ductular flow is stimulated by secretin and cholecystokinin. Endotoxins produced by Gram-negative bacterial infections will decrease bile salt-independent flow by inhibiting sodium/potassium ATPase activity (Spivak, 1985).

The total absence of glucuronyl transferase is known as Crigler-Najjar syndrome, type I, in which severe unconjugated hyperbilirubinemia is observed without evidence of a hemolytic anemia. It is an autosomal recessive disease that usually leads to neurologic disability secondary to kernicterus (see below). If glucuronyltransferase levels are reduced but not completely absent, the patient is said to have Crigler-Najjar syndrome type II. The mode of inheritance for this syndrome is unclear. An even milder form of Crigler-Najjar syndrome type II is Gilbert syndrome, which is thought to affect as many as 6% of the normal population. It is characterized by unconjugated hyperbilirubinemia with normal serum transaminases in an otherwise healthy child. Jaundice will occur during periods of fasting or with episodes of stress or fatigue. These episodes are self-resolving and the biochemical defect responsible for Gilbert syndrome may be similar to that for Crigler-Najjar syndrome type II. A patient showing conjugated (direct) hyperbilirubinemia in the setting of otherwise normal laboratory tests for liver function probably has either Dubin-Johnson or Rotor syndrome, both autosomal recessive disorders.

Diagnosis

Once a diagnosis of jaundice is suspected clinically on the basis of the child's skin color, the first step is to obtain a total and direct serum bilirubin concentration to determine whether the jaundice stems primarily from conjugated or unconjugated bilirubin. Once the type of bilirubinemia is detected, whether the jaundice represents a physiologic or a pathologic condition should be considered. Possible etiologies are listed in Table 7.9.

REFERENCES

Bell MJ, Ternberg JL, Bower RJ: The microbial flora and antimicrobial therapy of neonatal peritonitis. *J Pediatr Surg* 15:569, 1980.

Devries PA: The pathogenesis of gastroschisis and omphalocele. *J Pediatr Surg* 15:245, 1980.

Heathcote J, Deodhar KP, Scheuer PJ, et al: Intrahepatic cholestasis in childhood. *N Engl J Med* 295:801, 1979.

Jordan SC, Ament ME: Pancreatitis in children and adolescents. *J Pediatr* 91:211, 1977.

Kappas A, Drummond GS, Manola T, et al: Sn-Protoporphyrin use in the management of hyperbilirubinemia in term newborns with direct Coombs-positive ABO incompatibility. *Pediatrics* 81:485, 1988.

Maisels MJ, Gifford K, Antle CE, et al: Jaundice in the healthy newborn infant: A new approach to an old problem. *Pediatrics* 81:505, 1988.

Martin LW, Torres AM: Omphalocele and gastroschisis. *Surg Clin North Am* 65:1235, 1985.

McDougal WS, Izant RI, Zollinger RM: Primary peritonitis in infancy and childhood. *Ann Surg* 181:310, 1975.

Moore TC: Gastroschisis and omphalocele: Clinical differences. *Surgery* 82:561, 1977.

Moore TC, Nor K: An international survey of gastroschisis and omphalocele. *Pediatr Surg Int* 1:105, 1986.

Moosa AR: Diagnostic tests and procedures in acute pancreatitis. *N Engl J Med* 311:639, 1984.

Newman B, Teele RL: Ascites in the fetus, neonate and young child: Emphasis on ultrasonic evaluation. *Semin Ultrasound CT MR* 5:85, 1984.

Richter JM, Silverstein MD, Schapito R: Suspected obstructive jaundice: The decision analysis of diagnostic strategy. *Ann Intern Med* 99:46, 1983.

Scharschmidt BF, Goldberg HI, Schmid R: Approach to the patient with cholestatic jaundice. *N Engl J Med* 308:1515, 1983.

Schwartz DL: Congenital malformations of the gastrointestinal tract. In Silverberg M (ed): *Pediatric Gastroenterology*. New Hyde Park, NY, Medical Examination, 1983, p. 90.

Seidman EG, Deckelbaum RJ, Owen H, et al: Relapsing pancreatitis in association with Crohns disease. *J Pediatr Gastroenterol Nutr* 2:178, 1983.

Shwachman H, Lebenthal E, Khaw KT: Recurrent acute pancreatitis in patients with cystic fibrosis with normal pancreatic enzymes. *Pediatrics* 55:86, 1975.

Spivak W: Biliburin metabolism. *Pediatr Ann* 14:451, 1985.

Watson S, Giacoia GP: Cholestatis in infancy. *Clin Pediatr* 22:30, 1983.

Winship D, Butt J, Henstorf H, et al: Pancreatitis: Pancreatic pseudocysts and their complications. *Gastroenterology* 73:593, 1977.

Wyllie R, Arasu TS, Fitzgerald JF: Ascites pathophysiology and management. *J Pediatr* 97:167, 1980.

Diagnosis and Therapy of Specific Liver Diseases

6

APPROACH TO THE CHILD WITH LIVER DISEASE

Definition

A patient with a suspected liver disorder can be the subject of a rather complex and comprehensive diagnostic work-up to evaluate hepatic function. The history and physical examination form a foundation upon which biochemical, immunologic, viral and radiologic tests are added in order to provide a better classification and to identify hepatobiliary disease and dysfunction. (For a discussion of jaundice, see pages 466–467.)

Basic Science

Biochemical assays of hepatic tissue disease include aspartate aminotransferase (AST, formerly SGOT) and alanine aminotransferase (AAT, formerly SGPT), both of which are sensitive indicators of damage. While these enzymes are elevated in the setting of hepatic injury, they are not specific for a unique type of injury and their absolute values do not correlate with the extent of liver disease. SGOT elevations can represent damage to myocardium, skeletal muscle, liver, brain, pancreas, or kidney. (A CPK aldolase may be needed to evaluate the possibility of muscle disease.) On the other hand, in the presence of other indicators for chronic liver disease, the SGOT may remain a good indicator of disease activity. SGPT is also found in several organs, although its greatest activity remains in the liver, making it a more specific indicator of hepatocellular damage.

Cholestasis is present when conjugated serum bilirubin level is greater than 2.0 mg/dl, or when the conjugated serum bilirubin exceeds 30% of the total bilirubin. Intra- and extrahepatic cholestasis can also result in an elevated serum alkaline phosphatase, and intra- and extrahepatic obstruction cannot be distinguished on the basis of this enzymatic result. A total alkaline phosphatase represents a combination of liver, biliary tract, bone and intestinal isoenzymes, and fractionation of a total alkaline phosphatase into isoenzymes may be helpful if the elevation is not believed to be of hepatic origin. Other laboratory tests for cholestasis include assaying for γ-glutamyltransferase (GGT), a membrane-bound enzyme that has 80–90% of its activity in the biliary tract, and hence, can be useful as a cholestatic profile. High levels of GGT have been associated with obstructive biliary tract disease, including biliary atresia, α-1-antitrypsin deficiency, and cirrhosis. In acute viral hepatitis, GGT levels are usually normal or only minimally elevated, whereas they tend to be higher in cholestatic forms of liver disease. The specificity of GGT, however, remains low, with levels also being increased in pancreatitis, hyperthyroidism, and rheumatoid arthritis.

The ability of the liver to maintain adequate protein synthesis can be assayed by obtaining a serum albumin level. In acute liver disease a decrease in albumin is consistent with severe hepatocellular injury since the liver's reserve capacity to synthesize protein is considerable. Follow-up of serum albumin levels can also be helpful in assessing a patients prognosis. Chronic active hepatitis can be characterized by hypoalbuminemia in association with increased levels of γ-globulin, suggesting that serum protein electropheresis may provide a good quantitative measure of protein function of the liver in chronic liver disease. The ability of the liver to manufacture vitamin K-dependent factors, another indirect method of determining protein synthesis, can be obtained by measuring the prothrombin and partial thromboplastin times in acute, severe, chronic cholestatic liver disease. Ceruloplasm, another serum protein, is useful as a first screening test for Wilson disease.

α-Fetoprotein is an indicator of hepatic regeneration. It not only can represent a regenerating liver, but also the presence of neoplastic tissue. High levels of α-fetoprotein in a patient with chronic liver disease suggest the presence of a hepatoma. α-Fetoprotein is also elevated in some congenital hepatic diseases, including hereditary tyrosinemia type 1. If hepatic metastases are suspected 5-nucleotide phosphodiesterase isoenzyme 5 should be measured since its presence may be an early predictor of hepatic metastases that can serve as a marker for hepatoma.

Hepatobiliary excretory function, a useful adjunct to diagnosis of biliary atresia, is obtained through radionucleotide imaging or monitoring for biliary excretion of rose bengal labeled with ^{131}I or ^{125}I. Recently, rose bengal has been replaced with newer radiopharmaceuticals, including organic derivatives of amino diacetic acid labeled with 99-technetium, and hence, the origin of the H-IDA which is 99-mTC-n-(1,6-diethylacetinalide)-amino diacetic acid or BIDA 99-mTC-p-Butyl-amino-diacetic acid. Often, phenobarbital is given at a dose of 5 mg/kg/day for 5 days before the test to help stimulate biliary flow. The organic derivatives of amino diacetic acid provide readily available results, but the short half-life precludes imaging 18–24 hours after injection of the isotope, whereas the ^{125}I or ^{131}I tests can be made as long as 72 hours after the injection. Sensitivity and specificity are excellent with these tests.

Ultrasonography and CT also have a major role in the primary diagnosis of liver disease. Ultrasonography is particularly useful if biliary tract disease is suspected and is part of the work-up for a child with cholestatic jaundice, right upper quadrant pain, or a mass.

NEW DEVELOPMENTS

Nuclear magnetic resonance imaging is useful in diagnosis of hepatic disease. Although experience in childhood liver disease with this method of imaging is limited in 1988, magnetic resonance imaging permits two-dimensional images to be made through the use of very weak interactions with stable magnetic atomic nuclei which can have the property of nuclear spin. It is the magnetic spin becoming oriented in an external magnetic field that creates impulses which resonate, and by doing so, produce a measurable energy absorption. This measurable energy is then fed into a computer to generate an image thus permitting demonstration of focal fatty changes, measurement of metal composition as well as discrimination between normal and neoplastic hepatic tissue (Cohen, 1983). Another development is the use of positron emission tomography, which measures perfusion, metabolic distribution, and tissue metabolism of positron-emitting isotopes. This may permit localization of metabolically active hepatic tissue.

VIRAL HEPATITIS

Definition

Viral hepatitis is an infection of the liver that is caused by one of a group of hepatitis viruses. It can be acute and self-limited or chronic and progressive. A glossary of hepatitis nomenclature appears in Table 7.10. Epidemiologic and clinical characteristics are in Table 7.11.

Hepatitis A

Basic Science

Hepatitis A is caused by a ribonucleic acid member of the picornavirus family. The incubation period is 15–50 days during which time fecal excretion of the virus can be demonstrated. Once jaundice appears, fecal virus concentrations diminish. The virus has not been found in urine or other body fluids, and no chronic carrier state has been found.

Epidemiology

Approximately 22,000 cases of hepatitis A were reported in the United States in 1986. Most cases occur in young adults, and underreporting is probable. It is a problem in day care centers, which account for about 10% of cases in the United States (Balistreri, 1985).

Natural History

Hepatitis A is spread by fecal-oral contact. The onset is usually abrupt with fever, nausea, anorexia,

Table 7.10
Hepatitis Nomenclature[1]

Abbreviation	Term	Comments
Hepatitis A		
HAV	Hepatitis A virus	Etiologic agent of "infectious" hepatitis; a picornavirus; single serotype
Anti-HAV	Antibody to HAV	Detectable at oneset of symptoms; lifetime persistence
IgM anti-HAV	IgM class antibody to HAV	Indicates recent infection with hepatitis A; positive up to 4–6 months after infection
Hepatitis B		
HBV	Hepatitis B virus	Etiologic agent of "serum" or "long-incubation" hepatitis; also known as Dane particle
HBsAg	Hepatitis B surface antigen	Surface antigen(s) of HBV detectable in large quantity in serum; several subtypes identified
HBeAg	Hepatitis B e antigen	Soluble antigen; correlates with HBV replication, high titer HBV in serum, and infectivity of serum
HBcAg	Hepatitis B core antigen	No commercial test available
Anti-HBs	Antibody to HBsAg	Indicates past infection with and immunity to HBV, passive antibody from HBIG, or immune response from HBV vaccine
Anti-HBe	Antibody to HBeAg	Presence in serum of HBsAg carrier suggests lower titer of HBV
Anti-HBc	Antibody to HBcAg	Indicates past infection with HBV at some undefined time
IgM anti-HBc	IgM class antibody to HBcAg	Indicates recent infection with HBV; positive for 4–6 months after infection
Delta hepatitis		
δ virus	Delta virus	Etiologic agent of delta hepatitis; may only cause infection in presence of HBV
δ-Ag	Delta antigen	Detectable in early acute delta infection
Anti-δ	Antibody to delta antigen	Indicates past or present infection with delta virus
Non-A, non-B hepatitis		
NANB	Non-A, Non-B hepatitis	Diagnosis of exclusion. At least two candidate viruses; epidemiology parallels that of hepatitis B

Table 7.10 (Continued)
Hepatitis Nomenclature[1]

Abbreviation	Term	Comments
Epidemic non-A, non-B hepatitis		
Epidemic NANB	Epidemic non-A, non-B hepatitis	Causes large epidemics in Asia, North Africa; fecal-oral or waterborne
Immune globulins		
IG	Immune globulin (previously ISG, immune serum globulin, or γ-globulin)	Contains antibodies to HAV, low titer antibodies to HBV
HBIG	Hepatitis B immune globulin	Contains high titer antibodies to HBV

[1]Reproduced from CDC: *MMWR* 34:317, 1985.

abdominal discomfort, and jaundice. It is estimated that 90% of children are asymptomatic, but older children, in whom symptoms are most common, may complain of dull right upper quadrant pain which is aggravated by exercise. The urine is often dark orange and the skin and mucosal surfaces are yellow from hyperbilirubinemia. If obstruction of bile ducts is severe, stools may be light or even clay-colored. The duration of illness is about 2–3 weeks and recovery is heralded by a return of appetite and feeling of well-being.

Diagnosis

The diagnosis depends on acute and convalescent measurements of antibodies in sera; the presence of IgM class anti-HAV antibody during convalescence establishes the diagnosis and confers enduring immunity.

Both direct and indirect bilirubin levels are elevated, and serum transaminases rise (Fig. 7.11 illustrates the typical course of infection).

Prevention

Immune globulins contain antibodies against hepatitis A virus (HAV), and are protective if given early in the incubation period (first 2 weeks). Travelers to developing countries are advised to have pre-exposure prophylaxis with a single dose of 0.02 ml/kg immune globulin.

Hepatitis B

Basic Science

Hepatitis B virus (HBV) is a DNA virus. It has a number of antigens depicted in Figure 7.12. The incubation period is 45–160 days after exposure.

Epidemiology

Approximately 25,000 cases were reported in the United States in 1986. Children most at risk are those who require blood or blood products, or are offspring of

Table 7.11
Epidemiologic and Clinical Characteristics of Reported Cases of Viral Hepatitis, by Serologic Type, 1983, VHSP[1]

	Percentages of cases[2]		
	Hepatitis A N=7.854	Hepatitis B N=8.925	Non-A, non-B hepatitis N=2.960
Epidemiologic characteristics			
Child/employee in day care center	6.3	0.5	1.9
Contact of day care child/employee	9.8	1.5	3.7
Personal contact with hepatitis A	27.7	1.1	3.3
Employed as a foodhandler	6.1	3.4	4.5
Foodborne or waterborne outbreak	4.0	0.2	0.6
International travel	6.3	0.7	1.7
Personal contact with hepatitis B	1.7	14.8	4.9
Employed in medical/dental field	1.1	6.9	4.9
Association with dialysis/transplant	0.3	1.7	1.7
Blood transfusion	0.7	3.5	10.6
Hospitalized prior to illness	3.6	14.4	21.5
Surgery	1.6	6.7	11.6
Dental work	4.5	13.7	13.0
Drug abuse	2.7	12.7	10.9
Homosexual activity	1.6	8.7	2.1
Other percutaneous exposures	3.8	15.3	14.9
Clinical characteristics			
Jaundice	78.2	74.5	61.4
Hospitalized for hepatitis	33.2	44.4	45.6
Death as a result of hepatitis	0.6	1.6	2.0

[1]From CDC: *MMWR* 34:155, 1985.
[2]Note: Percentages are based on the number of persons who answered the question. For hepatitis A, the last 10 epidemiologic characteristics were answered by relatively few cases; therefore, the percentages are underestimated and cannot be accurately compared with the hepatitis B and non-A, non-B groups.

illicit drug users. Less than 3% of acute hepatitis B cases in the United States occur among children under age 14 years (CDC, 1987). It is estimated that 5–15% of the population in China and Southeast Asia carry the virus. Most of the population acquires infection at birth or in early childhood. An association has been made between chronic hepatitis B infection and hepatocellular carcinoma, which is an important cause of death in the Orient.

Natural History

The onset is insidious. Symptoms are those of acute hepatitis A, except for the more likely involvement of skin and joints. The virus is present in blood, saliva,

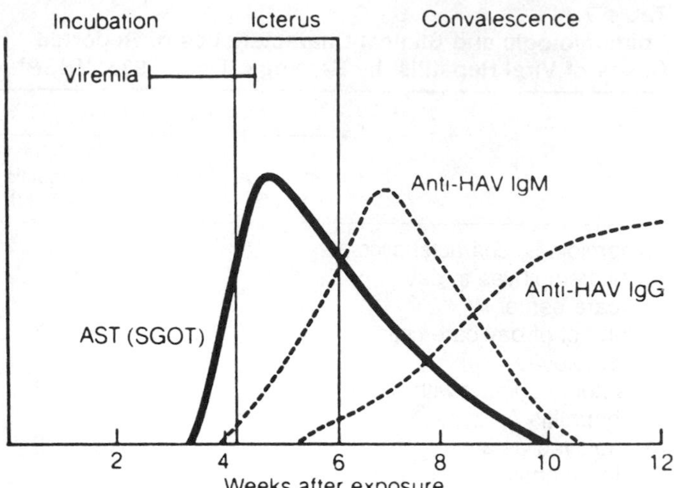

Figure 7.11. Typical course of hepatitis A infection. Icterus usually occurs 2–6 weeks after exposure, but is not present in all cases. The AST (SGOT) elevation precedes the development of clinical symptoms: values usually remain abnormal after serum bilirubin returns to normal. Viremia and fecal excretion of virus usually occur during the preicteric stage. Reproduced with permission from Balistreri WF: *Consultant,* p. 131–153, April 1984.

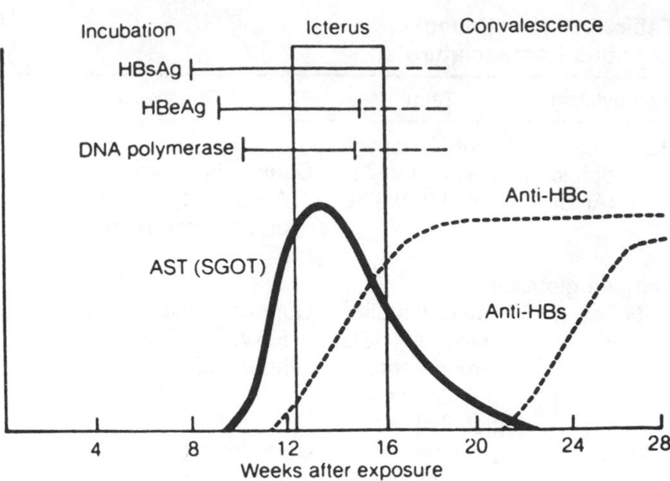

Figure 7.12. Typical course of hepatitis B infection. Icterus develops 12–16 weeks after infection and is preceded by an elevation of AST (SGOT) and the presence of HBsAg, HBeAg (in certain cases) and hepatitis B DNA polymerase in the serum. Icterus usually abates before AST returns to normal. Anti-HBc is usually found in serum long before anti-HBs. Reproduced with permission from Balistreri WF: *Consultant,* p. 131–153, April 1984.

and semen. Transmission is percutaneous or permucosal, and by sexual contact. Transmission by contaminated needles occurs in drug addicts, but transmission by transfusion is uncommon when blood is screened for hepatitis B surface antigen (HBsAg).

Diagnosis

The hepatitis B surface antigen (HBsAg) is the first serologic marker that becomes elevated during the incubation period, rising rapidly in the first 1–3 weeks of the presymptomatic stage and then reaching a peak at or shortly after the elevation of the aminotransferases. Usually, the HBsAg and aminotransferase levels decline together as the disease resolves.

Two months or more after the onset of clinical symptoms and signs, antibody to HBsAg can be detected in all but a few patients, but it does not become elevated until HBsAg declines. It is possible that a "window" occurs at which time the HBs antigen and the anti-HBs antibody cannot be detected, and the only marker for HBV infection will be the anti-HB core antibody. Nonetheless, when the anti-HBs does appear it is a marker for recovery and for immunity. Unfortunately, 5–10% of patients never produce anti-HBs and usually remain carriers of HBsAg. Anti-HBsAg is used following vaccine immunization to ensure that prolonged immunity has occurred.

Another viral antigen, HBeAg, is related to the core viral particle. It can rise shortly after the HBsAg and then will disappear within 1–2 months to be followed by antibodies to HBeAg that coincide with the peak of clinical signs and symptoms. HBeAg correlates well with viral replication and high infectivity.

Prevention

Hepatitis B vaccine is purified from human plasma and inactivated. Primary vaccination consists of three intramuscular doses with the second and third dose given 1 and 6 months apart after the first.

Hepatitis B immune globulin is given to infants of infected mothers at birth, to be followed by vaccine within the first week. Repeat doses of immune globulin are at 1 and 6 months.

Delta Hepatitis

Delta hepatitis, caused by the delta agent, differs from A and B. The agent is a defective RNA virus that cannot survive independently and requires the "helper" function of a DNA virus such as hepatitis B. Delta hepatitis can occur only in persons who have hepatitis B or are carriers.

Epidemiology

Delta infection occurs chiefly among drug addicts and hemophiliacs who are frequently exposed. It is endemic in southern Italy, and has been seen in northern Europe and the United States as well as parts of South America. In Worcester, Massachusetts in 1984, 200 drug addicts and their sexual partners were affected and 9 died (CDC, 1984). It is thought to participate in 20–30% of cases of chronic hepatitis B. Of American blood donors with serum hepatitis B surface antigen, 3–12% have antibodies to delta virus (Maggione et al, 1985).

Prognosis

In adults with delta hepatitis, over 50% of cases will progress to chronic active hepatitis and cirrhosis.

Hepatitis Non-A Non-B

Definition

Hepatitis non-A non-B (nAnB) remains a leading cause of human viral hepatitis, although little information is available concerning the disease in children. Hepatitis nAnB can only be differentiated from hepatitis B by serology. It remains a diagnosis of exclusion.

Basic Science

No information is available at present regarding the definitive viral structure or specific serologic markers.

Two viral agents may be responsible for this hepatitis. "Type 1" has an incubation period of about 6 weeks, followed by a clinical illness of 6 weeks' duration; whereas type 2 has a longer incubation period of up to 7 weeks with a duration of 18–20 weeks, although these observations require further confirmation.

Biopsy findings in liver include eosinophilic clumping in an irregular distribution within the cytoplasm; fatty change; marked sinusoidal activation; and a less intense portal and periportal inflammatory response than in hepatitis A or B.

Epidemiology

In adults, nAnB hepatitis represents 80–85% of post-transfusion hepatitis, with the remainder due to cytomegalovirus, Epstein-Barr, and hepatitis B virus. Epidemiologic data specific for children are lacking at the present time. Individuals subject to percutaneous blood exposure are also at risk.

Natural History

Most patients develop symptoms 5–10 weeks after exposure. Seventy-five percent of all patients with nAnB hepatitis will have jaundice, mild fatigue, and anorexia.

A most disturbing feature of nAnB hepatitis is the frequency of chronic liver disease, mostly chronic active hepatitis, with its possible progression to cirrhosis (see below). Predictors of chronicity include an anicteric rather than icteric acute illness; a large inoculum; anorexia, malaise and nausea; multiphasic pattern of aminotransferase elevation; and a peak SGOT level of over 300 in patients with anicteric disease.

The carrier state may exist long after biochemical resolution. There are more nAnB carriers than hepatitis B carriers in the United States.

Diagnosis

Clinical diagnosis depends on epidemiologic features and exclusion of hepatitis A and hepatitis B and other possible viral or toxic agents.

Treatment

The treatment of uncomplicated viral hepatitis is supportive. If vomiting is severe and dehydration is likely, oral hydration solutions or intravenous fluids may be needed. No drugs are indicated; rather, most drugs are contraindicated if they are metabolized by the liver.

Acute fulminant hepatitis, associated with hepatitis A or nAnB, involves high bilirubin and ammonia levels, and extremely elevated transaminase values (in the thousands). Encephalopathy, bleeding, edema, and ascites may ensue. The mortality is about 33%. Treatment is that used for liver failure (pp. 479).

Prevention

Thus far, immunoprophylaxis with hepatitis immune serum globulin and hepatitis B immune globulin has not been found to be effective. The carrier rate for nAnB hepatitis is reported to be 1–5% for blood donors.

Although immunoglobulin is effective in attenuating the illness, it does not completely prevent infection when blood is transfused, nor is it useful if administered before or immediately after transfusion. Therefore, immunoglobulin for prophylaxis is not recommended.

CHRONIC HEPATITIS

Chronic hepatitis is described by clinical and/or biochemical evidence of hepatic dysfunction and inflammation lasting for longer than 6 months, and is a known consequence of hepatitis B and nAnB infections, but does not occur with hepatitis A infection. Two types of chronic hepatitis occur: chronic persistent hepatitis and chronic active hepatitis, the diagnosis of each is based on biopsy findings. In chronic persistent hepatitis there is mild infiltration of the portal area with intact lobular architecture and no fibrosis, whereas chronic active hepatitis is characterized pathologically by "piecemeal" necrosis and collapse of lobular architecture with bridging necrosis and fibrosis.

Chronic Persistent Hepatitis

Definition

Chronic persistent hepatitis (CPH) represents a benign form of chronic hepatitis.

Basic Science

The development of the CPH state is not based solely on the persistence of hepatitis B virus since most children who are chronic carriers of HBsAg do not subsequently develop clinical or biochemical signs of chronic hepatitis.

Natural History

The child is usually asymptomatic or at times complains of fatigue, poor appetite, pain in the right upper quadrant, and fatty food intolerance, often following a bout of acute viral hepatitis.

Diagnosis

CPH may be diagnosed incidentally when liver function tests are found to be elevated. Physical examination may reveal mild hepatomegaly or, occasionally, a tender liver edge. Signs of chronic liver failure are absent with this disorder. Serum aminotransferases remain elevated at 2–4 times normal for years. The serum bilirubin level is usually normal or minimally increased. The serum immunoglobulin level is normal or mildly increased, in contrast to chronic active hepatitis which displays elevated levels of IgG. Serologically, these patients are often HB surface-antigen and HB core-positive but the e antigen is usually negative.

Definitive diagnosis is made by needle biopsy of the liver, which should be performed at least 6 months after abnormal liver functions have been first discovered, otherwise it is impossible to distinguish this condition from acute viral hepatitis. Biopsy findings are notable for expansion of the portal area, with mononuclear cells and minimal fibrosis. The portal area architecture is preserved.

Treatment

Therapy is not indicated for CPH.

Prognosis

The prognosis is excellent; most patients can be placed on a normal diet and follow normal daily activities. The clinical features of chronic liver disease and cirrhosis do not develop with CPH. Rarely, a patient may progress to mild chronic active hepatitis.

Chronic Active Hepatitis (Lupoid)

Definition

Chronic active hepatitis is a continuing inflammatory process of the liver progressing to severe irreversible destruction and death. There are two common types of chronic active hepatitis, either autoimmune (lupoid) or secondary to hepatitis B viral infection. In addition, nAnB and delta hepatitis can progress to chronic active hepatitis. Histologic and clinical descriptions identical to this disorder have been noted following the use of oxyphenatin, a laxative, methyldopa, and isoniazid, and also with α-1-antitrypsin deficiency and Wilson disease.

Basic Science

The pathophysiology leading to chronic active hepatitis has not yet been clarified. There appear to be hepatic plasma cell infiltrates, hypergammaglobulinemia, and multiple immunologic disturbances in patients with this disorder, and the response to anti-inflammatory and immunosuppressant medication in the autoimmune form of the disease supports the fact that immunologic factors play a role. On the other hand, it is still not clear what triggers the irreversible destruction of hepatocytes and whether immunologic findings are secondary to the primary viral infection. It is also not clear whether liver damage initiates the antigen-antibody reaction or that the liver is the primary end-organ in systemic autoimmune response for the autoimmune chronic active hepatitis.

Hepatitis B virus-induced chronic hepatitis may represent a combination of impaired host immune status and the ability of the virus to continue replicating in the liver. It has also been suggested that the association of delta agent with HBs antigen may increase the risk of the disorder (Maggione et al, 1985).

Epidemiology

Autoimmune chronic active hepatitis occurs most commonly in adolescent girls, with an overall ratio of 1:4, males to females. The virally induced disease occurs predominantly in adults but can also be seen in neonates born to B surface antigen-positive carrier mothers, adolescents who use intravenous drugs, children in institutional settings, and homosexuals.

Natural History

The age range for chronic active hepatitis is usually 5–16 years, with one study suggesting a median age of 13 years. The disease has usually been present for months or years before there is an insidious onset of malaise and jaundice, or the detection of hepatosplenomegaly on routine physical examination. Amenorrhea may occur and sexual development may be arrested. The return of menstrual flow often heralds disease remission.

A recognized acute illness may or may not have preceded evidence of liver dysfunction. Nonspecific symptoms such as malaise, anorexia, and weight loss may be present. A migrating arthritis is sometimes present. On examination, both liver and spleen are usually enlarged. Kidneys, colon, thyroid, and lymph nodes may also be involved and erythema nodosum may be the presenting finding. Later, bleeding may occur in association with thrombocytopenia and prothrombin deficiency.

Usually the HBV-induced form is not preceded by an obvious case of acute viral hepatitis. Instead, mild acute hepatitis is thought to persist for a long period of time.

Diagnosis

The serum albumin and alkaline phosphatase are usually normal, as are clotting studies initially. A striking feature of chronic active hepatitis is hypergammaglobulinemia, with IgG levels greater than 2000 mg/dl. In addition, antinuclear antibodies and antismooth muscle antibodies are often present, as well as a positive Coomb test. Serum albumin and alkaline phosphatase are usually normal. Transaminases are

Table 7.12
Hepatitis B Virus Postexposure Recommendations[1]

	HBIG		Vaccine	
Exposure	Dose	Recommended Timing	Dose	Recommended Timing
Perinatal	0.5 ml im	Within 12 hours of bath	0.5 ml (10 μg) im	Within 7 days[2] repeat at 1 and 6 months
Percutaneous	0.06 ml/kg im or 5 ml for adults	Single dose within 24 hours	1.0 ml (20 μg) im[3]	Within 7 days[2] repeat at 1 and 6 months
	or[4]			
	0.06 ml/kg im or 5 ml for adults	Within 24 hours repeat at 1 month		
Sexual	0.06 ml/kg im or 5 ml for adults	Within 14 days of sexual contact	[5]	

[1]Reproduced from CDC: *MMWR* June 1, 1984.
[2]The first dose can be given the same time as the HBIG dose but at a separate site.
[3]For persons under 10 years of age, use 0.5 ml (10 μg).
[4]For those who choose not to receive HB vaccine.
[5]Vaccine is recommended for homosexually active males and for regular sexual contacts of chronic HBV carriers.

often strikingly elevated. Bilirubin is mildly elevated. Leukopenia occurs early in the disease and late aplastic anemia may develop.

The diagnosis of HBsAg-positive chronic active hepatitis is confirmed by a liver biopsy and the presence of HBsAg since the biopsy picture alone is essentially identical to that seen in autoimmune chronic active hepatitis, with widespread areas of necrosis, pseudoacinar formation, and lymphocytic infiltration.

Treatment

Prednisone, 2 mg/kg/day up to 60 mg daily is effective for autoimmune chronic active hepatitis. When transaminase values are near normal, the dose can be reduced by about 5 mg/week until the maintenance dose of 10–15 mg/day is reached. For some patients, the drug can be given every other day with fewer side effects.

Treatment for hepatitis B virus disease is controversial. While steroids will diminish acute inflammation in autoimmune aspects of the disease, they may also increase viral replication and lead to exacerbating the condition, and therefore, are usually contraindicated.

Patients with HB surface antigen-positive disease may go into remission spontaneously, whereas those with the autoimmune type have a high mortality rate in the first 2 years of disease unless anti-inflammatory therapy is instituted. It is possible that the presence of e antigen determines whether patients with the HB type progress to cirrhosis and hepatic decompensation. These patients also are at an increased risk of developing primary hepatocellular carcinoma.

Prognosis

Almost all patients with the autoimmune disorder show an initial good response to corticosteroids. Long-term remissions have been reported in about 70% of patients. The others progress to cirrhosis.

The likelihood of an infant of an HBeAg- and HBeAg-positive mother becoming a chronic hepatitis B virus carrier is 90%, and as many as 25% may die of cirrhosis or hepatocellular carcinoma. If the mother is HBsAg-positive and HBeAg-negative, fewer than 25% of infants become infected. Even if perinatal infection does not occur, the infant should have prophylaxis against later acquisition of infection from family members.

Prevention

Prophylaxis against hepatitis B after exposure is indicated for infants born to antigen-positive mothers, after accidental percutaneous exposure, or after sexual abuse from an antigen-positive individual (Table 7.12). Fetal risk is shown in Table 7.13.

Table 7.13
Hepatitis in Pregnancy

Hepatitis	Carrier	Diagnosis	Fetal Risk of Illness	Fetal Risk to Be Carrier
A	No	Possible IgM	Negligible	None
B	Yes	HBsAg	Low 1st, 2nd trimesters	
		HBeAg	60% in 3rd	HBeAg + mothers 85% infant carriers (If HBeAb present, 25%)
D	——Similar to hepatitis B——		(undefined)	
NonA nonB	——Similar to hepatitis B——		Moderate especially in 3rd trimester	

WILSON DISEASE

Definition

Wilson disease is an autosomal recessive disorder that results in abnormal handling of copper by the liver and its accumulation in tissues.

Basic Science

The precise biochemical defect in Wilson disease remains unknown, although it probably exists either in the hepatic transport or storage of copper since absorption of copper has been found to be normal. Hepatic excretion of biliary copper is deficient. Ceruloplasmin, the copper-carrying protein in serum, is usually absent or low, probably secondary to the diminished availability of copper. Excess build-up in copper balance leads to excess deposition in other organs, including the brain, eyes, kidney and bones, with the manifestation of symptoms later in life.

Epidemiology

The prevalence rate of carriers remains 1/200–1/500 for this disease. A possibly related condition called Indian childhood cirrhosis is found in southeast Asia.

Natural History

A four-stage system has been used to describe the course of the disease in children (Nazer et al, 1983). Stage 1, which begins at birth, represents a period during which patients have a positive copper balance but are completely asymptomatic with only mild urinary excretion of copper and absence of Kayser-Fleischer rings (brown or gray-green pigment ring at the corneal limbus from deposition of copper in the Decemet membrane). Stage 2 occurs when the liver becomes saturated with copper and this stage is associated with hemolytic anemia and/or the onset of liver failure. The hemolysis is believed to be due to uptake of copper by red blood cells. Hepatitis is found in only 30–40% of patients in this stage. Kayser-Fleischer rings remain absent, although urinary excretion of copper is increased and ceruloplasmin levels may be normal or low. In stage 3, copper begins to accumulate in extrahepatic tissues including the eye, brain, and kidneys and Kayser-Fleischer rings will become visible. Urinary excretion of copper is marked and renal manifestations appear. In stage 4, the neurologic manifestations of the disease develop and the full spectrum of Wilson disease can be seen. Rarely is stage 3 or 4 present before age 4–5 years. The neurologic manifestations include clumsiness, dysarthria, behavioral disturbances, dystonia, fixed facial expressions, rigidity, and athetoid movements. The renal disorders can include renal tubular acidosis, reduced glomerular filtration rate, increased urate clearance, with decreased serum uric acid levels, amino aciduria, glycosuria, proteinuria, and hyperphosphaturia.

Diagnosis

Presenting symptoms can vary from mild lethargy, malaise, or abdominal pain to jaundice or even deteriorating school performance. Retrospective clinical series in the literature suggest a 2- to 5-year delay in diagnosis from time of onset of symptoms attributed to the disease (Nazer et al, 1983).

A family history, especially with respect to neurologic or psychiatric disease, may be useful in alerting the pediatrician to suspicion of Wilson disease.

The presence of copper in the lateral margin of the cornea is usually made by slit-lamp examination and, in the absence of overt cholestasis, is pathognomonic for Wilson disease. Nevertheless, Kayser-Fleischer rings may be absent and the disease still manifest.

Laboratory tests that may be helpful include the following: a serum ceruloplasmin at a reduced level suggests homo- or occasionally heterozygocity for the disease, although low serum ceruloplasmins may also occur in children with chronic active hepatitis or fulminating hepatic necrosis. A value of ceruloplasmin over 30 mg/dl will exclude Wilson disease. A serum copper is not useful since it may be normal or high even in those homozygous for the disease. Twenty-four-hour urine collections for copper excretion can be useful since patients with Wilson disease have elevated urinary copper, with values greater than 50 μg/24 hours. Cupriuria may also be found in chronic active hepatitis, biliary tract disease with cirrhosis, or direct contamination from a container that contains copper. In children with cupriuria who do not have Kayser-Fleischer rings, a liver biopsy is appropriate to quantitate the concentrations of hepatic copper and, thus, establish the diagnosis. Liver pathology may be suggestive of the disease but is not necessarily diagnostic, unless the copper concentration is elevated as well. Pathology specimens will reveal fatty vacuolization in degenerating liver cells, and later macrolobular or postnecrotic cirrhosis as well as bile duct proliferation.

Once the diagnosis has been established on the basis of the ophthalmologic examination and laboratory testing, other family members should also be subjected to eye examinations and laboratory tests. Asymptomatic relatives who have questionable findings, i.e., absence of Kayser-Fleischer rings, but suggestive laboratory or urine studies, should undergo a liver biopsy for histology and copper analysis.

Treatment

Therapy is designed to decrease the tissue copper concentration, thereby normalizing symptoms. The mainstay of treatment is d-penicillamine. This drug chelates copper and removes it by increasing urinary excretion, thus shifting equilibrium from tissue to plasma. The longer the delay in initiating treatment, the worse is the prognosis in reversing symptoms. Side effects of d-penicillamine include leukopenia, skin rash, and occasionally a lupus-like or nephrotic syndrome. It is useful also to reduce dietary intake of copper to no more than 1 mg/day. Foods to be avoided include chocolate, nuts, dried fruits, shellfish, dried beans and peas, whole wheat, and organ meats which are rich in copper. Penicillamine needs to be maintained throughout; periodic check-ups are advised to measure urinary copper excretion to ensure adequate compliance with medication.

The use of oral zinc therapy is also being considered as an alternative treatment for the disease, if penicillamine has failed (Brewer et al, 1983).

Prognosis

Without treatment the disease is fatal, with patients dying of chronic liver failure or neurologic disability. The earlier the disease is diagnosed and treatment is initiated, the better is the prognosis, with less functional impairment from any organ involvement. Liver transplantation remains controversial, with some patients apparently showing cure, but others having recurrence of symptoms.

The diagnosis should be considered in every child with chronic liver disease because of the importance of early diagnosis and treatment.

α-1-ANTITRYPSIN DEFICIENCY

Definition

α-1-Antitrypsin (see also pp. 260) is a glycoprotein that is produced by hepatocytes and is under the influence of two autosomally inherited, codominant alleles. It is a proteolytic enzyme inhibitor and also inhibits neutral proteases in neutrophils and acid proteases of alveolar macrophages. Deficiency states are associated with liver disease and emphysema.

Basic Science

The gene for α-1-antitrypsin has been isolated and is located on chromosome 14. Over 25 different alleles of α-1-antitrypsin have been reported to date. The PiM allele is the most common in the general population, giving a normal individual a PiMM phenotype, whereas the PiZZ phenotype is associated with complete deficiency of plasma α-1-antitrypsin. The heterozygote PiMZ has intermediate levels of α-1-antitrypsin, which may predispose patients to developing chronic liver disease. It is the PiZZ type—i.e., complete deficiency that is associated with significant hepatic and/or pulmonary (emphysema) pathology in children.

It appears that hepatocytes cannot secrete α-1-antitrypsin due to production of an abnormal protein within the cell. This protein causes the α-1-antitrypsin to aggregate within the hepatocyte cell and prevents excretion out of the cell. Although this material aggregates within the liver cell, it often may not result in liver damage and the mechanism by which the aggregation progresses to hepatocyte toxicity has yet to be elucidated. Many PiZZ neonates will show hepatic injury by 6 weeks of age, although α-1-antitrypsin deposits are rarely observed at this time and do not appear on biopsy until 8–10 weeks of age. According to another theory, the proteases released from other locations may overwhelm the reticuloendothelial system of the liver and, thus, injure the hepatocytes. This mechanism could also account for the lung disease since the lungs contain large concentration of elastin, which attract proteases to it. The mechanism for involvement of liver, or lung, or both in different children remains unclear at the present time.

At biopsy, the liver of a patient with α-1-antitrypsin deficiency shows eosinophilic-appearing cytoplasmic granules on hematoxylin and eosin stain. These granules, which are resistant to diastase, stain intensely with periodic acid-Schiff stain (PAS), and are concentrated in the hepatic cells, particularly in the periportal zones.

Epidemiology

α-1-Antitrypsin deficiency associated with the PiZZ phenotype occurs in 1/3000–1/5000 births. The heterozygote PiMZ phenotype is said to be present in 2.2–3% of the population, especially in northern Europeans. Of patients with α-1-antitrypsin deficiency, 10–20% develop liver disease as a complication. It is thought, however, that 5–35% of cases of pediatric liver disease are caused by α-1-antitrypsin deficiency (Sveger, 1984).

Natural History

In newborns and young infants, α-1-antitrypsin deficiency most often presents with cholestatic jaundice, usually persisting at age 3–12 weeks. In addition, there may be a history of mild failure-to-thrive, lethargy, and poor feeding. Physical examination is usually benign in these infants except for a mild enlargement of the liver and spleen. Usually more than half of these infants will have slow resolution of their jaundice over their first 6–8 months of life. Their inability to excrete bilirubin may mimic biliary atresia and require liver biopsy and/or cholangiography to clarify the diagnosis. Following the jaundice, hepatomegaly and decreased hepatic enzyme function persist for several years, subsequently progressing to a cirrhotic picture in many cases. At this time, the spleen will become enlarged because of portal hypertension and the patient will manifest symptoms and signs of chronic liver disease.

If the illness is not discovered during the neonatal and early infancy period, it is most likely to be detected in early childhood when a child presents with an enlarged liver as an isolated sign. Liver function tests in these children are abnormal, stressing the need to consider α-1-antitrypsin deficiency. If the disease is missed until children are older or adolescent, it most often presents as chronic liver disease, with a small liver, but with extreme splenomegaly. Hematemesis from esophageal varices often may be the presenting symptom in older patients. If a child presents with recurrent pulmonary symptoms including bronchitis and pneumonia, α-1-antitrypsin deficiency should also be considered and, if detected, the presence of liver disease should also be sought.

Diagnosis

An overall deficiency in α-1-antitrypsin can be detected by serum protein electropheresis, although phenotyping is required to determine whether the patient is homo- or heterozygous for the deficiency. Liver function is variable and studies are consistent with nonspecific hepatocellular injury during the icteric phase, when aminotransferase and alkaline phosphatase levels may be elevated. The aminotransferase levels may decline after the icteric phase and are not helpful during the cirrhotic phase.

NEW DEVELOPMENTS

Prenatal diagnosis is now available by analysis of fetal blood obtained at fetoscopy (Kidd et al, 1984). The only hope for complete cure at present is liver transplantation, which has been successfully performed on a small number of patients.

Treatment

Measures used for treatment of the neonate with cholestatic jaundice are appropriate. In addition, supportive therapy with cholysteramine, phenobarbital, medium chain triglycerides, and water-soluble vitamins are helpful. (See management of chronic liver failure for further information.) Enzyme replacement therapy has been beneficial in adults with emphysema and should be evaluated in infants with liver disease (Wewers et al, 1987).

Prognosis

If liver disease is noted in the neonatal period, cirrhosis can be expected in over 60% of those patients who survive infancy. Nevertheless, more recent findings suggest that the prognosis for PiZ infants with neonatal liver disease is better than was previously believed, although chances of complete recovery remain uncertain. In addition, the risk of developing hepatic carcinoma is increased.

If the patient with neonatal cholestasis has a clinical recovery after the first 6 months of life and has liver function tests that return to normal, the prognosis appears to be better. The liver biopsy remains the best prognostic tool, with the amount of portal fibrosis and ductular proliferation corresponding to the severity of subsequent cirrhosis. Monitoring liver function, while not diagnostic, may show a trend. Re-elevation of serum direct bilirubin also can correspond to a cirrhotic picture in the older children. In one study, the only clear-cut biochemical evidence of good outcome, with no overlap with an unfavorable outcome, was persistent normalization of liver function tests, although this occurs rarely (Sveger, 1984).

HEMOCHROMATOSIS

Definition

Primary hemochromatosis is characterized by excessive absorption of iron from the intestinal tract and storage in parenchymal cells. The classic triad of findings are bronzed skin, cirrhosis, and diabetes mellitus.

Epidemiology

The condition is 5–10 times more common in males and is usually not detected until the fourth or fifth decade. It is inherited as an autosomal recessive with the gene frequency of 3–8/1000 population. Primary hemochromatosis is associated with HLA types A3, B7, and B14. The locus for the hemochromatosis allele and the HLA loci on the short arm of chromosome 6 are linked (Cartwright et al, 1977). The youngest patient reported as of 1988 was 29 months old (Escobar et al, 1987).

Diagnosis

The diagnosis can be suspected on the basis of family history, particularly if a member had a hepatoma, which occurs in as many as 29% of patients. High serum ferritin (200–400 μg/L) and transferrin saturation (> 70%) are dependable screening tests. The definitive diagnostic test is a liver biopsy. CT scans of the liver may show increased density of liver and are useful to follow patients.

Treatment

The traditional treatment has been frequent phlebotomies. In children, 5–7 ml/kg of blood are removed every 7–10 days until iron loss equals intestinal absorption. Chelation therapy is used only when frequent venipunctures are difficult. Prevention of iron overload is aided by avoiding ascorbic acid and foods high in iron content.

Prognosis

The prognosis is improved if the condition is recognized and restriction of iron intake and phlebotomy are used to restore iron balance before liver damage is irreversible.

BILIARY ATRESIA

Definition

Biliary atresia characterized by a lack of patency of the extrahepatic biliary ducts represents a major cause of obstructive cholangiopathy in infants and children.

Basic Science

The sclerotic process in the disorder is panductular, affecting the intrahepatic as well as the extrahepatic biliary tree. In fact, intrahepatic biliary damage is often responsible for failure of the Kasai operation used to treat this disorder.

The condition is acquired in utero or in the perinatal period since infants with atresia have meconium that contains bile. No infectious agent has been identified, although many have been sought.

Epidemiology

The incidence of biliary atresia is about 1/15,000 live births. It is not familial and there is a slight predominance in females.

Natural History

Unless surgery is performed within the first 2–3 months of age, the diagnosis carries essentially 100% mortality within the first year of life. If untreated, the mean age of death is 10 months, with survival beyond 4 years of age being exceptional. Currently, with surgery performed before 2 months of age, biliary drainage has been observed in 75% of cases with a 5-year survival of 34%. Many long-term survivors are now in their third decade of life (Lilly and Karrer, 1985).

Diagnosis

The mainstay of diagnosis is to distinguish extrahepatic from intrahepatic cholestasis by use of laboratory tests, radiology, and liver biopsy. In differentiating extrahepatic biliary atresia from other metabolic diseases, a sweat test, α-1-antitrypsin level with Pi typing, titers for congenital infections, urine for reducing substances, and a hepatitis screen may be performed.

Radionucleotide imaging of hepatobiliary flow is most useful in distinguishing extra- and intrahepatic obstruction. Technetium-labeled aminodiacetic acid provides the best detail with reduced radiation exposure. Phenobarbital given for several days before the onset of the study enhances excretion by stimulating microsomal enzymes to improve the handling of bilirubin. If despite use of phenobarbital, repeated hepatobiliary imaging does not show patent bile ducts, a liver biopsy should be performed to make the diagnosis.

A percutaneous liver biopsy is most accurate if portal spaces are present on the specimen. Hepatitis is characterized on biopsy by lobular disarray, giant cell transformation, pseudoductular formation, and mononuclear lobular infiltration. Biliary atresia, on the other hand, is notable for bile duct proliferation, bile lakes, fibrosis, and portal inflammation. Dilated ducts can, but need not, be present in biliary atresia. Ultrasonographic demonstration of a normal gallblader supports the diagnosis of neonatal hepatitis, but does not rule out biliary atresia. Ultrasonography is not helpful in identifying the cause of jaundice if the gallbladder cannot be visualized. Regardless of the method of approach, work-up should be completed before an infant is age 6 weeks, and at the latest, 8 weeks of age.

Treatment

Surgical treatment includes an exploration and operative cholangiogram to identify landmarks for the Kasai procedure or a variant. The outcome of this procedure depends on the age of the patient and the pathology found. Risk factors for a poor outcome include an operation after 2 months of age, a history of ascending cholangitis, and portal hypertension (Altman, 1978).

Most infants have grossly nonpatent bile ducts from the liver hilus to the duodenum and, hence, have what is believed to be noncorrectable biliary atresia. For these patients, a hepatic portoenterostomy, the Kasai operation, is performed, during which the extrahepatic bile ducts are removed and bile drainage is established by an anastomosis of an intestinal conduit to the transected duct of the liver hilus. The success of this operation depends on the presence of microscopic patent biliary structures at the liver hilus. Postoperatively, jaundice may not resolve for 6–12 weeks.

Complications of surgery include increased risk for cholangitis owing to intrahepatic bile duct stasis, portal hypertension, and malnutrition. Cholangitis is manifest by fever, elevated white count, and increased evidence of biliary obstruction. Treatment is intravenous antibiotic coverage of abdominal flora for a period of 2–3 weeks. There is no evidence that antibiotic prophylaxis prevents cholangitis. Portal hypertension manifested by splenomegaly and, occasionally, variceal hemorrhages have been shown to occur in one-third of patients who have surgery. Usually these symptoms do not develop until a child is 1 or 2 years of age. More commonly, portal hypertension resolves and only rarely requires surgical intervention. A portacaval shunt has been necessary in only 10% of patients who have been alive 2–9 years after Kasai procedure. Endoscopic sclerotherapy may be useful in patients who have esophageal varices (Lilly and Karrer, 1985).

These patients routinely should receive aqueous preparations of fat-soluble vitamins D, A, E, and K.

Transplantation is now becoming a definitive treatment in these patients with use of immunosuppression with cyclosporine and prednisone. Survival is now 65–80% at 1 year after transplant, and some have survived for 11 years after surgery. Liver transplantation appears to be most appropriate for patients who achieve bile drainage through their Kasai procedure and, therefore, have prolonged survival, but develop intrahepatic ductular disease and worsening parenchymal liver damage (Perlmutter et al, 1985).

Prognosis

With widespread recognition of the importance of early operation, survival statistics have improved dramatically in the past 20 years. In the early postoperative years these patients often develop complications, but as they become older the complications become less frequent. They may also have a slower rate of growth and development between the ages of 8 and 24 months, but then have a good catch-up period.

ACUTE HEPATIC FAILURE

Definition

Fulminant hepatic failure occurs secondary to hepatocellular necrosis, in association with an encephalopathy. It implies either acute massive destruction of liver tissue or another process that causes rapid deterioration in function of a previously normal liver.

Basic Science

Acute hepatic failure in children is usually associated with B or nAnB, and, more rarely, hepatitis A, Epstein-Barr virus, or cytomegalovirus hepatitis. In neonates, it has been known to occur with systemic herpes infection and with adenovirus. Less common causes in children are toxins, Reye syndrome, and drugs, including acetaminophen, azathioprine, valproic acid, isoniazid, trimethoprim-sulfamethoxazole, dilantin, erythromycin estolate, rifampin, and halothane. The mechanisms triggering acute hepatic failure from viral infection are unknown, although coinfection with the delta agent is possible in hepatitis B infection (Partin, 1985a). It is still not clear why in some patients the livers regenerate completely after a viral infection and in others the livers show minimal regenerative properties, leading to fulminant necrosis and destruction.

Coma may be the result of release of γ-aminobutyric acid (GABA), an inhibitory neurotransmitter that is usually synthesized in the gut and removed by the liver via the portal circulation. In acute liver failure, however, GABA is not removed and an increase in its activity has been noted in the presynaptic neuronal connections in patients with hepatic failure. As a potent neuroinhibitor, GABA acts upon an increased number of neuroinhibitory receptor sites and induces brain depression and coma. If this theory is confirmed in subsequent studies, future research will be aimed at preventing hepatic coma by blocking the absorption of GABA from the gut, removing GABA from the blood, and providing a GABA receptor blocker (Jones et al, 1984).

Several other factors are thought to contribute to encephalopathy, most of which increase the production of ammonia. These include upper intestinal bleeding, which elevates ammonia via increased protein load through the intestine and also causes acute hypovolemia with compromise of hepatic function. Renal failure also produces an increase in urea which is a precursor of ammonia and infection, with increased tissue breakdown and hence increased protein load with associated dehydration, hypoxia and hypothermia all of which can add to the production of ammonia. Constipation, inappropriate protein loading with increased ammonia production, diuretics which produce hypokalemia and hypovolemia, and alkalosis which increases renal vein ammonia, all add to the ammonia load. In addition, prerenal azotemia and sedatives depress the CNS directly and may produce hypoxia by respiratory depression.

Natural History

The differential diagnosis of acute hepatic failure is extensive and includes infectious, metabolic, pharmacologic, toxicologic, ischemic, and hypoxic etiologies.

Any child who has hepatitis and develops severe vomiting, increased lethargy, profound anorexia, worsening jaundice, asterixis, and abnormal gait, on neurologic examination during the first 1–2 weeks should be considered to be on the verge of acute hepatic failure. The liver may increase and decrease in size and ascites and easy bruisability may also be associated with the syndrome. The encephalopathy that occurs has four clinical stages, as shown in Table 7.13.

Hyperventilation, hyperthermia, and hyperreflexia may also reflect CNS involvement. Death from this syndrome is usually either due to respiratory and circulatory failure, bleeding, infections, hypoglycemia, cerebral edema, renal failure, and/or pancreatitis; the encephalopathy is rarely the cause of death in these patients.

Diagnosis

Liver function tests, clotting studies, albumin and total proteins should be assessed. Electrolytes, calcium, phosphorus and BUN should also be obtained. Viral studies of hepatitis A, B, EBV, CMV, and, in infants, herpes and adenovirus should be obtained. Hyponatremia, prolonged prothrombin time, and hypoalbuminemia are all poor prognostic signs. An SGOT elevated 10- to 100-fold greater than normal or a bilirubin which can be even greater than 50 mg/dl direct are consistent with this syndrome. Ammonia is usually elevated, while the glucose is normal or increased. The CBC will show an elevated white blood cell count if there is extensive hepatocellular damage. If a hemolytic anemia is diagnosed, Wilson disease should be ruled out. Sodium, potassium, and BUN are decreased and there is usually a respiratory alkalosis. Elevation of BUN, creatinine, and a lowered calcium can occur as hepatorenal syndrome develops. Urinalysis should be normal except for bilirubinuria. A toxic screen should be examined to rule out any possible treatable causes.

Treatment

The goal of therapy is to support cerebral, renal, cardiac, and pulmonary function until hepatic regeneration can occur. This involves careful monitoring, intravenous alimentation, and fluid administration, respiratory support, control of cerebral edema, prevention and intervention for hepatorenal syndrome, prevention of bleeding disorders, and immediate therapy for potential infections. Routine medical therapy should include the use of neomycin and vitamin K, usually 5–10 mg/day, a high-carbohydrate, low-protein, low-sodium diet. There is no indication for prophylactic sedation unless complete control is needed to maintain adequate cerebral blood flow and prevent cerebral edema.

Treatment is generally supportive since no definitive cure has yet been found. If neurologic dysfunction occurs, attention should be directed toward relieving increased intracranial pressure.

Monitoring should include careful measurement of arterial blood pressure and other vital signs, urinary output, with placement of a urinary catheter, as well as central venous or pulmonary wedge pressure. EEG and intracranial pressure monitoring may become necessary as the CNS disease progresses. A nasogastric tube will prevent aspiration and can be used to monitor bleeding. Cimetidine may be added to suppress gastric acid secretion and hence avoid unnecessary bleeding.

Serum glucose should be kept between 100 and 300 and a 10% dextrose solution may be needed so that hepatic glycogen stores are not depleted. Hyperaldosteronism can result when the liver fails to degrade aldosterone and may lead to retention of fluid as edema and ascites. Hypoalbuminemia and inappropriate antidiuretic hormone will further increase fluid retention. Therefore, although fluid restriction and low-sodium intake should be used to minimize fluid retention, diuretics should be used carefully since they may lead to depletion of intravascular fluid and precipitate the hepatic renal syndrome. Serum sodium should be maintained over 130 mEq/L. If necessary, albumin followed by diuretics may be used to increase free water clearance. Hypokalemia may be secondary to kaluresis from secondary hyperaldosteronism and potassium supplements may be needed as well. Up to 120 mEq/m^2/day have been needed to replace potassium loss. Serum albumin should be maintained at 3.5 g/dl by infusing 1–1.5 g/kg of albumin every 6–8 hours, with care to avoid volume overexpansion.

The syndrome of inappropriate antidiuretic hormone may lead to pulmonary edema, although the mechanism for this edema is unclear. Positive pressure ventilation is a problem since it increases hepatic vein pressure, decreases flow out of the liver, and may lead to ischemic necrosis of the central lobules. Splanchnic blood flow may also be decreased. Hyperventilation may cause a further decrease since it increases splanchnic resistance resulting in a further fall in portal flow. Nevertheless, positive end-expiratory pressure and hyperventilation remain the mainstay of respiratory support for this syndrome.

Impending hepatic coma is best treated by avoiding electrolyte imbalances, with careful maintenance of potassium and phosphorus, avoiding hypotension and hypoglycemia, using sedatives with caution, and cleansing the gut with lactulose to alter gut flora and reduce production of ammonia. If hemorrhage does occur, platelets and coagulation factors should be administered as well as whole fresh blood. Epsilon aminocaproic acid has been used, but may predispose to microthrombi. Infections are usually related to respiratory tract, urinary tract, or intravenous line usage and are most often due to Gram-negative organisms. Paracentesis should be considered to rule out spontaneous bacterial peritonitis. Steroids have not been shown to improve the outcome in acute hepatic failure, since their use has been associated with life-threatening fungal infections, GI bleeding, and acute pancreatitis. Therapy with intravenous hepatitis B immune globulin has also been suggested, but has not been shown to be helpful.

CONTROVERSIES

Several therapeutic modalities, such as exchange transfusion, plasmapheresis, and charcoal hemoperfusion, have had mixed success. The exchange transfusions provide only temporary improvement and survival has not been influenced. Plasmapheresis has had similar success, although with fewer side effects than those attributed to exchange transfusions. Peritoneal dialysis and hemodialysis may remove ammonia, but they also produce fluid shifts and can precipitate hepatorenal syndrome, although there are anecdotal reported successes when these are combined with exchange transfusions. Charcoal hemoperfusion also has variable success and results in hypotension and destruction of platelets by the charcoal. Extracorporeal perfusion has not yet been successful. Hepatitis B surface antigen carriers have not benefitted from a liver transplant. Ultimately, the goal of therapy will be to design an artificial support system that will remove toxic compounds and replace needed activated compounds for sustenance of life.

Prognosis

Acute hepatic failure is associated with high mortality, up to 70–80% in adults when associated with severe hepatic encephalopathy. In children, the prognosis is more favorable. Survival has been noted to be as high as 47% in children between the ages of 11–20 years and up to 75% in the absence of hepatic coma. Liver biopsies performed months after survival are normal, although chronic active hepatitis may be seen in up to one-third of cases. Postnecrotic cirrhosis occurs in less than 10%. Patients with drug-induced hepatitis do better than those with viral, although again the development of hepatic encephalopathy indicates poor prognosis (Partin, 1985b).

HEPATIC ENCEPHALOPATHY

Definition

Hepatic encephalopathy is a clinical syndrome associated with severe hepatic insufficiency and characterized by changes in mental status that can resemble a neuropsychiatric disorder. The syndrome is sometimes known as hepatic coma.

Basic Science

Hepatic encephalopathy is thought to be secondary to an accumulation of toxic metabolites in the extracellular fluid. The failure of the liver to metabolize these substances occurs in end-stage liver disease. Associated changes can be identified in the blood brain barrier and in disturbed cerebral metabolism from impairment of sodium-potassium-ATPase activity in neuronal membranes.

The most significant alteration is an elevation in the plasma ammonia which can occur whenever metabolites are shunted past hepatic cells as in individuals with portacaval anastomosis. The production of ammonia is in the GI tract as a result of ingestion of protein or ammonium salts. Colonic bacteria and mucosal enzymes act on these substraits and liberate ammonia which is then transported through the portal circulation to the liver. The healthy liver converts the ammonia to urea through the urea cycle. When hepatic dysfunction is severe, ammonia cannot be metabolized so it enters the systemic circulation. The excess ammonia can be toxic to the brain.

One of the consequences of high circulating levels of ammonia is an increase in glucagon which leads to increased hepatic gluconeogenesis from amino acids and further increases ammonia production.

Another site of ammonia detoxification is the astrocytes in the brain which convert glutamic acids to form glutamine. In hepatic encephalopathy, elevated glutamine levels can be found in cerebrospinal fluid, which is thought to correlate with the degree of neurologic dysfunction. α-Ketoglutarate also rises as much as four-fold in patients with encephalopathy (Jones et al, 1984).

One system that is affected by hepatic failure is neurotransmission in the brain; false neurotransmitters including serotonin and histamine as well as catecholamines have been found elevated in spinal fluid and serum in hepatic encephalopathy.

Natural History

Initially, the symptoms are usually mild but can progress rapidly to frank coma unless the biochemical changes are reversed. In acute liver failure, the accumulation of metabolites may be very rapid and the course of encephalopathy measured in hours.

The earliest signs are irritability, restlessness, and confusion, followed by clouding of the sensorium. The patients may have a peculiar odor to their breath which is characteristic of advanced hepatic coma. Asterixis is a characteristic and prominent feature of hepatic encephalopathy, characterized by an involuntary clinching and unclinching of the fist around the examiner's finger.

Diagnosis

Once the clinical syndrome is recognized, the definitive diagnosis depends on the laboratory data which include a measurement of serum ammonia. The level may not be elevated since the level depends on the rate of production and metabolism of ammonia. It is useful, however, in following the clinical status of some individuals. Cerebrospinal fluid glutamine, the end product of cerebral ammonia metabolism is usually elevated, and when so, it is strongly indicative of hepatic encephalopathy.

The electroencephalogram may be useful in diagnosis since there is generalized slowing sometimes accompanied by high voltage and slow wave forms.

Treatment

One approach to treatment is an attempt to trap the ammonium ion in the gut to eliminate subsequent absorption. This can be accomplished to some extent with a synthetic disaccharide that is neither absorbed nor hydrolyzed in the upper GI tract, namely, lactulose (1, 4 galactosidofructose). The effect of the disaccharide is to acidify the intestinal lumen and allow the conversion of ammonia to the ammonium ion in the gut. This is followed by the movement of ammonia from the intracellular space to the extracellular space and then to the acid intestine which in effect traps the ammonium ion, and excretes it in the stool.

Another approach is neomycin, an antibiotic which has been used to decrease the concentration of urease-containing bacteria and, thus, decreasing the production of ammonia from proteins and amino acids. It can be given orally or by enema, with the knowledge that about 1–3% of the dose is absorbed when administered by these routes. If neomycin is ineffective, then oral ampicillin, kanamycin, or tetracycline may be effective.

In severe cases, more radical approaches to therapy include use of intravenous mannitol for control of cerebral edema, and exchange transfusion to reduce the concentration of ammonia.

Complications of treatment include electrolyte disorders, most commonly hypernatremia, secondary to the osmotic diarrhea associated with lactulose therapy.

For further discussion, see therapy of Reye syndrome (pp. 484).

REYE SYNDROME

Definition

In 1963, Reye and his colleagues in Australia described a syndrome characterized by acute encephalopathy in association with fatty degeneration of the liver and other organs. Since then, the syndrome has been found to encompass a wide clinical spectrum, with earlier diagnosis and aggressive management being necessary to improve prognosis.

Basic Science

The pathophysiology relating the encephalopathic picture with the fatty infiltration of the liver remains unclear. Nonetheless, specific metabolic and anatomic abnormalities have been found with the syndrome. Hyperammonemia is characteristic, thought to be secondary to dysfunction of the mitochondrial urea cycle enzymes. Moreover, it is believed that there is a generalized mitochondrial dysfunction in the liver and perhaps other organs as well leading to glycogen depletion, hypoglycemia, and fat mobilization and redeposition as a result of the energy deficit. Liver biopsy specimens of patients with Reye syndrome show microvesicular fat accumulation within the cytoplasm of the hepatocyte consistent with this theory. Cytotoxic cerebral edema without evidence of inflammation is observed.

If treated sucessfully these anatomic metabolic disturbances are transient and full recovery is possible.

The etiology for this syndrome appears to be multifactorial. It is possible that earlier cases might have represented congenital deficiencies of various enzymes in the urea cycle. Of greatest import is the increasing evidence associating aspirin usage with Reye syndrome (Hurwitz et al, 1985; 1987). The association is significant enough that the Centers for Disease Control, the Surgeon General, and the American Academy of Pediatrics have advised that use of salicylates be avoided in all children with viral infections, particularly varicella and/or influenza.

Epidemiology

The incidence of Reye syndrome in the United States varies greatly year by year (Fig. 7.13). The disease occurs primarily in children between the ages of 4 and 16 years, although it has been known to occur in infants. Usually there is an increased incidence of cases when antecedent viral illnesses are epidemic (e.g., in the winter months). It affects males and females in equal numbers. Middle class caucasian children living mainly in suburban and rural areas appear to be affected more than inner city children. However, infants in inner city, low socioeconomic populations appear to be more likely to develop the syndrome than infants in the suburban and rural areas (Huttenlocher and Trauner, 1978). These epidemiologic findings suggest that children in urban areas are exposed to some factor at an earlier age than are other children.

About 1 in every 2000 patients with influenza B and 1 in every 4000 patients with varicella virus will develop Reye syndrome. However, many cases that are mild and may go undetected (Corey et al, 1977; Lichtenstein et al, 1983).

Natural History

The onset of symptoms is almost always preceded by a prodromal viral illness (Lichtenstein et al, 1983). In children, this is usually a respiratory tract infection, but the syndrome can follow the infection with varicella, 3–5 days after the onset of the rash, or after an episode of infectious diarrhea. Fever is usually absent. Hepatomegaly may be present but it occurs in an anicteric setting. Focal neurologic signs are rare, although a generalized neurologic dysfunction is characteristic of the severe stages of the disease. In 1974, Lovejoy et al proposed a staging system that is currently recommended by the National Institutes of Health. The staging system appears in Table 7.14.

Diagnosis

The criteria for diagnosis include the following: (1) A characteristic history, suggestive of a preceding viral illness; (2) elevation in serum ammonia, which can also be prognostic, in that ammonia levels greater than 300 μg/dl have been associated with higher mortality (Corey et al, 1977); (3) abnormal liver function tests including elevated SGOT, and clotting studies; bilirubin levels are usually normal; in infants, blood glucose levels may be decreased (less than 60 ml/dl); (4) elimination of other possible explanations for the neurologic or biochemical abnormalities, including urea cycle disorders, other metabolic abnormalities such as systemic carnitine deficiency, fructose intolerance, medium-chain acyl-coA dehydrogenase (MCAD) deficiency, and ingestion of a toxin.

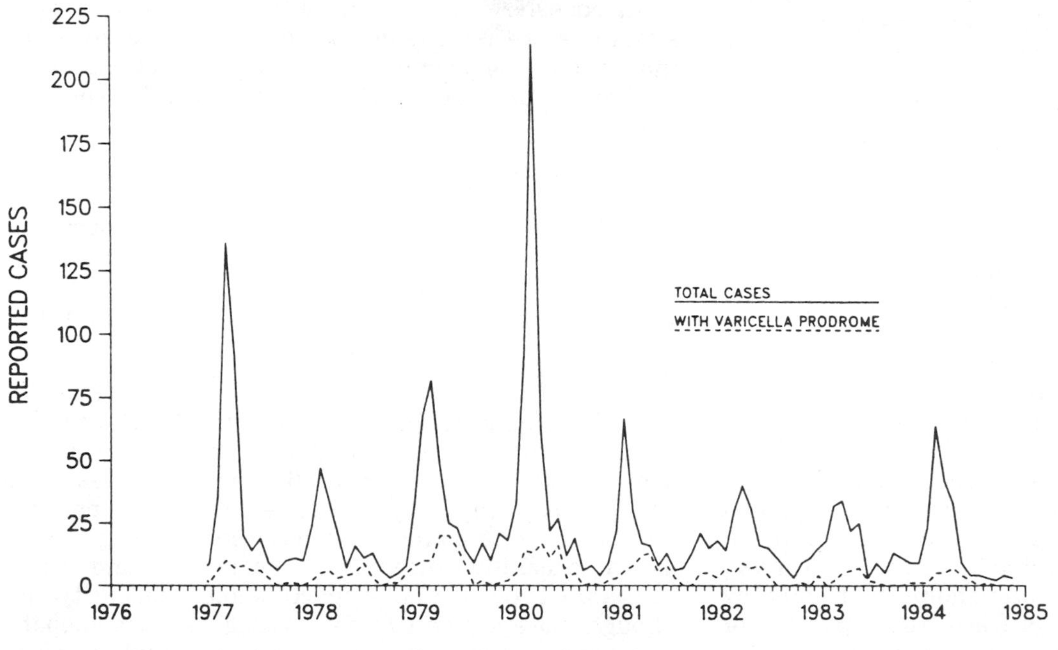

Figure 7.13. Cases of Reye syndrome by month of hospitalization. United States December 1976-November 1984. Reproduced with permission from CDC: *MMWR* Annual Summary 1984, p. 113.

Table 7.14
Stages of Reye Syndrome[1]

Stage	Criteria
I	Lethargy, vomiting, indifference
II	Delirium, combativeness, hyperventilation
III	Decorticate posturing, light coma, hypoventilation, intact pupillary responses
IV	Decerebrate posture, deep coma, loss of spontaneous ventilation, fixed dilated pupils
V	Seizures, flaccidity

[1]After Lovejoy et al, 1975.

Diagnostic work-up for a patient with suspected Reye syndrome should include the following: measurement of arterial ammonia, liver function tests including an SGOT, bilirubin, and amylase, complete blood count, clotting studies including prothrombin time and partial thromboplastin time, serum electrolytes, calcium, phosphorus, blood sugar, BUN creatinine, urinalysis, and toxic screen. A liver biopsy should be considered in patients, who present with recurrent Reye episodes, who are less than 1 year of age or over 16, or who present during nonepidemic periods. Serial arterial blood gases are obtained to monitor the metabolic acidosis and respiratory alkalosis that occur in this setting. In the early stages of the illness viral titers may be useful to identify an antecedent associated illness. If a patient is in stage 3 or 4 at the time of presentation, a lumbar puncture should be performed only if meningitis or encephalitis are likely (because of the presence of significant intracranial hypertension and the danger of cerebral herniation) and is contraindicated if a CT scan suggests elevated intracranial hypertension. Intracranial pressure monitoring should be instituted for those patients who are stage 3 or 4 since increases in intracranial pressure may not be detected by clinical examination (Rockoff and Pascucci, 1983). Such monitoring is done by the insertion of a subdural "bolt," since it need not be inserted into a very small or compressed ventricle. An EEG, or brain stem and cortical evoked potentials may be useful in assessing the degree of neurologic impairment.

Treatment

All patients require extensive and careful monitoring of input and output as well as daily weights. The patient should be given nothing by mouth, with parenteral support supplied by a 10% dextrose solution in quarter normal saline usually with 20 mEq KCl/L and 20 mEq potassium phosphate/L, given at a half maintenance rate, assuming adequate blood pressure. The goal is to restrict fluids but increase osmolality while maintaining a glucose level greater than 100 mg/dl (Partin, 1985b). If clotting studies are abnormal, vitamin K should be administered at a dose of 0.1 ml/kg im or slowly iv. Active bleeding should be treated by administration of 10 ml/kg of fresh-frozen plasma, or if needed, replacement blood. Hyperammonemia can be treated by the administration of lactulose, at a dose of 0.5 g/kg via nasogastric tube then 0.25 g/kg every 6–12 hours to decrease serum ammonia levels. Neomycin can also decrease serum ammonia.

If the patient is in stage 2, arterial and urinary catheters should be placed. Mannitol should be administered every 4–6 hours to help elevate serum osmolality to 300–320 mOsm/L. A patient in stage 3 or 4 should be anesthesized, intubated and sedated. Central venous pressure should be monitored and intracranial pressure monitoring devices should be inserted. The head should be placed in a midline position at a 30–45° angle which will improve cerebral venous return and help to diminish intracranial pressure. Serum osmolality should remain elevated with fluids appropriately restricted, use of diuretics, and by colloidal boluses to support intravascular volume when necessary. The Pa_{CO_2} should be maintained at 20–30 torr. This can be done by hyperventilation while minimizing positive end-expiratory pressure and mean airway pressure to avoid increasing intracranial pressure, and by supplying supplemental oxygen to keep the Pa_{O_2} greater than 100. Normothermia is usually maintained and hyperthermia prevented by the use of cooling blankets and, if necessary, vasodilation with thorazine derivatives. The goal of therapy is to maintain a mean cerebral perfusion pressure at 50–90 torr. This represents the difference between the mean arterial blood pressure and the intracranial pressure and requires that intracranial pressure be maintained at less than 15–20 torr.

Usually, barbiturates or hypothermia are removed first, with the barbiturates being weaned by 25% every 6–12 hours. If the patient can be weaned from a ventilator, the intracranial pressure monitor may be removed, and serum osmolality allowed to return to normal.

If intracranial pressure remains elevated despite these measures, high-dose barbiturates can be given intravenously. Complications of therapy in stage 3 Reye syndrome can include electrolyte imbalance, hyperosmolality, hypoglycemia, hemorrhage, infections, renal failure, seizures, pancreatitis, and intractable cerebral edema.

CONTROVERSY

The use of hypothermia to control intracranial pressure in this disease remains controversial. Other treatments of unproven value include hemodialysis, peritoneal dialysis, exchange transfusion, and steroids.

Prognosis

The prognosis for children with Reye syndrome continues to improve dramatically, with mortality formerly about 30% while in 1986, the rate was less than 5% (although this may also reflect that more patients in stage 1 are being included in the epidemiologic data). Death is usually caused by cerebral edema and uncontrollable intracranial hypertension. Morbidity, although more difficult to assess, suggests that hepatic and neurologic recovery is essentially complete except in those who are in stage 3 or 4, who may have some

CASE ILLUSTRATION 1

An 8-year-old female presented to the hospital disoriented and combative after 6 days of upper respiratory infection symptoms, 3 days of aspirin treatment, and 2 days of vomiting. Examination on arrival was notable for poor hydration, a symmetric neurologic examination, with intact cranial nerves, hyporeflexia, and upgoing toes. Initial laboratory values were notable for normal CBC and electrolytes, elevated liver function tests (except for a normal bilirubin), prolonged clotting studies, and an ammonia that reached a peak at 281 μg/dl. A toxic screen was normal. The prevailing opinion was that this patient's illness was most consistent with stage 2 Reye syndrome.

QUESTION AND COMMENT

What is the prognosis for this child and how should she be managed at this stage?

Since the patient was at a stage 2 status (see Table 7.14), her fluid was restricted initially and she was closely monitored neurologically, requiring treatment with mannitol once. Eighteen hours after admission, however, she became decorticate and her potentially increased intracranial pressure required more aggressive treatment, including hyperventilation, hyperosmolar agents, and an intracranial bolt to monitor intracranial pressure. An EEG confirmed that she had progressed to stage 3 Reye syndrome.

With respect to prognosis, a number of studies before the use of aggressive intracranial pressure management utilized clinical and EEG staging at the time of admission as an indicator of prognosis, with patients who were stage 3 or 4 showing poor survival or significant neurologic sequelae. With the advent of aggressive intracranial pressure management, however, survival has improved dramatically for stage 3 Reye syndrome patients. Other factors that do not bode well for a patient with the syndrome include the presence of seizures, persistent metabolic acidosis, an uncontrollable intracranial pressure, hyperosmolarity (none of which our patient had). One of the most helpful prognostic signs has been a peak ammonia level, with studies suggesting better prognosis for ammonia levels less than 300 μg/dl. Serial ammonia measurements early in a patient's course may be an indication for more aggressive management to improve prognosis.

As predicted, this patient demonstrated many of the "good" prognostic factors noted above, and within 72 hours after admission, her neurological status began to normalize both clinically and by EEG, and she was weaned from her intracranial pressure treatment. After a week in the hospital, her laboratory studies returned to baseline and she was discharged with normal ammonia and liver function tests.

CASE ILLUSTRATION 2

A 13-year-old female presented with vomiting and abdominal pain for 24 hours. She had had an upper respiratory infection and pharyngitis 6 days before admission, treated with aspirin, acetominophen, and decongestants, which had resolved before the onset of abdominal pain. Because of the fear of an acute abdomen, she was referred to the emergency room where, on examination, she was found to be irritable (believed to be secondary to lack of sleep), but fully oriented. Her examination was entirely benign except for dry mucus membrane secondary to dehydration. She received iv hydration for a presumptive gastritis while her laboratory values were pending. A CBC, electrolytes, blood sugar, BUN, creatinine, amylase, bilirubin, and urinalysis were all within normal limits. After 2 hours of hydration, the patient improved, stopped vomiting, denied abdominal pain, and was about to be discharged when the rest of her liver function tests were returned. The SGOT was 494 U/L and the SGPT was 930 U/L. Serum ammonia was 279 consistent with a diagnosis of Reye syndrome. She was then admitted and over the next few hours rapidly progressed from a state of alertness to one of obtundation (clinical stage 1 to clinical stage 3).

COMMENT

We mention this case because Reye syndrome is probably not considered sufficiently often in the differential diagnosis of vomiting in an adolescent female, although previous epidemics in 1973, 1974, 1977, and 1978 have shown the peak incidence of the disease between the ages of 11 and 14 years. In more than 2000 cases reported between 1973 and 1980 older children and adults were more apt to present with the upper respiratory infection prodrome than with varicella or an antecedent GI illness.

neurologic sequelae, including deficits in intelligence, visual motor integration, concept formation, and overall school performance. Older children who develop Reye syndrome appear to have more neurologic sequelae than do younger children. It is believed that earlier diagnosis secondary to increased clinical suspicion and subsequent vigorous management have dramatically improved the prognosis for children with Reye syndrome. Relapse, although infrequent, has been noted.

Prevention

Because of epidemiologic associations with viral disorders and aspirin usage, the medical community has been largely responsible for informing the public about the need to seek medical advice regarding treatment of flu, chickenpox, and use of aspirin.

LIVER TRANSPLANTATION

The advent of liver transplantation in 1967 as a therapeutic modality for patients with advanced chronic liver disease merits discussion. At present, most liver transplants are being performed on infants and children who have biliary atresia or inborn errors of metabolism.

The major development in the immunosuppression program has been the introduction of cyclosporine in 1980. In addition, improvements in procuring and preserving organs have added to better survival. New techniques have been developed so that donor organs can be preserved for periods of 8 hours, increasing the successful transplantation rate.

Cyclosporine in vitro inhibits the release and production of lymphokines from stimulated T cells, leading to a decrease in helper or cytotoxic effector cells. Suppressor cells, however, continue to be generated despite use of cyclosporine. In vivo, the drug has been found to suppress both cell-mediated and humoral immunity and helps to prevent both graft-versus-host and host-versus-graft-rejections, although the mechanisms for these effects currently remain unclear. It is used with prednisone to achieve long-term immunosuppression.

The number of institutions in the United States performing liver transplantation has increased dramatically over the past several years. The overall 1-year survival rate for children who received a liver transplant had increased from 30% in 1980 to over 60% in 1985 (Perlmutter et al, 1985).

Criteria for selection of patients include the following: (1) progressive jaundice with a total bilirubin level usually 15 mg/dl or more; (2) diminished hepatic synthetic function with uncorrectable clotting studies, despite use of vitamin K; (3) portal hypertension refractory to medical or surgical therapy; (4) hepatic encephalopathy that prevents an individual from functioning at his baseline normal level, despite full medical therapy with lactulose, neomycin, and a protein-restricted diet; (5) intractable cholestasis; (6) growth failure despite exhaustive nutritional therapy; and (7) an inability to maintain a reasonable quality of life as a result of liver disease. Contraindications to liver transplantation include the following: (1) advanced cardiac, pulmonary, or renal disease; (2) severe hypoxemia due to right-to-left shunts; (3) metastatic hepatobiliary malignancy; (4) an extrahepatic malignancy; (5) uncorrectable congenital anomalies; (6) sepsis; (7) portal vein thrombosis; (8) intrahepatobiliary sepsis, or the presence of hepatitis B surface antigen positivity (Zitelli et al, 1986; Malatak et al, 1987).

Complications after surgery include fluid and electrolyte imbalances and hepatic vascular thromboses that can be diagnosed by ultrasonography and radionucleotide scans. After several weeks, hepatitis is a problem from organisms such as cytomegalovirus, herpes, or viral hepatitis. The usual duration of hospitalization in our experience is about 6 weeks.

Follow-up should include evaluation for systemic hypertension of unknown etiology. Liver function tests are appropriate to monitor for signs of rejection.

With the onset of appropriate immunosuppression, better organ preservation, improved surgical techniques, survival rate remains at about 65% in children. However, repeat transplantation has been required in about one-third of children even after the introduction of cyclosporine, and in these children, the survival rate is 47% (Perlmutter et al, 1985).

REFERENCES

Abramson SJ, Treves S, Teele RL: The infant with possible biliary atresia, evaluation by ultrasound and nuclear medicine. *Pediatr Radiol* 12:1, 1982.

Altman RP: The portoenterostomy procedure for biliary atresia: A 5-year experience. *Ann Surg* 188:351, 1978.

Altman RP, Levy J: Biliary atresia. *Pediatr Ann* 14:481, 1985.

Balistreri WF: Neonatal cholestasis. In Liebenthal E (ed): *Textbook of Gastroenterology Nutrition in Infancy*. New York, Raven Press, 1981, p. 1081.

Balistreri WF: *Viral Hepatitis: Implications to Pediatric Practice.* Year Book of Pediatrics 1985. Chicago, Year Book Medical Publishers, 1985, p. 287.

Balistreri WF: Viral hepatitis. *Pediatr Clin North Am* 35:375,1988.

Brewer GJ, Hill GM, Prasad AS, et al: Oral zinc therapy for Wilson's disease. *Ann Intern Med* 99:314, 1983.

Cartwright GE, Edwards CQ, Kravitz K, et al: Hereditary hemochromatosis: Phenotypic expression of the disease. *N Engl J Med* 297:7, 1977.

CDC: Delta hepatitis—Massachusetts. *MMWR* p. 33, 1984.

CDC: Hepatitis B in an extended family—Alabama. *MMWR* 36:744, 1987.

CDC: Recommendations for protection against viral hepatitis. *MMWR* 34:313, 1985.

Chandra AS, Altman RP: Ductal remnants in extrahepatic biliary atresia: A histopathologic study with clinical correlation. *J Pediatr* 93:196, 1978.

Cohen SM: Application of nuclear magnetic resonance of the study of the liver, etiology and disease. *Hepatology* 3:738, 1983.

Corey L, Rubin RJ, Hattwick MAW: Reye Syndrome: Clinical progression and evaluation of therapy. *Pediatrics* 60:708, 1977.

DeLong GR, Glick TH: Encephalopathy of Reye's syndrome. *Pediatrics* 69:53, 1982.

Escobar GJ, Heyman MB, Smith WB, et al: Primary hemochromatosis in childhood. *Pediatrics* 80:549, 1987.

Fitzgerald JF, Clark JH, Angelides AG, et al: The prognostic significance of peak ammonia levels in Reye syndrome. *Pediatrics* 70:997, 1982.

Fraser CL, Arieff AI: Hepatic encephalopathy. *N Engl J Med* 313:865, 1985.

Garver RI, Marrex JF, Nueiwa T, et al: Alpha-1-antitrypsin deficiency and emphysema caused by homozygous inheritance of nonexpressing alpha-1-antitrypsin genes. *N Engl J Med* 314:762, 1986.

Hurwitz ES, Barrett MJ, Bregman D, et al: Public Health Service study of Reye's syndrome and medications. *N Engl J Med* 313:849, 1985.

Hurwitz ES, Barrett MJ, Bregman D, et al: Report of the main study. *JAMA* 257:1905, 1987.

Huttenlocher P, Trauner D: Reye syndrome in infancy. *Pediatrics* 62:84, 1978.

Javitt NB: Neonatal hepatitis and biliary atresia. US Public Health Service. Washington DC, DHEW Publication no. NIH 7901296, 1979.

Jones EA, Schafer DF, Ferenci P, et al: The neurobiology of hepatic encephalopathy. *Hepatology* 4:1235, 1984.

Kidd VJ, Golbus MS, Wallace RB, et al: Prenatal diagnosis of alpha-1-antitrypsin deficiency by direct analysis of the mutation site in the gene. *N Engl J Med* 310:639, 1984.

Latimer JS, Sharp HL: Alpha-1-antitrypsin deficiency in childhood. *Curr Probl Pediatr* 11:5, 1980.

Lichtenstein P, Heubi J, Daugherty C, et al: Grade 1 Reye syndrome: A frequent cause of vomiting and liver dysfunction after varicella and upper respiratory tract infection. *N Engl J Med* 309:133, 1983.

Lilly JR, Karrer FM: Contemporary surgery of biliary atresia. *Pediatr Clin North Am* 32:1233, 1985.

Lovejoy FH, Smith AL, Bresnan MJ: Clinical staging in Reyes syndrome. *Am J Dis Child* 128:36, 1974.

Madigan SM, Teele RL: Ultrasonography of the liver and biliary tree in children. *Semin Ultrasound CT MR* 5:68, 1984.

Maggione G, Bernard O, Hadchouel M, et al: Treatment of autoimmune chronic active hepatitis in childhood. *J Pediatr* 104:839, 1984.

Maggione G, Hadchouel M, Sessa F, et al: A retrospective study of the role of delta agent infection in children with HBsAg-positive chronic hepatitis. *Hepatology* 5:7, 1985.

Malatack JJ, Schaid DJ, Urbach AH, et al: Choosing a pediatric recipient for orthotopic liver transplantation. *J Pediatr* 111:479, 1987.

Manolaki AG, Larcher VF, Mowat AP, et al: The prelaparotomy diagnosis of extrahepatic biliary atresia. *Arch Dis Child* 58:591, 1983.

Morse JO: Alpha-1-antitrypsin deficiency, Parts I and II. *N Engl J Med* 299:1045, 1099, 1978.

Nazer H, Edrj EDE, Mowatt AP, et al: Wilson's disease in childhood: Variability of clinical presentation. *Clin Pediatr* 22:755, 1983.

Nebbia G, Hadchouel M, Odievere M, et al: Early assessment of evolution of liver diseases associated with alpha-1-antitrypsin deficiency in childhood. *J Pediatr* 102:661, 1983.

Partin JC: Acute hepatic failure in children. *Pediatr Ann* 14:446, 1985a.

Partin JC: Management of Reye syndrome: Need for early diagnosis and intravenous treatment of stage 1 noncomatose cases. *Pediatr Ann* 14:511, 1985b.

Perlmutter D, Vacanti J, Donaho EP, et al: Liver transplantation in pediatric patients. *Year Book of Pediatrics 1985*. Chicago, Year Book Medical, 1985, p. 77.

Poley JR: Practical approach to assessing liver function. *Pediatr Ann* 14:423, 1985.

Psacharopoulos H, Mowat AP, Davies M, et al: Fulminant and hepatic failure in childhood. *Arch Dis Child* 55:252, 1980.

Reye RDK, Morgan G, Baral J: Encephalopathy and fatty degeneration of the viscera. *Lancet* 2:749, 1963.

Rockoff MA, Pascucci RC: Reye syndrome. *Emerg Med Clin North Am* 1:87, 1983.

Rogers E, Rogers M: Fulminant and hepatic failure in hepatic encephalopathy. *Pediatr Clin North Am* 27:701, 1980.

Ruppin DC, Frydman MI, Lunzer MR: The value of serum gamma glutamyltransferase activity in the diagnosis of hepatobiliary disease. *Med J Austral* 69:421, 1982.

Sanders S, et al: Acute liver failure. In Wright R, et al (eds): *Liver and Biliary Disease*. London, WB Saunders, 1979, p. 569.

Shaywitz BA, Rothstein P, Venes JL: Monitoring and management of increased intracranial pressure in Reye syndrome: Results in 29 children. *Pediatrics* 66:198, 1980.

Smith FW, Mallard JR: NMR imaging and liver disease. *Br Med Bull* 40:194, 1984.

Starzl TE, Groth CG, Brettschneider L, et al: Orthotopic homotransplantation of the liver. *Ann Surg* 168:392, 1968.

Sveger T: The initial alpha-1-antitrypsin deficiency in early childhood. *Pediatrics* 62:22, 1978.

Sveger T: Prospective study of children with alpha-1-antitrypsin deficiency deficiency—8 year followup. *J Pediatr* 104:91, 1984.

Szmuness W, Stevens CE, Harley EJ, et al: Hepatitis B vaccine: Demonstration of efficacy in a controlled clinical trial in a high risk population in the United States. *N Engl J Med* 303:833, 1980.

Tonsgard JH, Huttenlocker PR, Thisted RA: Lactic acidemia in Reye's syndrome. *Pediatrics* 69:64, 1982.

Tray C: Acute hepatic failure. In Smith CA (ed): *The Critically Ill Child*. Philadelphia, WB Saunders, 1977, p. 117.

Van Caillie M, Morin C, Roy C, et al: Reye syndrome: Relapses and neurological sequelae. *Pediatrics* 59:244, 1977.

Vanthiel DH: Liver transplantation. *Pediatr Ann* 14:475, 1985.

Werlin SL, Grand RJ, Perman JA, et al: Diagnostic dilemmas of Wilson's disease: Diagnosis and treatment. *Pediatrics* 62:47, 1978.

Wewers MD, Casolaro MA, Sellers SE, et al: Replacement therapy for alpha-1-antitrypsin deficiency associated with emphysema. *N Engl J Med* 316:1055, 1987.

Zitelli BJ, Malatack JJ, Gartner JC, et al: Evaluation of the pediatric patient for liver transplantation. *Pediatrics* 78:559, 1986.

Approach to Gallbladder Disease 7

HYDROPS OF THE GALLBLADDER

Definition

Hydrops of the gallbladder indicates the presence of a distended gallbladder in the absence of any obstructive stone formation or any other acute infectious disease of the gallbladder and the presence of normal-sized extrahepatic bile ducts. It is most commonly found as a complication of mucocutaneous lymph node syndrome (Kawasaki disease).

Basic Science

The mechanisms by which hydrops arises have not yet been confirmed. Abnormality of the cystic duct involving either narrowing, twisting, or atresia have been reported as possible causes. Another theory suggests increased mucus secretion by the gallbladder, with ineffective emptying, which may predispose the gallbladder to becoming acutely distended and, thus, obstructed. In addition to its association with Kawasaki disease, it has also occurred following certain infectious illnesses, including staphlococcal and streptococcal disease, and leptospirosis, as well as in leukemia, nephrotic syndrome, and familial Mediterranean fever.

Epidemiology

Males develop the disease more often than females. It has a predilection for children of preschool age, although both neonates and older children have developed hydrops.

Natural History

The presenting complaint with hydrops is upper gastric or right-sided upper abdominal pain in association with nausea and vomiting, often mimicking an acute abdomen. Jaundice is rarely present and fever is usually slight or absent. Physical examination will reveal a mass in the right upper quadrant in more than half the cases.

Diagnosis

A child with fever, rash, and stigmata of Kawasaki disease should undergo ultrasonography to detect the presence of a hydrops if it is not palpable on physical examination. Ultrasonography will reveal a massively enlarged gallbladder with a normal bile duct.

Treatment

Treatment is usually supportive and consists of intravenous fluids followed by introduction of a low-fat diet which will lead to spontaneous resolution of the hydrops within 2–5 weeks. If the gallbladder is very large, mimicking an acute abdomen, drainage may be performed to avoid rupture. Only a small number of cases actually progress to rupture.

Prognosis

If detected early, prognosis is excellent, even without drainage or cholocystectomy. Perforation occurs rarely (as does bile peritonitis) and requires appropriate surgical and antibiotic regimens.

CHOLELITHIASIS

Gallstone formation, although infrequent in children, does occur. While in adults it is usually due to genetic factors and consists mostly of cholesterol gallstones, in children the disease is usually secondary to conditions such as a hemolytic anemia or a congenital anomaly of the biliary tract.

Basic Science

Gallstones occur in association with hemolysis, biliary malformations and, rarely, ileal resection, hepatic

CASE ILLUSTRATION

A 4-year-old black male presented with obstructive jaundice following a 10-day history of fever, cough, pharyngitis, vomiting, progressive right upper quadrant abdominal pain, and a leukocytosis despite treatment with antibiotics at his local hospital. On arrival, he had a temperature of 38°C, heart rate 130/min, respiratory rate 32/min, and blood pressure 100/66. An erythematous blanching macular rash was observed on the right upper back and axilla, but not elsewhere. There was scleral icterus. Throat showed moderate erythema. Abdominal examination was notable for a mass palpable 9 cm below the right costal margin. It was tender to palpation with an otherwise protuberant abdomen. There was no splenomegaly and stools were guaiac-negative. Scrotal edema as well as nonpitting edema of the hands and feet were also present.

Initial laboratory values were notable for hematocrit of 25.8%, white blood count of 40,200/mm^3, with 68% polys, 8% bands, and platelets of 786,000/mm^3, with a sedimentation rate of 65 mm/hr. Chemistries were normal except for total protein of 4.9 mg/dl, albumin of 2.2 mg/dl, SGOT 54 U/L, SGPT 39 U/L, and a bilirubin of 4.5 mg/dl total over 4.3 mg/dl direct. Alkaline phosphatase was 191 and urinalysis was notable for urobilinogen with a rare white blood cell. A heterophile test for mononucleosis was negative as were four sets of blood and stool cultures. Chest radiographs showed a small right middle lobe infiltrate. Ultrasonography of the abdomen on admission revealed a large cystic mass on the right upper quadrant extending below the umbilicus. The intrahepatic bile ducts and liver were normal. An extra "outpouching" from the cyst was noted and thought to be consistent with the gallbladder, making a large choledochal cyst the working diagnosis.

QUESTION AND COMMENT

How would you manage this patient?

With the fever, elevated white count, and right upper quadrant pain, ascending cholangitis or even pneumonia could not be ruled out and the decision was reached to treat with broad spectrum antibiotics for 2 weeks before attempting surgical exploration of the cyst.

During this interval, the patient symptomatically improved as the abdominal swelling and tenderness diminished. On the day before undergoing exploratory surgery, repeat ultrasonography was obtained which showed a marked decrease in the right upper quadrant mass which now had the orientation and configuration of a gallbladder making the diagnosis hydrops of the gallbladder rather than a choledochal cyst. Since the treatment of choice for a nonacutely distending hydrops is supportive medical therapy, the operation was cancelled.

We mention this case because hydrops of the gallbladder is not usually considered in the differential diagnosis of right upper quadrant abdominal pain in a previously well child. This patient had fever and a transient rash, but otherwise lacked most of the other clinical criteria needed to make the diagnosis of Kawasaki disease. Other diseases that have been reported in association with hydrops are leptosporosis, scarlet fever, familial Mediterranean fever, leukemia, and nephrotic syndrome, none of which could be documented in this patient. After 2 weeks of antibiotic therapy and observation, the patient was discharged on a low-fat diet and subsequently did well with no further occurrence of the hydrops.

cirrhosis, dehydration, infection, and total parenteral nutrition. Gallstones in children are rarely radiopaque. Gallstone formation in children on total parenteral nutrition probably results from decreased gallbladder contraction because of the absence of enteric feedings and hence an increase in bile stasis leading to stone formation.

The exact mechanism of gallstone formation is not known but it may be a combination of interacting processes, including dehydration, transient hepatic dysfunction, and hereditary, dietary, and inflammatory influences that affect the composition of bile. Spherocytosis, sickle cell anemia, and thalassemia have been associated with gallstone formation, but usually fewer than 10% of patients who carry these diseases will develop gallstones.

Epidemiology

Although rare in children, stones continue to be more prevalent in females. Cholecystitis often occurs in the setting of a recent pregnancy or birth control use in teenage girls, particularly those who are obese and have a family history of gallbladder disease. Clinical presentation is similar to that in adults. Although cholecystitis is of low incidence in teenage girls, it can result in great morbidity, with up to 35% of teenage girls in one series having complications, including jaundice, chemical pancreatitis, pancreatic pseudocysts, and a common duct stone.

Natural History

Cholelithiasis is usually characterized by intermittent colicky, abdominal pain, that can wax and wane, usually in the right upper quadrant. If the pain radiates to the lower quadrants, it may be confused with appendicitis. Multiple attacks are usual before the diagnosis is made. Anorexia, fatigue, listlessness, nausea, and vomiting may accompany the abdominal pain. Jaundice may be present, but is not diagnostic. Usually there is a delay between onset of symptoms and diagnosis, ranging from 1–5 years in children.

Strictures of the distal common bile duct are seen in patients with cystic fibrosis and liver disease. Abdominal pain and enlarged gallbladders are found in patients with strictures (Gaskin et al, 1988).

Diagnosis

Physical examination and routine laboratory findings are seldom useful in diagnosing gallstones. The CBC may be useful if a hemolytic disease is detected. Elevated liver function tests may be consistent with a diagnosis of cholangitis, but otherwise may remain normal, including alkaline phosphatase, since gallstones rarely result in significant obstruction. The mainstay of diagnosis is ultrasonography, since fewer than 15% of gallstones in children contain enough calcium to be radiopaque and, thus, most are radiolucent. In fact, ultrasonography has replaced the oral cholocystogram as a method of diagnosing gallstones. Ultrasonography carries a sensitivity of 98% and a specificity of about 95%, and is able to identify stones as small as 2 mm in size, making false-negative results very rare (Takiff and Fonkalsrud, 1984). Fasting levels of bile acids may be elevated with obstruction of the common duct.

Treatment

Cholecystectomy is the treatment of choice for symptomatic gallstones. It remains controversial, however, in the absence of symptoms to perform a cholecystectomy once gallstones have been visualized. Postoperatively, a T-tube transhepatic cholangiogram should be performed. If a retained stone is found, saline irrigation should be considered to flush the stone through or use of basket extraction 4–6 weeks after surgery when a fistulous tract is formed around the T-tube. If these methods are unsuccessful, endoscopic sphincterotomy may be worth a trial. The success and the risks of this procedure depend on the skill of the surgeon. Success with endoscopic sphincterotomy has been as high as 90% in adults, although complications have ranged from 8–10%, with a 1.5% mortality (Allen, 1983). Contraindications include acute pancreatitis, markedly abnormal clotting studies, stenosis extending above the intraduodenal portion of the common bile duct, evidence of proximal strictures in the hepatic ducts, or stones too large in diameter to pass through a maximum sphincterotomy.

In infants with cholelithiasis of the common bile duct, washing and external drainage of the biliary tract are adequate. Cholecystectomy is not indicated.

NEW DEVELOPMENTS

New procedures under investigation for removal of gallstones in children include the use of lasers, ultrasonic probes, and extracorporeal ultrasonic lithotripsy.

Prognosis

Prognosis after stone removal is excellent, with recurrence in fewer than 5% of children. If the common duct has been involved, however, there are some case reports of subsequent biliary cirrhosis persisting despite removal of the gallstone.

CHOLEDOCHAL CYSTS

Definition

A choledochal cyst is a congenital cystic dilatation of the common bile duct. Five types that have been defined are the following: type 1 involves the extrahepatic bile duct below the confluence of the hepatic ducts and above the pancreatic part of the common bile duct, and is usually sacular. Type 2 represents a diverticulum of the common bile duct. Type 3 is a choledochocele or cystic dilatation of an intraduodenal duct that can include the bile and pancreatic ducts. Type 4 are intra and extrahepatic cysts otherwise known as Caroli disease. Type 5 are intrahepatic cysts.

Basic Science

It is not clear whether choledochal cysts are congenital or acquired. One theory postulates atresia of the distal common bile duct with subsequent dilatation of the ducts above. Another theory suggests that there is a segmental muscle weakness in the wall of the common bile duct that is responsible for the dilatation. Others suggest that a distal obstruction around the duodenal ampulla may be hypoplastic and require pressures greater than normal to cause distention at the ampulla, thus, resulting in cystic formation proximal to the region of weakness. Weakness of the proximal region is thought to be due to an abnormal insertion of the common bile duct into the distal part of the pancreatic duct, such that reflux of pancreatic juices into this common channel causes inflammation, fibrosis, and stricture.

Epidemiology

Choledochal cysts account for less than 5% of gallbladder disease in children, if biliary atresia is excluded. Females outnumber males 4:1 and most patients are diagnosed before age 10 years, although very few are symptomatic before age 6 months (Barlow et al, 1976).

Natural History

Symptoms include intermittent jaundice, pain, and presence of a mass. The abdominal pain may be aching or colicky. It is usually in the right upper quadrant, but may also be in the epigastrium and can radiate to the back or right shoulder. The mass, if palpable, is usually felt in the right upper quadrant, and is cystic, and can be moved laterally but not vertically. The sicker the patient, the more likely that cholangitis is also present at the time of diagnosis.

Biliary cirrhosis with portal hypertension occurs very quickly in patients who have an obstruction secondary to a choledochal cyst. Moreover, ascending cholangitis may be a complication both before and after surgical repair.

Diagnosis

The most useful diagnostic tool is ultrasonography (Fig. 7.14*A*-*C*). The BIDA scan will confirm the continuity of the cyst with the biliary tract. Percutaneous transhepatic cholangiography may be useful in determining the size of the proximal biliary tree and whether there are any intrahepatic developmental abnormalities of the bile ducts. The endoscopic retrograde cholangiopancreatography (ERCP) can be useful for demonstrating any intraduodenal or intrapancreatic involvement from the cyst. Serum laboratory studies for this disorder are nondiagnostic.

If not visualized by radiographic studies, liver biopsy may demonstrate bile duct proliferation and fibrosis, biliary cirrhosis, or congenital hepatic fibrosis as early as 6–8 weeks of life in an infant with a choledochal cyst.

Treatment

Treatment is surgical, with removal of the cyst and reconstruction of normal anatomy. Failure to remove the cyst and simply to drain it or reanastomose it to the duodenum or jejunum may predispose the individual to a higher risk of biliary tract adenocarcinoma at a later date.

Prognosis

The prognosis for survival has advanced dramatically with improvement in surgical techniques. Mortality is now less than 10% as is morbidity, including postoperative cholangitis and stricture at the anastomosis site. Patients who have surgery for choledochal cysts before age 6 months usually carry a poor prognosis since the cysts usually occur in association with

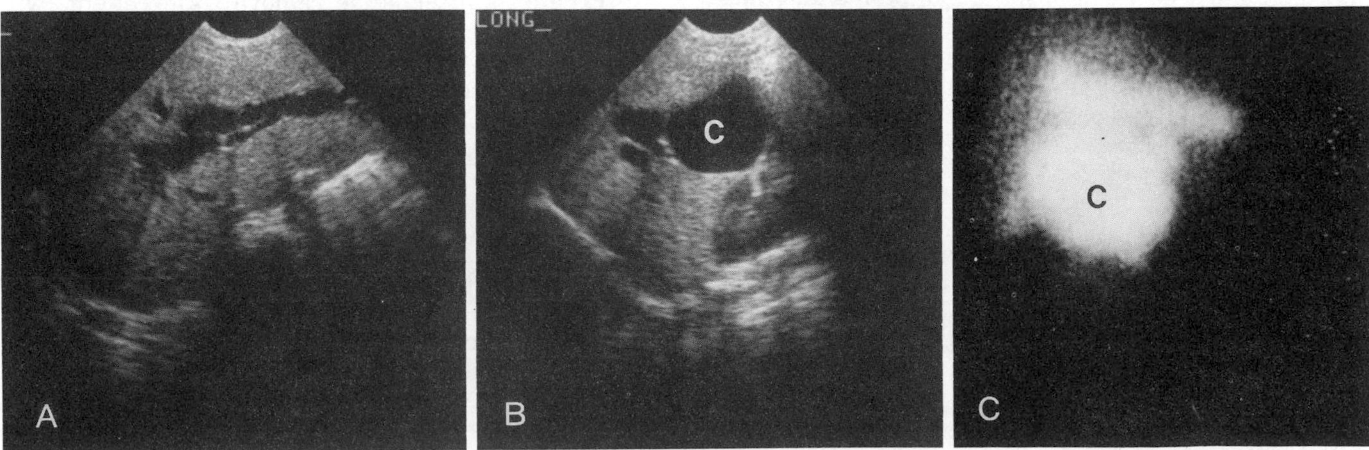

Figure 7.14. This child was admitted with signs of right upper abdominal pain and jaundice. The transverse ultrasonogram **(A)** shows dilated intrahepatic ducts. Longitudinal scan **(B)** demonstrates choledochal cyst connecting with the ducts. Radionuclide scan **(C)** confirms the diagnosis. *C* = choledochal cyst. Radionuclide scan courtesy of S. Treves, M.D., The Children's Hospital, Boston.

other congenital anomalies of the biliary system including biliary atresia. In young children or infants, they are also usually associated with biliary cirrhosis and portal hypertension and death can result from complications of chronic liver failure.

REFERENCES

Adye B, Ryan JA: Cholecystitis in teenage girls. *West J Med* 139:471, 1983.

Allen MJ, Thistle JL: Management of biliary duct stones. *Drug Ther* p. 17, July 1983.

Barlow B, Tabor E, Blanc W, et al: The choledochal cyst: A review of 19 cases. *J Pediatr* 89:934, 1976.

Crittenden SL, McKinley MJ: Choledochal cyst—clinical features and classification. *Am J Gastroenterol* 80:643, 1985.

Descos B, Bernard O, Brunell F, et al: Pigment gallstones of the common bile ducts in infants. *Hepatology* 4:678, 1984.

Gaskin KJ, Waters DLM, Howman-Giles R, et al: Liver disease and common bile duct stenosis in cystic fibrosis. *N Engl J Med* 318:340, 1988.

Holcomb GW, O'Neill JA: Cholelithiasis in common duct stenosis in children and adolescents. *Ann Surg* 191:626, 1980.

Kamari S, Lee WJ, Baron MG: Hydrops of the gallbladder in a child—diagnosis by ultrasonography. *Pediatrics* 63:295, 1979.

Krensky AM, Teele R, Watkins J, et al: Streptococcal antigenicity in mucocutaneous lymph node syndrome in hydropic gallbladders. *Pediatrics* 64:979, 1979.

Magilavy DB, Speert DP, Silver TM, et al: Mucocutaneous lymph node syndrome: Report of two cases complicated by gallbladder hydrops diagnosed by ultrasound. *Pediatrics* 61:699, 1978.

Powell CS,Sawyers JL, Reynolds VH: Management of adult choledochal cyst. *Ann Surg* 193:666, 1981.

Silverman A, Roy CC: *Pediatric Clinical Gastroenterology*. St. Louis, CV Mosby, 1983, p. 799.

Slovas TL, Hight DW, Philippart AI, et al: Synography in a diagnosis and management of hydrops of the gallbladder in children with mucocutaneous lymph node syndrome. *Pediatrics* 65:789, 1980.

Takiff H, Fonkalsrud EW: Gallbladder disease in childhood. *Am J Dis Child* 138:565, 1984.

LEWIS R. FIRST

Consultant
John Snyder

Section 8

Hematology

Introduction to Hematopoiesis

1

Definition

Hematopoiesis is the process whereby a pluripotent progenitor cell matures into a functional blood cell line. Medullary hematopoiesis refers to blood cell production via the bone marrow, whereas extramedullary hematopoiesis refers to this process in tissues other than the bone marrow. Hematopoiesis can be further classified as erythropoiesis, granulopoiesis (or myelopoiesis), and thrombopoiesis. Hematopoietic cells mature in the marrow outside sinusoidal beds which they then enter in order to be released into blood.

There are various ways to examine progenitor cells: morphologically, kinetically, or operationally as a colony-forming unit (CFU). Morphologically, progenitor cells appear to be small mononuclear cells similar to lymphoblasts, but fewer in number. Kinetically, a pool of progenitor cells can be viewed as being self-renewing, "stem" cells, able to give rise when necessary to further differentiated cells.

The operational definition of progenitor cell as a CFU was a result of in vitro assays of these cells. It became clear that in order for the stem cells to replicate and express their commitment to a cell line or lines they also required the addition of stimulating or growth factors. Moreover, the growth factors apparently could be equally restrictive in their biologic activities and target cells; some causing differentiation of all myeloid as well as macrophage, erythroid, and megakaryocytic progenitor cells, whereas others were more restricted, stimulating proliferation and development in only granulocytes, macrophage or eosinophil colony-forming cells (Metcalf, 1986).

Under the influence of the conducive hematopoietic microenvironment of the marrow, pluripotent stem cells can be irreversibly transformed to unipotent committed progenitors of erythropoiesis or granulopoiesis. Once committed, a humoral poietin, such as erythropoietin, can serve as the specific stimulus for a

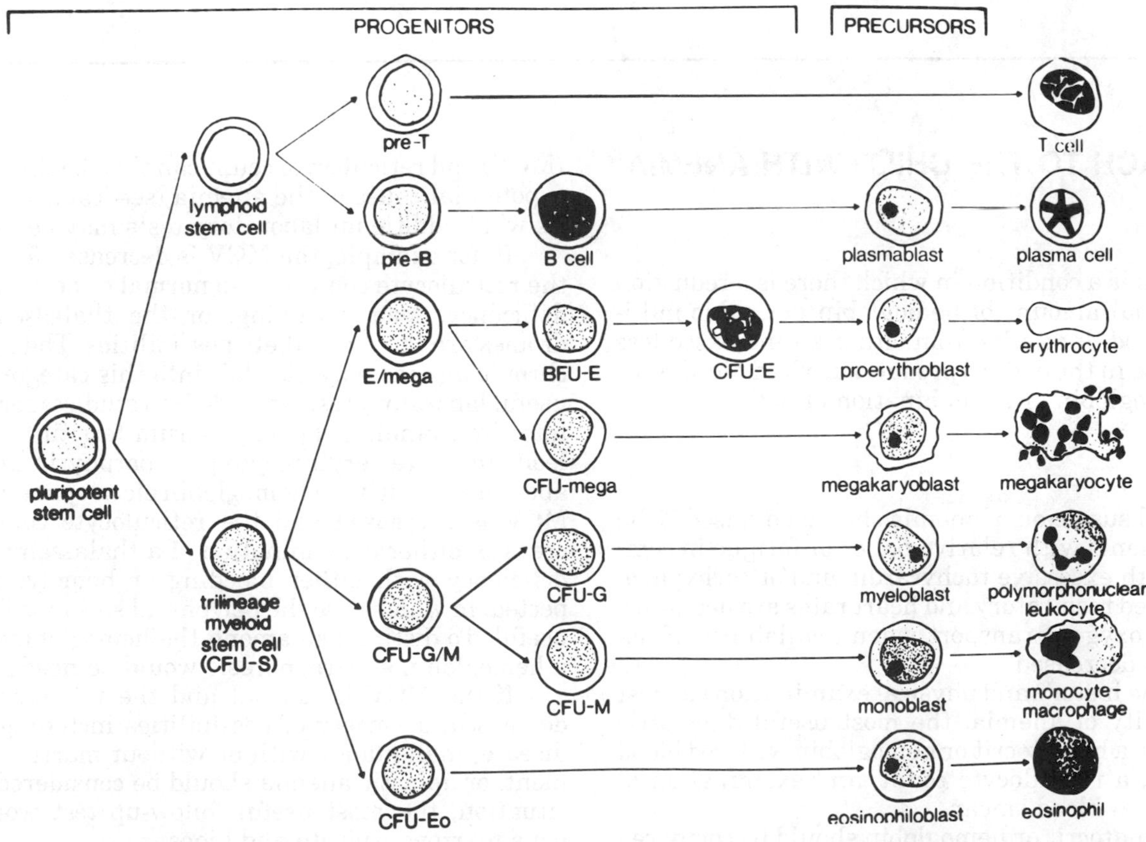

Figure 8.1. Schematic diagram of hematopoiesis. Reproduced with permission from Nathan DG, Oski FA: *Hematology of Infancy and Childhood.* Philadelphia, WB Saunders, 1987.

unipotent progenitor cell to become further committed to erythropoiesis.

A model of the cellular proliferation and differentiation that makes up hematopoiesis is shown in Figure 8.1, which shows how pluripotent hematopoietic stem cells begin the chain and give rise to lymphoid as well as myeloid elements and, subsequently, all the differentiated blood cells that enter the circulation. Cells that are more restricted in their potential to differentiate are referred to as committed progenitors and include the erythroid burst-forming units (BFU-E), the megakaryocyte site colony-forming units (CFU-MEG), the granulocyte-macrophage CFUs (CFU-G/M), and the eosinophilic CFUs (CFU-EOS). The erythroid burst-forming units differentiate to more mature erythroid CFUs known as CFU-Es. These give rise to pronormoblast and eventually to mature erythrocytes. Similarly, granulocyte-macrophage CFUs differentiate into colony-forming granulocyte and colony-forming macrophage unit cells, the progenitors of granulocytes and macrophages, respectively. This model serves as the backbone for the hematologic abnormalities discussed in the chapter that follows.

REFERENCES

Lipton JM, Nathan DG: The anatomy and physiology of hematopoiesis. In Nathan DG, Oski FA (eds): *Hematology of Infancy and Childhood*. Philadelphia, WB Saunders, 1987, p. 128.

Metcalf D: The molecular biology and functions of the granulocyte-macrophage colony-stimulating factors. *Blood* 67:257, 1986.

Quesenberry T, Levitt L: Hematopoietic stem cells. *N Engl J Med* 301:755, 819, 868, 1979.

Red Cell Disorders 2

APPROACH TO THE CHILD WITH ANEMIA

Definition

Anemia is a condition in which there is a reduction in the normal amount of hemoglobin per cubic millimeter of blood. It results from either an increased loss or a decrease in the overall production of red blood cells, and/or hemoglobin or a combination of both.

Diagnosis

Clinical suspicion of anemia should be raised if the patient presents with relative pallor or fatigue in combination with excessive tachycardia and/or tachypnea. The increased respiratory and heart rates are necessary to improve oxygen transport when availability of hemoglobin is decreased.

Once the history and physical examination suggest the possibility of anemia, the most useful diagnostic tests include a hematocrit or hemoglobin with red blood cell indices, a reticulocyte count, and examination of the peripheral blood smear.

The hematocrit or hemoglobin should be compared with a set of standards appropriate for age, as demonstrated in Table 8.1. The mean corpuscular volume (MCV) and reticulocyte count can then begin to suggest a potential cause of the anemia (see Table 8.2) as well as what additional laboratory tests may be needed.

If, for example, the MCV is decreased for age, and the reticulocyte count is also normal or decreased, iron deficiency, lead poisoning, or the thalassemia syndromes are the most likely possibilities. The anemia of chronic disease may also fall into this category. Other useful laboratory tests include iron studies (serum iron, total iron binding capacity, serum ferritin), a venous lead, and a free erythrocyte protoporphyrin and, if the above are negative, a hemoglobin electrophoresis. If the MCV is decreased and the reticulocyte count is increased, either a combination of a thalassemia or iron deficiency with either bleeding or hemolysis is suspected, in which case the peripheral smear will be most useful. To distinguish among the hemoglobinopathies, a hemoglobin electrophoresis would be needed.

If the MCV is normal and the reticulocytes are decreased, a variety of possibilities including chronic disease, malignancy with or without marrow involvement, or aplastic anemia should be considered. In this situation, the most useful follow-up test would be a bone marrow aspirate and biopsy.

A normal MCV with increased reticulocytes, however, suggests acute blood loss as the cause for the

Table 8.1
Average Normal Blood Values in Infancy and Childhood[1]

Age	Hemoglobin (g/dl)	RBC ($\times 10^{12}$/L)	Hematocrit (%)	MCV (fl)	MCH (pg)	MCHC (%)	Reticulocytes (%)
Cord Blood	16.8	5.25	63	120	34	31.7	3.2
1 day	19.0	5.14	61	119	36.9	31.6	3.2
3 days	18.7	5.11	62	116	36.5	31.1	3.8
7 days	17.9	4.86	56	118	36.2	32.0	0.5
2 weeks	17.3	4.80	54	112	36.8	32.1	0.5
3 weeks	15.6	4.20	46	111	37.1	33.9	0.8
4 weeks	14.2	4.00	43	105	35.5	33.5	0.6
2 months	10.7	3.40	31	93	31.5	34.1	1.8
3 months	11.3	3.70	33	88	30.5	34.8	0.7
6 months	12.3	4.60	36	78	27	34	1.4
8 months	12.1	4.6	36	77	26	34	1.1
10 months	11.9	4.6	36	77	26	34	1.0
1 year	11.6	4.6	35	77	25	33	0.9
2 years	11.7	4.7	35	78	25	33	1.0
4 years	12.6	4.7	37	80	27	34	1.0
6 years	12.7	4.7	38	80	27	33	1.0
8 years	12.9	4.7	39	80	27	33	1.0
10–12 years	13.0	4.8	39	80	27	33	1.0
Adult men	16.0	5.4	47	87	29	34	1.0
Adult women	14.0	4.8	42	87	29	34	1.0

[1]Based on standard sources and observations made at The New York Hospital–Cornell Medical Center. Reprinted with permission from Miller DR, Baehner R, McMillan C: In *Blood Diseases of Infancy & Childhood*, 5th edition. St. Louis, CV Mosby, 1984, p. 28.

anemia. Subsequent work-up should focus on possible causes for bleeding, including a menstrual history in adolescent females. Stool and urine in combination with the serum creatinine and BUN should also be examined to rule out hemolytic uremic syndrome.

Elevated MCV and decreased reticulocytes suggests either folate or vitamin B_{12} deficiency and a megaloblastic anemia, or chronic aplastic or hypoplastic anemia. Follow-up studies would include (in addition to an adequate nutritional history) a bone marrow biopsy and serum folate and B_{12} levels.

If the reticulocytes are increased in the setting of an elevated or normal MCV, hemolysis is likely. In this situation, a Coombs test can be useful to determine whether an isoimmune or autoimmune process is occurring.

A useful way to approach hemolytic anemias is to consider the red cell as being susceptible to hemolysis at any location from the outside of the cell to the inside (as shown in Table 8.3). From an external or environmental standpoint, trauma or burns can injure and cause hemolysis of red cells. Macroangiopathic injury from heart valves or hemangiomas, or microangiopathic changes within blood vessels, such as those associated with disseminated intravascular coagulation, also can lead to hemolysis. The peripheral smear in such situ-

Table 8.2
Diagnosing an Anemia

Mean Corpuscular Volume Decreased		Mean Corpuscular Volume Normal or Increased	
Reticulocytes Decreased or Normal	Reticulocytes Increased	Reticulocytes Decreased or Normal	Reticulocytes Increased
1. Iron deficiency	1. Combined iron deficiency with a. hemolysis, or b. bleeding	1. Chronic disease	1. Hemolysis
2. Thalassemia syndromes	2. Combined thalassemia trait with a. hemolysis, or b. bleeding	2. Malignancy	2. Active blood loss
3. Lead		3. Aplastic anemia	
4. Chronic disease		4. Folate or B_{12} deficiency	

Table 8.3
Approach to Hemolytic Anemia (a View from Outside to Inside the Red Cell)

External
Trauma
Burns
Vessels
Macroangiopathy
Hemangiomas
Heart valves
Microangiopathy
Disseminated intravascular coagulopathies
Organs
Hypersplenism
Plasma
Drugs
Infections
Antibodies
Toxins
Membranes
Hereditary spherocytosis
Hereditary elliptocytosis
Stomatocytosis
Paroxysmal nocturnal hemoglobinuria
Cytoplasm
Enzyme abnormalities (G6PD, pyruvate kinase deficiencies)
Hemoglobinopathies
Thalassemia
Hgb S,C,E
Unstable hemoglobins

ations would display helmets and fragmented red cells 50% of the time, and screening tests for disseminated intravascular coagulation (i.e., platelet count, serum fibrinogen and fibrin split products) might be useful to confirm the reason for the microangiopathic change. The spleen can capture red cells and prevent their release if hypersplenism occurs. In the plasma, hemolysis can occur on an immune basis secondary to drugs, various infectious organisms, or in the presence of autoantibodies. Hemolysis at the level of the cell membrane occurs in diseases such as spherocytosis, elliptocytosis, stomatocytosis, and paroxysmal nocturnal hemoglobinuria. Again the peripheral smear is most useful in making this diagnosis together with the Hamm test for paroxysmal nocturnal hemoglobinuria (see specific sections). Hemolysis at the level of the cell cytoplasm occurs with the enzyme disorders, including glucose-6-phosphate dehydrogenase deficiency and pyruvate kinase deficiency. Specific enzyme assays are available to test for these deficiencies. Finally, at the level of the hemoglobin itself hemolysis due to hemoglobinopathies may occur, the most common being sickle cell disease. Tests for these hemoglobinopathies are discussed in the appropriate section.

Treatment

Treatment depends on the cause underlying a specific anemia and is described under the appropriate disorders.

APLASTIC ANEMIAS

Definition

Aplastic anemias are a group of disorders characterized by peripheral blood pancytopenia, secondary to decreased bone marrow function with inadequate production of erythrocytes, granulocytes, and platelets. They can be constitutional in origin, but more often are acquired disorders secondary to exposure to drugs, chemicals, toxins, radiation, or infections; however, most often, there is no obvious cause. In addition, aplastic anemia has been associated with pregnancy and thymomas (Gale et al, 1981).

Basic Science

Four mechanisms are currently being studied as potential etiologies for bone marrow failure: (a) defective or absent stem cells; (b) abnormal hormonal or cellular control of stem cell proliferation; (c) abnormalities in the marrow micro-environment; and (d) immune suppression of the hematopoiesis (Camitta et al, 1982).

Evidence for the defect or absence of stem cells in humans has been provided by the success of bone marrow transplantation in producing normal hematopoiesis after transplantation of sufficient numbers of normal donor hematopoietic cells. Although there is less evidence to date for abnormal hematopoietic regulation by hormonal or cellular interaction causing poor stem cell proliferation, it has been confirmed that T-lymphocytes have promoted the growth of human erythroid stem cells. On the other hand, levels of erythropoietin and hormones that stimulate granulopoiesis are usually normal or even elevated in most patients with aplastic anemia.

Microenvironmental defects may play a role in aplastic anemia but may not be solely responsible for the lack of hematopoiesis since bone marrow transplantation patients are able to show hematopoiesis when donor marrow is transferred into recipient marrow that has been lethally irradiated. Evidence for immune suppression derives from the demonstration of antibodies cytotoxic to erythroid precursors in pure red cell aplasia, T-cell subsets that specifically suppress hematopoietic progenitor cell differentiation, autologous marrow recovery following immunosuppression despite an unsuccessful bone marrow transplantation, and failure of bone marrow transplantation to cure aplastic anemia in some identical twins who are HLA-compatible. It is still not clear, however, whether humoral or cell-mediated mechanisms are involved in depression of marrow growth in humans.

Understanding the mechanism responsible for an individual patient's aplasia will permit the most appropriate treatment. The precise mechanism by which drugs damage bone marrow and cause aplastic anemia, however, remains unknown. It is possible that some drugs are directly toxic to hematopoietic stem cells, whereas others exert their damage via immune mediated mechanisms. A list of agents most commonly associated with aplasia is given in Table 8.4.

CASE ILLUSTRATION

A 2-year-old girl was referred to our hospital for evaluation of a heart murmur. During the month before admission she had been increasingly irritable and less active, which her parents initially had attributed to "emotional upheaval" stemming from their move from California to Boston. Even after the family had settled down, the child's poor appetite, lethargy, and reluctance to walk persisted. She also developed low grade fevers over this period. She was seen by her pediatrician who noted a 3/6 systolic ejection murmur of the left sternal border and referred her to our hospital for further evaluation.

On physical examination, her temperature was 38.3° C, her weight was 10.4 kg. The physical examination was unremarkable except for the presence of the murmur as described. A chest radiograph and ECG were normal. The urinalysis was entirely unremarkable. CBC was notable for hematocrit of 27%, a white blood count of 8300, with 41% polys and 2% bands, 5% monos, 2% eos, an MCV of 80 and platelets of 200,000/mm^3. The reticulocyte count was 2.5%. Clotting studies were normal, stool guaiac was negative. Electrolytes, BUN, creatinine and liver function tests were within normal limits. A "monospot" was performed for evidence of mononucleosis and was negative. Her sedimentation rate was 65 mm/hr. Her smear was remarkable for the absence of toxic granulation or blasts, but did have "tear drop" red blood cells. Blood and urine cultures were negative and a PPD was unremarkable.

QUESTION AND COMMENT

What is the differential diagnosis for this 2-year-old girl who presents with fever, a heart murmur, mild normocytic anemia, an elevated sedimentation rate, and what further work-up is required?

If the anemia is considered as a clue in the setting of a normal MCV and low-normal reticulocyte count, the differential diagnosis includes the more chronic infectious diseases (subacute bacterial endocarditis, an occult bacterial infection or abscess, tuberculosis, persistent viral, fungal, or parasitic infection), other chronic illnesses such as a collagen vascular disease, inflammatory bowel disease, and/or malignancy. Such a differential would permit pursuit of a variety of options from in-hospital observation to bone and gallium scans, barium studies, ultrasonography, CT scans, and even biopsies.

Based on the patient's history, physical examination, and routine screening tests, an echocardiogram was performed that showed no structural abnormalities or heart valve vegetations, thus eliminating endocarditis as a possibility. The presence of the tear drops on the smear, however, was suggestive, albeit nonspecifically, of an infiltrative process in the bone marrow and a bone marrow biopsy was obtained. The biopsy showed clumps of cells with large pale blue cytoplasm consistent with metastatic infiltration, most likely secondary to either a neuroblastoma or a Wilms tumor. Subsequently, abdominal ultrasonography revealed a large prevertebral retroperitoneal mass encompassing the inferior vena cava and the aorta, which was highly consistent with and subsequently biopsy-proven to be a stage 4 neuroblastoma. The child subsequently underwent chemotherapy, which provided palliation, but she eventually died of her malignancy.

Chloramphenicol is one of the best categorized of the drugs that can produce either a dose-dependent or a dose-independent bone marrow toxicity. The dose-dependent aplasia appears to be mediated by inhibition of mitochondrial protein synthesis and iron incorporation into red blood cells. The dose-independent reaction is believed to reflect genetic predisposition to inhibition of DNA synthesis in stem cells.

Viruses have also been associated with aplastic anemia including Epstein-Barr virus, rubella, herpes, cytomegalovirus, and hepatitis (usually non-A, non-B, although hepatitis A and hepatitis B have also been involved in individual cases). It can be difficult to determine whether infection is the primary cause for an aplastic anemia, whether infection is secondary to aplasia-associated cytopenias, or whether the aplasia results from the use of antibiotics.

Table 8.4
Agents Commonly Associated with Aplasia

Benzene derivatives
Chemotherapeutic agents
Sulfur or nitrogen, mustard agents (e.g., busulfan, cyclophosphamide)
Antimetabolites (e.g., G-mercaptopurine, cytosine arabinoside)
Antimitotic agents (e.g., colchicine)
Some antimicrobial agents (e.g., chloramphenicol, quinacrine)
Gold compounds
Analgesics (phenylbutazone)

The congenital aplastic anemias include Fanconi anemia, Shwachman-Diamond syndrome, and dyskeratosis congenita, all of which typically occur in children under 10 years of age, with a male predominance. The mechanism of aplasia in these congenital disorders is unknown but, in the case of Fanconi anemia, is probably related to a defect in DNA repair (Alter, 1979).

Eventually, better insight into the pathophysiology of aplastic anemia will enable identification of patients who will recover spontaneously, those who need immunosuppressive therapy, or those who require bone marrow transplantation.

Epidemiology

The incidence of aplastic anemia varies widely depending on whether it is genetic or acquired, the age of the patient, and where the disease is occurring. For example, it is 2–5 times more frequent in the Far East than it is in North America or Europe. An increased incidence of consanguinity in patients with marrow aplasia is observed and it has been reported in twins. Twenty-five percent of patients are under 20 years of age and over one-third are over 60 years (Camitta, 1982).

The acquired aplastic anemias are estimated to occur in the pediatric population at roughly 1 case per million children per year, with a male-female ratio that is roughly 1:1 (Alter, 1979).

Aplastic anemia on a genetic basis occurs at a frequency one-third that of the acquired disorder. The most common form is Fanconi anemia, with more than 200 cases reported to date. Fanconi anemia is an autosomal recessive disease with a frequency of heterozygosity estimated to be 1/600. The male-female ratio is about 1.4:1.

Natural History

Patients whose aplastic anemia is acquired are characterized as having moderate to severe disease. Severe disease is characterized by at least two of the following: white blood cell counts less than 500/mm^3, platelet counts less than 20,000/mm^3, reticulocyte count less than 1% (after correction for hematocrit), and a hypocellular bone marrow. Patients who fail to meet these criteria are characterized as having mild or moderate disease, otherwise known as hypoplastic anemia.

The clinical presentation of a patient with acquired aplastic anemia will depend on the severity of the disorder. A decrease in platelets will lead to bleeding abnormalities, including petechiae, ecchymoses, and epistaxis. Neutropenia will often result in fever and bacterial infections (especially skin), whereas the anemia will present as pallor, fatigue, tachycardia, or heart failure.

Fanconi anemia is often associated at birth with congenital anomalies which are noted long before the hematologic problems begin (usually between ages 5 and 10 years). These patients may have melanin-like hyperpigmentation and café-au-lait spots. Thumbs may be absent, hypoplastic, or supernumerary with or without radial aplasia. If radial aplasia is present, however, thumbs are always hypoplastic or aplastic (Minagi and Steinbach, 1966). In addition, microcephaly, renal malformations, strabismus, hypogenitalism, mental retardation, and deafness have been associated with Fanconi anemia. Occasionally no anomalies are noted, but most patients will have at least one (Alter and Potter, 1983).

Another congenital form of aplastic anemia is dyskeratosis congenita. This is a rare ectodermal dysplasia and consists of hyperpigmentation of the face and neck, dystrophic nails, and mucous membrane leukoplakia. In addition, blocked lacrimal ducts, sparse hair, esophageal strictures, and hyperhydrotic palms may be present. Of the more than 50 cases that have been described, over one-half developed pancytopenia, usually in the second or third decades of life. Most cases are X-linked with a male-female ratio of 10:1. Anemia is the first sign of pancytopenia with this disorder. Malignancies are also frequent, especially squamous cell carcinomas, and are often the cause of death.

A third form of congenital form of aplasia is Shwachman-Diamond syndrome, which consists of exocrine pancreatic insufficiency and bone marrow failure. Most patients demonstrate neutropenia, usually in infancy, with pancytopenia developing later, during early childhood. More than 60 cases have been reported, with an autosomal recessive inheritance pattern, and a male-female ratio of 1:1. These patients often present with short stature and malabsorption. Metaphyseal dysostosis may be seen radiographically in one-third of the cases.

Another condition is pure red cell aplasia, which leads solely to anemia and reticulocytopenia. This condition can be seen with hemolytic disorders such as hereditary spherocytosis, sickle cell disease, or other hemolytic anemias, when it is referred to as an aplastic crisis. If the pure red cell aplasia is congenital, it is called Diamond-Blackfan anemia, with more than 200 cases described to date. In more than 90% of these patients, anemia is noted within the first year of life. The male-female ratio is 1:1. Ten percent of cases have been familial with both autosomal dominant and recessive inheritance patterns reported. Low birth weight may be a finding in these patients, and over one-third have some kind of physical abnormality, including short stature, web neck, or strabismus. Ten percent show abnormal thumbs, including duplications, triphalangeal, or other malformed digits. Bone marrow cellularity is normal, although erythroid hypoplasia is commonly seen. Serum erythropoietin levels are increased and it is believed from studies in vitro that there is a deficiency in the number of erythroid stem cells (Lipton et al, 1986).

A much more benign, self-limited red cell aplasia occurs under the designation transient erythroblastopenia of childhood. Children with this disorder experience anemia and reticulocytopenia on a transient basis, usually several weeks to months following a viral illness, when they present with pallor. Transient erythroblastopenia of childhood may be differentiated from congenital hypoplastic anemia as described below.

Diagnosis

Clinical onset of aplastic anemia is usually insidious. Initial findings may be nonspecific and dependent upon which of the three cell lines is most predominantly affected. Symptoms and signs can include: pallor, weakness, bleeding, purpura, fevers, and infections. A careful environmental history of any possible exposures to agents that have been associated with aplastic anemias can be useful. Physical examination is usually nonspecific, but is helpful in highlighting other diseases that can be confused in the differential diagnosis. For example, hepatomegaly, splenomegaly, or lymphadenopathy, are rare with this disorder, whereas they are more typical of other diseases, and in particular, malignancies.

A CBC with reticulocyte count and peripheral blood smear are mandatory in the diagnostic work-up. A high reticulocyte count would be more consistent with a hemolytic anemia, although marrow aplasia has been associated with paroxysmal nocturnal hemoglobinuria. The peripheral blood in acquired aplastic anemia will show normocytic or mildly macrocytic red cells. The fetal hemoglobin level also may be useful since it may be elevated during marrow failure, although the level of fetal hemoglobin does not serve as a prognostic factor. Platelets on the smear will be normal or small, unlike the large platelets commonly seen in idiopathic thrombocytopenic purpura.

The definitive diagnosis is obtained via bone marrow aspiration and biopsy. The aspirate can be more helpful for identification of individual cell types, whereas the biopsy is useful for evaluation of marrow cellularity and marrow architecture. Almost one-half of the biopsy specimens of patients with aplastic anemia show fibrinous exudates, plasma cell and lymphoid infiltrates, osteoporosis, and reticulin formation (Alter, 1978). Examination of the marrow helps to eliminate other possibilities for pancytopenia, including leukemia or tumor. In the acquired aplastic anemias, increased plasma iron, saturated transferrin, prolonged iron clearance with decreased turnover and utilization may be found, consistent with erythrocyte hypoproliferation. B_{12} and folate levels are usually normal or increased. Peripheral blood and bone marrow chromosome studies in the aquired aplasias are normal. Increased breaks and gaps, however, have been found to occur in marrow chromosomes in patients with Fanconi anemia. Radiologic examinations also are useful to search for some of the skeletal anomalies consistent with the Fanconi anemia.

The peripheral blood of a patient with Fanconi anemia shows anisocytosis and poikilocytosis in addition to the granulo-, thrombo-, and reticulocytopenia. The bone marrow specimens are similar to those seen in the acquired aplastic anemias. In patients with Shwachman-Diamond syndrome, bone marrow may be hypocellular or hypercellular and a maturation arrest in the neutrophil series is notable.

Patients with Diamond-Blackfan syndrome show increased levels of fetal hemoglobin even as adults. Bone marrow cellularity is usually normal in these patients, although severe erythroid hypoplasia can occur with the only detectable erythroid precursor being the proerythroblast.

In distinguishing Diamond-Blackfan syndrome from transient erythroblastopenia of childhood, it should be remembered that 90% of patients with Diamond-Blackfan syndrome are diagnosed before 1 year of age, whereas most children will have transient erythroblastopenia of childhood between the ages of 1 and 4 years. On physical examination, patients with Diamond-Blackfan syndrome may be small for age and have congenital anomalies, including abnormal thumbs, big head, hypertelorism, and micrognathia. Physical examination in patients with transient erythroblastopenia of childhood is normal. In the latter disorder, the MCV will only be increased during the recovery phase of the disease, whereas it is increased usually at diagnosis, during recovery, and during remission in patients with Diamond-Blackfan syndrome. In addition, it is only during recovery that hemoglobin F will be increased in children with transient erythroblastopenia, whereas it is almost always elevated in those with Diamond-Blackfan syndrome. Adenosine-deaminase activity is elevated in Diamond-Blackfan syndrome, but is not elevated in patients with transient erythroblastopenia of childhood (Oski, 1982).

Table 8.5 highlights some other differences and similarities of childhood bone marrow failure syndromes.

Treatment

If the aplastic anemia is known to be acquired, the first therapeutic measure should be removal of the agent suspected of causing the aplasia. Certain supportive measures should be instituted regardless of the etiology for the aplasia. For example, because of aspirin's association with platelet dysfunction, children needing fever control should be treated with acetaminophen. Moreover, because of the danger of persistent bleeding during menses, androgens or contraceptive agents may be needed.

When a patient is newly diagnosed as having aplastic anemia, histocompatibility studies should be performed immediately on the patient and siblings to determine whether the patient is a candidate for bone marrow transplantation. Before determining histocompatibility, transfusion support therapy should be given only in life-threatening situations. Furthermore, if needed, transfusions should be from unrelated donors rather than family members who may sensitize the patient against non-HLA-antigens that may be present in the donor's marrow but missing in the patient's. Red cells are usually given as frozen washed packed cells to minimize sensitization to white cells and platelets. Granulocyte transfusions should be used cautiously, because these transfusions can also increase the risk of sensitization not only to granulocytes but to platelets as well. They are certainly indicated in the setting of proven bacterial sepsis-unresponsive to antibiotics alone. If the platelet count can be kept above 10,000 and there is no evidence of ongoing bleeding, platelet transfusions should be withheld. Single donor transfusions will delay the development of sensitization to platelet antigens.

If patients fail to respond to transfusions of random single donor platelets, attempts can be made to transfuse the platelets from HLA-matched donors. Nevertheless, sensitization to non HLA-matched antigens again may occur and hamper a successful bone marrow transplantation.

Supportive therapy also includes the prevention and treatment of all infections in patients with aplastic anemia. Prophylactic antibiotics, reverse isolation, or total decontamination in laminar flow environments have all been utilized as prevention modalities (although none of these has been found to be more effective than the others). If fever should occur in these patients, broad spectrum antibiotics should be instituted immediately, with modification when results of bacteriologic, viral, and fungal cultures become available.

Table 8.5
Comparison of Childhood Bone Marrow Failure Syndromes

	Acquired	Fanconi	Dyskeratosis Congenita	Shwachman-Diamond	Diamond-Blackfan	Transient Erythroblastopenia of Childhood
M:F ratio	1	1.4	10	1	1	1.3
Genetics		Autosomal recessive	X-linked	Autosomal recessive	Autosomal recessive	
Age of onset of hemolytic disease (years)	All	5–10	10–20	Infancy	Infancy	1–4
Skin		Hyperpigmented	Reticular			
Stature		Short	Delicate	Short	Short	
Skeletal	1	Abnormal or absent thumb/radius		Metaphyseal dysostosis	Abnormal thumbs	
Other anomalies		Renal Strabismus Deafness Retardation	Nail dystrophy Leukoplakia Retardation Lacrimal-duct stenosis		Microcephaly Hypertelorism Micrognathia	
Birth weight	Normal	Low	Normal	Normal	Low	Normal
Bone marrow	Pancytopenia	Pancytopenia	Pancytopenia	Pancytopenia or maturation arrest	Decreased erythroblasts	Decreased erythroblasts
Peripheral blood	Pancytopenia	Pancytopenia and macrocytosis	Pancytopenia and macrocytosis	Neutropenia or pancytopenia	Anemia, macrocytosis	Anemia
Fetal hemoglobin	Normal	Increased	Increased	Increased	Increased	Normal
Chromosomes	Normal	Breaks	Normal	Normal	Normal	Normal
Prognosis	Poor	Poor	Poor	Fair	Fair–good	Excellent

A number of therapeutic measures have been tried in attempts to stimulate hematopoiesis, including the use of androgens, etiocholanolone, glucocorticoids, lithium, antilymphocyte globulin, and cyclophosphamide. While androgens have been found to enhance red cell production in many animal studies in vitro and in vivo, the success rate in humans has been variable. Some studies suggest that mild to moderate aplasia may be more responsive to the effects of androgens than is severe aplasia. A few patients with severe disease, however, definitely respond. Nonetheless, there is no controlled study demonstrating that androgens alter the long-term course in patients with mild aplastic anemia, nor has any androgen been found to be consistently effective or consistently superior to other androgens in patients with severe aplastic anemia. If androgen therapy is utilized, patients should be monitored for the possibility of hepatic toxicity and development of hepatic tumors. Virilization and fluid retention are also common complications (Camitta, 1982).

The usual oral androgen is oxymetholone given as 2–5 mg/kg/day until a response is achieved or for a maximum of 4–6 months. It is of interest that Fanconi anemia is the one disease in which androgen treatment has been found to be beneficial, with most patients responding initially. Unfortunately, however, these patients eventually become resistant to androgens or subsequently develop secondary malignancies following treatment with these agents.

Only a few studies report responses to glucocorticoids (Yoshida et al, 1986; Ozsoylo et al, 1984). In addition, glucocorticoids may predispose patients to infection, thus shortening their life span.

Lithium has been found to induce granulocytosis in normal patients, but unfortunately does not have a similar effect in patients with severe aplasia. If the pancytopenia is antibody-mediated, sporadic reports on single cases have suggested that plasmapheresis may be useful, but definitive evidence is lacking.

Various immunosuppressive treatment modalities have been tried in patients with aplastic anemia, particularly the use of antilymphocyte globulin or antithymocyte globulin. The results remain controversial, with some investigators failing to observe the beneficial effects reported by others. In addition, antilymphocyte globulin has many adverse effects, including fever, chills, rash, and serum sickness, as well as severe thrombocytopenia or anaphylaxis. Moreover, the efficacy of this agent is often unclear because patients are receiving other treatment concurrently or are undergoing bone marrow transplants at the same time. A randomized controlled trial is also needed to determine

CASE ILLUSTRATION

A 4-month-old male was seen by his pediatrician for evaluation of coryza and conjunctivitis of 4 days' duration. On examination, the child also appeared pale. A CBC was notable for hematocrit of 12%, prompting referral to our hospital for further evaluation. Physical examination was otherwise unremarkable except for the pallor. Review of the blood smear was notable for normochromic-normocytic red blood cells, with no evidence of hemolysis or bizarre cells. The MCV was 78, reticulocyte count was 0.1%. There was an adequate white blood cell count of 15,000/mm^3, with 40% polys, 47% lymphs, 2% atypical lymphs, and abundant platelets of 475,000/mm^3. The child did not appear dysmorphic or growth-retarded; he had no rash, stools were heme-negative, and urine was normal. His abdomen was benign, without masses or hepatosplenomegaly. He had a low-grade temperature of 100°F, but vital signs were otherwise normal. His past medical and family history was noncontributory. He had not been on any medication.

QUESTION AND COMMENT

What is the differential diagnosis of this child's anemia? How should he be treated?

The normocytic anemia with low reticulocyte count but an otherwise normal white blood cell and platelet line, classified this patient's disease process as being a pure erythrocyte aplasia. This was supported by absence of blood loss, hemolysis, splenic sequestration, underlying renal disease, rheumatic disease, or hyperthyroidism, all of which would usually provide a normal MCV, although with the blood loss and hemolysis, a higher reticulocyte count might have been expected. Lack of an elevated MCV discouraged the diagnosis of ineffective erythropoiesis due to impaired DNA synthesis, such as is found in B_{12} or folate deficiency. The MCV not being exceedingly low weighed against chronic states of diminished hemoglobin in red blood cells, such as in iron deficiency, lead intoxication, thalassemia, or chronic blood loss. Since the other cell lines remained intact, an infiltrative process such as leukemia or a storage disease also was less likely.

The most likely diagnosis appeared to be transient erythroblastopenia of childhood (TEC). This temporary benign cessation of red blood cell production usually occurs in association with a viral infection, typically 2–3 months before diagnosis, is fairly common in children ages 1 month to 6 years, and is self-limited—hence the term "transient" to distinguish it from the rare congenital type of red blood cell aplasia known as Diamond-Blackfan syndrome.

Certain characteristics help to distinguish TEC from Diamond-Blackfan syndrome. TEC has a much greater prevalence in infancy such that the number of children less than 1 year of age with TEC will still be substantially greater than those who present with Diamond-Blackfan syndrome. At least one-half of the patients with Diamond-Blackfan syndrome are small for age and at least one-third of them have congenital anomalies, including small head, micrognathia, hypertelorism, epicanthal folds, or abnormal thumbs. The TEC patients usually do not have congenital anomalies, as was the case with this child. While 70% of Diamond-Blackfan children will have a transiently normal MCV at the time of diagnosis, the typical pattern is one of a life-long macrocytosis. Children with TEC, however, usually have a normal MCV showing a macrocytosis only during the recovery phase.

Ultimately, time alone will distinguish between the two diseases. In TEC, complete recovery usually occurs within 1 month of diagnosis, and at the latest up to 4 months, whereas such recovery is not seen in Diamond-Blackfan syndrome. No therapy has been shown to hasten the recovery in TEC; occasionally, transfusions may be used if circulatory instability is seen. A bone marrow examination may be needed to rule out an infiltrative process initially and to demonstrate selective failure of the erythroid production in the presence of normal myelomonocytic and megakaryocytic progenitors.

This patient did undergo a bone marrow biopsy, which was found to be consistent with TEC. He required one transfusion, and was discharged to be followed by his pediatrician. He subsequently did well. It is hypothesized that an infectious agent plays a role in the etiology of this disease. Parvovirus has been demonstrated in patients with congenital hemolytic anemias who experience aplastic crises, and it may also play a role in TEC, although that has yet to be proven (Koduri et al, 1983).

whether antithymocyte globulin is an effective treatment. Recent evidence, however, does suggest that antithymocyte globulin may be useful in patients who are not candidates for bone marrow transplantation (Champlin et al, 1983). Cyclophosphamide has been less successful and is not recommended in patients with bone marrow failure except those who have unequivocal evidence of immune-mediated aplasia. Cyclosporine has been used in a few cases on an experimental basis and results are still inconclusive.

Recent studies evaluating the efficacy of recombinant human granulocyte macrophage colony stimulating factor and interleukin I may provide newer approaches to therapy (Lipton and Nathan, 1987).

The treatment of choice for children and young adults with aplastic anemia remains bone marrow transplantation, particularly if transfusions have not been given before the transplantation.

The major problems of bone marrow transplantation remain support of the suppressed recipient before engraftment, graft rejection, graft-versus-host disease, and treatment of opportunistic infections. While the survival for allogeneic bone marrow transplantation is 60% in children, the survival rate increases if the patient has an identical twin donor. Bone marrow transplantation has been used occasionally on patients with Fanconi anemia, assuming the related donor does not have the anemia with delayed expression.

The Shwachman-Diamond syndrome requires treatment with pancreatic enzymes for malabsorption and with antibiotics when there are neutropenia-related infections. Corticosteroids have been found along with androgens to improve the neutropenia. Bone marrow transplantation has not been needed for treatment of this syndrome.

Diamond-Blackfan anemia has been found to benefit from corticosteroid therapy, with the initial regimen consisting of prednisone, 2 mg/kg/day in divided doses until the hemoglobin reaches 10 g/dl. These patients can then be maintained on alternate-day tapered steroids, or if this fails, androgens can be added as is the case for Fanconi anemia. Unfortunately, because of its early presentation, multiple transfusions have been given to these patients, thus, making them poor candidates for bone marrow transplantation.

Patients with transient erythroblastopenia of childhood require careful observation so that their anemia does not become severe, but almost all will recover with increased reticulocyte responses without treatment.

Prognosis

The prognosis for patients with severe acquired aplastic anemia remains grave, with median survival usually less than 6 months and 80% of patients dying within 1–2 years. Those who survive usually need continued tranfusions of blood products (Camitta et al, 1982).

Several studies have been made in attempts to relate risk factors to prognosis. These risk factors include rapidity of onset, age, sex, degree of reticulocytopenia or anemia, MCV, neutropenia, thrombocytopenia, marrow cellularity, ultrastructural abnormalities, and ferrokinetics. None of these factors alone has predicted disease outcome. Multivariate analyses of combinations of these risk factors, however, suggest that male patients, who have more serious bleeding at presentation, and a longer interval from onset of symptoms to diagnosis, have a poorer prognosis.

The International Aplastic Anemia Study Group has established four criteria to identify severe aplastic anemia with an extremely poor prognosis. These include a neutrophil count of less than 500/mm^3, platelet count of less than 20,000/mm^3, reticulocyte count of less than 1% when corrected for hematocrit, and a bone marrow showing severe hypocellularity or moderate hypocellularity with less than 30% of the residual marrow being hematopoietic (Camitta et al, 1976).

Survival curves for aplastic anemia remain biphasic, with a rapid early mortality, followed by a much slower decline, and suggest that patients with severe aplastic anemia may have a better prognosis if they can be maintained long enough to permit their own hematopoietic recovery and they do not succumb to the complications of the disease. Long-term survivors of bone marrow transplantation have now been followed for over 10 years in complete remission.

IRON DEFICIENCY ANEMIA

Iron deficiency anemia is the most common preventable nutritional deficiency recognized in the first years of life. Increasing awareness of iron requirements and iron-supplemented formulas and other foods has diminished the prevalence of this condition, but continued surveillance is essential to well child care.

Definition

The anemia is hypochromic, microcytic, and of insidious onset in growing infants whose intake of iron is not adequate, or who have ongoing blood loss.

Basic Science

Iron is critical for carrying out a wide range of biologic functions. It is needed for certain metabolic and enzymatic processes, for growth, and is crucial in the structure of the hemoglobin molecule in that it is responsible for the transport of oxygen.

At term birth, the infant has about 0.5 g of iron; 0.8–1.5 mg of iron are needed each day for the first 15 years of life. The absorption of iron is more efficient from breast milk than from cow's milk, although breast milk contains very little iron. When cow's milk is given before 6 months of age without supplemental iron in formula or in solid foods, lack of intake and occult loss in stool lead predictably to anemia. When cow's milk is started after 9 months of age, iron deficiency anemia is rare. When iron-fortified formulas are used, anemia is virtually eliminated (Sadowitz and Oski, 1983).

Since most iron is in circulating hemoglobin, the amount at birth depends on duration of gestation, possible blood loss or deprivation at time of delivery from the timing of cord clamping, or the fetal to fetal transfusions through abnormal anastomoses in twin placentas. (One infant may be plethoric, the other anemic.)

The sequence of events that leads to iron deficiency begins with a decrease in stores. Circulating ferritin falls to less than 10 μg/ml. Serum iron falls, with an increase in total iron binding capacity. Free erythrocyte protoporphyrins increase, and hypochromia and microcytosis accompany the progressive anemia. In severe cases, intracellular iron-containing enzymes, such as monoamine oxidase, which is important in the CNS, become depleted. Iron deficiency may have deleterious effects on attention span, alertness, and learning ability (Oski, 1985).

There are three stages of development for iron deficiency. The first is characterized by depletion of iron stores, whereby iron reserves are lost but no decrease in iron supply to the developing red cell is observed. The second stage is that of deficient erythropoiesis, where the erythroid iron supply is decreased, although circulating hemoglobin still is not decreased significantly. The final stage is that of clinically noticeable iron deficiency anemia.

Epidemiology

The incidence of iron deficiency anemia varies from population to population and is dependent upon a variety of factors, including the age group of population being studied, ethnic composition, dietary habits, socioeconomic factors, presence of intestinal parasites, and methods used in determining iron deficiency. In the United States, over the past 20 years, studies have indicated that children between 6 and 36 months of age have an increased incidence of iron deficiency. This reaches a peak at 10–15 months of age with a prevalence of 30%, and then decreases to less than 5% by 36 months of age (Sadowitz and Oski, 1983). There is a higher prevalence of iron deficiency anemia in black versus white children, with the incidence being inversely proportional to economic status independent of ethnic group.

Diagnosis

Iron deficiency anemia can be suspected in premature infants who have not received supplemental iron. The onset occurs when growth is rapid in the face of finite iron reserves. Iron deficiency should be suspected in infants who have blood loss for any reason, but is most common with occult gastrointestinal bleeding in association with cow's milk feedings. Unless there is blood loss, term infants do not usually have a significant anemia before 6 months of age and, depending on dietary intake of iron, it may not be noted until 12–18 months.

Pallor is the most obvious sign. With hemoglobin levels of < 5 g/dl, cardiomegaly, tachycardia and systolic murmurs are common. Pica is common, and associated lead poisoning should be suspected. Occasionally, the spleen is mildly enlarged, but a large spleen should alert the physician to the possibility of a hemolyic process which may be associated with an intercurrent infection and aggravate the anemia.

The laboratory diagnosis of iron deficiency requires comparison with specific reference standards for hemoglobin, MCV, erythrocyte protoporphyrin, serum ferritin, and transferrin saturations. Moreover, other laboratory measurements can be useful depending on the stage of iron deficiency. For example, a patient less than 3 years of age in stage 1, or storage iron depletion, can be identified on the basis of a low serum ferritin or low transferrin saturation level. Stage 2, or iron-deficient erythropoiesis, can be identified by a low transferrin saturation level, elevated free erythrocyte protoporphyrin (FEP), and low blood cell indices. Finally, stage 3, clinical iron deficiency anemia, can be identified by the hemoglobin or hematocrit and a response to a therapeutic trial of iron, as discussed below.

In addition to the hematologic changes, serum iron levels in stage 3 are less than 30 μg/dl and percentage of saturation is below 15%. Serum ferritin levels parallel iron stores. Normal levels in children are 30–150 μg/dl. Levels below this indicate depletion of iron stores, making this assay a useful diagnostic test of iron deficiency.

Differential diagnosis of a microcytic anemia includes thalassemias and lead poisoning, which usually can be eliminated by history and physical examination. Laboratory tests useful for differentiating between thal trait and lead poisoning are shown in Table 8.6. It is not necessary to carry out a full set of laboratory determinations when the age, examination, and dietary history are compatible with iron deficiency. A good response to oral ferrous salts is signified by reticulocytosis by 48–72 hours, and an increase in hemoglobin by about a week. If no response is seen, a search for other causes of anemia is mandatory.

Iron deficiency anemia can be differentiated from lead intoxication by measuring a blood lead level or by using the FEP to hemoglobin ratio as a preliminary screen. If the ratio is in the range of 5.5–17.5 μg/g of hemoglobin, either iron deficiency anemia or lead intoxication is present; measurement of the lead level in the blood will distinguish between these possibilities. An FEP-hemoglobin ratio greater than 17.5 μg/g of hemoglobin, however, signifies lead intoxication with or without iron deficiency and this toxicity requires medical treatment. The only other disorder that can provide an elevated FEP-hemoglobin ratio is the rare genetic disorder erythropoietic protoporphyria, which is characterized by severe cutaneous photosensitivity. In addition, a ratio of less than 5.5 μg/g of hemoglobin is more consistent with a diagnosis of thalassemia trait rather than iron deficiency anemia.

Centrifugation of a hematocrit tube may be helpful. Serum from iron-deficient patients appears clear and colorless, whereas that from normal person appears straw-colored. A stool guaiac test should be done on all patients to detect possible GI bleeding.

Table 8.6
Differentiating the Causes of Microcytosis

	Mean Corpuscular Volume	Red Blood Cell Number	Morphology	Serum Iron/Total Iron Binding Capacity	Hemoglobin Electrophoresis	Free Erythrocyte Protoporphyrin	Lead Level	Family History
Iron deficiency	↓	→ or ↓	Nonspecific: hypochromic, bizarre forms, pencil-like	↓/↑	Nl or ↓ $HgbA_2$	↑	Nl	Neg
Thalassemia trait	↓	→ or ↑	Nonspecific: hypochromic, bizarre forms, targets	Nl/Nl	Nl or ↑ $HgbA_2$	sl ↑ or →	Nl	+/−
Lead poisoning	↓	↓ or → or ↑	Nonspecific: variable ± basophilic stippling	Nl/Nl; or ↓/↑	Nl	↑	↑	Neg

Treatment

A daily dose of 6 mg/kg of elemental iron administered as sulfate, gluconate, or fumarate will give an optimal response. Large amounts of milk may delay absorption; 1 pint a day is appropriate.

After a 1-month trial of iron, the hemoglobin value is expected to reach two-thirds of the normal value. If this is not the case, other causes of anemia should be considered. Reticulocytosis should reach a peak within 5–10 days after the institution of iron therapy, after which the hematocrit rises at a rate of 1%/day, or an average of 0.25–0.4 g of hemoglobin/dl/day. For outpatients, a therapeutic trial may precede a battery of diagnostic tests to confirm iron deficiency anemia. In the hospitalized patient, however, who may also be suffering from anemia of chronic disease or other causes, (another etiology for hypochromia), diagnostic tests such as the blood smear, serum ferritin, and an FEP-hemoglobin ratio might aid the diagnosis.

If anemia persists, and lack of compliance is possible, repletion of iron by intramuscular or intravenous injection of iron may be considered. The dose is calculated by adding the amount of iron necessary to raise the hemoglobin level to normal (e.g., 2.5 mg of elemental iron/kg to raise the hemoglobin concentration 1 g/dl) to the amount needed to replenish iron stores (10 mg of elemental iron/kg). An intramuscular injection is painful, however, and can lead to anaphylaxis, sterile abscesses, and permanent skin staining. Oral iron supplementation should continue usually for no longer than 6 months after the anemia has resolved and iron stores should be replete at that time.

Prevention

Infants should receive breast milk. If that is not available, iron-fortified formulas are indicated. Introduction of iron-containing solid foods by 4–6 months should be adequate. Cow's milk in excess is to be avoided since it is associated with GI bleeding which can aggravate the anemia. Fomon and associates (1981) suggest that whole milk should not be fed to infants before 140 days of age.

Screening for iron deficiency anemia is usually undertaken at 1 year although it might be performed sooner given the recent studies associating developmental delay with iron deficiency (Oski et al, 1983). A hemoglobin concentration of below 10 g/dl is considered indication for iron therapy. A rise of more than 0.5 g/dl within 3 weeks is considered a response.

MEMBRANE DEFECTS ANEMIA

Definition

Membrane defects anemia is a condition in which molecular defects in the composition of the red cell membrane alter the structural integrity of the membrane, ultimately resulting in a decreased red cell lifespan.

Basic Science

The red blood cell membrane is normally composed of a flimsy lipid bilayer supported by membrane proteins that combine to form an underlying skeleton. This skeleton can be described as a two-dimensional mesh of spectrin (one of these proteins) cross-linked by other proteins (e.g., "protein 4.1"), and short actin filaments. This skeleton is attached to the lipid bilayer through other proteins (ankyrin, protein 4.1) which attach to proteins dwelling in the bilayer ("protein 3", the glycophorins). This protein structure is the major determinant of membrane shape, strength, and flexibility and is shown in Figure 8.2 (Becker and Lux, 1985).

A defect in the formation of the membrane skeleton produces abnormal red cells, which lead to a spectrum of disease entities. The most common of these is hereditary spherocytosis, in which spherocytes are formed which are trapped more easily within the spleen than are normal cells, resulting in an anemia. In fact, the spleen can adversely affect hereditary spherocytes by either entrapping them, creating an environment detrimental to their metabolism or structure, or by enhancing phagocytic damage to these cells. Within the spleen, the low pH and decreased Po_2 may increase the rigidity of these cells.

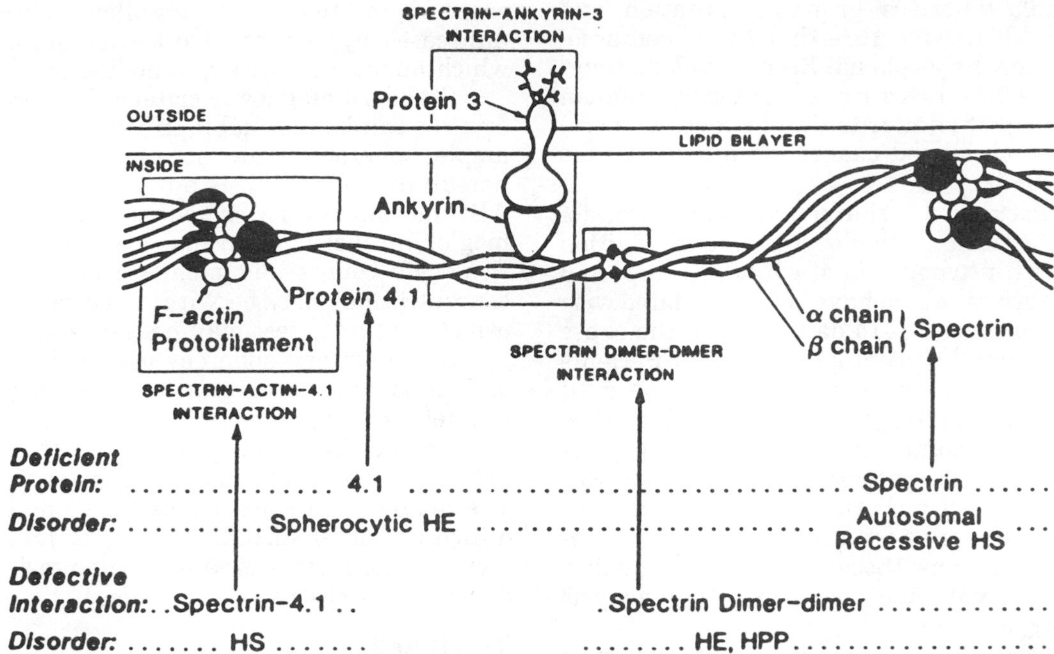

Figure 8.2. Schematic diagram of the red cell membrane. Reproduced with permission from Palek J, Lux SE: Red cell membrane skeletal defects in hereditary and acquired hemolytic anemias. *Semin Hematol* 20:189, 1983. Abbreviations: HS = hereditary spherocytosis; HE = hereditary elliptocytosis; HPP = hereditary pyropoikilocytosis.

The majority of membrane research today focuses on the primary molecular defect that leads to abnormal cellular physiology, change in red cell shape, hemolytic susceptibility, and increased splenic destruction of these cells. Since many observations are confirmed only in a subset of patients with a particular membrane disorder, it is likely that there is heterogeneity with regard to the specific molecular defect in these diseases. For example, although spectrin deficiency is found in all cases of hereditary spherocytosis, the specific defect may be in different steps of spectrin production.

Another red cell membrane disorder is hereditary elliptocytosis, again comprising a heterogeneous group of red cell disorders that result in an elliptically shaped red cell. This disorder is also thought to be a result of a primary genetic defect and the disease is clinically and pathophysiologically similar to hereditary spherocytosis. The five distinct clinical phenotypes of this disease are all believed to result from defects in the membrane skeleton. Most patients have a defect in the self-association of spectrin, although patients with protein 4.1 deficiency also have been described (Garbarz et al, 1984).

Epidemiology

Hereditary spherocytosis represents one of the most common inherited hemolytic anemias in childhood. The prevalence is 220 cases per million among a northern European white population (Morton et al, 1962). There are two modes of inheritance: a classical autosomal dominant pattern (80% of cases); and a much rarer, but more clinically severe, autosomal recessive type (20% of cases). The prevalence in white populations of hereditary elliptocytosis is not readily available due to lack of good epidemiologic data. It appears to be more common among Europeans and American blacks. Most patients with hereditary elliptocytosis have a dominant inheritance with complete penetrance, whereas patients with hereditary spherocytosis may have incomplete penetrance. An autosomal recessive variety of hereditary elliptocytosis has also been reported (Becker and Lux, 1985).

Natural History

The main features of hereditary spherocytosis are anemia, jaundice, and frequently mild splenomegaly, when the disease presents clinically. The disorder may be mild, moderate, or severe. Twenty-five percent of patients have mild disease, which presents without anemia, since RBC production easily compensates for the small degree of destruction. Hemolysis and splenomegaly are mild or absent in these patients, but can be exacerbated during illnesses that will result in splenomegaly (such as infectious mononucleosis) or at times of physiologic stress (such as vigorous exercise or pregnancy).

Patients with moderate hereditary spherocytosis will usually show mild to moderate anemia secondary to uncompensated hemolytic destruction, with intermittent periods of jaundice, usually again associated with viral infections. Splenomegaly is usually present in this form although the degree of splenic enlargement can vary.

A small percentage of patients with hereditary spherocytosis will have the severe type that requires transfusions for alleviation of the anemia. Complications include aplastic crises, growth retardation, and changes in facial bone structure that have been associated with marrow hyperplasia. Recent evidence suggests that the aplastic crises are often caused by a human parvovirus-like agent similar to that believed to be responsible for the childhood exanthem of fifth disease (Koduri et al, 1983).

The aplastic crises are characterized by fever, abdominal pain, vomiting, reticulocytopenia, in addition to the anemia, with hypoplasia of white cell lines and platelets. These crises, which have been associated with viral infections, last for 10–14 days and are the cause of death in a very small percentage of patients. Patients with the autosomal recessive subtype show the most severe clinical manifestations of the disease with marked anemia, massive splenomegaly, and frequent episodes of jaundice. The age at presentation is inversely correlated with the severity. Patients who present with the disease in infancy or early childhood are often moderately anemic, whereas those diagnosed in adolescence or adulthood will have a compensated hemolysis and little, if any, anemia.

Gallstones are the most common complication of hereditary spherocytosis, with their incidence rising from 5% to 40–50% in the second to fifth decades of life and even higher thereafter (Bates and Brown, 1952). Usually these are pigment stones characteristic of hemolytic anemias.

An additional skeletal membrane disorder is hereditary pyropoikilocytosis, a rare autosomal recessive disorder that manifests with severe hemolysis, marked poikilocytosis, and a characteristic sensitivity of red cells to heat, which results in their fragmentation. These patients usually present in the newborn period, and frequently have family members with hereditary elliptocytosis.

Diagnosis

If a patient presents with anemia, jaundice, and/or splenomegaly, a red cell membrane disorder should be considered in the differential. Since hemolysis is occurring, an elevated reticulocyte count is to be expected. This represents a much more reliable sign of hemolysis than does hyperbilirubinemia, which is only present in 50–60% of patients with red cell membrane disorders (Kruger and Burgert, 1966). Characteristic of the disorders is the spherocytic appearance of the red cells on peripheral blood smear. In 20–25% of patients (particularly those with moderate or severe forms of the disease) microspherocytes, the hyperchromic smaller spherocytes that result from multiple passes through the spleen, can be detected. The mean corpuscular hemoglobin concentration will be increased (greater than 36%) in more than half of patients with hereditary spherocytosis due to mild cellular dehydration. The most useful diagnostic test for hereditary spherocytosis is the incubated osmotic fragility test, which measures the ability of red cells to swell in hypotonic media. Since spherocytes have a decreased surface area to volume ratio, they are very fragile and burst easily. The incubation of these cells in the absence of glucose for 24 hours allows better detection of mild cases (by more rapid loss of membrane fragments), which might otherwise go undetected.

Standard diagnostic criteria for hereditary spherocytosis can be unreliable in newborn infants. For example, spherocytes are not only seen in infants with hereditary spherocytosis but also are characteristic of ABO incompatibility or neonatal sepsis. Moreover, hemoglobin concentration may not be decreased and reticulocyte counts and mean corpuscular hemoglobin concentrations may be within the normal range. The osmotic fragility test may not be reliable.

In hereditary spherocytosis, a bone marrow examination will show typical erythroid hyperplasia since the defect is expressed only in the circulating erythrocytes and, therefore, ineffective erythropoiesis does not contribute to the hemolysis noted in this disease. The diagnosis of spherocytosis may be confusing and difficult if other disorders are also present that will increase the surface area to volume ratio, such as iron deficiency or obstructive jaundice.

Treatment

The complications of red cell membrane defects can be markedly improved after a splenectomy; the hemolytic anemia will be less dramatic and red cell lifespan usually returns to normal after the surgical procedure. Nonetheless, the basic defect persists. At present, splenectomy is recommended for all patients with significant anemia, hemolysis (reticulocyte counts greater than 8%), or a history of gallstones occurring at a young age in either the patient or other affected family members. In patients who have mild compensated hemolysis (no anemia and reticulocyte count less than 6%), splenectomy is not currently recommended. The optimal time for the surgery is between the ages of 6 and 8 years, after the period of greatest susceptibility to childhood infections, but before the susceptibility to gallstone formation begins to increase. These children should be immunized with pneumococcal, meningococcal, and H-flu B vaccines before splenectomy, and then are usually maintained on prophylactic penicillin (250 mg bid) until late adolescence when prophylactic use of the drug might be discontinued (Schwartz et al, 1982).

The major risk of splenectomy is susceptibility to overwhelming infection, with sepsis occurring in 3.5% of splenectomized patients with hereditary spherocytosis; 60% of these individuals subsequently died from their infection (Singer, 1973). These studies, however, include a number of neonates and young children and, as noted above, risk is significantly decreased if splenectomy can be postponed until later childhood, and immunizations can be given before the procedure.

ENZYME DEFECT ANEMIAS

Definition

Enzyme defect anemias are hemolytic anemias associated with abnormal RBC metabolic defects.

Basic Science

Knowledge of the metabolism of normal red cells is a prerequisite for understanding the erythrocyte enzyme disorders. Mature RBCs are unique in that, unlike reticulocytes and earlier precursors, they do not contain mitochondria and microsomes and are, therefore, unable to synthesize protein. Hence, enzymes present in mature RBCs are "fixed" at the time of maturation when these cells are released into the circulation.

Since mature RBCs lack mitochondria, glucose, the main metabolic substrate for red cells, can be metabolized via two major pathways—the glycolytic pathway or the hexosemonophosphate shunt (as shown in Figure 8.3). An abnormality in the metabolism of glucose through either of these pathways results in hemolysis. Ninety-five percent of glucose that enters an RBC is usually metabolized through the glycolytic pathway to lactate, producing a small amount of adenosine triphosphate (ATP), which is important for active transport mechanisms, phosphorylation of membrane proteins, and even the maintenance of glycolysis itself. The overall result is a red cell that remains flexible so that it may change its shape during the passage through the microcirculation. When this flexibility is reduced, i.e., when ATP is not produced in sufficient amounts, red cells become less pliable and more prone to hemolysis and destruction. The most common defect causing glycolytic abnormalities is lack of pyruvate kinase activity, although other glycolytic enzyme deficiencies have been reported with a much lower incidence. These include deficiencies of glucose phosphate isomerase, hexokinase, phosphoglycerate kinase, phosphofructose kinase, and triose phosphate isomerase.

Only 5–10% of the glucose that enters the red cell is metabolized via the hexosemonophosphate shunt. Nevertheless, this shunt is responsible for the production of nicotinamide adenine dinucleotide phosphate (NADPH), which protects via glutathione the intracellular proteins in the red cell. Otherwise, these proteins can be attacked by oxidants such as the superoxide anion or hydrogen peroxide resulting in damage to the red cell. NADPH is crucial for the maintenance of high concentrations of reduced glutathione, which serves to prevent oxidant injury. Almost all cases of hemolysis associated with this pathway are due to a deficiency of the enzyme glucose-6-phosphate dehydrogenase (G6PD), which is required to generate the NADPH in the first step of the hexosemonophosphate shunt.

Hemolysis may also be associated with abnormalities of glutathione metabolism itself secondary to a deficiency in one of the two enzymes involved in its synthesis. Moreover, abnormalities of the RBC nucleotide metabolism, in particular pyrimidine 5'-nucleotidase deficiency, lead to accumulation of partially degraded messenger RNA in the red cell and the appearance of basophilic stippling when viewed under the microscope. Basophilic stippling also appears in lead intoxication because lead inhibits pyrimidine 5'-nucleotidase mimicking the situation in which the enzyme is lacking. The intracellular accumulation of partially degraded nucleic acids probably impairs survival of RBCs (Jennings et al, 1984).

The most common drugs associated with hemolysis in glucose-6-phosphate dehydrogenase (G6PD) defi-

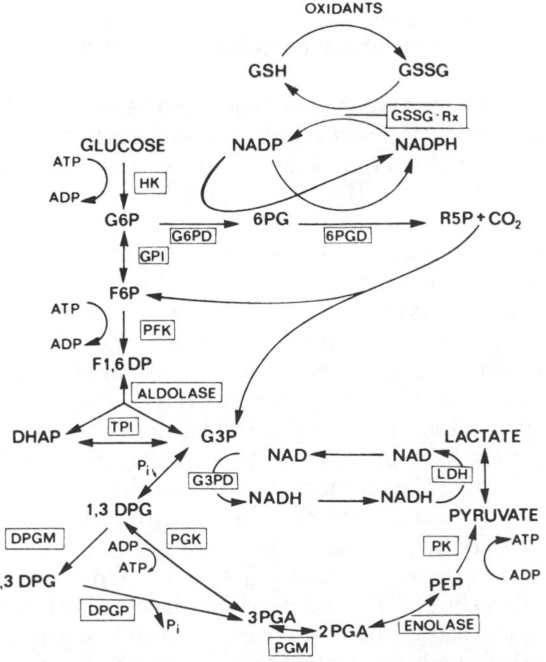

Erythrocyte glucose metabolism. Abbreviations of enzymes (boxed): HK, hexokinase; GPI, glucose-phosphate isomerase; PFK, phosphofructokinase; TPI, triose-phosphate isomerase; G3PD, glyceraldehyde-3-phosphate dehydrogenase; PGK, phosphoglycerate kinase; DPGM, diphosphoglyceromutase; DPGP, diphosphoglycerophosphatase; PGM, phosphoglyceromutase; PK, pyruvate kinase; LDH, lactic dehydrogenase; G6PD, glucose-6-phosphate dehydrogenase; 6GPD, 6-phosphogluconate dehydrogenase; GSSG-Rx, glutathione reductase. Abbreviations of substrates: G6P, glucose 6-phosphate; F6P, fructose 6-phosphate; F1,6DP, fructose-1,6-diphosphate; DHAP, dihydroxyacetone phosphate; G3P, glyceraldehyde-3-phosphate; 1,3DPG, 1,3-diphosphoglyceric acid; 2,3DPG, 2,3-diphosphoglyceric acid; 3PGA, 3-phosphoglyceric acid; 2PGA, 2-phosphoglyceric acid; PEP, phosphoenolpyruvate; 6PG, 6-phosphogluconate; R5P, ribulose-5-phosphate; GSH, reduced glutathione; GSSG, oxidized glutathione. Cofactors are given standard abbreviations: NAD, NADP, NADH, NADPH, and Pi (inorganic phosphate).

Figure 8.3. Erythrocyte glucose metabolism. Reproduced with permission from Lux SE: In Beck WS (ed): *Hematology*, 3rd edition. Cambridge, MIT Press, 1981, p. 216.

ciency are sulfonamides, some other antibiotics (e.g., chloramphenicol), and antimalarial drugs (Table 8.7). Although aspirin was thought to contribute, the viral infection requiring the aspirin is more likely to be the cause of the oxidant stress (Sullivan and Glader, 1980).

Epidemiology

Whereas G6PD deficiency affects millions of people worldwide, the next most common deficiency pyruvate kinase affects only hundreds or a few thousand. Most of the glycolytic enzyme defects, including pyruvate kinase, are autosomal recessive, except for phosphoglycerokinase deficiency, which is X-linked. G6PD deficiency carries an X-linked inheritance pattern and has the highest frequency of occurrence in Mediterranean countries, Africa and China. Over 150 G6PD variants have been reported to date, although only a few are of clinical importance. The normal enzyme is called $G6PD^{B}$ and is found in 99% of whites and 70% of American blacks. Another normal variant found in 20% of the additional blacks is $G6PD^{A+}$. The $G6PD^{A-}$ is the most common variant associated with hemolysis in the remaining 10% of American blacks and in many African populations. G6PD Mediterranean is another common variant observed among peoples in the Southern Mediterranean area, as well as in India and Southeast Asia.

Natural History

A glycolytic enzyme defect such as pyruvate kinase deficiency will present as chronic anemia, reticulocytosis, and often hyperbilirubinemia. Viral infections may increase the degree of hemolysis with this defect or may also suppress normal erythroid production. Thus, a decreased reticulocytosis may be evident while the bilirubin level remains unchanged or even decreases. Such hypoplastic crises can be a problem to the child who is dependent upon an increased production of RBCs to counteract his accelerated RBC destruction.

Patients with G6PD deficiency show a wide variability of clinical features depending on the particular biochemical type of G6PD present, the degree of the oxidant stress, and the sex of the individual. Most of these patients are not anemic and do not show hemolysis unless subjected to a severe oxidant stress, such as an infection or certain drugs. Moreover, in the most common form of G6PD deficiency, the $G6PD^{A-}$ subtype, the enzyme produced is the labile form with a very short half-life, such that while young red cells will have normal enzyme activity, older red cells will be grossly deficient. Hence, the degree of hemolysis is self-limited, only affecting an older population of red cells; when these cells have been lysed, hemolysis will stop, since the younger red cells do contain normal enzyme activity. Usually only 20–30% of the RBC population, representing the oldest RBCs in circulation are affected. Black females who carry the defect rarely show significant hemolysis unless there has been sufficient lyonization to the abnormal chromosome. Patients who have G6PD Mediterranean, the defect initially seen in peoples of the Mediterranean area, may develop a hemolytic crisis from the ingestion of fava beans, although only a small fraction of patients who carry this subtype will react in this way, suggesting that other factors may also be needed to trigger the hemolysis in this setting.

Table 8.7
Drugs Commonly Associated with Hemolysis in G6PD Deficiency

Antimalarials:	Primaquine, quinacrine, chloroquine
Analgesics:	Acetylsalicylic acid
Sulfonamides:	Sulfanilamide, salicylazosulfapyridine (azulfidine), sulfisoxazole (gantrisin)
Other Antibacterials:	Nitrofurantoin, chloramphenicol
Miscellaneous:	Dimercaprol (BAL), naphthalene, methylene blue, vitamin K, ascorbic acid

Diagnosis

A Coombs-negative hemolytic anemia that is not related to infection or drugs should raise suspicion of a glycolytic enzyme defect. A membrane or hemoglobin disorder should be ruled out. An enzyme defect anemia will be normochromic and normocytic with a nonspecific RBC morphology when viewed under the microscope. The definitive diagnosis of pyruvate kinase or other glycolytic enzyme deficiency requires spectrophotometric enzyme measurements in a special laboratory. Unfortunately, many of the affected cells have been destroyed by lysis at the time a sample is obtained. These already lysed cells cannot be analyzed in vitro, so that it may be useful to examine parents for their heterozygous state in order to define the enzyme deficiency.

A Coombs-negative hemolytic anemia associated with drugs or infection should also raise a suspicion for G6PD deficiency. A special stain of the peripheral blood such as methylviolet will reveal Heinz bodies on a peripheral smear. These represent intracellular precipitates of damaged hemoglobin. If splenic function is still intact, spherocytes or bite cells displaying areas where the spleen has removed or pitted the Heinz body may be seen. The definitive diagnosis is made by a spectrophotometric enzyme measurement or by use of an available screening kit. If hemolysis has occurred recently, a false-negative test may be obtained since most of the defective RBCs have already been removed by hemolysis. Thus, a waiting period of 2–3 months until the hemolytic crisis has passed may be required before retesting RBCs for the defective enzyme.

The most common screening test for G6PD deficiency involves NADPH-mediated dye decolorization or monitoring the reduction of methemoglobin in the presence of methylene blue, which would indicate the presence of NADPH. Unfortunately, usually 30–40% of cells must be abnormal for deficiency to be detected, al-

CASE ILLUSTRATION

A 15-month-old Egyptian male was referred for evaluation of anemia and a question of "blasts" on a peripheral smear. He had been well and living in the United States for 6 months until 3 weeks before admission to hospital, when he developed tonsillitis that was treated with ampicillin and acetaminophen. Two weeks before admission he began to show progressive pallor, prompting a visit to his pediatrician. There a hematocrit of 15% with an MCV of 94 fl was noted, as well as the fact that previous hematocrits had been normal 2 months before the visit. The white blood count was 49,000/mm^3, with the questionable smear as above and a platelet count of 405,000/mm^3. He was referred to us for further evaluation.

On examination, there was marked pallor without petechiae, lymphadenopathy, or hepatosplenomegaly. A repeat blood smear was notable for a large number of "bite cells" suggestive of a hemolytic picture and confirmed by a reticulocyte count of 15%, and an LDH greater than 1000 units, with otherwise normal liver function tests. There were "blasts" on the smear but these were felt to be normoblasts consistent with an RBC proliferative response. A Coombs test was negative, although cold agglutinins were weakly positive.

QUESTION AND COMMENT

What could be responsible for this child's hemolysis?

Although this patient was admitted to our oncology service on a presumptive diagnosis of hematologic malignancy, it quickly became apparent that the patient had a hemolytic process either on an autoimmune or enzymatic basis. A more careful history revealed a maternal cousin with G6PD deficiency.

In addition, a dietary history was notable for fava beans being introduced into the baby's diet within the past 3 weeks and pallor noted subsequently, again suggestive of G6PD deficiency (in which fava beans serve as an oxidizing agent to promote hemolysis).

In the presence of a large population of young red cells, enough G6PD activity may be present to pass the screening test in certain populations, for example, in blacks, who have a mild expression of the defect. In a patient of Egyptian descent, however, a defect in enzyme stability is quantitatively more severe and, thus, was confirmed easily by a G6PD screening test. Moreover, parental screening showed the patient's mother to be heterozygous for G6PD. It is not unusual for there to be a delay in presentation of a Mediterranean variant, until proper oxidant stress is introduced as was the situation in this case. With removal of the fava beans from the baby's diet, the child subsequently did well.

though more sensitive modifications of this test are being developed (Piomelli, 1987).

Treatment

For glycolytic defects, treatment is similar to that for chronic hemolytic anemia, with folic acid supplementation (1 mg/day), because of the increased folic acid requirements during erythropoiesis. Iron supplementation, however, is not necessary since the iron from hemolyzed cells can be recycled. Only if a hypoplastic crisis occurs, or if there is significant cardiovascular compromise from the hemolysis should transfusion be used. This is rare in children with glycolytic enzyme defects. Splenectomy may be performed in severely affected children since the spleen is responsible for destroying the enzymatically abnormal cell.

No specific therapeutic regimen is required for the hemolysis due to G6PD deficiency, although transfusion of RBCs may be useful when there is cardiovascular compromise. Usually therapy is directed toward removing the source of oxidant stress, be it infection or a particular drug.

SICKLE CELL DISEASE

Definition

Sickle cell disease constitutes a group of hemoglobinopathies in which there has been a mutation of the β-globin gene. It includes patients who have classic sickle cell anemia (homozygous SS disease), sickle hemoglobin C disease (S-C disease), and sickle cell-β-thalassemia (S-β thalassemia).

Basic Science

Classic sickle cell disease results from a single base mutation in a segment of nuclear DNA that codes for the β-globin gene. This mutation places a valine rather than glutamic acid in the sixth position in the globin chain. When this substitution is made, the deoxygenated sickle hemoglobin polymerizes, forming long rods that distort the cell and convert it from a biconcave into a sickle shape.

The clinical complications of this disease are a result of the inflexibility and fragility of the sickle red blood cells and include vaso-occlusive complications and a chronic hemolytic anemia. When sickle cells cannot revert to their normal biconcave shape, they become permanently trapped in small blood vessels, resulting in circulatory stasis and hypoxia which can then induce even more sickling.

Dehydration and hypertonicity can predispose to sickling and, in this setting, the extensive occlusion can result in tissue necrosis and, hence, the pain, referred to as the vaso-occlusive or painful crisis. The anemia that characterizes sickle cell disease is secondary to the abnormal fragility of the deformed cells, with red cells having a life-span as short as 20 days, owing to destruction occurring both in blood vessels and in the reticuloendothelial systems. Complications of this anemia may include complete suppression of erythrocyte production and splenic sequestration. Another problem under investigation is the extreme susceptibility to infection that is experienced by young sickle cell patients. Impaired or absent splenic function, abnormalities in the complement pathway, and a defect in granulocyte function have all been implicated in these patients, who succumb to life-threatening infections. Moreover, it is still unclear why some patients with sickle cell disease have only mild symptoms whereas others have severe clinical manifestations.

Deoxygenation with resultant sickling leads to a large increase in the viscosity of whole blood, with impairment of passage of the cell through the microcirculation. Irreversibly sickled cells comprise 0–40% of circulating cells in patients with sickle cell disease and are notable on a peripheral blood smear. The major determinant of sickling is the intraerythrocytic concentration of hemoglobin S. Dehydration, which can lead to an increase in the hemoglobin concentration, will increase the amount of sickling. Concurrent iron deficiency or α-thalassemia, on the other hand, conditions that diminish the concentration of hemoglobin in the red cell, may decrease the ability of red cells to undergo sickling. Other non-S hemoglobins may also retard the sickling process, particularly fetal hemoglobin, and to a lesser extent hemoglobin A. It has been shown that 5-azacytidine and hydroxyurea are able to increase hemoglobin F production in patients who have SS disease. The mechanism remains unclear, although some studies have suggested that these agents kill erythroid precursors (CFU-E cells) leading to utilization of earlier progenitors (BFU-E cells) that are able to produce hemoglobin F (Dover et al, 1986). Unfortunately, when the hydroxyurea treatment results in marrow toxicity (decreased reticulocyte counts and decreased CFU-E colony formation), the hemoglobin F production is less likely to increase.

Epidemiology

Sickle cell disease is found primarily in blacks and is most prevalent in areas of the world in which malaria is endemic. This is due to the protective effect of hemoglobin S against fatal malarial infections. If a parasite infects a red cell that contains sickle hemoglobin, the cell automatically undergoes sickling, sequesters the parasite, and destroys it along with its cell in the reticuloendothelial system. In equatorial Africa, the disease has been found in nearly 40% of some populations. Hence, the protective effect in the heterozygote must be balanced against the destructive effect in the homozygote, creating "balanced polymorphism," or a stable gene frequency. In American blacks, the prevalence of sickle trait has been found to be 7–10%, whereas the gene frequency in American whites has been estimated at 0.04–0.08% (Motulsky, 1973).

Natural History

The natural history of the disease varies significantly. In childhood, vaso-occlusive and anemic crises are common. Some patients have a vaso-occlusive crisis weekly or monthly, whereas others have no crises over a period of years. In older patients, the complications of chronic anemia and organ failure secondary to recurrent crises abound. Although patients with hemoglobin SS usually have more severe disease than do patients with SC or S-β-thal, all three of these disorders may give rise to complications in certain patients.

The earliest vaso-occlusive crisis has been reported to occur at 3 months of age when the hemoglobin F concentration begins to fall, and most patients have at least one crisis by 1 year of age. Usually these are characterized by extreme musculoskeletal pain, often involving the hands and feet at the initial presentation, due to symmetric infarction of metacarpals or metatarsals. In older children, the crises no longer involve the peripheral extremities but are often localized to back, abdomen, and the proximal aspects of the extremities.

The anemia in childhood can be complicated by a splenic sequestration crisis since, in younger children, splenic infarction has not yet occurred. Massive pooling of blood within the spleen can occur, leading to severe anemia and hypovolemic shock. Usually by 2–3 years of age the spleen is no longer palpable in children with SS disease secondary to repeated infarction.

An aplastic crisis is another complication which can occur after an infectious illness. Folic acid deficiency has been implicated as a potential factor in causing such crises, although is not the exclusive reason for their occurrence.

Complications characteristic of particular organ systems appear to affect children who have at least reached school age or adolescence. For example, 4–17% of patients with SS disease have a cerebrovascular accident, usually with a mean onset at age 10 years; these are responsible for about 16% of the fatalities in children. (Powars et al, 1978). Often, the cardiovascular system is stressed in patients with SS disease due to the impact of the anemia and cardiac enlargement. Systolic ejection murmurs are common. Renal pathology can result from low oxygen tension, acidosis, and hypertonicity characteristic of the environment within the renal medulla and then may be exacerbated by the sickling process, ultimately leading to loss of renal function. Patients with sickle cell disease experience enuresis, hematuria, salt-losing nephropathy, and recurrent urinary tract infections. In older patients, chronic renal failure can result and lead to hyperuricemia and gout.

A significant degree of intrapulmonary shunting can occur in patients with sickle cell disease, leading to a progressive chronic reduction in arterial oxygen as well as reduction in total lung capacity, vital capacity, and forced vital capacity. This decline in pulmonary function may be due to both pulmonary infarction from recurrent sickling and to recurrent infections.

The hepatobiliary system also can be affected by the disease. Children can suffer from intrahepatic sickling leading to hepatitis and elevated serum bilirubin, and, in older children and adults, cholelithiasis as well.

Some patients with sickle cell disease will develop skeletal abnormalities including avascular necrosis of the femoral head. An increased incidence of osteomyelitis that is often caused by salmonella is observed also. In addition, these patients may develop scoliosis and vertebral deformities.

In males, priapism is a frequent complication. Priapism can occur from obstruction of venous blood flow due to sickled cells within the erectile tissue of the corpus of the penis. Priapism usually occurs in sickle cell males before adolescence. Sexual maturation can be delayed several years in these patients. Women with sickle cell disease who become pregnant are susceptible to increased numbers of vaso-occlusive crises, pulmonary complications, eclampsia, and miscarriage.

Infections are usually due to encapsulated organisms and result from defective splenic function and deficient serum opsinizing activity. Patients with hemoglobin SC and sickle thalassemia appear to have only a slightly increased risk for overall infections as opposed to those with hemoglobin SS disease (Barrett-Connor, 1971; Buchanan et al, 1983).

Patients who have only the sickle cell trait usually do not manifest the vaso-occlusive crises and anemia commonly seen in those who are homozygous for the disease. On the other hand, the hyperosmolarity, acidosis, and hypoxia found in the medulla of the kidney of these patients can result in an abnormal urinary sediment that is found in a majority of patients. A few sickle trait patients will even experience gross hematuria, although without any impairment of renal function (Sears, 1978).

Diagnosis

The diagnosis of sickle cell anemia, if suspicion is raised, should be made during the newborn period by hemoglobin electrophoresis, which can determine the percentages of hemoglobin F, A, S, and C present at birth (Kolata, 1987).

In patients over 6 months of age, the peripheral blood smear will show 5–30% irreversibly sickled cells, polychromasia, targets, fragments, a rare nucleated RBC, and occasional Howell-Jolly bodies which are nuclear remnants near the red cell membranes, suggesting absent splenic function. Patients with sickle cell hemoglobin C disease will demonstrate target cells on their peripheral smear and only rare irreversibly sickled cells. Patients with sickle cell β-thalassemia will have microcytosis. White blood cell count may be elevated in these patients although the peripheral band count will be normal in the absence of infection. Platelet counts are usually slightly elevated or normal. Reticulocyte counts tend to be elevated which, in turn, causes the MCV to be elevated. If the latter value is low in sickle cell anemia, sickle cell β-thalassemia, α-thalassemia trait, or iron deficiency should be considered. Once the diagnosis has been made, routine complete blood counts, reticulocyte and platelet counts, liver function studies, renal function, and serum uric acid level can be helpful to monitor the course of the disease at regular intervals.

An intrauterine diagnosis of sickle cell anemia is possible by analysis of amniotic cells to demonstrate either normal or sickle globin DNA in the fetus (Orkin et al, 1982).

Treatment

Once the diagnosis has been made, the first line of treatment is preventive health maintenance. The single most important treatment is the use of prophylactic penicillin. As early as possible, attention should be given to adequate nutrition and immunization to prevent some of the future complications. It has been recommended that, in addition to prophylactic penicillin, infants be immunized with vaccines directed against encapsulated organisms to avoid the complications of life-threatening infection (Mills, 1985).

In addition, issues of delayed puberty and short stature should be anticipated and discussed to avoid the psychologic effects of such delayed growth on the child. Dental care should also be carefully monitored since increased erythropoiesis can result in malocclusion and require orthodontic care.

The child who has an uncomplicated vaso-occlusive crisis requires treatment for the pain as well as for any factors that have enhanced sickling, such as dehydration. Therefore, a child with a mild crisis should be encouraged to take adequate fluids by mouth, and take an appropriate analgesic dose of acetaminophen. If acetaminophen is insufficient for pain, narcotics should be administered. These can include acetaminophen with codeine, (about 1 mg/kg every 3–4 hours) or for more severe pain oral dilaudid (0.05 mg/kg every 3–4 hours). Usually, these symptoms should resolve within a few hours to a day.

Patients with a moderate vaso-occlusive crisis will usually avoid movement of the painful area, do not respond to oral analgesia, and generally have symptoms that have not resolved in several hours or days. These children require adequate hydration (intravenous fluids) and parenteral narcotics.

It should never be assumed that pain is simply due to vaso-occlusion unless other causes have been excluded. For example, chest pain might also represent a pulmonary infarct or infection in addition to vaso-occlusion. Bone pain may represent an osteomyelitis as well as a vaso-occlusive crisis.

Because of the failure of children with sickle cell disease to handle encapsulated organisms, children under the age of 3 years who have a temperature of 101°F or greater usually require admission to the hospital and administration of parenteral antibiotics pending the results of appropriate cultures.

The use of transfusion for vaso-occlusive therapy is effective only when it produces a significant reduction in the number of circulating sickle cells. Hence a simple blood transfusion actually may increase blood viscosity and enhance sickling. Exchange transfusions, therefore, are the most effective way to decrease the number of sickle cells. The complications of transfusion therapy have been discussed elsewhere (see Chapter 4) and if at all possible should be limited in these patients. Therefore many patients who are prone to recurrent episodes of vaso-occlusive crisis undergo a hypertransfusion therapy regimen instead. These transfusion programs strive to maintain hematocrits over 35% and suppress the patient's production of sickle cells. Iron overload, however, is still an unavoidable long-term complication of this therapy as is sensitization to blood antigens.

Currently, new therapies are focusing on ways to increase hemoglobin F via administration of antineoplastic agents such as 5-azacytidine and hydroxyurea. The mechanism whereby these agents increase fetal hemoglobin synthesis remains unclear at present (Dover et al, 1986).

Prevention

Screening of newborn infants for sickle cell disease now is routine in 10 states, and has been recommended by a panel of experts assembled by the National Institutes of Health (Kolata, 1987). The arguments are that early identification could alert parents and physicians to the need for prophylactic penicillin to prevent *S. pneumoniae* infections from ages 4 months to at least 5 years. Furthermore, symptoms would be recognized earlier and treated appropriately.

The ultimate prevention is prenatal diagnosis, and on the horizon, gene therapy (see pp. 790; Orkin et al, 1982).

THALASSEMIA

Definition

The thalassemias represent a heterogenous group of hereditary disorders characterized by decreased production of one or more globin chains and concomitant accumulation of other globin chains. The clinical spectrum of these disorders is dependent upon which of the globin chains is involved, and how toxic is the overproduction of other globin chains.

Basic Science

Regardless of the globin chain involved, a patient with thalassemia will produce erythrocytes that contain less hemoglobin, making them hypochromic as well as smaller than normal red cells. In addition, the excess normal globin chain that is manufactured accumulates as an unstable aggregate, which precipitates within the red cell and leads to significant destruction, both in the peripheral circulation and in the bone marrow. With the newest techniques in molecular biology, it has been possible to classify the thalassemias as more than simply defects in α-globin or β-globin chain production (see Section 13, Genetics, pp. 774–776).

The major problems in thalassemia usually stem from ongoing ineffective erythropoiesis. The body attempts to compensate for this severe anemia through excess extramedullary hematopoiesis, and frequent blood transfusions are needed to maintain an adequate hematocrit.

Epidemiology

The β-thalassemia genes were identified originally in the Mediterranean Basin, including the Middle East, and in India, Pakistan, Southeast Asia, and parts of Africa. Over the centuries, the disorder has migrated into other areas of the world. At present, persons of Italian, Greek, Oriental, and African descent have the widest incidence of β-thalassemia in North America. α-Thalassemia, on the other hand, is most common in Chinese and Southeast Asians, although has also been reported in people in the African, Middle Eastern, and Mediterranean areas.

Natural History

A patient who is heterozygous for a defective β-globin gene usually has minimal if any clinical symptoms, beyond a mild hypochromic microcytic anemia. Patients homozygous for β-thalassemia, however, are susceptible to severe anemia with a variety of clinical complications. The extramedullary hematopoiesis that results from the anemia leads not only to craniofacial deformities, but also to chronic sinusitis and impaired hearing due to cortical thinning and marrow hyperplasia. This same cortical thinning can result in pathologic fractures in weight-bearing bones if it continues untreated. It is not unusual to see hepatosplenomegaly in these patients as well. The chronic ineffective erythropoiesis that results leads to gallstones in some of the older children. In fact, 70% of thalassemic children over age 15 years will develop gallstones (Ohene-Frempong and Schwartz, 1980).

The excess transfusions that are needed result in an iron overload, with hemochromatosis being the major cause of morbidity and mortality; cardiac hemosiderosis remains the primary cause of death. Pericarditis, arrhythmias, and congestive heart failure all occur, particularly following a long history of transfusion therapy and iron overload. Iron usually further adds to the hepatomegaly, and may lead to hepatic fibrosis in patients of school age and, eventually, to cirrhosis in adolescents or older patients.

If patients require frequent transfusions, their growth may be normal until onset of puberty. Thereafter, height as well as endocrine development declines, so that most of these patients are below the 10th percentile at 21 years of age. It is believed that growth failure probably represents a combination of chronic anemia and excess iron deposition. The delayed or lack of sexual development in these patients is thought to be due to iron deposition impairing the pituitary and/or hypothalamus. Other endocrine dysfunctions also may occur, including hypothyroidism, hypoparathyroidism, and diabetes mellitus.

Diagnosis

Once a clinical suspicion is raised, diagnosis can be confirmed by observing the RBC smear and indices as well as by hemoglobin electrophoresis to quantitate the amounts of hemoglobin A_2 and hemoglobin F in the patient. Usually mean red cell volume and mean cell hemoglobin will be reduced in patients with thalassemia. If a suspicion is raised despite the absence of clinical symptoms, it is important to diagnose a patient carrying the heterozygous β-thalassemia trait since it may be useful for genetic and prenatal counseling, and because it will help to differentiate a patient who has iron deficiency anemia from one with β-thalassemia.

A child who is homozygous usually has less than 5 g/dl of hemoglobin, which is evident before the child is 2 years of age. The red cell indices again will demonstrate severe microcytosis and hypochromia, with a peripheral blood smear showing nucleated red cells, basophilic stippling, and aniso- and poikilocytes. The reticulocyte count in this disorder will be low because of ineffective erythropoiesis preventing the emergence of reticulocytes from the bone marrow.

In the homozygous form of β-thalassemia, levels of hemoglobin F represent 60% of the hemoglobin content of the red blood cells, owing to excess production of γ-chain. Again, the level of hemoglobin A_2 is also usually elevated as a proportion of the hemoglobin A present. It is the reduction in the ratio of β:α chains that confirms the diagnosis, with a ratio of β:α less than 0.25:1 consistent with the disorder.

Treatment

The mainstay of treatment is transfusion therapy and chelation therapy for the iron overload resulting from the transfusion therapy. In addition, splenectomy may be needed. Until the advent of transfusion therapy, most children with β-thalassemia did not live past age 4 years. Death was usually due to congestive heart failure from the severe anemia or intercurrent infections. With transfusion therapy, however, the prognosis has been improved so that some patients are now living through adolescence into adulthood.

The usual transfusion regimen is that of a "high" transfusion program with hemoglobin levels being maintained above 10 g/dl. Transfusion of hemoglobin to a high level provides improved physical well-being and improved growth and development at least until adolescence, less marked cardiomegaly and hepatomegaly, less craniofacial damage, and fewer intercurrent infections.

Usually patients require their first tranfusions when the hemoglobin level has fallen below 6 g/dl and, subsequently, a regular transfusion program is instituted to maintain hemoglobin levels no less than 10 g/dl. Generally children require transfusions at least every 2–4 weeks, with use of filtered, washed RBCs to reduce the chance of sensitization or febrile reactions (McGregor et al, 1983). More recently neocytes, young donor cells, have been given to these patients. Since the neocytes are only 15–30 days old, they should result in a substantial increase in the survival of the transfused cells, which prolongs the transfusion interval. The value of neocytes is not as yet resolved by clinical trial.

Because of the large amount of excess iron deposited in tissues from the transfusions, chelation therapy is necessary. At present, deferoxamine mesylate (Desferal) is given either continuously intravenously, or subcutaneously. The intramuscular route has been found to be less effective and is no longer used. The goal of a chelation program is to make urinary iron excretion exceed the amount of iron loading via transfusion. This usually requires daily subcutaneous infusions of deferoximine supplemented by intravenous administration. Most patients can receive infusions while asleep so that their normal daily activity is not interrupted. The usual regimen is to start chelation just before a transfusion, continue it as an intravenous infusion until after transfusion, and follow with subcutaneous infusion daily. A typical regimen for a child might call for deferoxamine at 40 mg/kg subcutaneously 8–10 hours/day, 6 days a week by portable infusion pump with 120 mg/kg given intravenously over 8 hours at the time of the transfusion (Festa, 1985).

Complications of chelation therapy are minimal. Localized irritation may occur at the site of an infusion and there are reports of hypertension if intravenous infusion is given at greater than 15 mg/kg/hour. Doses greater than 100 mg/kg/day have been associated with increased formation of cataracts, so ophthalmologic examinations should be done at least twice a year. The long range effects of chelation therapy have increased the life-spans of patients dramatically. Even adults who began deferoxamine therapy late showed reduced incidence of cardiac disease compared with those patients who did not begin chelation therapy at a similar age (Wolfe et al, 1985).

CONTROVERSIES

The use of vitamin C to supplement patients receiving chelation therapy remains controversial. Although it increases iron excretion in the urine by an unknown mechanism, increased cardiac toxicity has been reported in patients receiving more than 500 mg of vitamin C per day and deferoxamine. It is hoped that by limiting the dose of vitamin C to 100 mg daily and avoiding intramuscular infusion, the toxic interactions of vitamin C and iron can be avoided.

Likewise, although vitamin E is an antioxidant that can protect the RBC membrane against peroxidation by free radicals created by excess iron, no study has shown an improvement in the requirement for transfusions as a result of vitamin E supplementation, although it is frequently given at a dose of 10–15 units/kg/day divided tid.

If a transfusion program is not started early, at a young age, it is possible that splenomegaly can result from extramedullary hematopoiesis, bringing with it the risk of hypersplenism, leukopenia, and thrombocytopenia, and prompting a need for splenectomy. The risks of splenectomy, however, including susceptibility to life-threatening infection must be considered, so this procedure is usually delayed until the child is more than 5 years old, when the threat of overwhelming infection is reduced. Pneumococcal vaccines are recommended.

Bone marrow transplantation may be useful to replace genetically abnormal marrow with hematopoietically normal marrow stores, although more research is needed before this can become the definitive therapy (Lucarelli et al, 1983). The risks are very high. Other methods to increase the amount of fetal hemoglobin synthesis (e.g., 5-azacytidine, normally used as an antineoplastic agent for acute myelogenous leukemia [Ley et al, 1982]) continue to be explored.

Prognosis and Prevention

Improved transfusion regimens with chelation therapy have improved the prognosis for patients with thalassemias, although the complications of the therapy remain. Bone marrow transplantation may be a more definitive solution, but the ultimate solution, to increase the production of fetal hemoglobin or of β-globin, remains in the future.

Fetoscopy and amniocentesis can be performed at 18–22 weeks of gestation, or even in the first trimester of pregnancy with chorionic villus sampling, to permit diagnosis of homozygous β-thalassemia and allow parents the opportunity to discuss terminating the pregnancy. The risk of fetal loss with these procedures is minimal when they are carried out by a qualified obstetrician/gynecologist with experience in the procedure.

AUTOIMMUNE HEMOLYTIC ANEMIA

Definition

Autoimmune hemolytic anemia represents a condition in which an individual produces antibodies directed against his own RBC antigens, causing premature destruction of the red cells. There are two major types of antibodies that can cause hemolysis in humans, IgG and IgM; the ensuing disorders differ in mechanism, response to therapy, and prognosis. In addition, certain drugs can induce an immune hemolytic anemia.

Basic Science

The autoimmune hemolytic anemia that results from an IgM antibody-red cell interaction is referred to as a cold agglutinin disease. It is most commonly associated with an underlying *Mycoplasma* infection, although has also been known to occur with other infections, including infectious mononucleosis, cytomegalovirus, and mumps. It is not clear why anti-RBC antibodies arise following these infections, although some theories suggest cross-antigenicity between the organism and the human RBC membrane. In other cases, the anemia may be associated with an immunoproliferative disorder, such as leukemia, lymphoma, or a collagen vascular disease.

The IgM antibody that may be polyclonal with an infectious etiology is monoclonal in the immunoproliferative setting, usually directed against the I antigen on the RBC membrane. This affinity is most pronounced in the cold (0–10°C) and is much lower at higher temperatures. It may also be directed against the I antigen on the RBC membrane. Usually, the cold agglutinins will have no measurable activity directed against the red cell above 20°C, suggesting that the antigen is altered in the cold so as to increase its availability to the antibody. The extent of hemolysis depends on the titer of antibody available, the temperature at which the antibody is active, and the level of circulating C3B inactivator proteins in plasma (Schreiber and McDermott, 1978).

In the appropriate setting, interaction of the IgM antibody with the RBC surface brings about activation of the complement pathway. Once the complement pathway is activated, multiple C3B molecules are deposited on the RBC membrane surface. The cells are then attacked by macrophages containing specific receptors for detecting C3B-coated cells, and undergo phagocytosis, which becomes the major mechanism for hemolysis in the IgM-induced immune hemolytic anemia. In the absence of the classical complement pathway, IgM-coated red cells would have a normal survival. Further activation of the complement pathway leading to deposition of C8-C9 molecules can also lead to destruction of red cells independent of macrophages. If the C3B inactivator protein is present in the plasma, this may prevent a significant degree of hemolysis since it cleaves C3B to a less active molecule designated as C3D, which remains on the RBC surface but does not attract macrophages.

The IgG antibody reacts with the complement system quite differently, since it takes many IgG molecules on the RBC surface to bind and activate just one molecule of C1. Once activation has occurred, C3B molecules are deposited on the RBC surface and macrophages are attracted not only to C3B but to the IgG molecule as well. In fact, phagocytosis of RBCs by macrophages takes place even in the absence of C3B or even with an insufficient IgG to activate the complement pathway. Nevertheless, the combination of the IgG-directed macrophage clearance and the complement-activated clearance does accelerate hemolysis. Most of the macrophages directed against the IgM-coated erythrocytes are found in the liver, whereas the IgG-coated erythrocytes are cleared predominantly in the spleen.

In contrast to the IgM antibody, the IgG antibody functions maximally at 37°C and, hence, the disorder is referred to as a warm antibody-induced hemolytic anemia. Like the cold antibodies-induced anemia, it has been associated with immuno-proliferative disorders, various viral infections, as well as unknown causes. Many drug-induced immune hemolytic anemias also function through IgG antibodies.

There are three ways in which drug-induced immune hemolytic anemias can occur. The first is a hapten-type mechanism as seen in patients exposed to high doses of penicillin and possibly some cephalosporins. In this case, penicillin combines with the RBC surface and acts as a hapten and, thus, an antibody becomes directed against the penicillin-coated erythrocyte RBC membrane. This is usually an IgG response.

The second mechanism (known to occur with quinidine and sulfonamide) is referred to as an "innocent bystander" reaction. It appears that an IgM anti-quinidine antibody arises that results in activation of the classic complement pathway and deposition of C3 on the RBC surface not involved in the initial antibody reaction but leading to phagocytosis of the red cell nonetheless.

The third type (seen with α-methyldopa and its derivatives) is identical to IgG-induced immune hemolytic anemia.

If an IgG antibody is cold reacting, similar to the IgM, the disease is known as paroxysmal cold hemoglobinuria. In this situation, the antibody interacts with a P antigen of the P blood group system which is present in almost all human RBCs. The P antibody has been known to arise in three situations—(1) following viral infections, especially measles; (2) as an autoimmune process; and (3) in the setting of congenital or tertiary syphilis. Hemolysis in this disorder is intravascular and usually is due to the lytic action of complement.

Epidemiology

The prevalence of autoimmune hemolytic anemia is about 1 case per 75,000–80,000 persons in the general population. There is no known familial predisposition except in the setting of another autoimmune disorder such as systemic lupus erythematosus. The male-female ratio appears equal. Although the disease occurs primarily in adults, autoimmune hemolytic anemia has been reported in children as early as 1 month, particularly the IgG-induced hemolytic anemia. Peak incidence in children is usually in the first 4 years of life (Shreiber, 1980).

Natural History

Autoimmune hemolytic anemia may present subtly as progressive weakness or lightheadedness attributable to the anemia, or more dramatically, with jaundice or significant cardiovascular compromise due to the degree of destruction of red cells. Other symptoms may be due to underlying malignant disease or to an underlying systemic vasculitic condition.

Two main clinical patterns are apparent in children, an acute transient type and a prolonged chronic course. In the acute transient cases, hemoglobinuria is common as is a history of a prodromal acute infectious course. Full recovery usually occurs in less than 3 months, with steroid therapy usually being effective as discussed below. Most cases involve an IgG type of antibody.

In the chronic disorder, hemoglobinuria or an acute infectious prodrome is very uncommon and the onset is not as rapid as in the transient case. More than two-thirds of cases will have an underlying systemic disorder or be associated with thrombocytopenia or another immunologic difficiency. IgG- and IgM-type mechanisms have been reported and the course is prolonged for months or years. Steroid therapy has been less successful in these patients.

In paroxysmal cold hemoglobinuria, most patients experience hemolysis and hemoglobinuria.

Diagnosis

If clinical suspicion for a hemolytic anemia is raised, the diagnosis is confirmed by laboratory studies. Initially, an anemia with reticulocytosis should be documented. Examination of the peripheral blood smear can sometimes be notable for the presence of microspherocytes, these being more prominent in IgG- than in IgM-induced immune hemolytic anemia. Bone marrow examination usually reveals erythrocyte hyperplasia, assuming that the bone marrow itself has not been affected (e.g., the antibody may react with red cell precursors, a viral infection may suppress the bone marrow, or a neoplastic process may be infiltrating the bone marrow to prevent reticulocytosis).

A key diagnostic test is the direct Coombs test, a method of assaying for the presence of antibody and/or complement components on the red blood cell surface. In the Coombs assay, a patient's RBCs washed free of plasma proteins are mixed with a Coombs serum—an animal antihuman IgG agent that agglutinates RBCs in the presence of surface antibodies. If the red cells are agglutinated by an anti-IgG immunoglobulin, IgG is present on the surface of the red cell. If an anti-C3 reagent is used, the third component of complement on the surface of red cells can be assessed. Usually either IgG or IgG plus C3 will be identified if an IgG-induced immune hemolytic anemia is present. A cold agglutinin titer can also be useful if an IgM immune hemolytic anemia is suspected. The agglutinating activity of the patient's plasma is directed against normal ABO compatible red cells that contain the I antigen, with the titer being the highest dilution of antibody that can still agglutinate normal red cells. In patients with the IgM disease the titers will be greater than 1:1000.

In paroxysmal cold hemoglobinuria, the direct Coombs test is usually positive but is directed only against C3. The definitive test for paroxysmal cold hemoglobinuria is the test for Donath-Landsteiner antibody in which a patient's serum, a source of complement, and either normal red cells or those from a patient suspected of having paroxysmal nocturnal hemoglobinuria, are incubated initially at 4°C and then at 37°C. Usually, hemolysis will occur under these conditions but will not take place if the temperature is maintained at either 4°C or 37°C throughout the incubation (i.e., the hemolysis occurs during the rewarming process).

The indirect Coombs test detects antibody in serum in the absence of antibody on the red cell surface and will often suggest isoimmunization.

Treatment

Initial therapy should be aimed at any primary disorder identified (i.e., infectious, collagen vascular, or malignant). If the anemia is mild, only careful observation may be necessary. On the other hand, if the patient is symptomatic, therapy should be instituted. The hemolytic crisis may be resolved through the use of corticosteroids, (e.g., prednisone at doses of 1–2 mg/kg/day). These are especially effective in IgG-induced hemolytic anemia possibly by decreasing the production of abnormal IgG antibody, which results in an increase in hemoglobin within 2–4 weeks. Steroids cause the elution of IgG antibody from the RBC surface and thus improve erythrocyte survival; they also interfere with the macrophage IgG and C3B receptors responsible for the destruction of the RBC. Once a response to steroids is noted, a slow taper usually over several months follows. Corticosteroids have been found to be less effective in cold agglutinin IgM immune hemolytic anemias probably because of the large amounts of IgM and of C3B on the erythrocyte surface. These patients do best by avoiding cold which can precipitate their hemolytic crises.

If the patient does not respond to corticosteroid therapy, or requires excessive amounts of corticosteroids, or shows side effects, splenectomy should be considered, particularly in the IgG-induced immune hemolytic anemias since the IgG-coated cells are cleared through the spleen. Moreover, removal of spleen will decrease the amount of IgG anti-RBC antibody since there is a large B lymphocyte pool contained within the spleen. Again, splenectomy will not help a patient with a cold agglutinin disease since these cells are normally cleared in the liver.

Finally, immunosuppressive agents that decrease production of antibody may be tried, such as cyclophosphamide, azathioprine, and chlorambucil. These can also suppress normal bone marrow function, however, and complicate management. Moreover, these agents have only limited success in patients with cold agglutinin disease.

Danazol, a modified androgen with reduced masculinizing effects, has been found to be effective for the treatment of autoimmune hemolytic anemia regardless of the severity of the disorder, and even if other corticosteroids have failed. Danazol was found to be equally effective in patients with and without their spleen. In addition, danazol and lower doses of corticosteroids are believed to work synergistically, so that once the hemolysis lessens, the dose of corticosteroids can be reduced gradually and then discontinued, after which the dose of danazol can be lowered. Although the time required for maintenance with danazol is not yet known, it is currently recommended to continue treating with the agent for at least 1 year, since relapses are common after withdrawal of therapy within this period (Ahn et al, 1985).

Intravenous γ-globulin may be effective in a rare patient but is just beginning to be formally studied (Bussel et al, 1984).

The main treatment for paroxysmal cold hemoglobinuria is to avoid cold temperatures. If the disorder is chronic, corticosteroids may be useful. If it is short-lived or secondary to an acute viral infection, it should be self-resolving. Rarely a transfusion will be necessary, and if so, pp blood (rare) should be used to avoid reaction with a P antigen.

NEW DEVELOPMENTS

One of the most useful procedures for alleviation of IgM-induced hemolytic anemia has been plasmapheresis, which is able to reduce the level of cold agglutinins since IgM, a high molecular weight molecule, remains predominantly within intravascular spaces. It has also been found to be useful in some patients with IgG immune hemolytic anemia, particularly while waiting for other therapeutic modalities to show their effect. Transfusion therapy should be considered only when there is a life-threatening degree of anemia since these patients become increasingly difficult to crossmatch and the risk of receiving incompatible blood is increased. Washed red cells should be administered to minimize the possibility of a transfusion reaction (Schreiber and Gill, 1987).

Prognosis

Prognosis for a patient with immune hemolytic anemia is largely dependent upon the etiology. In children with IgG-induced hemolytic anemia, however, pharmacologic or surgical treatment can be useful in eliminating the disease, or at least reducing its severity, even if the etiology is not known.

Mortality is less than 10% in patients with the chronic disorders, and is usually secondary to an underlying disorder causing the hemolysis.

PAROXYSMAL NOCTURNAL HEMOGLOBINURIA

Definition

Paroxysmal nocturnal hemoglobinuria (PNH) is a disease of the hematopoietic stem cells that results in production of a clone of defective blood cells in all three circulating cell lines.

Basic Science

The defect in PNH is an abnormal membrane which can interact with components of the serum complement pathway so that the cell membrane becomes more susceptible than normal to the lytic action of complement. This membrane defect is due to absence of a regulatory molecule identified as decay accelerating factor (DAF), which normally, when present, will decrease the stability of the membrane for binding C3b and, therefore, activating complement (Nicholson-Weller et al, 1983). Usually the predominant manifestation as a result is hemolysis of red cells. Hence, this disorder is often classified among the hemolytic disorders.

Interestingly, the same defect on platelets may account for the thrombotic episodes in this disease, when C3 fixes to the platelet and activates it. In white cells, the excessive binding of C3 may account for a defect in chemotaxis, thus making these patients more susceptible to infections than are those without the disease.

Natural History

Children have rarely been reported to experience PNH, although 5–10% of children with aplastic anemia will develop the disorder as they recover from the aplasia (Rosse, 1978). There is great variability in the way in which PNH can present, usually due to the proportion of abnormal stem cells, and thus of red cells in the clone, which may vary from 1 to over 90%. Moreover, the stem cell abnormality may result in decreased hematopoiesis, with varied effects on any of the three cell lines. Overall, however, most patients with PNH will show hemolysis as a predominant clinical manifestation.

If only small to moderate proportions of red cells are hemolyzed, there may be no overt hemoglobinuria, despite the presence of a chronic hemolytic anemia. When the condition is severe, however, hemoglobinuria will result since the hemolysis is primarily intravascular. Hemosiderinuria is almost always found even when the hemoglobinuria is absent. For unclear reasons, the hemoglobinuria is most severe at night and may occur in paroxysms lasting several days especially after an acute infection. Because of hemoglobinuria and hemosiderinuria, these patients may develop iron deficiency as well.

Other conditions associated with PNH have included thrombocytopenia and granulocytopenia and a few patients have had unusual venous thromboses, including Budd-Chiari syndrome and cerebral and portal vein thromboses. In addition, children with PNH may experience abdominal pain, particularly early in the morning when severe hemolysis is occurring. These patients will be unable to swallow food and will complain of dysphagia as if food is caught at the esophageal-gastric junction. Abdominal pain further along the gastrointestinal tract occurs, perhaps due to thrombotic episodes or to excessive contraction of the small bowel.

Diagnosis

Diagnosis of PNH is established by demonstrating red cells that are unusually susceptible to the hemolytic action of complement, irrespective of how the complement pathway is being activated. The most reliable screening test is the sugar-water test, in which a low ionic strength solution of isotonic sucrose is used to aggregate serum globulins and, in turn, complement onto the red cell surface resulting in hemolysis. If this is abnormal, a more specific test, the Ham test, in which the alternative pathway of complement is activated by acidification of serum, is useful. In this case, the susceptible PNH cells will be hemolyzed more readily than normal cells. The abnormality can be quantitated by using antibody in excess and complement in limited quantities. Normally, a population of sensitized cells will require large amounts of complement to undergo lysis. On the other hand, cells from patients with PNH consist of two populations, one of which is virtually normal, while the other is markedly abnormal and requires as little as 1/25 the amount of complement for a similar degree of lysis. A third type of cell is often present in which there is only one-third to one-fifth as much complement required for lysis; the presence of each of these can be detected quantitatively, using excess antibody and a limited quantity of complement. Specific tests such as Decay Accelerating Factor that detect membrane proteins which may be defective or absent in PNH have been devised as tools to diagnose PNH.

Treatment

Anemia may require iron supplementation because of the large urinary losses of iron. Cortico- and androgenic steroids have also been found to be useful in some patients. If patients are symptomatic, transfusions of washed red cells may be necessary. These are immediate measures to alleviate the symptoms of the disease, but treating the underlying stem cell disorder is the treatment of choice. This has been accomplished by allogeneic bone marrow transplantation. Therefore, patients who have PNH and are unresponsive to medical management should undergo HLA typing in preparation for a potential transplant. If thrombosis occurs as a complication of PNH, it should be treated by anticoagulants, specifically coumadin.

Prognosis

With appropriate attention to the disease and its complications, patients can do well for many years. Sometimes the abnormal clone will disappear from the marrow of patients, particularly during recovery from aplastic anemia. In other patients, the abnormality may persist and in adults, death, when it occurs, is usually due to thrombosis, leukemic transformation, or rarely renal failure.

MEGALOBLASTIC ANEMIAS

Definition

Megaloblastic anemias of childhood usually stem from deficiency of vitamin B_{12} or folate, or from abnormalities in absorption, transport, or metabolism of these vitamins.

Megaloblasts are erythroid precursors with immature nuclei relative to cytoplasmic maturation. When there is megaloblastic maturation of red cells, it is the maturing erythroid precursors that are destroyed in the bone marrow, with defective RBCs released into the circulation. Hence, this anemia affects precursors rather than the mature erythrocytes themselves. Moreover, erythroid committed progenitor cells increase in number with a megaloblastic anemia. The defective mature red cells usually have a MCV greater than 105 μ^3. The megaloblastic morphology may also be observed in white cell lines characterized by multilobe neutrophils on peripheral smears.

Basic Science

Folate deficiency arises primarily from inadequate ingestion, absorption, or an increased requirement for the vitamin. The inadequate ingestion may result from the fact that cooking destroys the folate in food. Hence, not only a dietary history but how the food is prepared may be important in diagnosing this particular condition. Folate is absorbed in the monoglutamate form and impairment of absorption is usually due to the inhibition of the intestinal conjugase enzyme that cleaves polyglutamate to the monoglutamate. The enzyme is inhibited, owing to the presence of a heat-stable heat-activated conjugase inhibitor found in cooked vegetables, or because the intestinal pH becomes too acidic to allow the conjugase enzyme to work.

Although B_{12} deficiency may be due to inadequate intake, such as occurs with a pure vegetarian diet, the majority of patients in the United States suffer from inadequate absorption of the vitamin. Absorption normally occurs when B_{12} combines with intrinsic factors secreted by gastric parietal cells, and with nonintrinsic factor B_{12} binding proteins. Major malfunctions are usually due to either (1) a structural or functional gastric defect causing insufficient secretion of intrinsic factor, (2) an ileal defect resulting in inadequate absorption even when there is adequate intrinsic factor, or (3) a pancreatic disease in which the absorption of the vitamin is decreased, even though all the prerequisite factors are present. The condition in which there is insufficient secretion of intrinsic factor from unknown causes, although usually associated with gastric atrophy, is also known as pernicious anemia, and is most common in adults.

Deficiencies of B_{12} or folate may lead to reduction in the absorptive capability of the intestinal surface. This is because megaloblastosis represents impaired DNA synthesis which can affect all the dividing cells of the body, including those of the intestinal lumen, resulting in effective atrophy of absorptive cells which, in turn, leads to further malabsorption and the process essentially becomes self-perpetuating. Pancreatic disease will impair absorption if there is insufficient secretion of bicarbonate, since absorption only occurs in an alkaline environment, or if there is inadequate trypsin to cleave the nonintrinsic factor-binding proteins and allow intrinsic factor to bind exclusively to the vitamin prior to absorption.

In B_{12} or folate deficiency, very few cells of the body are in the resting state. Instead they are attempting to complete doubling their DNA, but are experiencing frequent maturation arrests in the synthesis phase of cell division, since B_{12} and folate are essential to the process. Since DNA replication and cell division are blocked while cytoplasm synthesis of proteins continues, a larger cell containing usually more than 1 unit of DNA, known as a megaloblastic cell is obtained. Because the ability to synthesize RNA is relatively unimpaired, the cytoplasm in the cell appears larger than the nucleus and more mature. The nucleus contains a finely particulate nuclear chromatin typical of the erythroid megaloblast, differentiating it from the normal erythroblast, which has coarsely clumped nuclear chromatin as its cytoplasm matures and begins to make hemoglobin.

It is possible to have combined nutritional anemias in which iron is deficient as well as B_{12} or folate. In these circumstances, the peripheral smear may not be characteristic for megaloblastic anemia, but may display a dimorphic picture of macro-ovalocytic progeny, and hypochromic microcytes. The presence of anemia from two underlying deficiencies may be confirmed by examining the bone marrow for the presence of hypersegmented polys as well as poor iron staining.

A primary defect characteristic of only B_{12} and not folate deficiency is an inability to synthesize myelin, which results in the development of a demyelinating neuropathy, beginning in peripheral nerves, progressing to the posterior and lateral columns of the spinal cord, and ultimately, to the cerebrum. This type of megaloblastic anemia requires specific treatment with B_{12}.

Natural History

Infants who are unable to utilize B_{12} and folate will usually develop a clinical manifestation of the deficiency in the first few weeks of life, whereas those with milder absorption defects will develop symptoms during later infancy and childhood and, occasionally, not until adolescence. Infants who are unable to absorb folate exclusively will develop symptoms of this deficiency at about 3 months of age, whereas those unable to absorb vitamin B_{12} will usually develop clinical symptoms after the sixth month, but most often before the third year of life.

Clearly, a megaloblastic disease should be considered in a patient who presents with the signs and symptoms of anemia. In megaloblastic diseases, leukopenia will seldom cause recurrent infections, whereas thrombocytopenia may occur in the most severe cases. Patients with megaloblastic anemias may also present with glossitis, dysphagia, weight loss, loss of appetite, or neurologic symptoms consistent with vitamin B_{12} deficiency (paresthesias and peripheral neuropathies). Often a loss of intellectual function and depression occurs in this setting, as well as degeneration of spinal cord function due to the lack of myelin formation.

Megaloblastic anemia due to nutritional folate deficiency is usually associated with conditions of increased demand. In particular, the neonate, patients with chronic hemolytic anemia, or those who are pregnant are most likely to develop this disorder if the patient has an unusual dietary pattern, such as having no fresh green vegetables. In infants and older children, this may be seen in chronic malabsorption states, such as in celiac or inflammatory bowel disease, or as a side-effect of medications that prevent folate utilization, such as dilantin or trimethoprim-sulfamethoxazole.

Diagnosis

Once suspected, a peripheral blood smear should be examined, to look for oval-shaped macrocytes or multilobed neutrophils. Only 25% of patients with an elevated MCV will show a characteristic blood smear. Hence, a bone marrow aspirate should be examined for megaloblastic changes. Finally, levels of vitamin B_{12} and folate in serum, and of folate in erythrocytes should be measured.

The serum folate level is very sensitive and can become low after only 3 weeks of a poor diet, whereas the red cell folate level reflects the tissue content of this vitamin. Therefore, a low red cell folate may be seen with B_{12} deficiency alone since B_{12} is required to keep folate in the cells. Hence, diagnosis of folate deficiency requires both a serum folate of less than 3 ng/ml and a red cell folate of less than 150 ng/ml.

If B_{12} deficiency is suspected secondary to an absence of intrinsic factor, a Shilling Test should be performed. This tests the ability of a patient to absorb radioactive B_{12} when it is given alone or when intrinsic factor is added. The test is carried out in two stages. In the first stage, a patient is given a small oral dose of radioactive B_{12}, followed by a large parenteral dose of nonradioactive B_{12}. This latter dose will bind to most available receptor sites in liver and other body tissues so that most of the radioactive dose is absorbed through the gastrointestinal tract, enters the blood stream, and is soon excreted in the urine since there are few binding sites available. The amount of radioactivity in a patient's 24-hour urine collection will then provide an index of the degree of malabsorption. If malabsorption is demonstrated in the first stage of the test, the patient is then given a dose of intrinsic factor in addition to the vitamin B_{12}. This constitutes the second stage. If absorption normalizes, it is clear that the patient lacks sufficient intrinsic factor of his own to absorb B_{12}.

If intrinsic factor fails to correct the defect, the problem lies either in the ileum or the pancreas. If pancreatic enzymes or bicarbonate is given with vitamin B_{12}, absorption should normalize if the defect is in the pancreas. If not, ileal malfunction is diagnosed by exclusion. Unfortunately, more than half the patients with pernicious anemia will still show an abnormal second stage test, even though the problem is lack of intrinsic factor. This is because, with the slow DNA synthesis characteristic of B_{12} deficiency, there is a consequent atrophy of the absorptive cells of the gut, and hence, despite the addition of intrinsic factor, absorption is still hampered. Therefore, if the results are equivocal in the second stage of the test, the patient should be started nonetheless on a regimen of B_{12} parenterally and have the test repeated 2 months later. If the test is now normal, it is clear that the patient's disease is pernicious anemia.

Other special studies may include the measurement of antibody to intrinsic factor in the serum, which can be found in 55–60% of patients with pernicious anemia.

Peripheral blood and bone marrow aspirates have also been used to provide biochemical evidence of megaloblastosis by showing impaired DNA synthesis. The deoxyuridine (dU) suppression test is used, which measures the ability of cultured lymphocytes or bone marrow cells to incorporate tritiated thymidine into DNA after preincubation in the presence and the absence of nonradioactive deoxyuridine. If folate and B_{12} activity are normal, nonradioactive deoxyuridine will be converted to thymidine and a reduced proportion of radioactive thymidine will be incorporated into DNA. If folate or B_{12} is deficient, then there will be a lesser degree of suppression of radioactive thymidine incorporation into DNA by deoxyuridine. If the addition of either folate or B_{12} normalizes results, the source for the deficiency is identified. This biochemical test has superseded the formerly used therapeutic trial in which sources of folate and B_{12} are eliminated for a period of 10 days, after which either B_{12} or folate is administered and reticulocyte counts and hemoglobin levels are re-evaluated 5–12 days later. The deoxyuridine suppression test can provide results on bone marrow cells in 1 day, and on peripheral blood lymphocytes in 4 days (Herbert et al, 1973).

Treatment

In contrast to iron deficiency, a therapeutic trial is rarely useful, since it is important to know whether B_{12} or folate or both are deficient. Once diagnosed, however, treatment should be started as soon as possible. Treatment for B_{12} deficiency is usually divided into primary and maintenance stages. In the primary therapeutic stage, a minimum of 1 μg/day of vitamin B_{12} is given parenterally for 10 days, with a minimum of 50–100 μg of folate if that is deficient, also. Reticulocytosis should begin within 3 days and should reach a peak by 1 week. Hemoglobin should normalize at the end of a month. These doses represent small, barely therapeutic doses of the single vitamins, and this regimen is used to avoid the possible danger of a too rapid conversion of the bone marrow to normoblastic. There are case reports of sudden deaths during treatment of patients with pernicious anemia, particularly in those patients who have been severely anemic. These deaths have been ascribed to severe hypokalemia as well as to thrombotic and embolic episodes.

If a patient lacks intrinsic factor or has a noncorrectable lesion of the ileum, resulting in malabsorption of B_{12} and folate, life-long maintenance therapy is necessary. Usually a minimum of 30 μg parenterally is given once a month to adults in the form of cyanocobalamin, although in Europe hydroxycobalamin is preferred for parenteral administration. There is no apparent difference between the two preparations. Oral preparations of B_{12} plus intrinsic factor are not recommended for long-term therapy in patients with pernicious anemia, since they result in unreliable absorption of B_{12}. Moreover, they would probably lead to the development of local intestinal antibodies to the exogenous intrinsic factor.

Patients with folate deficiency may be treated initially with 5–15 mg/day of folic acid for 7–14 days, followed by 2 mg orally twice weekly, or 0.05 mg once daily for several months until a new population of red cells is formed.

Transfusion therapy is rarely indicated in a megaloblastic anemia since the symptoms develop gradually rather than acutely. If a patient with a chronic disease develops severe anemia with megaloblastic components careful transfusion with packed red cells is indicated. Usually, 10 ml/kg up to 1 unit of packed cells will alleviate symptoms.

If iron deficiency is also detected, appropriate iron therapy should be instituted as well.

In children, most B_{12} deficiency is caused by abnormalities in B_{12} metabolism and is associated with homocystinuria. The most common of these B_{12} metabolism abnormalities is transcobalamin 2 deficiency. To prevent mental retardation, these patients normally are treated daily with large doses (1000 μg) of hydroxycobalamin (which can be utilized much more effectively than cyanocobalamin) either intramuscularly or perorally. This treatment should begin after collection of urine for determination of orotic acid, homocystine, methionine, cystathionine, and methylmalonic acid, and of blood for determination of B_{12}, folate, transcobalamin, homocystine, and methionine levels.

CONTROVERSY

Patients who have neoplastic disease and are malnourished develop folate or B_{12} deficiency. Whether such patients should be treated with the vitamins is unclear, since they may also encourage the development of the neoplasm. It appears, however, that these patients do improve if vitamin deficiencies are corrected and some studies suggest that they tolerate chemotherapy better than do those patients who are untreated with the vitamins. Nonetheless, it appears prudent at present to correct the deficiency in tumor patients with minimal doses of the vitamin, such as 500 μg/day of vitamin B_{12} orally (which will result in 5 μg/day being absorbed) (Cooper, 1984).

Prevention

Appropriate attention to diet, particularly under conditions of increased demand, is the best way to prevent the development of the megaloblastic nutritional anemias. Foods rich in folate include liver, meat, fresh vegetables, dried beans and fruits. Foods rich in B_{12} include dairy products and eggs.

POLYCYTHEMIA

Definition

Polycythemia describes a condition in which there is an elevated hematocrit or increase in red cell mass. A variety of arbitrary values have been used to define the disorder, with most common definitions giving peripheral venous hematocrit values greater than 65% as being diagnostic of the disease. Not all polycythemic patients have a hyperviscous state, however, nor are all hyperviscous infants polycythemic.

Basic Science

There is an inverse relationship between viscosity and the flow of a liquid. Therefore, if hyperviscosity is associated with polycythemia, the blood flow to various organ systems would be expected to decrease with the increase in hematocrit and blood viscosity. The expected complications are within the cardiopulmonary, GI, central nervous, renal, and musculoskeletal systems.

The polycythemia that most commonly affects infants is usually secondary to systemic hypoxemia which, in older children, is associated with chronic lung disease or cardiopulmonary right-to-left shunting. In addition, some congenital variants have been discovered (e.g., hemoglobin Chesapeake), in which abnormal hemoglobins with oxygen affinity higher than normal, decrease the unloading of oxygen to tissues and prompt an erythropoietin-mediated erythrocytosis. Tumors producing erythropoietin also can cause polycythemia. It is important to be certain that the polycythemia is real and is not the result of a contraction in plasma volume. In this case, the total number of red cells is not abnormally high, but the cells occupy a greater portion of the reduced total blood volume, such as can be seen in vomiting, diarrhea, and diuretic overdose.

For a discussion of neonatal polycythemia, its diagnosis and treatment, see Section 4.

Natural History and Epidemiology

Polycythemia vera is a primary polycythemia due to clonal expansion of an abnormal multipotent progenitor cell. It is uncommon in children, with less than 1% of patients being under 25 years of age. It is characterized clinically by headache, weakness, pruritis, and dizziness as a result of the increased blood viscosity and hypermetabolism.

Children with this disorder will appear plethoric, with most having splenomegaly and/or hepatomegaly. One-third will have elevated diastolic blood pressure. Leuco- and thrombocytoses are common. While erythropoietin is elevated in secondary or reactive polycythemia, it is usually normal or decreased in polycythemia vera.

Diagnosis

Unless a child is severely dehydrated, a hematocrit over 60% is consistent with the diagnosis of polycythemia and an increased red cell mass. Diagnostic confirmation rests with measurement of total red cell volume, (using radioactively labeled red cells), arterial blood oxygen saturation, and the oxygen pressure at which hemoglobin is 50% saturated (the P50 measurement).

Treatment

Phlebotomy alone is sufficient treatment for children with polycythemia vera to keep their hematocrits less than 60. In children, this should be done using isovolemic replacement solutions (with crystalloid or colloid) to maintain oxyhemoglobin flow. If chronic phlebotomy occurs, iron deficiency should be closely monitored, since it can readily occur in this setting. Chemotherapy and radioactive phosphorus have been used in adults with equal success in survival to phlebotomy, but have not been formally tested in children. (Wasserman, 1976).

In reactive polycythemia, the primary cause for the increased red cell mass should be sought since phlebotomy in this setting may hinder adequate delivery of oxygen.

Long-term survival with polycythemia vera is relatively common. The major cause of mortality and morbidity is due to vascular occlusive episodes. Bleeding, thrombosis, myelofibrosis, and transformation to acute leukemia have been reported in these patients, particularly those treated with alkylating agents.

METHEMOGLOBINEMIA

Definition

When the iron in hemoglobin is oxidized from the ferrous to the ferric state, it is unable to combine with oxygen, resulting in clinical cyanosis. In methemoglobinemia, it is this ferric-hemoglobin or methemoglobin that accumulates in the circulation.

Basic Science

Under normal circumstances methemoglobin is continually being formed in blood cells, but then is immediately reduced to hemoglobin. Normally the methemoglobin level does not exceed 1% of total hemoglobin. The reduction of methemoglobin occurs via two enzymatic reactions, either through an NADH cytochrome B5 reductase (Fig. 8.4) or an NADPH diaphorase catalyzed reaction.

If red cells are congenitally deficient in cytochrome B5 reductase or if they are exposed to excess oxidation stress, such as through toxins or drugs, methemoglobinemia will result. Red cells also contain an NADPH-dependent hemoglobin reductase system that normally does not function physiologically, but which can be induced in the presence of an exogenous electron carrier such as methylene blue. When methylene blue is present, the NADPH-dependent reductase system is found to be even more active than the NADH cytochrome B5 reductase.

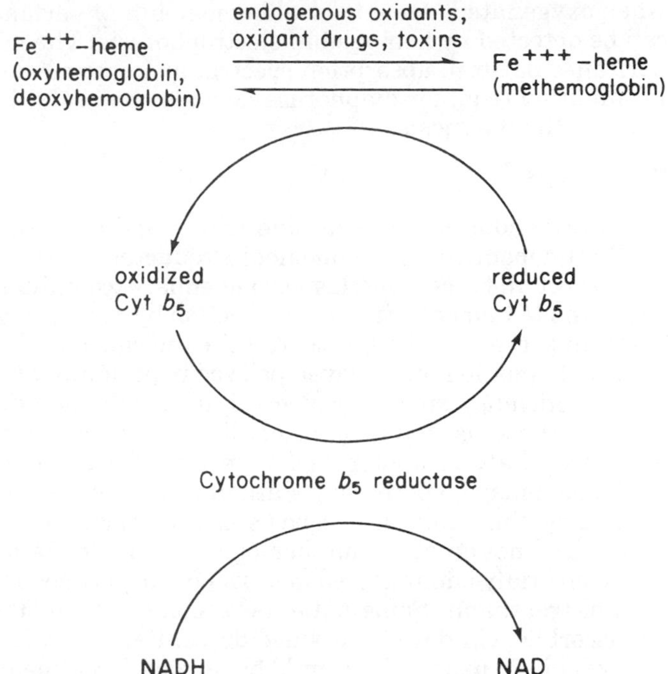

Figure 8.4. Methemoglobin metabolism. Reproduced with permission from Bunn HF: In Beck WS (ed): *Hematology,* 3rd edition. Cambridge, MIT Press, 1981, p. 139.

Abnormal hemoglobin variants, known as the M hemoglobins, can be responsible for generation of methemoglobin by allowing oxidation of iron to the ferric form in an affected globin chain.

Epidemiology

The inheritance pattern for the M hemoglobin is autosomal dominant. The inheritance pattern for the enzymatic deficiencies is usually autosomal recessive.

Natural History

Congenital methemoglobinemia is present if an enzyme deficiency or a hemoglobin M subtype exists at birth. Acquired methemoglobinemia comes from exposure to drugs or toxins, such as nitrates and other chemical agents, such as aniline, acetanilid, and sulfonamides. It has also been associated with severe dehydration and metabolic acidosis in young infants. If the methemoglobin level is in excess of 1.5 g/dl, i.e., 10% of the total hemoglobin, the patient will be visibly cyanotic. Normally cyanosis is not visible until the level of reduced hemoglobin reaches 5 g/dl. If the methemoglobin composes 35% of total hemoglobin, shortness of breath and headache can result. Seventy percent methemoglobin content is fatal.

Diagnosis

Methemoglobin appears as a chocolate-brown color in blood drawn from patients with the disease and, unlike a cyanotic blood sample, it will not become pink when oxygenated. An abnormal hemoglobin M variant can be detected by hemoglobin electrophoresis. The inheritance pattern, absorption spectra, and enzyme determination (e.g., for diaphorase) can also be useful in making the diagnosis.

Treatment

Intravenous methylene blue which activates the NADPH-dependent methemoglobin reductase system will correct all types of methemoglobinemia, except those due to the M hemoglobins, and correction by methylene blue can serve as a diagnostic test for the cause of the disease. It should not, however, be used in patients with G6PD deficiency since it can precipitate a hemolytic crisis in these patients. Occasionally, if the condition is severe, dialysis and/or exchange transfusion with fresh blood may be necessary. Patients with congenital methemoglobinemia on the basis of an enzyme deficiency, and not an abnormal hemoglobin, can be maintained on orally administered methylene blue as another form of treatment. Some patients respond to 200–500 mg ascorbic acid daily in divided doses. Patients with hemoglobin M usually have mild hemolysis. Treatment is, therefore, not indicated, nor is it possible.

PORPHYRIAS

Definition

The porphyrias represent a group of heterogeneous diseases characterized by abnormalities in heme biosynthesis. Porphyrins are intermediates in the synthetic pathway responsible for the formation of heme. Errors in the biosynthesis of these porphyrins (stemming from deficiencies of specific enzymes) result in abdominal pain, peripheral neuropathy, mental disturbances, as well as the skin photosensitivity. They can be inherited often on an autosomal dominant mode or as acquired defects. Two major groups of the porphyrias exist, erythropoietic or hepatic, depending on the major site of heme synthesis where the metabolic error occurs.

Basic Science

Heme synthesis is a complex process involving four mitochondrial and four cytoplasmic enzymes. Glycine and succinyl-coenzyme A first interact to form aminolevulinic acid (ALA), which is transformed enzymatically into porphobilinogen and then through several porphyrin intermediates, including uroporphyrinogen, coproporphyrinogen, protoporphyrinogen, uroporphyrinogen III, coproporphyrinogen III, protoporphyrinogen IX, and finally ending in the formation of heme. Hence, there are multiple steps in which abnormalities in the production or functioning of the eight enzymes can occur, leading to clinical disorders.

For example, acute intermittent porphyria (AIP) is a result of a partial defect of uroporphyrinogen I synthetase, the enzyme that is responsible for converting porphobilinogen to uroporphyrinogen I, an intermediate on the pathway to uroporphyrinogen III. It represents one of the hepatic porphyrias. In fact, all hepatic porphyrias will show increased levels of ALA synthetase owing to the deficiencies of the subsequent intermediates, which result in induction of ALA synthetase through negative feedback regulation. Congenital erythropoietic porphyria represents an imbalance between the activities of uroporphyrinogen I synthetase and uroporphyrinogen III cosynthetase resulting in overproduction of uroporphyrinogen I which cannot form heme, and with slightly decreased amounts of uroporphyrinogen III in the RBC. This autosomal recessive disorder results in a severe hemolytic anemia. In the noncongenital erythropoietic protoporphyria, the autosomal dominant defect is in ferochelatase, the enzyme responsible for converting protoporphyrin IX to the final form of heme.

The skin photosensitivity that occurs in these disorders is believed to be due to the increased accumulation of porphyrin intermediates. It leads to formation of oxygen-free radicals with destructive processes resulting in lysosomal release within skin tissue.

Epidemiology

About 1/30,000 people in the general population will be afflicted with one of the porphyrias (Elder, 1980).

Natural History

Although the porphyrias are often transmitted on the basis of a genetic pattern, clinical symptoms rarely appear before puberty, particularly in the hepatic form. Once they appear, however, they tend to persist throughout the patient's life. The symptoms may be divided into three categories: cutaneous, visceral, or neuropsychiatric. Tables 8.8 and 8.9 describe the clinical presentations of the erythropoietic and hepatic porphyrias.

Table 8.8
Erythropoietic Porphyrias

	Congenital Erythropoietic Porphyria	Protoporphyria
Inheritance	Autosomal recessive	Autosomal dominant
Age of onset	Infancy	Early childhood
Enzyme deficiency	Porphyrobilinogen deaminase and/or uroporphyrinogen III cosynthetase	Ferrochelatase
Signs and symptoms		
Cutaneous lesions	Yes	Yes
Visceral/neuro-psychiatric	No	No

Table 8.9
Hepatic Porphyrias

	Acute Intermittent Porphyria	Porphyria Variegata	Hereditary Coproporphyria	Porphyria Cutanea Tarda
Inheritance	Autosomal dominant	Autosomal dominant	Autosomal dominant	Autosomal dominant
Age of onset	Adolescence or adulthood	Adolescence or adulthood	Early childhood	Early childhood
Enzyme deficiency	Porphyrobilinogen deaminase	Protoporphyrinogen oxidase	Coproporphyrinogen oxidase	Uroporphyrinogen decarboxylase
Signs and symptoms				
Cutaneous lesions	No	Yes	Rarely	Yes
Visceral/ neuropsychiatric	Yes	Yes	Yes	No

The dermal lesions usually occur upon exposure to sunlight, whereas visceral and neurologic symptoms can be precipitated by an infection, pregnancy, menstruation, or certain drugs, such as barbiturates, sulfonamides, griseofulvin, and alcohol. An acute exacerbation in the absence of sunlight will present with colicky abdominal pain. The pain is usually located in the epigastrium or right lower quadrant, although it can be diffuse. Vomiting and constipation are usually associated with the attacks and fever and leukocytosis may occur also, so that it actually may mimic a surgically acute abdomen. Hypertension and tachycardia occur in more than half of these patients, whereas they are less likely if a surgical diagnosis is present. The neurologic symptoms can include weakness and paresthesias in the back and limb muscles or personality changes in which patients may appear depressed, nervous, hysterical, or simply "peculiar." The end of an attack may be heralded by return of normal blood pressure and pulse. The neurologic manifestations are believed to derive from demyelination of peripheral nerves or to cerebral demyelination.

Death is usually the result of quadraparesis with respiratory failure. Electrolyte disturbances are common with profound attacks, as evidenced by hypotonic serum characterized by hyponatremia and hypochloremia, hypotonic urine, and often hypocalcemia and hypomagnesemia.

The dermal lesions may appear as vesicles and edematous bullae on skin exposed to sunlight. They may be secondarily infected and often leave hyperpigmented chronic scarring. Hypertrichosis and a violaceous hue often develop in patients over the years with the dermatologic form of porphyria.

Diagnosis

If the symptom complex is suggestive, diagnosis of the prophyrias requires examination of urine and feces to ascertain increased excretion of porphyrin. Although the urine may be colorless, elevated levels of porphobilinogen may be present. Burgundy red urine is due to the presence of uroporphyrinogen. In the erythropoietic protoporphyrias blood can also be assayed for the presence of elevated porphyrins. Family members also should have their urine and feces inspected for the presence of elevated porphyrins. Laboratory analysis is required in order to pinpoint the specific enzymatic defect and, hence, the type of porphyria that exists within a given family. Diagnosis also can be made on skin samples.

Treatment

Treatment of an acute attack requires close monitoring of fluid and electrolyte balance. If neurologic symptoms occur monitoring for respiratory paralysis is required, with support equipment readily available. The use of heme infusions to decrease ALA synthetase has been associated (in clinical investigations) with dramatic improvement and is reserved for the most severe cases of porphyria (Bloomer and Pierach, 1982). Since many drugs and chemical agents can precipitate attacks, therapy must be approached cautiously. Morphine and chloral hydrate have been reported to be useful for control of pain.

In the long-term management, careful control of infections and avoidance of any drugs that can possibly precipitate an attack are critical. Attacks associated with the menstrual cycle often can be treated with birth control pills and other hormonal regulators, although they are contraindicated in families who also have dermal symptoms. Avoidance of exposure to sunlight is probably the best treatment for the skin lesions. Commercial sunscreen does not provide adequate protection.

Prognosis

With early diagnosis, appropriate fluid and dietary therapy, and avoidance of these contraindicated drugs, most patients have a good prognosis for survival and are able to obtain relief following acute visceral attacks.

REFERENCES

Ahn YS, Harrington WJ, Mylvaganam R, et al: Danazol therapy for autoimmune hemolytic anemia. *Ann Intern Med* 102:298, 1985.

Alter BP: Bone marrow failure in children. *Pediatr Ann* 8:444, 1979.

Alter BP, Potter NU: Long-term outcome in Fanconi's anemia: Description of 26 cases and review of the literature. In German J (ed): *Chromosome Mutation and Neoplasia.* New York, AR Liss, 1983, p. 43.

Barrett-Connor, E: Infection and sickle cell C disease. *Am J Med Sci* 262:162, 1971.

Bates GC, Brown CH: Incidence of gallbladder disease in chronic hemolytic anemia (spherocytosis). *Gastroenterology* 21:104, 1952.

Beaudry MA, Ferguson DJ, Pearse K, et al: Survival of a hydropic infant with homozygous alpha thalassemia 1. *J Pediatr* 108:713, 1986.

Becker PS, Lux SE: Hereditary spherocytosis and related disorders. *Clin Hematol* 14:15, 1985.

Beutler E: Red cell enzyme defects as nondiseases and as diseases. *Blood* 54:1, 1979.

Beutler E, Hartman K: Age related red cell enzymes in children with transient erythroblastopenia of children and with hemolytic anemia. *Pediatr Res* 19:44, 1985.

Bianchi DW, Beyer EC, Stark AR, et al: Normal long-term survival with alpha thalassemia. *J Pediatr* 108:716, 1986.

Black VD, Lubchenco LO: Neonatal polycythemia and hyperviscosity. *Pediatr Clin North Am* 29:1137, 1982.

Black VD, Lubchenco LO, Luckey DW, et al: Developmental and neurological sequelae of neonatal hyperviscosity syndrome. *Pediatrics* 69:426, 1982.

Bloomer JR, Pierach CA: Effect of hematin administration to patients with protoporphyria and liver disease. *Hepatology* 2:817, 1982.

Buchanan GR, Smith SJ, et al: Bacterial infection and splenic reticulo-endothelial function in children with hemoglobin SC disease. *Pediatrics* 72:93, 1983.

Bunn HF: Hemoglobin I: Structure and function. In Beck WS(ed): *Hematology.* Cambridge, MIT Press, 1985, p. 135.

Bussel JB, Cunningham-Rundles C, et al: Intravenous treatment of autoimmune hemolytic anemia with gamma-globulin. *Pediatr Res* 12:237A, 1984.

Camitta BM, Storb, R, Thomas ED: Aplastic anemia: Pathogenesis, diagnosis, treatment, and prognosis. *N Engl J Med* 306:645, 1982.

Camitta BM, Thomas ED, et al: Severe aplastic anemia: A prospective study of the effect of early marrow transplantation on acute mortality. *Blood* 48:63, 1976.

Carton RW: Pulmonary complications of sickle cell disease. *J Respir Dis* p 73, June 1986.

Cartwright GE, Edwards CQ, Kravitz K, et al: Hereditary hemachromatosis: Phenotypic expression of the disease. *N Eng J Med* 297:7, 1977.

Champlin R, Ho W, Gale RP: Antithymocyte globulin treatment in patients with aplastic anemia: A prospective randomized trial. *N Engl J Med* 308:113, 1983.

Chanarin I: Investigation and management of megaloblastic anemia. *Clin Hematol* 5:747, 1976.

Cooper BA: Megaloblastic anemia and disorders affecting utilization of vitamin B_{12} and folate in childhood. *Clin Hematol* 5:631, 1976.

Cooper BA: Megaloblastic anemia: when to suspect it, how to treat it. *Drug Ther Hosp* p. 55, April 1984.

Dover GJ, Humphries RK, Moore JG, et al: Hydroxyurea induction of hemoglobin F production in sickle cell disease: Relationship between cytoxicity and F cell production. *Blood* 67:735, 1986.

Elder GH: The porphyrias: Clinical chemistry, diagnosis, and methodology. *Clin Hematol* 9:371, 1980.

Escobar GJ, Heyman MB, Smith WB, et al: Primary hemachromatosis in childhood. *Pediatrics* 80:549, 1987.

Festa RS: Modern management of thalassemia. *Pediatr Ann* 14:597, 1985.

Fomon SJ, Ziegler EE, Nelson SE, et al: Cow milk feeding in infancy, gastrointestinal blood loss and iron nutritional status. *J Pediatr* 98:540, 1981.

Forget BG: Hemolytic anemias: Congenital and acquired. *Hosp Pract* p. 67, April 1980.

Gale RP, Champlin RE, Feig SA, et al: Aplastic anemia: Biology and treatment. *Ann Intern Med* 95:477, 1981.

Garbarz M, Dhermy D, et al: A variant of erythrocyte membrane skeletal protein band 4.1 associated with hereditary elliptocytosis. *Blood* 64:1006, 1984.

Goldstein M: The aplastic anemias. *Hosp Prac* p. 85, May 1980.

Gross GP, Hathaway WE, McGaughey HR: Hyperviscosity in the neonate. *J Pediatr* 82:1004, 1973.

Habibi B, Homberg JC, Schaison G, et al: Autoimmune hemolytic anemia in children: A review of 80 cases. *Am J Med* 56:61, 1974.

Herbert V, Tisman G, et al: The dU suppression test using I^{125} UdR to define megaloblastosis. *Br J Haematol* 24:711, 1973.

Jennings ML, Adams-Lackey M, et al: Peptides of human erythrocyte band 3 protein produced by extracellular papain cleavage. *J Biol Chem* 259:4652, 1984.

Kappas A, Sassa S, Anderson KE: The porphyrias. In Stanbury JB, et al (eds): *The Metabolic Basis of Inherited Disease,* 4th edition. New York, McGraw-Hill, 1983, p. 1301.

Koduri RPR, Patel AR, Anderson MJ, et al: Infection with Parvovirus-like virus and aplastic crisis in chronic hemolytic anemia. *Ann Intern Med* 98:930, 1983.

Kolata G: Panel urges newborn sickle cell screening. *Science* 236:259, 1987.

Krueger HC, Burgert EO: Hereditary spherocytosis in 100 children. *Mayo Clinic Proc* 41:821, 1966.

Labotka RJ, Mauer HS, Honig GR: Transient erythroblastopenia of childhood. *Am J Dis Child* 135:937, 1981.

Lanzkowsky P: Problems in the diagnosis of iron deficiency anemia. *Pediatr Ann* 14:618, 1985.

Ley TJ, DeSimone J, Anagnou NP, et al: 5-azacytadine selectively increases gammaglobin synthesis in a patient with beta plus thalassemia. *N Engl J Med* 307:1469, 1982.

Lipton JM, Kudisch M, Gross R, et al: Defective erythroid progenitor differentiation system in congenital hypoplastic (Diamond-Blackfan) anemia. *Blood* 67:962, 1986.

Lipton JM, Nathan DG: The anatomy and physiology of hematopoiesis. In Nathan DG, Oski FA (eds): *Hematology of Infancy and Childhood.* Philadelphia, WB Saunders, 1987, p. 144.

Lucarelli G, Izzi T, Polchi P, et al: Bone marrow transplantation in thalassemia. *Exp Hematol* 11:101, 1983.

Lux SE: Hemolytic anemias IV: Metabolic disorders. In Beck WS (ed): *Hematology.* Cambridge, MIT Press, 1985, p. 223.

Lux SE, Wolfe LC: Inherited disorders of the red cell membrane skeleton. *Pediatr Clin North Am* 27:463, 1980.

McGregor M, Harrison JF, et al: A study of the routine use of the imugard Ig 500 leucocyte removal filter, illustrating a possible cause of transfusion reactions and a method of prevention. *Clin Lab Haematol* 5:279, 1983.

McIntosh S, Rooks Y, Ritchey AK, et al: Fever in young children with sickle cell disease. *J Pediatr* 96:199, 1980.

Mentzer WC: Pyruvate kinase deficiency and disorders of glycolysis. In Nathan DG, Oski FA (eds): *Hematology of Infancy and Childhood,* 3rd edition. Philadelphia, WB Saunders, 1987, p. 545.

Mentzer WC, Wang WC: Sickle cell disease: Pathophysiology and diagnosis. *Pediatr Ann* 9:287, 1980.

Minagi H, Steinbach HL: Roentgen appearance of anomalies associated with hypoplastic anemias of childhood: Fanconi's anemia and cogenital hypoplastic anemia. *AJR* 97:100, 1966.

Mills ML: Life threatening complications of sickle cell disease in children. *JAMA* 254:1487, 1985.

Morton NE, Mackinney AA, et al: Genetics of spherocytosis. *Am J Hum Genet* 14:170, 1962.

Motulsky AG: Frequency of sickling disorders in US Blacks. *N Engl J Med* 288: 31, 1973.

Nicholson-Weller JA, March P, Rosenfeld SI, et al: Affected erythrocytes of patients with paroxysmal nocturnal hemoglobinuria are deficient in the complement regulatory protein, decay accelerating factor. *Proc Natl Acad Sci* 80:5066, 1983.

Ohene-Frempong K, Schwartz E: Clinical features of thalassemia. *Pediatr Clin North Am* 27:403, 1980.

Orkin SH, Little PF, et al: Improved detection of the sickle mutation by DNA analysis: Application to prenatal diagnosis. *N Engl J Med* 307:32, 1982.

Oski FA: Is bovine milk a health hazard? *Pediatrics* 75:(Suppl)182, 1985.

Oski FA: Transient erythroblastopenia. *Pediatr Rev* 4:25, 1982.

Oski FA, Honig AS, et al: Effect of iron therapy on behavior performance in nonanemic, iron-deficient infants. *Pediatrics* 71:877, 1983.

Ozsoylu S, Coskun T, et al: High dose intravenous glucocorticoid in the treatment of childhood acquired aplastic anemia. *Scand J Haematol* 33:309, 1984.

Palek J, Lux SE: Red cell membrane skeletal defects in hereditary and acquired hemolytic anemias. *Semin Hematol* 20:3, 189, 1983.

Piomelli S: G6PD deficiency and related disorders of the pentose pathway. In Nathan DG, Oski FA (eds): *Hematology of Infancy and Childhood*, 3rd edition, Philadelphia, WB Saunders, 1987, p. 583.

Powars D, Wilson B, et al. The natural history of stroke in sickle cell disease. *Am J Med* 65:461, 1978.

Reeves JD, Driggers DA, Lo EYT, et al: Screening for anemia in infants: Evidence in favor of using identical hemoglobin and red cell volume in infancy and childhood. *J Pediatr* 98:894, 1981.

Reeves JD, Vichinsky E, Addiego J, et al: Iron deficiency in health and disease. *Advances in Pediatrics 1984*. Chicago, Year Book Medical, 1983, p. 281.

Rosse WF: In Nathan DG, Oski F (eds): *Pediatric Hematology,* 2nd edition. Immune hemolytic anemia and paroxysmal nocturnal hemoglobinuria. Philadelphia, WB Saunders, 1981, p. 419.

Rosse WF: Paroxysmal nocturnal haemoglobinuria in aplastic anemia. *Clin Haematol* 7:541, 1978.

Sadowitz PD, Oski FA: Iron status and infant feeding practices in an urban ambulatory center. *Pediatrics* 72:33, 1983.

Schreiber AD: Autoimmune hemolytic anemia. *Pediatr Clin North Am* 27:253, 1980.

Schreiber AD, Gill FM: Autoimmune hemolytic anemia. In Nathan DG, Oski FA (eds): *Hematology of Infancy and Childhood*, 3rd edition. Philadelphia, WB Saunders, 1987, p. 413.

Schreiber AD, McDermott P: Effect on C36 inactivator on monocyte bound C3 coated crythrocytes. *Blood* 52:898, 1978.

Schröter W, Kahsnitz E: Diagnosis of hereditary spherocytosis in newborn infants. *J Pediatr* 103:460, 1983.

Schwartz PE, Sterioff S, et al: Postsplenectomy sepsis and mortality in adults. *JAMA* 248:2279, 1982.

Scott RB: The management of pain in children with sickle cell disease. In *Advances in the Pathophysiology, Diagnosis, and Treatment of Sickle Cell Disease*. New York, Alan R. Liss, 1982, p. 47.

Sears DA: The morbidity of sickle cell trait: A review of the literature. *Am J Med* 64:1021, 1978.

Singer DB: Postsplenectomy sepsis. In Rosenberg HS, Bolande RP (eds.): *Perspectives in Pediatric Pathology*, vol 1. Chicago, Year Book Medical Publishers, 1973, pp. 285.

Sullivan DW, Glader BE: Erythrocyte enzyme disorders in children. *Pediatr Clin North Am* 27:449, 1980.

Toback AC, Sassa S, Poh-Fitzpatrick MB, et al: Hepatoerythropoietic porphyria: clinical, biochemical, enzymatic studies in a three-generation family lineage. *N Engl J Med* 316:645, 1987.

Topley AM, Rogers DW, Stevens CG, et al: Acute splenic sequestration and hypersplenism in the first five years in homozygous sickle cell disease. *Arch Dis Child* 56:765, 1981.

Vichinsky EP, Lubin BH: Sickle cell anemia in related hemoglobinopathies. *Pediatr Clin North Am* 27:429, 1980.

Vichinsky EP, Lubin BH: Unstable hemoglobins, hemoglobins with altered oxygen affinity, and M hemoglobins. *Pediatr Clin North Am* 27:421, 1980.

Wang WC, Mentzer WC: Differentiation of transient erythroblastopenia of childhood. Congenital hypoplastic anemia. *J Pediatr* 88:784, 1976.

Wasserman LR: The treatment of polycythemia vera. *Semin Hematol* 13:57, 1976.

Wolfe LC, Lux SE: Nutritional anemias of childhood. *Pediatr Ann* 8:435, 1979.

Wolfe L, Olivieri N, Sallan S, et al: Prevention of cardiac disease by subcutaneous deferoxamine in patients with thalassemia major. *N Engl J Med* 312:1600, 1985.

Yoshida Y, Sakota H, et al: Lack of correlation between in vitro corticosteroid effect on hematopoietic colony formation and response to corticosteroid therapy in aplastic anemia. *Internat J Cell Cloning* 4:82, 1986.

White Cell Disorders 3

NEUTROPENIA

Definition

Neutropenia is the term used to define a decrease in the number of circulating polymorphonuclear leukocytes (PMNs). The quantitative definition depends on the age of the child with standards being a function of age and race of the child (Sadowitz and Oski, 1983).

Neutropenia is important because it results in an increased susceptibility to infection in children and, in turn, to the development of sepsis.

Basic Science

Two pathophysiological mechanisms are responsible for neutropenia, either decreased production or increased destruction of PMNs. A decrease in production can result from a defect in a progenitor cell, which fails to differentiate into PMNs. Examples of this disorder include the relatively benign "cyclic neutropenia" and the fatal disorder, reticular dysgenesis. Maturation arrest can also occur at a later stage of neutrophil development, such as the promyelocytic level as seen in Kostmann disease, another example of congenital decreased production. In addition, production may be hampered by metabolic defects, genetic predisposition, toxic exposure, or tumor infiltration. If the granulopoiesis is ineffective as occurs in Chédiak-Higashi syndrome, or due to nutritional deficiency from lack of B_{12} or folate, neutropenia can also occur. Increased destruction of PNMs can occur on an immune basis, giving rise to isoimmune or idiopathic immune neutropenia. Other underlying diseases, such as lupus, can also result in antibody formation directed against neutrophils. Certain drugs, such as the sulfa drugs, can also cross-react with and destroy neutrophils. Infections can result in neutropenia through both mechanisms noted above (i.e., decreased production and/or increased destruction of neutrophils). Endotoxins may deplete the reserve pool of PMNs in bone marrow via suppression of hematopoiesis, resulting in temporary or prolonged marrow failure, or there may be increased utilization of neutrophils to provide for excessive demargination of PMNs required for destroying infecting microbes.

Natural History

A description of some of the disorders associated with neutropenia follows.

Cyclic neutropenia represents a repetitive decrease in circulating PMNs usually accompanied by an associated monocytosis, with cycles lasting an average of 21 days (range of 14–24 days). Clinically, children may present with stomatitis and lymphadenitis. Some cases appear to be familial, believed to be on autosomal dominant basis, but others appear sporadically. No specific therapy has been reported although anecdotal case reports suggest that some patients may benefit from administration of steroids.

Reticular dysgenesis is a fatal disorder, secondary to failure of stem cells to differentiate into PMNs. In addition to abnormal myeloid precursors, patients show thymic hypoplasia, lymphopenia, and hypogammaglobulinemia.

Benign neutropenia comprises a heterogeneous group of disorders which have been reported to be genetically transmitted as well as sporadic in occurrence. PNM counts vary from 200–1500/mm^3, and hence, these patients usually have a benign course with occasional mild infections of skin and mucous membranes. It is possible that this disorder is due to abnormalities in the homeostatic mechanisms controlling mitosis of PMN precursors in the bone marrow. No treatment is usually necessary.

In *Kostmann disease* or severe congenital neutropenia, infants present at birth with PMN counts below 200/mm^3. These patients are susceptible to life-threatening infections. This type of neutropenia has been reported to be autosomal recessive in its genetic pattern, but sporadic cases have occurred also. Often bone marrow biopsies will show a maturation arrest at the promyelocyte level. Indeed bone marrow transplantation is the only therapeutic modality that has been anecdotally reported to be successful. Occasionally, this type of neutropenia may develop into acute myelogenous anemia.

A patient who develops neutropenia in association with metaphyseal chondrodysplasia, dwarfism, and/or pancreatic exocrine insufficiency, is likely to have *Shwachman-Diamond syndrome*. This is probably an autosomal recessive disorder, with PMN counts usually below 1000/mm^3, often associated with anemia and thrombocytopenia. Therapy is usually directed toward treating the malabsorption, although this does not improve the neutropenia. Notably these patients will have normal sweat tests in contrast to those with cystic fibrosis.

Chédiak-Higashi syndrome presents as an autosomal recessive disorder and, in addition to neutropenia, is associated with partial albinism, the presence of giant granules in the PMNs and other granule-containing cells, and frequent bacterial infections. The neutropenia is secondary to ineffective granulopoiesis, and it is most likely due to a defect in cellular membrane formation. Problems with chemotaxis, degranulation, and killing of bacteria have been resolved partially by administering ascorbic acid, but the neutropenia is not corrected.

Isoimmune neutropenia results from maternal sensitization to fetal neutrophil antigen during gestation, with placental crossing of an IgG directed against an infant's neutrophils. Usually by 7 weeks of age, based on the expected half-life of maternal IgG, neutrophil counts return to normal. Bone marrow examination reveals myeloid hyperplasia, but with depletion of mature neutrophil forms. These patients usually suffer from cutaneous infections and, more rarely, respiratory and urinary tract infections, or sepsis. Treatment for this disorder is mainly supportive, with administration of appropriate antibiotics. Rarely, infection appears to be life-threatening, transfusions with maternal neutrophils lacking the antigen to which the antibody is directed are given, or plasma exchange is performed to remove the maternal antibody.

Other patients may develop an autoimmune neutropenia on a nonisoimmune basis. Antibodies can be detected against neutrophil antigens. Physical examination may reveal slight to moderate splenomegaly and neutrophil counts, ranging from 0–1000/mm^3, which are associated with a monocytosis. Benign autoimmune neutropenia of childhood is a variation of this disorder, with the onset between 6 and 20 months of age, resolution in a year, and characterized by only mild infections. Occasionally, antineutrophil antibodies have been detected, and it is thought that the mechanism for this benign self-limited neutropenia has an immune basis. It is also possible that infections and/or toxic exposures can lead to neutropenia on an immune basis (Table 8.10; Weetman and Boxer, 1980). Other drugs, such as the phenothiazines, can cause direct marrow suppression, although complete recovery usually occurs if the offending agent is removed. Whether the mechanism by which drugs result in neutropenia represents an "innocent bystander" mechanism, or a drug-induced cell-mediated immune complex, similar to that seen for hemolytic anemias, is not clear.

Table 8.10
Infections and Drugs Associated with Neutropenia

Infections	Drugs
Bacterial	Antibacterial
Typhoid fever	Carbenicillin
Tuberculosis (disseminated)	Cephalosporins
Brucellosis	Chloramphenicol
Gram-negative sepsis	Penicillin (incl. semi-synthetic Pcns)
Viral	Sulfonilamides
Hepatitis	Vancomycin
Epstein-Barr	Antithyroid
Influenza	Propylthiouracil
Measles	Antirheumatic
Mumps	Gold
Rubella	Tranquilizing drugs
Roseola	Chlorpromazine
Varicella	Meprobamate
Polio	Promazine hydrochloride
Yellow fever	Antineoplastic agents
Psittacosis	Cyclophosphamide
Cytomegalovirus	Methotrexate
Rickettsial	6-Thioguanine
Rocky Mountain Spotted Fever	Cytosine arabinoside
Typhus	6-Mercaptopurine
Rickettsial pox	Adriamycin
Fungal	
Histoplasmosis	
Protozoal	
Malaria	
Leishmaniasis	

Diagnosis

In a patient with neutropenia from unclear causes, historical information should be obtained on possible exposure to drugs or toxins. Family history may also be useful pinpointing other family members with recurrent infections or, perhaps, even a history of low white blood cell counts. Neutropenia can be further suspected prior to obtaining the CBC, if lymphadenitis or hepatosplenomegaly are noted on physical examination. Serial white blood counts should be obtained once to twice weekly for 6–8 weeks to determine the pattern of chronicity of the neutropenia. On this basis, further laboratory tests may subsequently be ordered. If the patient is pancytopenic, a bone marrow examination is mandatory to decide whether an aplastic episode or an infiltrative process is occurring. Discontinuation of a medication followed by serial monitoring of white blood cell counts may be both diagnostic and therapeutic. Any evidence of growth failure or malabsorption should raise the possibility of an inherited disease associated with chronic neutropenia. If recurrent infections have been occurring, an immunoglobulin assay may be useful to rule out an agamma- or dysgammaglobulinemia. A nutritional assessment may be useful if folic acid, B_{12} or copper deficiency is suspected. Other autoimmune diseases can be evaluated by obtaining antinuclear antibodies or rheumatoid factor studies. If there is a history of recurrent infections or blood problems, other family members should have blood counts as well. Antineutrophil antibodies may be useful if autoimmune or isoimmune neutropenia is suspected. A complete listing of diagnostic tests available for the child with neutropenia appears in Table 8.11.

Treatment

If the absolute PMN count is ± 1000/mm^3 and the patient appears reasonably well, no therapy is indicated.

CONTROVERSY

Treatment is less clear-cut if the count is 500–1000/mm^3. Whether such patients could benefit from prophylactic antibiotics during this period remains controversial. A patient who develops a fever with a white

Table 8.11
Evaluation of the Child with Neutropenia[1]

Laboratory Analysis	Parameter Assessed	Associated Clinical Diagnosis
1. Serial absolute granulocyte determinations 2–3 times/week	Cycling of myelopoiesis Severity of persistent neutropenia	Cyclic neutropenia Chronic neutropenia
2. Bone marrow aspiration	Marrow cellularity and morphology Presence or absence of neutrophils and precursors Neutrophil maturation	Agranulocytosis Myeloid maturation arrest Megaloblastic or ineffective myelopoiesis Storage pool depletion
3. Hydrocortisone stimulation test Endotoxin stimulation test	Marrow granulocyte storage pool	Chronic neutropenia Chronic hereditary neutropenia Drug or toxin-induced hypoplasia Infection-induced hypoplasia Ineffective myelopoiesis Storage pool depletion secondary to increased peripheral utilization
4. Electronmicroscopy	Neutrophil subcellular morphology	Dysgranulopoiesis (congenital)
5. Colony-forming unit (CFUc) assay	Adequacy of myeloid committed stem cell compartment	Deficiency in CFUc Defective response to CSA Defective CFUc
6. Colony-stimulating activity (CSA) assay	Adequacy of CSA production	Lack of CSA Inhibitor of CSA effect Inhibition of CSA production
7. Antineutrophil antibody assay	Presence of neutrophil specific antibody	Autoimmune and isoimmune neutropenia
8. Rebuck skin window	Neutrophil mobilization	Agranulocytosis Chemotactic defects
9. ^{111}Indium survival	Neutrophil survival	Increased peripheral destruction Hypersplenism with sequestration
10. Antinuclear antibody determinations	Antibodies to nuclear components	Systemic lupus erythematosus Felty syndrome (rheumatoid arthritis, hypersplenism and neutropenia)
11. Serum copper	Nutritional copper status	Copper deficiency with neutropenia
12. Serum folate	Nutritional folate status	Folate deficiency with megaloblastic marrow
13. Serum vitamin B_{12}	Nutritional vitamin B_{12} status	Vitamin B_{12} deficiency with megaloblastic marrow
14. Exocrine pancreatic function	Overall nutritional status Adequacy of pancreatic enzymes from duodenal fluid	Shwachman-Diamond neutropenia
15. Serum muramidase	Serum muramidase levels	Increased mature neutrophil destruction Ineffective myelopoiesis
16. Serologic and culture screening for infection	Presence of active infection	Viral, bacterial, myobacterial or fungal infection
17. Immunologic evaluation	Quantitative immunoglobulins Skin test reactivity, including PPD Complement (C3; CH_{50}) T and B cell numbers Chemotactic assay Suppressor T cell assay	Hypogammaglobulinemia X-linked agammaglobulinemia Dysgammaglobulinemla types I and III Reticular dysgenesis Cartilage-hair hypoplasia Chemotactic defect with neutropenia

Table 8.11 (Continued)
Evaluation of the Child with Neutropenia[1]

Laboratory Analysis	Parameter Assessed	Associated Clinical Diagnosis
18. Sucrose hemolysis test	Sensitivity of erythrocyte membrane to complement activation	Paroxysmal nocturnal hemoglobinuria
19. Chromosome analysis	Chromosomal abnormalities	Fanconi syndrome
20. Radiographic bone survey	Bony abnormalities	Cartilage-hair hypoplasia Dyskeratosis congenita Fanconi syndrome Shwachman-Diamond syndrome Preleukemia
21. Plasma and urine amino acid screening	Amino acid abnormalities	Benign neutropenia Orotic aciduria: hyperglycinemia

[1]Reproduced with permission from Weetman RM, et al: *Pediatr Clin North Am* 27:361, 1980.

blood cell count below 500 PMNs/mm^3 requires broad spectrum antibiotics to protect against Gram-positive species, such as *Staphylococcus aureus,* as well as Gram-negative organisms, such as *Pseudomonas* species, which can occur in an immunosuppressed neutropenic patient. If the patient appears septic, granulocyte transfusions may also be useful. Steroids remain controversial as a treatment for the immunoneutropenias.

QUALITATIVE NEUTROPHIL DISORDERS

Definition

Qualitative neutrophil disorders are defined as conditions in which the neutrophils are present in appropriate numbers, but are unable to function normally. A child who has adequate numbers of circulating PMNs and normal or elevated levels of immunoglobulins and yet suffers from chronic and recurring bacterial or fungal infections should be suspected of having a qualitative neutrophil disorder.

Natural History

Patients who have defects in chemotaxis generally develop infections in sites that are constantly exposed to bacteria or fungi such as the cutaneous and subcutaneous tissues and their draining lymph nodes. Characteristic of these disorders are episodes of urticaria, icthyosis, atopic dermatitis, and chronic fungal infections. Patients may also suffer from chronic or recurrent otitis media, as well as chronic pneumonia and lung abscesses. *S. aureus* probably causes infection most frequently in these patients, although other organisms such as Gram-negative enterics and fungi also are frequent offenders. Patients who have recurrent severe staphylococcal abscesses as well as normal to elevated serum IgG levels with severe defects in neutrophil chemotaxis are referred to as having Job or hyper-IgE syndrome. It is believed that the histamine released from the mast cells triggered by the elevated levels of IgE hampers chemotaxis by raising the intracellular level of cyclic adenosine monophosphate.

Certain infectious organisms may themselves lead to less effective chemotaxis. For example, measles virus has been found to hamper chemotaxis as well as to suppress cellular immune responses. Burn patients have also been found to have limited chemotactic responsiveness, which is thought to be due to the thermal injury which releases granules within neutrophils that impair the ability of these neutrophils to respond to chemotactic stimuli. Poor chemotaxis may also occur with certain infections, hyperalimentation and malnutrition states, diabetes, Shwachman-Diamond syndrome, and in newborn infants. Deficiencies in complement factors C3A or C5A have been associated with chemotactic dysfunction in vitro. Serum inhibitors that act directly on the neutrophil and render it incapable of responding to chemotactic stimuli also may exist (Baehner, 1980).

If there is impaired opsonization of bacteria, life-threatening infections are often likely to occur, particularly those caused by encapsulated organisms, *S. aureus,* and enteric bacteria. The mechanism for impaired opsonization is thought to involve deficiencies in immunoglobulin and complement. For example, patients with sickle cell disease are believed to be defective in generation of the opsonizing C3 component through the alternative pathway of complement. In addition, it is possible that some patients have a rare disorder in which there is an actin dysfunction in the cell membrane preventing ingestion of an opsonized microbe.

One of the more common qualitative neutrophil disorders is an abnormality of degranulation referred to as the Chédiak-Higashi syndrome. It is an autosomal recessive disorder and is associated with partial oculocutaneous albinism, frequent pyrogenic infections and bleeding tendency, and abnormally large granules in peripheral neutrophils and other tissue cells that contain lysosomes. As patients get older, a lymphocytic and histiocytic infiltrate of lymphoreticular organs occurs, resulting in pancytopenia, lymphadenopathy, and hepatosplenomegaly. Most of the clinical signs of the disease are thought to be due to abnormal fusion of lysosomes to form giant lysosomes within cells. Hence, albinism results from the abnormal distribution of lysosomal melanin within retinal and skin cells. Skin, gastrointestinal, and respiratory infections are common when the underlying defect is a failure to transfer lysosomal content into phagocytic vacuoles, producing the large granules visible under the microscope. The more common organisms causing infection in Chédiak-Higashi syndrome are *Streptococcus pneumoniae* and *Haemophilus influenzae*.

In addition to degranulation, neutropenia can occur. Defects in chemotaxis are also common in Chédiak-Higashi syndrome. The chemotaxis problem results from an abnormality of the microtubule membrane-dependent function of the neutrophil.

Chronic granulomatous disease, an X-linked disorder, is the best known example of defective killing of organisms by neutrophils (see Section 16). Usually signs and symptoms of this disease develop within the first 2 years of life and initially present as recurrent infections, particularly of the skin or lymph node system. Subcutaneous abscesses in draining lymph nodes are common, as are pneumonia and lung abscesses as the disease progresses. An association is noted between antral obstruction of the stomach and chronic granulomatous disease.

The X-linked gene for chronic granulomatous disease has been identified, the carrier state can be detected in mothers, and antenatal diagnosis is possible. Diagnosis is made by specific examination of fetal DNA or the more classical nitroblue tetrazolium test. In this test neutrophils are stimulated in the presence of nitroblue tetrazolium to produce the superoxide anion which precipitates in the cell (see also pp. 1004).

The most likely offending organisms are catalase-positive organisms, fungus, although occasionally a catalase-negative organism such as streptococcus is at fault.

Diagnosis

The most useful diagnostic indicator for whether to pursue a work-up for qualitative neutrophil disorders is the frequency and nature of infections in the patient. For example, patients with defects in chemotaxis will usually have purulent infections confined to the skin, subcutaneous tissue or draining lymph nodes, and may occasionally develop upper respiratory infections, otitis media, pneumonia, and lung abscesses. Patients who have defects in opsonization, on the other hand, are likely to have more serious infections including sepsis, meningitis, and pneumonia from a wide variety of bacterial organisms. Patients with chronic granulomatous disease will rarely show infections from *H. influenzae, Pneumococcus, Streptococcus,* and *Meningococcus,* and the catalase-positive organisms are the usual offenders. A peripheral smear should be examined for morphologic abnormalities such as those seen in Chédiak-Higashi syndrome. If a neutrophil dysfunction is considered, selective laboratory tests are available for detection of the specific function. A hematologist can be consulted to decide on the most appropriate tests to detect the disorder.

Treatment

Treatment in Chédiak-Higashi syndrome is largely directed toward the specific infection, although bone marrow transplant is ultimately the treatment of choice. Treatment for chronic granulomatosis disease also consists of antibiotics appropriate for the infection. In severe life-threatening infections, infusions of neutrophils may be useful. The use of prophylactic trimetheprim-sulfamethoxosole or dicloxacillin has reduced the occurrence of infections in patients with this disorder. There are case reports of successful cure following bone marrow transplantation. Subcutaneous administration of γ-interferon has been effective in reversing the defect in catalase production in a few patients. It is presumed to affect a progenitor cell and subsequent generations of neutrophils, with a duration of effect of about 1 month (Orkin et al, 1988, personal communication).

REFERENCES

Babior BM: Oxygen-dependent microbial killing by phagocytes. *N Engl J Med* 298:659, 1978.

Baehner RL: Neutrophil dysfunction associated with states of chronic and recurrent infection. *Pediatr Clin North Am* 27:377, 1980.

Crowley CA, Curnutte JT, Rosin RE, et al: An inherited abnormality of neutrophil adhesion: Its genetic transmission and its association with a missing protein. *N Engl J Med* 302:1163, 1980.

Curnutte JT, Boxer LA: Disorders of granulopoiesis and granulocyte function. In Nathan DG, Oski FA (eds): *Hematology of Infancy and Childhood,* 3rd edition. Philadelphia, WB Saunders, 1987, p. 797.

Oski FA: Effective or low white blood cell count in children and adults. *Consultant* p. 93, January 1983.

Sadowitz PD, Oski FA: Differences in polymorphonuclear cell counts between healthy white and black infants: Response to meningitis. *Pediatrics* 72:405, 1983.

Stockman JA: Disorders of leukocytes. In Oski FA, Naiman JL, Stockman JA, et al (eds): *Hematologic Problems in the Newborn,* 3rd edition. Philadelphia, WB Saunders, 1982.

Weetman RM, Boxer LA: Childhood neutropenia. *Pediatr Clin North Am* 27:361, 1980.

Bleeding Disorders

4

APPROACH TO THE CHILD WITH BLEEDING DISORDERS

Definition

Spontaneous bleeding occurs in the absence of adequate hemostasis. Abnormalities in platelet or clotting factors can prevent hemostasis. The end result of any of these defects is hemorrhage.

Basic Science

Hemostasis is dependent upon four factors: (1) normal structure, resistance, and contractility of blood vessels; (2) normal platelet activity in terms of quantitative and qualitative functions; (3) an adequate coagulation system; and (4) clot stability. In order to understand the diagnostic tests needed to identify a bleeding disorder it is important to review the basic science of hemostasis.

Primary hemostasis occurs initially as a platelet-vessel interaction. When the vessel wall is damaged, there is usually a release of endothelial contents, including von Willebrand factor which serves as a platelet bridge, such that with exposure of subendothelium, platelets adhere to the vessel wall and then release adenosine diphosphate (ADP), allowing other platelets to aggregate. Following platelet aggregation, contractile proteins within platelets undergo contraction forming the primary hemostatic plug. Therefore, a variety of defects can occur in this phase of hemostasis, including failure of platelets to adhere to damaged tissue, failure of the platelets to release ADP and aggregate, or failure of the platelets to contract.

Disorders that have been associated with defects in platelet-vessel interaction include the hereditary thrombocytopenias (e.g., Bernard-Soulier), and von Willebrand disease in which a decreased von Willebrand factor cannot serve as the bridge for agglutination of platelets adherent to endothelial cells on vessel walls. The acquired thrombocytopenias can result in an insufficient number of platelets to supply adequate hemostasis. Aspirin can also inhibit platelet function and result in delayed defective secondary platelet aggregation.

The secondary phase of hemostasis is the activation of the coagulation system either through the intrinsic or extrinsic pathways illustrated in Figures 8.5 and 8.6. A variety of factor deficiencies in either of these pathways can result.

Epidemiology

See specific disorder.

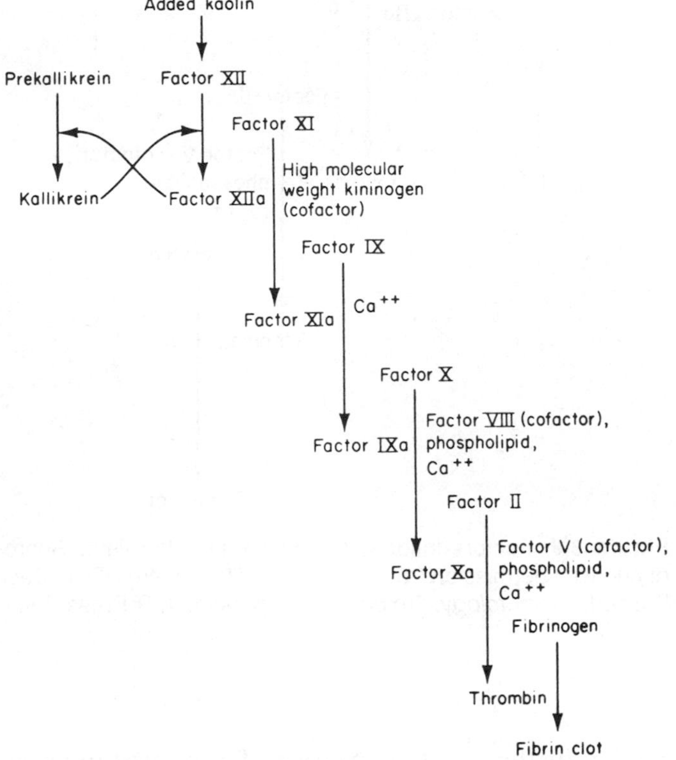

Figure 8.5. Factors influencing partial thromboplastin time. Reproduced with permission from Handin RJ, Rosenberg RD: In Beck WS (ed): *Hematology,* 3rd edition. Cambridge, MIT Press, 1981, p. 428.

Natural History

The history and physical examination may reveal whether bleeding is secondary to a coagulopathy or vascular and platelet abnormality. For example, petechiae and purpura are common findings in a vascular or platelet abnormality, as are superficial small multiple ecchymoses. On the other hand, large solitary ecchymoses or deep hematomas and hemarthroses are more characteristic of a coagulopathy. Moreover, epistaxis, menorrhagia, and GI bleeding, are seen more frequently with platelet disorders. Episodes of delayed onset bleeding after surgery or venipuncture, hematuria, or the presence of a positive family history are more consistent with a coagulopathy.

Diagnosis

In addition to obtaining a careful history and physical examination to identify the type of bleeding, useful information includes a detailed family history, a med-

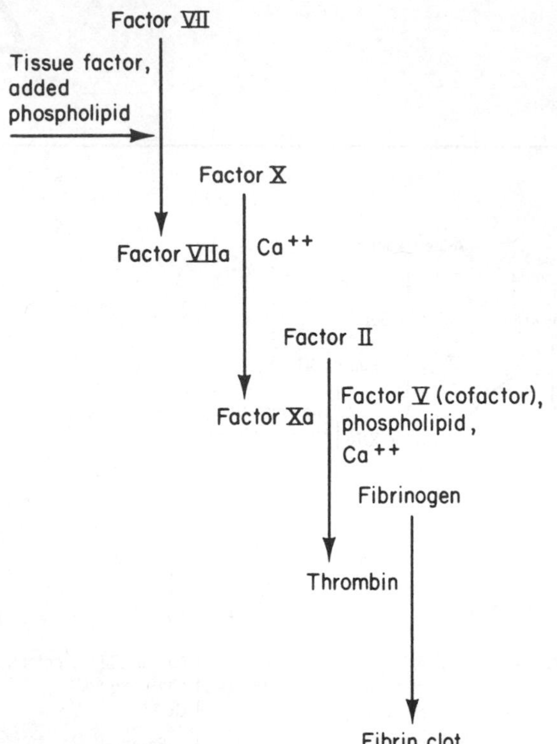

Figure 8.6. Factors influencing the prothrombin time. Reproduced with permission from Handin RJ, Rosenberg RD: In Beck WS (ed): *Hematology,* 3rd edition. Cambridge, MIT Press, 1981, p. 429.

ication history, and description of responses to everyday bleeding challenges. On the basis of this information, it should be possible to determine whether the defect most likely rests with vessel wall, platelets, or a coagulation abnormality. To confirm the suspicion, the following screening laboratory tests should be performed: a platelet count, a partial thromboplastin time (PTT), and a prothrombin time (PT). A bleeding time may also be useful in helping to identify a qualitative platelet defect, although there is great variation in how this particular test is performed and a lack of reliability. The peripheral smear can also be useful. Table 8.12 illustrates the differential diagnosis and approach to diagnosing a variety of bleeding disorders.

A second series of diagnostic tests should follow these screening tests if an abnormality is detected. For example, if the PTT is prolonged, a specific factor assay is usually necessary to identify the specific disorder. On the other hand, if only the bleeding time is prolonged, platelet function tests to determine the qualitative platelet disorder should be done. If platelet numbers are decreased, a bone marrow examination or antiplatelet antibodies might be assayed to determine the cause.

Treatment

See specific disorders.

Table 8.12
Differential Diagnosis of Bleeding by Screening Tests[1]

	Pl no.	PTT	PT	BT
Vascular abnormality	Nl	Nl	Nl	↑
Thrombocytopenia	↓	Nl	Nl	↑
Deficiency of Factors XII, XI, VIII, IX	Nl	↑	Nl	Nl
Deficiency of Factor VII	Nl	Nl	↑	Nl
Von Willebrand disease or qualitative platelet disorder	Nl, ↑, ↓	↑ in von Willebrand disease	Nl	↑
Deficiency of Factors X, V, II	Nl	↑	↑	Nl
Liver disease, DIC	Nl or ↓	Nl or ↑	↑	↑
Factor XIII deficiency	Nl	Nl	Nl	Nl

[1]Abbreviations: Pl no., platelet number; PTT, partial thromboplastin time; PT, prothrombin time; BT, bleeding time, Nl; normal.

THROMBOCYTOPENIA

Definition

Thrombocytopenia describes disorders in which there is a decrease in the quantity of circulating platelets in the blood stream. It can lead to abnormalities in coagulation and subsequently to hemorrhage.

Basic Science

Thrombocytopenia results from three different pathophysiologic mechanisms: (1) abnormalities in production of platelets; (2) abnormalities in distribution of platelets once produced; or (3) increased destruction of platelets. Decreased production can result from a hypoproliferative state such as would occur with damage to the bone marrow, either due to a congenital disorder, infections, or toxic exposure; theoretically, it could stem from a deficiency in thrombopoietin, which is thought to be a regulatory factor in the production of platelets or, indeed, from defects in other steps in the production cycle, or through marrow infiltration such as secondary to a tumor or storage disease.

Abnormal distribution can occur if the spleen sequesters a large number of platelets, resulting in a functional thrombocytopenia. Hypothermia has also been associated with abnormal distribution of platelets.

Increased destruction can result from overconsumption of platelets, via conditions such as disseminated intravascular coagulation, vasculitic conditions such as hemolytic uremic syndrome, the presence of prosthetic devices which can shear or consume platelets, through some inherited diseases, or through immune mediated mechanisms including isoimmune and idiopathic thrombocytopenic purpura (discussed in the next chapter).

CASE ILLUSTRATION

A 7-year-old black female began to complain of pain under one of her multiple thin tight hair braids. Over the course of the day the pain increased and the area became swollen and tender. The next day the scalp on that side was full, firm, and fluctuant. By the following day, the subcutaneous fluctuance extended to the other side of the head and on the following morning the entire scalp and forehead were distended, firm, and fluctuant. She was admitted to her local hospital where a CT scan demonstrated a large accumulation of subgaleal, although not intracranial, blood. Because a subgaleal hemorrhage is rarely seen outside of the neonatal period, a hematologic work-up was begun to see if there was a bleeding diathesis. Her hematocrit was 35%, PT and PTT were normal, platelet count was 250,000/mm^3, but the bleeding time was 15 minutes, significantly prolonged.

QUESTION AND COMMENT

What is the cause of this patient's bleeding disorder? What further diagnostic tests are necessary?

To sort out the pathogenesis of the coagulation disorder, a Factor VIII level was measured initially and was normal. Nonetheless, von Willebrand disease was considered since cases have been reported with normal PTT but long bleeding time. Following administration of cryoprecipitate, however, the bleeding time remained abnormal. The hematocrit dropped to 21%. On the third hospital day, the girl complained of pain behind her right eye and within an hour the eye had become extremely proptotic, chemotic, and showed severe limitation of extraocular movements. Examination of the right eye showed a flat optic disc, but venous engorgement, suggesting obstruction to venous outflow. Vision in the right eye was limited to only gross hand movements. In addition, the right pupil appeared "deafferented" i.e., constricted essentially to light on the left eye (suggesting an intact right third nerve motor response) but neither responded to direct light nor elicited consensual constriction on the left (a Marcus-Gunn pupil). A repeat head CT showed that the subgaleal blood had somehow eroded the periostium allowing it to stream into the apex of the orbit and cover the top of the globe. Immediate open drainage was clearly indicated. This was performed and successfully restored most of her vision.

With respect to the coagulation disorder, careful past medical history revealed that she had had hemostatic problems during an umbilical hernia repair as an infant. In addition, during the present episode the mother reported giving her aspirin for 3 days after the initial galeal bleeding, but before the eye involvement. Repeat laboratory values 3 days into her course for PT, PTT, and platelets were again normal with the hematocrit stabilizing at 20%, and at this stage, after 3–4 days without aspirin, the bleeding time was now normal at 5 minutes.

It is unlikely that this child's coagulation difficulties rested in the clotting cascade since her PT and PTT values were normal. Factor XIII at the terminus of the cascade necessary for fibrin clot stabilization is the only factor not measured by the PT or PTT, but such a deficiency is extremely rare and not characterized by an increased bleeding time. A defect in platelet subendothelial adhesion due to deficiency of von Willebrand factor is unlikely, given the normal PTT and Factor VIII level and a failure of cryoprecipitate to correct the bleeding time. That there was a primary defect in platelets themselves in the subendothelium is unlikely since the bleeding time corrected spontaneously.

The story, however, is consistent with secondary platelet dysfunction due to aspirin. The stress of hemorrhage requiring replacement by new, nonpoisoned platelets would result in a corrected bleeding time, and this may provide a partial explanation. Nonetheless, the initial subgaleal bleeding could still have resulted from subclinical deficiencies of certain factors (e.g., IX and XI) or primary platelet defect exacerbated by aspirin (e.g., a cyclooxygenase defect). She was, therefore, treated with fresh-frozen plasma, platelets, and transfusion with red blood cells prior to undergoing the surgical drainage necessary to restore most of her vision.

Natural History

The thrombocytopenic disorders occurring in the newborn period are discussed in Section 4, Neonatology. There are a variety of genetic familial forms of thrombocytopenia, most of which result in decreased production of platelets or production of defective platelets that have a decreased survival time in the circulation. Among these are Wiskott-Aldrich syndrome, an X-linked recessive disease in which the patient demonstrates thrombocytopenia, eczema, and recurrent infections. Patients with this disorder have small platelets which is believed to be secondary to membrane abnormalities of the megakaryocytes from which they are derived. Treatment for this disorder is bone marrow transplantation.

Bernard-Soulier syndrome is an autosomal recessive disease in which patients have a moderate to severe bleeding tendency associated with qualitative as well as quantitative platelet abnormalities. The May-Hegglin anomaly is an autosomal dominant disease and is characterized by the appearance of giant, often vacuolated, platelets in the peripheral blood smear. These patients generally have no bleeding tendencies.

Thrombocytopenia can occur in association with other exogenous events. For example, certain drugs and toxins can result in thrombocytopenia via a variety of mechanisms, some involving decreased production, although the majority involve immune mediated mechanisms of destruction. Thrombocytopenia also is associated with some of the microangiopathic diseases including hemolytic uremic syndrome, thrombotic thrombocytopenic purpura, and disseminated intravascular coagulation. Artificial heart valves have also been found to result in microangiopathic hemolytic anemias and thrombocytopenia due to the "Waring blender" syndrome or the shearing effect of platelets and red blood cells passing through the artificial valve. Patients with splenomegaly may demonstrate thrombocytopenia due to the increased pooling of platelets in the spleen. Certain infectious organisms have been associated with the disease, in particular meningococcemia, with subsequent microangiopathic changes as a result of disseminated intravascular coagulation. Some of the autoimmune disorders, including lupus, other collagen vascular diseases or even hyperthyroidism have been associated with thrombocytopenia. At other times thrombocytopenia has been the initial presentation heralding some of these immune disorders especially pediatric AIDS. Finally, infiltrative malignant diseases, as well as generalized marrow hypoplasia may initially present as thrombocytopenia.

A platelet count greater than 50,000/mm^3 is rarely associated with bleeding, whereas patients with values between 20,000 and 50,000 may develop some increased bruising with minor trauma. It is not until the platelet count is less than 20,000/mm^3 that spontaneous bruising regularly occurs. Risk of internal bleeding or cerebral bleeding is not greatly elevated until the platelet count is less than 20,000/mm^3.

Diagnosis

The diagnosis should be suspected in any patient who presents with spontaneous bleeding in the form of pinpoint hemorrhages known as petechiae or large unexplained bruises or ecchymoses scattered over the body. Trauma or vascular disorders such as Henoch-Schönlein purpura and qualitative platelet defects should also be considered in the differential diagnosis of bruising. Rarely do thrombocytopenic children present with large scale GI or CNS hemorrhages. A baseline laboratory evaluation should include a CBC, platelet count, PT, PTT, and examination of peripheral blood smear. Larger platelets on the peripheral blood smear may indicate the presence of younger platelets and may raise suggestion of active thrombopoiesis secondary to increased destruction of platelets. If the thrombocytopenia is severe enough to warrant treatment with steroids, a bone marrow examination should be performed since steroids may mask an infiltrative disorder, such as leukemia.

Treatment

See specific disorders for appropriate treatment. In general, only if there is significant evidence of ongoing bleeding is a platelet transfusion necessary. If there is evidence of hypersplenism, associated with transfusion dependency, splenectomy should be considered.

IDIOPATHIC THROMBOCYTOPENIC PURPURA

Definition

Idiopathic thrombocytopenic purpura is a quantitative platelet disorder in which a decreased peripheral platelet count occurs secondary to presumably immune-mediated early destruction of circulating platelets. If the disorder persists beyond 6 months after initial presentation, it is referred to as chronic, as opposed to acute idiopathic thrombocytopenic purpura.

Basic Science

Both acute and chronic idiopathic thrombocytopenic purpura are thought to result from the formation of an IgG directed against antigens on the platelet membrane. The specific cause for the formation of these antibodies is unknown. It appears that a proportion of antibodies directed against platelets is manufactured in the spleen. Regardless of the precipitating factor, the Fc portion of the bound IgG molecule apparently plays the key role in the eventual destruction of the platelet. Inhibiting or blocking the Fc receptor on reticuloendothelial cells as discussed under treatment is one mechanism by which these platelets may be prevented from being destroyed.

Thrombokinetic studies in patients with idiopathic thrombocytopenia purpura confirm the fact that megakaryopoiesis as well as platelet turnover are increased to as much as eight times normal. Platelet size and mean platelet diameter are increased, suggesting that a younger population of platelets is circulating during the course of the disease.

The antibody that is produced is usually nonspecifically directed against the platelet membrane at least in the initial phase of the disease, whereas in the chronic form of the disease the antibody is specifically directed against a platelet membrane glycoprotein. The main mechanism of clearance of platelets is through splenic macrophages and other cells in the reticuloendothelial system.

Epidemiology

Acute idiopathic thrombocytopenia purpura usually occurs in children below 10 years of age, whereas the chronic form is more common in older children. The male to female ratio is equal for the acute form, whereas it is 1:3 in the chronic form. Of all cases of the disorder in children, 85–90% are of the acute form. Annual incidence of symptomatic idiopathic thrombocytopenia purpura is 4/100,000 children (Shende, 1985).

Natural History

The most serious risk of bleeding in idiopathic thrombocytopenia purpura occurs when platelet counts are less than 20,000/mm^3. Patients presenting with the acute form usually give a history of preceding viral illness several weeks before the onset of the thrombocytopenia, whereas those patients with the chronic form will usually have a more insidious onset of their bleeding, although an intercurrent viral infection can reduce their platelet counts dramatically. Only one-third of the patients with the acute disorder will develop more severe bleeding episodes such as epistaxis, melena, and/or gross hematuria. Intracranial hemorrhage, which develops in 2% of patients, does not appear to depend on the age of patient or duration of thrombocytopenia (Shende, 1985). Usually, petechiae and ecchymoses are observed in an otherwise healthy child following a viral illness.

Diagnosis

The peripheral blood smear will show few if any platelets, and those that do appear will often be increased in size, suggesting that they are newly formed. It is important that other associated diseases or familial causes of thrombocytopenia are eliminated before the diagnosis is confirmed. This requires a bone marrow aspirate and biopsy, which should be obtained before any treatment is started. A bone marrow will usually show normal or increased numbers of megakaryocytes. Platelet kinetic studies, although not mandatory, will demonstrate reduced intravascular platelet survival and high turnover rates. While the diagnosis is being made, other underlying causes or possible precipitants of thrombocytopenia may be excluded by performing other immune studies, including HIV antibody, antinuclear antibodies, rheumatoid factor, direct and indirect Coombs test for immune mechanisms destroying the red cell line (as in Evans syndrome), and viral studies to detect a possible infectious cause.

A number of techniques will measure the presence of IgG on washed platelets from patients with this disease. At least three-quarters of patients will show elevated levels of platelet-associated IgG, although the specificity of this test is less than 50%, since other immune thrombocytopenic disorders will also be characterized by measurable platelet-associated IgG.

Treatment

The use of corticosteroids for treatment of acute idiopathic thrombocytopenia purpura is controversial. Nevertheless, a cooperative, randomized, double-blind study from Switzerland and southern Germany revealed that 90% of steroid-treated patients had attained a platelet count of 30,000/mm^3 within the first 10 days of treatment compared with only 45% of patients who were untreated. Furthermore, platelet counts of 100,000 were reached in 80% of steroid-treated patients by day 15, as compared with 30% of untreated patients (Sartorius, 1984).

At present, the current recommendation is not to withhold corticosteroid therapy from children with this disorder who present with thrombocytopenia and platelet counts under 30,000/mm^3 (Sartorius, 1984). In the study, serious complications of side effects of steroids were not encountered and, hence, the benefits outweighed the risks.

It is believed that corticosteroids inhibit removal of sensitized platelets by the reticuloendothelial system. The usual dosage is 1–2 mg/kg/day for 1 week, with a gradual taper and reduction by 0.5 mg/kg/week over a period of 2–4 weeks. Doses of prednisone are tapered regardless of platelet counts. If the platelet count again falls to less than 30,000/mm^3, a 2- to 4-week course of prednisone is repeated.

A number of reports document the efficacy of high-dose intravenous γ-globulin for treatment of chronic ITP. Intravenous γ-globulin is thought to provide a blockade of Fc receptors of the reticuloendothelial system, such that the rate of destruction of antibody-coated platelets is decreased. The usual dose is 400 mg/kg/day for 5 consecutive days. It is considered an alternative to splenectomy in these patients. Moreover, this treatment has also been found to be effective for some children who did not respond to splenectomy, permitting them to be weaned off immunosuppressant drugs. The use of intravenous γ-globulin in the acute form of the disease remains controversial and no controlled trials have been reported. It appears, however, that the effect of intravenous γ-globulin is transient and that it may be most useful around the time of surgical procedures or the splenectomy itself. Nevertheless, it has been successful in some children with the acute disorder (Warrier and Lusher, 1984).

Women with idiopathic thrombocytopenia who have problems with prolonged menstruation benefit from hormonal therapy to stop menstruation.

Platelet transfusions are rarely useful except when life-threatening bleeding occurs, since their half-life is quite short in patients with idiopathic thrombocytopenic purpura.

Splenectomy is reserved for special situations. These would include a life-threatening hemorrhage such as a cerebral or GI hemorrhage unresponsive to steroids and intravenous IgG. It is also indicated for patients who continue to have platelet counts less than 50,000/mm^3 for a year following diagnosis, despite adequate trials of corticosteroids or intravenous γ-globulin. Patients who undergo splenectomy should be given pneumococcal and meningococcal vaccines before the procedure so that they can mount an adequate immune response. Prophylactic penicillin is then maintained after the operation. These patients should be monitored for the onset of any febrile illness at which time parenteral antibiotics should be administered. Splenectomy is a successful treatment of chronic idiopathic thrombocytopenia purpura in 75% of patients, although 10–15% of patients will fail to achieve a remission and will remain thrombocytopenic (Russell and Maurer, 1984).

Splenectomy is advocated because the spleen remains one of the major sites responsible not only for destroying platelets but for production of the antiplatelet antibody. It is recommended that splenectomy be avoided in children under 2 years of age, because of the high risk of infection, but this may have to be weighed against the life-threatening hemorrhages that complicate the course in such children.

Danazol (an attenuated androgen) is frequently effective in patients who have failed to respond to splenectomy. In patients who fail to improve with Danazol, cyclophosphamide, vincristine, and other immunosuppressive chemotherapeutic agents are sometimes helpful (Ahn et al, 1983).

Prognosis

Spontaneous recovery occurs in 80–95% of patients with acute idiopathic thrombocytopenic purpura within 4 months (Shende, 1985). Moreover, only 10–15% of patients with the chronic form will fail to achieve permanent remission and will remain thrombocytopenic.

HEMOPHILIA

Definition

Hemophilia is a collective name for blood coagulation disorders secondary to deficiencies of either Factor VIII or Factor IX. Factor VIII deficiency is sometimes referred to as hemophilia A, whereas Factor IX deficiency is hemophilia B or Christmas' disease. Both hemophilia A and B are X-linked bleeding disorders.

Basic Science

Factors VIII and IX are plasma proteins found in the intrinsic pathway for blood coagulation and are necessary for the production of an insoluble fibrin clot when there is vascular injury. Factor VIII is a complex high molecular weight glycoprotein needed as a cofactor in the reaction in which Factor X is activated so that it can serve as a cofactor in the formation of thrombin from prothrombin. Factor VIII is synthesized in the liver and endothelial cells. Factor IX activates Factor X in the presence of Factors VIII, calcium, and platelets. If Factors VIII or IX are present in concentrations less than 20–30% of normal, a fibrin clot cannot be formed, resulting in a prolonged PTT, which results in the hemorrhagic manifestations in joints and muscles, and in subcutaneous sites. In patients with hemophilia it is possible to measure Factor VIII-related antigen, suggesting that the defect is not due to decreased production, but rather is the result of qualitative defects in its clotting function. On the other hand, if the Factor VIII antigen level is decreased, suggesting a quantitative abnormality, the patient is likely to have von Willebrand disease. A gene responsible for Factor VIII has been cloned, allowing the protein to be made by means of genetic engineering. Factor IX has also recently been cloned, although neither synthetic VIII nor IX is commercially available as of 1987 (see Section 13, Genetics, pp. 777).

Epidemiology

The overall prevalence of hemophilia is 20/100,000 males or 1/10,000 of the entire population. Factor VIII deficiency has been associated with 80–85% of cases of hemophilia, with the remainder accounted for by a Factor IX deficiency. The incidence is similar among all races worldwide (Karayalcin, 1985). Family history will be negative in one-third of cases. There is a high mutation rate for this disease.

Natural History

Clinical manifestations of Factor VIII and IX deficiency are essentially indistinguishable and, therefore, will be discussed together. Usually, patients are described as having severe, moderate, or mild hemophilia.

Severe hemophilia describes those patients whose factor levels of VIII or IX are less than 1% of those found in normal plasma. They represent two-thirds of the patients with hemophilia A and half of those with hemophilia B. Severe hemophilia is associated with recurrent or spontaneously occurring hemorrhages and will usually follow the most minor trauma. It is often diagnosed initially by prolonged bleeding after a circumcision. CNS hemorrhage is rare during the newborn period, although a few cases have been reported. Usually in severe cases subcutaneous bruising and ecchymoses will appear by 3–4 months of age, and certainly will be evident at 1 year of age when the child begins to walk. Large hematomas may follow intramuscular injections. Small lacerations may be followed by bleeding that persists for days, particularly in the oral mucosa. Musculoskeletal bleeding and hemarthroses begin to manifest themselves by 3–4 years of age, by which time diagnosis usually has been made, although musculoskeletal hemorrhages predominate in midchildhood and adolescence. It is only in adulthood that renal and GI bleeding present.

Patients with moderate hemophilia usually have 1–5% of the normal levels of factor. Although they may occasionally have a spontaneous hemorrhage, gross bleeding is more likely to follow some form of mild to moderate trauma.

Patients with mild hemophilia usually have 5–25% of the normal levels of factor and do not give evidence of hemorrhage unless there is moderate to severe trauma. Mild hemophilia may not be diagnosed until late childhood, adolescence, or even adulthood. Patients may only be identified by a slightly prolonged PTT on a routine examination obtained at the time of elective surgery. A high-risk female carrier usually will have 30–50% the normal level of Factor and may only manifest hemorrhage during gynecologic or obstetrical procedures.

Hemarthroses are common in the severe and moderate types of hemophilia and usually involve the knees, elbows, ankles, shoulders, hips, and wrists in descending order of frequency. Every time a hemarthrosis occurs inflammatory and hypertrophic changes result in the joint, which will eventually contribute to the erosion of cartilage and bone. Moreover, chronic synovitis may occur due to highly vascularized tissue at or near the joint surface and increase the possibility of repeated hemorrhage in the area. Thus, a vicious cycle can be set up which leads to repeated destruction of cartilage, resorption of bone, and eventually formation of bone cysts communicating with the joint space. The joint becomes less stable, leading to more frequent hemorrhages, not only in the joint itself but in the neighboring musculoskeletal areas as well. Eventually bony ankylosis of large joints can occur, and complete destruction of smaller joints may result, due to the thinner cortices of the smaller bones.

Other complications of the disease include intracranial bleeding (one of the most common causes of death before the availability of factor infusion), retropharyngeal or retroperitoneal bleeding, and bleeding into the vertebral canal. External compression or traction on the nerve from hemorrhage around the nerve area after intramuscular hemorrhage frequently leads to peripheral nerve lesions. The femoral nerve is most commonly involved following documented trauma to the area.

Five to 10% of patients with hemophilia A and about 3% of patients with hemophilia B will develop antibodies directed against the functional activity of factors. These are usually IgG immunoglobulins that destroy their own factor activity, and that of any infused factor concentrates as well. The antibodies or "inhibitors" bind to and inactivate the coagulant site on Factor VIII or IX. Notably, the incidence of severe bleeding in patients who have inhibitors is not increased. Two-thirds of patients will tend to mount an elevated response so that the titer is increased with each factor infusion, whereas other patients are referred to as "low responders" based on a chronically low antibody titer that rises only slightly after exposure to factor (Karayalcin, 1985).

Diagnosis

Hemophilia should be expected if there is a family history of prolonged bleeding. Laboratory studies are most useful for definitive diagnosis. PTT will be elevated, but definitive diagnosis rests with factor assays.

While a male child with hemophilia will have reduced levels of Factor VIII or IX, female carriers are much more difficult to detect since there is a wide range of normal levels for Factor VIII levels. Moreover, Factor levels can increase with exercise or pregnancy such that measurement of a Factor VIII level alone does not permit accurate diagnosis of the carrier state. Use of an antibody to Factor VIII, however, has helped greatly in the detection of carriers. One can detect for example that in noncarrier (normal) women, levels of Factor VIII coagulant activity are proportional to the concentration of Factor VIII-related antigen, whereas in carriers the Factor VIII antigen levels are normal whereas there is less Factor VIII coagulant activity able to be detected.

Carriers of Factor IX disease can be distinguished from normal women by use of the coagulant activity assay since 60% of these women will have less than 50% Factor IX activity as compared to normal women—a much greater gap than that found for carriers of Factor VIII (Panicucci et al, 1980).

Prenatal diagnosis is possible by the 12th to 14th week of pregnancy.

Treatment

Replacement of factor is currently the first line of treatment for management of hemorrhage in a hemophiliac. Cryoprecipitate is a protein that precipitates in fresh-frozen plasma that is thawed at 4°C and is rich in Factors VIII, fibrinogen, and Factor XIII. Blood banks capable of component fractionation will store cryoprecipitate at −20°C until it is needed; the advantage of this method is that it can concentrate Factor VIII 10-fold in 10 ml of plasma and results in 50–150% of Factor VIII being recovered from donor plasma. Since it is a single donor component it theoretically carries less risk for hepatitis and AIDS, although the fact that cryoprecipitate is heat-labile has made this an unfavorable therapy for hemophilia A, and does not allow for it to be easily administered at home.

Heat-treated lyopholized factor preparations, on the other hand, are the mainstay of home and often hospital therapy. Eighty-five percent of biologic activity is preserved in these factor preparations, and the heat-treatment lowers the risk of contracting AIDS. Factor IX concentrates also contain Factors II, VII, and X and have the same advantages as the Factor VIII concentrates.

The mainstay of hemophilia therapy is infusion of factor first if there is any suspicion of trauma or possible hemorrhage, followed by the diagnostic work-up to determine the precise nature of the injury. The dose of Factor VIII or IX for replacement depends on the severity of the bleeding that has ensued, although normally at least 20–30% normal factor activity is needed for normal hemostasis. Of note, Factor VIII has a half-life of 12 hours and Factor IX of 24 hours. Furthermore, 1 unit/kg of Factor VIII will increase the Factor VIII level 2%, whereas 1 unit/kg of Factor IX will only increase the Factor IX level by 1%. Despite its biologic half-life, at least half of Factor VIII will have disappeared by 4–8 hours, based on serologic detection, and Factor IX within 4–6 hours despite its longer biologic half-life.

An uncomplicated spontaneous hemorrhage into joint or muscle space usually requires an increase of at least 20% in the factor level or 20–25 units/kg. If the patient has hematoma in a more proximal joint (e.g., hip, knee, shoulder, elbow) or is undergoing dental extractions or elective surgery, factor levels of at least 25–50% are required. Patients who have undergone major multiple trauma, potential CNS bleeding, or major surgery, require factor levels of at least 100%. Once factor has been infused, analgesics can be used to help treat the pain of the hemarthrosis.

DDAVP (1-desamino-8-D-arginine-vasopressin acetate trihydrate) a synthetic analog of vasopressin has been shown to cause a marked increase in Factor VIII activity in patients with mild to moderate hemophilia over a brief period of time and is a useful adjunct to therapy for patients who require only one or few infusions for bleeding (Mannucci et al, 1981).

With chronic hemarthrosis, prophylactic infusions 2–3 times weekly to maintain factor above 25% normal are useful, in addition to a brief course of prednisone and intensive physical therapy of the lower extremity. If chronic inflammation persists after 6 months of therapy, a surgical synovectomy should be considered. In the acute manifestation of a hemarthrosis, ice and ace bandages may be helpful to assist the clotting mechanism. Occasionally, aspiration of the joint may be needed, with factor given both before and after the procedure, followed by placement of an ace bandage or splint.

The presence of inhibitors to factors should be suspected if the half-life of infused factors is decreased, there is decreased or no clinical response, or no correction of the PTT is observed following infusion of factor. Nonetheless, such patients with inhibitor can be treated by giving Factor IX (prothrombin complex or "proplex") concentrates. These contain variable levels of prothrombin, as well as of the activated forms of Factors VII, IX, and X, such that Factor VIII is bypassed since the product contains activated Factor X. This therapy does not always work. There have been reports of thrombotic complications in patients receiving proplex although most of these patients have had liver disease or have been Factor IX-deficient, requiring repeated doses of Factor IX concentrate. In addition, adolescents and young adults have developed myocardial infarcts after receiving large repeated doses of nonactivated Factor IX complex (Sullivan et al, 1984). If the patient has a low amount of inhibitor, less than 5 units/ml, Factor VIII infusions might be used in place of prothrombin complex concentrates.

One of the most useful aspects of treatment for hemophiliacs has been the institution of a home treatment program for the severe hemophiliacs, which permits parents of affected children over 3–4 years of age and, eventually, patients themselves when they reach adolescence to carry out venipuncture and instill factor at home. Usually, families are supplied with factor concentrates which can be stored in the refrigerator. Close telephone contact is maintained with the physician and nurse coordinator at the hospital. A comprehensive hospital team including hematologists, orthopedists, nurse practitioners, social workers, oral surgeons, physical therapists, genetic counselors, and psychologists or psychiatrists has also been useful to ensure continuity as well as management of care.

Prognosis and Prevention

Until recently, hemophiliacs with appropriate treatment and factor infusion were expected to have near-normal life expectancy. Mortality has been attributed to CNS bleeding or GI or retroperitoneal bleeding in adulthood. Morbidity has consisted of chronic arthropathy, renal disease in two-thirds of the adults with hemophilia, as well as pulmonary hemorrhage and hypertension.

Since multiple donors are required to make a concentrate, all children who have received concentrate are at risk of hepatitis. Currently, the major source of morbidity and mortality in hemophiliacs has been the increased number of AIDS cases among hemophilia patients since 1981. The highest risk was in 1982 (Evatt, 1984).

In 1987 in the United States, more than 60% of hemophiliacs over the age of 10 years are seropositive for HIV. Heat-treated Factor VIII concentrate is currently being used and the likelihood of HIV infection is expected to decrease. Specially purified monoclonal Factor VIII is expected to be more widely used in 1988.

VON WILLEBRAND DISEASE

Definition

Von Willebrand disease is an inherited, usually autosomal dominant, bleeding disorder characterized by defective primary hemostasis, secondary to abnormal platelet adhesion as well as by a prolonged bleeding time and a prolonged PTT.

Basic Science

Von Willebrand disease results from an abnormality in the production of a large glycoprotein referred to as von Willebrand factor (Fig. 8.7). Variants of the disease are due to quantitative as well as qualitative deficiencies of the factor. It is this factor that is responsible for normal adhesion of platelets to subendothelial surfaces, with platelets having receptor sites for this factor. Von Willebrand factor is also referred to as Factor VIII-related von Willebrand factor (FVIIIR:WF). It has been shown that von Willebrand factor is necessary to stabilize Factor VIII procoagulant activity (VIII:C), the plasma factor that is deficient in classic hemophilia. When von Willebrand factor is defective or deficient, the amount of circulating VIII:C will be low. Of note, von Willebrand factor also contains a ristocetin cofactor which is necessary for ristocetin-induced platelet agglutination, a test useful in making the diagnosis. A description of the types of variants of von Willebrand disease appears in Table 8.13.

Epidemiology

It is estimated that the prevalence is about one-half that of hemophilia A (i.e., 3–4/100,000 in the population; Bloom, 1980). There is no ethnic or racial association. Death due to hemorrhage is rare in these patients.

Natural History

Patients with von Willebrand syndrome disease have superficial bleeding involving the skin and mucous membranes consistent with the platelet defects. Early in life, epistaxis is a frequent complaint in presentation. In adolescents, menorrhagia and easy bruis-

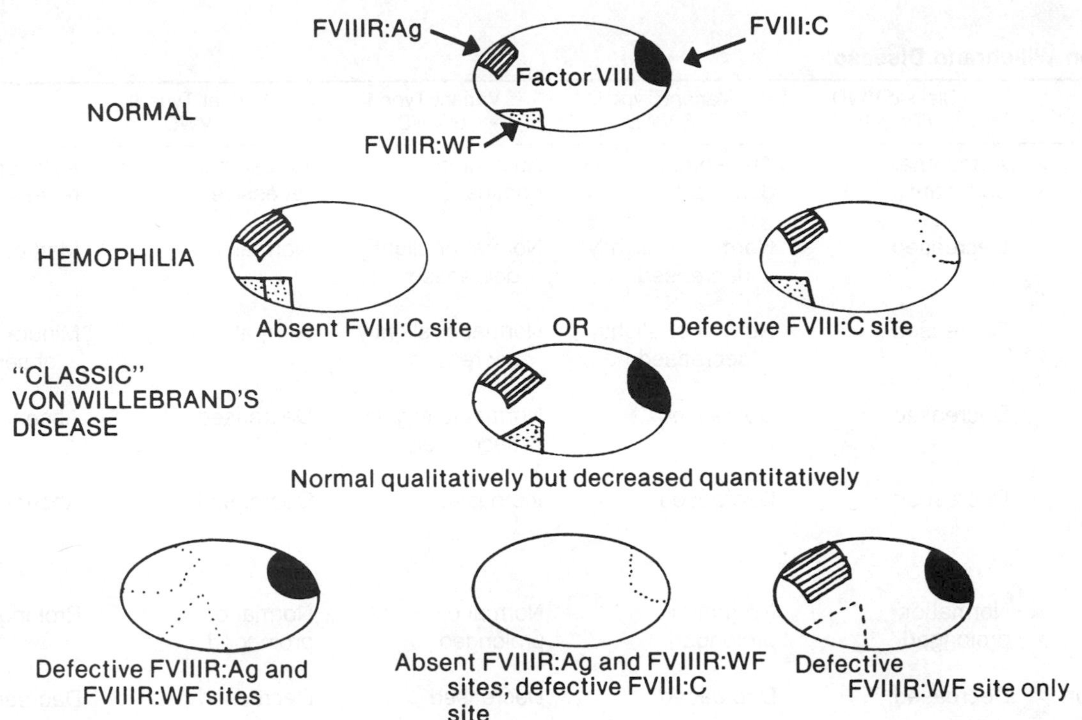

Figure 8.7. Diagram of the Factor VIII molecule in normal children as well as in patients with hemophilia A and von Willebrand disease. Reproduced with permission from Buchanan GR: *Pediatr Ann* 9:329, 1980.

ability may be noted. Hemarthroses are quite rare except in patients with very low Factor VIII activity, although postoperative hemorrhage can be a significant problem. Bleeding episodes tend to begin early in childhood and decrease with age.

Diagnosis

Once a bleeding disorder has been recognized, the family history is important since the disorder is autosomal dominant, although the severity may vary in different family members. A negative family history does not exclude a disease; it may simply mean that other family members may be mildly affected and asymptomatic.

Only the PTT and the bleeding time will usually be abnormal, although if the FVIII:C level is greater than 20–30%, the PTT may be within the normal range. Definitive diagnostic tests include assays for the FVIII:C, FVIIIR:AG assay, and the quantitative FVIIIR:WF assay measured in terms of the ristocetin cofactor, since ristocetin-induced platelet agglutination in platelet-rich plasma is usually absent or decreased in this disorder.

Treatment

Since most patients show only mild hemorrhagic symptoms, no treatment may be necessary. On the other hand, patients who are undergoing general surgery or who have severe epistaxes, menorrhagia or occasionally recurrent gastrointestinal bleeding will require therapeutic intervention.

The goal of therapy is to increase the levels of VIII:C and to reduce the bleeding time. Cryoprecipitate is the treatment of choice for severe hemorrhages and all major surgical procedures. It is usually administered anywhere from 1-14 days postoperatively or following major bleeding. Heat-treated Factor VIII preparations lack the Factor VIII R: WF multimeric complex and are not useful in this disorder.

Patients with mild hemorrhagic episodes and a mild form of the syndrome have been shown to benefit from administration of a nonvasoactive synthetic analog of vasopressin DDAVP. It has been found to cause a rise in Factor VIII and in von Willebrand factor in most patients and results in an increase in the concentration of all the polymers of von Willebrand factor. In the type II B form, DDAVP is contraindicated because there have been numerous reports of thrombocytopenia complicating therapy (Lusher, 1987).

Pregnancy results in increased levels of Factor VIII:C and von Willebrand factor in mild to moderate forms of the disease, so that delivery is possible without transfusion therapy.

Prognosis

Life-span of most patients with von Willebrand syndrome is normal, with a rare hemorrhagic death being reported.

Table 8.13
Variants of von Willebrand Disease[1]

	Classic VWD (Type I)	Variant Type II A VWD	Variant Type II B VWD	Variant Type II C VWD	Type III
Genetic transmission	Autosomal dominant	Autosomal dominant	Autosomal dominant	Autosomal recessive	Autosomal recessive
VIII:C	Decreased	Normal or slightly decreased	Normal or slightly decreased	Normal	Markedly decreased
VIIIR:AG	Decreased	Normal or slightly decreased	Normal or slightly decreased	Normal	Minute amounts or absent
VIIRCo	Decreased	Decreased	Normal to slightly decreased	Decreased	Absent
Platelet aggregation with ristocetin	Decreased	Decreased	Increased	Decreased	Absent
Bleeding time	Normal or prolonged	Normal or prolonged	Normal or prolonged	Normal or prolonged	Prolonged
Platelet retention	Decreased	Decreased	Decreased	Decreased	Decreased
Crossed immuno-electrophoresis	Normal rate of migration	Abnormal Arc	Abnormal Arc	Abnormal Arc	Variable (mostly abnormal)
Multimeric structure	Normal in plasma and platelets	Absence of large and intermediate multimers from plasma and platelets	Absence of only larger multimers from plasma, normal in platelets	Absence of only larger multimers from plasma, and platelets	Variable
Response to DDAVP	VIII:C, VIIIR:Ag and VIIIR:RCo increased BT:N	VIII:C VIIIR:Ag and VIIIR:RCo mildly increased BT:I	VIII:C VIIIR:Ag and VIIIR:RCo mildly increased BT:I[2]	VIII:C, VIIIR:Ag and VIIIR:RCo mildly increased BT:I	None

[1]Reproduced with permission from Karayalcin G: *Pediatr Ann* 14:655, 1985.
[2]May cause platelet aggregation; BT, bleeding time; N, complete correction; I = improved—not complete correction.

DISSEMINATED INTRAVASCULAR COAGULATION

Definition

Disseminated intravascular coagulation (DIC) is an acquired coagulation abnormality, resulting from activation and consumption of patient's plasma factors and platelets with various degrees of thrombosis and/or bleeding.

Basic Science

Activation of thrombin results in a change in the balance between fibrin formation and fibrinolytic action, with the end result being increased utilization of coagulation factors and platelets and increased risk of bleeding due to depletion of these factors.

The mechanism for the ultimate clinical finding of bleeding in DIC is due to one of the following three mechanisms: (1) the level of the plasma coagulation factor is depleted below normal hemostatic levels; (2) thrombocytopenia can occur and be severe enough to allow bleeding; (3) the fibrin-split products themselves can have abnormal effects on the coagulation mechanism.

Natural History

DIC may be seen in a variety of conditions including infection and septic shock, rickettsial, viral, and protozoal diseases, malignancies, hemangiomas, purpura fulminans, heat stroke, head injuries, transfusion reactions, respiratory distress syndrome in neonates, obstetrical conditions such as abruptio placenta, and/or necrotizing enterocolitis. Regardless of the underlying primary disease, patients usually present with bleeding as the major clinical symptom and/or thrombosis, although the thrombosis may not be clinically obvious. Bleeding usually occurs at multiple sites as petechiae of skin and mucous membranes, continued bleeding from venipuncture and cut-down sites, and occasionally, heavy bleeding from the GI tract or gross hematuria. CNS bleeding is rare.

Diagnosis

Once evidence of bleeding has been detected, diagnosis depends on screening tests. These include the platelet count, PTT, PT, and blood smear, and, in addition, measurement of the levels of fibrinogen and fibrin-split products.

In DIC, the platelet count will usually be less than 150,000, with prolonged PTT and PT. In addition, the blood smear will sometimes show a hemolytic picture with fragmented red cells. Finally, fibrinogen concentration will frequently be low and fibrin-split or degradation products are elevated in the serum.

While these findings may suggest the diagnosis, other tests provide additional supporting evidence for this diagnosis. The most specific test for DIC is the presence of increased fibrin degradation products, although this test is by no means absolutely diagnostic. One of the major differentials in diagnosing DIC is to distinguish it from fulminating liver disease, although this clinical distinction is frequently not possible.

Vitamin K deficiency will also result in prolonged PTs and PTTs, but in these patients, the fibrinogen and platelet count will be normal and fibrin-split products will not be present.

Treatment

The goals of treatment in DIC are to stop the bleeding and eliminate the possibility for fibrin deposition. Therefore, the initial treatment is to remove or treat the underlying cause triggering the coagulopathy. If this is not possible, or if it results in depletion of coagulation factors, transfusion of fresh-frozen plasma or platelets may be required. Only if the patient has a thrombotic component (e.g., "purpura fulminans," multifocal neurologic symptoms, acute renal failure) should anticoagulation therapy to interrupt the process be considered. The drug of choice is heparin since it has a quick onset of action and can be easily regulated and, if necessary, discontinued. Heparin is usually administered as a continuous infusion, with progress monitored for elevation in fibrinogen concentration. Complications of this therapy can include increased bleeding and thrombocytopenia.

APPROACH TO BLOOD PRODUCTS

Definition

A patient in need of a blood transfusion usually requires one of the many components contained in whole blood rather than whole blood itself. What follows is a description of the various types of transfusion therapy, and their advantages and disadvantages.

Basic Science

Whole blood collected from a donor usually contains an average of 450 ml of blood plus 63 ml of anticoagulant preservative. The hematocrit of whole blood is usually 40%. The anticoagulant preservative most commonly contains a mixture of trisodium citrate, a calcium-chelating agent, phosphate which maintains adequate levels of ATP in the blood, dextrose which serves as a source of energy for the red cells and preserves their levels of ATP, 2,3 diphosphoglyceric acid, and adenine which has recently been added as a means of preserving levels of ATP. Maintaining high levels of ATP helps preserve the sodium pump and the plasticity of the red cells. The presence of enhanced 2,3 diphosphoglyceric acid results in a rightward shift of the oxyhemoglobin dissociation curve and allows more oxygen to be dissociated from hemoglobin molecules and released into tissues.

When whole blood is allowed to settle or is centrifuged, resulting in the removal of about 250 ml of plasma, a unit of packed RBCs is produced. Packed cells will have a hematocrit of up to 80% in a volume of about 235 ml. Packed RBCs as described below may be useful in a patient who cannot tolerate a larger transfusion volume and yet requires enhancement of oxygen-carrying capacity.

Patients who have had repeated febrile nonhemolytic transfusion reactions secondary to factors contained in plasma, leukocytes, or platelets, benefit from having the RBCs frozen, thawed, and then washed thoroughly to remove the cryoprotective agent glycerol. These cells, packed cells and whole blood cells all require crossmatching before transfusion.

About 250 ml of plasma can be obtained from a unit of whole blood and contains albumin (3 g/dl) and various procoagulants, including fibrinogen, Factor VIII and coagulation Factors IX, as well as water and electrolytes. The plasma is frozen solid within 6 hours of collection to prevent deterioration of Factors V and VIII that usually occurs on storage at room temperature, and hence, fresh-frozen plasma can be useful when these procoagulants are needed in a patient. Plasma is also given according to ABO grouping, although Rh compatibility is not considered essential. It should be used within 6 hours of thawing in order to obtain maximum utilization of the coagulation factors that are heat-labile.

Leukocytes are usually derived from donor blood buffy coats or from single donors via plasmapheresis. Leukocyte concentrates once obtained also should be tested for ABO, Rh, hepatitis B surface antigen and syphilis. Leukocytes from a single donor are recommended when the recipient has been previously stimulated to produce antibodies (e.g., HLA directed), or when such stimulation would be detrimental as in candidates who have undergone transplantation.

Platelet concentrates can also be derived from multiple donor units or by plasmapheresis of a single donor. Platelet and leukocyte concentrates contain enough RBCs to result in Rh sensitization. Therefore, to avoid immune destruction of transfused platelets, these should be compatible with ABO, Rh, and HLA types in the recipient.

Table 8.14 summarizes information on volume, shelf-life, and uses of the most common blood products.

Transfusions can wreak havoc on the immune system if blood products are not carefully screened before administration. A major problem is alloimmunization in which both cellular and plasma antigens and transfused donor blood can subject the recipient to literally hundreds of known alloantigens. In addition, transfusion may result in immunosuppression with multiply transfused patients displaying decreased natural killer cell activity and increased circulating IA-positive T cells (Anderson, 1986).

Natural History

Complications of transfusion include febrile reactions usually attributed to leukoagglutinins or antibodies to substances in blood. These episodes can be minimized by the use of frozen washed red cells or "white cell poor" red cells. Sensitization to minor blood group antigens is also a frequent occurrence. Infection by certain viruses has been reduced by screening for infectious agents in the blood, usually performed by blood banks. This screening includes hepatitis B, hepatitis A, and human immunodeficiency virus (HIV). NonA-nonB hepatitis is the most common cause of hepatitis currently transmitted by blood from voluntary donors since there is still no appropriate assay for this disease.

Table 8.14
Common Blood Products

Product	Content	Uses	Volume	Shelf Life
Whole blood	Red cells White cells Platelets Plasma	Blood loss Neonatal exchange transfusion	500 ml	35 days
Red blood cells	Red cells White cells Plasma	Anemia	200–350 ml	35 days
Frozen-thawed red blood cells	Red cells Few white cells Platelets Plasma	Anemia Prevent immune reactions to white blood cells, platelets, plasma proteins Storage of rare bloods	170–190 ml	3 years frozen 24 hours thawed
Platelets	Platelets Few white blood cells Plasma	Bleeding with thrombocytopenia	20–50 ml	72 hours
White blood cells	White cells Platelets Few red cells	Infections in neutropenic pts.	50–300 ml	24 hours
Fresh frozen plasma	Clotting factors	Clotting disorders	220–250 ml	1 year frozen 6 hours thawed
Cryoprecipitate	Factors VIII, XIII Fibrinogen von Willebrand	VIII, XIII deficiencies von Willebrand factor deficiency Hypofibrinogenemia	10–25 ml	1 year frozen 6 hours thawed
Purified factors (heat-treated)	(1) Factor VIII (2) IX (also contains—II, VII, X)	VIII deficiency IX deficiency	Lyophilized powder Lyophilized powder	As per manufacturer As per manufacturer
Prothrombin complex concentrates	Activated procoagulants (Prothrombin, VII, IX, X & activated VIIa, IXa + Xa)	Inhibitor action of Factor VIII	Lyophilized powder	2 years
Albumin	5% or 25%	Plasma volume expansion	250–500 (5%) 50–100 cc (25%)	3 years

Finally, one of the most significant side effects of chronic transfusion therapy is iron overload. (This problem is discussed in the section on thalassemia.)

Patients who receive leukocyte transfusions will often have a history of febrile reactions and hence may require premedication with acetaminophen, intravenous hydrocortisone, or even intramuscular meperidine. Leukoagglutination may occur in pulmonary tissue, compromising respiratory status so that the transfusion has to be stopped.

As a result of the clinical effects of immune incompatibility following transfusion, a hemolytic reaction can occur either acutely or as a delayed reaction, as well as nonhemolytic effects including urticaria, anaphylaxis (especially to anti-IgA in the patient reacting with IgA in the blood product), fever usually secondary to interactions between donor leukocytes or platelets and recipient's antibodies, and pulmonary infiltrates (especially in blood products with either leukocytes or antileukocyte antibodies). Graft-versus-host disease may occur when immunocompetent cells are transfused into immunosuppressed hosts. Infectious complications include hepatitis B and A, which are much less frequent due to screening serology than non-A and non-B hepatitis. In addition cytomegalovirus and Epstein-Barr virus, and toxoplasmosis, have all been transmitted by blood products. A donor who has traveled to an area where malaria is endemic may end up donating the parasite to a host via a transfusion. Finally, and most important, acquired immune deficiency syndrome (AIDS) can be acquired via HIV exposure following blood product transfusion, although it is very rare now that blood banks are screening donors to ensure that there has been no exposure to HIV.

Treatment

Whole blood should be administered only if there is acute massive blood loss requiring replacement of more than 25% of the blood volume or during neonatal exchange transfusion. If blood loss has stopped, volume replacement can be achieved by the use of albumin or crystalloid fluid such as Ringer lactate, initially followed by packed RBC, with replacement of procoagulants or fresh-frozen plasma infused at a ratio of 1–2 units of fresh-frozen plasma for every 10 units of packed red blood cells. The use of fresh whole blood is recommended for exchange transfusions since these contain fewer older red cells, which would be destroyed. Packed RBCs are recommended in patients with anemia who are not actively hemorrhaging.

If leukocytes are being transfused, an adult dosage of 10^{10} granulocytes is considered appropriate therapy. Since the half-life of leukocytes is less than 12 hours, a rise in peripheral neutrophil count greater than 1000/mm^3 12 hours after the transfusion suggests the beginning of bone marrow recovery, although usually transfusions are continued for 3–5 days until blood cultures are negative, or for at least a week if blood cultures are positive. Indications for platelet therapy are discussed under thrombocytopenia.

REFERENCES

Ahn YS, Harrington WJ, Simon SR, et al: Danazol for the treatment of idiopathic thrombocytopenic purpura. *N Engl J Med* 308:1396, 1983.

Anderson KC: Blood component support. In *Department of Pediatric Hematology/Oncology Handbook 1986-87,* Children's Hospital and Dana Farber Cancer Institute, p 113.

Bloom AL: The von Willebrand syndrome. *Semin Hematol* 17:215, 1980.

Bowie EJW: Von Willebrand's disease: Clinical picture, diagnosis, and treatment. *Clin Lab Med* 4:303, 1984.

Buchanan GR: Hemophilia. *Pediatr Clin North Am* 27:309, 1980.

Buchanan GR: Von Willebrand's disease: A confusing disorder. *Pediatr Ann* 9:23, 1980.

CDC: Surveillance of hemophilia-associated acquired immunodeficiency syndrome. *MMWR* 35:669, 1986.

Corrigan JJ: Disseminated intravascular coagulopathy. *Pediatr Rev* 1:37, 1979.

Evatt BL, Chorbat AL: Acquired immunodeficiency syndrome (AIDS) in hemophilia. *Clin Lab Med* 4:333, 1984.

Imbach P, Barandun S, Hirt A, et al: Intravenous immunoglobulin for idiopathic thrombocytopenic purpura in childhood. *Am J Pediatr Hematol/Oncol* 6:171, 1984.

Karayalcin G: Current concepts in the management of hemophilia. *Pediatr Ann* 14:640, 1985.

Lawn RM, Vehar GA: The molecular genetics of hemophilia. *Scientif Am* p. 254, March 1986.

Lightsey AL: Thrombocytopenia in children. *Pediatr Clin North Am* 27:293, 1980.

Lilleyman JS: Idiopathic thrombocytopenic purpura—where do we stand? *Arch Dis Child* 59:701, 1984.

Lusher JM, Emami A, Ravindranath Y, et al: Idiopathic thrombocytopenic purpura in children: The case for management without corticosteroids. *Am J Pediatr Hematol/Oncol* 6:149, 1984.

Lusher JM: Diseases of coagulation: The fluid phase. In Nathan DG, Oski FA (eds): *Hematology of Infancy and Childhood*, 3rd edition. Philadelphia, WB Saunders, 1987, p. 1293.

Mann KG: The biochemistry of coagulation. *Clin Lab Med* 4:207, 1984.

Mannucci PM, Canciani ML, et al: Response of Factor VIII/von Willebrand factor in healthy subjects and patients with hemophilia A and von Willebrand's disease. *Br J Haematol* 47:283, 1981.

Montgomery RR, Hathaway WE: Acute bleeding emergencies. *Pediatr Clin North Am* 27:327, 1980.

Panicucci F, Segraponti A, Conte B, et al: Characterization of heterogeneity of hemophilia B for the detection of carriers. *Hemostasis* 9:310, 1980.

Russell EC, Maurer HM: Alternatives to splenectomy and the management of chronic idiopathic thrombocytopenic purpura in children. *Am J Pediatr Hematol/Oncol* 6:175, 1984.

Sartorius JA: Steroid treatment of idiopathic thrombocytopenic purpura in children: Preliminary results of a randomized cooperative study. *Am J Pediatr Hematol/Oncol* 6:165, 1984.

Shende A: Idiopathic thrombocytopenic purpura in children. *Pediatr Ann* 14:609, 1985.

Sirridge M: Laboratory evaluation of a bleeding patient. *Clin Lab Med* 4:285, 1984.

Stewart MJ: Inherited defects of platelet function. *Semin Hematol* 12:233, 1975.

Sullivan DW, Purdy LJ, et al: Fatal myocardial infarction following therapy with prothrombin complex concentrates in a young man with hemophilia A. *Pediatrics* 74:279, 1984.

Warrier I, Lusher JM: Intravenous gammaglobulin treatment for chronic idiopathic thrombocytopenic purpura in children. *Am J Med* 76:193, 1984.

LEWIS R. FIRST

Consultants
David G. Nathan
Orah S. Platt

Section 9

Oncology

Introduction to Oncology 1

Cancer is a general term for dysregulated growth of a tissue. Malignancy is used as a synonym to imply the possibility of a lethal condition from direct compromise of a vital organ due to cancerous cell growth or dissemination to distant organs (metastases) by the cancer.

Malignant growth depends on damage to the DNA of a previously differentiated cell. Dominant and recessive mutations, rearrangements of DNA, and point mutations alter the function of genes and permit neoplasia. In some instances, such as retinoblastoma, an hereditary predisposition to cancer is evident. Susceptibility to cancer is also associated with genetically impaired ability to repair damaged DNA (e.g., Bloom syndrome, xeroderma pigmentosum).

Tumor cells may show visible damage to chromosomes that includes translocations, deletions, and abnormal amplification of genes. Some of these chromosome changes have been associated with activation of proto-oncogenes. These "cancer" genes were first identified in retroviruses where they can account for the tumorigenicity of the virus. The proto-oncogenes represent normal cellular genes that have been conserved through evolution and have been copied into retroviral genomes by genetic recombination during the course of viral infection. Some retroviral oncogenes can induce more than one form of cancer, and each corresponding proto-oncogene likewise has become a suspect in human carcinogenesis.

Malignant cells acquire different properties which, in turn, affect their potential. Among the properties that produce disease are the capacity for proliferation, invasion of adjacent tissue, and metastasis. Doubtless a number of alterations in the cell's environment are essential for proliferation. For example, Folkman (1984) has characterized the role that angiogenesis plays in tumor growth.

Clearly, cancer can occur from many different causes. The risk of disease depends on a complex set of circumstances, many of which are under intense investigation in the 1980s (Bishop, 1987). For example, an excess of lymphomas occurs in children with primary or acquired immunodeficiency states. Viruses or other environmental factors may be important cofactors as well in the development of lymphomas in these patients (Filipovich et al, 1987).

Cancer has become an important cause of death for children. It is the third leading cause of death in the United States in children between the ages of 1 and 4 years, lagging behind injuries and congenital anomalies, and it rises to the second leading cause of death after injuries in individuals in the 5- to 19-year age group. There is a bimodal mortality rate among children with peaks between ages 1 and 4 years and then again between ages 15 and 19 years. This mortality rate also varies by race and gender. The rate for whites is higher than that for blacks and that for males is greater than that for females.

Fewer than 10,000 cases of childhood cancer are diagnosed in the United States each year, although the incidence rate has increased over the past 10 years. The incidence of these disorders for children under 15 years is shown in Figure 9.1. The most commonly diagnosed pediatric malignancies are leukemias and cancers of blood-forming organs, followed by tumors in the brain and nervous system, lymph nodes, bones, joints and cartilage, and those of endocrinologic origin.

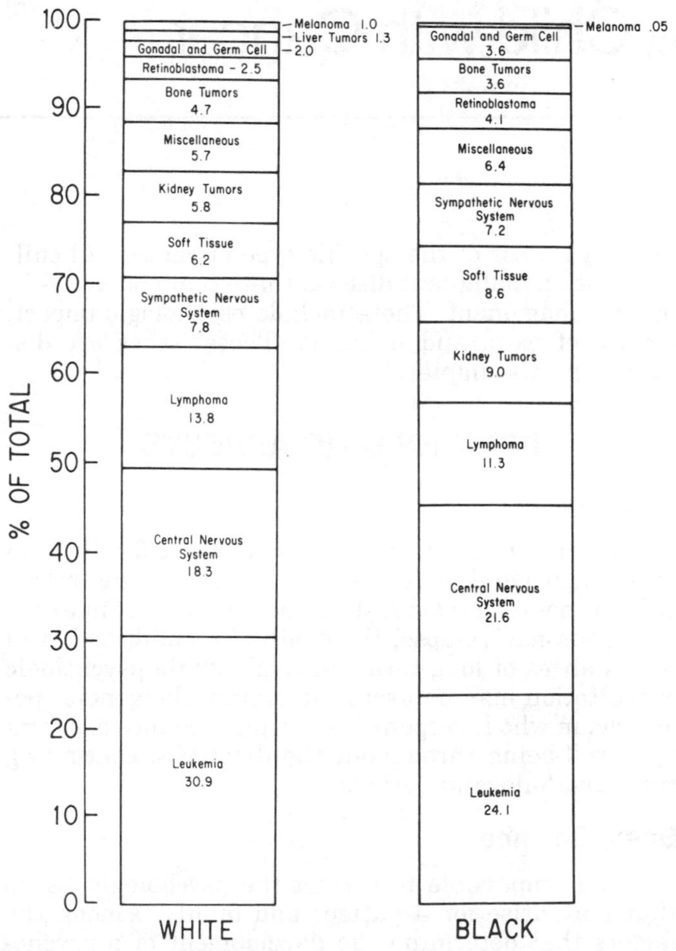

Figure 9.1. Cancer incidence for children ≤ 15 years of age by site and race. Data obtained from SEER program 1973–1976. Reproduced with permission from Pratt C: *Pediatr Clin North Am* 32:543, 1985.

Data collected by the Surveillance Epidemiology and End Results Program of the National Cancer Institute between 1978 and 1981 suggest an average prevalence of all childhood cancers of 18.1/100,000 for children between birth to age 4 years, 10.1/100,000 for those aged 5–9 years, 10.5/100,000 between ages 10 and 14 years, and 18.4/100,000 population between the ages of 15 and 19 years. While the incidence rate appears to have increased recently, the mortality rate for childhood cancers has declined by almost 50% over the past 30 years, although the decline varies for different age groups. The youngest children have shown the most dramatic improvement, with Wilms tumor and leukemia showing the greatest decline in mortality in children under age 5 years.

REFERENCES

Bishop JM: The molecular genetics of cancer. *Science* 235:305, 1987.

Filipovich AH, Heinitz KJ, Robinson LL, et al: The Immunodeficiency Cancer Registry: A research resource. *Am J Pediatr Hematol/Oncol* 9:183, 1987.

Folkman J: Toward a new understanding of vascular proliferative disease in children. *Pediatrics* 74:850, 1984.

Pratt CB: Some aspects of childhood cancer epidemiology. *Pediatr Clin North Am* 32:541, 1985.

Young JL Jr, Heise HW, Silverberg E, et al: Cancer incidence, survival, and mortality for children under 15 years of age. New York, American Cancer Society Professional Education Publication, Sept, 1978.

Approach to the General Management of a Child with Cancer

2

Regardless of the specific type of cancer, all children with a malignant disease share common issues in their management. These include psychologic impact, control of pain, and infection. These issues are discussed in this chapter.

PSYCHOLOGIC ASPECTS

Definition

There is no greater time of stress for a family than when their child is diagnosed as having a life-threatening illness. Moreover, stressful periods continue during remission, relapse, the death of a child, and even in instances of long-term survival. While psychologic consultation may be useful, it is often the general pediatrician who is responsible for maintenance of a family's well-being throughout the diagnosis, continuing care, and follow-up periods.

Basic Science

It is impossible to predict the psychologic issues that may arise for a patient and family. Among the factors that determine the development of a psychosocial crisis are baseline psychologic functioning for the child and family before the onset of illness, past experiences of the family with illness and loss, the course and prognosis of the disease, the age of the child, and the role of that child within that family structure. Families with pre-existing emotional problems are certainly at higher risk for psychosocial dysfunction when a malignancy is diagnosed than are more emotionally stable families.

Natural History, Diagnosis, and Treatment

The diagnosis of the child with cancer is only the start of what is going to be a long period of stress for that child and family. A pediatrician's role is to provide encouragement and support, and to be available for consultation at any time. Moreover, pediatricians must ensure effective communication between the oncology team and the family as well as with themselves.

Once treatment is ongoing, the side effects of therapy may become a prominent focus of behavioral difficulties for the child. Behavioral techniques may be needed to reduce the anticipation of side effects that the child grows to know and often to fear, including nausea, vomiting, and the anxiety of simply receiving the chemotherapy.

During this time of maintenance chemotherapy, the general pediatrician should continue to serve not only as a support for the family but also to ensure that health maintenance guidelines are still being followed, and that the child has adequate nutritional and developmental support. It is the pediatrician's job to ensure that normal family patterns are maintained, including relationships among family and friends, and that the child returns to school as soon as possible and is treated as normally as possible. Often it is useful for the pediatrician or the oncologist to speak to a child's class to assist the transition back into the schoolroom and to make sure that the child does not become isolated.

If a patient has a relapse of the malignancy following a period of prolonged remission, a multiplicity of emotional reactions can occur, including anger, guilt, fear, and resentment. If alternative therapies for relapse are available, they may have more severe side effects or be limited in success. If no alternative therapy is offered, the family must begin to think about palliative care, home supports, and dealing with the patient's declining clinical status. The pediatrician should attend not only to the child, but also to parents and to siblings during this period, since essentially the entire family is "the patient." Often, the general pediatrician will assist in the home management of terminally ill children, arranging for hospice care or visiting nurses so that the child may be made comfortable in his own environment rather than in a hospital setting.

At the time of death, it may be the pediatrician's role to guide the parents in how to deal with their loss, how to obtain an autopsy, or deal with the siblings of the deceased. A postdeath conference may provide a forum for discussing unresolved stressful issues within the family. A need for appropriate psychiatric referrals and follow-up can also be discerned at this time.

For a family, the period of grief can last for several years with recurrences thereafter. The pediatrician may continue to play a role throughout this time, particularly if there are other siblings involved in his care. The pediatrician can also help refer families to bereavement and support groups for parents of children who have also succumbed to an oncologic disease.

If the patient survives maintenance chemotherapy and goes into remission and even cure, family anxieties persist in regard to whether the disease will recur. The pediatrician is responsible for the health maintenance of these long-term survivors and should be aware of the late effects of the different therapeutic regimens utilized by the oncologist. These can hamper growth, intellectual function, reproductive function, and cause a variety of other complications discussed later in this chapter. In addition, there is an increased risk of secondary malignancy following some of these treatments.

It is often the pediatrician's job to assess when the family needs further support. In younger children, developmental regression, separation anxiety, and fear and unmanageable behavior are particularly common following a long-term hospitalization and may require psychologic or psychiatric assistance for behavior modification. In older children, fear of treatment, adjustment reactions to the treatment, depression and anger regarding their inability to deal with themselves in peer relationships may also result in a need for consultation.

Among therapeutic modalities often available to these patients are play therapy, behavioral modification and self-hypnosis, group therapy sessions, psychotherapy, and when needed, appropriate medication. It is important that the psychologic or psychiatric consultant be a part of the total team taking care of the patient and family so that again communication among all supports is open and unified.

PAIN

Definition

Oncology patients at some time during management, and perhaps throughout, will complain of pain. As described by Merskey (1979): "Pain is an unpleasant sensory and emotional experience associated with actual or potential tissue damage, or described in terms of such damage." This definition draws a distinction between the sensation of tissue injury, referred to as "nociception," and pain, which has both sensory and emotional aspects. Ongoing tissue injury is not necessary to perpetuate pain. For example, many forms of chronic neuropathic pain may be due to spontaneous neuronal excitability either in the peripheral or the central nervous system.

Basic Science

BIOLOGY OF NOCICEPTION

Specialized and free endings of thickly myelinated A-delta nerve fibers and unmyelinated C-fibers in the periphery respond to a variety of mechanical, chemical, and thermal stimuli with afferent impulses that are interpreted as painful. The A-delta fibers are responsible for mediating sharp and well-localized pain, while C-fibers transmit duller and more poorly localized pain, as well as pain due to pressure, heat, and chemical irritation. These neurons have cell bodies in the dorsal root ganglia. Proximal terminals of these neurons form synapses with projection neurons or interneurons in layers I (marginal layer), II (substantia gelatinosa), and V of the dorsal horn of the spinal cord. Projection axons ascend in the spinal cord in the spinothalamic and other tracts to form synapses in the thalamus and brain stem (periaqueductal grey, reticular formation, superior colliculus, and intercollicular nuclei). Fibers arising from these secondary neurons terminate in subcortical areas including the limbic system, as well as in the postcentral gyrus of the cortex. A diagram of the major pain pathways appears in Figure 9.2.

Chemical mediators implicated in peripheral sensitization of unmyelinated sensory afferents include bradykinin, prostaglandins, and potassium and hydrogen ions, among others. Several neuropeptides, including the undecapeptide substance P, have been proposed as neurotransmitters or neuromodulators involved in nociception that are released by sensory afferents in terminals in the dorsal horn of the spinal cord. At present, there is no simple description of the biochemical events in peripheral or spinal triggering of impulses related to nociception (Wall, 1984).

Several lines of evidence indicate that afferent transmission of impulses is modulated or "gated" at the level of the dorsal horn by afferent impulses from large A-α fibers as well as from descending inputs from the brain stem and other rostral sites. Several compounds,

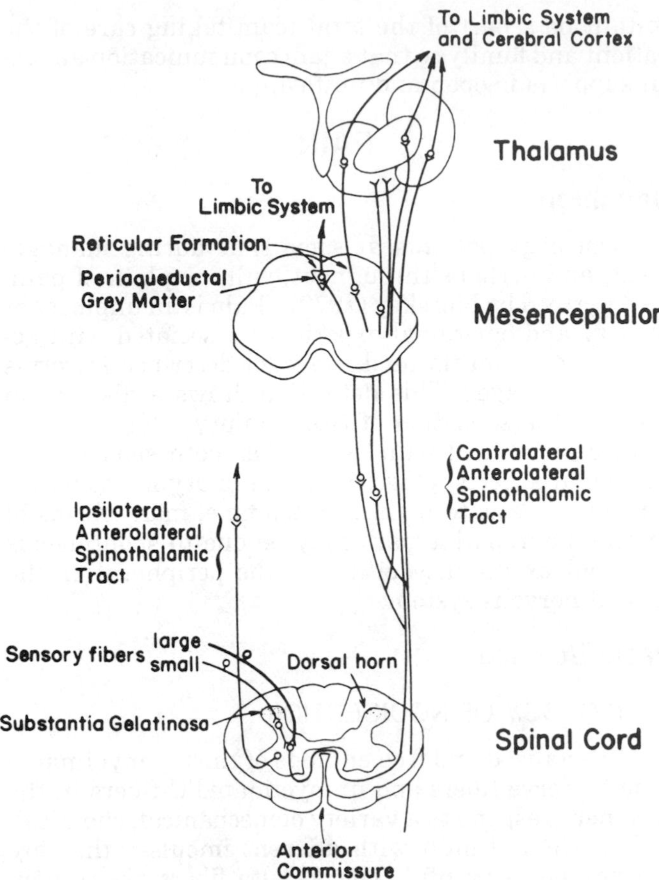

Figure 9.2. Diagram of the ascending pathways for pain perception. Reproduced with permission from Newburger PE, Sallan SE: *J Pediatr* 98:180, 1981.

including enkephalins, endorphins, norepinephrine, and serotonin, have been implicated in these descending control systems. Descending control of spinal and supraspinal gate mechanisms has been used to explain the influence of psychologic factors on pain perception and experience, and to interpret analgesia produced by transcutaneous nerve stimulation or acupuncture (Basbaum and Fields, 1984).

Although the basic pathways for pain perception appear to be developed in newborns, the meaning of pain and its affective components develop during early childhood. These aspects are based not only on the painful experiences of each individual child, but are affected markedly by family influences and child-rearing practices, the learning of coping strategies, and social and cultural factors. Thus, perception of pain as an unpleasant sensation may occur at birth, whereas the interpretation of pain as an emotional experience develops during early childhood (Anand and Hickey, 1987).

Contrary to widespread belief, there is evidence to suggest that pain threshold is lower in younger age groups than in older age groups. In addition, existing data do not support the widespread contention that children experience less acute pain following surgery than do adults (Beyer et al, 1983). Where subjective and behavioral pain scales have been employed, it appears that children experience pain as acutely as do adults in the immediate postoperative period, although it may resolve more rapidly.

From a psychologic perspective, pain threshold and tolerance depend upon the setting in which the pain is being perceived. The existence of pain may, in itself, suggest a loss of control for the child over the underlying disease, particularly in the hospital environment where it is difficult to direct the patient's attention away from the chronic illness. Nonetheless, there are methods for treating the child who presents with chronic pain.

Treatment

Pain may be due to the tumor directly, as with tumor infiltration of viscera, bone, or nerves or it may be associated with the cancer therapy, including painful procedures, mucositis, postoperative pain, or neuropathies.

Some guidelines for treatment are as follows:

1. Recognize that fear, anxiety, and depression are prominent in children with cancer and direct attention toward these factors. Where possible, employ relaxation, hypnosis, or involvement in activities. Often for younger children, fear of the disease or of dying is either too abstract to be verbalized or is made taboo by equally terrified parents. In this setting, the child's focusing on pain may be intensified by being unable to confront these other fears.
2. Physical measures, including ice massage and transcutaneous nerve stimulation may be helpful for many forms of localized pain. They are probably underutilized.
3. Flexibility in routes for narcotic administration is required. For patients with moderate pain who do not have severe nausea, oral narcotics may be effective. In other patients with nausea or severe mucositis, parenteral medications may be required. If a patient has available a central line or other easy intravenous access, continuous intravenous infusion may be the easiest route; if these are unavailable, continuous subcutaneous infusion may be more acceptable. For most kinds of ongoing pain, long-acting agents are desirable. For brief distressing procedures, such as bone-marrow aspiration, short-acting agents such as fentanyl are useful because they provide intense immediate effect with less sedation afterward. If oral premedication is used for a painful procedure, it must be given at least 90 minutes before the procedure.
4. When using oral narcotics, we recommend combining a long-acting agent, methadone, with a short-acting agent, usually either dilaudid, codeine, or oxycodone. The methadone is given on a fixed schedule *(not prn)* 3–4 times daily, providing a steady basal level of analgesia. If pain persists, dilaudid, codeine, or oxycodone (in combination with acetaminophen) may be taken as needed. If these short-acting medications are required for several days, sedation ensues, in which case the metha-

done dose is reduced. This algorithm helps to combat a common problem with methadone: the prolonged half-life makes titration to effect difficult. Slow release morphine preparations may be used instead of methadone.

5. Continuous intravenous or subcutaneous infusions generally contain morphine, dilaudid, methadone, or fentanyl. Meperidine should be avoided if chronic high doses are required since there is a risk of convulsions due to the metabolite normeperidine. Miser et al have reported good results with continuous intravenous (1980) and subcutaneous (1983) morphine infusions in children with cancer. For example, median effective morphine infusion rate was 0.06 mg/kg/hour for the subcutaneous route and 0.04–0.07 mg/kg/hour for the intravenous route, although there was substantial individual variation. It is not rare for children and especially adolescents to require up to 4–15 mg/kg/hour for pain in terminal malignancy. In the majority of children, these infusions will relieve pain adequately. In a very small number of patients, even when the infusion is titrated to the point of respiratory depression or sedation, pain relief is not adequate.
6. Adjunctive medications, including antidepressants, antiemetics, and stimulants are very useful, but their use should be tailored to the individual patient's needs and wishes. For example, some children find phenothiazines, butyrophenones, or cannabinoids so dysphoric that they would prefer to experience increased nausea; other children are calmed by these agents and find them very helpful for nausea.

   For many children who find narcotics excessively sedating, a small oral dose of dextroamphetamine (0.05–0.2 mg/kg) or methylphenidate in the morning and perhaps again at midday potentiates narcotic analgesia and combats sedation.

   For many children with anxiety, depression, or disturbed sleep, small doses of tricyclics such as amitriptyline at bedtime (0.5–1.5 mg/kg) potentiate narcotic analgesia and appear to improve mood and sleep patterns. As with adults, it is best to start with low doses and increase gradually as limited by dry mouth or morning somnolence.

   For children with neuralgia or deafferentation pain, in addition to transcutaneous nerve stimulation, either amitriptyline (especially for "burning pain"), phenytoin, or carbamazepine (especially for "shooting pain") should be tried. For the latter two agents, twice daily dosing is usually adequate, and plasma levels should approximate the lower end of the anticonvulsant range.

   Because children with cancer vary greatly in their associated complaints and need for adjunctive medications, we prefer to tailor a regimen individually rather than using a fixed combination of commercially prepared agents.
7. Anticipate and treat side effects, including nausea, pruritus, constipation, and urinary retention. If tolerance develops, increase doses appropriately.
8. The overwhelming majority of children with cancer can be made comfortable if the regimen outlined in steps 1–7 is optimized. Nevertheless, a small number of children, usually with widespread bony metastases or nerve root compression, remain in severe pain despite very large doses of narcotics. In these patients, consider lumbar epidural or subarachnoid catheter placement for administration of narcotics or local anesthetics, or consider neurolytic blocks and neurosurgical procedures. When blocks are utilized in patients receiving these large doses of narcotics, sudden deafferentation of the pain can make the patient become rapidly and profoundly narcotized. Epidural and subarachnoid catheters can be placed percutaneously or tunneled intraoperatively at any age by appropriately experienced personnel. Home administration of neuraxis medications by continuous infusion is now made practical in many areas by the availability of homecare companies and visiting nurses familiar with these techniques, which are now widely used in adults. If the above techniques fail to provide relief, neurosurgical consultation should be obtained for consideration of ablative or neurostimulatory procedures.
9. Sufficient treatment should not be limited by fear of addiction, especially in patients with terminal malignancy.

Since nausea and vomiting can also be debilitating and, in some respects, psychologically painful to the patient, they should also be well controlled pharmacologically before the onset of any chemotherapy. Prophylactic antiemetic therapy has been very helpful in reducing the potential side effects of nausea and vomiting. Phenothiazines are the drugs of choice for control of vomiting secondary to chemotherapy, with the most useful being thiethylperazine (Torecan), which is available for oral, intravenous, intramuscular or rectal administration. The dose is 10 mg for children 12 years of age or greater than 50 kg, whereas 5 mg are used in smaller children. It is not used if the child is under age 2 years, and will provide prophylactic protection if given on a regular basis around the clock, being tapered to an individual's own needs rather than a general every 6-hour schedule.

Other alternatives to Torecan include perphenazine (Trilafon), available for intravenous or oral administration and as a continuous infusion, prochlorperazine (Compazine), most useful in the younger children for sedation (but with very little antiemetic efficacy), and promethazine (Phenergan) which, again, is better for nausea and sedation than it is for vomiting.

Patients who receive the phenothiazine derivatives for antiemesis should be alerted to the possibility of extrapyramidal side effects which can occur up to 48 hours after the drug is discontinued, and are easily treated with the use of diphenhydramine.

Other alternatives for antiemesis include metaclopramide and the butyrophenones (droperidol and haloperidol). Second line agents would include the use of steroids, cannibinoid derivatives, and antihistamines provided that the latter are not used as single agent antiemetics.

An overall approach to adequate antiemetic therapy might include starting with Torecan or Trilafon and if there is no response, adding metaclopramide or droperidol. Once extrapyramidal reactions occur, a steroid like dexamethasone can be tried instead. If only a partial response occurs, dexamethasone might be added with any of the four drugs just mentioned, since combinations of other nonsteroid agents may only increase toxicity.

If anticipation of vomiting is more of a problem than the actual effect of the chemotherapeutic agent, lorazepam or diazepam may be indicated. Diphenhydramine should always be used with Torecan and Trilafon as well as with metaclopramide and droperidol to provide prophylaxis against dystonic reactions. In the small infant where some of these agents are contraindicated because the side effects outweigh their benefits, Phenergan might be tried first, with addition of diphenhydramine for poor response or if toxicity occurs. Behavioral modification techniques have also been used successfully to decrease anticipatory nausea and vomiting.

INFECTIOUS COMPLICATIONS

Definition

The cancer patient who is neutropenic and/or immunosuppressed is at increased risk for harboring infection. Since it is often difficult initially to establish that a fever is due to infection and does not stem from other causes, it is important that appropriate diagnostic and therapeutic management be initiated. Granulocytopenia, however, remains the most important risk factor associated with infection; indeed, in 80% of cancer patients, fevers were associated with granulocytopenia and of these, 75% were due to infection (Pizzo et al, 1982). In contrast, in patients without granulocytopenia, only 20% of fevers were due to infection. Any patient who presents, therefore, with fever above 101°F and a granulocyte count less than 1000/mm^3 should be started on empiric broad spectrum antibiotics. Any patient with fever who has been splenectomized, moreover, should be started on broad spectrum antibiotics regardless of granulocyte count.

Basic Science

Identification of the pathogens most likely to be present in an oncology patient with fever requires the following information:

1. The local epidemiology of organisms in the health care facility should be determined.
2. The effect of the underlying illness on the immune system should be assessed.

   For example, acute leukemia results in deficient granulocytes and leaves the patient susceptible to infection with *Pseudomonas* species and other Gram-negative rods as well as to *Staphylococcus aureus*. A patient with Hodgkin disease, on the other hand, can have defects in cellular immunity at time of diagnosis and may be susceptible to herpes viruses, bacterial illnesses, tuberculosis, and fungal infections such as *Cryptococcus*. The patient with multiple myeloma or chronic lymphocytic leukemia (extremely rare in childhood), presents with immunoglobulin defects and, therefore, is more susceptible to the encapsulated organisms of *Streptococcus pneumoniae* and *Haemophilus influenzae*.
3. The effects of chemotherapy should be considered. For example, induction therapy usually results in granulocytopenia, leaving the patient susceptible to infection with Gram-negative rods and *S. aureus*. During remission, there is a depression of cellular as well as humoral immunity that leaves the patient susceptible to infections with *Pneumocystis* or herpes viruses. During relapse, all mechanisms for combating infectious disease may be depressed and the patient can succumb to bacteria, fungus, protozoal, or viral infections.

Diagnosis

A careful physical examination is mandatory in these patients, although the inflammatory response may be impaired or not visible at all if there is significant granulocytopenia. For example, a cellulitis may demonstrate minimal erythema (which is normally suggestive of acute inflammation) because of the absence of inflammatory cells. In fact, any new pulmonary infiltrates or cellulitis that appear during recovery of the marrow from a chemotherapy treatment may suggest a delayed manifestation of a pre-existing infection and not a new superinfection. Funduscopic examination may be very useful in trying to isolate septic embolic lesions associated with fungal infections, cytomegalovirus, or toxoplasmosis. Fungal infections should be carefully looked for in both the nose and mouth, and if any nasal discharge is present, sinus radiographs should be obtained. Patients with poor dental hygiene are at increased risk for occult dental infections. Yellow plaques on the oral mucosa or esophagus may not always be due to *Candida* in these patients and should also be examined by Gram staining and cultured for viral infections such as herpes simplex. Finally, the anal area should be carefully inspected, since perirectal abscesses are common in patients with acute leukemia. A rectal examination is usually not recommended in the presence of neutropenia and thrombocytopenia.

Following a careful physical examination, laboratory work-up should include cultures of blood, urine, throat, stool, sputum, aspirates of any skin lesions or ear infections, and biopsy of any potentially necrotic lesions. A spinal puncture should be performed if symptoms point to the CNS or if fever has persisted without clear etiology. A chest radiograph is always indicated and, if symptoms are present, sinus and dental radiographs also should be obtained.

Despite a careful diagnostic work-up, the infectious agent often will not be identified at the time of presentation with fever. Therefore, broad spectrum antibiotic coverage is indicated, with a broad spectrum penicillin or cephalosporin and an aminoglycoside, to ensure coverage for Gram-negative organisms such as *Pseudomonas, Klebsiella, Escherichia coli,* as well as Gram-positive organisms, especially *S. aureus* and *Pneumococcus.* A cephalosporin and aminoglycoside may be used in patients allergic to penicillin or for organisms resistant to a broad spectrum penicillin. In 1988, we are using mezlocillin and gentamicin to provide such coverage. The use of trimethoprim-sulfamethoxazole may also be initiated if *Pneumocystis* is a possibility.

If after 48–72 hours the cultures are positive, therapy should be continued for a full course depending on the organism and the state of the patient's immune system. If cultures are negative at 72 hours and the patient's granulocytes have returned, antibiotics can be stopped but the patient should continue to have a work-up if fever persists.

If an infection is found subsequently, the use of a single agent or narrow spectrum antibiotics is sufficient given a normal granulocyte count. If, however, cultures are negative, granulocytopenia persists, and the fever responded to the original broad spectrum antibiotic, coverage should be continued until either the granulocytopenia resolves or 14 days of therapy have ensued.

If the patient remains persistently febrile and granulocytopenic, further cultures should be obtained every 1–2 days, and physical examinations and chest radiographs should be monitored closely; former cultures should be checked for evidence of fungus or organisms resistant to the current antibiotic regimen by routine surveillance cultures, and tests for fungal antigens if available. If any focus presents, it should be pursued aggressively, including a lung biopsy for pulmonary infiltrates.

In general, persistent fever or slow response to a focal infection does not necessitate empiric switching of or adding additional antibiotics. Switching should be based on cultures documenting resistance or any dramatic change in clinical status, for example, suggestive of Gram-negative sepsis. Among the antibiotics often added are vancomycin for the increasingly common *S. epidermidis,* clindamycin for broader coverage of anerobic organisms, or institution of trimethoprim-sulfamethoxazole for *Pneumocystis* or erythromycin for *Mycoplasma.* Empiric antifungal therapy (amphotericin B) should be instituted if the patient has 7–10 days of persistent fever and granulocytopenia despite broad spectrum antibiotics.

If the patient is granulocytopenic and afebrile but at risk for infection, certain prophylactic measures are recommended. For example, the patient should be placed in a single room, or with an uninfected roommate. Careful hand-washing by medical personnel is indicated. Oral nonabsorbable antibiotics to sterilize bowel flora and laminar flow room environments are not used routinely, except in the ultra high-risk groups, such as the bone marrow transplant patients. In many studies the use of trimethoprim-sulfamethoxazole on a prophylactic basis has been shown to reduce detectable bacteremias as well as a variety of focal infections, especially childhood otitis. Nevertheless, chronic use of Bactrim may also result in emergence of resistant organisms, more prolonged cytopenia, fungal superinfection, and toxicity to the drug itself. Therefore, trimethoprim-sulfamethoxazole prophylaxis is currently being recommended at our institution only in groups who are at high risk for *Pneumocystis* pneumonia (Siber, 1986). In other groups the decision is made on an individual basis.

Prophylactic oral antifungal agents have yet to be shown to be totally effective, although limited evidence does suggest that oral amphotericin B at a dose of greater than 1.5 g/day may reduce mucosal *Candida* infection. Nystatin and ketoconazole, however, have not been effective in preventing subsequent fungal infections in immunosuppressed patients.

The oncology patient who has not had chickenpox and develops active varicella infection should begin treatment with intravenous acyclovir at a dose of 500 mg/m^2 every 8 hours for 7 days. If the patient has been exposed and is without symptoms, varicella zoster immune globulin should be administered, ideally within 4 days of exposure, but certainly as early as possible. The dose is one vial per 10 kg intramuscularly up to a maximum of five vials. In the future, unexposed patients with a negative history of chickenpox who develop a malignancy may be candidates for varicella zoster vaccine trial.

Live viral vaccines should be withheld from children requiring routine immunization who are on chemotherapy. Instead, toxoids and killed vaccines should be administered. If the child is able to mount an appropriate immune response either between chemotherapeutic treatments or following the induction course of chemotherapy, routine immunizations should be given including DPT and inactivated polio vaccine. Measles, mumps, and rubella should be withheld from children on chemotherapy since these are live viral vaccines. Influenza vaccines, which are inactivated, may be administered and immunosuppressed children should receive this vaccine annually in the fall. The bacterial polysaccharide vaccines should also be administered to children after chemotherapeutic treatment, since usually the immune response to polysaccharide antigens is very poor during active chemotherapy.

REFERENCES

Anand KJS, Hickey PR: Pain and its effects in the human neonate and fetus. *N Engl J Med* 317:1321, 1987.

Basbaum AI, Fields HL: Endogenous pain control systems: Brain stem spinal pathways and endorphin circuitry. *Ann Rev Neurosci* 7:309, 1984.

Beyer JE, DeGood DE, Ashley LL, et al: Patterns of postoperative analgesic use with adults and children following cardiac surgery. *Pain* 7:71, 1983.

Colter JM, Schwartz AD: Psychological and social support of the patient and family. In Altman AJ, Schwartz AD (eds): *Malig-*

nant Diseases of Infancy, Childhood, and Adolescence. Philadelphia, WB Saunders, 1983.

Cronin C: Antiemetics. *Cancer Manual,* 7th edition. American Cancer Society, 1986, p. 102.

Gershon AA, Steinberg SP, Gelb L, et al: Live attenuated varicella vaccine: Efficacy for children with leukemia in remission. *JAMA* 252:355, 1984.

Koocher G, Berman S: Life-threatening and terminal illness in childhood. In Levine M, Carey W, Crocker A, et al (eds): *Developmental Behavioral Pediatrics*. Philadelphia, WB Saunders, 1983.

Lansky SB: Management of stressful periods of childhood cancer. *Pediatr Clin North Am* 32:625, 1985.

Melzack R, Wall PD: Pain mechanisms: A new therapy. *Science* 150:971, 1965.

Merskey H: Pain terms: A list with definitions and notes on usage. Recommended by the IASP Subcommittee on Taxonomy. *Pain* 6:249, 1979.

Meunier-Carpenter F: Chemoprophylaxis of fungal infections. *Am J Med* 76:652, 1984.

Miser AW, Dans DM, Hughes CS, et al: Continuous subcutaneous infusion of morphine in children with cancer. *Am J Dis Child* 137:383, 1983.

Miser AW, Miser JS, Clark BS: Continuous intravenous infusion of morphine sulfate for control of severe pain in children with terminal malignancy. *J Pediatr* 96:930, 1980.

Newburger PE, Sallan SE: Chronic pain: Principles of management. *J Pediatr* 98:180, 1981.

Patenaude A, Berman SJ: Psychological issues. *Pediatric Hematology-Oncology Handbook*. Boston, The Children's Hospital, Dana Farber Cancer Institute, 1986, p. 18.

Pizzo PA: Infectious complications in the child with cancer. 1. Pathophysiology of the compromised host in the initial evaluation and management of the febrile cancer patient. *J Pediatr* 98:341, 1981.

Pizzo PA: Infectious complications in the child with cancer. 2. Management of specific infectious orrganisms. *J Pediatr* 98:513, 1981.

Pizzo PA, Robichaud KJ, Gill FA, et al: Empiric antibiotic and antifungal therapy for cancer patients with prolonged fever and granulocytopenia. *Am J Med* 72:101, 1982

Sallan SE, Cronin CM: Nausea and vomiting. In Devita V, Helman S, Rosenberg S (eds): *Cancer Principles and Practice of Oncology*. Philadelphia, Toronto, JB Lippincott, 1982.

Siber G: Antimicrobial strategy in febrile cancer patients. *Department of Hematology/Oncology Handbook*. Boston, The Children's Hospital-Dana Farber Cancer Institute, 1986, p. 54.

Siber G: Virus infections. *Department of Hematology/Oncology Handbook*. Boston, The Children's Hospital-Dana Farber Cancer Institute, 1986, p. 79.

Wall PD: The painful consequences of perpetual injury. *J Hand Surg* 9:37, 1984.

Zeltzer L, LeBaron F, Zeltzer P: The effectiveness of behavioral intervention for reduction of nausea and vomiting in children and adolescents receiving chemotherapy. *J Clin Oncol* 2:683, 1984.

Leukemias 3

ACUTE LYMPHOBLASTIC LEUKEMIA

Definition

Acute lymphoblastic leukemia (ALL) is a malignant disease characterized by progressive infiltration of bone marrow and lymphatic organs by immature lymphoid cells known as lymphoblasts. It is the most common childhood malignancy.

Basic Science

The exact etiology of leukemia remains unknown, although environmental and genetic factors, viruses, and immunodeficiency states have been felt to be contributing factors to the disease. Regardless of etiology, it appears that childhood ALL is a heterogeneous disorder that can be classified morphologically, immunologically, biochemically, and cytogenetically. Morphologically, the French-American-British (FAB) Cooperative Working Group established a system for classifying ALL that is now almost universally accepted (Table 9.1).

Of note, 85% of patients have the L1 subtype of ALL, with less than 2% having L3 morphology, the remainder showing L2 morphology. In several studies, patients with L1 carry a higher remission induction rate and more prolonged remission duration and survival than those with L2 and L3, with the latter having the worst prognosis. It is not clear, however, how the morphologic differences between L1 and L2 relate to a biologic basis for prognosis. L3 is the Burkitt type leukemia which does have a unique biology. Therefore, other ways to classify the acute leukemias have been developed (Poplack, 1985).

Immunologically, ALL has been subclassified as being of T cell, B cell, early-B cell, undifferentiated, or what is referred to as common acute lymphocytic leukemia antigen positive (or CALLA). Approximately 60% of children have CALLA positive leukemia (pre-B), 15% are T-cell positive, 5% are undifferentiated ALL (neither T-, B-, nor CALLA-positive), approximately 15% are early pre-B-cell positive, with B-cell leukemia making up approximately 1% of all childhood leukemias. B-cell leukemia carries the worst prognosis, whereas

Table 9.1
The French-American-British (FAB) Classification of Acute Lymphoblastic Leukemia[1]

Cytologic Features	L_1	L_2	L_3
Cell size	Small cells predominate	Large, heterogeneous in size	Large and homogeneous
Nuclear chromalin	Homogeneous in any case	Variable—heterogeneous in any one case	Finely stippled and homogeneous
Nuclear shape	Regular, occasional clefting or indentation	Irregular, clefting and indentation common	Regular—oval to round
Nucleoli	Not visible, or small and inconspicuous	One or more present, often large	Prominent: one or more vesicular
Amount of cytoplasm	Scanty	Variable, often moderately abundant	Moderately abundant
Basophilia of cytoplasm	Slight or moderate, rarely intense	Variable, deep in some	Very deep
Cytoplasmic vacuolation	Variable	Variable	Often prominent

[1]Reproduced with permission from Bennett et al: *Br J Haematol* 47:553, 1981.

lymphoblasts that have CALLA antigen carry a more favorable prognosis (Sallen, 1987).

The T-cell leukemias are thought to be derived from three distinct stages of differentiation on the basis of monoclonal antibody studies corresponding to different stages of intrathymic differentiation.

Further adding to the heterogeneity of ALL subtypes have been cytogenetic studies which have demonstrated characteristic karyotypic abnormalities in leukemic cells. For example, T-cell ALL tends to demonstrate a t (11;14) (p 13; q 13) translocation. Other characteristic translocations have been associated with other immunologic subtypes (e.g., B-cell ALL is associated with 8 q-; 14 q+ translocation).

Biochemical enzymes have also been assessed in ALL and have shown to be useful markers. For example, terminal deoxynucleotidyl transferase (TdT) is an enzyme not usually found in mature lymphocytes but present in greater than 90% of cases of childhood ALL. Therefore, finding TdT can help to differentiate ALL from the acute nonlymphoblastic leukemias and helps to confirm the diagnosis of CNS or testicular relapse when routine histopathologic methods are equivocal. Unfortunately, TdT activity noted at diagnosis does not appear to correlate with prognosis. Other enzymes have also been identified to help in the identification of subtypes of ALL.

Epidemiology

There are approximately 1500 cases of ALL diagnosed in the United States each year, thus making it the most common childhood malignancy. It has a peak age incidence in whites between 2 and 6 years, although this has not been seen in blacks. The disease is only half as common in blacks as it is in whites, occurring with an annual incidence of 2.4/100,000 children relative to 4.2/100,000 for whites. It is more common in males than in females, but there is disparity increasing with increasing age. The median age of diagnosis is 4 years (Poplack, 1985).

Natural History

Clinical manifestations may be focal or systemic, minor or life-threatening—a reflection of the degree of bone marrow infiltration and extent of extramedullary spread. The usual clinical findings include the clinical signs and symptoms of anemia, thrombocytopenia, and neutropenia. Fever, lethargy, pallor, and fatigue, bleeding with petechiae or purpura and extramedullary spread characterized by hepatosplenomegaly, extremity and/or joint pain are classical presentations of the disease. Anorexia is common with duration of symptoms before presentation varying from days to weeks to months. The differential diagnosis of a child presenting with these symptoms is a broad one, and can include a variety of infectious as well as collagen vascular disorders that need to also be considered in the differential diagnosis.

Diagnosis

A peripheral blood count may be notable for anemia, thrombocytopenia, and/or neutropenia, with definitive diagnosis resting on a bone marrow biopsy and aspirate. Examination of the aspirate can give a prompt diagnosis. The marrow biopsy is done to assess cellularity and to obtain cells for special studies. Bone marrow findings of greater than 5% lymphoblasts are consistent with leukemia, although in an aspirate, a minimum of greater than 25% leukemic lymphoblasts are required to confirm the diagnosis. The pathologist may employ special stains to distinguish ALL from acute nonlymphoblastic leukemia, whereas most laboratories nowadays will utilize biochemical, immunologic, and cytogenetic markers to better characterize the type of ALL and, hence, influence therapy and prognosis.

Metabolic abnormalities may reflect the leukemic cell burden and be a result of excessive proliferation and destruction of leukemic cells. These metabolic abnormalities might include hyperuricemia from increased catabolism of purines, and if untreated may lead to a uric acid nephropathy and subsequent renal failure. Potassium, phosphate, and lactic acid dehydrogenase (LDH) levels may also be elevated in patients with high initial leukocyte counts. Serum calcium may be low to compensate for the elevated phosphate. Radiographic examination of the chest may reveal an anterior mediastinal mass in 5–10% of newly diagnosed children. CNS leukemia at diagnosis is unusual and occurs in less than 5% of children (Poplack, 1985).

Treatment

The heterogeneity of ALL requires different treatment regimens based upon various standard clinical and laboratory risk factors (age, WBC, etc) but also includes stratification for the different immunologic subtypes and chromosome abnormalities. For example, patients with T-cell disease, chromosome translocations, WBC > 100,000, a lymphoma-like presentation, or those who require a prolonged remission induction period tend to do poorly compared with the overall group (Sallan, 1987).

Treatment protocols today also take into account the risk of CNS relapse by including cranial irradiation, with the quantity of radiation being based on risk factors identified at time of diagnosis. The use of cranial radiation (without spinal radiation) in combination with intrathecal methotrexate appears to offer adequate preventative therapy for the possibility of CNS relapse. Intrathecal methotrexate appears to be adequate CNS prophylaxis for children with ALL who have standard risk features. The complications of cranial radiation are discussed under "Radiation Therapy" (see pp. 00).

Once remission induction has occurred, the patient is entered onto maintenance chemotherapy utilizing agents such as 6-mercaptopurine, methotrexate, L-asparaginase in addition to intermittent pulses of vincristine and prednisone. The choice of the appropriate maintenance chemotherapy is dependent again upon the patient's risk group of ALL (see below). Usually maintenance therapy is continued for a period of 2–3 years. Duration of therapy in remission has been arrived at empirically and shorter courses of treatment are currently being evaluated in prospective clinical trials.

The treatment regimen used at the Dana Farber Cancer Institute and The Children's Hospital in 1987 is a five-drug remission induction program (involving methotrexate, doxorubicin, vincristine, prednisone, and L-asparaginase), CNS prophylaxis with cranial irradiation, and intrathecal cytarabine and methotrexate, followed by 2 years of maintenance chemotherapy. Patients are divided into three risk groups. The very-high risk group include patients with a WBC > 100,000/mm^3. The high-risk group includes patients with one or more of the following adverse features: age below 2 years or above 9 years, a WBC count greater than 20,000 but less than 100,000/mm^3, the presence of T-cell immunologic markers, radiologic evidence of a thymic mass, and/or involvement of the CNS. The rest of the patients are put into a standard risk group. All patients are initially treated for the first 5 days with either high-dose or low-dose intravenous asparaginase. Following these 5 days, vincristine, prednisone, methotrexate, and doxorubicin are added. Cytarabine is injected into the CSF. Four weeks later, intrathecal cytarabine is replaced by intrathecal methotrexate and cranial irradiation is begun, as well as weekly therapy with asparaginase. Standard risk patients also receive 6-mercaptopurine, methotrexate, and vincristine-prednisone pulses. Very-high and high-risk patients receive doxorubicin with or without high-dose ara-c in addition to 6-mercaptopurine. Doxorubicin has only been found to be useful for very-high and high-risk patients. Follow-up studies suggest that both groups do well with this regimen.

Prognosis

Previously it was thought that clinical factors such as age less than 2 years or greater than 9 years, male sex, white blood counts greater than 20,000 were the only poor prognostic variables. Immunologic subtype, time to enter remission (>/= 1 month), and chromosome translocations are also predictive for long-term outcome. Eighty percent of children able to achieve remission at the end of a 1-month induction period and who have standard risk features will remain disease free 5 years out from therapy, compared to 50–60% of higher risk children. The 20% who will eventually relapse will usually do so within their first year off therapy (Sallen, 1987).

Sites of relapse are most likely to be bone marrow or in males testicular relapse, prompting most institutions to biopsy asymptomatic males either during or upon completion of a successful chemotherapy course. Patients with T-cell ALL are most likely to develop earlier testicular relapse. If testicular relapse occurs, treatment includes local radiotherapy and systemic chemotherapy. Subsequently, the patient may require androgen replacement and is left clinically sterile. If bone marrow relapse occurs, a repeat multiple drug reinduction regimen, in addition to CNS preventive therapy, is required.

With each marrow relapse the ability to obtain complete remission decreases. Therefore, for patients who do relapse following one treatment (especially within 2 years from remission) with chemotherapy and cranial radiation, the recommendation is that if the patient has an HLA-compatible donor, then bone marrow transplantation should be performed. A review of studies suggests that patients transplanted during a second remission fare better than those transplanted during subsequent ones, but not all patients who relapse have appropriate HLA-matched compatible donors.

Because survival has improved dramatically with the therapies mentioned above, new sequelae are being noticed in these patients, thought to be late complications of their initial treatment, and in particular, treatment associated with CNS prophylaxis. Studies suggesting psychomotor and intellectual impairment have led to decrease in the dosage of cranial radiation and intrathecal chemotherapy. Other complications of the therapy may include short stature, although in many patients catchup growth occurs following cessation of therapy. Large doses of anthracycline (e.g., doxorubicin) therapy may increase the risk for a cardiomyopathy, although this is now monitored closely. If testicular radiation is not required, most of these patients go on to have normal gonadal function, although information regarding the teratogenicity and immunogenicity of antileukemic chemotherapeutic agents has not yet been fully reported. Studies suggest, however, no evidence thus far for an increase in birth defects in children born to parents who have been previously treated for ALL (Blatt, 1980). The risk of second malignancy remains low, although a few reports do report brain tumors occurring in children who receive cranial irradiation for treatment of ALL. Physicians who are following the treatment of these patients should be aware of the potential complications and monitor the patients appropriately as they grow older, following their chemo- and radiation therapy.

ACUTE NONLYMPHOCYTIC LEUKEMIA

Definition

Acute nonlymphocytic leukemia (ANLL) or myelogenous leukemia (AML) is a primary malignant disease of the bone marrow characterized by a predominance of immature myeloid precursors.

Basic Science

The molecular etiology for the leukemic transformation in ANLL remains unclear, although it is believed that the poorly differentiated precursors (blasts) are derived from a single progenitor cell that undergoes malignant transformation and is capable of indefinite self-renewal. Evidence for a single cell of origin for ANLL is based on cytogenetic studies as well as studies done on black females who are heterozygous for two electrophoretic distinct G6PD enzymes. It has been shown that tumors arising from one cell will express only one enzyme type whereas a tumor arising from multiple cells will express both types of G6PD. Cases of ANLL (and ALL) that have been studied for this have shown only a single G6PD phenotype in the blasts. In addition, cytogenically 90% of children with ANLL have a clonal chromosomal abnormality in their leukemia blasts that disappears in remission and reappears at relapse, again suggesting clonal origin of these malignant cells (Kaneko et al, 1982).

Since the malignant transformation can occur at any point from the pluripotential stem cell to that of committed precursor, there are heterogeneous subtypes of ANLL with regard to cell of origin. Because of this, the French-American-British system has created conventional morphological and cytochemical methods that classify ANLL into six subtypes (Table 9.2).

From an immunologic standpoint, the cell surface phenotypes that have been useful to classify patients with ALL are not recognized on the ANLL blasts. However, there are monoclonal antibodies that react with myeloid blasts, although these are not specific for leukemic cells, but will also recognize antigens from normal myeloid progenitors and their progeny. Nonetheless, they may be useful for classifying the unusual case of a morphologically undifferentiated leukemia. Biochemical markers may also be useful in identifying this malignancy. For example, muramidase or lysozyme, a hydrolytic enzyme found in primary granules of primitive granulocytes and monocytes, will demonstrate elevated serum and urine levels if present in ANLL, particularly in the M5 and M4 subtypes. Tdt is another nuclear enzyme that is present in more than 90% of cases of ALL and absent in 95% of cases of ANLL, again helping in the differentiation between the two.

Table 9.2
The French-American-British (FAB) Classification of Acute Nonlymphocytic Leukemia[1]

FAB Class	Morphology	Cytogenetics
M1, M2 (AML)	Myeloblasts	8;21 translocation
M3 (APL)	Promyelocytes	15;17 translocation
M4 (AMML)	Myeloblasts, Monoblasts	1 inversion 16
M5 (AMoL)	Monoblasts	1;11, 9;11 translocation
M6	Abnormal erythroid Myeloblasts	No consistent change
M7	Megakaryoblasts	abnormal chromosome 21

[1]Modified from Poplack DG: *Pediatr Clin North Am* 32:669, 1985. Abbreviations: MP = myeloperoxidase, NSE = nonspecific esterase, PAS = periodic acidic-Schiff.

Epidemiology

ANLL represents 15–20% of leukemias in childhood with approximately 250–300 new cases in the United States each year. Unlike ALL, there are no peaks in incidence and the distribution of new onset cases remains constant from birth throughout childhood. This incidence is similar to that of Wilms tumor, soft tissue sarcomas, and lymphomas. While the pathophysiology of this disorder remains unknown, there are certain conditions that predispose children to having an increased risk for developing ANLL. These would include children who have been previously treated with alkylating agents for other tumors, children with certain heritable diseases, or chromosomal disorders, such as Down syndrome and Fanconi syndrome (Grier and Weinstein, 1985).

Natural History

The signs and symptoms of ANLL can be insidious or life-threatening, and are usually secondary to decreased normal hematopoiesis following infiltration, or from infiltration of organs other than the bone marrow. Anemia and thrombocytopenia are common with approximately 50% of newly diagnosed children having platelet counts less than 50,000. Those who have acute promyelocytic leukemia often present with disseminated intravascular coagulation with the granules in these malignant promyelocytes containing thromboplastin activity, thus, precipitating the coagulation abnormality.

Because the absolute granulocyte count is abnormal, patients may present with lingering bacterial infections, particularly those involving respiratory, dental, sinus, perirectal, urinary tract, and skin areas. Most patients will have white blood cell counts less than 50,000 at diagnosis, although 20% will usually demonstrate counts greater than 100,000. If the white count is greater than 200,000, then leukostasis occurs, with intravascular clumping of blasts and subsequent infarction of tissue. Leukostasis usually involves brain and lung and these patients may present with somnolence, stroke symptoms, or tachypnea, in the setting of hypoxia. Leukostasis is one presentation that requires emergency treatment as discussed below. Other organs that may show involvement are the liver and spleen as well as lymph node enlargement.

Occasionally, myeloblasts will form tumor masses anywhere in the body. Such tumor masses are referred to as chloromas, named for the greenish hue sometimes seen due to the presence of myeloperoxidase within the blasts. Chloromas have been found in the skin or the spinal cord and, less frequently, compressing the airway, again presenting as a medical emergency. Unlike ALL, testicular involvement with myeloblastic infiltration is a much rarer presentation. CNS involvement has been reported in a small number of patients who are usually asymptomatic for neurologic manifestations at the time of presentation. Patients with monocytic and myelomonocytic types usually have the highest incidence of CNS involvement.

Diagnosis

Definitive proof of the diagnosis rests in the bone marrow aspirate and biopsy following morphologic and histochemical analysis. Usually in an aspirate, greater than 30% myeloblasts in the bone marrow will confirm the diagnosis. Currently, chromosome abnormalities as well as cell surface markers are also sent to further subtype the malignancy and influence treatment and, in turn, prognosis. Biochemical enzyme studies may also be useful if the bone marrow does not clarify the situation.

Treatment

Initial treatment is directed toward recognizing and treating any life-threatening complications of the disease or even of the initial chemotherapy. This can include treatment of severe anemia, hemorrhage from the thrombocytopenia, disseminated intravascular coagulation, infection, or leukostasis. Following the onset of chemotherapy, the tumor lysis syndrome can occur, which is a result of the massive catabolism of DNA following destruction of a large mass of leukemic cells. Usually to prevent this from happening, hydration and alkinization of the urine with intravenous bicarbonate as well as the administration of allopurinol should be started even before beginning chemotherapy. Hydroxyurea can also be useful in the treatment of leukostasis.

Remission induction is usually achieved with the use of cytosine arabinoside and adriamycin or daunorubicin. Unfortunately, this regimen carries a narrow therapeutic index and results in prolonged periods of marrow hypoplasia in order to achieve remission. During this time, patients are extremely susceptible to infection and require antibiotics as well as blood component support to sustain them until their marrows begin to regenerate.

While CNS prophylaxis has been shown to be effective in preventing CNS relapse, clinical trials have not yet shown that children who receive CNS prophylaxis carry a better overall disease-free survival than those children who do not receive prophylaxis. Nonetheless, at present, CNS propyhylaxis continues to be used, in particular, the addition of intrathecal ara-C as the major agent providing the prophylaxis.

The most successful treatment to sustain a remission is the use of intensive maintenance therapy requiring patients to achieve moderate aplasia with each course. In addition, agents are presented in the form of sequential noncross-resistant therapy so as to circumvent the problem of drug resistance. The recent addition of a new effective antileukemic agent known as VP16 and very high-dose ara-C show promise of leading to prolonged remission in these patients. Approximately 40–50% of patients achieve a 4-year disease-free survival, although late relapses have been reported (Creutzig et al, 1985).

An alternative to continued chemotherapy following remission is to perform a bone marrow transplant if an HLA identical sibling exists. Fifty to 60% of the patients transplanted in first remission are surviving free of leukemia at 5 years (Grier et al, 1985). Unfortunately, transplantation mortality from this procedure is high due to graft-versus-host disease or interstitial pneumonia. The risks and benefits of undergoing bone marrow transplant rather than maintenance chemotherapy must be considered carefully after first remission. Since bone marrow transplantation in second remission or early relapse has been reported to provide an approximately 30% subsequent long-term survival, one current recommendation is to use chemotherapy following remission and, only if relapse occurs, undergo bone marrow transplantation. Most centers, however, recommend bone transplantation for the child who is in first remission and has an HLA-identical sibling. Once a patient has relapsed while on therapy, reinduction can be quite difficult. Combinations of high dose ara-C, VP16, AMSA, and 5-azacytadine are currently being used for this reinduction.

Prognosis

Currently, children who present with the monocytic subtype, or are under age 2 years, and/or have white blood counts greater than 100,000 have a poor prognosis. Other studies suggest that a more rapid induction of remission correlates with an increased chance for a long-term continuous remission (Baehner et al, 1981). Regardless of therapy used, overall survival 5 years following diagnosis remains at about 30–40%.

REFERENCES

Baehner RL, Kennedy A, Sather H, et al: Characteristics of children with acute nonlymphocytic leukemia and long term continuous remission: A report for Children's Cancer Study Group. *Med Pediatr Oncol* 9:393, 1981.

Bennett JM, Catovsky D, Daniel MT, et al: Morphologic classification of acute lymphoblastic leukemia: Correlation among observers and clinical observations. *Br J Hematol* 47:553, 1981.

Blatt J, Mulvihill JJ, Ziegler JL, et al: Pregnancy outcome following cancer chemotherapy. *Am J Med* 69:828, 1980.

Clavell LA, Gelber RD, et al: Four-agent induction and intensive asparaginase therapy for treatment of childhood acute lymphoblastic leukemia *N Engl J Med* 315:657, 1986.

Creutzig U, Ritter J, Riehm H, et al: Improved treatment results in childhood acute myelogenous leukemia. *Blood* 65:298, 1985.

Foon KA, Gale RP: Controversies in the therapy of acute myelogenous leukemia. *Am J Med* 72:963, 1982.

Grier HE, Weinstein HJ: Acute nonlymphocytic leukemia. *Pediatr Clin North Am* 32:653, 1985.

Kaneko Y, Rowley JD, Maurer HS, et al: Chromosome pattern in childhood acute nonlymphocytic leukemia. *Blood* 60:389, 1982.

Muller KB, Rosenthal DS, Weinstein HJ: Leukemia. *The Cancer Manual,* 7th ed. Chapter 29. Boston, American Cancer Society, 1986, p. 318.

Poplack DG: Acute lymphoblastic leukemia in childhood. *Pediatr Clin North Am* 32:669, 1985.

Sallan SE, Weinstein HJ: Childhood Acute Leukemias. In Nathan DG, Oski FA (eds): *Hematology of Infancy and Childhood.* Philadelphia, WB Saunders, 1987, p. 1028.

Sallan SE, Weinstein HJ, Nathan DG: The childhood leukemias. *J Pediatr* 99:676, 1981.

Weinstein H, Mayer RJ, Rosenthal DS, et al: Treatment of acute myelogenous leukemia in children and adults. *N Engl J Med* 303:473, 1980.

Weinstein HJ, Mayer RJ, Rosenthal DS, et al: Chemotherapy for acute myelogenous leukemia in children and adults: VAPA update. *Blood* 62:315, 1983.

Lymphomas 4

HODGKIN DISEASE

Definition

Hodgkin disease is a malignant lymphoma of unknown etiology that is diagnosed most commonly in lymph nodes, although the tumor has been found also in liver, spleen, lung, and bone marrow. Although genetic and/or environmental causes have been suggested for the disease, particularly in association with viral etiologies, no definitive agent or specific gene has been found to be associated with the disease at the present time.

Basic Science

Hodgkin disease is considered a histologic diagnosis with the essential feature being the presence of a multinucleated giant cell, known as the Reed-Sternberg cell. It is thought that this cell is derived from the interdigitating reticulum cell, which is a specialized cell found in the pericortex of lymph nodes. It is thought to be a malignant cell because it shows both aneuploidy and heterotransplantability. The Rye histologic classification of Hodgkin disease is shown in Table 9.3.

While lymphocyte predominance is associated more commonly with early stages of the disease and lymphocyte depletion and mixed cellularity with more advanced stages, it is the anatomic staging and the pattern of disease at presentation that are the most important factors in determining treatment response and outcome.

A variety of immunologic disturbances also have been associated with the disease. Initially cellular immunity is usually defective, which is believed to be due, in part, to active suppression of T-cell function by a circulating mononuclear cell. Humoral immunity is often compromised after splenectomy in Hodgkin disease. Patients are at increased risk for varicella, herpes zoster, protozoal, fungal and encapsulated bacterial infections. The T-cell defects recognized in Hodgkin disease may persist for prolonged periods following successful treatment (Kaplan, 1981).

Epidemiology

Hodgkin disease has an annual incidence in the United States in children under 15 years of age of 0.4/100,000. A unique bimodal age distribution is apparent with peaks between 15 and 34 years of age and again in those over 50 years of age. There is a male predominance in the earlier peak, while in the older peak both sexes are equally represented. Although there are re-

Table 9.3
The Rye Histologic Classification of Hodgkin Diseases[1]

Source	Pattern	Description
Lymphocyte predominant	Diffuse	Abundant lymphocytes, sparsely distributed granulocytes and plasma cells; only occasional Reed-Sternberg cells; no fibrosis
Mixed cellularity	Diffuse	Moderate numbers of lymphocytes, plasma cells, granulocytes; Reed-Sternberg cells readily identified; possible early diffuse fibrosis
Lymphocyte depleted	Diffuse	Stromal cells and lymphocytes depleted and replaced by fibrosis; bizarre Reed-Sternberg cells usually numerous
Nodular sclerosis	Nodular	Nodularity due to birefringent collagen bands; moderate numbers of lymphocytes, plasma cells, and granulocytes; "lacunar" Reed-Sternberg cells

[1]Modified from Lukes RJ, Crayer LF, Hall TC, et al: Report of the Nomenclature Committee. *Can Res* 26:111, 1966.

ports of clusters of cases, suggesting an infectious or environmental cause, there still is no strong evidence of person-to-person transmission. There is, however, a 7-fold increase in the risk of disease for siblings of patients with Hodgkin disease, although again it is not clear whether this is based on a currently undetermined genetic or environmental effect. Some HLA antigens (A1, B5, and B18) also have been associated with increased risk for the disease (Gilchrist and Evans, 1985).

Natural History

Most children who have Hodgkin disease will present with a painless, firm, enlarged, superficial lymph node, most commonly in cervical chain and supraclavicular areas. The disease rarely presents initially in Waldeyer ring and Peyer patches in the gut and in epitrochlear lymph nodes, in contrast to the non-Hodgkin lymphomas. Less than one-quarter of children will present initially with systemic symptoms, such as weight loss, night sweats, and fever. Usually such symptoms are associated with advanced stages of the disease. More rarely, obstructive respiratory symptoms or superior vena caval obstruction syndrome, secondary to a mediastinal mass, may be associated with the initial presentation of the disease (White, 1983).

Since treatment is highly dependent upon clinical stage, patients are usually classified on a four-stage system (Table 9.4). These stages along with the presence or absence of systemic symptoms noted above, are the most useful in terms of prognosis, and in selection of treatment, with the more advanced stage requiring more aggressive treatment and carrying a worse prognosis.

Diagnosis and Staging

Once the diagnosis of Hodgkin disease has been confirmed by lymph node biopsy, noninvasive studies including liver function tests, plain chest radiograph, as well as thoracic and abdominal computerized tomography, and a Gallium scan to identify for abnormal uptake in the liver, the spleen, or lymph nodes can all be useful in terms of clinical staging. Nevertheless, these tests can result in significant numbers of false-positive and false-negative values such that when laparotomy and splenectomy are performed for staging, 25% of these patients will be found to be in a different clinical stage, with a majority showing more advanced disease (Gilchrist and Evans, 1985). Therefore, unless it is clear that there is stage 4 disease on the basis of the noninvasive work-up, an exploratory laparotomy may be necessary in children to plan proper treatment

Table 9.4
The Four Stages of Hodgkin Disease[1]

Stage	Characteristics
Stage 1	Involvement of a single lymph node region or of a single extralymphatic organ or site
Stage 2	Involvement limited to one side of the diaphragm either of ≥2 lymph node region, or localized involvement of an extralymphatic site and ≥1 lymph node region
Stage 3	Involvement of lymph node regions on both sides of the diaphragm, which may include localized involvement of an extralymphatic site or spleen
Stage 4	Diffuse or disseminated involvement of ≥1 extralymphatic organ or any liver involvement, with or without associated lymph node involvement
Each case is further classified as:	
A	If asymptomatic
B	If any of the following are present: Unexplained weight loss of more than 10% of body weight in the preceding 6 months; Unexplained fever, with temperatures above 38°C; Night sweats

[1]Modified from Carbonne PP, Kaplan HS, Musshoff K, et al: *Can Res* 31:1860, 1977.

(especially if limited radiation therapy is the preferred treatment for early stage disease [1 and 2]).

Laparotomy usually includes a splenectomy and biopsy of abdominal nodes including splenic, splenic hilar, celiac, hepatic, periaortic, and mesenteric nodes. Iliac nodal areas may be included if they appear enlarged or abnormal by lymphangiography or CT scan. Liver biopsies are usually obtained in addition to bone marrow aspiration and biopsy.

Treatment

On the basis of laparotomy staging, the appropriate treatment modality is selected. For example, patients with localized Hodgkin disease without symptoms (stage 1A and 2A) have greater than 90% survival if treated solely with adequate doses of radiation to an extended field. The treatment for patients with stage 2B Hodgkin disease, however, remains more controversial; some institutions treat these patients with both radiation and chemotherapy, while others reserve chemotherapy for relapse only. The overall survival statistics (90%) are similar. Patients with a stage 1 or stage 2 Hodgkin disease with large mediastinal masses (> 1/3 transthoracic diameter) have only a 50% likelihood of relapse-free survival following extended field radiation. Hence, they are treated with combined chemotherapy plus radiation. The usual chemotherapeutic regimen for Hodgkin disease is referred to as MOPP, which represents the drugs nitrogen mustard, oncovine (vincristine), procarbazine, and prednisone (Kaplan, 1981).

Therapy for patients with stage 3A Hodgkin disease is also controversial. Those who have upper abdominal nodal involvement (splenic, plus or minus celiac or splenic hilar) tend to have 30–50% relapse-free survival following radiotherapy alone, whereas those with lower abdominal involvement have much poorer relapse-free survival rates and, hence, are usually treated with both extended field radiation therapy and chemotherapy. The patients who also have systemic symptoms (stage 3B) have slightly lower (70–75%) disease-free survival compared with the stage 3A patients after combined modality treatment.

About 80% of stage 4A patients who receive MOPP chemotherapy will have a complete remission and 60% of these are free of disease 10 years after cessation of treatment. Other combinations of drugs are found to be comparable to MOPP (i.e., adriamycin, bleomycin, vinblastine, diethyl-triazenoimidazole-carboxamide, designated "ABVD") and may improve prognosis in patients with advanced stages of Hodgkin disease (Gilchrist and Evans, 1985).

In addition, irradiation to areas of bulk nodal disease may also increase the success rate of treatment.

In younger children where delayed bone growth can be significant, the use of lower dose radiation in combination with chemotherapy has been found successful in the earlier stages of Hodgkin disease, where previously high-dose extended field radiation had been the recommended treatment. On the other hand, older children continue to be treated with extended field radiation for early stage disease to avoid the added risks of leukemogenesis and infertility from MOPP chemotherapy.

The complications of treatment in Hodgkin disease are receiving increased attention because over 80% of children are now long-term survivors. Sterility has been strongly associated with MOPP chemotherapy in almost all males and one-quarter of females treated with these agents, although the incidence may be lower in children treated before puberty. Younger children (< 10 years of age) treated with radiation develop abnormalities in bone and soft tissues within the radiation field, including a shortened sitting height as well as narrow intraclavicular distance and small neck. Radiation to the thyroid is associated with chemical hypothyroidism in 50–60% of patients. The staging laparotomy carries a postoperative mortality rate of 0.5% and, if splenectomy is induced, this may lead to increased risk for overwhelming sepsis if performed at a young age. Radiation pneumonitis, carditis, and pericarditis, more common a decade ago have decreased in frequency as complications, owing to more appropriate shielding of critical areas and adjustment of radiation doses (Mauch et al, 1983).

The most significant complication of therapy of Hodgkin disease has been the recent finding that these patients have an increased risk of developing a second malignancy. For example, acute nonlymphocytic leukemia has been shown to be a long-term complication of chemotherapy in patients who received MOPP with or without radiotherapy. The incidence of secondary non-Hodgkin lymphoma is also increased in these patients.

Prognosis and Follow-up

Prognosis is highly dependent upon stage at diagnosis. Patients who have been successfully treated require follow-up studies usually every 3 months within the first 2 years after completion of treatment, which is the prime time for relapse to occur. At present, overall 10-year survivals for patients with pathologically confirmed stage 1 to stage 3 ranges from 70–95%. Overall 5-year survival of patients with advanced stage 3 and 4 disease following chemotherapy alone is 65%, with disease-free survival at 10 years being 53% (Gilchrist and Evans, 1985). Survival is improved if radiation is added to the regimen for patients with stage 3 disease. Patients with systemic symptoms have a 10% lower survival rate than do those without such symptoms.

NON-HODGKIN LYMPHOMA

Definition

Non-Hodgkin lymphomas are a heterogeneous group of malignant tumors of lymphoreticular cell origin. They include all malignant lymphomas not classified as Hodgkin disease.

CASE ILLUSTRATION

An 8-year-old male with a past history of asthma presented with a 2-week history of progressive left cervical neck swelling. He was well until 1 month before admission, when he fell while holding a stick in his mouth scratching his posterior pharynx and uvula. He then remained well until 2 weeks before admission when he noted a lump on the left side of his neck. He was seen in the emergency room with an otherwise normal examination, a normal CBC except for 6% eosinophils and a sedimentation rate of 10 mm. The patient had a negative throat culture and normal chest radiograph, and was sent home on erythromycin for a presumptive cervical adenitis. Over the next 2 weeks, however, the neck mass continued to enlarge, prompting admission to the hospital. There was no history of fever, night sweats, weight loss, or exposure to cats or tuberculosis.

On examination, the patient was afebrile with heart rate of 128/min, respirations of 24/min, blood pressure 110/70. There was a 6 × 7 cm left submandibular mass that was nontender, firm, mobile without erythema, as well as several small lymph nodes in the right cervical chain and both axillae. There was no hepatosplenomegaly. Repeat laboratory studies were remarkable for a hematocrit of 37%, white blood count of 7400/mm^3, with 26% polys, 3% bands, 48% lymphs, 13% monos, 8% eos, and 1% atypical lymph, platelets of 355,000/mm^3, and a sedimentation rate of 24 mm.

QUESTION AND COMMENT

What is the differential diagnosis? What further diagnostic work-up is indicated?

It was initially thought that this patient's clinical presentation represented reactive hyperplasia secondary to the stick that was lodged in his pharynx for a period of time, or represented inflammation secondary to infection (e.g., viral, atypical mycobacteria, or even cat scratch disease despite a negative history). Studies suggest, however, that independent of location, if the node increases in size over a 2-week follow-up period as in our patient, or has not decreased in size over a full week despite antibiotics, or becomes firm and nonmobile, a biopsy is recommended (Knight et al, 1982).

A biopsy was performed shortly after admission in this patient and revealed pathology consistent with Hodgkin disease of the nodular sclerosing type. The patient subsequently underwent further staging laparotomy that confirmed stage 2A of Hodgkin disease.

Notably, the majority of Hodgkin disease in younger children is of the nodular sclerosing type, with less than 20% presenting with a constitutional symptom complex, and few being in stages 3 or 4 at time of diagnosis, as compared with 40% of an older (control) population, again consistent with a favorable prognosis.

The use of radiotherapy, however (with subsequent poor vertebral and rib growth) as well as of chemotherapy (with secondary oncogenesis, sterility, and/or immunosuppression), continues to remain a long-term complication despite the favorable cure rate in young children (Mauch et al, 1983).

Basic Science

The etiology for the malignant lymphomas continues to be essentially unknown. Although children with congenital or acquired immune deficiencies have an increased incidence of lymphoma, most children who develop non-Hodgkin lymphoma (NHL) have no detectable immune deficit at time of diagnosis. Viral etiologies have also been explored, since experimental work in animals has revealed a number of virus-induced lymphomas.

The Epstein-Barr virus has been most closely linked to development of human lymphoma and has been associated with the development of Burkitt lymphoma in Africa where the tumor is endemic. It is currently thought that Epstein-Barr virus infection results in polyclonal expansion of B lymphocytes in African children. The setting of malarial infection that can result in T-cell-mediated immunodeficiency, provides perfect conditions for unregulated B-cell growth, and hence, the increased incidence of Burkitt lymphoma. The fact that in areas outside Africa where Epstein-Barr virus infection is found the tumor is less prevalent suggests that an additional trigger mechanism affecting the immune system is needed, such as another B-lymphocyte tropic virus (Link, 1980).

Recent developments in cytogenetics and molecular biology have also aided definition of the pathogenesis of some non-Hodgkin lymphomas. For example, Burkitt lymphoma has been associated with chromosomal translocations in which genetic material from the distal segment of the long arm of chromosome 8 is translocated to chromosome 14 or occasionally to chromosomes 2 or 22. Interestingly, genetic coding for heavy chain, κ light chain, and λ light chains of immunoglobulin also reside on chromosomes 14, 2, and 22, respectively. As a result of these translocations, the c-myc oncogene, normally found on chromosome 8, is unregulated and most likely plays a major role in the clonal expansion of a B-cell line leading to the lymphoid neoplasia of Burkitt lymphoma (Croce and Norwell, 1985). Other lymphomas are currently being examined at the cytogenetic and molecular levels to determine whether translocations also play a role in tumor pathogenesis.

Many systems are used to classify the wide spectrum of pathologic heterogeneity in non-Hodgkin lymphoma. The best known and still most widely used is the classification into "nodular" and "diffuse" histology (Rappaport, 1966). While 50% of non-Hodgkin lymphoma in adults is of the nodular type, the vast majority of childhood non-Hodgkin lymphomas are classified as diffuse types with three major subtypes predominating—the diffuse lymphoblastic (30–40%), diffuse undifferentiated (30–40%), and diffuse histiocytic (15–20%) (Murphy, 1978).

The use of immunologic techniques has helped to classify further the different subtypes of non-Hodgkin lymphoma, particularly through the use of monoclonal antibodies to aid in the immunodiagnosis of these tumors. The majority of the lymphoblastic lymphomas are T-cell-derived, whereas the undifferentiated (Burkitt) lymphomas are B-cell-derived. The histiocytic lymphomas are largely B-cell but may be T-cell and are rarely true histiocytes (Foon and Todd, 1986).

Epidemiology

The malignant lymphomas represent the third most common malignancy of children in the United States, accounting for about 10% of all cases. The ratio of non-Hodgkin lymphoma to Hodgkin lymphoma is approximately 3:2, with the median age of children with non-Hodgkin lymphoma being 11 years (range 2–17) and with a male to female ratio of 2–3:1 (Link, 1980). As noted above, children with inherited or acquired immunodeficiency syndromes are estimated to be 100–10,000 times more likely to develop non-Hodgkin lymphoma than are age-matched controls.

Natural History

Unlike Hodgkin disease, only 10–15% of patients with non-Hodgkin lymphoma will present with primary peripheral lymph node involvement. These tumors have a propensity for extranodal involvement and will show early noncontiguous dissemination. Symptoms may be indistinguishable from those in a variety of childhood illnesses and can include pharyngitis, cough, abdominal pain, vomiting, and less often adenopathy, with symptoms usually lasting less than 4–6 weeks before diagnosis is made. Anterior mediastinal masses are frequently associated with adenopathy above the diaphragm and can be associated with respiratory difficulty or even obstruction of the superior vena cava.

Thirty to 40% of children present with abdominal pain or vomiting, with or without a palpable abdominal mass (Weinstein and Link, 1979). An ileocecal intussusception may also be the first diagnostic presentation, secondary to an intraluminal lymphoma within the intestine. Abdominal masses are usually rapidly enlarging, are rarely completely resectable at the time of diagnosis, and are of the undifferentiated Burkitt type. They are associated with a variety of metabolic abnormalities including hyperuricemia, hyperphosphatemia, and hyperkalemia. Acute renal failure can result from uric nephropathy and direct renal infiltration by these tumors can further compromise kidney function.

Overall, most children with non-Hodgkin lymphoma can be classified into two broad categories: those with localized disease in favorable sites (i.e., neck nodes, tonsils, limited ileal-cecal masses), and those with disease in unfavorable sites (e.g., anterior mediastinal masses) representing two-thirds of children and the majority of treatment failures.

Diagnosis

Definitive diagnosis of a non-Hodgkin lymphoma depends on histopathologic examination of the appropriate tissue obtained by biopsy, which should be subjected to immunophenotyping and cytogenetic analysis. As with Hodgkin disease, the clinical staging system based on pathologic and clinical evidence for tumor location is the most helpful in determining treatment and prognosis.

Since there is noncontiguous disease dissemination, an exploratory laparotomy for pathological staging is not indicated. Since the major thrust of treatment as outlined below is systemic chemotherapy, a search for occult disease is really unnecessary. Usually a laparotomy is reserved for those children who have abdominal presentations. In addition, CBC, reticulocyte, platelet counts, liver function tests, uric acid, calcium, phosphorus, BUN, creatinine, and electrolytes can be useful.

Although the CBC may demonstrate anemia or leukoerythroblastosis usually due to bone marrow infiltration, it is generally not very abnormal. Bone marrow aspirate and biopsy should be obtained and if the patient has greater than 25% blasts in the bone marrow in the presence of a lymphoblastic lymphoma the patient is classified and treated as a patient with acute lymphoblastic leukemia, since these two entities are not morphologically distinguishable in tissue sections or in bone marrow aspirates. Both children with T-cell ALL and lymphoblastic lymphoma tend to show relapse in the extramedullary sites, (the testes, the CNS, skin, and kidneys). From a radiologic standpoint, chest radiograph and abdominal ultrasonography, CT scan and radionucleotide examination may also be useful to help delineate tumor involvement. If pleural or ascitic fluid is present, it can be very useful in making the diagnosis, since these fluids will usually contain enormous numbers of malignant cells.

Treatment

Since there is great potential for rapid dissemination of these tumors from localized sites of disease, the mainstay of therapy is modeled after treatment for ALL, with current treatment programs achieving 50–80% 3-year relapse-free survival for all children with non-Hodgkin lymphoma (Link, 1980).

As with leukemia, achievement of remission is critical for long-term survival. Following induction, maintenance therapy is given for 6–24 months, with use of multiple agents to prevent the emergence of drug-resistant malignant clones. Prophylactic treatment for CNS relapse, a most common site in children, is incorporated into treatment protocols for non-Hodgkin lymphoma in children, with regimens similar to those for ALL. Children who have localized GI primaries carry a lower risk of primary meningeal relapse and, in some protocols, CNS prophylaxis has been omitted.

The role of radiotherapy in association with chemotherapy in assisting induction remains unproven at present, particularly in children with advanced stage non-Hodgkin lymphoma. In addition, radiotherapy has recently been shown not to be necessary in children with localized non-Hodgkin lymphoma, who also are being treated with combination chemotherapy.

As expected, certain histological subtypes respond better to particular chemotherapeutic regimens than do others.

The role of surgery in these patients is minimal. Surgery should be restricted to biopsy and resection of limited ileocecal undifferentiated lymphomas. Radiotherapy remains useful only in some protocols for CNS prophylaxis, which has been accepted for children in stage 3 and stage 4 lymphoblastic and undifferentiated lymphomas, but remains controversial for patients with histiocytic lymphomas. Usually cranial irradiation or intrathecal methotrexate alone provide adequate CNS prophylaxis. Only if there is a Burkitt lymphoma of the head and neck should CNS prophylaxis be used in children with stage 1 or stage 2 non-Hodgkin lymphoma.

Prognosis

At present, 90% of children with localized lymphoblastic lymphoma appear to be cured with chemotherapy (Jenkin, 1984). The prognosis for children with advanced abdominal B-cell undifferentiated lymphoma has improved dramatically during the past 5 years. Survival has increased from 40% to about 75%. Relapses almost always occur within the first 6–9 months after diagnosis. Failure to achieve remission occurs in fewer than 10% of patients and is associated with very short survival. Patients with Burkitt lymphoma and CNS involvement in particular carry the worst prognosis, with less than a 20% chance of survival over 5 years.

REFERENCES

Carbonne PP, Kaplan HS, Musshoff K, et al: Report of the committee on Hodgkin's disease staging classification. *Can Res* 31:1860, 1971.

Croce CM, Nowell PC: Molecular basis of human B cell neoplasia. *Blood* 65:1, 1985.

Desforges J, Rutherford C, Piro A: Medical progress in Hodgkin's disease. *N Engl J Med* 301:1212, 1979.

Donaldson SS, Kaplan HS: Complications of treatment of Hodgkin's disease in children. *Can Treat Rep* 66:977, 1982.

Foon KA, Todd RF III: Immunologic classification of leukemia and lymphoma. *Blood* 68:1, 1986.

Gilchrist GS, Evans RG: Contemporary issues in pediatric Hodgkin's disease. *Pediatr Clin North Am* 32:721, 1985.

Jenkin RDT, Anderson JR, et al: The treatment of localized non-Hodgkin's lymphoma in children: A report from the Children's Cancer Study Group. *J Clin Oncol* 2:88, 1984.

Kaplan HS: Hodgkin's disease: Biology, treatment, prognosis. *Blood* 57:813, 1981.

Knight PJ, Mulne AF, Vassy LE: When is lymph node biopsy indicated in children with a large peripheral node? *Pediatrics* 69:391, 1982.

Link MP: Non-Hodgkin's lymphoma in children. *Pediatr Clin North Am* 32:1699, 1980.

Lukes RJ, Craver LF, Hall TC, et al: Report of the nomenclature committee. *Can Res* 26:111, 1966.

Mauch P, Weinstein H, Botnick L, et al: An evaluation of long-term survival and treatment complications in children with Hodgkin's disease. *Cancer* 51:925, 1983.

Murphy SB: Current concepts in cancer: Childhood non-Hodgkin's lymphoma. *N Engl J Med* 299:1446, 1978.

Murphy SB: The lymphomas and lymphadenopathy. In Nathan DG, Oski FA (eds): *Hematology of Infancy and Childhood*, 3rd edition. Philadelphia, WB Saunders, 1987, p. 1086.

Rappaport H: Tumors of the hematopoietic system. In *Atlas of Tumor Pathology*. Section 3, Fascicle 8. Washington, DC, US Armed Forces Institute of Pathology, 1966.

Weinstein H, Link M: Non-Hodgkin's lymphoma in childhood. *Clin Hematol* 8:699, 1979.

White L: Patterns of Hodgkin's disease at diagnosis in young children. *Am J Pediatr Hematol/Oncol* 5:251, 1983.

Ziegler JL: Burkitt's lymphoma. *N Engl J Med* 300:735, 1981.

Histiocytic Proliferative Disorders

5

LANGERHANS CELL HISTIOCYTOSIS (Histiocytosis X)

Definition

Histiocytosis X (or reticuloendotheliosis) refers to a spectrum of histiocytic conditions. When it occurs at birth or during the first year of life, it is typically a fatal systemic disorder, known as *Letterer-Siwe* disease. Another variant is *Hand-Schuller-Christian* disease, which is characterized by otitis media, exophthalmos, and diabetes insipidus. At any age, single or multiple clusters of histiocytes and eosinophils may form granulomas, often in bone, but in other organs as well; this form of histiocytosis is called *eosinophilic granuloma.* A rare presentation of Letterer-Siwe disease can mimic severe combined immunodeficiency syndrome (SCIDS). Another rare histiocytic disorder referred to as familial erythrophagocytic lymphohistiocytosis occurs during the first year of life and is characterized by hepatosplenomegaly and CNS infiltration; it is a rapidly progressive and fatal disorder if untreated. Remissions can be achieved with chemotherapy, but no cures have been reported.

A malignant lymphoma-like disorder characterized by erythrophagocytosis, pancytopenia, lymphadenopathy, and fever has been referred to as malignant histiocytosis or histiocytic medullary reticulosis.

Basic Science

The grouping of these disorders with very different clinical manifestations was primarily on the basis of pathological evidence of a malignant or reactive histiocytosis. Reactive histiocytosis can be triggered by infection (as in congenital rubella) or immunodeficiency. The etiology of the various forms of histiocytosis remains obscure.

The severe forms of the syndrome have been seen in monozygotic twins, and in siblings in a manner that suggests an autosomal recessive inheritance (Juberg et al, 1970). Most cases are sporadic. No evidence has been found to suggest that the disorder is transmissible.

Nezelof et al (1973) have proposed the concept that the Langerhans cells, a subpopulation of the mononuclear-phagocytic system, proliferate. They may represent a malignant overgrowth of dendritic cells. These are the pathognomonic cells in the histiocytosis X syndrome and have unique cytoplasmic inclusions. In some cases, immunological abnormalities have been found that may be the consequence of viral illness, or a failure of regulation of mononuclear cells. These authors suggest that histiocytosis X be considered one kind of proliferative histiocytosis. Other categories of histiocytosis, according to Nezelof et al (1985) include a reactive and secondary response to chronic intracellular infection or an immune deficiency state. This kind of response can occur in association with Epstein-Barr virus infection. It presumably represents an altered immune state in familial lymphohistiocytosis.

Another category consists of dystrophic histiocytoses associated with storage of exogenous or endogenous lipid material. Included in this group would be Gaucher, Niemann-Pick, gangliosidosis, Wolman, Farber, and Tangier diseases.

Epidemiology

All forms of histiocytosis are rare. They have been noted in all races.

Natural History

Letterer-Siwe disease can mimic a number of serious disorders of infancy associated with fever, irritability, hepatosplenomegaly, lymphadenopathy, and skin lesions. No infectious agents have been incriminated in these infants, whose diagnosis depends on pathognomonic lesions in skin or lymph node biopsy. Hematologic findings may include anemia, thrombocytopenia, and a normal white cell count.

The cutaneous lesions can vary from discrete elevated 1- to 2-mm nodules over the trunk, to a widespread eczematous dermatitis, with or without petechiae. A crusted seborrheic dermatitis over the scalp is commonly the presenting symptom.

The course is usually progressively downhill, unless the infant is one of the few who responds to therapy. Intestinal malabsorption of unknown cause, and failure to gain weight are common problems. If the skin is the only organ involved, however, the prognosis is very good.

Hand-Schuller-Christian syndrome has a variable presentation. When the skeleton or skin are the primary organs involved, the course may be one of remissions, exacerbations, or recovery over years. When liver, spleen, lymph nodes, and marrow are involved, the syndrome more closely resembles Letterer-Siwe disease and has a grave prognosis.

Over age 5 years, the skeleton is the organ most severely involved. Granulomas can replace bone in calvarium, orbits, mandibles (with "floating" teeth loosened by granulomatous tissue around the roots) and appear in nearly all bones as single or multiple lesions. They may be asymptomatic and identified only by radiographic examination. Sometimes a soft nodule is palpable on the scalp. The lesions are osteolytic, with no evidence of new bone formation in the early stages. Eventually, they can heal completely.

Skin is affected in about one-third of patients, and can easily be misdiagnosed as eczema or seborrheic dermatitis. The external ear canal is involved frequently. Mastoid bone involvement also can erode the middle ear and establish a chronic otitis media that fails to respond to courses of antibiotics.

About 10–15% of patients have pulmonary infiltrates. The presenting finding may be pneumothorax. More often the infiltrates are asymptomatic and are seen on a chest radiograph taken as part of a bone survey.

Diabetes insipidus occurs with an acute onset in some individuals, as the granulomatous tissue surrounds the pituitary stalk and occludes the blood supply to the posterior lobe. When the disease involves the orbit, proptosis may occur, which together with punched-out bone lesions and diabetes insipidus constitutes the triad of symptoms (seen together in only about 10% of children).

Eosinophilic granulomas may occur as isolated bone lesions at any age. When found in childhood, they are rarely solitary for long, and more commonly (but not always) herald additional involvement.

Diagnosis

When the clinical syndromes suggest histiocytosis X, biopsy of a skin lesion, lymph node, liver, or bone marrow is in order although bone marrow involvement is rare. A solitary eosinophilic granuloma can be diagnosed by curettage, which may also be therapeutic.

The histologic findings are mononuclear infiltrates of papillary dermis, or clusters of mononuclear cells, giant cells, and eosinophils in other tissues. Necrosis of the cellular granuloma can occur. Some cells are xanthomatous or foamy and contain cholesterol (serum cholesterol levels are normal).

Treatment

The goal of treatment is to reduce the size of the lesions with the most benign intervention. Patients with disease in a single bone or occasionally multiple bones can be treated with surgical curettage if the lesions are easily accessible. Failure to respond, or further organ involvement is an indication for additional therapy with agents such as vinblastine or cyclophosphamide, in addition to prednisone. The latter agents can depress bone marrow and should not be used unless there is progressive involvement of liver and spleen or other viscera. Other chemotherapeutic regimens are used if vinblastine and prednisone fail. Chlorambucil is avoided due to the increased incidence of late (secondary) malignancy with this agent.

Lesions that endanger vital structures, such as in the orbit or mastoids, respond well to radiation therapy. Lesions in poorly accessible sites or those that recur after curettage should also be irradiated.

Prognosis

All lesions are potentially reversible except diabetes insipidus. Even that may reverse if radiation is started as soon as the diagnosis is established. The prognosis is dependent on extent of involvement, age at onset, number of organs involved, and degree of specific organ dysfunction.

Malignant Histiocytosis (Lymphohistiocytosis)

Definition

Malignant histiocytosis is a lymphoma-like disorder of the reticuloendothelial system. The liver, spleen, bone marrow, and lymph nodes become infiltrated with proliferating macrophages. Erythrophagocytosis is characteristic of the disease.

Epidemiology

This rare condition is seen mostly in adults, but can occur in the first decade of life. The familial syndrome of erythrophagocytic lymphohistiocytosis is another histiocytic disorder that may be confused with malignant histiocytosis.

Natural History

The presenting findings are usually fever, malaise, and failure to gain weight. Anemia, lymphadenopathy, hepatosplenomegaly, and pancytopenia are usually present. Pulmonary involvement is common. Erythrophagocytosis is prominent and may contribute to the refractory anemia.

The disease is progressive, and the mean survival from diagnosis to death is less than 6 months.

Diagnosis

Bone marrow aspiration or lymph node biopsy is essential for diagnosis.

Treatment

Combination chemotherapy with agents useful in non-Hodgkin lymphomas have resulted in remissions in the majority of patients and probable cures in some individuals.

REFERENCES

Avery ME, McAfee JG, Guild HG: The course and prognosis of reticuloendotheliosis (eosinophilic granuloma, Schuller-Christian disease, and Letterer-Siwe disease): A study of forty cases. *Am J Med* 22:636, 1957.

Case Record of Massachusetts General Hospital. Letterer-Siwe disease. *N Engl J Med* 313:874, 1985.

Greenberger JS, Crocker AC, Vawter G, et al: Results of treatment of 127 patients with systemic histiocytosis (Letterer-Siwe syndrome, Schuller-Christian syndrome and multifocal eosinophilic granuloma). *Medicine* 60:311, 1981.

Juberg RC, Kloepfer W, Oberman HA: Genetic determination of acute disseminated histiocytosis X (Letterer-Siwe syndrome). *Pediatrics* 45:753, 1970.

Nezelof C, Barbey S: Histiocytosis: Nosology and pathobiology. *Pediatr Pathol* 3:1, 1985.

Nezelof C, Basset F, Rousseau MF: Histiocytosis X: Histogenetic arguments for a Langerhans cell origin. *Biomedicine* 18:365, 1973.

Starling KA: Chemotherapy of histiocytosis. *Am J Pediatr Hematol/Oncol* 3:157, 1981.

Nervous System Tumors

6

Definition

Childhood nervous system tumors can be classified as being either infratentorial (cerebellar astrocytomas, medulloblastomas, brain stem gliomas) or supratentorial (pinealomas, ependymomas, glioblastomas, craniopharyngiomas).

Basic Science

There is great heterogeneity in the different types of brain tumors that can occur in a child, and hence each tumor requires separate treatment strategies depending on its biology, location, and therapeutic responsiveness. Because it is not possible to perform radical surgical resection and because the blood-brain barrier can significantly impair drug entry in normal brain tissue, there is limitation in the different types of therapy available for treatment of specific tumors. Basic science as it relates to a specific tumor is discussed under that subsection of this chapter.

Epidemiology

Neoplasms of the nervous system represent the most common solid tumors in children (15–20% of all childhood solid tumors) and are the second most common form of childhood cancer (20%). Two-thirds of childhood brain tumors occur in the posterior fossa with a peak age of 5–9 years. The annual incidence in children under 15 years is 2.4/100,000 with over 1200 new cases occurring each year (Young and Miller, 1975). Incidence and 5-year survival percentages are shown in Table 9.5.

Natural History

Brain tumors produce clinical signs and symptoms based on three mechanisms: (1) nonspecific effects of increased intracranial pressure, (2) secondary effects related to displacement of intracranial structures, and (3) the focal effects associated with direct involvement of the brain and cranial nerves. The clinical characteristics of increased intracranial pressure in a very young child can manifest as lethargy, alternating with irritability, vomiting, and listlessness. In older children, they can present as morning headache, morning vomiting, or lethargy. Signs of increased intracranial pressure in an infant can be demonstrated by finding split sutures or bulging fontanelle, whereas in an older child whose sutures have closed they may present as papilledema, a sixth cranial nerve or abducens palsy, nuchal rigidity, or head tilt. Clinical characteristics of specific tumors are given in Table 9.6.

Diagnosis

The presence of symptoms of increased intracranial pressure with a confirmatory finding of signs on physical examination represent the major criteria for suggesting the diagnosis of a brain tumor. A CT scan can give information regarding the degree of intracranial pressure, the amount of ventricular dilatation, evidence of a mass effect, the type of mass, presence of cerebral edema, bone erosion, or hemorrhage or infarction. With the advent of the CT scan, skull radiographs are no longer necessary, although they may provide initial clues if sutures are split or an empty or enlarged sella turcica or calcification is seen. If there is no finding to account for an increase in intracranial pressure, a lumbar puncture and myelogram should be performed to assess the possibility of spinal cord seeding. For example, approximately one-third of children (especially those under 5 years old) with medulloblastoma will show spinal cord disease as well. The documentation of metastatic spread will influence the treatment for patients with medulloblastoma and help measure effectiveness of subsequent chemotherapy.

Spinal fluid cytology, protein, and hormonal markers can be helpful in diagnosing and following the course of a tumor. Patients with medulloblastoma of stage T3 or greater should have a bone marrow aspirate and bone scan since bony involvement can occur in one-fifth of these patients. An EEG should be obtained if patients present after seizure activity. Angiography and pneumoencephalography are rarely used for diagnostic work-up with the advent of the CT scan, although an angiogram would be useful if an arteriovenous malformation is suspected or if the vascularity of the tumor needs to be determined before surgery. Most recently, the magnetic resonance imaging (MRI) scan has been found to be useful for evaluation and follow-up of children with brain stem gliomas (Gooding et al, 1984). The definitive diagnosis rests with tissue biopsy, which can be performed at the discretion of a neurosurgical consultant. Infratentorial tumors are much more difficult to biopsy, although by using a CT scan-guided technique, biopsies of brain stem tumors have been successfully obtained.

Treatment

Specific therapeutic modalities are discussed under the appropriate tumor type. Several general principles prevail regardless of the type of tumor diagnosed. For example, the best therapy is surgical resection if it is possible. By removing large numbers of malignant cells as well as necrotic areas with poor blood supply,

Table 9.5
Childhood Incidence and 5-Year Survival Percentages for Nervous System Tumors[1]

	Incidence	5-Year Survival
Medulloblastoma	25%	40%
Low-grade supratentorial astrocytoma	23%	69%
Cerebellar astrocytoma "Glioma A"	13%	91%
High-grade supratentorial astrocytoma	11%	35%
Brain stem gliomas	10%	17%
Ependymomas	9%	27%

[1]Data from SEER Registry 1973–1981.

the effectiveness of subsequent radiation and chemotherapy may be enhanced.

Following surgery, radiation therapy has historically been the treatment of choice, with tumor doses ranging from 5000–6000 rads in addition to craniospinal irradiation for tumors that are likely to metastasize to the spinal cord (medulloblastoma and ependymoma). Recently, increasing numbers of malignant tumors of the CNS have been treated by full craniospinal irradiation since this has been found to be most highly associated with long-range cure. Recurrent brain

Table 9.6
Clinical Characteristics of Specific Nervous System Tumors[1]

Tumor	Symptoms	Signs
Astrocytoma	Increased intracranial pressure (IIP)	Often few, depends on specific hemisphere location IIP
Medulloblastoma	IIP Head tilt Neck stiffness	IIP Truncal ataxia Nystagmus in all directions of gaze
Cerebellar astrocytoma	IIP Clumsiness to one side of body	IIP Ipsilateral limb ataxia Nystagmus when patient looks toward the lesion
Pontine glioma	IIP—later than others Head tilt Double vision Vertigo Gait disturbance	Multiple cranial nerve palsies, especially VI Ataxia IIP
Craniopharyngioma	IIP Visual disturbances Small stature Diabetes insipidus	IIP Bitemporal hemianopsia Skull films often diagnostic

[1]Courtesy of C. Kretschmar, M.D.

tumors have been found to show some response to chemotherapy. As of 1987, a number of cancer centers have begun to use chemotherapeutic regimens before radiation therapy since it is believed that "preradiation chemotherapy" can shrink gross tumors and, thus, enable later curative surgical resection and/or decrease the amount of radiation dosage to a child. Radiation may induce microvascular changes which can diminish uptake or delivery of drugs to CNS tumors. The maximal dose of a chemotherapeutic agent may be severely limited by bone marrow reserves following craniospinal irradiation. Finally, it is now clear that children under 2 years of age suffer some intellectual impairment following radiation therapy and for these infants, chemotherapy is a reasonable alternative (Allen, 1985).

New developments in therapy include more intensive preradiation drug combinations based on tumor sensitivities and potential toxicities, the use of radioactive implants, and antibody target chemotherapy.

ASTROCYTOMAS

Definition

Astrocytoma refers to a group of low-grade tumors derived from astrocytic glial cells that are usually located in the cerebellar hemispheres or less commonly above the tentorium or in the spinal cord. These are slowly growing tumors with slow infiltrative potential that are usually cystic and well encapsulated. If the tumor is not resectable, however, it becomes malignant on the basis of location since it will slowly expand into vital structures such as the brain stem, diencephalon, or optic chiasm.

Malignant astrocytomas or the most anaplastic form, glioblastoma multiforme, usually rise above the tentorium but can occur occasionally in the brain stem, and only rarely in the cerebellum. Although much rarer, these tumors carry a much poorer prognosis, with large infiltrating lesions causing major shifts in intracranial structure and episodes of increased intracranial pressure.

Basic Science

Gilles et al (1983) distinguish the benign cerebellar astrocytoma as a type A or glioma A subtype, and the more malignant and anaplastic astrocytomas as glioma B.

Epidemiology

Cerebellar astrocytomas constitute 10–30% of pediatric brain tumors.

Natural History

Glioma A cerebellar astrocytomas tend to have symptoms of long duration, whereas the more high grade astrocytomas (type B) have a clinical presentation relating primarily to their size, location, and rapidity of growth, with local seizures being the presenting symptom in over 30% of cases. Sometimes the presentation may suggest an intracerebral arterial malformation since the child can develop a sudden change in sensorium and rapid clinical deterioration.

Treatment

Cerebellar astrocytomas in children may be curable by surgery alone, and therefore, no adjuvant therapy is indicated. The glioma B tumors, however, cannot be completely resected and, therefore, radiotherapy is indicated. Recently, these tumors have been treated also with adjuvant chemotherapy, which has doubled the time of disease-free survival compared with radiation therapy and surgical resection alone. Complete cure, however, has yet to be achieved, with chemotherapy only postponing time to relapse (Gilles et al, 1983).

MEDULLOBLASTOMA

Definition

Medulloblastoma is the most common malignant brain tumor occurring in about 20–25% of children with brain tumors. Its normal site of origin is in the vermis of the cerebellum close to the fourth ventricle. It is thought that they are derived from neuroblasts or primitive neurons, such that their usual presentation is in midline position. Those that occasionally appear eccentrically along the cerebellar hemispheres, are believed to arise from the fetal granular layer. The tumors are solid, infiltrative, often tend to include the foramen magnum and can metastasize along the spinal cord via CSF.

Epidemiology

These tumors occur more frequently in males than in females and in infants than in older children or adults.

Natural History

Because of their predisposition to cause obstructive hydrocephalus, these tumors also present with symptoms of headache, lethargy, vomiting, and with ataxia if in a posterior cerebellar location.

Diagnosis

Diagnosis is usually made on the basis of the CT scan. Evidence for metatastic spread may be found by noting tumor cells in CSF. Once the tumor is suspected, all patients should be staged according to an operative staging system, which is useful for determining treatment and prognosis.

A myelogram, CSF examination, and a bone marrow aspirate will complete the diagnostic evaluation prior to therapy.

Treatment

The treatment of choice is surgical removal of as much tumor as possible, although surgery alone is not curative. The tumor is highly radiosensitive, occasionally radiocurable, and is also chemosensitive. Radiotherapy is administered to encompass the entire neuroaxis. Survival studies show that 30–50% of patients are disease-free in 10 years. If relapse occurs it is usually within the first 5 years of therapy. Children with invasive tumors or those who have metastases have greatly diminished survival statistics and are candidates for chemotherapy in addition to radiotherapy (although survival has not been greatly improved with the use of chemotherapeutic protocols to date) (Allen, 1985). Children who survive therapy are at increased risk for late effects of radiation, including learning disabilities, hypothyroidism, and growth failure.

Prognosis

Patients with disseminated disease at diagnosis have a poorer prognosis. In particular, children under age 4 years have a poor prognosis, not only because of the high incidence of metastatic disease at diagnosis, but also because radiation doses have been deliberately reduced in these children to avoid the late effects of the therapy (Jereb et al, 1982). Future research is being targeted at finding other methods of therapy for these patients.

EPENDYMOMAS

Definition

Ependymomas are tumors arising from ependymal cells, usually from the fourth ventricle, although tumors arising from other parts of the ventricular system have been described.

Epidemiology

Ependymomas constitute 8–10% of childhood posterior fossa tumors. They are the second most frequent cerebral hemisphere neoplasm.

Diagnosis

CT or MRI scans can localize these tumors. They are less contrast-enhancing than medulloblastomas.

Treatment

Therapy has traditionally been surgical resection and radiation therapy.

Prognosis

Low-grade ependymomas will have a 5-year survival approaching 80%, although the more high-grade differentiated tumors are fatal, with overall childhood survival being less than 30% (Gilles et al, 1983).

BRAIN STEM GLIOMAS

Definition

Brain stem gliomas are tumors of the pons and medulla. They can vary from a low-grade astrocytoma to highly malignant glioblastoma multiforme. It is probably the smallest tumor volume that can produce severe morbidity and early mortality. In many ways, it resembles the high-grade astrocytomas of adulthood (Littman et al, 1980).

Epidemiology

These tumors comprise 10–15% of primary brain tumors and 25% of the gliomas in children.

Natural History

These tumors usually present with cranial nerve dysfunction, long tract involvement, or ataxia before signs and symptoms of increased intracranial pressure appear. Vomiting is quite common at presentation. The degree of symptoms compared to the extent of tumor can be discordant producing few signs with extensive tumor (presumably a testimony to the infiltrative nature of the tumor).

Diagnosis

Diagnosis is made by clinical criteria, including history of progressive cranial dysfunction or gait disorder, neurologic examination remarkable for cranial nerve palsy, cerebellar, or pyramidal tract abnormalities. A CT or MRI scan reveals an intrinsic brain mass. While surgical incision is usually impossible, surgical confirmation by biopsy may still be reserved for those cases with lesions that appear cystic or where the differential diagnosis of an arterial-venous malformation, abscess, or encephalitis cannot be eliminated. Usually the potential risks of biopsy outweigh the benefits gained from examination of histologic tissue.

Treatment

Treatment of choice has traditionally been radiotherapy, although 5-year survival for a pontine glioma after radiation is still less than 30%. Chemotherapy may extend disease-free survival briefly in patients who have recurrent disease, but it has yet to make a substantial contribution to prolonging life in patients with high-grade astrocytoma-like tumors (Allen, 1985).

CRANIOPHARYNGIOMAS

Definition

The craniopharyngioma is derived from remnants of the embryonal structure, Rathke's pouch, which is a collection of squamous cells at the junction of the pituitary stalk with the gland. As it grows, it can compress adjacent structures and, thus, produce symptoms. The tumor is often cystic, containing a viscous cholesterol-rich fluid that resembles used motor oil. Calcification in the suprasellar area is common, as are abnormalities in the structure of the sella turcica. Histologically, these tumors are often benign, but their close proximity to vital structures makes them difficult to remove.

Epidemiology

These tumors are rare and account for less than 5% of brain tumors in children.

Natural History

The forward extension of this tumor compresses the optic chiasm and can produce bitemporal hemianopsia, which is commonly seen when this tumor presents. Upward extension will compress the third ventricle and can result subsequently in hydrocephalus and headache. Downward extension can compress the pituitary and yields a variety of endocrinologic abnormalities.

Diagnosis

Diagnosis can be expected on a plain radiograph revealing widening of the sella turcica or by CT scan.

Treatment

While optimal treatment is total excision, the closeness of these tumors to vital structures may make them difficult to remove, such that radiation therapy is the treatment of choice if complete excision cannot be achieved. The combination of radiation therapy after surgery leads to good to excellent disease-free survival and cure (Sung, 1982). Nonetheless, endocrine dysfunction is frequent and cognitive deficits secondary to the radiation therapy are not unusual.

OPTIC GLIOMA

Definition

Optic glioma represents a diffuse thickening of the optic nerve composed of mixed astrocytic and oligodendroglial elements. This tumor has a high association with neurofibromatosis.

Epidemiology

Fewer than 3% of brain tumors in children are optic gliomas.

Natural History

Presenting symptoms are usually diminished visual acuity and, in infants, a roving nystagmus. If the glioma involves the optic chiasm or both the optic nerve and chiasm it will frequently invade the hypothalamus and have a much poorer prognosis.

Diagnosis

The CT scan is most useful in making the diagnosis.

Treatment

Many of the optic gliomas are surgically removable and, if so, carry a good prognosis. Nevertheless, complete excision of a unilateral tumor which has already produced visual compromise usually results in unilateral blindness, despite the excellent long-term survival. Bilateral symptomatic tumors can respond to radiotherapy. The treatment of an asymptomatic or minimally symptomatic tumor is usually conservative, consisting of close observation.

PINEALOMAS

Definition

Pineal tumors represent the spectrum of benign dysgerminoma to the more malignant pinealblastoma. Some of the malignant germ cell tumors in the pineal region can be associated with increased serum or CSF β-human chorionic gonadotropin (β-HCG) or α-fetoprotein.

Epidemiology

These represent less than 4% of childhood brain tumors.

Natural History

Since these are midline tumors, a variety of endocrine dysfunctions can accompany their presentation, in addition to evidence for increased intracranial pressure. They should be considered in children with precocious puberty.

Diagnosis

Diagnosis may be suggested on the basis of elevated β-HCG and/or α-fetoprotein in serum or CSF, as well as by CT scan.

Treatment

It is important to request an early biopsy if feasible since the pure dysgerminoma will respond well to radiation, whereas the more malignant varieties require at least some preradiation chemotherapy (Packer et al, 1984).

These tumors are rarely resectable and, as a result, require radiation therapy and/or chemotherapy if a more

CASE ILLUSTRATION

A 12-year-old female was referred to our hospital for evaluation of "anorexia nervosa." Three years before admission she had begun to experience polydypsia, polyuria, headache, and vomiting. An evaluation for diabetes mellitus was "normal" and the family was placed in psychotherapy. Over the next 3 years, her symptoms continued, although she admitted that she voluntarily lost weight (40 pounds) and had begun exercising more. In the year before admission, her headaches and polydypsia appeared to subside spontaneously, although again she admitted to continuing to lose more weight intermittently. During the summer of her admission she was sent home from camp because of lethargy and disinterest in all activities, following a further 10-pound weight loss and a recurrence of her headaches and vomiting. During the 5 days before admission she demonstrated progressive lethargy, confusion, and bizarre thoughts bordering on hallucinations prompting the referral to our hospital.

She had never menstruated and denied self-induced vomiting, laxative abuse, or drug use of any kind. There was no history of head trauma or intense preoccupation with food preparation. She had normal electrolytes, CBC, and thyroid function tests, done at her physician's office before the admission.

Physical examination revealed a short, very thin but not cachectic female in no distress. Her temperature was 36.8° C, heart rate 90/min, respiration 20/min, blood pressure 92/60 without orthostasis. Her weight was 24 kg, in the 50th percentile for a 7-year-old. Her height was 51 inches, in the 50th percentile for a 9-year-old. She had sparse hair, dry skin, and mucous membranes, but showed evidence of subcutaneous fat, normal fundi, and no pubertal development. Her mental status was disoriented and confused intermittently, with confabulation noted. There was a question of a bitemporal visual field cut. A left upgrowing toe was noted without ataxia. Except for extreme muscle wasting, the remainder of the examination was normal.

QUESTION AND COMMENT

What further diagnostic work-up is in order?

A lateral skull film was obtained and showed a normal sella. A CT scan of the head, however, revealed a large mass in the suprasellar region, completely obstructing the third ventricle, with hydrocephalus.

Several features of this case are atypical to anorexia nervosa, including apparent onset before puberty, lack of preoccupation with food, variable emphasis on exercise, markedly delayed skeletal growth, absence of secondary sexual development, muscle wasting without loss of visible fat, and the findings on neurologic examination (Weller, 1982).

In retrospect, the patient probably did have diabetes insipidus 3 years before presentation, with normal electrolytes maintained because of an intact thirst mechanism, which only failed during the recent months. A hyperosmolar hypernatremic state was confirmed on admission. A slowly growing mass which does not erode the sella can be a hypothalamic tumor, pinealoma, or dysgerminoma. CSF and a serum HCG were elevated and CSF cytology was positive for dysgerminoma cells, consistent with an intracranial dysgerminoma. This patient underwent operative decompression from above, with prompt resolution of her mental status. She subsequently underwent radiotherapy, which can provide 65–85% long-term cure rates (Sung, 1978). She continues to do well 5 years after admission.

malignant subtype is diagnosed by biopsy. Placement of a ventricular peritoneal shunt to relieve elevated intracranial pressure, however, will allow peritoneal spread of these highly metastasizing tumors and, therefore, should be deferred as long as possible. If a shunt is to be placed before radiation therapy, chemotherapy should be included to reduce the risk of metastases.

REFERENCES

Allen JC: Childhood brain tumors: Current status of clinical trials in newly diagnosed and recurrent disease. *Pediatr Clin North Am* 32:633, 1985.

Becker LE, Yates AJ: Astrocytic tumors in children. In Finegold M(ed): *Pathology of Neoplasia in Children and Adolescents*. Philadelphia, WB Saunders, 1986, p. 373.

Cohen M, Duffner P, et al: SEER Registry results in children with brain tumors, 1973–81. *Proc Am Soc Clin Oncol* 3:79, 1984.

Gilles FH, Leviton A, Hedley-White EG, et al: Childhood brain tumor update. *Hum Pathol* 14:834, 1983.

Gooding CA, Brasch RC, et al: Nuclear magnetic resonance imaging of the brain in children. *J Pediatr* 104:589, 1984.

Herron GB: Hypothalamic tumor presenting as anorexia nervosa. *Am J Psychiatry* 133:580, 1976.

Jereb B, Reid A, et al: Patterns of failure in patients with medulloblastoma. *Cancer* 50:2941, 1982.

Littman P, Jarrett P, Bilaniuk L, et al: Pediatric brainstem glioma. *Cancer* 45:2787, 1980.

Packer RJ, Sutton LN, et al: Pineal region tumors of childhood. *Pediatrics* 74:97, 1984.

Rich TA, Cassady JR, et al: Radiation therapy for pineal and suprasellar germ cell tumors. *Cancer* 55:932, 1985.

Rose A, Matson DD: Benign intracranial hypertension in children. *Pediatrics* 39:227, 1967.

Sung D: Midline pineal tumors in supra-sellar germinomas: Highly curable by radiation. *Radiology* 128:745, 1978.

Sung DI: Suprasellar tumors in children. A review of clinical manifestations and managements. *Cancer* 50:1420, 1982.

Weller RA: Anorexia nervosa in a patient with an infiltrating tumor of the hypothalmus. *Am J Psychiatry* 139:824, 1982.

White JH: Clinical picture of atypical anorexia nervosa associated with hypothalamic tumors. *Am J Psychiatry* 134:223, 1977.

Young J, Miller R: Incidence of malignant tumors in U.S. children. *J Pediatr* 86:254, 1975.

Neuroblastoma 7

Definition

Neuroblastoma, the most common neoplasm of infancy, arises from neural crest cells usually in paraspinal sympathetic ganglia or the adrenal medulla. It shows unusual biologic behavior, ranging from spontaneous regression to fatal metastatic disease. The tumor may also spontaneously mature to a more benign form (ganglioneuroma).

Basic Science

The etiology remains unknown, although environmental and/or genetic factors probably play a role. Although specific chromosomal localization for the neuroblastoma gene has not been found as of 1987, cytogenetic studies reveal that these patients most frequently have deletions of the terminal part of chromosome 1, but at variable sites. In addition, amplified regions of DNA have been found related to the myc family of cellular oncogenes. Called N-myc, they are associated with the more aggressive forms of neuroblastoma, but not the milder ones (Israel, 1986).

The reason for the spontaneous remission and maturation that occur in the tumor remain unclear, although it is attributed in part to host immune defense mechanisms, even though no type of immunotherapy has been shown to be effective in treating this disease.

Epidemiology

Neuroblastomas represent 7% of all cases and 15% of all childhood cancer deaths and are more frequent in white than in black children. It is the most commonly diagnosed tumor in the first month and year of life (Bader and Miller, 1979).

Natural History

The clinical presentation of neuroblastoma is dependent upon the location of its primary site, with the abdomen being most common, followed by posterior mediastinum, neck, and lastly, pelvis or presacral region, which are rare. Major sites of metastatic disease include the liver, bone marrow, bone, and lymph nodes; pulmonary metastases are rare. Hence, in addition to common symptoms of irritability, loss of appetite, and fever, depending on the primary site, patients may present with an abdominal or neck mass, bone pain, proptosis, the Horner syndrome (with the neck mass), or paralysis from spinal cord compression. Other patients will have opsoclonus and myoclonus, which constitutes a paraneoplastic syndrome that remains an enigma. It does not always resolve after successful treatment of the neuroblastoma. Patients with neuroblastoma can present with severe secretory diarrhea due to excretion of vasoactive intestinal peptide made by the tumor (Lopez-Ibor and Schwartz, 1985).

One of the most useful prognostic variables is age. Infants under the age of 1 year have an extremely high rate of spontaneous regression and an overall 90% long-term survival. Patients over 2 years of age fare much more poorly with prognosis dependent upon the clinical stage of disease at time of diagnosis.

Diagnosis

Laboratory investigations are mandatory: these should include a CBC, liver function tests, chest radiograph (Fig. 9.3*A* and *B*), bone scan, bone marrow aspiration and biopsy, and body CT scan. Abdominal ultrasonography may be useful in the delineation of a suprarenal mass, which may then obviate the need for additional CT scanning if exploratory laporotomy is to follow. If liver involvement is suspected by ultrasonography or CT scan, a liver-spleen scan can be useful.

Patients with tumors in the abdomen may have downward and outward displacement of the kidney by adrenal tumors. Since more than 90% of patients will excrete catecholamines and metabolites in the urine, a freshly voided specimen should be evaluated for catecholamine or vanillylmandelic acid (VMA) and homovanillic acid (HVA), one of which is elevated in at least two-thirds of patients. This test is subject to false-positive or false-negative values and if the diagnosis is still under consideration, a 24-hour urine collection is required to measure true catecholamine excretion (Williams and Green, 1963). Once the tumor has been located, diagnosis should be confirmed by biopsy either of the primary or of a solid metastasis or by showing the presence of tumor cell clumps in the bone marrow together with elevated excretion of catecholamine metabolites in a 24-hour urine collection.

The goal of the diagnostic work-up is to stage the disease for determination of prognosis and treatment. The most widely used staging system is that of Evans et al (1987):

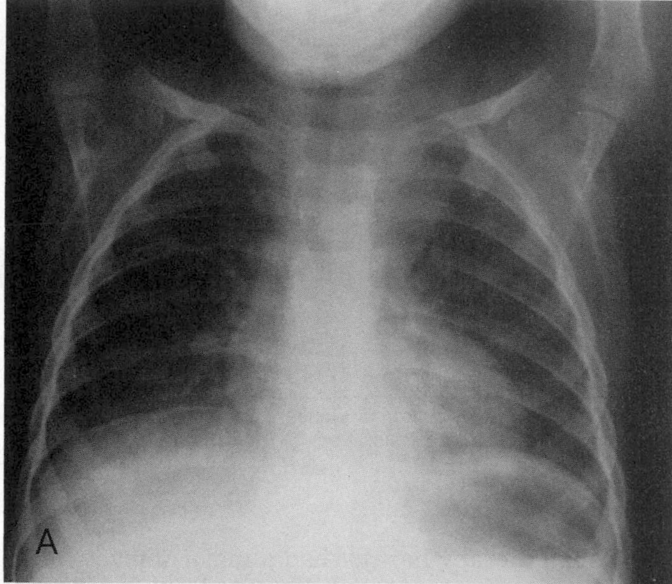

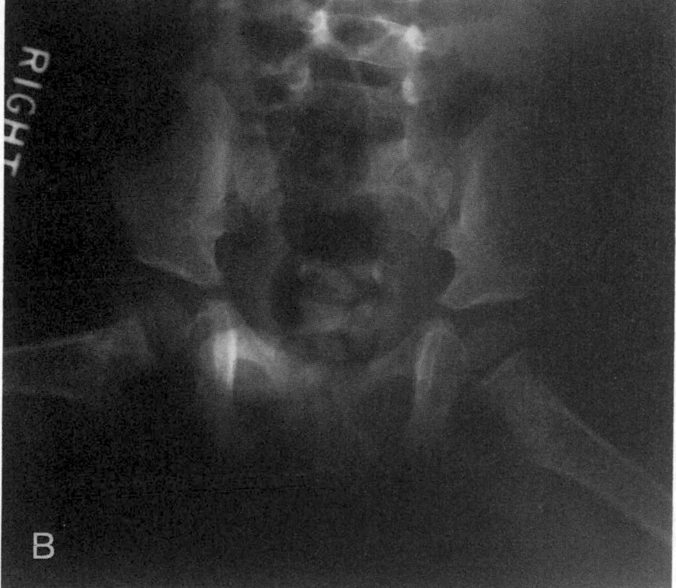

Figure 9.3. This 2½-year-old boy presented to the pediatrician with ecchymoses surrounding both eyes. The chest radiograph (**A**) shows paravertebral soft tissue masses—extensions from a primary retroperitoneal neuroblastoma. A cervical node was biopsied to establish the diagnosis. Note also the frayed metaphyses of proximal humeri that indicate metastatic involvement. Radiograph of pelvis taken 6 months later (**B**) shows obvious symmetrical metaphyseal destruction which is characteristic of this tumor.

Stage 1: A completely encapsulated and resected lesion

Stage 2: Regional disease on one side of the midline or localized spinal "dumbbell" tumors that extend with one end through a spinal frame and extradurally into the spinal canal causing cord compression and with the other end enter into the abdomen or chest

Stage 3: Tumors further defined as only those that are across the midline which push the aorta and vena cava to the side, demonstrate tumor firmly adherent to both sides of the midline or have positive nodes across the midline. A tumor that is readily resectable even though it hangs over the midline should be considered stage 2

Stage 4: Presence of distant metastases

Stage 4S: Class of infants who have stage 1 or 2 primary but also have metastases to liver, skin, and/or bone marrow, but not to bone

Table 9.7
Neuroblastoma Treatment Results by Age/Stage 1970–1980[1]

Stage	Age <1 Year	Age >1 Year	Total
1	5/5	2/2	7/7 (100%)
2	8/8	17/19	25/27 (93%)
3	9/10	5/7	14/17 (82%)
4	9/10	4/46	13/56 (23%)
4S	6/7	3/3	9/10 (90%)
Overall	37/40 (93%)	31/78 (40%)	68/118 (58%)

[1]Data obtained from Dana Farber Cancer Institute and The Children's Hospital, Boston, with permission from C. Kretschmar, M.D.

Treatment

Chemotherapy has not had a major impact on the long-term survival rate of children > 1 year with stage 4 neuroblastoma over the past 20 years, nor has it been shown to benefit children with early stage neuroblastoma (Evans et al, 1984). Resection of the primary lesion remains the treatment of choice for these patients. Infants with stage 1 or stage 2 require no further therapy after surgery. For the remainder of the children over age 1 year in stage 3 or 4, intensive chemotherapy and/or radiation therapy are recommended. Since the prognosis is so poor in patients with stage 4 disease, bone marrow transplantation has been used increasingly as an alternative therapeutic option. In the older patients, this therapy has prolonged disease-free survival time, but as of 1987 the impact upon 5-year survival is unknown. In particular, for patients over age 1 year with bony metastatic disease, bone marrow transplantation is now the treatment of choice. Of patients who undergo this procedure, which also includes much higher dose chemotherapy, about one-third are surviving 1–2 years following treatment. The purging of tumor cells from autologous bone marrow with monoclonal antibodies directed against the tumor is an experimental procedure, that requires further clinical studies (Treleaven et al, 1984).

Prognosis

The older the child and/or the more advanced the stage the worse the prognosis. Table 9.7 demonstrates how the stage and age are useful as prognostic tools. For example, there is only 10% survival for patients over 2 years of age who present in stage 4 neuroblastoma, whereas infants under the age of 1 year, with stage 3 or 4 disease do extremely well following aggressive surgery and chemotherapy. Moreover, stage 4S infants remain in remission and the majority will show spontaneous disease regression after surgery alone, without the need for radiation or chemotherapy (Evans et al, 1987). Some, however, will need chemotherapy. While therapy today may prolong disease-free survival, it has yet to produce long-term remission with patients in the more advanced stages. Evans et al (1987) suggest that age, stage of disease, serum ferritin (high levels ≥ 150 ng/ml carry a worse prognosis), and histologic type in combination allow prediction of good or poor prognosis. Overall survival in 124 children was 60% at 2 years. Therefore, genetic and immunologic therapeutic approaches to this disease are currently under study.

Some studies also have shown that prognosis depends on the location of the tumor. Mediastinal tumors carry the best prognosis and abdominal and adrenal tumors the worst, with neck and pelvis involvement in between (Kushner and Cheung, 1988). Interestingly, mediastinal primary tumor masses are most common in infants, so it is often difficult to separate age and stage in terms of prognosis.

REFERENCES

Bader KL, Miller RW: U.S. cancer incidence and mortality in the first year of life. *Am J Dis Child* 133:157, 1979.
Evans AE, D'Angio G, Seeger RC (eds): *Advances in Neuroblastoma Research*. New York, Academic Press, 1985.
Evans AE, D'Angio GJ, Koop CE: The role of multimodal therapy in patients with local and regional neuroblastoma. *J Pediatr Surg* 19:77, 1984.
Evans AE, D'Angio GJ, Propert K, et al: Prognostic factors in neuroblastoma. *Cancer* 59:1853, 1987.
Israel MA: The evolution of clinical molecular genetics. Neuroblastoma as a model tumor. *Am J Pediatr Hematol/Oncol* 8:163, 1986.
Kretschmar CS, Frantz CN, Rosen EM, et al: Improved prognosis for infants with stage I neuroblastoma. *J Clin Oncol* 2:799, 1984.
Kushner BH, Cheung N-K: Neuroblastoma. *Pediatr Ann* 17:269, 1988.
Lopez-Ibor B, Schwartz AD: Neuroblastoma. *Pediatr Clin North Am* 32:755, 1985.
Rosen EM, Cassady JR, Frantz CN, et al: Neuroblastoma: The Joint Center for Radiation Therapy/DFCI/Children's Hospital Experience. *J Clin Oncol* 2:719, 1984.
Treleaven JG, Ugelstad J, Philip T, et al: Removal of neuroblastoma cells from bone marrow with monoclonal antibodies conjugating to magnetic microspheres. *Lancet* 1:70, 1984.
Williams C, Green M: Homovanillic acid and vanillylmandelic acid in diagnosis of neuroblastoma. *JAMA* 183:836, 1963.

Renal Tumors

8

WILMS TUMOR

Definition

Wilms tumor (see pp. 781) is the common name for a malignant tumor of the kidney known as nephroblastoma. It is an embryonal tumor that may arise in utero.

Basic Science

The tumors usually contain stromal elements, tubular structures, and blastemal tissue. The histology can vary from differentiated to anaplastic, with the latter associated with a worse prognosis. Anaplastic changes occur in 12–15% of lesions.

Molecular biologic studies of Wilms tumor show homozygous loss of alleles at loci on both number 11 chromosomes. Chromosomes from lymphocytes in these patients show loss of genetic material on one chromosome 11 p. The homozygous loss of genetic material has also been detected in other childhood tumors including retinoblastoma and osteosarcoma. These loci have been referred to as recessive oncogenes. (Weissman et al, 1987).

Epidemiology

The annual incidence of Wilms tumor is 7.5/million children under age 15 years. The lesion has been diagnosed in the newborn although the usual age for diagnosis is 2–3 years.

The most common renal mass identified in newborn infants is a benign mesoblastic nephroma. In a series of 27 renal tumors in the neonate, 18 were mesoblastic nephromas and only four were Wilms (Hrabovsky et al, 1986).

Natural History and Diagnosis

Wilms tumor occurs in both heritable and sporadic forms. The heritable form is usually bilateral (but can be unilateral), and is inherited as an autosomal dominant trait with incomplete penetrance (Matsunaga, 1981). Inherited associated problems include aniridia, hemihypertrophy, hamartomas, and genitourinary defects.

The most common presentation is an abdominal mass. The tumor is deep in the flank and arises from the kidney. In 5–10% of cases, both kidneys are involved. Other signs may be hematuria or hypertension. Rarely, polycythemia is present from excess production of erythropoietin. The tumor has been found in association with Beckwith-Wiedemann syndrome.

About 15–20% of children present with metastases spread hematogerously, most commonly to the lung.

Radiologic evaluations should establish the presence of an intrarenal mass and a normally functioning and appearing contralateral kidney, document the patency of the inferior vena cava, and demonstrate the presence or absence of pulmonary metastases.

These evaluations can be accomplished with ultrasonography, followed by CT scans of the abdomen and lung.

Treatment

Nephrectomy is the primary treatment for Wilms tumor. At laparotomy, examination of opposite kidney, liver, spleen, and peritoneal surfaces is essential to search for metatases or bilateral Wilms tumors.

The decision for follow-up therapy depends on the stage of the tumor, as well as the pathology.

Stage 1: Tumor limited to kidney and resected completely.
Stage 2: Tumor extended beyond kidney and resected.
Stage 3: Residual nonhematogenous tumor confined to abdomen.
Stage 4: Tumor with hematogenous metastases to lung, liver, bone, or brain, and lymph node spread beyond the abdomen.
Stage 5: Tumor with bilateral renal involvement at diagnosis, or postdiagnosis.

Children with stage 1 disease and favorable histology usually receive nephrectomy alone, although chemotherapy may be added if the histology is unfavorable (e.g., anaplastic tumors). Those into stage 2 receive nephrectomy and chemotherapy. Children with stages 3–5 disease receive radiation in addition to nephrectomy and chemotherapy.

The most commonly used drugs are vincristine, actinomycin D, and doxorubicin. For children with anaplastic lesions, cyclophosphamide is added (Kosbrinsky et al, 1988).

Prognosis

Children with Wilms tumor should be evaluated in a center with experience with the disease, since modern treatment has greatly improved the outlook. The overall cure rate in 1984 was about 90% (Hrabovsky et al, 1986). Approximately 25% of patients with favorable histology but stage 4 disease and 50% of those with unfavorable histology and stages 2–5 will experience primary tumor progression or recurrence, although aggressive multi-

CASE ILLUSTRATION

A 1-day-old presented to our surgical service with a left-sided abdominal mass noted on routine physical examination. He was a full-term infant with an uncomplicated pregnancy, labor, and vaginal delivery, and good Apgar scores. Physical examination was entirely unremarkable, except for an 8 x 5 cm mass palpable in the left upper and lower quadrant, which was nontender and did not move with respiration. Baseline laboratory studies, including renal function and urinalyses were normal.

QUESTION AND COMMENT

What is the most likely cause of this mass and how should it be diagnosed?

The most common palpable masses in the newborn are usually of renal origin with hydronephrosis being the most common. Ultrasonography was performed which revealed a large, noncystic mass without evidence of normal renal outline. The right kidney and both ureters were normal. Renal scan was performed showing normal renal function, confirming the presence of a left kidney. Since an intrarenal (e.g., Wilms) versus an extrarenal (neuroblastoma) tumor could not be distinguished, an exploratory laparotomy was performed. A large renal mass was removed as part of a total nephrectomy with subsequent pathology confirming the presence of a mesoblastic nephroma. This is a benign renal tumor and actually is more common than Wilms in the neonate.

It is thought that congenital mesoblastic nephromas represent an early neoplastic step in the embryology of the kidney, with nephroblastoma (Wilms) representing a later step in the histopathologic spectrum of malignant transformation. In 11 cases of these tumors noted in our hospital over the past 50 years, local invasion has never been seen and nephrectomy alone has been the treatment of choice.

modal therapy can still produce a cure in some of these children (Kobrinsky et al, 1988).

In some patients, the "cure" has produced its own problems in later years. Severe spinal curvatures can occur from radiation injury early in life. Radiation pneumonitis, nephritis, and hepatitis are well documented but rare treatment complications.

NEW DEVELOPMENTS

The possibility that genetic information on chromosome 11 can control the malignant expression of Wilms tumor cells in tissue culture gained support from suppression of tumor formation by Wilms cells that had a normal human chromosome 11 inserted. Weissman et al (1987) conclude that "the Wilms tumor-suppressor gene would seem to regulate a late step in the progression to the malignant state rather than one of the initial preneoplastic stages."

CONGENITAL MESOBLASTIC NEPHROMA

Definition

Once confused with Wilms tumor, congenital mesoblastic nephroma is an isolated, usually benign tumor that presents in infancy as an enlarged kidney.

CASE ILLUSTRATION

A 5-year-old girl presented for evaluation with the sudden appearance of a left upper quadrant abdominal mass. She had been well until 5 months before admission when she presented with arthritis, a petechial lower extremity rash, and crampy abdominal pain, diagnosed as Henoch-Schönlein purpura. She responded to a bowel rest regimen utilizing parenteral alimentation and did well except for new onset of hypertension, controlled with diuril and aldactone. Two months before admission, her renal scan was normal. A month before admission, increased blood pressure was again noticed, but her examination was otherwise benign. BUN and creatinine as well as urinalyses were unremarkable. Plasma renin level and serum catecholamines were elevated. An arteriogram was scheduled. Several days before it was to be done the child's mother noted a bulge in the left side of the abdomen. Repeat physical examination revealed a firm, nontender 10–12 cm mass in the left upper quadrant.

QUESTION AND COMMENT

What further diagnostic work-up is necessary and what are the diagnostic possibilities?

Ultrasonography and intravenous pyelogram (IVP) were performed confirming an intrarenal mass, suggestive of a Wilms tumor. A CT scan of the chest showed multiple densities consistent with metastases and a left total nephrectomy, with para-aortic lymph nodes and liver biopsy was performed for staging of the presumptive Wilms tumor, subsequently confirmed by pathology.

While congenital anomalies such as aniridia and hemihypertrophy can serve as external markers for Wilms, we found no previous report of Henoch-Schönlein purpura predisposing to or associated with this malignancy. Moreover, the only reports of skin manifestations seen with the Wilms tumor have been of hemangiomas and multiple nevi, which were not seen in this patient (Simon et al, 1977).

Natural History

This dysplastic lesion has an exterior that demonstrates neither lobulation nor necrosis. It may infiltrate the perihilar connective tissues.

Diagnosis

The tumor has been diagnosed prenatally by ultrasonography, which is also the preferred method of postnatal diagnosis.

Hypercalcemia has been reported in association with mesoblastic nephromas (Vido et al, 1986). Levels up to 17 mg/dl with marked calciuria were accompanied by elevated urinary prostaglandins of the E series. All values returned to normal after the tumor mass was completely removed. The concentration of prostaglandin in the tumor was three times higher than in non-tumor tissue. Parathyroid hormone values were normal.

Treatment

Nephrectomy alone is adequate unless the tumor shows unusual aggressive features. Radiation and/or chemotherapy are rarely indicated.

REFERENCES

Allen RG: Tumor masses of the neonate. *Clin Perinatol* 5:115, 1978.

Bolande RP, Brough AJ, Izant RJ: Congenital mesoblastic nephroma of infancy: A report of eight cases and the relationship to Wilms' tumor. *Pediatrics* 40:272, 1967.

Chan HSL, Cheng MY, Mancur K, et al: Congenital mesoblastic nephroma: A clinicoradiologic study of 17 cases representing the pathologic spectrum of the disease. *J Pediatr* 111:64, 1987.

Henderson C, Torch EM: Differential diagnoses of abdominal masses in the neonate. *Pediatr Clin North Am* 24:557, 1977.

Hrabovsky EE, Othersen HB, deLorimier JFA, et al: Wilms' tumor in the neonate: A report from the national Wilms' tumor study. *J Pediatr Surg* 21:385, 1986.

Kobrinsky NL, Talgoy M, Shuckett B, et al: Wilms' tumor. *Pediatr Ann* 17:238, 1988.

Matsunaga E: Genetics of Wilms' tumor. *Hum Genet* 57:231, 1981.

Simon FA, Drutz JE, Corrier JN: Wilms' tumor in pigmented nevi. *J Pediatr* 90:40, 1977.

Snyder HM, Lack EE, Chetty-Baktavizian A, et al: Congenital mesoblastic nephroma: Relationship to other renal tumors of infancy. *J Urol* 126:513, 1981.

Vido L, Carli M, Rizzoni G, et al: Congenital mesoblastic nephroma with hypercalcemia. Pathogenetic role of prostaglandins. *Am J Pediatr Hematol Oncol* 8:149, 1986.

Weissman BE, Saxon PJ, Pasquale SR, et al: Introduction of a normal human chromosome 11 into a Wilms' tumor cell line controls its tumorigenic expression. *Science* 236:175, 1987.

Yunis JJ, Ramsay NKC: Familial occurrence of the aniridia-Wilms' tumor syndrome with children 11p13-14.1. *J Pediatr* 96:1027, 1980.

Bone and Soft Tissue Tumors 9

OSTEOSARCOMA

Definition

Osteosarcoma is a rare tumor found mostly in adolescents. It is a spindle-cell tumor that produces malignant osteoid or immature bone and has many histologic variants.

Basic Science

The cause is unknown. The tumor grows very rapidly with a median time to double its volume of 34 days (Shackney et al, 1978). The tumor is most common in growing bones; the peak incidence occurs during the period of maximal growth in adolescence.

It is possible that ionizing radiation to bone increases the likelihood of osteosarcoma. Genetic factors play a role, as evidenced by reports of 16 sets of siblings with the disease (Colyer, 1979). A relationship exists between hereditary bilateral retinoblastoma and the development of secondary osteosarcomas. Both tumors have been shown to have homozygous deletions on the long arm of chromosome 13.

Epidemiology

About 900 new cases of osteosarcoma are reported each year in the United States. Males are 1½–2 times more commonly affected than are females.

Natural History

The tumor is most common at sites of maximal bone growth, such as distal femur, proximal tibia and proximal humerus. Less than 10% of tumors are in the axial skeleton (skull, jaw, vertebrae, orbit, or pelvis).

The most common site of metastasis is the lung, where it may consist of a single (resectable) lesion. Other bones may show metastatses. Regional lymph nodes are rarely involved. The tumor may appear simultaneously at several sites.

The initial symptom is pain at the site of the lesion, which is often attributed to trauma. Its persistence and a palpable or visible tumor are the usual complaints. Occasionally, the presenting symptoms are pulmonary; pneumothorax may be the first finding.

Diagnosis

Plain radiographs of the involved site can be diagnostic. A "sunburst" sign may be seen representing extenstion of the tumor through the periosteum. In addition to radiographic findings suggesting the bone tumor, a work-up to evaluate metastases should be performed including radiographs of the chest and of the involved bone, bone scan, and a CT of the lungs and primary lesion. Both the CT and MRI scans can show the extent of cortical involvement, intramedullary spread, and soft tissue extension (Tebbi and Gaeta, 1988). Blood work should include a CBC, LDH, and alkaline phosphatase. Definitive diagnosis rests on an open biopsy of the bone tumor.

Treatment and Prognosis

Resection of the tumor is the first line of treatment. Usually an amputation is performed at 5–7 cm above the most proximal extent of the tumor. Limb-sparing resection with endoprostheses are used increasingly rather than amputation when in the opinion of the orthopedic surgeon the surgery can be performed safely with low risk of complications and/or metastases. Chemotherapy has been traditionally given after surgery, but the efficacy of its administration before surgery is under clinical study.

In the 10–20% of patients with visible metastases at the time of diagnosis, resection of all possible lesions and chemotherapy are undertaken albeit with knowledge that less than 20% will have long-term disease-free survival.

Before the era of aggressive chemotherapy (i.e., until the early 1970s), the prognosis was poor, with only 20% surviving 5 years after diagnosis and resection of the primary lesion. It was assumed that most patients had micrometastatic disease at the time of resection, so that, beginning in the 1970s, adjuvant chemotherapy was employed at the time of surgery. High-dose methotrexate with leucovorin rescue permits the antitumor effect of methotrexate without the serious side-effects. After 5 years of follow-up, the disease-free survival is 44% after adjuvant high-dose methotrexate (Goorin et al, 1985).

Combination chemotherapy including methotrexate with leucovorin rescue and doxorubicin has increased the 5-year survival to nearly 50%. Currently protocols with newer chemotherapeutic agents are under study, and appear to increase the overall survival rates of patients with nonmetastatic disease to 60–80% (Link et al, 1986).

EWING SARCOMA

Definition

Ewing sarcoma is the second most common bone tumor of childhood and adolescence. Ewing sarcoma belongs to a group of neoplasms referred to as "small round cell tumors," which includes neuroblastoma, rhabdomyosarcoma, non-Hodgkin lymphoma, and neuroectodermal tumors. In fact, it may be difficult to distinguish a Ewing sarcoma from other entities in this group.

Basic Science

Ewing sarcoma may exist in two pathologic forms: either (1) a classical Ewing sarcoma characterized by the presence of glycogen in the tumor cells, or (2) a tumor with histologic features identical to those of peripheral neuroectodermal tumors. Cytogenetic analysis of both types of tumor has revealed a translocation between chromosome 11 and 22, although further work is required to determine the importance of this translocation with regard to the occurrence or natural history of these tumors (Jaffe, 1985).

Epidemiology

More than half the patients with this tumor are between 10 and 20 years of age and two-thirds are under the age of 20 years. The tumor is rare in blacks. It is found more frequently in males than in females.

Natural History

Most patients present with pain at the site of the tumor, often followed by localized swelling. Systemic symptoms can occur such as weight loss and fever, especially in those who have metastatic disease at the time of presentation (roughly one-third of patients).

The most common site for a metastasis is the lung, followed by other bones and, less frequently, bone marrow. Lymph node spread does not appear to play a major role in dissemination. The most common sites for tumor occurrence include the upper end or midshaft of the femur or the pelvis. Tibia, fibula, humerus, scapula, clavicle, and ribs have also been described as sites for primary lesions.

Diagnosis begins with plain radiographs of the affected bone. Although no radiographic finding is pathognomonic of the tumor, the appearance of mixed lytic and blastic lesions associated with a soft tissue mass is consistent with the diagnosis. In addition, as the tumor elevates periosteum, multiple layers of subperiosteal reactive new bone may give an "onion skin" appearance on the radiograph, in direct contrast to the "sunburst" appearance associated with osteogenic sarcoma. Definitive diagnosis rests with proper biopsy, preferably of the soft tissue mass containing tumor rather than of bone to minimize the increased risk of a post-biopsy fracture. In addition, the use of a CT scan of the bone and a bone scan, CT scan of the lung, and a bone marrow aspirate and biopsy, are essential for metastatic work-up.

Treatment

Treatment consists of combined local control and adjuvant chemotherapy. Localized therapy alone will result in a 5-year survival rate of less than 20%, with the majority of patients having relapses in distant sites. Therefore, systemic therapy is mandatory in addition to local control of the tumor by radiation therapy or sometimes surgery. The use of whole bone irradiation remains controversial since it can affect the further growth of the child or adolescent. Complications of radiotherapy include joint deformities, fractures, soft tissue changes, and a second malignant neoplasm.

The use of adjuvant chemotherapy in combination with localized radiation has been found to increase the disease-free survival rate to 50–75% for all patients with nonmetastatic Ewing sarcoma (Rosen et al, 1981).

Most patients are treated initially with a four-drug regimen that includes vincristine, adriamycin, cytoxan, and actinomycin D, before institution of radiotherapy. Experimental protocols include total body irradiation in addition to chemotherapy, followed by autologous bone marrow infusion. The role of aggressive surgery remains controversial, with some studies suggesting that disease free survival is increased with complete excision of the tumor. Surgery is indicated if the soft tissue mass is small and if the tumor involves only the clavicle, ribs, or fibula and, hence, the bone can be removed without significant functional loss.

The younger the patient, the more incapacitating and complicated are the long-term results of radiation therapy. In fact, some studies suggest that in children under 8 years, amputation of the involved bone is preferable to radiotherapy. Secondary malignancies that have appeared following radiotherapy and chemotherapy include osteogenic sarcoma in the irradiated bone, with an actuarial incidence as high as 10–20%. It is not clear yet whether decreasing the radiation dose will decrease this incidence.

Prognosis

Prognosis varies widely according to presentation. Patients with overt metastases do worse, as do those with location of the primary in the pelvis. Patients with distal disease involving the hands and feet or distal long bones tend to have a better prognosis than do those who have proximal long bone involvement. An elevated lactate dehydrogenase formerly thought to signify a poor prognosis is probably a nonspecific associated indicator of the presence of a tumor (Glaubigerder et al, 1980). Leptomeningeal CNS involvement is rare and, hence, CNS prophylaxis is not recommended for this tumor.

RHABDOMYOSARCOMA

Definition

Rhabdomyosarcoma is a soft tissue sarcoma derived from unsegmented mesoderm that accounts for approximately 5% of solid tumors in children. It is the most common soft tissue sarcoma in children.

Basic Science

Rhabdomyosarcomas are usually subdivided into three types: (1) embryonal, (2) alveolar, and (3) pleomorphic cell. The embryonal subtype makes up more than half of the childhood rhabdomyosarcomas and consists of primitive round and spindle-shaped cells showing little myoblastic differentiation. The term sarcoma botyroides refers to the classic embryonal rhabdomyosarcoma that grossly appears as a grape-like mass.

The alveolar subtype is the second most common and is distinguished by histology reminiscent of pulmonary alveoli, in which tumor cells and multinucleated giant cells line septa and extend into open "alveolar" spaces. This type is more common in older children and is more likely to arise in the extremity and retroperitoneal sites. It carries a worse prognosis than the embryonal type and has a higher likelihood of lymph nodal spread.

The pleomorphic rhabdomyosarcoma consists of compact yet haphazardly arranged spindle and multinucleated giant cells and is rarely seen in children. The etiology of these tumors remains unknown. Cytogenetic studies and molecular biology techniques applied to the rhabdomyosarcoma are still in the early stage and have yet to reveal significant insight into the derivation of this tumor.

Epidemiology

Rhabdomyosarcomas are three times more common in whites than nonwhites with an annual incidence in the United States of 4.4 per million white children and 1.3 per million black children under age 15 years (Maurer et al, 1977). There is an increased association with neurofibromatosis and with a family history of soft tissue sarcomas and breast cancer. There is a biphasic age incidence with peaks occuring either between ages 2 and 4 years and then again between ages 16 and 20 years. There is a slight male predominance. No definitive environmental factors have yet been revealed. The early peak is usually due to the occurrence of tumors in the head and neck region and the genito-urinary tract, while the late peak is usually composed of tumors of the trunk and extremities (Miser and Pizzo, 1985).

Natural History

Rhabdomyosarcoma presents most commonly in the extraorbital head and neck sites or the genitourinary sites (each approximately one-third of the time) with the remainder of tumors occurring in the orbit or in the trunk or extremity. Essentially it can occur at any anatomic site where striated muscle or its mesenchymal anlage exist. The extraorbital head and neck tumors occur usually in the middle ear, perinasal sinuses, and parotid region and will present as asymptomatic masses, polyps, or chronic infections, such as sinusitis or otitis externa, parotitis, or isolated cranial nerve palsies (especially the seventh cranial nerve). The abdominal or genitourinary masses rarely present asymptomatically and are usually associated with urethral or vaginal polypoid projections or acute urinary retention, in addition to being a palpable abdominal mass. The trunk and extremity can also reveal a rhabdomyosarcoma as an asymptomatic mass, but because of the tendency for these tumors to disseminate rapidly, it may also present as metastatic disease in lungs, bones, bone marrow, or distant lymph nodes.

Diagnosis

Desmin, an intermediate protein, has been shown to be a useful diagnostic biologic marker in differentiating a rhabdomyosarcoma from other round cell tumors with high specificity (Actmansberger et al, 1985). The definitive diagnostic examination, however, is biopsy of suspected tumor. Since up to 20% of patients will present with metastatic disease, investigation of potential metastatic sites is also in order at the time of diagnosis. Therefore, staging studies should be obtained in addition to biopsy of the suspected tumor including chest radiograph and lung CT, CT scan or MRI of the primary tumor site, bone scan, and bone marrow aspiration and biopsy. Depending upon the primary tumor site and anticipated subsequent therapy, regional lymph nodes may sometimes also require biopsy. The most commonly used staging classification for therapeutic purposes is that of postoperative findings devised by the Intergroup Rhabdomyosarcoma Study (IRS) (Maurer, 1975). The IRS staging includes: (a) group 1: localized, completely resected disease; (b) group 2: total gross resection with regional Spread noted; (c) group 3: incomplete gross resection or biopsy; (d) group 4: distant metastatic disease present.

Treatment

Treatment consists of biopsy and limited surgical resection of the tumor, followed by radiation and chemotherapy. Patients with a genitourinary rhabdomyosarcoma who do not achieve a pathologic complete remission after combined treatment modalities are then subject to a radical surgical procedure. If a uterine or cervical rhabdomyosarcoma is present, then an abdominal hysterectomy is the initial surgical procedure of choice. Of note, patients with group 1 or completely resected tumors with clear margins usually do not require radiation therapy but need adjuvant chemotherapy. Vincristine, actinomycin-D, and cyclophosphamide remain the most commonly used chemotherapeutic agents (Malogolowkin and Ortega, 1988).

Prognosis

Prognosis is dependent upon primary site, stage at presentation, and histologic subclassification of disease. Children with group 1 or group 2 disease have an 80–90% survival rate, whereas group 3 (unresectable) patients have a 50–60% survival rate, and group 4 (metastatic) have a 10–20% survival rate 5 years following diagnosis. Patients with the alveolar or monomorphous round cell histology have a significantly worse overall survival stage for stage than those patients with the embryonal subtype. Moreover, children with trunk and extremity tumors often have unfavorable histology and, as such, carry a poor prognosis. Patients who relapse will rarely survive even if the relapse is local (Raney et al, 1983). Recently, there has been an increase in secondary malignancies in rhabdomyosarcoma patients, including AML and other solid tumors. Close follow-up of these patients is mandatory.

REFERENCES

Actmansberger M, Weber K, Droste R, et al: Desmin is a specific marker for rhabdomyosarcomas of human and rat origin. *Am J Pathol* 118:85, 1985.

Colyer RA: Osteogenic sarcoma in siblings. *Johns Hopkins Med J* 145:131, 1979.

Glaubigerder DL, Makuch R, Schwarz J, et al: Determination of prognostic factors and their influence in therapeutic results in patients with Ewing's sarcoma. *Cancer* 45:2213, 1980.

Goorin AM, Abelson HT, Frei E: Osteosarcoma: Fifteen years later. *N Engl J Med* 313:1637, 1985.

Green DM, Jaffe N: Progress and controversy in the treatment of childhood rhabdomyosarcoma. *Can Treat Rev* 5:7, 1978.

Jaffe N: Advances in the management of malignant bone tumors in children and adolescents. *Pediatr Clin North Am* 32:801, 1985.

Link MP, Goorin AM, Miser AW, et al: The effect of adjuvant chemotherapy on relapse free survival in patients with osteosarcoma of the extremity. *N Engl J Med* 314:1600, 1986.

Malogolowkin MH, Ortega JA: Rhabdomyosarcomia of childhood. *Pediatr Ann* 17:251, 1988.

Maurer HM: The Intergroup Rhabdomyosarcoma Study: Objectives and clinical staging classification. *J Pediatr Surg* 10:977, 1975.

Maurer HM, Moon T, Donaldson M, et al: The Intergroup Rhabdomyosarcoma Study: A preliminary report. *Cancer* 40:2015, 1977.

Miser JS, Pizzo PA: Soft tissue sarcomas in childhood. *Pediatr Clin North Am* 32:779, 1985.

Raney RB, Crist WM, Maurer HM, et al: Prognosis of children with soft tissue sarcoma who relapse after achieving a complete response. *Cancer* 52:44, 1983.

Rosen G, Caparros B, Nirenberg A, et al: Ewing's sarcoma: 10 year experience with adjuvant chemotherapy. *Cancer* 47:2204, 1981.

Schackney SE, McCormack GW, Cucharal GI Jr: Growth rate patterns of solid tumors and their relation to responsiveness to therapy: An analytical review. *Ann Intern Med* 89:107, 1978.

Tebbi CK, Gaeta J: Osteosarcoma *Pediatr Ann* 17:286, 1988.

Trent J, Casper J, Meltzer P, et al: Nonrandom chromosome alterations in rhabdomyosarcoma. *Can Genet-Cytogen* 16:189, 1985.

Eye Tumors 10

RETINOBLASTOMA

Definition

Retinoblastoma is an intraocular malignancy of childhood. For an historic review, see Albert (1987).

Basic Science

About 40% of retinoblastomas are inherited as autosomal dominant with penetrance of 20–95%. The probability of bilateral retinoblastoma in hereditary cases is over 90%, and in sporadic cases, 18–30%. Offspring of patients with unilateral disease have a 7–10% risk of developing retinoblastoma (Cavenee et al, 1986).

Hereditary forms may be associated with partial deletions of the long arm of chromosome 13. (Deletion 13 q 14 is most common in association with severe malformations such as microcephaly.) Deletions have also been found at several other sites, including 13 q 31–32 and 13 q 33–34. A gene has been isolated that is expressed in normal cells, but is absent in retinoblastoma cells. Such a gene can be thought of as a recessive oncogene, the absence of which allows tumors to form (Friend et al, 1986; 1988).

Epidemiology

Retinoblastoma occurs once in 17,000–34,000 live births. It is the most common intraocular malignancy of childhood, and the eighth most common tumor.

Diagnosis

The tumor may be present at birth, but is most commonly diagnosed between 1 and 2 years of age. The tumor arises in the retina from one or more sites, and may extend into the vitreous. Further expansion into the anterior chamber may lead to glaucoma and inflammation. The tumor may extend along the optic nerve to the subarachnoid space and choroid plexus, and hematogenous spread can occur.

The first sign is usually a white pupil. About 20% of infants will have a fixed strabismus. Orbital cellulitis, glaucoma, and heterochromia may be the presenting signs.

Ocular ultrasonography is indicated to help distinguish vitreous lesions from retinoblastoma. CT scans can, likewise, localize tumors and detect calcification (Arrigg et al, 1983).

Treatment

Large tumors in one eye in sporadic cases are treated by enucleation. Small unilateral tumors respond to radiation therapy. Bilateral tumors are treated by irradiation and chemotherapy. Small tumors may be treated locally with cryotherapy, photocoagulation, or radon-seed implantation. Photocoagulation is best directed around the tumor to destroy its blood supply and, if successful, the tumor will regress. The results can be followed with fluorescein angiography.

CONTROVERSY

The indications for chemotherapy remain controversial. If metastatic disease is present, combinations of vincristine, cyclophosphamide, and adriamycin have been used.

Prognosis

The overall prognosis for survival from this tumor is excellent. Patients with familial types of retinoblastoma are at risk of multifocal lesions in either eye. A high percentage of survivors of hereditary retinoblastoma will develop potentially fatal second cancers (most commonly sarcomas), although 50% will arise out of the treatment field (Abramson et al, 1976).

Prevention

A pediatrician who examines eyes of infants should always ascertain whether the red reflex is present. If not, an ophthalmologist should be consulted immediately. A more careful examination of the retina should take place in the first months of life. If there is a positive family history, an ophthalmologist should follow the infant.

Advances have been reported in prediction of familial predisposition to the disease with use of DNA markers close to the retinoblastoma locus on chromosome 13 (Cavenee et al, 1986). Early diagnosis has occurred when karyotype analysis for dysmorphic features has shown a band 13 q 14 deletion which prompted an ophthalmic examination (Seidman et al, 1987).

REFERENCES

Abramson DH, Ellsworth RM, Zimmerman LE: Non-ocular cancer in retinoblastoma survivors. *Trans Am Acad Ophthalmol Otolaryngol* 81:454, 1976.

Albert DM: Historic review of retinoblastoma. *Ophthalmology* 94:654, 1987.

Arrigg PC, Hedges TR, Char DH: Computed tomography in the diagnosis of retinoblastoma. *Br J Ophthalmol* 67:588, 1983.

Cavenee WK, Murphree AL, Shull MM, et al: Prediction of familial predispostion to retinoblastoma. *N Engl J Med* 314:1201, 1986.

Friend SH, Bernards R, Rogelj S, et al: A human DNA segment with properties that predispose to retinoblastoma and osteosarcoma. *Nature,* October 16, 1986.

Friend SH, Dryja TP, Weinberg RA: Oncogenes and tumor-suppressing genes. *N Engl J Med* 318:618, 1988.

Lee WH, Murphree AL, Benedict WF: Expression and amplification of N-myc gene in primary retinoblastoma. *Nature* 309:458, 1984.
Murphree AL, Benedict WF: Retinoblastoma: Clues to human oncogenesis. *Science* 223:1028, 1984.
Seidman DJ, Shields JA, Augsburger JJ, et al: Early diagnosis of retinoblastoma based on dysmorphic features and karyotype analysis. *Ophthalmology* 94:663, 1987.
Shields JA, Augsburger JJ, Donoso LA: Recent developments related to retinoblastoma. *J Pediatr Ophthalmol Strabis* 23:148, 1986.

Chemotherapy 11

Definition

Chemotherapeutic agents are drugs directed against proliferating neoplasms. The selection of which particular chemotherapeutic agent to use is a function of the tumor being treated, the expected benefits versus risks of the agent being used, and the overall general condition of the patient.

Basic Science

Most chemotherapeutic agents are more effective when the tumor cell burden is small. The lethal action of most agents follows first order kinetics; that is, an effective dose will kill a fixed percentage of tumor cells not a fixed number. Hence, numerous applications of treatment may be needed before the maximal benefit is achieved. Most agents are effective against dividing rather than resting cells. In fact, agents can be divided into those that are (1) cell cycle-specific in that they kill more dividing than resting cells, (2) phase-specific in that they kill during a particular phase of the cell cycle, such as mitosis, or (3) cycle phase-nonspecific in that they kill both resting and dividing cells equally well. The site of action of the most common chemotherapeutic agents is shown in Figure 9.4.

The toxic side effects of chemotherapy are those that occur when the agents affect normal as well as neoplastic cells. The cells that divide rapidly, such as those of the GI tract and bone marrow, are the most sensitive to its effects and hence are the sites of most of the complications of this therapy.

One of the more recent developments has been the Goldie-Coldman model that explains the rationale of using more than one agent. This model is founded on the hypothesis that curability is related to the time of appearance of a singly or multiply resistant cell line. Therefore, multiple drug resistance can be prevented by using as many effective agents as possible at the highest doses tolerated as a first line treatment. Multiple agent therapy has been useful in the treatment of leukemias, lymphomas, and other solid tumors.

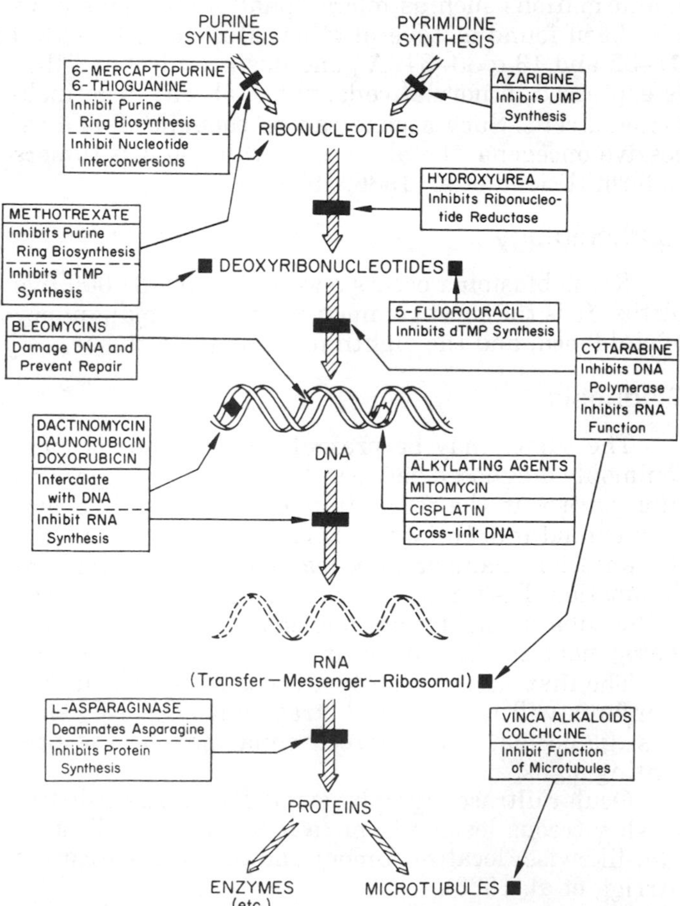

Figure 9.4. Summary of the mechanisms and sites of action of chemotherapeutic agents in neoplastic disease. Reproduced with permisssion from Calabresi P, Parks RE: In Goodman AG, Goodman LS, Gilman A (eds): *Pharmacological Basis of Therapeutics,* 6th edition. New York, Macmillan, 1980.

CASE ILLUSTRATION

A 9-year old developed the onset of seizures while being treated for leukemia. Three months before admission, she was diagnosed with ALL and started on the high-risk arm of the Dana Farber Cancer Institute protocol because of her high peripheral white blood count. Induction chemotherapy was complicated only by fever and neutropenia without documented infection. She went into remission and was undergoing intensified maintenance chemotherapy with vincristine, prednisone, 6-mercaptopurine, and L-asparaginase. During the week before admission, she experienced generalized body aches, which were attributed to vincristine neurotoxicity and had been placed on erythromycin for a left otitis. She was admitted for symptomatic control of her pain which was achieved with minimal doses of meperidine and received her usual dose of L-asparaginase on the third day of hospitalization. Twelve hours afterward, she complained of severe frontal headache, moderate periumbilical pain, and lethargy, and her parents thought she was "not herself."

On examination, she was found to alternate between being combative and lethargic, with poorly visualized eye grounds and no other focal findings. During the examination, she had a right-sided and generalized tonic clonic seizure that was self-resolved, became clearly combative afterward, and then had recurrent seizure activity despite anticonvulsive therapy, prompting transfer to the intensive care unit.

Laboratory studies at that time included hematocrit of 33, a white blood count of 6000/mm^3, with 97% polys, and 2% bands, platelets of 400,000/mm^3. She had normal electrolytes, calcium, magnesium, BUN, creatinine, glucose, clotting studies, and fibrinogen. A CT scan showed no mass effect, blood, or edema. A lumbar puncture was performed and was entirely normal. Liver function tests were remarkable for an SGOT of 45 U/L, an SGPT of 54 U/L, and an ammonia of 298 mg/dl.

Thirty-six hours later, her ammonia was 382 mg/dl, and she began to demonstrate posturing.

QUESTION AND COMMENT

What is the cause of her hyperammonemia and how should she be treated?

The patient was treated on an emergency basis with L-asparagine with dramatic results. One hour after the start of the infusion of 5 g/day of L-asparagine, her ammonia dropped to 157 mg/dl and over the next 2 days it further declined to 109 mg/dl, before it stabilized. Her mental status lagged behind the biochemical changes, but subsequently also normalized.

Seizures and alteration of mental status during chemotherapy for ALL are well-recognized and are usually due to thrombotic and hemorrhagic consequences of the L-asparaginase (Priest et al, 1982) typically occurring, as was the case here, after the completion of a month's course of the drug. However, the negative CT and nonfocal neurologic examination even after the seizure effectively ruled out this diagnosis. Less dramatic mental status changes of lethargy and confusion have been reported in up to 33% of children receiving L-asparaginase and are correlated with the EEG changes which mimic those seen in hepatic coma, and are presumably due to alteration of CNS amino acids or inhibition of protein synthesis, according to some authors (Cairo, 1982). More severe organic brain syndrome has also been reported, which typically occurs later in the course of therapy, which has a poor-dose response relationship to L-asparaginase. Hyperammonemia has been intermittently reported in children receiving this drug.

L-Asparaginase is known to reduce blood and CSF L-asparagine concentrations to zero for weeks after therapy and to cleave asparagine and glutamine to aspartate, glutamate, and ammonia. This may account, therefore, for some of the hyperammonemia that this patient experienced. Whether other amino acids are significantly affected via transamination or whether important urea cycle intermediates are depleted is unknown. From limited studies, the hyperammonemia and severe organic brain syndrome of L-asparaginase therapy can last from days to weeks. The infusion of L-asparagine has been used in small numbers of patients to treat the neurologic dysfunction and hyperammonemia and, similar to this patient, improved their course dramatically (Howland, 1974). These trials in our experience suggest that depletion of L-asparagine may interfere directly with the urea cycle activity; they further suggest new strategies for treatment of hyperammonemia secondary to other etiologies.

The scheduling and route of administration of chemotherapeutic drugs have evolved from clinical investigation. Some tumors have been found to respond to high-dose pulse therapy, whereas others seem to respond to continuous use of lower doses of the same drugs. Usually tumors with slow tumor cell turnover benefit from continuous low-dose therapy, whereas tumors that are rapid growing respond better to pulse therapy. The administration of chemotherapeutic drugs has been facilitated in the past 10 years with the use of the central venous catheter, which allows delivery of continuous infusions with less discomfort and fewer cutaneous side effects. Likewise, injections of chemotherapeutic agents into the CSF via subcutaneous reservoirs connected to ventricular catheters such as the Ommaya reservoir have become much more practical for administering intrathecal medications.

How long treatment should be administered for optimal benefit remains a subject of study in childhood malignancies. At present, Wilms tumor and nonlymphoblastic non-Hodgkin lymphoma with good prognostic markers are examples of childhood tumors that do not require prolonged treatment. Moreover, acute lymphoblastic leukemia with good prognostic markers may not need therapy beyond 2–3 years. Children with acute nonlymphocytic leukemia may not need more than 1 year of therapy.

Among the most difficult groups to treat with chemotherapy are neonates and infants since vascular access, nutrition, and growth and development may complicate the routine use of chemotherapeutic agents.

Common toxicities of major chemotherapeutic agents can include myelosuppression, nausea and vomiting, mucositis, and alopecia. Less common complications of some agents include nephrotoxicity (e.g., with methotrexate and cisplatinum), cardiomyopathy (e.g., with adriamycin and daunorubicin), pulmonary fibrosis (e.g., with bleomycin), and peripheral neuropathy (e.g., with vincristine and vinblastine).

The long-term effects of chemotherapy on growth and development in children continue to be a concern to oncologists. Other long-term complications can include: endocrinologic abnormalities, infertility, teratogenic effects in offspring, or an increase in the incidence of secondary malignancy. These risks must be weighed against the benefits of combating a malignancy in a child.

REFERENCES

Bleyer WA: Cancer chemotherapy in infants and children. *Pediatr Clin North Am* 32:557, 1985.

Cairo MS: Adverse reactions to l-asparaginase. *Am J Pediatr Hematol/Oncol* 4:335, 1982.

Howland J: Asparagine to reverse neurologic dysfunction associated with l-asparaginase. *J Pscyhiatric Res* 10:105, 1974.

Kaufman SD, Hetzel PC, Zimbler H: Overall principles of cancer management in chemotherapy. *Cancer Manual,* 7th edition. Boston, American Cancer Society, 1986, p. 69.

Ohnuma T, Howland JF, Freeman A: Biochemical and pharmacologic studies with asparaginase. *J Can Res* 30:2297, 1978.

Priest JR, Ramsay NK, Steinherz PG: A syndrome of thrombosis and hemorrhage complicating l-asparaginase therapy for acute childhood ALL. *J Pediatr* 100:984, 1982.

Radiation Therapy 12

Definition

Radiation therapy generally refers to the localized form of treatment directed against a malignancy. The exception to this is total body irradiation used for bone marrow transplantation programs. A tumor is considered radiocurable if it can be permanantly controlled by irradiation without undue morbidity. It is considered radioresponsive if there is a rapid decrease in tumor size with only moderate doses of radiation. Radioresponsive tumors are not necessarily radiocurable. Radiosensitivity is a measure of cell killing per given amount of radiation and can only be measured in vitro.

The unit of radiation absorbed is referred to as a rad and equals 100 ergs absorbed per gram of tissue. Fractionation refers to separation of a radiotherapy course into multiple dosage increments to allow repopulation repair and recovery for normal tissue. Skin-sparing refers to the ability of the megavoltage beams of radiation to penetrate beneath the skin and result in fewer epidermal and dermal complications secondary to radiation therapy.

Basic Science

Various forms of radiation therapy are available currently. Ionizing radiation can be produced by a wide variety of sources. Currently, most children are treated by external beam therapy. These external beams are produced by linear accelerators which result in high energy protons referred to as x-rays. These megavoltage beams provide only low doses to superficial tissues as they penetrate into deeper tissues. This results in skin sparing and reduces the amount of epidermal and dermal burn that was associated when radiation was given in the kilovoltage rather than in the megavoltage range. Placing a radioisotope into a intracavitary space is known as a radiation implant. These are used infrequently in children, although they have been used in the treatment of some brain tumors. Superficial skin tumors have been found to respond well to electron beam therapy, since electrons lose energy more rapidly and, therefore, tend to have a much weaker penetration.

The relationship between radiation dose and cell killing appears to be a sigmoid alone in that initially small doses result in relatively few killed cells, whereas at slightly higher doses small increments can produce relatively much greater cell killing. At highest dosage, large numbers of malignant cells can be killed, but large amounts of normal tissue also are destroyed. Following radiation therapy, tissues undergo repair and become repopulated by progeny of surviving cells normal and malignant. In addition, there can be a redistribution of cells through the phases of the cell cycle, with the newly dividing cells being more radiosensitive than others. Radioresistant hypoxic tumor cells may become more oxygenated and, thus, radiosensitive by redistribution of blood flow patterns secondary to radiation-induced cell killing in tumor shrinkage. Daily radiotherapy programs have evolved in attempts to optimize the effects of these four processes of repair, repopulation, redistribution, and tumor reoxygenation.

Natural History

The overall goal of radiation therapy is to treat the tumor and spare normal tissues from long-term complications of the therapy. This requires detailed treatment planning. The tumor must be precisely localized on the basis not only of physical examination but of other radiologic procedures such as computed tomography (CT scans). The symmetry of distribution is important since the radiation can affect the growth of a child. Immobilization of the patient is crucial to ensure adequate delivery of the appropriate dose in the appropriate location. In younger children, sedation or daily anesthesia may be required to provide such immobilization. Once localization is complete, the radiotherapy team then decides on the appropriate treatment plan, i.e., which is the best beam distribution with minimal dose to normal tissues. The use of radiation fields at right angles to each other and the use of multiple arcs and 360° rotations of the external beam are helpful.

Radiotherapy is useful for a variety of pediatric malignancies. For example, Hodgkin disease and some of the non-Hodgkin lymphomas are very responsive to radiation therapy. Unfortunately, the initial enthusiasm for radiation treatment of pediatric tumors has declined to some extent with the development of secondary cancers occurring even up to 30 years following initial treatment. Many tumors require a combination of radiation, chemotherapy, and surgical therapy, which has its own complications. For example, while radiation therapy and actinomycin D in combination appear to be synergistic, increased incidence of both lung and liver toxicity has been observed when this combination has been used for treatment of Wilms tumor. When adriamycin is used in combination with radiation, esophagitis and severe cardiotoxicity have been reported. The separation of these modalities reduced toxicity of both of these agents. Combined use of cytoxan and radiation therapy has led to an increased incidence of cystitis. Systemic methotrexate therapy with radiation has been associated with an increased likelihood of severe, potentially fatal, leukoencephalopathy, although this has not been seen with intrathecal methotrexate and radiation therapy (Table 9.8) (Byrd, 1985).

Table 9.8
Complications of Radiation Therapy

Site Irradiated	Complications
Mediastinum	Pericarditis
Head and neck[1]	Range of endocrinologic disorders stemming from effects on hypothalamic pituitary axis, e.g., growth hormone deficiency; panhypopituitarism
Thyroid	Hypothyroidism Thyroid carcinoma as secondary malignancy
Gonads	Fertility problems
Gastrointestinal	Malabsorption and altered digestive enzyme activity affecting growth and development; rarely esophageal strictures or intestinal obstruction
Right upper quadrant	Liver damage, generally fibrosis, which can lead to hepatic failure and death
Skeletal system	Epiphyseal, metaphyseal, or diaphyseal injury; abnormal periosteal activity and growth arrest
Pulmonary system	Interstitial pneumonitis and pulmonary fibrosis
Kidney (if not appropriately shielded above 1500 rad)	Nephritis

[1] CNS prophylaxis for acute lymphoblastic leukemia also can cause similar complications.

Secondary malignancies, although appearing less frequently following the use of megavoltage radiation, still occur (Coleman, 1982). Leukemias, bone sarcomas and thyroid cancer have been the most common secondary malignancies reported. Moreover, the combination of chemotherapy with radiotherapy may increase the likelihood of developing a second malignancy. Continuous improvements in the methods of administering radiation therapy are being designed, with the hope of minimizing some of the above complications.

REFERENCES

Byrd R: Late effects of treatment of cancer in children. *Pediatr Clin North Am* 32:835, 1985.

Coleman CN: Adverse effects of cancer therapy: Risk of secondary neoplasms. *Am J Pediatr Hematol/Oncol* 4:103, 1982.

Coleman CN, Howes AE: Overall principles of cancer management: Radiation therapy. Chapter 6, *Cancer Manual,* 7th edition. Boston, American Cancer Society, 1986, p. 57.

Hellman S: Principles of radiation therapy. In Devita VT Jr, Hellman S, Rosenberg SA (eds): *Cancer Principles and Practice of Oncology.* Philadelphia, JB Lipincott, 1985, p. 227.

Bone Marrow Transplantation 13

Definition

Bone marrow transplantation has become an accepted therapeutic option for patients with a variety of diseases. Its usefulness has been proven for selected leukemias and some other malignancies as well as for a number of nonmalignant hematologic and immunodeficiency diseases. Three types of bone marrow transplants currently are being performed. Autologous transplants are those in which the infused cells are the patient's own that have been previously collected and sometimes pretreated in vitro. Syngeneic transplants are those in which an identical twin serves as donor. Allogeneic transplants, the most common type, utilize a genetically nonidentical donor who has the same histocompatibility antigens as the recipient.

Basic Science

The major histocompatibility or human leukocyte antigen (HLA) complex is located on the short arm of chromosome 6. These antigens are responsible for regulating the immune response, allowing distinction between self and nonself, and hence determining whether an allograft will be successful. Considerable polymorphism exists in the genes of the HLA complex allowing HLA antigens to vary greatly among individuals. There are two major classes of HLA antigens. The class I antigens labeled HLA-A, HLA-B, and HLA-C, are found on essentially all cells in the body with the A and B antigens being strong transplantation antigens, so that incompatibility will result in a major rejection response. Class II antigens, on the other hand, have a more restricted distribution and are found on monocytes, B cells, and activated T cells. Serologic techniques can be used to type HLA A, B, and C antigens and compatibility can be demonstrated at the HLA-D or Class II locus by noting nonreactivity in mixed leukocyte cultures (MLC). The HLA-A, B, C genes as well as the HLA-D and DR, another class II antigen gene, are usually inherited as a single haplotype unit. Since a child will inherit one haplotype from each parent, there is a one in four chance that two siblings will have the same two identical haplotypes and thus be considered a perfect histocompatibility match. A mismatch between either the class I or the class II antigens will produce a cytotoxic response that will result in either rejection of the graft by the recipient or, if the graft is rich in immunocompetent cells, reaction against the recipient and subsequent graft-versus-host disease. If the immune system of the recipient has been suppressed, graft rejection rarely occurs. On the other hand, in diseases where the immune system is left relatively intact, such as in aplastic anemia, graft rejection can be a major problem. Graft-versus-host disease can occur in any recipient of an allogeneic transplant, even when HLA-matched sibling donors are used, since there are presumably as yet unidentified or unmatched histocompatibility antigens.

Epidemiology

Human bone marrow transplants were first performed in the 1950s, although only in the past 15 years have they finally been added to chemotherapy, radiation therapy, and surgery for tumor management. Currently, more than 10,000 bone marrow transplants have been performed worldwide.

Natural History

Children are ideal candidates for bone marrow transplantation since they are better able to withstand the rigors of the process. Children whose malignancies or diseases cannot be cured by other means are likely to be candidates for bone marrow transplantation. The malignancies that are appropriate for bone marrow transplantation are discussed under the specific disorders.

Once a potential recipient has been identified, HLA typing of all siblings and parents should be performed in order to see if there is a suitable donor. A sibling is most likely to match the recipient, followed by other relatives, and, least likely, a nonrelated histocompatible donor.

Before the actual transplant, most patients undergo a combination of high-dose chemotherapy and total body irradiation with the hope of producing immunosuppression. This will allow donor marrow to engraft and, at the same time, minimizes chances of graft rejection and eradicates any existing malignancy. The exact dosage and method of administration for radiation as well as for chemotherapy continues to be modified based on success and complication rates of this therapy.

The donor bone marrow is obtained by multiple needle aspirations of the iliac crests under general anesthesia. This usually supplies the cell dose of at least 1–3 $\times$ 10^8 cells/kg, or about 400–800 cc of bone marrow. The marrow is then filtered through screens to remove spicules and then immediately infused intravenously to the recipient in a manner similar to a blood transfusion. There have been no fatalities and little morbidity in donor aspirations, the only risks being from anesthesia or infection.

Engraftment usually occurs beginning in the second week after the transplant. Before this time, the recipient should be supported with blood products and parenteral alimentation and usually parenteral antibiotics to avoid the possibility of infection. During this "pre-engraftment" period, the effects of the pretransplant regimen become clinically evident as the recipient may develop fevers, nausea, diarrhea, mucositis, and dermal erythema from the pretransplant conditioning. If the transplant is successful, complete engraftment should be evident by 3 months after transplantation, although full immunologic recovery may take up to a full year. During the pre-engraftment period, the patient is usually placed in an infection-free environment using reverse isolation or laminar airflow and is given antibiotic prophylaxis.

There are several complications of bone marrow transplantation.

1. Infections. Gram-positive or Gram-negative sepsis and fungal infections typically occur in patients with granulocytopenia before engraftment. Following engraftment, full immune function returns much more slowly, as noted above, and therefore, the patient remains at risk for developing infections secondary to viruses, fungi, Gram-positive and encapsulated organisms, and *Pneumocystis carinii*. The incidence of opportunistic infections has been slightly decreased with the institution of trimethoprim-sulfamethoxazole prophylaxis for *Pneumocystis* and the use of acyclovir for herpetic infections (Meyers et al, 1988).

2. Interstitial pneumonia. During the first 3–5 months after transplantation, patients are at greatest risk for developing interstitial pneumonitis, which is usually due to a combination of infections and noninfectious causes such as irradiation therapy used before transplantation. Infection with cytomegalovirus, the most common agent for the infectious pneumonitis carries an extremely high mortality rate. The use of fractionated doses of radiation before transplantation has helped to reduce the incidence of noninfectious pneumonitis.

3. Graft-versus-host disease (see also Section 16). Graft-versus-host disease is one of the most common complications of marrow engraftment, and occurs in both acute and chronic forms. The incidence and severity of the acute disorder is lower in children than in adults. It usually results from immunocompetent donor T lymphocytes that are transferred in the marrow infusion. Apparently in acute graft-versus-host disease there is a T-cell imbalance, with decreased helper and increased suppressor cells. The target organs for acute disease are skin, GI tract, and liver. It usually occurs within the first 100 days after transplantation, and the severe acute form is associated with a 10–20% mortality.

Chronic graft-versus-host disease is seen in about one-third of allogeneic transplants. It can either evolve from the acute disorder or appear de novo. This disorder is characterized by skin lesions similar to those of scleroderma, as well as gastrointestinal involvement including esophagitis, enteritis, and hepatitis. Chronic graft-versus-host disease results in abnormal immune function; these patients are unable to produce specific antibodies due to lack of T- and B-cell cooperation. Infections with encapsulated organisms are common in both acute and chronic disease and can occur in even the perfect HLA-matched donor-recipient combination.

Treatment for graft-versus-host disease includes nonspecific immunosuppression with methotrexate for the first 100 days after engraftment, although its efficacy remains controversial. It is thought that the addition of steroids and antithymocyte-globulin to the methotrexate regimen has reduced the incidence of the disease, but has not decreased mortality. Moreover, the use of methotrexate may delay engraftment.

One approach has been the ex vivo elimination of T cells from the donor marrow before infusion, which may be the best method of prevention for the future (Quinn, 1985). Acute graft-versus-host disease also has been found to sometimes respond to the use of steroids or antithymocyte-globulin, although it is still not clear what the mechanism is for the response. The chronic disorder can be treated with prednisone and azathioprine, which has also been found to decrease the mortality rate. Cyclosporin A is also useful in prevention and has some efficacy in the treatment of established graft-versus-host disease.

4. Veno-occlusive disease of the liver. Although this problem is more common in patients with prior liver disease, it can occur in any patient. As a result of thrombotic obstructive lesions of the small hepatic vein, patients present with jaundice, ascites, and at least half of them progress to fatal hepatic failure.

5. Recurrence of original malignancy. Patients who are not truly in remission, or those who have had more than two remissions at the time of transplant are at increased risk for recurrence of their initial malignancy. These recurrences usually occur in recipient rather than donor cells.

6. Late complications. High-dose irradiation can result in cataracts, and in endocrinologic dysfunction, including hypothyroidism, sterility, and growth abnormalities. Cranial irradiation or methotrexate therapy may influence cerebral development in children undergoing transplants. The incidence of secondary malignancies following bone marrow transplantation remains unknown at this time.

Treatment

Among the malignant diseases that have responded to bone marrow transplantation are acute lymphoblastic leukemia, acute nonlymphocytic leukemia, chronic myelogenous leukemia, non-Hodgkin lymphoma, and neuroblastoma. In the nonmalignant category, patients with severe combined immunodeficiency, Wiskott-Aldrich syndrome, severe aplastic anemia, osteopetrosis, Fanconi anemia, congenital hypoplastic anemia, as well as infiltrative diseases such as Gaucher disease have benefited from bone marrow transplantation. Chronic granulomatus disease, Diamond-Blackfan syndrome, and thalassemia also have responded to bone marrow transplantation.

Future use of T-cell depletion is targeted to decrease the incidence of graft-versus-host disease. In addition, T-cell depletion may permit engraftment between partially and totally mismatched donors and recipients. Alternatively, attempts are being made to use autologous bone marrow transplantation, in which the recipient's own marrow is obtained, the patient is then treated with supralethal doses of irradiation and chemotherapy after which the marrow is reinfused into the patient (Champlin and Gale, 1984). Since some malignant cells are likely to remain at the time of marrow harvesting, it will also be important to be able to purge this marrow of the residual malignant cells in order to improve disease-free survival with autologous bone marrow transplantation.

REFERENCES

Champlin RE, Gale RP: Bone marrow transplation the treatment of hematologic malignancies in solid tumors: Critical review of syngeneic autogogous and allogeneic transplants. *Can Treat Rep* 68:145, 1984.

Grouse LD: Bone marrow transplantation a life-saving applied art. An interview with E. Donnall Thomas, MD. *JAMA* 249:2528, 1983.

Kamani N: Bone marrow transplantation of pediatric hematologic disorders. *Pediat Ann* 14:661, 1985.

Meyers JD, Reed EC, Shepp DH, etal: Acyclovir for prevention of cytomegalovirus infection and disease after allogeneic marrow transplanatation. *N Engl J Med* 318:70, 1988.

Quinn JJ: Bone marrow transplantation in the management of childhood cancer. *Pediatr Clin North Am* 32:811, 1985.

Rappeport JM, Smith BR, Parkman R, et al: Application of bone marrow transplantation in genetic diseases. *Clin Hematol* 12:755, 1983.

Current Trends and Future Directions 14

Garrett M. Brodeur
Alan L. Schwartz

Most cancers in children probably are not caused solely by environmental exposure and, as such, are not preventable. A subset of individuals can be identified as having genetic predisposition to develop specific malignant diseases, and these individuals can be followed carefully to detect tumors early. However, such approaches are not practical for the majority of cases which are sporadic, or for heritable cases which represent new mutations (i.e., a negative family history).

The emphasis of clinical and laboratory research has to be placed on early detection and treatment, and on reducing the short- and long-term consequences of therapy. Successful treatment of cancer with the conventional approaches of surgery, radiation and chemotherapy, apparently has reached a plateau, so radically new approaches to treatment are required. To develop these, it will be necessary to understand better the mechanisms of tumorigenesis, tumor progression, and drug resistance.

Currently, bone marrow transplantation offers hope for cure in subsets of individuals who might otherwise have little chance of survival. Allogeneic marrow transplantation from HLA-matched siblings is becoming one of the preferred approaches to management of patients with acute nonlymphoblastic leukemia, as well as certain other myeloproliferative disorders. Autologous marrow transplantation, preceded by purging the marrow of malignant cells with one or a panel of monoclonal antibodies, appears to be a promising approach to the management of very poor risk patients with neuroblastoma and selected other solid tumors. Nevertheless, marrow transplantation and its attendant treatment have substantial morbidity and mortality, especially from graft-versus-host disease, so there is considerable cost in both human and financial terms. While marrow transplantation seems to be a short-term solution to the treatment of certain diseases, more specific and less toxic therapy would clearly be preferable.

There appear to be three main areas in which future improvements in the understanding and treatment of malignant diseases may come. These include pharmacology, immunology, and molecular biology. Preliminary information in all of these areas has come to light in recent years and may soon provide valuable tools for the diagnosis and treatment of cancer.

The bane of clinical oncology today is drug resistance. While literally dozens of chemotherapeutic agents are available, with different mechanisms of action and toxicities, the effective agents are quickly exhausted in almost half of the patients treated. Some respond initially, only to have recurrences later whether therapy is continued or not, and the recurrent disease is usually refractory to further treatment. Clearly, a better understanding of how malignant cells become resistant to drugs may assist us in the development of better drugs or the more effective delivery of available agents. Mechanisms include altered drug entry or efflux from the cell, altered binding specificities, as well as gene amplification or overexpression of the target protein.

An important advance in this area is the recent identification of a family of genes whose products confer resistance to a variety of seemingly unrelated drugs. This multidrug-resistant family of proteins (also called mdr-1, p-glycoprotein, gp170) appears to cause the rapid efflux from the cell of chemotherapeutic agents that have different mechanisms of action but bear some structural relatedness. An understanding of how the expression or amplification of these proteins occurs may suggest ways to administer drugs without enhancing their expression. Aternatively, identifying individuals whose tumors have or develop enhanced mdr-1 expression will spare those individuals exposure to agents to which they will not respond. These individuals then can be treated by alternative or even unconventional approaches.

Another important area involves new methods of drug delivery. The amount of a specific drug that can be administered is usually limited by some organ-specific host toxicity, such as bone marrow suppression, nephrotoxicity, etc. If a greater portion of drug could be delivered to the tumor, the therapeutic index could be greatly increased, thereby enhancing effectiveness, decreasing toxicity, or both. This may be accomplished by linking drugs to: (a) tumor-specific monoclonal antibodies (see below); (b) ligands that bind to receptors that are relatively abundant on tumor cells; or (c) liposomes that may fuse preferentially to tumor cells.

New agents represent a third frontier for cancer pharmacology. It is possible that third and fourth generation anthracyclines, or platinum analogs, and the like will offer some improvement. Also, some new types of antimetabolites, alkylating agents, DNA intercalators, or antimitotics may be effective. However, conventional approaches appear to have reached a plateau, and further improvements in the above areas are likely to offer only modest improvements. Radically new, cancer-specific agents will probably be required to make more substantial headway. Understanding the cellular and molecular biology of the cancer cell and how its genetic program has gone awry will likely provide insights into new approaches, such as inducing differentiation or triggering regression of certain tumors, such as neuroblastoma or certain leukemias.

Cancer immunology currently is a rapidly expanding field. Virtually every leukemia classification relies heavily on a panel of monoclonal and polyclonal antibodies to determine the leukemia cell type. Antibodies to relatively tissue-specific proteins (e.g., myoglobin, glial-associated protein) are useful in sorting out the "small, round blue cell tumors of childhood" which frequently pose diagnostic dilemmas. Indeed, panels of monoclonal antibodies which are relatively tumor specific and nonreactive with normal marrow are being used to purge marrow of contaminating malignant cells in preparation for autologous marrow transplantation. Finally, there are some promising efforts to use monoclonal antibodies that are radioactively labeled (e.g., with I^{131}) for diagnostic imaging. Successful diagnostic imaging could be readily scaled up in order to provide a means of targeted radiation therapy.

A number of attempts have been made to develop a successful approach to immunotherapy, but few have been very effective to date. With respect to monoclonal antibodies, there are problems with species differences between the host and the source of antibody, cross-reactivity of the antibodies with other tissues, adequate delivery of antibody to the center of bulky tumors, modulation of the tumor cell membrane, etc. In addition, it is not clear which is the best method of effecting cell kill (e.g., complement-mediated cell lysis; delivery of a chemotherapeutic agent, radioisotope, or toxin). A better understanding of the normal function of the immune system may overcome these obstacles.

Other approaches that enhance the immune response of the patient may prove more effective. These include active or passive immunization, as well as the delivery of immunoregulatory molecules or lymphokines, such as the interferons or interleukins. A variation on this approach employs the extracorporeal activation of "killer" leukocytes (lymphokine-activated killer, or LAK, cells) from an individual patient to enhance the patient's cellular response to his/her own malignant cells. Indeed, a focus on enhancement of the patient's own cellular immunity to his/her tumor may be more effective than the antibody approach, given the key role that cellular immunity is thought to play in the immune surveillance of cancer.

In the long run, advances in the molecular biology of cancer offer the greatest potential for understanding cancer development and progression, as well as the greatest hope for more effective and less toxic treatment. At least two major classes of cancer-related genes appear to play a role in tumorigenesis. The best characterized are known as oncogenes or proto-oncogenes, which are the cellular counterparts of retroviral oncogenes in animals. Currently at least 40 proto-oncogenes have been identified by homology with their retroviral counterparts, by DNA transfection, or by association with tumor-specific chromosome rearrangements. Oncogenes can be activated by increasing their number per cell, increasing the expression of a single-copy gene, or by structural alteration or modification of the gene or its product.

One of the more striking examples of oncogene activation is amplification of the N-myc oncogene in neuroblastomas. This oncogene is amplified from 3- to 300-fold in about a third of all neuroblastomas at the time of diagnosis. N-myc amplification is found almost exclusively in patients with extensive or metastatic disease. Indeed, the presence of amplification in these patients is associated with rapid tumor progression and a poor prognosis. This represents the first example of an association between basic research on oncogenes and clinical outcome, although there will undoubtedly be others.

The second important class of cancer-related genes contains those variously known as suppressor genes, regulatory genes or antioncogenes. Their existence was postulated to explain the genetic predisposition to retinoblastoma in certain families and the association with a specific, constitutional chromosome deletion in some cases. Subsets of individuals with other tumors, such as Wilms tumor, also with a heritable predisposition were identified. The basis for this predisposition has been explained by the inheritance of a defective or deleted copy of a suppressor gene. Since this represents one of a pair of alleles, a tumor develops if the second allele is inactivated in any cell of the target tissue. In sporadic cases, it presumably takes inactivation of both suppressor alleles in the same cell of the target tissue for a tumor to develop.

The existence of suppressor genes was hypothesized based on genetic analysis of populations with a given malignancy, as well as the specific constitutional chromosome deletions with which they were associated. There is now substantially more evidence from the suppression of tumorigenicity in somatic cell hybrids, as well as from the molecular analysis of both hereditary and sporadic tumors with DNA probes for specific regions of particular chromosomes. These probes can be used to identify individuals who are genetically predisposed in selected families. Indeed, there is recent evidence that a portion of the retinoblastoma predisposition locus may have been cloned. The development of a battery of probes for these suppressor genes should be very useful in determining diagnosis and predisposition, and possibly even prognosis.

Other DNA probes have become available that identify tumor-specific rearrangements, first identified as cytogenetic rearrangements, such as the 9;22 translocation in chronic myelogenous leukemia, resulting in the bcr-abl hybrid gene and protein. In addition, there are probes for relatively tissue-specific gene rearrangements, such as immunoglobulin genes in B-lymphocytes and T-cell receptor genes in T-lymphocytes. These provide us with powerful additional tools in the diagnosis and classification of malignant diseases.

Moreover, it is possible that a better understanding of oncogene function and activation, suppressor gene function and inactivation, as well as other tumor-specific genetic changes, will provide insight into how cancer develops or progresses. This, in turn, may suggest ways in which the altered genetic program can be subverted to halt the relentless progress of malignant cell growth. Clearly, only a subpopulation of the malignant cells is capable of sustaining this continued growth. Therefore, a concerted effort to reprogram these cells toward death, differentiation, or quiescence may be the most effective and least toxic approach to cancer treatment in the future. Recombinant DNA technology may not only provide a means of identifying the important genes and how they are controlled, but it may also provide a means of producing biologic reagents that may be useful in treatment or prevention. It is reasonable to assume that our first efforts in this regard may be possible in the next 5–10 years.

REFERENCES

Ames GFL: The basis of multidrug resistance in mammalian cells: Homology with bacterial transport. *Cell* 47:323, 1986.

Berger NA: Cancer chemotherapy: New strategies for success. *J Clin Invest* 78:1131, 1986.

Brodeur GM: Involvement of oncogenes and suppressor genes in human neoplasia. *Adv Pediatr* 34:1, 1987.

Brodt P: Tumor immunology—three decades in review. *Ann Rev Microbiol* 37:447, 1983.

Cavenee WK, Murphree AL, Shull MM, et al: Prediction of familial predisposition to retinoblastoma. *N Engl J Med* 314:1202, 1986.

Foon KA, Todd RF III: Immunologic classification of leukemia and lymphoma. *Blood* 68:1, 1986.

Frankel AE, Houston LL, Issell BF: Prospects for immunotoxin therapy in cancer. *Ann Rev Med* 37:125, 1986.

Friend SH, Bernards R, Rogelj S, et al: A human DNA segment with properties of the gene that predisposes to retinoblastoma and osteosarcoma. *Nature* 323:643, 1986.

Goldie JH, Coldman AJ: The genetic origin of drug resistance in neoplasms: Implications for systemic therapy. *Can Res* 44:3643, 1984.

Levy R, Miller RA: Biological and clinical implications of lymphocyte hybridomas: Tumor therapy with monoclonal antibodies. *Ann Rev Med* 34:107, 1983.

Matthay KK, Heath TD, Badger CC, et al: Antibody-directed liposomes: Comparison of various ligands for association, endocytosis and drug delivery. *Can Res* 46:4904, 1986.

Oldham RK: Biological response modifiers. *J Natl Cancer Inst* 70:789, 1983.

Pastan I, Willingham MC, FitzGerald DJP: Immunotoxins. *Cell* 47:641, 1986.

Rosenberg SA, Lotze MT, Muul LM, et al: Observations on the systemic administration of autologous lymphokine activated killer cells and recombinant interleukin-2. *N Engl J Med* 313:1485, 1985.

Sager R: Genetic suppression of tumor formation: A new frontier in cancer research. *Can Res* 46:1573, 1986.

Schimke RT: Gene amplification, drug resistance, and cancer. *Can Res* 44:1735, 1984.

Seeger RC, Brodeur GM, Sather H, et al: Association of multiple copies of the N-myc oncogene with rapid progression of neuroblastomas. *N Engl J Med* 313:1111, 1985.

Varmus HE: The molecular genetics of cellular oncogenes. *Ann Rev Genet* 18:553, 1984.

Weissman BE, Stanbridge EJ: Complementation of the tumorigenic phenotype in human cell hybrids. *J Natl Cancer Inst* 70:667, 1983.

LEWIS R. FIRST
CHARLES BERDE
ALAN L. SCHWARTZ
GARRETT M. BRODEUR

Consultants
Howard Weinstein
David G. Nathan

Section 10

Nephrology

Pediatric nephrology is one of the newest and most rapidly expanding subspecialties. In common with many clinical specialties, new technology has illuminated and permitted more detailed categorization of specific entities, such as glomerular and tubular disorders. Imaging has been enhanced with ultrasonography, CT scans, radionuclide scans, and angiography. Management of chronic renal failure has been revolutionized by hemodialysis and renal transplantation. Advances in immunology and immunopathology, and the use of electron microscopy and freeze fracture microscopy have further defined some of the mechanisms of renal pathology.

In the following pages, we have summarized some of the salient points that the general pediatrician needs to know as an approach to renal disease. Renal tumors will be discussed under oncology.

Evaluation of Renal Function

1

There are several ways of assessing renal function. The simplest is the analysis of a sample of urine. The sample may be obtained randomly or after various test procedures. Timed urine samples coupled with analyses of specific substances in the sample can provide information regarding urinary clearance rates. More sophisticated tests include renal biopsy and radiographs of the kidney after administration of specific contrast agents.

URINALYSIS

Careful analysis of urine is required in many circumstances. These include periodic checks at well-child visits for any urinary tract symptoms and in the presence of unexplained vomiting and/or diarrhea. The daily excretion of urine depends on fluid intake: in infants, it is 200–400 ml/24 hours; in children, 500–1000 ml/24 hours; and in adolescents, 700–1500 ml/24 hours.

The analysis of urine should include observation of color and odor, measurement of the pH and specific gravity or osmolarity, and testing for the presence of solutes such as sugars, protein, and ketones. In addition, the urine should be centrifuged and the sediment inspected for the presence of cells, bacteria, or crystals.

Odor

The most common abnormal *odor* of urine results from acidosis and dehydration. Some rare hereditary metabolic diseases may be recognized in infancy by the characteristic odor of the urine. Branched-chain ketoaciduria (leucine, isoleucine, and valine) produces an odor of maple syrup in urine, hence, the name maple syrup urine disease. For those individuals unfamiliar with maple syrup, burnt sugar has a similar odor. Phenylketonuria produces a musty smell. Hypertyrosinemia and hypermethioninemia produce unpleasant odors like rancid butter. The urine of isovaleric acidemia smells like sweaty socks.

The pH of urine normally ranges between 5.0 and 6.5.

Color

The *color* of urine comes from the yellow pigment urochrome. Blood will give a red or brown color. If the urine is red, and the supernatant fraction is clear after centrifugation, the blood is generally from the lower urinary tract. If the urine is brownish or rust colored, and the supernatant fraction remains the same color, the blood is probably renal in origin. In the newborn infant, rust-colored urine is most likely to be due to the presence of urates, which can be readily distinguished by microscopic examination of the sediment. Very pale color usually denotes dilute urine with low specific gravity, except in diabetes (or other conditions with glycosuria) when glucose can raise the specific gravity without changing the color of urine. Dark yellow color can indicate concentrated urine or the presence of bile pigments. If a urine sample turns red on standing, porphyrins are likely to be present. If the diaper stains blue after a few hours of being wet, it indicates excessive indole production from degradation of tryptophan in the intestine (a familial disorder with hypercalcemia know as blue diaper syndrome).

Glucose and protein are most often measured with commercially available dipsticks. The glucose dipstick uses glucose oxidase and is, therefore, specific for glucose, and does not detect galactose and fructose. If total reducing substances are to be measured, a copper sulfate solution (Benedict solution) is appropriate. Protein dipsticks will detect protein in a concentration of 20 mg/dl or more. Excessive excretion of amino acids can be measured by paper chromatography and is important in screening for hereditary metabolic diseases. Nitrite dipsticks are positive in the presence of bacteria: the first voided specimen in the morning is preferable for testing since bacteria will have had time to incubate in the bladder producing measured amounts of nitrates. The test correlates with urine cultures in about 80% of cases, but does not detect coccal infections.

Microscopic examination of sediment after centrifugation at 800–1000 rpm for 5 minutes can be informative about the location and type of urinary tract pathology. Large epithelial cells are usually from the bladder. When mixed with polymorphonuclear leukocytes, bladder infection is likely. A fresh specimen under a cover slip may show motile bacteria and, thus, establish the presence of infection. The organisms can be further identified by Gram stain and culture.

Fresh red blood cells that retain normal morphology almost certainly have originated in the lower urinary tract (bladder or urethra). On the other hand, red blood cells that originate in the kidney, as in glomerulonephritis, and have been exposed to the osmotic, pH and other change of tubular fluid, will appear small, crenated, and damaged.

Red blood cell casts are, on the average, about 4 red cell diameters in width. The presence of red cells and red cell casts generally indicates some type of glomerulonephritis. If the red cells are dysmorphic and the casts are wider than average, the probability of tubular injury and chronic renal damage is high. Granular casts represent degenerating red or white cells; unstained granular casts from red cells have a brownish hue. These casts have presumably been in the collecting duct longer than casts with discrete cells. Casts form when Tamm-Horsfall protein, which is formed in the loop of Henle, precipitates in the collecting duct and traps cells and other debris. Hyaline casts indicate the presence of proteinuria. Waxy casts are more refractile than hyaline casts and indicate renal failure.

White cells can appear in urine in reponse to inflammation anywhere in the urinary tract. White cell casts, however, can come only from the renal collecting duct. More than 5 white cells per high power field is considered abnormal.

Crystals in urine may provide a lead to a metabolic diagnosis. Crystals that can be readily identified include cystine, calcium oxalate, phosphate, and uric acid. Crystals frequently are seen in normal urine especially when urine pH is at the extremes of the normal range. For example, triple phosphates are precipitated in alkaline urine. In acid urine, uric acid appears as a red rhomboid prism, and urates are amorphous brown clumps, needles or fans. Cystine is readily recognized by its hexagonal configuration (like a benzene ring), and its presence may indicate cystinuria (see pp. 00).

Excretion of electrolytes and other metabolites in urine can be assessed by timed urine collections. For example, normal calcium values in urine are 5 mg/kg/24 hours when calcium intake is less than 500 mg/24 hours. Elevated values are found in metabolically induced calcium nephrolithiasis, after treatment with furosemide, and in hyperparathyroidism. Sodium excretion depends on intake, and can reach 250 $mEq/m^3/24$ hours. Similarly, potassium excretion can reach 250 $mEq/m^3/24$ hours, or be as low as 20 $mEq/m^3/24$ hours. Potassium excretion greater than intake is found in metabolic acidosis, diuretic therapy, and hyperadrenalism. Urinary oxalate excretion is elevated in an inborn error of oxalate metabolism, and in other conditions characterized by nephrolithiasis. Normal values are under 40 mg/24 hours.

Specific Test of Renal Function: Glomerular Filtration Rate

The glomerular filtrate rate (GFR) is the volume of plasma filtrate formed per unit time. Normally about 20% of renal plasma flow is filtered. The GFR is measured most accurately by inulin (a fructose polymer of 5000 molecular weight), which is freely filtered but neither absorbed nor excreted by the renal tubules. Plasma (P) and urine (U) concentrations during constant infusion and urine volume (V) per unit time permit calculation of GFR, which equals UV/P.

More commonly, however, glomerular filtration is estimated by clearance of endogenous creatinine over a 12- to 24-hour period.

$$\text{GFR (cc/min)} = \frac{\text{creatinine excreted (mg)}}{\text{plasma creatinine (mg/cc)} \cdot \text{min}}$$

Serum creatinine levels are also helpful, with values in infants of 0.3 mg/dl, values of 0.6 mg/dl in children, and in adults, less than 1.5 mg/dl. Phosphate clearance is discussed on page 632.

Concentrating Ability of Kidney

Urine osmolality depends on fluid intake and renal concentrating ability. After fluid restriction (4 hours in an infant or 8–12 hours in a child), urine osmolality is an appropriate measure of tubular function. Osmolalities over 600 are rare in infants, except if they are severely dehydrated, when values can reach 1000 mOsm/L. After a 12-hour period of fluid restriction osmolality in the normal child reaches 900 mOsm/L (specific gravity 1.024) or more (range 870–1310).

Impaired concentrating ability is found in chronic renal failure from any cause, sickle cell disease, hypokalemia, hypercalcemia, distal renal tubular acidosis, and nephrogenic diabetes insipidus.

Renal Biopsy

Renal biopsy is most helpful in distinguishing different types of glomerular disease. Percutaneous biopsy can permit monitoring of the course of disease and its response to treatment. It should be done only by experienced physicians who have access to immunopathologic techniques and electron microscopy. It is contraindicated in the presence of a bleeding disorder.

ACID-BASE DISORDERS

Definition

Disorders that result in a hydrogen ion concentration in extracellular fluid that is outside the normal narrow range (pH 7.35–7.45) are considered to be disturbances in acid-base balance.

Basic Science

pH is defined as the negative logarithm of the $[H^+]$ when the latter is given as equivalents per liter. The pH of the blood of a normal person is 7.4 (alkaline). However, large amounts of acid (any compound that can give up a hydrogen ion) are produced daily from two major sources: (1) some 13,000–20,000 mMoles of CO_2 as the result of oxidative metabolism and (2) 40–60 mMoles of inorganic and organic acids that are not derived from CO_2. The CO_2 generated dissolves in water to form carbonic acid which dissociates to ions of hydrogen and bicarbonate:

$$CO_2 + H_2O \rightleftharpoons H_2CO_3 \rightleftharpoons H^+ + HCO_3^-$$

Sulfuric acid is produced from catabolism of protein and phosphoric acid is a byproduct of phospholipid catabolism. Because these acids are not volatile or in equilibrium with a volatile component they are known as fixed acids. A diet high in meat produces large amounts of fixed acids. In certain states, other acids such as lactic (exercise and hypoxia) and acetoacetic acid and β-hydroxybutyric acid (diabetes mellitus) are produced.

The body must be protected from these large amounts of acids. Several lines of defense are available. First, the acid can be buffered directly.

Strong acid + Buffer salt
$\rightleftharpoons$ Neutral salt + Weak acid

For example:

$$\underbrace{H^+\ Cl^-}_{\text{strong acid}} + \underbrace{Na^+ + HCO_3^-}_{\text{buffer salt}} \rightleftharpoons \underbrace{Na^+ + Cl^-}_{\text{neutral salt}} + \underbrace{H_2CO_3}_{\text{weak acid}}$$

This reaction minimizes but does not prevent a drop in pH. The carbonic acid can dissociate to CO_2 and H_2O if the CO_2 can be removed continuously (shifting equilibrium). This brings into play the second line of defense: the lungs. As a result of the lower pH of the blood, alveolar ventilation is increased and the excess CO_2 is excreted by the lungs. Though the lungs can restore the pH almost to normal within a few minutes, the stores of body buffer have been depleted. As the concentration of HCO_3^- falls, the third line of defense comes into play: the kidney. The process of renal excretion of H^+ and replenishment of HCO_3^- stores is much slower than the first two lines of defense, requiring hours to days rather than seconds to minutes.

Like Na^+ and other small solutes, HCO_3^- is freely filtered by the glomeruli. Approximately 99.9% of this filtered HCO_3^- is reabsorbed in the tubules. In addition, new HCO_3^- is formed within renal cells and added to the blood. H^+ is excreted in urine as the acid salt NaH_2PO_4 or in combination with NH_3 to form neutral NH_4^+ salts.

An exogenous acid load is distributed equally throughout the extracellular fluid in about 20–30 minutes. Some of it moves into cells, where buffering is accomplished by sodium and potassium proton exchange and by chloride-bicarbonate exchange. In fact, with continued infusion of acid, cellular buffering can be twice that of extracellular buffering.

Respiratory compensation starts as soon as the chemoreceptors detect the acidosis. By stimulating alveolar ventilation, carbon dioxide is removed, thus minimizing the fall in pH. The time required for full respiratory compensation of a sustained metabolic acidosis is from 12–24 hours. If the acidosis is then corrected by removal of cause or infusion of bicarbonate, CO_2 will increase in the extracellular fluid and further stimulate ventilation. If the lungs are abnormal and respiratory compensation is limited, CO_2 will increase in the extracellular fluid and the fall in pH will be more severe since CO_2 production may exceed the capacity for loss through ventilation (Fig. 10.1).

In contrast, renal compensation is a relatively slow process that requires several days to adapt. In individuals with chronic lung disease and sustained elevated P_{CO_2}, renal retention of bicarbonate results in a chronic compensated respiratory acidosis. If the condition of lungs suddenly improves, as in children with cystic fibrosis who may receive intensive physical therapy

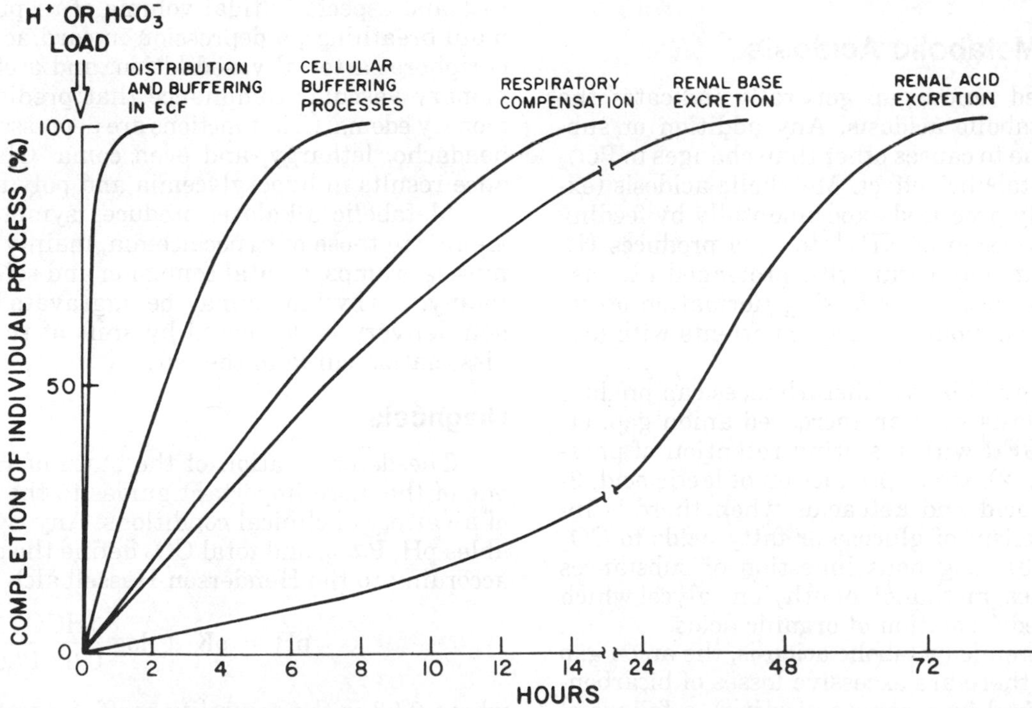

Figure 10.1. Time course of acid-base compensatory mechanisms. In response to a metabolic acid or alkaline load, individual approaches to completion of the extracellular buffering mechanisms, cellular events, and respiratory and renal regulatory processes are presented as functions of time. Reproduced with permission from Cogan MG, Rector FC: Acid base disorders. In Brenner BM, Rector FC (eds): *The Kidney,* 3rd edition. Chap 13. Philadelphia, WB Saunders, 1986.

and bronchodilatation, the P_{CO_2} can fall within hours, but the renal release of bicarbonate may take several days. Thus, they can become alkalotic for a short period.

Renal excretion of bicarbonate is impaired when chloride and potassium are depleted such as occurs from GI losses of these ions. In fact, potassium depletion alone could be associated with a metabolic alkalosis. Thus, in situations such as pyloric stenosis in which vomiting has continued for days, a profound metabolic alkalosis can be present. Correction requires administration of both chloride and potassium (see Case Illustration).

Anion Gap

Sodium is the principal cation in extracellular fluids. The sum of plasma chloride plus bicarbonate concentrations is less than the serum sodium concentration; the remaining anions required for electroneutrality are referred to as unmeasured anions or as the anion gap.

$$\text{Anion Gap} = Na^+ - (Cl^- + HCO_3^-)$$

The anion gap includes phosphates, sulfates, lactates, ketoacids, and negatively charged protein molecules, principally albumin. The normal gap is 8–16 mEq/L.

The presence of a normal anion gap implies that the GFR is sufficient to excrete sulfates and phosphates, that there is no endogenous overproduction of organic acids, and that there has not been ingestion of substances that lead to organic acid accumulation.

Metabolic Acidosis

An increased anion gap generally indicates the presence of metabolic acidosis. Any addition or subtraction of H^+ due to causes other than changes in P_{CO_2} is termed a "metabolic" effect. Metabolic acidosis (excess H^+) is easily produced experimentally by feeding NH_4Cl; the conversion of NH_4^+ to urea produces H^+ Physiologically it may occur with prolonged exercise (accumulation of lactate) or fasting (formation of ketone bodies). It commonly occurs in patients with kidney failure.

Basically, three kinds of disturbances can produce a metabolic acidosis with an increased anion gap: (1) a reduction in GFR with resulting retention of phosphate or sulfate, (2) excess production of lactic acid, β-hydroxybutyric acid and ketoacids when there is incomplete metabolism of glucose or fatty acids to CO_2 and H_2O, and (3) exogenous ingestion of substances such as salicylates, methanol, or ethylene glycol which leads to increased formation of organic acids.

In hyperchloremic metabolic acidosis, the anion gap is normal when there are excessive losses of bicarbonate (diarrhea, renal bicarbonate wasting), a failure of bicarbonate regeneration (renal tubular acidosis), or the ingestion of acidifying salts (ammonium hydrochloride).

Metabolic Alkalosis

While metabolic alkalosis may be initiated by the loss of H^+ from the body (i.e., vomiting) the maintenance of sustained metabolic alkalosis requires that the net rate of renal bicarbonate reabsorption and/or renal bicarbonate generation be greater than normal. The primary cause of metabolic alkalosis may be intrarenal, because of increased rate of renal bicarbonate generation, or net acid excretion.

A high concentration of bicarbonate in serum indicates either a primary metabolic alkalosis or a chronic respiratory acidosis (compensated). The causes of metabolic alkalosis are many, but in toto are much less common than causes of metabolic acidosis. Excessive bicarbonate loads are usually caused by medical administration of excessive citrate (transfusions in infants) or antacids. Excessive milk intake can lead to a high serum calcium, reduced glomerular filtration, and impaired renal bicarbonate excretion (milk alkali syndrome).

Metabolic alkalosis in children most frequently results from potassium and chloride losses through vomiting, and acid losses from gastric drainage.

Finally, chronic potassium wasting will result in a metabolic alkalosis. Examples include Bartter syndrome and hormonal causes such as primary aldosteronism, estrogen therapy, and hyperadrenocortical activity (Cushing syndrome).

Natural History

The symptoms of acidemia include an increase in rate and especially tidal volume of respiration (Kussmaul breathing), a depression in cardiac contractility, peripheral arterial vasodilation, and a change in pulmonary vascular compliance that predisposes to pulmonary edema. CNS functions are depressed and produce headache, lethargy, and even coma. Glucose intolerance results in hyperglycemia and polyuria.

Metabolic alkalosis produces symptoms that are similar to those of hypocalcemia, mainly paresthesias, muscle cramps, mental confusion and seizures, or even tetany. Arrhythmias may be aggravated. Tissue oxygen delivery is decreased by shift of the hemoglobin dissociation curve to the left.

Diagnosis

The determination of the state of H^+ balance is one of the more important guides to the management of a variety of clinical conditions. Any two of the variables pH, P_{CO_2}, and total CO_2 define the other in blood according to the Henderson-Hasselbalch equation:

$$pH = pK + \log \frac{[HCO_3^-]}{0.03\ P_{CO_2}}$$

where 0.03 is the solubility coefficient of CO_2 and pK is the carbonic acid dissociation constant.

The determination of blood gases (pH, P_{CO_2}, P_{O_2}) from which total CO_2 is calculated is important. A low value of total CO_2 is usually the result of a metabolic acidosis, although it may be due to a respiratory alkalosis (Fig. 10.2). The normal value for infants is 22–24 mEq/L and for older children 24–27 mEq/L.

Other data are important also. Serum electrolytes will give information that can be used in determining the anion gap. For example, a normal individual with a Na^+ = 140 mEq/L; K^+ = 4 mEq/L; Cl^- = 103 mEq/L and HCO_3^- = 27 mEq/L has a total of 144 mEq/L cations and 130 mEq/L anions; or an anion gap of 10 mEq/L, a normal value. Some examples of diagnostic problems follow.

CASE 1

Arterial pH 7.58; PCO_2 = 28 mm Hg; total CO_2 = 25.5 mEq/L.

The high pH indicates an alkalosis and the PCO_2 is remarkably low. This suggests a respiratory alkalosis. The value for total CO_2 ("bicarbonate") is slightly higher than the normal for the measured PCO_2 (Fig. 10.2) suggesting a possible slight metabolic alkalosis also. Diagnosis: hyperventilation.

CASE 2

Venous total CO_2 = 8 mEq/L; Na^+ 119 mEq/L; Cl^- = 87 mEq/L. The low total CO_2 suggests metabolic acidosis. The high anion gap (119 − 87 − 8 = 24) makes

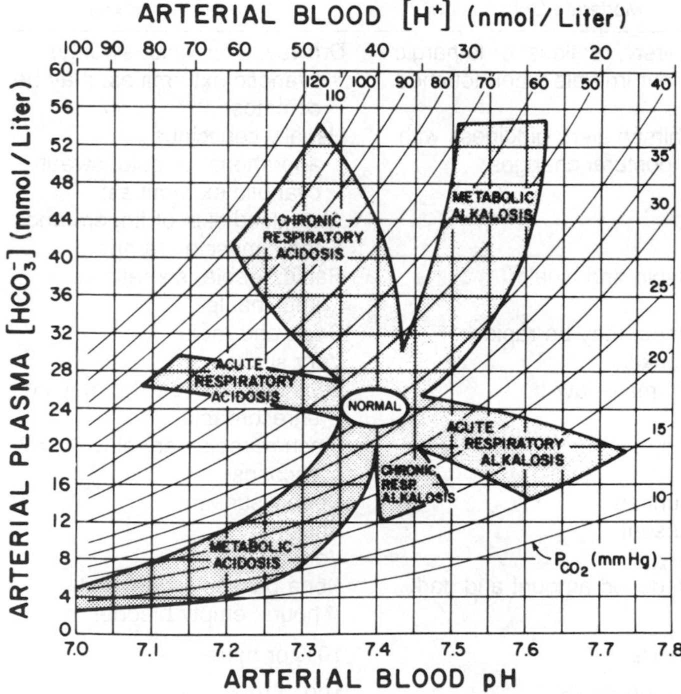

Figure 10.2. Acid-base nomogram. Shown are 95% confidence limits of the normal respiratory and metabolic compensations for primary acid-base disturbances. Reproduced with permission from Cogan MG, Rector FC: Acid base disorders. In Brenner BM, Rector FC (eds): *The Kidney,* 3rd edition. Chap 13. Philadelphia, WB Saunders, 1986.

diabetes a likely possibility. The arterial pH = 7.14; PCO_2 = 19 mm Hg; both values fall within the typical range for primary metabolic acidosis. Diagnosis: diabetes mellitus with ketoacidosis.

CASE 3

Arterial pH 7.46; PCO_2 = 56 mm Hg; total CO_2 40 mEq/L. The pH is slightly elevated, suggesting a mild alkalosis. Is it mild because the primary cause is mild or because of compensation? The high PCO_2 suggests compensated metabolic alkalosis. Diagnosis: persistent vomiting.

Treatment

FLUID THERAPY

Most acid-base disorders accompany depletion of extracellular fluid known as dehydration, and can be corrected by oral therapy. Even patients with acute dehydration can respond to appropriate oral rehydration solutions that have a 1:1 molar ratio of sodium to glucose, with added potassium, such as the World Health Organization's (WHO) prescription (20 g/L glucose, 90 mEq/L Na^+, 20 mEq/L K^+, 30 mEq/L bicarbonate with an osmolarity of 330 mOsm/L). This solution is usually well-tolerated by even infants who have been vomiting. When dehydration is mild, 50 ml/kg should be given within 4 hours, and when dehydration is more severe, 100–150 ml/kg over 6 hours is recommended, given slowly at brief intervals as tolerated. Commercially available ready-made solutions widely used in the United States contain 50 mEq/L Na^+ and substitute citrate for bicarbonate (Hirschhorn, 1980; Herzog et al, 1987).

For the few instances in which parenteral fluid therapy is required, the usual approach is to calculate requirements on the basis of estimated deficits, ongoing losses, and subsequent maintenance needs. Supplemental fluids are needed occasionally to promote diuresis in the presence of certain poisons. When the pH falls below 7.20, parenteral alkali (usually bicarbonate) should be provided.

The basic principle that underlies the calculation of fluid and electrolyte requirements is estimation of caloric expenditure. Once known, the requirement for maintenance for each 100 kcal metabolized is 125 ml H_2O, 3.2 mEq Na^+, and 2.4 mEq K^+ to replace normal losses. Since endogenous water is produced continuously, the actual replacement volume is slightly less, and hence, usual values are 115 ml H_2O, 3 mEq/L Na^+, and 2.5 mEq/L K^+ for each 100 kcal metabolized. These figures are based on careful studies of basal metabolism in infants and children of different weights.

Adjustments are required to replace ongoing losses, as in diarrhea, gastric drainage, excessive sweating, body temperature (12% increase in basal rate for each 1°C elevation) or a similar decrease for each 1°C depression in body temperature. The crudest estimate of calorie needs comes from an assessment of calories needed for activity. A patient in bed can require up to 30% fewer calories to compensate for reduced activity.

Despite the imprecision of estimates of needs, maintenance fluids can be prescribed initially by a simple relationship that, in the presence of normal renal function and no unusual losses, meets most requirements.

Body weight (kg)	Calorie expenditures per day
<10	100 kcal/kg
10–20	1000 kcal + 50 cal/kg for each kg above 10
> 20	1500 kcal/ + 20 cal/kg for each kg above 20

Water requirements are approximately 115–125 ml for each 100 kcal metabolized.

Deficit therapy will depend on knowledge of the type, underlying cause, and duration of the deficit. Acute losses are less well tolerated than are more chronic ones. The degree of dehydration can be estimated by reference to Table 10.1. In general, the second column shows the mildest stage of dehydration, which involves loss of less than 5% of body weight; the third column shows moderate dehydration, 6–9% loss of body weight, or 60–90 ml/kg deficit; the fourth column represents severe dehydration with >100 ml/kg deficit. Initial deficit therapy may require up to 20–30 ml/kg administered intravenously within an hour or less to individuals who are severely dehydrated. Isotonic saline with 5% glucose is appropriate to start therapy, but the solution then requires modification depending on the underlying condition and blood electrolyte determinations. Potassium should not be administered until it is known that the kidneys are functioning.

Although it has been traditional to omit oral feedings in diarrheal states, "to give the bowel a rest" or to reduce stimulation of the gastrocolic reflex, that dictum is being challenged, particularly in situations of chronic malnutrition. In some infants, survival is limited by their caloric deficits, and early replacement of calories with breast milk (if available) for infants, or with easily digested prepared formulas, rice water, or coconut milk is advised as soon as deficits are met or about 6–8 hours after initiation of therapy. When appetite returns, infants over 4–6 months can drink juices and eat easily digestible foods such as bananas. Fish and eggs are suitable, but coarse fruits, vegetables, and whole grain cereals should be avoided.

Table 10.1
Assessment of Dehydration and Fluid Deficit[1]

Signs and Symptoms	Mild Dehydration	Moderate Dehydration	Severe Dehydration
General appearance and condition Infants and young children	Thirsty; alert; restless	Thirsty; restless, or lethargic but irritable when touched	Drowsy; limp, cold, sweaty, cyanotic extremities; may be comatose
Older children and adults	Thirsty; alert; restless	Thirsty; alert; giddiness with postural changes	Usually conscious; apprehensive; cold; sweaty cyanotic extremities; wrinkled skin of fingers and toes; muscle cramps
Radial pulse[2]	Normal rate and volume	Rapid and weak	Rapid, feeble, sometimes impalpable
Respiration	Normal	Deep, may be rapid	Deep and rapid
Anterior fontanelle[3,4]	Normal	Sunken	Very sunken
Systolic blood pressure[5]	Normal	Normal—low	Less than 80 mm Hg; may be unrecordable
Skin elasticity[3,6]	Pinch retracts immediately	Pinch retracts slowly	Pinch retracts very slowly (>2 seconds)
Eyes[3]	Normal	Sunken	Deeply sunken
Tears	Present	Absent	Absent
Mucous membranes[7]	Moist	Dry	Very dry
Urine flow[3]	Normal	Reduced amount and dark	None passed for several hours; empty bladder
% body weight loss	4–5%	6–9%	10% or more
Estimated fluid deficit	45–50 ml/kg	60–90 ml/kg	100–110 ml/kg

[1]Reproduced with permission from WHO: A Manual for the treatment of acute diarrhoea. WHO, 1211 Geneva 27, Switzerland.
[2]If radial pulse cannot be felt, listen to heart with stethoscope.
[3]Particularly useful in infants for assessment of dehydration and monitoring of rehydration.
[4]Useful in infants until fontanelle closes at 6–18 months of age. After closure there is a slight depression in some children.
[5]Difficult to assess in infants.
[6]Not useful in marasmic malnutrition or obesity.
[7]Dryness of mouth can be palpated with a clean finger. Mouth may always be dry in a child who habitually breathes by mouth. Mouth may be wet in a dehydrated patient due to vomiting or drinking.
[8]A marasmic baby or one receiving hypotonic fluids may pass good urine volumes in the presence of dehydration.

CASE ILLUSTRATION 1

A 1-month-old, 4-kg male was brought to the emergency room by his mother, who reported a 1-week history of progressive projectile vomiting, lethargy, and decreasing urine output.

Physical examination revealed a well-developed, lethargic male, with tachycardia (160/min), normal respirations (32/min), and normal blood pressure (60/palpation). Decreased skin turgor, dry mucous membranes, and a sunken fontanelle were noted. The abdomen was scaphoid with prominent peristaltic waves that were left to right across the upper abdomen.

Laboratory examination revealed a normal hematocrit, white blood count, and differential. Urinalysis was remarkable for: specific gravity 1.035, pH 5. Serum electrolytes revealed: Na^+ = 134 mEq/L, Cl^- = 90 mEq/L, K^+ = 2.8 mEq/L. An arterial blood gas in room air was obtained: Po_2 = 80 mm Hg, Pco_2 = 45 mm Hg, pH = 7.50, HCO_3^- = 34 mEq/L, anion gap = 10 mEq/L. Urine electrolytes revealed urine Na^+ = 10 mEq/L, urine K^+ = 35 mEq/L.

An abdominal radiograph showed a distended stomach and barium swallow revealed delayed gastric emptying and a narrow pylorus.

Assessment of this child's history, physical examination, and laboratory evaluation yielded the following probable diagnoses:

1. Pyloric stenosis
2. Mild (5%) hyponatremic dehydration
3. Metabolic alkalosis
4. Hypokalemia

Prolonged vomiting due to the gastric outlet obstruction led to depletion of total body water and sodium, contraction of the extracellular fluid compartment, and a resultant mild (5%) dehydration. In addition, steady loss of gastric fluids rich in H^+ led to a secondary loss of urinary potassium and total body potassium depletion. The loss of hydrogen ion via vomiting, contraction of the extracellular fluid compartment, and intracellular potassium depletion all combined to maintain a state of metabolic alkalosis in this child.

The infant was given half-strength physiologic saline in 5% glucose at a rate of 10 ml/kg over the first hour intravenously, then 150 ml/kg/day. Potassium chloride (KCl, 40 mEq/L) was added to the solution when urine output began. After the infant appeared well hydrated, maintenance fluids were given at a rate of 100 ml/kg/day with 30 mEq of NaCl/L and 30 mEq of KCl/L. During the first day the infant received nothing by mouth, and had an oral-gastric tube in place to decompress the stomach. An elective pyloromyotomy was performed once the infant was stabilized.

CASE ILLUSTRATION 2

A 3-day-old, 3.5-kg female infant developed the insidious onset of tachypnea and vomiting. Prenatal, perinatal, and early neonatal history were unremarkable. Obstetric history revealed that the full-term product of the mother's last pregnancy died early in the neonatal period. The infant had been feeding on a casein-based formula since the first day of life.

Physical examination revealed a tachypneic, lethargic female. Respiratory rate was 68/min, pulse 170/min, blood pressure 60/palpation. Skin turgor was normal, as was mucous membrane hydration and tension of the anterior fontanelle. Breath sounds were clear to auscultation. Abdominal examination revealed mild hepatomegaly and a normal spleen.

Laboratory examination revealed: chest film = normal lungs and normal cardiothymic silhouette. Urinalysis = pH 5, 4+ ketonuria. Arterial blood gas in room air revealed Po_2 = 84 mm Hg, Pco_2 = 20 mm Hg, pH = 7.40, HCO_3^- = 12. Serum electrolyte values were Na^+ = 140 mEq/L, Cl^- 106 mEq/L, K^+ 3.5 mEq/L, anion gap = 22 mEq/L. Serum ammonia was 200 μMol/L (normal 12–55 μMol/L). Urine amino acid/organic acid analysis revealed extreme elevations of propionic acid.

Assessment of this infant's history and family history, physical examination, and laboratory examination supported the following diagnoses:

1. Propionic acidemia
2. High anion gap metabolic acidosis
3. Respiratory alkalosis

The absence of propionyl-CoA carboxylase activity in this infant had led to the accumulation of propionic acid and ketones in both serum and urine, as well as hyperammonemia. Increased protein intake and postnatal catabolism increased the rate of production of organic acids in this setting. Accumulation of organic acids and ketones induced a state of metabolic acidosis with increased anions that were unaccounted for; thus, a high anion gap was observed. Of note, despite the profound metabolic acidosis, normal serum pH was preserved, suggesting that a second primary acid-base disturbance coexisted in this infant, specifically, a primary respiratory alkalosis. The usual respiratory compensation for the metabolic acidosis had been further stimulated by the state of hyperammonemia and resultant central hyperventilation. The acid-base nomogram (Fig. 10.2) substantiated the conclusion that the observed pH, Pco_2, and HCO_3^- must have been due to two separate acid-base disorders: metabolic acidosis *plus* respiratory alkalosis.

Therapy in this child was focused upon reducing the production of acid and ammonia. Thus, feedings were withheld until the acid-base derangements were corrected. Then a low-protein diet was slowly instituted, while maintenance iv therapy was continued with 30 mEq of NaCl/L in 10% dextrose water, with 20 mEq KCl/L at 120 ml/kg/day. A decision to treat the metabolic acidosis with sodium bicarbonate should include consideration of the pH, particularly in a mixed acid-base disorder. A normal pH, such as that initially observed in this case, would not warrant parenteral $NaHCO_3$ replacement. As protein restriction is instituted, reclamation and regeneration of HCO_3^- in the kidney will gradually restore serum HCO_3^- and anion gap to normal values. Of note, however, if the primary respiratory alkalosis were to abate, a pH of 7.15–7.20 might be observed. Metabolic acidosis accompanied by acidemia below 7.20 would then warrant therapy with parenteral bicarbonate.

DISORDERS OF SODIUM BALANCE

Hyponatremia

Definition

A condition in which the concentration of serum sodium is reduced by either excessive water retention or sodium losses is defined as hyponatremia.

Natural History

Hyponatremia can be associated with dehydration if sodium losses have exceeded water losses. This occurs in some diarrheal disorders and can lead to profound shock, as water shifts from extracellular spaces into cells.

Dilutional hyponatremia follows excessive water intake, either orally or intravenously, in the absence of adequate sodium intake. Excessive sodium losses may occur in urine, especially in premature infants who are prone to hyponatremia.

Edema from any cause, including malnutrition, may be complicated by hyponatremia.

Disorders of vasopressin (antidiuretic hormone) production can result in hyponatremia (see pp. 819). Whenever the hormone is released, as a result of reduction in plasma volume, pain, anxiety, or by drug stimulation, water retention occurs, with the possibility of dilutional hyponatremia.

Chronic infection, classically tuberculous meningitis, produces chronic hyponatremia. The low spinal fluid chloride is a reflection of this state.

Hyponatremia may occur in individuals with cystic fibrosis who perspire profusely, because the relatively high electrolyte concentrations in their sweat can deplete body stores of sodium.

Treatment

Profound hyponatremia and shock require emergency expansion of blood volume with single-donor plasma, whole blood (if the patient is anemic), or 5% albumin, 20 ml/kg in 20 minutes. If the serum sodium is low, sodium should be added in amounts calculated to replace half the deficit over 45 minutes. This often requires 3% or 5% NaCl, which must be given cautiously.

To calculate the sodium deficit, assume total body water = 0.7 weight. (For a newborn, the value is closer to 0.8; for a child, it varies from 0.6–0.7 and for adults, the range is even greater.) Normal serum sodium [Na^+] = 140 mEq/L minus measured serum sodium is the deficit per liter. The deficit per liter times body weight (kg) × 0.7 is the absolute deficit. Subsequent NaCl administration should proceed more slowly, to be determined by circulatory status and serum levels. Restoration to normal values should require 12–24 hours; 0.45% NaCl with 5% glucose and potassium acetate or chloride (20 mEq/L) is an appropriate solution. If the patient is hyponatremic but not in shock, the initial hydrating solution would depend on the degree of sodium deficit. One-half the deficit could be replaced in the first hour, and the remainder over 12–24 hours. If an additional volume deficit is present, isotonic saline is appropriate (see Case Illustration 1).

CASE ILLUSTRATION 1

A 1-year-old infant was brought to the emergency room with a 3-day history of vomiting and diarrhea. Physical examination revealed a markedly dehydrated child whose vital signs included: blood pressure = 70 mm Hg by palpation, pulse = 160/min, respiration = 32/min. The infant weighed 9 kg. He was given 20 ml/kg or 200 ml 0.9% saline iv in 1 hour. By that time, the laboratory values were available and revealed: Na^+ = 120 mEq/L, K^+ = 4.1 mEq/L, Cl^- = 88 mEq/L, HCO_3^- = 18 mEq/L.

He was presumed to be about 10% dehydrated, indicating that his usual weight was 10 kg and total fluid loss was 1 L. His usual total body water was 10 × 0.6 = 6 L. Therefore, his current (dehydrated) total body water was 6 L − 1 L = 5 L. The sodium deficit in his dehydrated state was 5 L (140 mEq/L − 120 mEq/L) = 5 L × (20 mEq/L) = 100 mEq. In addition, he had a deficit of 1 L which should be isotonic, thus, indicating a further Na^+ deficit of 1 L × 140 mEq/L or 140 mEq. Overall, his Na^+ deficit was 100 mEq + 140 mEq = 240 mEq and his fluid deficit was 1 L.

CASE ILLUSTRATION 2

A 1-year-old infant was brought to the emergency room with a 3-day history of diarrhea and fever. His only intake had been boiled skim milk. Physical examination revealed a moderately dehydrated infant whose vital signs included: pulse = 120/min, respiration = 28/min, blood pressure = 100 mm Hg (by palpation). He weighed 9 kg. He was given 200 ml 0.9% NaCl iv during the first hour. At that time, the laboratory values were available and revealed: Na^+ = 170 mEq/L, K^+ = 4.3 mEq/L, Cl^- = 126.

He appeared 10% dehydrated, indicating that his usual weight was 10 kg and fluid loss was 1 L. His normal total body water was 0.6 × 10 = 6 L. Thus his current (dehydrated) total body water was 6 L − 1 L = 5 L. His current total body sodium was 5 L × 170 mEq/L = 850 mEq and his usual (ideal) total body sodium was 6 L × 140 = 840 mEq. Thus, he had no Na^+ deficit, but had a 1-L fluid deficit.

His iv fluid was changed to 5% dextrose water in one-quarter physiologic saline with 20 mEq KCl/L at 60 ml/hour, in order to replace the water deficit over 36–48 hours. Serum sodium was checked every 4 hours.

QUESTION AND COMMENT

What is the purpose of adding glucose to the solution when the patient is hyperosmolar?

Rapid decrease in NaCl concentration may promote a shift of water into the brain. The relatively slow metabolism of glucose will reduce the rate of rehydration of brain cells and lessen the risk of cerebral edema. The added potassium serves the same purpose.

Hypernatremia

Definition

Excessive intake of sodium with respect to water, or abnormal water losses will lead to hypernatremia (an elevation in serum sodium above the normal range).

Natural History

Some diarrheal states are characterized by excessive losses of water in the stool. The situation is aggravated by a history of vomiting and reduced water intake. Other causes of hypernatremia include hyperthermia or excessive sweating. Individuals with nephrogenic diabetes insipidus are prone to hypernatremia.

Excessive salt intake can occur from inappropriate intravenous therapy, or salt poisoning from feeding of hyperosmolar solutions.

Treatment

If serum sodium levels are over 180 mEq/L, the danger of cerebral edema and hemorrhages with seizures is sufficient to justify peritoneal dialysis. Simultaneously, an iv maintenance solution of 2–5% glucose, 25 mEq/L Na^+, and 40 mEq/L K^+ at a rate of about 150 ml/kg/24 hours is appropriate for infants once urine output is established. One ampule of 10% calcium gluconate should be added to every 500 ml of solution (Finberg et al, 1982).

Less severe hypernatremia is treated with a solution containing sodium and glucose. Glucose and water alone are not used so as to avoid water intoxication. A solution of 20–40 mEq/L of NaCl is advised to avoid sudden decreases in serum sodium and potential cerebral edema. The intravenous solution should also contain 2–5% glucose and potassium acetate or chloride, 30–40 mEq/L with 20 ml of a 10% solution of calcium gluconate per liter.

The amounts given depend on the degree of dehydration and sodium excess as illustrated under hyponatremia. Slow correction over 24–48 hours is appropriate when the patient is not in shock and shows gradual improvement. Most of the misadventures in correction of hypernatremia result from haste in restoring laboratory values to normal. An improving patient is sending a message.

REFERENCES

Cogan MG, Rector FC: Acid base disorders. In Brenner BM, Rector FC (eds): *The Kidney,* 3rd edition. Philadelphia, WB Saunders, 1986.

Finberg L, Kravath RE, Fleischman AR: *Water and Electrolytes in Pediatrics.* Philadelphia, WB Saunders, 1982.

Herzog LW, Bitnoney WG, Grand RJ: High sodium rehydration solutions in well-nourished outpatients. *Acta Paediatr Scand* 76:306, 1987.

Hirschhorn N: The treatment of acute diarrhea in children: An historical and physiological perspective. *Am J Clin Nutr* 33:637, 1980.

Pizarro D, Posada G, Mata L: Treatment of 242 neonates with dehydrating diarrhea with an oral glucose-electrolyte solution. *J Pediatr* 102:153, 1983.

Hypertension 2

Definition

Hypertension in childhood is usually defined as blood pressure levels above the 95th percentile for size and age. Thus, in neonates, the smaller the infant, the lower the blood pressure. Mean pressures for 1- to 2-kg infants are 35–40 mm Hg, for infants 2–3 kg 40–50 mm Hg, and infants weighing over 3 kg 50–55 mm Hg. Values 10–15 mm Hg higher than these mean values, if sustained, would be considered hypertension and should stimulate an investigation.

For children of various ages, upper limits of normal blood pressure are shown in Table 10.2 and Figure 10.3*A*-*D* (panel).

Basic Science

CONTROL OF BLOOD PRESSURE

The renin-angiotensin-aldosterone system (RAS) has the major role in regulation of arterial blood pressure. Changes in dietary sodium and potassium intake result in changes in aldosterone and angiotension II levels. Changes in intrarenal physical factors also affect sodium and potassium excretion and modulate the release of renal renin. Further regulation of the RAS comes from the atrial natriuretic peptide, vasopressin, and catecholamines. Atrial natriuretic peptide released from the atria under multiple stimuli related to in-

Table 10.2
Classification of Hypertension by Age Group[1]

Age Group	Significant Hypertension (mm Hg)	Severe Hypertension (mm Hg)
New born		
7 days	Systolic BP ≥96	Systolic BP ≥106
8–30 days	Systolic BP ≥104	Systolic BP ≥110
Infant (<2 yr)	Systolic BP ≥112	Systolic BP ≥118
	Diastolic BP ≥74	Diastolic BP ≥82
Children (3–5 yr)	Systolic BP ≥116	Systolic BP ≥124
	Diastolic BP ≥76	Diastolic BP ≥84
Children (6–9 yr)	Systolic BP ≥122	Systolic BP ≥130
	Diastolic BP ≥78	Diastolic BP ≥86
Children (10–12 yr)	Systolic BP ≥126	Systolic BP ≥134
	Diastolic BP ≥82	Diastolic BP ≥90
Adolescents (13–15 yr)	Systolic BP ≥136	Systolic BP ≥144
	Diastolic BP ≥86	Diastolic BP ≥92
Adolescents (16–18 yr)	Systolic BP ≥142	Systolic BP ≥150
	Diastolic BP ≥92	Diastolic BP ≥98

[1]Reproduced with permission from Report of The Second Task Force on Blood Pressure Control in Children—1987. *Pediatrics* 79:1, 1987.

creased vascular volume, promotes diuresis and lowering of blood pressure, and appears to inhibit renin release (Laragh, 1985).

Epidemiology

The spectrum of hypertension in childhood varies with age. Between 1 and 2.5% of infants in intensive care nurseries will be hypertensive. Less than 2% of hospitalized infants are hypertensive. By adolescence the numbers are higher, especially among blacks, but true incidence is not known.

Natural History

Renal vascular disease and coarctation are the most common causes of hypertension in infants in the first year of life. Renovascular disease in young infants may be associated with emboli from clots at the site of indwelling umbilical artery catheters. Other vascular causes of increased blood pressure are congenital renal artery stenosis, coarctation of the aorta, and renal vein thrombosis. In young children, renal abnormalities such as polycystic kidney disease, hydronephrosis, neuropathies, or hemolytic uremic syndrome account for 80% of secondary hypertension, with renovascular causes accounting for 10%. Occasionally, hypertension is associated with increased intracranial pressure, neuroblastoma, primary aldosteronism, or adrenal hyperplasia.

Most older children with high blood pressure do not have a structural or recognized hormonal explanation for it. Lauer et al (1985), in an extensive study of Iowa school children, showed a relationship between height, weight, age, and blood pressure. High blood pressure for age is associated with precocious height and/or excessive body weight. True high blood pressure for a given height, on the other hand, is more common in short children. Lauer et al (1985) suggest that a factor exists that relates to blood pressure independent of height and weight but is related to age.

Diagnosis

Hypertension in infants is recognized more readily when monitors are attached to umbilical artery catheters. Measurement in infants not requiring such monitoring is best done with a 4 × 9 cm cuff around the upper arm, which is used with an oscillometric device or to a Doppler transducer (Colan et al, 1983). In older children, appropriately sized blood pressure cuffs are available. They should occupy about two-thirds of the distance from elbow to shoulder and the inner bladder should extend more than halfway around the arm.

The question of who should be evaluated for the possible causes of hypertension (in the absence of symptoms) depends on reasons for ascertainment of blood pressure and knowledge of the individual's height and weight. If hypertension is found on routine screening, The Second Task Force on Blood Pressure Control in Children recommends that any patients with blood pressures over the 95th percentile for age be evaluated regardless of body size (Tables 10.3 and 10.4).

The signs and symptoms of hypertension are usually inapparent until such problems as congestive failure develop. The symptoms include irritability, tachypnea, vomiting, diarrhea, and even seizures. Signs are cardiac enlargement, hepatomegaly, and hypertonicity.

The appropriate evaluation of a child with hypertension depends both on age and severity of blood pressure elevation. If primary hypertension is suspected on the basis of negative physical findings, age, and family history, a urinalysis and urine culture, creatinine electrolytes, and CO_2, as well as consideration of evaluation of cardiac function by echocardiogram, are all that is warranted at first. If secondary hypertension is suspected, evaluation ought to rule out renal and renovascular disease by screening anatomic studies such as ultrasound and radionuclide scans and, in some cases, arteriography. If endocrine hypertension is suspected, the evaluation may include studies of catecholamine metabolism, steroid metabolism, or thyroid function.

Treatment

Surgical treatment of anatomical problems with sustained hypertension is indicated as soon as they are identified, if technically possible. In other cases, medical management is required. For mild hypertension, medications are usually not indicated. Weight control and moderate reduction in dietary sodium to a no-added salt diet, together with a program of dynamic exercise may be helpful. When hypertension is marked or when mild blood pressure increase does not respond to nonpharmacologic measures, medication is indicated to prevent left ventricular hypertrophy and damage to kidney and brain. Multiple agents are available and include diuretics, adrenergic inhibitors, and vasodila-

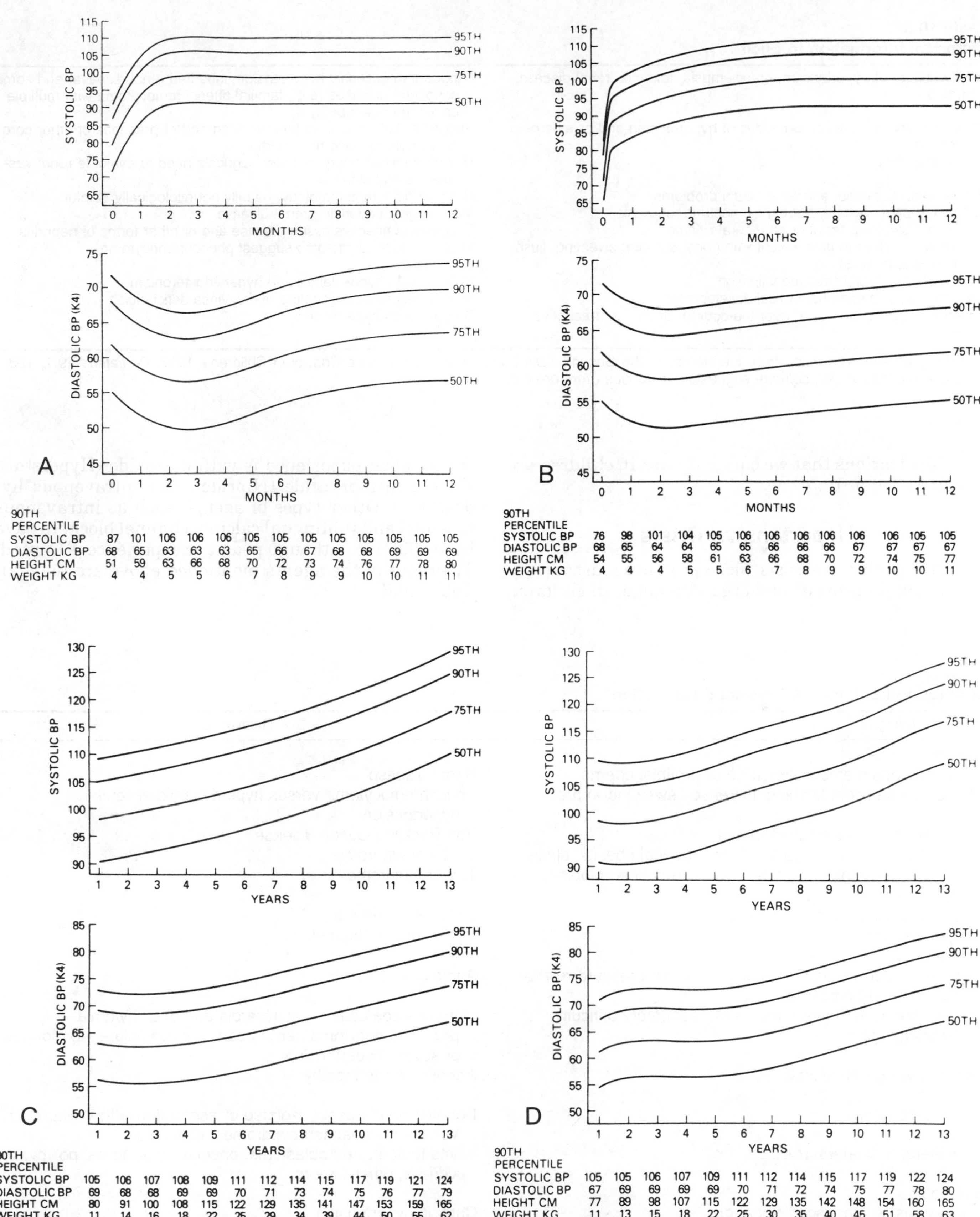

A

90TH PERCENTILE													
SYSTOLIC BP	87	101	106	106	106	105	105	105	105	105	105	105	105
DIASTOLIC BP	68	65	63	63	63	65	66	67	68	68	69	69	69
HEIGHT CM	51	59	63	66	68	70	72	73	74	76	77	78	80
WEIGHT KG	4	4	5	5	6	7	8	9	9	10	10	11	11

B

90TH PERCENTILE													
SYSTOLIC BP	76	98	101	104	105	106	106	106	106	106	106	105	105
DIASTOLIC BP	68	65	64	64	65	65	66	66	66	67	67	67	67
HEIGHT CM	54	55	56	58	61	63	66	68	70	72	74	75	77
WEIGHT KG	4	4	4	5	5	6	7	8	9	9	10	10	11

C

90TH PERCENTILE													
SYSTOLIC BP	105	106	107	108	109	111	112	114	115	117	119	121	124
DIASTOLIC BP	69	68	68	69	69	70	71	73	74	75	76	77	79
HEIGHT CM	80	91	100	108	115	122	129	135	141	147	153	159	165
WEIGHT KG	11	14	16	18	22	25	29	34	39	44	50	55	62

D

90TH PERCENTILE													
SYSTOLIC BP	105	105	106	107	109	111	112	114	115	117	119	122	124
DIASTOLIC BP	67	69	69	69	69	70	71	72	74	75	77	78	80
HEIGHT CM	77	89	98	107	115	122	129	135	142	148	154	160	165
WEIGHT KG	11	13	15	18	22	25	30	35	40	45	51	58	63

Figure 10.3. Age-specific percentiles of blood pressure measurements. Reproduced with permission from Report of The Second Task Force on Blood Pressure Control in Children—1987. *Pediatrics* 79:1, 1987.

Table 10.3
Historical Information to Elicit[1]

Historical information	Possibilities
Family history of hypertension, preeclampsia, toxemia, renal disease, tumors	Important in essential hypertension, inherited renal disease, and some endocrine diseases (e.g., familial pheochromocytoma with multiple endocrine adenopathy II)
Family history of early complications of hypertension and/or atherosclerosis	Suggests likely course of hypertension and/or presence of other coronary artery disease risk factors
Neonatal history	Use of umbilical artery catheter suggests need to evaluate renal vasculature and kidneys
Headaches, dizziness, epistaxis, visual problems	Nonspecific symptomatology, usually not etiologically helpful
Abdominal pain, dysuria, frequency, nocturia, enuresis	May suggest underlying renal disease
Joint pains/swelling, facial or peripheral edema	Suggests connective tissue disease and/or other forms of nephritis
Weight loss, failure to gain weight with good appetite, sweating, flushing, fevers, palpitations	In combination, symptoms suggest pheochromocytoma
Muscle cramps, weakness, constipation	May suggest hypokalemia and hyperaldosteronism
Age of onset of menarche, sexual development	May be helpful in suggesting hydroxylase deficiencies
Ingestion of prescription and over-the-counter drugs, contraceptives, illicit drugs	Drug-induced hypertension

[1]Reproduced with permission from the Report of the Second Task Force on Blood Pressure Control in Children—1987. *Pediatrics* 79:1, 1987. Historical information (*left column*) suggests possibilities (*right column*).

tors. Medications that we currently use in children are shown in Table 10.5.

Hypertensive Crisis

In hypertensive crisis, blood pressure must rapidly be lowered to prevent end-organ damage. In children, the greatest experience is with diazoxide (Hyperstat), sodium nitroprusside (Nipride), and intravenous hydralazine. Other types of agents, such as intravenous labetolol and sublingual calcium channel blockers have been effective, although pediatric experience is limited. The doses of the agents mentioned above are listed in Table 10.6.

Table 10.4
Findings to Look for on Physical Examination[1]

Physical Findings	Relevance
General	
Pale mucous membranes, facial or pretibial edema	Renal disease
Pallor, evanescent flushing, increased sweating at rest	Pheochromocytoma versus hyperdynamic essential hypertension
Café-au-lait spots, neurofibromas	Von Recklinghausen disease
Moon face, hirsutism, buffalo hump, truncal obesity, striae	Cushing syndrome
Webbing of the neck, low hairline, wide-spaced nipples, wide carrying angle	Turner syndrome
Elfin facies, poor growth, retardation	Williams syndrome
Thyroid enlargement	Hyper- or hypothyroidism
Cardiovascular	
Absent or delayed femoral pulses, low leg pressure relative to arm blood pressure	Aortic coarctation
Heart size, rate, rhythm, murmurs, respiratory difficulty, hepatomegaly	Murmur—coarctation; tachycardia and/or arrhythmia—pheochromocytoma; large heart or heart failure—prolonged or severe hypertension
Bruits over great vessels	Arteritis or arteriopathy
Abdomen	
Epigastric bruit	Renovascular disease isolated or associated with Williams or Von Recklinghausen syndromes, or arteritis
Unilateral or bilateral masses	Wilms tumour, neuroblastoma, pheochromocytoma, polycystic kidneys, other tumors
Neurologic	
Hypertensive funduscopic changes	Chronic hypertension
Bell palsy	Chronic hypertension
Neurologic deficits (e.g., hemiparesis)	Chronic or severe acute hypertension with stroke

[1]Reproduced with permission from The Second Task Force on Blood Pressure Control in Children—1987. *Pediatrics* 79:1, 1987.

Table 10.5
Antihypertensive Medications[1,2]

	Dose	No. of Times/Day	Route
Diuretics			
Hydrochlorothiazide (Hydrodiuril, Esidrix)	1–2 mg/kg	2	Oral
Chlorthalidone (Hygroton)	0.5–2 mg/kg	1	Oral
Furosemide (Lasix)	0.5–2 mg/kg	2	Oral, IV
Spironolactone (Aldactone)	1–2 mg/kg	2	Oral
Triameterene (Dyrenium)	1–2 mg/kg	2	Oral
Adrenergic inhibitors			
β-adrenergic antagonists			
Metoprolol (Lopressor)	1–4 mg/kg	2	Oral
Atenolol (Tenormin)	1–2 mg/kg	1	Oral
Propranolol (Inderal)	1–3 mg/kg	3	Oral
Central adrenergic inhibitors			
Methyldopa (Aldomet)	5–10 mg/kg	2	Oral, IV
Clonidine (Catapres)	0.05–0.40 mg	2	Oral
Guanabenz (Wytensin)	0.03–0.08 mg/kg	2	Oral
α_1-Adrenergic antagonist			
Prazosin hydrochloride (Minipress)	0.5–7 mg	3	Oral
Vasodilators			
Hydralazine (Apresoline)	1–5 mg/kg	2 or 3	Oral, IM, IV (drip)
Minoxidil (Loniten)	0.1–1.0 mg/kg	2	Oral
Diazoxide (Hyperstat)[3]	3–5 mg/kg/dose		IV (bolus)
Nitroprusside (Nipride)[3]	1–8 μg/kg/min		IV (drip)
Angiotensin-converting enzyme inhibitor			
Captopril			
<6 months of age	0.05–0.5 mg/kg	3	
>6 months of age	0.5–2.0 mg/kg	3	Oral

[1]Reproduced with permission from Report of The Second Task Force in Blood Pressure Control in Children—1987. *Pediatrics* 79:1, 1987.
[2]Not to exceed usual adult dosage with all drugs.
[3]Primary use is in hypertensive emergencies.

Table 10.6
Drugs Most Effective in Hypertensive Crisis

Drug	Dose	Route	Comment
Diazoxide	3–5 mg/kg	IV bolus	Patient may become profoundly hypotensive
Sodium nitroprusside	0.5 to 8 ug/kg/min	IV drip	Titrated easily, agent is light sensitive, toxic by-product
Hydralazine	0.15–1 mg/kg for parental dose	IV or IM	Slower effect, may be used with other agents
Nifedipine	? in child	Sublingual	Smooth decrease in blood pressure
Labetalol	? in child	IV	α- and β-adrenergic inhibitor

CASE ILLUSTRATION 1

A 4-year-old black female was seen in clinic for her annual check-up. Blood pressure was 120/85 mm Hg. Family history was positive for maternal hypertension, which was controlled with medication. No abnormalities were found on urinalysis, intravenous pyelography, or blood chemistries. A 24-hour urine for vanillylmandelic acid (VMA) showed normal levels. A renal scan was normal. Physical examination was also within normal limits. A repeat blood pressure, resting quietly, was 115/70 mm Hg in the arms, and 125/80 mm Hg in both legs.

She was started on a low-salt diet and diuretics. Within a few weeks her blood pressure was 105/65 mm Hg, which is within the normal range for her age. The child followed monthly at the clinic for presumed essential hypertension.

QUESTIONS AND COMMENTS

Can children have essential hypertension?

Yes. Even 2-year-old infants in families of hypertensives have been found to have higher than expected blood pressures (Zimmer and Kass, 1971).

What is the cause of essential hypertension?

Abnormalities in the renal handling of sodium loads and, perhaps, abnormal angiotensin II may be involved. Essential hypertension is probably due to a variety of problems and is properly considered a syndrome. Occasional individuals who develop end-stage renal disease from untreated essential hypertension, and who have renal transplants, experience reversal of the hypertension, and even reversal of vascular damage to retinal and heart vessels.

CASE ILLUSTRATION 2

A 14-year-old white male, known to have tuberous sclerosis complicated by seizures, subaortic stenosis, and mild hypertension, had the sudden onset of right flank pain, with fevers up to 38.5°C. The pain had been intermittent for about a week, with an occasional sharp, piercing quality that lasted minutes to hours. Although the youngster was active in skiing and ice hockey, he recalled no unusual trauma to the flank. Because of persistence of the symptoms and some increase in lethargy, he was admitted to the hospital for evaluation.

On review of his past history, it was clear that his seizures were well-controlled by dilantin and that he had a successful resection of his membranous subaortic stenosis in 1979. His tuberous sclerosis had been diagnosed at the age of 12 months on the basis of multiple "ash leaf" lesions on the back and extremities. His past hypertension was well-controlled by atenolol and his adenoma subaceum had been treated successfully with laser therapy in 1983.

A physical examination showed a 14-year-old of normal height and weight with a blood pressure of 130/80 mm Hg. The most remarkable finding was a tender mass about 4 × 6 cm in the right lower quadrant. He also had significant right costovetebral angle tenderness. A urine analysis had a specific gravity of 1.014 and no cells, bacteria, or casts. Repeat urine cultures and blood culture were negative for bacteria. The white count was 14,600/mm^3, 73% polys, 22% lymphs, 2% monos, 2% eos, 1% atypical lymph, sodium was 141/mEq/L, chloride 97 mEq/L, potassium 4.4 mEq/L, CO_2 27 mEq/L, BUN 7 mg/dl, calcium 0.5 mg/dl, blood sugar 91, hematocrit was 36%, sedimentation rate 52 mm/hour, test for infectious mononucleosis was negative.

Renal ultrasonography revealed that both kidneys were enlarged and the left kidney had multiple punctate lesions. The right kidney had a large aneurysm in which the blood could be seen to be moving in a counterclockwise manner. Angiography confirmed the vascular nature of the mass within the kidney.

QUESTIONS AND COMMENTS

What was the likely diagnosis in this situation?

Angiomyolipomas in the kidney are characteristic of tuberous sclerosis and probably existed in both kidneys in this youngster. Nearly 80% of individuals with tuberous sclerosis at some time or other develop renal tumors or vascular lesions.

The major question concerns the treatment of the aneurysm which was probably compressing normal kidney on the right and presumably caused the symptoms. At the time of angiography, a coil was placed in the aneurysm which promoted thrombosis.

What is the prognosis for this youngster?

Fortunately, the thrombosis in the dilated aneurysm did not further compromise renal function. In fact, the kidney returned to near-normal size and the blood pressure and fever likewise normalized over the subsequent weeks. The ultimate prognosis is unknown.

Should this child be restricted in any way in the future?

Frequent follow-up is in order and prompt attention to any symptoms that could be referable to the kidneys is appropriate. On the other hand, this active youngster was encouraged to continue his full sports activity on the assumption that he no longer had an aneurysm nor hypertension and was not at special risk of injury.

REFERENCES

Colan SD, Fujii A, Borow KM, et al: Noninvasive determination of systolic, diastolic and end-systolic blood pressure in neonates, infants and young children: Comparison with antral aortic pressure measurements. *Am J Cardiol* 52:867, 1983.

Ingelfinger JR: *Pediatric Hypertension.* Philadelphia, WB Saunders, 1982.

Laragh JH: Atrial natriuretic hormone, the renin-aldosterone axis, and blood pressure-electrolyte homeostatis. *N Engl J Med* 313:1330, 1985.

Lauer RM, Burns TL, Clarke WR: Assessing children's blood pressure—considerations of age and body size: The Muscatine study. *Pediatrics* 75:1081, 1985.

Task Force on Blood Pressure Control in Children: Report of the Second Task Force on Blood Pressure Control in Children—1987. *Pediatrics* 79:1, 1987.

Zimmer SH, Kass E: Familial aggregation of blood pressure in childhood. *N Engl J Med* 254:401, 1971.

Genitourinary Tract 3

URINARY TRACT INFECTIONS

Definition

Infection may involve any portion of the urinary tract from urethra to renal cortex. In general, infections of the urethra and bladder are considered to be in the lower urinary tract, and infection in the kidney is in the upper tract. Most urinary tract infections are bacterial. The diagnosis is made by documenting bacteriuria, which is considered significant when 100,000 organisms/mm^3 of a single organism are present in one or more clean-voided specimens of urine. Any growth from a urine specimen obtained by bladder puncture is diagnostic. Overt urinary tract infections are those in which medical advice is sought because the child has symptoms. Covert bacteriuria is identified on routine urinalysis or screening programs.

Acute pyelonephritis is characterized by chills, fever, flank pain, and tenderness. Chronic atrophic pyelonephritis is almost always due to recurrent episodes of ascending infection with involvement of the renal parenchyma. Infections restricted to the bladder are termed cystitis, and to the urethra, urethritis.

Basic Science

The route by which organisms reach the urinary tract is hematogenous in less than 3% of individuals of all ages; ascending infection occurs in 97%. The major organisms capable of hematogenous spread are *Staphylococcus aureus, Salmonella* species, *Pseudomonas aeruginosa,* and *Candida* species. Organisms responsible for ascending infection are most commonly *Escherichia coli* (about 90%), *Proteus mirabilis,* and other *Enterobacteriaceae*. The exceptions are uncircumcised male infants who most commonly are infected with staphylococcal species. *Chlamydia trachomatis, Ureaplasma urealyticum,* and *Mycoplasma hominis* may be more common than was appreciated formerly because of difficulties in identification.

It is apparent that most urinary tract infections are caused by relatively few O-serotypes of *E. coli* that are normally resident in the bowel. Surface properties of these strains differ and probably account for their invasiveness. Surface pili interact specifically with uroepithelial cell receptors and explain the adherence of the bacteria with cell surfaces.

Adenovirus types 11 and 21 have been associated with cases of hemorrhagic cystitis in school children. Immunocompromised children have developed renal failure in the presence of Bk polyomavirus in the renal parenchyma and urine. With improved diagnostic techniques, a larger role for viruses in the pathogenesis of urinary tract infections will doubtless emerge.

The normal bladder can usually clear itself of organisms within 2–3 days of their introduction presumably by voiding, by bacteriostatic action of urine, or by intrinsic mucosal defense mechanisms. Factors that promote the establishment of infection include the accumulation of residual urine, foreign bodies or stones, and pre-existing inflammation.

VESICOURETERAL REFLUX

Reflux of urine from bladder to ureters and kidneys is usually present if bacteria reach the kidneys by the ascending route. The vesicoureteral junction is normally competent at all ages. Reflux is prevented by the angulation of the ureter as it enters the bladder where it runs an intramural submucosal course which is compressed during micturition. Primary (congenital) reflux most often occurs when the intramural segment is too short, either because of an embryonic displacement of the ureteric bud, or developmental delay in lengthening.

Secondary reflux results from deformation of the ureterovesical junction (UVJ) by a paraureteral diverticulum, surgery, trauma, or, in the event of a neuropathic bladder. Both types of reflux are accentuated by inhibition of ureteral peristalsis from bacterial endotoxin or oliguria. Obstruction at the junction can affect the rate of urine flow and the extent of reflux.

Vesicoureteral reflux is the most common diagnosis in children presenting with urinary tract infections. Thirty to 50% of them will show reflux on a voiding cystourethrogram.

Reflux has been reported in two consecutive generations; however, the mode of inheritance appears to be multifactorial. Of asymptomatic siblings, 45% were found to reflux when evaluated by radionuclide cystography (Van den Abbeele et al, 1987).

The severity of reflux may be graded as follows:

Grade I:	Reflux partly up the ureter
Grade II:	Reflux up to pelvis and calyces without dilation
Grade III:	Same as II with dilation
Grade IV:	Tortuosity of ureters
Grade V:	Gross dilation of pelvis and calyces.

Epidemiology

The prevalence of asymptomatic urinary tract infections on school entry is between 1 and 2% in girls and less than 0.05% in males. About one-third of the children with asymptomatic bacteriuria will have some degree of ureterovesical reflux.

In a study of 100 infants ages 5 days to 8 months with significant bacteriuria, a male preponderance was evident in the first 3 months of life (75% males), but at 3–8 months, only 11% were males. Ninety-five percent of affected males were uncircumcised (Ginsburg and McCracken, 1982). Sepsis was documented in 20 of 91 infants whose blood was cultured.

Natural History

In infancy, bacteriuria may be the first indication of congenital obstruction or reflux. Uncircumsized males with urinary infection have a similar increase in congenital urinary tract anomalies (Lincoln and Winberg, 1964; Abbott, 1972). After infancy, asymptomatic bacteriuria is found in about 1.2% of girls and rarely in boys. Bacteriuria may recur in nearly 80% of school girls after a first attack, and 20% of them have vesicoureteral reflux (Kunin, 1970).

The clinical presentation of acute pyelonephritis is characterized in older children by chills, high fever, flank or abdominal pain, and tenderness. Likewise, older children with cystitis have the classical symptoms of frequency, burning with voiding, and suprapubic discomfort. Infants and young children usually have nonspecific symptoms of fever, failure to gain weight, abdominal pain and vomiting, and diarrhea. Frequency and dysuria are uncommon.

Diagnosis

Evaluation of a history of previous urinary tract disease or predisposing conditions such as diabetes, renal stones, recent instrumentation, chronic constipation, child abuse, sexual activity, and neurologic disorders is a first and essential step to diagnosis.

Examination of urine should include a Gram stain of a dried drop of uncentrifuged urine. If positive for bacteria, there is an 80–90% chance of significant numbers of bacteria (over 100,000 colonies/ml) on quantitative culture. Commercially available dipstick or dipslide methods are useful for office screening. Pyuria may or may not be present. If squamous epithelial cells are present, contamination is likely and repeat testing is necessary.

METHODS OF COLLECTION OF URINE

In infants, suprapubic aspiration of a full bladder is the best approach to documentation of infection. In older children, thorough washing and rinsing of external genitalia, followed by attachment of a bag may be adequate and is particularly valuable if negative. Midstream specimens can be collected in children who are toilet-trained.

Any infant or child with documented bacteriuria deserves radiologic investigation. A voiding cystogram is indispensible since it can verify or rule out reflux, which is the most common finding. If negative, ultrasonography can follow to document normal kidneys or to identify a dilated urinary tract. Intravenous urography should follow a voiding cystourethrogram, if this study shows significant reflux.

Treatment

Treatment of pyelonephritis in infancy or severely ill patients is usually initiated with intravenous broad spectrum antibiotic parenteral therapy until afebrile, followed by a 1- to 3-month course of oral therapy in low dosage. For most children, oral therapy for uncomplicated urinary tract infection (absence of anatomic abnormalities) is usually with sulfasoxazole (120–150 mg/kg four times a day, or amoxicillin 25–50 mg/kg 3–4 times a day for 14 days). Repeat culture is necessary before treatment is stopped.

Prevention

For recurrent infections and especially in children with mild to moderate reflux, long-term prophylaxis (for at least a year) with trimethoprim sulfamethoxazole given once a day has been found to lessen the likelihood of recurrences and renal injury (Smellie et al, 1976). Prophylaxis must be continued until reflux has subsided. Training the child to empty the bladder completely and frequently and ensure adequate fluid intake and regular bowel habits is important in reducing recurrent infections.

SURGERY AND CONTROVERSY

The history of surgical therapy for reflux reimplantation of ureters into the bladder, has swung like a pendulum from enthusiasm to wariness to moderation. All of this has occurred while the surgical results have progressively improved, so that reflux can be cured in over 90% of children. The initial wave of enthusiasm was questioned by Smellie and others who demonstrated spontaneous cessation of reflux in well over half the children followed without surgery. In addition, in those children who were prevented from any further episodes of infection by prophylactic doses of antibiotics, normal renal growth without parenchymal scars was seen. The sequelae of chronic pyelonephritis (or reflux nephropathy as it is often called) are significant. Once established, hypertension and renal failure may present years later. Since prevention is the key, if a nonoperative approach is adopted, a surveillance program must be carefully followed. The indications generally accepted for surgical correction are as follows:

1. High grade of reflux with upper tract dilatation.
2. Persistent or progressive hydronephrosis and/or renal scarring.
3. Persistent reflux after full growth maturation.
4. Recurrent urinary tract infection despite antibiotic prophylaxis and effective bladder emptying.

Because of the high incidence of this anomaly, surgical and medical treatment plans will continue to be weighed against each other. If medical management is under-

CASE ILLUSTRATION 1

A 3-month-old white female presented with a 6-hour history of fever and irritability. The mother's pregnancy and delivery were uncomplicated, as was the infant's neonatal course. At home she was nursing well and had been entirely normal until the day before admission when she was slow to feed. On the evening of admission she was very irritable and frequent diaper changes were required. Her temperature was 39.5°C.

The family history was negative for known renal abnormalities. On physical examination she was irritable but alert, well-developed, and had a blood pressure of 112 mm Hg systolic, pulse was 164/min, respiratory rate was 50/min. The physical examination was entirely normal and the kidneys were not palpable. External genitalia were unremarkable.

Laboratory studies revealed a hematocrit of 36%, white count 7700/mm^3, 47% neutrophils, 38% lymphs, 11% basophils, 3% monocytes, 1% atypical lymph, sodium 134 mEq/L, potassium 5.1 mEq/L, chloride 101 mEq/L, BUN 8 mg/dl, calcium 10.2 mg/dl, creatinine 0.2 mg/dl, urine analysis 3–5 white blood cells per high powered field, 3+ bacteria, Gram stain of unspun specimen showed Gram-negative rods, specific gravity 1.010, pH 5.9, 1+ protein.

The infant presumably had a Gram-negative urinary tract infection and intravenous ampicillin and gentamicin were instituted. Cultures of the blood and spinal fluid were negative, but those of urine grew *E. coli* sensitive to gentamicin. She was, therefore, continued on that drug alone, with blood levels monitored and maintained within a therapeutic range. Repeat urine collected by suprapubic tap after 36 hours on antibiotics was sterile. She was continued for a 5-day course of intravenous gentamicin and discharged on a 7-day course of oral trimethroprim-sulfasoxazole at home.

QUESTION AND COMMENT

Should this child's urinary tract be studied?

Our answer was an unequivocal "yes" since this must have been a retrograde infection and there was a 25% chance of an anatomical abnormality (especially reflux) being the reason for the infection. One month after the infection cleared, she had a normal voiding cystourethrogram and normal ultrasonographic examination of the kidneys. Therefore, she was not given prophylactic antibiotic therapy. She has had no recurrences in the subsequent year. The cause of this initial infection is thus unknown.

CASE ILLUSTRATION 2

A 3-year-old white male was well until he presented with pain on voiding, frequency, and fever. Urine analysis showed a specific gravity of 1.017, 2% protein, 12–15 red cells, numerous white blood cells, and no casts per high powered field. A Gram stain of the urine showed Gram-negative rods and culture grew more than 100,000 colonies of *E. coli.* He was treated as an outpatient for 10 days with trimethroprim-sulfasoxazole and recovered. However, 2 months later there was a recurrence with a culture again positive for *E. coli.* Creatinine was 0.4 mg/dl, BUN 15 mg/dl. At this point, an investigation was undertaken and revealed that he had grade 2 vesicoureteral reflux on the right side. An intravenous pyleogram was normal. Nitrofurantoin at bedtime daily was prescribed for prophylaxis against infection and subsequent urine cultures were negative.

QUESTION AND COMMENT

Should this patient have been investigated with his first urinary tract infection?

We think that an investigation with a voiding cystourethrogram should have been undertaken at the time of the first infection since reflux represents the greatest potential risk to the kidney in the presence of urinary infection. An intravenous pyleogram or ultrasound and cystourethrogram could have been done 2–4 weeks after treatment was begun. Children with grade I or grade II reflux are given prophylactic antibiotic therapy which has been shown to be effective in preventing pyelonephritis and renal scarring. If the reflux had been grade IV or there had been recurrent infections despite antibiotics we would have recommended reimplantation of the ureter, which is nearly always effective in correcting reflux.

taken, close surveillance to ensure compliance is essential. The Birmingham controlled trial of medical and surgical management of children with reflux showed no significant difference (Birmingham Reflux Study Group, 1987).

Prognosis

Bacteriuria with reflux may result in injury to the kidney with further scarring. Most, but not all, of the renal damage occurs by age 5 years; symptomless bacteriuria and reflux may remain with normal kidney growth in children over age 5 years. About one-third of a group of children ages 1 week to 12 years seen at University College Hospital, London with urinary tract infections had vesicoureteric reflux, and half of these had renal scarring. On follow-up after 4–20 years, about 1/6 with renal scars had hypertension. The likelihood of hypertension is reduced if infections can be controlled by chemoprophylaxis (Smellie and Prescod, 1986).

REFERENCES

Abbott GD: Neonatal bacteriuria: A prospective study in 1,460 infants. *Br Med J* 1:267, 1972.

Birmingham Reflux Study Group: Prospective trial of operative versus non-operative treatment of severe vesicoureteric reflux in children: Five years' observation. *Br Med J* 295:237, 1987.

Ginsburg CM, McCracken GH: Urinary tract infections in young infants. *Pediatrics* 69:409, 1982.

Hodson CJ, Edwards O: Chronic pyelonephritis and vesicoureterine reflux. *Clin Radiol* 11:219, 1960.

Kunin CM: The natural history of recurrent bacteriuria in school age children. *N Engl J Med* 282:1443, 1970.

Lebowitz RL, Olbing H, Park Kulainen KU, et al: International system of radiographic grading of vesicoureteral reflux. *Pediatr Radiol* 15:105, 1985.
Levitt SB, Weiss RA: Vesicoureteral reflux. In Kelalis PP, King LR, Belman AB (eds): *Clinical Pediatric Urology*. 2nd edition. Philadelphia, WB Saunders, 1985, p. 355.
Lincoln K, Winberg J: Studies of urinary tract infections in infancy and childhood. II. Quantitative estimation of bacteriuria in unselected neonates with special reference to the occurrence of asymptomatic infections. *Acta Paediatr Scand* 53:30, 1964.
Rubin RH, Tolkoff-Rubin NE, Cotran RS: Urinary tract infection, pyelonephritis and reflux nephropathy. In Brenner BM, Rector FC (eds): *The Kidney,* 3rd edition. Philadelphia, WB Saunders, 1986.
Smellie JM, Gruneberg RN, Leahey A, et al: Long term low dose cotrimoxazole in prophylaxis of childhood urinary tract infection: Clinical aspects. *Br Med J* 2:203, 1976.
Smellie JM, Edwards D, Normand ICS, et al: Effect of VUR on renal growth in children with urinary tract infection. *Arch Dis Child* 56:593, 1981.
Smellie JM, Katz G, Gruneberg RN: Controlled trial of prophylactic treatment in childhood urinary tract infection. *Lancet* 2:175, 1978.
Smellie JM, Normand ICS: Bacteriuria, reflux and renal scarring. *Arch Dis Child* 50:581, 1975.
Smellie JM, Normand ICS: Urinary tract infections in children 1985. *Postgrad Med J* 61:895, 1985.
Smellie JM, Prescod N: Natural history of overt urinary infection in childhood. In Asscher AW, Brumfitt W (eds): *Microbiologic Diseases in Nephrology*. New York, John Wiley & Sons, 1986, p. 243.
Stansfeld JM: The measurement and meaning of pyuria. *Arch Dis Child* 37:257, 1982.
Van den Abbeele AD, Treves ST, Lebowitz RL, et al: Vesicoureteral reflux in asymptomatic siblings of patients with known reflux: Radionuclide cystograph. *Pediatrics* 79:147, 1987.

Approach to Renal Masses 4

Renal masses may be detected on physical examination of the newborn or may already have been diagnosed as such on prenatal ultrasonography. In the 0- to 1-year-old with a retroperitoneal mass, the kidney is the most common site of origin.

Occasionally a renal mass may be diagnosed clinically after a baby has signs of urinary tract infection: fevers, vomiting, bacteriuria, poor feeding, and weight gain. Renal ultrasonography should follow plain abdominal films in the evaluation of a retroperitoneal mass. Depending on the appearance on ultrasonograms, any necessary further studies can be selected. For example, the child with a prenatal scan showing a cystic mass in the renal fossa would have postnatal ultrasonography to determine if the mass is a multicystic dysplastic kidney, hydronephrosis, or a cystic adrenal mass displacing kidney. If a multicystic dysplastic kidney is identified on an ultrasonogram radionuclide, scintigraphy should follow to prove that no functioning renal tissue is present. If hydronephrosis with or without hydroureter is found, voiding cystourethrogram (VCUG) should be carried out to document presence or absence of vesicoureteral reflux. If severe reflux is present, an intravenous urogram (IVU) is performed while the baby has an indwelling bladder catheter to prevent simulation of function by reflux of opacified urine. A cystic adrenal mass should be identified as such, because a normal kidney can be found inferior to the mass. Attention is then drawn from the urinary tract and toward lesions of the adrenal. Solid renal masses are uncommon in the neonate (Fig. 10.4) and evaluation following the preliminary ultrasonogram depends on the size of the mass, the presence or absence of similar lesions in the other kidney, renal venous or inferior vena caval displacement, clot, or tumor and the associated clinical features (Berger et al, 1980). IVU, radionuclide scans, CT, angiography, and follow-up ultrasonograms might be indicated depending on the likelihood of the mass being nephroblastomatosis, mesonephric blastoma, Wilms tumor or an ischemic kidney from renal venous thrombosis.

HYDRONEPHROSIS

Hydronephrosis (see pp. 781) signifies dilatation of renal pelvis and calyces (Fig 10.5). It does not necessarily connote obstruction, although most cases of hydronephrosis are obstructive in origin. Vesicoureteral reflux, megacalyces, and prune-belly syndrome are associated with hydronephrosis of varying degrees in the absence of obstruction.

The detection of hydronephrosis has increased with the use of ultrasonography in prenatal screening. The most common conditions found were ureteropelvic junction obstruction (41%), obstruction of distal ureter, usually megaureter (23%), upper-pole hydronephrosis

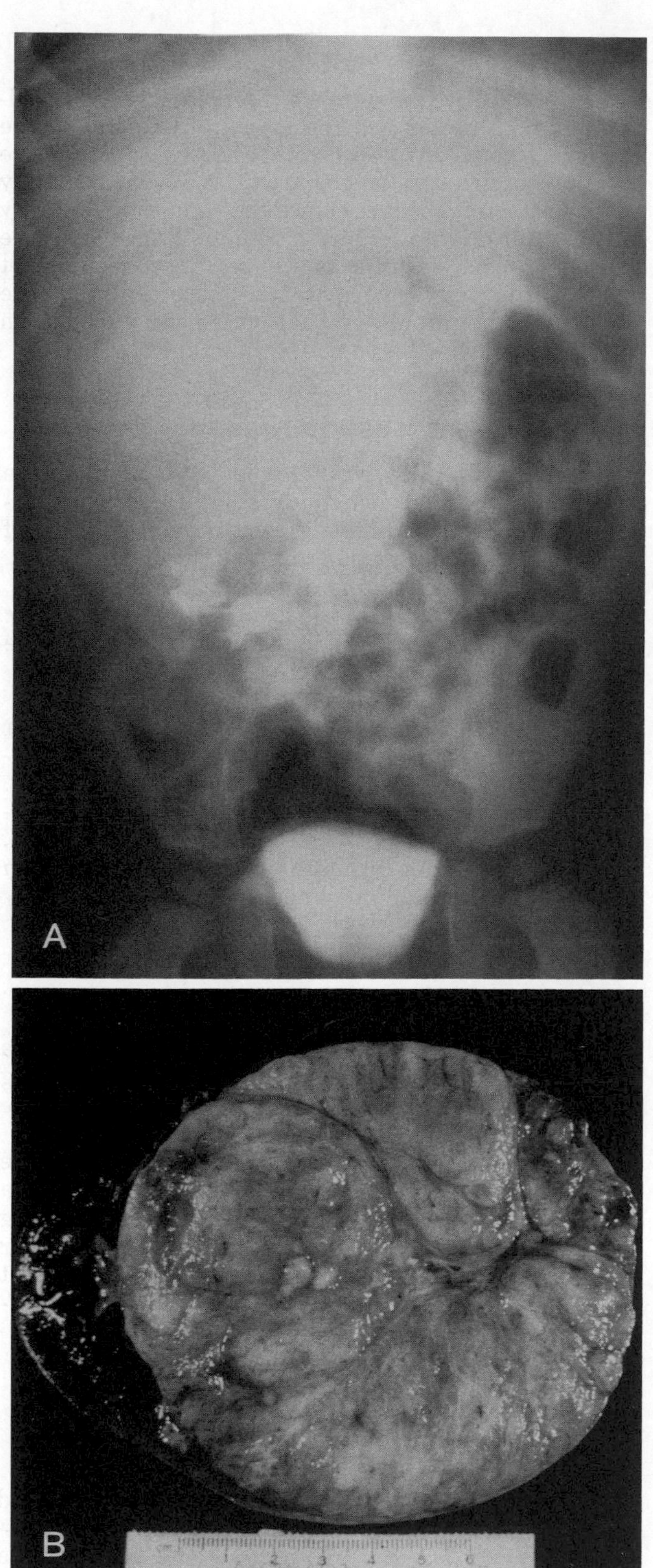

Figure 10.4. A. This baby presented with a unilateral flank mass. IVU shows displacement of the renal collecting system by a huge soft-tissue mass. On further work-up, inferior vena cava was patent and the left kidney was normal. **B.** Although unusual in the first year of life, this mass proved to be a Wilms tumor, well encapsulated as seen on this surgical specimen.

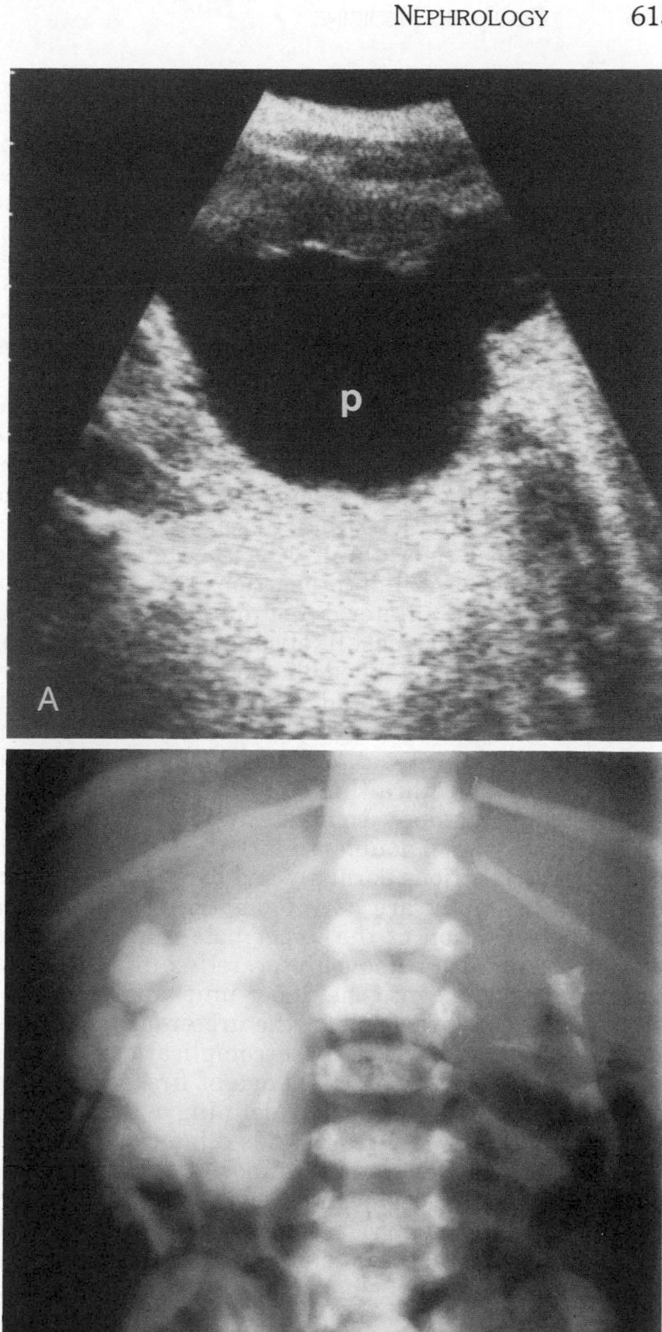

Figure 10.5. A. Prone longitudinal scan of the kidney shows dilated renal pelvis *(p)* and calyces. The prenatal scan of this child had shown hydronephrosis, confirmed by this follow-up study. No dilation of the ureter was present; this appearance is typical of obstruction at the ureteropelvic junction. **B.** IVU shows good function of both kidneys with pelvocalyceal dilation on the right confirming the diagnosis of obstruction at the ureteropelvic junction.

associated with duplex anomalies (13%), and posterior urethral valves(10%) (Brown et al, 1987).

Ureteropelvic obstruction is a common sequela of congenital stenosis at the junction of the proximal ureter with the renal pelvis. The baby may present because of abnormal prenatal scan, flank mass, or urinary infection. In uncomplicated cases, the dilatation is restricted to the upper collecting system. A dilated ureter is not present on ultrasonograms or IVU. Delay in function of the affected kidney (IVU, radionuclide scans) is present if the obstruction is severe.

Primary megaureter is characterized by unilateral dilatation of renal pelvis, calyces and ureter, in the absence of vesicoureteral reflux. Since prenatal scanning was introduced, this anomaly (obstruction at the ureterovesical junction from fibrous replacement of normal ureteric musculature) has become recognized as responsible for a high proportion of cases of hydronephrosis. When bilateral hydroureteronephrosis is present in a boy, the most likely diagnosis is a posterior urethral valve. A distended bladder, decreased urinary stream or dribbling should suggest the diagnosis. In such patients, ultrasonography usually can demonstrate the thickened wall of bladder and often, the dilated posterior urethra (Fig. 10.6).

The duplex kidney (complete duplication of the collecting system with double ureters inserting into bladder) usually functions normally and babies and children with this anomaly are asymptomatic. Complications include obstruction of the upper pole unit associated with ureterocele or ectopic ureter, reflux into the lower unit, rarely reflux into the upper unit, and rarely obstruction of the lower pole at the ureteropelvic or ureterovesical junction. All these complications present the radiologist with the challenge of first identifying the hydronephrosis and then defining which unit is involved and for what reason it is dilated.

The neurogenic bladder (almost always in babies with meningomyelocele) may be associated with hydronephrosis secondary to reflux or obstruction. Our usual initial evaluation includes a VCUG and a renal ultrasonogram after the baby has had corrective spinal and shunt surgery.

Treatment

After the diagnosis of hydronephrosis and its cause are made, treatment includes relief of obstruction if present (permanently by surgery or temporarily by percutaneous drainage of the renal collecting system) and medical therapy of concurrent infection. Untreated obstruction results in decreased function and propensity toward infection because of stasis of urine.

Severe vesicoureteral reflux is treated surgically by reimplanting the offending distal ureter. Minor degrees of reflux may be followed without surgical intervention as long as renal growth is normal and infections do not occur.

Posterior urethral valves most commonly can be treated by fulguration or resection transurethrally through a cystoscope.

CONTROVERSY

Now that hydronephrosis can be diagnosed by ultrasonography after the 16th week of fetal life, some urologists have advocated fetal surgery to drain the distended portions of the urinary tract. We would rarely advocate such procedures since the condition is hardly ever life-threatening. Once a fetus is known to have hydronephrosis, we prefer to wait for spontaneous onset of labor and deliver in a tertiary care center where complete radiographic evaluation can be undertaken after birth (Lebowitz, personal communication).

Horseshoe Kidney

Horseshoe kidney results when a segment of the developing renal parenchyma fuses during embryogenesis. The joining isthmus is usually inferior (90% of cases) and located anterior to the aorta or vena cava. Some renal parenchyma is usually in the isthmus.

Partial obstruction at the level of the ureteropelvic junction can occur, and, when it exists, may predispose to infection or parenchymal damage.

The condition is unlikely to be detected in the absence of infection or imaging examinations for other reasons. The diagnosis can be made with ultrasonography, intravenous pyelography, or radionuclide scans.

No treatment is usually required unless the obstruction is severe or associated with renal infection. More frequent routine urinalysis should be done to search for bacteria in individuals known to have any urinary tract anomaly.

Ectopic Kidney

During embryogenesis, the kidney ascends from a low position to its permanent site. It is not surprising that arrest in ascent can occur at any level, so that one kidney may be in the pelvis or lower abdomen.

Ectopic kidneys may be prone to infection, and are often detected during imaging studies. Occasionally, a mass can be felt on abdominal examination. Screening for and treatment of infections are appropriate. No other interventions are necessary unless there is upper tract infection, significant obstruction, or associated vesicoureteral reflux.

RENAL CYSTIC DISEASES

Definition

Renal cystic diseases include a variety of inherited and acquired disorders, occurring separately or in association with specific syndromes, and involving a number of pathogenetic mechanisms. They can be loosely grouped into five categories: (1) polycystic kidney diseases, (2) cysts associated with other inheritable syndromes, (3) medullary cystic diseases, (4) localized or segmental cysts, and (5) renal cystic dysplasia (see Table 10.7).

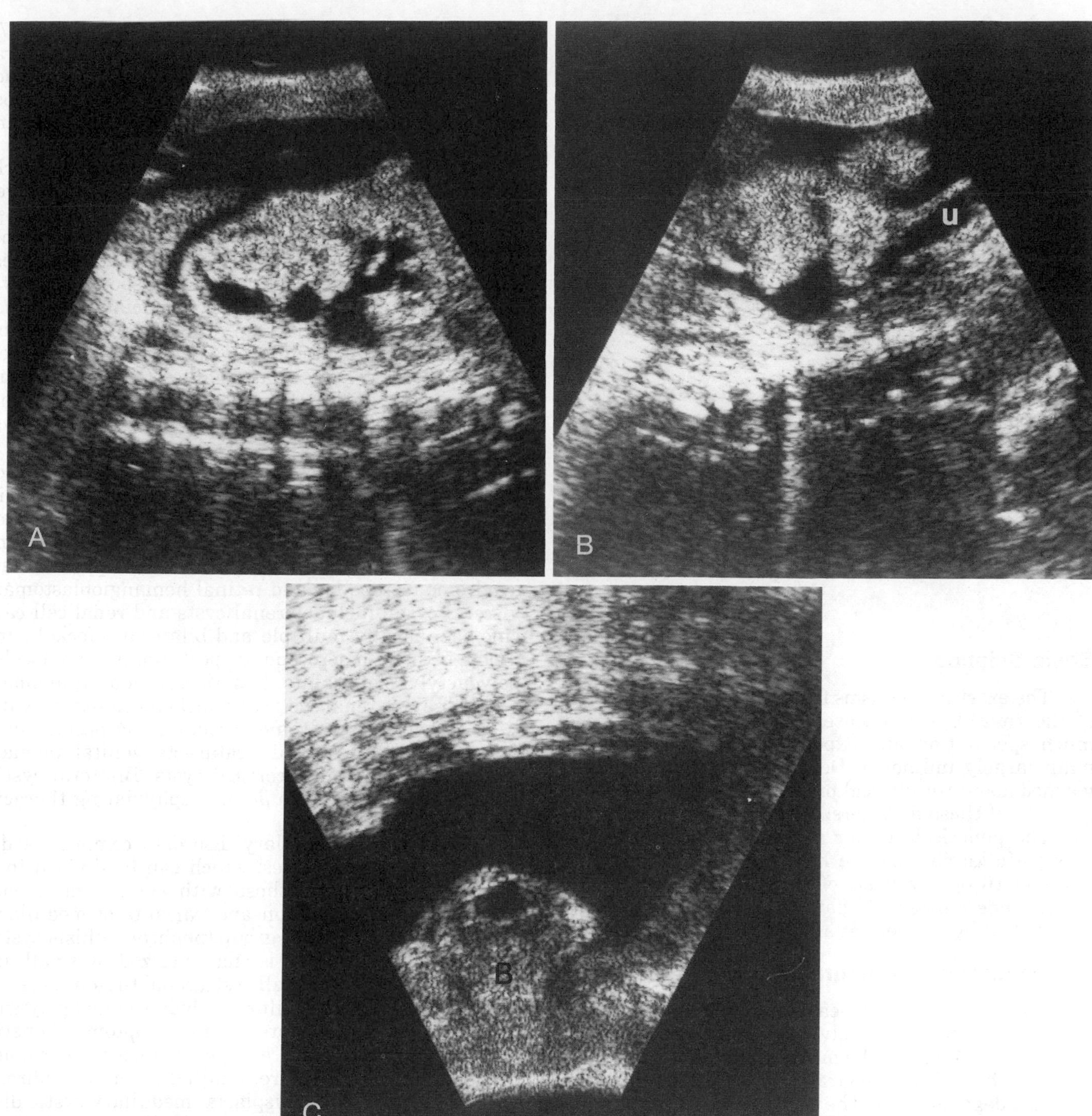

Figure 10.6. This baby boy presented with oliguria and abdominal distention. The scans are diagnostic of obstruction at the bladder neck, typically from posterior urethral valves as in this case. The ascites shown on these scans is urine. This usually results from forniceal tears in the kidneys that allow urine to escape into retroperitoneal space and then to dissect intraperitoneally. **A.** Prone longitudinal scan of the right kidney shows a dilated calyceal system, echogenic renal parenchyma, and ascites outlining edge of liver and lateral renal border. **B.** Longitudinal scan of left kidney is similar with dilation of left ureter *(U)* also present. **C.** Perineal scan of the bladder *(B)* shows the thickened wall of bladder (from urethral obstruction by valve) outlined by ascites.

Table 10.7
Renal Cystic Diseases

Polycystic kidney disease
Autosomal dominant polycystic disease
Autosomal recessive polycystic disease
Cysts associated with other inheritable syndromes
Tuberous sclerosis complex
von Hippel-Lindau disease
Meckel syndrome
Zellweger cerebrohepatorenal syndrome
Jeune asphyxiating thoracic dysplasia
Medullary cystic diseases
Nephronopthisis-cystic medulla complex
Familial juvenile nephronopthisis
Renal-retinal dysplasia
Medullary cystic disease
Localized or segmental renal cysts
Cystic renal dysplasia
Aplastic cystic dysplasia
Multicystic dysplasia
Diffuse and segmental cystic dysplasia
Cystic dysplasia associated with lower urinary tract obstruction
Acquired cystic disease (dialysis patients)

Basic Science

The exact mechanisms for the development of many of the renal cystic diseases have been the source of much speculation and experimentation, but still remain largely unknown. Despite this, much has been learned about the clinical presentation, pathology, and genetics of these disorders.

The genetic locus for autosomal dominant adult polycystic kidney disease has been assigned to chromosome 16 on the basis of genetic linkage to the α-globin gene cluster. Prenatal diagnosis has been accomplished by Reeders et al in 1986.

Epidemiology and Natural History

Polycystic kidney disease includes a spectrum of inheritable disorders involving both kidneys. The disease is identifiable by the mode of transmission of both kidneys, their clinical characteristics, and appearance of cystic degeneration. The most common form, adult polycystic disease, is more properly designated by its pattern of inheritance as autosomal dominant polycystic disease. Cysts are found in both cortex and medulla. Fluid in the cysts provides evidence of functional cells in the cyst wall. Proximal cysts have fluid that resembles serum, whereas distal cyst liquid has lower sodium and chloride concentrations, and higher potassium, hydrogen ion, creatinine, and urea concentration.

About 25% of individuals do not know of its occurrence in relatives, which may mean that it can exist in mild degree and not be detected, or that there is a high rate of spontaneous mutations. Presumably acquired in utero, it presents symptomatically in the fourth and fifth decades of life with the most common clinical features including bilateral flank masses (Fig. 10.7), hypertension, hematuria, and progressive deterioration of renal function. Other significant pathologic findings include pancreatic and liver cysts, and most important, cerebral artery aneurysms which account for about 10% of the related deaths.

Infantile polycystic kidney disease, more properly termed autosomal recessive polycystic disease, involves a spectrum of clinically and morphologically overlapping disorders. It occurs in 1/4000–1/8000 live births, with a higher incidence in autopsy series. It may present in infancy, with greatly enlarged, spongy kidneys, severe renal failure, and often is associated with maternal oligohydramnios, respiratory insufficiency, and Potter facies. In older children (so-called juvenile type), the kidneys are somewhat smaller, the renal failure more variable in its progression, and, most significant, hepatic fibrosis with portal hypertension and liver dysfunction predominate.

Renal cystic disease is present as a component of several hereditary syndromes. Tuberous sclerosis (mental retardation, seizures, sebaceous adenomas of the skin) is associated with renal cystic disease, angiomyolipomas, and renal failure. Von Hippel-Lindau syndrome (cerebellar and retinal hemangioblastomas, visceral cysts) includes renal cysts and renal cell carcinomas, usually multiple and bilateral. Meckel syndrome involves macrocephaly, posterior encephalocele, polydactyly, cleft palate, hepatic and genital anomalies, and severe renal cystic dysplasia incompatible with life. Zellweger syndrome (cerebrohepatorenal syndrome) includes hypotonia, cataracts, genital anomalies and multiple renal cortical cysts. Bilateral cystic dysplasia is also seen in Jeune asphyxiating thoracic dysplasia.

Cystic renal medullary disorders comprise a diverse group of syndromes, which can be divided into two major categories; those with significant abnormalities of renal function and variants of medullary sponge kidney. The first group (nephronopthisis-cystic renal medulla complex) is characterized by small, irregular kidneys with small cysts, renal tubular defects, and progressive renal failure. Polydypsia and polyuria are the most common presenting symptoms. Genetic patterns of transmission and penetrance are variable. Included in this group are: familial juvenile nephronopthisis, renal-retinal dysplasia, medullary cystic disease, and Alstrom syndrome (diabetes mellitus, neuropathy, obesity, and renal concentrating defect). The second category, medullary sponge kidney, is a relatively common disorder (1/5000), and is often asymptomatic. The most common presenting complaint is that of renal stones with colic or hematuria (Cantani et al, 1986).

Localized and segmental renal cysts represent a group of acquired abnormalities. Most are simple or retention cysts. They may be solitary, multiple, unilateral, or bilateral. Acquired cystic renal disease is becoming increasingly recognized in association with chronic dialysis. The process develops in kidneys scarred from glomerulonephritis, atherosclerosis, interstitial

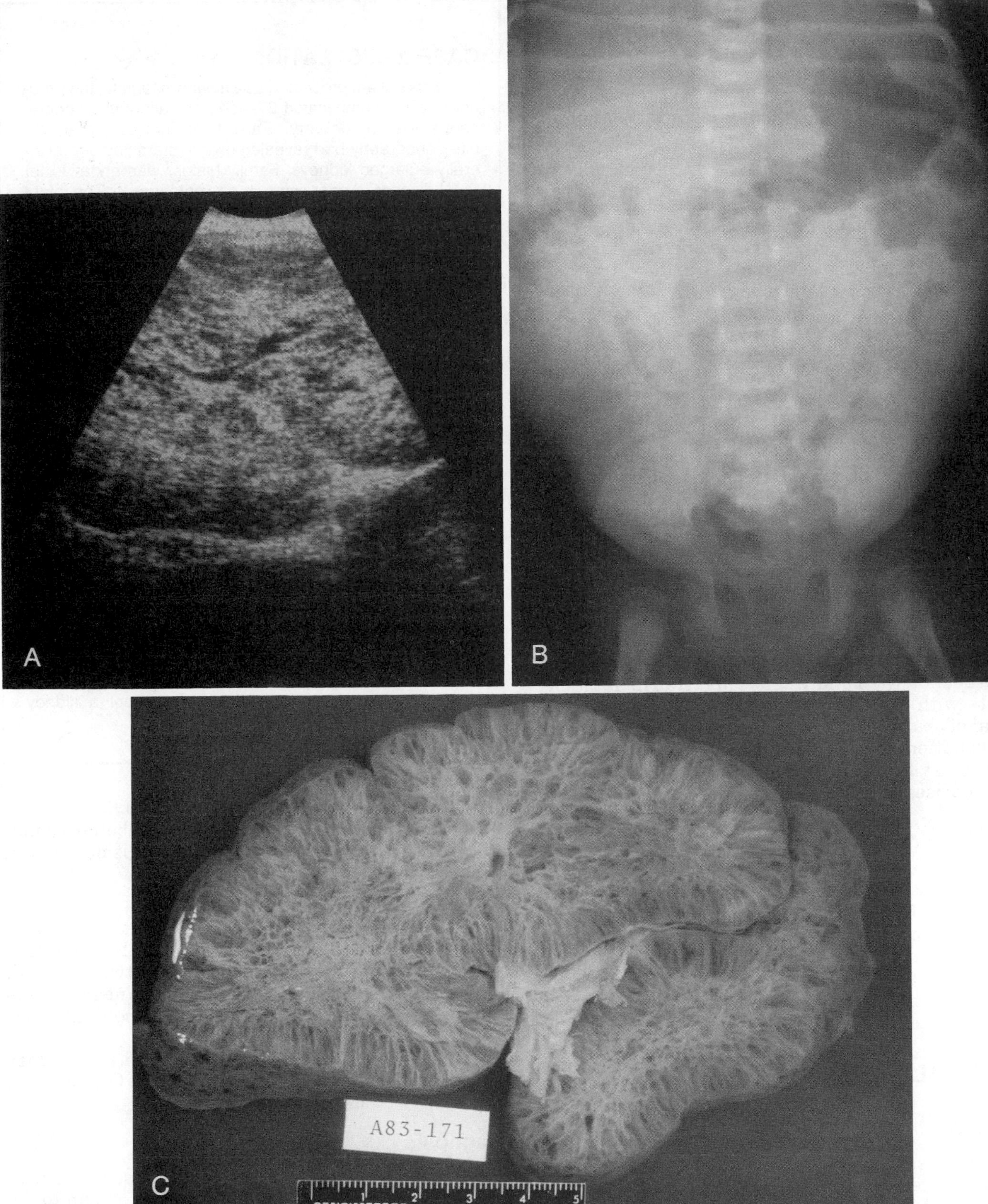

Figure 10.7. **A.** This baby was born with bilateral flank masses palpated on clinical examination. The ultrasonogram shows a portion of the large right kidney. The multiple echoes are reflections of multiple small cystic spaces in this baby with infantile polycystic kidneys. **B.** IVU shows gross enlargement of the kidneys with a striated nephrogram typical of uptake in the radially arrayed tubules of infantile polycystic kidneys. **C.** Postmortem section of the right kidney shows the diffuse polycystic involvement.

nephritis, and other renal diseases. About 15% of these cystic kidneys will develop a malignancy.

Cystic renal dysplasia refers to a large group of renal abnormalities caused by maldevelopment or arrest of cytodifferentiation early in embryogenesis. This may present as aplastic cystic dysplasia with bilateral involvement and Potter syndrome. The most common form of cystic dysplasia in childhood is unilateral multicystic dysplasia which is more common on the left side. This entity presents as a unilateral abdominal mass in infancy or on prenatal ultrasonography. Cystic dysplasia may be segmental or generalized and is often seen in association with severe lower urinary tract obstruction or reflux (see Controversy).

Diagnosis

The diagnosis of cystic disease of the kidney can be made most readily by an imaging study of the kidney such as intravenous urography or in cases of renal failure either ultrasonography or CT. The radiologic finding of ectatic or cystic tubules in the pyramids with or without stones is characteristic of medullary sponge kidney.

Treatment

Treatment for dominantly inherited polycystic disease is medical and symptomatic until end-stage renal failure occurs, after which dialysis or renal transplantation is a potential option. Therapeutic considerations for the neonate with recessive polycystic disease are few except for the child eligible for transplantation. Patients with medullary sponge kidney may require removal of obstructing stones that pass into the ureter. Dialysis patients who show changes of acquired cystic disease must be monitored for malignancy and, if a question arises, nephrectomy should be performed.

CONTROVERSY

The management of a unilateral multicystic dysplastic kidney (the most common abdominal mass in the newborn) has usually been to resect it. The argument for resection is to confirm the diagnosis and to eliminate the small risk of malignant change or infection and the 15% risk of hypertension (Hartman et al, 1986). However, serial follow-up with ultrasonography may be an alternative in some infants.

CASE ILLUSTRATION

This patient presented as a newborn female, the product of an uncomplicated 37-week gestation with spontaneous vaginal delivery. Early third trimester maternal ultrasonography had revealed oligohydramnios and bilaterally enlarged kidneys. Family history was negative for renal disease. Apgar score at 1 minute was 4. The infant required intubation and ventilation. Physical examination revealed gross abdominal distention with bilateral flank masses. Chest film revealed a right pneumothorax. Moderate renal insufficiency (creatinine 1.2 mg/dl) and severe hypertension were present. Renal ultrasonography (Fig. 10.7*A*) showed grossly enlarged, highly echogenic kidneys compatible with recessive polycystic kidney disease. IVU confirmed these findings (Fig. 10.7*B*). The infant was followed closely, but medical management became more difficult with poor control of hypertension and deteriorating renal function.

Following an apparent upper respiratory infection, she began coughing and became apneic. Resuscitation was instituted; however, neurologic function was not evident. The baby was pronounced dead at 9 months of age. Postmortem examination revealed pulmonary dysplastic changes as well as acute inflammation. Grossly enlarged kidneys compatible with the clinical diagnosis of inherited polycystic kidney disease were found (Fig. 10.7*C*).

COMMENT

In some infants with minimal renal function, it is possible to maintain growth with strict dietary control (occasionally, dialysis) until the infant can accept a kidney transplant.

RENAL VASCULAR THROMBOSIS

Definition

Renal vascular occlusions can occur in any renal vessel and interfere with blood flow.

Epidemiology

Venous thrombosis occurs mostly in the first year of life in association with dehydration or sepsis. Infants of diabetic mothers, with or without polycythemia, are prone to venous thrombosis in kidneys and other organs as well (Oppenheimer and Esterly, 1965).

Arterial occlusions can occur with emboli from umbilical arterial catheters. The prevalence is not known.

Natural History

Renal vein thrombosis with calcification has been found in stillborn infants. More commonly, the condition develops postnatally, with males at twice the risk of females. The clinical status of an infant may deteriorate suddenly with hematuria, metabolic acidosis, and hypertension or shock.

In about 60% of infants, an enlarged firm kidney is palpable. Edema is not usually present. Oliguria and anuria may occur.

Diagnosis

Hematuria, an abdominal flank mass, and sudden clinical deterioration should alert the physician to the possibility of renal vascular thrombosis. Radionuclide scans reveal diminished perfusion and poor excretion, if any, on the involved side. Ultrasonography will show an enlarged kidney and, occasionally, the clot within renal vein extending into the interior vena cava. Hematuria, proteinuria, and hypertension are commonly present in renal artery thrombosis. Azotemia and oliguria may occur. The kidneys may be enlarged, but usually are not palpable. Blood urea and creatinine may be normal or elevated. Radionuclide scans are useful to delineate the extent of infarct.

Treatment

Renal vein thrombosis is so rare that prospective controlled studies of medical versus surgical management are not feasible. Reports of good outcome with supportive therapy alone, and return of renal function have encouraged medical management. The outlook for bilateral disease with hypertension is so grave, an attempt to remove thrombi may sometimes be indicated. Peritoneal dialysis and heparin infusions for at least 5 days are favored by most nephrologists. Meticulous attention to fluid and electrolyte balance provides the best hope of survival in renal artery thrombosis. Occasionally with unilateral disease and hypertension, nephrectomy is in order. Antihypertensive agents are needed for elevated pressures.

Prognosis

The outlook depends on the extent of thrombosis. Renal atrophy may be a late result.

RENAL CORTICAL AND MEDULLARY NECROSIS

This disorder is seen in association with severe asphyxia, shock, sepsis, and other serious illnesses. It causes anuria or oliguria with a few cells and low levels of protein.

The diagnosis is suggested by anuria, and the associated evidence of renal damage, including hypertension. The blood urea nitrogen and creatinine are elevated. After several days, a period of polyuria and sodium wasting occur. The kidneys are poorly visualized by intravenous pyelography or radionuclide scans.

The treatment is supportive.

The prognosis depends on the associated disease and the extent of intravascular coagulation. Late sequelae can lead to renal failure. In a review of 16 infants, 2–35 days of age, Chevalier et al (1984) reported 9 infants with renal failure secondary to perinatal asphyxia. Ischemic renal failure was found to have a poor prognosis if anuria had been present for 4 or more days and no renal uptake of nuclide was observed.

REFERENCES

Belman AB, Susmano DF, Burden JJ, et al: Nonoperative treatment of unilateral thrombosis in the newborn. *JAMA* 211:1165, 1970.

Berger PE, Munschauer RW, Kuhn JP: Computed tomography and ultrasound of renal and perirenal diseases in infants and children. *Pediatr Radiol* 9:91, 1980.

Bernstein J: Heritable cystic disorders of the kidney. *Pediatr Clin North Am* 18:435, 1971.

Brown T, Mandell J, Lebowitz RL: Neonatal hydronephrosis in the era of ultrasonography. *AJR* 148:959, 1987.

Cantani A, Bamonte G, Ceccolli D, et al: Familial juvenile nephronophthisis: A review and differential diagnosis. *Clin Pediatr* 25:90, 1986.

Chevalier RL, Campbell F, et al: Prognostic factors in neonatal acute renal failure. *Pediatrics* 74:265, 1984.

DeKlerk PP, Marshall FF, Jeffs RD: Multicystic dysplastic kidney. *J Urol* 118:306, 1977.

Feiner HD, Katz LA, Gallo GR: Acquired cystic disease of the kidney in chronic dialysis patients. *Urology* 17:260, 1981.

Frideman J: Cystic diseases of the kidney. In Emery AEH, Rimoin DG (eds): *Principles and Practice of Medical Genetics*. New York, Churchill-Livingstone, 1983.

Gardner KD Jr: *Cystic Diseases of the Kidney*. New York, Wiley Biomedical, John Wiley and Sons, 1976.

Hartman GE, Smolik LM, Shochat SJ: The dilemma of the multicystic dysplastic kidney. *Am J Dis Child* 140:925, 1986.

Lebowitz RL: The detection of vesicoureteral reflux in the child. *Invest Radiol* 21:519, 1986.

Lebowitz RL, Teele RL: Fetal and neonatal hydronephrosis. *Urol Radiol* 5:185, 1983.

Oppenheimer EH, Esterly JR: Thrombosis in the newborn, comparison between infants of diabetic and non-diabetic mothers. *J Pediatr* 67:549, 1965.

Osthanondh V, Potter EL: Pathogenesis of polycystic kidneys. *Arch Pathol* 77:474, 1964.

Reeders ST, Zerres K, Gal A, et al: Prenatal diagnosis of autosomal dominant polycystic kidney disease with a DNA probe. *Lancet* 2:6, 1986.

Welling LW, Grantham JJ: Cystic and developmental diseases of the kidney. In Brenner BM, Rector FC (eds): *The Kidney,* 3rd edition. Philadelphia, WB Saunders, 1986.

Renal Agenesis and Dysgenesis

5

Definition

Renal agenesis may be unilateral or bilateral (Potter syndrome), sporadic or hereditary (Potter, 1946). Dysgenesis or hypoplasia may be severe, with only a kidney remnant remaining. A kidney is called dysgenetic when its weight is at least 2 standard deviations below average.

Epidemiology

Agenesis or dysgenesis of one or both kidneys was found in 1/6369 births at The Boston Hospital for Women in the 1970s. The true incidence in terms of a population of individuals is probably lower since high risk pregnancies were referred to that hospital.

Natural History

The absence of urine production by the fetus with renal agenesis does not cause uremia since blood clearance is achieved by the placenta. Thus, fetal growth occurs, although the average birth weights are 2 kg and oligohydramnios is present. Lung hypoplasia may coexist as an independent embryologic insult or, more likely, as the consequence of lack of amniotic liquid. Extrarenal anomalies may exist in other organs, such as limbs, in association with oligohydramnios. The fetal surface of the placenta has plaques described as amnion nodosum. The facies of the affected infants, who are usually male, show widely spaced eyes, a depressed nasal bridge, receding chin, and posteriorly rotated asymmetrical low-set ears.

Death often occurs in the first days of life from renal or pulmonary failure.

Treatment

Until recently, chronic renal failure at birth was considered to be a fatal condition. Recent developments in dialysis, nutrition and renal transplantation have improved this prognosis. Genetic counseling is important, since family members may have less severe renal malformations. In an ultrasonographic study of 41 relatives of affected infants, 9% were found to have asymptomatic renal malformations, the most frequent of which was unilateral renal agenesis (Roodhooft et al, 1984).

REFERENCES

Bell ET: *Diseases of the Kidney,* 2nd edition. Philadelphia, Lea & Febiger, 1951.

Potter EL: Bilateral renal agenesis. *J Pediatr* 29:68, 1946.

Roodhooft AM, Birnholz JC, Holmes LB: Familial nature of congenital absence and severe dysgenesis of both kidneys. *N Engl J Med* 310:1341, 1984.

Glomerulonephritis—Approach to Hematuria

6

Any child with gross or microscopic hematuria requires a systematic investigation to ascertain whether the problem is a benign microhematuria or a more serious manifestation of chronic renal disease or neoplasm.

Initially, the history should ascertain any familial renal disease, recent febrile illness, or trauma, or exercise-induced hematuria. The first round of laboratory investigations should include urinalysis and urine culture, 24-hour calcium excretion, blood count, blood urea nitrogen, serum creatinine, serum albumin, antistreptolysin titer, and assay of complement C3. Dipsticks should be given parents for twice daily testing at home to determine the possible effect of exercise. These initial studies may establish that the hematuria is benign, particularly if they are all normal, and no proteinuria is present in a concentrated specimen. A normal intravenous pyelogram or ultrasound examination is an additional requirement for the diagnosis, since Wilms tumor can present with hematuria alone.

If serum complement is persistently low, either acute or chronic glomerulonephritis is likely.

Asymptomatic gross hematuria should alert the physician to the possibility that the bladder is the site of bleeding, from tumor, or a foreign body (hemorrhagic cystitis would not be asymptomatic). Cystoscopy may be indicated to find the site of bleeding. Occasionally renal stones are asymptomatic and cause hematuria. If that possibility exists, ultrasonography and computerized tomography can localize the stone.

Hematuria in the absence of proteinuria is often self-limited and of unknown etiology in about half the cases. Stapleton and others (1984) found that urinary calcium excretion is elevated in about a third of children with otherwise unexplained hematuria. More than 4 mg of calcium per kg in a 24-hour period is defined as hypercalciuria. Calcium oxalate crystals may be seen under light microscopy of the urine sediment. Since children with hypercalciuria are at risk of stones, increased intake of fluids and moderate sodium restriction is recommended. (Calcium excretion increases with high sodium intake.) In most children, the hematuria resolves.

Symptomatic hematuria associated with proteinuria and edema or hypertension can be a manifestation of acute or chronic glomerulonephritis or nephrosis. The best single test to distinguish the disorders is measurement of serum complement, which is depressed in acute poststreptococcal glomerulonephritis. If hypocomplementemia persists for more than 6 weeks, a renal biopsy is appropriate to identify the basis for the chronic glomerulonephritis.

NEPHROPATHY WITH HENOCH-SCHÖNLEIN PURPURA

Henoch-Schönlein purpura involves skin, GI tract, and joints. Renal manifestations are present in over 20% of children and are more common in older children. The condition is thought to be an immunologic response, although no single stimulus has been identified. It has been seen most often in the winter and has occurred in clusters (CDC, 1988; see pp. 445–445).

Natural History

In most instances, characteristic petechial-purpuric rash follows an upper respiratory infection. The rash is most evident over extensor surfaces of the lower legs and arms. Melena and abdominal pain occur about the same time and may be severe. Migratory arthritis may occur at any time. Renal involvement may precede or follow the other symptoms.

The renal findings are either microscopic or gross hematuria, with or without protein. Transient azotemia may occur, but hypertension is not common. Serum complement components are depressed in about one-third of children during the acute presentation. Of these children, 1–5% progress to end-stage renal disease over several months to years.

Diagnosis

The combination of purpura, abdominal pain, and migratory arthritis establish the diagnosis. The renal involvement is mainly characterized by mild hematuria. Differentiation from the hemolytic uremic syndrome is by presence of a microangiopathic hemolytic anemia and acute renal failure in the latter.

Treatment

Supportive treatment only is appropriate for Henoch-Schönlein purpura. Prednisone may give relief if the arthritis is severe.

RAPIDLY PROGRESSIVE ACUTE GLOMERULONEPHRITIS

When a child does not recover from apparent acute poststreptococcal glomerulonephritis, and has persistent abnormalities in the urine, the phrase "rapidly progressing disease" is used to designate a group of conditions that can only be distinguished by biopsy. Differentiation depends on examination of the tissue with immunofluorescence. Under light microscopy, glomeruli may show crescents, from whence the name crescentic glomerulonephritis derives. Early agressive treatment with high doses of glucocorticoids can lead to an improvement in renal function (McEnery and Strife, 1984).

ACUTE POSTSTREPTOCOCCAL GLOMERULONEPHRITIS

Definition

This form of glomerulonephritis follows a pharyngeal or cutaneous infection with certain serotypes of group A β-hemolytic streptococci, and is sometimes called poststreptococcal glomerulonephritis. (Other forms of acute glomerulonephritis are discussed under the associated systemic disease such as Henoch-Schönlein purpura and disseminated lupus erythematosus.)

Basic Science

The latent period of 5–21 days from streptococcal infection (chiefly with types 12 or 49) to evidence of glomerulonephritis supports the probability of immune mechanisms as important in pathogenesis. Serum complement (C3) is depressed, and immunopathologic and electron microscopic findings are similar to those in immune-induced renal disease in animals. IgG and complement C3 are deposited on the epithelial side of the glomerular basement membrane.

Epidemiology

Poststreptococcal glomerulonephritis is the most common form of acute glomerulonephritis. It appears most often in children aged 7–10 years. The incidence is not known, although the impression is widely held that in the United States it is much less common than it was in the 1940s and 1950s. It is more common in

Africa and Southeast Asia. Boys are affected twice as often as girls.

Natural History

Most of the time, a history can be obtained of pharyngitis or impetigo about 10 days before the abrupt presentation of dark urine. Mild periorbital and peripheral edema may be present, as may flank or abdominal pain and low-grade fever. Acute hypertension is associated with headache, vomiting, and (rarely) seizures. If hypertension is severe, heart failure may occur, with symptoms of tachypnea, dyspnea, and the finding of hepatomegaly and pulmonary edema.

The acute phase lasts about a week, after which urine output increases, edema decreases and blood pressure gradually falls. Gross hematuria lasts about a week but microscopic hematuria can persist for several months.

Diagnosis

The urine shows red cells and red cell casts, and mildly elevated protein levels (about 30–100 mg/dl). In peripheral blood, a mild anemia and leukocytosis may be present. The erythrocyte sedimentation rate is elevated, and serum C3 levels are down for about 10 days, but are normal by 4–5 weeks. The antistreptolysin titer is often elevated.

A renal biopsy is not indicated unless the course is unusually prolonged, or the diagnosis is in doubt.

Treatment

If the *Streptococcus* is still present, a course of penicillin is indicated. Other treatment should be directed to the complications of the associated hypertension or oliguria. Rigid salt restriction and avoidance of excess fluid intake early in the course of illness may prevent hypertension.

Prognosis

Complete recovery is expected in almost all instances. Second attacks are rare, but can occur with a different nephritogenic strain of *Streptococcus.*

Prevention

Prompt treatment of cutaneous streptococcal infections with penicillin apparently reduces the risk of

CASE ILLUSTRATION (from Case Records of Massachusetts General Hospital. *N Engl J Med* 308:1343, 1983.

A 12-year-old boy presented at the hospital with renal failure. Two weeks earlier, he had had a streptococcal pharyngitis treated with ampicillin and cephalexin because of possible penicillin sensitivity. During the next few days he developed a petechial rash over the lower legs and arthralgia in multiple joints. The blood pressure was 140/90 mm Hg and urinary sediment had innumerable red cell and hyaline casts. White count was 13,000 mm^3 with 94% neutrophils.

Subsequent laboratory studies on admission revealed urine specific gravity 1.011 and 3+ protein. Red cells and granular casts were present. Hematocrit was 32%, white count 19,000/mm^3, with 87% neutrophils. Platelet count was 275,000/mm^3 and erythrocyte sedimentation rate 8 mm/hour. Urea nitrogen was 75 mg/dl, creatinine 3.6 mg/dl, calcium 7.8 mg/dl, and phosphorus 6.7 mg/dl. Total protein was 4.3 g, (albumin 1.8, globulin 2.5)/100 ml. Sodium was 130 mEq/L, potassium 3.7 mEq/L, chloride 102 mEq/L and carbon dioxide 20 mEq/L. Serum osmolality was 297 mOsm/L. Urine creatinine was 280 mg/dl, sodium 7 mEq/L and potassium 68 mEq/L. Chest radiographs were normal, but abdominal films showed air-fluid levels in the small bowel. Stool was 1+ for occult blood. Urine volume fell to 210 ml/24 hours.

Serum complement (CH 50 and C4) were 63 u/ml and 8 mg/dl, respectively (both reduced). C3 was at the lower limit of normal, 78 mg. A test for antinuclear antibodies was negative.

Renal biopsy showed extensive and severe tubular damage and hypercellularity and reduction in capillary lumens in all glomeruli. No crescents were seen in the specimen. Immunofluorescence showed scattered deposits of C3, IgG, and Clq along the glomerular basement membranes. The histologic picture was characteristic of postinfectious glomerulonephritis.

Over the next month, the child had additional bouts of purpura and joint pains suggestive of continuing vasculitis. The symptoms responded to glucocorticoid therapy, which was tapered and discontinued after 6 weeks.

A second course of steroids was required for recurrence of symptoms, with a repeat response. Four months later he was well, with a normal urinalysis.

QUESTIONS AND COMMENTS

What would your initial diagnosis have been, and what might have made you consider another?

The initial symptom complex was that of Henoch-Schönlein purpura. Unusual findings were the marked proteinuria and casts, both red cell and granular, which would have been unlikely in an allergic purpura and were more consistent with a postinfectious nephritis. Evidence of involvement of the classical pathway of complement activation limits the differential diagnosis to acute poststreptococcal glomerulonephritis, lupus nephritis, membranoproliferative nephritis, subacute bacterial endocarditis with nephritis, and "shunt" nephritis.

Was the renal biopsy helpful?

It was consistent with the clinical diagnosis and was probably indicated given the severity of the clinical course and the unusual degree of proteinuria.

glomerulonephritis. Treatment of pharyngeal streptococcal infections is appropriate, although no evidence shows a reduction in the likelihood of glomerulonephritis.

OTHER INFECTIONS ASSOCIATED WITH GLOMERULONEPHRITIS

Patients with subacute bacterial endocarditis and staphylococcal septicemia may develop a rapidly progressive glomerulonephritis. It is associated with immune complexes and reverses when the infection is cleared.

Glomerulonephritis may occur with other infections, although it is very rare in childhood.

REFERENCES

CDC: *MMWR* Henoch-Schönlein purpura—Connecticut. 37:121, 1988.
McEnery PT, Strife CF: Chronic glomerulonephritis in children. In Tune MB, Mendoza SA (eds): *Pediatric Nephrology* New York, Churchill Livingstone, 1984, p. 231.
Stapleton FB, Roy S, Noe HN, et al: Hypertension in children with hematuria. *N Engl J Med* 310:1345, 1984.

Approach to Proteinuria 7

Definition

The average protein concentration in urine is less than 5 mg/dl. Amounts greater than that can be detected by standard clinical laboratory tests and are usually considered indicative of diffuse disturbance in the permeability of the glomerular basement membrane. (The exception is production of large amounts of low molecular weight serum proteins that can cross a normal basement membrane, as in multiple myeloma.)

Basic Science

The normal glomerular capillary wall permits filtration of large amounts of water and electrolytes, but severely limits the movement of macromolecules that include all but the smallest plasma proteins. In addition, the glomerular basement membrane has a relatively dense concentration of negative charges that repel plasma proteins (Chang et al, 1975). If injured, there is a reduction in negative charge that permits serum proteins to cross into urine generally in proportion to their molecular weight and configuration.

Reduction in serum proteins reduces colloid osmotic pressure. Albumin is the principal protein that affects capillary dynamics since it is present in nearly twice the concentration of globulins and is of the order of 69,000 molecular weight, while globulin averages 140,000, and fibrinogen 400,000. Their relative concentrations are:

albumin	4.5 g/dl
globulins	2.5 g/dl
fibrinogen	0.3 g/dl

The reduction in colloid osmotic pressure permits fluid loss from intravascular to extracellular space and edema formation in accordance with Starling's law: mean capillary hydrostatic pressure + tissue colloid osmotic pressure = tissue pressure + plasma colloid osmotic pressure. In other words, at equilibrium the sum of the forces that move fluid out of the vascular bed must equal the sum of forces directed toward moving fluid into it. Normally, mean capillary hydrostatic pressure is 25 mm Hg and plasma colloid osmotic pressure is 28 mm Hg. Tissue pressure is thought to be near 0, or even a few mm Hg subatmospheric, and tissue colloid osmotic pressure averages 4 mm Hg.

Although the reduction in plasma oncotic pressure is associated with edema, the presence of hypoalbuminemia does not always result in edema. For example, in the rare clinical syndrome of congenital analbuminemia, edema is not always present (Benhold et al, 1960). It is probable that in the presence of low levels of albumin, compensation occurs by reduction in interstitial fluid oncotic pressure and an increase in pericapillary lymph flow.

Perpetuation of edema depends on increased renal sodium retention, which is signalled by a reduction in intravascular volume and activation of the renin-angiotension-aldosterone axis.

Natural History

Causes of loss of protein in urine can be benign, such as so-called "exercise" proteinuria, and postural or orthostatic proteinuria. Occasionally traces of protein are found in dehydrated children, especially when they are febrile. If proteinuria is persistent and no other abnormalities in the urine sediment are present, a check for orthostatic proteinuria is appropriate. This is best done by examination of the first specimen voided immediately on awakening in the morning. If the concentration of protein is not greater than 10 mg/dl but protein is present later in the day (in a specimen of similar specific gravity), the diagnosis of postural proteinuria is established. If protein appears intermittently through the day, a relationship to vigorous exercise should be sought (Walker and Solez, 1984). Follow-up studies confirm that this condition is benign (Mery et al, 1961).

Far more commonly, proteinuria (Table 10.8) is the result of diffuse glomerular injury. When it is sufficient to cause edema, the resulting events are called the nephrotic syndrome. The characteristic features are edema, hypoalbuminemia, proteinuria, hypercholesterolemia, and hyperlipemia. Gammaglobulins are depressed, but other globulin fractions are elevated. Plasma volume may be lowered and aldosterone production increased (so that more sodium and water are reabsorbed from the renal tubule).

Diagnosis

Evaluation of proteinuria requires that the urine have a specific gravity of over 1.010, and preferably be the first voided morning specimen. Examination should be done soon after voiding and include a microscopic examination for cells, casts, lipids and bacteria. A 24-hour urine collection to measure protein output is important.

Protein clearance techniques have revealed two types of proteinuria termed selective and nonselective.

Table 10.8
Disorders Associated with Proteinuria

Benign:	
Exercise	
Febrile	<100 mg/day
Orthostatic	
Glomerular diseases	>100 mg/day
Nephrosis	
Membranous glomerulonephritis	
Membranoproliferative glomerulonephritis	
Acute glomerulonephritis	
Focal glomerular sclerosis	
Glomerular disease with systemic illness	
Systemic lupus erythematosus	
Anaphylactoid purpura	
Sickle cell disease	
Subacute bacterial endocarditis	
Goodpasture syndrome	
Diabetes	
Preeclampsia	
Amyloidosis	
Renal vein thrombosis	
Toxic nephropathies	

In the nonselective type, larger plasma proteins such as IgG constitute a significant fraction of excreted protein. This observation can be used to calculate a selectivity index, which is the ratio of IgG to albumin clearance. When the ratio is over 0.1, proteinuria is nonselective. Patients with selective proteinuria are more likely to respond to corticosteroids; hence a therapeutic trial would be indicated. With less selective proteinuria, a biopsy would be a more useful predictor of response to steroids. In minimal change nephrotic syndrome, the massive selective albuminuria is thought to represent a disorder of electrostatic barrier function.

NEPHROTIC SYNDROMES

Definition

Nephrotic syndromes are characterized by significant proteinuria, and reduction in serum albumin and total serum proteins as well as an increase in α-2 globulin. Clinically, the syndromes are characterized by massive edema. Serum lipid levels, including cholesterol are elevated. Arbitrarily, nephrotic syndromes are defined as conditions in which there is more than 50 mg/kg/day of proteinuria with serum albumin levels below 3 g/dl.

Basic Science

Primary nephrotic syndromes can be classified according to their pathological lesions, which also correlate with the differing clinical courses. Minimal change nephrotic syndrome is defined by the absence of abnormalities in the glomeruli as seen under light microscopy (allowing only for an occasional sclerosed glomerulus or slight focal tubular atrophy). With electron microscopy, fusion of the glomerular foot processes can be seen.

Focal glomerulosclerosis is defined by the presence of some completely sclerosed glomeruli with accompanying tubular atrophy and interstitial inflammation. The number of sclerosed glomeruli required to make this diagnosis is not specified by the International Study of Kidney Disease of Children (1978), but differences in therapeutic responses have been described when more than 5% of glomeruli were affected (Kohaut et al, 1981).

Mesangial proliferation is defined as an increase in mesangial cells and fibrils, to the extent of 4 or more cells per mesangial zone. Capillary walls are thickened, and a fibrinoid deposit can be seen on the epithelial aspect of the basement membrane. Immunofluorescent studies reveal anti-IgG and anti-BiC deposits along the walls of the glomerular capillaries.

Pathogenesis of Nephrotic Syndrome (Type I, Minimal Change)

Both clinical observations and laboratory studies link immunological abnormalities with nephrosis.

(Schnaper and Aune, 1987). Clinically, the susceptibility of patients to infections (especially pneumococcal), remissions after rubeola which modifies cell-mediated immunity, exacerbations with poison ivy, and various manifestations of atopy suggested a relationship between the immune system and minimal change nephrotic syndrome. T-cell dysfunction can be shown in numerous laboratory tests. Humoral immunity is also impaired, with a decrease in IgG from impaired synthesis, and a decrease in EAC rosette-forming cells. Immediate-type hypersensitivity is increased and serum IgE levels may be elevated. Finally the syndrome is associated with certain histocompatibility types, HLA B12, DRw7, and B8, B13, and B18.

Some of the reported associations may not pertain to the pathogenesis of nephrosis and a number of abnormalities may be secondary to other manifestations of the nephrotic state. The sequence of abnormalities and the primary lesion remain unknown, hence the persistence of the name idiopathic nephrotic syndrome.

Natural History

Minimal change nephrotic syndrome accounts for about 85% of cases, more than half of which are recognized before the age of 4 years, and two-thirds of them before the age of 5 years. More than two-thirds of the patients are boys.

The symptoms are usually of gradual onset, often after a mild upper respiratory infection. The first sign is often periorbital puffiness in the morning, which subsides during the day. Edema may then be noticed in the abdomen and later in the feet. Often swelling is the only complaint, but some children have a loss of appetite and produce more concentrated urine, which may foam in the toilet bowl because of dissolved protein. (See individual disorders for their respective natural courses.)

Proteinuria is selective. Microscopic hematuria is present in about one-third of the cases. Rarely does the blood urea nitrogen or blood pressure rise. Serum complement (C′3) is normal. This form of nephrosis sometimes subsides spontaneously and almost always is responsive to corticosteroids.

Treatment

GENERAL ASPECTS

Edema is the most obvious and debilitating aspect of nephrosis. If mild to moderate in extent, it will usually be improved by sodium restriction. Diuretics are neither helpful nor indicated since most children will be hypovolemic. If the edema is severe, hydrochlorothiazide may be used provided that electrolytes and cardiac status are observed closely. If hyponatremia occurs, reduction in fluid intake is preferable to use of diuretics. Elevation of plasma oncotic pressure with albumin administration can provide temporary relief, but such treatment should be used only in the presence of anasarca.

Scrupulous attention to skin care is essential in edematous children to prevent skin breakdown and infection.

Maintenance of nutrition may be difficult in edematous children who are prone to vomiting and diarrhea. They should be encouraged to eat even small portions and to drink milk to maintain positive caloric balance. If they are unable to do so, supplemental alimentation is indicated. Adequate calcium intake is important since vitamin D-binding globulin may be lost in the urine. Supplements of oral calcium and vitamins are needed.

Since relapses are most commonly triggered by infections, and infections are poorly tolerated by nephrotic patients, avoidance of exposure is very important. For this reason, arrangements for home care may be preferable to hospitalization. Instructions about the risk of infection from family members and friends cannot be overemphasized.

DRUGS

Prednisone is the most effective immunosuppressive drug and is given in a dose of about 1–2 mg/kg/24 hours. Most children have a remission, defined as protein-free urine for at least 3 days, within the first 2 weeks of therapy. Treatment is continued daily for 1–2 weeks beyond remission, then every other day up to 12 additional weeks. Nearly 80% of children will have a relapse, but will respond to another course of prednisone. For the group that does not respond, an alternate-day dose of prednisone for 3–6 months is advised since most will respond eventually (or have a spontaneous remission). Nonresponders or steroid-dependent patients are candidates for cytotoxic therapy with chlorambucil or cytoxan.

Type 2 Nephrotic Syndrome (Focal Glomerular Sclerosis)

This form of the nephrotic syndrome can appear at any age, but is most common in the first 5 years of life. It may be familial.

Natural History

This syndrome takes its name from the characteristic histology, which is the only definitive way to distinguish it from the other types. It differs clinically from minimal lesion disease by having a higher incidence of microscopic hematuria in about one-third of the patients. Blood pressure and blood urea nitrogen may be elevated.

This group of patients is particularly prone to intercurrent infections, which can include septicemia, pneumonia, peritonitis, urinary tract infection, and lymphangitis.

Treatment

The response to steroids is unpredictable, but more than one-half of the patients will fail to have a good diuresis and are then treated with other cytotoxic agents, such as chlorambucil or cyclophosphamide. About a third of patients so treated will have a remission, although some proteinuria may persist.

Overall, the prognosis is poor and many of the individuals develop renal failure within 6 years of diagnosis. Only about one-quarter of the patients will sustain a remission and have normal renal function.

Group 3 Nephrotic Syndrome (Mesangial Proliferation)

This condition is sometimes called extramembraneous glomerulonephritis or membranoproliferative glomerulonephritis (MPGN) with a nephrotic syndrome.

Natural History

This particular nephropathy occurs in children of all ages. It should be considered whenever nephrosis occurs beyond age 7 years, or when clinical improvement does not occur after 1 month of steroid therapy. The nephrotic syndrome is usually present in association with macroscopic hematuria, although occasionally only microscopic hematuria is observed. Hypertension occurs in about one-third of patients.

Diagnosis

The diagnosis depends on identification of glomerular ultrastructural changes on renal biopsy. The mildest changes are subendothelial deposits of immune complexes with an intact glomerular basement membrane. More advanced lesions include thickening of the basement membrane and the most marked changes are disruption of the basement membrane and subendothelial and subepithelial deposits. No evidence of inflammation is present. Over time, glomerulosclerosis develops.

The immune complexes consist of IgG, IgM, C3, Clq, and C4. Serum complement levels are depressed.

Treatment

MPGN has been so difficult to treat that many physicians have opted for supportive therapy only; the drugs that were tried have variable effects and often considerable toxicity. The problem is that it has not been possible to distinguish the individuals who will have a complete spontaneous remission from those who will progress to renal failure.

High-dose prednisone given on alternate days has improved survival according to McEnery et al (1986). Optimal results were obtained if prednisone was started within a year of onset of symptoms. The dose was 2.0–2.5 mg/kg every 48 hours up to a maximum of 80 mg. Results were evaluated by comparison with previous published experiences; renal survival at 10 years of follow-up was 90% when treatment was initiated with 1 year of onset.

Relapses are often associated with infection and marked by gross hematuria and the nephrotic syndrome.

The side-effects of high-dose prednisone have included growth delay which was most marked in boys. Small posterior subcapsular cataracts developed in 18% of the 51 patients in McEnery's series.

Prognosis

About 10% of individuals with biopsy-proven membranoproliferative changes develop renal failure within 2 years if untreated. About 50% will develop renal failure by 10 years. The other half will sustain a permanent remission without treatment.

Congenital Nephrotic Syndrome

The condition defined as congenital nephrotic syndrome is hereditary and is transmitted as an autosomal recessive trait. It is characterized by proteinuria at or shortly after birth.

Basic Science

There is a pseudocystic dilatation of the proximal tubules that resembles a rosary chain on light microscopy. The tubular cells are hyperplastic at the site of the dilation and, rarely, atrophic. Immunofluorescent studies are usually negative. This is distinguished from microcystic disease since most all the glomeruli are involved, with abnormalities in the glomerular basement membranes, foot processes, and sclerosis of glomerular tufts.

The etiology is unknown. The absence of heparin-sulfate anionic sites in the glomerular basement membrane raises the possibility of an underlying defect in proteoglycan synthesis in some patients (Vernier et al, 1983).

Epidemiology

Congenital nephrosis has been found most commonly in Finland, or in families of Finnish extraction in other parts of the world. The gene frequency is estimated to be 1/200 Finns. It has occurred in only one of a pair of dizygotic twins.

Natural History

Infants with the congenital nephrotic syndrome are frequently born prematurely and first identified by a very large placenta, which may weigh more than 25% of the weight of the infant.

The babies themselves have wide-set eyes and low-set ears and the cartilage of the nose and ears is said to be soft. Edema may be present at birth, but more commonly appears in the first 4 weeks of life. Abdominal distention from ascites is very common and may be accompanied by dilation of the veins in the abdominal wall. Often the infants have an intense diarrhea which may be associated with further protein loss and malnutrition. Blood pressure in this condition is almost always normal. Growth is usually profoundly retarded.

The course is progressive, and most children die of sepsis or thrombotic complications in the first year of life.

Diagnosis

The laboratory investigations reveal hypoproteinemia with the albumin and γ-globulin levels low and a considerable elevation of the α-2 lipoprotein levels. Cholesterol rises and complement fractions fall as the disease progresses. A rise in blood urea and creatinine levels occurs late. Other causes of familial congenital nephrosis that require evaluation in differential diagnosis include congenital syphilis, malaria, toxoplasmosis, and possibly cytomegalovirus. Some forms of interstitial kidney disease with glomerulosclerosis are found in pseudohermaphrodites who eventually develop Wilms tumor (Drash syndrome). Nephrosis can be a part of the nail patella syndrome, congenital rubella, or maternal mercury poisoning.

Treatment

Steroids are ineffective and often are tolerated poorly. The only treatment is symptomatic—diuretics for the edema, antibiotics for infection, maintenance of normal fluid and electrolyte balance, and optimal nutritional intake that may require nasogastric feeding. The infants may require added calcium to prevent hypocalcemia and rickets.

Nephrectomy and management with dialysis prevent urinary protein loss, and are recommended at 2–6 months of age, before frank renal failure develops.

The infants can be maintained on chronic dialysis until renal transplantation. The time of transplantation depends on sufficient growth to permit the donor kidney to be transplanted into the peritoneal cavity. The disease does not reappear in the transplanted kidney.

Prevention

Pathologic changes of congenital nephrosis have been seen in a 19-week fetus. A rise in amniotic fluid α-fetoprotein occurs before then and, thus, is valuable for prenatal diagnosis.

CASE ILLUSTRATION

A 2.2-kg male infant was born after a normal pregnancy at 37 weeks' gestation. Both parents were of northern European ancestry, but were not from Finland. On initial examination the infant was normal except for a gastroschisis which prompted transfer to The Children's Hospital. A routine urinalysis showed proteinuria which progressed to 2 g/24 hours by 1 month of age. Initial ultrasonograms showed normal sized kidneys, but they were clearly enlarged by 1 month.

The course was complicated by the staged repair of the gastroschisis, respiratory compromise, and the need for mechanical ventilation. In order to promote growth, he was fed through a central venous catheter. He became colonized with *Candida parasipilosis,* which was treated with a course of amphotericin B. Management of renal and respiratory failure was complicated, and renal transplantation was not an option with the compromised abdominal cavity. The infant survived 8 months before death with *Staphylococcus epidermidis* bacteremia and *C. parasipilosis* fungemia.

QUESTION AND COMMENT

If the child had not had a major defect in the anterior abdominal wall, when would nephrectomy have been recommended?

Once the infant is stabilized after birth, and is nursing well, the timing of nephrectomy should be based on the magnitude of the selective proteinuria. The purpose of nephrectomy is to reduce protein losses. Peritoneal dialysis or hemodialysis in a young infant has its own risks and would not be undertaken until essential. In general, nephrectomy is recommended at 2–6 months, and renal transplantation as soon as the abdominal cavity can accept a donor kidney.

REFERENCES

Benhold H, Klaus D, Scheurlen PG: Volume regulation and renal function in analbuminemia. *Lancet* 2:1169, 1960.

Brenner BM, Rector FC (eds): *The Kidney,* 3rd edition. Philadelphia, WB Saunders, 1986, p. 901.

Chang RLS, Deen WB, Robertson CR, et al: Permselectivity of the glomerular capillary wall. III Restricted transport of polyanions. *Kidney Int* 8:212, 1975.

International Study of Kidney Disease in Children: Nephrotic syndrome in children: Prediction of histopathology from clinical and laboratory characteristics at the time of diagnosis. *Kidney Internat* 13:159, 1978.

International Study of Kidney Disease in Children: The primary nephrotic syndrome in children. Identification of patients with minimal change nephrotic syndrome for initial response to prednisone. *J Pediatr* 98:561, 1981.

Kohaut EC, Edwards GA, Hill LL, et al: Focal glomerulosclerosis: Extent of involvement related to steroid resistance. *Am J Clin Pathol* 75:181, 1981.

McEnery PT, McAdams AJ, West CD: The effect of prednisone in a high-dose, alternate-day regimen on the natural history of idiopathic membranoproliferative glomerulonephritis. *Medicine* 64:401, 1986.

Melvin T, Sibley R, Michael AF: Nephrotic Syndrome. In Tune BM, Mendoza SA (eds): *Pediatric Nephrology.* New York, Churchill Livingstone, 1984.

Mery JP, Berger J, Milhand A, et al: La proteinurie orthostatique. A propos de 300 observations. *Rev Pract (Paris)* II:3115, 1961.

Robson AM, Giangiacoma J, Keinstra RA, et al: Normal glomerular premeability and its modification by minimal change nephrotic syndrome. *J Clin Invest* 54:1190, 1974.

Schnaper HW, Aune TM: Steroid-sensitive mechanism of soluble immune response suppressor production in steroid-responsive nephrotic syndrome. *J Clin Invest* 79:257, 1987.

Vernier RL, Klein DJ, Sisson SP, et al: Heparin-sulfate-rich anionic sites in the human glomerular basement membrane: Decreased concentration in congenital nephrotic syndrome. *N Engl J Med* 309:1001, 1983.

Pediatric Urolithiasis

8

Definition

Urolithiasis may be divided arbitrarily into several classes based on stone composition, metabolic causes, site of origin, symptomatology and the presence or absence of obstruction, infection, or foreign body. One simple way to consider stones is as primary (no complicating structural factors) or secondary (due to obstructed and/or infected urinary tracts; see Table 10.9).

Basic Science

Biochemical studies have shown that urinary tract stones are composed of a mucoprotein matrix and crystals of varying composition and configuration. The major crystalline components are: calcium oxalate, magnesium ammonium phosphate (struvite), calcium phosphate, uric acid, and cystine.

Natural History

Several factors, including urinary pH, solute load, and activity of urinary inhibitors, influence crystal formation. Therefore, in addition to metabolic imbalances, the state of hydration is critical for initiation of stone formation. Secondary factors, including obstruction with stasis, and infections with urea-splitting organisms, can also be important. Infected stones most commonly associated with obstruction usually consist of struvite.

Table 10.9
Classification of Urolithiasis

- Renal tubular syndrome
  - Renal tubular acidosis
  - Cystinuria
- Enzyme disorders
  - Primary hyperoxaluria
  - Xanthuria
- Hypercalciuric states
  - Primary hyperparathyroidism
  - Sarcoidosis
  - Hypervitaminosis D
  - Milk-alkali syndrome
  - Neoplasms
  - Infantile hypercalcemia
  - Immobilization
- Uric acid lithiasis
  - Hereditary hyperuricosuria
  - Myeloproliferative disorders
  - Oxaluria from increased absorption (intestinal disease)
- Idiopathic renal lithiasis
- Infected and obstructed urolithiasis
- Endemic calculi

Metabolic factors can be important. Uric acid lithiasis is rare in children, but can present as a complication of treatment for myeloproliferative disorders. Hyperoxaluria occurs in inflammatory bowel disease from increased absorption oxalate and may result in calcium oxalate stones. The reason for increased absorption is thought to be from binding of intestinal calcium to fat, leaving oxalate in its soluble (hence, absorbable) form. Idiopathic renal lithiasis is a term often used in the past for poorly understood metabolic disorders. Many patients so designated have been shown to have more subtle defects, such as absorptive or renal leak hypercalciuria, as a cause of recurrent stone formation. Inherited disorders of metabolism such as hyperoxaluria or cystinuria must also be excluded.

Environmental factors may play a role in the development of stone disease. Children immobilized after trauma or surgery are at risk for calcium urolithiasis. A predisposition to calculi is endemic in developing countries, especially in Southeast Asia, and usually presents as bladder stones, with symptoms of frequency, urgency, and pain on voiding.

Diagnosis

Gross hematuria, urosepsis, abdominal or flank pain, and renal colic are the most common presenting symptoms. Painless hematuria in childhood may occur as a premonitory sign to later symptomatic calcium urolithiasis. Special attention must be paid to past medical history, such as immobilization, excess vitamin D or calcium intake, or prior medical intervention. Laboratory investigation should include examination of urine sediment for crystals and infection; collection of urine for calcium, phosphate, uric acid, and oxalate levels; cyanide nitroprusside screening of urine for cystine; radiographic studies for stone localization; and screening for electrolyte abnormalities, hypercalcemia, or hyperuricemia in serum.

Treatment

Prevention and treatment will depend on the underlying metabolic defect, if any, and the degree of obstruction created by the stone. Renal tubular acidosis is treated by oral alkalinization, cystinuria requires hydration, alkalinization, and occassionaly administration of D-penicillamine, which acts to bind cystine in the gut. Medical experience with treating enzymatic defects such as hyperoxaluria has not been extremely successful. For hypercalciuria, increasing fluid intake, reducing excess calcium intake, and use of thiazide diuretics are very helpful. With high grade, symptomatic obstructing stones and/or infected stones associated with underlying obstruction, surgical therapy may be indicated. New techniques, including percutaneous extraction or dissolution, and extracorporeal shock wave lithotripsy have proved useful in children and reduced the need for open operative therapy in many (Androulakakis et al, 1982). The latter therapy (ESWL) can be used in children as long as the lung fields are shielded to prevent hemoptysis. The child is anesthetized and placed in a water bath. A number of shocks are administered that result in fragmentation of the calculi in most cases. The new modality has replaced open operative intervention in most instances (Kramolowsky et al, 1987).

Prognosis

The prognosis depends on the ability to identify and treat the underlying disorder.

REFERENCES

Androulakakis PA, Baratt TM, Ransley PG, et al: Urinary calculi in children: A 5 to 15 year followup with particular reference to recurrent and residual stones. *Br J Urol* 54:176, 1982.

Bennett AH, Colodny AH: Urinary tract calculi in children. *J Urol* 109:318, 1973.

Malek RS, Kelalis PP: Pediatric nephrolithiasis. *J Urol* 113:545, 1975.

Kramolowsky EV, Willoughby BL, Loening SA: Extracorporeal shock wave lithotripsy in children. *J Urol* 137:939, 1987.

Roy S III, Stapleton FB, Noe HN, et al: Hematuria preceding renal calculus formation in children with hypercalciuria. *J Pediatr* 99:712, 1981.

Renal Tubular Disorders

9

The renal tubule is central to the maintenance of the volume and composition of body fluids. It is also the site of action of aldosterone and vasopressin, and of production of renin and 1, 25 hydroxy-vitamin D_3. The major inherited disorders of tubule function affect phosphate and amino acid transport, glucose reabsorption, and movement of hydrogen ions and water.

The hallmarks of renal tubular dysfunction are retention of toxic substances or excessive losses of substances in the urine.

RENAL TUBULAR ACIDOSIS

Definition

Renal tubular acidosis (RTA) is a condition characterized by sustained metabolic acidosis, urine pH >5.4, and hyperchloremia.

The first cases described were in infants who had a transient form of renal tubular acidosis that is no longer observed (Lightwood, 1963). The condition that is observed in infants is associated with a permanent defect in urine acidification (Caruana and Buckalew, 1988).

Basic Science

Primary RTA can stem from an inability of the distal tubule to establish a hydrogen ion gradient between blood and tubule urine, regardless of the degree of metabolic acidosis. The pH of the urine cannot be reduced below 5.4. The cellular basis of this defect is not known.

Another form of primary RTA, called proximal RTA, results from failure of bicarbonate resorption in the proximal tubule. It is distinguished from distal RTA by large urinary bicarbonate losses, and a poor response to alkali therapy.

Most instances of RTA are secondary to other conditions that impair renal tubular function as listed in Table 10.10.

Epidemiology

Distal RTA can be inherited as an autosomal dominant condition, although sporadic cases occur. A few families have been documented to have a deficiency in the enzyme carbonic anhydrase. The incidence of primary RTA is not known, although both distal and proximal defects on an hereditary basis are unusual.

Table 10.10
Causes of Renal Tubular Acidosis[1]

Distal Type	Proximal Type
Primary	Primary
Sporadic, with infantile or later onset	Sporadic, with infantile or later onset
Hereditary, with infantile or later onset	Hereditary, with infantile or later onset
Hereditary, associated with nerve deafness	
Secondary[2]	Secondary[3]
Amphotericine B	Cystinosis
Hyperimmunoglobulinemia	Galactosemia
Renal transplantation	Heavy metals (lead, cadmium)
Medullary nephrocalcinosis due to hypercalcemia hyperparathyroidism, or vitamin D intoxication	Hereditary fructose intolerance
	Primary or secondary hyperparathyroidism
Toluene sniffing	Hyperimmunoglobulinemia
Ehlers-Danlos syndrome	Vitamin D deficiency rickets
Obstructive uropathy	Wilson disease
Lithium salts	Lowe syndrome
	Tyrosinosis
	Outdated tetracycline
	Leigh syndrome
	Renal vascular accidents in the newborn period

[1]Reproduced with permission from Drummond, KN: Renal tubular acidosis. In Behrman RE, Vaughn VC (eds): *Nelson's Textbook of Pediatrics*. Philadelphia, WB Saunders, 1983, p. 1344.
[2]Distal renal tubular acidosis has been reported rarely in other conditions; most are listed in the references.
[3]Many of these disorders are expressed as the Fanconi syndrome of proximal renal tubular dysfunction and, thus, are associated with generalized aminoaciduria, glycosuria, hyperkaliuria, uricosuria, hypercalciuria, and phosphaturia, in addition to bicarbonaturia.

Natural History

Regardless of etiology, a predictable chain of events follows either deficient acidification of urine or bicarbonate wasting. The higher the urine pH, the more bicarbonate will be present. Loss of bicarbonate anion must be accompanied by loss of cations, mainly sodium and potassium. Loss of sodium leads to reduction in extracellular volume and secondary hyperaldosteronism, which promotes further loss of potassium. The consequence is a hypokalemic, hyperchloremic metabolic acidosis. Hypercalciuria, only observed in distal RTA, leads to nephrocalcinosis and osteomalacia, and retarded bone age. The deposition of calcium in the kidney may accentuate tubular dysfunction.

Diagnosis

In children, the presenting complaint is often growth retardation but the diagnosis may be suspected if a metabolic acidosis is sustained, or rickets are noted clinically or radiographically. Only later do the metabolic defects produce symptoms. Hyperkalemia can lead to muscle weakness and cardiac arrhythmias, polyuria, and isosthenuria. If acidemia is severe, anorexia, vomiting, hyperventilation, and vascular collapse may ensue.

Biochemical changes are exemplified by a low plasma pH with a urinary pH usually between 6.5 and 7.5. In distal tubular acidosis, urinary calcium levels reach 10–20 mg/kg/day.

Early diagnosis is of great importance since alkali therapy is so effective. The condition should always be considered in infants and children whose growth is impaired.

Treatment

The essence of treatment is administration of alkali in sufficient amounts to correct the acidosis. Potassium may be needed to restore deficits. The maintenance bicarbonate intake is 2–3 mEq/kg/day in distal RTA, but higher intake may be required. Children can be maintained on a solution of sodium and potassium citrate. Once the acidosis is corrected, the children grow normally. Treatment, which is lifelong, reverses nephrocalcinosis and osteopenia.

DEFECTS IN PHOSPHATE TRANSPORT

Basic Science

The most important regulators of phosphate excretion are plasma parathormone concentration and dietary phosphate intake. Changes in glomerular filtration rate and plasma phosphate concentration initiate the regulatory events that change parathormone concentration. An increase in parathormone inhibits distal phosphate reabsorption. Dietary phosphate restriction increases renal reabsorptive capacity. Conversely, dietary phosphate excess limits the ability of the kidney to reabsorb phosphate. Vitamin D and its metabolites enhance net phosphate resorption.

Acute hyperphosphatemia can occur with use of phosphate enemas, in acute renal failure, especially with rhabdomyolysis, and during chemotherapy for lymphomas and leukemia. It can induce a fall in plasma calcium with precipitation of calcium phosphate in soft tissues.

Chronic hyperphosphatemia occurs in chronic renal failure or hypoparathyroidism. Calcium levels fall from reduced production of 1, 25 $(OH)_2$ D_3, and bone resorption is inhibited.

Defects in renal phosphate transport constitute one feature of Fanconi syndrome, which includes phosphaturia, a generalized aminoaciduria, and renal glycosuria (see below). Other rare situations in which hypophosphatemia occurs are vitamin D-resistant rickets, vitamin D-deficiency rickets, and vitamin D-dependent rickets, in which secondary hyperparathyroidism is observed.

DEFECTS IN AMINO ACID TRANSPORT (AMINOACIDURIA)

Excess amino acids in urine may result from a metabolic defect, or a renal tubular defect, or both.

Basic Science

Amino acids are filtered by the glomerulus and are normally 95–99% resorbed in the proximal convoluted tubule. The mechanisms have been well-studied in tissue slices and isolated tubules. Briefly, amino acids move against an electrochemical gradient and show stereospecificity. L-forms are better reabsorbed than are D-forms, for example.

Many agents that cause defective resorption of amino acids (including heavy metals, such as lead and cystine) inhibit sulfhydryl-requiring enzymes. Cystinosis is the most common cause of generalized aminoaciduria in children. Glycogen storage disease, galactosemia, and hereditary fructose intolerance cause renal tubular damage that is reflected by aminoaciduria.

FANCONI SYNDROME

Definition

Three findings are required to make the diagnosis: generalized aminoaciduria, renal glycosuria, and renal phosphaturia. Defective renal tubular reabsorption of water, sodium, potassium, bicarbonate, and organic acids is usually present. The syndrome has many causes, the most common of which is cystinosis.

Natural History

Cystinosis is a recessively inherited disorder of cystine metabolism, in which cystine is accumulated in lysosomes and is not transported to the cytosol. Free cystine concentrations in plasma are normal.

Most affected children are normal for about 6 months. Thereafter, polyuria and recurrent fever and dehydration (a diabetes insipidus-like picture) ensue. As renal tubular failure advances hypophosphatemic rickets and poor growth become prominent. Most children remain below the third percentile for height and weight for life.

Other organ involvement includes deposits of cystine in the cornea and thyroid, but the CNS is spared.

Eventually glomerular dysfunction progresses, and end-stage renal failure occurs before 10 years of age.

One form of cystinosis is benign, because even though the cornea and bone marrow may be involved, the kidney is spared. Other individuals have late onset or adolescent cystinosis. These individuals have milder disease than those whose onset was in the first year of life. All forms of the disease follow an autosomal recessive pattern of inheritance.

Diagnosis

Slit-lamp examination of the cornea is the most useful test once aminoaciduria has been demonstrated and heavy metal poisoning has been ruled out.

Treatment

Attention to the metabolic disturbances can improve general well-being. Adequate fluid intake and maintenance of optimal pH with a potassium-containing alkalinizing mixture such as sodium, potassium citrate, and 10,000–15,000 units of vitamin D daily can prevent many complications. Eventually, however, renal failure will require dialysis and transplantation. Renal function can be restored, but deposition of crystals in the cornea progresses.

DEFECTS IN CARBOHYDRATE RESORPTION

Definition

Renal glucosuria is a renal proximal tubular defect that prevents resorption of filtered glucose. Glucosuria is present with a normal blood sugar.

Natural History

These individuals are detected by routine urinalysis since they are asymptomatic. The only importance of the condition is to be sure affected individuals are not mistaken for diabetics.

For a discussion of hereditary fructose intolerance, see page 919.

WATER TRANSPORT

Nephrogenic Diabetes Insipidus

This disorder of the renal tubule is characterized by failure to respond to the pituitary antidiuretic hormone, vasopressin. It may be inherited as an X-linked recessive trait, occurring mainly in males, or it can be acquired by either sex as a consequence of other diseases such as chronic renal disease, hypercalcemia, amyloidosis, or the result of drug therapy, especially lithium. It is characterized by polydipsia and polyuria.

Basic Science

Arginine vasopressin is released from the posterior pituitary in response to increased plasma osmolality and decreased plasma volume. Vasopressin binds by a specific receptor to the cells that line the collecting duct and the distal tubule. It stimulates production of adenylate cyclase which, in turn, increases cyclic adenosine monophosphate (AMP) levels. The net result is increased water reabsorption, by mechanisms that remain to be elucidated. The defect in nephrogenic diabetes insipidus is thought to be defective generation of cyclic AMP in response to vasopressin, which results in failure of tubular water resorption.

Epidemiology

The rare congenital variety of nephrogenic diabetes insipidus was presumably brought to North America by the Ulster clan from Scotland in 1761. The disorder has an X-linked autosomal dominant pattern of inheritance with male predominance. Most female heterozygotes show a partial defect in concentrating urine.

Natural History

Polyuria develops soon after birth, but may not be noticed until the infant displays other symptoms such as fever and dehydration. Thirst is intense, and older children are rarely without their thermos bottles. Enlarged bladders are common in these children. Growth failure and mental retardation may occur, presumably as a consequence of episodes of dehydration and hypernatremia, and poor caloric intake.

CASE ILLUSTRATION

The patient was the 2.7-kg baby boy of a full-term uncomplicated pregnancy. The baby did well in the nursery but, at home, the mother noted that he drank only water and had a poor appetite. At the age of 9 months the baby was admitted to the hospital with a history of vomiting, diarrhea, and failure to thrive, as well as recurrent fevers. Urine specific gravities were consistently 1.003, except after a solute load when the specific gravity rose to 1.013. No diagnosis was made at this time.

At the age of 4 years, the child was again admitted and a repeat evaluation for polydipsia, polyuria, and short stature was performed. Once again, urine specific gravities were consistently 1.002–1.004 and urine osmolality averaged 82 mOsm/kg H_2O. Serum osmolality was 298 mOsm/kg H_2O and serum sodium was 142. Neither water deprivation nor pitressin therapy resulted in any change in urine osmolality. A diagnosis of nephrogenic diabetes insipidus was made.

The patient was placed on a low solute diet with Polycose (a glucose polymer of 900 mOsm/kg water) and Lipomil added for extra calories. On this regimen, his growth averaged 5 cm/year. After age 7 years, the patient followed his diet erratically. He urinated roughly 10–12 times per day and twice each night. His fluid turnover was estimated to be at least 10 liters each day. At age 14 years, he showed signs of puberty and began his adolescent growth spurt. His final adult height is 154 cm.

At present, the patient is 21 years old, married, and has two children. There are no other members of his family with diabetes insipidus. He has complained over the past several years of back pain relieved by urination. Otherwise he feels his diabetes insipidus is under good control on a high calorie, low protein, low salt diet.

This patient is leading a productive happy life despite a large fluid turnover. He is followed yearly with particular attention to renal function. Although he is short, his height is not too inappropriate, because of genetically short parents.

Diagnosis

Urine osmolality is usually under 50 mOsm, and does not increase after fluid restriction or vasopressin.

A water deprivation test (usually 4 hours is sufficient) will reveal the presence of diabetes insipidus. Continuous excretion of dilute urine after the administration of vasopressin establishes the diagnosis of nephrogenic diabetes insipidus. These patients excrete a hypotonic urine despite 15-fold variations in plasma vasopressin levels.

Treatment

Solute restriction and diuretics that promote negative sodium balance such as hydrochlorthiazide in doses of 1–2 mg/kg/day are of some help. Indomethacin, 1–2 mg/kg/24 hours, may be synergistic with thiazides and is effective in some cases.

NEW DEVELOPMENTS

A natriuretic peptide isolated from atrial muscle and called atrial natriuretic peptide has recently been described (deBold et al, 1981). It appears to be a factor in the complex neurohumoral mechanisms that regulate sodium and water balance. Release of the hormone is stimulated by atrial distention, epinephrine, arginine vasopressin, and acetylcholine. The half-life of the peptides in the blood is on the order of minutes. Binding to specific receptors in kidney, blood vessels, and adrenal cortex has been demonstrated (deBold, 1985).

The response of the intact animal to an increase in atrial natriuretic factor is a rapid diuresis of short duration, and depressant effects on aldosterone and renin secretion. The factor probably has an inhibitory effect on adenylate cyclase, thus producing a temporary nephrogenic diabetes insipidus. Inhibition of secretion of natriuretic peptide should follow from low blood volume. The role of this factor in nephrogenic diabetes insipidus remains to be elucidated.

Prognosis

The above modes of therapy, if followed carefully, will permit normal growth and weight gain. Unfortunately, in our experience the diet is difficult for patients to manage, particularly older children.

Despite rigorous medical management, these patients require a high water intake, even during the night. Bed wetting is often a problem, even in the older child. Dilation of the bladder and even the upper urinary tract may occur in older children and adults who attempt to go for longer periods of time without urinating. The disorder is lifelong.

REFERENCES

Anderson B: Regulation of water intake. *Physiol Rev* 58:582, 1978.

Caruana RJ, Buckalew VM: The syndrome of distal (Type 1) renal tubular acidosis. *Medicine* 67:84, 1988.

deBold AJ: Atrial natriuretic factor: A hormone produced by the heart. *Science* 230:767, 1985.

deBold AJ, Borenstein HB, Veress AT, Sonnenberg HA: A rapid and potent natriuretic response to intravenous injection of atrial myocardial extract in rats. *Life Sci* 28:89, 1981.

Drummond KN: Renal tubular acidosis. In Behrman RE, Vaughan VC (eds): *Nelson's Textbook of Pediatrics*. Philadelphia, WB Saunders, 1983, p. 1344.

Lightwood R, Butler N: Decline in primary infantile renal acidosis: Aetiological implications. *Br Med J* 1:855, 1963.

Schneider JA: Hereditary disorders of tubular function. In Tune BM, Mendoza SA (eds): *Pediatric Nephrology*. New York, Churchill Livingstone, 1984, p. 85.

Prune Belly Syndrome 10

Definition

The typical triad of prune belly syndrome consists of abdominal muscle deficiency, urinary tract dilation, and cryptorchidism. Synonyms for the syndrome include Eagle-Barrett syndrome, abdominal muscular deficiency syndrome, triad syndrome, and mesenchymal dysplasia syndrome.

Basic Science

The cause of prune belly syndrome is unknown. Its appearance is usually sporadic and the syndrome has been associated with chromosomal anomalies.

Epidemiology

This syndrome occurs approximately once in every 35,000–50,000 live births. Ninety-five percent of the reported cases are in males.

Natural History

Prune belly syndrome presents with various degrees of severity. In its most severe form, the syndrome may be detected prenatally with oligohydramnios. Postnatally, severe renal and pulmonary dysplasia result in stillbirth or neonatal death. Patent urachus and urethral atresia are often found in this setting. Moderate disease is manifested by lax abdominal wall, cryptorchidism, and hydronephrosis with mild to moderate renal insufficiency (Fig. 10.8). Milder presentations involve minimal mesenchymal abnormalities with slight hydronephrosis and normal renal function.

Diagnosis

The diagnosis of prune belly syndrome is most obviously made with the finding of an infant with the wrinkled, prune-like appearance of the thin abdominal wall, and the bilaterally nonpalpable testicles. Diagnostic studies of the urinary tract reveal hydronephrosis with irregular renal contours, deformed calyces, and tortuous ureters. The bladder is often very large, and irregular, with a urachal diverticulum seen at the dome, and a funnelled, open bladder neck. Reflux is also present in a majority of children with this syndrome.

Treatment

Immediately after birth, studies of general renal function are performed as baseline data. Pneumothorax may occur and should be promptly diagnosed and treated. Infants with mild to moderate degrees of renal functional abnormalities should not require intervention unless urosepsis or progressive deterioration occurs. Temporary urinary diversion will often allow stabilization in these situations. Primary urinary tract reconstruction early in life is sometimes indicated and has been reported as successful in cases with persistent infection and urinary stasis. Orchiopexy is often performed as a staged procedure and requires excellent technique to achieve satisfactory results.

Prognosis

The overall reported mortality rate is 20% neonatal death, 20–30% dying within 1 year after birth,

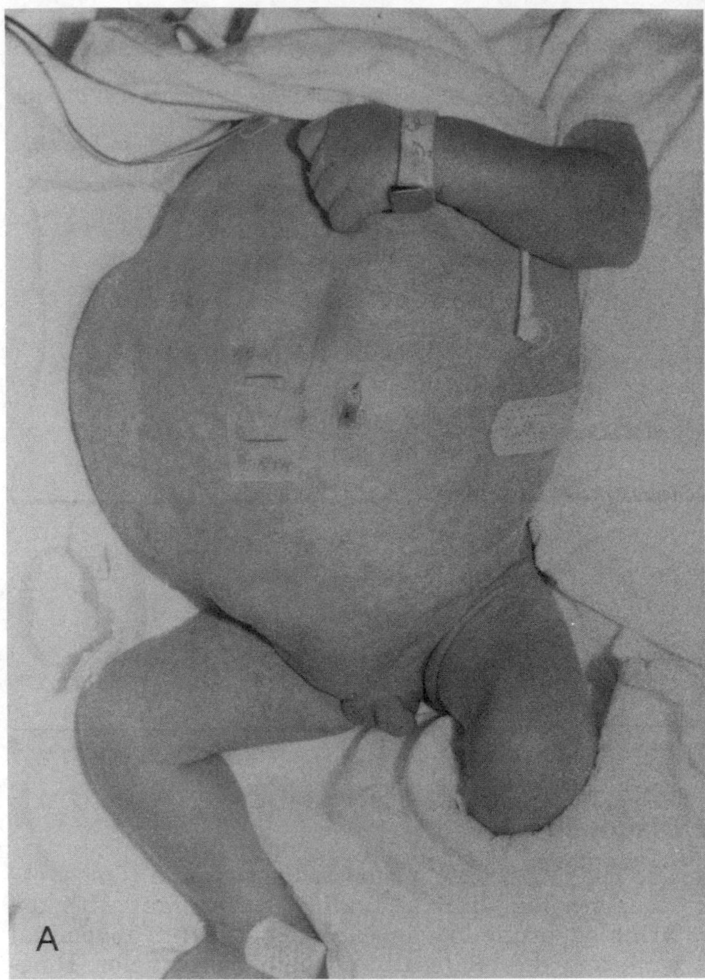

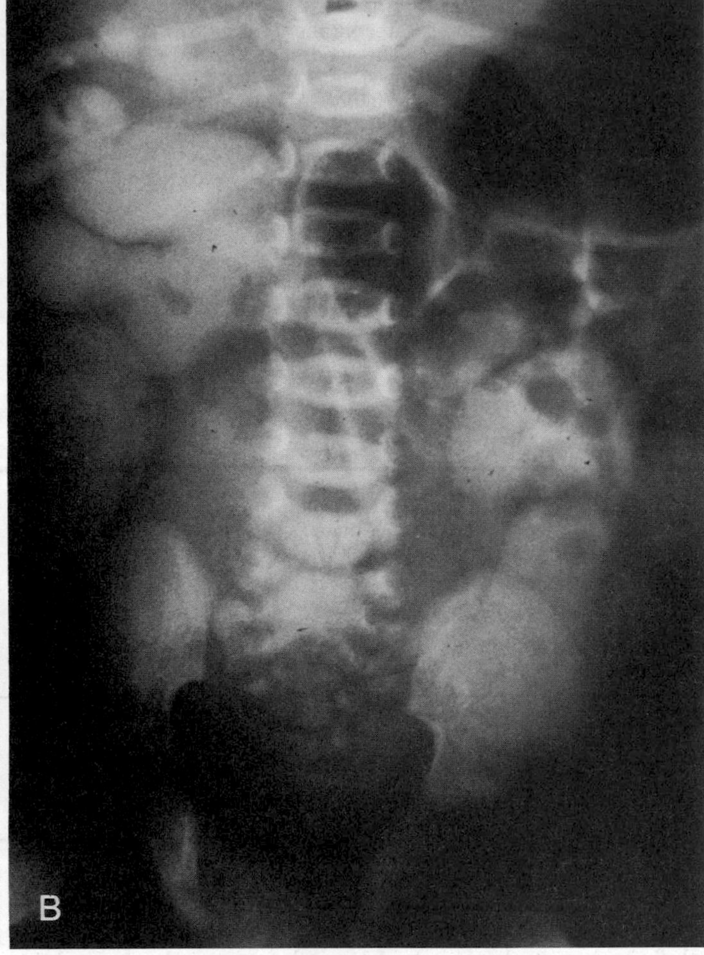

Figure 10.8. A. This photograph of a newborn male with prune belly syndrome demonstrates the lax abdominal musculature with wrinkled skin that is typical of this disease. **B.** IVU shows the hydronephrosis and tortuous megaureters associated with the syndrome. The bladder is large but poorly defined because it is filled with urine that has not yet opacified.

CASE ILLUSTRATION

This newborn male was the product of an uncomplicated gestation and vaginal delivery. The child was referred for evaluation of anatomic features of "prune belly syndrome." Physical examination revealed an infant with a lax abdominal wall with multiple skin creases, obvious herniation of visceral contents, which were covered by skin and subcutaneous tissues, and undescended testes. Radiographs of the abdomen revealed a floppy abdominal wall with some flaring of the ribs. Intravenous urogram revealed gross bilateral hydronephrosis and a large bladder. Serum creatinine remained elevated at 1.2 mg/dl. Electrolytes were within normal limits. Urine culture was negative. The child was observed and over the next several weeks, creatinine fell to 0.7, and then to 0.4 mg/dl. No surgical intervention was undertaken and the child continued to grow at around the fifth percentile. Future plans include elective bilateral orchiopexy.

and an additional 15–20% dead by the third year. Those with mild to moderate disease may have later problems with respiratory infections and/or renal functional abnormalities. Many, however, will have a satisfactory long-term outlook.

REFERENCES

Duckett JW: The prune-belly syndrome. In Kelalis PP, King LR (eds): *Clinical Pediatric Urology*. Philadelphia, WB Saunders, 1976, pp. 615–635.

Nunn IN, Stephens FD: The triad syndrome: A composite anomaly of the abdominal wall, urinary system and testes. *J Urol* 86:782, 1961.

Woodward JR, Parrott TS: Orchiopexy in the prune belly syndrome. *Br J Urol* 50:348, 1978.

Woodward JR, Parrott TS: Reconstruction of the urinary tract in prune belly syndrome. *J Urol* 119:824, 1978.

Hemolytic-Uremic Syndrome 11

Definition

Hemolytic-uremic syndrome (HUS) consists of acute renal failure, a microangiopathic hemolytic anemia, and thrombocytopenia. It can also be associated with abdominal pain, bloody diarrhea, and frank colitis. HUS represents a syndrome that can have multiple causes.

Basic Science

The major mechanism of injury in HUS appears to be damage to endothelial cells located principally in glomerular capillaries but also in renal arterioles and other organs. The current hypothesis for the mechanism of endothelial injury is that it is an inherited or acquired disturbance in prostacyclin metabolism, either the lack of a plasma factor needed for prostacyclin production, the presence of an inhibitor, or increased metabolism of prostacyclin (Remuzzi et al, 1980). Other mechanisms being explored include activation of an alternative complement pathway, inhibition of glomerular fibrinolysis, oxidant stress to vascular endothelium and erythrocytes, and/or endotoxemia leading to vascular endothelial damage (Gonzalo et al, 1981; Bergstein et al, 1982; O'Regan et al, 1980).

While the cause for this endothelial injury is not clear, once it has occurred, local deposits of fibrin and platelets are detected at the sites of injury. These fibrin deposits subsequently lead to increased platelet aggregation, consumption, and red cell injury with the peripheral findings of the thrombotic microangiopathic changes. No internal defect in red cell enzymes or membranes has been associated with the syndrome; normal red cells infused into a patient with HUS have a shortened half-life, whereas red cells from a patient with HUS infused into a normal person remain intact. HUS represents part of the continuum of the pathogenetic mechanisms that produce thrombotic thrombocytopenic purpura (TTP), with the differences being predominantly in the extent and distribution of vascular changes. In HUS, the damage is usually confined to the kidneys and is self-limited. In TTP, the onset is usually in late adulthood, with neurologic abnormalities and widespread involvement of other organs being more common.

Coagulation abnormalities are often detected within 24 hours of onset. Most notably, the fibrinogen level is elevated rather than reduced as in disseminated intravascular coagulation. The prothrombin time (PT) and partial thromboplastin time (PTT) are frequently normal and the platelet count may not correlate with evidence of intravascular coagulation.

The thrombocytopenia that results has been attributed to consumption of platelets during intravascular coagulation, aggregation in the kidneys as a result of a localized intravascular coagulation, or simply adhesion to the damaged endothelial lining. However, radionucleotide-labeled platelets have not been detected around the kidneys in patients with HUS. Therefore, the most likely mechanism appears to be that platelets are damaged by fibrin strands in the microvessels of the kidney and are subsequently destroyed in the reticuloendothelial system of the spleen and liver. The same endothelial changes in the vascular lining of the colon as well as the kidney are thought to be responsible for the colitis that occurs. With severe microvascular injury, the colitis can develop into areas of necrosis, submucosal hemorrhage, fibrinoid necrosis of small arterioles, and extensive thromboses. In extreme cases a pseudomembranous enterocolitis and a toxic megacolon can result.

NEW DEVELOPMENTS

It is possible that a strain of *Escherichia coli* that produces vero-cell cytotoxin has a role in both classic HUS in younger children and the hemorrhagic colitis of older patients (Drummond, 1985). The toxin is identical to the toxin of some shigellae that have been associated with HUS and raises the possibility of a role of an endotoxin in the pathogenesis. In addition, certain clinical pathological correlations have been established that suggest that if the damage is primarily glomerular as distinct from arterial, a more classic HUS results and carries a good prognosis. Predominantly arterial microangiopathy appears to occur in older children and adults and results in more severe cases of hypertension, renal damage, and poor prognosis.

Epidemiology

Eighty percent of childhood cases have been reported to occur in children under 3 years old (Loirat et al, 1984). The ratio of males to females is 1:1. Sibling involvement has been reported with two different types of familial cases, each type established on the basis of onset, geographic area, and mortality. It appears that siblings whose onset occurred within a short time of each other (suggesting an environmental influence) have better prognoses than those whose onsets are more than a year apart, the latter suggesting a genetic influence. The mode of inheritance is not known.

Natural History

There are several different forms of HUS. The classic or prototypical form occurs principally in infants under 3 years of age, usually as isolated cases or in summer outbreaks. It is responsible for most cases in North America. It presents with a prodrome of bloody diarrhea followed by a symptom-free interval of 1–10 days before the onset of the anemia and anuria. It is predominantly characterized by glomerular thrombotic microangiopathy. Abnormalities in prostacyclin function are absent. The prognosis for this condition is good if standard treatment for acute renal failure is administered.

A postinfectious form usually follows infection with *Shigella dysenteriae 1, Streptococcus pneumoniae, Salmonella typhiminimum,* and some viruses. These cases are not limited to younger children. Endotoxemia and disseminated intravascular coagulation can be present. Hereditary forms may present in infancy or in adulthood and be recurrent. In these forms, the microangiopathy predominantly involves renal arterioles and hypertension is severe. In these situations, patients may lack the factor needed for adequate prostacyclin production or may have an inhibitor that prevents production.

A fourth form demonstrates evidence of immune pathogenesis that may also be familial. It is characterized by a low plasma C3, activation of the alternative complement pathway, C3 deposits on the glomerular membrane, and, in some cases, a plasma C3 nephritic factor.

Finally, there are forms of HUS associated with other illnesses or precipitating factors including systemic lupus erythematosus, scleroderma, radiation to the kidneys, immunosuppresive drugs, oral contraceptives, or pregnancy. In these cases, the microangiopathy is predominantly arterial and the prognosis is usually poor.

The child with the more "classic" disease may have had a flu-like illness or diarrhea before presenting looking pale and frequently showing petechiae. Lethargy and irritability are frequent findings. Jaundice is uncommon. Neurologic manifestations are rare in the younger children, but cerebral infarcts can occur. Nephrophathy can present as hematuria, proteinuria, edema, oliguria, anuria, and hypertension. Acute complications of HUS are usually those associated with acute renal failure and its treatment. These can include hyperkalemia, metabolic acidosis, hypocalcemia, hypertension, encephalopathy, infection, inanition, bleeding, cardiac failure, and dehydration. The acute phase lasts about a week, but can persist for a month or more before renal function returns.

Diagnosis

Diagnosis is made when acute renal failure, hemolytic anemia, and thrombocytopenia are present. Hemoglobin levels will usually be from 3–10 g/dl. Examination of peripheral blood will show fragmented cells or schistocytes as the predominant form. Reticulocytes are elevated. The Coombs test is usually negative and enzymatic defects of red blood cells have not been found. Haptoglobin concentration is decreased consistent with intravascular hemolysis. The white count is often markedly elevated and the platelet count is usually under 140,000 but rarely will fall below 20,000. It will usually remain low for 1–2 weeks. The fibrinogen level can often be elevated rather than reduced with normal PT and PTT times. Notably, the platelet count need not correlate with evidence of intravascular coagulation. Elevation of BUN, serum creatinine, uric acid, potassium, phosphorus, hydrogen ion, and lipid concentrations may occur with a decrease in serum calcium, bicarbonate, and albumin levels. Hypertension can also be present at the onset or after a volume infusion.

Early hemodialysis or peritoneal dialysis is the mainstay of therapy since it prevents serious metabolic problems in this multisystem disease.

Treatment

A variety of treatment modalities have been explored including the use of heparin and other anticoagulants, steroids, exchange transfusion, plasmapheresis, splenectomy, fibrinolytic agents (such as streptokinase, urokinase), aspirin, and dipyridamole. Reports on the use of anticoagulants remain conflicting and experimental therapeutic trials have usually been

CASE ILLUSTRATION

A 3-year-old white female was well until 4 days before admission when she developed frequent red loose watery stools and some vomiting. She also apparently had diffuse abdominal pain for the 2 days before she was admitted to the hospital. On admission, she was afebrile, pale, and irritable with a blood pressure of 108/60 mm Hg. The physical examination was remarkable for mild dehydration but otherwise no specific findings. The laboratory, however, revealed a hematocrit of 22% and platelets of 39,000 mm^3. Her BUN was 46 mg/dl, and creatinine 0.8 mg/dl. She became anuric shortly after admission and was maintained with meticulous fluid management and infusion of high carbohydrate loads to decrease ureagenesis through endogenous protein catabolism. Nonetheless, her BUN rose to 110 mg/dl and creatinine was 7.7 mg/dl. She was started on peritoneal dialysis and continued for 48 hours. At that time she began to produce urine and her platelet count returned to normal. Over the subsequent week, her renal function returned to normal and she was discharged. She has remained well.

COMMENT

This patient presented a fairly typical course including a colitis that preceded the onset of evidence of anemia or uremia.

Although many forms of therapy, including heparin, salicylates, and exchange transfusion have been reported, no convincing evidence suggests that these interventions are helpful. Most of the patients will recover with the kind of supportive care this child received and have no persistent renal dysfunction.

uncontrolled or have too few individuals to permit definitive claims. At present, plasma infusion to replace the missing plasma components, plasmapheresis (either to replace a factor or remove a toxic factor), and exchange transfusion are used in serious cases (Gillor et al, 1983). γ-Gobulin infusions look promising.

It is to be hoped that, if verotoxin proves to be the proposed causative factor for the majority of cases in younger children, the administration of a hyperimmune globulin-containing antitoxin may be the next step. To date, the most successful results are obtained by early vigorous supportive care of the acute renal failure.

Prognosis

Mortality during the acute phase of HUS ranges from 7–10% (Loirat et al, 1984). Serious renal defects are believed to occur in at least 20% of cases. Factors associated with a better prognosis include younger age, presentation in the summer months, and in those patients requiring dialysis, a short prodromal diarrhea has been associated with a better outcome, especially among males (Trompetter et al, 1983). Five-year follow-up suggests that over 60% of children demonstrate no functional sequelae and less than 5% require chronic hemodialysis (Loirat et al, 1984).

REFERENCES

Bergstein JM, Kuederli U, Bang NU: Plasma inhibitor of glomerular fibrinolysis in hemolytic uremic syndrome. *Am J Med* 73:322, 1982.

Dolislager D, Tune B: The hemolytic uremic syndrome: Spectrum of severity and significance of prodrome. *Am J Dis Child* 132:55, 1978.

Drummond KN: Hemolytic uremic syndrome then and now. *N Engl J Med* 312:116, 1985.

Gillor A, Bulla M, Roth B, et al: Plasmapheresis as a therapeutic measure in hemolytic uremic syndrome in children. *Klin Wochenschr* 61:363, 1983.

Gonzalo A, Mampaso F, Gallego N, et al: Hemolytic uremic syndrome with hypocomplementemia and deposits of IGM and C3 in the involved renal tissue. *Clin Nephrol* 16:193, 1981.

Grupe WE: Clinical pathological conference. *N Engl J Med* 304:715, 1982.

Kaplan BS, Thomson PD, de Chadarevian JP. The hemolytic uremic syndrome. *Pediatr Clin North Am* 23:761, 1970.

Kaplan BS, Drummond KN: The hemolytic uremic syndrome as a syndrome. *N Engl J Med* 298:964, 1978.

Loirat C, Sonsino E, Moreno AV, et al: Hemolytic uremic syndrome: An analysis of the natural history and prognostic features. *Acta Pediatr Scand* 73:505, 1984.

O'Regan S, Chesney RW, Kaplan BS, et al: Red cell membrane phospholipid abnormalities in hemolytic uremic syndrome. *Clin Nephrol* 15:14, 1980.

Remuzzi G, Mecca G, Livio M, et al: Prostacycline generation by cultured endothelial cells in hemolytic uremic syndrome. *Lancet* 1:656, 1980.

Trompetter RS, Schwartz R, Chantler C, et al: Hemolytic uremic syndrome: An analysis of prognostic features. *Arch Dis Child* 58:101, 1983.

Acute Renal Failure 12

Definition

Acute renal failure is a sudden and usually reversible decrease in glomerular filtration rate (GFR) that results in alterations in regulation of fluid and electrolyte balance and in accumulation of metabolic toxins.

Etiology

A frequent cause of acute renal failure in childhood is the hemolytic uremic syndrome. Acute glomerulonephritis, either poststreptococcal, membranoproliferative glomerulonephritis or nephritis, that is, rapidly progressive or secondary to lupus, can either lead directly to acute renal failure, or, in conjunction with a concomitant nephrotic syndrome, can lead to renal hypoperfusion and acute tubular necrosis. Other causes of acute tubular necrosis in children include sepsis, multiple trauma, and operative procedures, especially cardiac surgery. Additionally, tumor chemotherapy can result in massive tumor lysis and acute urate nephropathy. Acute obstruction with stone or tumor is very rare in children.

Diagnosis

The most reliable and readily available guide to GFR is the serum creatinine level. Creatinine production day-to-day is constant and only massive rhabdomyolysis or multiple trauma will lead to increased creatinine production. Excretion of creatinine is solely renal, primarily by glomerular filtration. Therefore, serum concentration of creatinine will reflect the GFR. If the patient is completely anuric, creatinine will increase by 2 mg/dl/day.

Urine output is a poor guide to renal function since prerenal states with marked urine concentration may lead to oliguria in the face of a normal GFR. Conversely, high output in acute tubular necrosis may indicate the failure of tubular resorption of the glomerular filtrate and leave the patient with a very high urine output in the face of poor GFR.

A baby or child in acute renal failure of unknown cause can be scanned by ultrasonography, which may show anatomic abnormalities of parenchyma or collecting system. Inferior vena cava, aorta, and, in some cases, renal veins and arteries can be visualized by this technique.

Radionuclide studies can be directed toward evaluating GFR and renal blood flow and its distribution. Tc-99m-labeled DTPA (technetium-99m stannous diethylenetriaminepentacetic acid), which is chiefly filtered through glomeruli, is injected intravenously and its flow detected on sequential scans by gamma camera. This study shows perfusion of the kidneys, and provides an estimate of GFR that correlates with the rate that radionuclide is washed out into collecting systems. Obstruction to outflow results in retention of radionuclide in the collecting system. Tc-99m-labeled DMSA (dimercaptosuccinic acid) binds to the proximal convoluted tubules and is particularly useful in demonstrating cortical mass, scars or masses. The fractional distribution of Tc-99m-DMSA between right and left kidneys correlates with blood flow to the kidneys.

Treatment

Since most episodes of acute renal failure are temporary and renal function recovers, it is essential that supportive treatment is excellent. If the patient becomes fully anuric, conservative medical management without dialysis should be able to maintain satisfactory metabolic status for 7–10 days. Thus, dialysis is rarely an emergency measure.

Fluid and Electrolyte Balance. Fluids generally are adjusted to keep the patient's weight stable and allow the patient to lose about 0.5% of body weight per day. This is ordinarily achieved through insensible losses plus urine output. Sodium is generally restricted to daily losses in the urine. Little or no potassium is allowed. If potassium is not provided, in the absence of excretion the serum potassium should increase by about .75 mEq/L/day through cellular catabolism. Therefore, there is generally a need for potassium to be removed through an exchange, given orally or rectally. Emergency treatment for hyperkalemia, including sodium bicarbonate infusions, glucose and insulin, and calcium infusion temporarily will decrease the extracellular fluid potassium or stabilize the myocardium, but they will not lead to a removal of total body potassium.

Calcium, Phosphorus and Magnesium Balance. Most patients with acute renal failure develop hyperphosphatemia because of decreased excretion of phosphate. Frequently this leads, either directly or indirectly, to hypocalcemia. Additionally, serum magnesium levels often increase. Rarely do these abnormalities present life-threatening conditions. Conservative measures (aluminum hydroxide to lower the serum phosphate, supplemental calcium, and 1,25-hydroxy vitamin D to increase the serum calcium) are usually directed at long-term management and are rarely necessary in the acute setting.

Metabolic Acidosis. Because of the decreased acid excretion and bicarbonate regeneration, patients with acute renal failure generally develop a metabolic acidosis. This situation can exacerbate other abnormalities by affecting cellular metabolism. Treatment usually entails sodium bicarbonate infusions either orally or intravenously. This treatment must be used judiciously since it can exacerbate sodium overload. THAM (tris-buffer) is indicated only in severe situations. Diuretics are obviously ineffective in this setting.

Nutrition. Maintenance of stable nutritional balance is extremely important in the recovery process, but is often overlooked in the treatment of the metabolic abnormalities. If the patient with acute renal failure is placed in a catabolic position because of insufficient nutritional intake, the recovery process will be complicated and prolonged. Early studies had suggested that provision of sufficient calories and essential amino acids led to a decreased urea generation rate and, thus, forestalled the requirement for dialysis. Essential amino acids, on the other hand, have led to serious metabolic complications in children. It seems more reasonable to supply a low sodium, low potassium, low phosphate diet either orally or parenterally with moderate amounts of protein (about 0.5 g/kg/day) to promote an anabolic state.

DIALYSIS

Indications for dialysis include: severe fluid and sodium overload, pulmonary edema or severe hypertension, metabolic acidosis intractable to treatment, hyperkalemia uncontrolled by conservative measures, and a BUN concentration greater than 150 mg/dl. The choice of the method of dialysis is usually based upon availability. Hemodialysis is generally more efficient, quicker, and more easily controlled. Peritoneal dialysis is technically easier and is more readily available in most hospitals (Fildes et al, 1986).

Peritoneal Dialysis

The technique of peritoneal dialysis has been perfected over the past 2 decades. A Silastic catheter is placed percutaneously or by means of a minor surgical procedure into the peritoneal space. Dialysate in volumes of 20–50 ml/kg body weight is instilled and allowed to dwell for 20–30 minutes; the cycle is then

CASE ILLUSTRATION

A 4-year-old girl suffered multiple trauma as a result of falling 50 feet from a bridge into a river. On arrival at an emergency room, she had hypothermia and was unconscious. Assessment at that time established that she had a concussion, a torn femoral artery, acute renal failure, pulmonary edema, and multiple fractures of arms and legs, perforation of the small intestine and contusions of the liver. Immediate treatment entailed intubation and ventilation, gradual warming, and surgical repair of the femoral artery. Because of the hyperkalemia secondary to tissue destruction, a femoral catheter was placed and hemodialysis was initiated immediately. Hyperkalemia and pulmonary edema resolved after the first two treatments, within 12 hours. She underwent laparotomy for peritonitis and a temporary colostomy was performed. Urine output was less than 100 ml/day for the first 2 weeks. Her hemodialysis treatments were repeated twice within the next 24 hours and then she was placed on maintenance hemodialysis four times per week. Standard intravenous alimentation was begun on the third hospital day, but quickly led to hypophosphatemia and hypercalcemia. The solutions were adjusted appropriately and she was given 80 cal/kg and 1.5 g of protein/kg/day in 750 ml of fluid per day. She was extubated in 3 days, regained consciousness in 5 days, and renal function after 4 weeks. The colostomy was closed at 3 months and she had regained full renal function at the time of discharge 3 months after admission.

COMMENT

Major trauma is a recognized cause of acute tubular necrosis and renal failure since the kidney is susceptible to ischemic injury in association with shock, asphyxia, and heart failure. Mild ischemia leads to a transient loss of tubular concentrating ability. A more severe injury, as in this patient, leads to azotemia and hyperkalemia. Acute tubular necrosis is highly variable lasting from 1 day to 3 months.

repeated. The first treatment generally lasts for 24–36 hours and is discontinued. In some centers, the patient is treated with continuous long-dwell procedures or with overnight exchanges by utilizing an automated cycling machine. Major complications of peritoneal dialysis include peritonitis, failure of the procedure to provide effective ultrafiltration, and functional problems from placement of the catheter.

Hemodialysis

An access for hemodialysis is usually attained through a subclavian or femoral catheter, often dual-lumen. The dialysis treatment must be individualized based upon the patient's size and metabolic requirements. Clearance and ultrafiltration are controlled separately. The primary complication of acute hemodialysis is a disequilibrium syndrome secondary to correcting the metabolic abnormalities too rapidly. Also, problems with the catheter and infections are major complications.

REFERENCES

Feld LG, Springate JE, Fildes RD: Acute renal failure. I. Pathophysiology and diagnosis. *J Pediatr* 109:401, 1986.

Fildes RD, Springate JE, Feld LG: Acute renal failure. II. Management of suspected and established disease. *J Pediatr* 109:567, 1986.

Kon V, Ichikawa I: Research seminar: Physiology of acute renal failure. *J Pediatr* 105:351, 1984.

Chronic Renal Failure 13

Definition

Chronic renal failure is the irreversible loss of more than 50% of the glomerular filtration rate (GFR) resulting in metabolic derangements and accumulation of uremic toxins. Chronic renal failure is invariably progressive.

Etiology

Table 10.11 lists the usual causes of chronic renal failure in childhood.

COMPLICATIONS OF CHRONIC RENAL FAILURE

In addition to the accumulation of nitrogenous waste products (urea, creatinine, uric acid, etc), multiple metabolic abnormalities result from chronic renal failure.

The deficiency of 1-hydroxylation of vitamin D produces hypocalcemia and secondary hyperparathyroidism. Insufficient phosphate excretion and chronic acidosis contribute to osteosclerosis.

Renal osteodystrophy, chronic malnutrition, and multiple abnormalities of cellular metabolism contribute to marked reduction, or occasionally, total cessation of linear growth.

Fluid and salt overload secondary to decreased excretion and hyperreninemia secondary to abnormalities of interrenal blood flow lead to sustained elevations of blood pressure.

Decreased production of erythropoietin produces a hypoplastic anemia. Fortunately, a new treatment is in the offering since, in preliminary trials, recombinant erythropoietin has been effective.

Seizure disorders, learning disabilities, and cerebral atrophy are frequently seen in chronic renal failure.

Treatment

Treatment usually follows stages as the chronic renal failure progresses.

CONSERVATIVE TREATMENT

Usually conservative treatment is required when the serum creatinine exceeds 2 mg/dl and is generally sufficient until the creatinine reaches 8–12 mg/dl. Unless the patient has a salt-losing nephropathy (e.g., secondary to obstructive uropathy), salt and fluid intake is restricted to prevent fluid overload, edema, and hypertension. Diuretics may be used but their efficacy is hampered by a significantly lowered GFR. Hypertension may be treated with vasodilators (hydralazine), β-blockers (propranolol) or angiotensin antagonists (captopril). Nutrition is controlled usually with provision of a low phosphate, low potassium diet which provides 80–100% of the recommended daily allowance (RDA) of calories and 1–1.5 g/kg/day of protein. Protein-restricted diets are counterproductive since they may exacerbate growth failure. Hydroxylated vitamin D and calcium supplements are given; aluminum hydroxide and/or calcium carbonate are given to reduce absorption of dietary phosphorus.

DIALYSIS

When the GFR is less than 10% of normal and the patient has overt symptoms of uremia (anorexia, fatigue), dialysis is indicated.

Hemodialysis is the standard form of chronic dialysis for adults, but becomes technically more difficult

Table 10.11
Primary Diagnosis Leading to Chronic Renal Failure[1]

Disease Category		No.	(% Total)
Congenital/hereditary	57		(48%)
Hypoplasia-dysplasia		25	
Obstructive uropathy		18	
Nephronophthisis		4	
Alport syndrome		3	
Cystinosis		3	
Prune belly syndrome		2	
Polycystic kidney disease		1	
Tuberous sclerosis		1	
Glomerulonephritis	43		(36%)
Chronic GN (unclassified)		13	
Membranoproliferative GN		11	
Focal segmental sclerosing GN		10	
Rapidly progressive GN		4	
Mesangioproliferative GN		3	
Anaphylactoid purpura GN		1	
Systemic lupus GN		1	
Chronic tubulointerstitial	8		(6%)
Chronic interstitial nephritis		8	
Vascular	6		(5%)
Hypertensive glomerulosclerosis		2	
Renal vein thrombosis		2	
Polyarteritis nodosa		1	
Hemolytic uremic syndrome		1	
Other	6		(5%)
Wilms tumor		2	
Drug-induced		2	
Unknown		1	
Diabetes		1	
Total		120	

[1]GN, glomerulonephritis.

CASE ILLUSTRATION

The patient was a 6-month-old girl who was well until an abdominal mass was felt at a routine examination. Exploratory laparotomy revealed a neuroblastoma. Complications of surgery led to loss of both kidneys and to loss of a moderate amount of small bowel. Therefore, continuous ambulatory peritoneal dialysis was initiated, but the patient developed monilia peritonitis, which was treated with intraperitoneal amphotericin for 3 days, and intravenous amphotericin for 3 more weeks. A Thomas femoral shunt was placed and the patient was treated with hemodialysis four times per week. Intravenous hyperalimentation was instituted and continued through the next 6 months. The patient grew reasonably well and, when there was no sign of recurrence of tumor at age 1 year, the patient underwent a renal transplant from her mother. The match between mother and daughter was quite good and the mixed lymphocyte culture was nonreactive, indicating a very low potential for cell-mediated reactivity by the patient against her mother's cells. The patient was treated postoperatively with prednisone and azathioprine and 6 months after the transplant, when the prednisone was reduced to an alternate-day schedule, she began to grow at a normal rate. The patient is currently 6 years old, has had significant catch-up growth and has developed normally. Currently the renal function also is normal. She remains on azathioprine 2 mg/kg/day and prednisone 0.5 mg/kg every other day.

QUESTIONS AND COMMENTS

Is there a lower age limit for renal transplantation?

Renal transplantation is so successful that virtually any child with chronic renal failure should be considered as a candidate, regardless of age, size, or etiology of renal failure. If the graft functions well and the immunosuppression can be reduced to low maintenance levels, the child can grow and develop normally. Nonetheless, because of the potential for chronic rejection and, thus, the need for containing immunosuppression, the child must be seen and evaluated periodically. If possible, we postpone transplantation until 1 year of age when the infant is large enough to accept an adult kidney.

How do you monitor renal function?

BUN and creatinine are measured every month; a urinalysis is performed every 6 months and renal ultrasonography is done once a year.

Is infection a problem?

The major concern is varicella. If exposed, the patient would be given varicella immune globulin. If infected, she would receive intravenous acylovir. She has not been immunized because the potential danger of immunization in an immunosuppressed child is unknown.

with small patients. Vascular access, via shunt or arteriovenous fistula, or by subclavian catheter is generally the limiting factor. Patients usually receive 2- to 4-hour treatments three times per week. In addition to the other complications of chronic renal failure, the major complications of chronic hemodialysis include access infection and obstruction, iron overload from chronic transfusion, and disruption of school and family life by the treatment schedule. Even so, the 5-year patient survival for hemodialysis should be at least 90%.

Peritoneal dialysis (continuous ambulatory peritoneal dialysis or CAPD) is technically easier and favored by many pediatric centers. Dialysate is instilled into the peritoneal space through a permanently implanted catheter and left to dwell 2–6 hours; that fluid is replaced with another exchange of fresh dialysate and the cycle is repeated. Sometimes the exchanges are performed overnight by an automatic cycler. The advantages of CAPD include independence from the dialysis center, less need for transfusions, and better control of acidosis. Complications include peritonitis, failure to continue treatments secondary to peritoneal scarring or patient fatigue and slightly higher morbidity and mortality than are found in hemodialysis.

Renal transplantation is the undisputed preferred treatment for children with chronic renal failure. Even though renal transplant cannot be considered a "cure" (since rejection is always possible and long-term immunosuppression is necessary), a well-functioning transplant provides normal renal function and permits normal growth and development. The size of the graft is not important, so adult kidneys can be used for all except the smallest infants. Transplants from living related donors, usually "half-matched" parents as donors, with pretreatment with donor-specific blood transfusions, can yield 90% 5-year graft survival. Cadaver donor transplants generally are not as successful but can provide excellent outcome for many patients. The results from transplantation with infant cadaver donors are discouraging. Immunosuppression for pediatric patients is similar to that for adults: prednisone, azathioprine, antilymphocyte serum, and cyclosporin have all been used. Most patients require some prednisone, but improved growth is generally achieved with alternate-day dosage.

Earlier transplantation, before growth is stunted, improves the chances of normal height. In a follow-up study of nine infants who received transplants, So et al (1987) concluded that normal growth and development is possible post-transplant, but does not always occur if the underlying disease recurs.

The infant with chronic renal failure presents multiple technical problems with dialysis and transplantation, primarily because of small size. Although it had been thought until just recently that there was no treatment possible for these unfortunate children, recent studies have shown that aggressive conservative management can produce positive nitrogen balance and growth, even if the glomerular filtration rate is reduced significantly. Continuous ambulatory peritoneal dialysis can be performed in very small infants if necessary. These patients can be permitted to grow so that generally by 1 year of age they have achieved 7–10 kg. At that point, renal transplant from living related donors is possible and frequently very successful.

REFERENCES

Avner ED, Harmon WE, Grupe WE, et al: Mortality of chronic hemodialysis and renal transplantation in pediatric end-stage renal disease. *Pediatrics* 67:412, 1981.

Nevins T, Chang PN, Mauer SM: Renal transplantation in the very young child. In Tune BM, Mendoza SA, Brenner BM, et al (eds): *Pediatric Nephrology*. New York, Churchill Livingstone, 1984, pp. 381–397.

So SKS, Chang PN, Najarian JS, et al: Growth and development in infants after renal transplantation. *J Pediatr* 110:343, 1987

Circumcision 14

Definition

Circumcision is the excision of foreskin that covers the glans penis. This procedure, which began as an ancient Semitic ritual, became almost routine in this country in the post-World War II period. Socioeconomic and medical questions have arisen regarding this practice.

Epidemiology

In the 1970s, about 85% of male infants were circumcised in the United States; in 1984, the number had dropped to 70% (Wiswell et al, 1987).

Natural History

At birth, the foreskin normally covers the glans penis completely, and extends beyond the tip and tapers to a narrow point. The foreskin cannot be retracted for the first several months of age. By 1 year of age, 50% are retractable and 96% are retractable by school age.

Complications of circumcision include surgical trauma to the penis, ulceration of the meatus from ammoniacal urine, infection that can be local or systemic, and rarely, gangrene of the penis from prolonged ischemia. Infants with hemorrhagic disorders may first be identified by excessive bleeding from circumcision. Overall, however, complications are thought to be less from circumcision than almost any other surgical procedure.

The arguments for circumcision include reduced risk of penile carcinoma later in life, and less cervical cancer in wives of circumcised men. It is thought that penile hygiene is just as effective. The frequency of foreskin problems is about double in noncircumcised infants as in those circumcised in infancy. Balanitis, defined as redness and swelling with or without pus occurs in 6% of circumcised and 3% of uncircumcised infants according to a retrospective study (Herzog and Alvarez, 1986). Conversely, urinary tract infections in infants are more common in uncircumcised males (Anderson and Smey, 1985; Wiswell and Roscelli, 1986).

Treatment

If circumcision is performed in the newborn period, most often a bell-clamp is used for hemostasis. Although anesthetics are not usually given, a penile dorsal nerve block with xylocaine is safe and effective. Sedation is regularly given, as is a pacifier. After the newborn period, general or regional anesthesia is required.

RECOMMENDATION

The American Academy of Pediatrics task force recommended in 1975 that routine neonatal circumcision be discontinued and that physicians "provide parents with information pertaining to the long-term effects of circumcision and noncircumcision." Despite this advice, the frequency of circumcision in the United States is essentially the same as before 1975.

Consideration should be given to religious, cultural, and other factors that might justify circumcision in some instances. The risks of both circumcision and noncircumcision are so few that the medical considerations assume less importance than do the social ones.

REFERENCES

Anderson GF, Smey P: Current concepts in the management of common urologic problems in infants and children. *Pediatr Clin North Am* 32:1133, 1985.

Gairdner D: The fate of the foreskin. *Br Med J* 2:1443, 1949.

Herzog LW, Alvarez SR: The frequency of foreskin problems in uncircumcised children. *Am J Dis Child* 140:254, 1986.

Kirya C, Werthmann MW: Neonatal circumcision and penile dorsal nerve block—a painless procedure. *J Pediatr* 92:998, 1978.

Shulman J, Ben-Hur N, Neuman Z: Surgical complications of circumcision. *Am J Dis Child* 107:149, 1964.

Thompson HC, King LR, Knox E, et al: Report of the ad hoc task force on circumcision. *Pediatrics* 56:610, 1975.

Wiswell TE, Enzenauer RW, Holton ME, et al: Declining frequency of circumcision: Implications for changes in the absolute incidence of male to female sex ratio of urinary tract infections in early infancy. *Pediatrics* 79:338, 1987.

Wiswell TE, Roscelli JD: Corroborative evidence for the decreased incidence of urinary tract infections in circumcised male infants. *Pediatrics* 78:96, 1986.

Congenital Disorders of the Male Genitalia 15

Definition

Congenital abnormalities of the male phallus and scrotum include a number of disorders of development influenced by androgenic stimulation in utero. These structures include the phallic urethra, corpora cavernosa (erectile bodies), and glans penis (Table 10.12).

Table 10.12
Congenital Abnormalities of Male Genitalia

- Phallus
  - Chordee without urethral abnormality
    - Dorsal
    - Ventral
  - Penile torsion
  - Microphallus
- Phallic urethra
  - Hypospadias (with or without chordee)
    - Glandular
    - Coronal
    - Penile shaft
    - Penoscrotal
    - Perineal
  - Episadius
    1. Proximal (with or without exstrophy)
    2. Distal
- Scrotum and contents
  - Cryptorchidism
  - Monorchidism
  - Anorchidism
  - Bifid scrotum

Basic Science

The phallic structures are formed under the influence of testosterone produced by the fetal testes. The penis develops from the genital tubercules that fuse to form the corpora cavernosa and glans penis. With infolding of the urogenital folds the phallic urethra is formed. The genital swelling lateral to the tubercule migrates downward to form the scrotum. The testes migrate into the scrotum in the last trimester. These structures are present in their completed form by 16 weeks of gestation. The elements necessary for normal development include the Y chromosome, H-Y antigen, fetal gonad, intact steroidogenic enzymes, and end-organ androgen receptors.

Epidemiology

The most common abnormalities of the male external genitalia are hypospadias—0.8% (Sweet et al, 1974), and undescended testicles—3% of babies at term and 0.8% at 1 year (Scorer and Farrington, 1971; see Endocrinology, Section 14, pp. 874). Chordee without hypospadias, penile torsion, epispadias, and microphallus are uncommon disorders. Monorchidism occurs 1/5000 males and is four times as common as is anorchidism (Goldberg et al, 1974).

Natural History

Disorders of the phallus include hypospadias, epispadias, curvature of the penis, and micropenis. Hypospadius, the most common abnormality, presents as a urethral meatal opening on the ventral aspect of the phallus, with absence of the ventral foreskin, giving the appearance of a "dorsal hood." It varies in degree, ranging from mild or glandular hypospadias to the more severe or perineal urethral meatal position. The milder forms constitute the majority of findings.

The more severe forms are usually associated with ventral curvature of the penis termed "chordee." Chordee can be present with the milder forms and even without hypospadias. Epispadius is a rare anomaly associated with exstrophy of the bladder and, even more rarely, it presents as an isolated finding. The urethral meatus is placed dorsally at the penopubic angle or more distally. Incontinence is a frequent problem with this anomaly. Micropenis is a small, normally formed organ, often associated with hypogonadotrophic states.

Disorders of the scrotal contents include cryptorchidism (undescended testes), monorchidism, anorchidism, and the bifid scrotum. Monorchism (one testicle absent) or anorchism are much rarer than undescended testes. Monorchidism implies loss of the testis at sometime during embryonic development. It must be distinguished from cryptorchidism because the latter has a malignant potential. Ambiguities of the scrotal wall, mainly bifid scrotum, are seen in severe cases of hypospadius and imply a failure of complete androgenization of the external genitalia.

Diagnosis

The diagnosis of external genitalial anomalies is not usually difficult. The only diagnostic problem arises when severe hypospadias and/or intersex anomalies are present (pp. 874). Care must be taken in these cases, before gender assignment, to know the genotypic as well as phenotypic sex. Chromosomal studies as well as hormonal levels are often helpful.

In the case of bilaterally nonpalpable testes, the presence of anorchia must be excluded. Stimulation with human chorionic gonadotropin and measuring serum testosterone levels along with baseline gonadotropins will distinguish between these two entities.

Treatment

Surgical reconstruction of hypospadias, epispadias, and penile curvature usually begins at around 6 months of age. In most cases, this can be accomplished in one procedure. Micropenis is first evaluated by testosterone injections and if response is seen, then subsequent treatment is given (pp. 876). If no response is noted, then gender reassignment should be considered, if the child is seen in the neonatal period.

In cases of monorchism or anorchism, placement of testicular prostheses (and androgen replacement in the latter case) is recommended.

Prognosis

Excellent results are possible with reconstructive procedures of the external genitalia. The current trend is toward earlier surgery (under 1 year) for psychosocial reasons.

SCROTAL PAIN AND/OR SWELLING

Definition

Painful scrotal swelling is a common childhood problem, often termed the "acute scrotum." It can be caused by a variety of inciting events (Table 10.13), but in most cases, torsion of the spermatic cord must be ruled out. Torsion of an appendage of the testis or epididymis may mimic these findings. Epididymitis is very rare in the prepubertal period, but must be considered in the sexually active teenager. Orchitis is usually associated with a viral illness such as mumps. Scrotal trauma may result in disruption of the tunical covering of the testes and/or a hematocele.

Nonpainful swelling in children will most often be due to hernia or hydrocele; in older children, a varicocele may be palpable in the left hemiscrotum.

Basic Science

The underlying cause for many of these lesions is an anatomic abnormality. Torsion of the spermatic cord is due to abnormal fixation of the testicle to the overlying tunical covering. Hernia and hydrocele are due to failure of the processus vaginalis to obliterate. Varicoceles are almost always on the left side, because of the perpendicular insertion of the left spermatic vein into the renal vein. In young children, bacterial epididymitis is most often secondary to urethral instrumentation or rarely associated with a renal duplication anomaly. Viral epididymitis *(Chlamydia)* is sexually transmitted as is gonococcal disease.

Epidemiology

The exact incidence of torsion of the spermatic cord is unknown, but it accounts for more morbidity than all the other etiologies of an acute scrotum combined. Hernias are more common in premature infants and occur in 1–4% of all newborn males (Harper et al, 1975). Hydroceles are often seen at birth, but most will resolve by 1 year of age. Varicoceles were found in 16% of 1072 teenaged males (Oster, 1971). Epididymitis and orchitis are extremely rare in the prepubertal, nonsexually active child. Testicular or paratesticular tumors are also very unusual in this age group.

Table 10.13
Causes of Scrotal Pain and/or Swelling

Torsion of the spermatic cord
Torsion of the testis or epididymis
Incarceration/strangulation of inguinal hernia
Epididymitis
Orchitis
Trauma
Varicocele
Testicular or paratesticular tumor

Natural History

The child with the acute onset of swelling and discoloration of the scrotal wall and/or contents is considered a diagnostic and treatment emergency. The time to irreversible injury due to ischemia from torsion of the spermatic cord is only a few hours. In any case of torsion, the subsequent risk of contralateral occurrence is significant.

Hernia and hydrocele are usually present at birth. Incarceration of a preexisting hernia is a potentially dangerous event, and is usually evident by history and physical examination. Varicoceles are not usually found until immediately pre- or postpubescence age. Varicoceles are sometimes associated with impaired testicular growth on the affected side.

Diagnosis

Although the differential list of etiologies of scrotal swelling and pain is long, the diagnosis is one that must be made swiftly and definitively. Associated signs and symptoms may include abdominal tenderness, fever, leukocytosis, and nausea or vomiting. With the presentation of an acute scrotum, surgical exploration is usually mandatory. Scrotal nuclear scanning is relatively accurate in the diagnosis of torsion, but it is usually reserved for a very delayed presentation or in cases where another diagnosis is strongly entertained.

Occasionally, the diagnosis of torsion of a testicular appendage can be made reliably if the child is seen early and a "blue dot" is evident. Traumatic injury to the testicle or scrotum is usually identifiable by history, but minor trauma may mask torsion. Severe traumatic injuries to the scrotum should be evaluated with ultrasonography to help determine the extent of testicular damage.

In the rare child with epididymitis, symptoms of dysuria, frequency, or urethral discharge may be present as well as findings of pyuria or bacteriuria. Urinalysis and/or urine culture is important whenever acute scrotal swelling is evaluated.

Causes of nonpainful swelling of scrotal contents are, as already mentioned, usually evident by history and physical examination. Testicular tumors are rare, but can be evaluated effectively by palpation and scrotal ultrasonography.

Treatment

The treatment of testicular torsion is prompt scrotal exploration and detorsion. If the testicle is viable, bilateral orchiopexy with nonabsorbent sutures is performed. If the testicle is necrotic, removal with placement of a prothesis is recommended. If the pain and discomfort associated with torsion of an appendage is not severe, conservative management is satisfactory. If the diagnosis is in doubt or significant discomfort is present, exploration and removal of the appendage is performed.

Hernias are approached through an inguinal incision, with reduction and repair of the defect. Care must be taken in cases of incarceration to make sure the involved bowel is viable. In cases of testicular or paratesticular tumors, inguinal orchiectomy is mandatory, followed in some cases by intraperitoneal lymphadenectomy and/or chemotherapy. Scrotal trauma, if severe, should be explored in order to preserve the maximal amount of testicular tissue. In cases of epididymitis, appropriate antibiotic coverage should continue until the swelling and tenderness subside. Uroradiographic studies should be performed to rule out an underlying anatomic abnormality.

Prognosis

Torsion of the spermatic cord may lead to ischemic injury with loss of hormonal and spermatic function. The risk to the contralateral testicle makes appropriate diagnosis and therapy even more important. The testicular appendages serve no known physiological function. Testicular tumors, although rare, can be malignant and require aggressive treatment and follow-up.

REFERENCES

Allen TD: Microphallus. Clinical and endocrinologic characteristics. *J Urol* 119:750, 1978.

Belman AB, Kass EJ: Hypospadias repair in children under one year of age. *J Urol* 128:1273, 1982.

Goldberg LM, Skaist LB, Morrow JW: Congenital absence of testes; anorchism and monorchism. *J Urol* 111:840, 1974.

Harper RG, Garcia A, Sia C: Inguinal hernia. A common problem of premature infants weighing 1000 gms or less at birth. *Pediatrics* 56:112, 1975.

Knight PJ, Vassey LE: The diagnosis and treatment of the acute scrotum in children and adolescents. *Ann Surg* 200:664, 1984.

Oster J: Varicocele in children and adolescents: An investigation of the incidence among Danish school children. *Scand J Urol Nephrol* 5:27, 1971.

Scorer GC, Farrington GH: *Congenital Deformities of the Testis and Epidiymis*. London, Butterworth, 1971.

Sweet RA, Schrott HG, Kurland R, et al: Study of the incidence of hypospadias in Rochester, Minnesota, 1940–1970, and a case-control comparison of possible etiologic factors. *Mayo Clin Proc* 49:52, 1974.

Hydrometrocolpos

16

Definition

Hydrometrocolpos is a collection of fluid in the vagina, which is obstructed. Distention of the uterus is commonly associated.

Epidemiology

The condition is rare, but represents about 6% of abdominal masses that present in newborn infants. It is the third most common abdominal mass.

Natural History

Excessive vaginal secretions from transplacental estrogen stimulation are common. Endometrial stimulation can also occur, with pseudomenstruation. If the vagina is obstructed, the secretions may accumulate and distend the vagina and uterus. Obstruction may be from distal vaginal atresia, urogenital sinus anomaly, or an imperforate hymen.

Diagnosis

The most common presentation is a bulging at the vaginal orifice. Rarely, if undetected, massive uterine enlargement can cause respiratory distress or even intestinal obstruction. The anatomy can be elucidated by ultrasonography. Urinary tract abnormalities may be associated.

Treatment

An imperforate hymen should be incised at the apex of the bulge. Relief of obstruction is curative. If a urogenital sinus or distal vaginal atresia is present, endoscopic drainage from below is usually adequate. Reconstruction may be needed later.

REFERENCE

Hahn-Pedersen J, Kvist N, Nielson OH: Hydrometrocolpos: Current views on pathogenesis and management. *J Urol* 132:537, 1984.

MARY ELLEN AVERY
JAMES MANDELL
WILLIAM HARMON
CHARLES SIMMONS
LEWIS R. FIRST

Consultants
Julie Ingelfinger
Dorothy Villee

Section 11

Gynecology

Medical care of the child and adolescent often involves attention to gynecologic complaints. In the prepubertal child, vaginitis, vulvitis, labial adhesions, bleeding, and sexual abuse may require evaluation. In the adolescent, vulvovaginal infections, sexually transmitted diseases, menstrual problems, pregnancy, and contraception are common concerns. The health care provider who regularly sees the child or adolescent is in the best position to know about the general medical history, psychosocial adjustment and family issues, and to have established rapport with that child. Knowledge of correct techniques for examination and treatment and of resources for referral is essential to good health care for the child and adolescent.

Gynecologic Evaluation of the Prepubertal Child

1

The examination of the child with a gynecologic complaint should include a general physical examination to look for signs of puberty, adenopathy, pharyngitis, and skin disease. In the child with vulvar irritation, the scalp (especially behind the ears) and the skin creases should be inspected for dermatitis. The inguinal areas should be carefully palpated for a hernia, gonad, or adenopathy. The genital examination should include inspection of the external genitalia with the child supine (feet together, knees apart) by pulling the labia gently forward (Fig. 11.1). The anterior vagina can be visualized and the hymenal ring examined for evidence of trauma by using an otoscope to provide appropriate magnification and light. Small lacerations of the hymen, attenuation and dilatation of the hymen, and adhesions from the hymen to the vagina may be visualized and may suggest the possibility of sexual abuse (Figs. 11.2 and 11.3). Friability at the posterior forchette as the labia are separated appears to be more common in sexually molested children than in normal children but also may occur in the child with vulvitis (Emans et al, 1987). The normal clitoral glans is 2 mm in width. Although rare in the prepubertal child, lichen sclerosis produces a characteristic atropic, white figure-of-eight pattern around the vagina and anus; excoriations, macerations, secondary infection, and small hemorrhages resulting from minor trauma may be on the vulva.

After initial inspection of the vulva, the physician should examine the child in the knee-chest position to allow visualization of the upper vagina and cervix again by using an otoscope (Emans, 1981; Emans, 1986; Emans and Goldstein, 1980; Emans and Goldstein, 1982; Fig. 11.4). Foreign bodies such as wads of toilet paper, safety pins, or magic marker tips may be seen when the patient is in this position. When the presenting complaint is vaginal irritation or discharge, a specific diagnosis is more likely in girls who have visible discharge during this examination than in those who do not (Paradise et al, 1982). If the initial examination is normal, the child has no visible discharge, and the history is not suggestive of a specific infection, the child can be treated with sitz baths and appropriate hygienic measures (see p. 656).

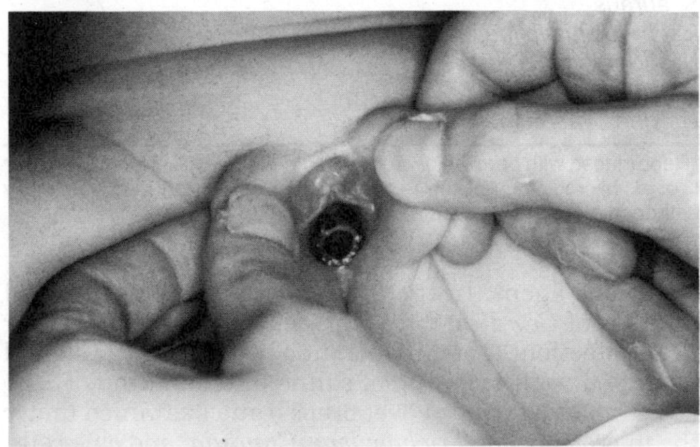

Figure 11.1. Genital evaluation of the prepubertal child supine. Reproduced with permission from Emans SJ, Goldstein DP: *Pediatric and Adolescent Gynecology*, Little, Brown & Co., Boston, 1982.

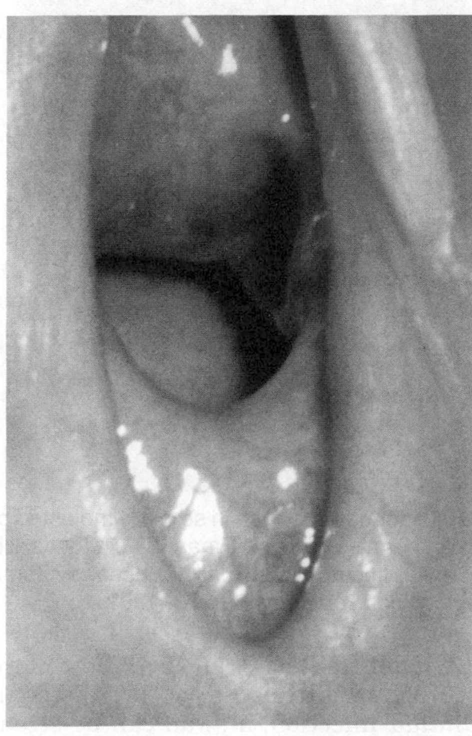

Figure 11.2. Normal hymen in 4-year-old child. Reproduced with permission from Emans SJ, Woods ER, Flagg NT, et al: Genital findings in sexually abused, symptomatic, and asymptomatic, girls. *Pediatrics* 79:778, 1987.

In the child with persistent or purulent discharge, cultures and so-called "wet preps" of the discharge should be evaluated (Fig. 11.5). A small plastic Clinitest dropper or a saline-moistened Calgiswab should be used to obtain samples. If multiple samples are needed, a small amount of saline can be squeezed into the vagina with the Clinitest dropper and aspirated back. A swab should be planted directly onto media appropriate for culturing *Neisseria gonorrhoeae* (Thayer-Martin Jembec) and another swab sent to a bacteriology laboratory for planting on GU media (blood, McConkey, and chocolate agar). The normal flora of the vagina are shown in

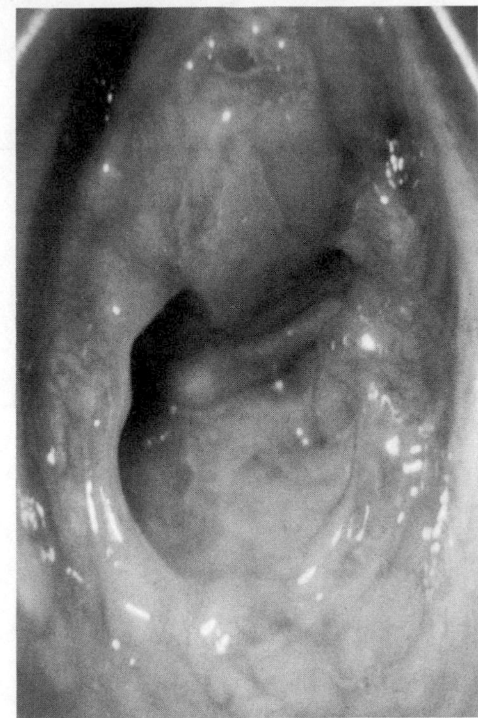

Figure 11.3. Attenuated hymen in sexually molested child. Reproduced with permission from Emans SJ, Woods ER, Flagg NT, et al: Genital findings in sexually abused, syptomatic, and asymptomatic, girls. *Pediatrics* 79:778, 1987.

Table 11.1 (Hammerschlag et al, 1978). In children with vaginal itching, a white discharge, or a history suggestive of *Candida* infection, a swab can be streaked directly onto Biggy agar (Fig. 11.6) and incubated in the office laboratory to determine whether *Candida* is the

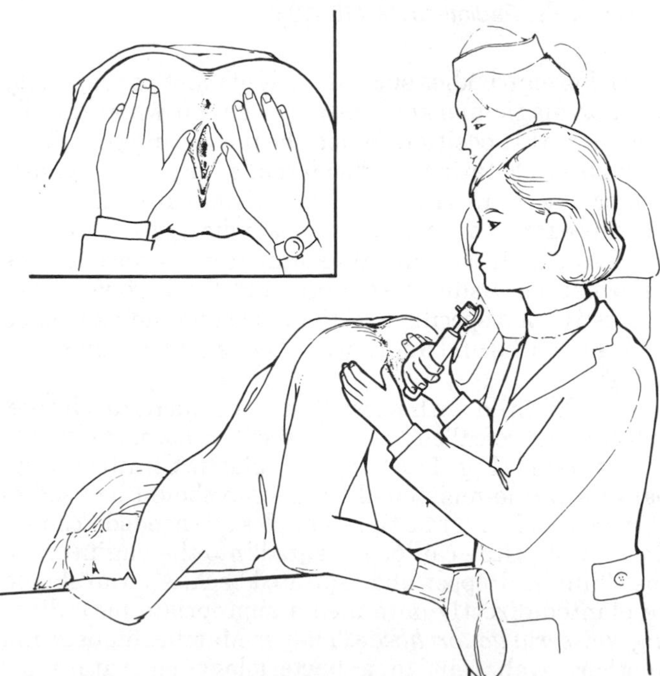

Figure 11.4. Knee-chest position for visualization of the vagina in the prepubertal child.

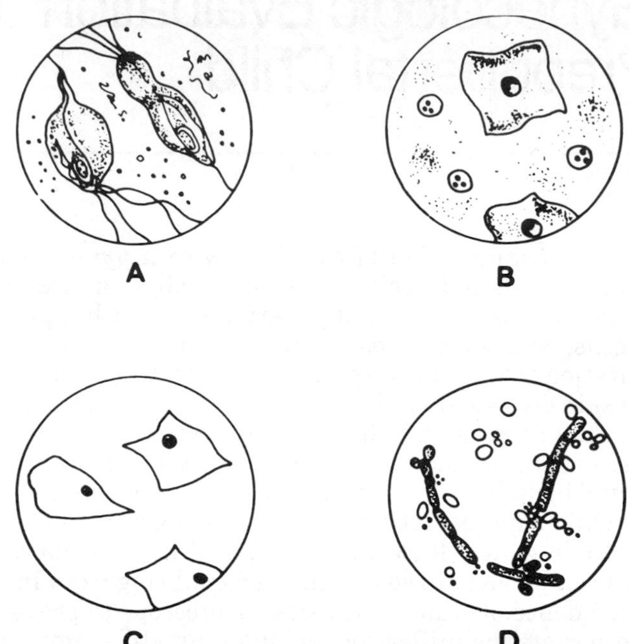

Figure 11.5. Wet preparations. **A.** *Trichomonas.* **B.** Nonspecific vaginitis. **C.** Leukorrhea. **D.** *Candida.* **A, B,** and **C** are saline preparations; **D** is a KOH preparation. Reproduced with permission from Emans SJ, Goldstein DP: *Pediatric and Adolescent Gynecology.* Boston, Little, Brown & Co., 1982.

Table 11.1
Normal Flora of the Vagina in Girls, Ages 2 Months to 15 Years[1]

Organism	Percent of Patients
Diphtheroids	78
Staphylococcus epidermis	73
α-Hemolytic streptococci	39
Lactobacilli	39
Nonhemolytic streptococci	34
Escherichia coli	34
Klebsiella	15
Group D Streptococcus	8.5
S. aureus	7
Haemophilus influenzae	5
Pseudomonas aeruginosa	5
Proteus	5
Gardnerella vaginalis	13.5

[1] Reproduced with permission from Hammerschlag MR, Albert S, Resner I, et al: Microbiology of the vagina in children: Normal and potentially pathogenic organisms. *Pediatrics* 62:57, 1978.

infectious agent. In the absence of symptoms, a small number of *Candida* may represent colonization rather than infection. A small amount of the discharge should be mixed with one drop of saline and one drop of 10% KOH on a glass slide ("wet preps") and examined under the microscope for *Trichomonas, Candida,* and clue cells. The presence of a characteristic amine odor when the discharge is mixed with 10% KOH (positive "whiff" test) suggests *Gardnerella vaginalis* (also termed "nonspecific" vaginitis or NSV). A Gram stain of a purulent

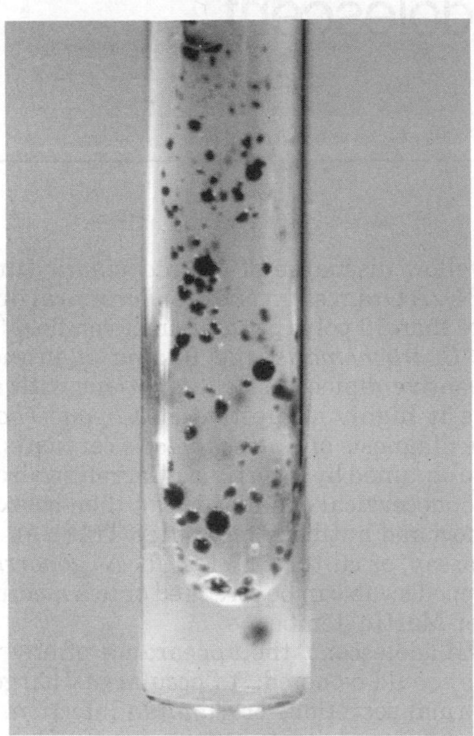

Figure 11.6. Biggy agar with multiple colonies of *Candida*. Reproduced with permission from Emans SJ: Vulvovaginitis in the child and adolescent. *Pediatr Rev* 8:12, 1986.

discharge can be helpful in making a presumptive diagnosis of *N. gonorrhoeae,* although a culture is always necessary because occasionally other *Neisseria* may cause vaginitis in the prepubertal child.

As more is learned about the incidence of *Chlamydia trachomatis* in children with vulvovaginal symptoms and normal children, the use of either the rapid monoclonal antibody test to detect antigen or culture will become important in its detection. For the moment, culture should be the preferred method because of the implication for sexual abuse. Vaginal colonization acquired at birth may persist to 1 year of age (Schacter et al, 1986). Beyond that, sexually acquired infection should be suspected (Ingram et al, 1986). Since *C. trachomatis* is an intracellular organism, the vagina or perihymenal area of the prepubertal child should be gently scraped with a Dacron urethral swab to obtain epithelial cells.

Girls with vulvar or anal pruritus should be screened for pinworms. Because the rectal examination is sometimes uncomfortable for the child, it should be performed last. The child should be in lithotomy position with knees apart and feet together. A bimanual rectoabdominal examination can be used to detect a mass or foreign body and to milk any discharge forward. Radiograph and ultrasound of the abdomen or pelvis are rarely indicated except when the question of a mass, an ovarian cyst, an abscess, or ectopic ureter is raised. The foreign bodies found most frequently in the vagina are wads of toilet paper and these are not radiopaque.

For children in whom an adequate examination is not possible because of poor cooperation or because the vagina does not gape open in knee chest position, a brief assessment under general anesthesia may be necessary. This is particularly true in girls with vaginal bleeding and persistent discharge and those under age 2 years.

REFERENCES

Emans SJ: Vulvovaginitis in children and adolescents. *Pediatr Rev* 2:319, 1981.

Emans SJ: Vulvovaginitis in the child and adolescent. *Pediatr Rev* 8:12, 1986.

Emans SJ, Goldstein DP: *Pediatric and Adolescent Gynecology*. Boston, Little, Brown & Co., 1982.

Emans SJ, Goldstein DP: The gynecologic examination of the prepubertal child with vulvovaginitis: Use of the knee-chest position. *Pediatrics* 65:758, 1980.

Emans SJ, Woods ER, Flagg N, et al: Genital findings in sexually abused, symptomatic and asymptomatic girls. *Pediatrics* 79:778, 1987.

Hammerschlag MR, Albert S, Rosner I, et al: Microbiology of the vagina in children: Normal and potentially pathogenic organisms. *Pediatrics* 62:57, 1978.

Ingram DL, White ST, Occhiuti AR, et al: Childhood vaginal infections: Association with *Chlamydia trachomatis* with sexual contact. *Pediatr Infect Dis* 5:226, 1986.

Paradise JE, Compos JM, Friedman HM, et al: Vulvovaginitis in premenarchal girls: Clinical features and diagnostic evaluation. *Pediatrics* 70:193, 1982.

Schacter J, Grossman M, Sweet R, et al: Prospective study of perinatal transmission of *Chlamydia trachomatis*. *JAMA* 255:3374, 1986.

Gynecologic Evaluation of the Adolescent

2

The gynecologic examination of the adolescent needs to be undertaken with special sensitivity. After an explanation of the pelvic examination, the adolescent should be given a gown and a drape. The health care provider should explain each part of the examination as it is done. A general physical examination including a breast examination is done first. The pelvic examination begins with observation of the external genitalia. The Tanner Stage of pubic hair (see pp. 872) and size of the clitoris are noted (the width of the normal glans is <5 mm). The size of the hymenal opening and the degree of estrogen effect are assessed. A well-estrogenized vagina is moist and light pink, whereas a poorly estrogenized vagina is red and the mucosa appears thin. In a virginal young teenager with a tight hymen and vaginal discharge, a small amount of the discharge can be obtained by gently inserting a cotton-tipped applicator through the hymenal ring. If the hymen is 1 finger-breadth wide, a virginal speculum (the Huffman speculum) can be inserted gently. Visualizing the cervix with use of a speculum is easier if the position of the cervix has first been located by a one-finger vaginal examination. With the speculum in place, the size and shape of the cervix and the presence of discharge are assessed. The portio of the cervix may be pink (squamous cells with the squamocolumnar junction inside the cervical os) or, more commonly, a reddened area is visible because the squamocolumnar junction is on the portio. This ectropion or ectopy (sometimes called an "erosion" in the past) represents columnar cells. Use of birth control pills and in utero exposure to diethylstilbestrol is often associated with a prominent ectropion. All sexually active adolescents should have a Pap smear annually and be screened for sexually transmitted infections *(N. gonorrhoeae* and *C. trachomatis)* every 6–12 months. *Chlamydia trachomatis* cervicitis is common in adolescent oral contraceptive users, in part because if barrier contraception is not used, the cervix is exposed to sexually transmitted infections, but also because the ectopy often persists under the influence of contraceptive hormones and is easily colonized with *Chlamydia* (Stamm and Holmes, 1984; Shafer et al, 1984; Shafer et al, 1985; Washington et al. 1985; Brunham et al, 1984; Kiviat et al, 1985). Sexually active adolescents appear to be three times more likely to have chlamydial infections than do women over age 20 years. Thus, it is important for the physician to look for the presence of a mucopurulent cervical discharge and edema and friability of the ectropion (signs of *C. trachomatis)* in the sexually active teenager.

A cotton-tipped applicator should then be swirled in the endocervix and examined for the presence of typical yellow discharge of *C. trachomatis* (Brunham et al, 1984). A Gram stain of the endocervical discharge with more than 10 polys per oil immersion field (1000X), suggests *C. trachomatis*; the finding of intracellular Gram-negative diplococci in the patient with cervical discharge is highly suggestive of *N. gonorrhoeae.* To make the diagnosis of *C. trachomatis* cervicitis, a sample can be obtained by inserting a Dacron swab or brush into the endocervical canal; this can then be examined by a monoclonal antibody test (MicroTrak), an enzyme immunoassay, or culture. To test for *N. gonorrhoeae,* a cotton-tipped swab can be streaked onto a medium such as Thayer-Martin Jembec.

In the adolescent, the appearance of any vaginal discharge should be noted. A floccular discharge is typical of normal secretions or *Candida* infection. A sample of the discharge should be tested with pH paper and wet preps and whiff test (as described in the previous section) should be performed.

Normal vaginal pH is less than 4.5; pH is increased in patients with *Trichomonas* and NSV. On the saline-wet preparation, an increased number of white cells suggests cervicitis or *Trichomonas.* Clue cells (vaginal epithelial cells to which such a large number of organisms are attached that the entire cell border is obscured) suggest NSV. A Gram stain of the vaginal secretions can be very helpful because the normal vaginal Gram stain contains lactobacilli. In the adolescent with an itchy, undiagnosed vaginitis, secretions should be streaked on Biggy agar to aid detection of *Candida.*

After the speculum is removed, the uterus and adnexae should be palpated by bimanual one- or two-finger vaginal abdominal examination. A rectovaginal-abdominal examination allows palpation of a retroverted uterus and the uterosacral ligaments. In the adolescent with severe dysmenorrhea, tenderness along the uterosacral ligaments may suggest endometriosis.

REFERENCES

Brunham RC, Paavonen J, Stevens CE, et al: Mucopurulent cervicitis—The ignored counterpart in women of urethritis in men. *N Engl J Med* 311:1, 1984.

Kiviat NB, Petersen M, Kinney-Thomas E, et al: Cytologic manifestations of cervical and vaginal infections. II. Confirmation of *Chlamydia trachomatis* infection by direct immunofluorescence using monoclonal antibodies. *JAMA* 253:997, 1985.

Shafer MA, Beck A, Blain B, et al: *Chlamydia trachomatis*: Important relationships to race, contraception, lower genital tract infection, and Papanicolaou smear. *J Pediatr* 104:141, 1984.

Shafer MA, Sweet RL, Ohm-Smith MJ: Microbiology of the lower genital tract in postmenarchal adolescent girls: Differences by sexual activity, contraception, and presence of nonspecific vaginitis. *J Pediatr* 107:974, 1985.

Stamm WE, Holmes KK: *Chlamydia trachomatis* infections of the adult. In Holmes KK, Mardh PA, Sparling PF, et al (eds): *Sexually Transmitted Diseases.* New York, McGraw Hill Book Co., 1984.

Washington AE, Gove S, Schachter J, et al: Oral contraceptives, *Chlamydia trachomatis* infection, and pelvic inflammatory disease. *JAMA* 253:2246, 1985.

Vaginal Disorders 3

VULVOVAGINITIS IN THE PREPUBERTAL CHILD

Definition

Infection of the vulva and/or vagina is termed vulvovaginitis.

Natural History

The prepubertal girl is particularly susceptible to nonspecific irritation of the vulvovaginal area, but also can have specific infections from respiratory or enteric pathogens or sexually acquired organisms (Altchek, 1984; Emans and Goldstein, 1980). Because of poor hygiene, the lack of protective hair and labial fat pads, and lack of estrogenization, the vulvar skin is susceptible to irritation and is easily traumatized by topical medications, soaps, and clothing. In some girls, the vulvar inflammation may progress and cause a secondary vaginitis. The child may also acquire a primary vaginal infection and the discharge may cause maceration of the vulva and a secondary vulvitis. A "nonspecific vulvovaginitis" accounts for 25–75% of the diagnoses in children seen in referral centers for evaluation of vulvovaginitis. This term applies to children whose vaginal cultures grow normal flora or Gram- negative enteric organisms (usually *Escherichia coli*) and who have no other etiology for the vaginitis. Nonspecific irritation occurs frequently in children with pinworm infestations who have scratched the anus and vulva and contaminated the vagina. Factors which appear to promote nonspecific vulvar irritation include irritant or allergic contact, the wearing of tight-fitting nylon clothes, obesity, skin disease, masturbation, sexual abuse, labial agglutination, reflux of urine into the vagina, neutral pH of the vagina (6.5–7.5), and either a high hymenal opening which does not allow normal drainage or gaping hymenal ring which allows easy contamination of vagina. Children susceptible to recurrent vulvovaginitis may have other factors that promote adherence of bacteria to epithelial cells. The role of toxigenic or invasive strains of *E. coli* and other enteric organisms such as *Campylobacter* has not been investigated.

The specific infections seen in prepubertal children include Group A streptococcus, *S. pneumoniae, N. meningitidis, Shigella, Yersinia, Candida*; nonspecific vaginitis associated with *Gardnerella vaginalis* (NSV), *N. gonorrhoeae, C. trachomatis,* herpes simplex, and *Trichomonas* (Murphy and Nelson, 1979; Watkins and Quan, 1984; Hammerschlag et al, 1985; Bump, 1985). *Staphylococcus aureus* and *Haemophilus influenzae* can occur as normal flora but also appear to be responsible for some cases of vaginitis. *S. aureus* can be associated with impetiginous lesions on the vulva and buttocks.

Other causes of vulvovaginal complaints are vaginal foreign bodies, vaginal and cervical polyps and tumors, urethral prolapse, systemic illnesses (measles, chickenpox, scarlet fever), anatomic anomalies (for example, double vagina with a fistula, ectopic ureter), and vulvar skin disease (seborrhea, psoriasis, atopic dermatitis, lichen sclerosis, scabies). Occasionally, children have psychosomatic vaginal complaints; these usually generate great concern from the mother.

Children with specific infections usually present with a purulent, persistent discharge and respond to appropriate antibiotic treatment. Children with nonspecific vulvovaginitis may have recurrences with changes in clothing and hygiene.

Diagnosis

The possible diagnoses described in Table 11.2 should be considered in the child presenting with vulvovaginal symptoms. Most children have scant or mucoid discharge associated with nonspecific vulvitis or pinworm infestation and do not require extensive evaluation. A brief external examination in the office and instructions to the mother and child on improved hygiene or the treatment of pinworms is all that is needed.

Table 11.2
Etiology of Vulvovaginitis in the Prepubertal Child

- Nonspecific vulvovaginitis
- Specific infections
  - Group A β streptococcus
  - *S. pneumoniae*
  - *N. meningitidis*
  - *Candida*
  - *Shigella*
  - *S. aureus*
  - *H. influenzae*
  - *N. gonorrhoeae*
  - Condyloma accuminatum
  - *Gardnerella vaginalis*
  - Herpes
  - *Trichomonas*
  - *C. trachomatis*
- Pinworms
- Foreign body
- Polyps, tumors
- Systemic illiness
  - Measles
  - Chickenpox
  - Scarlet fever
  - Steven-Johnson syndrome
- Vulvar skin disease
  - Seborrhea
  - Psoriasis
  - Atopic dermatitis
  - Lichen sclerosis
  - Scabies
- Trauma
- Psychosomatic vaginal complaints
- Miscellaneous
  - Draining pelvic abscess
  - Prolapsed urethra
  - Ectopic ureter

Any child with a persistent, purulent or recurrent vaginal discharge deserves a thorough assessment. Information on hygiene, use of soaps, bubblebaths, and other irritants, the presence of pinworms, the duration, quantity, and character of the discharge and any infections in family members and patient may give some clue to the diagnosis. A green or bloody discharge and a recent onset of a purulent discharge are most likely to be associated with a specific pathogen or foreign body (Emans and Goldstein, 1980; Paradise et al, 1982). Itching and redness are usually nonspecific signs of irritation. Any history of atopic dermatitis or allergies in the patient or family should be elicited. Information on caretakers that might give a clue to ongoing sexual abuse should be sought. The parent should be asked about behavioral changes, nightmares, and fears as well as abdominal pain, headaches, and enuresis, all of which may suggest abuse. The child should be asked both when the history is taken and later during the examination about the possibility of someone having touched her in the vaginal area.

The examination, wet preparations, and cultures (see p. 652) described above, should allow the physician to make a definitive diagnosis.

Treatment

Treatment of nonspecific vulvovaginitis includes specific measures to improve hygiene; avoidance of leotards, nylon tights, jeans, sleepers, and wool; double rinsing of cotton underwear; tepid sitz baths either without soap applied to the vulva or sparing use of bland soap; and handwashing. After the bath, the child should pat dry the vulva or air dry it with the legs spread apart; a hair dryer on cool setting can aid the drying. In persistent cases of nonspecific vaginitis oral antibiotics (amoxicillin or a cephalosporin) may be given for 10 days. Occasionally, topical estrogen cream is warranted to thicken the vagina and vulva and make it more resistant to infection. In children with persisting symptoms, if an adequate examination is not possible, a brief examination under anesthesia in an ambulatory operating room should be done to exclude the possibility of a foreign body or tumor and to obtain additional cultures.

The treatment of specific infections is outlined in Table 11.3, Group A streptococci, *S. pneumoniae, N. gonorrhoeae,* and *C. trachomatis* are treated with the appropriate oral antibiotic. *Candida* vaginal infections are treated with topical nystatin, miconazole, or clotrimazole cream. Rarely is it necessary or practical to use intravaginal medication in the young child. Small perianal condylomata can be treated with podophyllin

Table 11.3
Treatment of Vulvovaginitis in the Prepubertal Child

Etiology	Treatment
Group A β streptococcus *S. pneumoniae*	Pen Vee K 125–250 mg qid for 10 days
C. trachomatis	Erythromycin 50 mg/kg/day po for 10 days
N. gonorrhoeae	Amoxicillin 50 mg/kg po single dose or procaine penicillin G 100,000 units/kg i.m. + probenecid 25 mg/kg po (max 1 g) or Ceftriaxone 125 mg i.m.
Candida	Topical nystatin, miconazole, or clotrimazole cream
Shigella	Trimethoprim/sulfamethoxazole 8 mg/40 mg/kg day po for 7 days
S. aureus	Cephalexin 25–50 mg/kg/day for 7–10 days Dicloxacillin 12.5–25 mg/kg/day for 7–10 days
H. influenzae	Amoxicillin 20–40 mg/kg/day for 7 days
Trichomonas	Metronidazole 125 mg (15 mg/kg/day) tid for 7–10 days

CASE ILLUSTRATION

A 4½-year-old girl was evaluated for a complaint of green vaginal discharge for the past week. The mother and the girl denied a history of bubble bath use, recent streptococcal infections in the family, sexual abuse, and pruritis. During the daytime, the girl had been cared for by a neighborhood woman for the past year.

Physical examination revealed a cooperative child. Inspection of the vulva showed perihymenal erythema. The hymen was slightly attenuated and green discharge was evident. In knee chest position the vagina and cervix could be seen and discharge was present. No foreign bodies were seen. Rectal examination was negative and cultures were taken. Wet preps of the discharge showed numerous polymorphonuclear leukocytes but no yeast or clue cells. The whiff test was negative.

Two days later, the culture grew *N. gonorrhoeae* and the mother was asked to bring the girl back to the office. The discharge was still present and a culture for *C. trachomatis* was taken. The child still denied the possibility of sexual contact. She was treated with single dose amoxicillin and probenecid. The test for *Chlamydia* was also positive and she was given a 10-day course of erythromycin. Although both mother and child denied the possibility of sexual abuse, the child abuse authorities were notified of the positive gonorrhea culture and the strong suspicion of sexual abuse. The child was also referred to a mental health professional experienced in sexual abuse history for an evaluation. Over the course of several sessions, the child admitted that the 14-year-old son of the babysitter had abused her on five or six occasions and through doll play she was able to demonstrate attempted vulvar coitus. She had been threatened by the boy to secrecy, and therefore, had been previously unwilling to tell the story.

QUESTIONS AND COMMENTS

Should all children with vaginal discharge be cultured?

Although many children have transient erythema of the vulva and scant mucoid vaginal discharge which responds to simple hygienic measures, a persistent, recurrent, or purulent discharge requires adequate cultures. Denial of a history of sexual abuse does not negate the possibility of sexually transmitted infection.

Should *Chlamydia trachomatis* be evaluated in sexually abused children?

With increasing availability of methods for antigen detection and cultures, pediatricians can be expected to find more *Chlamydia* infections in prepubertal children. It is particularly important that children with other sexually transmitted diseases such as gonorrhea be cultured for *Chlamydia* (Ingram et al, 1986). Cultures are preferred until the sensitivity and specificity of antigen detection methods in prepubertal children are known.

Is sexual abuse possible with normal dimensions of the hymenal ring?

Most children with a history of sexual molestation have had touching or vulvar coitus and, thus, in most cases there are no signs of penetration or laceration of the hymenal ring. In cases of chronic ongoing digital manipulation, there may be attenuation and rounding of the lower hymenal border or transsections of the hymen.

in tincture of benzoin; however, large lesions and rectal and hymenal lesions require laser treatment under general anesthesia.

Since the mother frequently has concerns about the cause of the vaginitis out of proportion to the problem, it is important for the pediatrician to do a careful examination and outline a treatment program to the child and mother. Since mothers sometimes fear damage to the reproductive tract, the benign nature of recurrent nonspecific vaginitis should be emphasized.

Prognosis

Most children with specific infections are cured promptly. Children with nonspecific vulvovaginitis may have recurrences, especially with upper respiratory infections or with poor hygiene. Recurrences may respond to improved hygienic measures and sitz baths or may require a course of antibiotics.

Prevention

Vulvovaginal irritants should be avoided, as outlined in the treatment of nonspecific vaginitis.

LABIAL ADHESIONS

Definition

Agglutination of the labia minora in prepubertal girls is designated labial adhesion.

Basic Science

Labial adhesions occur primarily in infants and girls between age 3 months and 6 years but the adhesions may occasionally persist to the time of puberty. The cause is unknown but may be related to vulvar inflammation.

Epidemiology

Minor agglutination of the labia minora may occur in 4–20% of girls, but the incidence of significant agglutination is considerably less.

Natural History

Minor labial agglutination at the posterior forchette may disappear without therapy or progress to significant agglutination. It is possible, although unproven, that poor hygiene and vulvar irritation are responsible for this difference in outcome. Although extensive labial adhesions may disappear spontaneously, especially during estrogenization at puberty, persistent, thick labial adhesions completely covering the vaginal orifice causing poor drainage of the vaginal secretions and reflux of urine into the vagina often require therapy.

Diagnosis and Treatment

Visual inspection of the vulva at the time of routine physical examination may reveal asymptomatic labial adhesions, or the mother may have brought the child to the pediatrician because the "vagina appeared absent" (Fig. 11.7). The treatment of labial adhesions remains controversial. Spontaneous separation may occur, particularly with small labial adhesions at the posterior forchette.

If the opening in the adhesion is large enough for vaginal and urinary drainage, the labia may be lubricated with a bland ointment (Vaseline or A & D ointment) and gently separated by the mother over several weeks. For adhesions that impair vaginal or urinary drainage, the most effective treatment is application of an estrogen-containing cream (Premarin cream) applied twice daily for 2 weeks and then at bedtime for another 1–2 weeks. After separation, the labia should be gently opened and a bland ointment applied each night at bedtime for 6–12 months to prevent recurrences. Forced separation is traumatic for the child and often causes the adhesions to form again.

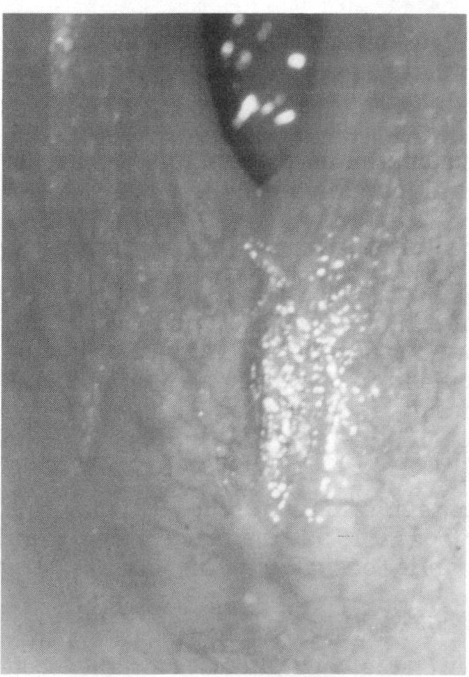

Figure 11.7. Labial adhesions.

Prognosis

Labial adhesions are usually benign, although they can impair vaginal and urinary drainage and may require treatment.

Prevention

It is possible but unknown whether improved hygienic measures will prevent this problem.

VAGINAL BLEEDING IN PREPUBERTAL CHILD

Definition

A prepubertal girl with the complaint of "blood in the underwear" is often assumed to have "vaginal bleeding" although the source may be the uterus, vagina, urethra, perihymenal area, or rectum.

Basic Science

In the neonate, vaginal bleeding may occur several days to several weeks after delivery, as a result of withdrawal from exposure in utero to maternal hormones. In the young child, vaginal bleeding may result from vaginitis, trauma (straddle injuries, sexual abuse), hemangiomas, polyps, foreign body, tumor, precocious puberty, and blood dyscrasias. Urethral prolapse may mimic vaginal bleeding.

Epidemiology

The incidence is unknown.

Natural History

The natural history depends upon the cause of the bleeding.

Diagnosis

The child with the complaint of vaginal bleeding should have a general physical examination for other signs of trauma, bleeding, or precocious development and a careful genital examination. If the child shows a growth spurt, breast development or vaginal estrogenization, she should be evaluated for precocious or pseudoprecocious puberty. If excoriations are noted around the vulva or anus, pinworms should be considered. Visualization of the vagina and cervix is crucial to exclude the possibility of a foreign body, polyps, or tumor. A foreign body should be suspected in girls with bleeding and purulent discharge (Paradise and Willis 1985). Vaginal inspection can usually be accomplished adequately in the knee-chest position (see pp. 652), but if not, examination under anesthesia is necessary.

Treatment

Treatment depends upon the cause of the problem. Vaginitis and pinworm infections can be treated (pp.

1127). Foreign bodies may be removed in the office or under anesthesia; lacerations frequently require suturing under general anesthesia. The rare tumor needs referral to a teaching center for therapy.

Prognosis and prevention depend upon the nature of the diagnosis.

CASE ILLUSTRATION

A 6-year-old girl presented with intermittent vaginal bleeding for 3 weeks. She had had a 2-month history of a small amount of green vaginal discharge and now had intermittent spotting. Her mother had brought her underwear which showed a dime-sized spot of fresh blood. The girl denied a history of trauma or sexual abuse. She had no history of bubble bath use, medication, or diarrhea.

Physical examination revealed a normal hymenal ring with several punctate hemorrhagic areas in the perihymenal area. Knee-chest examination showed scant discharge and wet preparations revealed white cells. Cultures for *N. gonorrhoeae* and *C. trachomatis* were negative. Vaginal culture grew *Shigella sonnei* resistant to ampicillin. The patient was treated with sulfamethazole/trimethoprim with resolution of her symptoms. Follow-up vaginal and stool cultures were negative. Epidemiologic studies revealed that the child had attended a day camp 2 months earlier where eight other children had developed *Shigella* diarrhea.

QUESTIONS AND COMMENTS

Should trauma or sexual abuse have been suspected on the basis of the initial examination?

Because of the frequency of sexual abuse, the clinician should always be highly suspicious of the possibility. However, vaginitis especially if associated with scratching by the child or maceration can present with bleeding.

How does *Shigella* vaginitis present to the clinician?

Vaginal infection with *Shigella* commonly causes a mucopurulent or bloody discharge, and the introitus may show small areas of superficial hemorrhage. A history of diarrhea is present in only one-fourth of patients.

VAGINAL DISCHARGE IN THE ADOLESCENT

Basic Science

The adolescent with vaginitis is likely to have a specific etiology for the discharge. The three most common causes are *Candida, Trichomonas,* and NSV. Normal vaginal discharge or leukorrhea is mucoid and white and can be irritating if the underwear is nonabsorbent. *C. trachomatis* and *N. gonorrhoeae* cause cervicitis which may present as a vaginal discharge.

Candida vaginitis, seen both in virginal and sexually active adolescents, can occur before or after menarche and, thus, should be considered in an adolescent who has a pruritic white discharge. Predisposing factors for *Candida* vaginitis include diabetes, use of antibiotics, immunosuppressive drugs, or corticosteroids, pregnancy, obesity, and possibly oral contraceptive usage.

Trichomonas and NSV are primarily sexually acquired infections.

Epidemiology

In sexually active girls, *Trichomonas* is found in 11%, *N. gonorrhoeae* in 1–13%, and *C. trachomatis* in 6–22%. *Candida* is a common cause of vaginitis in virginal and sexually active girls. Although *Gardnerella vaginalis* can be isolated from 30–40% of adolescents, the complex alteration of vaginal flora associated with NSV is considered to be sexually acquired. Data on vaginal flora of adolescents has been recently published (Shafer et al, 1985; Bump et al, 1986).

Diagnosis

The diagnosis is made from the appearance of the discharge, the wet preps, vaginal pH, and cultures. The office procedures are outlined.

The adolescent with *Candida* vaginitis usually complains of a white discharge and itching, especially prominent before and after the menstrual period. On examination, the vulva may be erythematous and the discharge thick, white, and curdy. The 10% KOH prep is 80–90% accurate in making the diagnosis of *Candida* in the symptomatic patient. A Biggy culture should be obtained in questionable cases since, otherwise, an adolescent with nonspecific or allergic itching may be recurrently treated with antifungal creams.

The adolescent with *Trichomonas* typically complains of an irritating, odorous discharge, and sometimes dysuria. On examination, yellow or green bubbly discharge can be seen. The vagina and cervix may be red and inflamed; punctate hemorrhages (strawberry spots) are occasionally visible on the cervix. Flagellated organisms and white cells are seen on wet prep in greater than 75% of symptomatic women with purulent discharge. However, in patients seen in STD clinics without regard to symptoms, the wet smear detects only about 50% of those detected by culture. The Pap smear appears to detect about 70% of those found on culture. Cultures, thus, provide the most sensitive method of detection but appropriate culture techniques are not generally available to the practitioner.

NSV, also termed *G. vaginalis,* associated vaginosis, or bacterial vaginosis has been the subject of much controversy over the years, because *G. vaginalis* and "clue cells" can occur in asymptomatic women. Based largely on work by Holmes and associates, it is currently thought that NSV involves a complex alteration in microbial flora with an increase in the concentration of *G. vaginalis* and anaerobic bacteria, a decrease in lactobacilli, and an increase in organic acids produced by the abnormal flora (Holmes, 1984). Colonization with *G. vaginalis* generally is not related to sexual activity, but bacterial vaginosis is correlated with sexual experience as well as previous *Trichomonas* infection. The odor noted by the patient and during the whiff test results from increased amines volatilized by KOH and is increased with the presence of seminal fluid. The diagnosis in the symptomatic patient, thus, should be based on three or four criteria: (1) a gray to white homogeneous thin discharge adherent to the vaginal wall, (2) vaginal fluid pH >4.5, (3) a positive whiff test, (4) clue cells representing 20% of all vaginal epithelial cells. The absence of lactobacilli on wet prep or Gram stain and the presence of Gram-variable coccobacilli and curved Gram-negative rods provides confirmatory evidence.

N. gonorrhoeae may occur as an asymptomatic cervical, rectal, or pharyngeal infection in the sexually active teenager. Symptomatic infections include cervicitis, urethritis, proctitis, pharyngitis, arthritis, pelvic inflammatory disease, and rarely, meningitis or endocarditis. Thus, the patient with a gynecologic infection may present with vaginal discharge, dysuria, dyspareunia, or pelvic pain. The diagnosis of *N. gonorrhoeae* cervical infection can be suspected on the basis of a Gram stain of the endocervical discharge demonstrating Gram-negative intracellular diplococci but should be confirmed by culture on appropriate media.

Adolescents infected with *C. trachomatis* may be asymptomatic or present with dysuria-pyuria, vaginal discharge, irregular bleeding, or pelvic pain. *C. trachomatis* is a major cause of cervicitis and pelvic inflammatory disease. The diagnosis should be suspected if the cervix is friable with a mucopurulent discharge, a cotton-tipped applicator twirled in the endocervix shows a characteristic yellow color, or a Gram stain of the endocervical discharge shows 10 polymorphonuclear leukocytes per high power field (1000×) (Washington et al, 1985; Shafer et al, 1984; Brunham et al, 1984). Diagnostic tests include monoclonal antibody test (MicroTrak), enzyme immunoassays, and culture.

Table 11.4 has references to other sexually transmitted diseases and this chapter (pp. 662 and 663) discusses genital herpes and condylomata acuminata.

Treatment

Treatment is outlined in Table 11.5.

For *Candida,* single dose vaginal clotrimazole or a 3-day course of one of the other antifungal agents appears to be the simplest treatment. Recurrences should be treated with a 7-day course of antifungal cream; a 1- to 2-day course following each menstrual period, or at any sign of itching; or 1 applicatorful once a week ("always on Sunday"). Because of potential toxicity, ketoconazole should probably not be used in the adolescent with recurrent *Candida* vaginitis until more data are available. Oral antifungal medication aimed at eliminating rectal carriage of *Candida* does not seem to prevent recurrences. Sexual partners should be examined for *Candida* genital infections although sexual transmission does not appear to be the usual source of reinfection. The patient with recurrent *Candida* vaginitis should be screened for diabetes.

Table 11.4
Sexually Transmitted Diseases

Disease or Organism	Refer to Page
AIDS	1039
Chlamydia trachomatis	1105
Gonorrhea (*N. gonorrhoeae*)	1067
Genital herpes simplex	663
Viral hepatitis	470
Parasitic skin infections	1121
Scabies	1169
Mycoplasma hominis	1110
Syphilis	1101
Trichomoniasis	659
Condylomata acuminata (genital warts)	662

Table 11.5
Treatment of the Adolescent with Vaginitis

Candida	Clotrimazole 500 mg vaginal tab for 1 day, or Clotrimazole 200 mg vaginally HS for 3 days, or Clotrimazole 1% cream HS for 7 days, or Miconazole 2% cream HS for 7 days, or Miconazole 200 ng vaginally HS for 3 days, or Butoconazole cream HS for 3 days Mycostatin cream bid for 14 days
Trichomonas	Metronidazole 2 g single dose
NSV-*G. vaginalis*	Metronidazole 500 mg bid for 7 days Ampicillin 500 mg qid for 7 days (less effective)
N. gonorrhoeae (uncomplicated cervical, urethral, rectal infection)	Amoxicillin 3.0 g *or* ampicillin 3.5 g po *or* aqueous procaine penicillin G (APPG) 4.8 million units IM + Probenecid 1.0 g po *or* Ceftriaxone 250 mg IM FOLLOWED BY Doxycycline 100 mg po bid for 7 days or Tetracycline 500 mg qid for 7 days *or* Erythromycin base or stearate 500 mg po qid for 7 days
C. trachomatis	Doxycycline 100 mg po bid for 7 days or Tetracycline 500 mg po qid for 7 days or Erythromycin base or stearate 500 mg po qid for 7 days or 250 mg po qid for 14 days

CASE ILLUSTRATION 1

A 13-year-old adolescent came to the office for evaluation of a recurrent white discharge. She had had her menarche at age 12½ years of age and had had menses approximately every month without dysmenorrhea. The discharge began about 1 year before her menarche and she had been treated with miconazole on four occasions. Occasionally, the discharge had been irritating and pruritic, but usually, a white mucoid discharge was apparent on her underwear. She denied having been sexually active.

Physical examination revealed a healthy 13-year-old. Inspection of the external genitalia showed Tanner IV pubic hair with a well-estrogenized virginal introitus with copious white discharge visible at the hymenal ring. Samples of the discharge were obtained with cotton-tipped swabs and a culture was plated on Biggy agar for yeast. The wet preps showed many epithelial cells without evidence of inflammation. No *Candida* were seen on wet prep and the Biggy agar was negative at 7 days.

The diagnosis was leukorrhea and the patient was treated with reassurance, attention to hygiene, and the use of panty shields as needed.

QUESTIONS AND COMMENTS

What is the most likely cause of vaginal discharge in a 13-year-old virginal patient?

The primary cause of discharge is normal leukorrhea, the desquamation of vaginal cells and cervical mucus associated with the high estrogen levels of early adolescence. The discharge occasionally may be mildly irritating and pruritic, but adolescents should not be treated with antifungal creams without an adequate evaluation. The other likely cause of pruritic vaginal discharge in the young adolescent group is *Candida*. The KOH prep is usually positive in the symptomatic patient.

Does a 13-year-old with vaginal discharge need a full pelvic examination with a speculum?

The 13-year-old virginal patient can often be evaluated by obtaining small samples of the discharge on a cotton-tipped swab inserted gently through the hymenal ring into the vagina. However, any patient with unusual discharge or foul odor, and any sexually active patient should have an adequate speculum examination.

CASE ILLUSTRATION 2

A 12-year-old adolescent came to the Gynecology Clinic for evaluation of a foul-smelling vaginal discharge. She had had her menarche 4 months before the visit. Shortly thereafter, she had developed a foul-smelling yellowish discharge. She had been seen at another clinic where she had allowed only a partial pelvic examination. Wet preparations of the discharge had been negative for *Candida* and positive for white cells and clue cells. The discharge was noted to be malodorous; no foreign bodies could be palpated within the vagina. Bimanual rectoabdominal examination had been difficult because of poor relaxation. The patient denied the use of tampons and she had no history of sexual activity. She was treated with hygiene and oral metronidazole, 500 mg, twice a day for 1 week with clearing of the discharge.

With her next menstrual period the discharge recurred, and the patient was seen in the Gynecology Clinic. At this time, the discharge was purulent and foul smelling with an increased number of white cells and some clue cells. On bimanual examination, a questionable fullness in the right adnexa was palpated. Ultrasonography revealed a mass in the right adnexa with fluid and debris and agenesis of the right kidney. At surgery, the patient had a bicornuate uterus; a small right uterine horn emptied into an obstructed vaginal pouch which communicated through a small opening into the vagina. The patient had a uterine metroplasty and fenestration of the blind vaginal pouch. She did well at follow-up.

QUESTIONS AND COMMENTS

What should make the physician think of the possibility of a uterine anomaly?

The occurrence of a foul-smelling discharge in association with the onset of menarche in a patient without a foreign body or history of sexual activity should be evaluated for the possibility of a uterine anomaly. The finding of agenesis of the right kidney on ultrasound should alert the physician to the probability that the mass found in the right adenexa is likely to be an obstructed müllerian anomaly. In adolescents, scanning the kidneys at the same time as the pelvis when an abnormality is found is extremely useful.

Why did the patient initially respond to metronidazole?

Because the infection within the vaginal pouch was probably caused by anaerobes, a temporary response to metronidazole could be expected. These symptoms, however, recurred with the onset of the next menses when the uterine horn drained within the pouch again and became infected.

Treatment of *Trichomonas* should include the sexual partner. Although reinfection is the usual cause of "persistent" *Trichomonas* in the adolescent, rare *Trichomonas* isolates have acquired a significant degree of resistance to metronidazole. Resistant organisms have responded to higher doses of metronidazole over a longer course. Metronidazole should not be given during the first trimester of pregnancy and only during the second and third trimesters if benefits clearly outweigh potential risks.

The drug of choice for treatment of NSV is metronidazole. The most effective dosage is still under study. Metronidazole, 500 mg twice a day for 7 days, is clearly effective; a single dose of 2 g has a variable efficacy rate (67–90%). Single dose treatment may appear effective at 7–10 days after treatment but symptoms may recur by 3 weeks after treatment (Swedberg et al, 1985). A recent report of use of 2 g on day 1 and 2 g on day 3 may offer another potential regimen to

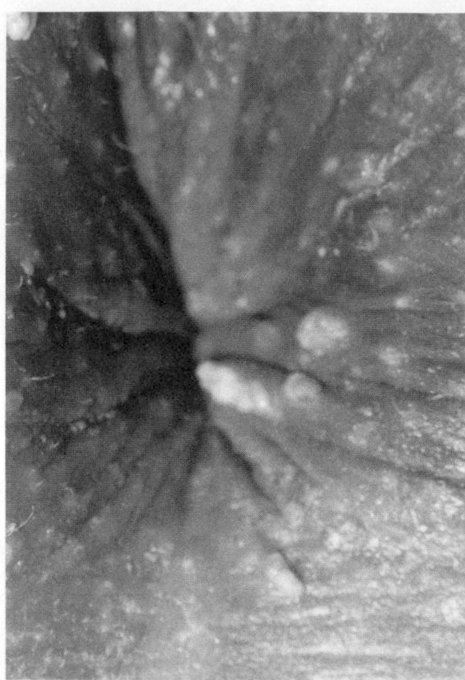

Figure 11.8. Perianal condyloma.

minimize the dosage of this medicine (Jerve et al, 1984). Ampicillin therapy, although less effective than metronidazole, is an alternative for pregnant women. Asymptomatic patients with clue cells need not be treated. The sexual partner appears to need treatment only in a patient with recurrent symptoms.

The treatment of uncomplicated cervical infections with *N. gonorrhoeae* should consider the high probability of coexisting *C. trachomatis* infection and the prevalence of penicillin-resistant and penicillinase-producing *N. gonorrhoeae*. Recommended therapies are shown in Table 11.5. A serology for syphilis should be drawn before treatment. Contacts should be cultured and treated. Patients should return for test-of-cure 3–7 days after therapy.

The treatment of *C. trachomatis* cervical or urethral infection is ahown in Table 11.5. Contacts should be cultured and treated. Follow-up cultures are recommended.

Pelvic inflammatory disease treatment is discussed on page 670.

Prognosis

The initial cure of these infections is excellent. However, patients with *Candida* may have recurrences. Patients with *Trichomonas* may have reinfections if partners are not adequately treated. The factors involved in recurrences for NSV have not been fully elucidated.

Prevention

Since many vaginal infections seen in adolescents are sexually transmitted, a number of factors including abstinence, monogamous relationships, and barrier contraception can lessen the risk. Adolescents must have improved access to confidential medical care. The risks of infections including AIDS (see pp. 1039) should be discussed with all adolescents. Screening tests which are both sensitive and specific in asymptomatic and symptomatic patients need further refinement. The development of new antibiotics and antviral agents effective in shorter courses should improve compliance and decrease recurrences.

CONDYLOMATA ACUMINATA

Definition

Condylomata acuminata are anogenital warts caused by human papilloma virus (HPV).

Natural History

Both children and adolescents may have anogenital warts caused by HPV. In the adolescent, the virus is sexually transmitted and the incubation period may be between 6 weeks and 8 months. The warts may occur on the vagina, cervix, vulva, anus, or rarely, mouth. In the young child, genital warts may occur from exposure to virus during delivery, from close physical contact, or from sexual abuse. A prepubertal child with genital warts should be examined for other sexually transmitted diseases and evaluated by a mental health provider experienced in obtaining histories of sexual abuse.

Although condylomata acuminata may disappear spontaneously, most require treatment because of possible spread to other areas of the anogenital tract and to partners.

Diagnosis

The diagnosis is made by inspection (Fig. 11.8 and 11.9). Secondary syphilis should be excluded by the appropriate serologic test for syphilis. Children and adolescents should be evaluated for other sexually transmitted diseases such as *C. trachomatis, N. gonorrhoeae,* NSV, and *Trichomonas*. A coexisting vulvovaginitis can make the successful treatment of the warts more difficult.

Treatment

In the prepubertal child, a few small anal warts may be treated with podophyllin resin, 10–25%, in tincture of benzoin, with special care to avoid the normal skin. Extensive condylomata or those involving the hymen or vulva require treatment with laser or cautery under general anesthesia.

In the adolescent, podophyllin resin or trichloroacetic acid can be applied to small vulvar or anal lesions. If the lesions are numerous, a few can be treated each week. Podophyllin should be washed off 2–4 hours after the therapy. Additional treatments are given every week. Podophyllin is contraindicated during pregnancy. Condylomata that involve the urethra, vagina,

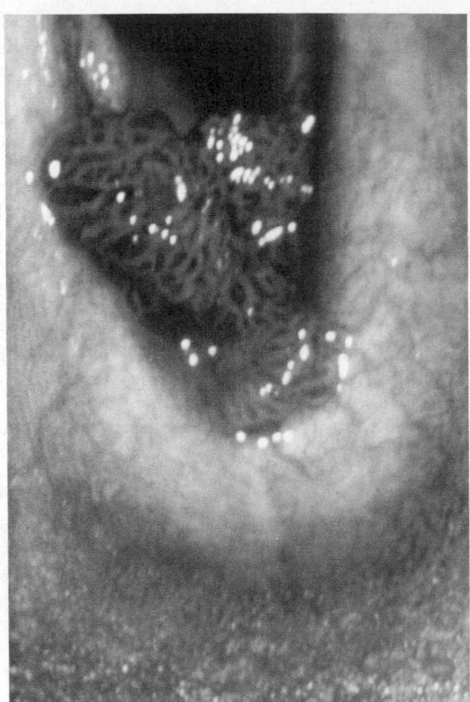

Figure 11.9. Condyloma acuminata on hymen of prepubertal child. Reproduced from Emans, *Pediatr Rev* 8:12, 1986.

or cervix, or are large should be treated with cryocautery, excision, trichloroacetic acid, or laser. Warts may recur, especially in patients with extensive lesions. For persistent or recurrent perianal or periurethral warts, the rectum should be examined with an anoscope and the urethra with a cystoscope. A Pap smear should be obtained from all adolescents with condylomata.

Prognosis

Condylomata acuminata may recur and need further therapy. Recurrence appears more likely in patients with virus in the skin adjacent to the wart.

Because of the association of certain types of HPV and cervical dysplasia, cervical carcinoma in situ, and possibly vulvar carcinoma, adolescents who have had condylomata require careful observation and follow-up by Pap smear.

Prevention

In small children, improved hygiene on the part of caretakers and more important, the prevention of childhood sexual abuse should reduce the incidence of this problem. In adolescents, the avoidance of multiple partners should lessen the exposure to this virus.

HERPES SIMPLEX GENITAL INFECTIONS

Definition

A herpes simplex genital infection is an infection (vulva, vagina, cervix) resulting from contact with type 1 or type 2 herpes simplex.

Epidemiology

An estimated 5 million Americans have genital herpes with approximately 300,000 new cases each year. The number of private patient visits for newly diagnosed herpes has increased 7.5-fold from 1966–1981 (Becker, 1985).

Natural History

Herpes simplex genital infections are sexually acquired. Primary infections with either type 1 or 2 (more commonly 2) occur in patients with no antibodies to either type. In patients with antibodies (usually to type 1), the first known genital infection is termed *nonprimary first episode*. Patients with *recurrent* genital infections are more likely to have type 2 infections.

Local symptoms include pain, dysuria, itching, discharge, cervicitis, vulvitis, and inguinal adenopathy. Systemic symptoms often occur in primary episodes and may include fever, headache, malaise, myalgia, aseptic meningitis, and urinary and bowel retention.

Shedding of virus lasts 11–12 days and healing takes 10–21 days in primary infections versus 4–5 days for healing in current infections. Nonprimary episodes have an intermediate time course. The virus remains latent between infections. Patients may become infected without symptoms.

Diagnosis

The diagnosis of genital herpes is usually apparent on inspection. A smear (Tzanck prep) may show characteristic multinucleated giant cells. Tissue culture of vesicles and ulcers from a patient with a first episode has the highest yield and can determine the type of herpes (Corey et al, 1983a).

Treatment

No currently approved treatment can eradicate the latent state within the body. Oral acyclovir can shorten the duration of symptoms and viral shedding in primary infections and reduce the number of recurrences in women with frequently recurring, troublesome genital lesions. Once the medication is stopped, recurrences reappear. Long-term safety is unknown and the question of resistant strains has not been fully answered. Symptomatic relief with sitz baths and oral analgesics can be helpful. Patients should avoid sexual contact while they have active lesions.

Prognosis

Some patients have a single episode of genital herpes without recurrence; others experience frequent, painful recurrences. Strategies for preventing infection of the neonate at the time of delivery are controversial.

Prevention

Prevention of all sexually transmitted infections is similar. Condoms play less of a role because of the sites of the ulcers.

REFERENCES

Altchek A: Pediatric vulvovaginitis. *J Reproduc Med* 29:359, 1984.

Becker TM, Blount JH, Guinan ME: Genital herpes infections in private practice in the United States, 1966–1981. *JAMA* 253:1601, 1985.

Bump RC: *Chlamydia trachomatis* as a cause of prepubertal vaginitis. *Obstet Gynecol* 65:384, 1985.

Corey L, Adams H, Brown ZA: Genital herpes simplex infections: Clinical manifestations, course, and complications. *Ann Intern Med* 98:958, 1983a.

Corey L, Holmes KK: Genital herpes simplex virus infections: Current concepts in diagnosis, therapy, and prevention. *Ann Intern Med* 98:973, 1983b.

Crum CP, Ikenberg H, Richart RM, et al: Human papillomavirus type 16 and early cervical neoplasia. *N Engl J Med* 310:880, 1984.

Emans SJ, Goldstein DP: The gynecologic examination of the prepubertal child with vulvovaginitis: Use of the knee-chest position. *Pediatrics* 65:758, 1980.

Ferenczy A, Mitro M, Nagai N, et al: Latent papillomavirus and recurring genital warts. *N Engl J Med* 31:784, 1985.

Hammerschlag MR, Cummings M, Doraiswamy B, et al: Nonspecific vaginitis following sexual abuse in children. *Pediatrics* 75:1028, 1985.

Holmes KK: Lower genital tract infections in women: Cystitis/urethritis, vulvovaginitis, and cervicitis. In Holmes KK, Mardh PA, Sparling PF, et al (eds): *Sexually Transmitted Diseases*. New York, McGraw Hill, 1984.

Ingram DL, White ST, Occhiuti AR, et al: Childhood vaginal infections: Association with *Chlamydia trachomatis* with sexual contact. *Pediatr Infect Dis* 5:226, 1986.

Jerve F, Berdal TB, Bohman P, et al: Metronidazole in the treatment of nonspecific vaginitis (NSV). *Br J Ven Dis* 60:171, 1984.

Murphy TV, Nelson JD: *Shigella* vaginitis: Report of 38 patients and review of the literature. *Pediatrics* 63:511, 1979.

Neinstein LS, Goldenring J, Carpenter S: Nonsexual transmission of sexually transmitted diseases: An infrequent occurrence. *Pediatrics* 74:67, 1984.

Paradise JE, Compos JM, Friedman HM, et al: Vulvovaginitis in premenarchal girls: Clinical features and diagnostic evaluation. *Pediatrics* 70:193, 1982.

Paradise JE, Willis ED: Probability of vaginal foreign body in girls with genital complaints. *Am J Dis Child* 139:472, 1985.

Pinsonneault O, Goldstein DP: Obstructing malformation of the uterus and vagina. *Fertil Steril* 44:241, 1985.

Seidel J, Zonana J, Totten E: Condylomata acuminata as a sign of sexual abuse in children. *J Pediatr* 94:553, 1979.

Swedberg J, Steinea JF, Deiss F, et al: Comparison of single dose vs one week course of metronidazole for symptomatic bacterial vaginosis. *JAMA* 254:1046, 1985.

Watkins S, Quan L: Vulvovaginitis caused by *Yersinia enterocolitica*. *Pediatr Infect Dis* 3:444, 1984.

Gynecologic Evaluation of the Sexually Abused Child and Adolescent 4

Definition

Sexual abuse is defined as the involvement of developmentally immature children or adolescents in sexual activities that they do not fully comprehend, to which they are unable to give informed consent, or that violates taboos of family relationships. Sexual abuse may include exhibitionism, fondling and manipulation, genital viewing or genital contact, and vaginal or rectal penetration.

Epidemiology

From 10–25% of adult women give a history of sexual abuse occurring during their childhood or adolescence (Russell, 1984; Finkelhor, 1980; DeJong et al, 1983).

Natural History

Although single episodes of rape of a child or adolescent by a stranger occur, the majority of cases of sexual abuse involve a long-standing relationship between a known individual, frequently a relative, and a child, often with repeated encounters over months to years. The sexual abuse may be uncovered by sudden disclosure or during an evaluation for behavioral changes, psychosomatic complaints, vulvovaginal symptoms, sexually transmitted diseases, or pregnancy.

Diagnosis

The medical evaluation of the sexually abused child and adolescent is but one component of an important psychosocial assessment of the family and child. Most hospitals have rape protocols which are established to document and preserve medical-legal evidence of abuse (Duenhoelter et al, 1978; Sarles, 1982; Tilelli et al, 1980; Woodling and Kossoris, 1981; Rimsza and Niggemann, 1982).

In acute situations in which the sexual abuse occurred within 1 week of the visit to the emergency ward, specimens should be collected by using the rape kit. The child's general appearance and emotional state should be assessed; any clothing worn at the time of the episode should be collected. A general physical examination should be done to look for evidence of other trauma, and a Wood lamp should be used to detect semen.

In the prepubertal child, the genital examination requires careful inspection of the hymenal ring under magnification of an otoscope or a colposcope to identify any attenuation or transsection of the hymen, synechiae from hymen to vagina, and scarring of the posterior forchette. Friability as the labia are separated should be noted. The size of the hymenal opening should be measured in millimeters in transverse and anteroposterior direction. The vagina should be visualized in knee-chest position (see pp. 652) to exclude the possibility of discharge or foreign bodies. Reflex dilatation of the anus may occur in children who have been repeatedly sodomized. A specimen should then be collected from the vagina to culture for *N. gonorrhoeae* and *C. trachomatis*.

In the adolescent, the lithotomy position should be used for the examination and collection of specimens. A small Huffman speculum can usually be inserted without trauma through the hymenal ring of adolescent girls. Evidence of transsection of the hymenal ring or other genital trauma should be evaluated. Cultures for *N. gonorrhoeae* and *C. trachomatis* are taken from the endocervix. In the child and adolescent, wet mounts are done to look for sperm and *Trichomonas*. Fixed slides should be preserved. Swabs of the vagina, vulva, or any area showing fluorescense with the Wood lamp should be saved for the police laboratory for testing for acid phosphatase, p-30, and MHS-5. The rectum and throat should be cultured for *N. gonorrhoeae*. A rectal examination to assess rectal tone should be done last. A bimanual examination is essential in the adolescent to exclude cervical or adnexal tenderness or pregnancy. Serum should be collected for a serology for syphilis, and a pregnancy test should be done at the time of the evaluation of pubertal patients and 3 weeks later. If the patient was not treated with antibiotics at the time of a rape, repeat cultures for *N. gonorrhoeae* and *C. trachomatis* should be obtained at follow-up evaluation 1 week after the rape. Wet preparations should be reevaluated for *Trichomonas* and NSV infections (see pp. 652). HIV testing should be offered.

Although some children and adolescents are seen within hours to a few days of the sexual abuse, many girls are seen weeks to months after the episode. A detailed medical assessment and cultures for sexually transmitted diseases are required. The perineum should be carefully examined for evidence of old trauma. In a recent study, only 34% of sexually abused children had abnormal findings on physical examination (Emans et al, 1987). The likelihood of detecting evidence of penetration, nongenital trauma, or genital trauma increases with age of the patient, in part, because the episodes in adolescents are more likely to be single-episode rapes with strangers. The presence or absence of findings should be relayed to the family and to the child and the intactness of the child should be emphasized.

Treatment

Prophylaxis may include antibiotics for *N. gonorrhoeae* and *C. trachomatis* in rape cases. In situations involving long-standing abuse in the asymptomatic patient, treatment can await culture results. In postmenarchal patients seen within 48–72 hours of a rape, "morning-after" treatment with Ovral should be offered as therapy (see pp. 678). Stool softeners or Pyridium may be indicated; tetanus toxoid should be given along the guidelines of the American Academy of Pediatrics.

Since the most important sequelae of sexual abuse are psychologic, long-term support for the patient and her family are essential.

REFERENCES

DeJong AR, Hewada AR, Emmett GA: Epidemiologic variations in childhood sexual abuse. *Child Abuse Negl* 7:155, 1983.

Duenhoelter JH, Stone IC, Santos-Ramos R, et al: Detection of seminal fluid constituents after alleged sexual assault. *J Forensic Sci* 4:824, 1978.

Emans SJ, Woods ER, Flagg N, et al: Genital findings in sexually abused, symptomatic and asymptomatic girls. *Pediatrics* 79:778, 1987.

Finkelhor D: Sex among sibships: A survey on prevalence, rarity, and effects. *Arch Sex Behav* 3:171, 1980.

Rimsza ME, Niggemann EA: Medical evaluation of sexually abused children: A review of 311 cases. *Pediatrics* 69:8, 1982.

Russell DE: The prevalence and seriousness of incestuous abuse: Stepfathers vs biological fathers. *Child Abuse Negl* 8:15, 1984.

Sarles RM: Sexual abuse and rape. *Pediatr Rev* 4:93, 1982.

Tilelli J, Turek D, Jaffe A: Sexual abuse of children. *N Engl J Med* 302:319, 1980.

Woodling BA, Kossoris PD: Sexual misuse: Rape, molestation, and incest. *Pediatr Clin North Am* 28:481, 1981.

Dysfunctional Uterine Bleeding

5

Definition

Abnormal uterine bleeding caused by anovulation is termed dysfunctional uterine bleeding.

Basic Science

Dysfunctional uterine bleeding occurs because of acyclic hormonal stimulation of the endometrium secondary to anovulation or aberrations in ovulation such as abnormal follicular or luteal phases. The unopposed secretion of estrogen induces endometrial hyperproliferation and the lack of progesterone inhibits endometrial stability.

Epidemiology

Because physiologic anovulation is most common in perimenarchal girls, dysfunctional uterine bleeding is observed most frequently in this group. The incidence of anovulation is 55–82% in the first year postmenarche and 0–40% 4–5.5 years postmenarche (Lemarchard-Beraud, et al, 1982; Apter et al, 1978; Apter, 1980; Claessens and Cowell, 1981).

Natural History

With increasing time after menarche, most adolescents begin to experience increasingly regular cycles. Anovulatory cycles may persist in various conditions, which are also associated with secondary amenorrhea (see pp. 890), including stress and polycystic ovarian disease.

Diagnosis

Evaluation of the adolescent with dysfunctional uterine bleeding requires a general physical examination for consideration of important medical diagnoses (see Table 11.6) and a pelvic examination before a conclusion can be reached. Laboratory tests include a CBC, differential, and assessment of platelets (by smear or count) and, if menorrhagia is severe, a prothrombin time, a partial thromboplastin time, and a bleeding time to rule out an unsuspected coagulopathy (for example, von Willebrand disease). Girls with menorrhagia from the time of menarche are especially likely to have a bleeding disorder. In the sexually active adolescent, a pregnancy test, sedimentation rate, and endocervical cultures for *N. gonorrhoeae* and *C. trachomatis* should be included. Ultrasonography should be used to confirm clinical suspicion or in patients in whom an adequate bimanual examination is difficult. In patients who have persistent dysfunctional uterine bleeding, endocrine studies including thyroid function tests, blood sugar, and appropriate screening for polycystic ovary syndrome should be assessed (see pp. 887; Emans and Goldstein, 1982).

Table 11.6
Differential Diagnosis of Dysfunctional Uterine Bleeding

1. Anovulatory cycles
2. Disorders of pregnancy—threatened, incomplete or missed abortion; ectopic pregnancy; trophoblastic disease.
3. Blood dyscrasias and clotting disorders
4. Endocrine—hypo- or hyperthyroidism, adrenal disease, diabetes mellitus
5. Uterine—polyps, cancer, congenital anomalies, breakthrough bleeding on oral contraceptive pills, IUD use, endometritis
6. Vaginal—adenosis, cancer
7. Ovarian—tumor, polycystic ovary syndrome, pelvic inflammatory disease, ovarian failure
8. Systemic diseases
9. Trauma
10. Foreign body

Treatment

Patients with mild dysfunctional bleeding (cycles slightly shortened and menses prolonged) should be observed after adequate evaluation. Iron supplements should be prescribed for girls with persistent heavy flow. Antiprostaglandin therapy may be helpful in reducing flow.

In patients with mild to moderate bleeding and disruption of cycles but a near-normal hematocrit, medroxyprogesterone (Provera) should be given, 10 mg for 10 days each cycle, or 1–3 cycles of oral contraceptive therapy (e.g., OrthoNovum or Norinyl 1/35 or 1/50 once or twice daily). Oral contraceptive therapy is especially useful in girls with significant disruption of their cycles, those bleeding at the time of evaluation, and those in need of contraception.

For the patient with severe dysfunctional bleeding who presents with hemorrhage and anemia, initial therapy should include either OrthoNovum (Norinyl) 2 mg (two tablets OrthoNovum or Norinyl 1/50) or Ovral one tablet every 4 hours until bleeding subsides (usually within 24–36 hours), then q6h for 24 hours, q8h for 48 hours, then one tablet once or twice a day for the remaining 15 days. In cases of severe bleeding at the time of admission to the hospital, treatment can be initiated by administration of Premarin 25 mg i.v. ev-

CASE ILLUSTRATION

A 13-year-old girl came to the clinic with a history of having had menarche 6 months ago followed by menses lasting for 8–10 days and occurring every 16–22 days. She had been bleeding for 10 days on the day of her visit. Her general physical examination and pelvic examination were normal. Her hematocrit was 34% and clotting studies were normal. She was started on Norinyl 1+50 twice a day and bleeding rapidly stopped. She experienced no breakthrough bleeding and no nausea. Four days after completing a 21-day pill cycle, she had light withdrawal flow. Her hematocrit rose to 38% after 3 weeks of oral iron. She was subsequently treated with cyclic doses of medroxyprogesterone (Provera) 10 mg on days 14–23 of the next three cycles and has had normal withdrawal flow. After discontinuing the Provera therapy, she began to have normal cycles every 25–30 days.

QUESTIONS AND COMMENTS

Should a 13-year-old with dysfunctional uterine bleeding have a pelvic examination?

Although most perimenarchal girls are having vaginal bleeding because of anovulatory cycles, organic pathology including pregnancy, pelvic inflammatory disease, ovarian cysts, and tumors should be excluded. A pelvic examination is generally atraumatic if it is done with a small Huffman speculum followed by a gentle one-finger vaginal-abdominal or rectal-abdominal examination.

Would this patient be managed differently if she were sexually active?

A sexually active adolescent should have laboratory tests to exclude pregnancy and pelvic inflammatory disease. Cervical cultures for *C. trachomatis* and *N. gonorrhoeae* should be obtained, and a Pap smear should be done at a later visit when she is not bleeding. A low-dose oral contraceptive should be continued for birth control.

What should be done if the patient experiences significant nausea from the hormonal therapy?

The nausea associated with hormonal medications is most striking in the first few days of pill-taking; antiemetics such as chlorpromazine 5–10 mg given 1–2 hours before the dose of hormones can be helpful in alleviating these symptoms. If the symptoms are persistent, once a day Norinyl (OrthoNovum) 1+50 or Ovral, a lower dose pill containing 30–35 μg of estrogen, or norethindrone alone may be sufficient to control the bleeding. In cases of significant nausea, even as little as 10 days of oral contraceptives may be sufficient to control the problem and then the patient can be switched to medroxyprogesterone on a cyclic schedule.

When is ultrasonography indicated?

Ultrasonography is indicated when adequate bimanual examination is not possible, a pelvic mass is palpated, or a uterine anomaly is suspected because of spinal and renal anomalies.

For the diagnosis of primary and secondary amenorrhea and oligomenorrhea, see page 890.

ery 4 hours for not more than three doses. Antiemetics are often required with these doses of estrogen. After the initial course of oral contraceptives, the patient should be cycled for two or three additional cycles on an oral contraceptive pill with 35–50 μg of estrogen or, if not tolerated, medroxyprogesterone 10 mg, (Provera) for 10 days each cycle. If hormonal therapy fails to ameliorate the problem within 24–36 hours, dilatation and currettage is indicated. More radical surgery is rarely required.

Prognosis

Most patients with perimenarchal dysfunctional uterine bleeding will begin to have regular ovulatory cycles once normal maturation of the hypothalamic-pituitary-ovarian axis has occurred. In the meantime, iron replacement and emotional support are important. Endocrine evaluation should be undertaken if ovulatory cycles fail to establish.

REFERENCES

Anderson AB, Haynes PJ, Guillebaud J, et al: Reduction of menstrual blood-loss by prostaglandin-synthetase inhibitors. *Lancet* 1:774, 1976.

Apter D: Serum steroids and pituitary hormones in female puberty: A partly longitudinal study. *Clin Endocrinol* 12:107, 1980.

Apter D, Viinikka L, Vihko R: Hormonal patterns of adolescent cycles. *J Clin Endocrinol Metabol* 47:944, 1978.

Claessens EA, Cowell CA: Dysfunctional uterine bleeding in the adolescent. *Pediatr Clin North Am* 28:369, 1981.

Emans SJ, Goldstein DP: *Pediatric and Adolescent Gynecology*. Boston, Little, Brown & Co., 1982.

Lemarchard-Beraud T, Zufferey M, Reymond M, et al: Maturation of the hypothalamo-pituitary-ovarian axis in adolescent girls. *J Clin Endocrinol Metabol* 54:241, 1982.

Acute and Chronic Pain in the Adolescent Girl

6

Definition

The adolescent girl with an acute episode of pelvic pain necessitates aggressive diagnosis and management, because of the possibility of a life-threatening condition.

Chronic pelvic pain implies a time course of weeks to months, often without an obvious diagnosis. Usually the adolescent has experienced three or more months of constant or intermittent cyclic or acyclic pelvic pain.

Basic Science

The differential diagnosis of acute pelvic pain in the adolescent girl is shown in Table 11.7. The gynecologic causes include infection, rupture of an ovarian cyst or endometrioma, torsion, mittelschmerz, and dysmenorrhea. Symptoms associated with infection usually occur over several days, whereas pain with torsion or rupture usually occurs abruptly. However, patients with intermittent or partial torsion may experience crampy pelvic pain for days to weeks before the acute episode. GI causes include appendicitis, gastroenteritis, mesenteric adenitis, volvulus, intestinal obstruction, and trauma. Urinary causes include urinary tract infection and renal stones.

Chronic pelvic pain is a frequent complaint among adolescents and can be related to a number of gynecologic and nongynecologic problems as well as psychosomatic issues. Since the list of differential diagnoses is long (Table 11.8), it is particularly important for the physician to take an adequate history and perform a complete physical examination including a pelvic examination before ordering laboratory tests or reaching a conclusion.

Diagnosis

ACUTE PELVIC PAIN

The diagnosis of acute pelvic pain should include a careful history of the location and radiation of the pain; factors which relieve or exacerbate the pain; the date of the last menstrual period; and associated gastrointestinal, urinary, or musculoskeletal symptoms. A past history of previous pelvic pain and/or surgical pro-

Table 11.7
Differential Diagnosis of Acute Pelvic Pain in Adolescent Girls

- Gynecologic causes
  - Infection—pelvic inflammatory disease, postabortion endometritis
  - Rupture of follicular cyst, corpus luteum cyst, endometrioma, tumor, or ectopic pregnancy; mittelschmerz
  - Torsion of ovarian cyst, ovarian tumor, or Fallopian tube
  - Dysmenorrhea
- Gastrointestinal causes
  - Appendicitis
  - Gastroenteritis
  - Mesenteric adenitis
  - Intestinal obstruction
  - Trauma
  - Intestinal perforation
  - Bowel spasm
  - Inflammatory bowel disease
  - Meckel diverticulum
- Urinary tract causes
  - Infection
  - Calculi
- Orthopedic causes
  - Slipped capital-femoral epiphysis
  - Bone and joint infections in sacrum, ilium, and hip
  - Vertebral osteomyelitis
  - Psoas and iliacus abscess

Table 11.8
Differential Diagnosis of Chronic Pelvic Pain in Adolescent Girls

- Gynecologic causes
  - Dysmenorrhea
  - Mittelschmerz
  - Endometriosis
  - Chronic pelvic inflammatory disease
  - Ovarian cyst
  - Genital tract malformation
  - Pelvic congestion and pelvic serositis
  - Postoperative adhesions
- Gastrointestinal causes
  - Constipation
  - Bowel spasm
  - Fecolith of the appendix
  - Inflammatory bowel disease
  - Dietary intolerance (e.g., lactose intolerance)
- Urinary tract causes
  - Urinary tract infection
  - Hydronephrosis and obstructing lesions
- Orthopedic causes
  - Herniated intervertebral disc
  - Chronic slipped capital-femoral epiphysis,
  - Osteitis pubis
  - Neoplasms of pelvis and lower spine
  - Stress fractures of pelvis
  - Spondylolysis
- Psychosomatic

cedures should be noted. The pertinent family and social history should be elicited to ascertain if stress might be a contributing factor.

Evaluation should include a complete physical examination with particular attention to the following: careful palpation of the abdomen for evidence of masses, tenderness, or organomegaly; any signs of peritoneal irritation; and evaluation of the range of motion in the hips and back (a limited range of motion may indicate a skeletal source of referred pain) and tests of the sacroiliac joints. Depending upon the age of the patient and the size of the hymenal opening, a bimanual vaginal-abdominal, rectal-abdominal, or rectovaginal-abdominal examination in lithotomy position should be done to assess the size of the uterus and any ovarian or adnexal tenderness. Vaginal or cervical pathology should be assessed by speculum examination in all sexually active girls and in virginal girls if the examination can be accomplished without trauma. Cultures for *C. trachomatis* and *N. gonorrhoeae* should be obtained in all girls who might be sexually active.

Laboratory tests should include a complete blood count with differential and erythrocyte sedimentation rate, a urinalysis and urine culture, cervical cultures, and a stool specimen for occult blood. A serum pregnancy test is advisable if there is a possibility of pregnancy or ectopic pregnancy.

Pelvic inflammatory disease (PID) is a likely possiblity in the sexually active adolescent presenting with pelvic pain, especially during or at the end of her menses. The criteria for clinical diagnosis include abdominal tenderness, tenderness on motion of the cervix, and adnexal tenderness *plus* at least one of the following: Gram stain positive for Gram-negative intracellular diplococci; temperature greater than 38°C; white blood count greater than 10,000; purulent material obtained by culdocentesis or laparoscopy; pelvic abscess or inflammatory complex by bimanual or ultrasound. In patients with genital infection, lower abdominal pain, and pelvic tenderness, the clinical diagnosis of PID is confirmed 60–70% of the time. In patients with these findings plus a sedimentation rate greater than 15 mm/hour, temperature greater than 38° C, and adnexal masses, the clinical diagnosis is confirmed in 96% of cases. Inasmuch as most patients will not present with all these signs, therapy should be started as early as possible to avoid long-term sequelae.

A genital malformation should be considered in girls with unilateral renal agenesis or spinal anomalies. In adolescents in whom either a pelvic mass is palpated or an adequate bimanual pelvic examination is not possible, ultrasonography can aid in the diagnosis of pelvic pathology. However, it is important to remember normal adolescents may have 1- to 2-cm functional follicular ovarian cysts. Endometriosis and infection cannot be excluded by normal ultrasonography. GI and skeletal radiographs, bone scans, and other radiological studies should be done as clinically indicated. Depending on the evaluation of symptoms and urgency of the problem, laparoscopy or laparotomy may be required for a definitive diagnosis.

CHRONIC PELVIC PAIN

The diagnosis of chronic pelvic pain is very similar in many respects to that for acute pelvic pain; except that the tempo of the investigation is slowed and accurate assessment of family and social issues and the impact of the pain on the life of the teenager are extremely important. Many teenagers will have missed significant time in school; reluctance to return to school may intensify the bowel spasm that resulted in the initial pain and subsequent absences. Nevertheless, if an adolescent's complaints have not been assessed thoroughly she may feel that her symptoms have not been taken seriously by the physician. A recommendation "to see a counselor" may be interpreted by the adolescent as "the pain is all in your head." The family may then seek other medical opinions. Thus, the physician should reassure the adolescent girl that all efforts will be made to provide a diagnosis, and deal with the problem.

The diagnosis of chronic pelvic pain requires careful evaluation and history as described for "acute pelvic pain" above. A complete physical examination including a pelvic examination and musculoskeletal evaluation should be performed. Laboratory tests should include a complete blood count, sedimentation rate, urinalysis, urine culture, stool for occult blood, and, in the sexually active adolescent, cervical cultures for *C. trachomatis* and *N. gonorrhoeae*. Pelvic ultrasonography, upper GI series, barium enema, and urologic studies should be performed as needed. For adolescents with significant *pelvic* pain (not vague abdominal pain), laparoscopy has become an invaluable aid to making a definitive diagnosis (Goldstein et al, 1979). Laparoscopy allows the physician to make or confirm a specific diagnosis, to take biopsies, to lyse adhesions, if present, and to aspirate cysts. In patients in whom chronic PID has been excluded by history, the major cause of pelvic pain is endometriosis. The typical complaint is of increasingly severe dysmenorrhea, which is unresponsive to antiprostaglandin therapy or oral contraceptive suppression. The pain may be exacerbated at midcycle and 3–4 days premenstrually; occasionally pain occurs throughout the cycle. Genital anomalies with obstruction may cause pelvic pain and should be suspected in girls with spinal or renal anomalies (Duncan et al, 1979; Pinsonneault and Goldstein, 1985). The laparoscopic findings in 282 adolescents with chronic pelvic pain seen at The Children's Hospital between 1974 and 1983 are shown in Table 11.9 (Pinsonneault and Goldstein, in press, 1988), and the age-related incidence of laparoscopic findings in 129 adolescents is noted in Table 11.10. Although a normal examination was seen in 25% of 282 adolescents, the value of the negative laparoscopy should not be underestimated since in three-fourths of these adolescents, chronic pelvic pain resolved. Adolescents who have had previous pelvic surgery or venereal disease and remain anxious about the status of their reproductive tract are reassured by evidence of the normal status of their pelvis.

Treatment

Treatment depends upon the diagnosis and ranges from reassurance to antibiotics to surgery. PID requires prompt therapy. Because of the polymicrobial etiology of this disease, antibiotic coverage should take into account probable pathogens. Adolescents should receive strong consideration for hospitalization because of potential noncompliance and long-term sequelae including pain and infertility. The best antibiotic combination for inpatient therapy has not been thoroughly investigated but includes cefoxitin plus doxycycline *or* clindamycin plus gentamicin. Ambulatory treatment is initiated with ceftriaxone intramuscularly (or other single dose treatment) followed by doxycycline. The reader should consult up-to-date CDC recommendations. Endometriosis is treated with fulguration of the endometrial implants; amenorrhea and pseudopregnancy induced by oral contraceptive hormones; danazol; or, in some cases, conservative laparotomy, depending upon the stage of the endometriosis found at laparoscopy. Recurrence of endometriosis remains a problem for many adolescents.

DYSMENORRHEA

Definition

Cyclic pelvic pain occurring with menses is designated dysmenorrhea.

Basic Science

Pickles et al (1965) was the first to suggest that dysmenorrhea might be related to a "menstrual stimulant" found in human menstrual fluid that induced smooth muscle contractions. This substance was later found to be a mixture of prostaglandins $F_2\alpha$ and E_2. Jet washings, endometrial sampling, and collection of menstrual fluid on tampons have generally confirmed higher prostaglandin levels in women with primary dysmenorrhea than those without symptoms. The prostaglandin hypothesis has been further confirmed by the observation that inhibitors of prostaglandin synthetase relieve dysmenorrhea and the associated symptoms in a substantial percentage of adolescent and adult women (Chan et al, 1971; Chan et al, 1979; Alvin and Litt, 1982). The currently used prostaglandin drugs include the nonsteroidal anti-inflammatory agents such as naproxen, naproxen sodium, ibuprofen, and mefenamic acid. The effectiveness of oral contraceptives in relieving dysmenorrhea appears to be related to their antiovulatory action and their ability to produce endometrial hypoplasia and diminished prostaglandin synthesis.

Secondary dysmenorrhea may be caused by endometriosis, genital anomalies, adhesions, and the use of intrauterine devices for contraception.

Table 11.9
Laparoscopic Diagnosis in 282 Adolescents with Chronic Pelvic Pain, The Children's Hospital, Boston, 1974–1983[1]

	No. of Patients	
Endometriosis	126	(45%)
Postoperative adhesions	37	(13%)
Serositis	15	(5%)
Ovarian cyst	14	(5%)
Uterine malformation	15	(5%)
Others[2]	4	(2%)
No pathology	71	(25%)

[1]Reproduced with permission from Pinsonneault O, Goldstein DP: The role of laparoscopy in the diagnosis of chronic pelvic pain in adolescent females. *J Reproduc Med* (in press) 1988.
[2]Ileitis, infarcted hydatid of Morgagni, pelvic congestion.

Epidemiology

In the data from the National Health Examination Survey for 12- to 17-year-old girls, 59.7% of 1611 adolescents reported dysmenorrhea, and 14% frequently missed school because of cramps (Klein and Litt, 1981). In a survey of private school girls (mean age 15.5 ± 1.1 years), dysmenorrhea was reported as mild by 32%, moderate by 15%, and severe by 6% (Wilson et al, 1984).

Natural History

Adolescents often have 1 or 2 years free of dysmenorrhea. As the number of ovulatory cycles increase with increasing gynecologic age, dysmenorrhea becomes more common. Some adolescents, however, have dysmenorrhea from their first menstrual cycle.

Diagnosis

In assessing the adolescent with dysmenorrhea, the physician needs to elicit the menstrual history, including the duration of flow, the regularity of the cycles, and the timing of the menstrual cramps. Most adolescents with functional menstrual cramps have pain for 1 or 2 days at the beginning of the cycle. The patient should be asked about associated symptoms including pallor, syncope, nausea, vomiting and diarrhea, and whether she misses school or other activities at the time of her cramps. Prior use of over-the-counter and prescription medications should be discussed and the mother-daughter interaction should be assessed.

In the virginal adolescent with mild dysmenorrhea, a general physical examination including routine assessment of external genitalia is sufficient. In the adolescent with mild to severe cramps, a bimanual vaginal-abdominal or rectoabdominal examination should be done to exclude abnormal masses and adnexal or uterosacral tenderness or nodularity which might suggest endometriosis.

Treatment

Treatment of dysmenorrhea is aimed at symptomatic improvement. In patients with mild dysmenorrhea, over-the-counter medications including aspirin, ibuprofen, and Midol are available. For some patients, aspirin therapy may be accompanied by an increase in menstrual flow (Klein et al, 1981). If aspirin or low doses (200 mg) of ibuprofen are not successful or the cramps are moderate to severe, the options include naproxen 250 mg, two or three times daily; naproxen sodium, 550 mg given immediately and 275 mg every 6 hours; ibuprofen, 400–800 mg three to four times a day; or mefenamic acid, 500 mg given immediately and then 250 mg every 6 hours. For most patients, effective relief can be obtained by taking the medication at the first sign of cramps or bleeding and then for 1–3 days. In patients with severe nausea and vomiting at the onset of menses or significant premenstrual cramps, antiprostaglandin therapy can be started in advance of the menstrual period, provided the patient is not at risk for pregnancy. Antiprostaglandin drugs should be avoided in patients with known or suspected ulcer disease, gastrointestinal bleeding, clotting disorders, and those with aspirin-induced asthma or anaphylaxis. Acetaminophen with codeine (15–30 mg) can be used in the rare adolescent who cannot tolerate antiprostaglandin therapy; however, the codeine may cause dizziness and nausea.

A return visit should be scheduled every 3–6 months to assess the effectiveness of the medication and to establish physician-patient rapport. In patients who fail to respond to antiprostaglandin medications or are sexually active, suppression with oral contraceptives is a reasonable option (see pp. 675). A pelvic examination should be performed before oral contraceptives are prescribed. Cramps are usually substantially, if not completely, relieved by suppression of ovulation and scantier flow. If severe cramps persist despite ovulation suppression *or* the initial pelvic examination reveals tenderness or nodularity along the uterosacral ligaments or posterior cul-de-sac, laparoscopy should be done to evaluate the possibility of endometriosis or other organic causes for the severe dysmenorrhea.

Prognosis

Adolescents may continue to have dysmenorrhea throughout their adolescent and young adult years. Many notice a waxing and waning of the symptoms, however, and may require changes in medication with increasing age. Adolescents who become sexually active and have severe dysmenorrhea are good candidates for therapy with oral contraceptive pills. Patients with increasing cramps not responsive to medical therapy may have endometriosis, which should be investigated in order to preserve reproductive potential.

CASE ILLUSTRATION

A 14-year-old adolescent came to her pediatrician's office with a history of increasingly severe menstrual cramps and nausea during the first 2 days of her cycle. Her menarche was at age 12 years. She had had regular menses about every 30 days and for the past 6 months she had had moderately severe menstrual cramps keeping her home from school for 2 days each month. She had tried several over-the-counter medications which did not relieve her symptoms. Her general examination, including rectoabdominal examination, was normal and she was given a prescription for an antiprostaglandin medication to be taken at the first sign of her menstrual periods and then for 2 days. She had dramatic relief for her menstrual cramps.

QUESTIONS AND COMMENTS

Do adolescents need a pelvic examination for dysmenorrhea?

In patients with moderate to severe dysmenorrhea, a modified pelvic examination is important to assess the possibility of organic disease. A brief examination is nontraumatic in the adolescent if details of the procedure and its importance in diagnosing and managing her complaint are carefully explained.

When should oral contraceptives be prescribed for this type of patient?

In the patient who fails to respond to maximal doses of several different antiprostaglandins, a 3-month course of ovulation suppression should be tried to assess the effect on relieving menstrual cramps. If the patient fails to respond to antiprostaglandins or oral contraceptives or has nodularity or tenderness on physical examination, endometriosis is likely and laparoscopy is indicated. Patients with renal agenesis or spinal anomalies should be assessed for the possibility of a müllerian anomaly causing dysmenorrhea.

Table 11.10
Age-Related Incidence of Laparoscopic Findings in 129 Adolescents with Chronic Pelvic Pain, The Children's Hospital, Boston, 1980–1983[1]

	Age in Years				
	11–13	14–15	16–17	18–19	20–21
	No. of Patients	No. of Patients	No. of Patients	No. of Patients	No. of Patients
Endometriosis	2 (12%)[2]	9 (28%)	21 (40%)	17 (45%)	7 (54%)
Postoperative adhesions	1 (6%)	4 (13%)	7 (13%)	5 (13%)	2 (15%)
Serositis	5 (29%)	4 (13%)	0 (0%)	2 (5%)	0 (0%)
Ovarian cyst	2 (12%)	2 (6%)	3 (5%)	2 (5%)	0 (0%)
Uterine malformation	1 (6%)	0 (0%)	1 (2%)	0 (0%)	1 (8%)
Others	0 (0%)	1 (3%)	2 (4%)	1 (3%)	1 (0%)
No pathology	6 (35%)	12 (37%)	19 (36%)	11 (29%)	3 (23%)

[1]Reproduced with permission from Pinsonneault O, Goldstein DP: The role of laparoscopy in the diagnosis of chronic pelvic pain in adolescent females. *J Reproduc Med* (in press) 1988.
[2]Percentage refers to the number within each age group.

REFERENCES

Alvin PE, Litt IF: Current status of the etiology and management of dysmenorrhea in adolescence. *Pediatrics* 70:516, 1982.

Chan WY, Dawood MY, Fuchs F: Prostaglandins in primary dysmenorrhea. Comparison of prophylactic and nonprophylactic treatment with ibuprofen and use of oral contraceptives. *Am J Med* 70:535, 1971.

Chan WY, Dawood MY, Fuchs F: Relief of dysmenorrhea with the prostaglandin synthetase inhibitor ibuprofen: Effect on prostaglandin levels in menstrual fluid. *Am J Obstet Gynecol* 135:102, 1979.

Duncan DA, Shapiro LF, Stangel JJ, et al: The MURCS association: Mullerian duct aplasia, renal aplasia, and cervicothoracic somite dysplasia. *J Pediatr* 95:399, 1979.

Goldstein DB, deCholnoky C, Leventhal J, et al: New insights into the old problem of chronic pelvic pain. *J Pediatr Surg* 14:675, 1979.

Klein JR, Litt IF: Epidemiology of adolescent dysmenorrhea. *Pediatrics* 68:661, 1981.

Klein JR, Litt IF, Rosenberg A, et al: The effect of aspirin on dysmenorrhea in adolescents. *J Pediatr* 98:987, 1981.

Pickles VR, Hall WJ, Best FA, et al: Prostaglandins in endometrium and menstrual fluid from normal and dysmenorrheic subjects. *Br J Obstet Gynaecol* 72:185, 1965.

Pinsonneault O, Goldstein DP: Obstructing malformations of the uterus and vagina. *Fertil Steril* 44:241, 1985.

Pinsonneault O, Goldstein DP: The role of laparoscopy in the diagnosis of chronic pelvis pain in adolescent females. *J Reproduc Med* (in press).

Wilson C, Emans SJ, Mansfield J, et al: The relationships of calculated percent body fat, sports participation, age, and place of residence on menstrual patterns in healthy adolescent girls at an independent New England high school. *J Adol Health Care* 5:248, 1984.

In Utero Exposure to Diethylstilbestrol 7

From the mid-1940s to the early 1970s diethylstilbestrol (DES) and other nonsteroidal estrogens were given to pregnant women with the hope of preventing miscarriage. An estimated 2–4 million children, thus, were exposed to DES in utero.

Basic Science

In the early 1970s, Herbst and coworkers reported an association between maternal use of DES and the later development of clear cell adenocarcinoma of the vagina and cervix in female offspring (Herbst et al, 1971; Herbst et al, 1974). Several years later, Herbst and other investigators demonstrated an association between maternal DES use and the presence in offspring of vaginal adenosis, malformations of the cervix and vagina, and other abnormalities of the lower genital tract (Herbst, 1975; Burke and Antonioli, 1974; Sherman et al, 1974). An increased risk of premature births and ectopic pregnancy has also been reported (Berger and Goldstein, 1980; Barnes et al, 1980; Herbst et al, 1980; Goldstein, 1978; DeCherney et al, 1981). Although more than 500 cases of clear cell adenocarcinoma with a peak age of mid to late adolescence have been reported to the Registry, the risk appears to be extremely small: 0.014–0.14% (Mattingly and Stafl, 1976).

Exposure to DES is commonly associated with an increased incidence of benign vaginal adenosis, often termed vaginal epithelial changes (VEC). Exposure to DES apparently interferes with normal differentiation and development of the cervix and vagina, so that columnar epithelium persists on the portio of the cervix and in the vagina, resulting in a large cervical ectopy in most DES-exposed girls. Other changes include a cervical-vaginal hood, pseudopolypoid formation, vaginal membranes and septi, and hypoplasia of the cervix. Uterine abnormalities include a T-shaped appearance of the endometrial cavity, constricting bands in the cavity, and hypoplasia (Kaufman et al, 1977). These cervical and uterine abnormalities appear to cause increased problems in pregnancy, including premature birth, tubal pregnancy, and possibly miscarriage.

In boys exposed in utero to DES, abnormalities such as epididymal cysts, testicular hypoplasia, cryptorchidism, microphallus, urethral stenosis, hypospadias, varicoceles, and pathologic semen have been reported (Bibbo et al, 1977; Gill et al, 1979). However, a recent study has concluded that the risk of urogenital abnormalities is not increased and the potential impact on the health and fertility of young males is minimal (Leary et al, 1984).

Diagnosis

Given the number of patients potentially exposed to DES in utero, it is important to determine the maternal drug history in all adolescents. Girls with a known maternal history of treatment with even minimal amounts of DES or other nonsteroidal estrogen should be referred for gynecologic evaluation at menarche or at age 14 years. The primary health provider can be helpful to the adolescent by suggesting the use of tampons before the examination and by providing counseling and facts about DES.

The gynecologic examination for the teenager exposed to DES consists of careful palpation of the vagina and cervix and speculum examination to visualize the vagina and cervix. Cytologic samples are taken from the portio of the cervix, the vagina, and the endocervix along with iodine staining of the vagina and cervix. Colposcopy is very helpful in assessment and directing biopsies.

Males exposed to DES in utero should have particular attention paid to evaluation of the scrotum and testes during routine physical examinations. Semen analysis is probably indicated only in males with infertility problems.

Treatment

Definitive surgical therapy is required for adenocarcinoma of the cervix or vagina. Benign adenosis and anatomical changes of the cervix should be followed by observation and by cytologic examination at least annually. Cervical vaginal hoods and ectropions tend to decrease in extent and sometimes disappear over the course of the years of follow-up. Since the majority of young women exposed to DES can carry pregnancy to full term, hysterosalpingography is indicated only in patients who have a preterm pregnancy. Pregnancies in DES-exposed patients should be followed closely to detect ectopic pregnancy and threatened miscarriage resulting from cervical incompetence.

Prognosis

Overall, the prognosis of DES-exposed patients appears excellent. The possible increased risk of squamous cell carcinoma in the areas of adenosis is controversial. Although a recent study found the incidence of cervical dysplasia in DES-exposed patients to be higher, there was a difference in the frequency of a history of herpes (Robbey et al, 1984; CDC, 1986). Increased exposure to papilloma virus also may play a role.

REFERENCES

Barnes AB, Colton T, Gundersen J, et al: Fertility and outcome of pregnancy in women exposed in utero to diethylstilbestrol. *N Engl J Med* 302:609, 1980.

Berger MJ, Goldstein DP: Impaired reproductive performance in DES-exposed women. *Obstet Gynecol* 55:25, 1980.

Bibbo M, Gill WB, Azizi F, et al: Follow-up study of male and female offspring of DES-exposed mothers. *Obstet Gynecol* 49:1, 1977.

Burke L, Antonioli D: Vaginal adenosis: Correlation of colposcopic and pathologic findings. *Obstet Gynecol* 44:257, 1974.

CDC: Report of the Recommendation of the 1985 DES Task Force of The United States Department of Health and Human Services. *JAMA* 255:1849, 1986.

DeCherney AH, Cholst I, Naftolin F: Structure and function of the Fallopian tubes following exposure to DES during gestation. *Fertil Steril* 36:741, 1981.

Gil WB, Schumacher GF, Bibbo M, et al: Association of diethylstilbestrol exposure in utero with cryptorchidism, testicular hypoplasia, and semen abnormalities. *J Urol* 122:36, 1979.

Goldstein DP: Incompetent cervix in offspring exposed to diethylstilbestrol in utero. *Obstet Gynecol* 52:73S, 1978.

Herbst A: A prospective comparison of exposed female offspring with unexposed controls. *N Engl J Med* 292:334, 1975.

Herbst A, Robboy SJ, Scully RE, et al: Clear cell adenocarcinoma. *Am J Obstet Gynecol* 119:713, 1974.

Herbst A, Ulfelder H, Poskanzer DC: Adenocarcinoma of the vagina. *N Engl J Med* 284:878, 1971.

Herbst AL, Hubby MM, Blough RR, et al: A comparison of pregnancy experience in DES-exposed and DES-unexposed daughters. *J Reproduc Med* 24:62, 1980.

Kaufman RH, Binder GL, Gray PM, et al: Upper genital tract changes associated with exposure in utero to diethylstilbestrol. *Am J Obstet Gynecol* 128:51, 1977.

Leary FJ, Reseguie LJ, Kurland LT, et al: Males exposed in utero to diethylstilbestrol. *JAMA* 252:2984, 1984.

Mattingly RE, Stafl A: Cancer risk in diethylstilbestrol-exposed offspring. *Am J Obstet Gynecol* 126:543, 1976.

Robbey SJ, Noller KJ, OBrien P, et al: Increased incidence of cervical and vaginal dysplasia in 3980 diethylstilbestrol-exposed young women. Experience of the National Collaborative Diethylstilbestrol Adenosis Project. *JAMA* 252:2979, 1984.

Sherman AI, Goldrath M, Berlin A, et al: Cervical-vaginal adenosis after in utero exposure to synthetic estrogens. *Obstet Gynecol* 44:531, 1974.

Breast Examination and Lesions

8

Between the ages of 9 and 13 years, the vast majority of adolescent girls begin their pubertal breast development. Because breast development is often regarded as a sign of femininity, mothers and daughters often worry inordinately about minor asymmetry or small breast development. In addition, because of widespread publicity on cancer of the breast, any breast lump may cause tremendous anxiety to a teenager and her mother, even though malignancy is extremely rare in persons under age 20 years.

Although there is controversy on the appropriate age to begin self-examination, most adolescent girls benefit from learning the techniques during their routine physical examination (Hein et al, 1982; Goldstein and Miler, 1982), particularly since this arrangement often makes the adolescent feel more at ease as the examiner palpates for any abnormalities. Instruction for self-examination includes: (1) looking in the mirror for asymmetry while undressing for a shower; (2) examining the breast while standing up in the shower (soap on her hands facilitates the examination); and (3) re-examining the breasts while supine before falling asleep that night. The adolescent is taught to begin at the outermost edges of the breast, pressing gently in circular motions clockwise starting at 12 o'clock. The motion is repeated by moving inward an inch for each circle until the nipple is examined. During the physical examination, the physician uses a similar technique while the patient is supine. The breast tissue can also be palpated in a straight line from the margin inward clockwise around the breast. The hand is held so that the flat portion of the fingers are moved in a rotatory fashion to detect abnormal masses and the areola is compressed to assess any abnormal discharge. The breasts are staged using the Tanner Staging (see pp. 872). If asymmetry or disorders of the breast are a concern, exact measurements of the areola, breast tissue, and overall dimensions of the breast should be recorded in the office notes. In the young patient with no history of asymmetry or breast masses, examination with the patient in the sitting position can be omitted and the examination performed on the patient supine.

Asymmetry of glandular development is often seen in adolescents, especially at the initiation of development. This asymmetry often becomes less prominent by the end of full breast development (3–5 years). The initial breast bud may appear as a tender lump on one side, but it may be 6 months to a year before the other breast bud begins to develop. Asymmetry of the areola during development often suggests that there will be significant asymmetry of glandular maturation as well. If the degree of asymmetry is mild, the use of slightly padded bras can improve the self-image of an adolescent who is anxious about the asymmetry. If the asymmetry is marked at the end of development (ages 14–18 years), the patient may wish to discuss the risks and benefits of cosmetic surgery. Success is often dramatic and the self-image of the adolescent is usually improved.

True hypertrophy of the breast (so called virginal hypertrophy) may cause the breast to enlarge beyond the normal growth period, resulting in back pain and kyphosis. Surgical reduction can be offered once growth has ceased.

Lack of development of the breast tissue may result from amastia (congenital absence of glandular tissue) or delayed development from gonadal dysgenesis, hypogonadotrophic hypogonadism, systemic illness, or rarely, from androgen excess (congenital adrenal hyperplasia; see pp. 855). Early breast development is discussed on page 872, Table 14.1.

Accessory nipples or breasts occur in 1–2% of healthy children; the accessory areola may appear as a "mole" beneath the breast on the embryologic milk line between the axilla and the groin. No therapy is usually necessary. Engorgement of accessory breasts may occur during pregnancy and lactation.

Nipple discharge is rare during adolescence. Occasionally, a small amount of yellow, clear serous material can be expressed in early adolescence. The more usual clinical problem is galactorrhea, discharge of a milky substance (see pp. 890). A blood-tinged discharge should prompt a search for an intraductal papilloma or rarely carcinoma. Occasionally, a periareolar gland of Montgomery will drain a small amount of brownish fluid for several weeks, but usually no treatment is necessary.

The normal adolescent often has very dense "lumpy" breasts which may become increasingly nodular and painful premenstrually.

Fibroadenomas, the most common cause of persistent breast masses in the adolescent, are typically firm, rubbery and mobile, with a clearly defined edge (Daniel and Mathews, 1968; Sandison and Walker, 1968; Tarbey et al, 1975; Goldstein and Miler, 1982). The size may remain unchanged or increase over the course of several cycles. Occasionally, giant fibroadenomas occur during adolescence and present as breast asymmetry; the overlying skin is typically taut, with dilatation of the superficial veins. If the patient detects an abnormal mass, she should be seen promptly. Unless a diagnosis such as an abscess or trauma is clear-cut, the adolescent should be seen again after her next menstrual period to assess the natural history of the mass. On the second visit, if aspiration of a persistent discrete mass is negative or the mass is enlarging and a source of considerable anxiety, an excision biopsy should be done.

Contusion of the breast may result in a poorly defined mass which may take weeks to resolve and occasionally may leave an ill-defined palpable mass. If a discrete mass is found immediately after trauma, it is probably a pre-existing lesion, especially if it is sharply delineated and nontender.

Infection in the breast is uncommon, except in the newborn girl and the lactating adolescent or woman. However, occasionally in adolescent girls, periareolar abscesses may occur at the base of a hair root. Administration of antibiotics and incision and drainage are indicated.

REFERENCES

Daniel WA, Mathews MD: Tumors of the breast in adolescent females. *Pediatrics* 41:743, 1968.

Goldstein DP, Miler V: Breast masses in adolescent females. *Clin Pediatr* 21:17, 1982.

Hein K, Dell R, Cohen MI: Self-detection of a breast mass in adolescent females. *J Adol Health Care* 3:15, 1982.

Sandison AT, Walker JC: Diseases of the adolescent breast. *Br J Surg* 35:443, 1968.

Tarbey WJ, Buntain WL, Dudgeon DKL: The surgical management of pediatric breast masses. *Pediatrics* 56:736, 1975.

Contraception for the Adolescent 9

Although many physicians caring for adolescents still feel ambivalent about providing sex education and contraceptive advice to their patients, it is clear that more teenagers are engaging in intercourse at earlier ages and, thus, remain at risk of pregnancy. The denial of contraceptive services or the requirement for parental involvement will increase the number of unwanted pregnancies rather than decrease the number of sexually active adolescents. Sex education in schools and at home, peer counseling, and addressing the issue of the sexual messages in magazines and movies are more likely to alleviate the problems associated in early premarital sexual intercourse. Thus, the adolescent should be asked about menses and sexual history at each visit to her health care provider. A teenager who is 14 or 15 years old will rarely make a specific request for contraceptives from her primary provider unless she knows that the topic can be discussed confidentially. A college student of 18 or 19 years of age is much more likely to seek gynecologic care on her own and deal with the issue of contraception.

In providing good medical care to the sexually active adolescent, the physician should obtain a complete medical history and determine if there are any specific contraindications to the use of a particular form of birth control. If the patient has already practiced birth control, she may be more apt to comply with the method chosen. The degree to which one or both partners can take responsibility for avoiding an unwanted pregnancy should be assessed. Multiple partners, low evaluation of personal health, and feelings of hopelessness have been associated with noncompliance with oral contraceptives (Durant et al, 1984). The future plans of the adolescent should be assessed since those bound for college are more likely to be compliant with appropriate birth control measures (Scher et al, 1982). In contrast, the 15-year-old adolescent who has dropped out of school and has no future plans may have ambivalent feelings about whether a pregnancy can give her adult status and help her to move out of her home.

Before prescribing contraceptives, the physician should discuss the risks of being sexually active, including the emotional consequences, sexually transmitted diseases, and pregnancy. The possibility of parental involvement should be assessed with the adolescent, particularly since many adolescents can share the information with a parent, particularly her mother. Payment for the visit and laboratory tests and issues of confidentiality should be discussed early in the provision of contraceptive services.

METHODS OF CONTRACEPTION

The methods of contraception and the theoretical and actual pregnancy rates are listed in Table 11.11. Although exact figures of rates vary with studies and methods of calculation (Corson et al, 1985; Grimes, 1986; Vessey et al, 1982), noncompliance is a major issue for adolescents and accounts for a failure rate with oral contraceptive pills that may be as high as 9–13 pregnancies/100 women years of use. The teenager should feel that she has actively participated in choosing a contraceptive method that best fits her lifestyle. All forms of birth control should be discussed. Physicians should not impose their preferences on the adolescent, and should realize that method-switching is common (Hirsch and Zelnik, 1985). For example, the health care provider may feel that a diaphragm is the best form of birth control, but this method may be inappropriate for a 15-year-old who does not feel comfortable inserting tampons.

Adolescent females and males should be alerted to the risk of HIV infection and other sexually transmitted diseases. Prevention by avoiding exposure is the best strategy to prevent all sexually transmitted diseases. Abstinence, or intercourse with one faithful uninfected partner are totally effective. Condoms should be used with each act of sexual intercourse to reduce the risk of infection. Latex condoms are effective mechanical barriers to HIV, herpes simplex, cytomegalovirus, hepatitis B virus and *Clamydia trachomatis* as well as *N. gonorrhoeae*. Vaginal use of spermicides offers some protection from HIV. The safety and efficacy of spermicides in prevention of sexually transmitted infections of the anal canal and oropharynx is not known.

Some practical points recommended by CDC (1988) are to handle condoms with care to avoid puncture, use latex condoms stored in a cool, dry place out of direct sunlight, use adequate lubrication, leave space for semen but avoid air trapping, and never reuse a condom.

Table 11.11
Pregnancy Rates per 100 Women-Years of Use for Different Contraceptive Methods

	Theoretical	Use
Oral contraceptives	0.16–0.27	0.7–2.4
Progestin only—mini-pill	1.2	1.5–3.0
Progestasert IUD	1.3	2.1
Diaphragm	3	4–20
Condom	3.6	4–20
Cervical cap		8–17
Sponge		13–18
Contraceptive foams and suppositories		3–20
Condom and foam	1	5

ORAL CONTRACEPTIVES

Most teenagers choose the oral contraceptive pill. A list of common birth control pills is shown in Table 11.12. In our clinic, the compliance rate at 3 months for an upper socioeconomic group of adolescents was 84% and for a clinic population was 48%. In spite of the availability of contraceptive services, many teenagers remain at risk for pregnancy (Emans et al, 1987).

Side effects of the oral contraceptive pills include weight gain, blood pressure elevation, headaches, nausea, vomiting, mood change, acne, amenorrhea, and breakthrough bleeding. Although weight gain with the new low-dose pills appears to be uncommon, weight is

Table 11.12
Commonly Used Oral Contraceptives

Drug	Estrogen (μg)	Progestin (mg)
Norinyl or Ortho-Novum 1/50	Mestranol 50	Norethindrone 1.0
Demulen 1/50	Ethinyl estradiol 50	Ethynodiol diacetate 1.0
Ovral	Ethinyl estradiol 50	Norgestrel 1.0
Norlestrin 1/50	Ethinyl estradiol 50	Norethindrone acetate 1.0
Ovcon-50	Ethinyl estradiol 50	Norethindrone 1.0
Norinyl or Ortho-Novum 1/35	Ethinyl estradiol 35	Norethindrone 1.0
Brevicon or Modicon	Ethinyl estradiol 35	Norethindrone 0.5
Ovcon 35	Ethinyl estradiol 35	Norethindrone 0.4
Ortho-Novum 10/11	Ethinyl estradiol 35	Norethindrone 0.5 for 10 days
	Ethinyl estradiol 35	Norethindrone 1.0 for 11 days
Ortho-Novum 7/7/7	Ethinyl estradiol 35	Norethindrone 0.5 for 7 days
	Ethinyl estradiol 35	Norethindrone 0.75 for 7 days
	Ethinyl estradiol 35	Norethindrone 1.0 for 7 days
Tri-Norinyl	Ethinyl estradiol 35	Norethindrone 0.5 for 7 days
	Ethinyl estradiol 35	Norethindrone 1.0 for 9 days
	Ethinyl estradiol 35	Norethindrone 0.5 for 5 days
TriPhasil or TriLevlen	Ethinyl estradiol 30	Levonorgestrel 0.05 for 6 days
	Ethinyl estradiol 40	Levonorgestrel .075 for 5 days
	Ethinyl estradiol 30	Levonorgestrel .125 for 10 days
LoOvral	Ethinyl estradiol 30	Norgestrel 0.3
Nordette	Ethinyl estradiol 30	Levonorgestrel 0.15
Loestrin 1.5/30	Ethinyl estradiol 30	Norethindrone acetate 1.5
Loestrin 1/20	Ethinyl estradiol 20	Norethindrone acetate 1.0
Mini-pills		
Ovrette		Norgestrel .075
Nor QD or MicroNor		Norethindrone .35

a major concern for most adolescents and should be monitored at each visit. Patients with pre-existing hypertension should not be given the pill, and those who develop hypertension should discontinue its use. Although in some patients migraine headaches may be exacerbated by the pill, in others, particularly those on the low-dose pills, headaches may be decreased. Teenagers who develop significant headaches, or, especially exacerbation of pre-existing migraine headaches, require a lower dosage or an alternative form of contraception. A prior history of migraine associated with ophthalmoplegia or hemiparesis is a contraindication to pill use. Nausea or vomiting can occasionally occur during the first few days after initiation of pill use but generally lessens with subsequent days. Taking the pill after dinner or at bedtime with food rather than in the early morning may alleviate nausea. Persistent nausea may require lowering the estrogen dosage of the pill.

The occurrence of mood changes on the pill remains controversial. Occasionally, an adolescent does appear to have an increase in depressive symptoms or the onset of emotional lability which improves when the pill is discontinued or the dosage is altered. Increase in acne may occur with progestin-dominant pills and can be alleviated by changing to a more estrogenic pill.

Alterations in menstrual cycles occur commonly with pill use. Menses typically become lighter, because of endometrial hypoplasia, and the likelihood of iron deficiency is diminished (Grace et al, 1982). Dysmenorrhea may also be substantially relieved. Amenorrhea on the pill is common, especially in long-term users. If this occurs, pregnancy should be excluded, after which the same pill can be continued, or, if withdrawal bleeding is important for the patient, a more estrogenic pill can be prescribed. Amenorrhea after the pill is discontinued (postpill amenorrhea) is uncommon (1%) and usually occurs in patients with a prior history of menstrual dysfunction, especially those with polycystic ovary syndrome and those patients who have lost weight or become involved in endurance sports while on the pill; most patients will spontaneously resume their cycles. If cycles have not returned within 6 months after pill use, endocrinologic evaluation for causes of amenorrhea as outlined on page 889 should be undertaken.

Depending on the estrogen-progestin dosage, the oral contraceptive pill may alter glucose tolerance and lipid levels (Wahl et al, 1983; Powell et al, 1984). Thus, the least amount of estrogen (30–35 μg) and progestin potency should be prescribed to avoid affecting lipid metabolism. Because of the effects of the pill on glucose tolerance, barrier forms of contraception are preferable in the diabetic adolescent, but the risks and benefits should be weighed for each individual since the young adolescent may be unwilling to use a barrier form of contraception.

Liver function may be altered in patients with inherited or acquired defects of hepatic function; and adolescents with a history of recurrent cholestatic jaundice of pregnancy should not be given the pill. Pill use also should be avoided in patients with active hepatitis and symptoms of gall bladder disease. An absolute increase in thyroxine (T_4) and a decrease in resin triiodothyronine (resin T_3) occur secondary to increase in thyroid-binding globulin. There is no alteration in free T_4 or in the clinical status of the adolescent.

Adolescents with epilepsy rarely experience an increase in seizures related to oral contraceptive usage; in general the pills containing 35–50 μg of estrogen are well tolerated. Since anticonvulsant medications increase the metabolism of contraceptive steroids, the risk of pill failure is greater than in normal individuals and, thus, the occurrence of breakthrough bleeding may signify inadequate levels of contraceptive steroids. Other medications, such as Rifampin, have also been shown to have important interactions, and a back-up method is required. Although still debated, usage of antibiotics such as ampicillin and tetracycline may impair contraceptive efficacy.

The most serious side effects of oral contraceptives are thromboembolic disease, cardiovascular accidents, pulmonary embolism, mesenteric artery thrombosis, retinal artery thrombosis, and myocardial infarction (Slone et al, 1981; Stadel, 1981). Fortunately, these side effects appear to be mainly age-related. The highest risk of cardiovascular events is in smokers over age 35 years. Risk factors such as diabetes and obesity also appear to increase the possibility of these serious consequences. Thus, it is important for the adolescent to read the package insert carefully, and the physician should discuss the possible serious consequences of pill use. In order to minimize the risk of thromboembolism, pill use should be stopped 4 weeks before elective surgery requiring bed rest, especially if immobilization in plaster casts is necessary.

The possible association of cancer and pill use remains a subject of investigation. There appears to be no excess risk of breast cancer and a probable decrease in ovarian and endometrial cancer with pill use (Lipnick et al, 1986; Weiss and Saywetz, 1980; CDC, 1984). The relationship of carcinoma in situ of the cervix to pill use has not been totally settled, in part because pill users may have higher rates of sexual activity, an increased number of partners and, by not using a barrier method, greater exposure to papilloma virus and other potential risk factors. An increased risk of dysplasia, or an increase in the progression of dysplasia may be the result of these multiple factors. Sexually active adolescents on oral contraceptives should have annual Pap smears and any abnormal smear or atypical cervical lesions should be referred appropriately.

Adolescents who are planning to use the pill should have a complete medical history and physical examination including blood pressure, breast and pelvic examinations, appropriate laboratory studies including a urinalysis, hemoglobin level, and Pap smear with screening for *N. gonorrhoeae* and *C. trachomatis*. Cholesterol, high density lipid (HDL) cholesterol and triglyceride levels should be obtained on patients with a family history of early myocardial infarction. Patients should be encouraged to give up smoking even though the mortality risk is not substantially increased in adolescents. A pill low in estrogen and progestin should be selected, such as Norinyl 1+35, Ortho-Novum 1/35, Tri-Norinyl, Ortho-Novum 7/7/7, Tri-Phasil or Tri-Levlen. The possible occurrence of breakthrough bleeding should be explained and a detailed instruction sheet should be given to the patient. A return visit should be made for 3 months ahead. At that time, the blood pressure and weight should be monitored and any side effects noted. Adolescents should have return visits at least every 6 months specifically to assure compliance, answer questions, and deal with ongoing medical and social issues. For patients who are less likely to comply with instructions or those with increased risk factors, more frequent visits should be scheduled.

The mini-pill is a progestin-only pill, which results in a higher pregnancy rate and a higher incidence of breakthrough bleeding. It is useful primarily in patients who cannot tolerate estrogen.

INTRAUTERINE DEVICES

In the past 10 years, the intrauterine device has fallen into significant disfavor for use among nulliparous adolescents because of the risk of pelvic inflammatory disease and infertility (Kaufman et al, 1983). The Progestasert and CuT 380A are the current options.

BARRIER CONTRACEPTION

Barrier forms of contraception have become increasingly popular, especially among older adolescents and young adults. The risks of pelvic inflammatory disease and cervical neoplasia appear to be diminished by barrier use. Although the theoretical efficacy of diaphragms among married women in their 30s is excellent, the efficacy is substantially lower in adolescent populations. In general, this method should be used only by the extremely motivated, mature adolescent who is able to cope with the increased risk of an unplanned pregnancy. Visual aids such as the Omni Health communicator cassettes are helpful in teaching the adolescent proper techniques of insertion and removal of the diaphragm. The major advantage of the diaphragm is the lack of medical side effects, except for allergy to the cream. The risk of urinary tract infections appears to be increased (Fihn et al, 1985) and toxic shock has occurred rarely in association with diaphragm use (Wilson, 1983).

Another device is a cervical cap, fitted to the cervix and held in place by suction. (Tietze et al, 1953). Clinical trials on some of the devices have been disappointing. The newest female barrier contraceptive is the Today sponge which has the advantage of over-the-counter availability and "one size fits all." The pregnancy rate is higher than with diaphragm use, and the sponge should be used with a condom for maximum protection. The problems with the sponge have included odor, disintegration of the sponge, difficulty in removal, and rare cases of toxic shock usually associated with the use of the sponge during the menstrual cycle.

Intravaginal spermicides should be used with a condom to increase efficacy. Spermicides include vaginal creams, jellies, foams, and suppositories; most contain Nonoxyl-9. The condom remains an excellent barrier method because it can diminish the risk of sexually transmitted diseases and can increase the responsibility of young men for birth control.

Developing technologies should soon make available injectable progestins and progestin-containing implants. Research in luteinizing hormone-releasing hormone (LHRH) analogues and progesterone antagonists continues.

POSTCOITAL CONTRACEPTION

Postcoital contraception has gradually shifted from the use of high-dose estrogens, including conjugated estrogen 15–25 mg twice a day for 5 days and ethinyl estradiol 2–2.5 mg twice a day for 5 days, to Yuzpe regimen which utilizes Ovral, two tablets within 72 hours (preferably 12–24 hours) of unprotected intercourse, followed by two tablets 12 hours later (Yuzpe and Lancee, 1977).

Clearly, the most important issue in providing contraception is adequate education and compliance. Adolescents appear to be more likely to seek contraception as they become older, more cognizant of future plans, and if they can identify a contraceptive program that meets their needs. Friends, families, and physicians may all help in directing an adolescent to come to terms with her sexuality and the need for contraception. Inreasing commitment in a relationship or a pregnancy scare may help the adolescent seek contraceptive services. Once the adolescent enters the health care sector, the issue of compliance becomes of paramount importance. Although numerous studies have examined issues that influence compliance, adolescents from diverse ethnic and socioeconomic groups may respond quite differently. Peer counseling appears to be particularly effective in high-risk low-income groups. Contraceptive services available within a high school also appear to have a dramatic impact on lowering pregnancy rates and increasing access to services. The individual health care provider should set aside extra time for counseling adolescents.

REFERENCES

CDC: Condoms for prevention of sexually transmitted diseases. *MMWR* 37:133, 1988.

CDC: Human immunodeficiency virus infection in the United States: A review of current knowledge *MMWR* (Suppl 36): 1987.

CDC: Oral contraceptives and the risk of breast cancer in young women. *MMWR* 33:353, 1984.

Corson SL, Derman RJ, Tyrer LB: *Fertility Control.* Boston, Little, Brown & Co., 1985.

Durant RH, Joy MS, Linder CW, et al: Influence of psychosocial factors on adolescent compliance with oral contraceptives. *J Adol Health Care* 5:1, 1984.

Fihn SD, Latham RH, Roberts P, et al: Association between diaphragm use and urinary tract infection. *JAMA* 254:240, 1985.

Emans SJ, Grace E, Woods ER, et al: Adolescents' compliance with the use of oral contraceptives. *JAMA* 257:3377, 1987.

Grace EM, Emans SJ, Drum DE: Hematologic abnormalities in adolescents who take oral contraceptive pills. *J Pediatr* 101:771, 1982.

Grimes D: Reversible contraception for the 1980s. *JAMA* 255:69, 1986.

Hirsh MB, Zelnik M: Contraceptive method switching among American female adolescents, 1979. *J Adol Health Care* 17:53, 1985.

Kaufman DW, Watson J, Rosenberg L, et al: The effect of different types of intrauterine devices on the risk of pelvic inflammatory disease. *JAMA* 250:759, 1983.

Lipnick RJ, Buring JE, Hennekins CH, et al: Oral contraceptives and breast cancer. *JAMA* 255:58, 1986.

Powell MG, Hedlin AM, Cerskus I, et al: Effects of oral contraceptives in lipoprotein lipids: A prospective study. *Obstet Gynecol* 63:764, 1984.

Scher PW, Emans SJ, Grace EM: Factors associated with compliance to oral contraceptives use in an adolescent population. *J Adol Health Care* 3:120, 1982.

Slone D, Shapiro S, Kaufman DW, et al: Risk of myocardial infarction in relation to current and discontinued use of oral contraceptives. *N Engl J Med* 305:420, 1981.

Stadel BV: Oral contraceptives and cardiovascular disease. *N Engl J Med* 305:612, 1981.

Tietze C, Lehfeldt H, Liebermann HHG: The effectiveness of the cervical cap as a contraceptive method. *Am J Obstet Gynecol* 66:904, 1953.

Vessey M, Lawless M, Yeates D: Efficacy of different methods of contraceptive methods. *Lancet* 1:841, 1982.

Wahl P, Walden C, Knopp R, et al: Effect of estrogen/progestin potency on lipid/lipoprotein cholesterol. *N Engl J Med* 308:862, 1983.

Weiss NS, Saywetz TA: Incidence of endometrial cancer in relation to the use of contraceptives. *N Engl J Med* 302:551, 1980.

Wilson CD: Toxic shock syndrome and diaphragm use. *J Adol Health Care* 4:290, 1983.

Yuzpe AA, Lancee WJ: Ethinyl estradiol and dl-norgestrel as a postcoital contraceptive. *Fertil Steril* 28:932, 1977.

School-Age Pregnancy 10

The past two decades have witnessed major changes in sexual mores, contraceptive technology, the acceptance of single parent families, and availability of induced abortion. Adolescent pregnancy and epidemic venereal disease are currently major child health problems in the United States. In a survey of metropolitan adolescents, Zelnik and Kantner (1980) found that the reported sexual activity among 15- to 19-year-old adolescent girls increased from 30% in 1971 to 50% in 1979. In 1980, there were 921,696 pregnancies among 15- to 19-year-old girls with about 500,000 ending in live births, and 23,010 pregnancies in girls under 15 years (CDC, 1985). Teenage fertility in the United States is considerably higher than in the great majority of developed countries (Jones et al, 1985).

Unfortunately, adolescents may lack the persistence and responsibility necessary for effective contraceptive use even though they may have chosen to become sexually active. Making an appointment in a family planning clinic and use of contraception implies acknowledgment of planned sexual activity and the adolescent may risk discovery by the parent. In a large survey of 1200 teenagers interviewed on their first visit to a family planning clinic, Zabin and Clark (1981) found that 36% already suspected pregnancy, 58% were already sexually active, and only 14% were seeking protection before first intercourse. Only 8% of sexually active adolescents came to the clinic within 3 months of initiation of sexual activity. The reasons given for delay in seeking help in the clinic included "I just didn't get around to it," "I was afraid my family would find out if I came," and "I didn't have sex frequently enough to get pregnant." Others feared the pelvic examination or the possibility of adverse effects from prescription contraceptives.

The limitation in cognitive development in a young adolescent often makes it impossible for him or her to consider the feelings and values of the partner, that a pregnancy can result, and that contraception is necessary. Although for older adolescents risk-taking is less haphazard and their consequences are more clearly connected, many continue to deny possible consequences of lack of contraceptive use. Often, the longer that an adolescent is sexually active without experiencing pregnancy, the more the risk-taking behavior is reinforced. Adolescents are usually unaware that with increasing gynecologic age, the chance of regular ovulatory cycles and, thus, fertility is greater. In addition, adolescents are often reluctant to destroy the spontaneity of intercourse by planning ahead. Those in the older age group (between 18 and 22 years) are more likely to plan for sexual intercourse, to obtain information on birth control before intercourse, and to be capable of mature relationships. Access to contraceptives has been difficult for many adolescents; even those who do obtain prescription contraceptives often discontinue effective methods in spite of continued sexual activity.

Given the frequency of premarital pregnancy in adolescent girls, increased research on motivation for and the impact of pregnancy at the various stages of adolescence are needed. Although the 13-year-old pregnant adolescent is distinctly different from the 18- or 19-year-old young woman who has completed high school, statistics and studies have tended to include such individuals in the category of "adolescent pregnancy." Among the causes of adolescent pregnancy are lack of contraception because of denial of fertility and inability to plan ahead, lack of access to an acceptable clinic, death or loss of a family member, emotional deprivation in which the adolescent girl anticipates a nurturing figure in the child, and attempts to foster a relationship with a boyfriend. Feelings of despair, worthlessness, and chronic school failure appear to be more common among those who choose to carry a pregnancy to term. Moreover, very little is known about the motivation or needs of the male adolescent.

Identifying adolescents at risk to future pregnancies is difficult. In a predominantly black population in North Carolina, Vernon and colleagues (1983) found that a combination of three factors—(1) a family that would be pleased by a pregnancy, (2) a boyfriend listed as the girl's closest friend, and (3) four or more sisters—predicted a pregnancy in 57% of young women who became pregnant in the next year. The specificity of these factors, however, was only 65%. The relationship of low self-esteem and pregnancy remains controversial (Nadelson et al, 1980; Freeman et al, 1984; McAnarney, 1983). The boyfriend who may wish to father a child in order to fulfill his own role within a peer group may undermine attempts at effective contraception.

Adolescents who receive adequate prenatal care can have good obstetric outcomes and improved contraceptive compliance after delivery. Unfortunately, only about 20% of pregnant adolescents are involved in special programs aimed at meeting their needs. In addition, the needs of 13- to 15-year-old patients are very different from those of 18- to 19-year-old patients, and many programs combine them into a single adolescent pregnancy clinic. Adolescent mothers obviously require long-term aid since social isolation and depression can be causes as well as consequences of early child-bearing (McAnarney et al, 1978; Gabrielson et al, 1970). The provision of contraceptives, infant day care within a high school, and social and nutritional services can make a dramatic impact on the morbidity associated with school-age pregnancies. Since a second pregnancy with closely spaced children appears to limit sharply options for the adolescent in terms of school achievement, independence from welfare and other goals, an adolescent's best hope is adequate contraception following delivery of her child.

The options for an unplanned pregnancy are abortion or continuing to term (acceptance or adoption). A nonjudgmental counselor ideally should be available to

CASE ILLUSTRATION

E.B. was a 15-year-old adolescent who came to the clinic for a physical examination and gynecologic assessment. She was in the ninth grade at a suburban high school and her parents were both professionals. Her parents had been concerned about increased rebellious behavior and had been worried that she might run away or become pregnant. They described her as having been running with "a fast crowd" and cutting classes. Because of these problems, they had begun family counseling. During the visit, E.B. admitted that she had been sexually active for the past 6 months with her 19-year-old boyfriend. The risks of sexually transmitted diseases and pregnancy were discussed with E.B. and she decided to begin taking oral contraceptives. E.B. was erratic in keeping her return appointments and 14 months after the initial prescription she discontinued the oral contraceptives because she "ran out of pills" and had broken up with her boyfriend. Three months later she came to clinic for a regular appointment. Her menstrual period was overdue by 10 days and her urine pregnancy test was positive. E.B. had had a single episode of unprotected intercourse 3½ weeks before the visit, but she had not considered the possibility of pregnancy at the time of the appointment. On questioning, she had had breast soreness for 1 week. E.B. was counseled about the options, and she decided to have an abortion. Both parents were supportive of the decision, although quite angry at E.B. for the unplanned pregnancy.

QUESTIONS AND COMMENTS

Why had E.B. failed to continue to take contraceptives?

Many adolescents stop taking oral contraceptives if they break up with a boyfriend, experience minor side-effects, or run out of the prescription. Adolescents often have difficulty with long-range planning and may not restart oral contraceptives in advance of a new relationship. Unfortunately, the developmental age of the patient may not be compatible with consistent contraceptive use.

How should physicians involve families?

In each situation, the physician needs to assess with the adolescent the possibility of involving parents. The physician also needs to be knowledgeable about the applicable statutes in each state. Although teenage girls often find that their mothers are significantly more supportive than they thought, there are many cases in which involvement of the parents is not in the best interest of the adolescent.

Do adolescents always think of pregnancy as a consequence of their actions?

Adolescents may come for a routine appointment with no prior thought of the possibility of pregnancy. They may also present with complaints of nausea, vomiting, abdominal pain, syncope, dizziness, or constipation, and the diagnosis may be pregnancy. Denial of having missed a period or the possibility of pregnancy may further confuse the physician who does not consider this diagnosis.

each adolescent to help her assess the meaning of the pregnancy, her feelings about the options, her long-term goals and plans, and her psychologic strengths and defenses. Nadelson et al (1980) found that teenagers selecting abortion appeared to be remarkably similar to a peer group of nonpregnant high school students in terms of focusing on the importance of finishing school, the impracticality of caring for a child, and the need to take responsibility for their actions. In contrast, adolescents who carried their pregnancies to term often felt that they had "no real choice" and were significantly less able to search for an active solution to the unplanned pregnancy.

DIAGNOSIS OF PREGNANCY

Any adolescent whose menstrual cycle is overdue or who is concerned about the diagnosis of pregnancy should have a urine pregnancy test. In addition, pregnancy should be considered in the differential diagnosis of patients presenting with constipation, nausea, vomiting, dizziness, or syncope. The technology of urine and blood tests is rapidly evolving with increased sensitivity to low levels of human chorionic gonadotropin (HCG). Physicians should have kits for "rapid urine" pregnancy tests available in their offices and should be knowledgeable about laboratory resources for sending urine and blood specimens for sensitive assays, including quantitative β-subunit HCG when abnormalities of pregnancy such as ectopic pregnancy are being considered. The results of urine and blood tests should always be correlated with a physical examination including a pelvic examination.

REFERENCES

CDC: Teenage pregnancy and fertility trend—United States, 1974 and 1980. *JAMA* 253:3064, 1985.

Freeman EW, Rickels K, Higgins GR: Urban black adolescents who obtain contraceptive services before or after their first pregnancy. *J Adol Health Care* 5:183, 1984.

Gabrielson IW, Klerman LV, Currie JB, et al: Suicide attempts in a population pregnant as teenagers. *Am J Public Health* 12:2289, 1970.

Jones EF, Forrest JD, Goldman N, et al: Teenage pregnancy in developed countries: Determinants and policy implications. *Fam Plann Perspect* 17:53, 1985.

McAnarney ER, Roghmann KJ, Adams BN, et al: Obstetric, neonatal, and psychosocial outcomes of pregnant adolescents. *Pediatrics* 61:199, 1978.

McAnarney ER: *Premature Adolescent Pregnancy and Parenthood.* New York, Grune & Stratton, 1983.

Nadelson CC, Notman MT, Gillon JW: Sexual knowledge and attitudes of adolescents: Relationship to contraceptive use. *Obstet Gynecol* 55:340, 1980.

Vernon ME, Green JA, Frothingham TE: Teenage pregnancy: A prospective study of self-esteem and other sociodemographic factors. *Pediatrics* 72:632, 1983.

Zabin LS, Clark SD: Why they delay: A study of teenage family planning clinic patients. *Fam Plann Perspect* 13:205, 1981.

Zelnik M, Kantner JF: Sexual activity, contraceptive use and pregnancy among metropolitan-area teenagers: 1971-1979. *Fam Plann Perspect* 12:230, 1980.

S. JEAN EMANS

Section 12

Neurology

In this section, we propose to discuss a point of view, a general stance, that should be taken when brain disease is suspected in a child. We view this as the most important step in proper neurologic diagnosis, and thus, the essential foundation for all rational therapy. The diseases of the nervous system are best approached by the physician with an eye to determining the localization, in space and time, of the dysfunction. Armed with this knowledge, the examination can be tailored in such a way as to gather useful information. Subsequent to this directed examination, a differential diagnosis can be approached with less trepidation.

This section is divided into two parts: the first part encompasses common problems the general pediatrician sees in daily practice—clinical syndromes, rather than disease states. Patients present with headaches, dizziness, or gait disturbance, not with migraines, paroxysmal vertigo, or cerebellitis.

We then propose to review major categories of pediatric neurologic disease, to serve as a reference guide to the many syndromes and diseases briefly discussed in the first half of the section.

We do not claim this approach as an original one, as it clearly stems from the tradition of clinical medicine in general, and the teaching and writings of Raymond Adams and Maurice Victor in particular. The reader is referred to the preface of Drs. Adams' and Victor's textbook for an explanation of this mode of presentation as it applies to neurology (1985). We would add certain amendments to that approach which are peculiar to pediatric neurology. In addition to the idea of localization in space (thus, implying a knowledge of neuroanatomy), the concept of localization in time becomes important as well (thus implying a knowledge of neuroembryology and neural development). We will not review these relevant disciplines in isolation; instead, we shall discuss relevant aspects of anatomy, physiology, embryology, or development as they present themselves in the course of understanding the various neurologic syndromes.

Neurologic Evaluation

1

The nervous system is a highly structured organ and, hence, lesions can be localized spatially. This anatomic localization is the central tool of the neurologic examination. The organization of the nervous system can be projected on two axes, the rostrocaudal and the dorsoventral. Phylogenetically simpler nervous systems are organized into a number of homologous segments, each specifically designed for its location. In the human, this is best seen in the spinal cord, where each segment is defined by a spinal root that addresses a specific body locus. To a lesser extent, this segmentation is preserved in the brain stem, where the cranial nerves serve to identify the location of the segment. The diencephalon and the telencephalon have undergone such dramatic phylogenetic change that identification of segments is impossible (Brodal, 1981).

History

This is by far the most important aspect of the neurologic evaluation. The format of how the history is taken is different for each patient, not only because of the range of ages, but also because neurologic disease may impair the individual's ability to understand or respond to questions. Indeed, this becomes an important diagnostic clue.

The history should consist of the following elements: (1) A detailed history of the present illness; information about the time course of a symptom or dysfunction such as mode of onset, whether it is continuous or intermittent, and related observations often provide the basis for diagnosis. (2) Information about the gestation, labor, and delivery of the child; particular reference to drug usage or illness during the pregnancy and the medical condition of the neonate should be made. (3) History of any neurologic or non-neurologic diseases in siblings or other close relatives. (4) Any history of previous illness or of substance abuse should be noted. (5) Close attention must be paid to social conditions and occupational exposures.

Physical Examination

The neurologic examination of the child is dependent upon the maturity of the nervous system and, hence, the age of the child. For instance, many of the findings present in a normal preterm neonate would be considered abnormal in a 10-month-old child. Even though no further generation of neurons occurs after birth, myelination and synaptogenesis continue well into young adulthood. The early neurologic examination is primarily concerned with the demonstration of certain reflexes that disappear as the nervous system develops. The persistence of these reflexes past the age at which they would be expected to disappear is a sign of neurologic abnormality.

EXAMINATION OF THE NEONATE

Neonates spend much of their time sleeping and it is usually in this state that the examiner finds the child. If possible, the examination should be carried out in a warm, quiet environment. It is at this age more than any other that observation is the dominant feature in the physical examination.

The state of the child should be assessed before handling. This provides information regarding respiratory rate and pattern, as well as spontaneous movements including eye motion. Asymmetries in motion would suggest a hemiparesis or monoparesis. Clonic motion (i.e., repetitive purposeless motion) suggests seizure activity and the exact location and amplitude of the movements should be observed.

Next, the blanket is removed and the resting posture of the child noted. A normal term neonate should assume a flexed posture with the hips and knees flexed so as to bring the knees toward the abdomen and the arms flexed across the chest. If the legs are in a persistent extended posture, this is suggestive of a lesion somewhere in the corticospinal-anterior horn cell-muscle pathway. Again, asymmetries of posture are important; any spontaneous activity should be further scrutinized at this point.

The infant is then placed in the supine position with the head straight up (as described later, tilting the head to one side may introduce asymmetries of tone and posture). The skull is examined for asymmetries, as well as the presence of a cephalohematoma or caput succedaneum. Next, the fontanelle should be palpated and the size and tension noted. In a quiet infant in the supine position, a bulging fontanelle suggests increased intracranial pressure. The face should be scrutinized for asymmetries suggestive of a facial palsy.

Next, the child should be undressed. Again, refinement and extension of previous observations of posture and movement should be made. If the child is still asleep, an assessment of the level of consciousness is made by holding the baby's thorax and shaking gently. A normal infant should respond to this stimulus. The examination should now progress from procedures that are the least disturbing to those found more disturbing by the child.

Tone and deep tendon reflexes should be assessed in all four limbs, with careful attention to asymmetries and the presence of hypotonia. At this age, both central and peripheral motor lesions are expressed as hypotonia. The plantar reflex is elicited by drawing the thumbnail up the lateral aspect of foot. It is crucial that the infant be quiet for this procedure as the natural movements of the foot and leg can easily obscure the action.

The traction response is elicited by grasping the infant's wrists and gently pulling to a sitting position. One hand can be used to grasp both wrists, with the other available to support the head if there is exaggerated lag. The control of head position as well as the presence and symmetry of the elbow flexion should be observed.

If the head is slowly turned toward one shoulder with the infant in the supine position, there may be extension of the elbow on the "jaw" side and flexion of the contralateral elbow. This is called the tonic neck reflex. It may be present or absent in the neonate, but is usually seen at age 2–3 months. An obligate reflex, i.e., the posture is maintained as long as the head is turned, is a sign of central dysfunction. Asymmetries in the reflex are also abnormal.

The child should now be held with the examiner's hands under the arms. If the child is held vertically, normal axial tone should prevent a feeling that the child is slipping through the hands. If this is not so, hypotonia should be suspected. The posture of the legs is important, as scissoring or persistently extended posturing suggests a corticospinal lesion. The placing response can be elicited by lifting the child so the dorsum of the foot contacts the edge of the examining table. The appropriate response is flexion at the hip and knee so as to place the foot on the table.

The Moro reflex is observed with any abrupt stimulus such as if the child is held at a 45 degree angle and the head and trunk are allowed to fall a short distance. The presence and symmetry of the response should be ascertained. The complete response is abduction of the arms at the shoulder and flexion of the elbows. The child is now placed in the prone position and observed for head control.

Finally, the fundi, pupils, and extraocular motion should be examined. If the child is held supine at about 45 degrees and gently swung from side to side, a vestibulo-ocular reflex with correctional saccades can be seen. The head circumference should be measured.

EXAMINATION OF THE OLDER CHILD

As the nervous system develops, examination of the child gradually changes focus from testing reflexes to ability to comply with standardized commands. The examination of the older child closely follows that of the adult.

Briefly, the examination should begin with an assessment of the mental state, which should include level of consciousness, attention, language, memory, and spatial skills.

The cranial nerves are examined next, including testing of smell, the fundi, and ocular structures. Gaze should be examined in all four quadrants and both saccadic and smooth pursuit movements should be seen. The pupils should be examined for size, contour, and reaction, both consensually and directly to light. It is important to examine pupils in a darkened room to maximize the likelihood of detecting an oculosympathetic palsy or Horner syndrome. When convergence is tested, the pupils should be observed for constriction. Facial symmetry, movement, and sensation test the seventh and fifth cranial nerve. Finally, the gag, tongue motion, and power of the sternocleidomastoid and trapezius muscles should be examined.

Examination of the motor system should include power of each major muscle group, as well as tone, bulk, and deep-tendon reflexes. The plantar reflex can be elicited by stroking the lateral aspect of the sole of the foot with a sharp object.

Sensation to light touch, pin prick, vibration, and position sense should be tested. In addition, two-point discrimination and tests of stereognosis and graphesthesia can give information of sensory function. The function of rapid alternating movements is impaired in cerebellar dysfunction, but may also be impaired in lesions of the corticospinal tract. An assessment of gait completes the examination.

Laboratory and Neuroradiologic Evaluation

The history and physical examination are the central tools of neurologic evaluation. Potential diagnoses can then be confirmed and refined by the use of a few selected laboratory and neuroradiologic tests.

EXAMINATION OF THE CEREBROSPINAL FLUID

Careful examination of the cerebrospinal fluid (CSF) is an important test for inflammatory and infectious disorders and may also aid in the diagnosis of some neoplastic conditions. The CSF should be examined for:

General Appearance. This includes degree of opacity and color. Normal CSF is clear and colorless. This can best be evaluated by holding the tube of CSF up to a white background and comparing it to a tube of water. Haziness suggests pleocytosis (usually greater than 200 cells/mm^3). The presence of more than 1000 red blood cells/mm^3 usually imparts a pinkish tinge to the fluid.

Often, the procedure of lumbar puncture introduces red cells into the CSF, a so-called traumatic tap. A true subarachnoid hemorrhage can be distinguished from a traumatic tap. In a traumatic tap:

1. The number of red cells decreases as more fluid is collected.
2. Normal CSF pressure is present.
3. There is formation of clots and fibrinous webs.
4. There is absence of xanthochromia (a yellow discoloration, see below).

If the tap is traumatic and the hemogram is normal, the addition of 1000 red cells to the CSF is usually accompanied by one white cell.

Xanthochromia may be caused by hemolysis of red cells, hyperbilirubinemia (with subsequent diffusion of both conjugated and unconjugated bilirubin into the CSF), protein (usually greater than 150 mg/dl), hypercarotenemia, and hemoglobinemia.

Cellularity. Normal CSF contains fewer than 5 monos or lymphs/mm^3. The presence of more than 5 cells, or of any polys, suggests an inflammatory process involving the meninges or adjacent structures. The presence of neoplastic cells suggests a tumor involving the meninges. Parenchymal tumors of the brain, in the absence of meningeal spread, seldom shed their cells into the CSF.

Protein. Normal CSF contains less than 45 mg of total protein/dl (in younger patients, the level may be considerably lower). Most of the protein is albumin, although a clinically important fraction is made up of γ-globulins. Usually this fraction is less than 12% of the total protein. γ-globulins may be elevated in multiple sclerosis, subacute sclerosing panencephalitis (SSPE), viral meningoencephalitis, and neurosyphilis. SSPE and multiple sclerosis generate a small number of specific idiotypes of γ-globulin that may be measured by using protein electrophoresis (oligoclonal banding).

Glucose. The CSF glucose has a roughly linear relationship to plasma glucose, being about two-thirds of the value. This value is somewhat decreased with profound hypoglycemia. The presence of low CSF glucose (hypoglycorrhachia) suggests infection (fungal, tubercular, or pyogenic), diffuse neoplastic invasion of the meninges, sarcoidosis, or the early phase of subarachnoid hemorrhage.

COMPUTERIZED AXIAL TOMOGRAPHY (CAT SCANNING)

The assistance of computer analysis to the procedure of classic tomography allows generation of multiple cross-sectional images of the head that demarcate regions of different density (Fig. 12.1). Hence, bone, CSF, white and gray matter, and blood can be differentiated. The greatest clinical value of CAT scanning is the demonstration of mass lesions (including tumors, hemorrhages, and infarcts) and congenital abnormalities of brain development. It has also proven useful in imaging similar pathology in the spinal cord. In the neonate, the use of *echoencephalography* through the anterior fontanelle may define subdural collections, hydrocephalus, and developmental abnormalities and may be carried out at the cribside.

MAGNETIC RESONANCE IMAGING (MRI SCANNING)

This technique (using Nuclear Magnetic Resonance, NMR) also generates cross-sectional images of the brain or spinal cord. Instead of using ionizing X-radiation, it takes advantage of the fact that spinning electrons will line up parallel to a magnetic field. The images are devoid of any bone image and, hence, are of particular use in imaging the posterior fossa, where bone artifact limits CAT scan resolution. Although still in its formative years, the increased resolution and lack of known hazard make it a superior form of imaging over CAT scanning in some, if not all, types of neuropathology (Andreasen, 1988).

ANGIOGRAPHY

The introduction of a radiopaque dye into a blood vessel, followed by conventional radiography allows imaging of the architecture of the arterial or venous tree. This is of particular importance in the evaluation of patients with infarcts, nontraumatic subarachnoid hemorrhage, or for preoperative analysis of tumor patients.

MYELOGRAPHY

The subarachnoid space may be seen by introducing a radiopaque dye via a lumbar puncture needle, followed by conventional radiography or CAT scanning. This is of particular use in the definition of herniated intervertebral disks, arteriovenous malformations of the spinal cord, and of spinal cord tumors.

ELECTROENCEPHALOGRAPHY

The placement of electrodes on the scalp with subsequent amplification of the signal to a pen writer allows observation of waveforms of brain activity. This procedure is useful in the evaluation of many different types of CNS disease, and the specific abnormalities seen will be described under those diseases. It is particularly useful in the diagnosis of seizure disorders and metabolic diseases.

EVOKED POTENTIALS

Small changes in brainwave activity can be seen after sensory stimulation, if the larger EEG background is averaged out. The pattern of the waveform gives information about the sensory system tested. This type of analysis is termed "evoked potential." The visual system may be tested by using a shifting checkerboard pattern (PSVER; pattern shift visual evoked response) or a flash of light. Congenital and acquired lesions from many etiologies may result in an abnormality in the size and latency of the response.

The use of "clicks" as a stimulus gives information about the auditory system in the brain stem (brain stem auditory-evoked response; BAER).

Finally, somatosensory stimuli may be applied to the arm or leg and the resulting potential (SSEP; somatosensory evoked potential) gives information about the integrity of the peripheral nerves, spinal cord and brain components of the sensory path.

Other laboratory studies such as electromyography and tissue biopsy will be discussed under the appropriate disease sections.

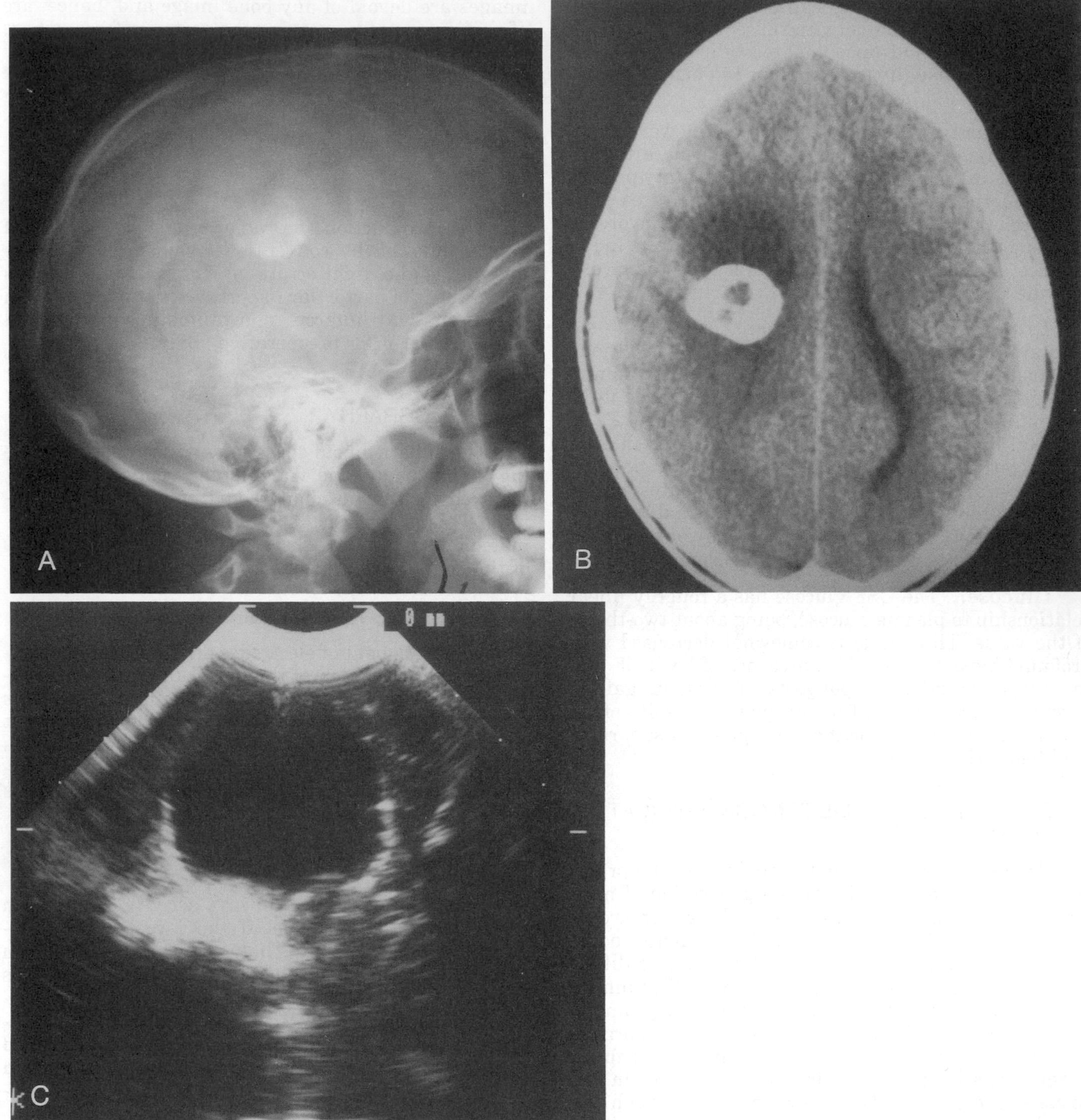

Figure 12.1 A, B, and C. This 15-year-old was originally referred to an orthopedic surgeon for complaints of difficulty walking. It was obvious on physical examination that the motor deficit affected the entire right side. A plain radiograph of skull showed calcification which was demonstrated more fully on CT scan **(B)** as being part of a solid/cystic tumor deep in the left cerebral hemisphere. At surgery, the mass could not be identified as it caused no change in the gyral pattern over the surface. Intraoperative ultrasonography **(C)** showed the cystic and calcific portions of the mass and the shortest surgical path through normal brain. Low grade astrocytoma was the final pathologic diagnosis.

REFERENCES

Adams RD, Victor M: Principles of Neurology, 3rd edition. New York, McGraw-Hill, 1985.

Andreasen NC: Brain imaging: Applications in psychiatry. *Science* 239:1381, 1988.

Brodal A: *Neurological Anatomy in Relation to Clinical Medicine,* 3rd edition. New York, Oxford, 1981.

Chiappa KH: *Evoked Potentials in Clinical Neurology*. New York, Raven Press, 1983.

Fenichel G: *Neonatal Neurology,* 2nd edition. London, Churchill Livingstone, 1986.

Fishman RA: *Cerebrospinal Fluid in Diseases of the Nervous System.* Philadelphia, WB Saunders, 1980.

Niedermeyer E, DaSilva FL: *Electroencephalography*. Baltimore, Urban and Schwarzenberg, 1982.

Neurologic Problems 2

MACROCEPHALY

Definition

Macrocephaly implies a head circumference greater than 2 standard deviations above the mean. This is a feature of pathology rather than a disease in itself.

Basic Science

Primary megalencephaly, a form of macrocephaly, is a developmental anomaly that results in an increase in volume of all neural elements. Histopathologically, it is characterized by abnormal migration of cortical neurons with heterotopias, disorganization of both white and gray matter, and defective cortical lamination. It is often familial, with an autosomal dominant inheritance. It is clinically expressed as a syndrome of mental retardation, seizures and bilateral corticospinal and cerebellar dysfunction, which may also be associated with neurofibromatosis, multiple hemangiomata, and other cutaneous anomalies. Primary megalencephaly may also occur with no perturbation of the cortical architecture and normal intelligence.

Natural History

The normal growth of the intracranial contents and, hence, head circumference is delicately controlled. Increased head circumference suggests either that the normal intracranial contents are large, such as hydrocephalus or megalencephaly, or that an abnormal space-occupying mass such as a subdural collection of liquid is present.

In the first 6 months of life, macrocephaly could result from hydrocephalus, subdural collections, or megalencephaly. In the late infantile period (from 6 months to 2 years), other considerations are Dandy-Walker syndrome, pseudotumor cerebri, and megalencephalies. The megalencephalies may be secondary to leukodystrophies (Canavan or Alexander disease), phakomatoses, lipidoses, or achondroplasia. Megalencephaly may also be a primary condition.

Diagnosis

Examination of the head is obviously important in evaluation of macrocephaly. In an infant, the increase in volume may express itself as a bulging anterior fontanelle. Later on, as the cranial sutures begin to fuse, increased intracranial volume may result in "Macewen sign"—a "cracked pot" sound on percussion of the skull. In addition, the sutures may be widely spaced. Bulging parietally is suggestive of porencephaly or a subdural collection, while frontal bossing or downward eye deviations may be seen in obstructive hydrocephalus. A CT scan or MRI is an essential part of the evaluation of macrocephaly.

HYDROCEPHALUS

Definition

Hydrocephalic progressive ventricular dilation is a cause of macrocephaly and it also reflects an underlying pathology. The causes of hydrocephalus may be physiologically classified into three groups: (1) increased CSF production; (2) obstruction to flow within the ventricular system (noncommunicating hydrocephalus); and (3) decreased absorption at the level of the arachnoid granulations (communicating hydrocephalus).

Basic Science

Increased CSF production is seen in choroid plexus papillomas, benign tumors of the choroid plexus that account for 1–4% of childhood intracranial tumors. They usually present in the first year of life with hydrocephalus, often with acute intraventricular hemorrhage. It is a cause of infant papilledema, a rare finding at this age.

The syndrome of obstruction to flow within the ventricular system has been termed *noncommunicating hydrocephalus*. In infants, intraventricular hemorrhage can obstruct outflow of spinal fluid from the fourth ventricle. Mass lesions compressing the ventricular system (aneurysms of the vein of Galen) may compress the aqueduct, leading to obstructive hydrocephalus or to disease within the system itself. Aqueductal stenosis is a developmental anomaly of the aqueduct and is associated with anomalies of nearby structures, such as fusion of the quadrigeminal bodies, oculomotor nuclei, or more caudal defects of neural tube closure. It is the most common site of obstruction in congenital hydrocephalus.

Aqueductal obstruction secondary to a gliosis may be seen as a sequela of perinatal infection or subarachnoid hemorrhage, or as part of von Recklinghausen disease.

Obstruction may occur at the level of the fourth ventricle, as a result of Chiari malformation (inferior displacement of medulla and fourth ventricle into the upper cervical canal and a variety of bony defects) or Dandy-Walker syndrome.

Communicating hydrocephalus represents about one-third of all childhood hydrocephalus and physiologically indicates a failure of CSF absorption at the level of the arachnoid granulations. It commonly follows bacterial or fungal meningitis or subarachnoid hemorrhage. A rare cause is diffuse meningeal infiltration by lymphoma or leukemia.

Diagnosis

Suspicion of raised intracranial pressure in infants is first aroused by the presence of a full or tense anterior fontanelle. In children, widening of the sutures seen on skull radiographs is an important sign. The most important diagnostic step is an accurate measurement of the occipitofrontal circumference of the head. Serial measurements plotted on a graph of normal head growth are most helpful. A head circumference in the 90th percentile may not cause concern if it stops on the same percentile. A head circumference that moves across percentile lines requires an explanation. Knowledge of parents' head sizes and shapes is also helpful since infants may inherit relatively large heads.

Transillumination with a standard light source and soft rubber adaptor that conforms to the contour of the infant's skull can provide valuable information on regional collections of excess fluid. With hydranencephaly, the whole cranial vault is transilluminated and, thus, establishes the diagnosis. Although transillumination remains a useful adjunct to the physical examination, if ultrasonography and CT scanning are available, these should be used for a more definitive diagnosis (Fig. 12.2).

Treatment

Raised intracranial pressure should be lowered. In premature infants with intraventricular hemorrhage, daily lumbar punctures to remove excess fluid were advocated in the past, but in a controlled study Mantovani et al (1980) failed to show any beneficial effect on mortality or risk of hydrocephalus. If the head is rapidly growing, external ventriculostomy or placement of a ventriculoperitoneal shunt is appropriate.

Progressive hydrocephalus after meningitis or subarachnoid hemorrhage may require a ventriculostomy and, if drainage continues, a more permanent shunt.

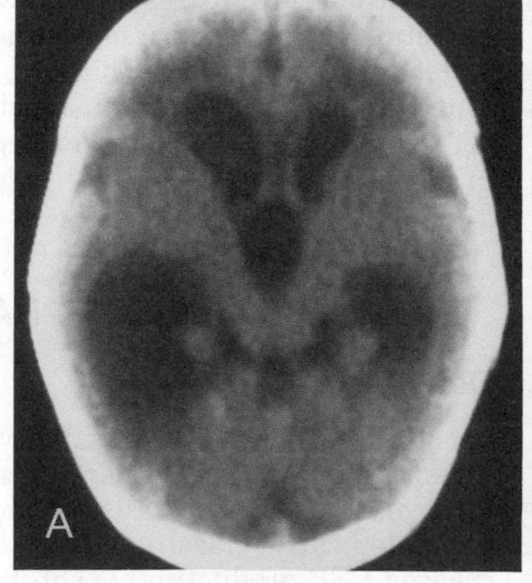

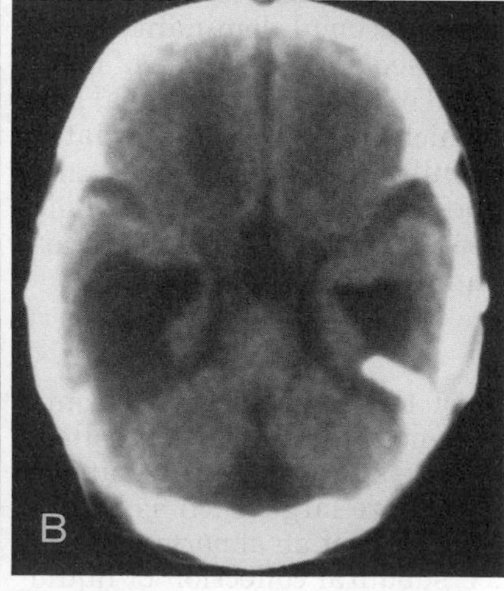

Figure 12.2 A and B. Hydrocephalus was diagnosed on third-trimester ultrasonography and the baby was referred for confirmatory CT scan. Ventriculomegaly of third and lateral ventricles (but a normal fourth ventricle), associated with periventricular white matter changes indicated that obstruction at the aqueduct was the likely diagnosis. The baby was immediately referred for ventriculoperitoneal shunting to decompress the ventricular system.

When the hydrocephalus is secondary to a malformation, the shunt will have to be in place throughout life in more than 90% of infants. Frequent revisions will be required as the infant grows.

Prognosis

Among infants whose hydrocephalus was recognized and treated early, and who survived to age 2 years, more than half had no major dysfunction in the series from Sweden. Twenty-five percent had cerebral palsy, 20% severe mental retardation (Fennell et al, 1987).

PSEUDOTUMOR CEREBRI (BENIGN INTRACRANIAL HYPERTENSION)

Definition

Pseudotumor cerebri is an increase in intracranial pressure in the absence of space-occupying lesion.

Basic Science

This symptom complex can follow middle ear infection or mild head injuries. It has also been seen after changes in steroid therapy or oral contraceptives. Hypervitaminosis A and tetracycline have been implicated. Lateral sinus thrombosis is the most common single abnormality. In some instances, the etiology is obscure.

Natural History

The increase in volume of CSF from any cause produces intermittent headaches, blurred vision, vomiting, and diplopia. The level of consciousness in pseudotumor cerebri is usually normal. The duration of increased intracranial pressure is, on average, about 2–3 months. Recurrences have been noted in about 10% of patients.

Diagnosis

The diagnosis is made after exclusion of a space-occupying lesion by CT scan. The CSF is usually normal although a few white cells may be present.

Treatment

Osmotic diuretics, steroids, and carbonic anhydrase inhibitors have been tried, although their efficacy is not always evident. Repeated, careful lumbar punctures may also be successful. Careful monitoring of visual fields is also indicated.

Prognosis

The disorder is self-limited.

HEADACHE

Definition

A headache is a common symptom of many pathologies both within and outside the CNS. Although most headaches are expressions of benign disease, some represent a cardinal feature of more sinister pathology.

Basic Science

Observations made during cranial surgery have illustrated the rather limited number of structures that are sensitive to pain. They include the fifth, ninth, and tenth cranial nerves and the roots of the first three cervical spinal nerves, the basally located dura and pia arachnoid maters and the blood vessels within them; the skin, scalp, and muscular tissue that surround the skull and the periosteum of the skull; and finally the eye, ear, and nasal passages. It is important to realize that stimulation of these structures provides the only source of pain in the head. The brain parenchyma itself as well as the choroid plexuses and distal blood vessels have no nociception.

Diagnosis

The clinical evaluation of the headache patient centers on a detailed history and physical examination. It is important to question both the parents and the child as to the nature of the disorder. Information should be obtained on the quality of the pain. For example, a pulsatile pain suggests a vascular etiology. The location of the pain is particularly important. If significant pain is localized in the face, sinus, ocular, and neck pathology should be considered as well as affections of the fifth cranial nerve (trigeminal neuralgia, zoster, or tumor) and cluster headache. Acute ocular pathology may present with periorbital and occipital pain. Disease of the cervical vertebral column, spinal roots, or meninges may reveal itself with neck pain that then involves the occipital head region.

More important is the time course of the headache. The acute onset of a severe headache should always suggest subarachnoid hemorrhage. Meningeal infection usually has a more gradual onset, over hours or days. As with any somatic pain, the history of present illness is not complete without discussing aggravating and ameliorating factors. For instance, the headache that accompanies a third ventricle cyst usually has a prominent postural component, being precipitated by lying down or standing up. The headache that follows lumbar puncture is usually much worse on sitting or standing. Migraine headaches may be triggered by certain foods such as cheese, red wine, or chocolate.

Migraine

Definition

Two patterns of migraine headaches have been described: a "common" variety that presents as a pulsatile unilateral or bilateral headache often with nausea and vomiting, but without any neurologic features, and a "classic" variety where the headache is preceded by transient neurologic dysfunction.

Epidemiology

Migraine headache represents a significant percentage of headaches in children. It is thought to be a hereditary disorder with an autosomal dominant inheritance and a variable penetrance. Boys are afflicted about twice as often as girls.

Natural History

Nearly 20% of patients with migraine report that their first attack was in the first 5 years of life (Barlow, 1984). Classic migraine often begins in the morning, when the patient may sense a change in mood or appetite. This may last up to a day. The actual attack is ushered in by visual abnormalities such as zigzag white lines (fortification spectra or teichopsia) that sweep across the visual field leaving a scotoma. The visual field deficits are almost always bilateral and homonymous suggesting primary visual cortex dysfunction. Other neurologic dysfunction such as paresthesias, weakness, confusion, or aphasia may also occur. If there is a spread of the symptoms from one part of the body to another, it is invariably slow, over a matter of minutes (in contrast to seizures that march over seconds). This neurologic dysfunction may last up to 30 minutes and gradually is replaced by a unilateral, pulsatile headache that may last for hours to days. Rarely, the headache is continuous for days on end, a disorder termed status migrainus (Table 12.1).

Migraine is variable, both with regard to the neurologic dysfunction and the headache. Certain variants are common enough to be described in their own right. One of these is the so-called "hemiplegic" variant, where hemiplegia occurs and outlasts the headache phase. These usually run in families, begin in childhood and recur, often every few weeks. The hemiplegia may involve alternate sides, and usually affects the face and arm more than the leg. If the dominant hemisphere is involved, an aphasia may accompany the corticospinal dysfunction. These patients often require brain imaging with CT or MRI and EEG to rule out other disorders. Rarely, the ictus is followed by a permanent deficit, suggesting cerebral infarction secondary to migraine.

Table 12.1
Characteristics of Migraine

Symptom	Percent of Individuals
Nausea, vomiting, abdominal pain	70–100
Family history	50–90
Antecedent history of motion sickness	50
Aura	50
Visual	
Somatosensory	
Other	
Unilateral/retro-orbital pain	25–50

Another variant is termed the "ophthalmoplegic" variant and is characterized by an oculomotor palsy during the migraine. The patient has a unilateral ptosis, and ophthalmoplegia involving the medial, inferior and superior recti, and inferior oblique muscles. The parasympathetic fibers serving the pupillary light reflex are rarely involved. The disorder may outlast the headache by days or weeks and, occasionally, may become permanent.

One of the most dramatic variants is the "confusional" migraine. The child experiences an agitated confusional state often with combative behavior. The attack may last up to 20 hours, but may be as brief as 10 minutes. This form may occur after trivial closed head trauma, when it must be differentiated from intracranial contusion. The EEG may show unilateral temporal or occipital slowing, or be generally slowed.

Finally, episodic brain stem and cerebellar dysfunction may accompany migraine and has been termed "vertebrobasilar" migraine. Occasionally, brief loss of consciousness is found with this disorder.

Treatment

Treatment of migraine is usually successful: if there are frequent attacks, prophylactic therapy is advised; if the migraine attacks occur less than five or so times per month, each attack may be treated separately.

The mainstay of *prophylactic* therapy is propranolol, a nonspecific beta-adrenergic antagonist. The dose used is usually 2 mg/kg in three divided doses. Because of adverse reactions, mainly bradycardia, hypotension, fatigue, or exacerbation of reactive airways disease, the medication should be started at less than one-half the therapeutic dose and increased gradually.

More recently, the use of amitriptyline in older children has proved helpful. This tricyclic drug acts to inhibit the uptake of serotonin in the spinal cord and brain stem and thereby enhance the body's own analgesic mechanisms. The starting dose should be 10 or 25 mg at night, and the dose should be increased by 25-mg increments every 5 or 7 days to a maximum dose of about 150 mg. Adverse effects reflecting the muscarinic antagonist activity of the drug and limiting its use in higher doses are common. These include blurred vision, dry mouth, memory difficulties and constipation. Other medications that have been used successfully include pizotifen (1–3 mg daily) and cyproheptadine (2–5 mg daily).

Methysergide has been advocated as a prophylactic medicine for migraine, but the retroperitoneal fibrosis and other fibrotic syndromes limit its use to periods of less than 6 months. The dose used is 2 mg three times a day, after meals.

Recent studies suggest that calcium channel antagonists may also be effective in preventing migraines.

Treatment of the *acute migraine* is a different problem. Acetaminophen or aspirin may provide relief in mild cases, but often are not sufficient. Two specific antimigraine drugs are available: ergotamine and isometheptene. Ergotamine, taken 2 mg sublingually at the onset of the headache or visual dysfunction and then again in 20 minutes if no relief is experienced, is the drug of choice. Although it has been suggested that ergotamine may exacerbate a hemiplegia or hemianopia, this has not been proved.

Tension Headache

This disorder is characterized by a diffuse, dull, nonpulsatile ache that is usually bilateral and is associated by a sense of fullness or stiffness in the head or neck. It is common in adults and in pediatric practice is seen in adolescents. The headache has a gradual onset and may persist for many hours, days, or weeks. It may occur alternating with actual migraine attacks. It is treated with acetaminophen, aspirin, or Fiorinal.

Headache as a Manifestation of Neuropathology

Headaches are the cardinal feature of a subarachnoid hemorrhage. The classic presentation is of a hyperacute onset of a severe headache with neck stiffness and pain. The patient appears ill and may become confused or develop other neurologic features. In contrast to migraine, the neurologic features develop during or after the headache. A CT scan may show subarachnoid blood usually around the basal cisterns and provide the diagnosis. If the scan is normal, a lumbar puncture must be performed.

Meningeal irritation in acute bacterial or viral meningitis also presents with headache and stiffness in the neck. The onset is more leisurely than in subarachnoid hemorrhage, and the patient may have fea-

CASE ILLUSTRATION

A 12-year-old male presented to our emergency room with a sudden onset of gait unsteadiness, vertigo, confusion, nausea, vomiting, and a throbbing headache. He reported no fevers, experienced no head trauma, and denied any ingestion. He did admit to headaches in the past, with visual symptoms, nausea, and weakness. Family history was significant for migraines. Social history was remarkable for the recent traumatic divorce of his parents. He had a history of "acting out" in the past.

On physical examination he was lethargic but easily arousable. When awake he was inattentive and mildly dysarthric. Vital signs including blood pressure were stable. Examination was also notable for unremitting, horizontal, bidirectional, and upbeating nystagmus, unaffected by movement and enhanced by fixation. Extraocular movements were full and conjugate. Pupils were 3 mm and reactive. Vision was sharp and normally colored. There were no other cranial nerve abnormalities. Gait was severely ataxic, with the patient able to walk only with support. Movements were dysmetric, but strength, tone, and bulk were normal. Sensation was intact. Deep tendon reflexes were brisk but symmetrically so. There were three beats of clonus at both ankles and upgrowing toes bilaterally. Remainder of the examination was entirely normal, including a supple neck with no meningismis.

QUESTION AND COMMENT

What is the most helpful finding in the above physical examination, and what is the differential diagnosis that this finding suggests for this patient?

Of the multiple neurologic findings given, the one that has the greatest localizing value and the least easily feigned is nystagmus. In evaluating nystagmus one should attempt to determine whether its origin is peripheral (i.e., emanating from the vestibular-labyrynthine apparatus) or centrally (coming from the brain stem). Peripheral nystagmus, although seen in some neoplastic processes such as an acoustic neuroma, will usually carry a benign prognosis, often spontaneously resolving over time. Central nystagmus, however, although often due to a transient condition such as drug toxicity or a basilar artery migraine can also represent a more permanent condition such as a posterior fossa tumor or bleed or vertebrobasilar arterial insufficiency, multiple sclerosis and Arnold-Chiari malformation, encephalitis, or a degenerative process.

Peripheral nystagmus will be worsened by head motion and suppressed by fixation of gaze. Gait may be unsteady but there are usually no other cerebellar signs. Central nystagmus seems to be unaffected by motion and enhanced by fixation. It is often associated with evidence of cerebellar, brain stem, cranial nerve, or long tract involvement. There may also be signs of increased intracranial pressure. Both peripheral and central nystagmus may be rotary, horizontal, or vertical, although vertical alone is usually indicative of the central focus and downbeating nystagmus is said to be virtually pathognomonic of the Arnold-Chiari malformation.

This patient's nystagmus was central in origin. The most common cause of this constellation of symptoms in children is basilar artery migraine. Affecting the vertebrobasilar arterial tree, basilar artery migraines are characterized by transient disturbances in function of the brain stem, cerebellum, and occipital cortex, followed by severe pulsatile, bilateral headaches, vomiting, and ultimately by complete and rapid (within minutes to hours) clearing of all these signs. There are often transient aberrations of consciousness, paresthesias, and long tract signs. Typical headache may be absent in as many as 20% of cases, but a family history for migraine is solicited in more than 90% and, thus, is an important diagnostic clue. Children with basilar arterial migraines will often go on to develop the common migraine in reaching adolescence. Certainly basilar artery migraines could account for this child's findings, in that they resolved by the following morning. On the other hand, this patient's toxic screen was also positive for butalbital, a barbiturate, which can give a picture similar to basilar artery migraine including nystagmus.

tures of an infection, such as fever, elevated white count, and metabolic acidosis.

Intracranial neoplasms may present as a headache disorder, often with neurologic symptoms and signs that are not intermittent. Rarely, a neoplasm or arteriovenous malformation may present with a headache resembling a migraine.

Pseudotumor cerebri is a condition characterized by headache, bilateral papilledema, and occasionally, an abducens palsy or inferior quadrantanopsia. The CT shows diffuse swelling of the brain parenchyma with slit ventricles and no mass lesions. Lumbar puncture reveals increased opening pressure, greater than 250 mm H_2O and often greater than 400 mm H_2O. The CSF analysis is normal (see pp. 619).

DEVELOPMENTAL DELAY

The child who fails to achieve developmental milestones within the "windows" prescribed by any of a number of standard instruments is a cause of concern for families and daycare/school personnel. Developmental delay is also a major source of discomfort for the pediatrician, and frequently prompts a neurologic consultation. The major aspects of development that require evaluation are gross and fine motor skills, language, and personal-social development.

The presence or absence, appropriate or inappropriate, of certain motor responses is most useful in the infant (Table 12.2). For older children, the emphasis should shift to more cognitively based skills.

Delayed Walking and Gait Disturbance

Definition

Delayed walking is a condition where development in other domains is not delayed, but the child has not started walking. *Gait disturbance* is present when the child stops walking but appears otherwise apparently intact neurologically.

It is important to ask the family whether other family members have been "late walkers." Nevertheless, although it may be comforting to know that the child's father was also a late walker, many of the indolent myopathies are dominant in their transmission seem to be variable in their penetrance and should not be overlooked.

Table 12.2
Developmental Responses[1] in the First 12 Months of Life

Response	Appears	Disappears
Moro	Birth	4–5 months
Palmar grasp	Birth	3–4 months
Step and place	2–4 weeks	Dissolves into standing
Asymmetric tonic neck	2–3 weeks	5–6 months
	(should never be obligate or unilateral)	
Parachute	6–7 months	Persists

[1]Although these are often designated as "developmental reflexes" we prefer to use "developmental responses," which more accurately reflects these complex activities.

The following questions should be borne in mind.

1. Are the child's legs hypotonic and do they appear weak? Is there muscle dysfunction elsewhere, suggesting a widespread myopathic process? Useful screening tests are serum creatinine phosphokinase and aldolase and thyroid function.
2. Are the deep tendon reflexes diminished or absent? Are there fasciculations and fibrillations of the tongue? These suggest spinal muscular atrophy and nerve conduction studies and muscle biopsy would be appropriate.
3. Is there sensory dysfunction and diminished reflexes in the distal hands and feet, suggesting a neuropathic process? Electrophysiologic studies would be useful.
4. Are there sphincteric disturbances, such as bladder or bowel dysfunction (a constantly wet diaper or a patulous anal sphincter), suggesting the possibility of spinal cord disease? Anatomic imaging of the cord would be appropriate.
5. Are there cutaneous signs (e.g., a tuft of hair over the lumbosacral spine, which may indicate spinal dysraphism) or a bruit over the spinal column (which may signify an underlying arteriovenous malformation)? Again, anatomic imaging of the cord would be appropriate.

Spinal Cord Lesion

In the child who ceases walking but otherwise appears normal, the crucial issue is whether the child has a spinal cord lesion. The cardinal signs of spinal cord disease are: (1) detectable level at which sensation appears to stop; (2) detectable level at which motor performance stops; (3) no involvement of the facial musculature; (4) bowel or bladder dysfunction.

In addressing points 1 and 2 it should be borne in mind that the fibers emanating from primary motor cortex in the cerebral hemispheres that control the legs are closely applied to the lateral ventricles; hence, acute dilatation of the lateral ventricles can produce a syndrome that appears to be spinal in its localization (acute paraplegia or paraparesis with urinary dysfunction). The lack of sensory involvement is a useful diagnostic criterion.

Spinal cord dysfunction in the child may be acquired or congenital. In the past, spinal cord disruption and transsection was relatively common during difficult breech deliveries. The advent of modern obstetrical techniques has essentially eliminated this particular acquired lesion. Currently, the most common cause of acquired spinal cord disease in children is compression. Compression may be epidural, intradural but extra-arachnoid, intra-arachnoid but extramedullary, or intramedullary in its localization (Table 12.3). These differences are clinically useful, as they can distinguish very different etiologic processes. The differential diagnosis of cord compression given various centripetal localizations is presented in Table 12.4. Management

Table 12.3
Signs and Symptoms of Spinal Cord Compression

Symptoms
- Stops walking
- Changes in bowel and bladder function (constipation most frequent bowel symptom; urinary frequency may increase or decrease)
- Back pain
- Paresthesias in the legs

Early Signs
- Loss of sensation in the lower extremities (pinprick and vibration often first)
- Deep tendon reflexes are first diminished and then increased with time
- Tenderness over the spine at the level of the lesion
- In infants and toddlers, a sweat level may be useful to establish an autonomic deficit

Late Signs
- Clear sensory level
- Clear muscle weakness
- Increased deep tendon reflexes with Babinski sign
- Sphincter disturbances

of these conditions is usually neurosurgical or through radiotherapy.

Another acquired spinal cord disease is acute or subacute transverse myelitis, usually preceded by a very typical infrascapular pain and often progressing quite rapidly. Most are thoracic in localization; they are often parainfectious, occurring after a viral illness (varicella, mononucleosis). The examination is similar to that of an intramedullary spinal cord process; myelography or MRI is usually required to rule out a cord lesion.

Discitis, an inflammation of the nucleus pulposus of the intervertebral disk, is usually seen in young children (less than 5 years of age), and has symptoms and signs that are similar to other extramedullary compression syndromes. It is usually lumbar in its localization.

Table 12.4
Spinal Cord Compression by Centripetal Localization

Epidural
- Metastatic disease (including leukemic deposits and lymphoma)
- Hematoma (factor deficiency states)
- Abscess
- Bony abnormalities (especially remember C1-C2 subluxation in Down syndrome)

Intradural but Extra-Arachnoid
- Neurofibroma

Intra-Arachnoid but Extramedullary
- "Drop" metastases from primary CNS tumor (ependymoma, medulloblastoma)
- Dermoid cyst

Intramedullary
- Glioma
- Ependymoma
- Syringomyelia

Striking the patient's head lightly commonly produces pain at the involved site. Treatment is conservative, with bedrest and antibiotics.

Congenital spinal cord anomalies are presented in Table 12.5; they produce spinal cord syndromes at the level of involvement. The treatment is usually surgical, with "aggressive conservative" team management by neurosurgeons, orthopedic surgeons, urologists, and physical and occupational therapists greatly decreasing the long-term morbidity and mortality of these patients (see pp. 720).

SPEECH AND LANGUAGE DELAY

Definition

Language is that set of operations whereby the CNS takes in information in any of a variety of modalities, transforms it in some way, and then expresses that transformation to others. Speech is the most commonly used method of transmitting that information, although it is not the only way. Thus, language is a more encompassing concept than is speech. There are any number of people who have grave speech disorders, but who cannot be said to be entirely without language (the deaf, for example). Although this division is somewhat simplistic, and also glosses over the complex interaction between speech and language in the developing infant, it is nonetheless a useful construct for clinical practice. Furthermore, definition of speech or language delay requires a framework of the progression of language development in the normal child.

The Denver Developmental Screening test (DDST) is most often used for delineating a framework for addressing the issue of a speech or language disorder. Examination of the original Frankenburg and Dodds data permits construction of projected developmental milestones for speech and language behavior. Thus, a table of the ages by which a given percentage of children ultimately deemed normal have acquired a given language or speech behavior is helpful. Tables 12.6 and 12.7 are modifications of such an approach, after Wright (Swaiman and Wright, 1982).

More detailed tools for assessment of early language are the Early Language Milestone Scale (ELM) or Receptive-Expressive Emergent Language Scale

Table 12.5
Congenital Abnormalities of the Spinal Cord

Bony Abnormalities Only
- Spina bifida occulta (underlying cord not involved)

Bony Abnormality with Underlying Cord Pathology
- Diastematomyelia and other dysraphic states

Meninges Involved
- Meningocele

Meninges and Cord Involved
- Myelomeningocele (cord and meninges protrude through bony defect)

Table 12.6
Progression of Language Development[1]

Language Behavior	Age by which 90% of Normal Children Acquire
Vocalizes	6 months
Laughs and squeals	
Localizes sound direction	12 months
Imitates sounds	
Mama, dada (nonspecific)	
Mama, dada (specific)	14 months
Three words in addition to mama, dada	21 months
Points to body part on command	24 months
Two-word phrases	30 months
Names simple pictures	
Follows directions	36 months
First and last name	48 months

[1]After Swaiman and Wright: Swaiman KF, Wright FS: *Practice of Pediatric Neurology*, 2nd edition. St. Louis, CV Mosby, 1982.

Table 12.7
Progression of Speech Development (Consonants)

Consonant	Position	Age by which 90% of Normal Children Acquire
b	initial	
d	initial	
h	initial	
p	initial	
m	initial and final	
w	initial	2 years
b	final	
f	initial	
g	initial	
k	initial	
n	initial and final	
p	final	
t	initial	3 years
f	final	
j	initial	
l	initial	
ng	final	
y	initial	4 years
d	final	
g	final	
k	final	
s	initial	
th	initial	
v	initial	5 years
l	final	
ng (soft)	final	
th	final	
v	final	6 years
s	final	7 years

[1]After Swaiman and Wright: Swaiman KF, Wright FS: *Practice of Pediatric Neurology*, 2nd edition. St. Louis, CV Mosby, 1982.

(REEL). They can be administered in an office practice (Coplan, 1983).

Diagnosis

As noted in previous sections, the performance in other domains of behavior should be considered in evaluating delay in language acquisition. Such a delay in a child with Down syndrome is conceptually less troubling than the delay in a child who is otherwise developing along a more usual course.

It should be determined whether the child displays problems with language or speech, or demonstrates elements of both. The presence of other, nonlinguistic oromotor problems (excessive drooling, difficulties learning to suck through a straw, trouble blowing out candles) suggest speech as the major problem, particularly if coupled with the parental observation that the child "just seems to understand everything." On the other hand, the child with minimal eye contact, poor articulation of needs both verbally and gesturally, and diminished capacity to execute simple commands certainly leads to consideration of a primary language disorder.

The single most important item in the differential diagnosis of language and speech delay is hearing impairment. This is the most common cause of language delay in most North American series, and also is treatable in many instances. Parental assurance that the child "startles or pays attention" when called is not a reliable assessment, as many other cues are often available to the child. Few practicing pediatricians appear to be aware of this important fact; indeed, 75% of the 60 children referred by practicing pediatricians to the Department of Neurology at The Children's Hospital Boston for evaluation of language or speech delay over the last 2 years had not been screened with a hearing evaluation before referral (seven proved to have significant hearing impairment). Thus, hearing tests are crucial to the rational management of speech and language delay.

Speech disorders may be divided somewhat artificially into anterior (articulation) and posterior (voice) problems, and Table 12.8 shows the most common disorders seen in clinical practice. Developmental dyslalia may be the consequence of tongue tie; it is useful to remember that most tongue ties noted at birth resolve sufficiently by the fourth or fifth month of life so that speech is not affected. Dysarthria is to talking what ataxia is to walking, a disorder of control and modulation. It is often associated with an underlying disorder of neural control, or may be seen as an effect of medication (such as phenobarbital). Oromotor apraxia may be viewed as a derangement of the sequential organization of orobuccal movements; as such it is certainly "neurologic" in its origin. It also affects other uses of the mouth (drooling and dysfunctional sucking through straws are often seen in this group of children). It may produce a striking delay in the acquisition of any language or speech behavior, and hence, may reduce the child's interactive capacities to the extent that many are erroneously labeled "autistic." Finally, dysrhythmia (stuttering) is frequently seen transiently and

Table 12.8
Differential Diagnosis of Speech and Language Disorders

Mental retardation
Hearing Impairment
Speech disorders
- Anterior problems (articulation)
  - Dyslalia
  - Dysarthria
  - Oromotor apraxia
  - Dysrhythmia
- Posterior problems (voice)
  - Cleft palate
  - Dysphonia secondary to vocal cord pathology
  - Palatopharyngeal incompetence

Language disorders
- Acquired language disorders
  - Stroke
  - Post-traumatic
  - Acquired epileptic aphasia
- Congenital (developmental) disorders of language

often resolves spontaneously. The presence of secondary motor signs (tics, grimacing, abdominal contractions) is an indication for referral to a speech-language pathologist.

Voice disorders are more obviously physical, as can be seen from Table 12.8 and often reside in the province of the otolaryngologist.

Language disorders may be conceptually divided into acquired and congenital. Stroke is the most common cause of an acquired language disorder in a child, just as it is in an adult, but the causes of stroke are obviously quite different (see pp. 731). In most series, trauma is the second leading cause of acquired language disorder in the child. The phenomena seen in childhood-acquired language disorders differ greatly from those described classically; in most right-handed children a lesion anywhere in the left hemisphere produces a syndrome similar to a Broca's aphasia in the adult. Most posterior left hemisphere lesions in the child produce "anterior" aphasia syndromes. Moreover, Hecaen has observed that speaking immediately after a stroke was the best prognosticator of long-term recovery, whereas mutism had an unfavorable effect with respect to long-term outcome (a finding distinctly different from that seen in the adult population). This demonstrates that childhood aphasia occurs against a backdrop of incomplete language acquisition and incomplete cerebral lateralization and localization.

The syndrome of Landau and Kleffner, acquired ictal aphasia, although interesting from the perspective it provides on the mechanisms of language in the child is very rare (Bishop, 1985).

SCHOOL PERFORMANCE AND LEARNING DISORDERS

Definition

A child is considered to be learning disabled or underachieving if school performance is poor in the absence of major physical, neurologic, or psychiatric pathology, and the child has adequate knowledge of the language of instruction, adequate exposure to school, and otherwise normal intelligence. The last-mentioned point is crucial; the child's overall cognitive capacities should be tested, preferably through the administration of a standardized psychological instrument. The pediatrician can act as the child's advocate by ensuring that an adequate assessment of cognitive function has been performed (Rutter, 1983; Levine and Jordan, 1987).

Diagnosis

It is important to make certain that no physical disability is preventing the child from learning. Hence, a medical history (with attention to prenatal and perinatal risk factors for later cognitive difficulties), a family history (with attention to any relevant family history of similar troubles), and a physical examination are essential. Vision and hearing should be examined; consultation with a specialist should be obtained if there is any question of difficulties in these areas. If the child is said to "space out" (a common referral from a school, in our experience), hyperventilation in the office may precipitate an absence seizure. Even if this does not occur, an EEG is usually warranted, as partial seizures with complex symptomatology also may have this presentation and are not potentiated by hyperventilation. Abnormalities on the "classic" neurologic examination may argue for neurologic consultation, imaging of the brain, or both. The presence of "soft signs" is certainly common among learning disabled children, but is neither particularly sensitive nor specific. Many normal children manifest these signs of minor neurologic dysfunction, and a significant percentage of learning disabled children have normal "extended" neurologic examinations.

Therefore, when all the above questions have been answered, a multidisciplinary evaluation process combining services of speech-language pathologists, special educators, physical and/or occupational therapists, or psychologists can give a better picture of the child than any one discipline alone. Pediatricians may need to act as the coordinator and advocate for their patients based upon the collective findings.

"Attention deficit hyperactivity disorder" also requires discussion, as its treatment involves the physician directly. This collection of behaviors is a syndrome rather than a specific diagnosis. Many children demonstrate such behavior (distractibility, motor overactivity with short attention span) on the basis of underlying emotional or psychologic issues; this behavior is also often seen in brain-damaged children (children with cerebral palsy, for example). A significant subset of these children, however, have these difficulties on a "constitutional" basis, in which heredity and sex play major roles. Most studies indicate that boys outnumber girls by a ratio of 3–4:1, and there is usually a strong family history of other males with this disorder. Various rating scales to assist in the diagnosis and rational follow-up of these children have been promulgated; we prefer the Conners Rating Scale, which

COMMENTARY: A NEUROLOGIST'S PERSPECTIVE

Pediatricians have long been involved with school systems and have served as consultants to special education programs regarding the medical and developmental aspects of children with unexpected failure in school. Given the recent societal changes that have fostered and institutionalized special education (Public Law 94–142 and its various stage counterparts), as well as the shrinking tax base to support public education of children, the pediatrician is now called upon to pass judgment on "organic" nature of a child's problem in school. The pediatrician may also be subjected to pressure to restrict administration of pharmacologic agents for the treatment of hyperactivity and related attentional disorders, from parents horrified by stories in the lay press regarding the dangers of such medication ("Ritalin made my son a zombie"), or conversely from advocates from overtaxed school systems who hope that medication will allow a "hyper" child to stay in his (cost-efficient) mainstream classroom and avoid a specialized (expensive) resource room. This area is made all the more troublesome by the nexus of the political, ethical, and pedagogic dilemmas. That so much has been written in the medical and neurologic literature regarding learning disabilities, and that so little light has been shed on these problems is testimony to the lack of understanding of the behavioral neurology of children.

has both a parent and teacher version, for the assessment of such children. In our experience, a boy with a positive family history, Conners score in excess of 15, normal medical history, and examination revealing only "soft signs," has a 70–80% chance of responding favorably to medication if behavioral approaches fail. Nevertheless, only about 30% of those children referred for attention deficit disorder fit these criteria (see also pp. 71—Section 2).

Treatment

The mainstay of therapy for the child is still behavioral; small, structured classroom environments with clear guidance and expectations that do not change suddenly or dramatically, limit-setting, and the avoidance of overstimulating, distracting educational aids are most useful. If these fail to produce adequate improvement, and the child meets most of the criteria noted above, an empiric trial of medication may be in order.

CONTROVERSY

Medication must always be viewed as an adjunct and as empiric in nature, given the lack of any reliable clinical marker. Stimulants, used judiciously and cautiously, are the treatment of choice. Methylphenidate offers the advantages of a short half-life, ready bioavailability, and relatively few side-effects. With careful monitoring of weight and height, we have not found a convincing case of irreversible growth failure among the patients seen in the Learning Disabilities Clinic at The Children's Hospital Boston, over the last 5 years. Should methylphenidate produce unacceptable anorexia or insomnia (common side-effects), it may be replaced by pemoline. While the use of low-dose tricyclic agents (desipramine) has received much publicity recently, its utility in school-age children is still under investigation. Anecdotal evidence suggests that the major tranquilizers and lithium carbonate are of benefit in cases recalcitrant to conventional therapy; such cases merit subspecialty referral unless the pediatrician is comfortable with the use of such drugs.

Dyslexia

Definition

Difficulty in learning to identify printed words in an otherwise normally intelligent child is considered a specific reading disability, or dyslexia. In other words, it represents the gap between IQ and academic achievement. Dyslexia is, however, more than failure to learn to read, as recent neuropsychologic studies have demonstrated. Language and motor deficits exist in this population as well. Precise, nonexclusionary definitions of dyslexia are still unavailable (Shaywitz and Waxman, 1987).

Basic Science

Some new techniques such as brain electrical activity mapping (BEAM) show that left hemisphere functioning is qualitatively different in children with reading difficulties. Studies of brains of male dyslexia subjects postmortem show an absence of the normal asymmetry in the language regions. Abnormal position of neurons in the left cerebral cortex was also associated with dyslexia. These preliminary observations suggest a developmental basis for dyslexia, but deserve further study (Galaburda et al, 1985).

Epidemiology

The problem is widespread, but its actual prevalence is unknown because of lack of a specific measure or objective test of dyslexia. It is estimated that as many as 10% of the population may manifest the syndrome. It is usually agreed, however, that reading difficulties are more common in boys, by a ratio of 4:1 to 10:1. Dyslexia occurs more often in identical than in dissimilar twins, and is considered in some cases to be an autosomal dominant with variable penetrance (Smith et al, 1983).

Natural History

Reading difficulties are first suggested by prolonged persistence of mirror writing (which normally disappears by age 6 or 7 years). An otherwise normally bright child has continued difficulty reading, although speech usually seems normal to parents. Dyslexics are slower and less accurate in naming letters or words and even common objects; they may have trouble understanding sentences or embedded changes (Chall, 1983).

The condition is lifelong, but often well-compensated. Many scientists, architects, and artists have special competence in understanding spatial relationships even though they remain slow readers.

Treatment

Continuing controversy persists around the treatment of this poorly defined condition. At this time, intensive special education intervention and sympathetic understanding that the problem is not "laziness" or failure to fulfill a potential seem to be the best approach.

FLOPPY INFANT

Definition

The evaluation of the hypotonic infant centers on the anatomic localization of the dysfunction. Hypotonia is a clinical expression of motor system dysfunction. The motor system includes the primary motor cortex, the corticospinal tract, the anterior horn cell in the spinal cord, the α-motor neuron, the neuromuscular junction, and the muscle itself. Hypotonia may result from dysfunction at any of these levels. The clinical examination and laboratory evaluation make the anatomic and, hence, etiologic diagnosis.

Basic Science/Natural History

Dysfunction of the *cortex or telencephalic corticospinal tract* is the most common cause of infant hypotonia. It usually reflects perinatal ischemic-anoxic encephalopathy and is commonly referred to as atonic cerebral palsy. The infant often has delayed development of language and social skills or has seizures as other manifestations of cortical dysfunction. Alternatively, dysgenesis of the cerebrum, including some syndromes such as trisomy 21, Prader-Willi syndrome, or degenerative diseases (lipidoses or leukodystrophies) will result in corticospinal dysfunction.

The next anatomic level is the *spinal cord.* The hallmark of disease in this location is preservation of cortical function and the presence of bilateral sensory dysfunction often with a clear-cut level. Etiologies include trauma, maldevelopment including dysraphic states, or infection.

Werdnig-Hoffmann disease is a degenerative disease of the *anterior horn cells* that presents with arreflexia and hypotonia. Other diseases of these cells include type II glycogen storage disease (Pompe disease or acid maltase deficiency) and poliomyelitis.

Lesions within the peripheral nerve as isolated causes of hypotonia are rare. They include acute inflammatory demyelinating neuropathy (the Guillain-Barre syndrome) and the polyneuropathies that accompany Krabbe and metachromatic leukodystrophies.

Disorders of the *neuromuscular junction* that present with hypotonia include transient neonatal myasthenia in infants of myasthenic mothers as well as congenital myasthenia due to inborn errors in acetylcholine release or nicotinic receptor function. Certain aminoglycoside antibiotics may produce a neuromuscular syndrome similar to myasthenia. Infantile botulism also may resemble myasthenia.

Other disorders of the *muscle* itself must be considered, including the congenital myopathies (nemaline, central core, etc), myotonic dystrophy, and congenital muscular dystrophy.

Systemic causes of hypotonia include cardiac failure, hypercalcemia, hypothyroidism, renal acidosis, and collagen dysfunctions (Ehlers-Danlos syndrome).

Diagnosis

A chief distinguishing feature of neuromuscular disorders is the alertness and responsiveness of the flaccid infant in contrast to the lethargy and stupor associated with cerebral dysfunction. The laboratory evaluation of the hypotonic infant depends on the clinical suspicion as to the anatomic localization of the lesion. Central causes are best evaluated with CT or MRI, and EEG. Myelopathy usually requires a myelogram, while disorders of the anterior horn cell and peripheral nerve are best evaluated with electromyography and nerve conduction studies.

To elucidate neuromuscular dysfunction, other laboratory studies include measurement of serum creatine phosphokinase (CPK), which is elevated in some muscular dystrophies. The CSF may have an elevated protein in infection and polyneuropathies. An ECG will be abnormal in type II glycogen storage disease (Pompe disease).

SEIZURES

Convulsive disorders of childhood form a large part of clinical practice for the pediatric neurologist, and are among the neurologic conditions most frequently encountered in general pediatric practice. While EEG techniques are undoubtedly useful in the diagnosis and management of these conditions, it is important to have a system of classifying paroxysmal events that depends only upon clinical criteria—information the physician can obtain through a careful history and examination.

While many attempts have been made to classify seizures on the basis of any number of criteria, a simplified modification of the International League against Epilepsy's International Classification of Epilepsies strikes us as the least unwieldy approach proposed to date (Adams et al, 1985), and is presented in Table 12.9.

Partial Seizures

Definition

The term "partial" refers to the notion that the entire brain is not involved in the epileptic phenomenon during these seizures, and thus, there is neither a complete loss of consciousness nor loss of contact with the environment. That is, while children may seem confused or agitated during some varieties of partial seizures, they do not lose consciousness as occurs in the

Table 12.9
Classification of Seizures

Partial Seizures
  Simple symptomatology
    Motor
    Sensory
    Autonomic
  Complex symptomatology
  Secondary generalization
Generalized Seizures
  Absence
  Myoclonic
  Tonic, clonic, and tonic-clonic
  Akinetic
  Atypical absence
  Mixed
  Infantile spasms
Febrile Convulsions
Others
  Neonatal seizures

generalized epilepsies. This is often correlated with EEG changes that are limited to certain regions of the brain. Several types of partial seizures are commonly encountered in practice (indeed, partial seizures make up roughly 60% of the seizures seen in pediatric practice).

Partial Seizures with Simple Symptomatology

Basic Science/Natural History

Focal electrical discharges in either motor or sensory cortex will produce localized, limited changes in the child, the nature of the phenomena depending upon the location of the discharges. Common examples include adversive seizures (in which the child turns head and eyes away from the discharging focus in the brain), simple motor seizures (which may progress in an orderly fashion up the motor strip, involving hand, arm, face, and then leg on the involved side, a phenomenon known as "jacksonian march" and often associated with focal pathology in the brain), or benign rolandic (sylvian) seizures.

The last-mentioned are frightening events for parent and child. The seizure itself consists of a feeling of numbness or tingling in the mouth, tongue, and lips, with subsequent mutism and drooling because of dysfunction of the orobuccal musculature. Children do not lose consciousness during these spells, and are, thus, often quite afraid. These episodes often occur in the evening, just before or after bedtime for most children, who will often run to find their parents, and point to their mouths, unable to speak. The seizure then progresses to involve the rest of the face, arms, and occasionally the body. The episode resolves, usually without any appreciable postictal state, in minutes.

Epidemiology

The peak rate of onset is in the last half of the first decade (where it represents roughly a quarter of all new seizure disorders); the disorder seems to be autosomal dominant with incomplete penetrance.

Diagnosis

The EEG is often alarmingly focal, with spikes over the midtemporal to central region, exacerbated by sleep or drowsiness. Nonetheless, this is one of the most benign forms of epilepsy in terms of long-term prognosis.

Treatment

Treatments of choice are carbamazepine, diphenylhydantoin, or phenobarbital.

Prognosis

Essentially all children outgrow these attacks by age 16 years, with a low rate of progression into other more generalized seizure disorders (which distinguishes them from absence seizures).

Partial Seizures with Complex Symptomatology

Basic Science/Natural History

These seizures, previously referred to as "psychomotor" or "temporal lobe" seizures are characterized by the clouding of consciousness (often some sort of confusional state), with an associated aura, usually a feeling of anxiety but other hallucinatory experiences are described by many patients: deja vu, jamais vu, unpleasant odors (uncinate fits, which in some series have a high rate of associated tumor in the uncus), or visual phenomena have all been well-documented in children. These give way either to the cessation of all activity for a time, followed by repetitive, automatized motor phenomena, or directly by these automatisms (lipsmacking, fumbling with garments, or chewing). Although these spells occasionally become generalized, the majority terminate and are followed by a postictal confusional state and amnesia for the seizure itself. Partial complex status has been described in children and must be included in the differential diagnosis of a confusional state. Much has been made of the association between partial complex seizures and behavioral disorders. Although many patients in the midst of a partial complex seizure will be confused, and some patients will be violent if attempts are made to obstruct or restrain them, true aggression (directed violent behavior) is not seen as an ictal phenomenon, according to most reviews and systematic studies. The association between partial complex seizures with temporal lobe foci and certain interictal personality disorders, well-documented and frequently seen in the adult, is not commonly seen in pediatric practice.

Diagnosis

Focal pathology is often present in individuals with partial complex seizures and consideration should be given to anatomic study in addition to EEG examination.

Treatment

Treatments of choice include carbamazepine, diphenylhydantoin, and phenobarbital.

Generalized Seizures

Definition

As the name implies, the presentation of these seizures usually involves the entire body at once, and usually implies a loss of or extreme alteration of consciousness. While any partial seizure may evolve into secondary generalization, the seizure types that are generalized from the outset will be considered here.

Absence Seizures

Basic Science/Natural History

These spells, often referred to as "petit mal" epilepsy in the old nomenclature, consist of the abrupt loss of consciousness without aura, with a mild loss of tone but usually without a fall, and often with associated motor phenomena (eyelid fluttering and motor automatisms, the former at the same 3 Hz frequency as the cortical discharges). The seizure stops as quickly as it started; patients are often not aware that they were "out" unless the train of conversation has radically altered around them. These spells start in the second half of the first decade of life, and usually become very frequent until treatment is instituted (20–30 spells/day). They are often associated with a decline in school performance, presumably secondary to the frequent interruptions in consciousness rather than to any associated dementing state, as the school performance usually returns to its premorbid state upon institution of anticonvulsant therapy.

Epidemiology

The condition is frequently inherited in a dominant fashion; it is more common in females.

While originally considered to be a "benign" form of childhood epilepsy with little risk of adult convulsive disorder, it has been recognized that an appreciable number of children with childhood absence seizures will progress to have generalized clonic convulsions in adult life.

Treatment

The treatments of choice include the suximides and valproic acid; the diones have fallen out of favor as first-line therapeutic considerations.

Tonic-Clonic Seizures

Definition

Tonic events (a brief increase in muscle tone throughout the body), clonic events (the regular shaking of various parts of the body, usually the extremities), and tonic-clonic events are all well-known seizure types. The common name for these sorts of events is "grand mal" epilepsy. They may, in many instances, represent partial seizures that have generalized (extended) secondarily.

Epidemiology

They represent roughly 10% of seizures encountered in pediatric clinical practice.

Diagnosis

They may be associated with focal pathology, and therefore a focal neurologic examination or a focal discharge on an interictal EEG should lead to consideration of anatomic study by CT or MRI scan. It should be remembered that a Todd paresis (hemi- or monoplegia transiently seen after a seizure) is frequently encountered in children and does not signify the same high likelihood of focal pathology observed in adults.

Treatment

The treatments of choice for generalized tonic-clonic fits include phenobarbital, diphenylhydantoin, and carbamazepine.

Myoclonic Seizures

Definition

Myoclonus, the rather rapid jerking of a group of muscles, may be seen as a seizure equivalent, or as part of another disorder of the nervous system, often a movement disorder or degenerative disease. Numerous attempts have been made to classify myoclonus into either cortical, subcortical, brain stem, and spinal subtypes, or epileptic (further subdivided into the myoclonus and myoclonic epilepsies) and nonepileptic types.

Natural History

Myoclonus is seen frequently in the so-called "Lennox-Gastaut syndrome," a seizure disorder of childhood associated with multiple seizure patterns (akinetic, atypical absence, and generalized tonic-clonic), subnormal intelligence, and a very disorganized EEG. Myoclonus may also be seen as an isolated phenomenon, as in the myoclonic epilepsy of Janz. This type of seizure, which usually presents in the second decade, is characterized by single or repetitive myoclonic jerks of the extremities, without associated loss of consciousness. The patient does not usually fall, but will often drop objects being held at the time of the attack. Emotional stress, alcohol, and sleep deprivation all exacerbate or potentiate these attacks. The disorder may become associated with absence or tonic-clonic seizures as the patient ages.

Treatment

Most patients are readily controlled on valproic acid and diphenylhydantoin or clonazepam and diphenylhydantoin, but most require anticonvulsant therapy for long periods of time.

Infantile Spasms

Definition

Infantile spasms may either reflect underlying neurologic pathology ("symptomatic infantile spasms") or be seen in isolation ("cryptogenic infantile spasms"). They consist of a sudden flexion at the waist with associated arm extension ("salaam attacks") often seen in succession; other manifestations may include sudden extensor postures ("cheerleader spells"), or a sudden contraction of all muscle groups ("blitzkrampfe").

Natural History

The age of onset is usually between 3 and 8 months of life, and the condition is often misdiagnosed as colic.

The conditions associated with symptomatic infantile spasms include tuberous sclerosis, the metabolic encephalopathies of infancy (especially phenylketonuria, nonketotic hyperglycinemia, and maple syrup urine disease), postinfectious encephalopathies (especially the TORCH infections), Aicardi syndrome (females with agenesis of the corpus callosum, chorioretinitis, retinal colombomata, and mental retardation), Down syndrome, and stroke.

Diagnosis

Most infants manifest a typical EEG pattern (hypsarrhythmia, with spike-wave, spike, and polyspike components, burst suppression, and decremental discharge phenomena) shortly after the onset of clinical spells.

Treatment

Treatment is still controversial, as there has been clinical experience suggesting that long-term treatment with ACTH not only controls seizure, but also improves the prognosis for normal mental development (which is otherwise compromised in a significant portion of children with either symptomatic or cryptogenic infantile spasms). Current recommendations in most centers are for treatment with ACTH in cryptogenic cases, where the mental outcome is most directly tied to speed and adequacy of seizure control, and more routine anticonvulsant treatment (valproic acid or clonazepam) for symptomatic cases, where mental outcome is more closely associated with the underlying neurologic diagnosis. Physicians in most centers believe that the risk of long-term ACTH therapy (about 6–8 months of treatment) is not warranted in symptomatic cases, where normalization of the EEG may not improve outcome. The only exception has been in Down syndrome, where speed and adequacy of seizure control do seem to be linked to improved outcome.

Simple Febrile Convulsions

Definition

Febrile seizures are simple, generalized convulsions, usually clonic, which present between 6 months and 6 years of age (most commonly between 18 months and 3 years), that are associated with a febrile illness that otherwise does not involve the nervous system. They are, by definition, brief (usually under 15 minutes) and usually single. They occur when the temperature is rising and is at least 38°C.

Epidemiology

Febrile seizures occur in roughly 2–4% of the population. Family history is positive in over 40% of cases. Nelson and Ellenberg (1976) have noted three significant risk factors for subsequent afebrile convulsions: a family history of epilepsy, antecedent neurologic or developmental abnormalities, and the occurrence of a complex febrile convulsion (prolonged, focal, or repetitive). The absence of risk factors was associated with a 2% incidence of subsequent epilepsy, the presence of a single risk factor increased the incidence to 3%, whereas two or three risk factors increased this to 13%.

Treatment

The first step is to undress the child, and possibly use tepid sponging to lower body temperature. No further treatment is required, unless a source of infection is found, in which case antibiotics may be indicated. Acetominophen is appropriate as long as fever persists.

Prevention

Intermittent barbiturate therapy (phenobarbital during febrile ailments) is not effective. Effective therapies include chronic administration of phenobarbital or valproic acid. The effect of intermittent oral diazepam (i.e., during febrile episodes) is currently under study in the United States (Rosman, personal communication).

CONTROVERSY

The question of whether a child should be placed on anticonvulsant medication after a single febrile convulsion has to be individualized on the basis of risk factors. If any abnormal neurologic findings are present, even if transient, long-term (about 2 years) anticonvulsant therapy is appropriate. Similarly a family history of seizures would be a significant risk factor and a reason to initiate therapy.

The question of treatment of recurrent febrile seizures remains debatable. Half of them will recur within

6 months and 90% within 30 months. In the absence of any risk factors, some physicians will permit two febrile seizures before embarking on 2 years of anticonvulsant therapy. Others prefer to treat the first seizure.

If the seizure is complex (see Case Illustration), most physicians recommend long-term therapy with phenobarbital to achieve a blood level of 15 μg/ml, or if it is not tolerated, valproic acid. Liver function should be followed if a child is on valproic acid since fatal hepatitis has been reported.

Cyclic Vomiting

A syndrome of recurrent episodes of nausea and vomiting, with associated pallor and no demonstrable gastroenterologic, endocrine, or structural neurologic cause, has been described in children. The relationship between this condition and migraine is not entirely clear, although it has been noted that a disproportionate number of children with this syndrome develop migraine headaches in adult life, and that there is a strong family history of migraine headaches in many children with cyclic vomiting. It has been our experience that the same drugs that have proved useful for juvenile migraine are helpful in this condition (barbiturates, diphenylhydantoin, and cyproheptadine being first choices, with propranolol also demonstrating efficacy).

Breath-Holding Spells

Definition/Natural History

This syndrome may present in one of two types: cyanotic or pallid. The majority of infants present between 6 and 18 months of age, and 90% cease having these spells by the sixth birthday. The cyanotic spell is preceded by an emotional upset. The child follows with a prolonged inspiratory phase, and appears to hold his or her breath, then turns quite blue (hence the name) and loses consciousness. The loss of consciousness is presumably from low cerebral blood flow or low P_{O_2}.

In the pallid variety, the child is frightened or startled, and quite rapidly loses consciousness (more rapidly than in the cyanotic variety). The loss of consciousness is presumably from a decrease in cerebral blood flow that is vagally mediated. Ocular compression during ECG recording frequently demonstrates prolonged asystole, arguing for vagal oversensitivity or overactivity. Both types of episodes are associated with a strong history of similar episodes in other family members, and individuals with such spells in infancy are often "ready fainters" in adult life.

There is no relationship between these spells and epilepsy, nor is there increased incidence of these spells among the retarded. Increased incidence of certain be-

CASE ILLUSTRATION

M.M. was nearly 4 years old when she was brought to the emergency room at 3:30 AM one weekday. She had been in her usual state of good health upon retiring the night before. Her father had come to her room at 3:00 AM to find her "moaning and thrashing about." She then turned her head to the right, and began to "twitch" on the right side of her body, arm and then leg. She made "horrible gurgling noises," and then began "to shake all over." Her father called the emergency rescue number, and returned to find his daughter still shaking. He noticed that he had first come in at 3:00, the twitching had started on the right side at 3:01, and his daughter was still seizing, and she continued to seize until arrival at Boston Children's Hospital at 3:30 AM. As she was being cared for in the emergency room initially (with intravenous anticonvulsants and supplemental oxygen), the seizing abated. Her initial examination was remarkable for stupor and a mild right hemiparesis, as well as a rectal temperature of 102°F. Laboratory evaluation was unremarkable, including examination of the CSF. The child's level of consciousness improved gradually over 2 hours, and the hemiparesis resolved over the next 12 hours. Imaging studies of the brain (CT scan and MRI) were unrevealing. She was discharged on phenobarbital. An EEG 6 weeks later was normal. Follow-up is planned for every 3 months for 2 years; if she remains well, phenobarbital will be discontinued.

COMMENTS

The case illustrates several important points about febrile convulsions. By definition, the case illustrated would not be considered a simple febrile convulsion, given its focal onset, the duration of the seizure activity (greater than 15 minutes), the prolonged postictal state and, perhaps, the excessive postictal focality to the neurologic examination. Since the child was febrile upon arrival to the hospital, this event should be viewed as a seizure precipitated by fever, or a complex febrile seizure. The focality of onset would classify this event at the time of presentation as a partial seizure with secondary generalization, and would argue for investigation of the CSF, as was performed, as well as imaging studies of the brain in order to rule out focal pathology. While studies had demonstrated that the risk of seizures after typical febrile convulsions was increased (Nelson and Ellenberg, 1976; Annegers et al, 1979), a recent study also demonstrated that for children with a single complex feature (focal seizure, prolonged seizure, or repeated episodes within the same episode), the risk of subsequent unprovoked seizure was increased from 2.4% to between 6 and 8%; the presence of two features increased the risk to 17–22%, and three features increased the risk to 49%. The presence of all three complex features was strongly associated with subsequent partial complex epilepsy (Annegers et al, 1987). For these reasons, this child was discharged on phenobarbital, 5 mg/kg/day in a single dose, to be continued for at least 2 years.

havioral characteristics among these children (limit-testing, stubborn, aggressive personality traits) have all been described.

Treatment

The treatment of breath-holding spells is mainly parental reassurance and behavior modification of the precipitating events and response to these events. Anticonvulsant medications are not effective; atropine and belladonna may prevent or attenuate pallid breath-holding spells but are usually impractical because of the side effects. Correction of underlying anemia and any other conditions that also may stimulate the vagus (e.g., gastroesophageal reflux) may help diminish the frequency and severity of pallid spells.

Status Epilepticus

Definition

Status epilepticus is a condition characterized by generalized or lateralized seizures that persist for 30 minutes or more, without complete recovery of consciousness between seizures.

Natural History

There are multiple etiologies of status epilepticus; the two most common in pediatric practice are: (1) a decrease in serum levels of anticonvulsant medication in a known epileptic because of intercurrent systemic infection with associated fever, decreased absorption of medications, and decreased transit time in the gut; and (2) a similar decrease in serum levels because of noncompliance. The former represent about 30% of cases and the latter about 25%.

Diagnosis

When a child is brought to the emergency room convulsing, the usual ABCs of supportive care must be assured (airway, breathing, and circulation, rather than "accuse, blame, and criticize"). At the same time, a member of the team taking care of the child should perform a very targeted examination and obtain a very targeted history. What medications was the child taking? When were they last taken? Are there signs of major neurologic problems; i.e., head trauma, petechiae, needle tracks, pupillary asymmetry or unreactivity, fundoscopic abnormalities, hemiparesis, or a focal signature to the seizure?

After the airway has been secured, and the pulse and blood pressure established as satisfactory, venous access should be obtained if possible, but consideration should be given to obtaining the following tests before treatment: blood sugar, Ca, Mg, Na, K, Cl, TCO_2; BUN, creatinine; liver function tests and NH_3; complete blood count with differential, platelet count, prothrombin time, partial thromboplastin time, blood cultures, if febrile; anticonvulsant levels; toxic screen; lead level and/or free erythrocyte protoporphyrin; and blood gases.

While the choice of therapy is under consideration, it is appropriate to administer 50% dextrose in water, and to give the patient some extra oxygen (remember, the cortex utilizes glucose and status creates enormous cellular energy demands).

Treatment

The major therapeutic options for the treatment of status epilepticus are: barbiturates, short-acting benzodiazepines, diphenylhydantoin, and combinations of these drugs; valproate; and anesthesia.

Principles for the use of these agents are included in tabular form. Certain points should be borne in mind when choosing which agents to use.

1. More children are hurt or killed from overtreatment of seizures than from the seizures themselves. Thus, it is important to consider known side-effects of a particular agent (such as respiratory depression), and to be prepared to deal with them.
2. Benzodiazepines and barbiturates can produce synergistic respiratory depression; their use together requires extreme caution and close observation of the child for at least 8 hours after the administration of this combination.
3. Pre-existing respiratory or cardiac illness may necessitate rapid termination of seizures.
4. If at all possible, therapy should spare subsequent mental status, so that this may be followed.
5. Most physicians and all parents want seizures stopped immediately.
6. For the practicing physician, it is prudent to choose a certain approach, and then habitually to use it. This permits familiarity with all the side-effects and interactions that a given drug can produce, and also allows for a certain automaticity of action during a particularly acute emergency (see Table 12.10).

Prognosis

Although contemporary intensive care and acute care medicine has improved the outcome in many cases of status compared to Gowers experience (when roughly 25% of individuals with status died in the course of an episode), it can still be a fatal event and should be taken seriously.

COMA

Definition

If consciousness is defined as "the state of awareness of the self and the environment" (Plum et al, 1980), and is further defined as having two primary components (content and level of arousal), then the level of arousal is the salient issue in the understanding of coma and other related alterations of consciousness. In these states, we are not concerned so much with the content of what the child is thinking as with the level of arousal. This is a distinction with a material differ-

Table 12.10
Seizure Medications

Therapeutic Agent	Loading dose	Administration Time	Onset of Action	Half-life	Disadvantages
Benzodiazepines					
Diazepam	0.1 mg/kg, maximum 5 mg	1 mg/min	Rapid, 1–3 min	20 min anticonvulsant; prolonged respiratory effects	Hypotension and respiratory depression in some cases; *rarely* clonic status converted to tonic status, requiring major intervention
Lorazepam	4–8 mg iv school age children; 0–05 mg/kg for younger children		Rapid, 1–3 min	Up to 16 hours	Same as diazepam
Diphenylhydantoin (DPH)	15–20 mg/kg	1 mg/kg/min ¼ vol. of solution without dextrose	≤15 min	18–36 hours	If administered too quickly may produce cardiac difficulties, especially rhythm disturbances
Barbiturates	10–20 mg/kg, in two divided doses, 30 min apart	5–15 min, while respirations and BP are monitored	Slow, 15–45 min	40–120 hours	Subsequent use of diazepam problematic; difficult to follow mental status
Paraldehyde	0.4 ml/kg to maximum of 8 ml delivered per rectum in 1–2 vol. oil. May be repeated up to 4 times in 24 hr		Rapid, about 5 min		Possible synergistic respiratory depression with barbiturates
Combination therapy	Combination of short-onset agent (e.g., diazepam or paraldehyde) followed by a long-acting (e.g., DPH) is often effective: control is established quickly, effect on respiration is low, and mental status is not obscured for long periods				

ence, in that the structures that subserve level of arousal in the human are different from those that subserve content of consciousness.

Plum and Posner define *coma* as "a state of unarousable psychologic unresponsiveness in which the subject lies with the eyes closed" and exhibits no psychologically understandable response to external stimuli or internal need. *Stupor* is defined as "a deep sleep or behaviorally similar unresponsiveness from which subjects can be aroused only by vigorous and repeated stimulation." It is our contention that other terms to describe conditions between stupor and full arousal be avoided, as there is no general agreement on their meaning (i.e., one person's obtundation is another person's lethargy).

Basic Science

Broadly speaking, two neural structures are required for consciousness: the cerebral cortex, and the ascending reticular activating system (ARAS), a collection of neurons centered in the upper brain stem (particularly the midbrain) with widespread projections throughout the cortex. Thus, an alteration of level of consciousness may come about through either cortical or brain stem involvement (i.e., bihemispheric or brain stem). The examination and investigation of the comatose child, thus, should be organized so that this question may be answered.

Diagnosis

In common with all neurologic problems, understanding the anatomy of consciousness is very important. Observation of the respiratory status is most helpful. Cheyne-Stokes respirations (cyclic breathing marked by gradual increases in respiration followed by gradual decrease and then apnea prior to recycling) while of poor localizing value, are frequently seen in bihemispheric disease. Central neurogenic hyperventilation (rapid, regular hyperventilation without apparent metabolic cause) usually signifies brain stem localization. Apneustic breathing (a prolonged inspiratory phase with apnea in expiration, cycling at a rate of 1–1½/minute) usually implies pontine pathology. Ataxic breathing (death rattle), without any clear pattern, implies medullary damage, and requires intubation as respiratory failure is imminent.

The neurologic examination should focus on the distinction between hemispheric and brain stem pa-

GUIDELINES FOR THE DETERMINATION OF BRAIN DEATH IN CHILDREN[1]

The criteria outlined are useful in determining brain death in infants and children. In term newborns (> 38 weeks), the criteria are useful 7 days after the neurologic insult. The newborn is clinically difficult to evaluate after perinatal insults. This relates to many factors including difficulties of clinical assessment, determination of proximate cause of coma, and certainty of the validity of laboratory tests. These problems are accentuated in a premature infant. However, after an interval, currently suggested as the first 7 days after the insult in a term newborn, the extent and reversibilitity of neurologic injury can be determined by the physical examination and laboratory studies.

History

The critical initial assessment is the clinical history and examination. The most important factor is determination of the proximate cause of coma to ensure absence of remediable or reversible conditions. Most difficulties with the determination of death on the basis of neurologic criteria have resulted from overlooking this basic fact. Especially important are detection of toxic and metabolic disorders, sedative-hypnotic drugs, paralytic agents, hypothermia, hypotension, and surgically remediable conditions. The physical examination is necessary to determine the failure of brain function.

Physical Examination Criteria

1. Coma and apnea must coexist. The patient must exhibit complete loss of consciousness, vocalization, and volitional activity.

2. Absence of brain stem function as defined by:

(a) Midposition or fully dilated pupils which do not respond to light. Drugs may influence and invalidate pupillary assessment.

(b) Absence of spontaneous eye movements and those induced by oculocephalic and caloric (oculovestibular) testing.

(c) Absence of movement of bulbar musculature including facial and oropharyngeal muscles. The corneal, gag, cough, sucking, and rooting reflexes are absent.

(d) Respiratory movements are absent with the patient off the respirator. Apnea testing using standardized methods can be performed, but is done after other criteria are met.

3. The patient must not be significantly hypothermic or hypotensive for age.

4. Flaccid tone and absence of spontaneous or induced movements, excluding spinal cord events such as reflex withdrawal or spinal myoclonus, should exist.

5. The examination should remain consistent with brain death throughout the observation and testing period.

Observaton Periods According to Age

The recommended observation period depends on the age of the patient and the laboratory tests utilized.

7 days to 2 months

The Task Force recommends two examinations and electroencephalograms (EEGs) separated by at least 48 hours.

2 months to 1 year

The Task Force recommends two examinations and EEGs separated by at least 24 hours. A repeat examination and EEG are not necessary if a concomitant radionuclide angiographic (CRAG) study demonstrates no visualization of cerebral arteries.

Over 1 year

When an irreversible cause exists, laboratory testing is not required and the Task Force recommends an observation period of at least 12 hours. There are conditions, particularly hypoxic-ischemic encephalopathy, in which it is difficult to assess the extent and reversibility of brain damage. This is particulary true if the first examination is performed soon after the acute event. Therefore, in this situation, the Task Force recommends a more prolonged period of at least 24 hours of observation. The observation period may be reduced if the EEG demonstrates electrocerebral silence or the CRAG does not visualize cerebral arteries.

Laboratory Testing

Electroencephalography

Electroencephalography to document electrocerebral silence should, if performed, be done over a 30-minute period using standardized techniques for brain death determinations. In small children it may not be possible to meet the standard requirement for 10 cm electrode separation. The interelectrode distance should be decreased proportional to the patient's head size. Drug concentrations should be insufficient to suppress EEG activity.

Angiography

A cerebral radionuclide angiogram (CRAG) confirms cerebral death by demonstrating the lack of visualization of the cerebral circulation. A technically satisfactory CRAG that demonstrates arrest of carotid circulation at the base of the skull and absence of intracranial arterial circulation can be considered confirmatory of brain death, even though there may be some visualization of the intracranial venous sinuses. The value of this study in infants under 2 months is under investigation. Contrast angiography can document lack of effective blood flow to the brain.

COMMENT

No set of guidelines for brain death in infants has found uniform acceptance or "official standing." Problems exist with the statements from the Task Force inasmuch as an isoelectric EEG in the first 24 hours of age may be compatible with recovery, and conversely, residual EEG activity can be recorded hours after clinical brain death. We agree with Freeman and Ferry (1988) that brain death in infants remains a clinical diagnosis "to be made at the bedside, by knowledgeable physicians who, in concert with grieving families, make the most agonizing of all life's events (the death of a child) as bearable as possible for all concerned."

[1] Reproduced with permission from Task Force for Determination of Brain Death in Children: *Pediatr Neurol* 3:242, 1987.

thology. The frontal eye fields, which control saccadic eye movements, may be damaged in cases of hemispheric disease-producing coma. Thus, if the patient's eyes deviate to one side, a hemispheric lesion on that side is likely, since the contralateral frontal eye field is acting unopposed. This simple observation may truncate the formal examination.

The fundi should be examined carefully for any signs of raised intracranial pressure and/or hemorrhage. The pupillary responses are obviously most important. Reactive pupils suggest that the midbrain is intact. Fixed midposition pupils (3.5 mm) imply midbrain pathology, and small fixed pupils are either secondary to opiate overdosage or pontine pathology. Unilateral dilatation of the pupil ("blown pupil") implies third nerve compression secondary to herniation of the uncus. Reactive pupils without extraocular movements are seen in hypoglycemia or barbiturate overdosage. Dilatation of the pupil to painful stimuli (the ciliospinal reflex) implies that the lower brain stem is still intact.

Given the location of the ocular motor nuclei, examination of the extraocular movements is usually most helpful in determining the status of the midbrain. If spontaneous, conjugate or dysconjugate roving eye movements can be seen in all directions, the midbrain must be intact and the coma must, therefore, be hemispheric in origin. If this is not noted, and a cervical spine injury is unlikely, one can attempt to elicit the oculocephalic response ("Doll eyes"). A quick lateral displacement of the head should result in the eyes moving in the direction opposite to the head. Failure to elicit this response suggests either barbiturate intoxication or pontine/midbrain damage. The intactness of this response indicates a hemispheric localization of the coma.

If oculocephalic responses cannot be elicited, attempts should be made to elicit caloric responses. After establishing that the tympanic membranes are intact, the head is elevated 30 degrees off the horizontal (to align the semicircular canals with gravity). Then 50 ml of ice-cold saline are injected into the ear; an awake patient would become violently nauseated, and have brisk nystagmus with the fast phase away from the stimulated ear. If the patient demonstrates a tonic deviation toward the stimulated ear but no fast phase away, this suggests hemispheric pathology with intact brain stem. If there is no response the injection should be repeated. Failure to respond to 100 ml (total) of ice-cold water implies dysfunction at the brain stem level.

While motor signs may be helpful in extreme cases ("decorticate" and "decerebrate" posturing), it must be remembered that the neuroanatomy of motor responses does not correspond to the neuroanatomy of consciousness, and thus, may lead to erroneous conclusions.

Having established the localization of coma, diagnostic investigations can proceed. In children, hemispheric coma is almost always due to intoxication or diffuse dysfunction secondary to infection or parainfectious pathology. Brain stem coma is much more likely to be associated with focal, structural pathology, and therefore, argues for prompt imaging and neurosurgical consultation (see Injuries; Fig. 12.3).

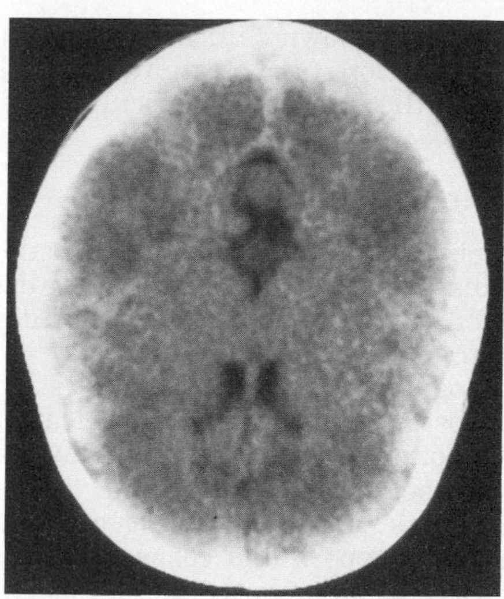

Figure 12.3. This baby had been admitted at 1 month of age for spiral fracture of midshaft of right humerus, an injury very suspicious for having been inflicted by parents or babysitter. Presentation at the emergency room at 3.5 months of age was obviously preceded by another episode of abuse. The baby was seizing, had retinal hemorrhages, and, on the CT scan, had bilateral diffuse areas of low density indicating cerebral edema. This baby had an abrupt neurologic decline and died shortly after admission.

ATAXIA

Definition

Ataxia refers to a disorder of the coordination of movement. It is commonly used to signify a movement disorder that results from dysfunction of the cerebellum or its connections. Strictly speaking, ataxia can result from lesions elsewhere in the motor system, such as the corticospinal tract, or in the sensory system, particularly the dorsal columns of the spinal cord. In this chapter, however, ataxia will be used to refer to cerebellar ataxia. This disorder is characterized by several findings: (1) incoordination of limb motion resulting in dysmetria, an action tremor and dysdiadochokinesis (inability to execute rapid alternating movements smoothly); (2) the loss of muscle tone; and (3) inability to maintain posture and axial stability.

Basic Science

The somatotopic arrangement of the cerebellar output is less strict than that of the primary motor sensory cortex, which makes localization of lesions within the cerebellum difficult. There is some evidence that limb ataxia without postural difficulties is more likely to reflect lesions within the hemisphere of the cerebellum.

On the other hand, lesions in the midline of the cerebellum, i.e., the vermis, tend to give rise to axial difficulties. This is shown clinically in truncal ataxia: the inability to sit or stand straight. Often the gait is wide-based and the patient has difficulty in walking in a straight line.

Natural History

The cerebellum is the site of considerable pathology in CNS disease, which is usually generalized. These can be broken down into the acute, the intermittent, and the progressive ataxias.

The etiology of *acute* cerebellar ataxia includes infection and postinfectious causes, intoxication, infarction and hemorrhage, seizure, migraine, and acute demyelinating polyneuropathy.

Viral agents such as poliovirus type I, influenza A and B, echovirus type 9 and coxsackie B have been implicated. Occasionally, varicella infection may cause the syndrome, often within 3–7 days of the exanthem.

Other causes should be considered in the differential. Intoxication with phenytoin, ethanol, cytosine arabinoside, and thallium may primarily affect the cerebellum. Hemorrhage and infarction of the cerebellum may present with acute ataxia and often proceed quickly to obtundation as the posterior fossa swells. This is an indication for rapid neurosurgical decompression.

Acute cerebellar ataxia may reflect viral infection of the cerebellum or a postviral autoimmune attack on the cerebellum. It can be seen at all ages, but usually occurs between 1 and 2 years of age. The most dramatic clinical sign is the acute onset of truncal ataxia with dysarthria and nystagmus. Limb ataxia and hypotonia are seen less often. About half the patients will have experienced a nonspecific viral syndrome within the 3 weeks preceding the attack. Analysis of the CSF shows a mild pleocytosis and elevated protein in some cases. The prognosis is good with about two-thirds of the patients recovering within 2 months. The remaining one-third of children will have persistent neurologic findings.

Occult neuroblastoma may present with ataxia as part of the myoclonus-opsoclonus. These patients have multidirectional darting eye movements and myoclonic jerks of the limbs and face. The urine must be screened for vanilylmandelic acid and radiologic examinations of the chest and kidneys must be made to search for the tumor. It is thought that the nervous system manifestations represent a remote effect of the tumor and are referred to as paraneoplastic.

Finally, acute demyelinating polyneuropathy may present as the "Miller Fisher Variant," with ataxia, ophthalmoplegia, and areflexia. Some of these patients will develop the profound weakness of limb and truncal muscles that is characteristic of the disease.

Diagnosis

Dysmetria refers to the inability to guide the limb to a target. This may be shown by asking the patient to guide his finger from his nose to your finger (the finger-to-nose test). It is important that the elbow is held away from the body, as cerebellar movement disorders tend to involve the proximal limb muscles more than the distal ones. In the lower limbs, the analogous test is the heel-to-shin test, where the patient is asked to place his heel on the contralateral knee and then run it down his shin. Both these tests will show dysmetria. Moreover, a tremor at the end of the executed movement with its amplitude orthogonal to the line of motion may be seen. This is referred to as an intention, kinetic, or action tremor and is suggestive of cerebellar dysfunction.

Dysdiadochokinesia is the inability to execute rapid alternating movements smoothly. Tasks such as repeatedly slapping the palm then the dorsum of the hand on the thigh quickly are often difficult in patients with ataxia.

Occasionally, particularly with acute lesions, limb hypotonia ipsilateral to a cerebellar lesion may be seen.

Intermittent ataxia may be the presenting sign of childhood multiple sclerosis. Other features of lesions disseminated in time and space, such as optic neuritis and spasticity provide the diagnosis. In addition, certain metabolic states may present with intermittent ataxia. Maple syrup urine disease is an heredofamilial degenerative disease caused by a defect in oxidative decarboxylation of branched-chain ketoacids. It usually presents in the first week of life with opisthotonos, respiratory irregularity, and seizures. However, there is a variant that presents between 6 and 9 months of age with intermittent ataxia, seizures, drowsiness, and behavioral changes that are triggered by infection or other stressors. The diagnosis is made by noting the characteristic odor of the urine and showing a positive dinitrophenylhydrazine test. The attacks are treated by restriction of dietary branched-chain amino acids.

Hartnup disease presents with intermittent ataxia, behavioral changes, photosensitive dermatitis, and renal aminoaciduria. The abnormal urine amino acid pattern in the face of a normal serum pattern is diagnostic of the disease. Nicotinic acid (25 mg/day) may improve the symptoms.

Other metabolic causes include pyruvate dehydrogenase deficiency and arginosuccinate aciduria. In addition, the designation of familial intermittent cerebellar ataxia has been given to a disease for which no metabolic lesion has yet been found.

Many diseases may present as a *progressive ataxia*. Subdural hematomas and tumors within the posterior fossa, present with the gradual onset of ataxia, headache (often occipital in location), nausea and vomiting, and papilledema. The child also may have neck stiffness and head tilt. It is mandatory that all children with ataxia have a high-resolution CT scan of the head, with emphasis on the posterior fossa, or an MRI.

A number of degenerative diseases primarily affect cerebellar function. Ataxia-telangiectasia is a phakomatosis that presents with ataxia, choreoathetosis, and telangiectasias of the skin and conjuctivae. This is the second most common cause of progressive ataxia in children under 10 years of age, after posterior fossa tumors. These patients are at increased risk for lymphoproliferative neoplasia and sinopulmonary infections. Family members who are presumably heterozygotes also have an increased risk of breast and other cancers (Swift et al, 1987). The diagnosis is usually clinical, but patients characteristically have altered cellular immunity and decreased serum levels of IgA and IgE with high levels of IgM, IgG_1 and IgG_3 (see pp. 743).

Friedreich ataxia is an autosomal recessive disease that presents before puberty with gait ataxia or scoliosis, followed within 2 years with the rapid progression of limb ataxia, loss of vibration and position sense, and areflexia. An associated cardiomyopathy is the most common cause of death.

Finally, metabolic diseases may cause a progressive ataxia. These include abetalipoproteinemia, Refsum disease, biotinidase deficiency, and certain urea cycle abnormalities. It may also be the presenting feature of metachromatic leukodystrophy, Wilson disease and multiple sclerosis (see Section 15).

CASE ILLUSTRATION

A 7-year-old female presented with acute onset of inability to walk. She had been well except for an episode of meningitis at 1 year of age (presumed meningococcal) with no sequelae, until upper respiratory symptoms began 2 days before admission. On the morning of presentation she complained of the "room spinning" and proceeded to develop vomiting and inability to walk over the next few hours. She presented to her pediatrician afebrile, with a physical examination normal, except for a mild otitis and truncal ataxia without weakness, which became progressive over a period of hours prompting her referral to our hospital.

Physical examination was remarkable for a child with persistent vomiting, normal mental status, profound truncal ataxia, normal fundi, no nystagmus, and no weakness. Electrolytes were normal. CBC was remarkable for a white blood cell count of 20,000/mm^3, with a marked left shift. CT scan and lumbar puncture were both within normal limits.

QUESTIONS AND COMMENT

What is this child's diagnosis and how should she be managed?

This patient's presentation was typical for that of acute cerebellar ataxia: the abrupt onset of ataxia, rapid deterioration of gait, vomiting, tremulousness, and mild lethargy are common in this disorder, with nystagmus, weakness, and major alterations of consciousness being more unusual. The disease occurs primarily in children ages 1–5 years, either 1–2 weeks following a mild illness or during an infection. The tempo of the illness is rapid, with mild maximal dysfunction typically 24–48 hours after onset, and with recovery just as quickly. Laboratory findings are helpful only to exclude other processes and are usually normal except for a minimal CSF lymphocytosis, which this patient did not demonstrate. Identified etiologic agents include varicella, Epstein-Barr virus, echo 9, coxsackie, polio virus, adenovirus, and *Mycoplasma pneumoniae.*

This child was admitted for complete bed rest and over the next 24 hours basically recovered full normal neurologic function. The prognosis, however, is not uniformly good with this disorder, with up to 35% of hospitalized patients showing persistent cerebellar signs.

REFERENCES

Ad hoc committee on brain death, The Children's Hospital, Boston: Determination of brain death. *J Pediatr* 110:15, 1987.

Adams RD, Victor M: *Principles of Neurology,* 3rd edition. New York, McGraw-Hill, 1985, p. 234.

Annegers JF, Hauser WA, Elveback LR, et al: The risk of epilepsy following febrile convulsions. *Neurology* 29:297, 1979.

Annegers JF, Hauser WA, Shirts SB, et al: Factors prognostic of unprovoked seizures after febrile convulsions. *N Engl J Med* 316:493, 1987.

Barlow CF: *Headaches and Migraine in Childhood.* Philadelphia, JB Lippincott Co, 1984.

Bell WE, McCormick WF: Acute cerebellar ataxia of childhood. In: *Neurologic Infections in Children,* 2nd edition. Philadelphia, WB Saunders, 1981, p. 677.

Bishop DVM: Age of onset and outcome in acquired dysphagia with convulsive disorder (Landau-Kleffner syndrome). *Dev Med Child Neurol* 27:705, 1985.

Boder E, Sedgwick RP: Ataxia-telangiectasia. A familial syndrome of progressive syndrome of cerebellar ataxia, oculocutaneous telangiectasia and frequent pulmonary infection. *Pediatrics* 21:526, 1958.

Brown LW: Infant botulism. *Adv Pediatr* 28:141, 1981.

Capute AJ, Shapiro BK, and Palmer FB: Marking the milestones of language development. *Contemp Pediatr* 4:24, 1987.

Chall JS: *Stages of Reading Development.* New York, McGraw-Hill, 1983.

Coplan J: Evaluation of a child with delayed speech or language. *Pediatr Ann* 14:203, 1985.

Diamond S, Dalessio DJ (eds): *The Practicing Physician's Approach to Headaches,* 3rd edition. Baltimore, Williams & Wilkins, 1982.

Dubowitz V: The floppy infant. *Clinics in Developmental Medicine,* Spastics Intl Med Pub No 76. London, Heineman Co, 1980.

Fenichel G: Migraine in children. *Neurol Clin* 3:77, 1985.

Fennell E, Hagberg B, Hagberg G, et al: Epidemiology of infantile hydrocephalus in Sweden. *Acta Paediatr Scand* 76:411, 1987.

Freeman JM, Ferry PC: New brain death guidelines in children: Further confusion. *Pediatrics* 81:301, 1988.

Galaburda AM, Sherman GF, Rosen GD, et al: Developmental dyslexia. Four consecutive cases with cortical anomalies. *Am Neurol* 18:222, 1985.

Gilman S, Bloedel JR, Lechtenberg R: *Disorders of the Cerebellum.* Philadelphia, FA Davis, 1981.

Levine MD, Jordan NC: Learning disorders: The neurodevelopmental underpinnings. *Contemp Pediatr* 4:16, 1987.

Levine MD, Oberklaid F, Meltzer LJ: Developmental output failure: A study of low productivity in school age children. *Pediatrics* 67:18, 1981.

Lombroso CT, Lerman P: Breath-holding spells (acyanotic and pallid infantile syncope). *Pediatrics* 39:563, 1967.

Lorber J, Priestly BL: Children with large heads. *Dev Med Child Neurol* 23:474, 1981.

Mantovani JF, Pasternak JF, Mathew O, et al: Failure of daily lumbar puncture to prevent hydrocephalus following intraventricular hemorrhage. *J Pediatr* 97:278, 1980.

Matson DD, Crofton FDL: Papilloma of choroid plexus in childhood. *J Neurosurg* 17:1002, 1960.

Mattis S, French J, Rapin I: Dyslexia in children and young adults: Three independent syndromes. *Dev Med Child Neurol* 17:150, 1978.

McComb JG: Recent research into the nature of cerebrospinal fluid formation and absorption. *J Neurosurg* 59:369, 1983.

Menkes JH: Diseases of the motor unit. In Avery ME, Taeusch HW (eds): *Diseases of the Newborn*. Philadelphia, WB Saunders Co., 1984.

Nelson KB, Ellenberg JH: Predictors of epilepsy in children who have experienced febrile seizures. *N Engl J Med* 295:1029, 1976.

Norman RM: Malformations of the nervous system, birth injury and diseases of early life. In Greenfield JF (ed): *Neuropathology*. London, Edward Arnold, 1967.

Plum F, Posner JB: *The Diagnosis of Stupor and Coma,* 3rd edition. Philadelphia, FA Davis, 1980.

Pomarede R: Endocrine aspects of tumoral markers in intracranial germinoma. *J Pediatr* 101:374, 1982.

Rosen FS: Case Records of the Massachusetts General Hospital. *N Engl J Med* 316:91, 1987.

Rutter M: *Developmental Neuropsychiatry*. New York, Guilford Press, 1983.

Shaywitz BA, Waxman SG: Dyslexia (editorial). *N Engl J Med* 316:1268, 1987.

Smith S, Kimberling W, Pennington BF, et al: Specific reading disability: Identification of an inherited form through linkage analysis. *Science* 219:1345, 1983.

Stumpf DA: The inherited ataxias. *Neurol Clin* 3:47, 1985.

Swift M, Reitnauer PJ, Morrell D, et al: Breast and other cancers in families with ataxia-telangiectasia. *N Engl J Med* 316:1289, 1987.

Vellutino FR: Dyslexia. *Sci Am* 256:34, 1987.

Wilson R, Morris JG Jr, Snyder JD, et al: Clinical characteristics of infant botulism in the United States: A study of the non-California cases. *Pediatr Infect Dis* 1:148, 1982.

Wolff HG: In Dalessio DJ (ed): *Headache and Other Head Pain,* 4th edition. New York, Oxford University Press, 1983.

Nervous System Disorders 3

MOVEMENT DISORDERS

Definition

The term "movement disorder" is often used by convention to describe those derangements of voluntary movement in which the burden of pathophysiology is believed to reside in the deep grey nuclei of the brain. That is, these are extrapyramidal disorders. Dysfunctions of voluntary movement are also produced by damage to the pyramidal system (spasticity); these will not be discussed here nor will those movement disorders that seem to be mediated by dysfunction of the cerebellum and cerebellar outflow tracts (dysmetria and many of the ataxias).

It is useful to group the disorders by their phenotype, rather than by their presumed anatomic substrate, as patients may present with chorea, for example, rather than dysfunction of their basal ganglia as the major complaint.

Choreiform Movement Disorders of Childhood

Chorea is defined as an involuntary, jerky movement, usually involving distal structures (fingers, hands, feet) that are quite rapid and interrupt any ongoing voluntary movement. Older children often learn to "cover up" their choreiform movements by subsuming them into a seemingly purposeful movement (a hand jerk that becomes a gesture to straighten the hair). Chorea is exacerbated by cold, agitation, and psychologic distress, and, like most extrapyramidal movement disorders, it tends to disappear during sleep.

Sydenham Chorea

This disorder was first described by Sydenham in 1684; its relationship to rheumatic fever was first suggested in 1780 by Stoll. The disorder is characterized by hypotonia, emotional lability, and choreiform movements of the face, extremities, and trunk. The clinical variability of the disorder is great, and children may be mute and bedridden because of profound hypotonia and nearly continuous facial grimacing, or they may have been erroneously labeled as "fresh and hyperactive." Useful clinical signs include lack of persistence of motor movements on voluntary or command performance (the "chameleon tongue": withdrawn almost immediately upon protrusion), and the tendency for the hands to drift outward when held above the head ("pronator sign").

CASE ILLUSTRATION

An 11-year old girl was referred to our emergency room for evaluation of a 2-week history of gradually worsening abnormal eye movements and sudden jerking movements of the head. She was entirely well until 1 month before the visit when an impetiginous skin lesion appeared, which progressively worsened over the next 3 weeks. The child was then seen by her pediatrician who diagnosed bullous impetigo, and started the child on the appropriate antibiotic. The lesion resolved. Approximately 1 week following the antibiotic course, however, the parents noticed occasional darting lateral eye movements. These became increasingly more noticeable and seemed to include quick random jerking movements of the head and neck, which increased with stress and subsided in sleep. She was somewhat more tired but there were no reports of altered mental status, deterioration of school performance, lapses in posture, consciousness, obvious seizures, difficulty swallowing, change in bowel or bladder habits, coprolalia, or exercise intolerance. There were no rashes or arthralgias nor was there a history of pharyngitis. Family history was noncontributory.

Examination initially was remarkable for an otherwise well-appearing, well-developed, prepubescent girl with mild but clearly evident choreiform movements of the head, neck, trunk, arms, and fingers. The legs were quiet. There were facial grimaces with contortions of the mouth, darting tongue movements, and occasional sudden bidirectional deviation of the eyes. Her mental status was normal. Speech was clear and appropriate. Cranial nerves were intact. Gait coordination, strength, and reflexes were normal. Tone was diminished slightly in the arms, but normal in the legs. Significantly there was no rash, subcutaneous nodules, arthritis, pharyngitis, or fever. An ECG and chest radiograph were entirely normal. Sedimentation rate was 13 mm, and an antistreptococcal antibody titer was not elevated. A C-reactive protein was negative as was antinuclear antibody (ANA).

QUESTION AND COMMENT

What is the differential diagnosis and how should this patient be treated?

The differential diagnosis of chorea in this girl is an extensive one, and includes encephalopathy, lupus, Wilson disease, Tourette syndrome, juvenile Huntington disease, a variety of familial choreiform diseases, and of course, Sydenham chorea. The unremarkable family history, negative ANA, absence of dysmorphology or previous neurologic disease, and physical examination make all but the last of these highly unlikely. However, the lack of historical or laboratory evidence of either a prior strep pharyngitis or acute rheumatic fever seems to make clinching the diagnosis of Sydenham chorea also a difficult one. It is important to remember that impetigo or streptococcal infections of the skin have never been incriminated as etiologic in rheumatic fever.

The diagnostic dilemma in this child, however, would probably have not stopped seasoned clinicians of yesteryear who knew that chorea, especially in prepubescent females, may be the sole manifestation of rheumatic fever and that during the often prolonged 1- to 6-month latent period from pharyngitis to chorea antistreptococcal antibodies and acute phase reactants frequently will return to normal at least one-third of the time. Active arthritis and chorea never coexist and a clear pharyngitis history is often unobtainable. On the other hand, it is also important to remember that almost one-third of patients with pure chorea will ultimately develop carditis and, therefore, all such cases of chorea for which no alternative explanation is available should receive antistreptococcal prophylaxis. Such was the case with this particular patient. She received 1.2 million units of benzathine penicillin, IM, and will continue to do so monthly for life. In the absence of active carditis or arthritis, aspirin therapy was not instituted. Since the chorea was not disabling, haloperidol treatment for such choreiform symptoms was also withheld.

Sydenham chorea is rather rare in developed countries at present, as there has been a significant decline over the past 2 decades. Over the past 5 years, we see one or two cases annually on the neurology service at The Children's Hospital, Boston, usually in recent immigrants to the United States from southeast Asia.

The differential diagnosis is considered in Table 12.11.

Treatment

While Sydenham urged bleeding and purging, the current therapy of choice for the severely afflicted child is haloperidol. Steroids and ACTH have supporters, but their efficacy is not clear at present. Salicylates and chlorpromazine have also been reported to be of benefit. Since roughly one-third of children with Sydenham chorea eventually develop valvular heart disease, careful consideration to a course of antibiotic therapy must be given.

Table 12.11
Choreiform Disorders of Childhood

Choreiform Disorders of Childhood
Sydenham chorea
Tic disorders
Choreoathetoid cerebral palsy
Benign familial choreoathetosis
Drug intoxication (diphenylhydantoin, phenothiazines, reserpine, birth control pills, isoniazid)
Paroxysmal choreoathetosis (kinesogenic and dystonic)
Lesch-Nyhan syndrome (see pp. 972)
Hyperalaninemia
Ataxia-telangiectasia
Lipidoses (see pp. 743)
Huntington disease

Huntington Disease

Definition

Huntington disease is characterized by an autosomal dominant, seemingly completely penetrant transmission of dementia and a choreiform movement disorder. The disorder was actually first described by Waters in 1841, but Huntington became associated with this disorder because of his rather exhaustive description and keen interest in the subject.

Basic Science

Gusella et al (1983) reported the association of the gene for Huntington disease with a polymorphic marker on the short arm of chromosome 4, which may allow for prenatal diagnosis and, eventually, gene therapy. The genetic defect is thought to have originated from a common source; new mutations are possibly nonexistent (Martin and Gusella, 1986).

Epidemiology

The disorder occurs in approximately 1:24,000 individuals in the United States.

Natural History

The usual presentation is between 35 and 40 years of age, but 5% of cases present before the 15th birthday. For unclear reasons, earlier presentation is more frequent in tropical and subtropical climates.

The clinical presentation in childhood is quite different from the adult form, in that most juveniles appear Parkinsonian rather than choreoathetoid. Seizures are also common in childhood. Table 12.12 is from Menkes (1985), who pooled 28 cases from Jervis (1963) and Markham and Knox (1965). Dementia was usually the presenting sign, although often it was not recognized until a second sign occurred. Given the pediatric clinical manifestations, the differential diagnosis includes all the choreiform disorders and also Wilson disease (see pp. 476), Hallervorden-Spatz disease, and dystonia musculorum deformans.

No treatment other than control of seizures is effective.

Benign Familial Choreoathetosis

This is an autosomal dominant condition with variable penetrance. While the movement disorder is generally progressive with age, and usually presents during the second decade of life, the illness is not associated with dementia, distinguishing it from Huntington disease. The inheritance pattern distinguishes the disorder from Sydenham chorea.

Table 12.12
Clinical Features of Juvenile Huntington Disease[1]

Feature	Number of Cases = 28
Age of onset	
< 5 years	7
5–10 years	21
Hyperkinesia and/or choreoathetosis	13
Rigidity	19
Seizures	13
Dementia	22
Ataxia and/or dysmetria	5

[1]Data from Menkes, 1985.

Paroxysmal Kinesogenic Choreoathetosis

First described by Mount and Reback, the disorder appears to have a high spontaneous mutation rate; although certain families have a clear autosomal dominant history, many cases seem to be sporadic. The movements may be small and easily hidden in a volitional "cover-up," or may be quite violent and throw the patient across the room. The movements occur quite frequently, up to hundreds of times daily, but are all quite short-lived. As the name implies, movements most often occur during the initiation of a sudden voluntary movement. The disorder is usually well-controlled with modest doses of diphenylhydantoin.

Paroxysmal Dystonic Choreoathetosis

This disorder is distinguished from paroxysmal kinesogenic choreoathetosis by its completely penetrant autosomal dominant transmission, and its occurring as "attacks" which last for 30–60 minutes, but usually once daily or less frequently. It is rather insensitive to pharmacologic management.

Fahr Disease (Familial Calcification of the Basal Ganglia)

This term undoubtedly subsumes several genetic disorders, all associated with progressive calcification of the basal ganglia. There appears to be an autosomal recessive form with juvenile dementia, microcephaly, and choreoathetosis, as well as an autosomal dominant form, with dementia in the fourth or fifth decade and choreoathetosis. There are also families described with apparently asymptomatic calcification of the basal ganglia; their relationship to either of these two entities is obscure.

Hallervorden-Spatz Disease

Hallervorden and Spatz described a disorder of gait which was progressive and fundamentally dystonic, but which was associated with pes equinovarus deformity of the feet, dementia, and choreoathetosis. Spasticity, rigidity, retinitis pigmentosa, and optic atrophy have all been noted since the original description. The onset is usually before the end of the first decade.

Dystonic Movement Disorders of Childhood

Dystonia is used to describe a slow, spasmodic, twisting movement, usually of the extremities.

Dystonia Musculorum Deformans

First described by Schwalbe in 1908, the condition was originally considered as a variant of hysteria. It is characterized by slow, writhing, spasmodic movements which are usually distal (a plantar flexion-inversion posture of the foot is the most common presenting sign). While the movements are intermittent at first, they tend to coalesce as the disorder progresses. As in most movement disorders, the abnormal movements remit in sleep. An autosomal recessive form has been described in Swedes and Franco-Americans, and a variably penetrant autosomal dominant form has been described in Ashkenazim.

Trihexyphenidyl, levodopa, and levodopa in combination with a decarboxylase blocker have all been reported to be successful; in recalcitrant cases, thalamectomy (usually cryosurgical) has been used with some benefit. It has significant side effects as a therapy and, of late, has been limited to use in unilateral cases.

Tic Disorders of Childhood

Definition

Tics are complex, stereotyped multiple muscle group movements that are quite rapid and frequently migratory. While many individuals manifest an occasional tic at some point in their lives, there are disorders in which the frequency and severity of the abnormal movements merit medical attention.

Epidemiology

Tics occur in 10–35% of all children and are, thus, by far the most common of movement disorders. Boys are affected about three times as frequently as girls. In half the cases they are present in other family members.

Natural History

Tics can begin at any age in childhood, with the mean age of onset at 7 years. Most tics disappear within a few months. Chronic tic disorders can involve echolalia (repeating the words of others) or coprolalia (the involuntary utterance of obscenities). Severe repetitive movements such as hand-wringing in Rett syndrome reflect major neurologic dysfunction.

Treatment

No medications are helpful in the treatment of transient tics. Recognition that such tics are self-limited and, therefore, not bringing them to attention is the best course. Operant conditioning is often useful.

Gilles de la Tourette Syndrome (Tourette Syndrome)

First described in 1885 by Gilles de la Tourette, this disorder is characterized by frequent, migratory tics and associated behavioral disturbances. The disorder usually presents in males (3:1 or 4:1, depending upon the series) between the ages of 5 and 10 years; there is a tendency for the disorder to abate during the third or fourth decade. There seems to be a greater-than-chance association with "obsessive-compulsive disorder" and attentional disorders (Pauls et al, 1986). In some pedigrees, Tourette syndrome appears to be an autosomal dominant condition, but identical twins are sometimes discordant for the syndrome (Eldridge and Denckla, 1986).

As the disorder is not in itself dangerous, except for the social consequences of the tics and associated phenomena (coprolalia and copropraxia), therapy should be guided by how disabled the child is rendered by the movements (Erenberg et al, 1985). Behavior modification and operant conditioning have been very successful in mild forms. In more severe cases, haloperidol or clonidine may be used (Leckman et al, 1986). In our experience, clonazepam usually produces unacceptable sedation. Pimozide has recently been released in the United States, and may prove useful as an alternative therapy. It has been found as efficacious as haloperidol, and with just as few significant side effects.

DEGENERATIVE DISEASES

Definition

These diseases comprise a heterogeneous collection of pathologies that are characterized by specific patterns of cell death. They are often genetically transmitted and deserve the larger appellation "heredodegenerative diseases." The nature of the genetic abnormality is not known in most of these diseases; however, it is only a matter of time before this changes. Some of these diseases are discussed under movement disorders (i.e., Huntington disease). The heredodegenerative diseases that affect the peripheral nervous system are discussed under neuromuscular pathology.

Degenerative Diseases of the Brain Stem, Cerebellum, and Spinal Cord

These diseases specifically affect the more inferior parts of the CNS and are characterized by programmed cell death with subsequent gliosis. Usually, a family history of the clinical entity is found.

Friedreich Ataxia

Definition

This autosomal recessive disorder is characterized by ataxia, scoliosis, loss of position and vibration sense, and areflexia (Stumpf, 1985).

Basic Science

Friedreich ataxia is one of the best delineated of the heredodegenerative diseases, yet the underlying etiology of the pathology is not known. It has been suggested that an abnormality in mitochondrial malic enzyme is involved (Stumpf, 1982).

The pathologic changes are found mainly in the posterior columns, corticospinal and spinocerebellar tracts, where the fibers are lost and replaced by gliotic scar. The Purkinje cells in the superior vermis of the cerebellum and the inferior olivary nuclei are atrophied. Histopathologic examination of the heart shows myocardial cell loss with fibrosis, and an infiltrate of macrophages.

Natural History

The most common initial finding is a gait disorder that usually begins before puberty, although it may appear up to 25 years of age. Scoliosis may accompany this initial finding, and will inevitably be present as the disease progresses. After the initial presentation, there is a rapid deterioration involving limb ataxia, loss of position and vibration sense, and areflexia. The fully developed syndrome includes orthopedic deformities such as pes cavus, hammer toes, and kyphoscoliosis. Optic atrophy and retinitis pigmentosa are common. About 40% of Friedreich ataxia patients will develop diabetes mellitus, thought to be secondary to degeneration of the pancreatic β cells. The most lethal sequela of the disease is the cardiomyopathy, which eventually occurs in all patients. Initially it is a hypertrophic form that may involve the septum more than the free wall (a form of asymmetric septal hypertrophy). The ECG may show T-wave abnormalities suggestive of a myocarditis (Boyer et al, 1962).

Diagnosis

Visual evoked potentials will often show decreased amplitude and increased latency. The CT scan is normal until late in the disease when it shows atrophy of the cerebellar vermis and cortex. The EEG is usually normal. Electrodiagnostic studies of the peripheral nerves reveal a profound sensory neuropathy with absent or slow nerve conduction and reduced or absent sensory action potentials. The motor nerve conduction and electromyogram are normal.

Prognosis

The disease is relentlessly progressive and leads to death, usually from heart failure, between ages 26 and 36 years. No therapy is known, although some believe that thyrotropin-releasing hormone may improve the cerebellar findings transiently (Sobue et al, 1978).

Metachromatic Leukodystrophy (Sulfatide Lipidosis)

Definition

Metachromatic leukodystrophy is the result of an inborn error of metabolism. The activity of arylsulfatase A is reduced so that sulfatide accumulates in myelin of the CNS and peripheral nerves. The disorder is autosomal recessive.

Natural History

The onset is usually before the first birthday but may occur later. The child initially experiences disturbance of gait. Spasticity and Babinski responses are present. Flaccid weakness and atrophy of distal muscles is common.

Diagnosis

Reduced activity of aryl sulfatase A may be found in renal tubular cells from urinary sediment, fibroblasts, or white blood cells. CSF protein is often elevated.

Treatment

Until recently, only supportive care was possible. Enzyme replacement is theoretically possible with bone marrow transplantation. At least one patient, a sibling of one who died from the disease, was given a transplant as soon as she showed signs of the disease, and has developed normally over the subsequent year at least.

Prevention

Prenatal diagnosis is possible.

Krabbe Disease (Cerebroside Lipidosis)

Definition

Krabbe disease is a disorder of early infancy characterized by lack of myelin and multinucleated giant cells (globoid cells) in the white matter. The disorder is an autosomal recessive lysosomal storage disease.

Natural History

The illness can be suspected in an infant who has swallowing problems and is hyperreflexic. Most infants fail to develop and appear unaware of their environment. They require tube feedings. The duration of life is usually under 2 years.

Diagnosis

Galactocerebrosidase is deficient in white blood cells. Spinal fluid protein is increased. Prenatal diagnosis is possible by enzymatic assay of cultured fibroblasts from amniotic fluid (Suzuki, 1971).

Treatment

Supportive care is all that is available. However, bone marrow transplantation in a mouse strain with galactosylcermidase deficiency induced a partial remyelination of the CNS. No attempts to carry out this procedure in humans has been reported as of 1988 (Hoogerbrugge et al, 1988).

Subacute Necrotizing Encephalomyelitis (Leigh Syndrome)

Definition

Leigh syndrome is a rapidly progressive degenerative syndrome characterized by somnolence, blindness, deafness, spasticity, and peripheral neuropathy (Leigh, 1951). It is inherited as an autosomal recessive disorder.

Basic Science

Pathologic findings include spongy degeneration of the gray matter of brain stem, basal ganglia, thalamus, and spinal cord. Astrocytosis and capillary proliferation are prominent especially surrounding the ventricles. Disorders of mitochondrial function increase brain lactate and may be the primary defects (Evans, 1981; Robinson et al, 1987).

Natural History

The onset is in infancy and may be marked by vomiting, hypotonia or spasticity, and seizures. Nystagmus and extraocular palsies are common as vision is lost. Respirations may become periodic and apneic spells are common.

Diagnosis

CSF and blood lactate and pyruvate levels are elevated. (Normal CSF lactate is 11.7 ± 2.7 mg/dl.) Fibroblast cultures show deficient cytochrome oxidase activity.

Treatment

Only supportive measures can be recommended as of 1987.

DEMYELINATING DISEASES

Multiple Sclerosis

Definition

Multiple sclerosis (MS) is a demyelinating disorder that usually presents about age 30 years, but can occur as early as age 2 years. Evidence of two or more lesions in the white matter is considered diagnostic.

Epidemiology

The disorder is about twice as common in women, and in individuals under age 14 years, the female-male ratio is 3:1. A positive family history is present in about 20%. The prevalence of MS in individuals under age 10 years is 1.5/1000 in a Canadian survey (Duquette et al, 1988).

Natural History

Presenting symptoms can differ, but in general, involve afferent structures of the CNS. Optic neuritis, diplopia, blurred vision, disorders of gait, transverse myelitis, and sphincter problems have been reported at onset. Complete recovery is the rule after the initial symptom. Relapses are probable. In some children, the course is progressive, but slower than in adults.

Diagnosis

The clinical course is suggestive of the diagnosis. CT scans or MRI of the CNS can demonstrate the lesions. The CSF may show elevated IgG levels, but in nearly 40% of patients levels were below 14% (normal adult levels; Duquette et al, 1988).

Treatment

Acute exacerbations may respond to a 2-week course of ACTH. Physiotherapy is helpful if muscle spasticity is present. If bladder dysfunction occurs, frequent emptying may be required to reduce residual urine and infection.

Prognosis

The course is unpredictable. Some children are symptom-free for years after the initial episode.

Schilder Disease (Diffuse Cerebral Sclerosis)

Definition

Schilder disease is a sporadic, chronic (sometimes acute) demyelinating disorder that occurs most commonly in late childhood. The name has been applied to a number of demyelinating conditions which accumulate sudanophilic lipids in the demyelinated areas.

Natural History

Like multiple sclerosis, the findings can be protean. The onset is usually between ages 5 and 12 years. Cortical blindness, spastic hemiplegia, deafness, aphasia, or seizures may herald the disorder or occur during the relentless course. Dementia, coma, and death may occur within weeks or months after onset.

Diagnosis

Definitive diagnosis can be made only pathologically when demyelination of white matter and sparing of subcortical U fibers is characteristic. The CSF may show a lymphocytic pleocytosis and elevated protein. CSF pressure may be elevated.

Treatment

Treatment to lower CSF pressure may be needed. Otherwise, no specific therapy is known.

Adrenoleukodystrophy

Definition

Adrenoleukodystrophy is a genetically determined disease that is characterized by progressive central demyelination and adrenal cortical deficiency.

Basic Science

Characterized as a peroxisomal disorder, affected individuals have an impaired ability to degrade saturated long-chain unbranched fatty acids, especially hexacosanoate (C26:0). Adrenal cortical cells and Schwann cells contain characteristic lamellar cytoplasmic inclusions, consisting of cholesterol esterified with the long chain saturated fatty acids. Other tissues and body fluids also show increased levels of these fatty acids. The gene has been mapped to X chromosome region Xq28, in the same region as the genes for hemophilia and color blindness.

Epidemiology

The condition is rare, although Moser et al (1984) reviewed 303 cases from 217 kindreds. It has been reported in all races.

Natural History

A rare neonatal form of the disorder is an autosomal recessive disease that presents with hypotonia and severe developmental delay. Seizures are prominent. Since only 15 cases have been reported as of 1984, the range of findings is not known. Retinal degeneration was a feature of most cases, and liver dysfunction is often noted. Death occurs in infancy.

The more common X-linked disorder has its onset in childhood (after age 3 years) with adrenal insufficiency preceding neurologic findings in the younger group, and neurologic abnormalities preceding adrenal insufficiency in the older group which includes adults. The outstanding features are the gradual onset and steadily progressive dementia, impaired hearing, and vision and paralysis. The lesions are frequently asymmetrical.

Diagnosis

Assay of very-long-chain fatty acids in plasma or cultured fibroblasts establishes the diagnosis. Addison disease is indistinguishable from that of later onset (see pp. 864). Prenatal diagnosis is possible from fibroblasts obtained by amniocentesis.

Treatment

Attempts at dietary restriction of C26:0 have been unsuccessful in lowering the tissue levels or alleviating the neurologic symptoms. Glucocorticoids can correct the adrenal insufficiency but not the neurologic abnormalities. At least one bone marrow transplant did not deter the progression of the neurologic symptoms, although the plasma levels fell by 60%.

Prognosis

In the limited experience to date, nearly all symptomatic individuals have shown a progressive deterioration.

Rett Syndrome

Definition

Rett syndrome (first described in 1966) is a progressive encephalopathy characterized by ataxia, autistic behavior, and cerebral atrophy observed only in girls. It is one of the leading causes of progressive dementia in girls (Opitz et al, 1986).

Epidemiology

This condition was first described in Vienna in 1966, and has been recognized more frequently in Sweden and Scotland, although cases have been reported in other countries. The prevalence is estimated to be 0.65–0.67/10,000 girls in Sweden. Cases reported as of 1985 have all been Caucasian. No occurrence of the syndrome in full siblings has been reported, although two half-sisters were affected (Hagberg et al, 1983). The empiric recurrence risk is less than 1%.

Natural History

Development is normal for the first months of life, with gradual deterioration beginning about 1 year of age, but may be as early as 4 months. The deterioration usually accelerates and is marked by bizarre behavioral changes and loss of purposeful use of the hands (with characteristic hand-washing or hand-wringing gestures), jerky ataxia of the trunk, and vasomotor instability. Excessive inappropriate laughter or autistic withdrawal are components of the dementia. Hypertension was noted in at least one patient who had renal artery stenosis.

The course is one of progressive deterioration. Spastic signs and convulsions tend to be of later onset than loss of purposeful hand use (Al-Mateen et al, 1986).

Diagnosis

No pathognomonic metabolic changes have been documented. The diagnosis is made on the clinical findings and progressive course. The ECG is typically abnormal with generalized slow-wave activity and epileptiform abnormalities.

Treatment

Only supportive measures can be recommended as of 1988.

Prognosis

The disorder is compatible with life into the 30s. In the early teen years, upper neuron damage leads to muscle wasting and decreases mobility. Difficulty swallowing becomes a major problem and may necessitate gavage feeding (MacLeod P: personal communication, Queens University, Kingston, Canada).

OTHER RARE DEGENERATIVE DISORDERS

Olivopontocerebellar Atrophy

This heterogeneous group of diseases has in common degeneration within the cerebellum, pons, and olivary nuclei. The initial description of the disorder pathologically by Dejerine and Thomas (1900) was of a sporadic disorder. It has become evident, however, that the disorder follows an autosomal dominant inheritance pattern in the majority of cases. A classification of the disorders into five types by Konigsmark and Weiner (1970) has clarified the heterogeneity of the clinical presentation.

The most common presentation occurs in early adulthood with progressive cerebellar ataxia and loss of vibration and position sense, with facial palsies and dysphagia. This corresponds to the type IV disease. The type I or Menzel cerebellar ataxia presents between teenage years and middle life with a gait disorder and dysarthria.

Biochemical examination of those with the type IV disease has shown a partial defect in glutamate dehydrogenase in about 40% (Plaitakis et al, 1984). There is no known therapy.

Ramsay Hunt Syndrome (Dentatorubral Atrophy)

This is a rare disorder which combines myoclonus and ataxia. It usually manifests with ataxia in teenaged patients. Myoclonus follows after a variable interval. Occasionally, mental retardation is part of the syndrome. The differential diagnosis should include the myoclonic epilepsies that invariably have mental retardation with myoclonus and the late-infantile form of neuronal ceroid lipofuscinosis. It is unclear whether the Ramsay Hunt syndrome is a single disease. The pathology shows degeneration of the dentate nucleus, spinocerebellar tracts, and rarefaction of the dentatorubral tract and superior cerebellar peduncle (Bird and Shaw, 1978). Cerebral cortical degeneration is often seen, but cardiomyopathy or corticospinal tract disease is not part of the pathology. These later two findings should suggest Friedreich ataxia.

Joseph Disease

This disorder occurs in patients of Portugese descent from the Azores. The age of onset of the symptoms is variable, but may involve the adolescent population. The symptoms include a progressive ataxia with features of corticospinal involvement such as hyperrefexia, spasticity and extensor plantar reflexes. Often some aspect of extrapyramidal dysfunction is present resulting in bradykinesia and rigidity. Some patients have a peripheral neuropathy accompanying the CNS dysfunction. The pattern of inheritance is autosomal dominant. Histopathologic examination reveals degeneration of the dentate nuclei, spinocerebellar tracts, anterior horn cells, substantia nigra, and oculomotor nuclei.

Familial Spastic Paraplegia

This is, relatively speaking, a common childhood system degeneration that primarily involves the spinal cord. It has an autosomal dominant or, less commonly, an autosomal recessive mode of inheritance. It presents with the gradual onset of a painless spasticity involving the lower extremities accompanied by weakness and extensor plantar reflexes. Muscular atrophy is not a prominent finding, and position and vibration sense are intact. The bladder and bowel are involved late in the disease. The age of onset is in the teenage years, although onset is earlier for the recessive form. In addition, the recessive form is rapidly progressive, whereas the dominant form may stabilize until adulthood. In the terminal stages of the disease, the spasticity involves the upper extremities and the patient is bedridden with no control over autonomic spinal cord function.

A number of complicated forms have been described with wasting of the small hand muscles, ophthalmoplegia, ataxia, or optic atrophy. It is mandatory that a myelogram or MRI be done to exclude a tumor either within or compressing the spinal cord. There is no therapy for the disease itself, but meticulous supportive treatment improves the quality of life.

Histopathologic examination reveals degeneration of the corticospinal tracts especially below the cervical spine, and, to a lesser degree, in the posterior columns, spinocerebellar tracts, and dorsal root ganglia.

Fazio-Londe Disease

This rare disorder is characterized by a progressive bulbar palsy that has its onset usually in early childhood and progresses over 10 years to death. The clinical picture is one of facial diplegia, dysarthria, dysphonia, and dysphagia. Occasionally, extensor plantar reflexes are seen, imitating the clinical picture of a late onset Werdnig-Hoffmann disease. In others, the posterior columns of the spinal cord degenerate. It is essential that a pontine glioma or multiple sclerosis be excluded in the patient with this presentation.

Leber Disease (Hereditary Optic Atrophy)

This degenerative disease of the optic nerves presents with the gradual onset of bilateral visual blurring with large central scotomas. Occasionally, the onset is sudden, with pain in or above the eye. This sudden onset is reminiscent of acute optic neuritis. Rarely, the onset is of a unilateral disorder, but both eyes are involved eventually. The vision deteriorates over weeks to months, but the peripheral fields are maintained. Blue-yellow color vision seems to be lost much more than red-yellow. Fundic examination initially shows blurred disc margins, which eventually give way to bilateral optic atrophy.

The histopathology shows degeneration of the papillomacular bundles and the central aspects of the optic nerves and tracts to the lateral geniculate nucleus. The inheritance of the disorder suggests a mitochondrial disease with mothers passing the disease to their children, but males never doing so (Nikoskelainen et al, 1987).

As is common in heredodegenerative diseases, other forms of Leber disease with different pathologies have been described. This includes corticospinal cerebellar dysfunction.

Progressive Hereditary Nerve Deafness

Progressive loss of hearing usually is found in the company of other heredodegenerative diseases. It has been described with Friedreich ataxia, hereditary motor and sensory neuropathy type I and II (Charcot-Marie-Tooth disease), and with hereditary sensory neuropathies. In addition, retinitis pigmentosa either by itself, or as part of Refsum disease may be associated with a progressive hearing loss. Nondegenerative causes of hearing loss must be excluded.

Progressive Facial Hemiatrophy

This striking disease has its onset usually in early childhood and has as its hallmark the progressive wasting of the bone and soft tissue of one side of the face. For unknown reasons, the onset may be triggered by trivial trauma to the face. The hair of the eyelashes and eyebrows and even of the scalp may be involved, but trigeminal and facial nerves function normally. The neurologic sequelae of the disease include corticospinal tract dysfunction and seizures. CT scans are usually normal, but may show generalized atrophy or calcifications contralateral to the facial atrophy.

MALFORMATIONS OF THE CENTRAL NERVOUS SYSTEM

The development of the human CNS is an awesome event, and it is a wonder that it proceeds without error in so many children. Although the details and mechanisms of neuroembryology are not known, the gross organogenetic steps in human nervous system development can be identified (Moore, 1982). It is important that the general pediatrician be able to identify the pathology of this event, as it accounts for 75% of fetal deaths and 40% of deaths within the first year of life. This chapter will briefly review normal development and then describe the known abnormalities.

The neural folds close to form the neural tube at about 3 weeks' gestation. This process begins in the cervical region and extends in both directions, completing the closure by the fourth week. This is followed by a folding of the neural tube at the cranial and cervical flexures. At this point, the primordial nervous system is a fluid-filled tube with two bends in it. Abnormalities at this stage will give rise to an open nervous system such as is seen in spina bifida, myelomeningocoele and Chiari malformations, or more drastically, actual anencephaly.

During the 5th week, the telencephalic vesicles evaginate to form the primordial brain proper. In addition, the roof of the fourth ventricle (formed at the apex of the cranial flexure) is thinned, allowing flow of CSF. It is this last event that, when abnormal, gives rise to the Dandy-Walker syndrome. Holoprosencephaly is thought to arise from abnormal evagination of the telencephalic vesicles.

The 7th week sees the evagination of the olfactory vesicles from the developing telencephalon and the formation of the pigmented epithelium of the retina. The two histopathologic correlates of abnormal development are arhinencephaly and aniridia, respectively.

The 8th to 15th weeks are an important period for further development of the cerebral cortex. The presumptive cortical neurons are found in a number of layers adjacent to the fluid-filled ventricular system (in the so-called neurons that eventually come to lie in the innermost layer of the cortex migrating first (inside-out pattern of migration). It is thought that the migration occurs along radially aligned glial cells that are transiently found during this stage of development. This migration occurs in both the cerebrum and cerebellum. Abnormalities of cortical migration include heterotopias and abnormalities of gyral architecture such as lissencephaly and pachygyria.

The cortical migrations are complete by the 16th to 20th weeks and the nervous system now fine-tunes its connectivity. It is at this stage that the thalamocortical synapses are made and a number of pre-existing cells undergo a programmed natural cell death. The remaining intrauterine development is concerned with myelination and synaptic branching, as well as with the development of non-neuronal brain elements.

The chapter will divide the anomalies of CNS development into three categories: (1) the disorders of neural tube formation and closure; (2) the disorders of cranial nerve development; and (3) the disorders of cellular migration.

DISORDERS OF NEURAL TUBE FORMATION AND CLOSURE

Microcephaly

Definition

Head circumference is considered too small (microcephaly) when it is more than 2 standard deviations below the mean for age, race, and sex. An abnormally small head denotes a small brain except in the situation of premature closure of sutures. Primary microcephaly is the result of anomalous brain development in the first two trimesters; secondary microcephaly results from disease in the last 2 months of gestation.

Primary microcephaly may be an autosomal recessive disorder. The sibling recurrence risk was 19% in a series from Scotland (Tolmie et al, 1987). Affected patients are mentally retarded but often trainable, and exhibit problems with motor coordination. About one-third have seizures. Visual defects are frequent and include cataracts. The external skull is characterized by a narrow receding forehead and a flat occiput.

Anencephaly is the most common major CNS anomaly. It occurs in females more often than in males and does not show simple Mendelian inheritance. There is a 3–5% chance of anencephaly in the next child if one child has the disorder, but probably a 10% chance of some anomaly of neural tube closure, such as encephalocele or spina bifida. The cephalad neural folds do not form a tube, and subsequently the brain and calvaria fail to develop. About half of the infants are stillborn. Liveborn infants may breathe normally and survive for hours or days (we have no experience with ventilatory support for these infants and do not know how long they could survive it). Certain brain stem reflex movements may be intact.

Antenatal diagnosis may be made by assaying the α-fetoprotein (AFP) in maternal blood or amniotic fluid. Levels of greater than 1000 ng/ml suggest an open neural tube defect, such as anencephaly, bifid cranium, or open spina bifida. It is thought that supplementation of the maternal diet with folate may decrease the incidence of this devastating anomaly. Prenatal ultrasonography can establish the diagnosis (see Fig. 13.14, Genetics, pp. 783). Genetic counseling is essential to alert the family to available prenatal diagnosis (Sadovnick et al, 1987).

Hydranencephaly

Definition

Hydranencephaly is characterized by the failure of development of both cerebral hemispheres and corpus striatum which are reduced to membranous sacs covered by intact meninges containing clear, protein-rich CSF. A number of abnormalities can be present in basal ganglia, brain stem, cerebellum, and pituitary fossa.

Basic Science

Although it is not possible to establish the pathogenesis in most cases, the probable associated events include intrauterine infection, occlusion of both internal carotid arteries, or a severe developmental defect.

Natural History

The infants may appear normal on first evaluation, but careful examination will usually reveal poor affect, irritability, poor sucking and increased muscle tone. Survival is possible for several months, but developmental landmarks are not achieved.

Diagnosis

Once the abnormality is suspected, transillumination of the skull will reveal the absence of brain tissue. An EEG is virtually flat, and CT scans can elucidate the extent of the defect.

Treatment and Prognosis

Supportive care to provide comfort to the infant and solace to the parents is all that is possible.

Agenesis of the Corpus Callosum

Definition

The corpus callosum results from formation of the major telencephalic commissure, which results in complete separation of the hemispheres, except in the region of the anterior commissure and lamina terminalis. The lateral ventricles are displaced laterally and the third ventricle is displaced dorsally. In early infancy, hydrocephalus may be the sole manifestation of partial agenesis of the corpus callosum in association with subarachnoid cysts.

Agenesis of the corpus callosum may be found with anomalies of contiguous structures or as part of other syndromes such as faciotelencephalopathy or Aicardi syndrome. When found in conjunction with anomalous development of contiguous structures it is associated with partial or complete absence of the cingulate lobe, with simplification of the medial hemispheres and absence of the septum pellucidum.

Epidemiology

Most cases are sporadic, although a few examples of X-linked recessive inheritance are known.

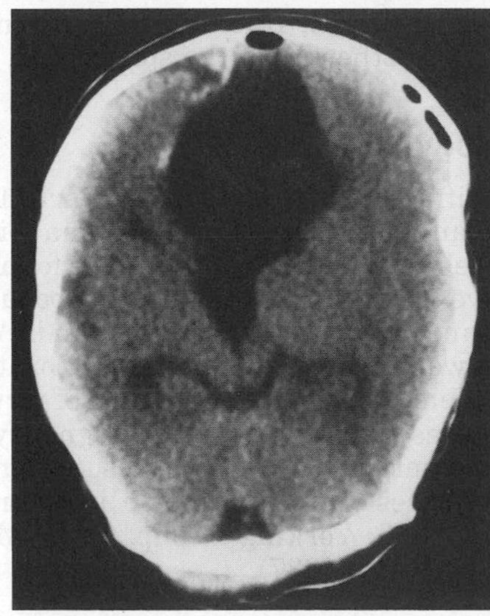

Figure 12.4. This infant has a right hemispheric and right paramedian cyst associated with agenesis of corpus callosum. Agenesis of corpus callosum is frequently a marker for other anomalies including cortical heterotopia, arachnoid cysts, or Dandy-Walker malformation. The variable clinical presentation depends on the underlying abnormality. This infant was found to have an abnormal increase in head circumference in the first weeks of life. The CT scan was performed at 3 weeks of age after the mother noted asymmetry of the forehead. A shunt was placed in the cyst and drained into the peritoneal cavity. At age 13 months, a revised shunt was working well and the cyst was much reduced in size. The child walks, says words, and is neurologically and developmentally normal.

Diagnosis

The clinical presentation shows difficulty with visually guided reaching and bimanual tasks (probably reflecting abnormal premotor cortical development), mental retardation, and seizures.

Agenesis of the corpus callosum is central to the diagnosis of Aicardi syndrome. The patients (uniformly female) suffer from severe mental retardation, a profound seizure disorder, and chorioretinal lacunae.

The CT scan provides definitive diagnosis by showing the characteristic anomalies of the ventricles (Larsen and Osborn, 1982; Fig. 12.4).

Spina Bifida

Failure of fusion of the posterior skull will result in *cranium bifidum,* just as failure of fusion of the vertebral bodies will result in *spina bifida.* The enclosed neural tissue may herniate through the defect, resulting in an encephalocele (brain tissue), meningocele (meninges alone), or meningomyelocele (meninges, spinal cord, and spinal roots). The term spina bifida cystica has been used to describe the latter two conditions. The usual location of spina bifida cystica is lumbosacral, where the posterior neuropore was located. Occult spina bifida is often associated with dermal dimples, sinuses, lipomas, or abnormal filum terminale with tethering of the spinal cord.

Epidemiology

Spina bifida occulta is found in nearly 15% of the population and is asymptomatic. Spina bifida with meningomyelocele, or myelodysplasia is found in 0.13–4.0/1000 live births depending on the population. It, along with anencephaly, is most common in Wales and Ireland. If a woman has had an infant with either anencephaly or meningomyelocele, the risk of recurrence of either is increased in a subsequent pregnancy. Increasing use of prenatal diagnosis has resulted in abortion of affected fetuses with a reduction in the number of cases (EUROCAT Working Group, 1987; Myrianthopoulos and Melnick, 1987).

Natural History

The clinical manifestations of spina bifida depend on the extent of nervous system herniation and the location along the neuraxis. The lesions often are lumbosacral in location and present with a flaccid bladder and hypotonic paraplegia. A Chiari malformation may accompany the lesion and result in hydrocephalus and posterior fossa abnormalities.

Treatment

The approach to treatment of lumbar and sacral defects is to consider the condition a surgical emergency and cover the defect to reduce the likelihood of meningitis. In many centers, including ours, all defects are aggressively treated. In some societies, infants with major defects with total paralysis and absent bladder control are not treated.

The lifelong management of these patients requires a multidisciplinary approach toward health care maintenance. One of the major concerns is to prevent urinary tract infections and hydrocephalus. Careful evaluation of bladder and bladder sphincter function is required. Intermittent catheterization to empty the bladder is the most effective intervention. If that fails, vesicotomy may be required. If sphincter activity is present, the Crede maneuver is contraindicated since it stimulates sphincter activity.

Orthopedic interventions may be helpful to maintain muscle balance to facilitate walking with crutches. Kyphosis is very common and segmental fixation of the spine with rods can greatly improve the ability to sit upright or stand.

Neurosurgical procedures may be required if the child's function deteriorates with growth. Sometimes, the spinal cord is tethered by scar tissue, and surgical release can prevent further destruction of nervous tissue.

Throughout the child's life, special attention must be given to psychological, social, and educational supports.

Prognosis

The prognosis relates to the size of the defect, the level, the extent of involvement of the spinal cord and associated malformations such as the Arnold-Chiari syndrome. Prognosis is also dependent on muscle strength, intelligence, and motivation. Early efforts at health maintenance and continuing care by experienced personnel can greatly improve adaptation to the handicap. In general, infants with sacral lesions have better than 50% chance of later ambulation. Those with upper lumbar and thoracic lesions have less than a 10% chance of ambulation.

Another manifestation of abnormal neural tube closure is a number of anomalies collectively known as the *Chiari malformations*. This disorder is characterized by maldevelopment of the posterior fossa with displacement of the caudal medulla and cerebellar tonsils below the foramen magnum and hydrocephalus. The basal skull is not formed normally and shows platybasia, basilar invagination, and atlantoaxial dislocation as well as fusion of the cervical vertebrae (Klippel-Feil anomaly, see below). The clinical presentation is one of a posterior fossa mass with ataxia, downbeating nystagmus, and lower cranial neuropathies. Often, syringomyelia, syringobulbia or diastematomyelia are also found.

Agenesis of the sacrum is usually found with maldevelopment of the lumbosacral spinal cord. As in spina bifida cystica, the clinical presentation is one of an atonic bladder and hypotonic paraplegia. It is seen in about 1% of infants of diabetic mothers.

Spinal dysraphism may also present with *neurodermal sinuses*. This refers to a continuity between the skin proper and the central neuraxis. As in other dysraphic states, the most common locations are the positions of the posterior and anterior neuropores, that is, the lumbosacral region and the occiput. The sinus may be a portal for infection. The treatment is exploration and obliteration of the sinus (Fig. 12.5).

Malformations of Vertebrae

There exist a group of disorders of development of the rostral cervical vertebrae and base of the skull. These include *platybasia, Klippel-Feil syndrome*, and *cleidocranial dysostosis*.

Definition

Platybasia is an autosomal dominantly inherited anomaly with variable penetrance. The disorder results in stenosis of the foramen magnum and upward displacement of the odontoid process. The base of the skull is flattened and displaced upward.

Basic Science/Natural History

The neurologic abnormalities are a result of compression of the caudal posterior fossa structures such as the medulla and cerebellum, as well as the rostralmost cervical spinal cord.

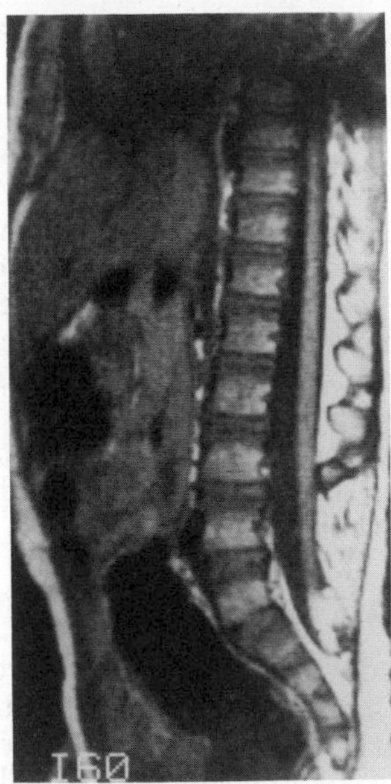

Figure 12.5. This is a magnetic resonance image of a tethered spinal cord in a 2-year-old girl who had been born with anal atresia. Postoperatively, she had urinary retention and was found to have a neurogenic bladder. The image is a T1-weighted midsagittal section of the spine. The conus is low placed and a high density mass can be seen adjacent to it. The diagnosis is dysraphism with a lipomeningomyelocoele. The dilated rectosigmoid colon is visible. In these patients, an evaluation of the cerebellar tonsil by MRI is indicated to search for a Chiari malformation.

The clinical presentation is one of a foramen magnum syndrome with evolving quadriparesis, cerebellar ataxia and downbeat nystagmus. It usually presents in the teenage or early adult years. It may accompany more striking anomalies in this area such as the Chiari malformation.

Diagnosis

Plain radiographs of the upper cervical spine will show the upward displacement of the odontoid process and the narrowed foramen magnum. The diagnostic procedure of choice is the MRI scan which, when reconstructed in the sagittal plane, will show the compression of the lower posterior fossa structures.

Treatment

Neurosurgical decompression of the area is the only treatment.

The Klippel-Feil syndrome is a developmental anomaly of the upper cervical vertebral column characterized by a reduction in the number, or fusion, of vertebrae. As in many other anomalies of this area, it may be associated with other developmental disorders such as congenital heart disease, deafness, or spina bifida. The clinical presentation reflects subacute or chronic progressive cervical myelopathy with a spastic quadriparesis, loss of bowel and bladder control, and, occasionally, cervical radicular dysfunction. The children have short necks with reduced mobility and a low hairline. The diagnosis is made with cervical radiographs which show atlanto-occipital, cervical, or cervicothoracic fusion with a reduction in the number of vertebrae or the presence of hemivertebrae. The treatment is decompressive cervical laminectomy.

Cleidocranial dysostosis is a rare autosomal dominant condition that reflects developmental anomalies of the clavicles, skull, and vertebral columns. The clavicles are rudimentary, the forehead is broad, and there is often mental retardation reflecting anomalous cerebral development.

The *faciotelencephalopathies* are a heterogeneous group of anomalies that result from abnormalities of the cerebral vesicle at the rostralmost end of the neural tube. The vesicle fails to cleave and expand, resulting in midline defects in the brain and face. The normal cleavage is thought to occur at about 23 days' gestation within rather a limited period of time, which may account for its rarity as a developmental anomaly. It may be associated with chromosomal abnormalities such as trisomy 13, 18. Like any developmental anomaly, it may be secondary to an environmental insult that occurs at the specific time of development. Hence, it has been associated with infections and systemic diseases such as toxoplasmosis, syphilis, cytomegalic inclusion disease, and diabetes mellitus. There is controversy in terms of whether these environmental factors can act without inducing aneuploidy.

The most striking form of faciotelencephalopathy is holoprosencephaly. In this disorder, there is a single large ventricle, an undivided single thalamus, and absence of the inferior frontal and temporal neocortex and mesocortex. The olfactory cortex is absent. The brain stem and cerebellum and the primary idiotypic motor and sensory cortices are intact. The septum pellucidum is absent, and multifocal abnormalities of cortical migration such as heterotopias occur. The abnormality of induction of the entodermal anlage for facial development results in a median cleft in the frontonasal face. This may express itself as cyclopia, or simply a cleft lip and palate with orbital hypotelorism.

As might be expected, the clinical picture is heterogeneous, but includes mental retardation, seizure disorder, hydrocephalus, and anosmia.

CRANIAL VAULT DISORDERS

Craniosynostoses

Definition

Craniosynostosis refers to premature closure of one or more cranial sutures and leads to developmental problems depending on their location. Scaphocephaly is the term given to premature closure of the sagittal suture; brachycephaly is closure of the coronal suture; oxycephaly is closure of sagittal and coronal sutures; and plagiocephaly refers to closure of a single (unilateral) suture.

Basic Science

Growth of the cranial vault is perpendicular to the sutures; thus, sagittal suture fusion prevents lateral growth and coronal suture fusion restricts anteroposterior growth. The reasons for premature closure of sutures are unknown.

Epidemiology

The condition is sometimes familial, but more often sporadic. Some craniosynostoses are associated with other malformations, especially of the facial structures (Crouzon disease) and may have dominant inheritance.

Natural History

Asymmetry of the skull may be apparent in the newborn infant, or in the first months of life. The anterior fontanelle may bulge and frontal bossing be present. Ocular complications, including exophthalmos, nystagmus, and strabismus are commonly seen. Deafness and anosmia have been seen in Crouzon disease.

Diagnosis

Skull radiographs are essential to establish which sutures are fused. Increased digital impressions are seen in the skull from local pressure on the internal table (Fig. 12.6). The base of the skull may be shortened. In the most severe of the malformations premature closure of coronal, lambdoid, and squamosal sutures leads to bulging of the frontal and temporal regions (clover leaf skull).

Treatment

Early operation is advocated to prevent further deformity and brain damage. A new suture line is created by removal of the closed suture. If facial deformities are present, they too should be corrected if possible. Major advances have been made in craniofacial reconstructions in the past decade. A patient who has a malformation should be referred to a center with teams of plastic surgeons, neurosurgeons, and dental surgeons experienced in their management.

CELLULAR MIGRATION DISORDERS

In normal development of the cerebral and cerebellar cortices, the neurons migrate out to the cortex from a periventricular zone. This delicate process begins in the 8th week and continues until the 20th week. As noted in previous sections, if the primary neural tube is not properly developed, migration anomalies are common. This section will consider only those disorders thought to result from a primary abnormality of cellular migration with normal organ induction.

Schizencephaly is a disorder that results in bilateral symmetric clefts extending from the ventricular cavity to the surface of the hemisphere. The cleft region

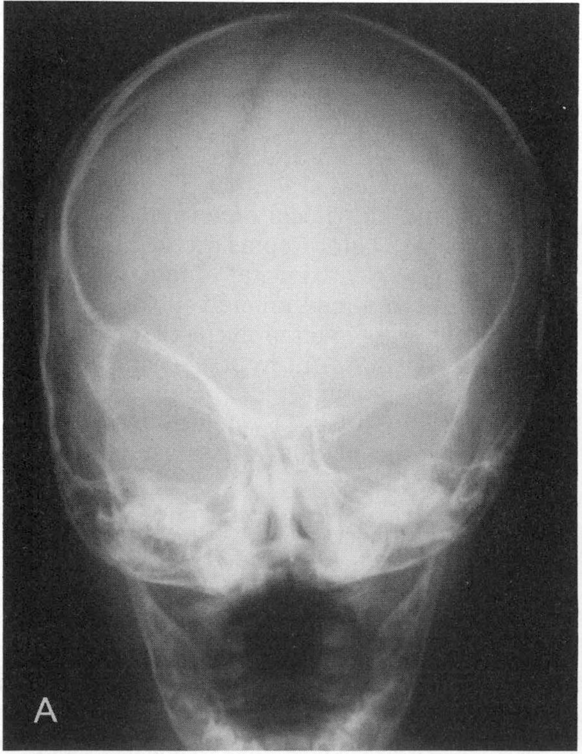

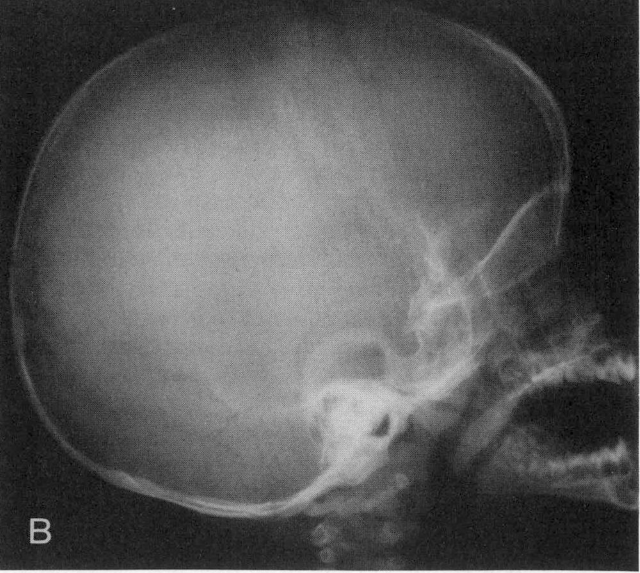

Figure 12.6 A and B. This baby was seen by an ophthalmologist because of an abnormal appearance to the right eye. The AP and lateral radiographs were obtained when it was obvious that the shape of her orbits was unusual. The radiographs show right coronal synostosis as the cause of harlequin or "mephistophelian" right eye. Sagittal synostosis is the more common variety and is usually treated for cosmetic reasons. Children with bilateral cranial synostosis may also have Apert or Crouzon syndrome. Unilateral synostosis, as in this case, needs surgical creation of a neosuture in order to preserve proper vision.

shows poor development and there are abnormalities in sulcal development such as lissencephaly (see below) and heterotopias. This anomaly probably occurs very early in the phase of cellular migration.

The clinical picture is one of mental retardation, seizures, microcephaly, and hemi- or quadriparesis. The diagnosis is made by CT scan or MRI.

Lissencephaly is a disorder of sulcal generation that results in a smooth brain without significant sulcalation. The surface is that of a 2-month fetus and reflects the abnormal cellular migration. The anomaly probably occurs slightly later than does schizencephaly, before 12 weeks. Like schizencephaly, it may be accompanied by other disorders of cellular migration. The clinical presentation is identical to schizencephaly.

Pachygyria or *macrogyria* refers to an abnormality characterized by a few gyri that appear coarse in gross architecture. The defect is not one in primary sulcalation, such as lissencephaly, but one of secondary or tertiary sulcalation. Hence, the disorder may be more lateralized and tends to reflect insult later in development, around the 18th to 20th week.

Micropolygyria refers to the presence of an excess of secondary and tertiary gyri with the surface of the brain resembling a prune. The isocortex is maldeveloped showing only four rather than six layers, with poor lamination and an excess of columnarization. This disorder reflects abnormal migration and, as expected, may be associated with heterotopias. The clinical picture again comprises the triad of mental retardation, seizures, and spastic quadriparesis.

The mechanism of the *Dandy-Walker malformation* is unknown. It is characterized by hypoplasia of the cerebellar vermis, a posterior fossa cyst, and, usually, hydrocephalus. It may be associated with callosal agenesis, polymicrogyria, heterotopias, and cardiovascular anomalies. The clinical picture is one of nystagmus, ataxia, and a bulging occiput.

Möbius syndrome is a developmental anomaly of the facial nerve. It is not familial. The pathology is characterized by partial or complete absence of the facial nuclei, hypoplasia of the facial nerve, and facial musculature wasting. There may be an associated gaze paresis. The disorder is usually asymmetric, and may be associated with clubfoot or a spastic diplegia.

REFERENCES

Al-Mateen M, Philipart M, Shield WD: Rett syndrome. A commonly overlooked progressive encephalopathy in girls. *Am J Dis Child* 140:761, 1986.

Bird TD, Shaw CM: Progressive myoclonus and epilepsy with dentatorubral degeneration: A clinicopathological study of the Ramsay-Hunt syndrome. *J Neurol Neurosurg Psychiatry* 41:140, 1978.

Boyer SH, et al: Cardiac aspects of Friedreich's ataxia. *Circulation* 25:493, 1962.

Critchley M, Greenfield JG: Olivopontocerebellar atrophy. *Brain* 71:343, 1948.

Dejerine J, Thomas A: L'atrophie olivo-ponto-cérébelleuse. *Nouv Icon Salpet* 13:330, 1900.

Duquette P, Murray TJ, Pleines J, et al: Multiple sclerosis in childhood: Clinical profile in 125 patients. *J Pediatr* 111:359, 1987.

Eldridge R, Denckla M: Gilles de la Tourette syndrome: Etiologic considerations. *Rev Neurol (Paris)* 142:833, 1986.

Erenberg G, Cruse RP, Rothner AD: Gilles de la Tourette syndrome. Effects of stimulant drugs. *Neurology* 35:1345, 1985.

EUROCRAT Working Group: Prevalence of neural tube defects in 16 regions of Europe, 1980–1983. *Int J Epidemiol* 16:246, 1987.

Evans OB: Pyruvate decarboxylase deficiency in subacute necrotizing encephalomyelopathy. *Arch Neurol* 38:515, 1981.

Gusella JF, Wexler NS, Connealy PM, et al: A polymorphic DNA marker genetically linked to Huntington's disease. *Nature* 306:234, 1983.

Hagberg B: Rett's syndrome. Prevalence and impact on progressive severe mental retardation in girls. *Acta Paediatr Scand* 74:405, 1985.

Hagberg B, Aicardi J, Dias K, et al: A progressive syndrome of autism, dementia, ataxia, and loss of purposeful hand use in girls: Rett's syndrome: Report of 35 cases. *Ann Neurol* 14:471, 1983.

Hoogerbrugge PM, Suzuki K, Sukuki K, et al: Donor-derived cells in the central nervous system of twitcher mice after bone marrow transplantation. *Science* 239:1035, 1988.

Jervis GA: Huntington's chorea in childhood. *Arch Neurol* 9:244, 1963.

Konigsmark BW, Weiner LP: The olivopontocerebellar atrophies. A review. *Medicine* 49:227, 1970.

Larsen PD, Osborn AG: Computed tomographic evaluation of corpus callosum agenesis and associated malformations. *J Comput Tomogr* 6:225, 1982.

Leckman JF, Ort S, Caruso KA, et al: Rebound phenomena in Tourette syndrome after withdrawal of clonidine. *Arch Gen Psychiatr* 43:1168, 1986.

Leigh D: Subacute necrotizing encephalomyelopathy in an infant. *J Neurol Neurosurg Psychiatry* 14:216, 1951.

Markham CH, Knox JW: Observations in Huntington's chorea. *J Pediatr* 67:46, 1965.

Markowitz M, Gordis L: *Rheumatic Fever*. Philadelphia, WB Saunders, 1972, p 147.

Martin JB, Gusella JF: Huntington's disease. Pathogenesis and management. *N Engl J Med* 315:1267, 1986.

Menkes JH: *Textbook of Child Neurology*. Philadelphia, Lea & Febiger, 1985.

Moore K: *The Developing Human. Clinically Oriented Embryology*, 3rd edition. Philadelphia, WB Saunders, 1982.

Moser HW, Moser AE, Singh, I, et al: Adrenolenkodystrophy: Survey of 303 cases: Biochemistry, diagnosis, and therapy. *Ann Neurol* 16:628, 1984.

Myrianthopoulos NC, Melnick M: Studies in neural tube defects. I. Epidemiological and etiologic aspects. *Am J Med Genet* 26:783, 1987.

Nikoskelainen EK, Savontaus ML, Wanne OP, et al: Lebev's hereditary optic neuroretinopathy, a maternally inherited disease. A genealogic study in four pedigrees. *Arch Ophthalmol* 105:665, 1987.

Opitz JM, Reynolds JF, Spano LM, et al (eds): *The Rett Syndrome*. New York, Alan R. Liss, 1986.

Pauls DL, Towbin KE, Leckman JF, et al: Gilles de la Tourette syndrome and obsessive-compulsive disorder. *Arch Gen Psychiatr* 43:1180, 1986.

Plaitakis A, et al: Neurologic disorders associated with deficiency of glutamate dehydrogenase. *Ann Neurol* 15:144, 1984.

Robinson BH, DeMeirleir L, Glerum M, et al: Clinical presentation of mitochondrial respiratory chain defects in NADH coenzyme Q reductase and cytochrome oxidase: Clues to pathogenesis of Leigh disease. *J Pediatr* 110:216, 1987.

Sadovnick AD, Baird PA, Hall JG, et al: Use of genetic counselling services for neural tube defects. *Am J Med Genet* 26:811, 1987.

Sobue I, et al: Effects of thyrotropin-releasing hormone on ataxia in spinocerebellar degenerations. In: *Spinocerebellar Degenerations*. Tokyo, University of Tokyo Press, 1978.

Stumpf DA: The inherited ataxias. *Neurol Clin* 3:47, 1985.

Stumpf DA: Friedreich's Ataxia III. Mitochondrial malic enzyme deficiency. *Neurology* 32:221, 1982.

Suzuki Y, Suzuki K: Krabbe's globoid cell leukodystrophy: Deficiency of galactocerebrosidase in serum, leukocytes and fibroblasts. *Science* 171:73, 1971.

Tolmie JL, McNay M, Stephenson JB, et al: Microcephaly: Genetic counselling and antenatal diagnosis after birth of an affected child. *Am J Med Genet* 27:583, 1987.

Neurologic Disorders of the Neonate

4

Some acute neurologic diseases of the newborn period or rather with those aspects of neurologic disease that present acutely in that period are discussed in Section 4, Neonatology. We will, therefore, emphasize the long-term consequences of those disorders, and then discuss several common neurologic problems of the first year of life.

The age at which an infant is evaluated provides critical information, since some infants may seem hypertonic, but become less so in time. This is especially notable for very low birth weight infants who at 2 years (corrected age) may be diagnosed as having spastic cerebral palsy, but are normal at 5 years of age (Kitchen et al, 1987).

While it is dangerous to consider cerebral palsy as a "diagnosis" in the proper neurologic sense, nonetheless, certain syndromes of infants resulting from troubled gestations, labors, and deliveries are seen frequently enough in clinical practice to merit discussion.

Spastic Diplegia

The hallmark is bilateral spastic involvement of the legs, with tight heel cords, brisk deep tendon reflexes at the knees and ankles, and Babinski sign. In the infant, stroking adduction and internal rotation of the legs may be seen upon suspension under the arms (a posture suggesting upper motor neuron dysfunction, also known as "scissoring"). Sphincter disturbances are unusual. Spastic diplegia may present quite floridly before the end of the first year of life, or may not be recognized until well on in the first decade.

The differential diagnosis includes spinal cord pathology (distinguished from spastic diplegia by the sensory findings inherent in cord disease), hydrocephalus involving the lateral ventricles (distinguished from spastic diplegia by the frequency of urinary symptoms in hydrocephalus, as well as headache in acute cases), and a parasagittal mass. Spastic diplegia is often associated with normal cognitive function, or at least the lack of severe retardation commonly seen in other syndromes. The question of an over-representation of milder forms of cognitive dysfunction in this group has not been satisfactorily settled. Seizures are usually not a significant problem.

Spastic Quadriplegia

This is clearly the syndrome most often associated with "cerebral palsy." These children have spastic involvement of the extremities, and often of the orobuccal musculature, rendering swallowing and talking difficult. Mental retardation and seizure disorders are common in this group, and active multidisciplinary management by orthopedic surgeons, physical and occupational therapists, and neurologists is usually indicated. The association between this syndrome, spastic diplegia, and the pathologic conditions of periventricular leukomalacia remains to be elucidated.

Spastic Hemiplegia

This syndrome is usually not documented medically until 15–18 months of life, although observant parents will have made the observation of asymmetric use of the extremities as early as 4–6 months (Cohen and Duffner, 1981). The disorder begins as a flaccid disuse and hemiparesis, which gradually becomes spastic. Most children learn to walk, usually after the 18th month of life (90% of those who eventually walk do so by the third birthday). Tizard et al (1954) demonstrated cortical sensory abnormalities in roughly two-thirds of patients with this syndrome; seizures occur in 50% of these children and, therefore, the diagnosis warrants an EEG to assess the individual risk of seizures. While the classic observation has been that the hemisphere involved did not predict intellectual or cognitive outcome, a more recent study has indicated a poorer prognosis for language development in those children with right hemisphere involvement (Nass et al, 1985).

Extrapyramidal or Choreoathetoid Cerebral Palsy

While this syndrome was classically associated with those children who suffered kernicterus and, therefore, had preferential injury of the basal ganglia, recent studies have indicated that low birth weight is a more important contemporary risk factor (Hagberg et al, 1975; Kyllerman et al, 1982). This is based on the essential disappearance of kernicterus in the developed world, as well as the increased survival of low birth weight infants. The syndrome is clinically similar to other choreoathetoid disorders with the frequent co-occurrence of dystonic and spastic elements as well (see pp. 707). Kyllerman et al (1982) indicate that over two-thirds of children with this syndrome have IQs in excess of 90; their striking movement disorder and associated dysarthria often lead to an erroneous impression of underlying retardation. Walking is delayed in this group, with the mean age of independent ambulation occurring around 2½ years. The persistence of the asymmetric tonic neck response is a poor prognostic sign for the development of independent ambulation. Contemporary management includes consideration of augmentative communication strategies (communication boards, microcomputer-assisted devices).

Hypotonic Cerebral Palsy

While most children with one of the above-noted syndromes begin life significantly hypotonic, a small group persist in their diminished tone beyond the second birthday. The differential diagnosis at this stage includes disorders of muscle and neuromuscular transmission, as well as spinal muscular atrophy. In contradistinction to those disease processes, however, these children demonstrate increased deep tendon reflexes, sometimes leading to consideration of the leukodystrophies as an alternative diagnosis, but the nerve conduction times are not altered. As these children age, they frequently manifest ataxia and dysmetria; a small group will also demonstrate extrapyramidal movement disorders. Seizures are unusual in this group; one-third are retarded. (Approaches to orthopedic management of cerebral palsy is discussed on pp. 1298).

OTHER SYNDROMES OF THE NEWBORN

Spinal Cord Trauma

Spinal cord trauma, usually as a result of a difficult breech delivery, is much less common in contemporary practice given the advances in obstetrics over the past two decades.

Facial Nerve Palsy

This is the most common traumatic injury of the cranial nerves among newborns, occurring in about 0.25% of newborns according to one series (McHugh et al, 1969). The degree of paresis may be complete loss of function of all three branches of the facial nerve, or weakness limited to a few branches. Recovery may begin within a week or it may take as long as several months. The cause is usually compression of the facial nerve distal to the stylomastoid foramen by the maternal sacral prominence; forceps injuries also occur. Although electrodiagnostic procedures may be able to predict outcome accurately, it has been our experience that they are sufficiently uncomfortable so that the event is unpleasant for physician, parent, and child alike. Treatment is conservative, with taping of the eyelid during sleep and methylcellulose eyedrops to avoid corneal injury.

Branchial Plexus Injury

Erb palsy, the injury of the fifth and sixth cervical roots, usually occurs after a traction injury of the plexus during a breech delivery or in the presence of significant cephalopelvic disproportion. The injury is usually edema and hemorrhage secondary to the stretching, rather than complete avulsion. The clinical presentation is usually paralysis of the deltoid, spinati, biceps, and brachioradialis on the affected side leading to wrist flexion, forearm pronation, elbow extension, and shoulder adduction and internal rotation. The biceps reflex is absent or diminished with respect to the triceps; electromyography and nerve conduction studies in children 2–3 weeks of age will document the localization, and help in the prognosis, as truly isolated lesions of the upper plexus generally have a good outcome. Therapy is conservative, with range-of-motion exercises and avoidance of immobilization.

A lower plexus lesion, Klumpke palsy, is less common, as its outcome is generally less favorable. The injury is also usually a result of traction; hence "yanking" a child by the arm may produce this if the force is sufficient, which must be kept in mind in suspicious circumstances. The clinical presentation is one of weakness of the wrist flexors and intrinsic muscles of the hand. A Horner syndrome is not uncommon, secondary to co-occurring cervical sympathetic nerve injury. (It is noteworthy that congenital or early Horner syndromes are associated with iris hypopigmentation.)

Torticollis

"Wryneck" is produced by asymmetric contraction of one sternocleidomastoid muscle. The head deviates toward the injured or dysfunctional muscle, while the chin points in the opposite direction (thus, the child faces away from the injured muscle). The most usual pediatric presentation is congenital, due to injury of the sternocleidomastoid during delivery, with hemorrhage and fibrosis of the muscle. Therapy is usually conservative (physical therapy and massage); surgical therapy should be avoided.

Acquired torticollis must be distinguished from a head tilt secondary to a fourth nerve palsy (the latter may be difficult to ascertain without careful examination of the eye for intortion/extortion on movement). Both may be associated with infratentorial tumors and, therefore, imaging of the posterior fossa is mandatory.

REFERENCES

Cohen ME, Duffner PK: Prognostic indicators in hemiparetic cerebral palsy. *Ann Neurol* 9:353, 1981.

Hagberg B, Hagberg G, Olow I: The changing panorama of cerebral palsy in Sweden, 1954-1970. II: Analysis of the various syndromes. *Acta Paediatr Scand* 64:193, 1975.

Hagberg B, Hagberg, G, Olow I: The changing panorama of cerebral palsy in Sweden. IV: Epidemiological trends 1959-1978. *Acta Paediatr Scand* 73:433, 1984.

Kitchen WH, Ford GW, Rickards AL, et al: Children of birth weight < 1000 g: Changing outcome between 2 and 5 years. *J Pediatr* 110:283, 1987.

Kyllerman M, et al: Dyskinetic cerebral palsy I: Clinical categories, associated neurologic abnormalities and incidences. *Acta Paediatr Scand* 71:543, 1982.

McHugh HE, Sowden KA, Levitt MN: Facial paralysis and muscle agenesis in the newborn. *Arch Otolaryngol* 89:131, 1969.

Nass R, Koch DA, Janowsky J, et al: Differential effects of left versus right brain injury on intelligence. Child Neurology Society Meeting, October 1985. *Ann Neurol* 18:393, 1985.

Tizard JP, Paine RS, Crothers B: Disturbances of sensation in children with hemiplegia. *JAMA* 155:628, 1954.

Autoimmune and Postinfectious Disorders

5

Certain disorders of the nervous system are thought to be mediated or potentiated by a dysfunctional response of the body's normal immune mechanism. Some diseases that are considered as "autoimmune," even though definitive evidence is not yet available, are included here. Others that are clearly autoimmune (e.g., myasthenia gravis) or likely to be autoimmune (e.g., Sydenham chorea), are discussed elsewhere in more appropriate sections.

POSTINFECTIOUS AND POSTVACCINAL VASCULOMYELINOPATHY

Definition

This condition, sometimes referred to as acute disseminated encephalomyelitis, was first recognized in the 18th century. It is usually a monophasic illness, with a rapid onset and course. Although slowly progressive, chronic and recurrent forms have all been reported, they are rather rare.

Basic Science and Natural History

The preceding illness may be one of the major viral exanthems of childhood, or may be a rather mild viral syndrome. After a latent period of 7–21 days, the child develops clouding of the sensorium. Seizures are common in some forms (postmeasles and postrubella). Ataxia is seen commonly in postvaricella, but rarely in other forms. Cranial nerve signs and involuntary choreoathetoid movements are reported in roughly 10% of cases, regardless of the precipitating illness.

Diagnosis

Peripheral nerve involvement, clinically silent but readily demonstrated with electromyography and nerve conduction studies, helps to distinguish troublesome cases with subtle preceding illnesses from multiple sclerosis (an uncommon disorder in childhood).

The CSF usually displays a pleocytosis (mononuclear) with elevated protein but normal glucose. IgG is often elevated; oligoclonal banding may be detected in one-quarter to one-third of cases.

Imaging reveals lesions in the white matter that are lucent on CT scan, as well as occasional cortical mantle lesions.

Treatment

Treatment is conservative and supportive, although some have advocated administration of steroids or ACTH. Plasmapheresis also has been reported to be of benefit in some cases.

Acute Hemorrhagic Leukoencephalitis

The illness also occurs after an infection, usually a nonspecific viral syndrome. It is characterized by the rapid evolution of stupor and alteration of the mental status, with frequent focal neurologic findings (hemiparesis, aphasia). The CSF reveals a lymphocytic pleocytosis and elevated protein. There is a peripheral leukocytosis also. The disease can be quite serious, and may be attenuated by early and prompt therapy with steroids. Pathologic examination reveals a necrotizing vasculitic process with preferential involvement of small veins and capillaries, and attendant small hemorrhages.

Landry-Guillain-Barré-Strohl Syndrome

This disorder, also known as acute infectious polyneuritis, while not unequivocally autoimmune in nature, is included in this section by general convention. The clinical history usually includes a preceding viral illness (often respiratory), followed in 3–7 days by mild sensory disturbance in the feet. The patient then experiences a progressive, ascending weakness which is usually distal, but may be proximal in about 15% of patients. The paralysis may involve the respiratory muscles, and special care should be taken to monitor the vital capacity carefully. The patient is areflexic, and demonstrates diminished position, vibration, pain, and touch modalities progressively. Autonomic involvement, with cardiac rhythm disturbances and chaotic blood pressures, may be seen. Within 7–10 days of onset of the neurologic syndrome, a marked elevation of the CSF protein without a pleocytosis (albuminocytologic dissociation) may be seen. The disease is usually maximal by the 14th day; recovery is usually over 2–4 months, although longer periods have been described. The outcome in children is usually good.

A variant of this disease, in which a progressive ophthalmoplegia and ataxia with an associated areflexia is seen, may occur after a viral illness. The toes are often upgoing, and while CSF protein may be elevated, a pleocytosis is also seen. The relationship between this variant and brain stem encephalitis is controversial.

A relapsing form of the disease, described in adults, has also been seen in children.

Bell Palsy

An acute paralysis of the seventh cranial nerve after a viral illness, with frequent loss of taste on the anterior two-thirds of the tongue on the involved side, is well-recognized. The evolution is fairly rapid, and recovery usually occurs within 2 months. The differential diagnosis of an isolated peripheral seventh nerve palsy includes tumor, diabetes mellitus, sarcoid, hypertension, postinfectious and postvaccinal palsies, otic herpes zoster, and histiocytosis X. Treatment no longer includes consideration of decompression of the nerve, which is of no demonstrable benefit in children. Steroid therapy, if introduced early in the illness, may attenuate the course somewhat. Conservative therapy to prevent corneal injury (methylcellulose eyedrops and patching the eye at night) should be used as well.

"Slow Virus" and Chronic Viral Infections of Childhood

Definition

Creutzfeldt-Jakob disease is a slow virus infection of the CNS that leads to pyramidal and extrapyramidal signs, dementia, and death.

Epidemiology

The disorder is indistinguishable from Kuru, and is transmitted by inoculation of brain tissue from affected humans. In the case of Kuru, the epidemic in New Guinea ceased when ingestion of human brain was discontinued. In the United States, at least four cases resulted from growth hormone derived from human pituitaries.

Natural History

The latency between exposure and onset of disease may be as long as 18 years. The earliest symptoms are mental disturbance, progressing to dementia within a few months. The entire brain is affected, so that pyramidal, extrapyramidal, and cerebellar signs may be present.

Diagnosis

The history of exposure and relentless downhill clinical course suggest the diagnosis. Confirmation comes from finding noninflammatory spongiform changes and gliosis on biopsy or autopsy.

Treatment

Treatment is supportive only.

Prevention

The greatest care is needed in handling the tissues or instruments or needles in contact with infected brain and, perhaps, other tissues.

Subacute Sclerosing Panencephalitis (SSPE)

Definition

Subacute sclerosing panencephalitis (SSPE) is a very rare complication of measles characterized by mental deterioration, myoclonic seizures and, eventually, death. It can follow immunization with live virus vaccine, but much less frequently than after natural infection.

Basic Science

This complication of measles is thought to represent a persistence of the virus in an incomplete form in brain tissue. The reasons for susceptibility of a given individual are not known, although partial C4 deficiency has been associated with SSPE (Rittner et al, 1984).

Epidemiology

This grave complication occurs in only about 1/100,000 cases of natural measles. The risk is greater if measles occurs in the first year of life. (The last six cases seen at The Children's Hospital, Boston, were acquired in South America or the Caribbean basin.)

Natural History

The signs of SSPE can appear at most any age, but are most common at 8–14 years. School failure is an early sign, accompanied by emotional lability and loss of higher cerebral functions. Later, myoclonic jerks that may become generalized are seen. Finally, the child becomes rigid and immobile.

Diagnosis

The onset of symptoms may occur many years after the measles infection, and may be insidious, with behavioral, motor, or intellectual impairment (average age is 7 years). The EEG has a striking periodicity (5–15 seconds with correlated bursts and suppression). The spinal fluid may show elevated globulins with measles complement fixing or hemagglutinating antibodies.

Treatment

Treatment is supportive only. Antiviral agents have not been found effective, nor has immunosuppression with steroids.

Prognosis

The prognosis is uniformly fatal, usually within 2 years of onset of symptoms.

Prevention

Administration of measles vaccine reduces the likelihood of SSPE (*CDC,* 1977).

Rubella Panencephalitis

A disease similar to SSPE and with a similar course and outcome has now been reported in at least 10 boys suffering from congenital or acquired rubella. Symptoms appear at 4–14 years after the initial infection (Menkes, 1985).

Progressive Infantile Encephalopathy (AIDS)

Definition

Although it is too soon in 1988 to know the full extent or range of course of AIDS-associated encephalopathy, enough experience has accumulated to make it evident that CNS dysfunction can be the presenting symptom and fatal consequence of HIV infection of the brain in infants.

Epidemiology

CNS dysfunction is one of the most frequent complications of AIDS in infancy. Belman et al (1988) documented manifestations of CNS infection in 61 of 68 infants and children.

Natural History

Developmental regression at the onset of HIV infection may first present as loss of motor and intellectual functions often associated with a spastic diplegia. Failure of the head to grow normally is one of the most frequent findings. The onset is in the first months of life, and may be the first or only manifestations of infection. Apathy, irritability, clumsiness, myoclonic jerks, and increased deep tendon reflexes are all characteristic. CT scan shows characteristic deep white matter calcifications.

The course is steadily progressive, with death usually associated with other manifestations of the illness, or concurrent infections with other organisms within the first 2 years.

Diagnosis

HIV serology is positive, and the organism may be isolated from CSF. Immunodeficiency need not be evident at the onset of neurologic symptoms. Pathologic examination of brain shows atrophy of cerebral white matter and subacute encephalitis. CT scans of brain during life and EEG may be abnormal, but can be normal even with advanced symptoms.

Treatment

No drugs are known to be effective, but a physician who has an affected infant should ascertain the most recent results with the new drugs under evaluation. Intravenous γ-globulin is administered monthly to help prevent and treat intercurrent infections.

Prevention

See page 678.

CASE ILLUSTRATION

A black female infant presented at 9 months of age with a 5-week history of intermittent fever and recurrent explosive yellow diarrhea. She was born after a 38-week gestation to a 26-year-old gravida 3 para 2 mother with a birth weight of 2.3 kg. The mother was an intravenous drug addict who shared a needle with the father who had been diagnosed 2 years earlier with AIDS-related complex. The mother was HIV antibody negative and hepatitis-B negative antenatally; both mother and infant were HIV-negative at 2½ months postnatally.

The infant had poor weight gain and recurrent thrush for several months. She had facial eczema and recently had regressed so that she could no longer crawl or stand with support.

On admission, her weight was 6.4 kg (less than the third percentile), length 69 cm (25th percentile), and head circumference 43 cm (less than second percentile). Temperature was 39.7°C and pulse 144/min.

She was alert but irritable, slightly jaundiced, and had a blanching erythematous maculopapular rash over the face and trunk. She had extensive oropharyngeal thrush. Breath sounds were harsh and she coughed occasionally. The liver edge was palpable at 3 cm below the costal margin.

Significant laboratory findings were a hemoglobin of 10 g, hematocrit 30, WBC 5000/mm^3 (59% polys, 4% blasts, 26% lymphs, 6% monos, 2% eos, 3% atypical lymphs). Serum electrolytes were normal, glucose 144 mg/dl, SGPT 215 U/ml, SGOT 340 U/ml, LDH 480 U/ml, CPK U/ml, bilirubin 1.1–1.0 mg/dl. Total proteins were 5.8 mg/dl. CSF proteins were 21 mg/dl, glucose 109 mg/dl. A CT scan of the head showed widening of the subarachnoid space and moderate ventricular enlargement consistent with diffuse cerebral atrophy.

All cultures for bacteria and parasites were negative. *Candida albicans* was present in the mouth. HIV antibody was found by ELISA screen and confirmed by Western blot.

She improved after hospitalization and a course of chloramphenicol. Two months later, she was readmitted because of respiratory distress and increased tone in the lower extremities, Tracheal aspirate was negative for *P. carinii,* but tracheal lavage revealed the organism. She was given trimethoprim-sulfamethoxazole and pentamidine but without improvement. She died on hospital day 10.

Autopsy revealed extensive consolidation of both lungs with giant cells consistent with *P. carinii* infection. The brain showed diffuse atrophy; panencephalitis and mineralization of small vessels were widespread.

COMMENT

This infant presumably acquired HIV infection from her drug-addicted mother who was HIV-positive by the infant's second admission at age 1 year. Both mother and infant were HIV-negative 2 months after delivery.

Tropical Spastic Paraparesis

Definition

Tropical spastic paraparesis is a progressive paralytic disorder that affects principally the lower limbs.

Basic Science

Tropical spastic paraparesis is one of the myelopathies that has been linked to retrovirus HTLV-I. In 1985, French workers found that 60% of patients on Martinique had antibodies to HTLV-I, whereas only 4% of controls had evidence of infection. These observations have been extended and confirmed so that the linkage of HTLV-I and tropical spastic paraparesis is accepted.

Epidemiology

The disorder is said to be "common" in the tropics and, perhaps, in Japan. It may occur elsewhere and has not been recognized.

Natural History

The major findings are progressive weakness, atrophy, paralysis, then contractures of lower limbs. The upper body is less affected and the brain is spared.

Diagnosis

The diagnosis depends on serologic evidence of HTLV-I antibody. The virus has not been isolated from these patients (as of mid-1987).

Treatment

Treatment is supportive only.

Prevention

It is not clear how this virus is spread, hence, prevention is not possible. No vaccines are available.

REFERENCES

Belman AL, Diamond G, Dickson D, et al: Pediatric acquired immunodeficiency syndrome. Neurologic syndromes. *Am J Dis Child* 142:29, 1988.

Brown P, Gajdusek DC, Gibbs CJ, et al: Potential epidemic of Creutzfeldt-Jakob disease from human growth hormone therapy. *N Engl J Med* 313:728, 1985.

CDC: Subacute sclerosing panencephalitis and measles. *MMWR* 26:309, 1977.

Davis SL, Halsted CC, Levy N, et al: Acquired immune deficiency syndrome presenting as progressive infantile encephalopathy. *J Pediatr* 110:884, 1987.

Duffy P, Wolf J, Collins G, et al: Person-to-person transmission of Creutzfeldt-Jakob disease. *N Engl J Med* 290:692, 1974.

Gadjusek DC: Unconventional viruses and the origin and disappearance of Kuru. *Science* 197:943, 1977.

Johnson RT: Myelopathies and retroviral infections. *Ann Neurol* 21:113, 1987.

Marx JL: Leukemia virus linked to nerve disease. In: Research News. *Science* 236:1059, 1987.

McArthur JC: Neurologic manifestations of AIDS. *Medicine* 66:407, 1987.

Menkes JH: *Textbook of Child Neurology*. Philadelphia, Lea & Febiger, 1985, pp. 390.

Rittner C, et al: Partial C4 deficiency in subacute sclerosing panencephalitis. *Immunogenetics* 20:407, 1984.

Nutritional Diseases 6

Nutritional disease states, resulting either from insufficient intake of necessary food substances or from impaired absorption and utilization of those substances, are a frequent cause of neurologic disease in the adult. There are also nutritionally induced disorders of the nervous system in the child that are quite important worldwide, although relatively uncommon in North America.

Infantile Beriberi

This disorder, which presents between 2 and 5 months of age, is seen in infants who have not yet been weaned. It is an acute disease which is predominantly cardiovascular in its symptomatology, but also may show bulbar and cortical signs (seizures, ophthalmoplegia, nystagmus, facial spasm, and aphonia have all been

Table 12.13
Malabsorptive States Associated with Neurologic Disease

Defect	Substance	Neurologic Signs
Gastric lesion		
Pernicious anemia	Vitamin B_{12}	Combined systems degeneration
Intrinsic factor deficiency	Vitamin B_{12}	Combined systems degeneration
Partial gastrectomy	Vitamin B_{12}	Combined systems degeneration
	Vitamin D	Myopathy
Small intestine		
Proximal	Vitamin D	Myopathy
Distal	Vitamin B_{12}	Combined systems degeneration
Blind loop	Vitamin B_{12}	Combined systems degeneration
Miscellaneous congenital	Neutral amino acids	Hartnup disease
	Methionine	"Oast-house" urine
	Folic acid	Retardation, seizures, ataxia
	Tryptophan	"Blue diaper"
Chylomicron formation	Fat-soluble vitamins	Bassen-Kornzweig
Villous infiltration	Fats	CNS Whipple
Cystic fibrosis	Fat-soluble vitamins, especially Vitamin E	Posterior column degeneration
Intrinsic liver disease	Fat-soluble vitamins, especially Vitamin E	Posterior column degeneration

From Adams & Victor, 1985.

described). It is seen in infants of mothers without beriberi, and mothers with beriberi have been reported to bear normal children, which has led to the suggestion that the disease may be due to a toxic factor in breast milk (Adams et al, 1985). No data exist regarding levels of thiamine in the breast milk of mothers of affected infants. The ailment responds dramatically to the administration of thiamine. Adams and Victor have reported cases that at autopsy appear similar to Wernicke encephalopathy (Adams et al, 1985).

Protein-Calorie Malnutrition

Protein-calorie malnutrition (see also pp. 87) may be divided into two clinical syndromes, which may overlap in some instances: kwashiorkor and marasmus. Kwashiorkor occurs in infants up to the time of weaning and consists of edema and/or ascites (secondary to hypoalbuminemia), depigmentation and loss of hair, and profound growth retardation. If these infants are rescued, they often present with motor signs of spasticity, rigidity, and tremor in the early stages of recovery. Marasmus is seen in infants already weaned, and consists of cachexia, irritability, and growth retardation (see pp. 88).

Brain weight itself is not diminished in these syndromes, but there is evidence suggesting deficient dendritic branching and reduced myelination. Most studies indicate that the majority of infants rescued recover normal intellectual functioning, but all studies indicate a significant minority with permanent retardation. The age by which recovery must occur to ensure a better neurologic prognosis is not clear.

Malabsorptive States

Table 12.13 demonstrates those medical conditions associated with defective absorption of vitamins, amino acids, or fats that produce neurologic disease.

REFERENCES

Adams RD, Victor M: *Principles of Neurology,* 3rd edition. New York, McGraw-Hill, 1985, p. 234.

Cerebrovascular Disease

7

Definition

Cerebrovascular disorders are a heterogeneous group of diseases that affect the CNS secondary to primary pathology within the blood vessels, usually arteries. In adults, the neural consequences of atherosclerotic arteriopathy constitute the most common neurologic disease. This disease is quite rare in children and, hence, cerebrovascular disease is not common. Nevertheless, congenital lesions such as arteriovenous malformations, fibromuscular dysplasia, or the vasculopathy of tuberous sclerosis may cause artery thrombosis with occlusion and subsequent infarction. In addition, inflammation within the vessel wall, a condition called vasculitis or arteritis, may cause occlusion of the lumen. Finally, emboli from heart or great vessels may lodge in intracranial vessels and cause stroke.

Basic Science

The brain is supplied by two parallel systems that communicate with each other in a basal anastomosis called the circle of Willis. The anterior or carotid system supplies about 80% of the CNS and, hence, constitutes 80% of the blood flow. The other 20% is carried by the vertebrobasilar or posterior circulation.

Nervous system dysfunction in cerebrovascular disease is due to tissue ischemia. It is now known that this dysfunction is graded rather than all-or-none. When tissue perfusion is reduced, the extraction of oxygen increases without neural dysfunction. This is asymptomatic clinically, although sophisticated brain imaging by positron emission tomography (PET) can identify the abnormality. As the perfusion is further compromised, the neurons lose the ability to release neurotransmitters, resulting in clinical dysfunction. The neurons are not dead at this time and, if normal perfusion is restored, they return to normal functioning. The tissue is "stunned." Further reduction in perfusion results in the inability to maintain membrane ion gradients, with subsequent irreversible death of the cell. This chapter will discuss the various causes of cerebrovascular disease.

Natural History

The brain may be subject to *emboli* that originate in the heart. This usually occurs in the setting of congenital cardiac disease, rheumatic valvulitis, or bacterial endocarditis. The emboli usually lodge in one of the branches of the middle cerebral artery, giving rise to a hemiparesis, hemisensory loss and various disorders of cognitive function.

Fat embolism may occur after fractures of the pelvis or long bones. The neurologic deficit is seen with a petechial rash involving the upper trunk, and tachypnea from multiple pulmonary infarcts. The emboli usually occur within 2 days of the fracture.

Diagnosis

Cerebral hemorrhage usually presents as an acute onset of a profound neurologic deficit with headache, nausea, and, often, vomiting. The patient may have a decreased level of consciousness. A CT scan is diagnostic. A search for possible causes should proceed at a measured pace so as to avoid added stress.

Treatment

Rest and control of seizures is essential. Subsequent treatment is preventive and consists of anticoagulation with heparin followed by coumadin. In the setting of bacterial endocarditis, localized bacterial arteritis accompanies the embolus, with subsequent fragility of the vessel wall. Hence, anticoagulation is contraindicated because of the risk of cerebral hemorrhage.

Other Conditions Associated with Cerebral Ischemia

Stroke may accompany *carotid or vertebral artery dissections*. The pathophysiology of this condition is unclear, but it is thought that trauma, even of a mild degree, causes a small intimal tear in the artery, with subsequent tracking of blood under arterial pressure into a space within the media of the vessel. As a result, the true lumen of the vessel is compromised and stroke may occur secondary to profound stenosis or artery-to-artery embolism. The clinical picture is one of the sudden onset of pain involving the neck and face, followed within hours by a stroke that may be in the anterior (carotid dissection) or the posterior circulation (vertebral dissection). If the dissection involves the carotid artery, an ipsilateral 12th nerve palsy and Horner syndrome may be seen and indicate nerve dysfunction within the carotid sheath. Angiography reveals a characteristic tapering of the extracranial vessel and may even show the embolus lodged in a branch vessel further upstream. The treatment of this condition is controversial, but some have suggested anticoagulation for 6 weeks, followed by repeat angiography. If the angiogram has normalized, the anticoagulation is then stopped.

A condition in infants that is characterized by recurrent cerebral hemorrhage is called *moyamoya* disease and is seen most often in Asians. In North America, it has been seen as a result of early cranial irradiation. A family history is positive in 10% of patients. The cause is unknown. Hemorrhage tends to be intraventricular and intraparenchymal and is rarely primarily subarachnoid. The disease involves a progressive narrowing of carotids and anterior and middle cerebral arteries, with compensatory dilation of smaller arteries. The process eventually runs its course, although survivors may have subarachnoid hemorrhage from aneurysms as adults. The treatment consists of administration of aspirin and steroids, although the response is unpredictable. Revascularization surgery has given promising results in the Toronto experience (Olds et al, 1987).

Fibromuscular dysplasia is an idiopathic disorder that affects the renal, cephalic (usually extracranial carotid) and visceral arterial systems. The pathologic lesions are multifocal and are characterized by smooth muscle hyperplasia and rarefaction of the elastic tissue resulting in disorganization of the arterial wall. The neurologic disease results from local stenosis or embolus to more distal vasculature. Coincident saccular aneurysms may cause subarachnoid hemorrhage.

Migraine may be associated with permanent deficits, which are thought to result from cerebral infarction secondary to vasospasm. Nevertheless, the direct evidence for vasospasm is sparse at best. It has been shown that there exists a decrease in cerebral blood flow in classic migraine patients. However, the blood flow reductions documented have not been low enough to result consistently in permanent neural damage. It may be concluded that whereas stroke may accompany migraine, the mechanism of the infarction is unknown.

Stroke can be seen in early adulthood where it is often expressed as a familial disorder with abnormalities in lipoprotein metabolism in concert with coronary artery disease.

Homocysteinuria, an inborn error of methionine metabolism, is clinically expressed as mental retardation, ectopia lentis and a thromboembolic tendency. Blood vessels show intimal fibrosis with fraying of the elastic membranes. This vasculopathy, combined with a putative increase in platelet adhesiveness, results in multiple thromboembolic events involving cerebral, pulmonary, coronary, and renal vessels (see Section 15, Metabolism).

Clinically, this results in stroke at an early age, usually within 9 months. CT can localize the thrombosis (Schwab et al, 1987). Certain bony abnormalities are seen, such as codfish vertebrae, scoliosis, and osteoporosis. The metabolic diagnosis is made by testing the urine with a cyanide-nitroprusside reagent, or by demonstrating increased urinary homocysteine and decreased serum methionine.

BRAIN ABSCESS

Definition

A brain abscess is a localized collection of pus with surrounding inflammation within the brain substance.

Basic Science

Bacteria enter the brain via the blood stream from a distant infection, or by direct spread from a contiguous infection such as the paranasal sinus. Older children with right to left shunts associated with cyanotic congenital heart disease are most at risk of septic emboli. Cystic fibrosis patients are also at increased risk of brain abscess (Fischer et al, 1979).

The most common organisms are *Staphylococcus aureus,* anaerobic streptococci, β-hemolytic streptococci, α-hemolytic streptococci, and pneumococci. Gram-negative rods and fungi can also produce abscesses, as can protozoa such as *Entamoeba histolytica.* Multiple abscesses occur in 6% of patients.

Diagnosis

Any child with cyanotic congenital heart disease, fever, and any neurologic signs should have a CT scan as soon as possible (Fig. 12.7). Symptoms vary from the nonspecific headache and vomiting to blurred vision, and hemiparesis, depending on location of the abscess. Peripheral blood counts are of little value. Lumbar punctures are contraindicated. An EEG nearly always shows a focal slowing with phase reversals.

Treatment

Antibiotic therapy is sufficient in the early stages of an abscess. Once pus accumulates, surgical aspiration is required.

VENOUS OCCLUSIONS

Thrombosis of cerebral veins may follow infections such as meningitis or mastoiditis or may be the result of hemoconcentration as in polycythemia or profound dehydration.

The signs are those of cerebral edema including headache, stupor, and, in infants, a bulging fontanelle. If the thrombosis involves cortical veins, infarction of brain tissue may occur. Seizures are common; focal seizures which are difficult to control should always lead to the consideration of cerebral venous thrombosis as a possibility. In *cavernous sinus thrombosis,* proptosis of the eye on the affected side is likely. Local pyogenic infections of the sinuses are the most common associated findings.

Diagnosis

The diagnosis of cerebral venous thrombosis is based on clinical findings and confirmed by cerebral angiography.

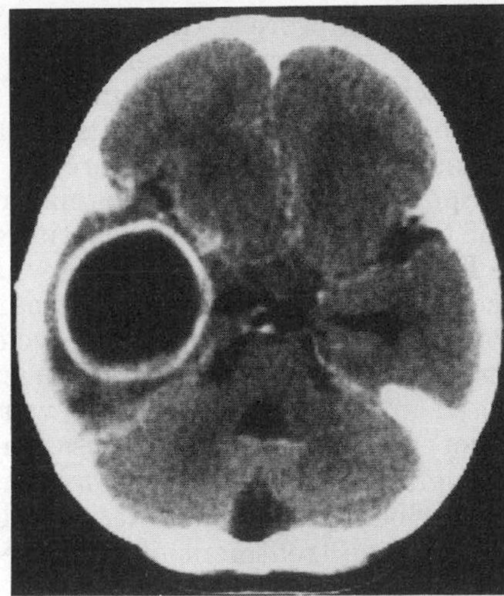

Figure 12.7. This 13-year-old boy who had congenital cyanotic heart disease (right to left shunt) presented with focal seizures and fever. His CT scan, done on admission, shows a cystic lesion in the left cerebral hemisphere enclosed by rim of tissue. Intravenous contrast had been administered before the scan; thus, the ring of the lesion is enhanced. This is typical in cases of brain abscess where the rim is hypervascular.

Treatment

Increased CSF pressure requires mannitol or dexamethasone. Localized infection requires antibiotics and surgical drainage of mastoids or sinuses.

REFERENCES

Abbott MH, Folstein SE, Abbey H, et al: Psychiatric manifestations of homocysteinuria due to cystathionine beta-synthase deficiency: Prevalence, natural history, and relationship to neurologic impairment and vitamin B6-responsiveness. *Am J Med Genet* 26:959, 1986.

Fischer EG, Schwachman H, Wepsic JG: Brain abscess and cystic fibrosis. *J Pediatr* 95:385, 1979.

Golden GS: Stroke syndromes in childhood. *Neurol Clin* 3:59, 1985.

Olds MV, Griebel RW, Hoffman HJ, et al: The surgical treatment of childhood moyamoya disease. *J Neurosurg* 66:675, 1987.

Pearl PL: Childhood stroke following intraoral trauma. *J Pediatr* 110:574, 1987.

Purvin V, Dunn DW, Edwards M: MRI and cerebral venous thrombosis. *Comput Radiol* 11:75, 1987.

Schwab SJ, Peyster RG, Grill CB: CT of cerebral venous thrombosis in a child with homocysteinuria. *Pediatr Radiol* 17:244, 1987.

Peripheral Nervous System Disorders 8

NEUROPATHIES

Most peripheral neuropathies that present in childhood are symmetric, unlike the common presentation of mononeuropathy in the adult. Diagnosis rests largely on localization of the lesion in space and time. Based on the symptoms, a lesion may be characterized as primarily neuropathic, radiculoneuropathic, or radicular. The next question is whether it appears to be a widespread process (i.e., symmetric and polyneuropathic, or isolated and mononeuropathic), and whether it is sensory, motor, or sensorimotor in its predilection, and if the damage to the nerve is demyelinating or axonal. The time course of the illness itself will prove helpful. For example, if it is known that a child presents with a chronic, symmetric, demyelinating, sensorimotor neuropathy, a proper diagnosis is virtually established; confirmation depends on examination and, perhaps, the electrodiagnostic laboratory.

Hereditary Neuropathies

Many of the neuropathic illnesses of childhood are genetically transmitted. These have been subdivided into several clinical categories based upon their localization. The hereditary motor sensory neuropathies (HMSN) and the hereditary sensory neuropathies (HSN) are two widely accepted subdivisions of this class of disease.

Hereditary Motor Sensory Neuropathies

The demyelinating motor sensory neuropathy described by Charcot and Marie, as well as by Tooth, and known by their names, is now considered to be the paradigm of the hereditory motor sensory neuropathies, and is known as type I. Type II is an axonal disease, and may actually have the burden of its pathology in the anterior horn cell. Type III is Dejerine-Sottas disease, the hypertrophic form of this illness (with striking "onion bulb" formation in the nerves). Type IV is Refsum disease, a disorder of phytanic acid metabolism, already discussed in the section on metabolic disorders. Types I and II are transmitted as autosomal dominant traits, whereas type III is autosomal recessive.

Hereditary motor sensory neuropathy type I usually presents in the second or third decade, but cases have been reported as early as the first half of the first decade. Pes cavus is the usual presenting sign, and gait disturbance the usual presenting symptom. Indeed, 30% of children presenting to The Children's Hospital, Boston, for evaluation of pes cavus have been diagnosed as having HMSN type I (Jones, personal communication). As the disease progresses, there is increasing involvement of the intrinsic muscles of the feet, and there may also be involvement of the anterior tibial compartment. The majority of these patients remain quite functional and, therefore, it behooves the physician to be positive and encouraging. Conservative management with bracing is usually the extent of orthopedic intervention.

Hereditary Sensory Neuropathies

While many subtypes of hereditary sensory neuropathy have been described to date, only type I is commonly encountered. This disorder, which has been described in autosomal recessive and dominant forms, usually presents late in the first decade of life. The underlying process is one of axonal damage to the small unmyelinated fibers that carry pain and temperature sensation. There is, therefore, a dissociated sensory loss (i.e., preferential sparing of the larger myelinated fibers that carry position, vibration, and touch sensations), which is reminiscent of a syrinx. Hence, the temporal course of the illness becomes important. Since this is a neuropathic process, the feet are involved first, and only later are the upper extremities involved. This presentation would be extremely unusual in a syrinx, which is more commonly cervical in its localization and, therefore, usually involves arm before leg.

The important feature to recognize in the management of this condition is the repetitive trauma to which the feet are subjected, and from which they are not protected because of the damage to pain-transmitting nerve fibers. That is, a vicious cycle is created wherein trauma produces painless injuries which are not protected and, therefore, become worse. Charcot joints are not uncommon in this illness, and osteomyelitis of the metatarsals from extension of a cellulitis is also well-described. Thus, constant surveillance of the feet and aggressive treatment of any infection are of paramount importance.

Spinocerebellar Degenerations

These conditions have been discussed in the section on degenerative disorders of the nervous system.

Metabolic Diseases Presenting with Neuropathies

Several rare metabolic disorders preferentially afflict the peripheral nervous system (Refsum disease, the leukodystrophies). The reader is referred to the section on metabolic disorders.

Compressive Neuropathies and Entrapment Syndromes

Compression, usually due to an ill-fitting orthopedic appliance in a thin individual, has been described in children as well as in adults. Entrapment syndromes, such as those seen in the adult, are also encountered in adolescent practice (Hallett et al, 1983).

REFERENCE

Hallett M, Dawson DM, Millender LH: *Entrapment Neuropathies*. Boston: Little, Brown & Co., 1983.

Muscle and Neuromuscular Function Disorders

9

Although myopathies, anterior horn cell diseases, or neuromuscular junction disorders constitute some of the more striking aspects of pediatric neurologic practice, they are encountered relatively infrequently. In many instances, however, they are the most acutely ill patients the neurologist sees, given their predisposition for complicating intercurrent illnesses and the frequency of respiratory involvement; therefore the common subtypes in each classification will be considered in some detail.

As already discussed, the primary issue in neurologic diagnosis is localization. Motor dysfunction may occur at any level in the nervous system, from the primary motor cortex down to the muscle itself. In other sections, cortical disorders, which can produce motor dysfunction (e.g., cerebral palsy) and spinal cord processes (cord compression, for instance) have been considered, as well as neuropathic processes. In the section below, processes affecting the anterior horn cell, the neuromuscular junction, and the muscle are discussed.

Anterior Horn Cell Disorders

Definition

The anterior horn cell may be afflicted by viral infections, such as poliomyelitis (see pp. 1045), or by a degenerative process. These disorders are designated as conditions of spinal muscular atrophy.

This group of disorders, including various subtypes which present at different ages in infancy and early childhood, is transmitted in an autosomal recessive fashion. It is associated with a loss of anterior horn cells in the spinal cord, although there are some suggestions that this may not be the location of the primary metabolic defect (Probst et al, 1981). The affected infant may have been perceived as a "quiet baby" during gestation, and quickening may have occurred late. If the afflicted child represents the mother's first child, the lack of any standard of comparison may thwart the utility of this observation. The infant may present in the neonatal period with arthrogryposis (the most severely affected, as the lack of muscle tone in utero produces contractures), or, more commonly, as severely hypotonic. The infant is usually areflexic, but early in the course of the illness a few scattered deep tendon reflexes may be present. Fasciculations, and fibrillations of the tongue, may be noted. With time, the muscles of respiration become involved, and diaphragmatic breathing becomes prominent. There is no involvement of smooth muscle, sensation, or intellect. Severely affected infants diagnosed shortly after birth rarely survive beyond the first birthday; later, diagnosis is compatible with longer survival. A related subtype, Wohlfart-Kugelberg-Welander disease, presents later in the first decade and is not inconsistent with survival into adulthood. An autosomal dominant form has been described. Death in all forms of spinal muscular atrophy is usually due to respiratory insufficiency.

Diagnosis

The diagnosis is confirmed by electromyography/nerve conduction studies, which demonstrate denervation without sensory involvement, and muscle biopsy, which shows evidence of denervation atrophy. The muscle biopsy early in the first year of life may be similar to intrinsic muscle disease, and the creatine phosphokinase also may be elevated to the range of 300–500 units at early stages.

Neuromuscular Junction Disorders

Disordered transmission across the neuromuscular junction is an uncommon cause of motor dysfunction in the child. The relevant processes include myasthenia gravis (properly considered as an autoimmune disease but included here as it most frequently presents as a neuromuscular disorder) and toxic effects from bacteria *(Clostridium tetani* and *C. botulinum),* reptile and arachnid venoms, and antibiotic blockade. Myasthenia gravis will be discussed as a paradigm.

Myasthenia Gravis

Definition

Myasthenia gravis is an autoimmune disease characterized by sustained production of antibodies to the nicotinic acetylcholine receptor at the neuromuscular junction.

Three conditions must be considered in clinical pediatric practice: neonatal, congenital, and juvenile myasthenia.

Basic Science

Myasthenia results from blockage of transmission of nerve impulses at some of the neuromuscular junctions. The problem is a reduction in acetylcholine receptors because of the discrete (and reversible) loss of receptors from circulating antibodies. Antibodies directed against the receptors can be demonstrated in the serum of about 80% of patients. Presumably, the receptor site that accepts acetylcholine is blocked by the antibody.

Among effective medications are anticholinesterase agents, such as pyridostigmine bromide (Mestinon), and immunosuppressive agents, such as prednisone and cyclosporine.

Neonatal myasthenia is a transient condition seen in roughly one-seventh of the infants of myasthenic mothers. It represents passive transmission of acetylcholine receptor antibodies from mother to child. The onset is usually 24–72 hours after birth, and the usual presentation is bulbar weakness (weak suck, cry, and swallow). Half the infants are hypotonic as well.

The duration of the illness is up to 5 weeks. The severe cases respond to acetylcholinesterase inhibitors; severity of illness is not correlated with acetylcholine antibody titers (Lefvert et al, 1983).

Congenital myasthenia presents in an infant with no maternal history of myasthenia gravis, and is probably not an autoimmune process, but rather represents structural or ultrastructural anomalies of the neuromuscular junction. Five subtypes have been noted to date: (1) a sporadic form that is a congenital deficiency of acetylcholine esterase; (2) an autosomal recessive defect in acetylcholine resynthesis; (3) an autosomal recessive defect in acetylcholine mobilization; (4) an autosomal dominant abnormally-prolonged open-time of acetylcholine-ion channels; (5) a familial form of unclear inheritance with a decreased number of receptors and distorted endplate morphology.

As expected, this population is variable in its presentation. The majority of cases present before the second birthday, and many had decreased fetal movements. They present with bulbar symptoms, but these are not as severe as those in children with neonatal myasthenia. Spontaneous remissions have been noted in some forms, but the usual course is lifelong and poorly responsive to treatment with inhibitors of acetylcholine esterase (Kuban, personal communication).

Juvenile myasthenia is fundamentally a female disorder (estimates on sex ratios vary, with figures between 2:1 and 6:1 cited). The presentation is usually in the brain stem, as noted in Table 12.14 (Millichap and Dodge, 1960). About half of all patients experience one or more remissions in their illness. A significant minority have associated autoimmune diseases (juvenile rheumatoid arthritis, juvenile-onset diabetes mellitus, thyroid disease).

Table 12.14
Clinical Features of Juvenile Myasthenia Gravis[1]

	Cases
Ptosis	32/35
Diplopia	30/35
Facial weakness	29/35
Dysphonia	29/35
Arm weakness	29/35
Leg weakness	29/35
Chewing weakness	22/35
External ophthalmoplegia	18/35
Respiratory difficulties	12/35

[1]Data from Millichap and Dodge, 1960.

Diagnosis

The diagnosis is made by history (variable fatiguing weakness, worse over the course of the day), and confirmed by edrophonium examination (0.2 mg/kg administered intravenously, up to a dose of 10 mg, with ECG monitoring and atropine 0.01 mg/kg at the ready); resolution of index signs with edrophonium is compelling evidence for the diagnosis of myasthenia. The presence of acetylcholine receptor antibodies is not universal; electromyographic studies with single-fiber technique also may be useful if readily available (Cornblath, 1986).

Treatment

Symptomatic treatment with acetylcholinesterase inhibitors may be helpful if the case is mild. More severe cases may respond to steroids (1–2 mg/kg prednisone daily); this treatment is associated with a nearly obligate decline in muscle strength during the early phases of treatment, and thus, the patient should be carefully monitored, preferably as an inpatient. For more recalcitrant cases, immunosuppressive therapies (cyclosporine), plasmapheresis, or thymectomy may be considered. While the cumulative 15-year remission rate with the last-mentioned technique is rather good, the experience with juveniles is limited (Drachman, 1987).

Myopathies

The primary muscle diseases of childhood may be considered under the following categories: congenital myopathies, the muscular dystrophies, and the myotonic disorders.

Congenital Myopathies

As discussed above, the floppy infant may have an underlying disorder of muscle. Although such infants are usually floppy, they have preserved deep tendon reflexes; the muscle enzymes may not show striking elevation and the electromyogram may also be unrevealing. Muscle biopsy may show any of several subtle derangements of architecture, and these syndromes are distinguished on the basis of their histology.

The commonly encountered congenital myopathies are presented in Table 12.15.

Central Core Disease

Definition

Central core disease is a congenital, nonprogressive myopathy characterized by proximal muscle weakness and hypotonia.

Basic Science

The microscopic appearance is characteristic. The central muscle cores lack oxidative enzyme and phosphorylase reactivity (Shuaib et al, 1987).

Table 12.15
Clinical and Pathologic Features of Congenital Myopathies

Type	Clinical Features	Pathology
Nemaline	Autosomal dominant (AD) Autosomal recessive (AR) Skeletal abnormalities Respiratory difficulty	Rod bodies of Z-band
Central core	AD or sporadic Congenital hip dislocation	Central area of muscle fiber without mitochondria
Centronuclear (Myotubular)	AD with variable penetrance	Central nuclei
Multicore (Minicore)	Nonprogressive, proximal	Multiple areas of fiber disruption
Mitochondrial	Quite variable: MELAS, MERRF, and Kearns-Sayre Syndromes	Ragged red fibers

Epidemiology

Central core disease was first described by Shy and Magee in 1956, and as of 1987 about 75 cases have been described in the English literature. The disorder is familial and may be autosomal dominant or sporadic.

Natural History

Most cases present as "floppy babies" in infancy with generalized hypotonia and proximal muscle weakness. Deep tendon reflexes are reduced or absent. Associated skeletal defects include congenital dislocated hips and, in older children, kyphoscoliosis and pes cavus. However, many patients do not have myopathic features, but present with cardiac abnormalities (arrhythmias and mitral valve prolapse) or malignant hyperthermia. The latter condition was present in all 11 patients reported by Shuaib et al (1987).

Diagnosis

The diagnosis depends on histologic evidence of central cores in muscle that lack oxidative enzyme activity demonstrated by reaction to NADH dehydrogenase. Muscle strips from affected individuals can be tested in vitro for response to halothane to determine susceptibility to malignant hyperthermia.

Treatment

Attention to orthopedic problems, and their prevention, is essential in these individuals.

Prognosis

The condition is not progressive and may not be diagnosed until middle age. A 59-year-old woman was diagnosed on the basis of family history and susceptibility to malignant hyperthermia.

Muscular Dystrophies

Muscular dystrophies are distinguished from the congenital myopathies by their progressive course and evidence of destructive changes of the muscle on pathologic examination. These disorders may be fatal and present as the insidious progression of proximal weakness without sensory or sphincter involvement. Careful questioning regarding family history, particularly for males who died at a young age, may be fruitful.

The clinical characteristics of the commonly encountered dystrophies are outlined in Table 12.16.

Duchenne Muscular Dystrophy (Pseudohypertrophic Muscular Dystrophy)

Definition

Duchenne muscular dystrophy is a progressive hypertrophy of muscle associated with fatty infiltration and weakness.

Basic Science

The condition is most common in males and displays an X-linked pattern of inheritance in about half the cases. Chromosomal translocations can result (rarely) in expression of the disease in females. Sporadic occurrences are presumably mutations.

The gene for Duchenne muscular dystrophy was isolated and cloned in 1987. The gene has about 1–2 million base pairs, which makes it one of the largest yet identified. The gene codes a protein, dystrophin, that is expressed in normal muscle cells but not in muscle from mice with Duchenne muscular dystrophy (Hoffman et al, 1987) (see pp. 777).

Epidemiology

The disorder affects 1/3500 males.

Natural History

Affected infants may have delayed motor milestones, a waddling gait, and difficulty climbing. The calf muscles, in particular, increase in mass and are firm to palpation.

Table 12.16
Clinical and Pathologic Features of the Muscular Dystrophies

Type	Clinical Features	Pathology
Duchenne	Sex-linked recessive Onset 3–6 years Pseudohypertrophy Diminished IQs Cardiac involvement Rapid decline Death by age 20 years usual	Severe dystrophic changes Striking CPK Elevation early on
Becker	Sex-linked recessive Onset variable More benign course	Less marked changes Milder CPK rise
Facioscapulohumeral	Autosomal dominant Onset 7–12 years Minor disability Cannot pucker	Mild myopathic changes CPK usually normal
Limb-girdle	Autosomal recessive, some autosomal dominant Onset 5–10 years Disabled by 30s or 40s Cardiac involvement rare	Myopathic changes CPK usually normal

CASE ILLUSTRATION

A 2-year-old boy was referred to our hospital for evaluation of hepatomegaly and elevated liver function tests. He was well until 1 month before admission, when he was hospitalized elsewhere for gastroenteritis and dehydration. At that time his liver was felt to be enlarged and liver function tests were obtained. The SGOT was noted to peak at over 1000 U and an SGPT was in the 500s, although the bilirubin, alkaline phosphatase, and hepatitis screen were normal. The patient improved clinically but was referred to our hospital for further evaluation of the enlarged liver and abnormal laboratory values.

Initial examination was notable for a temperature of 38.3°C, but otherwise normal vital signs. The liver was down 3 cm, with a 10-cm span, and a spleen tip was palpable 1 cm below the left costal margin. Height, weight, and head circumference were appropriate for age, and the rest of the examination was initially felt to be unremarkable. Liver function tests were repeated and revealed an SGOT of 123 U, an SGPT of 253 U, an LDH of 353 U, with normal bilirubin and alkaline phosphatase clotting studies.

QUESTION AND COMMENT

What is the diagnosis and what further laboratory tests might be of help?

The differential diagnosis at this point was that of hepatomegaly in an otherwise previously healthy male. While infectious etiologies need to be considered, particularly viral etiologies, one also needs to evaluate the possibility of storage diseases, such as the less symptomatic glycogen storage diseases, infiltrative processes, or toxins (although the history was noncontributory for this possibility). An ultrasound was performed and showed a borderline enlarged liver and normal spleen.

Just when it appeared that the child might remain a diagnostic dilemma, a CPK returned at 5880 U, and it became clear that muscle rather than liver was making the significant contribution to the enzyme elevations. In fact, on repeat careful neurologic examination, the calves appeared slightly larger and firmer than one might expect. Moreover, strength was slightly diminished in the deltoids and iliopsoas muscles, although the patient did not do a classical Gower's maneuver, or have a gait disturbance. A subsequent electromyogram and muscle biopsy, however, confirmed the diagnosis of Duchenne muscular dystrophy.

We mention this case because usually an elevated SGPT with SGOT point to liver pathology, although, as demonstrated here, a muscle disorder can also present this way. It is hypothesized that enzyme release into serum is secondary to an abnormal permeability of the muscle cell membrane, followed by necrosis and muscle degeneration. As muscle mass diminishes with more necrotic fibers (as the child gets older), one sees a progressive decrease in serum enzyme activity. It is probable that without his viral gastroenteritis prompting initial studies, the diagnosis of muscular dystrophy (especially with a negative family history and normal developmental milestones to date) would have gone undetected for at least several more months. Of note, a check of mother's CPK was normal, although the normal finding is often seen in female carriers when they reach adulthood.

Gower sign is usually present: on rising from the floor, the child rolls to the prone position, kneels, then pushes his hands against his shins, knees, and finally thighs to assist in attaining a standing position.

The disease is progressive, so that few children can walk after age 12 years, and death from respiratory complications occurs in the teenage years or early 20s. Aspiration pneumonia from pharyngeal weakness is commonly the terminal event. Cardiomyopathy may be present. Mental deficiency is present to some degree in about 25% of patients.

Diagnosis

Serum creatinine phosphokinase is elevated as much as 10-fold, even in infancy. Electromyograms reveal decreased amplitude and duration of motor unit potentials. On biopsy, the muscle fibers vary in size and some have degenerated and have been replaced by fat and connective tissue.

The respiratory status should be evaluated with serial pulmonary function tests. The vital capacity and peak expiratory flow rates are most helpful in following a patient.

Treatment

No treatment for the basic disease is known, but children need very careful management in several areas.

Among the general aspects of management of children with muscular dystrophy are weight control to prevent the added burden of obesity and physiotherapy to prevent contractures and encourage walking. More than half the children with muscular dystrophy develop scoliosis and require careful orthopedic evaluation (Smith et al, 1987). Although some physicians advocate breathing exercises to strengthen respiratory muscles, little evidence justifies the effort required. Swimming remains one of the best exercises for accessory muscles of respiration. Ventilatory support can prolong life when respiratory muscles are involved.

Prevention

The identification of the muscular dystrophy gene on the X-chromosome makes prenatal diagnosis possible for families with affected children. This probe is thought to be about 95% accurate in identifying affected fetuses (Darras et al, 1987).

Myotonic Disorders

Myotonia is the phenomenon of being unable to relax a muscle after contraction. It can be seen with hand grip (the handshake that "won't let go"), or in other voluntary acts (upgaze); it may also be elicited with percussion (in children, we favor percussion of the thenar eminence or the belly of the finger extensors).

Myotonic Muscular Dystrophy

Myotonic muscular dystrophy, the most common form of muscular dystrophy, is inherited as an autosomal dominant trait located on chromosome 19. Most commonly, the onset is in late adolescence or adulthood, with wasting of facial muscles and a straight smile. Myotonia is present and most commonly demonstrated by a tightly clenched fist and inability to extend the fingers for several seconds after the command (Westrom et al, 1986).

Congenital myotonic dystrophy is characterized by early onset of hypotonia of the facial and neck muscles, disturbances in swallowing, respiratory difficulties, and arthrogryposia that occurs in about 10–20% of affected individuals. Half of the affected infants die in the first year. A history of hydramnios, prematurity, and abnormalities of labor are common. Ventricular dilation may be present in the newborn (Regev et al, 1987). Mental retardation is often severe, and present in about 80% of patients.

In affected individuals with the congenital form who survive infancy, a number of other problems may occur. These include cataracts, cardiac arrhythmias, frontal baldness, loss of body hair, and testicular atrophy. About 20% of patients develop an insulin-resistant form of diabetes mellitus.

The most characteristic aspects are facial diplegia and generalized hypotonia.

Diagnosis

Myotonic discharges may be seen on electromyogram. Nerve conduction is normal, as is CPK. The metabolic defect is unknown as of 1988.

Muscle pathology in the congenital form shows a disturbance in maturation with incomplete differentiation of fibers.

Treatment

Only general supportive measures are helpful.

Prevention

Since there are no documented cases of new mutations, and the mode of transmission is autosomal dominant, a family history is always positive. Linkage studies have established the gene to be on chromosome 19, and restriction fragment length polymorphisms have been found sufficiently tightly linked to be useful in prenatal diagnosis with the use of two probes. The error in carrier detection is less than 1%. Thus, both carrier detection and prenatal diagnosis are possible.

Myotonia congenita (Thomsen disease) is an autosomal dominant condition, with myotonia without weakness as the salient clinical feature. Indeed, individuals with this condition may be quite well-muscled. There is a tendency to be quite slow at the initiation of strenuous muscle activity (for example, a patient was referred to us because of difficulty in initiating the game "duck-duck-goose" in nursery school). It is not progressive.

Paramyotonic conditions include those diseases in which myotonia can be elicited after exposure to the cold (paramyotonia of Eulenburg), or in a periodic fashion, often associated with abnormalities of potassium metabolism (the hypokalemic and hyperkalemic periodic paralyses).

PERIODIC PARALYSES

Definition

A group of illnesses characterized by episodes of intermittent weakness with full recovery in between have different etiologies. Hyperkalemic periodic paralysis, hypokalemic periodic paralysis, paroxysmal myoglobinuria, and McArdle disease all qualify as periodic paralyses.

Hyperkalemic Periodic Paralysis

Epidemiology

This disorder is inherited as a dominant trait, and is most severe in males.

Natural History

The onset is in infancy or early childhood, and weakness, especially in the legs, appears after strenuous exercise. Attacks last several hours. Eyelid lag on downward gaze is characteristic.

Diagnosis

The serum potassium is elevated during an attack. An oral potassium load of 2–3 g may cause an attack.

Treatment

Acetozolamide is effective in preventing attacks.

Hypokalemic Periodic Paralysis (Familial Periodic Paralysis)

Natural History

The onset of this disorder is in late childhood and it is more severe in males. Heavy exercise and large carbohydrate intake can precipitate weakness, especially in the morning. The limbs, and sometimes muscles of respiration are affected for 24 hours or longer.

Diagnosis

Serum potassium is low, often 2 mEq/L.

Treatment

Potassium chloride (2–3 g/dose orally) or acetazolamide reduce the likelihood of attack.

Paroxysmal Myoglobinuria

Natural History

Muscle breakdown after exercise can produce myoglobinuria and paralysis in affected family members. (Dominant or sex-linked inheritance has been described.)

Diagnosis

Myoglobin makes the urine dark red or brown and produces a positive benzidine test.

Treatment

Treatment is supportive only, with adequate hydration to prevent renal damage.

REFERENCES

Chamberlain JS, Pearlman JA, Muzny DM, et al: Expression of the murine Duchenne muscular dystrophy gene in muscle and brain. *Science* 239:1416, 1988.

Cornblath D: Disorders of neuromuscular transmission in infants and children. *Muscle Nerve* 9:606, 1986.

Darras BT, Harper JF, Francke U: Prenatal diagnosis and detection of carriers with DNA probes in Duchenne's muscular dystrophy. *N Engl J Med* 316:985, 1987.

Drachman DB: Present and future treatment of myasthenia gravis. *N Engl J Med* 316:743, 1987.

Grob D, Brunner NG, Namba T: The natural course of myasthenia gravis and effect of therapeutic measures. *Ann NY Acad Sci* 377:652, 1981.

Hoffman EP, Brown RH, Kunkel LM: Dystrophin: The protein product of the Duchenne muscular dystrophy locus. *Cell* 51:919, 1987.

Koenig M, Hoffman EP, Bertelson CJ, et al: Complete cloning of the Duchenne muscular dystrophy (DMD) cDNA and preliminary genomic organization of the DMD gene in normal and affected individuals. *Cell* 50:509, 1987.

Lefvert AK, Osterman PO: Newborn infants to myasthenic mothers: A clinical study and an investigation of acetylcholine receptor antibodies in 17 children. *Neurology* 33:133, 1983.

Millichap JG, Dodge PR: Diagnosis and treatment of myasthenia gravis in infancy, childhood and adolescence. *Neurology* 10:1007, 1960.

Probst A, Ulrich J, Bischoff A, et al: Sensory ganglioneuropathy in infantile spinal muscular atrophy. Light and electronmicroscopy findings in 2 cases. *Neuropediatrics* 12:215, 1981.

Regev R, deVries LS, Heckmatt JZ, et al: Cerebral ventricular dilation in congenital myotonic dystrophy. *J Pediatr* 111:372, 1987.

Shuaib A, Paasuke RT, Brownell KW: Central core disease: Clinical features in 13 patients. *Medicine* 66:389, 1987.

Smith PEM, Calverley PMA, Edwards RHT, et al: Practical problems in the respiratory care of patients with muscular dystrophy. *N Engl J Med* 316:1197, 1987.

Sun SF, Binder J, Streib E, et al: Myotonic dystrophy: Obstetric and neonatal complications. *South Med J* 78:823, 1985.

Tindall RSA, Rollins JA, Phillips JT: Preliminary results of a double-blind, randomized, placebo-controlled trial of cyclosporine in myasthenia gravis. *N Engl J Med* 316:719, 1987.

Westrom G, Bensch J, Schollin J: Congenital myotonic dystrophy. Incidence, clinical aspects and early prognosis. *Acta Paediatr Scand* 75:849, 1986.

Phakomatoses (Neurocutaneous Disorders) 10

The phakomatoses are a group of clinical entities characterized by abnormalities in the nervous system and skin. The developmental mechanism of these disorders is unknown; they usually present in childhood, but may be clinically quiescent into adulthood. The diseases that fall under this category are *neurofibromatosis, tuberous sclerosis, ataxia-telangiectasia, von Hippel-Lindau disease,* and *Sturge-Weber disease.*

NEUROFIBROMATOSES (VON RECKLINGHAUSEN DISEASE)

For a review of current research on neurofibromatoses (NF), see Rubenstein et al, 1986.

Definition

The neurofibromatoses are a set of disorders characterized mainly by the tendency to develop tumors along nerves. There are two major clinical forms which are genetically distinct. NF-1 (von Recklinghausen NF, peripheral NF) is associated with the occurrence of café-au-lait spots on the skin, and neurofibromas along peripheral nerves. Tumors of the CNS, skeletal dysplasias, learning disabilities, and malignant schwannoma may also occur. NF-2 is associated with the development of bilateral acoustic neuromas, and occasionally schwannomas along other nerves, meningiomas, and gliomas. Genetic linkage studies have recently shown that the locus for NF-1 is on chromosome 17 (Seizinger et al, 1987; Barker et al, 1987); the gene for NF-2 is probably on chromosome 22 (Seizinger et al, 1987).

Epidemiology

NF-1 affects approximately 1/4000 people, making it the most common single gene defect that affects the CNS. The mode of genetic transmission is autosomal dominant. About half the cases are familial and the remainder occur sporadically and presumably represent new mutations. NF-2 is much less common, affecting about 1/50,000. It is also an autosomal dominant trait.

Natural History

The most common presenting feature of NF-1 is multiple café-au-lait spots, which usually become apparent during the first year of life. In a child, more than six spots measuring at least 0.5 cm should raise strong suspicion of NF-1. Rarely, children with this condition are born with deformities such as bowing or pseudoarthrosis of the tibia, absence of the sphenoid wing, or a large plexiform neurofibroma. Neurofibromas usually do not appear until late childhood or adolescence. When the tumors are subcutaneous, they are palpable as soft nodules. They may occur along any peripheral nerve and may cause symptoms due to nerve or spinal cord compression. An appreciable number of children with NF-1 develop gliomas along the optic nerves or chiasm, although these rarely become symptomatic or require treatment. Malignant gliomas and schwannomas can occur, but are rare. Spinal deformities, particularly scoliosis, occur relatively commonly. Hypertension in children with NF-1 may be due to renal artery stenosis. Learning disabilities are especially common in people with NF-1, and are often the major medical burden posed to an individual with the disorder.

NF-2 usually does not present until the second or third decade, but affected individuals virtually all eventually develop bilateral acoustic neuromas. These may present with tinnitus, problems with balance, or hearing loss. Schwannomas along other cranial or peripheral nerves, meningiomas, and gliomas are also seen in this disorder (Martuza and Eldridge, 1988).

Diagnosis

Diagnosis is based on clinical features. The following diagnostic criteria were proposed by an NIH Consensus Development Conference on Neurofibromatosis in 1987 (Fig. 12.8).

Neurofibromatosis 1

The diagnostic criteria for NF-1 are met in an individual if two or more of the following are found:

Six or more café-au-lait macules. These should be over 5 mm in greatest diameter in prepubertal individuals and over 15 mm in greatest diameter in postpubertal individuals;
Two or more neurofibromas of any type or one plexiform neurofibroma;
Multiple freckles in the axillary or inguinal regions;
Optic glioma;
Two or more Lisch nodules (iris hamartomas);
A distinctive osseous lesion such as sphenoid dysplasias or thinning of long bone cortex with or without pseudarthrosis;
A first-degree relative (parent, sibling, or offspring) with NF-1 by the above criteria;

Other disorders of pigmentation such as McCune-Albright or leopard syndrome can be confused with NF-1.

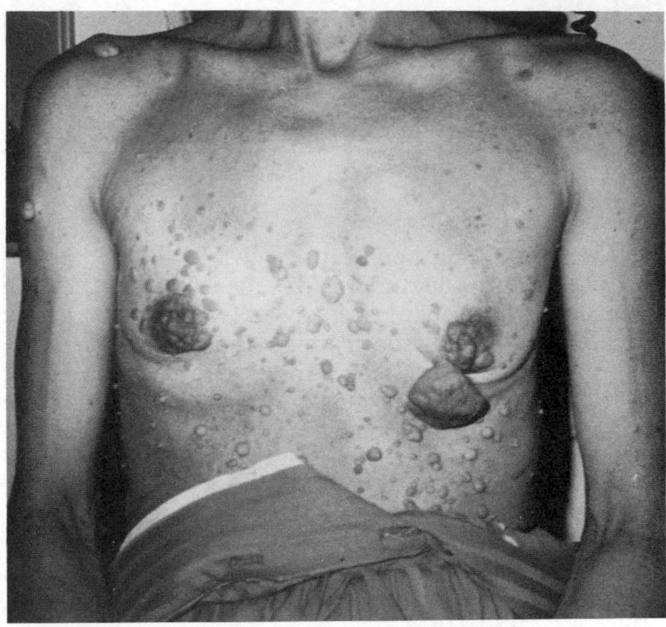

Figure 12.8. Multiple subcutaneous neurofibromas are evident mostly over the thorax of this adolescent male. Photograph courtesy of Dr. Bruce Korf.

Neurofibromatosis 2

The criteria for NF-2 are met by an individual who has:

Bilateral eighth nerve masses seen with appropriate imaging techniques (e.g., CT or MRI).

A first degree relative with NF-2 and either unilateral eighth nerve mass or two of the following:

plexiform neurofibroma;
neurofibroma of another type;
meningioma;
glioma;
schwannoma;
presenile posterior cataract.

Treatment

There is no primary treatment for either form of neurofibromatosis. In NF-1, treatment is directed toward local resection of symptomatic lesions. Affected individuals should be monitored closely for signs of scoliosis, hypertension, visual disturbance, and learning disabilities. People with NF-2 should have periodic monitoring of eighth nerve function, best done using brain stem auditory-evoked potentials, in conjunction with MRI scanning if needed. Early detection of acoustic neuromas can permit resection of tumors with at least partial preservation of hearing.

Prognosis

Life span for people with either form is usually normal, except in individuals who develop malignant tumors. The degree of expression of NF-1 varies widely from person to person, even within a family. There is no clearly documented difference in expression based on maternal or paternal transmission. For information for families write to National Neurofibromatosis Foundation, Inc., Suite 7-S, 141 Fifth Avenue, New York, NY 10010.

Prevention

Genetic counseling requires examination of parents. If one parent is affected (based on above clinical criteria), the risk of recurrence in a sibling is 1 in 2. If neither parent is affected, the patient represents a new mutation. Prenatal diagnosis is not possible as of 1988.

Tuberous Sclerosis

Definition

Tuberous sclerosis is a dominantly inherited condition characterized by sclerotic patches (tubers) scattered throughout the brain, and also affecting eyes, skin, kidneys, bones, heart, and lungs.

Epidemiology

The disorder is inherited as a dominant trait; about 50% of cases appear to be new mutations. It is thought to affect 1/30,000 individuals. Expression is variable.

Natural History

This disorder can present in infancy with myoclonic seizures or later with grand mal or psychomotor seizures and is sometimes associated with severe mental deficiency. About 6% of patients develop "giant cell astrocytoma," an expansion of a subependymal nodule.

CASE ILLUSTRATION

A boy was noted at the time of birth to have severe bowing of the left lower leg. Examination at that time did not reveal cutaneous stigmata of neurofibromatosis. Café-au-lait spots became apparent after the first few weeks of life, however, and at age 6 months he had seven spots measuring at least 0.5 cm. No cutaneous neurofibromas were seen, and there were no iris Lisch nodules. The bowed left leg was placed in a brace. On careful examination of both parents, the mother was found to have 15 café-au-lait spots, freckles within the axillae, and three small skin nodules resembling neurofibromas. A slit-lamp examination revealed iris Lisch nodules. She had previously been told that the skin spots were just "birth marks" of no consequence and had not been aware that she had neurofibromatosis. The couple was subsequently counseled that they had a 50% recurrence risk for the condition in any future child, and that specific complications in other affected offspring cannot be predicted.

A characteristic skin lesion is adenoma sebaceum, red or brown nodules in a butterfly distribution over nose and cheeks. They appear after age 2 years, and by adolescence are present in over 80% of patients. (The name is inappropriate since the lesions do not involve the sebaceous glands, but are rather hamartomas.) Hypopigmented white leaf macules from a few millimeters to centimeters in diameter may be found on the arms, legs, or trunk, and are best seen under a Wood light. They are sharply demarcated, and may be single or multiple (see Section 18, Dermatology).

The disease may be of little consequence if it involves only skin, or it can be associated with severe convulsions and retardation. Affected individuals are at risk of rhabdomyoma of the heart and angiomyolipoma or cysts of the kidney (see pp. 618, Section 10, Nephrology).

Retinal lesions are present in about half the patients and appear as white or yellow raised areas near the edge of the optic disc. They are malformations of the nerve fibers in the retina (glioma-angiomas).

In older patients, particularly females, progressive pulmonary lymphangiomatosis may result in pulmonary failure.

Treatment

Convulsions are managed with anticonvulsant medication. Surgical excision of symptomatic tumors may be appropriate. Pertussis vaccine should be withheld in these infants as they are prone to convulsions (Gomez et al, 1982).

Sturge-Weber Disease

Definition

Sturge-Weber disease is characterized by a port-wine nevus involving the face, seizures, intracranial calcifications, and mental retardation. The central pathologic lesion is a meningeal angiomatosis that tends to involve the occipitoparietal region and is associated with a cutaneous port-wine angioma of the ipsilateral face. The cortex underlying the angiomatosis is atrophic and calcified.

Natural History

The port-wine stain is present at birth and involves the skin innervated by the first division of the trigeminal nerve. Angiomas involving only the second or third trigeminal divisions are not associated with neurologic disturbances. An angioma may be seen in the ipsilateral choroid membrane and give rise to congenital glaucoma and buphthalmos. The facial nevus may be bilateral.

Mental retardation is seen in about 80% of patients. Seizures are very common and almost always occur before 1 year of age. Fixed neurologic deficits are ultimately present in about one-third of patients. They take the form of a homonymous hemianopia and hemiparesis.

Plain skull radiographs may show the intracranial calcifications, which are best imaged with CT scans. MRI scans, while less efficient at showing the calcium, will show the cerebral atrophy underneath the angiomatosis.

Prognosis

Unfortunately, the disease is progressive, with seizures, and worsening of the motor and cognitive deficits. Often the seizures are difficult to control with anticonvulsants and surgical resection of the abnormal tissue is required.

Von Hippel-Lindau Disease

Von Hippel-Lindau disease is an autosomal dominant disorder with variable expression. It is characterized by the association of cerebellar hemangioblastomas with retinal hemangiomas, renal carcinoma, and cysts of the pancreas. The disease often presents in the second decade of life with intraocular or cerebellar hemorrhage. Other lesions associated with the syndrome are hepatic cysts, epididymitis, meningiomas, pheochromocytomas, and polycythemia. The CSF protein is often elevated.

Ataxia Telangiectasia

Ataxia-telangiectasia is autosomal recessive, with an estimated gene frequency of 2.8%. Pathophysiologically, it is characterized by defective DNA repair mechanisms resulting in frequent chromosomal breaks, and a series of immunologic abnormalities (low IgA and IgE).

Clinically, it presents as a progressive cerebellar ataxia with choreoathetosis and nystagmus. Later in the disease hypotonia, weakness, and hyporeflexia may develop. Telangiectasias are found involving the bulbar conjuctivae and in exposed skin areas. Children with the disease are at increased risk for recurrent sinopulmonary infections, lymphoproliferative diseases, and a peculiar form of diabetes mellitus characterized by peripheral insulin resistance, hyperinsulinemia, hyperglycemia, and little or no glucosuria or ketosis. The general clinical course is one of a progressive disease with no specific therapy.

Patients with ataxia-telangiectasis have a high risk of developing lymphomas, breast cancer, and a variety of other tumors. The risk of cancer is 2 to 3 times that expected in heterozygotes (Swift et al, 1987).

REFERENCES

Barker D, Wright E, Nguyen K, et al: Gene for von Recklinghausen neurofibromatosis is in the pericentromeric regions of chromosome 17. *Science* 236:1100, 1987.

Gomez MR, Kuntz NL, Westmoreland BF, et al: Tuberous sclerosis, early onset of seizures and mental subnormality: Study of discordant homozygous twins. *Neurology* 32:604, 1982.

Martuza RL, Eldridge R: Neurofibromatosis 2 (bilateral acoustic neurofibromatosis). *N Engl J Med* 318:684, 1988.

Riccardi VM, Eichner JE: *Neurofibromatosis: Phenotype, Natural History and Pathogenesis*. Baltimore, Johns Hopkins University Press, 1986.

Riccardi VM, Wald JS: Discounting an adverse maternal effect on severity of neurofibromatosis. *Pediatrics* 79:386, 1987.

Rubenstein AE, Bunge RP, Housman DE (eds): Neurofibromatosis. *Ann NY Acad Sci* 466:1, 1986.

Seizinger BR, Rouleau G, Ozelius LJ, et al: Common pathogenetic mechanism for three tumor types in bilateral acoustic neurofibromatosis. *Science* 236:317, 1987.

Swift M, Morrell D, Cromartie E, et al: The incidence and gene frequency of ataxia-telangiectasia in the United States. *Am J Hum Genet* 39:573, 1986.

Swift M, Reitnauer PJ, Morrell D, et al: Breast and other cancers in families with ataxia-telangiectasia. *N Engl J Med* 316:1289, 1987.

Other Disorders 11

FAMILIAL DYSAUTONOMIA (RILEY-DAY SYNDROME)

Definition

Familial dysautonomia occurs in infants born to parents of Ashkenazi Jewish ancestry, and is characterized by deficient sensory input and evidence of autonomic nervous system dysfunction.

Basic Science

The peripheral nerves have been found to have a deficit in the number of the small unmyelinated fibers that normally carry pain sensation, temperature, and taste sensations. There is also a deficit of some of the large myelinated fibers which carry afferent impulses from muscle spindles and, thus, proprioceptive information. Although evident in some infants with dysautonomia, these abnormalities are not universally present.

Disturbed autonomic function is sometimes reflected in the absence of dopamine betahydroxylase in the plasma and a diminution in urinary vanillylmandelic acid. None of these biochemical or pathologic findings is pathognomonic of the condition.

Natural History

In early infancy, an absence of tearing and sometimes corneal anesthesia may be noted. Corneal injury may be common because of the dryness. Skin blotching is frequently present, with patches of redness appearing transiently. Unexplained or erratic fevers have been described, although, occasionally, they are associated with pneumonias which appear to be increased in occurrence. Over a period of time it will be evident that there is retardation in both body growth and often in mental development. Episodic vomiting can be prominent as can breath-holding spells. As the youngsters reach adolescence many have significant spinal curvatures, probably because of inadequate appreciation of proprioceptive information. Deep tendon reflexes are usually diminished or absent.

The condition can present with such severity that the infants may die in the first year of life from overwhelming pulmonary infections and chronic pulmonary failure. Individuals with a less severe manifestation can be carried to adulthood with careful medical supervision and special education.

School performance may be below intellectual capacity, partly because speech may be delayed. When present, the speech sometimes has a nasal quality. Some improvement may take place with time. Some individuals have functioned well in regular school and several have attended college (Welton et al, 1979).

Puberty is often delayed, particularly in the females. At least two dysautonomic women have given birth to apparently normal offspring (Porges et al, 1978).

Diagnosis

Three tests are widely used for the diagnosis of familial dysautonomia:

1. Histamine Test: A 1:10,000 dilution of histamine phosphate injected intradermally in normal individuals usually produces pain, erythema, a central wheal and an axon flare 1–3 cm in radius that persists 1–10 minutes. In the dysautonomic patient, the same intradermal injection is not associated with significant pain. A wheal may develop, but flares are absent or minimal.

2. Mecholyl Test: A 2½% solution of Mecholyl in the conjunctival sac produces a contraction of the pupil in almost all patients with familial dysautonomia. There is no observable affect on the normal pupil. This test is best perfomed by applying one drop of the solution to one eye, with the other eye serving as a control. The size of the pupils can then be compared at 5-minute intervals for 20–30 minutes.
3. Absence of fungiform papillae on the tongue: The normal tongue has clearly visible red dots about 1 mm in diameter, which are richly vascularized fungiform papillae, along the tip and sides of the tongue. The tongue of a child with dysautonomia is smooth and pale because of the absence of these papillae.

Treatment

The most life-threatening aspect of the illness is the tendency to chronic pulmonary disease, some of which may well be related to swallowing difficulties and the recurrent vomiting with associated aspiration. Each episode of fever deserves full investigation, despite the difficulties stemming from evaluation of such frequent episodes. If the cornea is involved, artificial tears can be very helpful. Spinal curvature should dictate appropriate bracing. Developmental problems may require special education.

The lack of appropriate sensory input can be of continuing concern for the growing child. Swimming is contraindicated under all circumstances since these youngsters have a diminished awareness of impending hypoxia or hypercarbia, and some have drowned while swimming under water. The relative indifference to pain can lead to serious injury and should be taken into consideration when advising affected individuals about participation in contact sports.

Prognosis

About one-third of the patients followed by Axelrod et al in New York were 20 years old or older, with the oldest being age 38 years in 1982. The cause of death in the younger group was primarily pneumonia (44%) with cardiorespiratory arrest occurring in 40%. Drowning was cited as the cause of death in 4% (Axelrod and Abularrage, 1982).

COUNSELING PARENTS

Parents of a child with dysautonomia will need extensive education about the manifestations of the disease and advice on the management of the child, including confronting the characteristic emotional lability. The parents should be informed that the frequency of the carrier state is about 1% of Ashkenazi Jews and the inheritance is autosomal recessive. Unfortunately, there is no method of prenatal diagnosis available as of 1987. For up-to-date information, consult the Dysautonomia Association, 370 Lexington Avenue, New York, NY 10016.

CONGENITAL HEMIHYPERTROPHY/ HEMIATROPHY

Definition

This condition describes relative overgrowth of one side of the body. It is thought to result from unequal division of cells in the zygote.

Epidemiology

Females are more often affected than males; the right side is more affected than the left. The larger bones are longer and thicker on the affected side.

Diagnosis

The assymmetry is occasionally evident at birth, but may become more pronounced with later growth. A search for other abnormalities is essential, since aniridia, Wilm tumor, cryptorchidism, hypospadias, and polydactylyly have been described in association with hemihypertrophy. Vascular abnormalities (hemiangiomas, etc) are common.

Treatment

Shoe lifts are used to equalize the leg length. If the size discrepancy is great, orthopedic consultation is appropriate to consider surgical intervention.

REFERENCES

Aguayo AJ, Nair CP, Bray GM, et al: Peripheral nerve abnormalities in the Riley-Day Syndrome. *Arch Neurol* 24:106. 1971.

Axelrod FB, Porges RF, Sein ME: Neonatal recognition of familial dysautonomia. *J Pediatr* 110:947, 1987.

Axelrod FB, Abularrage JJ: Familial dysautonomia: A prospective study of survival. *J Pediatr* 101:234, 1982.

Porges RF, Axelrod FB, Richards M: Pregnancy in familial dysautonomia. *Am J Obstet Gynecol* 132:485, 1978.

Riley CM, Day RL: Central autonomic dysfunction with defective lacrimation. I. Report of five cases. *Pediatrics* 3:468, 1949.

Welton W, Clayson D, Axelrod FB, et al: Intellectual development and familial dysautonomia. *Pediatrics* 63:708, 1979.

DAVID URION
K. JAMES SABRY
BRUCE KORF
MARY ELLEN AVERY

Section 13

Genetics

Clinical Genetics

1

GENERAL PRINCIPLES

"Just as our present knowledge and practice of medicine relies on a sophisticated knowledge of human anatomy, physiology, and biochemistry, so will dealing with disease in the future demand a detailed understanding of the molecular anatomy, physiology, and biochemistry of the human genome" (Paul Berg, Nobel Prize Lecture, 1980).

Within the field of pediatrics, there has been no greater explosion of knowledge than in the area of genetics. Basic developments in the laboratory have resulted in molecular comprehension of the pathophysiology of many of the inherited disorders that affect children. Recombinant DNA technology has had such far-reaching effects that it has essentially revolutionized the approach to all disease and not strictly "genetic" diseases. Many of the principles discussed in this section will be cross-referenced to other sections where useful. It is one aim of this section to provide pediatricians who entered medical school before 1975 with an understanding of fundamental molecular genetics and its relevance to clinical pediatrics.

Although individual genetic disorders may be relatively rare, the sum of all genetic disorders has a significant effect on morbidity and mortality at all ages (Nadler, 1981). Several studies have documented the frequency of genetic disease in both general pediatric hospitals and tertiary referral centers (Hall et al, 1978; Day and Holmes 1973; Scriver et al, 1973). In a review of 4115 general pediatric medical records, Hall and associates categorized diagnoses as to: (I) clearly genetic disorders (single gene and chromosomal abnormalities), (II) multifactorial disorders (e.g., cleft palate, congenital dislocation of the hip); (III) developmental anomalies (e.g., imperforate anus, renal anomalies); (IV) familial disorders (e.g., prematurity, cancer, glomerulonephritis); and (V) nongenetic disorders (e.g., trauma, infection, feeding problems). Of all admissions, 4.5% had category I, clearly genetic disorders, 22.1% had category II, multifactorial conditions, 13.6% had category III, developmental anomalies, 13.2% had category IV, familial disorders, and 46.6% had category V, nongenetic disorders. The first three categories comprise conditions that fall within the traditional realm of genetics—40.2% of pediatric admissions in this study. Patients with clearly genetic disorders were also found to have, on average, four times as many hospitalizations as those with nongenetic disorders (Hall et al, 1978).

Genetic Counseling

Genetic counseling should be considered an integral component of the genetic approach to human disease. Genetic counseling may be defined as "the process by which patients or relatives at risk of a disorder that may be hereditary are advised of the consequences of the disorder, the probability of developing or transmitting it, and of the ways in which this may be prevented or ameliorated" (Harper, 1983). The fundamental goal of genetic counseling is to provide information to the patient or family but in order to do this accurately, several steps must be followed (Table 13.1).

In most cases, the initiation of genetic counseling begins with an affected individual who is known as the proband or index case. *It is incumbent upon the person performing the genetic counseling to confirm the diagnosis of the proband.* This may be done by a direct physical examination of the proband or by obtaining copies of the relevant medical records. Once a diagnosis is made, the counselor can proceed to the next step, which is risk estimation. Risk is defined as a number, P, the probability that the disorder will occur or recur. Before the risk can be calculated, a thorough family history must be obtained. The importance of this cannot be overemphasized (see following case). A pedigree is constructed with use of conventional symbols (Fig. 13.1). If the questions asked of the proband's family are specific rather than general, they are more likely to result in useful information. While taking a family history, special attention should be paid to neonatal or childhood deaths occurring within the family, previous infants with birth defects, children or adults with mental retardation or deafness, women with multiple miscarriages, or adults with tallness or shortness of stature. A complete history should also include information on allergies, malignancy, coronary artery disease, diabetes, hypertension, as well as any other findings pertinent to the proband's disorder. As evidenced in the case below, parental consanguinity must be ruled out.

During discussions with the proband's family, it is helpful to keep in mind certain definitions. Autosomal dominant traits vary more frequently in their clinical expression than do autosomal recessive traits. Thus, it is important to examine all siblings and both parents to rule out *variable expression.* As an example, a child diagnosed as having neurofibromatosis may have clinically normal parents. On detailed physical examination, however, one of the parents may have multiple *café-au-lait* spots. The recurrence risk for neurofibromatosis in a sibling is then 50%. If the parental examinations and the family history are negative, the child is considered a new mutation and the recurrence

Table 13.1
Elements of Genetic Counseling[1]

Diagnosis	Clinical assessment of affected individual(s) Confirmation from records
Risk estimation	Recording of family history Recognition of specific patterns of inheritance Interaction with other information to give specific risk estimate
Communication	Adequate time Ability to relate to others Timing of counseling
Follow-up	Availability of treatment Other preventive measures Information on the nature of the disorder

[1]Modified from Harper PS: Genetic counseling and prenatal diagnosis. *Br Med Bull* 39:302, 1983.

risk is 0%. *Penetrance* refers to the frequency of appearance of a phenotype when a mutant gene is present. The phenotype is present (penetrant) or absent (nonpenetrant). *Pleiotropy* means that there are multiple phenotypic effects of the same gene or pair of genes. With neurofibromatosis again as an example, the neurofibromatosis gene may have effects on the skin, peripheral nerves, eyes, brain, and skeletal system. In *genetic heterogeneity,* different genes or different mechanisms may result in similar phenotypes. Patients with Turner syndrome and Noonan syndrome resemble each other but, in the former, the patient lacks part or all of an X chromosome and in the latter, the chromosome number is normal. Noonan syndrome is frequently transmitted in an autosomal dominant manner.

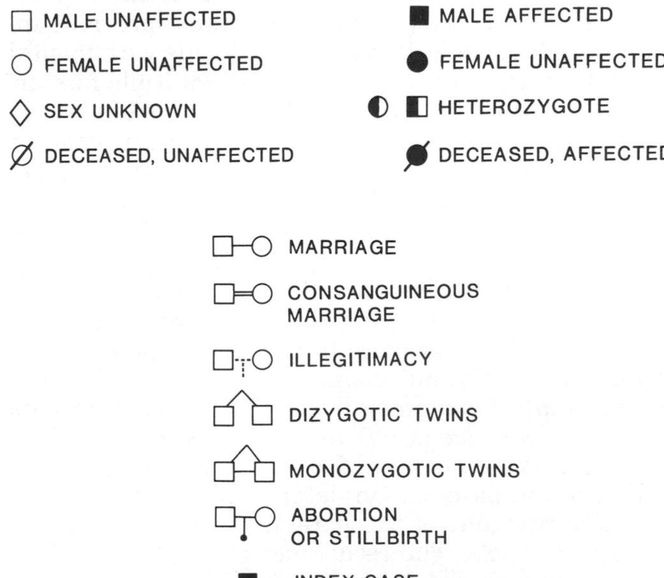

Figure 13.1. Symbols used in the construction of a genetic pedigree.

After obtaining the relevant family details and commencing analysis of the pedigree, it is important to note whether there is more than one affected person in the family. Evidence of vertical (parent-to-child) transmission is more characteristic of an autosomal dominant pattern of inheritance, whereas a horizontal pattern (multiple affected offspring in the same generation) is more typical of an autosomal recessive form of inheritance. Evidence of male-to-male transmission is incompatible with an X-linked pattern of inheritance. The counselor should keep in mind that first degree relatives share one-half of their genes; examples are parents, siblings, and children. Second degree relatives share one-quarter of their genes; these would include grandparents, grandchildren, uncles, aunts, nieces, nephews, and half siblings. Third degree relatives share one-eighth of their genes and include great-grandparents, great-grandchildren, and first cousins.

The calculation of the risk relies not only on the information obtained from the family history and pedigree analysis, but on laboratory testing where appropriate. As an example, a young woman who is concerned about a family history of Duchenne muscular dystrophy requests genetic counseling. Her maternal uncle and brother had confirmed diagnoses of this disorder. By pedigree analysis, the young woman has a 50% *a priori* risk of being a carrier, but this number may be modified as a result of CPK (creatine phosphokinase) testing and DNA-based analyses (see Chapter 3).

Communication is a key element in the successful provision of genetic counseling. Important factors include: sufficient time for counseling, privacy, ability to listen, and the relationship between the timing of counseling and diagnosis (Harper, 1983). It is quite common for parents to "forget" the exact recurrence risk when they are told simultaneously that their child has a devastating disease. It is often helpful to follow a counseling session with a written record to the counselees to document what has been discussed.

Finally, genetic counseling must include a discussion of what is available for treatment, prevention, prenatal diagnosis, or modification of the particular disorder.

Given the cumulative impact of genetic disease on the general pediatric population, it is surprising that genetic counseling does not play a larger role in pediatric health care. Riccardi et al (1978) reviewed medical records from 478 patients with one of 10 genetic disorders. Of the affected families, 84% had a recurrence risk of greater than 1% for siblings or offspring of the index case. Yet in only two cases (0.4%) was genetic counseling offered. It is the responsibility of the primary care pediatrician to ensure that if the patient has a genetic disease, genetic counseling is provided and documented in the medical record.

Single Gene (Mendelian Disorders)

Single gene disorders arise from the presence of a mutant gene or pair of genes. Many of the disorders inherited in this manner occur infrequently, but as a

CASE ILLUSTRATION

A 4-year, 5-month-old male was referred to The Children's Hospital, Boston because of failure to thrive, developmental delay, and renal tubular acidosis. He was seen by multiple subspecialists, all of whom took a cursory family history. The pedigree was drawn as shown in Figure 13.2*A*. The genetics service was asked to examine the child because his friendly personality, small stature, and "cute," elfin-like facies suggested a diagnosis of Williams syndrome. A complete family history was obtained and revealed that the mother had been married twice and that her second husband was her first cousin. The pedigree was corrected and redrawn as shown in Figure 13.2*B*.

The patient's physical examination was not compatible with a diagnosis of Williams syndrome. Given the history of parental consanguinity, the diagnosis of an autosomal recessively inherited inborn error of metabolism became more likely. By using McKusick's catalog of *Mendelian Inheritance in Man* (see below) it became possible to look for a syndrome that was recessively inherited and had as its clinical manifestations failure to thrive and renal tubular acidosis. Carbonic anhydrase II deficiency was suggested and confirmed by characteristic intracranial calcifications, osteopetrosis on long bone films, and diagnostic serum enzyme levels (Sly et al, 1985).

Carbonic anhydrase II deficiency is an extremely rare disorder. Most pediatricians would not include it in their differential diagnosis of renal tubular acidosis. The key point, however, is that the discovery of parental consanguinity by taking a precise family history changed the approach to this case, and ultimately led to the diagnosis.

INITIAL PEDIGREE:

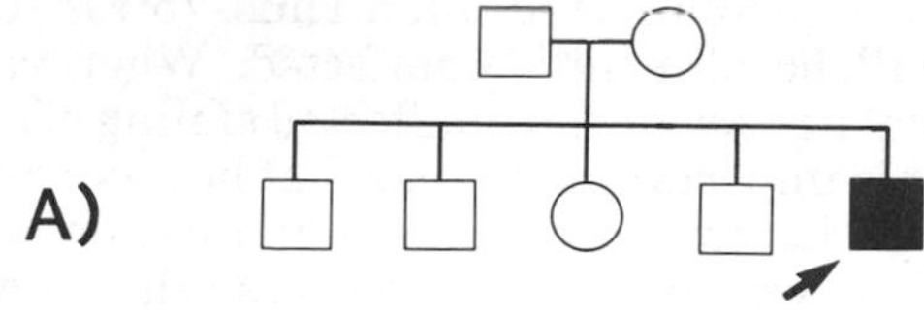

CORRECTED PEDIGREE:

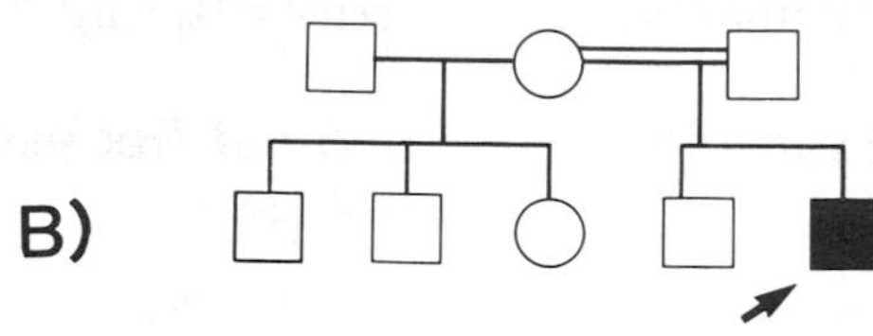

Figure 13.2. Consanguineous pedigree as described in the case illustration.

group they affect at least 1% of liveborn infants and account for 8.5% of childhood deaths and 7.1% of perinatal deaths (Costa et al, 1985). Monogenic disorders are well-known to pediatricians, who are familiar with the X-linked pattern of inheritance in hemophilia, the autosomal recessive inheritance in phenylketonuria, and the autosomal dominant inheritance in achondroplasia. The categorization of these patterns of inheritance is the result of experiments performed on garden peas during the 19th century by the Austrian monk, Gregor Mendel. Mendel studied certain physical characteristics of pea plants which we now know are determined by genes. Alternative forms of genes are called *alleles*. If a given allele has a frequency of greater than 1% in the population, it is known as a *polymorphism*. In Mendel's honor, monogenic disorders are frequently referred to as "Mendelian diseases." Only recently has an exception been found to the Mendelian inheritance patterns in single gene disorders. Abnormalities in the genes of the mitochondria are transmitted directly from mother to child (see below). A catalog of Mendelian variation in man was compiled and is continuously updated online by McKusick. As of 1986, a total of 1906 variants were of confirmed monogenic etiology. Of these, 1172 are inherited as autosomal dominants, 610 as autosomal recessives, and 124 as X-linked variants (McKusick, 1986a).

The diploid human genome consists of 6 x 10^9 base pairs of deoxyribonucleic acid (DNA), half of which is contributed by the DNA in the nucleus of the maternal ovum, and the other half of which is contributed by the DNA in the nucleus of the paternal sperm. In the human, nuclear DNA is coiled and modified into 46 chromosomes. There are 23 pairs of chromosomes, which are subdivided into 22 pairs of autosomes and one pair of sex chromosomes. Each gene, or segment of DNA, has a particular position, or *locus,* on a chromosome. Since chromosomes exist in pairs, the homologous chromosome normally contains a corresponding gene at the same locus. If an individual has two identical genes at that locus, he is referred to as a *homozygote*. If the individual has different variants of the same gene (alleles) at that locus, he is referred to as a *heterozygote*. When discussing Mendelian inheritance in man, however, it is important to note that the terms "dominant" and "recessive" refer to the observable phenotype, not the genotype.

Autosomal Recessive Inheritance

Conditions that are inherited in an autosomal recessive manner may be characterized in certain ways. Individuals who are affected are homozygous for the particular gene involved in the disorder. In most cases, the affected individual has clinically normal parents who are heterozygotes (carriers) at that locus. As discussed earlier, on pedigree analysis, it is usually apparent that there is a horizontal pattern to the affected individuals, if any pattern exists. Practically speaking, however, in the days of limited family size, the affected individual is usually the first person to come to clinical attention. In autosomal recessive disorders, males and females are equally affected in terms of frequency and severity. The recurrence risks for two heterozygote (carrier) parents are 25% for a homozygote affected child,

25% for a homozygote unaffected child, and 50% for a heterozygote unaffected child. Thus, 75% of future children will be clinically unaffected. When calculating recurrence risks for the unaffected sibling of an affected child, it is important to realize that he has a 66% chance of being a heterozygote. This is because he is clinically normal, so we can rule out the possibility that he is an affected homozygote. Individuals with identical autosomal recessive phenotypes who mate will have only affected offspring; conversely, affected individuals who mate with noncarrier unaffected individuals will have clinically unaffected but carrier offspring.

Examples of Autosomal Recessive Phenotypes

Tay-Sachs Disease

Tay-Sachs disease is a good example of the roughly one-quarter of the diseases inherited in an autosomal recessive manner that are associated with abnormalities in enzyme activity (Rosenberg, 1979). The clinical features in this syndrome are the result of a deficiency in the lysosomal enzyme, hexosaminidase A, which is important in the degradation of the sphingolipid G_{M2} ganglioside. Sphingolipids are key components of nerve cell membranes. When normal metabolism of G_{M2} ganglioside does not occur, its accumulation in neuronal tissue results in the phenotype of blindness, seizures, and psychomotor deterioration.

All individuals, regardless of ethnic background, are heterozygotes (carriers) for 4–8 genes that are potentially harmful in a homozygous condition. Under usual circumstances, two unrelated people will differ in the particular mutant genes they carry. Certain ethnic groups, however, have a higher heterozygote frequency for certain mutant genes and, therefore, at higher risk of certain conditions in their offspring. In a large survey of American Jews of Northeastern European ancestry, 1/27 people were found to be a carrier of the Tay-Sachs gene. In contrast, the heterozygote frequency among non-Jews (with the exception of a small group of French Canadians) is 1/300 people (Kolodny, 1979). The increased carrier frequency in this ethnic group combined with the availability of a simple and accurate method of heterozygote detection has enabled couples at risk for an affected child with Tay-Sachs disease to be identified. Prenatal diagnosis for this condition is available.

Cystic Fibrosis

Cystic fibrosis is the most frequent lethal genetic disease of childhood. Its incidence in Caucasian populations has been estimated between 1/1800 (based on presymptomatic screening of meconium in newborns) (Stephan et al, 1975) and 1/2500 (based on autopsy records) (McCrae, 1983). In persons of northern European background, the carrier (heterozygote) rate, therefore, is between 1/20 and 1/25. Since cystic fibrosis is so common among the general population, it is unlikely that two carrier parents would be consanguineous. Initially, evidence for cystic fibrosis being inherited in an autosomal recessive manner was based on the documented 25% recurrence in siblings of known affected patients (Danks et al, 1965). More recently, by use of DNA-based linkage analysis, the cystic fibrosis gene has been shown to travel in a Mendelian manner very closely linked to an oncogene (White et al, 1985). Several investigators have mapped the cystic fibrosis gene to human chromosome number 7 (White et al, 1985; Tsui et al, 1985; Knowlton et al, 1985; Wainwright et al, 1985).

The protean clinical manifestations of cystic fibrosis include chronic bronchitis, chronic pulmonary infection, malabsorption due to pancreatic dysfunction, meconium ileus, abnormal sweat electrolyte content, cor pulmonale, diabetes mellitus, and male sterility (see pp. 248). The disorder affects all exocrine glands but the primary molecular defect is not known. Prenatal diagnosis is currently available by use of monoclonal antibodies against intestinal alkaline phosphatase present in amniotic fluid. Affected fetuses characteristically have abnormal meconium passage in utero and, therefore, have depressed levels of intestinal alkaline phosphatase (Brock et al, 1985). It is likely that DNA-based analysis of fetal cells will become the standard means of performing prenatal diagnosis for cystic fibrosis in pregnancies at risk (Farrall et al, 1986).

Autosomal Dominant Disorders

Autosomal dominant inheritance may be distinguished from autosomal recessive inheritance in that the mutant gene is inherited from only one parent. Upon pedigree analysis, there is likely to be a vertical pattern of transmission; that is, the abnormal phenotype may be traced through parents and grandparents rather than brothers and sisters. In general, autosomal dominant disorders are less severe clinically than are autosomal recessive disorders. They are more compatible with survival into adulthood and reproduction. If reproductive fitness is unaffected by the mutant gene, the majority of new cases will derive from affected parents. If, on the other hand, the clinical phenotype is severe, affected persons are unlikely to reproduce, and the abnormal gene will be maintained in the population by new mutation. Advanced paternal age has been correlated with an increased incidence of fresh dominant mutations, even when corrected for advanced maternal age (Jones et al, 1975). In autosomal dominant disorders, when an affected person mates with an unaffected person, 50% of their offspring will inherit the mutant phenotype. Two individuals affected with the same dominant phenotype who mate have, in addition, a 25% risk of their offspring inheriting the abnormal gene from both parents. The "homozygote" for the dominant disorder is, in general, more severely affected, and in many cases, this condition is lethal. Autosomal dominant disorders affect males and females equally. They tend to be more variable in their clinical expression than do recessive disorders. In a study of the effects of Mendelian disease on human health, autosomal dominant disorders were shown to have a trimodal age of onset (with peaks occurring during morphogenesis, infancy, and adult life). In contrast, autosomal recessive and X-linked disorders had unimodal onsets that were almost all expressed by puberty (Costa et al, 1985).

Examples of Autosomal Dominant Phenotypes

Marfan Syndrome

The Marfan syndrome is one of the more common autosomal dominant disorders, with a prevalence of four to six cases per 100,000 people. The clinical manifestations of the disorder are diverse (pleiotropic) and expressed in many different ways. The classic physical findings include skeletal abnormalities (inappropriately long limbs, arachnodactyly, pectus deformity, and joint laxity), ocular abnormalities (ectopia lentis), and cardiovascular abnormalities (aortic and mitral valve regurgitation, aortic aneurysms). The diagnosis may be made at birth or not until early adulthood. Since there are no laboratory tests available at the present time to confirm a clinical impression of the Marfan syndrome, the diagnosis is made on the basis of a positive family history, and the presence of characteristic ocular, cardiovascular, and skeletal findings (Pyeritz and McKusick, 1979). Unfortunately, in mildly affected patients, the classic criteria for diagnosis may not be fulfilled. This is an example of the clinical heterogeneity typical of autosomal dominant disorders. In the majority of patients affected with the Marfan syndrome there is a positive family history, but 15% of cases appear to be sporadic. For the new mutations the average paternal age has been shown to be increased (Murdoch et al, 1972). Prenatal diagnosis relies on the use of ultrasonography to document an increased femur length relative to the cranial biparietal diameter as well as any cardiac valvular abnormalities. The precise biochemical defect in the disorder is not known but is presumably related to the structure of collagen. Treatment consists of β-adrenergic blocking agents to prevent the occurrence of aortic root dilatation, which has a high incidence of associated morbidity (see Section 23).

Neurofibromatosis

Neurofibromatosis is a progressive, multisystemic disorder which affects 1/3000 people of both sexes and all races equally. The cardinal clinical features that establish the diagnosis include *café-au-lait* spots, multiple neurofibromas, and the presence of Lisch nodules (pigmented iris hamartomas). Other abnormalities may include: macrocephaly, hearing loss, CNS tumors, intellectual handicap, speech impediment, seizures, kyphoscoliosis, and pseudarthroses or malignant neoplasms, but due to the tremendous variability in clinical expression of the mutant gene, none of these findings are constant (Riccardi, 1981). Although most patients affected with neurofibromatosis appear to live to reproductive age, at least half of the index cases derive from new mutational events, making the neurofibromatosis gene one of the most common spontaneous mutations in man (Crowe et al, 1956). The underlying biologic defect in neurofibromatosis is not understood, although the gene has recently been shown to be linked to the nerve growth factor receptor gene on chromosome 17 (Seizinger et al, 1987; Barker et al, 1987). At the present time, management consists of genetic counseling and surgical intervention (Riccardi, 1981). Prenatal diagnosis is not available. For a more complete discussion of the clinical aspects of neurofibromatosis, see page 741.

X-linked Inheritance

An impressive number of clinical conditions have been mapped to the X chromosome (Fig. 13.3). X-linked disorders are similar to autosomal dominant disorders in that they are clinically variable. What makes them unusual is that males and females differ in the number of X chromosomes they possess. Females have two X chromosomes and are heterozygotes for genes present on the X chromosome. In somatic cells, however, only one X chromosome is expressed and the other is inactivated—a phenomenon known as *lyonization.* Since males have only one X chromosome, they are *hemizygotes* for genes present on that chromosome. Thus, in males, the mutant gene and the phenotype are either present or absent. An unaffected male cannot transmit the mutant gene or the phenotype to his offspring. An affected male, however, will transmit the gene to *all* of his daughters (who will be heterozygote carriers) and *none* of his sons. A heterozygote female carrier will, on the average, transmit the mutant gene to one-half of her sons (who will manifest the phenotype). If an affected male mates with a heterozygote carrier female, one-half of their sons will be affected, but the X chromosome containing the mutant gene will be inherited from the mother. Homozygous daughters arising from such a mating will be as severely affected clinically as their hemizygous brothers. Not all affected males with X-linked disorders have mothers who are heterozygote carriers. In some affected males, the abnormal gene originates by mutation. In fact, in diseases where the affected male does not survive long enough to reproduce, there is likely to be an increased incidence of new mutations responsible for the aberrant gene.

X-linked disorders may be subdivided further by phenotype into X-linked dominant, X-linked recessive, or X-linked lethal. In X-linked dominant conditions, the mutant gene will be expressed phenotypically even if another X chromosome is present and contains a normal homologous gene. In X-linked recessive disorders, the mutant gene is only expressed phenotypically in the hemizygous or homozygous state (usually this occurs in males but females could be homozygous or have another X chromosome that is structurally abnormal). In X-linked lethal conditions, the disorder is only seen clinically in females. Presumably, in hemizygous males, the presence of the mutant gene is incompatible with survival.

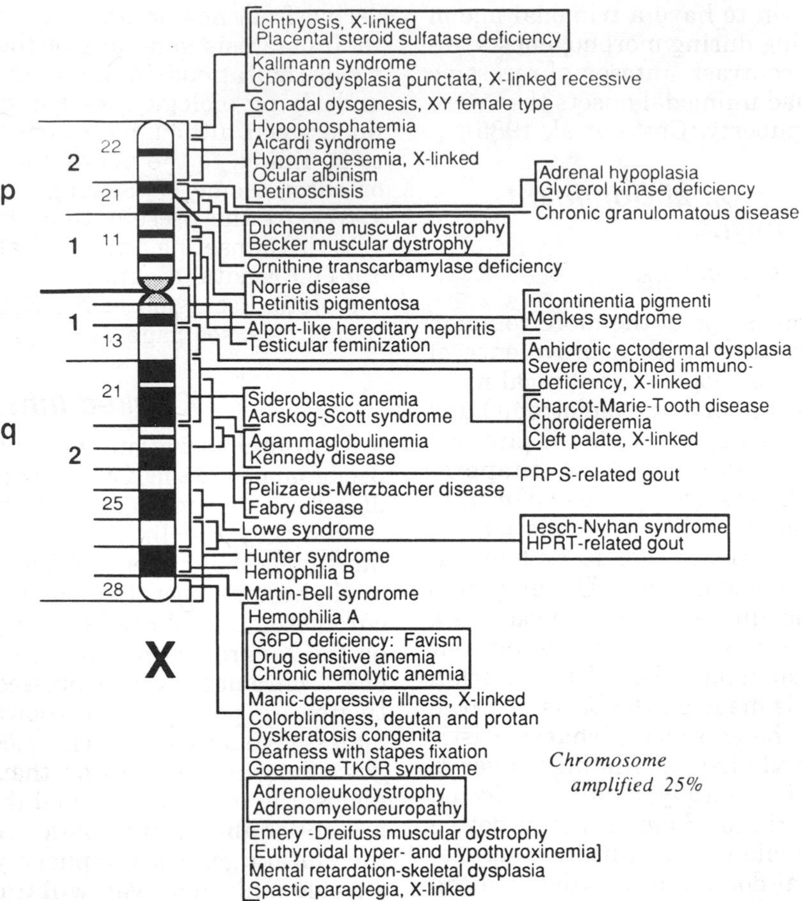

Figure 13.3. The morbid anatomy of the human X chromosome (McKusick VR, *Medicine* 66:237, 1987).

Example of X-linked Dominant Disorders

Vitamin D-Resistant (Renal Hypophosphatemic) Rickets

Renal hypophosphatemic rickets is caused by an isolated defect in phosphate reabsorption in the proximal tubule of the kidney associated with a relatively low serum 1,25-dihydroxy-vitamin D_3 (calcitriol) concentration (Chan et al, 1985). Clinical findings in this condition include childhood rickets, hypophosphatemia, short stature, bone deformities, spontaneous dental abscesses, and osteomalacia in adulthood. The X-linked dominant mode of transmission has been supported by numerous large family studies (Chan et al, 1985). Interestingly, as in all dominant disorders, there is some degree of variability of expression of the phenotype. Not all affected adults will manifest rachitic symptoms but they will uniformly have low fasting serum phosphorus levels. In this disorder, affected males will pass the mutant gene to all of their daughters but none of their sons. Although the heterozygous daughters will all be affected, they will have less severe clinical symptoms than their hemizygous fathers because of random inactivation of one of their X chromosomes. In only some of their cells will the X chromosome containing the mutant gene be the one that is actively expressed. Affected females transmit the mutant gene to one-half of their offspring, independent of sex. Prenatal diagnosis for this condition is not available as affected infants are clinically normal at birth because placental phosphate transport is probably normal.

Examples of X-linked Recessive Disorders

Hemophilia A

Hemophilia A (Factor VIII deficiency) is a well-known X-linked recessive disorder affecting 1/10,000 liveborn males. Factor VIII is a plasma protein essential for the formation of a fibrin clot at the site of vascular injury. Affected individuals are classified as severe, moderate, or mild by their baseline Factor VIII level as compared with normals. Clinical symptoms may include: subcutaneous ecchymoses, hematomas following intramuscular injections, oral mucosal membrane bleeding, and musculoskeletal hemorrhages. Central nervous system bleeding develops in about 3% of affected patients and is a major source of morbidity and mortality (Buchanan, 1980). The diagnosis is suggested by a prolonged partial thromboplastin time but specific functional Factor VIII assays are necessary for confirmation. In about two-thirds of cases, there is a positive family history of hemophilia. The other cases represent new mutations. Affected females have been described but the majority of them have had cytogenetic or DNA abnormalities of their other X chromosome. Recently, DNA probes that map close to the gene for hemophilia have been used to diagnose both the carrier state in females and the affected state in male fetuses (Harper et al, 1984; Antonarakis et al,1985). Hemophilia A has been shown at the molecular level to be a very heterogeneous disorder (see pp. 538).

Lowe Syndrome (Oculocerebrorenal Syndrome)

Lowe syndrome is an X-linked recessive disorder of metabolism that results in abnormalities of the eye, nervous system, and kidneys. Specifically, the ocular defects include cataracts, glaucoma, and nystagmus. Neurologic defects include mental retardation, generalized muscular hypotonia, absent deep tendon reflexes, and hyperactivity. There is renal tubular dysfunction which causes a generalized aminoaciduria, albuminuria, and organic aciduria. Affected males fail to thrive. The X-linked recessive pattern of inheritance has been proven by the nearly exclusive occurrence of the syndrome in males and the high incidence of cataracts in mothers of affected patients. Mothers of affected males have been shown to have asymptomatic fine lenticular abnormalities on slit-lamp examination (Delleman et al, 1977). In addition, ornithine loading has resulted in generalized aminoaciduria in carrier females. The biochemical defect in this syndrome has been postulated to be due to inadequate sulfation of cellular glycosaminoglycans (Yamashina et al, 1983). Affected males have not been known to reproduce.

Examples of X-linked Lethal Conditions

Aicardi Syndrome

Over 100 cases are now known of this syndrome, which essentially occurs only in females. It is thought to be due to a mutant gene on the X chromosome that is lethal in a hemizygote male. Interestingly, a case of Aicardi syndrome has been described in a male with Klinefelter syndrome whose chromosome constitution was 47, XXY (Hopkins et al, 1979). The X chromosome mutation in Aicardi syndrome presumably occurs spontaneously as the family history is always negative and the disease has never been reported in siblings. Salient clinical features of the syndrome include: a distinctive pathognomonic chorioretinopathy consisting of areas of atrophy in the pigment epithelium, infantile flexor spasms beginning shortly after birth, agenesis of the corpus callosum, mental retardation, a characteristic EEG pattern with an asynchronous burst suppression pattern, cortical heterotopia, microophthalmos, and facial asymmetry (Dennis and Bower, 1972). Affected infants may have a limited life span. No affected female has ever reproduced.

Orofacial-Digital Syndrome, Type I

In orofacial-digital syndrome, type I, there are many cases reported in the literature of mother-to-daughter transmission. The overwhelming majority of affected patients are female, although there have been two males described with phenotypic features of the syndrome—one was chromosomally normal and the other was 47,XXY. Most geneticists agree that the inheritance pattern is X-linked, with lethality in males. Autosomal dominant inheritance with sex limitation of expression has been postulated but never proven. An additional argument for X-linked lethal inheritance is the fact that, in families with more than one affected female, there is an increased incidence of spontaneous abortions. The clinical features of the syndrome are not life-threatening and include: a very distinctive facies consisting of a midline cleft of the upper lip, cleft tongue and palate, multiple frenulae of the buccal mucosa, broad nasal bridge with hypoplasia of the nasal alar cartilages, patchy alopecia, digital abnormalities, and mild mental retardation in 25–35% of affected girls (Gorlin and Psaume, 1962). Affected females should be counseled regarding: (a) A 50% recurrence risk in their daughters, (b) the possibility of an altered sex ratio in their living offspring due to in utero loss of affected male fetuses, and (c) the strong probability that liveborn sons will be unaffected clinically.

Y-linked Inheritance

Relatively few genes have been definitively mapped to the Y chromosome. These include genes for H-Y antigen, tooth size, stature, and spermatogenesis factor 3 (McKusick, 1986b). No diseases have, as yet, been proven to be transmitted via the Y chromosome. Obviously, genes on the Y chromosome can only be transmitted from father to son.

Response to Treatment in Mendelian Disorders

The impact of Mendelian (single gene) disease upon life span, reproductive capability, somatic growth, intellectual development, learning ability, capacity to work, and cosmetic appearance was assessed in a recent study of 351 randomly selected gene disorders. The success of treatment for these disorders was later analyzed. The response to treatment was minimal in that life span was increased in 15% of diseases, reproductive capability in 11%, and social adaptation in 6%. In a defined subpopulation of diseases due to inborn errors of metabolism, where the mutant gene product was known, treatment completely eradicated symptoms in 12% of diseases; gave a partial response in 40%, and no response to treatment in 48% of diseases (Hayes et al, 1984). The treatment was most effective when the normal gene product could be delivered to its normal site of action or when dietary or environmental changes restored normal physiology (Hayes et al, 1984).

Single Gene (Non-Mendelian) Disorders

Mitochondrial Inheritance

The preceding sections have described Mendelian inheritance where abnormal phenotypes are the result of transmission of mutant genes in the nucleus from generation to generation. Not all DNA, however, resides in the nucleus. It is now known that mitochondria possess their own chromosome, which is capable of autonomous replication and independent protein synthesis. At least 37 genes have been mapped to the mitochondrial chromosome, 13 of which code for enzymes important in oxidative phosphorylation (McKusick, 1986b). In higher animals, including man, the ovum contributes substantially more cytoplasm to the zygote than does the sperm at fertilization. The sperm mitochondria degenerate upon penetration of the ovum (Nikoskelainen, 1984). Thus, mitochondria in offspring are always exclusively maternally derived. This was elegantly shown by the study of DNA polymorphisms (see Chapter 3) in mitochondrial DNA. Peripheral blood platelets were used as a source of mitochondrial DNA because these cells are anucleate. In families where each of the parents demonstrated different restriction endonuclease patterns in their mitochondrial DNA, the progeny always inherited the maternal pattern (Giles et al, 1980). Thus, in diseases characterized by abnormalities of mitochondrial structure or metabolism, a non-Mendelian (maternal) pattern of inheritance might be predicted. Such is the case in two disorders, Leber optic atrophy and mitochondrial cytopathy. Since this is an active area of research, it seems likely that other disorders will be added to the list.

Examples of Mitochondrial Inheritance

Mitochondrial Cytopathy

Mitochondrial cytopathy is a familial disorder. Signs and symptoms include ophthalmoplegia, CNS abnormalities, short stature, diabetes, cardiomyopathy, hypoplastic anemia, and renal tubular dysfunction. On skeletal muscle biopsy, aggregates of abnormal mitochondria are seen. Mitochondrial enzymes have been shown to be deficient in this syndrome. A recent multigenerational review of 30 families affected with mitochondrial cytopathy showed exclusive maternal transmission in 27/30. The results were believed to be consistent with mitochondrial transmission of mitochondrial cytopathy (Egger and Wilson, 1983).

Leber Optic Atrophy

Leber optic atrophy is an intraocular neuroretinopathy which results in acute or subacute visual loss in otherwise healthy young people. The majority of affected patients are male but 14% of those affected are female. The pathology may be secondary to a defect in the metabolism of cyanide. This detoxification of cyanide is catalyzed by the mitochondrial enzyme, thiosulfur-transferase. Evidence in favor of mitochondrial transmission of the disease is that men have never been shown to pass the disease to their offspring; the disease is always transmitted via carrier women. What is not known, however, is why there is an unequal sex ratio in persons clinically manifesting symptoms (Nikoskelainen, 1984) (see p. 717).

Multifactorial Inheritance

Multifactorial inheritance refers to the interaction between an individual's genetic background and environmental factors such as socioeconomic status, diet, or geography. Counseling regarding recurrence risks is more difficult for multifactorial inheritance than for the Mendelian single gene disorders. On average, a recurrence risk of 5% is usually quoted, but for many of the more common birth defects (congenital hip dislocation, hypospadias, neural tube defects) empiric data obtained from large population surveys are available and should be used.

REFERENCES

Antonarakis SE, Waber PG, Kittur SD, et al: Hemophilia A: Detection of molecular defects and of carriers by DNA analysis. *N Engl J Med* 313:842, 1985.

Barker D, Wright E, Nguyen K, et al: Gene for von Recklinghausen neurofibromatosis is in the pericentromeric region of chromosome 17. *Science* 236:1100, 1987.

Berg P: Dissections and reconstructions of genes and chromosomes. *Science* 213:296, 1981.

Brock DJH, Barron L, Bedgood D, et al: Prospective prenatal diagnosis of cystic fibrosis. *Lancet* 1:1175, 1985.

Buchanan GR: Hemophilia. *Pediatr Clin North Am* 27:309, 1980.

Chan JCM, Alon U, Hirschman GM: Renal hypophosphatemic rickets. *J Pediatr* 106:533, 1985.

Costa T, Scriver CR, Childs B: The effect of Mendelian disease on human health: A measurement. *Am J Med Genet* 21:231, 1985.

Crowe FW, Schull WJ, Neel JV: *A Clinical, Pathological, and Genetic Study of Multiple Neurofibromatosis*. Springfield, IL, Charles C Thomas, 1956.

Danks DM, Allan J, Anderson CM: Genetic study of fibrocystic disease of the pancreas. *Ann Hum Genet* 28:323, 1965.

Day N, Holmes LB: The incidence of genetic disease in a university hospital population. *Am J Hum Genet* 25:237, 1973.

Delleman JW, Bleeker-Wagemakers EM, van Veelen AW: Opacities of the lens indicating carrier status in the oculo-cerebro-renal (Lowe) syndrome. *J Pediatr Ophthalmol* 14:205, 1977.

Dennis J, Bower BD: The Aicardi syndrome. *Dev Med Child Neurol* 14:382, 1972.

Egger J, Wilson J: Mitochondrial inheritance in a mitochondrially mediated disease. *N Engl J Med* 309:142, 1983.

Farrall M, Rodeck CH, Stanier P, et al: First trimester prenatal diagnosis of cystic fibrosis with linked DNA probes. *Lancet* 1:1402, 1986.

Giles RE, Blanc H, Cann HM, et al: Maternal inheritance of human mitochondrial DNA. *Proc Natl Acad Sci USA* 77:6715, 1980.

Gorlin RJ, Psaume J: Orodigitofacial dysostosis—a new syndrome. *J Pediatr* 61:520, 1962.

Hall JG, Powers EK, McIlvaine RT, et al: The frequency and financial burden of genetic disease in a pediatric hospital. *Am J Med Genet* 1:417, 1978.

Harper PS: Genetic counseling and prenatal diagnosis. *Br Med Bull* 39:302, 1983.

Harper K, Pembrey ME, Davies KE, et al: A clinically useful DNA probe closely linked to haemophilia A. *Lancet* 2:6, 1984.

Hayes A, Costa T, Scriver CR, et al: The effect of Mendelian disease on human health: Response to treatment. *Am J Med Genet* 21:243, 1984.

Hopkins IJ, Humphrey I, Keith CG, et al: The Aicardi syndrome in a 47,XXY male. *Austral Pediatr J* 15:278, 1979.

Jones KL, Smith DW, Harvey MAS, et al: Older paternal age and fresh gene mutation: data on additional disorders. *J Pediatr* 86:84, 1975.

Knowlton RG, Cohen-Haguenauer O, Van Cong N: A polymorphic DNA marker linked to cystic fibrosis is located on chromosome 7. *Nature* 318:380, 1985.

Kolodny EH: Tay Sachs disease. In: Goodman RM, Motulsky AG (eds): *Genetic Diseases Among Ashkenazi Jews*. New York, Raven Press, 1979, p. 221.

McCrae WM: Cystic fibrosis. In Emery AH, Rimoin DL (eds): *Principles and Practice of Medical Genetics*. New York, Churchill Livingstone, 1983, p. 899.

McKusick VA: *Mendelian Inheritance in Man*, 7th edition. Baltimore, Johns Hopkins University Press, 1986a.

McKusick VA: The morbid anatomy of the human genome: A review of gene mapping in clinical medicine. *Medicine* 65:1, 1986b.

Murdoch JL, Walker BA, McKusick VA: Parental age effects on the occurrence of new mutations for the Marfan syndrome. *Ann Hum Genet* 35:331, 1972.

Nadler HL: Role of the general pediatrician in genetics. *Pediatr Rev* 3:5, 1981.

Nikoskelainen E: New aspects of the genetic, etiologic, and clinical puzzle of Leber's disease. *Neurology* 34:1482, 1984.

Pyeritz RE, McKusick VA: The Marfan syndrome: Diagnosis and management. *N Engl J Med* 300:772, 1979.

Riccardi VM: Von Recklinghausen neurofibromatosis. *N Engl J Med* 305:1617, 1981.

Riccardi VM, Cohen A, Chen MT: Genetic counseling as part of hospital care. *Am J Public Health* 68:652, 1978.

Rosenberg LE: Progress in understanding autosomal recessive diseases. In Goodman RM, Motulsky AG (eds): *Genetic Diseases Among Ashkenazi Jews*. New York, Raven Press, 1979, p. 108.

Scriver CR, Neal JL, Saginur R, et al: The frequency of genetic disease and congenital malformations among patients in a pediatric hospital. *Can Med Assoc J* 108:1111, 1973.

Seizinger BR, Rouleau GA, Ozelius LJ, et al: Genetic linkage of von Recklinghausen neurofibromatosis to the nerve growth factor receptor gene. *Cell* 49:589, 1987.

Sly WS, Whyte MP, Sundaram V, et al: Carbonic anhydrase II deficiency in 12 families with the autosomal recessive syndrome of osteopetrosis with renal tubular acidosis and cerebral calcification. *N Engl J Med* 313:139, 1985.

Stephan U, Busch EW, Kollberg H, et al: Cystic fibrosis detection by means of a test-strip. *Pediatrics* 55:35, 1975.

Tsui LC, Buchwald M, Barker D, et al: Cystic fibrosis locus defined by a genetically linked polymorphic DNA marker. *Science* 230:1054, 1985.

Wainwright BJ, Scambler PJ, Schmidtke J: Localization of cystic fibrosis locus to human chromosome 7 cen - q 22. *Nature* 318:384, 1985.

White R, Woodward S, Leppert M, et al: A closely linked genetic marker for cystic fibrosis. *Nature* 318:382, 1985.

Yamashina I, Yoshida H, Fukui S, et al: Biochemical studies on Lowe's syndrome. *Molec Cell Biochem* 52:107, 1983.

Cytogenetics 2

Normal Karyotype

Cytogenetic disease is the result of visible, quantitative changes in the human genome. The normal human karyotype consists of 46 chromosomes, as shown in Figure 13.4. There are 22 pairs of autosomes and one pair of sex chromosomes. Normal females have two X chromosomes and normal males have an X chromosome and a Y chromosome. A chromosome is actually a single long DNA molecule which has various proteins attached to it.

Chromosomes may be studied in almost any nucleated cell, but the easiest to obtain are peripheral blood leukocytes. Depending upon the age of the patient, a venous blood sample of between 1 and 10 ml is collected in a green top tube containing heparin. The blood is then incubated with a culture medium including phytohemagglutinin, which stimulates cell division. After a 2- to 3-day incubation, the chromosomes are "harvested" by adding colcemid to arrest cells in mitosis. A hypotonic solution is added to spread out the chromosomes. Chromosomes are analyzed with a light microscope. Under 10X magnification, metaphases suitable for cytogenetic analysis are selected and are then studied in detail at 100X. Chromosomes consist of two parallel sister chromatids held together by a centromere. The position of the centromere is constant for each chromosome and is an important part of its identification. Acrocentric chromosomes have their centromere near the tip. Metacentrics have their centromere in the middle of the chromosome.

Banding Techniques

When a karyotype is ordered, the patient's chromosomes are analyzed and grouped according to size, position of the centromere, and banding pattern with certain stains. The pairs of autosomes are numbered 1–22, in order of decreasing size. In the past, they were grouped according to similar appearance and given letters A through G. Banding techniques currently allow precise identification of individual chromosomes. In the standard metaphase karyotype, 440 separate bands may be observed (Michels, 1985). A chromosome band is the

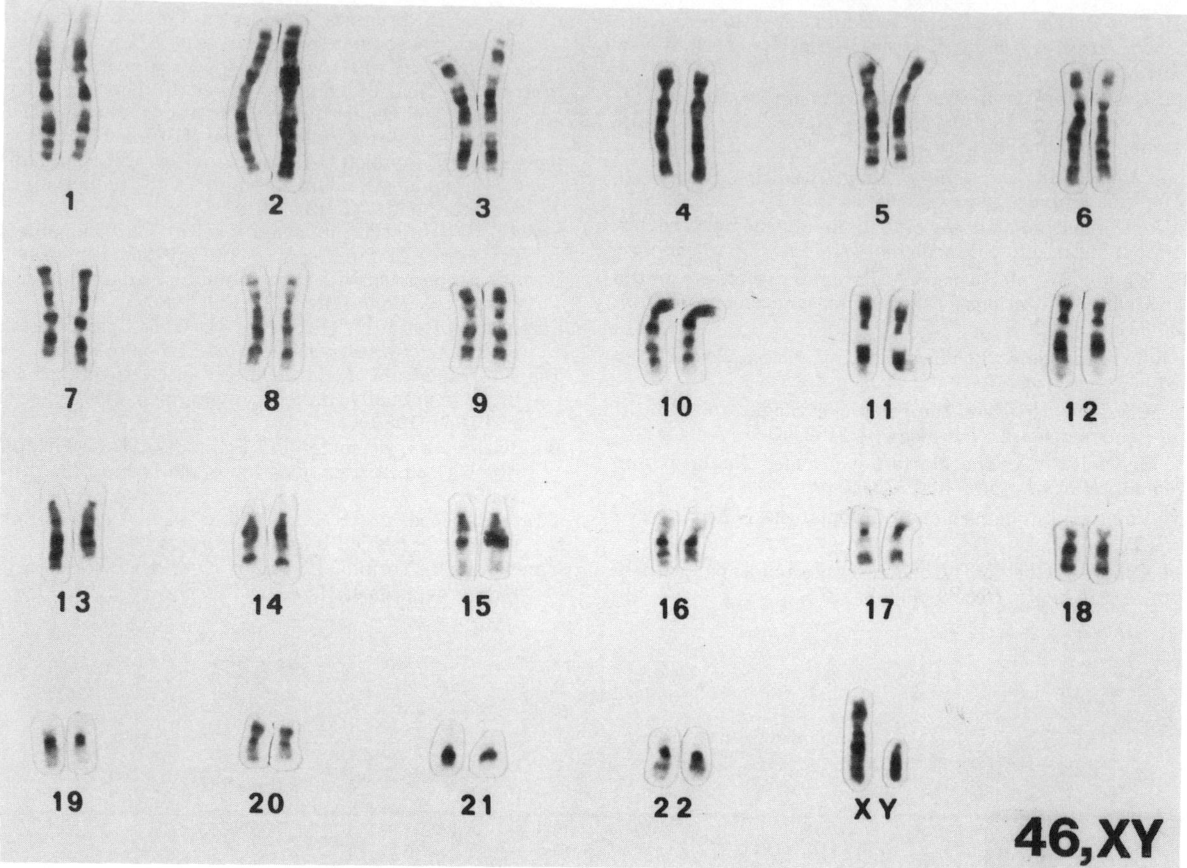

Figure 13.4. Giemsa banded normal male karyotype (photograph courtesy of Dr. Mary Sandstrom and Brigham and Women's Hospital Cytogenetics Laboratory).

part of the chromosome that can be differentiated from its neighboring segments by appearing darker or lighter. A summary of the different banding techniques is given in Table 13.2. Each segment of a chromosome is defined by a chromosome number, arm designation (p = short arm, q = long arm), region number, and band number (example = 15 q 11; Fig. 13.5).

The indications for performing a chromosome analysis are summarized in Table 13.3.

Incidence of Abnormalities in Newborns

In a study of 11,148 consecutive live births, 8.6/1000 were shown to have a chromosomal abnormality (Nielsen et al, 1981). Of these, 2.6/1000 had a sex chromosome abnormality, 2.2/1000 had an extra autosome, and 3.8/1000 had balanced translocations or inversions. In studies of stillbirths and abortuses, the rate is much higher.

NUMERICAL ABERRATIONS

Aneuploidy describes abnormalities in the number of chromosomes present. Usually this is the result of *nondisjunction* in either the first or second parental meiotic division during gametogenesis. Homologous chromosomes normally migrate to separate daughter cells, but occasionally they end up in the same daughter cell. After fertilization, one daughter cell contains one whole chromosome in excess (*trisomy*) and the other

Table 13.2
Banding Techniques[1]

Type	Description
"Q" (quinacrine)	Fluorescent derivatives of quinacrine followed by microscopic examination in ultraviolet light; useful for study of the Y chromosome and the region around the centromere of chromosome 3
"R" (reverse)	Staining after heat denaturation; useful to study the tips of chromosomes
"G" (giemsa)	Staining after ionic or enzymatic treatment
"C"	Staining of centromeres
"T"	Staining of telomeres
"Nor-silver stain"	Staining of the nucleolar organizers present on the short arm of the acrocentric chromosomes

[1]Modified from deGrouchy J, Turleau C: *Clinical Atlas of Human Chromosomes*. New York, John Wiley and Sons, 1984, p. 418.

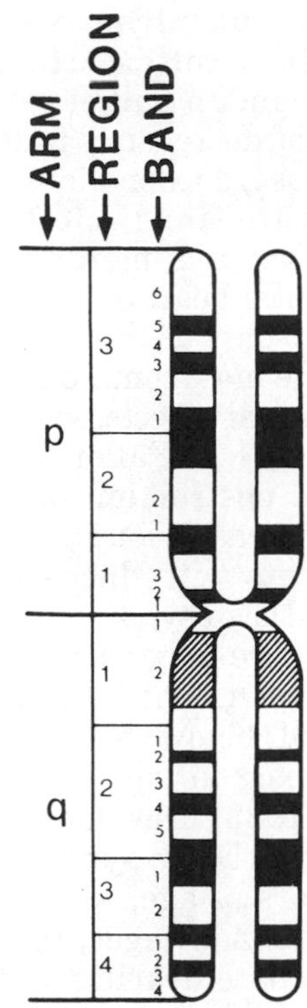

Figure 13.5. Each segment of a chromosome may be identified by an arm letter, region, and band number.

Table 13.3
Indications for Chromosome Analysis

Prenatal Diagnosis
Maternal age greater than 35 years
Family history of chromosome abnormality
Previous child with chromosome abnormality
Family history of X-linked disorder
Stillbirth with Anomalies
Infant or Child
Multiple congenital anomalies
Psychomotor retardation with dysmorphic features
Ambiguous genitalia
Adolescents
Female with short stature
Female with primary amenorrhea
Male with delayed puberty
Adults
Infertile couples
Couples with two or more spontaneous abortions
Family history of specific cancer
Question of chromosomal breakage syndrome

daughter cell is missing one chromosome (*monosomy*). In general, monosomy is lethal in embryonic life, whereas trisomy is somewhat more compatible with survival through at least part of the pregnancy.

Polyploidy refers to a multiple of the normal haploid chromosome number (23). Thus, triploid infants have 69 chromosomes and tetraploid infants have 92 chromosomes. Both conditions are incompatible with prolonged extrauterine survival. Polyploidy is the result of fertilization of the ovum with two or three sperm.

Mosaicism is the presence of two or more cell lines with different karyotypes in the same person. This develops when nondisjunction occurs after fertilization. If one of the cell lines contains a normal complement of chromosomes, the clinical manifestations of the syndrome will be lessened.

Autosomes

The most common examples of aneuploidy compatible with life are trisomy 21, trisomy 18, and trisomy 13. The trisomies 8, 9, and 14 have also been reported but the survivors tend to be mosaic with a normal cell line.

Trisomy 21 (Down Syndrome)

Definition

Trisomy 21 is a syndrome of multiple malformations, characteristic physical appearance (Fig. 13.6), and mental retardation due to an extra copy of chromosome 21.

Basic Science

Although the disorder was first described clinically in 1866 by the British surgeon John Langdon Down (Scoggin and Patterson, 1982), it was not until 1959 that Lejeune reported that Down syndrome patients had an extra acrocentric G group chromosome (Zellweger, 1977). Chromosome 21 represents 1.5% of the haploid genome. The portion of the chromosome that is responsible for the syndrome's phenotype is the distal long arm, bands q 22 to q ter. It has been estimated that there are about 750 genes in this region (Shapiro, 1983). The clinical manifestations are presumed to be due to gene dosage (three copies of these genes are present instead of two) but the biochemical mechanisms involved are currently unknown. Ninety-four percent of patients have the full trisomy, 4% have a translocation between number 21 and another chromosome, and 2% are mosaics (Zellweger, 1977). In the most common situation (full trisomy), the extra chromosome 21 is the result of parental nondisjunction. Although the incidence of nondisjunction increases with advanced maternal age, the extra chromosome has been shown to originate from the mother only 80% of the time (Juberg and Mowrey, 1983).

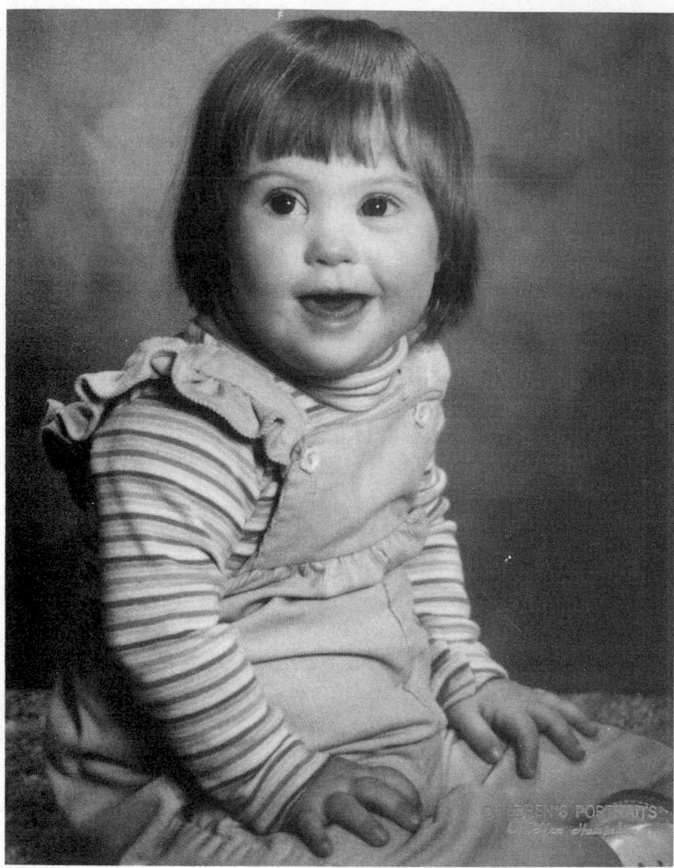

Figure 13.6. A young girl with Down syndrome demonstrating the flattened facies, upslanting palpebral fissures, epicanthal folds, flattened nasal bridge and brachydactyly (photograph courtesy of Dr. Allen C. Crocker). Her personal progress has been assisted by a program that includes developmental stimulation and family support. She will require special educational and vocational training.

Epidemiology

The incidence of trisomy 21 is 1/800 to 1/1000 live births. The prevalence of 1/3000 in the general population reflects the high infant mortality rate (Zellweger, 1977).

Natural History

Trisomy 21 is highly lethal in fetal life; 65% of conceptuses do not survive to term (Zellweger, 1977). A study of aborted trisomy 21 fetuses has shown that there is a recognizable fetal phenotype consisting of growth retardation, septal cardiac defects, simian crease, and clinodactyly (Stephens and Shepard, 1980). Affected fetuses have decreased motor activity in utero. The umbilical cord is significantly shorter than in normal controls (Moessinger et al, 1986). Newborns with trisomy 21 are typically lethargic and poor feeders. Hall has described 10 cardinal signs of Down syndrome in neonates: slanting palpebral fissures, small dysplastic ears, excess nuchal skin, flattened facies, simian crease, dysplastic middle phalanx of the fifth finger, hyperextensible joints, muscular hypotonia, dysplastic pelvis, and absent Moro reflex (Hall, 1964). Major malformations are found in half of patients with Down syndrome. In order of decreasing frequency, they are: congenital heart disease, duodenal obstruction, club foot, cataracts, imperforate anus, cleft lip and palate, Hirschsprung disease, and meningomyelocele (Zellweger, 1977). Congenital heart disease is found in 28.5% of newborns with trisomy 21 but 63.5% of necropsies (Zellweger, 1977). The most common cardiac anomalies are atrioventricular canal defects, ventricular and atrial septal defects, tetralogy of Fallot, and patent ductus arteriosus. Duodenal obstruction (due to atresia, stenosis, or annular pancreas) is found in 2–3% of patients. Conversely, in patients with duodenal obstruction at birth, one-third have Down syndrome (Zellweger, 1977).

In trisomy 21, there is generalized retardation in growth and development. The height of affected individuals is usually 2 SD below the mean for age. Special growth charts now exist for children with Down Syndrome (Cronk et al, 1988). Developmental delay is apparent in infancy. Most Down syndrome children walk between 2 and 4 years of age, while the average age for speech is 4–6 years (Zellweger, 1977). Frequent serous otitis may exacerbate hearing and speech difficulties. Down syndrome children are at risk for atlantoaxial joint instability. Secondary sexual development is essentially normal in both sexes, but males are infertile due to testicular interstitial fibrosis and hypoplasia of seminiferous tubules (Zellweger, 1977). Some females have become pregnant. Compared with normal controls, patients with trisomy 21 have an increased incidence of primary congenital hypothyroidism (Fort et al, 1984), thyroiditis, and diabetes mellitus. The 10- to 30-fold increased incidence of leukemia is well documented (Robison et al, 1984).

Down syndrome adults age prematurely and may develop senile dementia in the fourth decade of life. Neuropathologic studies have revealed a striking similarity between the brains of adults with Down syndrome and the brains from phenotypically normal adults with Alzheimer disease. In both disorders decreased cerebral metabolism of glucose is observed as well as decreased concentrations of neurotransmitters in brain tissue, and decreased amounts of the enzyme choline acetyltransferase in the brain (Fishman, 1986). The gene encoding the amino acid sequence of the amyloid β peptide found in senile plaques from brains with Alzheimer disease and Down syndrome maps to chromosome 21 (Tanzi et al, 1987).

Diagnosis

The diagnosis may be suggested by the finding of duodenal obstruction or atrioventricular canal defect on prenatal ultrasonography. In such cases, prenatal karyotype is indicated. Most commonly, the affected infant is born after an unremarkable pregnancy, and it is the physical appearance that alerts delivery room personnel to the possibility of Down syndrome. Once the question has been raised, a banded karyotype is necessary to confirm or refute the diagnosis. In the rare event of a translocation, parental chromosomes should be studied.

Treatment

Bowel obstruction and congenital heart disease may be treated surgically. Congestive heart failure is treated with digoxin and diuretics. Primary hypothyroidism is managed with thyroid replacement. Leukemia is treated with conventional chemotherapy. Frequent monitoring for serous otitis is indicated. A screening lateral cervical roentgenogram should be performed at age 6 years to rule out atlantoaxial joint instability before participation in sports involving stress on the head. Infant stimulation, physical therapy, and speech therapy are warranted. Megadose vitamin and mineral supplementation has not been shown to increase intelligence (Smith et al, 1984).

NEW DEVELOPMENTS

The presence of double satellites on silver staining of parental acrocentric chromosomes has been considered by some to confer an increased risk of offspring with Down syndrome (Jackson-Cook et al, 1985). Fluorescent chromosome 21 DNA probes have been developed to screen rapidly uncultured amniotic fluid cells for the presence of trisomy 21 (Julien et al, 1986).

Prognosis

Mortality is high in fetal and neonatal life. In a study of 1341 patients with Down syndrome from British Columbia, an increased likelihood of survival was correlated with the absence of congenital heart disease. Survival to age 1 year was 76.3% for the patients with congenital heart disease and 90.7% for the patients without heart disease (Baird and Sadovnick, 1987). Survival to adulthood is complicated by premature senility.

Prevention

The disease may be detected prenatally by fetal karyotype of cells obtained at chorionic villus biopsy or amniocentesis. The disorder may be prevented by selective termination of affected fetuses. The recurrence risk for full trisomy 21, independent of maternal age, is 1%. No increased risk of trisomy 21 has been shown in siblings, nieces, nephews, aunts, or uncles of the proband with trisomy 21 (Abuelo et al, 1986). A low maternal serum α-fetoprotein may be present if the fetus has Down syndrome (see pp. 786).

Trisomy 18 (Edwards Syndrome)

Definition

Trisomy 18 is a syndrome of multiple malformations resulting from the presence of an extra number 18 chromosome.

Basic Science

The existence of the extra chromosome 18 is due to meiotic nondisjunction, the incidence of which increases with advanced maternal age. It is not known precisely how the presence of the extra chromosome influences organogenesis. Many of the anomalies characteristic of the syndrome reflect developmental arrest early in gestation.

Epidemiology

Different studies have placed the incidence between 0.3/1000 live births (Edwards et al, 1960) and 1/6766 live births (Taylor, 1968).

Natural History

The syndrome is more common at conception than at birth. One study of the natural history of trisomy 18 fetuses showed that the live birth rate was only 30% of the rate found at amniocentesis (Schreinemachers et al, 1982). Most trisomy 18 fetuses are growth-retarded. The average birth weight is 2.18 kg (Warkany et al, 1966). There is a predominance of affected females. The characteristic malformations, found in more than 50% of cases, are: prominent occiput, low-set malformed ears, micrognathia, clenched hands with overlapping of the index and fifth fingers, short sternum, inguinal and umbilical hernias, cardiac defects, short dorsiflexed halluces, and rocker bottom feet. Over 130 abnormalities have been described (Muller and deJong, 1986). Malformations of the CNS are less common in trisomy 18 than trisomy 13 (Warkany et al, 1966). In a postmortem study of cardiac findings in cases of trisomy 18, 87% had a membranous ventricular septal defect, 73% had a patent ductus arteriosus, and 80% had an abnormally high takeoff of the right coronary ostium. In addition, the valvular tissue was noted to be dysplastic and resembled primitive fetal mesenchyme (Matsuoka et al, 1983). Affected infants with trisomy 18 are mentally retarded. There is a characteristic dermatoglyphic pattern, consisting of at least three and as many as 10 low arches on the fingertips (Taylor, 1968).

Diagnosis

The diagnosis may be suspected at ultrasonography by the presence of polyhydramnios, growth retardation, cardiac defects, or micrognathia (Benacerraf et al, 1986). The diagnosis is made by karyotype, preferably a banded one. If the clinical findings are strongly suggestive of trisomy 18 yet the chromosome results are normal, there are two possibilities: the patient either is a mosaic, or has one of the syndromes that overlap with trisomy 18. These are: (a) Pena-Shokeir, type I: a syndrome of intrauterine growth retardation, pulmonary hypoplasia, scalp edema, decreased fetal movement, and multiple congenital contractures; and (b) cerebro-oculo-facial-skeletal syndrome: microcephaly, microphthalmia, cataracts, prominent nasal root, and joint contractures (Pena and Shokeir, 1974). These syndromes are distinguished from trisomy 18 by their normal chromosomes and autosomal recessive pattern of inheritance.

Treatment

Since the life span of infants with trisomy 18 is so limited (see Prognosis, below) treatment should be judged accordingly. Surgical emergencies (such as tracheoesophageal fistula) may need to be treated to allow the infant to survive until a diagnosis can be made. Infants with mosaic trisomy 18 may survive long enough to require repair of cardiac defects. When an infant is born and is presumed to have trisomy 18, early involvement of a genetics service will help in providing family support and continuity of care.

Prognosis

Less than 4% of affected patients survive to their first birthday. In one study, the median life expectancy for a live born infant was 5 days (range 1 hour to 18 months) (Carter et al, 1985). Longer survivors are all mentally retarded. A patient who survived to 13 years of age has been reported. Her clinical findings included progressive scoliosis, limb hypertonicity, frequent respiratory infections, and a developmental age of 3 months (Mehta et al, 1986).

Prevention

Trisomy 18 may be diagnosed by prenatal karyotype of fetal cells obtained at amniocentesis or chorionic villus biopsy. The condition may be prevented by termination of affected fetuses. There is a recurrence risk of 1%, independent of maternal age but the incidence of the syndrome increases with advanced maternal age. A low serum maternal α-fetoprotein may be seen in fetuses with trisomy 18.

Trisomy 13 (Patau Syndrome)

Definition

Trisomy 13 is a constellation of congenital anomalies resulting from the presence of an extra number 13 chromosome, either whole or translocated onto another chromosome.

Basic Science

About 80% of patients with trisomy 13 have the full trisomy (47, XX or 47, XY + 13), which is due to meiotic nondisjunction. Trisomy 13 does not increase with advanced maternal age as sharply as does trisomy 18 or 21 (Schreinemachers et al, 1982). The other 20% have either mosaic trisomy 13 or trisomy 13 due to a translocation. Robertsonian translocations occur between D and G group (acrocentric) chromosomes. Fusion occurs at the centromeres and this results in loss of chromosomal material from both short arms. Robertsonian translocations are the most common kind of balanced translocation in the normal population (1/1000) (Hodes et al, 1978). They predispose individuals to produce offspring with trisomy 13 or 21.

It is not known how the presence of the extra chromosome 13 disrupts organogenesis.

Epidemiology

The reported frequency of trisomy 13 live births varies from 1/2206 to 1/7602 (Taylor, 1968).

Natural History

Fetuses with trisomy 13 are more active in utero than are fetuses with trisomy 18. They are not dramatically growth-retarded. Although the average birth weight is 2.48 kg (Warkany et al, 1966), many affected patients are normal in size. The sex ratio of affected infants is probably equal. The most common physical findings include: scalp defects (often confused with scalp lacerations made by fetal scalp electrodes) (Fig. 13.7), microcephaly, microphthalmia, cleft lip and palate, congenital heart disease, inguinal and umbilical hernias, omphalocele, cryptorchidism, micropenis, polycystic kidneys, polydactyly, and capillary hemangiomata. CNS anomalies frequently found are: holoprosencephaly, absent olfactory nerves, absent or small optic nerves, and an abnormally small corpus callosum (Taylor, 1968). In a series of 76 cases, cardiac malformations were found in 82% and renal anomalies were found in 60% (Hodes et al, 1978). Infants who survive the perinatal period are always retarded.

Diagnosis

The diagnosis may be suggested by the finding of holoprosencephaly or cleft lip and palate with cardiac anomalies on prenatal ultrasonography (Benacerraf et al, 1986). If the diagnosis of trisomy 13 is suspected, a banded chromosome study must be performed. If the infant has a translocation, the parents' chromosomes should be studied to give accurate figures for risk of recurrence. If the chromosomes are normal, the patient

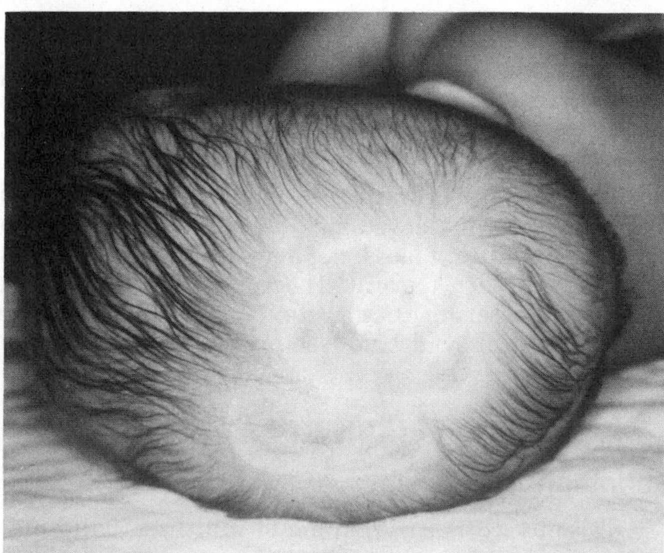

Figure 13.7. Large scalp defect seen in an infant with trisomy 13.

may be a mosaic trisomy 13 or possibly have the Meckel-Gruber syndrome. Findings in Meckel-Gruber syndrome include: polycystic kidneys (seen in 100% of patients), encephalocoele (80%), polydactyly (70%), and cleft lip and palate (30%) (Miller, 1983). It is important to diagnose the Meckel-Gruber syndrome, as it is inherited as an autosomal recessive disorder and carries a recurrence risk of 25%.

Treatment

Since the life span of infants with trisomy 13 is severely limited (see Prognosis, below) most treatment is directed toward comfort measures. In rare cases, surgical treatment may be necessary to allow an infant to survive long enough until a definitive diagnosis can be made. When an infant suspected to have trisomy 13 is born, early involvement of a genetics service will assist in providing family support and continuity of care.

Prognosis

The prognosis for infants with trisomy 13 is poor. The mean survival time is 89 days (Taylor, 1968) and all are retarded. Survival is related to the severity of cardiac and brain anomalies.

Prevention

The recurrence risk for a nondisjunction type of full trisomy, independent of maternal age, is 1%. If the infant is shown to have a translocation but the parental chromosomes are normal, the recurrence risk is less than 1%. If one of the parents has a balanced translocation, there is a 20% risk of spontaneous abortion and a 5% risk of a liveborn infant with trisomy 13. An exception to this would be a balanced Robertsonian translocation between both parental number 13 chromosomes. In this case, no normal offspring could be produced. Trisomy 13 may be prevented by prenatal diagnosis via fetal karyotype obtained at chorionic villus biopsy or amniocentesis.

Trisomy 8

In trisomy 8, there is a high incidence of mosaicism in those who survive beyond the perinatal period. The craniofacial dysmorphism may be quite mild—abnormalities include a wide nose and thick lower lip. Osteoarticular abnormalities are common but organ malformations are rare. Mental retardation may be mild or absent (Berry et al, 1978; Riccardi, 1977).

Trisomy 9

Infants with trisomy 9 have severe mental retardation and failure-to-thrive. Craniofacial features include microcephaly, high forehead, microphthalmia, and retromicrognathia. Dislocation of the hips, knees, and elbows exists. Congenital heart disease is common. Mosaicism is present in 50% of cases (Katayama et al, 1980; Qazi et al, 1977).

Trisomy 14

Trisomy 14 usually exists in the mosaic state. Infants have intrauterine growth retardation, microcephaly, a broad nose, cleft palate, micrognathia, short stature, congenital heart disease, and severe retardation (Kaplan et al, 1986). A 13½-year-old girl has been described with this karyotype (Johnson et al, 1979).

Sex Chromosomes

Aneuploidy for the sex chromosomes (45, X; 47, XXY; 47, XYY) occurs quite frequently. The clinical manifestations of these syndromes are discussed in Section 14, Endocrinology.

STRUCTURAL ABERRATIONS

Deletions

The presence of a deletion implies that, at some point, the chromosome has broken and some of the genetic material has been lost. Hence, individuals with a deletion are monosomic for the genes present on that chromosome.

Prader-Labhart-Willi syndrome is an example of a well-known disorder that has an associated cytogenetic deletion present in about 50% of cases. Other syndromes include Langer-Giedion (deletion of 8 q 24), Miller-Dieker (deletion of 17 p 13), and DiGeorge (deletion 22 q 11).

Rarer syndromes are known by the missing segment. Discussed below are $4p^-$, $5p^-$, $9p^-$, $18p^-$, and $18q^-$.

$4p^-$ (Wolf-Hirschhorn Syndrome)

This deletion occurs de novo in 90% of cases. In 10% of cases, there is parental translocation or mosaicism. Affected infants have intrauterine growth retardation, microcephaly, scalp defects, and a characteristic "greek warrior helmet" facies. There is hypospadias in males. Fifty percent of patients have congenital heart disease. The life expectancy is not known (Guthrie et al, 1971; Lurie et al, 1980; Miller et al, 1970).

$5p^-$ (Cri Du Chat Syndrome)

This is a clinically and cytogenetically heterogeneous syndrome with an incidence of 1/50,000 live births. The syndrome received its name because affected newborns have a distinct, shrill, cat-like cry which may be due to a hypoplastic larynx. Patients with the syndrome are only mildly dysmorphic, are mentally retarded, may have frequent upper respiratory infections and otitis, but have a normal life expectancy. Associated malformations are rare (Breg et al, 1970; Niebuhr, 1978; Wilkins et al, 1983).

$9p^-$

This syndrome is due to the deletion of material distal to band 9p 22. Infants have a striking appearance consisting of trigonocephaly (triangular-shaped head), midface hypoplasia, upward slanting palpebral fissures, arched eyebrows, and epicanthal folds. There is an increased incidence of cardiac malformations, omphalocele, and hernias. Infants have a normal birth weight and length. The average IQ is 30–60. A normal life span is expected (Deroover et al, 1978; Funderburk et al, 1979).

$18p^-$

Patients with this chromosome constitution have CNS malformations, mental retardation (IQ 25–75), large floppy ears, frequent dental caries, a characteristic posture with widespread legs and a forward lean, and small stature. IgA is decreased or absent in 50% of cases. Life expectancy is not shortened (Schinzel et al, 1974).

$18q^-$

In this syndrome, muscular hypotonia, microcephaly, a depressed midface, a carp-like mouth, and abnormal genitalia are present. Mental retardation is variable. In one-third of cases, IgA is deficient. Ten percent of affected newborns die in the first few months of life. At least one female with the syndrome has reproduced (Schinzel et al, 1975).

Prader-Labhart-Willi Syndrome

Definition

Prader-Labhart-Willi is a syndrome of mental retardation, infantile hypotonia, early childhood obesity, short stature, hypogonadism, and small hands and feet.

Basic Science

The clinical findings in the syndrome were described in 1956 but it was not until 1981 that the syndrome was shown to be associated with a specific deletion on the long arm of chromosome 15 (Ledbetter et al, 1981). By use of high resolution prophase banding techniques, the deleted segment was demonstrated to be between bands 15 q 11 and 15 q 13. Other chromosome abnormalities found less commonly in Prader-Labhart-Willi syndrome include apparently balanced translocations involving chromosome 15, mosaicism for abnormalities of chromosome 15, and marker chromosomes containing duplicated segments of chromosome 15 (Ledbetter, et al 1982). About half of patients have normal chromosomes. This could be explained by the presence of a submicroscopic deletion, undetected mosaicism, or etiologic heterogeneity (Ledbetter et al, 1982). In a study of 15 cases where the patient had a deleted chromosome 15, the parental chromosomes were normal but the deleted chromosome was always paternal in origin (Butler et al, 1986). The explanation proposed for this phenomenon was that in the male, the continual proliferation of gametes during adult life is more susceptible to environmental insult than in the female, where oocytes are essentially arrested in meiosis.

The biochemical basis of the disorder is unknown as of 1988.

Epidemiology

Prader-Labhart-Willi patients represent 1% of all mentally retarded persons (Butler et al, 1986). The incidence of the disorder is 1/25,000 live births (Butler et al, 1986). Ninety-five percent of patients are Caucasian and of European descent (Butler et al, 1986).

Natural History

Compared with a previously normal pregnancy, decreased fetal movements in a Prader-Labhart-Willi pregnancy may be noted by the mother. Breech presentation is common. Sixty-five percent of affected infants are born prematurely (Butler et al, 1986). All patients exhibit infantile hypotonia but have good underlying muscle bulk. There is a poor cry and a weak suck. Most infants require gavage feeding. There is no increased incidence of respiratory problems. A characteristic facies is present, consisting of a high forehead, almond-shaped eyes, strabismus, and prominent nasal bridge (Fig. 13.8). Development is delayed. The average IQ of affected children is 70 (Laurance, 1985). The typical personality is described as friendly and happy. Between 2 and 4 years (range 6 months to 6 years) the child develops a voracious appetite and becomes obese. Body fat is distributed more to the lower trunk, buttocks, and thighs than to the face or upper

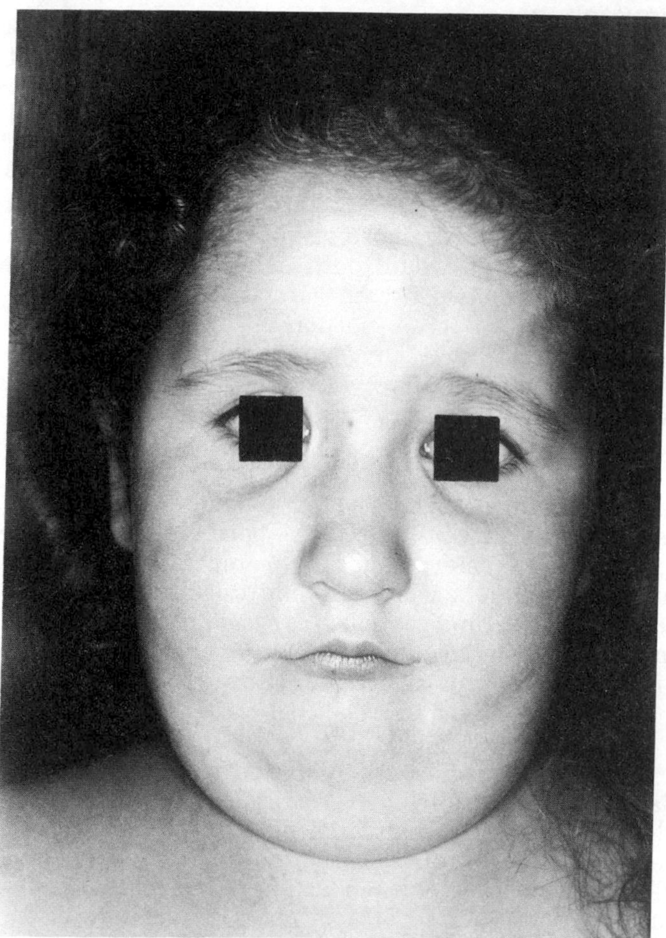

Figure 13.8. Seven-year-old female with the Prader-Labhart-Willi syndrome. Note obesity and dysmorphic features (photograph courtesy of Dr. Lawrence Kaplan).

trunk. Stature remains below the third percentile for age. The hands and feet are typically quite small. Males have micropenis and cryptorchidism or abnormal testes. Females have poorly developed labia majora. In both sexes, pubic hair is sparse. There have been no reports of reproduction in either sex. Other problems include persistent skin sores, frequent dental caries, and scoliosis.

Diagnosis

Prader-Labhart-Willi syndrome is a clinical diagnosis. The symptoms essential for diagnosis are infantile hypotonia, hypogonadism, obesity, developmental delay, dysmorphic facial features, and short stature (Mattei et al, 1983). The diagnosis should be considered in an infant with generalized hypotonia and poor feeding or a child with obesity. The average age at diagnosis is 7 years 2 months (Butler et al, 1986). Twenty-five percent of patients are diagnosed by 3 years and 11% are diagnosed in adulthood (Butler et al, 1986). Banded prometaphase chromosome studies should be performed to look for abnormalities in chromosome 15. Muscle biopsies, electroencephalogram, and electromyogram studies have been normal in affected patients. The differential diagnosis includes Laurence-Moon-Biedl syndrome and adiposogenital dystrophy.

Treatment

The overwhelming problem in Prader-Labhart-Willi syndrome is the obesity and difficulty in limiting food access. The treatment is severe dietary restriction, which has an improved chance of success if instituted early in childhood. Appetite suppressants have not been shown to be helpful (Laurance, 1985). Other treatment may include corrective surgery for scoliosis or strabismus. Orchidopexy is not recommended (Laurance, 1985).

Prognosis

Morbid obesity interferes with mobility and most adults become bedridden. Death ensues in early adulthood from cardiopulmonary insufficiency (Laurance, 1985). Although most patients are retarded, many learn to read.

Prevention

The inheritance pattern of this disorder has been described as both sporadic and autosomal recessive. Theoretically, in cases where the proband has a cytogenetic abnormality, prenatal diagnosis would be available for a subsequent pregnancy.

For further information for patients and families, contact:

The Prader-Willi Syndrome Association
P.O. Box 392
Long Lake, Minnesota 55356.

CASE ILLUSTRATION

After a pregnancy complicated by maternal streptococcal infection and second trimester vaginal bleeding, a 1200-g male infant was born at 32 weeks' gestation. His neonatal course was remarkable for jaundice, a 2-week oxygen requirement, and gavage feeding for 3½ months. At discharge he continued to have a poor suck and slow weight gain. At age 4½ months he was readmitted to the hospital for dehydration and failure-to-thrive. His parents described him as a "very good baby" but in the hospital it was noted that he was lethargic, slept excessively for age, and had poor muscle tone. The failure-to-thrive was, at that point, diagnosed as being on a primary neurologic basis. At age 3½ years he began to overeat. This progressed to compulsive overeating and obesity. At age 8 years the patient was found by a trash can eating garbage. At age 10 years, a diagnosis of Prader-Labhart-Willi syndrome was made, and the patient was started on strict dietary and behavior modification. At age 12 years, he was tested psychologically and scored at the 6½ year-level.

COMMENT

The diagnosis of Prader-Labhart-Willi syndrome should be considered in any full-term infant with a poor suck in the absence of evidence of perinatal insult. This case was complicated by the fact that the boy was premature and, initially, would have required gavage feeding. By a post-conceptional age of 35–36 weeks, however, a normal infant should suck well enough to take a bottle. The requirement of gavage feeding for 3½ months is sufficiently unusual to warrant a work-up. The lethargy and infantile hypotonia were also early clues to this child's diagnosis. The major benefit of making an early diagnosis in this syndrome is to institute early dietary therapy, which is better accepted by the younger patient than the older one. Weight control has been shown to reduce the morbidity in this syndrome.

Translocations

Translocations involve a reciprocal exchange of material between 2 chromosomes. Robertsonian translocations are quite frequent in the normal population and are due to fusion at the centromere between 2 acrocentric chromosomes, with consequent loss of the short arms. Although individuals with Robertsonian translocations are phenotypically normal, they are at risk for producing offspring with trisomy 13 or 21. Translocations between other chromosomes may have no consequence if they are "balanced," but again, abnormalities during meiosis may give rise to offspring with duplications or deficiencies.

Chromosome Breakage

Certain syndromes are characterized by spontaneous chromosome breakage and abnormalities in DNA repair mechanisms. The better-known examples of these phenomena are: Bloom syndrome, ataxia telangiectasia (see pp. 708), xeroderma pigmentosum (see pp. 1163), and Fanconi anemia. Fanconi anemia is discussed below.

Fanconi Anemia

Definition

Fanconi anemia is a syndrome of variable congenital anomalies, progressive pancytopenia occurring during childhood, and spontaneous chromosome breakage which worsens after in vitro exposure to bifunctional alkylating agents.

Basic Science

Fanconi anemia is the most common inherited aplastic anemia. The disease is inherited as a Mendelian autosomal recessive. The association between bone marrow failure and the congenital anomalies is not understood but is presumed to be related to simultaneous developmental events occurring between 25 and 34 days of gestation. Cultures of bone marrow cells from Fanconi patients reveal markedly decreased or absent progenitor cells (CFU-C, CKU-E, BFU-E) (Alter and Potter, 1983). The biochemical basis for the enhanced sensitivity to bifunctional alkylating agents is unknown, but is hypothesized to be due to abnormal DNA repair mechanisms (Auerbach et al, 1985). Recent experiments have shown that the subcellular distribution of topoisomerase (a DNA-related enzyme) is different in placental cells taken from affected patients as compared with normals. In Fanconi cells, the DNA topoisomerase activity is high in the cytoplasm where it is produced, but low in the nucleus where it is needed for DNA repair (Schroeder, 1982).

Epidemiology

The incidence is unknown. The frequency of heterozygote carriers of the disorder has been estimated at 1/300 (Auerbach et al, 1985). The disease affects all ethnic groups.

Natural History

The usual presenting symptoms are pallor, fatigue, bleeding, or easy bruisability occurring in mid childhood. Review of the history reveals that the child was small for gestational age and may have had congenital anomalies. In one review of 155 patients with Fanconi anemia, 76% of probands had hyperpigmentation and/or café-au-lait spots, 65% had short stature for age, 40% had thumb anomalies (aplasia, hypoplasia, supernumerary), 30% were microcephalic, 31% had renal anomalies (absent kidney, duplication of the kidney or collecting system, renal ectopia, or horseshoe kidney), 28% had skeletal malformations, 23% had strabismus, 20% had hyperreflexia, 19% had microphthalmia, 18% showed mental retardation, 12% manifested ear anomalies and/or deafness, and 7% had congenital heart disease (Alter and Potter, 1983). In a study of 44 affected siblings of probands, 25% had no dysmorphic features (Glanz and Fraser, 1982). Affected children develop progressive pancytopenia and eventually bone marrow failure. Leukopenia predisposes to multiple infections. Fanconi patients develop acute nonlymphatic leukemias, hepatocellular carcinomas, and squamous cell carcinomas. Leukemia is the terminal event in 5–10% of patients with Fanconi anemia (Alter and Potter, 1983).

Diagnosis

The anemia rarely presents at birth. The median age for clinical diagnosis in males is 6 years, and in females is 7½ years. Ninety percent of males are diagnosed by age 12 years and 90% of females by age 14 years (Alter and Potter, 1983). The most specific laboratory finding is in the metaphase chromosomes of affected individuals. Typical abnormalities include chromatid breaks, gaps, chromosome rearrangements, endoreduplication, or formation of triradials or quadriradials (Alter and Potter, 1983). These abnormalities will increase greatly in number after the patient's cells have been exposed to DNA crosslinking agents, mitomycin C or diepoxybutane. Because of the low mitotic index often seen in cells from patients with Fanconi anemia, additional methods of diagnosis have been developed involving flow cytometry and DNA histograms (Kaiser et al, 1982).

Although not specific for Fanconi anemia, the hematologic findings at the time of diagnosis may include: macrocytosis, mild poikilocytosis, mild anisocytosis, leukopenia, thrombocytopenia, and reticulocytopenia. The stressed hypocellular bone marrow will produce erythrocytes with fetal-like qualities (expressing i surface antigen and containing fetal hemoglobin) (Alter and Potter, 1983).

Treatment

The treatment is mainly supportive with transfusions of red cells, white cells, and platelets (Alter and Potter, 1983). Splenectomy is not indicated. Androgen therapy with oxymetholone results in improved blood counts, but causes masculinization and may cause hepatoma formation. Bone marrow transplantation is complicated by an unusual sensitivity to the chemotherapeutic agents used to prepare the marrow for the transplant as well as a severe problem with graft-versus-host disease (Deeg et al, 1983).

Prognosis

Survival of affected patients has been prolonged by androgen therapy. In older studies, an overall mortality of 80% by 12 years was reported (Alter and Potter, 1983). The cause of death in Fanconi patients is usually bleeding, infection, or malignancy.

Prevention

Prenatal diagnosis for the condition is available. Cells from the fetus are obtained at amniocentesis or chorionic villus biopsy, exposed to diepoxybutane, and monitored for chromosome breakage. This method has been successful in determining the status of 30 fetuses

CASE ILLUSTRATION

A 4-year, 7-month old male presented to the emergency room with a nosebleed. Review of his medical history revealed that he was born after an uncomplicated pregnancy of 38 weeks duration and weighed 2.28 kg at birth. He had several congenital anomalies including (1) occipital encephalocele, (2) cleft palate, (3) hydrocephalus, (4) extra mesenchymal tissue at the tip of his nose, (5) absent thumbs bilaterally, (6) right radial aplasia with bowed ulna, (7) bilateral renal dysplasia, and (8) rib anomalies. He remained small and was brought to the hospital repeatedly with evidence of bruising. Because of this, he was placed in a foster home at the age of 18 months on suspicion of child abuse. He was returned to his natural mother at age 3½ years.

At the time of presentation for the nosebleed, the child's physical examination was notable for the congenital anomalies described above, multiple café-au-lait spots on the trunk and neck, and scattered petechiae along both upper extremities. A complete blood count in the emergency room showed a white count of 2200, a hematocrit of 29.6%, a hemoglobin of 10.3 g/dl, a platelet count of 25,000/mm^3, and an MCV of 105 μm^3. A diagnosis of Fanconi anemia was made and subsequently confirmed by cytogenetic studies. The child has been followed closely to detect the development of hepatic or hematologic malignancy.

COMMENT

In light of the social history, the child's medical record was reviewed and, surprisingly, revealed that a platelet count was not performed at the time the child was placed in foster care. At age 3 years, during elective hand surgery, a platelet count of 84,000/mm^3 was documented but not followed up. Although the hematologic manifestations of Fanconi anemia may be subtle in early childhood, a child who presents with repeated bruising due to an organic cause is likely to have some abnormalities on a complete blood count. Had the presence of the radial aplasia (or the other congenital anomalies) suggested a diagnosis of Fanconi anemia to the pediatrician, this child would not have been removed from his natural home, and the family would have been spared much psychologic trauma.

(Auerbach et al, 1985). Since the condition is inherited as an autosomal recessive, there is a 25% recurrence risk for families with one affected child.

Fragile Sites

Fragile sites can appear as nonstaining gaps or dislocated segments present in the chromosomes. They have been shown to occur in many chromosomes, but thus far have only been linked with clinical pathology in a common form of mental retardation, the fragile X syndrome.

Fragile X-linked Mental Retardation (Martin-Bell Syndrome)

Definition

Fragile X syndrome is an inherited condition which occurs mainly, although not exclusively, in males. It is the second most common cause of mental retardation after Down syndrome. Affected individuals have various degrees of mental retardation and may have certain physical and/or behavioral traits. Karyotype analysis reveals that, in a certain percentage of cells, one X chromosome will have a narrowing or break at band Xq 27.

Basic Science

Fragile sites are defined as nonstaining gaps of variable widths involving both chromatids (Michels, 1985). Thus far, 21 fragile sites have been described in human chromosomes (Michels, 1985), but the only one with known clinical significance is at Xq 27. The underlying biochemical cause of the fragility is unknown. The inheritance pattern of the fragile X syndrome was initially believed to be X-linked recessive, but this has been challenged by the increasing evidence of transmission through normal males (Webb et al, 1981; Froster-Iskenius et al, 1986).

Epidemiology

The fragile X syndrome has been estimated to affect 1 in every 1000–2000 liveborn males (Carmi et al, 1984). In an Australian population of 1977 intellectually handicapped persons, the prevalence rate for fragile X syndrome was 1:2610 for males and 1:4221 for females (Turner et al, 1986). In institutions for the severely retarded, between 2 and 6% of the males may have a fragile X chromosome (Michels, 1985). The fragile X syndrome occurs with equal frequency among all racial and ethnic groups (Chudley and Hagerman, 1987).

Natural History

No specific congenital anomalies are associated with the syndrome. The degree of retardation seen in males varies from profound to borderline. One-third of carrier females may be retarded (Fryns, 1986). Some males are intellectually normal. Carrier females are phenotypically normal. Affected males may have a characteristic facial appearance consisting of a large head size, high prominent forehead, prominent jaw (prognathia), and large protruding ears (Fig. 13.9). Stature is shorter than average. The most specific finding in males is macroorchidism, which is usually postpubertal, but has been described in an affected infant of 5 months (Carmi et al, 1984). Absence of these physical features in males does not eliminate the diagnosis. Fragile X males are generally pleasant and socially engaging, although they may avoid eye contact and appear nervous or "fidgety." In addition, a typical speech pattern is present, which is described as rapid and repetitive. A significant as-

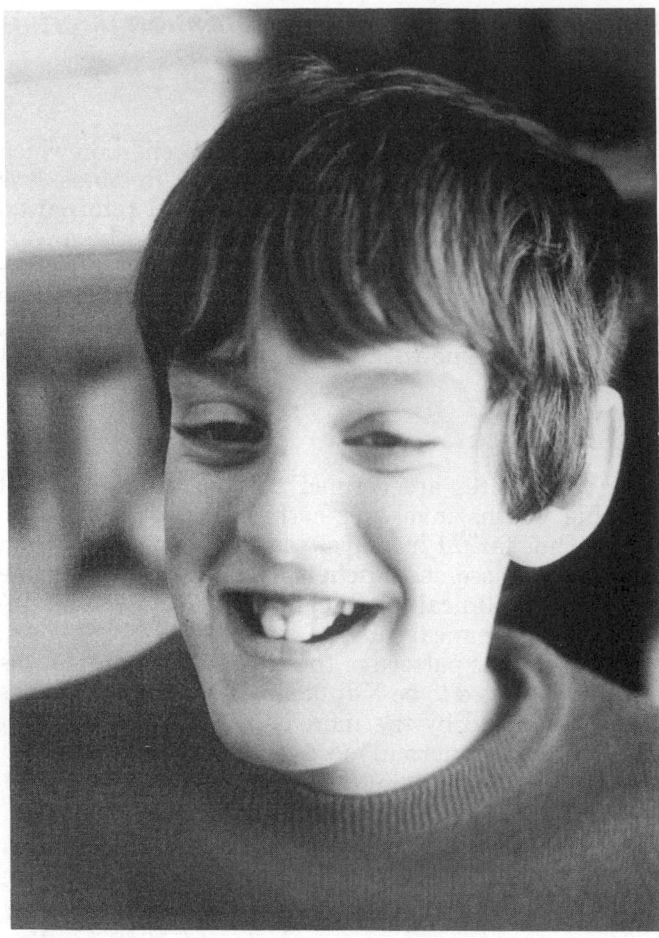

Figure 13.9. Ten-year-old male with Fragile X syndrome. A prominent jaw and large ears are present (photograph courtesy of Dr. David Meryash).

sociation exists between fragile X and autism (Chudley and Hagerman, 1987).

Diagnosis

The diagnosis is made by the demonstration of the fragile X chromosome in metaphase spreads under light microscopy. Peripheral blood lymphocytes must be cultured in medium that is deficient in folic acid and thymidine. Since this is not the routine culturing medium used by cytogenetics laboratories, the referral slip should read "rule out fragile X." The fragile X is never expressed in all cells in vitro. An affected male will have 3–60% fragile X positive cells. Female heterozygote carriers will have 0–80% fragile X positive cells (Michels, 1985) but advanced age will decrease the percentage of cells expressing the abnormal X (Turner et al, 1980b). A correlation has been shown between the number of cells expressing the fragile X and the likelihood of intellectual handicap in females (Turner, 1986). The fragile X is more readily expressed in peripheral lymphocytes than in skin fibroblasts or amniocytes.

Treatment

No major medical problems are associated with the syndrome. The macro-orchidism is not on an endocrine basis (Turner et al, 1980a). Treatment with 10 mg folic acid daily has possibly produced improvement in psychologic testing and behavior (Hagerman et al, 1986). There has been a suggestion that use of trimethoprim-sulfa antibiotics (a folic acid inhibitor) causes clinical deterioration (Hecht and Glover, 1983). The most effective treatment consists of special education, speech therapy, and vocational counseling. Phenothiazines have been used in adults to control violent temper outbursts (Chudley and Hagerman, 1987).

Prognosis

Affected individuals have a normal life span and are not predisposed to any particular illnesses.

Prevention

Initially, fetal sex determination with selective termination of male fetuses was the method of prenatal diagnosis. Now that it has been shown that one-third of carrier females are retarded, efforts are being focused on demonstration of the fragile X in the peripheral lymphocytes obtained from umbilical venous blood at 18 weeks' gestation, with selective termination of pregnancy. DNA-based diagnosis has been hampered by an unusually high frequency of recombination in this region of the X chromosome (Davies et al, 1985; Chudley and Hagerman, 1987).

REFERENCES

Abuelo D, Barsel-Bowers G, Busch W, et al: Risk for trisomy 21 in offspring of individuals who have relatives with trisomy 21. *Am J Med Genet* 25:365, 1986.

Alter BP, Potter NU: Long term outcome in Fanconi's anemia: Description of 26 cases and review of the literature. In German J (ed): *Chromosome Mutation and Neoplasia*. New York, Alan Liss, Inc. 1983, pp 43–62.

Auerbach AD, Sagi M, Adler B: Fanconi anemia: Prenatal diagnosis in 30 fetuses at risk. *Pediatrics* 76:794, 1985.

Baird PA, Sadovnick AD: Life expectancy in Down syndrome. *J Pediatr* 110:849, 1987.

Benacerraf BR, Frigoletto FD Jr, Greene MF: Abnormal facial features and extremities in human trisomy syndromes: Prenatal US appearance. *Radiology* 159:243, 1986.

Berry AC, Mutton DE, Lewis DGM: Mosaicism and the trisomy 8 syndrome. *Clin Genet* 14:105, 1978.

Breg WR, Steele MW, Miller OJ, et al: The cri du chat syndrome in adolescents and adults: Clinical findings in 13 older patients with partial deletion of the short arm of chromosome no. 5. *J Pediatr* 77:782, 1970.

Butler MG, Meaney J, Palmer CG: Clinical and cytogenetic survey of 39 individuals with Prader-Labhart-Willi syndrome. *Am J Med Genet* 23:793, 1986.

Carmi R, Meryash DL, Wood J, et al: Fragile X syndrome ascertained by the presence of macro-orchidism in a 5-month old infant. *Pediatrics* 74:883, 1984.

Carter PE, Pearn JH, Bell J, et al: Survival in trisomy 18. *Clin Genet* 27:59, 1985.

Chudley AE, Hagerman RJ: Fragile X syndrome. *J Pediatr* 110:821, 1987.

Cronk C, Crocker AC, Pueschel SM, et al: Growth charts for children with Down Syndrome: 1 month to 18 years of age. *Pediatrics* 81:102, 1988.

Davies KE, Mattei MG, Mattei JF, et al: Linkage studies of X-linked mental retardation: High frequency of recombination in the telomeric region of the human X chromosome. *Hum Genet* 70:249, 1985.

Deeg HJ, Storb R, Thomas ED, et al: Fanconi's anemia treated by allogeneic marrow transplantation. *Blood* 61:954, 1983.

Deroover J, Fryns JP, Parlovi C, et al: Partial monosomy of the short arm of chromosome 9. A distinct clinical entity. *Hum Genet* 44:195, 1978.

Edwards JH, Harnden DG, Cameron AH, et al: A new trisomic syndrome. *Lancet* 1:787, 1960.

Fishman MA: Will the study of Down syndrome solve the riddle of Alzheimer disease? *J Pediatr* 108:627, 1986.

Fort P, Lifshitz F, Bellisario R, et al: Abnormalities of thyroid function in infants with Down syndrome. *J Pediatr* 104:545, 1984.

Froster-Iskenius U, McGillivray BC, Dill FJ, et al: Normal male carriers in the Fra (X) form of X-linked mental retardation (Martin-Bell syndrome). *Am J Med Genet* 23:619, 1986.

Fryns JP: The female and the fragile X. A study of 144 obligate female carriers. *Am J Med Genet* 23:157, 1986.

Funderburk SJ, Sparkes RS, Klisak I, et al: The 9p- syndrome. *J Med Genet* 16:75, 1979.

Glanz A, Fraser FC: Spectrum of anomalies in Fanconi anemia. *J Med Genet* 19:412, 1982.

Guthrie RD, Aase JM, Asper AC, et al: The 4p- syndrome. A clinically recognizable chromosomal deletion syndrome. *Am J Dis Child* 122:421, 1971.

Hagerman RJ, Jackson AW, Levitas A, et al: Oral folic acid versus placebo in the treatment of males with the fragile X syndrome. *Am J Med Genet* 23:241, 1986.

Hall B: Mongolism in newborns. A clinical and cytogenetic study. *Acta Paediatr Scand* (Suppl) 154:1, 1964.

Hecht F, Glover TW: Antibiotics containing trimethoprim and the fragile X chromosome. *N Engl J Med* 308:285, 1983.

Hodes ME, Cole J, Palmer CG, et al: Clinical experience with trisomies 18 and 13. *J Med Genet* 15:48, 1978.

Jackson-Cook CK, Flannery DB, Corey LA: Nucleolar organizer region variants as a risk factor for Down Syndrome. *Am J Hum Genet* 37:1049, 1985.

Johnson VP, Aceto T Jr, and Likness C: Trisomy 14 mosaicism: Case report and review. *Am J Med Genet* 3:331, 1979.

Juberg RC, Mowrey PN: Origin of nondisjunction in trisomy 21 syndrome: All studies compiled, parental age analysis, and international comparisons. *Am J Med Genet* 16:111, 1983.

Julien C, Bazin A, Guyot B, et al: Rapid prenatal diagnosis of Down's syndrome with in-situ hybridisation of fluorescent DNA probes. *Lancet* 2:863, 1986.

Kaiser TN, Lojewski A, Dougherty C, et al: Flow cytometric characterization of the response of Fanconi's anemia cells to mitomycin C treatment. *Cytometry* 2:291, 1982.

Kaplan LC, Wayne A, Crowell S, et al: Trisomy 14 mosaicism in a liveborn male: Clinical report and review of the literature. *Am J Med Genet* 23:925, 1986.

Katayama KP, Wilkinson EJ, Hermann J, et al: Clinical delineation of trisomy 9 syndrome. *Obstet Gynecol* 56:665, 1980.

Laurance BM: The Prader Willi syndrome. *Maternal Child Health* 10:106, 1985.

Ledbetter DH, Mascarello JT, Riccardi VM, et al: Chromosome 15 abnormalities and the Prader-Willi syndrome: A followup report of 40 cases. *Am J Hum Genet* 34:278, 1982.

Ledbetter DH, Riccardi VM, Airhart SD: Deletions of chromosome 15 as a cause of the Prader-Willi syndrome. *N Engl J Med* 304:325, 1981.

Lurie IW, Lazjuk GI, Ussova YL: The Wolf-Hirschhorn syndrome. *Clin Genet* 17:375, 1980.

Matsuoka R, Misugi K, Goto A, et al: Congenital heart anomalies in the trisomy 18 syndrome, with reference to congenital polyvalvular disease. *Am J Med Genet* 14:657, 1983.

Mattei JF, Mattei MG, Giraud F: Prader-Willi syndrome and chromosome 15. *Hum Genet* 64:356, 1983.

Mehta L, Shannon RS, Duckett DP, et al: Trisomy 18 in a 13-year-old girl. *J Med Genet* 23:256, 1986.

Michels VV: Fragile sites on human chromosomes: Description and clinical significance. *Mayo Clin Proc* 60:690, 1985.

Miller OJ, Breg WR, Warburton D: Partial deletion of the short arm of chromosome no. 4 (4p-). *J Pediatr* 77:792, 1970.

Miller WA: Case records of the Massachusetts General Hospital. *N Engl J Med* 308:642, 1983.

Moessinger AC, Mills JL, Harley EE, et al: Umbilical cord length in Down's syndrome. *Am J Dis Child* 140:1276, 1986.

Muller LM, deJong G: Prenatal ultrasonographic features of the Pena-Shokeir I syndrome and the trisomy 18 syndrome. *Am J Med Genet* 25:119, 1986.

Niebuhr E: The cri du chat syndrome. Epidemiology, cytogenetics, and clinical features. *Hum Genet* 44:227, 1978.

Nielsen J, Hansen KB, Sillesen I: Chromosome abnormalities in newborn children. Physical aspects. *Hum Genet* 59:194, 1981.

Pena SDJ, Shokeir MHK: Autosomal recessive cerebro-oculo-facio-skeletal (COFS) syndrome. *Clin Genet* 5:285, 1974.

Qazi QH, Masakawa A, Madahar C, et al: Trisomy 9 syndrome. *Clin Genet* 12:221, 1977.

Riccardi VM: Trisomy 8: An international study of 70 patients. *Birth Defects, Original Article Series* XIII-3C:171, 1977.

Robison LL, Nesbit ME Jr, Sather HN: Down syndrome and acute leukemia in children: A 10-year retrospective survey from Children's Cancer Study Group. *J Pediatr* 105:235, 1984.

Schinzel A, Schmid W, Luscher U, et al: Structural aberrations of chromosome 18. I. The 18 p- syndrome. *Arch Genetik* 47:1, 1974.

Schinzel A, Hayaski K, Schmid W: Structural aberrations of chromosome 18. II. The 18q- syndrome. Report of three cases. *Humangenetik* 26:123, 1975.

Schreinemachers DM, Cross PK, Hook EB: Rates of trisomies 21, 18, 13 and other chromosome abnormalities in about 20,000 prenatal studies compared with estimated rates in live births. *Hum Genet* 61:318, 1982.

Schroeder TM: Genetically determined chromosome instability syndromes. *Cytogenet Cell Genet* 33:119, 1982.

Scoggin CH, Patterson D: Down's syndrome as a model disease. *Arch Intern Med* 142:462, 1982.

Shapiro BL: Down syndrome—a disruption of homeostasis. *Am J Med Genet* 14:241, 1983.

Smith GF, Spiker D, Peterson CP, et al: Use of megadoses of vitamins with minerals in Down syndrome. *J Pediatr* 105:228, 1984.

Stephens TD, Shepard TH: The Down syndrome in the fetus. *Teratology* 22:37, 1980.

Tanzi RE, Gusella JF, Watkins PC, et al: Amyloid beta protein gene: cDNA, mRNA distribution, and genetic linkage near Alzheimer locus. *Science* 235:880, 1987.

Taylor AI: Autosomal trisomy syndromes: A detailed study of 27 cases of Edwards' syndrome and 27 cases of Patau's syndrome. *J Med Genet* 5:227, 1968.

Turner G, Brookwell R, Daniel A, et al: Heterozygous expression of X-linked mental retardation and X-chromosome marker fra (X) (q27). *N Engl J Med* 303:662, 1980.

Turner G, Daniel A, Frost M: X-linked mental retardation, macro-orchidism, and the Xq 27 fragile site. *J Pediatr* 96:837, 1980.

Turner G, Robinson H, Laing S, et al: Preventive screening for the fragile X syndrome. *N Engl J Med* 315:607, 1986.

Warkany J, Passarge E, Smith LB: Congenital malformations in autosomal trisomy syndromes. *Am J Dis Child* 112:502, 1966.

Webb GC, Rogers JG, Pitt DB, et al: Transmission of fragile (X) (q27) from a male. *Lancet* 2:1231, 1981.

Wilkins LE, Brown JA, Nance WE, et al: Clinical heterogeneity in 80 home-reared children with cri du chat syndrome. *J Pediatr* 102:528, 1983.

Zellweger H: Down syndrome. In Vinken PJ, Bruyn GW (eds): *Handbook of Clinical Neurology,* Volume 31: Congenital Malformations of the Brain and Skull. Amsterdam, North Holland Publishing Co., 1977.

Molecular Genetics

3

"The presence of a genetic disease implies an abnormality in, or absence of, at least 1 specific sequence of bases (a gene) in the patient's DNA. In theory, the application of molecular biology to genetic disease can offer diagnosis (by analysis of the affected sequence), understanding of pathogenesis (by relating the DNA lesion to a defective gene product), and cure (by repair or replacement of the relevant stretch of DNA)" (Steel, 1984).

Advances in molecular biology and genetics have led to a detailed understanding of the molecular pathophysiology in diseases as diverse as β-thalassemia, α-1-antitrypsin deficiency, and phenylketonuria. It is important and appropriate to include a chapter on molecular genetics in a textbook of pediatrics because most of the disorders in which the abnormal gene has been cloned are diseases of childhood. In addition, it is the pediatrician who is prescribing some of the "fruits of labor" of recombinant DNA technology—human growth hormone, somatostatin, and insulin. In the following pages, therefore, a brief background in clinically relevant molecular genetics will be given. Should the reader require more information at any point, a series of recent references is provided at the end of the chapter.

An appreciation of genes necessitates a familiarity with the molecule that genes are made of: deoxyribonucleic acid, or DNA. DNA contains and transmits the genetic information essential for cellular growth, differentiation, and reproduction. The molecule itself is a helical structure consisting of two strands of deoxyribose sugars linked by covalent phosphodiester bonds. One of four nucleotide bases is attached to each sugar. These bases are adenine, guanine, cytosine, and thymine. Since DNA is double stranded, each base forms a hydrogen bond with the nucleotide base directly opposite. The bonding is very specific—adenine (A) will only pair with thymine (T), and guanine (G) will only pair with cytosine (C).

DNA replication, or duplication of DNA prior to cell division, is dependent on specific and accurate base pairing. When replication commences, the two DNA strands unwind so that each one serves as a template for the new molecule. The new nucleotides are aligned opposite their complementary partners and are joined by the enzyme DNA polymerase. DNA replication is termed "semi-conservative" as each new molecule contains one old and one newly synthesized strand.

DNA synthesis does not lead directly to protein synthesis. There are multiple intermediate steps involving another molecule, ribonucleic acid (RNA) (Fig. 13.10). RNA differs from DNA in that it is single stranded, contains a ribose sugar, and has the base uracil substituted for thymine. Uracil, like thymine, pairs only with adenine (Miller, 1981).

In a process known as transcription, "unwound" DNA present on a chromosome in the nucleus acts as a template for RNA synthesis. This messenger RNA (mRNA) then travels into the cytoplasm where, on the ribosomes, it directs the incorporation of amino acids into polypeptide chains. In a process known as translation, small molecules of transfer RNA (tRNA) bring amino acids to the ribosome for protein synthesis. Each amino acid is encoded by a set of three nucleotides read in sequence (Miller, 1981). Since there are four potential bases in each of the three positions, there are 64 potential "codes." There are roughly 20 essential amino acids and each one is encoded by more than one triplet base sequence. For example, the amino acid glycine is coded by the bases CGU, GGC, GGA, and GGG. There

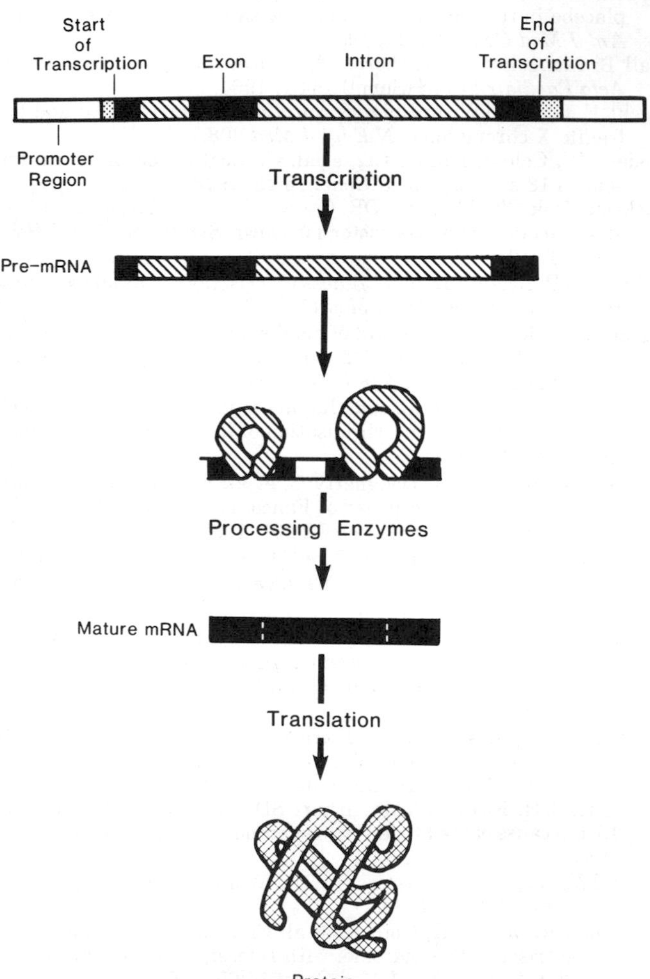

Figure 13.10. The steps involved in transcription of DNA to pre-mRNA, and the translation of mature mRNA to protein.

are special sequences called promoters, which define where the reading of the code should begin. In addition, there are sequences known as "nonsense" or "termination" mutations where reading of a particular triplet causes cessation of protein synthesis.

Once a polypeptide chain has been formed, additional processing steps may be necessary to create a functional protein. These may include glycosylation, cleavage, or assembly of multiple subunits.

Recent studies have shown an important difference between prokaryotes, organisms such as bacteria which do not have separate nuclei, and eukaryotes, higher organisms in which genetic information is present in a discrete nucleus. In prokaryotes, the DNA is transcribed into mRNA where it is used directly for protein synthesis. In eukaryotes, however, it has been shown that the DNA sequences coding for proteins (known as exons) are often interrupted by long DNA sequences (known as introns or intervening sequences) which have no known function (Miller, 1981). During transcription, the entire DNA sequence, including introns, is made into mRNA. This "pre mRNA" is then further processed in the nucleus such that introns are excised and the exons are joined together (Leder, 1978). Mature mRNA may be considered the essential protein-coding component of a gene. It is important for the clinician to recognize the complexity of this process. For most genes, the introns are collectively as long as the exons, affording multiple opportunities for error in transcription. Each of the intron-exon boundaries is an additional potential site of mutation (Kazazian, 1985). It has been estimated that only 1% of the total DNA in the nucleus ends up as mature mRNA for protein synthesis. Another 1% of the nuclear DNA codes for ribosomal and transfer RNA (Williamson, 1983). The role of the other 98% of nuclear DNA is currently a matter of speculation.

Preparation of Genomic DNA

Genomic DNA is only the DNA contained in the chromosomes in the nucleus of a cell. As discussed earlier (see p. 756), mitochondrial DNA is not genomic DNA.

Genomic DNA can be prepared from any nucleated cell. Peripheral leukocytes are the most commonly used source of DNA; however, fibroblasts grown from a skin biopsy, amniotic fluid cells grown in culture, and placental (chorionic) villus tissue are equally useful. Ten to 20 ml of venous blood (depending on the age of the child), collected in a purple top tube (ethylene-diamine-tetra-acetic acid [EDTA] as anticoagulant) should provide enough DNA for analysis. Routinely, 25–60 μg of DNA is obtained from each milliliter of whole blood (Antonarakis et al, 1982). Once the DNA is prepared, it may be stored for years.

Recombinant DNA technology and clinically relevant DNA studies were made possible by the discovery of *restriction endonucleases,* enzymes that can digest double stranded human DNA. They are part of a naturally occurring defense mechanism in bacteria. Their usual purpose is to cleave invading viral DNA. They function by recognizing and cutting a very specific DNA sequence 4–8 base pairs long. An example is EcoRI which recognizes the sequence:

G ↓ AATTC
CTTAA ↑ G

The fact that some of the enzymes cleave the DNA in an unequal fashion has been exploited in various cloning techniques (see pp. 778). Over 200 restriction endonucleases are now known; about half of them are available commercially.

Southern Blot

Most clinical diagnoses are made via the Southern blot, which is an autoradiograph of human DNA that has been incubated with a piece of DNA known as a *probe.* A probe is a single stranded short segment of DNA which has been chemically modified such that some of its individual nucleotides are radioactive (the isotope is usually ^{32}P). The probe has been constructed so that its gene sequence or location on a chromosome is usually known. Because single stranded DNA will pair with a complementary base sequence of DNA or RNA, the probe is used to generate information about an unknown segment of DNA. At this point, it would not be unreasonable to ask why it would not be simpler to determine the gene sequence on a patient's DNA and compare that with the "normal" person's DNA without resorting to the use of probes? The reasons are two-fold: (1) with 6×10^9 base pairs of DNA in the diploid human genome, sequencing the DNA of one individual would take years; and (2) it is now appreciated that there is a tremendous amount of variation in DNA sequences in completely normal people. It has been estimated that each individual has 10^7 clinically silent variations in his or her DNA (Kazazian, 1985). Another way of stating this is that along each DNA molecule, at about every 200–300 base pairs, the DNA sequence may differ from individual to individual but the change does not result in clinical pathology. These changes are also known as *DNA polymorphisms,* meaning that the variation is present in at least 1% of the population and is transmitted from generation to generation in a Mendelian manner. DNA polymorphisms are useful clinically to trace the inheritance of certain gene segments through families.

The Southern blot is generated as follows: (see Fig. 13.11) genomic double stranded DNA which has been previously prepared from an individual is incubated with one of the many available restriction endonucleases. The enzyme will cut only at the site of certain specific base sequences. Since the base sequences vary from person to person, the enzyme will cut at different points in different people. The cut DNA is then placed in an agarose gel and subjected to electrophoresis. The smallest fragments will migrate the farthest toward the anode. After electrophoresis, the gel is soaked in alkali to denature the double stranded DNA into single stranded DNA. The DNA is then transferred from the agarose to a nitrocellulose filter paper and baked onto

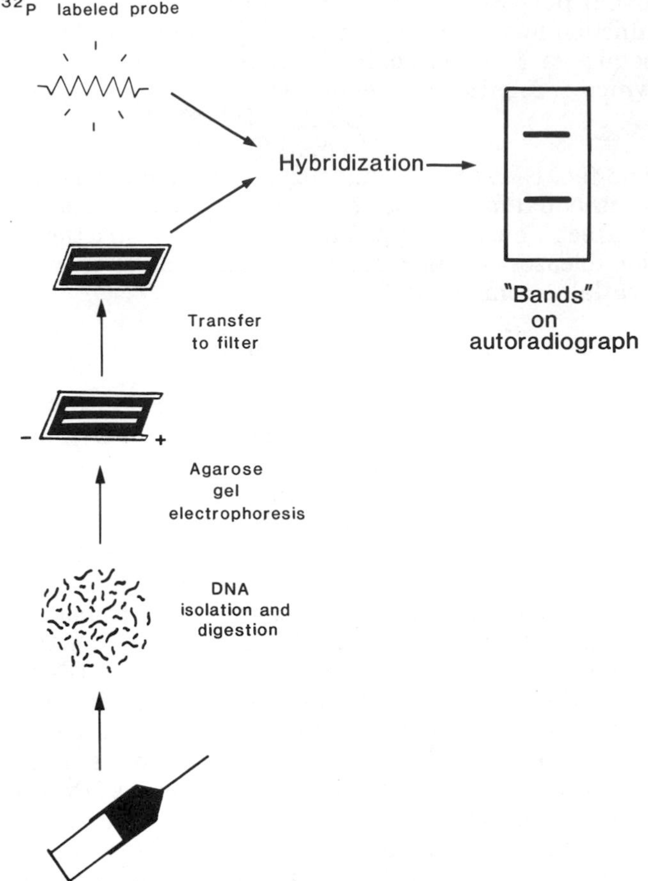

Figure 13.11. Preparation of a Southern blot, beginning with DNA isolation from venous blood. See text for details.

the filter paper. Gene studies are then performed by placing the filter paper containing the patient's DNA in a bag containing radioactive probe. If the patient's DNA is complementary to the probe (in other words, if base pairing occurs and hydrogen bonds form to make double stranded DNA) then *hybridization* takes place and a black band is visualized on the resulting autoradiograph. If hybridization occurs, we can infer the patient's DNA sequence because we know that the patient's bases are complementary to the known base sequences in the probe.

Before discussing how Southern blots have been utilized to make clinical diagnoses in pediatrics, it seems appropriate at this point to define two other terms: Northern blots and Western blots. Southern blots were named for Dr. E. M. Southern, the investigator who originated the technique. In a pun on the name "Southern," "Northern" blots were coined to describe RNA hybridization with complementary DNA. Similarly, "Western" blots describe the binding of antibody to protein antigen on a nitrocellulose gel transfer (Steel, 1984). Clinicians may be familiar with Western blots as part of the diagnosis of human T-cell leukemia virus (HTLV-III) infection.

Use of Southern Blots in Diagnosis of Genetic Disease

The understanding of the molecular basis of genetic disease would be much simpler if pathology could be correlated with the loss of all or part of the normal gene sequence for a particular protein. Unfortunately, as molecular methods have evolved to study the bases of various inherited diseases, it has become clear that the disease state can be the result of whole or partial gene deletions, single base mutations, insertion of bases into normal sequences, duplications of regions of a gene, and many other phenomena. A disease such as β-thalassemia which has a fairly classic clinical presentation, has been shown to be very heterogeneous on the molecular level. Over 200 mutations are known to exist in the gene for β-globin which is present on chromosome 11 (Kazazian, 1985).

Because of the variety of molecular defects present in a given genetic disease, a series of different strategies have been developed to identify the affected patient on a Southern blot. In *direct detection* of the mutation, the normal gene sequence and/or the mutant gene sequence is known and can be specifically searched for in the patient. For example, in diseases such as sickle cell anemia and α-1-antitrypsin deficiency, where the disease state is known to result from a single base mutation in the protein coding sequence, oligonucleotide probes have been created to detect the mutation site directly. Oligonucleotide probes are pieces of chemically synthesized DNA, usually 18–19 bases long, which are made to hybridize at the exact site of the known mutation in the disease state. In the *indirect detection* of a mutation, the mutant gene sequence is not known, but a DNA sequence closely linked physically to the gene is used as a marker for the abnormal gene. This so-called *linkage analysis* relies on the assumption that if two genes are located close to one another on a chromosome, they will be inherited together more frequently than by chance alone. If, however, crossing over occurs (this is an exchange of DNA between homologous chromosomes during meiosis) between the DNA marker and the disease gene they will no longer be inherited as a pair—*recombination* has taken place. To be useful for clinical diagnosis a DNA marker must be physically very close to the disease locus–i.e., recombination must occur rarely. Another name for this type of study is *restriction fragment length polymorphism*, abbreviated RFLP. Different restriction enzymes will generate different fragments of DNA based on the various gene sequences in members of a family. One difficulty in performing linkage analyses is that simply looking at the Southern blot will not determine who in the family is normal and who is affected. Complete family studies are needed to establish a pattern linking the DNA marker with the abnormal gene.

RELEVANCE OF MOLECULAR GENETICS TO PEDIATRIC DISEASES

In this section, only a limited number of the pediatric diseases that have been studied at the molecular level can be discussed. Emphasis is on the more common or well-known disorders. The reader is referred to a review article summarizing the disorders diagnosed by recombinant DNA technology (Cooper and Schmidtke, 1986).

Phenylketonuria (PKU)

Phenylketonuria is one of the more common inborn errors of metabolism encountered by the general pediatrician. The disease is typically, but not exclusively, due to a severe deficiency of the hepatic enzyme, phenylalanine hydroxylase, which normally catalyzes the conversion of phenylalanine to tyrosine. An infant born with PKU will become progressively mentally retarded as toxic intermediary metabolites accumulate. As a result of neonatal screening for the condition, affected newborns are now identified early in life and may achieve normal intellectual development with a permanent diet low in phenyalanine. PKU affects 1/10,000 Caucasian newborns. The disease is inherited as a Mendelian autosomal recessive, with the carrier frequency in Caucasians being about 1/50. The clinical manifestations of PKU are discussed further on page 925.

Molecular Genetics of Phenylketonuria

The gene for phenylalanine hydroxylase has been cloned and extensively analyzed on a molecular basis. The gene is quite large, on the order of 90–100 kilobase pairs in length (1 kilobase = 1000 base pairs). The gene contains multiple introns and a minimum of 10 exons. The gene has been mapped to the long arm of the human chromosome number 12 (Lidsky et al, 1985). A genetic probe has been synthesized that is complementary to the mRNA (message) for human phenylalanine hydroxylase. This DNA probe has been used to detect the presence of phenylalanine hydroxylase mRNA in persons affected with PKU (Woo et al, 1983b). One of the first conclusions from molecular genetic studies in PKU patients, therefore, was that the disease state did not result from deletion of the entire normal gene for phenylalanine hydroxylase. Recently, the molecular defect for the mutant phenylalanine hydroxylase allele in 38% of a Danish PKU population has been shown to be a single base substitution from G to A in intron 12. This mutation causes intron 12 to be eliminated from the mature mRNA and the resultant protein product is unstable (DiLella et al, 1986). In other ethnic groups, clinically useful tests have been developed that take advantage of the extensive variation in DNA sequences (polymorphisms) within the phenylalanine hydroxylase gene in normal individuals. These variations, seen on Southern blots, do not represent the actual PKU mutation but they can be used as a powerful tool to track the abnormal gene through families. Since phenylalanine hydroxylase is specific to liver and is not expressed in fibroblasts, prenatal diagnosis by enzyme analysis of amniocytes was not possible in the past. Current methods enable the use of amniocytes as a source of fetal genomic DNA. The restriction fragment patterns produced by digestion with 10 different enzymes are compared among family members (see Case Illustration). With these techniques, prenatal diagnosis can be performed in about 90% of families who have at least one child affected with PKU (Lidsky et al, 1985).

> **CASE ILLUSTRATION**
>
> An example of how restriction fragment length polymorphisms can be used to trace the mutant gene in a family is given here. A family with one affected PKU child wants to know if a subsequent pregnancy will result in another affected child. Peripheral blood from both parents, the child affected with PKU, and a child unaffected with PKU are obtained. Genomic DNA is prepared and a small part of the DNA is digested with the enzyme Sph I. This enzyme creates an 11.0-kilobase (kb) band in all people, and either a 9.7 kb, a 7.0 kb, or a combination of those two bands on a Southern blot (see Fig. 13.12). This family is informative because each parent is heterozygous, having a 9.7-kb band and a 7.0-kb band. The affected child is homozygous for the 9.7-kb band, so the PKU gene in this family (but not all families) is associated with the 9.7-kb band. The unaffected child happens to be a homozygote for the 7.0-kb band, so he is clinically normal and does not even carry the trait for PKU. Prenatal diagnosis is feasible in this family. If the fetus is a homozygote for the 9.7-kb band, he will be diagnosed as affected. All other combinations of bands (homozygous for 7.0 kb, heterozygous 9.7 kb/7.0 kb) result in clinically unaffected offspring.

α-1-Antitrypsin Deficiency

α-1-Antitrypsin is a serum glycoprotein that functions as a major inhibitor of neutrophil elastase. Persons with a genetic deficiency of α-1-antitrypsin develop severe emphysema because the unimpeded elastase will

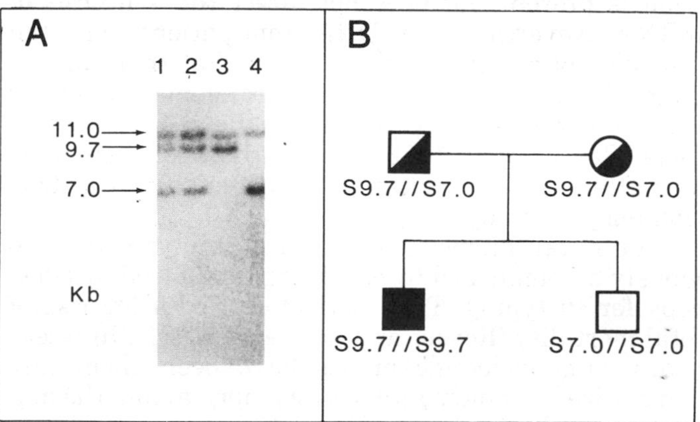

Figure 13.12. Southern blot and pedigree analysis of a family with phenylketonuria by Sph I restriction fragment length polymorphism in phenylalanine hydroxylase gene: lane 1, father's DNA: lane 2, mother's DNA: lane 3, affected child's DNA: lane 4, unaffected sibling's DNA. Reprinted with permission from *Pediatrics* 74:412, 1984.

slowly destroy the connective tissue elements of the lower respiratory tract. Screening of 200,000 newborns has shown that the deficiency exists in 1 in 1666 Caucasians (Sveger, 1976). In about 20% of affected infants, neonatal hepatitis and potentially fatal cirrhosis occurs. The pathogenesis of the liver disease is not known.

α-1-Antitrypsin consists of a single polypeptide chain. Over 30 different variants of the molecule have been classified on the basis of their electrophoretic mobility in starch gels. Most of the variants are the result of a single amino acid substitution. α-1-Antitrypsin genes are inherited as co-dominant alleles, meaning that both parental contributions are expressed equally. The most common normal allele is Pi (protease inhibitor) ^{M}, which has a gene frequency of greater than 85% in Caucasians of Northern European extraction (Gadek 1983). The major mutant alleles are Pi^{Z} and Pi^{S}. The Pi^{Z} gene is found in 1–2% of Northern Europeans but in 8.2% of New Zealand Maoris (Gadek and Crystal, 1983). Persons who are homozygous for the Z allele have a serum level of α-1-antitrypsin that is 10–15% of normal (Woo et al, 1983a). The clinical deficiency state is inherited in an autosomal recessive pattern.

The gene for α-1-Antitrypsin consists of 5 exons within a 10-kb segment on chromosome 14 (Garver et al, 1986). The Pi^{ZZ} phenotype is caused by a single amino acid substitution from glutamic acid to lysine at residue 342 in the protein. Sequence analysis has shown the amino acid change to be the result of a point mutation from guanine to adenine. In cells from patients with the Pi^{ZZ} phenotype, the mutant gene is transcribed, the mRNA is translated, and a protein is produced that differs from the normal Pi^{MM} phenotype by one amino acid. The clinical symptoms, however, derive from the inability of hepatocytes to process and secrete the mutant proteins in normal amounts (Garver et al, 1986). A rarer form of α-1-antitrypsin deficiency is caused by the Pi null-null phenotype, where affected patients have no detectable α-1-antitrypsin. Recent molecular genetic studies have shown that the α-1-antitrypsin gene is present but does not direct the synthesis of mRNA. Nevertheless in DNA from patients with the null phenotype, it has been shown that there are no major deletions, additions, or rearrangement in either the promoter region or exons in the α-1-antitrypsin gene (Garver et al, 1986). Hence, there is likely to be a small but critical mutation not detectable by restriction enzyme analysis.

Prenatal diagnosis of the Pi^{ZZ} genotype was previously accomplished by obtaining fetal blood by fetoscopy for Pi typing. This method carried a 5% risk of fetal mortality (Rocker and Lawrence, 1981). In recent years, oligonucleotide probes have been chemically synthesized complementary to the normal and the mutant gene. The probes consist of 19 bases and are constructed to have: 9 bases—mutation site—9 bases. When fetal DNA from amniotic fluid cells or chorionic villi is incubated with the two probes, only 1 will be complementary and produce a band on the Southern blot. This technique has been used to diagnose with certainty persons with MM, MZ, and ZZ genotypes (Kidd et al, 1984).

Hemoglobinopathies

Prior to the advent of molecular genetic techniques, prenatal diagnosis of the hemoglobinopathies relied on globin chain analysis of fetal blood obtained at second trimester fetoscopy. DNA analysis of the α- and β-globin genes has not only contributed greatly to the understanding of the pathophysiology of the globin disorders but has enabled prenatal diagnosis to be offered via safer methods as early as 9 weeks of gestation.

α-Thalassemia

The molecular basis of α-thalassemia is relatively straightforward. Each genetically normal individual has 2 α-globin genes on each chromosome 16, for a total of 4 α genes. The normal genotype, by convention, is written α α/α α. In general, the molecular defect causing the disease state of homozygous α-thalassemia is a deletion that can occur in various locations along the α gene. The α-globin gene has 3 exons and 2 introns and exists as part of a complex that includes a pseudo α gene and 2 α-like genes, ζ 1 and ζ 2. The complete nucleotide sequence for the α-globin gene is known. Rare examples of clinical pathology have been reported where the α-globin gene is intact, but there is an absence of functional α chains because of a single nucleotide mutation or an abnormality in RNA processing (Kan, 1983). The overwhelming majority of cases, however, are due to gene deletions. Clinical severity is inversely proportional to the number of remaining α-globin genes. In other words, 1/4 deleted α-genes results in a "silent carrier state" without microcytosis or anemia. A subtle clinical finding may be 1–2% Hb Bart (γ_4) on electrophoresis of hemoglobin from cord blood, but not adult blood (Lehmann, 1970). The molecular mechanisms involved in the loss of a single α-globin gene on a chromosome include deletion of the gene, a single nucleotide mutation in which a termination codon mutates to a glutamine codon and elongates the α-chain by 31 amino acids (producing Hb Constant Spring), or an intron mutation that affects mRNA precursor processing. Interestingly, the loss of one α-globin locus on a chromosome is a fairly common event in some of the world's populations and may confer some evolutionary protective advantage.

Deletions or abnormalities in 2/4 α-globin genes are referred to as "α-thalassemia trait." There are racial and ethnic differences in the distribution of these defects per chromosome. In American blacks and Ashkenazi jews, there is usually one deletion on each chromosome (genotype written: -α/-α) whereas in Orientals it is more common to find both deletions occurring on the same chromosome (genotype written: --/α α). Carriers of α-thalassemia trait are clinically asymptomatic but may have a mild microcytic anemia. Electrophoresis of hemoglobin in cord blood usually reveals a 2–10% level of Bart hemoglobin. Abnormalities in 3/4 α-globin genes (genotype written: --/- α) result in a condition known as hemoglobin H disease. Hemoglobin H is a tetramer of 4 β-globin chains that is unstable and precipitates upon oxidation. This results in a hemolytic anemia which is generally well-tolerated because the single remaining α-gene can direct the production of enough normal α chains. Hemoglobin H disease has been reported to be associated with mental retardation (Weatherall et al, 1981).

Of all the α-globin disorders, the most serious one occurs when all 4 α-globin genes are deleted (genotype written: --/--). The affected fetus produces no α chains. Its hemoglobin composition consists of Hb Bart (γ_4), Hb Portland (ζ_2, ϵ_2), and HbH (β_4). Until recently, this condition was thought to be incompatible with life because the affected fetus became severely anemic and hydropic in utero. Two recent reports have described premature infants with homozygous α-thalassemia who received aggressive transfusion therapy and survived (Beaudry et al, 1986, Bianchi et al, 1986). Prenatal diagnosis is available on chorionic villi or amniotic fluid cells by use of a cloned probe for the α-globin gene. A blank lane seen on the Southern blot indicates absence of α genes (see Fig. 13.13) and is consistent with a diagnosis of homozygous α-thalassemia or hydrops fetalis.

β-Thalassemia

β-thalassemia is a good example of a single disease with relative homogeneity in clinical presentation, yet the underlying molecular mechanisms are many and varied. Each person has one β-globin gene on the short arm of each chromosome 11. The β-globin gene exists as part of a complex which includes the ϵ and γ-globin genes important for hemoglobin synthesis during embryonic and fetal life. Two pseudo β genes and a δ gene are additionally present on each chromosome 11. Each individual has only two β-globin genes, so that they are either homozygous or heterozygous for mutations.

Since the molecular basis of β-thalassemia is so heterogeneous, it is helpful to review the steps in the normal transcription of β-globin genes in order to understand where mutations can occur. The β-globin gene (as well as the α-globin gene) contains 3 exons and 2 introns. Initially, the entire gene, including exons and introns, is transcribed to make a precursor mRNA. This "pre mRNA" is modified so that residues are added to both ends of the polypeptide chains (processes called "capping" and "tailing" or "polyadenylation"). Subsequently, certain nucleotides are methylated and the entire chain is "spliced" such that the introns are removed and the exons are rejoined. The mature mRNA moves to the cytoplasm where it directs protein synthesis (Kan, 1983).

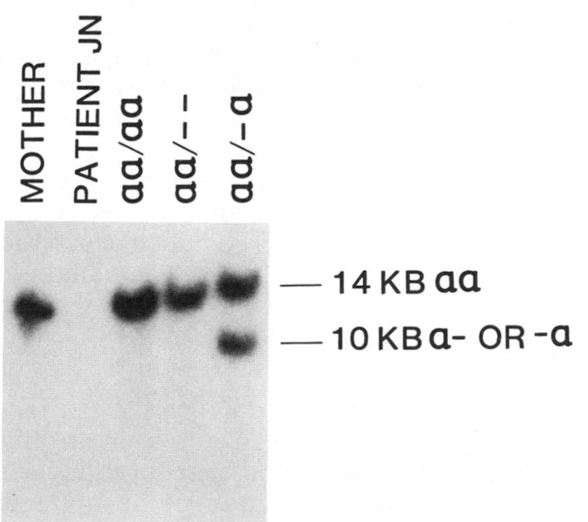

Figure 13.13. Southern blot analysis showing complete absence of alpha globin genes in patient JN. Genomic DNA from the patient, her mother, and controls was digested with the restriction endonuclease Bam HI. Reprinted with permission from *J Pediatr* 108:716, 1986.

Gene deletion is the most common molecular etiology in α-thalassemia, yet it is infrequent in β-thalassemia. The majority of people affected with β-thalassemia have an intact β-globin structural gene. An exception is the Asian-Indian type of β-thalassemia which is a deletion of 619 nucleotides, starting at the second intron and continuing into the coding region of the β-globin gene (Weatherall, 1985).

Although at least 30 clinically significant abnormalities in the β-globin genes of thalassemics have been described (Weatherall, 1985), the molecular lesions have been divided into two main categories. In β^o thalassemia, no β chains are produced. In β^+ thalassemia, some β chains are synthesized, but the overall production is reduced in comparison with normal individuals. In general, the β-thalassemia mutations cause nonfunctional globin mRNA to be produced, to interfere with the post-translational processing of mRNA, or prevent the normal transcription of the globin gene. This occurs on a molecular basis by frameshift mutations, nucleotide substitutions, deletions, chain terminator (nonsense) mutations, defective RNA splicing in introns, exons, junctions, or at polyadenylation sites, or mutations in regulatory areas.

The most common mutation affecting about two-thirds of Greeks and one-third of Italians with β-thalassemia is the result of a single base substitution (G to A) in the first intron of the β-globin gene (IVS-1). This creates a different splicing signal, forming an abnormally processed RNA which is unstable (Orkin et al, 1983). Unfortunately, initial attempts at prenatal diagnosis were unsuccessful because the single base change in the DNA did not alter restriction enzyme recognition sites. More recently, however, oligonucleotide probes (see pp. 774) have been developed that hybridize to either the normal β-globin IVS-1 gene or the common mutant Mediterranean β-globin IVS-1 gene, facilitating accurate genotype identification for prenatal diagnosis. Another oligonucleotide probe has been developed for the common mutation present in over 95% of thalassemics of Sardinian origin. In this ethnic group, the normal codon for glutamine (CAG) at position 39 of the β-globin gene has a single base change to TAG, which is a stop codon and terminates the β-globin chain prematurely (Pirastu et al, 1983). Prenatal diagnosis and selective termination of affected fetuses has resulted in a 60% reduction in the Sardinian thalassemic birth rate over 5 years (Modell et al, 1984).

Although collectively many mutations give rise to β-thalassemia, it is a general principle that certain mutations are characteristic of specific ethnic groups or geographic areas. As evidenced above, prenatal diagnosis is easily performed if the parents are carriers of the common mutations. An alternative (although more complicated) method is to analyze parental and familial DNA for restriction enzyme polymorphisms located within the β-globin gene. The linkage of these DNA markers with the mutant gene ideally should be determined before considering pregnancy (Orkin, 1984). The clinical manifestations of β-thalassemia are described more fully on pages 514–516.

Sickle Cell Anemia

The clinical disease of sickle cell anemia occurs because the affected person is homozygous for the sickle cell allele at the β-globin gene locus (Saiki, 1985). It is now known that the S allele is the result of a single nucleotide mutation from A to T in the second position of the sixth codon of the β-globin gene. There is an amino acid change from glutamic acid to valine in the protein end product. This DNA substitution from A to T alters a base sequence that is normally recognized and cleaved by three different restriction enzymes: Mnl I, Dde I, and Mst II (Orkin, 1984). Dde I and Mnl I enzyme restriction sites are fairly frequent within the human genome. Digestion of human DNA with either of these enzymes generates multiple small fragments that are not technically suitable for diagnostic Southern blots. Since the enzyme Mst II has a 7-base recognition site (C-C-T-N-A-G-G, where N = any base) it cleaves the DNA at less frequent intervals and creates a 1.1-kb DNA fragment from the A allele and a 1.3-kb fragment from the S allele. This latter assay has been successfully utilized in the prenatal diagnosis of sickle cell (SS) anemia (Orkin, 1982), but unfortunately, it will not detect the presence of the C allele in sickle SC disease. This mutation derives from a nucleotide substitution of GAG to AAG, glycine to lysine in the sixth codon of the β-globin gene, and does not alter the Mst II recognition site. In families with SC disease it is more appropriate to use oligonucleotide probes to detect the mutant C allele. As discussed earlier, under appropriate hybridization conditions, only perfectly matched oligonucleotide-DNA combinations will form stable double stranded DNA molecules. Thus, if a single nucleotide mismatch exists, a duplex will not form. Nonadecanucleotide probes have been developed that are complementary to the known gene sequences in the normal (A) allele, S allele, and C allele (Conner et al, 1983). These chemically synthesized probes also have been used to provide accurate prenatal diagnosis of sickle cell disease. Even more recently, techniques have been described that provide fetal genotype analyses in less than 1 day and require significantly less than 1 μg of genomic DNA (Saiki et al, 1985, Saiki et al, 1986). The clinical spectrum of sickle cell disease is discussed on page 511. The frequency of sickle cell trait (HgB AS) in American blacks is 8% (Rucknagel, 1974), so theoretically, 1 in 625 black pregnancies is at risk for producing a homozygous affected infant.

Ornithine Transcarbamylase Deficiency

Ornithine transcarbamylase (OTC) is a hepatic mitochondrial enzyme that catalyzes urea biosynthesis and ammonia detoxification. Deficiency of the enzyme is inherited as an X-linked recessive condition which is usually lethal in hemizygous males. Affected males experience severe protein intolerance and toxic ammonia levels during the neonatal period after commencement of feeding. Carrier heterozygote females may have clinical symptoms related to partial enzyme deficiency depending on the extent of random inactivation of their normal X chromosome. In other words, if the "active" X chromosome is the one carrying the deficiency, the hepatocytes may be unable to metabolize protein normally. Such women may have a history of protein intolerance or even cerebral dysfunction (Batshaw et al, 1980). The disorder is discussed more fully on page 944.

The gene for ornithine transcarbamylase has been mapped to the mid-short arm of the X chromosome, at band Xp 21 (McKusick, 1986). Although the majority of the gene has been cloned, the exact length is not known. It is estimated that the gene is at least 25–30 kb in length (Rozen et al, 1985). In a study of 15 affected males with OTC deficiency, only one showed a partial deletion of the gene on a Southern blot. The remainder of the patients were indistinguishable from normal controls (Rozen et al, 1985). It is now assumed, however, that most of the clinically significant OTC mutations are the result of single base changes, minor deletions, or insertions.

Prior to DNA analysis, prenatal diagnosis by amniocentesis was uninformative. Ornithine transcarbamylase, being a hepatic enzyme, is not expressed in amniocytes. In addition, the amniotic fluid of affected males does not show any unusual metabolites (Rozen et al, 1985). Although fetal liver biopsy for determination of OTC activity in hepatocytes has been performed (Old et al, 1985), this procedure carries considerable morbidity. Fetal DNA analysis combined with family studies offers a safer and potentially more accurate means of diagnosis. Several restriction fragment length polymorphisms have been identified at the OTC locus, and these are being used to identify the X chromosome carrying the mutant gene. A case has already been described where OTC deficiency in the fetus was excluded prenatally by direct gene analysis (Old et al, 1985).

Lesch-Nyhan Syndrome

Lesch-Nyhan syndrome results from an inherited X-linked recessive absence or near total deficiency of the enzyme hypoxanthineguanine phosphoribosyltransferase (abbreviated HPRT). This enzyme is important in the synthesis of purines and plays a critical role in brain metabolism. Although the disorder is rare, occurring in 1/100,000 births, its unusual symptoms are well-known to pediatricians. They include: mental retardation, microcephaly, compulsive self-mutilation of the oral mucosa and distal phalanges, spasticity, and choreoathetosis. Partial deficiency of HPRT leads to overproduction of uric acid which may cause a severe form of hereditary gout with or without mild CNS symptoms. Females heterozygous for HPRT deficiency may develop gout after menopause. These "carriers" are hyperuricemic throughout their lives, but endogenous estrogens present before menopause have a uricosuric effect and minimize symptoms. Unlike many inherited disorders, such as sickle cell anemia where the heterozygote has a selective advantage in resistance to malaria infection, the heterozygote in HPRT deficiency has no discernible genetic advantage. There is a high new mutation rate, and no particular ethnic group is associated with the disease.

HPRT is coded by a single structural gene, which has been mapped to the terminal portion of the X chromosome, band Xq 26 (McKusick, 1986). The gene has been cloned, and consists of 9 exons, for a total length of about 34 kb (Wilson and Kelley, 1984). The coding portion of the gene, the mature mRNA, is only about 1.6 kb in length. The molecular mechanisms underlying HPRT deficiency are diverse, because of the large size of the gene and the high new mutation rate (Yang et al, 1984). Several structural variants of HPRT have been shown to be due to single amino acid substitutions, which are the result of a single base change (Wilson et al, 1983). Other molecular phenotypes described thus far have included complete and partial deletions of the gene, insertion of additional genetic material within the gene, and an internal duplication of exons 1 and 3. Eighteen percent of cases have been shown to be the result of a gene deletion (Yang et al, 1984).

Because HPRT is encoded by a single gene and the absence of the enzyme causes such a severe disease, Lesch-Nyhan syndrome has been considered a potential candidate for gene therapy. Bone marrow transplantation has been attempted, but even proven engraftment with peripheral blood leukocytes containing normal levels of HPRT did not result in clinical improvement in an affected patient (Parkman, 1986). The human gene for HPRT has been transferred to and expressed in bone marrow cells by use of a retrovirus (Gruber et al, 1985). Obviously, clinical improvement will be related to successful delivery of the normal HPRT gene to the CNS. Clinical trials are in the planning stage. Prenatal diagnosis, however, is currently available for the condition.

Hemophilia A

Hemophilia A is the most common inherited disease of blood coagulation, affecting about 1 in 10,000 live male births. The inheritance pattern is X-linked recessive (see pp. 754). The abnormal gene causes a deficiency or abnormality in its protein product, clotting factor VIII:C. The factor VIII:C gene is enormous, consisting of 26 exons and 25 introns. It encodes for a protein that is composed of 2351 amino acids (Antonarakis et al, 1985). For purposes of comparison, the β-globin gene is comprised of 3 exons and 2 introns. Relatively speaking, the β-globin gene is small, and yet over 30 molecular defects that cause β-thalassemia have been described. Since the factor VIII:C gene is over 100 times larger than is the β-globin gene, a corresponding increase in the number of molecular opportunities for mutation would be expected. To date, however, only three mechanisms have been documented as the cause of the hemophilia A mutation within individual families: (1) a large (80 kb) deletion within the factor VIII:C gene; (2) a single nucleotide change (C to T) in exon 18 of the factor VIII:C gene, creating a "stop" codon instead of amino acid 1960 in the protein product; and (3) an underlying nucleotide change that results in a different restriction fragment length polymorphism as compared with normals (Antonarakis et al, 1985). In the great majority of affected families, the underlying molecular defect has not been identified. Although prenatal diagnosis has traditionally been offered via fetal blood sampling at fetoscopy, or more recently, peripheral umbilical venous sampling, efforts are being directed at identification of hemophiliacs by fetal DNA testing in the first trimester. Thus far, probes cloned from part of the factor VIII:C gene and so-called "anonymous" DNA probes (St 14 and Dx 13) which map very close to the factor VIII:C gene have been utilized to provide carrier testing in female relatives of hemophiliacs (Janco et al, 1986).

Duchenne Muscular Dystrophy

Duchenne muscular dystrophy is the most common X-linked recessive disorder occurring in humans, with an incidence of 1/4000 live male births (Moser, 1984). About 600 affected males are born in the United States each year. Although they are clinically normal during the neonatal period, muscular weakness becomes apparent during the early childhood years. This progresses to severe wasting and death in the second or third decade of life. Affected males do not reproduce; thus the gene is maintained in the population by carrier females and a very high mutation rate.

The gene for Duchenne muscular dystrophy (DMD) has been mapped to the short arm of the X chromosome, band Xp 21 (Monaco et al, 1986). The complete gene has been cloned. It has a minimum of 60 exons, spans approximately 2000 kb in length, and is the largest human gene to be identified thus far (Koenig et al, 1987). Its large size potentially explains the frequency of the disease and the high incidence of new mutations (Moser, 1984). Subfragments of the transcript of the DMD gene have been used as a probe for the molecular analysis of the defect in affected males. In 104 samples of DNA from unrelated boys, about 50% showed deletions of part of the DMD gene (Koenig et al, 1987).

The biochemical basis for the disorder is beginning to be understood. The protein product of the DMD gene has been identified in human muscle (Hoffman et al, 1987). It has been named *dystrophin*. Dystrophin represents 0.002% of total striated muscle protein. Muscle tissue from DMD males and the animal model, the mdx mouse, contains no detectable dystrophin.

Although current treatment for this unrelenting disorder is mainly supportive, the discovery of dystrophin will undoubtedly lead to new and more specific therapy. Carrier detection, prenatal diagnosis of affected males, and selected pregnancy termination is possible. Prior to the development of molecular probes for DNA sequences linked to the DMD locus, carrier detection depended on classic pedigree analysis and creatine phosphokinase measurement (CPK) (Pembrey et al, 1984). CPK is a muscle enzyme which is strongly elevated in affected males and mildly elevated in carrier females. At the present time, clinical medicine is benefitting from the new molecular probes available. DNA-based prenatal diagnosis has already been described for this condition (Bakker et at, 1985; Cole et al, 1988); (see p. 737).

CLONING

Cloning may be thought of as a means of making thousands of copies of an isolated piece of DNA by inserting that piece of DNA into a simple, rapidly dividing organism (usually the bacterium, *Escherichia coli*). The inserted, foreign DNA replicates along with the host bacterial DNA.

The strategy for cloning a fragment of DNA may be simply summarized as follows: (1) If a particular protein product is desired (for example, the peptide hormone, insulin) the gene for that product must be isolated. The gene may be defined as a "sequence of nucleotides that gives rise to a messenger RNA from which a corresponding sequence of amino acids is translated" (Murray, 1984). Total cellular mRNA may be isolated from a cell known to be expressing the gene of interest, and a complementary DNA (cDNA) strand may be chemically synthesized for insertion into the bacterium. Alternatively, if the amino acid sequence of the desired protein is known, the RNA and DNA sequences may be inferred from the genetic code.

Three different methods are used to ensure incorporation and replication of the foreign DNA. The simplest involves the use of plasmids, which are short circular lengths of DNA that replicate independently of host bacterial DNA (Steel, 1984). Clinicians may be familiar with plasmids as the originators of resistance (R factors) to various antibiotics. With use of restriction endonucleases, the DNA molecule to be cloned is cleaved in an unequal manner, leaving two fragments with "sticky ends." The plasmid may then be cut with the same enzyme and mixed with the isolated DNA to form a new, larger, "recombinant" DNA molecule. The plasmids are modified such that the restriction endonuclease sites are within the gene loci coding for antibiotic resistance. Thus, recombinant molecules may be selected by growth or absence of growth in the presence of certain antibiotics (Cederbaum, 1984). Another *vector,* or carrier of foreign DNA, is a bacterial virus known as a phage. Phage are more difficult to work with than are plasmids, but they can accommodate larger segments of foreign DNA (Steel, 1984). The basic principles involved in insertion of the DNA into phage are the same as with plasmids. A third vector has been artificially created to combine properties of plasmid and phage and is known as a cosmid.

What clinically useful products have been generated by use of the above techniques?

Human growth hormone sequences were cloned from mRNA extracted from the pituitary tumors removed from patients with acromegaly. Complementary DNA was synthesized. The human growth hormone gene sequences were linked to a tryptophan gene of *E. coli.* A protein was synthesized by the bacteria that contained 70% of the amino acids specified by the growth hormone gene (Martial et al, 1979). Insulin has been synthesized by similar techniques, and is now available commercially. Nucleotide sequence determination in cloned copies of hepatitis B viral DNA has facilitated the analysis of the arrangement of specific antigen genes within its genome. This has resulted in isolation and expression of the segments of DNA that code for hepatitis B surface antigen (Murray, 1984). A genetically engineered hepatitis B vaccine is on the horizon.

REFERENCES

Antonarakis SE, Phillips JA III, Kazazian HH: Genetic diseases: Diagnosis by restriction endonuclease analysis. *J Pediatr* 100:845, 1982.

Antonarakis SE, Waber PG, Kittur SD, et al: Hemophilia A: Detection of molecular defects and of carriers by DNA analysis. *N Engl J Med* 313:842, 1985.

Bakker E, Goor N, Wrogemann K, et al: Prenatal diagnosis and carrier detection of Duchenne muscular dystrophy with closely linked RFLPs. *Lancet* 1:655, 1985.

Batshaw ML, Roan Y, Jung AL, et al: Cerebral dysfunction in asymptomatic carriers of ornithine transcarbamylase deficiency. *N Engl J Med* 302:482, 1980.

Beaudry MA, Ferguson DJ, Pearse K, et al: Survival of a hydropic infant with homozygous alpha-thalassemia 1. *J Pediatr* 108:713, 1986.

Bianchi DW, Beyer EC, Stark AR, et al: Normal long-term survival with alpha-thalassemia. *J Pediatr* 108:716, 1986.

Cederbaum SD: Introduction to recombinant DNA. *Pediatrics* 74:408, 1984.

Cole CG, Walker A, Coyne A, et al: Prenatal testing for Duchenne and Becker muscular dystrophy. *Lancet* 1:262, 1988.

Conner BJ, Reyes AA, Morin C, et al: Detection of sickle-cell β-S globin allele by hybridization with synthetic oligonucleotides. *Proc Natl Acad Sci USA* 80:278, 1983.

Cooper DN, Schmidtke J: Diagnosis of genetic disease using recombinant DNA. *Hum Genet* 73:1, 1986.

DiLella AG, Marvit J, Lidsky AS, et al: Tight linkage between a splicing mutation and a specific DNA haplotype in phenylketonuria. *Nature* 322:799, 1986

Gadek JE, Crystal RG: Alpha-1-antitrypsin deficiency. In Stanbury JB, Wyngaarden JB, Fredrickson DS, et al (eds): *The Metabolic Basis of Inherited Disease*, 5th edition. New York, McGraw Hill, 1983, p. 1450.

Garver RI, Mornex JF, Nukiwa T, et al: Alpha-1-antitrypsin deficiency and emphysema caused by homozygous inheritance of non-expressing alpha-1-antitrypsin genes. *N Engl J Med* 314:762, 1986.

Gruber HE, Finley KD, Hershberg RM, et al: Retroviral vector-mediated gene transfer into human hematopoietic progenitor cells. *Science* 230:1057, 1985.

Hoffman EP, Brown RH Jr, Kunkel LM: Dystrophin: The protein product of the Duchenne muscular dystrophy locus. *Cell* 51:919, 1987.

Janco RL, Phillips JA III, Orlando P, et al: Carrier testing strategy in hemophilia A. *Lancet* 1:148, 1986.

Kan YW: The thalassemias. In Stanbury JB, Wyngaarden JB, Frederickson DS, et al (eds): *The Metabolic Basis of Inherited Disease,* 5th ed. New York, McGraw-Hill, 1983, p. 1711.

Kazazian HH: The nature of mutation. *Hosp Prac* p 55, February 1985.

Kidd VJ, Golbus MS, Wallace RB, et al: Prenatal diagnosis of alpha-1-antitrypsin deficiency by direct analysis of the mutation site in the gene. *N Engl J Med* 310:639, 1984.

Koenig M, Hoffman EP, Bertelson CJ, et al: Complete cloning of the Duchenne muscular dystrophy (DMD), cDNA and preliminary genomic organization of the DMD gene in normal and affected individuals. *Cell* 50:509, 1987.

Leder P: Discontinuous genes. *N Engl J Med* 298:1079, 1978.

Lehmann H: Different types of alpha-thalassemia and significance of hemoglobin Bart's in neonates. *Lancet* 2:78, 1970.

Lidsky AS, Ledley FD, DiLella AG, et al: Extensive restriction site polymorphism at the human phenylalanine hydroxylase locus and application in prenatal diagnosis of phenylketonuria. *Am J Hum Genet* 37:619, 1985.

Martial JA, Hallewell RA, Baxter JD, et al: Human growth hormone: Complementary DNA cloning and expression in bacteria. *Science* 205:602, 1979.

McKusick VA: The morbid anatomy of the human genome: A review of gene mapping in clinical medicine. *Medicine* 65:1, 1986.

Miller WL: Recombinant DNA and the pediatrician. *J Pediatr* 99:1, 1981.

Modell B, Ward RHT, Rodeck C, et al: Effect of fetal diagnostic testing on birth rate of thalassemia major in Britain. *Lancet* 2:1383, 1984.

Monaco AP, Neve RL, Colletti-Feener C, et al: Isolation of candidate cDNAs for portions of the Duchenne muscular dystrophy gene. *Nature* 323:646, 1986.

Moser H: Duchenne muscular dystrophy: Pathogenetic aspects and genetic prevention. *Hum Genet* 66:17, 1984.

Murray K: New routes to drugs, diagnostic agents, and vaccines. *Lancet* 2:1194, 1984.

Old JM, Purvis-Smith S, Wilcken B, et al: Prenatal exclusion of ornithine transcarbamylase deficiency by direct gene analysis. *Lancet* 1:73, 1985.

Orkin SH: Prenatal diagnosis of hemoglobin disorders by DNA analysis. *Blood* 63:249, 1984.

Orkin SH, Little PFR, Kazazian HH Jr, et al: Improved detection of the sickle mutation by DNA analysis. *N Engl J Med* 307:32, 1982.

Orkin SH, Markham AF, Kazazian HH Jr: Direct detection of the common Mediterranean beta-thalassemia gene with synthetic DNA probes. *J Clin Invest* 71:775, 1983.

Parkman R: The application of bone marrow transplantation to the treatment of genetic diseases. *Science* 232:1373, 1986.

Pembrey ME, Davies KE, Winter RM, et al: Clinical use of DNA markers linked to the gene for Duchenne muscular dystrophy. *Arch Dis Child* 59:208, 1984.

Pirastu M, Kan Y-W, Cao A, et al: Prenatal diagnosis of beta thalassemia. Detection of a single nucleotide mutation in DNA. *N Engl J Med* 309:284, 1983.

Rocker I, Lawrence KM: An assessment of fetoscopy. In Rocker I, Lawrence KM (eds): *Fetoscopy*. Amsterdam, Elsevier/North-Holland, 1981, p 301.

Rozen R, Fox J, Fenton WA, et al: Gene detection and restriction fragment length polymorphisms at the human ornithine transcarbamylase locus. *Nature* 313:815, 1985.

Rucknagel DL: The genetics of sickle cell anemia and related syndromes. *Arch Intern Med* 133:595, 1974.

Saiki RK, Bugawan TL, Horn GT, et al: Analysis of enzymatically amplified beta-globin and HLA-DQ alpha DNA with allele-specific oligonucleotide probes. *Nature* 324:163, 1986.

Saiki RK, Scharf S, Faloona F, et al: Enzymatic amplification of beta-globin genomic sequences and restriction site analysis for diagnosis of sickle cell anemia. *Science* 230:1350, 1985.

Steel CM: DNA in medicine: The tools. *Lancet* 2:908, 1984.

Sveger T: Liver disease in alpha-1-antitrypsin deficiency detected by screening of 200,000 infants. *N Engl J Med* 294:1316, 1976.

Weatherall DJ: The molecular pathology of single gene disorders. In Weatherall DJ: *The New Genetics and Clinical Practice*, 2nd ed. Oxford, Oxford University Press, 1985, pp 66–90.

Weatherall DJ: The molecular pathology of single gene disorders. In Weatherall DJ: *The New Genetics and Clinical Practice*, 2nd edition. Oxford, Oxford University Press, 1985, pp. 66–90.

Williamson R: Molecular biology in relation to medical genetics. In Emery AH, Rimoin DL (eds): *Principles and Practice of Medical Genetics*. New York, Churchill Livingstone, 1983, p. 16.

Wilson JM, Kelley JN: Molecular genetics of the HPRT-deficiency syndromes. *Hosp Prac* May:81, 1984.

Wilson JM, Young AB, Kelley WN: Hypoxanthine-guanine phosphoribosyltransferase deficiency. *N Engl J Med* 309:900, 1983.

Woo SLC: Prenatal diagnosis and carrier detection of classic phenylketonuria by gene analysis. *Pediatrics* 74:412, 1984.

Woo SLC, Kidd VJ, Pam ZK, et al: Alpha-1-antitrypsin deficiency and pulmonary emphysema: Identification of recessive homozygotes by direct analysis of the mutation site in the chromosomal gene. In Caskey CT, White RL (eds): *Banbury Report 14: Recombinant DNA Applications to Human Disease.* Cold Spring Harbor Laboratory: 1983, p. 105.

Woo SLC, Lidsky AS, Guttler F, et al: Cloned human phenylalanine hydroxylase gene allows prenatal diagnosis and carrier detection of classical phenylketonuria. *Nature* 306:151, 1983.

Yang TP, Patel PI, Chinault AC, et al: Molecular evidence for new mutation at the HPRT locus in Lesch-Nyhan patients. *Nature* 310:412, 1984.

Oncogenetics

4

INHERITED PREDISPOSITION TO NEOPLASTIC DISEASE

A multitude of chromosome abnormalities, single gene disorders, and polygenic conditions predispose to childhood malignancy. As discussed earlier (see Chapter 2), single gene conditions such as ataxia telangiectasia and xeroderma pigmentosum are associated with defective DNA repair. Thus, tumors characteristically develop in affected individuals exposed to ultraviolet light and/or X-irradiation. Other single gene disorders, for example, neurofibromatosis, are associated with an increased incidence of tumors such as meningioma, glioma, schwannoma, or pheochromocytoma, but the relationship between the single gene and tumor development is less straightforward. Chromosomal abnormalities, in general, have long been observed to be associated with neoplasia. An old example is the Philadelphia chromosome, now known to be the result of a reciprocal translocation between the long arms of chromosomes 22 and 9, and typically found in the peripheral lymphocytes of patients with chronic myelogenous leukemia. Patients with aneuploidy, such as trisomy 21, have at least a 10-fold higher risk of developing leukemia than does the general population (Littlefield, 1984). Disorders of the sex chromosomes (XO/XY gonadal dysgenesis or testicular feminization) are associated with the development of gonadoblastoma if the testes are allowed to remain in an intra-abdominal location.

In this chapter, two examples are given of predisposition to neoplastic disease being inherited as a Mendelian trait. Prior to that, however, a brief introduction to the concept of *oncogenes* is useful.

Oncogenes were first identified in tumors and were shown to cause neoplastic transformation of cells in vitro. They were thought to be related to retroviral infection and were postulated to be the genes that caused cancer. Subsequently, oncogenes have been shown to be important coding genes present in all eukaryotic cells. Their sequences have been carefully conserved throughout evolution. More than 30 of them have been identified, and the great majority have been mapped to human chromosomal locations (Gordon, 1985). When the oncogenes have been transcribed and translated into protein products, the substances produced tend to be those involved in the control of orderly cell division. Thus, in its normal location, an oncogene may be thought of as "a unit of genetic information that specifies a protein that promotes mitosis" (Gordon, 1985). If, however, the oncogene is mutated, amplified, or moved to a location other than its normal one, its effects will change. An example of this is the translocation of the normal *c-myc* oncogene present on the long arm of chromosome 8 to the long arm of chromosome 14, near an area of active transcription of the gene for heavy chain immunoglobins. This translocation activates the *c-myc* gene, promoting disorderly cell division, and resulting in the genesis of Burkitt lymphoma. The molecular biological phenomenon of oncogene activation has already had an important clinical application: a correlation has been shown between the increased amplification of the *N-myc* oncogene and an advanced clinical stage of malignancy (Brodeur et al, 1984).

An important theory regarding the development of malignancy is Knudson's "two mutational event" hypothesis. A mutational event may be defined as a single nucleotide change occurring within a gene, a chromosomal rearrangement, or even viral or environmental damage to the genome. According to the theory, it takes two such events to generate a tumor. In the case of hereditary tumors, however, an individual is born with the first mutation present. Thus, only one additional event in a susceptible cell type is necessary for neoplastic change (Knudson et al, 1975). Two examples—retinoblastoma and Wilms tumor—illustrate and validate this hypothesis.

Retinoblastoma

Retinoblastoma is the most frequent intraocular tumor found in young children and neonates, occurring in 1/15,000 live births (Shields and Augsburger, 1981). The tumor presents with equal frequency among all races and both sexes. The disease can occur in two forms—either as a sporadic event, or as an inherited, almost fully penetrant, autosomal dominant trait. Characteristically, the inherited tumors present bilaterally or multifocally in infancy, whereas the sporadic tumors are unilateral and tend to present in the toddler-preschool years. About 10% of affected patients have a positive family history of the disease, while 30% of patients have a negative family history but a history of multifocal disease. Together, these groups comprise the 40% of patients able to transmit the disease to their own offspring (Dryja et al, 1984). Persons who have the disease and survive have an additional 15% chance of developing an independent, second primary malignancy, most commonly, osteogenic sarcoma (Shields and Augsburger, 1981).

Cytogenetic studies performed in the 1960s and 1970s revealed a nonrandom association between deletions of the long arm of chromosome 13 and retinoblastoma. Subsequently, the involved band was shown to be 13q 14 (Wilson et al, 1977), although 95% of affected patients had normal karyotypes when their peripheral lymphocytes were studied (Dryja et al, 1983). In 1980, a quantitative assay for esterase D, an enzyme found in most human tissues but with unknown biological function, was developed. This assay facilitated mapping of the gene for that enzyme to chromosome 13, band q 14. Studies of patients with structural defects of chromosome 13 showed a close linkage between esterase D and the locus for retinoblastoma (Sparkes et al, 1980).

Using the molecular genetic techniques described in Chapter 3 it has become possible to understand the genetic factors that promote tumorigenesis at the cellular level in retinoblastoma. When DNA is extracted from tumor cells in enucleated eyes and probed with a set of cloned DNA fragments homologous to loci on chromosome 13, restriction fragment length polymorphisms have revealed a difference between the tumor DNA and the constitutional (peripheral blood) DNA from the same person. In four of eight patients, Dryja and colleagues determined that the tumor loci were homozygous at the long arm of chromosome 13 but the constitutional DNA was heterozygous at the equivalent loci (Dryja et al, 1984). Homozygosity of the tumor occurred in both the sporadic and inherited forms of the disease. Thus, development of homozygosity for a mutant gene on chromosome 13 may be a fundamental event in the oncogenesis of retinoblastoma (Dryja et al, 1984). Interestingly, these molecular studies have shed new light on Knudson's two-mutation hypothesis regarding tumorigenesis, and may explain the difference between the multifocality of hereditary tumors and the unifocality of sporadic tumors. In the hereditary tumors, a mutation should be present in one of the two chromosome 13s in the individual's constitutional DNA. Thus, any subsequent mutational event (the second hit) resulting in homozygosity for that inherited mutation would form a tumor in a susceptible cell. Events that could account for the development of homozygosity include: loss of the normal chromosome 13 due to mitotic nondisjunction (see Chapter 2), reduplication of the mutant chromosome, or some sort of mitotic recombination between the retinoblastoma locus and the centromere (Cavenee et al, 1983). There is now evidence to suggest that the retinoblastoma gene has been cloned (Friend et al, 1986).

Since surgical treatment has been so successful in curing patients affected with retinoblastoma, many people are now surviving to adulthood and reproducing. Progeny of persons with the hereditary form of retinoblastoma are at a 50% risk of developing the disease themselves. Current clinical practice is to perform multiple ophthalmologic examinations under general anesthesia for infants who have a 50% risk of developing retinoblastoma. An important and fascinating clinical application of the molecular studies is to use restriction fragment length polymorphisms present in constitutional DNA to identify those infants likely to develop or likely to be free from the disease (Cavenee et al, 1986; Wiggs et al, 1988). In other words, each parent has two chromosome 13s. By definition, one of the parents is affected with the hereditary form of retinoblastoma. One of the four parental chromosomes, therefore, contains the mutant retinoblastoma allele. If that chromosome is present in the child then he will fall into a high risk category for the development of retinoblastoma. If, however, the child does not inherit the chromosome 13 containing the mutant allele, he will fall into a lower risk category and may be spared unnecessary exposures to general anesthesia (see p. 582).

Wilms tumor

Wilms tumor is a nephroblastoma with an incidence of 1/10,000 children (Van Heyningen et al, 1985). It accounts for 15% of all childhood neoplasms (Schimke, 1981). It has been estimated from epidemiologic data that up to one-third of cases represents an inherited form of the disease. The recent improvement in treatment and survival of affected patients, however, will enable more family pedigrees to be analyzed for inheritance patterns (Littlefield, 1984). The majority of Wilms tumors are sporadic (see pp. 577).

In 1–2% of Wilms tumor patients, there is concurrent aniridia (Narahara et al, 1984). Aniridia may be defined as a congenital absence of the iris which usually leads to blindness. It may be inherited as an isolated anomaly in an autosomal dominant manner. In patients with the "sporadic" occurrence of aniridia, about one-third will develop Wilms tumor (Van Heyningen et al, 1985). This so-called Wilms tumor-aniridia association is genetic and can be accompanied by other malformations including genitourinary anomalies, mental retardation, microcephaly, and hemihypertrophy. When studied with appropriate high resolution cytogenetic techniques, most patients with Wilms tumor-aniridia association have a deletion of at least part of band p 13 on the short arm of one of their number 11 chromosomes. These deletions overlap a cluster of individual, but closely linked, genes important in the development of the kidney, eye, and genitourinary tract (Glaser et al, 1986). It has been suggested that this gene complex additionally contains a recessive oncogene, necessary for Wilms tumor formation. Inheritance of the deletion of band 11 p 13 in an autosomal dominant pattern is potentially the first of two steps in nephroblastoma oncogenesis.

In a manner analogous to retinoblastoma, Wilms tumor DNA has been shown—even in sporadic, isolated cases—to be homozygous for certain alleles on the short arm of chromosome 11 (Fearon et al, 1984; Orkin et al, 1984). In addition, two tumors have been shown to be hemizygous for the C-Harvey-ras 1 oncogene, which also maps to the short arm of chromosome 11. Hemizygosity for C-H-ras 1, resulting from submicroscopic deletions of chromosome 11, is possibly related to tumor development (Reeve et al, 1984). Most recently, the gene for the β subunit of follicle-stimulating hormone (FSH) has been shown to be deleted in the leucocyte DNA from 4 of 4 patients with Wilms tumor-aniridia association (Glaser et al, 1986), indicating very tight linkage with the Wilms tumor-aniridia gene complex. The chromosome 11 segment containing the catalase gene, the beta subunit of FSH gene, and the Wilms-aniridia complex has been estimated to encompass 3000–6000 kb of DNA.

The cytogenetic, molecular, and biochemical abnormalities described in the constitutional and tumor DNA of patients with Wilms tumor are likely to lend themselves to both prenatal diagnosis of the condition and identification of children at high risk for developing the disease.

REFERENCES

Brodeur GM, Seeger RC, Schwab M, et al: Amplification of N-myc in untreated human neuroblastomas correlates with advanced disease stage. *Science* 224:1121, 1984.

Cavenee WK, Dryja TP, Phillips RA, et al: Expression of recessive alleles by chromosomal mechanisms in retinoblastoma. *Nature* 305:779, 1983.

Cavenee WK, Murphree AL, Shull MM, et al: Prediction of familial predisposition to retinoblastoma. *N Engl J Med* 314:1201, 1986.

Dryja TP, Bruns GAP, Orkin SH, et al: Isolation of DNA fragments from chromosome 13. *Retina* 3:121, 1983.

Dryja TP, Cavenee W, White R, et al: Homozygosity of chromosome 13 in retinoblastoma. *N Engl J Med* 310:550, 1984.

Fearon ER, Vogelstein B, Feinberg AP: Somatic deletion and duplication of genes on chromosome 11 in Wilms' tumours. *Nature* 309:176, 1984.

Friend SH, Bernards R, Rogelj S, et al: A human DNA segment with properties of the gene that predisposes to retinoblastoma and osteosarcoma. *Nature* 323:643, 1986.

Glaser T, Lewis WH, Bruns GAP, et al: The beta subunit of follicle-stimulating hormone is deleted in patients with aniridia and Wilms' tumour, allowing a further definition of the WAGR locus. *Nature* 321:882, 1986.

Gordon H: Oncogenes. *Mayo Clin Proc* 60:697, 1985.

Knudson AG Jr, Hethcote WH, Brown BW: Mutation and childhood cancer: A probabilistic model for the incidence of retinoblastoma. *Proc Nat Acad Sci USA* 72:5116, 1975.

Littlefield JW: Genes, chromosomes, and cancer. *J Pediatr* 104:489, 1984.

Narahara K, Kikkawa K, Kimira S, et al: Regional mapping of catalase and Wilms' tumor-aniridia, genitourinary abnormalities, and mental retardation triad loci to the chromosome segment 11 p 1305 p 1306. *Hum Genet* 66:181, 1984.

Orkin SH, Goldman DS, Sallan SE: Development of homozygosity for chromosome 11 p markers in Wilms' tumor. *Nature* 309:172, 1984.

Reeve AE, Housiaux PJ, Gardner RJM, et al: Loss of a Harvey ras allele in sporadic Wilms' tumour. *Nature* 309:174, 1984.

Schimke RN: Genetics and cancer in children: Current concepts. In: *Genetic Issues in Pediatric and Obstetric Practice*. Chicago, Year Book, 1981, p. 413.

Shields JA, Augsburger JJ: Current approaches to the diagnosis and management of retinoblastoma. *Surv Ophthalmol* 25:347, 1981.

Sparkes RS, Sparkes MC, Wilson MG, et al: Regional assignment of genes for human esterase D and retinoblastoma to chromosome band 13q 14. *Science* 208:1042, 1980.

Van Heyningen V, Boyd PA, Seawright A, et al: Molecular analysis of chromosome 11 deletions in aniridia-Wilms tumor syndrome. *Proc Natl Acad Sci USA* 82:8592, 1985.

Wiggs J, Nordenskjold M, Yandell D, et al: Prediction of the risk of hereditary retinoblastoma, using DNA polymorphisms within the retinoblastoma gene. *N Engl J Med* 318:151, 1988.

Wilson MG, Ebbin AJ, Towner JW, et al: Chromosomal anomalies in patients with retinoblastoma. *Clin Genet* 12:1, 1977.

Prenatal Diagnosis and Fetal Therapy 5

Just as the biologic limit of viability is being pushed back into earlier points in gestation, so too is the pediatrician's involvement with the very young patient. Formerly, the pediatrician's therapeutic role began when the obstetrician handed over the newborn infant in the delivery room. That role, however, is changing. With the advent of sophisticated fetal monitoring and increasingly diverse prenatal diagnostic techniques, the pediatrician is being called upon more frequently to participate in the planning of medical treatment for a fetus who is still in utero. Alternatively, in the delivery room, the pediatrician may be presented with information such as: "this mother had a high serum α-fetoprotein level" or "antenatal ultrasonography showed bilateral ureteral dilatation." The interpretation of these antenatal tests necessitates inclusion of a chapter on prenatal diagnosis and fetal therapy in this textbook of pediatrics.

ULTRASONOGRAPHY

Ultrasonographic (ultrasound) imaging is currently the state of the art noninvasive means of assessing fetal anatomy and the intrauterine environment. Ultrasonography was first used in obstetrics in 1958 (Donald et al, 1958) and since that time, no adverse effects secondary to its use in humans have been documented. Initially, the indications for ultrasonographic study during pregnancy included measurement of biparietal diameter (BPD) and placental localization. More recently, however, ultrasonographic studies have been utilized to document fetal anatomy as well as physiology. Real-time imaging allows a dynamic evaluation of fetal well-being, including fetal urine production, fetal swallowing movements, and visualization of cardiac contractility. The fetal biophysical profile has been developed as a noninvasive screening test for the high-risk fetus. Parameters analyzed include fetal muscular tone, fetal movements, fetal breathing, amount of amniotic fluid, and sonographic qualities of the placenta.

Although ultrasonographic studies have not received a blanket recommendation as a routine screening test in all United States pregnancies, many obstetricians advocate an antenatal awareness of fetal malformations in order to manage labor and delivery effectively and plan for neonatal treatment. In a recent review article, it was stated that 40% of obstetric practices have all of their patients undergo scanning at least once during their pregnancy (Hill et al, 1983). Screening for the presence of congenital anomalies is best done at 16–18 weeks' gestation (Lange, 1985).

In the subsequent paragraphs, specific fetal pathological conditions and the relative accuracy of ultrasonographic imaging in their diagnosis will be discussed. One of the more useful aspects of ultrasonographic study, however, is in the serial measurement of fetal growth as an indication of fetal health. Traditionally, growth parameters have included biparietal diameter, head circumference, abdominal circumference, and femur length (Campbell and Pearce, 1983). More recently, in utero standards (similar to pediatric postnatal growth curves) have been developed for biparietal diameter, occipitofrontal diameter, thoracic diameter, abdominal circumference, size of iliac bones, stomach size, bladder size, length of long bones, spinal canal dimensions, size of ventricular horns, and intermalar as well as interethmoidal distances (Elejalde and Elejalde, 1986). Such serial measurements enable a distinction to be made between two subgroups of growth-retarded fetuses. In one, initial fetal growth is normal, but in the third trimester there is slowing and eventual cessation of growth. With this pattern there is an increased brain-to-abdomen ratio that occurs when the underlying cause is inadequate placental perfusion. Such neonates will appear wasted and may suffer from hypoglycemia, but the long-range prognosis is good. This contrasts with the fetus whose symmetric growth retardation is noted early in the second trimester. The etiology here is more likely to be genetic, chromosomal, or infectious. This type of fetal growth pattern carries a poorer prognosis for normal postnatal growth and development (Campbell and Pearce, 1983). Asymmetry in any of the fetal measurements may enable a diagnosis of microcephaly (in the case of the head) or dwarfism (in the case of the limbs) to be made.

Common Malformations Detectable by Ultrasonography

In about 3–5% of all live births in the United States, a congenital anomaly is present. This amounts to about 150,000 infants annually. Of the affected infants, about 10% have malformations involving the head or spine (Hill et al, 1983). The most common craniospinal defects detectable by ultrasonography include: anencephaly, spina bifida, hydrocephalus, microcephaly, encephalocele, brain cysts and tumors, and holoprosencephaly. On an ultrasonographic study, anencephaly appears as a large defect or absence of the skull (Fig. 13.14), absence of the cerebral hemispheres, and a grossly malformed brain remnant (Hill et al, 1983). The diagnosis can be made reliably as early as 12 weeks' gestation, allowing the mother the option of first trimester termination of pregnancy. The disorder is incompatible with life. Spina bifida, one of the most common birth defects in the general population, is a herniation of the meninges or spinal cord through an absent dorsal aspect of the vertebra. Real-time imaging enables the site and extent of the lesion to be described with great accuracy (Campbell and Pearce, 1983). In addition, although the majority of fetuses with spina bifida have pathologically dilated ventricles, the biparietal diameter of the skull tends to be small for gestational age (Campbell and Pearce, 1983; Nicolaides et al, 1986). The diagnosis of encephalocele refers to the protrusion of brain matter and/or meninges through a defect of the skull. An important consideration in the differential diagnosis of encephalocele is Meckel-Gruber syndrome, which has many physical findings in common with trisomy 13 (see pp. 762) and is generally fatal in the neonatal period.

Fetal gastrointestinal malformations are likewise common in the general population, occurring 6/1000

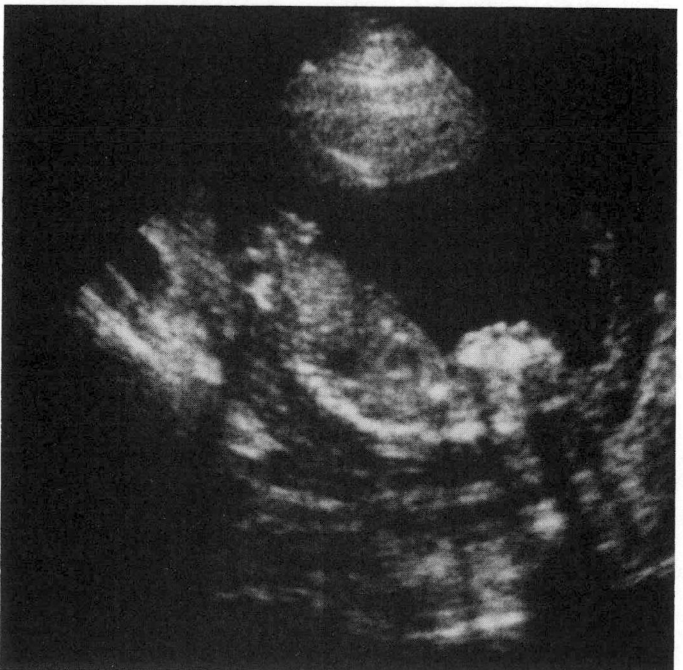

Figure 13.14. Ultrasonagraphic appearance of a fetus with anencephaly (photograph courtesy of Dr. Beryl Benacerraf).

births (Barss et al, 1985). Diagnoses that can be made by ultrasonographic study include bowel obstruction (esophageal atresia, duodenal atresia or stenosis, ileal or jejeunal atresia, annular pancreas), omphalocele, gastroschisis, and diaphragmatic hernia. The decrease in fetal swallowing seen in cases of bowel obstruction can lead to polyhydramnios. Affected pregnancies are likely to be referred for evaluation by an ultrasonographer because of a discrepancy between the size of the uterus and the gestational dating. Roughly one-third of fetuses with gastrointestinal anomalies will have associated malformations (Barss et al, 1985). Thus, a thorough fetal anatomic survey should be undertaken before assigning a diagnosis or prognosis. In addition, fetal karyotyping should be performed if the anomalies include duodenal atresia or omphalocele because of the high rates of associated chromosomal abnormalities.

With the use of real-time imaging, identification of the kidneys is possible at 14 weeks' gestation. The large size of the adrenals in fetal life as well as the presence of perirenal fat can make the diagnosis of renal agenesis difficult. Oligohydramnios is an indication of poor renal function. Other diagnoses made on ultrasonographic study include polycystic kidneys, solitary renal cysts, hydronephrosis, obstructive uropathy, and prune-belly syndrome.

Detailed ultrasonographic examination of the heart is possible at 20 weeks' gestation. The presence of four cardiac chambers, the position and size of the great vessels and their valves, the orientation and movement of the two atrioventricular valves, and the thickness of the ventricular walls and intraventricular septum may all be documented. Cardiac structural anomalies diagnosed prenatally include hypoplastic left heart, single atrium, single ventricle, double outlet right ventricle, tricuspid atresia, pulmonic or aortic stenosis, tetralogy of Fallot, Ebstein anomaly, and ventricular septal defect. In addition, pericardial effusion and cardiac arrhythmias may be studied.

Other organ systems important in antenatal ultrasonographic examination include the skeletal system (achondroplasia, thanatophoric dwarfism, diastrophic dysplasia, limb anomalies) and the face and neck (cleft lip and palate, micrognathia, cystic hygroma). It has been suggested that a particular combination of abnormal facial features and skeletal findings on ultrasonographic study is seen in fetuses with trisomy 13 or 18 (Benacerraf et al, 1986). The presence of cystic hygroma may be seen in Turner syndrome, Noonan syndrome, fetal alcohol syndrome, familial pterygium colli, or chromosome abnormalities (Chervenak et al, 1983). Hydrops fetalis may be caused by immune disorders, cardiac dysrhythmias, viral infections, chromosome abnormalities, or inborn metabolic errors, among other etiologies. Fetal sex can be reliably determined by ultrasonographic visualization of the external genitalia by the fifth month of pregnancy (Birnholz 1983). Although this point in gestation may be too late to allow selective termination of pregnancy in families affected by X-linked disorders, the information is useful in interpretation of antenatal pulmonary indices in preterm fetuses.

At this point, it seems appropriate to ask two questions: (1) what is the accuracy of ultrasonographic diagnosis and (2) what is the benefit to the patient and/or family to know the diagnosis antenatally? Several studies have attempted to answer the first question. Sabbagha and associates studied 596 women at high risk for birth defects (Sabbagha et al, 1985). Eighty-one fetuses (13.6%) had fetal anomalies diagnosed prenatally. On follow-up, there were four false-abnormal findings (0.6%) and three false-normal results (0.5%). The authors concluded that accuracy of ultrasonographic examination depended upon the expertise of the examiner, prevalence of the anomaly in specific geographic locations, "prescreening" studies of the obstetric patients involved, and the length of time of the postpartum follow-up. An even larger study by Campbell and colleagues reported 244 correct diagnoses in 1737 referrals, with six false-abnormal results (0.3%) and 17 false-normal results (0.9%) (Campbell and Pearce, 1983). In over 100 reported cases of anencephaly, however, there have been no false-positive diagnoses (Chervenak et al, 1986). The accuracy and limitations of fetal ultrasonography were addressed in a study correlating anatomic findings at autopsy with prenatal ultrasonographic diagnoses. Fifty-two malformations were correctly diagnosed prenatally, but 90 additional malformations were not. Of importance, nine diagnosed abnormalities could not be confirmed at autopsy (Rutledge et al, 1986). This information should be considered when decisions regarding management of pregnancy are being made.

The risks versus benefits of receiving ultrasonographic screening in low-risk pregnancies were studied by Bakketeig et al (1984) in 1009 Norwegian women between 19 and 32 weeks' gestation. Among the 510 women in the study group, there were slightly fewer post-term inductions, fewer low birth weight babies, and an earlier diagnosis of twins, but the results were not statistically significant. Medical intervention became more active for the small for gestational age babies in the study group. No adverse effects of ultrasonography were demonstrated (Bakketeig et al, 1984). The presumed advantages of antenatal diagnosis of fetal anomalies include: (1) improved neonatal medical and surgical management at delivery; (2) allowing the parents the option of termination if the anomalies are detected early enough in pregnancy; (3) giving the parents time to adjust to the diagnosis if the anomalies are detected late in gestation; and (4) in rare cases, in utero treatment is a possibility. Fetal therapy is discussed in more detail on pages 789–790.

Finally, ultrasonography is not only of potential benefit as a diagnostic test. Continuous ultrasonographic guidance during procedures such as amniocentesis, chorionic villus sampling, percutaneous umbilical cord sampling has already been shown to improve the safety and efficacy of such methods of prenatal diagnosis (Chervenak et al, 1986).

α-FETOPROTEIN

α-Fetoprotein (AFP) is one of the major glycoproteins produced by the fetus. Although its physical and biochemical properties are similar to that of albumin, its precise physiologic role is unknown (Bergstrand, 1986). Since its protein structure shows strong evolutionary conservation, it is assumed that the role is an essential one.

Human AFP is first made in the yolk sac and is detectable by 4 weeks' gestation (Bergstrand, 1986). Subsequently, it is made in the fetal liver, passes into the fetal serum, is excreted into fetal urine, and mixes with amniotic fluid. Before keratinization occurs at 20 weeks' gestation, some AFP diffuses directly from the fetal skin into the amniotic fluid. The fetal serum concentration is measured in mg/ml and reaches a peak at 13 weeks' gestation. The amniotic fluid levels are measured in μg/ml and rise to a maximum of between 13 and 15 weeks' gestation. Although fetal concentrations decrease at this point in pregnancy, placental permeability for the protein increases, so maternal serum levels rise until 32 weeks' gestation. Maternal serum AFP has been shown to be exclusively fetal in origin (Crandall, 1981) and is measured in ng/ml.

The clinical utility of AFP as a screening test for open neural tube defects was first demonstrated in 1972 (Brock, 1983). At the time, it was reasoned that AFP would be found in high concentrations in the amniotic fluid of fetuses who had a defect that caused leakage between the fetal circulation and the amniotic fluid (Brock, 1983). This was subsequently confirmed, and it was additionally shown that in the affected pregnancies there was a rise in the AFP detected by radioimmunoassay (Ferguson-Smith, 1983). In 1977, a collaborative study of 18,000 singleton and 150 twin pregnancies between 16 and 18 weeks' gestation was performed in the United Kingdom. To allow comparison among laboratories, results were expressed as multiples of the median (MoM) and showed that 4.5% of the serum samples had AFP levels greater than 2.5 multiples of the median. After repeat samples were drawn, 3.5% remained elevated. Ultrasonography revealed incorrect gestational dates, twins, or fetal demise in 1.5% of the pregnancies with elevated AFP. Ultimately, 2% of the screened population came to amniocentesis for amniotic fluid analysis. A total of 30 neural tube defects were identified (Crandall, 1981). The detection rate was 88% for anencephaly and 79% for open spina bifida (Ferguson-Smith, 1983).

The incidence of neural tube defects in the United States is about 1/1000 live births (Crandall, 1981). The relative frequency of this birth defect has led to the development of screening programs for maternal serum AFP as part of routine prenatal care in the United States. In most laboratories, if the first sample is greater than 2.5 MoM, a second sample is requested. If both samples are elevated, the patient proceeds to ultrasonographic examination and amniocentesis. If the initial sample is greater than 3.0 MoM, it is recommended that the patient has an ultrasonographic examination as soon as possible. Recently, it has been determined that maternal weight exerts a dilutional effect on the maternal levels of AFP. Thus, maternal weight is necessary for calculation of AFP concentration.

Although serum AFP screening was developed for the detection of neural tube defects, an increased maternal level may signify a variety of conditions. The most common cause of an abnormally elevated result, seen in 15–20% of patients, is an incorrectly underestimated gestational age. In a further 25% of patients with elevated values, there is either a threatened abortion or multiple pregnancy (Ferguson-Smith, 1983). Ultrasonographic examination is critical in distinguishing these causes from the rest of the differential diagnosis, given in Table 13.4.

As discussed above, after two elevated values of serum AFP, the patient usually undergoes amniocentesis to assay amniotic fluid AFP. The fluid is also tested for the presence of acetylcholinesterase, which is highly specific for neural tube defects. There are a few rare situations where maternal serum screening is usually not performed, and the patient has amniotic fluid AFP assayed directly. The indications are the following: (1) The birth of a previous child with a neural tube defect (3% risk of recurrence). If two previous children have had neural tube defects, the risk increases to 12–15% (Crandall, 1981). (2) One parent has a neural tube defect (3% risk of recurrence). (3) A previous child has had Finnish congenital nephrosis (25% recurrence risk) or Meckel-Gruber syndrome (encephalocele, omphalocele) (25% recurrence risk).

In 1984, an association was noted between low maternal serum AFP values and fetal chromosomal abnormalities (Merkatz et al, 1984). Although the relationship is still being explored, it appears that women under age 35 years with maternal serum AFP values of less than 0.5 MoM have, on average, a risk of 1:180 for having a fetus with trisomy 13, 18, or 21. This risk

Table 13.4
Differential Diagnosis for Elevated Maternal Serum AFP at 16–18 Weeks' Gestation

Incorrect gestational dates
Multiple pregnancy
Threatened/missed abortion/ectopic pregnancy
Ventral wall defects—gastroschisis, omphalocele
GI malformations
Open neural tube defects
Turner syndrome
Cystic hygroma
Renal agenesis
Polycystic kidneys
Finnish congenital nephrosis
Epidermolysis bullosa
Lesions of placenta and umbilical cord
Rh isoimmunization
Hereditary persistence of AFP (autosomal dominant trait)
Acardiac monster

is higher than is the risk of amniocentesis. By offering fetal cytogenetic studies to the women with the low AFP levels, it is anticipated that 20% of fetal trisomies will be detected (Doran et al, 1986). The explanation for the low levels of AFP seen in fetal trisomies appears to be related to the generalized retardation in growth, immaturity of the fetal liver, and decreased production. Low levels of AFP predominate in the situation where fetal trisomy coexists with neural tube or ventral wall defect (Macri et al, 1986).

AFP screening plays an important role in the detection of birth defects. It is critical, however, to remember that a normal AFP level does not guarantee a normal baby. In contrast, an elevated level, with a normal ultrasonography and amniotic fluid level, may be present in an otherwise normal pregnancy.

AMNIOCENTESIS

Amniocentesis is the procedure whereby amniotic fluid is removed from the pregnant uterus, usually during the second trimester, for the purpose of obtaining information about the fetus. Both the cellular constituents and the biochemical components—AFP, acetylcholinesterase, bilirubin, lecithin, sphingomyelin, and phosphatidylcholine—can be analyzed. In this section, however, amniocentesis will be discussed only in the context of prenatal genetic diagnosis.

The actual technique of amniocentesis is relatively straightforward. Before the procedure, a genetic counseling session is scheduled to review the family history, indications for the test, and the potential risks and benefits to be expected. Amniocentesis is usually performed between 16 and 18 weeks' gestation. At the time of the amniocentesis, a real-time ultrasonographic examination is performed to determine (1) fetal viability, (2) gestational age, (3) placental location, (4) volume of amniotic fluid, (5) existence of multiple pregnancies, and (6) presence of fetal anatomic defects. A 22-gauge spinal needle is then inserted into the womb and about 20 ml of amniotic fluid are withdrawn. Removal of this amount of fluid does not harm the fetus, as under normal conditions, one-third of the amniotic fluid volume is replaced each hour (Gosden, 1983).

The fluid is then processed as follows: the cells are gently centrifuged, the supernatant liquid is poured off, and the cells are resuspended in a tissue culture medium designed to keep the pH between 6.7 and 7.3 (Gosden, 1983). The cells are grown on coverslips or flasks with flat surfaces to promote adherence. Since the majority of cells obtained at amniocentesis are nonviable, it usually takes a minimum of 2 weeks to culture enough living cells for cytogenetic, biochemical, or DNA analysis. The supernatant fraction, in contrast, may be assayed immediately.

The utilization of amniocentesis has increased dramatically since the results of the first large-scale randomized United States and Canadian trials were published in the mid-1970s (NICHD National Registry, 1976; Simpson et al, 1976). Amniocentesis is now considered the "gold standard" with which newer methods of prenatal diagnosis, such as chorionic villus biopsy, are compared. The cytogenetic indications for the procedure are: (1) maternal age ≥ 35 years at the time of conception because of the known increased risk of bearing a child with a chromosome abnormality; (2) previous child with a chromosome abnormality; (3) a parent with a balanced chromosome translocation; (4) a mother with a family history of an X-linked disorder; (5) a low or a high maternal serum AFP; and (6) family history of neural tube defects (see discussion under AFP, p. 785). The basis for metabolic diagnosis is that cultured amniocytes will show abnormal levels of enzyme activity or toxic metabolites characteristic of specific disease states. The DNA contained in the nucleus of the amniocyte will be representative of all the cells in the fetus, if maternal contamination has been excluded.

In a series of 3000 amniocenteses performed at a single institution over 8 years, amniotic fluid was obtained on the first attempt in 99.3% of cases (Golbus et al, 1979). The frequency of cytogenetic abnormalities detected varied on the basis of indications for testing. Thus, 2.4% of 2404 women with advanced maternal age, 1.2% of 240 women who had a previous infant with trisomy 21, and 9.1% of 55 women with "other" cytogenetic problems had chromosomally abnormal fetuses. Mosaicism, defined as the presence of two or more distinct karyotypes in multiple culture flasks, was seen in 0.4% of cases (Golbus et al, 1979). In this series, there were 14 diagnostic errors/3000 cases. Eight resulted in the incorrect determination of fetal sex. These were due to contamination with maternal cells, slide labeling errors, and secretarial typing errors. In six cases, the errors had serious medical consequences. Similar error rates were reported in the NIH collaborative study (NICHD Registry, 1976).

As with any invasive procedure, the safety of amniocentesis has been scrutinized from the beginning. The NIH collaborative study initially reported a 2% rate of immediate complications following the procedure. These complications included amniotic fluid leakage, vaginal bleeding, premature labor, and chorioamnionitis. There were no differences seen between the study group and controls in the spontaneous abortion rate following the test. A more recent prospective randomized trial of 4606 Danish women, ages 25–34 years, with low risk of genetic disease, found a 1.7% rate of spontaneous abortion following amniocentesis versus a 0.7% rate in a control group (Tabor et al, 1986). The study was criticized, however, because an 18-gauge rather than 22-gauge needle was used to obtain the fluid. Another consideration is the individual expertise of the physician performing the amniocentesis. It has been shown that the risk of spontaneous abortion following the procedure decreases sharply as the obstetrician becomes more experienced with the technique (Verjaal et al, 1981). Additionally, it has been recommended that amniocentesis be performed under continuous ultrasonographic guidance, because 10% of the time the fetus moves directly under the intended path of the needle in the 30–60 seconds between localization and needle insertion (Benacerraf and Frigoletto, 1983). Most institutions in the United States currently quote a 0.5–1.0% serious complication rate following amniocentesis. The diagnostic accuracy rate of greater than 99% is unmatched by most other laboratory tests. Low maternal serum AFP levels are defining a new group of women at risk for fetal chromosome abnormalities independent of maternal age. Finally, research efforts are being directed at offering amniocentesis between 11 and 14 weeks' gestation so that results become available earlier in the second trimester (Hanson et al, 1987). The technique of first trimester prenatal diagnosis is discussed in the next section on chorionic villus biopsy.

CHORIONIC VILLUS SAMPLING

As discussed in the previous section, amniocentesis is a safe and accurate means of providing prenatal diagnosis. Its main disadvantage derives from the fact that the procedure is performed during the second trimester of pregnancy. The majority of the desquamated fetal fibroblasts within the amniotic fluid are dead or dying; hence, additional time is required for cell culture. In actual practice, this means that results are generally communicated to the patient around 19–20 weeks' gestation. If a termination of the pregnancy is then elected, the mother must be hospitalized as an inpatient and experience the psychologic and physiologic stress of labor and delivery. Recently, interest has developed in the technique of chorionic villus sampling as a means of identifying genetic abnormalities during the first trimester of pregnancy, allowing patients to opt for a simpler and safer earlier termination. Initial studies performed in the 1960s and early 1970s (Mohr, 1968; Kullander and Sandahl, 1973) were disappointing because of technical problems. With the advent of improved ultrasonography, many of the technical problems have been resolved (Kazy et al, 1982). Chorionic villus sampling has been offered to patients in the United States since 1983.

Chorionic villus sampling is ideally performed between the ninth and eleventh weeks of gestation. At this point in pregnancy, the chorion has differentiated into the *chorion frondosum,* a branched, coral-like structure that interfaces with the maternal decidua, and the *chorion laeve,* a smoother structure that covers the fetus. Since the cells of the chorion frondosum are dividing actively, metaphases may be examined directly. Thus, cytogenetic abnormalities or fetal sex can be detected within hours of the sampling. DNA-based diagnostic methods (see Chapter 3) which require milligram amounts of fetal tissue may proceed directly from chorionic villus sampling without intervening time for cell culture. Chorionic villus tissue similarly can be utilized immediately for enzyme assays to detect inherited metabolic diseases.

The procedure of chorionic villus sampling itself is relatively simple and painless. Before the sampling, a detailed ultrasonographic examination is performed to document fetal size and viability, and to locate the placenta. Under aseptic conditions, a flexible catheter is passed either transcervically or transabdominally under continuous ultrasonographic guidance. A syringe filled with sterile tissue culture medium is attached to the catheter and the sample is obtained by simple suction. About 10–50 mg of chorion are obtained. A geneticist will then immediately check the aspirated tissue for contamination with maternal decidua. If the sample appears adequate for diagnosis, the patient is able to return to her normal activities.

As of February 1988, an international registry reported that 41,521 patients had undergone chorionic villus sampling in continuing pregnancies. Of these, 1382 had fetal losses after the procedure (= 3.54%, Jackson, 1988). Thus far, 22,737 infants have been delivered without report of any major birth defects related to the procedure (Barela et al, 1986). Diagnoses already described or theoretically possible with chorionic villus sampling are shown in Table 13.5.

A prospective, randomized, multicenter NIH-sponsored trial is currently comparing amniocentesis versus chorionic villus sampling. Complications of chorionic villus sampling may be divided temporally into immediate, short-term, and long-term (Table 13.6). Immediate complications include failure to obtain fetal tissue. This situation occurs, on the average, 2.7% of the time but with increased individual experience, falls to 1% (Jackson, 1985). Other potential complications include fetal membrane damage and fetal bleeding. Controversy exists over whether chorionic villus sampling causes an increased rate of spontaneous loss following the procedure. When patients undergoing chorionic villus sampling are compared with age-matched patients who have a normal pregnancy documented on ultrasonographic examination at 9 weeks' gestation, there is an increased rate of fetal loss (Gilmore and McNay, 1985). In addition, there appears to be a 0.3% risk of acute localized maternal infection which may result in septic abortion (Brambati and Varotto, 1985). What is more worrisome, however, are the two reports of serious maternal sepsis, shock, and (in one case) renal failure and hysterectomy following the villus sampling (Blakemore et al, 1985; Barela et al, 1986). By assaying maternal serum AFP before and after the procedure, investigators have shown feto-maternal hemorrhage to occur in 63% of chorionic villus samplings (Blakemore et al, 1985). Rh immunization is indicated after chorionic villus sampling, but the risk of immunizing the mother against other fetal antigens is unknown. Issues raised regarding diagnostic accuracy of chorionic villus sampling include: potential contamination with maternal decidua, poor quality of banded metaphases on direct preparations, and chromosomal mosaicism. The latter problem appears to be a biologic one and is not a technical artifact. In one study, chorion, amnion, and cord blood samples were studied in 46 human conceptuses. In two of 46, a chromosomal mosaicism was found but it was expressed exclusively on the chorionic cells (Kalousek and Dill, 1983).

In summary, chorionic villus sampling has the inherent advantage over amniocentesis in that results

Table 13.5
Diagnoses Made by Chorionic Villus Sampling[1]

DNA-based Diagnosis
- Hemophilia
- Duchenne muscular dystrophy
- α-1-Antitrypsin deficiency
- Lesch-Nyhan syndrome
- Hemoglobinopathies
- PKU
- OTC deficiency

Chromosome Abnormalities
- Trisomy 21
- Trisomy 18
- Trisomy 13
- Turner syndrome
- Klinefelter syndrome
- Fanconi anemia

Metabolic Assays
- Adenosine deaminase deficiency
- Adrenoleukodystrophy
- Argininosuccinic aciduria
- Citrullinemia
- Cystinosis
- Fabry disease
- Farber disease
- Gaucher disease
- G_{m1} gangliosidosis
- G_{m2} gangliosidosis (Tay-Sachs disease)
- Homocystinuria
- Krabbe disease
- Lesch-Nyhan syndrome
- α-Mannosidosis
- β-Mannosidosis
- Maple syrup urine disease
- Menkes syndrome
- Metachromatic leukodystrophy
- Methylmalonic aciduria
- Mucolipidosis II (I-cell disease)
- Mucopolysaccharidoses
  - Ia (Hurler syndrome)
  - II (Hunter syndrome)
  - III (Sanfilippo syndrome)
  - IV (Morquio syndrome)
  - VI (Maroteaux-Lamy)
  - VII (β-glucuronidase deficiency)
- Multiple sulfatase deficiency
- Niemann-Pick disease
- Pompe disease
- Wolman disease
- Zellweger syndrome

[1]See Gustavii et al: First trimester diagnosis on chorionic villi obtained by direct vision technique. *Hum Genet* 65:373, 1984.

are available within the first trimester. The procedure is still relatively new, and precise information regarding safety and accuracy are not yet available on large numbers of patients.

FETAL THERAPY

With the increased utilization of the prenatal diagnostic tests discussed in the preceding sections, opportunities for fetal therapy have expanded. "Fetal therapy" here is defined in a broad sense, referring to changes in medical or surgical management that result from information obtained on antenatal tests. The "treatment" may be as simple as changing the timing, mode, or place of delivery of the infant. The therapy may also be medical—an example is the in utero transfusion of erythrocytes to a fetus with *erythroblastosis fetalis*. Treatment may be dietary, as well. In pregnant women with phenylketonuria, a diet low in phenylalanine begun before conception has been shown to prevent birth defects. In only rare instances is in utero surgical correction of a fetal anatomic defect possible as a means of therapy.

Table 13.6
Complications of Chorionic Villus Sampling

Immediate
- Failure to obtain fetal tissue (1–2.7% depending on experience)
- Fetal membrane damage (l%)
- Fetal bleeding

Short-Term
- Increased incidence of spontaneous abortion following procedure
- Risk of infection
- Contamination with maternal decidua
- Quality of banded metaphases
- Chromosomal mosaicism/fetal-villus discrepancy

Long-Term
- Fetus
  - Risk of inducing fetal anomalies
  - Risk of increased prematurity
  - Long-term effects on growth and development
- Mother
  - Risk of immunization against fetal antigens (Rh, ABO, etc.)
  - Sepsis, shock, renal failure

Fetal Medical Treatment

Numerous examples of medications given to the mother to replace or enhance factors missing or diminished in the fetus are present in the medical literature. The above examples of low phenylalanine diet and erythrocyte transfusions fall into this category. Fetuses determined antenatally (on the basis of HLA typing of fetal tissue) to have congenital adrenal hyperplasia are treated with corticosteroids given to the mother. Fetuses with evidence of congestive heart failure secondary to cardiac dysrhythmias are treated with digitalis administered to the mother. Betamethasone, a glucocorticoid that crosses the placenta, is given to enhance fetal pulmonary maturation in fetuses who are at risk for premature delivery. At least two cases of inborn errors of metabolism—B_{12}-responsive methylmalonic acidemia and biotin-dependent multiple carboxylase deficiency—have been treated by giving the mothers massive doses of B_{12} and biotin, respectively (Adzick et al, 1985).

Fetal Surgical Treatment

The overwhelming majority of fetal anatomic malformations that are surgically correctable are best managed by term delivery and conventional postpartum repair (Adzick et al, 1985). The advantage of diagnosing such malformations antenatally is that delivery can be planned to occur at a tertiary medical center, in the presence of appropriate specialists. Examples of malformations best treated after birth are given in Table 13.7. Certain malformations may necessitate cesarean section to minimize maternal uterine trauma and/or fetal organ damage and to lower the risk of infection. Examples of these situations include conjoined twins, exceptionally large hydrocephalus, and large, ruptured neural tube defects.

The rationale behind more aggressive surgical intervention is that more severe, possibly irreversible fetal damage will occur if treatment is delayed until delivery at term. Two approaches have been taken. One is to deliver the fetus prematurely and proceed with ex utero repair, despite increased risks of pulmonary disease, and technical and anesthetic complications. In utero intestinal volvulus with perforation and bowel ischemia has been managed in this manner (Baxi et al, 1983). The other approach is to perform in utero fetal surgery to correct a malformation which, if successfully rectified, will allow normal fetal development to proceed. At the present time, there is clinical fetal human experience in repair of obstructive uropathies and obstructive hydrocephalus. Congenital diaphragmatic hernia has been repaired in laboratory animals.

In the diagnosis and management of fetal urinary tract obstruction it is important to assess renal function as well as renal anatomy. The volume of amniotic fluid is a key physiological indicator of the amount of fetal urine production. Normal fetal urine is hypotonic, whereas human fetuses with obstructive uropathy and consequent renal dysplasia produce isotonic urine (Adzick et al, 1985). Normal amniotic fluid volume predicts the presence of at least one functioning kidney, but oligohydramnios is a marker for severe impairment (Harrison et al, 1981). Anatomically, it is important to determine whether the malformation(s) is (are) unilateral or bilateral and whether the lesion is surgically reparable (obstruction) or not (multicystic disease). If the fetal urinary tract obstruction is relieved, normal fetal urine production will ensue, amniotic fluid dynamics will be normal, and pulmonary development will proceed normally. A technique for placement of a long-term vesicoamniotic catheter has been developed. Between 1982 and 1985, 73 such catheters were placed in fetuses and reported to an international registry. Thirty of 73 fetuses (41%) survived. There was a procedure-related death rate of 4.6%. Impressively, only two of the 30 survivors have chronic illness (Manning et al, 1986).

Obstruction to the flow of CSF will eventually create increased intracranial pressure, ventricular dilatation, compression of the cerebral cortex, and damage to neurological function. Here, also, a technique of in utero ventriculoamniotic shunting has been developed for fetuses shown to have progressive hydrocephalus by serial ultrasonographic monitoring of ventricular size. Although 34 of 44 (83%) reported fetuses survived, there was a 10% procedure-related death rate. Of the survivors, 53% are seriously neurologically handicapped, 12% have a moderate neurologic handicap, and 35% are developing normally (Manning et al, 1986).

Congenital diaphragmatic hernia deserves mention because it carries a high mortality risk (80%), the prenatal diagnosis of the condition is accurate, there is a physiological marker for poor prognosis (polyhydramnios), and surgical techniques for repair of the defect in lambs have been developed. Since herniation of abdominal viscera into the thorax impedes normal pulmonary development and it is the pulmonary hypoplasia that contributes greatly to the neonatal mortality, repair of the defect between 22 and 28 weeks' gestation may allow sufficient pulmonary growth to occur to permit postnatal survival (Adzick et al, 1985).

Clearly, in utero fetal surgery is still in its early stages of development, but it has great future prospects for the treatment of birth defects.

Table 13.7
Malformations Detectable in Utero but Best Corrected after Delivery at Term[1]

Esophageal, duodenal, jejeunal-ileal, and anorectal atresias
Meconium ileus
Enteric cysts and duplications
Small intact omphalocele
Small intact meningocele, myelomeningocele, and spina bifida
Unilateral multicystic dysplastic kidney
Craniofacial, extremity, and chest wall deformities
Cystic hygroma
Small sacrococcygeal teratoma
Ovarian cysts

[1]Reproduced with permission from Adzick NS, Flake AW, Harrison MR: Recent advances in prenatal diagnosis and treatment. *Pediatr Clin North Am* 32:1103, 1985.

REFERENCES

Adzick NS, Flake AW, Harrison MR: Recent advances in prenatal diagnosis and treatment. *Pediatr Clin North Am* 32:1103, 1985.

Bakketeig LS, Jacobsen G, Brodtkorb KJ, et al: Randomised controlled trial of ultrasonographic screening in pregnancy. *Lancet* 2:207, 1984.

Barela AI, Kleinman GE, Golditch IM, et al: Septic shock with renal failure after chorionic villus sampling. *Am J Obstet Gynecol* 154:1100, 1986.

Barss VA, Benacerraf BR, Frigoletto FD Jr: Antenatal sonographic diagnosis of fetal gastrointestinal malformations. *Pediatrics* 76:445, 1985.

Baxi LV, Yeh M-N, Blanc WA, et al: Antepartum diagnosis and management of in utero intestinal volvulus with perforation. *N Engl J Med* 308:1519, 1983.

Benacerraf BR, Frigoletto FD Jr, Greene MF: Abnormal facial features and extremities in human trisomy syndromes: Prenatal US appearance. *Radiology* 159:243, 1986.

Benacerraf BR, Frigoletto FD: Amniocentesis under continuous ul-

trasound guidance: A series of 232 cases. *Obstet Gynecol* 62:760, 1983.
Bergstrand CG: Alphafetoprotein in pediatrics. *Acta Paediatr Scand* 75:1, 1986.
Birnholz JC: Determination of fetal sex. *N Engl J Med* 309:942, 1983.
Blakemore KJ, Mahoney MJ, Hobbins JC: Infection and chorionic villus sampling. *Lancet* 2:338, 1985.
Brambati B, Varotto F: Infection and chorionic villus sampling. *Lancet* 2:609, 1985.
Brock DJH: Amniotic fluid tests for fetal neural tube defects. *Br Med Bull* 39:373, 1983.
Campbell S, Pearce JM: Ultrasound visualization of congenital malformations. *Br Med Bull* 39:322, 1983.
Chervenak FA, Isaacson G, Blakemore KJ, et al: Fetal cystic hygroma: Cause and natural history. *N Engl J Med* 309:822, 1983.
Chervenak FA, Isaacson G, Mahoney MJ: Advances in the diagnosis of fetal defects. *N Engl J Med* 315:305, 1986.
Crandall BF: Alphafetoprotein: The diagnosis of neural tube defects. *Pediatr Ann* 10:39, 1981.
Donald I, MacVicar J, Brown TG: Investigation of abdominal masses by pulsed ultrasound. *Lancet* 1:1188, 1958.
Doran TA, Cadesky K, Wong PY, et al: Maternal serum alphafetoprotein and fetal autosomal trisomies. *Am J Obstet Gynecol* 154:277, 1986.
Elejalde BR, Elejalde MM: The prenatal growth of the human body determined by the measurement of bones and organs by ultrasonography. *Am J Med Genet* 24:575, 1986.
Ferguson-Smith MA: The reduction of anencephalic and spina bifida births by maternal serum alphafetoprotein screening. *Br Med Bull* 39:365, 1983.
Gilmore DH, McNay MB: Spontaneous fetal loss rate in early pregnancy. *Lancet* 1:107, 1985.
Golbus MS, Loughman WD, Epstein CJ, et al: Prenatal genetic diagnosis in 3000 amniocentesis. *N Engl J Med* 300:157, 1979.
Gosden CM: Amniotic fluid cell types and culture. *Br Med Bull* 39:348, 1983.
Hanson FW, Zorn EM, Tennant FR, et al: Amniocentesis before 15 weeks' gestation: Outcome, risks, and technical problems. *Am J Obstet Gynecol* 156:1524, 1987.
Harrison MR, Filly RA, Parer JT, et al: Management of the fetus with a urinary tract malformation. *JAMA* 246:635, 1981.
Hill LM, Breckle R, Gehrking WC: The prenatal detection of congenital malformations by ultrasonography. *Mayo Clin Proc* 58:805, 1983.
Jackson LG: *CVS Newsletter*. February, 1988.
Jackson LG: First trimester diagnosis of fetal genetic disorders. *Hosp Pract* p. 39, March 15, 1985.
Kalousek DK, Dill FJ: Chromosomal mosaicism confined to the placenta in human conceptions. *Science* 221:665, 1983.
Kazy Z, Rozovsky IS, Bakharev VA: Chorion biopsy in early pregnancy: A method of early prenatal diagnosis for inherited disorders. *Prenat Diag* 2:39, 1982.
Kullander S, Sandahl B: Fetal chromosome analysis after transcervical placental biopsies during early pregnancy. *Acta Obstet Gynecol Scand* 52:355, 1973.
Lange IR: Congenital anomalies: Detection and strategies for management. *Semin Perinatol* 9:151, 1985.
Macri JN, Buchnan PD, Gold MP: Low alphafetoprotein and trisomy. *Lancet* 2:405, 1986.
Manning FA, Harrison MR, Rodeck C, et al: Catheter shunts for fetal hydronephrosis and hydrocephalus. *N Engl J Med* 315:336, 1986.
Merkatz IR, Nitowsky HM, Macri JM, et al: An association between low maternal serum alphafetoprotein and fetal chromosomal abnormalities. *Am J Obstet Gynecol* 148:886, 1984.
Mohr J: Fetal genetic diagnosis: Development of techniques for early sampling of fetal cells. *Acta Pathol Microbiol Scand* 73:73, 1968.
Nicolaides KH, Gabbe SG, Campbell S, et al: Ultrasound screening for spina bifida: Cranial and cerebellar signs. *Lancet* 2:72, 1986.
NICHD National Registry for Amniocentesis Study Group: Midtrimester amniocentesis for prenatal diagnosis—safety and accuracy. *JAMA* 236:1471, 1976.
Rutledge JC, Weinberg AG, Friedman JM, et al: Anatomic correlates of ultrasonographic prenatal diagnoses. *Prenat Diag* 6:51, 1986.
Sabbagha RE, Sheikh Z, Tanura RK, et al: Predictive value, sensitivity, and specificity of ultrasonic targeted imaging for fetal anomalies in gravid women at high risk for birth defects. *Am J Obstet Gynecol* 152:822, 1985.
Simpson NE, Dallaire L, Miller JR, et al: Prenatal diagnosis of genetic disease in Canada: Report of a collaborative study. *CMA J* 115:739, 1976.
Tabor A, Madsen M, Obel EB: Randomized controlled trial of genetic amniocentesis in 4606 low-risk women. *Lancet* 1:1287, 1986.
Verjaal M, Leschot NJ, Treffers PE: Risk of amniocentesis and laboratory findings in a series of 1500 prenatal diagnoses. *Prenat Diag* 1:173, 1981.

Gene Therapy 6

Gene therapy may be thought of as the ultimate application of the recombinant DNA technology discussed in Chapter 3. Disorders formerly considered "untreatable" or "only hypothetically treatable" now have the real potential of being cured or symptomatically improved with the advent of gene therapy. In affected individuals whose own cells possess mutant copies of a particular gene, gene therapy may be defined as the delivery of normal genes to that person. For the purposes of this chapter, gene therapy is not considered equivalent to "therapy given in genetic disorders," which is mainly symptomatic. As examples, the low phenylalanine diet given to patients with phenylketonuria or the pharmacologic stimulation of fetal hemoglobin by cytarabine or hydroxyurea in patients with sickle cell anemia are not gene therapy.

Gene therapy theoretically could be performed early in embryonic or fetal life, in which case many subsequently differentiating cells, including the germ line, would contain copies of the inserted normal gene. This form of germ line therapy would have the potential of transmitting the altered genes to the next generation. At the present time, germ line therapy in humans is considered technically difficult and ethically inappropriate (Anderson, 1984). Somatic gene therapy, on the other hand, involves the delivery of the normal gene to a specific somatic target cell population, with the goal of clinical improvement in a debilitating disease. Since the inserted genes are localized to the target cells, the germ line is not affected, and any changes that occur are limited to the affected patient himself.

The following criteria have been established for the development of therapeutic techniques: (1) the new gene can be physically inserted into target cells and will remain there long enough to exert an effect; (2) the new gene will be expressed in the cell at an appropriate level; and (3) the new gene will not harm the cell or the animal (Anderson, 1984). The best candidates for gene therapy appear to be those diseases that are due to a defective enzyme or protein that functions inside the cell where the regulation of the gene is not essential.

Currently, the two types of human tissue being studied for gene transfer include the bone marrow and skin. Of the two, there is more clinical experience with bone marrow. Bone marrow has the advantage of being easily accessible for sampling, in vitro manipulation, and reinfusion (Williams and Orkin, 1986). In addition, the target stem cell population has the potential for further differentiation. The various methods attempted thus far for transferring the cloned genes into the target cells have included: (1) retroviral mediated transfer, (2) chemical uptake by addition of calcium phosphorus, (3) fusion of DNA-loaded vesicles with the target cell membrane, and (4) physical gene transfer by microinjection or electroporation (Anderson, 1984). Retroviruses are RNA viruses that use the enzyme reverse transcriptase to transcribe their viral genome into DNA. Studies with defective retroviruses have had the most success in obtaining gene expression. When compared with wild-type retroviruses, the defective retroviruses differ in that the sequences essential for virus production have been removed to permit insertion of foreign DNA (Williams and Orkin, 1986). Retrovirus-mediated gene transfer is efficient—100% of the target cells can be infected and will be integrated within the host genome.

BONE MARROW TRANSPLANTATION

Bone marrow transplantation is considered "gene therapy" because the normal gene is being transferred to the affected patient in one of two ways: either the normal gene is transplanted via an allogeneic but histocompatible donor or the affected patient's autologous bone marrow is removed, the normal gene is inserted in vitro, and the bone marrow is returned after therapy. Autologous transfected bone marrow is especially attractive as a mode of therapy because there is virtually no possibility of immune rejection of the marrow. Theoretically, there is always a small chance that the inserted gene might modify the expression of a cell-surface antigen on the bone marrow cells, making them appear "foreign" to the host, but this is unlikely. Autologous gene therapy can only be attempted if the single gene responsible for the disease state has been characterized and is available as a complementary DNA clone (Parkman, 1986). Autologous bone marrow transplantation has the obvious advantage of avoiding the need for a compatible donor. Results thus far have shown that there is less clinical correction obtained with autologous bone marrow transplantation as compared with engraftment of normal allogeneic bone marrow (Parkman, 1986). In a recent review article, Parkman classified some of the genetic diseases potentially treatable by bone marrow transplantation (Table 13.8). In class I, the expression of the genetic defect is restricted to lymphoid cells. In class II, the expression of the defect is restricted to lymphoid and hematopoietic cells. In class III, the defect is restricted to hematopoietic cells alone. In class IV, the genetic defect is generalized, but the clinical symptomatology is restricted to the lymphohematopoietic system. Class V defects are similar, with the addition of CNS involvement. Class VI defects are not expressed in lymphohematopoietic cells and are not treatable by bone marrow transplantation.

Three disorders are commonly mentioned as realistic candidates for gene therapy and autologous bone marrow transplant. Adenosine deaminase (ADA) deficiency and purine nucleoside phosphorylase (PNP) deficiency cause a serious clinical immunodeficiency state. The third disorder is Lesch-Nyhan syndrome, also known as hypoxanthine guanine phosphoribosyltransferase (HGPRT) deficiency. This last disease, discussed more fully on page 972 results in severe mental retardation and debilitating self-mutilatory behavior. The first two disorders are considered class IV, generalized enzymatic deficiencies in which symptomatology is limited to the lymphohematopoietic system. Delivery of the normal gene and subsequently the normal enzyme theoretically benefits the patient by producing degradation of accumulated substrate. ADA and PNP deficiencies have already been clinically corrected by allogeneic bone marrow transplantation (Parkman, 1986). In addition, the genes for ADA and PNP have been cloned. In at least one cell line from a patient with immunodeficiency, it has been shown that the loss of ADA enzyme function is due to a point mutation in a coding gene (Bonthron et al, 1985). HGPRT deficiency presents a bigger therapeutic challenge because so much of its symptomatology is related to accumulation of abnormal metabolites in the CNS. Establishment of normal enzyme levels in the bone marrow might effect some generalized clinical improvement, but delivery of the enzyme past the blood-brain barrier is a problem. The gene for HGPRT has been successfully transferred into human bone marrow cells by retroviruses (Gruber et al, 1985), although proven allogeneic bone marrow en-

Table 13.8
Classification of Some of the Genetic Diseases that May be Treated by Bone Marrow Transplantation (BMT)[1]

Class I	Class II	Class III	Class IV	Class V	Class VI
Expression					
Expression of genetic defect restricted to lymphoid cells	Expression of genetic defect restricted to lymphoid and hematopoitic cells	Expression of genetic defect restricted to hematopoietic cells	Generalized genetic defect; clinical symptomatology restricted to lympho-hematopoietic cells	Generalized genetic defect; generalized clinical symptomatology with or without CNS involvement	Lympho-hematopoietic cells do not express the normal gene product
Treatment					
Correctable by BMT	Correctable by BMT	Correctable by BMT	May be correctable by BMT	May be correctable by BMT	Not Correctable by BMT
Disease					
Severe combined immune deficiency (non-ADA deficient)[2]	Wiskott-Aldrich syndrome[2]	Thalassemia[2]	Gaucher's disease[2,3]	Adrenoleuko-dystrophy[2]	Cystic fibrosis
	Chediak-Higashi syndrome[2]	Granulocyte actin deficiency[2]	Adenosine deaminase deficiency[2,3]	Metachromatic leukodystrophy[2]	Hemophilia
gpL-115 deficiency[2]		Chronic granulocyte disease[2]	Nucleotide phosphorylase deficiency[2,3]	Krabbe disease	Phenylketonuria
X-linked agamma-globulinemia		Infantile agranulo-cystosis[2]	Fanconi anemia[2]	Mucopolysacchar-idosis[2,3]	
		Sickle cell disease[2] Osteopetrosis[2]		Lesch-Nyhan syndrome[2,3]	

[1]Reprinted with permission from Parkman R: The application of bone marrow transplantation to the treatment of genetic diseases. *Science* 232:1373, 1986.
[2]Diseases for which allogeneic bone marrow transplantation has been attempted.
[3]Candidate diseases for gene therapy.

graftment with establishment of normal peripheral blood levels of HGPRT in a patient with Lesch-Nyhan syndrome did not produce clinical improvement (Parkman, 1986).

The prospect of gene therapy is generating interest and excitement on the part of molecular biologists, clinical geneticists, and primary care physicians. At the present time, clinical application is being limited to disease states where the clinical phenotype is severely debilitating, other therapeutic options are unavailable, the gene for the disease is known and cloned, regulation of the enzyme or protein produced is not essential, and delivery of the normal gene to the bone marrow potentially will produce symptomatic improvement. In the future, as techniques are modified and clinical experience accrues, the indications for gene therapy undoubtedly will be broadened.

REFERENCES

Anderson WF: Prospects for human gene therapy. *Science* 226:401, 1984.

Bonthron DT, Markham AF, Ginsburg D, et al: Identification of a point mutation in the adenosine deaminase gene responsible for immunodeficiency. *J Clin Invest* 76:894, 1985.

Gruber HE, Finley KD, Hershberg RM, et al: Retroviral vector-mediated gene transfer into human hematopoietic progenitor cells. *Science* 230:1057, 1985.

Parkman R: The application of bone marrow transplantation to the treatment of genetic diseases. *Science* 232:1373, 1986.

Williams DA, Orkin SH: Somatic gene therapy: Current status and future prospects. *J Clin Invest* 77:1053, 1986.

DIANA W. BIANCHI

Section 14

Endocrinology

Two great systems act to transmit information and regulate function in the human body: the nervous system, which transmits electrical impulses; and the circulatory system, which carries chemical messengers formed in the endocrine glands of the body. An exception to this general rule is the hypothalamus where chemical messengers, or hormones, are formed within neurons but are transported to the target cells by a plexus of blood vessels.

Mechanism of Hormone Action

1

HORMONES

Definition

Hormones are substances that are formed by one group of cells in the organism, secreted into the blood stream, and carried to other cells where, at very low concentrations, they manifest their effects. Hormones can be divided into two main types, protein and nonprotein, and the latter can be subdivided into the steroid hormones and those that are derivatives of amino acids.

The paracrine system involves the synthesis of specific substances by one cell and the subsequent action of the substance on other nearby tissues. Substances such as prostaglandins and related molecules are formed locally and exert their effects on surrounding cells. Certain hormones exert local regulatory control: for example, the action of testosterone in fetal life on the wolffian duct and the action of the müllerian-inhibiting factor on the müllerian duct (pp. 870). This type of local action by prostaglandins and some hormones involves diffusion of the substance from its site of origin through the extracellular space to its target cell or tissue.

Control within a cell of its own function is called autocrine regulation or autoregulation. In the thyroid gland, for example, the follicular cells are capable of modifying several aspects of their own function, most important being the responsiveness to thyroid-stimulating hormone (TSH) (pp. 826).

Regulation of Secretion

The output of any hormone from an endocrine gland can be stimulated or suppressed by other hormones or regulatory factors. The production of many hormones (such as cortisol, thyroid hormone, and the sex hormones) is under the influence of tropic hormones from the anterior pituitary gland. These, in turn, are regulated by factors from the hypothalamus. Thus, for example, as the hypothalamus elaborates more thyrotropin-releasing hormone (TRH) the thyrotrophs of the anterior pituitary are stimulated to make and secrete more TSH. The latter circulates in the peripheral blood and eventually acts on the thyroid gland to enhance production of thyroid hormone. It is the circulating level of thyroid hormone that serves as a signal to the pituitary to increase or decrease production of TSH. Evidently, thyroid hormones induce the synthesis of a protein that, in turn, somehow inhibits the pituitary response to TRH. This kind of control is called negative feedback and many endocrine glands are so regulated. In some cases, as with cortisol and its tropic hormone adrenocorticotropic hormone (ACTH), the negative feedback has a greater effect on the hypothalamus than on the pituitary.

Parathyroid-stimulating hormone (PTH) secretion is controlled directly by the level of circulating Ca^{++}. This is a simpler form of negative feedback since the product, Ca^{++}, directly inhibits the formation of the stimulator, PTH. As the amount of PTH secreted increases, bone resorption is stimulated and Ca^{++} is released into the circulation. As the Ca^{++} concentration rises it eventually reaches a level that shuts off PTH production allowing bone resorption to decline and the blood levels of Ca^{++} to fall gradually. When the Ca^{++} concentration reaches a nadir the parathyroid gland is stimulated to release more PTH.

For each endocrine system, there are varying degrees of complexity in the feedback systems that regulate hormone production. In the reproductive system, an important positive feedback effect of estrogen on luteinizing hormone (LH) release occurs at the time of ovulation (pp. 873). Frequently, one hormone will affect the production of another hormone. For example, thyroid hormone enhances growth hormone (GH) production. The control of hormone secretion is exquisitely tuned to the needs of the organism.

Processing of Hormones

Hormones are commonly formed from larger precursor molecules. Generally, a preprotein is formed which contains an N-terminal sequence of amino acids that functions as a signal to move the protein from the rough endoplasmic reticulum, where it is synthesized, to the intracisternal space from which it will move to the Golgi apparatus. The molecule is then further processed and incorporated into secretory granules and extruded from the cell. For PTH and insulin, removal of the signal segment leaves a prohormone that is still larger than the final active molecule. Sometimes prohormones, like proinsulin, are released into the blood stream, especially in abnormal states. In addition to processing of large prohormones to smaller biologically active hormones, other modifications of the hormone molecules may occur. Those hormones that are secreted as glycoproteins have their carbohydrate moieties added in the Golgi apparatus after the polypeptide chain has been synthesized.

Receptors

Hormones act on target cells by interacting with specific receptors (Kaplan, 1984; Csaba, 1984). The receptors of the protein hormones are located on the cell membrane, whereas receptors for most of the nonprotein hormones are intracellular. Hormone specificity for a target cell is imposed by the specificity of the receptor. Once the hormone binds to its receptor a complex series of reactions is initiated by which the cell responds to hormone stimulation. Examples of these hormone-receptor actions are given in Figure 14.1.

In contrast to the protein hormones, most nonprotein hormones do not have plasma membrane receptors. Rather, their receptors are located within the nucleus of the cell and the hormone-receptor complex interacts directly with chromosomal acceptors (Fig. 14.1). Characteristically, such interaction results in altered gene expression. Depending upon the system, specific DNA is "read out" and mRNA for that message is increased in the cell. The result is enhanced synthesis of specific proteins coded for by the specific mRNAs. Such hormone action is very important for growth and differentiation of cells and tissues.

Peptide and Polypeptide Hormones

These hormones include the neuroendocrine peptides (Guillemin, 1985) such as TRH, gonadotropin-releasing hormone (GnRH), corticotropin-releasing hormone (CRH), growth hormone-releasing hormone (GHRH), and somatostatin, and the protein hormones from the anterior pituitary: ACTH, GH, TSH, follicle-stimulating hormone (FSH), LH, and melanocyte-stimulating hormone (MSH); the pancreatic islets: insulin, glucagon; the parathyroid glands: PTH; the medullary cells of the thyroid: calcitonin; and the gonads: inhibin. Many of these hormones exert their effects by increasing intracellular cyclic adenosine monophosphate (cAMP) in their respective target cells. The binding of the hormone to its specific membrane receptor leads to activation of membrane-bound adenylate cyclase, which catalyzes the conversion of adenosine triphosphate (ATP) to cAMP (Fig.14.1).

Adenylate Cyclase

Adenylate cyclase is found in the plasma membranes of essentially all tissues of vertebrates as well as many invertebrate species. Hormonal activation of adenylate cyclase is tissue-specific; in a given tissue only certain hormones are capable of activation. For example, glucagon stimulates adenylate cyclase of the liver cell, increasing the intracellular concentration of cAMP.

The plasma membrane, which covers the outer surface of the cell, contains all of the components of the

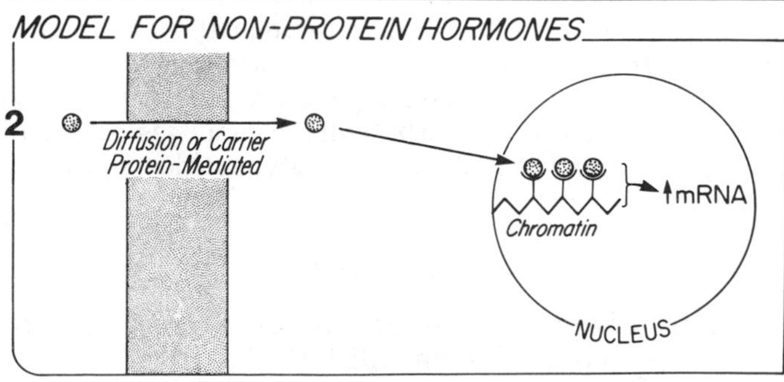

Figure 14.1. Mechanism of hormone action. The interaction of hormones with receptors is depicted at both the cell membrane level and the nuclear level. Protein hormones and catecholamines are bound by specific receptors on the plasma membrane of the cell. The resulting hormone-receptor complex then interacts with the regulatory unit of adenylate cyclase catalyzing GDP/GTP exchange. The regulatory unit (often called the G or N protein) can interact with both the receptor and the catalytic unit of adenylate cyclase, probably shuttling from one to the other depending upon the presence of hormone and the nature of the guanine nucleotide bound to the regulatory unit. Release of GDP and substitution of it by GTP on the regulatory unit allows direct activation of the catalytic unit of adenylate cyclase and subsequent increase in cyclic AMP within the cell. The regulatory unit under other circumstances may inhibit the catalytic unit or it may act on cell processes independently of the catalytic unit.

Other hormones, acting independently of adenylate cyclase may interact with membrane receptors to alter Ca^{++} flux or to initiate activation (often via phosphorylation) of intracellular proteins. For example, Inositol phospholipids in the cell membrane are hydrolyzed in response to hormone-receptor stimulation. The resulting diacyl glycerol and inositol triphospate serve as second messengers to alter intracellular Ca^{++} concentration and to activate a specific type of protein kinase (C).

Most protein hormone-receptor complexes are internalized after the initial membrane response, but the biological significance of this is unknown.

Nonprotein hormones (except for the catecholamines) pass through the cell membrane by diffusion and/or carrier protein-mediated transport. Once within the cell, these hormones bind to nuclear receptors. The hormone-receptor complex then binds to chromatin resulting in altered gene expression.

target cell that are involved in the initial steps in the action of peptide hormones: i.e., the receptor, regulatory unit and catalytic unit of adenylate cyclase. Methods are now available to measure directly the binding of hormone to its receptor. It has become evident that the concentration and affinity of the receptors change rapidly in response to intracellular and extracellular signals. For example, the binding of insulin to its receptor is pH- and temperature-dependent. ACTH binding to its receptors has a strong inverse relation with the Ca^{++} concentration in the medium.

The adenylate cyclase system is composed of two parts, a regulatory unit (N or G protein) and a catalytic unit (Aurbach, 1982). The latter is responsible for the generation of cAMP. Recently it has been shown that there are actually two regulatory components of the adenylate cyclase system; a stimulatory (G_s) and an inhibitory (G_i) component (Gilman, 1984). Each regulatory component is a heterodimer of α and β subunits. The subunit of each protein contains a high affinity guanine nucleotide-binding site. When guanine dinucleotide phosphate (GDP) is attached to the subunit of the regulatory unit it is inactive. Hormone bound to receptor leads to dissociation from the regulatory unit of GDP and its replacement by GTP (Hughes, 1983). The regulatory unit (actually the subunit of G_s) with GTP bound activates the catalytic unit of adenylate cyclase and confers on it high affinity for its substrate, Mg^{++}·ATP, which is rapidly converted to cAMP (Fig. 14.1). Patients with pseudohypoparathyroidism type I suffer from a deficiency of the regulatory unit of adenylate cyclase and have subnormal responses to several hormones (pp. 846).

The adenylate cyclase system can be inhibited by a comparable series of actions involving the G_i component. Most hormonal action on adenylate cyclase, however, involves stimulation rather than inhibition of the enzyme.

Protein Kinase

The cAMP generated by activation of adenylate cyclase serves as a "second messenger" in hormone response. It is capable of activating a single group of closely related soluble and membrane-bound enzymes known as cAMP-dependent protein kinases. These protein kinases also have regulatory and catalytic subunits. In the absence of cAMP, the regulatory subunit is bound to the catalytic unit and the latter is inactive. With cAMP bound to it the regulatory unit dissociates from the catalytic unit, which is now active.

A "kinase" is an enzyme that phosphorylates its substrate. For example, glucagon stimulates liver cell adenylate cyclase and the level of cAMP rises, cAMP-dependent kinases are activated, and certain key enzymes in glycogen metabolism are phosphorylated. The enzymes that promote glycogenolysis are active in their phosphorylated form. Thus, glucagon stimulates glycogen breakdown and raises the concentration of glucose in the blood. Enzymes involved in glycogen synthesis are inactive when phosphorylated; therefore, the phosphorylation of enzymes that is stimulated by glucagon also results in decreased glycogen synthesis. Glucagon acts both to stimulate glycogen breakdown and to decrease glycogen synthesis.

Cyclic AMP is inactivated by hydrolysis to 5′-AMP. This reaction is catalyzed by cyclic nucleotide phosphodiesterase. Hormones, such as insulin and ACTH, enhance the activity of this phosphodiesterase, while steroids reduce its activity.

Hormones such as insulin and prolactin appear to have a "second messenger" which is not cAMP. Evidence suggests that it is a soluble protein, the identity of which protein is yet unknown (Czech, 1984; Kelly et al, 1984). Calcium also plays a key role in many cellular processes via its interaction with calmodulin (pp. 841). The effects of cAMP and Ca^{++} as second messengers are often intertwined. Some forms of adenylate cyclase and phosphodiesterase are Ca^{++}-sensitive.

Derivatives of Amino Acids

Both thyroid hormone and the catecholamines are derivatives of the amino acid tyrosine. Their modes of action are distinctly different. Epinephrine interacts with adrenergic receptors on the cell membrane (pp. 855) and, in consequence, alters the activity of adenylate cyclase in a manner similar to that of peptide hormones. Thyroid hormones bind to nuclear receptors increasing the synthesis of specific mRNAs and the production of specific proteins.

The catecholamines, like the peptide hormones, are water soluble. They are low molecular weight substances that contain a catechol nucleus and an amine group. Dopamine serves as a precursor of norepinephrine and also functions as a neurotransmitter in areas of the brain. Norepinephrine is present mainly in the sympathetic nerves and acts locally in several tissues as a neurotransmitter. Epinephrine is primarily synthesized in the adrenal medulla and acts as a hormone on distant target glands after its release from the adrenal gland.

In contrast, thyroid hormones belong to the class of lipid-soluble hormones. Thyroxine and to a lesser extent triiodothyronine are carried in the blood bound reversibly to thyroid-binding globulin (TBG) and thyroid-binding prealbumin (TBPA). The binding proteins are clearly distinct from the target cell receptors. Binding proteins are not biologically essential since extreme elevations or total absence has little consequence. Only the free hormones that readily traverse the cell membrane interact with their specific receptors; these receptors are found in a wide range of target cells (pp. 827).

Steroid Hormones

Like the thyroid hormones, steroids are lipid-soluble; they are carried in the blood stream bound to protein carriers and readily cross the outer cell membrane to enter the target cell where specific receptors are intracellular. A considerable amount of research has been devoted to the study of steroid receptors, particularly the estrogen receptor. Until recently, most investigators believed the steroid receptor resided in the cytoplasm and that the steroid-receptor complex was then translocated to the nucleus where it bound to a specific acceptor. This event brought about changes in gene expression, with increased production of specific mRNAs and their proteins. More recent evidence suggests that the estrogen receptor resides in the nucleus (Welshons et al, 1984; King and Greene, 1984). If so, there are really only two major classes of receptors: those on cell membranes, which are specific for protein hormones and catecholamines, and those within the nucleus, which are specific for thyroid and steroid hormones (Fig. 14.1).

Classes of Steroids

There are six general categories of steroid hormones: vitamin D and its derivatives, glucocorticoids, mineralocorticoids, estrogens, progestins, and androgens. They are all products of cholesterol and all but vitamin D (pp. 843) are synthesized via a common metabolic pathway (pp. 853). Because of their lipid solubility, these hormones have limited solubility in aqueous media such as blood. Thus, as with thyroid hormone, they bind reversibly to one or more plasma proteins. In humans, transcortin (corticosteroid-binding globulin, CBG) has high affinity for both progesterone and cortisol. Sex hormone binding globulin (SHBG) binds dihydrotestosterone, testosterone, and estradiol with high affinity. The binding proteins act as a reservoir for plasma hormone. Clinically, consideration of binding proteins is most important as they affect measurements of hormone levels in blood. Typically, total hormone is measured rather than the concentration of free hormone.

Receptors

Glucocorticoids act on many tissues as evidenced by the presence of their receptors on a wide range of cell types. The sex hormones have receptors in a narrower spectrum of target cells. Androgen action is expressed through two sets of distinct receptors; one which binds testosterone strongly (testis, kidney) and another which binds dihydrotestosterone with higher affinity than testosterone (prostate, seminal vesicles).

ACTH

The regulator of glucocorticoid production is the hormone ACTH secreted by the corticotrophs of the anterior pituitary. This protein hormone activates the adenylate cyclase of the adrenal cortex. As mentioned previously, the increased cAMP activates cAMP-dependent protein kinases, which then act to phosphorylate key proteins in the cell. Presumably, these phosphorylated proteins, directly or indirectly, stimulate the rate-limiting step in steroidogenesis (pp. 853) and also induce adrenocortical growth.

Gonadotropins

The secretion of the sex hormones is dependent upon the actions of FSH and LH on gonadal cells. The mode of action is similar to that of ACTH, that is, via stimulation of adenylate cyclase. Under normal conditions, maximal sex hormone synthesis is evoked when only a small fraction of LH receptors are occupied. Hence, there is an excess of LH receptors.

The tropic hormones of the anterior pituitary are secreted in a pulsatile manner. Recent studies have shown that GnRH and other hypothalamic hormones are secreted in a pulsatile fashion also. Indeed, this pulsatile pattern of secretion of GnRH appears to be fundamental for the control of gonadotropin secretion. Continuous infusion of GnRH in experimental animals fails to stimulate the gonadotropes to secrete FSH and LH.

The very nature of the biosynthesis of steroid hormones, involving many enzymatic steps, and the complexity of the hypothalamic pituitary regulation of this synthesis, generate many clinical conditions of a similar nature but varying etiology (pp. 870). The problem may reside in the hypothalamus or in the pituitary, at any one of the enzymatic steps of biosynthesis or at the receptor level. Thus, a knowledge of hormone synthesis, regulation, and action is essential for proper clinical appraisal of the patient with endocrine dysfunction.

Prostaglandins

Because of the enormous amount of literature on prostaglandins and their interrelationship with the endocrine system, a brief survey of this unique group of cyclic fatty acids will be given. They are derived from essential fatty acids, particularly arachidonic acid, in response to a host of stimuli. Once synthesized, prostaglandins are released locally. They are rapidly inactivated and, therefore, their action is short-lived. The biological activity of these molecules is closely linked to changes in cAMP, the same prostaglandin stimulating adenyl cyclase in one tissue and inhibiting it in another. Prostaglandins have effects on cAMP in almost every cell in the body.

The prostaglandins apparently play a major role in inflammatory and hypersensitivity reactions. Injury leads to tissue release of arachidonic acid and subsequent synthesis of prostaglandins. They may also serve as modulating factors in the cellular response to the polypeptide and amine hormones. They can mimic TSH action on the thyroid or inhibit it. They have been implicated in the cyclic release of LH.

The pathway of biosynthesis of prostaglandins and the thromboxanes is shown in Figure 14.2.

The therapeutic implications of the prostaglandins are enormous. They have been used to induce labor and as abortifacients. Inhibition of prostaglandin synthesis by indomethacin leads to a high incidence of closure of patent ductus arteriosus, obviating the need for surgery in many instances. Their effects on peripheral arteriolar dilatation may make them important antihypertensive agents in the future.

Summary

The endocrine system is involved in the control of many aspects of growth and development. Although

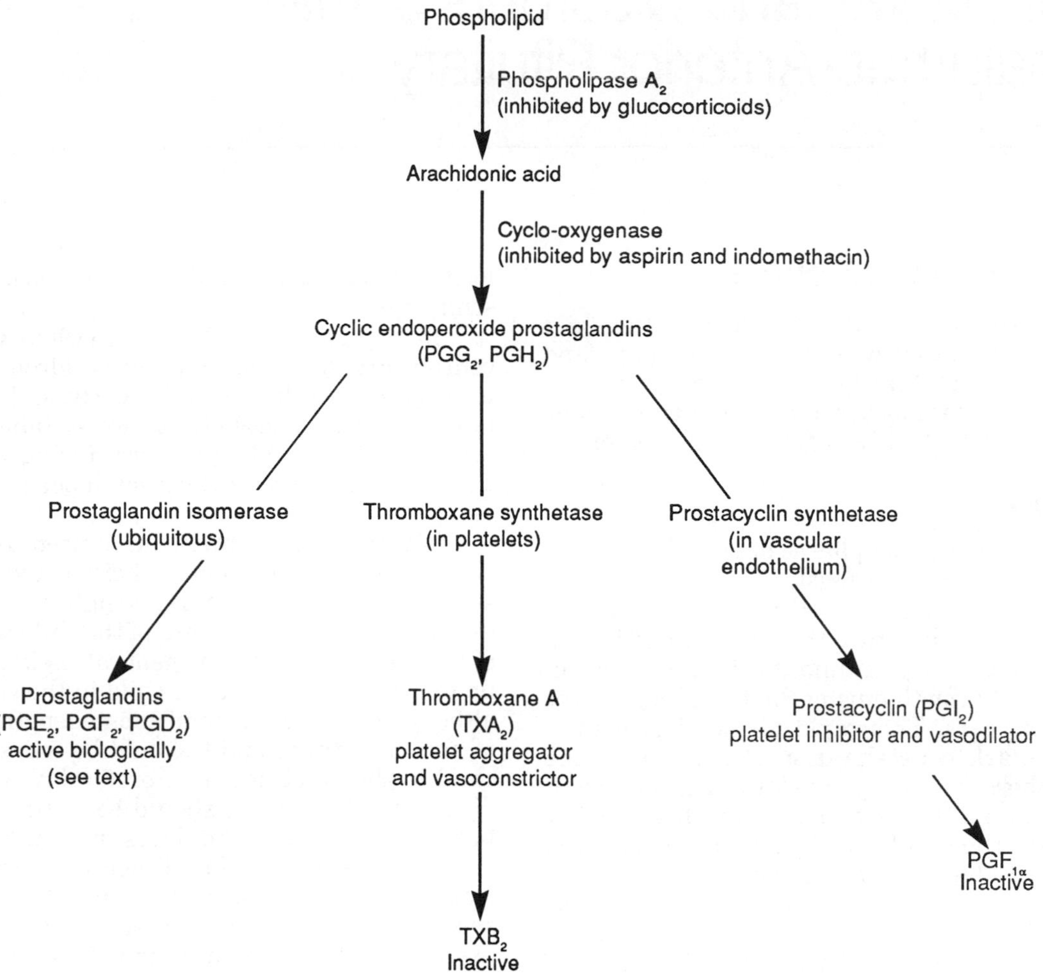

Figure 14.2. Biosynthesis of prostaglandins and thromboxanes.

there are many different kinds of hormones, the basic mechanism of action is via either membrane perturbation with transmission of signals which subsequently alter the form and activity of intracellular enzymes or via direct interaction with nuclear genetic material and subsequent increase in synthesis of specific mRNAs. By either metabolic or genetic means the target cell of the hormone is activated to perform a specific function, such as the secretion of a product. The specificity of the hormonal action resides in the specific receptors for that hormone which are located on the cell membrane or within the cell.

REFERENCES

Aurbach GD: Polypeptide and amine hormone regulation of adenylate cyclase. *Ann Rev Physiol* 44:653, 1982.

Csaba G: The present state in the phylogeny and ontogeny of hormone receptors. *Hormone Metab Res* 16:329, 1984.

Czech MP: New perspectives on the mechanism of insulin action. *Rec Progr Horm Res* 40:347, 1984.

Gilman AG: Guanine nucleotide-binding regulatory proteins and dual control of adenylate cyclase. *J Clin Invest* 73:1, 1984.

Guillemin R: The language of polypeptides and the wisdom of the body. *Physiologist* 28:391, 1985.

Hughes SM: Are guanine nucleotide binding proteins a distinct class of regulatory proteins? *FEBS Lett* 164:1, 1983.

Kaplan SA: Cell receptors. *Am J Dis Child* 138:1140, 1984.

Kelly PA, Djiane J, Katoh M, et al: The interaction of prolactin with its receptors in target tissues and its mechanism of action. *Rec Progr Horm Res* 40:379, 1984.

King WJ, Greene GL: Monoclonal antibodies localize oestrogen receptor in the nuclei of target cells. *Nature* 307:745, 1984.

Szego CM: Mechanisms of hormone action: Parallels in receptor-mediated signal propagation for steroid and peptide effectors. *Life Sci* 35:2383, 1984.

Welshons WV, Lieberman ME, Gorski J: Nuclear localization of unoccupied oestrogen receptors. *Nature* 307:747, 1984.

Normal Growth and Disorders of the Hypothalamus-Anterior Pituitary

2

NORMAL GROWTH

Growth represents the process whereby the child gets bigger in association with changes in shape and in body composition and in the distribution of various tisses. Different tissues mature at different rates; thus, the growth of a child is a highly complex series of changes.

Natural History

There are three distinct phases of growth. In utero and in infancy growth is very fast. For example, there is more than a doubling of birth weight and a 50% increase in birth length within the first year of life. In very small prematurely born infants there may be an accelerated rate of growth during the first 6 months or even for 1 or 2 years. This rapid phase of growth is followed by a marked deceleration of growth. In the second phase, there is a steady but slower rate of growth between ages 2 and 10 years, with a gradual further decline in rate in the prepubertal years. Finally, in the third or pubertal phase, growth is rapid.

One of the most vexing problems that pediatricians face is the child who is very short and may have a treatable disorder of growth. Therefore, a firm knowledge of normal growth is essential.

Diagnosis

Standardized growth curves are available for plotting heights and weights. The 50th centile at a given age is that height at which 50% of children fall above the curve and 50% below the curve. Of all children, 3% will fall below the third centile and another 3% will fall above the 97th centile.

Unfortunately, a given centile on the growth curves based upon cross-sectional data does not resemble the actual growth curve of any individual child. In other words, the practicing physician who is following the growth of a patient may find the growth points deviating from the norm and suspect an abnormality of growth that does not exist. One reason is that such data do not allow for individual differences in rate of maturation at adolescence. Longitudinal data can provide curves that will be followed more closely by normal individuals. The Bayer and Bayley growth curves are very helpful in this regard (see Fig. 14.5*A* and *B*). Growth data from an individual child will often fit the Bayer and Bailey curves better than those of the National Center. It is also helpful to use the incremental curve at the bottom of the Bayer and Bayley charts. In plotting yearly height velocity, increments should cover not less than 0.85 year and not more than 1.15 years. Velocities calculated over shorter periods may reflect seasonal effects.

In the Tanner and Davies (1985) growth charts, centiles are given not only for children growing at an average tempo, but also for early and late maturers (see Fig. 14.7). These charts are suitable for following an individual child's progress during observation or treatment throughout the growth period, including puberty.

Whatever the growth curve used by the pediatrician, serial measurement of height (two or more measurements 3 months apart), weight, and bone age are essential for the assessment of the child with a question of disordered growth. In general, height is measured up to 2 or 3 years with the child in the supine position, although many recommend supine lengths until 6 years of age. Standing height should be measured with the child in the erect position, preferably by use of a stadiometer. The patient should be in bare feet with the heels, buttocks, and shoulders in contact with the stadiometer. Heels are placed together with medial malleoli touching. Lordosis is reduced by relaxing the shoulders and applying pressure to the abdomen. The external auditory meatus and the outer angle of the eye should be horizontal. Variation among observers of measurements obtained in this fashion should be no more than 0.3 cm. Recumbent length is measured with the child lying on a meter stick mounted in a wood frame. A sliding wooden block is positioned at the top of the head with the feet resting on the bottom of the frame. The length is read off the meter stick at the position of the wooden block. Recumbent length is 1–2 cm greater than standing height.

Linear Growth

The peak velocity of growth in length is reached in midtrimester of gestation. From birth until age 4 or 5 years the rate of linear growth decelerates rapidly. Linear growth velocities, which are as high as 30 cm per year in the first 2 months of life, decline to one-third of this rate by 2 months of life and continue to decline thereafter (Tanner and Whitehouse, 1976). The decline becomes gradually less so that from age 5 or 6 years up to the beginning of the adolescent growth spurt the velocity of linear growth is practically constant (5–6 cm/yr).

The absolute height or centile of the growing child at any one time is less important than the pattern of growth. If the growth rate is below the norm for that age the child will progressively fall further below his centile. Height can also be evaluated by use of standard deviations (SDs) from the mean. A child should maintain the same SD from the mean unless there is a problem in growth or the tempo of growth has changed. At adrenarche and just before and during the adolescent growth spurt the rate of linear growth changes normally. Another period of change in rate of growth is the first year of life. The linear growth of about two-thirds of normal infants crosses centile lines during the first 12–18 months of life, the number shifting upward on the curve being roughly equal to the number shifting downward (Smith et al, 1976).

Genetic influences play an important role in stature. In assessing growth of the child, the parents' heights should be plotted on the right side of the growth chart (adult values). It is important to correct for the sex difference in height. Thus, when plotting the growth data of a boy the mother's height must be corrected by adding 13 cm to her adult height value before it is recorded on the boy's growth chart. On a girl's chart the father's height should have 13 cm subtracted. From the parents' heights (corrected appropriately), one can calculate the mean parental centile. Ninety-five percent (2 SD) of the population of children of given parents will be within centiles that are 10 cm on either side of the mean parental centile (Tanner and Davies, 1985).

Most body measurements follow approximately the growth curve for height. For example, most skeletal and muscular dimensions grow in this manner, as do internal organs such as liver, spleen and kidney. The exceptions are the brain and skull (rapid growth postnatally, levelling off around age 6 years), the reproductive organs, the lymphoid tissues (which reach the peak amount before adolescence and then decline), and subcutaneous fat.

Although there are differences in height between blacks and whites, for the American black and white populations these differences are considered inconsequential and a single growth curve can be used for both. The mean height and weight of Americans of Oriental extraction is less than those of whites and these differences may be clinically significant (Barr et al, 1972). There are definite racial differences in body proportions.

Seasonal variation in linear growth may occur. Children may grow faster in height in spring and summer than in autumn and winter.

Irrespective of where the child's height is found to plot on the growth curve, if the increment in growth over the recent 6–12 months is normal it is most unlikely that an active disorder impairing growth exists in the individual. Therefore, it is the rate at which a child grows that is important in growth assessment. Generally, measurement should be made over a period of a year with values at 3-monthly intervals.

Weight

In much the same fashion as linear growth is followed, a child's weight should be measured and plotted on standard weight charts. The first peak velocity in weight is shortly before, or at, birth. This is followed by a gradual decrease of velocity during the long interval between weaning and puberty.

Weight changes are important as an index in acute illness or starvation, but in chronic growth disorders height is a better index. Because it is easy to measure, weight has come to have disproportionate importance in growth disorders. Nevertheless, it represents the sum of many different tissues and, thus, it is harder to interpret a weight chart than a height one. In general, weight should be interpreted in relationship to height rather than to chronological age. A child who is 2 SD below the mean in weight has an appropriate weight if that child is 2 SD below the mean for height also. Another way of expressing comparisons of height and weight is to use height ages and weight ages. A child whose height and weight values are on the 50th centile has a height age and weight age equal to his chronological age. If the values lie above or below the 50th centile curve, the height age and weight age can be determined by drawing a horizontal line from the growth point to the 50th centile line and reading off the corresponding age. Most patients with endocrine disorders of growth have a normal or above normal weight for height. When the weight is considerably less than that appropriate for the height, attention should be directed toward the detection of malabsorption syndromes and systemic illnesses.

The use of height ages and weight ages is subject to limitations. For example, a normal child growing along the third centile will by definition have a delayed height age for chronologic age. If the height age is compared to the bone age, however, the normal child will be found to have an appropriate height for bone maturation. Thus, height age can be a useful concept for comparisons with bone age, but otherwise has limited value. Weight age also can be less helpful than defining how overweight or underweight the child is for height by use of SDs for each age.

Osseous Development

The major factor contributing to growth is the lengthening of the skeleton. Measurement of epiphyseal center development or bone age has great value in assessing growth disorders. In principle, any part of the skeleton could be used, but, in practice, the hand and wrist form the most convenient area. Using the radiographs of 100 normal children, Greulick and Pyle compiled the Radiographic Atlas of Skeletal Development of the Hand and Wrist, published in 1959 by the Stanford University Press. The standard hand films of males differ from those of females, especially in the adolescent years. From comparisons with standard films an evaluation of bone maturity can be made. The hand and wrist provide useful information only from about 18 months onward, so other parts of the skeleton (legs and feet) have to be used from birth to about 18 months.

Another index of osseous maturity is the age of eruption of teeth. Deciduous dentition erupts at 6 months to 2 years. Permanent dentition appears at about 6–13 years. Skeletal maturity and dental maturity, however, are not closely related. Each system seems to measure separate kinds of maturation.

A strong positive correlation exists between bone age and percentage of mature height achieved at any age. Children of a given height with the least advanced bone age tend to become taller adults than those whose skeletal development is more mature.

Several tables exist for predicting adult height from a comparison of height and bone age (Zachmann et al, 1978), but for several reasons such predictions are only rough estimates. First it is difficult to interpret the bone age, even for experienced observers. For example, there may be discrepancies of maturation between different epiphyseal centers and often the development of the carpal bones does not correlate well with that of the phalanges. Tanner has introduced a system whereby the observer compares each bone individually with standard radiographs of normal children (Tanner et al, 1975). Each of several bones is given a maturity score and the final bone age represents a summation of individual scores. The method allows for discrepancies in the degree of maturation of various epiphyseal centers. If properly used, this method reduces the error of bone age measurement considerably. Another source of error in predicting adult height is the discordance between skeletal maturation and growth which is likely to occur in children with sexual precocity. In general, it is safest to plot the child's height and extrapolate the value horizontally to the age on the growth chart that is equal to the bone age. If this extrapolated point falls between the 5th and 95th centiles, then a guarded prediction of adult stature can be given. The closer the point is to the 50th centile the more likely the predicted height will be achieved. It should be remembered that height prediction is often inaccurate in children with pathological growth patterns.

The correlation of length at birth with adult height is only about 0.3 since size at birth reflects uterine conditions much more than fetal genotype. Postnatally the correlation coefficients between height at a given age and adult height rise steeply and by age 3 years they are about 0.8. Therefore adult height can be predicted from height at age 3 years with an error which may amount to as much as 8 cm either way. At puberty the correlations diminish because some children mature early and some late. If bone age is taken into account the correlation is improved.

ROLE OF HORMONES IN NORMAL GROWTH

Basic Science

Most of the hormones involved in growth (GH, thyroid hormone, glucocorticoids, sex hormones, and somatomedins) are partially or completely regulated by the secretions of the hypothalamus (Fig. 14.3). Releasing or inhibiting factors synthesized in the hypothalamic neurons are secreted in pulses into the median eminence from whence they are carried by the pituitary portal system to the cells of the anterior pituitary. The factors involved in controlling pituitary synthesis and secretion of GH (GHRH, somatostatin (St)), TSH (TRH), ACTH (CRH), and sex hormones (GnRH) have been isolated, purified, and their structures have been determined. St, TRH, and GnRH are available for clinical studies. CRH and GHRH are currently available only in research centers. All are small peptides that can be synthesized with relative ease.

Once the appropriate releasing factor binds to the receptor on its pituitary target cell, hormonal activation of adenylate cyclase occurs and a chain of cellular events is started that results in the biosynthesis and release of pituitary hormones. The inhibiting factors, St and dopamine, inhibit the release of the appropriate pituitary hormones (GH, prolactin).

These pituitary trophic hormones act on their respective target tissues to cause synthesis and release of the final hormone: Somatomedin C (SmC), GH, thyroid hormones (TSH), glucocorticoids (ACTH), and sex hormones (LH, FSH).

The final hormone products exert a negative feedback effect on the hypothalamus and/or pituitary gland, thus controlling formation of the releasing factors and the pituitary tropic hormones.

Growth Hormone

GH is necessary for normal growth from birth to adulthood. Although GH is produced in the fetal pituitary and the blood levels of GH rise with the growth of the fetus, there is no evidence that this hormone is necessary for fetal growth. Anencephalic babies born without a pituitary gland and babies subsequently shown to be deficient in GH are normal in size at birth. There is a correlation between neonatal serum SmC levels and birth weight, birth length, and placental weight (D'Ercole and Underwood, 1981). Thus, GH or GH-like peptides such as prolactin or human placental lactogen (hPL) may stimulate the synthesis of Sm and play an indirect role in fetal growth. In the human fetus SmC in serum rises progressively during pregnancy and the values correlate directly with maternal levels of hPL.

Children who lack GH grow at a much slower rate and achieve an adult height of about 130 cm, but with normal proportions. GH is species-specific and only human GH is active in promoting growth in GH-deficient children. Besides its effect on linear growth, GH is required for growth of bone mass, for skeletal maturation, and probably is needed for replication of muscle and adipose tissue cells. It also has a lipolytic action.

GH is a potent anabolic agent promoting increase in growth of virtually all tissues of the body. Many of its effects are mediated by various growth factors called Sms. For example, when GH is administered to GH-deficient animals in vivo, it enhances incorporation of precursors (sulfate and thymidine) into cartilage. This effect could not be demonstrated in vitro; therefore, it was proposed that GH does not act directly on target tissues, but rather via Sms. Recent studies suggest that GH can act directly on bone explants in vitro causing

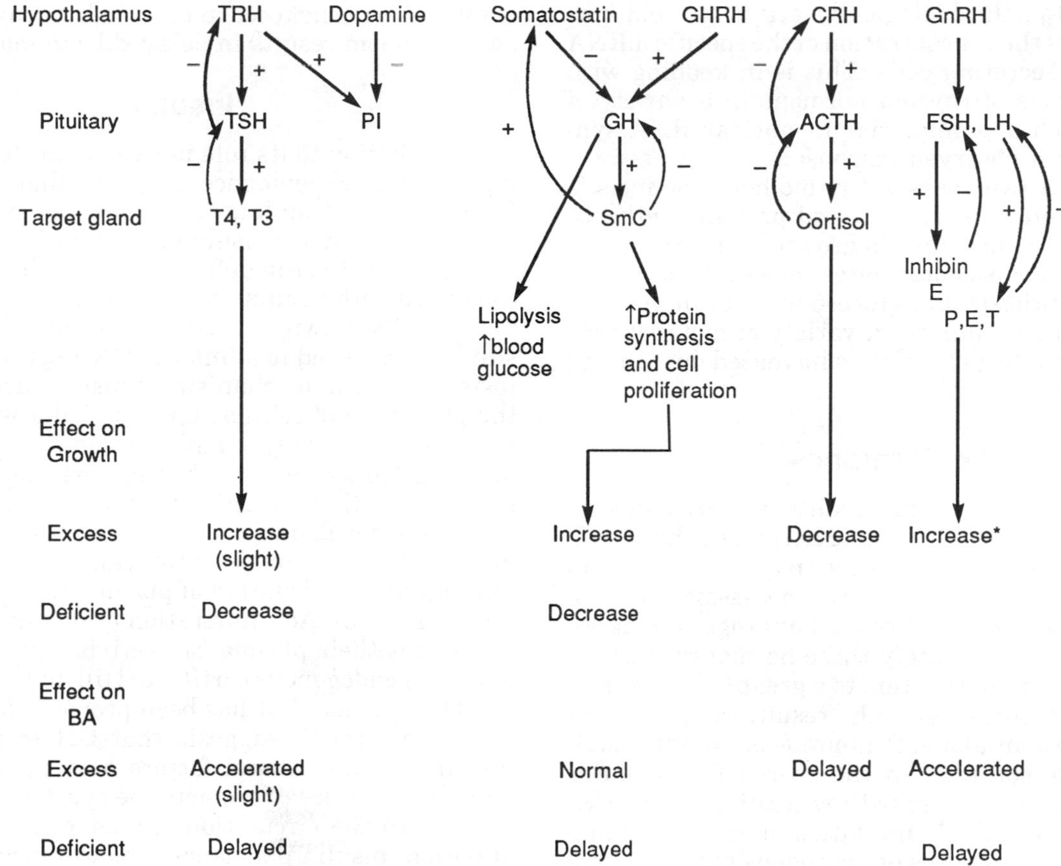

Figure 14.3. Hypothalamic factors act positively or negatively upon the anterior pituitary to regulate the synthesis and release of trophic hormones. The latter act upon target tissues to produce hormones which alter growth and bone materation. The specific affect depends upon whether the hormones are present in excessive or deficient amounts. Positive (+) and negative (−) feedback exists in these systems. Abbreviations: E = estrogen, P = progesterone, T = testosterone. *Accompanied by accelerated bone maturation resulting in compromised adult height.

an increase in the synthesis and secretion of Sm into the media of the explants (Stracke et al, 1984). The terms Sm and insulin-like growth factor (IGF) are now used as synonyms for the same class of growth-promoting polypeptides. Human serum contains two main types of IGF: IGFI, which is identical to SmC (Klapper et al, 1983) and IGFII, a slightly different molecule. The three-dimensional structures of IGFI, IGFII, and insulin are essentially identical. Their biological responses are mediated by interaction with the insulin receptor or with specific IGF receptors, depending on the tissue.

Unlike insulin, the IGFs are tightly bound to carrier proteins in the serum. Thus, clinical measurements of Sm levels remain remarkably stable because of the long biologic half-life in the presence of carrier proteins. No obvious diurnal rhythm has been observed. Overnight fasting does not alter values significantly. IGFI-related peptides reach a peak during puberty and fall during old age.

It is well established that production of IGFI-related peptides is regulated by GH; the tropic hormone for the IGFII peptides is as yet unknown. The biologic effects of GH can be divided into those mediated via Sm production and those that are direct and can be demonstrated in vitro. Among the latter is the GH-stimulated amino acid uptake and protein synthesis in liver and muscle.

In addition to the Sms (or IGF peptides) many other growth factors are present in tissues and blood. Factors such as epidermal growth factor, erythropoietin, nerve growth factor, platelet-derived growth factor, and fibroblast pneumocyte factor are all involved in growth of one or more tissues and all are influenced by one or another of the classical hormones.

Thyroid Hormone

Thyroid hormones do not appear to play any significant role in the growth of the human fetus; however, they are essential for protein synthesis in the brain and for the proper development of nerve cells as well as for normal osseous development. Children who have postnatal thyroid deficiency show increasingly slow body growth and delayed skeletal and dental maturation. Severe hypothyroidism results in nearly complete growth arrest.

Thyroid hormone itself enhances protein synthesis and also influences growth at the pituitary level by regulating the synthesis and secretion of GH. Triiodothyronine (T_3), the biologically active thyroid hormone, increases the concentration of the specific mRNA for GH in GH-secreting cells. This is in keeping with the known effects of thyroid hormone in a variety of tissues in which a prompt rise in nuclear RNA synthesis is the first observed response.

The cellular responses to thyroid hormone include increased oxygen consumption and protein synthesis, both of which are important in growth of the organism. Thyroid hormone also potentiates the effects of insulin on glycogen synthesis and glucose uptake. In general, thyroid hormone stimulates a variety of metabolic reactions, the net effect of which is increased growth and development of the organism.

Sex Hormones

Testosterone and its metabolite dihydrotestosterone (DHT) are powerful anabolic hormones that accelerate linear growth and weight gain and increase lean muscle mass. The presence of GH is necessary for these effects. There is also evidence that androgens enhance GH secretion. Unfortunately these hormones increase the rate of skeletal maturation to a greater degree than they accelerate linear growth, resulting in compromised growth potential and diminution of eventual adult stature. Efforts continue in the search for synthetic androgens that promote growth without producing virilization and excessive stimulation of epiphyseal maturation. Very small doses of androgens may be useful for stimulating growth in girls with Turner syndrome (pp. 882).

Estrogens in physiologic amounts stimulate growth and epiphyseal maturation, but most evidence suggests that their pharmacologic effect on somatic growth is inhibitory. The growth spurt seen in girls at puberty may be due in part to androgens released by the adrenal and ovary. Estrogens increase basal plasma GH levels and enhance the GH responses to provocative stimuli. Recent studies on patients with Turner syndrome suggest that very low doses of estrogen may stimulate growth, whereas large doses are inhibitory (pp. 884). Certainly administration of pharmacologic doses of estrogen to excessively tall girls leads to attenuation of their growth rates, rapid acceleration of epiphyseal maturation and fusion, and a decrease in their predicted adult stature (pp. 816).

Glucocorticoids

Glucocorticoids are very effective inhibitors of growth in the immature organism. It takes only 2 or 3 times the average daily secretion of cortisol to arrest growth; only severe hypothyroidism can bring about a comparable growth arrest. GH administered in conjunction with glucocorticoid will not reverse the growth retardation. These effects are not limited to the skeleton, for glucocorticoids inhibit thymidine incorporation into DNA in a variety of tissues. With restoration of normal hormonal balance, catch-up growth will occur, providing that sexual maturation and fusion of the epiphyses have not occurred. As in hypothyroidism, hypercortisolism results in delayed bone maturation.

Insulin

In addition to its role in carbohydrate metabolism (pp. 894) much evidence suggests that insulin may function as a stimulator of growth, as exemplified by the oversized hyperinsulinemic infant born to a diabetic mother. Insulin deficiency or insulin resistance is associated with intrauterine growth failure (Hill, 1978).

In cells grown in vitro high concentrations of insulin are required to stimulate DNA synthesis and mitosis. The basic mechanism of insulin action, that is, the promotion of cellular uptake of glucose and amino acids (pp. 894) may simply provide the energy and building blocks for growth, thus making insulin promote rather than directly stimulate growth.

In the developing fetus insulin may play a role via Sms. Pig fetuses made chronically hyperinsulinemic had significant elevation of plasma Sm activity (Spencer et al, 1983). Administration of insulin to fetal rabbits raises their plasma Sm activity, as well as their growth of endogenous cartilage (Hill and Milner, 1980).

One scheme that has been proposed for the role of insulin in growth suggests that GH in concert with insulin and nutritional factors acts on the liver and other body tissues to promote the synthesis and release of Sm into the circulation. Under conditions of malnutrition, insulin deficiency, and/or glucocorticoid excess, the liver appears to release reduced levels of Sm and increased levels of Sm inhibitors. Therefore, if cells are malnourished and insulin-deficient, growth may be poor despite normal or elevated levels of GH.

SHORT STATURE

Definition

Children whose heights lie below the third centile are arbitrarily considered to have short stature. Any child who is growing at a subnormal rate for age, whatever centile he may occupy, requires investigation.

Diagnosis

Most children who are seen by the pediatrician for short stature are perfectly normal and comprise the 3% of children whose stature lies below the third centile. If the child is within normal limits for his parents, he is probably normal, unless one or the other of his parents has a growth disorder. Ideally both parents' heights should be measured also since their estimates of heights are notoriously inaccurate.

The differential diagnosis of short stature is considered based on the scheme represented in Figure 14.4. From that figure, it is clear that the first differential requirement is to distinguish those children who are disproportionately short from those who are short but have normal proportions. It is extremely important to have accurate ratios of upper to lower body segments of the child, which involves measuring either a sitting

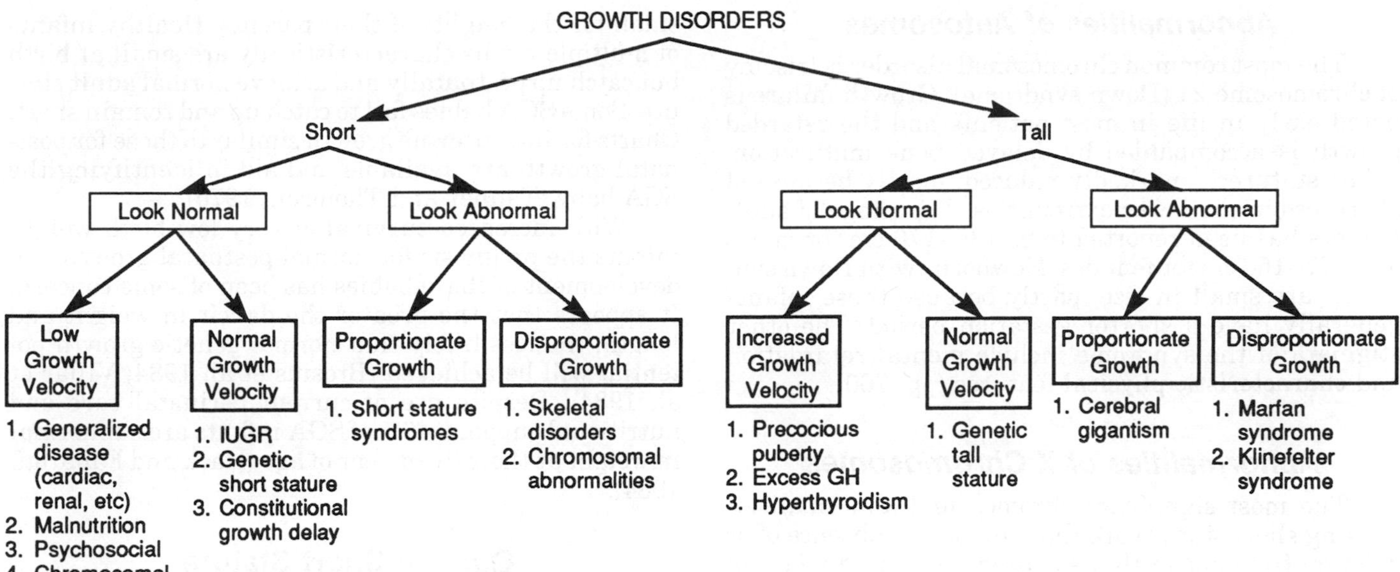

Figure 14.4. Differential diagnosis of growth disorders.

height and subtracting that value from the total for the lower measure, or measuring accurately the distance from the top of the symphysis pubis to the base of the feet and subtracting this lower value from the total height to obtain the upper segment length. In addition, the distance between finger tips of the laterally extended arms should be measured (arm span).

PRIMARY DISORDERS OF GROWTH

In general, these disturbances begin before birth and are readily discernible in the newborn infant. They can be considered under the headings of skeletal disorders, chromosomal disorders, intrauterine growth retardation, genetic short stature, and finally, a miscellaneous group of short stature syndromes.

Skeletal Disorders

Definition

Children born with skeletal disorders associated with short stature have disporportionate growth of bones. The classical disproportionate child is the achondroplastic dwarf.

Basic Science

This disorder is due to the mutation of a single gene and is inherited as an autosomal dominant. Most cases, however, are the result of a new mutation without prior family history of the disorder. Apparently the gene is particularly unstable and subject to mutation. Hypochondroplasia is also inherited as a dominant gene.

Natural History

Children and adults with achondroplasia have short upper arms and thighs, a normal length back, a large head and a characteristic face with depressed nasal bridge, a small nose, and a large forehead. Their muscles are well developed. They have normal intelligence and health.

Hypochondroplasia resembles a milder form of achondroplasia, but the two disorders are different and do not occur in the same family. In this condition, only the limbs are short and the shortened legs are responsible for the short stature. The face is normal so that hypochondroplasiacs often pass as very short normals. In both achondroplasia and hypochondroplasia bony changes are seen on radiographs, but the findings in achondroplasia are much more marked and characteristic.

Some disorders of metabolism produce skeletal abnormalities and short stature. For example, the mucopolysaccharidoses are characterized by diffuse involvement of the skeletal system including the epiphyses, the metaphyses, and the diaphyses and many are associated with abnormalities of bone growth. Abnormalities of trunk growth in Morquio disease lead to severe kyphosis and scoliosis.

It is impossible to discuss all the skeletal dysplasias (which number well over 50), but the pediatrician must consider them in the differential diagnosis of the disproportionately short child (Beighton, 1978). Careful review of bone films by the radiologist is essential in diagnosing these rare conditions.

Chromosomal Abnormalities

In general, the growth in patients with certain chromosomal abnormalities is retarded but the bodily proportions may be normal or only mildly disproportionate. Careful measurements to detect disproportions are often necessary, but physical stigmata are frequently present and make the diagnosis relatively easy.

Abnormalities of Autosomes

The most common chromosomal disorder is trisomy of chromosome 21 (Down syndrome). Growth failure is noted early in life in most patients and the retarded growth is accompanied by delayed bone maturation. Adult stature is markedly reduced, mostly because of shortness in the lower extremities. The range of adult heights has been reported to be 135–170 cm for males and 127–158 cm for females. Newborns with Down syndrome are small in size, partly because these infants generally have a shorter gestation period. The other stigmata of the syndrome include mental retardation and characteristic physical features (pp. 760).

Abnormalities of X Chromosomes

The most significant chromosomal abnormalities causing short stature are those involving absence of or deletion from one of the sex chromosomes. The lack of the second X chromosome produces Turner syndrome (pp. 882). The phenotype of the Turner patient is female and it behooves the practicing pediatrician to consider this diagnosis in any girl with growth retardation. The patient may have none, some, or all of the stigmata of Turner; therefore, a karyotype should be obtained in all short girls with retarded growth rate.

In many cases, the only sign of Turner syndrome is slow growth. Girls with this syndrome frequently have abnormally short limbs and a high upper to lower segment ratio. They fail to undergo the adolescent growth spurt and frequently exhibit progressive slowing of their growth.

The most common variants of Turner syndrome presenting with few somatic stigmata other than short stature are isochrome abnormalities involving the long arm of the X chromosome, deletions of a portion of the X chromosome, or mosaic patterns.

Klinefelter syndrome (XXY) is another common chromosomal anomaly, but growth is generally excessive. This syndrome is discussed in detail elsewhere (pp. 878).

Intrauterine Growth Retardation (IUGR)

Infants born after a normal gestational period with a birth weight of less than 2000 g or those born before term whose size is small for gestational age (SGA) belong in this category of growth disorders. The causes of fetal growth retardation (see also pp. 160) are many and include factors peculiar to the fetus (chromosomal and genetic abnormalities, congenital infections, and congenital anomalies), to the placenta (abnormal implantation, vascular malformations or disease), and to the mother (malnutrition, toxemia, severe diabetes mellitus, drugs, uterine malformations).

The baby who is SGA is below the centile limits for weight at that particular gestational age. The majority of these children, especially those born at term, develop within the normal centiles, although they do not fulfill their genetic potential and appear somewhat small for the heights of their parents. Healthy infants of multiple births characteristically are small at birth but catch up postnatally and achieve normal adult stature. Some SGA babies fail to catch up and remain short. Charts for intrauterine growth similar to those for postnatal growth are available and aid in identifying the SGA baby (Tanner and Thomson, 1970).

With increased survival of very low birth weight infants the prognosis for normal postnatal growth and development of these babies has been of some concern. It appears that the greater the deficit in weight and length, the less likely that normal genetic growth potential will be achieved (Brosius et al, 1984; Villar et al, 1984). Despite use of current perinatal care and nutritional support, 46% of SGA infants are subnormal in weight at their third year of age (Hack and Fanaroff, 1984).

Genetic Short Stature

Basic Science

The inheritance of growth potential is multifactorial. Unfortunately, in the past, the diagnosis of genetic or familial short stature was made when the pediatrician was confronted with a short child of short parents and did not pay careful attention to the possibility that the parents might have a genetic disorder of growth (Fig. 14.5*A* and *B*. With more accurate hormone assays now available it is becoming evident that many cases of so-called genetic short stature represent disorders of synthesis of biologically active GH and the Sms. For example, the striking short stature seen among the African pygmies has been recently investigated. Results show that the pygmies represent an example of a selective Sm deficiency. Serum levels of radioimmunoassayable IGFI levels are low, whereas IGFII values are normal (Merimee et al, 1981). Although they are small, pygmies do not have the characteristic appearance found in GH deficiency. Their maturation occurs at the normal rate and their GH levels are normal. Therefore, a selective IGFI deficiency is characterized by inhibition of skeletal growth only.

With respect to height, each parent usually contributes equally to each offspring. The union of Bantus of normal height and pygmies tends to produce individuals of intermediate height (Tanner, 1978). In other parts of the world similar results are often found: one tall and one short parent tend to have a child of intermediate height.

Since growth is modulated by hormones and environmental factors, very short families should receive an appropriate investigation of these modulators. The designation of genetic short stature should be reserved for those individuals in whom all other causes of growth retardation have been excluded. When such a diagnosis is made the question of GH therapy is usually raised. Several recent studies have shown that healthy short children with normal GH secretion responded to exogenous GH with increased rate of linear growth (Gertner et al, 1984). At present, the policy is to reserve

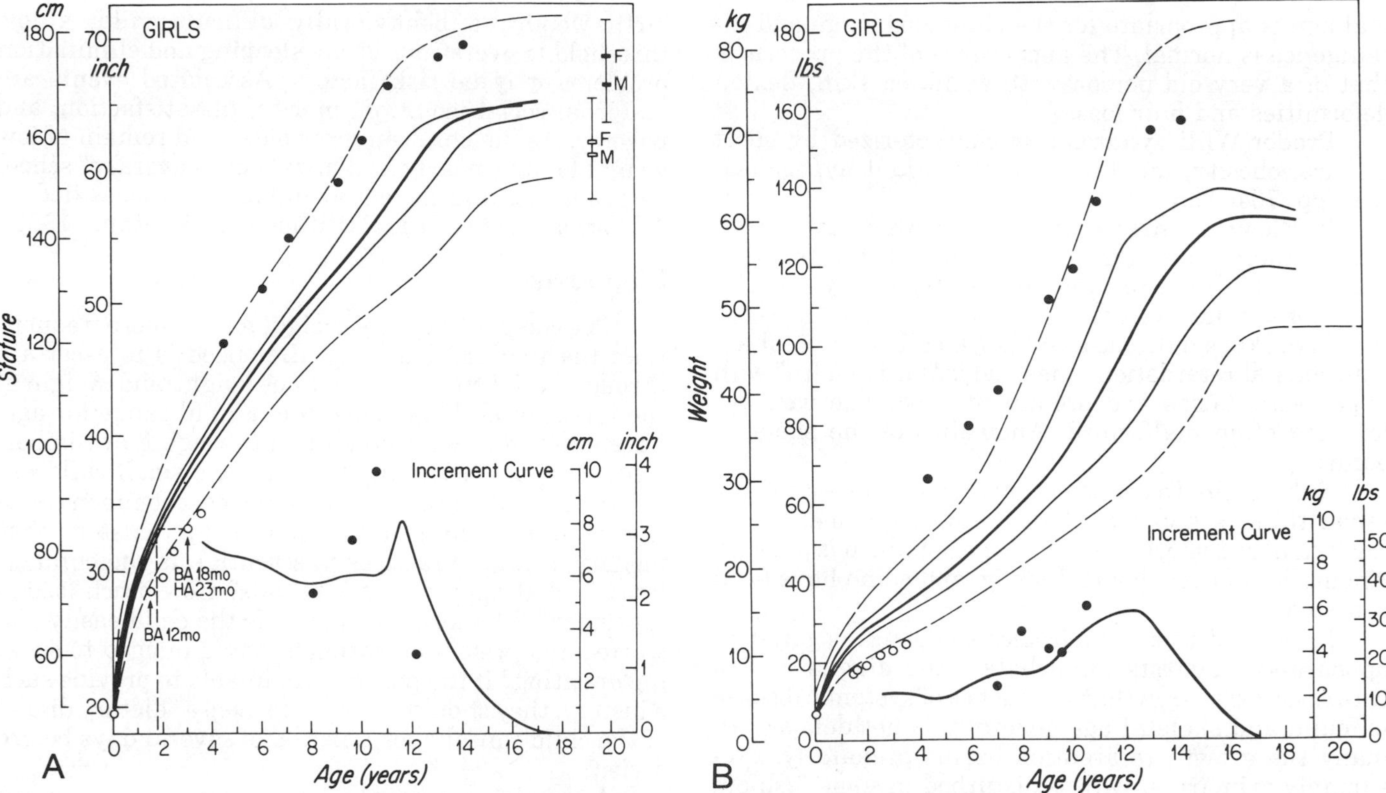

Figure 14.5A and B. Genetic patterns of growth. Growth in height **(A)** and weight **(B)** of a patient with genetic short stature *(open circles)* and of a patient with genetic tall stature *(closed circles)* plotted on Bayer and Bayley growth charts. The *dashed lines* of the growth chart represent the smallest and the tallest girls in the study.

The growth points of the genetically short and tall girls adhere to the appropriate longitudinal centile lines. The increment curve for height shows an earlier growth spurt for the tall girl than is seen in girls of average height. Accelerated weight gain occurred at adrenarche (age 8 years) and with the pubertal growth spurt in this girl. Parental heights are plotted to the right of the height curve and the bars represent 2 SD above and below mean parental heights. In each case the father's height has been corrected for the female growth chart.

As expected, the genetically small girl had a BA (12 months) much closer to her height age (23 months) than to her chronologic age (39 months). Her growth would be expected to follow her present centile line, giving her an adult height appropriate for her genetic potential.

human GH for those children demonstrated to lack biologically active GH (see Controversy, pp. 814).

Miscellaneous Short Stature Syndromes

Several short stature syndromes have been described that are of unknown etiology and classical phenotype. They are rare and there is no known effective therapy for their poor growth. One, Noonan syndrome, has a phenotype like that of Turner syndrome except that it is seen more often in males than females. These patients have a normal karyotype, short stature, and physical findings such as low set ears and low hair line, webbing of the neck, skeletal abnormalities, small penis and cyryptorchidism. Mental retardation is present in about half. Congenital heart lesions may be present on the right side in contrast to the left-sided heart defects in Turner syndrome.

The Russell-Silver syndrome is characterized by intrauterine growth retardation, triangular shaped face, frontal bossing, craniofacial dysostosis, and disproportionately short limbs. There is often asymmetry involving various parts of the body, clinodactyly, cafe-au-lait areas of the skin, and syndactyly of the toes. Pubertal development may be early. Other features of the syndrome include: mental retardation, dislocation of the hips, radius, and the ulna, hypoglycemia, renal anomalies and hypospadias. Patients who have these findings are probably a heterogeneous group. Some achieve normal adult height; others remain small. Some have normal psychomotor development; others are delayed (Saal et al, 1985).

Progeria is extremely rare, with an estimated incidence of 1 in 8 million live births. The child may appear normal at birth but by 6 months to 1 year a progressive loss of hair and subcutaneous fat occurs. Growth in height and weight decrease and the final height is that of a 5-year-old and the weight is that of a 3-year-old. Rapidly progressing atherosclerosis of the coronary arteries, aorta, and other large vessels brings about death in the teens, usually of coronary artery disease with myocardial infarction and fibrosis. Skeletal age is appropriate for the chronologic age and intelligence is normal. The appearance of the progeric is that of a very old person with wrinkled skin, flexion deformities and hair loss.

Prader-Willi syndrome is characterized by short stature, obesity, mental retardation, and hypogonadism (pp. 764–765).

In Bloom syndrome there is growth delay and facial erythema. Intelligence is normal. There is a tendency for development of malignancy of the lymphoreticular system.

In Seckel syndrome there is typically microcephaly with mental retardation. The head is "bird-headed" with hypoplastic facies and prominent nose. The ears are low and often malformed. Anomalies of the skeleton occur.

Rubinstein-Taybi syndrome is characterized by broad thumbs and toes, facial anomalies, mental retardation, and short stature. Cryptorchidism is present. Anomalies of eyes, heart, kidney, and spine have been reported.

In each of these syndromes the striking physical appearance suggests immediately the diagnosis of a rare disorder of growth. No evidence of systemic disease is found and skeletal age generally is not delayed. In many the growth retardation begins prenatally. Presumably primary growth is disturbed in some fashion, generating dysmorphic features as well as stunted growth. There is no known therapy for these conditions.

It is impossible to discuss all of the short stature syndromes; however, a book such as David Smith's *Recognizable Patterns of Human Malformation*, (2nd edition, Philadelphia, W.B. Saunders, 1976) can be very helpful in sorting out the features of a given patient.

SECONDARY DISORDERS OF GROWTH: NONENDOCRINE

Approach to "Failure-to-Thrive"

Definition

"Failure-to-thrive" is a term frequently used to describe infants or young children whose weights are persistently below the third percentile for age on standardized growth charts. The phrase "failure to gain weight" appropriately would be more descriptive. Nonorganic failure-to-thrive has been described as "a disease stemming from a distortion in the reciprocal interaction of infant with caregivers" (Rosenn et al, 1980).

Epidemiology

The label failure-to-thrive is currently given to 3–5% of infants under age 1 year admitted to the hospital (Mitchell et al, 1980). About 70–80% of cases stem from nonorganic etiology (Homer and Ludwig, 1981).

Natural History

Recognition of risk factors is essential to alert the physician to the possibility of poor weight gain. Low birth weight, a behaviorally difficult child, a low threshold to overstimulation, sleeping and elimination problems may be risk factors. Associated events are maternal social isolation, marital dissatisfaction, and poverty. As the children grow older and remain of low weight for age, nearly half have "below average" school performance, and an equal number are classified as "abnormal personalities" (Bithoney and Ratbun, 1983).

Diagnosis

The complaint of poor weight gain is more frequent than the finding. Thus, the first need is to ascertain through serial measurements of height and weight if the infant or child is below the normal range for age. Parental and sibling heights and weights are important, since small parents tend to have small children

Since inadequate intake is the most common cause of poor weight gain, a complete dietary history that includes feeding practices is essential. Is the child offered food at appropriate intervals? How much food is consumed? Who feeds the child? Is the child easily distracted and prefers attention or being hugged to sucking or eating? If the parents are unable to provide such a history, they should be asked to keep a "dietary diary" of the child's intake for a period of several days before a visit.

A complete medical history is also needed to assess possible dysfunction in any organ system. Only after a full history including consideration of feeding practices are laboratory tests in order.

Baseline laboratory tests include CBC, urine, and examination of stools (for evidence of infection or malabsorption). In some settings, a blood lead level, tuberculin test, or sweat test may be appropriate.

Treatment

Regardless of etiology, the best treatment is early recognition and mobilization of appropriate resources (be they medical, social, nutritional, or psychologic) for parental support. Clearly, medical problems should be addressed. Cognitive stimulation and optimal nutritional intake can reverse the problem, or at least significantly help. If inadequate intake is diagnosed, frequent weight checks to ensure maintenance of adequate calories and to lend support to the family can be useful.

Indications for hospitalization include: (1) Severe malnutrition or dehydration; (2) failure of outpatient management; (3) evidence of child abuse or neglect; or (4) extreme parental anxiety that requires time to permit a constructive physician-parent-child relationship (Bithoney and Rathbun, 1983).

The following sections focus in more detail on some of the organic disorders that may be associated with growth delay.

Malnutrition

Malnutrition (see Section 3) is by far the most common cause of growth failure throughout the world. Even in developed countries the economically deprived may have undernutrition of a sufficient degree to interfere with normal growth. In marasmus, the intake of both calories and protein is insufficient, resulting in loss of subcutaneous fat and muscle wasting. In kwashiorkor, caloric intake may be close to normal but the quantity and quality of dietary protein is inadequate. Permanent stunting of growth occurs in children with severe malnutrition.

Full-blown marasmus and kwashiorkor are relatively easy to diagnose. The diagnosis of modest nutritional deficiency is more difficult. Such a diagnosis is important, however, since restoration of normal caloric and protein intake can result in catch-up growth unless undernutrition has been prolonged or has occurred very early in life. There are two ways in which catch-up growth can occur. In one form of catch-up the velocity of growth increases to such an extent that the original growth curve is attained and thereafter growth proceeds normally. In the second form of catch-up the growth velocity is increased but not to a sufficient degree to attain the original growth curve. Sexual maturation is delayed, however, and growth continues for a longer time so that in the end catch-up is achieved. There may be a mix of these two responses in the calorically deprived child after restored nutritional intake. In malnourished children the serum levels of GH may be elevated, but the serum Sm concentrations are low.

Recent studies have shown that growth retardation may be associated with deficiencies of specific dietary components, such as zinc and iron. Zinc deficiency in the United States seems confined to individuals with absorptive disturbances or those sustained by parenteral nutrition containing inadequate amounts of zinc. Zinc deficiency is a very unlikely cause of growth failure in the otherwise healthy individual. Iron deficiency is discussed (on page 104).

Gastrointestinal Disorders

Disorders of the gastrointestinal tract associated with malabsorption often cause impairment of growth, as exemplified by celiac disease (gluten enteropathy). Although symptoms such as diarrhea and abdominal distention are associated with this disorder, an occasional patient will present with few if any gastrointestinal symptoms. Growth failure may be the presenting complaint (Fig. 14.6). Indeed, in patients for whom there is no explanation for growth failure, jejunal biopsy should be considered even though there is no clinical evidence for celiac disease. Children with celiac disease have normal GH responses to provocative stimuli but low Sm activity in serum. The fact that Sm does not rise with GH administration in these patients but does increase with gluten-free diet suggests that the GH resistance is on the basis of malabsorption secondary to the celiac disease. Children with Crohn disease (regional enteritis) may suffer marked growth delay for months or years before typical symptoms such as diarrhea occur. Studies of the diets of children with chronic

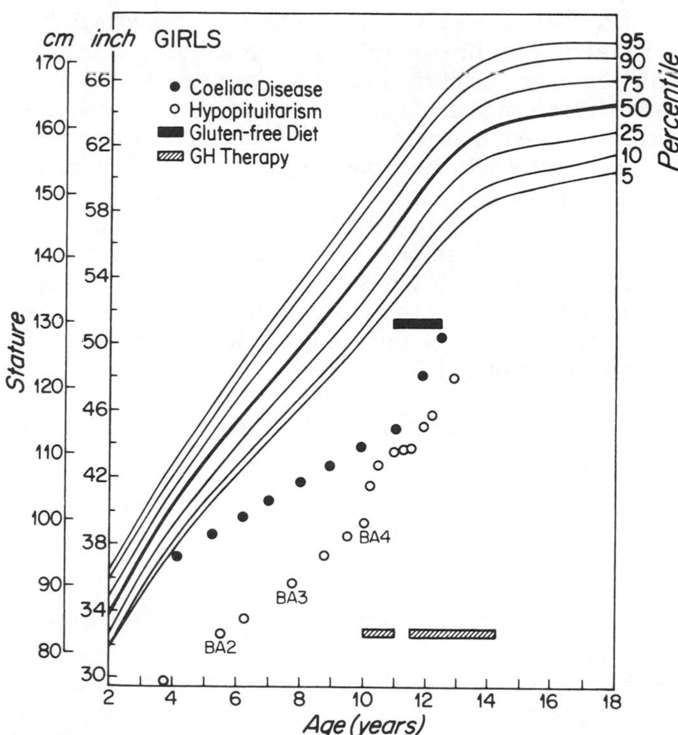

Figure 14.6. Linear growth of a patient with hypopituitarism (see case illustration) and of a patient with celiac disease. The latter had no gastrointestinal symptoms and was seen only for growth failure. On a gluten-free diet her linear growth rate accelerated and her weight which had been low prior to the diet increased.

inflammatory bowel disease show that these children have a low caloric intake and are in negative nitrogen and caloric balance.

Gastrointestinal involvement in patients with cystic fibrosis can cause impairment of growth, and the growth failure may be the most prominent manifestation of the disease.

Chronic Renal Disease

Disorders of the kidney that bring about chronic renal insufficiency can cause profound growth failure (see pp. 642). Clinical signs and symptoms may be minimal in the early stages, so that all short patients in whom growth failure is unexplained should have renal function evaluated.

Among the causes of the growth failure in renal disease are several severe biochemical disturbances such as acidosis, disturbances of body fluid tonicity, hyperphosphatemia, hypocalcemia, impaired synthesis of 1,25-dihydroxyvitamin D, anemia, and hypertension. Any and all of these disturbances as well as reduced intake of protein and calories may contribute to impaired growth. In general, growth failure from renal disease is most evident in infancy and early childhood.

Studies of the hormonal aspects of growth failure in renal disease have established certain relationships.

Studies of the hormonal aspects of growth failure in renal disease have established certain relationships. Thus, insulin resistance is present in uremic patients. Growth factors do not appear to be in short supply, and serum Sm levels are usually elevated in chronic renal failure. Glucocorticoids, used in treatment of renal disease, are profound growth depressants. The decrease in 1,25-dihydroxyvitamin D synthesis in patients with renal disease results in impaired formation and remodeling of bone (pp. 843). Clearly biochemical and hormonal imbalance secondary to the renal disease plus impaired nutrition result in a milieu in which normal growth cannot be achieved.

Cardiac Diseases

Growth retardation is a frequent accompaniment of congenital heart disease (see Section 6). It is more prevalent in those patients who are cyanotic. There is a general trend for growth failure to be more severe if congestive heart failure occurs early. Corrective surgery is not always accompanied by accelerated growth since the heart lesion may be just one expression of a more general damage to the fetus. Heart lesions in Down syndrome and Turner syndrome serve as examples of general cellular damage and impaired growth in the developing fetus.

Psychosocial Impaired Growth

There is clear evidence that in some children psychologic stress causes relative failure to grow by inhibiting the secretion of GH (see Section 2). When the stress is removed, secretion of GH resumes. Catch-up growth occurs that is indistinguishable from the catch-up after treatment with GH in the GH-deficient child.

Depressed growth in infants may be the result of failure of the parent to provide adequate mothering and nutrition. In this condition, GH, rather than being suppressed, is often normal or even abnormally high. Caloric deprivation is the major cause of this growth failure. An adverse environment may affect the appetite of the child or create disturbances of gastrointestinal function with resulting impaired absorption (Ellerstein and Ostrov, 1985). There is probably a whole spectrum of growth failure secondary to psychosocial stress. At one end of this spectrum suppression of GH secretion is the primary mechanism for growth failure and nutritional deficiency is a relatively minor factor. At the other end of the spectrum, nutritional deprivation predominates and GH secretion is normal.

The possibility of psychosocially impaired growth should always be considered if no cause for growth retardation can be found. Bizarre behavior, such as drinking water from toilet bowls or fish tanks or eating from garbage cans, should alert the physician to the presence of psychosocial stress in the child's environment. The diagnosis may require hospitalization or foster home care where caloric intake and weight gain can be monitored. Most children will show accelerated weight gain within 2 weeks of hospitalization if the failure to thrive is nonorganic in nature.

Constitutional Growth Delay

Growth retardation because of a slower than normal rate of maturation is called constitutional growth delay (pp. 877, 881, and Fig. 14.7) or growth retardation with delayed adolescence. Constitutional growth delay is most commonly seen in boys and accounts for the majority of short boys seen in the clinic. The rate of growth is normal for the bone age but height age and bone age are delayed by 2–4 years and the onset of pubertal development is delayed similarly. Frequently one of the parents, or some other family member, gives a history of delayed development. The mother may say her menarche was at age 15 or 16 years instead of the more usual 12–14 years.

This kind of growth retardation is not abnormal; the child simply resembles the father or mother. It is, however, extremely important to ascertain that pituitary function is normal. Mild or transient hypopituitarism can give a picture not unlike that of constitutional growth delay (pp. 880). As many as 20% of 105 adolescent children with growth and pubertal delays had sluggish GH responses to provocative stimuli, but when tested after the onset of puberty, almost all had normal GH secretion (Gourmelen et al, 1979). Therefore, some children with delayed development may have mild hypopituitarism, which disappears as puberty progresses.

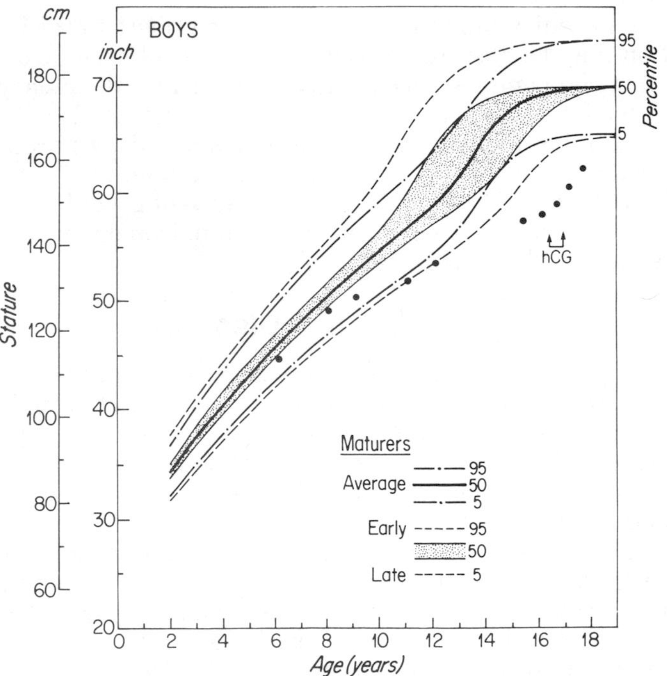

Figure 14.7. Constitutional growth delay. Growth in height of a boy with constitutional growth delay plotted on Tanner growth curve. This patient had no signs of puberty when he was seen in the clinic at 16 years of age. He was otherwise healthy with a normal endocrine status. His father had also had delay in onset of puberty. Administration of hCG for 6 months brought about early signs of puberty and accelerated linear growth. When therapy was stopped the patient continued to mature and grow at a normal rate.

Boys with delayed sexual development and short stature often have feelings of physical and social inadequacy. If the patient is already showing early signs of testicular enlargement, reassurance that the process of development has started may be sufficient. If the delay is severe and the psychologic symptoms are sufficiently disturbing, short term treatment with androgens or human chorionic gonadotropin (hCG) can be considered (pp. 877–878).

Metabolic Disorders Associated with Growth Failure

Several disorders of metabolism are associated with growth failure. For example, many of the glycogen storage diseases are characterized by impaired growth, which can be corrected by a regimen of frequent glucose feedings. A more detailed discussion of these metabolic disorders can be found in Section 15.

SECONDARY DISORDERS OF GROWTH–ENDOCRINE

Growth Hormone Deficiency

Definition

A deficiency of GH is defined as a state of decreased GH secretion by the pituitary or diminished action of GH on the target organ. This condition may result from impaired pituitary function, hypothalamic dysfunction, or target cell unresponsiveness to GH.

The most common form of GH deficiency is that associated with idiopathic hypopituitarism. Pituitary dysfunction may involve diminished secretion of one or more hormones, but the most common single deficiency is that of GH. Less frequently, secretions of TSH and ACTH are impaired. Involvement of the gonadotropins cannot be ascertained clinically until puberty, but roughly half of GH-deficient children will fail to show signs of development at the age of puberty.

Basic Science

Human GH is a single chain polypeptide consisting of 191 amino acids, with a molecular weight of about 21,500. It is formed in the somatotrophs of the anterior pituitary gland. The formation and secretion of GH is regulated by GHRH and St, both peptides formed in hypothalamic neurons and released in the median eminence where the portal blood vessel system carries them to the somatotrophs in the pituitary. GHRH has now been isolated and is available for clinical use in some centers. St not only inhibits GH secretion induced by several stimuli (sleep, arginine, insulin, etc) but also blocks TRH-induced TSH release. It does not, however, block TRH-induced prolactin release or the basal secretion of FSH, LH, TSH, and ACTH or the GnRH-induced release of LH and FSH.

Secretion of GH occurs in a series of irregular bursts throughout the day and night. Factors such as sleep, exercise, a rapid fall in blood glucose concentration, administration of amino acids, and stress can bring about bursts of GH release. Sleep associated GH release occurs whenever the subject sleeps, whether day or night, and is closely associated with the development of slow wave rhythm in sleep.

In the newborn, serum GH levels are high but after a few weeks they fall to levels found in the resting child and adult. In rats it has been shown that there is a sex difference in the level and periodicity of GH release with males having higher, less frequent peaks and lower nadirs of GH than females (Jansson et al, 1985). These sex differences also may exist in the human since fasting GH levels in the sera of adult women are higher than those found in adult men. Treatment of males with estrogens results in an increase in their fasting GH concentration to levels found in females.

Neurotransmitters play an important role in the regulation of GH secretion. The administration of 500 mg of L-DOPA by mouth leads to the secretion of GH between 45 minutes and 2 hours later. Serotonin also appears to be involved in the regulation of GH secretion. Administration of 5-hydroxytryptophan, a serotonin precursor, increases GH release.

Epidemiology

Most examples of idiopathic hypopituitarism are spontaneous, but about 3% of patients with GH deficiency have brothers or sisters with the disorder. In a very few cases one of the parents is affected. Since most GH disorders are autosomal recessive many of the sporadic cases of GH deficiency may have a genetic etiology. With new techniques of genotyping, and use of DNA from leukocytes it is becoming possible to categorize various genetic growth disorders more accurately (Phillips, 1985).

GH deficiency is four times as common in boys as in girls. It has been estimated to occur in about 1 of every 10,000 live births in the United Kingdon (Tanner, 1978). These children have a high incidence of perinatal problems (Craft et al, 1980). For example, there is an increased incidence of breech births, forceps deliveries, early vaginal bleeding, and either prolonged or very short labor with children subsequently found to have idiopathic GH deficiency. Abnormal deliveries and history of perinatal asphyxia have been observed in as many as 50–60% of children with GH deficiency.

Primary pituitary failure is associated with a variety of developmental defects. The pituitary gland may be hypoplastic or completely absent (anencephaly). Midline defects of the embryo may be associated with malformations of the pituitary. Pituitary destruction may also be secondary to trauma, intrasellar tumors, histiocytosis, and therapeutic radiation of the CNS.

Pituitary hypofunction secondary to hypothalamic damage may be caused by infections, granulomata, hydrocephalus, and hypothalamic tumors such as craniopharyngioma, hamartoma, and neurofibroma.

The prototype of the GH-resistant syndromes is Laron dwarfism, a familial disorder believed to have an autosomal recessive mode of transmission (Laron, 1974). Most affected patients are of Middle Eastern extraction and are the products of consanguineous marriages. Instead of low GH levels, these children have elevated basal serum GH concentration and exaggerated GH responses to provocative stimuli. The Sm concentrations in serum are low and do not increase in response to human GH (hGH).

A variant of GH resistance has been described in which patients have the clinical picture of GH deficiency, elevated GH concentrations, and low levels of Sm in serum. These patients are able to raise serum Sm concentrations and to exhibit linear growth response to administration of hGH. Presumably these patients have an abnormal GH molecule which is immunologically but not biologically active (Kowarski et al, 1978).

Another form of dwarfism was described in a child with normal GH responses but with increased levels of Sm (based on bioassay, receptor assay, and radioimmunoassay). Presumably this represents a defect in end-organ responsiveness to Sm (Lanes et al, 1980).

Natural History

Patients with GH deficiency usually appear normal at birth with appropriate weight and length. Impairment of linear growth first manifests itself in the first or second year of life. There is a tendency to obesity and the full-blown picture is one of a short chubby child of normal proportions. Hypoglycemia is a frequent finding in infancy, which may be due to concomitant deficiency in ACTH, but GH deficiency alone can cause hypoglycemia. The tendency to hypoglycemia tends to disappear after the second year of life.

The linear growth curve of the child with GH deficiency deviates progressively from the normal curve (Fig. 14.6). Growth rates are almost always less than 5 cm/year and are commonly as slow as 3 cm/year. Bone age is delayed but is roughly equal to height age. Skeletal proportions are normal for age. Although head circumference is within the normal range for age, the growth of facial bones is retarded, producing a disparity between the size of the face and the calvaria. Dental eruption is delayed.

Boys born with GH deficiency often have small genitalia and subsequent pubertal development may be delayed even if gonadotropin function is intact. GH deficiency occurring later in childhood may manifest itself only as retarded growth. The child is likely to be overweight. Rarely is there clinical evidence of hypothyroidism; however, serum thyroid hormone concentrations are frequently below normal or in the low-normal range.

Patients with multiple hormonal deficiencies of the anterior pituitary may show only mild symptoms other than growth retardation. Hypoglycemia should always suggest ACTH deficiency and growth retardation may suggest GH and/or thyroid hormone deficiency. Clinical evidence of gonadotropin deficiency before puberty will only be evident if hypogonadotropinism existed prenatally.

Children with hypopituitarism secondary to a brain tumor may have symptoms related to the primary lesion. Headaches, vomiting, visual symptoms, or field defects are some of the signs which should alert the physician to this possibility.

Diagnosis

The diagnosis of GH deficiency is best made on the basis of the growth data. Resting levels of GH are normally low and are not helpful in this regard. Provocative testing (Table 14.1) is laborious and expensive and, therefore, many endocrinologists utilize an exercise screening test first. Among the tests widely used is the exercise stimulation test. The child is asked to exercise vigorously (running up and down stairs) for 15–20 minutes after an overnight or 4-hour fast. The serum level of GH after exercise is compared with that before exercise. A rise of 7 ng/ml or more is considered normal; however, only about 50% of normal children respond adequately in the exercise test and therefore, a failure to respond is not necessarily abnormal. Those short children who have a normal GH exercise test may have growth retardation secondary to the production of a biologically inactive GH. Any child who continues to grow subnormally despite a normal immunoreactive GH response to exercise should be considered for a trial of GH therapy.

Sleep induces a rise in serum GH. The patient can be admitted overnight to the hospital. An intravenous (i.v.) line is placed in the evening and blood samples are drawn every 20 minutes through the night. Other pituitary hormones can be measured from the same blood sample so that a more complete survey of hormone deficiency can be performed. Generally serum is analyzed for glucose, insulin, cortisol, LH, FSH, and GH; thyroid hormone is analyzed in the initial blood sample. This test is expensive and involves overnight hospitalization; however, it can be combined with provocative tests performed the next morning after fasting and provide a more complete picture of the integrity of the hypothalamic-pituitary axis.

The provocative stimuli most commonly used are listed in Table 14.1. Probably one of the most reliable is the induction of hypoglycemia with intravenous insulin, but this test is also the one most likely to evoke side effects. The risk of symptomatic hypoglycemia although small is very real and necessitates the presence of a physician to monitor closely the progress of the test. An i.v. line should be in place and concentrated glucose should be available for treatment of severe hypoglycemia. The nadir of blood glucose generally occurs 20–30 minutes after i.v. insulin, but the GH response is observed later. Usually blood samples are drawn every 15 minutes for 2½ hours after insulin administration, and blood glucose is monitored by use of Chemstrips throughout the procedure. The test is useful also for determining if the patient has a deficiency of ACTH

Table 14.1
Clinical Tests of Growth Hormone Secretion

	Test Conditions	GH Response[1]
Screening Tests		
1. Exercise	Fasting (4–8 hr), vigorous exercise for 15–20 min	20–40 min after exercise is begun
2. Sleep	Blood sampling throughout the night	Peaks of GH with deep sleep
Provocative Tests		
1. Insulin	O.05–0.10 U/kg IV of regular insulin; 50% fall in blood glucose for adequate test	Rise in GH at 45–75 min
2. Glucagon	0.03 mg/kg intramuscular or subcutaneous (max = 1 mg)	Rise in GH at 120–180 min
3. Argine	5–10% solution L-arginine hydrochloride, 0.5 g/kg infused over 30 min	Rise in GH at 60–120 min
4. L-DOPA	0.5 g/1.73 m^2 by mouth	Rise in GH at 45–120 min
5. Clonidine	4 μg/kg by mouth	Rise in GH at 60–120 min

[1]Propranolol may be used to augment the GH responses to the provocative stimuli. A dose of 0.75 mg/kg by mouth should be given 60 min before glucagon, insulin, or arginine.

since hypoglycemia is a stimulus for ACTH secretion. Samples obtained during the test are sent to the laboratory for determinations of glucose, GH, and cortisol concentrations. LH, FSH, and thyroid hormone levels should be checked in the initial blood sample.

Arginine is an excellent stimulus for GH secretion; however, it must be administered intravenously, necessitating the placement of a second i.v. line. Glucagon, or glucagon preceded by propranolol to augment the response, is another stimulant used widely, as is L-DOPA. A significant percentage of single provocative tests will give false positive results; therefore, at least two different tests should be performed, usually on the same day, one after the other. We have found that insulin-induced hypoglycemia followed by a glucagon test is a good combination of provocative stimuli.

Recently, GHRH has become available in some centers but its use in differentiating primary pituitary failure from failure secondary to hypothalamic dysfunction remains to be defined. TRH is more readily available to test pituitary responsiveness to hypothalamic factors; a TRH test is simple to perform and may provide valuable information in regard to the function of the hypothalamic-pituitary axis (pp. 828).

There is a poor correlation between levels of serum SmC and growth rate. Very low values (< 0.25 U/ml) should be of some concern; however, it must be remembered that SmC values correlate more with state of maturity than with chronological age. The boy with delayed development, for example, may have a low SmC and perfectly normal GH secretion. Malnutrition also lowers SmC values.

In those patients with demonstrated hypopituitarism the etiology of the condition should be sought (Table 14.2). Skull radiographs or CAT scans may demonstrate a CNS lesion. Ophthalmologic examination may reveal previously unsuspected ocular field defects, pointing to involvement of the optic chiasm or tracts. Recently, nuclear magnetic resonance (NMR) techniques have been introduced for finer anatomic evaluation of CNS tumors. Other tests of pituitary function are summarized in Table 14.2.

Table 14.2
Tests for Pituitary Function in Patients with Possible Hypopituitarism[1]

Test	Interpretation
Skull radiograph	Look for calcification of a tumor and enlarged sella size
CAT scan	Look for intra- or suprasellar mass
Visual fields	Evidence of optic chiasm involvement
T_4, FT_4 index, TSH	If low, secondary hypothyroidism
Metapyrone test (see Chapter 6)	Poor ACTH response suggests decreased pituitary reserve of ACTH
Fasting AM serum cortisol (± serum cortisol post-ACTH, 0.25 mg cosyntropin intramuscular or IV)	Baseline cortisol should be >5 μg/dl with a rise 45 min after ACTH of >7 μg/dl
GH responses to stimuli	See Table 14.1

[1]In addition to the above, the physician may also wish to check serum concentrations of prolactin and gonadotropins. If possible, a 24-hour urine collection can be obtained for 24-hour 17-KS, and 17-hydroxysteroids (see Chapter 6).

Treatment

The definitive treatment of GH deficiency is the administration of hGH. The usual therapeutic dose is 0.1–0.2 U/kg of body weight given subcutaneously two or three times a week. This schedule of dosage is not physiologic and in those few patients who respond poorly or inadequately, a more physiologic pulsatile administration of GH or GnRH may be required for normal growth (Gelato et al, 1985). The hGH used for therapy in the past has been obtained by extraction of the hormone from human pituitary glands; however, recently three cases of Creutzfeldt-Jakob disease were reported in patients who had previously been treated in the 1960s and 1970s with hGH extracted from human pituitaries (Brown et al, 1985). Distribution of human pituitary GH has been halted and commercial suppliers of hGH have taken their products off the market. The FDA has recently approved Protropin, the Genentech recombinant DNA GH preparation, for clinical use. This preparation has been undergoing clinical trials since 1981. These trials show that Protropin is therapeutically equivalent to GH of human pituitary origin. About 30% of all patients treated with Protropin developed persistent antibodies to GH; however, these antibodies do not usually interfere with the growth response to Protropin GH.

In general, young children respond to GH therapy better than adolescents; the obese respond better than the thin; and severely GH-deficient children respond better than those with partial deficiencies. Invariably the response to GH therapy declines with time and several months of rest from treatment may bring about renewed growth response (Fig. 14.6). Larger doses of GH produce more rapid growth and as bacterial hGH (Protropin) becomes increasingly available it may be possible to use greater amounts of GH in treating children with retarded growth.

If the patient has a low serum T_4 (pp. 827), therapy with thyroid hormone should be instituted concomitantly with the hGH. GH therapy in the hypopituitary patient may actually induce TSH deficiency. The response to GH of children who are hypothyroid is poor and unless the deficiency of thyroid hormone is corrected growth will remain subnormal. Therapy for hypoadrenalism is rarely needed and since cortisol is such a profound depressant of growth, cortisol therapy should be avoided unless there is clear-cut evidence of adrenal insufficiency. It should be kept in mind, however, that the patient with marginal adrenal function may require glucocorticoids under conditions of severe stress (surgery, high fever, etc).

If the patient shows no signs of pubertal development by age 15 or 16 years, and especially if there is concomitant poor growth response to GH therapy, small doses of sex hormones may be used in conjunction with the hGH to augment the rate of growth (Craft and Underwood, 1984). In boys, testosterone enanthate doses as low as 50 mg/month intramuscularly may more than double the growth rate. Bone age should be followed closely and all efforts to prevent excessive bone maturation should be employed, particularly in the very short child. In those patients showing signs of early or normal sexual development, consideration should be given to extending the growing period by delaying sexual development with the use of GnRH analogues (pp. 886).

CONTROVERSY

Parents of short children exert considerable pressure on physicians to treat their children with hGH to improve growth. Several studies have now shown that whereas normal (by all known standards) children may respond to hGH administration with increased linear growth, no evidence of increased mature height has been reported. Compensatory deceleration of growth has been observed in GH-deficient patients who are taken off GH therapy. Worse still, there is considerable doubt whether even the response in height velocity during the entire first year is predictive of the final outcome. In treated GH deficient patients, the strongest correlation of final adult height is with parental height, just as in normal stature (Tanner, 1985). Continuous GH therapy in normal short children may ultimately enhance adult stature, but as yet the appropriate studies have not been performed. Over the coming years, as information is obtained about long-term effects of GH in normal very short children, we should be able to determine more clearly the advisability of treating such individuals. Until such studies are performed in large clinical centers with appropriate controls, the use of GH in normal short children cannot be recommended.

Prognosis

The prognosis in terms of final height for the child with deficiencies of pituitary hormones depends upon the completeness of the replacement therapy and the age at which therapy is started. When instituted early, replacement therapy can enable the child to achieve his full growth potential. Catch-up growth will occur; the younger the child, the more complete the catch-up. Growth deficits in later childhood are more difficult to correct. Very often puberty will supervene and bone maturation will accelerate, thus shortening the time available for catch-up. In the extremely short child, the physician may wish to consider delaying pubertal development (pp. 886) in order to provide additional time for GH-induced growth to occur.

Hypercortisolism

Excess amounts of glucocorticoids, whether endogenously formed or exogenously administered, will suppress linear growth. In the patient with hypopituitarism in which there is an ACTH deficiency as well as GH deficiency it may be necessary to give glucocorticoid therapy. If the ACTH deficiency is mild, as it often is, serum cortisol values will be normal but there will be diminished pituitary reserves of ACTH for stressful situations. Glucocorticoid therapy can be used in such

CASE ILLUSTRATION (Fig. 14.6)

The patient was first seen at 19 months of age for slow growth. She was the 3.2-kg product of a full-term pregnancy. She had been healthy with a normal development except for linear growth. She did, however, have a skull fracture at age 13 months and was hospitalized for 2 days, without complications. In the clinic her length was 65.5 cm (3rd centile) and her weight was 6.8 kg (3rd centile). Her bone age was 9 months which was comparable to her height age (6 months). Her weight was appropriate for her height. Her mother's height was 157 cm and her father's was 170 cm. Two male siblings had heights between the 3rd and 10th centiles. A great-aunt had an adult height of 148 cm. Urinalysis, WBC, Hb, and Hct were normal. Skull radiographs and brain scan were normal except for a somewhat small sella turcica.

The patient was followed in the endocrine clinic over several years during which time all tests of hormone function were normal except for low concentrations of GH in the serum. Her appearance was that of a normally proportioned small girl. When hGH became available for clinical use the patient was studied further for evidence of GH deficiency. Exercise and provocative stimuli produced no rise in the low baseline levels of serum GH. At the age of 10 years she was started on 4 units of hGH three times a week administered intramuscularly. Her linear growth rate before therapy was 2.5–3.0 cm/year and on GH treatment it accelerated to 10 cm/year (Fig. 14.6). During a 6-month period without GH, growth was arrested, but reinstitution of therapy accelerated growth once more.

This girl showed no signs of sexual development by age 15 years and was started on estrogen therapy at that time. Throughout her clinical course bone ages remained appropriate for her height age. Her weight at all times was appropriate for her height.

In retrospect, it seems possible that the brain trauma secondary to the head injury and fracture at 13 months of age was the cause of her subsequent hypopituitarism. Her growth retardation began at that time.

patients during periods of stress (surgery, high fever). If the ACTH deficiency is moderate or severe, the physician should be careful to treat with no more than replacement amounts of cortisol to avoid growth suppression.

Children with nonendocrine disorders requiring large doses of glucocorticoids will usually show significant growth impairment. If the amount of glucocorticoids can be reduced or they can be administered every other day it is often possible to restore growth to normal or near normal.

Endogenous hypersecretion of cortisol may be secondary to an adrenal tumor, to an ACTH-secreting tumor of the pituitary gland, to hypothalamic dysfunction in which CRH is secreted in excessive amounts, or to an ACTH-secreting or CRH-secreting tumor elsewhere in the body. The disorders of glucocorticoid production are discussed in Chapter 6. The clinical picture in all children with excess cortisol (Cushing syndrome) is the same, however, and from the standpoint of growth the salient features are arrested linear growth (unless sex hormones are produced) and excessive weight gain (p. 861).

Pseudohypoparathyroidism Type I

This inherited disorder is characterized by short stature, obesity, and bony anomalies. There is increased production of (parathyroid hormone) PTH but deficient end-organ responsiveness to the hormone. For details of this disorder and a case history, see Chapter 5.

Sex Hormone Deficiency

Children with hypopituitarism including gonadotropin deficiency will fail to grow normally at adolescence even if all other hormone deficiencies have been rectified. Much as in the child with constitutional growth delay, and for the same reasons, the growth pattern deviates from the norm at this age. In the absence of sex hormones the normal adolescent growth spurt does not occur. In the child with known deficiencies of other pituitary hormones, a test of gonadotropin release after administration of GnRH should be performed (pp. 880). In general, children with hypopituitarism who are receiving GH and/or thyroid hormone for growth, and who have not shown signs of development by age 15 years should be considered for treatment with low doses of sex hormones.

Tanner (1978) makes the point that GH stimulates leg growth more than trunk growth and that delaying sexual maturation to achieve greater stature under GH treatment may result in increasing disproportion of the upper and lower body segments with sitting height falling progressively behind leg length. Such are the body proportions of the eunuch. Testosterone stimulates trunk growth somewhat more than leg growth, so that starting testosterone therapy before the body proportions deviate too much is wise. The patient may lose a small amount in total stature, but will end up with more normal body proportions. Estrogens are less effective stimulators of truncal growth than is testosterone; even so, administering estrogens before body proportions get too abnormal will achieve more normal body proportions at the cost of some total height. These become real issues for the physician treating the hypogonadal adolescent. Some of our patients have achieved a very satisfactory height under prolonged GH therapy with delay of sex hormone treatment, but in retrospect better body proportions might have been achieved with earlier sex hormone treatment. Details of treatment regimens are given in Chapter 7.

EXCESSIVE GROWTH

Definition

An accelerated rate of linear growth (Fig. 14.5) above the norm for the individual in question results in excessive growth.

Genetic Tall Stature

Epidemiology

The majority of patients seeking medical advice for tallness are genetically tall (Fig. 14.5). They nearly always have tall parents and most are girls who are themselves anxious about being very tall or who have mothers who remember the problems of the tall girl and want their daughters to be saved from this embarrassment.

Diagnosis

The physical examination of such an individual is normal and plotting the growth points of the patient and the parent shows invariably that the subject will achieve an adult stature appropriate for her genetic inheritance.

A bone age is helpful in estimating final height. Those girls who are estimated to achieve an adult stature of over 6 feet and who wish to be treated may be considered for therapy.

Treatment

The treatment involves the daily administration of 10 mg of conjugated estrogen or 0.15–0.3 mg of ethinyl estradiol over a long period of time until the epiphyses fuse. Depending upon how early treatment is begun a reduction of 2–7 cm in adult height can be expected. There are side-effects which include acceleration of puberty, nausea, irregular menses, hypertension, and weight gain. More serious side effects are rare.

Most physicians do not treat tall girls with estrogens, because of the possible long-term adverse effects. Those who elect to treat these girls should start ideally at a relatively young age (bone age at or below 12 years) if sufficient reduction in stature is to be achieved. The patient must be followed carefully to detect any side-effects of the estrogen.

Klinefelter Syndrome

This syndrome is discussed in detail in Chapter 7. A few comments, however, are appropriate in regard to growth.

This form of hypergonadotropic hypogonadism (pp. 878) is generally associated with excessive long-bone growth which begins before puberty. The linear growth of the long bones in the lower extremities is greater than it is in the upper extremities. This results in an arm span to height ratio of 1 or less. This ratio is different from that in eunuchoidal individuals whose long bones in both upper and lower extremities grow in a comparable fashion, resulting in an arm span at least 2 inches greater than the height and an arm span to height ratio greater than 1.

Since these patients have a chromosomal abnormality (karyotype 47,XXY) it is assumed that these skeletal growth differences are related to the abnormal sex chromosome constitution in the osseous tissue. It should be remembered that in Turner syndrome, where the second X chromosome is missing, growth is severely retarded. The exact mechanism of the growth abnormalities in both Turner syndrome and in Klinefelter syndrome is unknown.

Marfan Syndrome

These patients are usually well above average in height, but are not outside the normal range (pp. 753). They have long limbs and narrow hands with slender fingers (arachnodactyly). Their arm spans are greater than their heights and the lower segment is significantly greater than the upper segment. Other clinical features include hyperextensible joints, kyphoscoliosis, rib cage deformities and dislocation of the lens. Death from dissecting aortic aneurysm occurs in early adult life. The cause of the disorder is unknown.

Homocystinuria

Diagnosis

Patients with this disorder may have a similar appearance to the patients with Marfan syndrome (pp. 753). They are distinguished by the presence of mental retardation and excretion of large amounts of homocystine in the urine.

Growth Hormone Excess

Definition

Excess GH is defined as an elevation of the mean GH level, usually greater than 10 ng/ml, accompanied by signs and symptoms of excess hormone.

Basic Science

Typically, excessive GH production is caused by somatotropic adenomas of the pituitary gland (eosinophilic or chromophobic), which are usually small and are confined within the sella turcica. The signs of GH excess will depend upon the age at which the tumor arises. Before closure of the epiphyses excess GH will produce accelerated linear growth resulting in gigantism. There is overgrowth of soft tissues as well. The most famous patient with GH excess was Robert Wadlow, known as the "Alton Giant", who reached the adult height of 8 feet 11 inches and weight of 475 pounds. Excess GH after fusion of the epiphyses results in acromegaly.

Epidemiology

The condition can occur at any age but is most common between the third and fifth decades of life. It has been estimated, however, that as many as one-sixth of all patients show the earliest signs of GH excess between ages 10 and 20 years. This diagnosis is rarely made in children.

Natural History

The earliest signs of GH excess after closure of the epiphyses involve the face, hands, and feet. There is coarsening of the facial features and soft tissue swelling of the feet and hands. The patient may remember needing increasing sizes in rings, gloves, or shoes. The changes are gradual and it is only by looking at a series of pictures over the years that the differences are readily detected.

Body hair is increased as are the size and function of sebaceous and sweat glands. Perspiration may be excessive and the odor offensive. Most organs, including the thyroid, are enlarged.

Bony proliferation is seen on radiographs of the hands as cortical thickening and distal tufting. The bony changes in the skull are particularly striking, with lengthening and thickening of the mandible giving the "lantern jaw" appearance. The sinuses may be enlarged to a remarkable degree.

Impaired glucose tolerance is present in nearly half the cases of acromegaly, but clinical diabetes mellitus occurs in only about 10%. Insulin resistance is present in all patients and may be severe in rare instances.

Goiter may be present secondary to enlargement of the thyroid gland, but thyroid function is generally normal.

Diagnosis

Often the plasma GH level will be only slightly elevated, or even within the high normal range. Frequent sampling of blood over a 24-hour period may show peaks of GH secretion. In some instances glucose administration will produce a paradoxical rise in GH in contrast to the normal fall of GH with hyperglycemia. A plasma level of GH of over 10 ng/ml 90 minutes after administration of 75 g of glucose by mouth (adult dose) supports the diagnosis of acromegaly. In addition, elevation of Sm levels may be helpful in making the diagnosis.

If the tumor has enlarged and compressed other areas of the pituitary gland there may be evidence of thyroid and gonadal deficiency. ACTH secretion is usually adequate to maintain basal cortisol secretion but a metyrapone test (pp. 862) may reveal decreased ACTH reserve. Prolactin levels may be elevated.

Radiographs of the skull, hands, and feet are very helpful in making the diagnosis of acromegaly. CAT scans of the area of the sella turcica may show the tumor.

Treatment

Transphenoidal microsurgery is the treatment of choice in removal of the pituitary microadenoma. If the tumor is large, craniotomy or radiation therapy may be appropriate.

Prognosis

Very few cases in children have been followed since the introduction of the newer techniques of transphenoidal microsurgery. Even if removal of the adenoma is successful other areas of the pituitary may be permanently damaged and hormone replacement therapy may have to be continued indefinitely.

Cerebral Gigantism: Sotos Syndrome

Children with cerebral gigantism are tall, usually above the 90th centile for length and weight at birth (Sotos, 1964). They continue to grow rapidly for the first few years of life. Clinical features include prominent forehead, large elongated head, high arched palate, hypertelorism, large ears and jaw, coarse facial features, and pointed chin. Most are mentally retarded. Bone age is usually advanced and, therefore, final adult height may not be excessive. Endocrine function is normal in these children. The cause of the disorder is unknown.

Fetal Gigantism

Other syndromes characterized by early overgrowth include the syndromes of Weaver-Smith, Beckwith-Wiedemann, and Marshall-Smith (Amir et al, 1984). All show evidence of excessive growth in utero and either delayed or retarded psychomotor development. There are characteristic bony deformities in each and the bone age is advanced. There is no evidence of endocrine abnormality in these children although some infants with Beckwith-Wiedemann syndrome have hypoglycemia in the first days of life. Tests of carbohydrate tolerance and histologic examination of the pancreas suggest that hyperinsulinemia may be responsible for the hypoglycemia.

The infant of the diabetic mother is another example of fetal overgrowth. Details of this entity are to be found on page 151.

Hyperthyroidism

Linear growth may be accelerated somewhat in hyperthyroidism (pp. 835) and the bone age may be advanced. These changes are generally small and are readily reversed by treatment.

Precocious Secretion of Sex Hormones

Acceleration of linear growth invariably occurs simultaneously with signs of premature sexual development or inappropriate virilization (pp. 885). The rapid growth is accompanied by a rate of bone maturation greater than that expected for chronologic age. Height velocity approaches that expected for the stage of sexual development and bone age. The final adult stature is diminished. Synthetic analogues of GnRH are now available in some centers for the treatment of idiopathic central precocity (pp. 886). Where excess sex hormones are secondary to tumor of the gonad, adrenal, or hypothalamus, a surgical approach should be employed whenever possible. Details of the approach to the diagnosis and treatment of sexual precocity are found in Chapters 6 and 7.

Summary

Disorders of growth are among the more common problems seen by pediatricians. All organs and systems can affect growth and development, but the special regulatory role of the endocrine system makes the differential diagnosis of abnormal growth extremely challenging. In general, patients who are overweight for height are more likely to have an endocrine problem than are those who are underweight. The hormones most frequently involved are GH, thyroid hormone, glucocorticoids, and sex hormones. Constitutional growth delay (delayed pubertal development) is one of the most common problems seen in the adolescent boy. Parental history is often helpful in making this diagnosis.

In the young child with adequate nutrition whose linear growth rate is decreasing, a careful work-up for evidence of GH and/or thyroid hormone deficiency is mandatory. Even the genetically short child with normal GH by radioimmunoassay may have a biologically inactive hormone. Sm levels if high are helpful in diagnosis, but a low SmC level is not necessarily abnormal in the prepubescent child. In all conditions careful monitoring of linear growth and weight changes, as well as appropriate diagnostic tests should enable the pediatrician to decide if the patient has a hormonal deficiency.

REFERENCES

Amir N, Gross-Kieselstein E, Hirsch HJ, et al: Weaver-Smith syndrome. *Am J Dis Child* 138:1113, 1984.

Barr GD, Allen CM, Shinefield HR: Height and weight of 7500 children of three skin colors. *Am J Dis Child* 124:866, 1972.

Beighton P: *Inherited Disorders of the Skeleton.* New York, Churchill Livingston, 1978.

Berwick D: Non-organic failure-to-thrive. *Pediatr Rev* 1:265, 1980.

Bithoney WG, Rathbun JM: Failure to thrive. In Levine M, et al: *Developmental-Behavioral Pediatrics.* Philadelphia, WB Saunders, 1983, p. 557.

Brosius KK, Ritter DA, Kenny JD: Postnatal growth curve of the infant with extremely low birth weight who was fed enterally. *Pediatrics* 74:778, 1984.

Brown P, Gajdusek DC, Gibbs CJ Jr, Asher DM: Potential epidemic of Creutzfeldt-Jakob disease from human growth hormone therapy. *N Engl J Med* 313:728, 1985.

Craft WH, et al: High incidence of perinatal insult in children with idiopathic hypopituitarism. *J Pediatr* 96:397, 1980.

Craft WH, Underwood LE: Effect of androgens on plasma somatomedin-C/IGF-1 responses to growth hormone. *Clin Endocrinol* 20:549, 1984.

D'Ercole AJ, Underwood LE: Growth factors in fetal growth and development. In Novy MJ, Resko JA (eds): *Fetal Endocrinology.* New York, Academic Press, 1981, p.155.

Ellerstein NS, Ostrov BE: Growth patterns in children hospitalized because of caloric-deprivation failure to thrive. *Am J Dis Child* 139:164, 1985.

Gelato MC, Ross JL, Malozowski S, et al: Effects of pulsatile administration of growth hormone (GH)-releasing hormone on short term linear growth in children with GH deficiency. *J Clin Endocrinol Metabol* 61:444, 1985.

Gertner JM, Genel M, Gianfredi SP, et al: Prospective clinical trial of human growth hormone in short children without growth hormone deficiency. *J Pediatr* 104:172, 1984.

Gourmelen M, Pham-Huu-Trung MT, Girard F: Transient partial human growth hormone deficiency in prepubertal children with delay of growth. *Pediatr Res* 13:221, 1979.

Hack M, Fanaroff AA: The outcome of growth failure associated with preterm birth. *Clin Obstet Gynecol* 27:647, 1984.

Hill DE: The effect of insulin on fetal growth. *Semin Perinatol* 2:319, 1978.

Hill DJ, Milner RDG: Increased somatomedin and cartilage metabolic activity in rabbit fetuses injected with insulin in utero. *Diabetologia* 19:143, 1980.

Homer C, Ludwig S: Categorization of etiology of failure to thrive. *Am J Dis Child* 135:848, 1981.

Jansson J, Eden S, Isaksson O: Sexual dimorphism in the control of growth hormone secretion. *Endocrinol Rev* 6:128, 1985.

Klapper DG, Svoboda ME, Van Wyk JJ: Sequence analysis of somatomedin C: confirmation of identify with insulin-like growth factor I. *Endocrinology* 112:2215, 1983.

Knittle JL, Timmers K, Ginsberg-Fellner F, et al: The growth of adipose tissue in children and adolescents. Cross-sectional and longitudinal studies of adipose cell number and size. *J Clin Invest* 63:239, 1979.

Kowarski A, Schneider J, Ben-Galim E, et al: Growth failure with normal serum radioimmunoassayable growth hormone and low somatomedin activity: Somatomedin restoration and growth acceleration after exogenous growth hormone. *J Clin Endocrinol Metabol* 47:461, 1978.

Lanes R, Plotnick LP, Spencer EM, et al: Dwarfism associated with normal serum growth hormone and increased bioassayable, receptorassayable and immunoassayable somatomedin. *J Clin Endocrinol Metabol* 50:485, 1980.

Laron Z: Syndrome of familial dwarfism and high plasma immunoreactive growth hormone. *Isr J Med Sci* 10:1247, 1974.

Merimee TJ, Zapf J, Froesch ER: Dwarfism in the pygmy. An isolated deficiency of insulin-like growth factor I. *N Engl J Med* 305:965, 1981.

Mitchell W, Gorrell R, Greenberg R: Failure to thrive: A study in a primary care setting. *Pediatrics* 65:971, 1980.

Phillips JA III. Genetic diagnosis: Differentiating growth disorders. *Hosp Pract* 20:85, 1985.

Pollitt E: Failure to thrive: Socioeconomic, dietary intake, and mother-child interaction data. *Fed Proc* 34:1593, 1975.

Rosenfield RI, Furlanetto R, Bock D: Relationship of somatomedin-C concentrations to pubertal changes. *J Pediatr* 103:723, 1983.

Rosenn DW, Loeb LS, Jura MB: Differentiation of organic from non-organic failure to thrive syndrome in infancy. *Pediatrics* 66:698, 1980.

Saal HM, Pagon RA, Pepin MG: Reevaluation of Russell-Silver syndrome. *J Pediatr* 107:733, 1985.

Smith DW, Truog W, Rogers JE, et al: Shifting linear growth during infancy: Illustration of genetic factors in growth from fetal life through infancy. *J Pediatr* 89:225, 1976.

Sotos JF, Dodge PR, Muirhead D, et al: Cerebral gigantism in childhood. *N Engl J Med* 271:109, 1964.

Spencer GSG, Hill DJ, Garssen GJ, et al: Somatomedin activity and growth hormone levels in body fluids of the fetal pig: Effect of chronic hyperinsulinaemia. *J Endocrinol* 96:107, 1983.

Stracke H, Schulz A, Moeller D, et al: Effect of growth hormone on osteoblasts and demonstration of somatomedin C/IGF I in bone organ culture. *Acta Endocrinol* 107:16, 1984.

Tanner JM: *Fetus into Man.* Cambridge, MA, Harvard University Press, 1978.

Tanner JM: Problems in assessing the efficacy of growth promoting substances: The role of height prediction. *Growth Genet Hormone* 1:1, 1985.

Tanner JM, Davies PSW: Clinical longitudinal standards for height and height velocity for North American children. *J Pediatr* 107:317, 1985.

Tanner JM, Thomson AM: Standards for birth weight at gestation periods from 32-42 weeks allowing for maternal height and weight. *Arch Dis Child* 45:566, 1970.

Tanner JM, Whitehouse RH: Clinical longitudinal standards for height, weight, height velocity, weight velocity and the stages of puberty. *Arch Dis Child* 51:170, 1976.

Tanner JM, Whitehouse RH, Marshall WA, et al: *Assessment of Skeletal Maturity and Prediction of Adult Height.* London, Academic Press, 1975.

Villar J, Smeriglio V, Martorell R, Brown CH, Klein RE: Heterogeneous growth and mental development of intrauterine growth retarded infants during the first three years of life. *Pediatrics* 74:783, 1984.

Zachmann M, Sobradillo B, Framk M, et al: Bayley-Pinneau, Roche-Wainer-Thissen and Tanner height predictions in normal children and in patients with various pathologic conditions. *J Pediatr* 93:749, 1978.

Posterior Pituitary Disorders 3

Definition

Clinical disorders of the posterior pituitary are limited to those conditions characterized by either excessive or deficient secretion of vasopressin or deficient response of target cells to the biologically active hormone. No clinical disorders of oxytocin secretion have been recognized.

Basic Science

The posterior pituitary or neurohypophysis is derived from the floor of the diencephalon. In the human it secretes the two nonapeptides oxytocin and arginine vasopressin (VP, also called antidiuretic hormone). The hormones are synthesized in hypothalamic nuclei and are then transported along the neurohypophyseal tract to the posterior pituitary where they are stored and released under central control (Brownstein et al, 1980). VP nerve endings also terminate in the primary plexus of the pituitary portal system. Thus, neurohypophyseal neurons may have a role in the regulation of anterior pituitary hormones as well as secretion in the neural lobe. The hypothalamic nuclei involved in the synthesis of oxytocin and vasopressin are the supraoptic and paraventricular nuclei of the anterior hypothalamus. The former lies just above the optic chiasm and the latter lies ventral to the thalamus and adjacent to the third ventricle. The nuclei have a very close anatomic and functional relationship to the area of the hypothalamus controlling thirst which is located next to the area of temperature control. Slightly more posterior are the areas controlling hunger and satiety. Thus, in a relatively small area of the hypothalamus are neurons that perceive and respond to a variety of somatic signals relating to temperature, osmotic and caloric balance of the organism. Lesions in this area of the brain, or deficiencies of specific peptides can produce clinical abnormalities relating to these functions.

HORMONES OF THE POSTERIOR PITUITARY

Most of the cells of the supraoptic nucleus contain VP but some contain oxytocin. Somewhat fewer (but still a majority) of the cells in the paraventricular nucleus also contain VP. The hormones are transported in membrane-bound vesicles through the axons to the neurohypophysis. Both VP and oxytocin contain nine amino acids; both have a Cys-Cys bridge in the 1–6 position and they differ in only two of the nine amino acids.

In addition to the nonapeptides, the posterior pituitary is rich in proteins called neurophysins that have a special property of binding both oxytocin and VP by covalent bonds. VP and oxytocin are each associated with a distinct neurophysin now recognized to be part of common precursor hormones, propressophysin and prooxyphysin (Russell et al, 1980). The prohormones are transported in membrane-bound vesicles through the axons to the neural lobe where they are stored and later released (Verbolis and Robinson, 1983). Processing of the prohormones to VP, oxytocin and the two neurophysins takes place in the vesicles during transport. Nerve action potentials in the cell body are propagated along the axon and trigger hormone discharge. VP and oxytocin leave the cell together with neurophysin in a fixed ratio. The neurohypophyseal neurons are directly controlled by cholinergic and nonadrenergic neurotransmitters and by several neuropeptides (Sklar and Schrier, 1983).

Vasopressin

VP secretion is influenced by a number of stimuli. All stimuli initiate release of VP through depolarization of the neurohypophyseal neurons. Osmoreceptors, located near the supraoptic nuclei and the thirst center influence both drinking behavior and VP secretion. Increases of serum osmotic pressure by only 1 or 2% result in VP release and increased osmolality of urine. VP release is also influenced by intravascular volume. Stretch receptors in the left atrium inhibit the release of VP during hypervolemia, while baroreceptors located in the carotid sinus stimulate VP release during hypotension. These volume signals are mediated via the vagus nerve.

Once secreted, VP circulates in unbound form in the plasma; its half-life is about 15–20 minutes. VP receptors are present on the plasma membrane of the cells of the collecting duct of the kidney. Interaction with the receptor stimulates adenylate cyclase and a chain of events which results in greater porosity of the luminal (urine) side of the collecting duct epithelium with passive reabsorption of water and urea. For example, during hydropenia the interstitium of the medulla of the kidney is hypertonic and tubular fluid entering the medullary collecting duct is isotonic; therefore, an osmotic gradient is present between the collecting duct lumen and the medullary interstitium. In the presence of VP, water movement occurs across the collecting duct lumen into the interstitium and vasa recta of the medullary circulation, resulting in concentration of the solute remaining in the urine. In the human, maximal urinary concentrating ability depends upon the degree of medullary hypertonicity as well as on the presence of adequate amounts of VP.

Glucocorticoids modulate the "set point" of neurohypophyseal control. Adrenal insufficiency lowers it and thereby induces a relative increase in VP secretion.

Oxytocin

Oxytocin is involved primarily in milk ejection. It binds to myoepithelial cells of the mammary gland and thereby causes contraction of the smooth muscle. It is secreted in response to stimulation of the nerve endings in the nipple.

The uterus-contracting property of oxytocin has been used for the induction of labor; however, a role for the hormone in normal labor has not been established. Labor occurs normally in women with oxytocin deficiency.

NEUROGENIC DIABETES INSIPIDUS

Definition

Neurogenic diabetes insipidus (DI) is a clinical condition of VP deficiency associated with an inability to form concentrated urine.

Basic Science

Central (neurogenic) DI results from a spectrum of deficiencies from mild partial defects to complete absence of VP synthesis. The disorder may be familial or, more commonly, may be due to a lesion in the hypothalamic-pituitary area. The lesions may be secondary to tumors, head trauma, neurosurgery, or sequelae of a CNS infection. Disorders such as leukemia or histiocytosis may involve this area and cause DI.

Epidemiology

There are many causes of the clinical syndrome of DI (Table 14.3). The true incidence of each is unknown, but all should be considered rare.

Natural History

The severity of the symptoms will depend upon the completeness of the VP deficiency, the diet, renal function, presence of an intact sensation of thirst, and integrity of the anterior pituitary.

Craniopharyngioma is a relatively common cause of central DI in children, not usually as an initial symptom complex, but secondary to the surgery and/or radiation therapy of the tumor. Any tumor of the hypothalamus, third ventricle, optic nerve, or pituitary gland may result in endocrine dysfunction. DI may be the first recognizable sign of an intracranial tumor and may antedate neurological symptoms by several years. Periodic evaluation for CNS tumor is mandatory in any child with unexplained DI. Nevertheless, the most common presentation for CNS tumors is with symptoms of raised intracranial pressure or of visual problems consequent upon compression of the optic chiasm. DI is a frequent sequela of operations to these areas, because of the removal or interruption of the tract from the supraoptic nuclei to the posterior pituitary gland. After the postoperative period it is not uncommon for secretory function of the supraoptic nuclei to resume. Only 10% of the neurosecretory neurons must remain intact to avoid central DI. Although transient DI may accompany any injury to the neurohypophysis, permanent DI generally occurs only after neurohypophyseal damage high in the pituitary stalk.

A rare clinical syndrome of DI associated with diabetes mellitus, optic atrophy, and neurosensory hear-

Table 14.3
Causes of Diabetes Insipidus

- Central (neurogenic) DI
  - Genetic
  - Trauma (neurosurgical, radiation, accidental)
  - Secondary to tumors of hypothalamus
    - Glioma
    - Germinoma
    - Cyst
    - Craniopharyngioma
  - Histiocytosis X
  - Infection (viral, bacterial, parasitic, fungal)
  - Vascular (aneurysm, thrombosis, embolus)
- Psychogenic water drinker
- Renal tubular deficiency
  - Nephrogenic DI
  - Hypokalemia
  - Hypercalcemia
  - Chronic renal failure

ing loss has been recognized (Wolfram syndrome). The order of appearance of the various components varies (Dreyer et al, 1982).

DI may also occur in the newborn infant following asphyxia, intraventricular hemorrhage, sepsis, and meningitis.

The major symptoms of DI are polyuria, thirst, and polydipsia. The volume of urine excreted may vary from only a few liters per day in the case of a partial deficiency of hormone, to a maximum of nearly 18 liters daily, the average volume of glomerular filtrate delivered to collecting ducts in the total absence of VP. The onset of DI is often abrupt, the patient or parents being able to pinpoint the exact moment. In the previously toilet-trained child nocturia and enuresis may be the first clues. Excessive crying, growth failure, and fever of unknown origin are commonly seen in the infant with DI. In the older child, anorexia is common. Children with DI perspire little or not at all. The skin is dry and pale.

DI secondary to head trauma or surgery in the hypothalamic-pituitary area may be transient or permanent. Transient polyuria may begin 1–3 days after trauma or surgery and lasts from 1–7 days. This variety of DI is probably related to the onset and resolution of local edema.

Permanent polyuria may begin within the first 2 or 3 days after trauma or surgery to the head and is secondary to marked hypothalamic damage. There may be a triphasic pattern of DI beginning with polyuria within 2 or 3 days after the trauma and lasting 1–7 days. This is followed by a period of normal urinary output for 1–7 days and then by permanent polyuria. The interphase of normal urine output is probably due to release of stored VP. When the VP is completely exhausted, permanent DI ensues.

The familial form of DI varies in severity. Usually affected members of a family show some evidence of residual VP secretion and may be asymptomatic in early life. Patients may come to medical attention only years after symptoms of polyuria and polydipsia are first observed. Younger children may be brought to the physician because of persistent bed-wetting. Both autosomal dominant and X-linked inheritance have been described, the autosomal inheritance being more frequent.

In patients whose DI begins in childhood considerable dilatation of the urinary bladder, ureters, and renal pelvis may occur.

Diagnosis

DI must be separated from other polyuric states (Table 14.4). Serum and urine solutes should be measured for evidence of excess substances (glucose, mannitol, urea) which may cause an osmotic diuresis. Measurements of serum concentrations of creatinine and electrolytes will help discover alterations in glomerular filtration rate, hypokalemia, and hypercalcemia. A history of recent head trauma, intracranial surgery, or neurological deficits (bitemporal hemianopsia), which point to a midline tumor would suggest DI as the cause of the polyuria.

Table 14.4
Causes of Polyuria

Damage to the hypothalamic-neurohypophyseal system, DI
Excessive thirst, compulsive water drinking
Psychogenic
Hypothalamic lesion(s)
Decreased renal responsiveness to VP, nephrogenic DI
Osmotic diuresis
Diabetes mellitus
Chronic renal insufficiency

Making the diagnosis of DI hinges on the demonstration that urinary osmolality is inappropriately low when serum osmolality is raised. Classically in DI the urine specific gravity is 1.005 or less and the urinary osmolality is less than 200 mOsm/kg H_2O. The patient with complete DI has polyuria of at least 10–12 L/day with a urinary osmolality below 100 mOsm/kg H_2O. Serum sodium concentration and osmolality are elevated.

Often an initial evaluation of the child with suspected DI can be performed by the mother at home. She is instructed to collect each urine sample through a 24-hour period in separate bottles. The volume and time of each sample can be recorded and an aliquot placed in a test tube for subsequent measurement of specific gravity and/or osmolality. The mother should also record volumes and times of fluid intake. The log and urine samples are brought in the next day and values for 24-hour fluid intake and output as well as urine osmolalities throughout the period can be ascertained. Such data are invaluable in evaluating the patient with partial or complete DI. Figures depicting the relationship between urine and plasma osmolalities in normal children and patients with DI have been published (Richman et al, 1981). These are very helpful in the initial evaluation of the patient and in interpreting results of fluid deprivation.

Distinguishing true DI from compulsive water drinking may be difficult. Psychogenic polydipsia is seldom seen in childhood and generally these compulsive water drinkers deny the classical history found in most patients with DI, such as sudden onset of symptoms, persistent need to drink during the night, and preference for iced water. Their serum sodium and osmolality values are usually in the low normal range even upon awakening. Occasionally the chronic excess water consumption may have decreased or abolished the renal concentration gradient. In such instances urine concentration after water deprivation initially will be suboptimal. A 24-hour urine volume greater than 18 liters, a random serum osmolality value below 285 mOsm/kg H_2O, or a history of episodic polyuria are all suggestive of compulsive water drinking.

Basal levels of VP depend upon the state of hydration. Therefore, tests of VP secretion must rely on stimulation-suppression testing to evaluate VP control mechanisms. The basis of most tests for neurogenic DI rests on the ability of the kidney to excrete a hypertonic urine after an osmotic stimulus. The simplest way to achieve hypertonicity of body fluids is by water deprivation.

Water Deprivation Test

The water deprivation test (Miller et al, 1970) is begun in the morning either after a light breakfast or no breakfast at all, but no restriction on fluids overnight before the test. In the morning the bladder is emptied and the urine is discarded. All intake of food and fluids is stopped and 1 hour later the patient is weighed and samples of urine and blood are obtained for determinations of osmolality and sodium concentration. Hourly determination of weight and urine osmolality are obtained thereafter until two urine osmolalities vary by less than 30 mOsm/kg H_2O or when 3–5% of body weight is lost. Final blood and urine samples are analyzed at that point. In most instances, the water deprivation test is followed by the administration of VP to test responsiveness to the hormone.

In general, the time required to achieve a maximal urine concentration varies from 4–18 hours; most tests are conducted for 8 hours. A final urine/serum osmolality greater than 1.5 and/or a change in the ratio of 1.0 or more indicates normal ability to concentrate urine. In normal persons the plasma osmolality should remain in the normal range (about 295 mOsm/kg H_2O) and the urine should be concentrated to an osmolality of about 800 mOsm/kg H_2O. In true DI the plasma osmolality will rise, whereas the urine osmolality will not rise and the U/P ratio will be less than 1. In compulsive water drinking the ability to concentrate urine may be compromised, but the urine osmolality will rise and the U/P ratio should approach 1.9. It will certainly exceed 1.

Thus, the persistent excretion of dilute urine, a rise in serum sodium (>145 mEq/L) and serum osmolality (>290 mOsm/kg), and a weight loss of 3–5% suggest the presence of DI.

The results of the water deprivation test may be difficult to assess in patients with a partial deficiency of DI. Direct measurements of serum VP may be helpful, but such assays have only recently become available and care must be taken in interpreting the results (Zerbe and Robertson, 1981).

Patients with a diminished sensation of thirst and a diminished release of VP in response to osmotic stimulation may show inconclusive results in the water deprivation test. Since these individuals have normal VP production and storage and the volume receptor mechanism for VP release is intact, the hypovolemia which can occur during the test will stimulate VP release. In these patients osmotic urine-concentrating ability may be tested by increasing plasma osmolality while normal blood volume is maintained. This is usually accomplished by administering hypertonic saline (Hickey and Hare, 1944). With continued administration of the saline progressive hypernatremia ensues; however, these patients cannot respond to the osmotic stimulus with sufficient secretion of VP to concentrate the urine. In addition they have no thirst response to the hypernatremia. Normal subjects will have an antidiuresis within 30 minutes of the onset of the saline infusion. Patients with DI show an increase in urine volume and a fall in urine osmolality. This test should not be performed in children with nephrogenic DI. Severe hypernatremia may ensue requiring large amounts of solute-free water to correct.

Vasopressin Test

The water deprivation test is usually followed immediately by the administration of VP to test responsiveness to the hormone. This test must be administered under careful supervision so that water intoxication in patients with primary polydipsia is avoided. Either aqueous Pitressin (0.1 U/kg body weight) given intramuscularly or 1-desamino-8-D-arginine vasopressin (DDAVP) (20 μg) given intranasally should be followed promptly by a reduction in urine output and a subsequent increase in urine osmolality in VP-sensitive patients. A patient with nephrogenic DI will show no response.

Treatment

The treatment for DI is the administration of VP. Several preparations of the hormone are available. A short acting aqueous preparation (Pitressin) is of value in short-term treatment. Intermittent intramuscular injections of 0.1–1.0 ml are usually effective and last for 4–6 hours. The higher doses may produce side effects.

Pitressin tannate in oil (PTO), like Pitressin, is obtained from animal pituitaries, but has a longer duration of action. It is given intramuscularly in doses of 0.25–1.0 ml. The ampule of hormone should be warmed and agitated so that the active hormone, which appears as a brownish material at the bottom, will be suspended. Usually the entire contents of the ampule (1 ml) can be given. The duration of action is variable (24–72 hours) and the preparation is, therefore, a potential cause of water intoxication. It should be avoided in children under 3 years of age, and in older children careful monitoring of its use may be necessary in the early stages of treatment.

Nasal sprays are also available. Lysine-8-VP nasal spray is cleared from the blood within 4 hours after application. It is useful in patients for whom use of longer acting preparations would present significant risk of water intoxication. The synthetic analogue, DDAVP, is the drug of choice as hormone replacement in DI. The modification of the molecule gives the analogue a longer duration of action (8–24 hours) and greatly diminished vasopressor activity. Nasal insufflation of DDAVP, 2.5–10 μg (0.025–0.10 ml) once or twice daily, will usually restore the amount of fluid ingested and the urine volume to normal. The required dosage is variable and is unrelated to age and body size. The percent absorption from the nasal mucosa decreases as the dosage is increased. Upper respiratory infections or allergic rhinitis associated with excess mucus may interfere with hormone absorption. A disadvantage of DDAVP is the expense of the preparation when compared to the cost of PTO. Thus, it is wise to start with a small dose and increase in increments of 2.5 μg as needed. Side effects of DDAVP are uncommon. Headaches may occur and at large dosages (40 μg) increased blood pressure has been reported. In infants and in patients with a disturbed mechanism for thirst, continuous use can be associated with water intoxication. With children who can be managed on a single daily dose of DDAVP the dose should be given in the evening so that sleep is not interrupted. Often the single dose will carry the child until the next afternoon or evening. In some cases twice daily doses are necessary.

Certain nonhormonal preparations are helpful in the treatment of partial DI. Chlorpropamide is one such agent. Its antidiuretic action is three-fold: it amplifies the response of medullary adenylate cyclase to VP, stimulates adenylate cyclase directly, and antagonizes prostaglandins, which inhibit the activity of adenylate cyclase. The recommended dose of 150 mg/m^2 of body surface is given once daily. Among the effects of the drug is a rise in insulin secretion with resulting hypoglycemia. This is rarely a problem unless the dose that is given is excessive or unless there is concomitant deficiency of hormones of the anterior pituitary.

Those patients with CNS lesions who have disturbances of the thirst center as well as DI will require very careful management of water balance (Andersson and Rundgren, 1982). The patient must be instructed in regard to daily fluid intake required.

Patients with DI and inadequate water intake become water depleted and hypernatremic with ensuing hypertonic encephalopathy. The brain adjusts to the hypertonicity in part by increasing intracellular solute content. If repletion of water occurs too rapidly the dilution of extracellular fluid will cause translocation of water into cells to achieve osmotic equilibrium. The result is cellular swelling and cerebral edema. A good rule of thumb is to reduce the concentration of sodium in serum to normal over 36–48 hours, or a reduction of 1 mEq sodium/L of serum every 2 hours.

CONTROVERSY

There is a difference of opinion over the hormonal treatment of the patient with DI who is receiving IV fluids postoperatively or who has acute gastrointestinal disorders. The options are to maintain antidiuresis or to eliminate VP therapy entirely. Certainly in the infant there is real danger of water intoxication, especially under conditions of full antidiuresis and i.v. fluids. A slight excess of fluid over a short period of time can lead to convulsions and other CNS evidence of water intoxication. Water requirements under full antidiuresis are very restrictive (ca 1.6 L/m^2/24 hours for infants with normal activity and diet). Since normal infants on formula receive about 2.5 L of water/m^2/24 hours, it is obvious that a period free of VP activity is required daily to prevent water intoxication. Thus, whether or not VP is used, a very careful hourly record of fluid intake and output is required. Twice daily body weights, serum electrolytes, and BUN measurements should be obtained.

Our preference is to avoid the use of VP in infants until 2 weeks after surgery or until the acute intestinal disorder is resolved. The fluid regimen is adjusted such that the hourly intake is matched to urine output, with the following limits: minimal fluid 0.8 L/m^2/day, maximal fluid (assuming diet solute 500 mOsm/m^2/day) 2.3 L/m^2/day. The maximal fluid allotment can be liberalized if the child is thirsty and water is being excreted. Sodium intake is kept within the range of 5–30 mEq/m^2/day and potassium 30–100 mEq/m^2/day. The lower limit of water intake is required for insensible loss and the excretion of solute. The sodium restriction decreases solute load and, therefore, water requirements.

Other groups prefer to maintain the patient under constant antidiuresis, which can be induced with DDAVP, or with i.v. infusion of aqueous VP, 0.5 U/kg of body weight/minute. The volume of IV fluids should be reduced initially to about 0.8 L/m^2/day and thereafter be adjusted according to observed changes in urine and serum osmolarity and sodium concentrations obtained at 12-hour intervals.

Prognosis

Partial or complete DI can be managed very successfully with hormonal replacement therapy or drugs that amplify the action of VP produced in small amounts. Those underlying lesions responsible for the DI may cause other pituitary hormone deficiencies, necessitating additional hormonal replacement regimens. The risk of water intoxication has been alluded to and the patient must be instructed to watch for prodromal signs such as headache. Occasionally disturbances of the thirst center accompany DI and seriously complicate the management of water balance in these patients.

SYNDROME OF INAPPROPRIATE SECRETION OF ANTIDIURETIC HORMONE

Definition

This syndrome (SIADH) represents a condition in which secretion of VP persists despite hypotonicity of plasma (hence the name inappropriate). It is characterized by fluid retention.

Basic Science

The syndrome may result from stimulation of VP secretion in the course of specific diseases, most commonly CNS (tumor, infection, inflammation, trauma, hemorrhage) or pulmonary (viral and bacterial pneumonias) disease; aberrant production of VP by a tumor; or it may occur secondary to drugs that cause increased release of VP, enhance the action of VP on the kidney,

CASE ILLUSTRATION

A 4-year-old boy was seen in the clinic with a 3-week history of urinating and drinking all the time. The mother counted 17 trips to the bathroom in 1 day. The patient had been perfectly healthy except for occasional asthma attacks. He had had no head injuries of any type. The parents tried restricting fluids but the child became uncontrollable and tried to drink from the toilet bowl. The boy had been toilet-trained but over the past 3 weeks he had been wetting the bed each night. Otherwise the child remained perfectly healthy with no behavioral problems.

The mother had been diagnosed as having epilepsy the previous year. There was no family history of DI, kidney disease, or endocrine disorders. The paternal grandfather had mild adult-onset diabetes mellitus, controlled with diet.

The physical examination was completely normal. Urinalysis on admission revealed a specific gravity of 1.005 with no sugar, acetone, or albumin present. Serum electrolytes were normal. BUN was 12.

The child was admitted for observation and evaluation. Radiographs of the skull, chest, and wrist were reported as showing no abnormalities. A neurologic evaluation revealed no evidence of a CNS lesion. Thyroid and adrenal functions were normal. Growth and bone age were appropriate for chronologic age. Urine output averaged 150 ml/hour and fluid intake matched this output. Urine S.G. were very low (1.001–1.005) throughout a 36-hour observation period and remained low after an 8-hour period of water deprivation (a shorter period would have been acceptable if the child was excessively thirsty). Immediately after the water deprivation test the urine osmolality was 110 mOsm/kg H_2O. Administration of aqueous pitressin raised the urine osmolality to 850 mOsm/kg H_2O and lowered the plasma osmolality to 285 mOsm/kg H_2O.

The diagnosis of idiopathic DI was made and 2.5 μg (0.025 ml) of DDAVP were administered twice a day. Subsequently the dose had to be increased to 5 μg (0.05 ml) twice daily to maintain the patient symptom-free.

Over several years of follow-up the child has shown no evidence of a CNS lesion nor other endocrine deficiencies. He continues to require DDAVP but is otherwise perfectly heatlhy.

This child represents a straightforward case of central DI. Such children require lifelong follow-up since manifestations of a CNS lesion may occur many years after the diagnosis of DI has been made.

For a discussion of nephrogenic DI, see page 633.

or promote renal water reabsorption independently of VP. Chlorpropamide, carbamazepine, analgesics and barbiturates induce VP secretion. Chemotherapeutic agents such as vincristine and cytoxan can cause SIADH.

Natural History

The symptoms of SIADH are related to water retention and eventual water intoxication. Usually weight gain is accompanied by anorexia and lethargy. The patient may complain of headache and show signs of irritability. When the serum sodium concentration falls below 120 mEq/L more severe symptoms including nausea, vomiting, confusion, convulsions, and coma may ensue. Symptoms are more likely to be severe in acute water intoxication. In chronic hyponatremia, patients may be asymptomatic even with serum sodium concentrations below 125 mEq/L.

Diagnosis

The diagnosis is established by the finding of hypoosmolality of serum accompanied by urine that is less than maximally dilute and with persistent urinary excretion of sodium. Serum concentrations of sodium, urea, creatinine, uric acid, and albumin are low. The concentration of sodium in the urine is high (>30 mEq/L).

Treatment

SIADH should be treated with fluid restriction. In patients in whom the hyponatremia has occurred rapidly and is life-threatening a more rapid form of therapy is necessary. Either the infusion of hypertonic saline (slow, IV, 3% saline, 5 ml/kg) and/or the administration of furosemide will bring about a rise in serum sodium concentration and a concurrent water diuresis. No attempt should be made to correct the hyponatremia rapidly, since central pontine myelinolysis has been produced with this maneuver in experimental models (Norenberg and Leslie, 1982). Demethylchlortetracycline, a drug that interferes with the renal action of VP, has been used for long-term treatment of chronic SIADH in adults.

Summary

Polyuria and polydipsia are common symptoms in clinical practice. Among the causes of these disorders is insufficient or absent production of vasopressin (antidiuretic hormone) by the paraventricular and supraoptic nuclei of the hypothalamus. Injury to these areas of the brain can produce partial or complete neurogenic DI. Even with normal secretion of VP, some patients have a genetic lack of the VP receptor in the kidney, which causes lack of response to the hormone. This form of DI is nephrogenic.

Finally, inappropriate release of VP in the presence of hypotonic plasma produces a clinical syndrome of water intoxication. The normal release of and response to VP is essential for the maintenance of fluid balance.

REFERENCES

Andersson B, Rundgren M: Thirst and its disorders. *Annu Rev Med* 33:231, 1982.

Brownstein MJ, Russell JT, Gainer H: Synthesis, transport and release of posterior pituitary hormones. *Science* 207:373, 1980.

Crigler JF Jr: Diabetes insipidus. *Curr Pediatr Ther* 11:319, 1984.

Dreyer M, Rudiger HW, Bujara K, et al: The syndrome of diabetes insipidus, diabetes mellitus, optic atrophy, deafness, and other abnormalities. (DIDMOAD-Syndrome).*Klin Wochenschr* 60:471, 1982.

Hickey RC, Hare K: The renal excretion of chloride and water in diabetes insipidus. *J Clin Invest* 23:768, 1944.

Miller M, Moses AM, Streeten DH: Recognition of partial defects in antidiuretic hormone secretion. *Ann Intern Med* 73:721, 1970.

Norenberg MD, Leslie KO: Correction of hyponatremia and central pontine myelinolysis. *Am J Med* 73:882, 1982.

Richman RA, Post EM, Notman DD, et al: Simplifying the diagnosis of diabetes insipidus in children. *Am J Dis Child* 135:839, 1981.

Russell JT, Brownstein MJ, Gainer H: Biosynthesis of vasopressin, oxytocin, and neurophysins: Isolation and characterization of two common precursors (propressophysin and prooxyphysin. *Endocrinology* 107:1880, 1980.

Sklar AH, Schrier RW: Central nervous system mediators of vasopressin release. *Physiol Rev* 63:1243, 1983.

Verbalis JG, Robinson AG: Characterization of neurophysin-vasopressin prohormones in human posterior pituitary tissue. *J Clin Endocrinol Metabol* 57:115, 1983.

Zerbe RL, Robertson GL: A comparison of plasma vasopressin measurements with a standard indirect test in the differential diagnosis of polyuria. *N Engl J Med* 305:1539, 1981.

Thyroid Gland

4

Definition

Because of the pre-eminent role of the thyroid hormone in growth and differentiation, disorders of thyroid function often manifest themselves as abnormalities of linear growth, weight, and bone maturation. The signs and symptoms of thyroid dysfunction can be very subtle and the diagnosis of hypothyroidism in particular can be missed easily.

Basic Science

The anlage of the thyroid gland appears at about the 3- to 4-mm stage of the embryo (about 16–17 days of gestation). The primordium of the thyroid appears as a proliferation of endoderm of foregut in the pharyngeal floor. Subsequently (4–5 weeks) this thickened anlage migrates to its location over the thyroid cartilage. Thyroid tissue also arises laterally from the fourth branchial pouch. Much of this tissue undergoes cystic degeneration; however, some may contribute to the normal thyroid gland. The stalk, which connects the thyroid gland to the pharyngeal floor (the thyroglossal duct), undergoes elongation as the thyroid migrates caudad. With time, the thyroglossal duct gradually disappears, except for cells of the lower portion which may remain to form the pyramidal lobe of the thyroid gland.

In humans, the ultimobranchial body (a distinct structure in submammmalian vertebrates derived from the fifth branchial pouch) and the medial portion of the fourth branchial pouch become incorporated into the lateral lobes of the thyroid and form the calcitonin-secreting parafollicular cells or C cells. These C cells are derived from ectodermal neural crest precursors that migrate ventrally into the branchial pouch. Thus, their origin is neural whereas the thyroid follicular cells which form thyroid hormone are endodermal in origin.

The follicular cells of the thyroid gland line the follicles, which are filled with colloid. The parafollicular or C cells never reach the colloid space, but remain in the periphery of the follicles.

The thyroid gland begins to function around the eighth week of gestation. Thyroglobulin is produced and, by 10 weeks, iodine trapping is evident in the thyroid. By the twelfth week thyroid hormone is produced and colloid appears in the lumen of the follicle. The major thyroid hormone produced by the fetus is thyroxine (T_4). Conversion of T_4 to 3,5,3′-triiodothyronine (T_3) is low in the fetus, whereas conversion of T_4 to 3,3′, 5′-triiodothyronine (reverse T_3; rT_3) occurs readily and levels of rT_3 in fetal fluids are higher than those for T_3. After the 18th to 20th week of gestation serum T_4 levels increase progressively until term. Serum T_3 levels in the fetus increase from 30 weeks of gestation to term, while the serum levels of rT_3 fall (Fisher and Klein, 1981).

Iodide crosses the placenta readily; however, thyroid hormones do not cross to any degree so that the fetus is dependent upon hormones from its own thyroid gland. A chorionic thyrotropin in placenta has been described but its role in fetal thyroid function is unknown.

Iodide

One of the most important and unique functions of the thyroid gland is to concentrate and store iodide. For the thyroid gland to synthesize adequate amounts of thyroid hormone, iodide must enter the gland more rapidly than would be possible by simple diffusion. There is a transport mechanism that achieves this end. The exact biochemical mechanism of the transport is unknown; however, like other active transport mechanisms, iodide transport in the thyroid is an energy-requiring process and is closely related to the function of the Na^+/K^+-dependent adenosine triphosphatase (ATPase) system. ATPase, acting on adenosine triphosphate (ATP) at the cell membrane, may make phosphate bond energy available for iodide transport. Iodide transport is enhanced by thyroid-stimulating hormone (TSH) and decreased by hypophysectomy. It is also influenced by the glandular content of organic iodide in an autoregulatory manner. The ability of the thyroid gland to concentrate iodide is shared by the salivary, mammary, and gastric glands and by the choroid plexus.

Synthesis of Thyroid Hormones

Once trapped within the thyroid gland, iodide is rapidly oxidized into organic iodine. This process is coupled to the transport process so that very little inorganic iodide is found within the thyroid cells.

The first step in organification of iodide is oxidation of the iodide ion to iodine, probably mediated by a peroxidase (Fig. 14.8). The product may be I^+ or a free radical of iodine and it is the intermediate that is incorporated into the tyrosyl residues of thyroglobulin. The latter is the major protein synthesized by the thyroid cell. It is a large glycoprotein with a molecular weight of 660,000. The iodination of thyroglobulin is believed to occur at the interface of the follicular cell and the lumen of the colloid space where the thyroid peroxidase is located. Both mono- and diiodotyrosines are formed in the thyroglobulin molecule and these, in turn, can condense to form T_3 (monoiodotyrosine coupled with diiodotyrosine) and thyroxine (two diiodotyrosines condense). T_4 is preferentially formed over T_3. The condensing process is activated by peroxidase and once the coupling is complete the finished thyroglobulin molecule is transported into the colloid space of the follicle where it is stored. Some of the thyroglobulin is secreted into the blood stream and provides a marker for the presence of thyroid tissue.

About one-quarter of iodide in the thyroid gland is in the form of T_4, about 3% as T_3, and the rest as mono- and diiodotyrosine. T_4 and T_3 are liberated from thyroglobulin by proteolytic cleavage within the follicular cell (Fig. 14.7). The thyroglobulin in the colloid is taken into the follicular cells by endocytosis. Droplets containing thyroglobulin can be seen within the cells. These droplets subsequently fuse with cellular lysosomes and thyroglobulin is hydrolyzed, releasing T_4 and T_3. Any monoiodotyrosine or diiodotyrosine released in this hydrolysis is deiodinated and the iodine is reused.

Regulation of Thyroid Hormone Synthesis

The synthesis and release of T_4 and T_3 are controlled by TSH from the anterior pituitary. TSH is synthesized by a special cell in the pituitary called the thyrotroph. The hormone is a glycoprotein of 28,000 daltons and like other glycoprotein hormones (luteinizing hormone [LH], follicle-stimulating hormone [FSH]) it is composed of an α and a β subunit. The α units of these hormones are identical, but each β subunit is unique and confers specificity on the hormone. There are now highly specific and sensitive radioimmunoassays for TSH in blood. The normal range is 0.5–4.5 μunits/ml. There are fluctuations in serum TSH every hour or 2 suggesting a pulsatile release from the thyrotroph. Its effect on the thyroid follicular cell is to enhance all steps involved in the synthesis and release of thyroid hormones. TSH binds to a specific membrane receptor activating adenylate cyclase to increase the intracellular level of cyclic adenosine monophosphate (cAMP). Apparently a calcium-calmodulin complex is involved in the regulation of TSH-stimulated human thyroid adenylate cyclase (Lakey et al, 1985).

The synthesis and release of TSH is governed by two major factors: (1) thyrotropin-releasing hormone (TRH) from the hypothalamus, which is stimulatory,

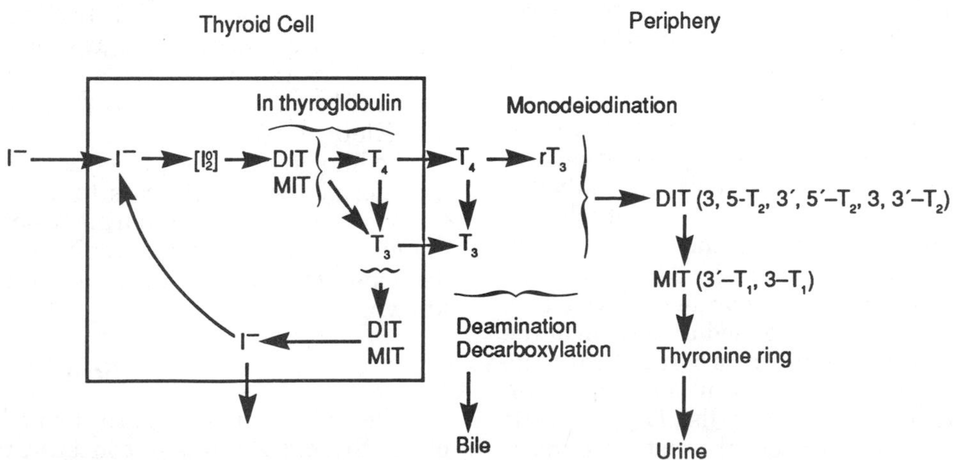

Figure 14.8. Synthesis and metabolism of thyroid hormones.

and (2) thyroid hormone in the blood, which is inhibitory. TRH is a tripeptide, pyro-glutamyl-histidyl-prolinamide, which is found throughout the CNS and in the gut. TRH in the blood stream has a half-life of 5½ minutes and appropriate doses (200–500 μg) will cause a rise in serum TSH, with a peak at 30 minutes. TRH also causes serum levels of prolactin to rise.

The response of thyrotroph to TRH is decreased by any increase in serum T_4 concentration. The thyrotroph can convert T_4 to T_3 and contains high affinity nuclear receptors for T_3. Therefore, feedback inhibition of TSH secretion by thyroid hormones is probably mediated at the nuclear level. There may also be a decrease in TRH receptors induced by thyroid hormones. When T_4 concentration in the blood is low the response of thyrotrophs to TRH is exaggerated.

Metabolism of Thyroid Hormones

Over 80% of T_3 is produced peripherally. T_4 formed in the thyroid gland can be metabolized peripherally by monodeiodinating enzymes. One of these, a 5′-monodeiodinase, removes an iodine atom, from the outer ring of the T_4 molecule to yield 3,5,3′-T_3; the other, a 5-monodeiodinase, removes an iodine atom from the inner ring to yield 3,3,5′-triiodothyronine (reverse T_3; rT_3). About one-third of the T_4 produced in the thyroid gland is converted peripherally to T_3 and another third to rT_3. T_3 and rT_3 can be further deiodinated to yield diiodthyronines and these, in turn, can be metabolized to monoiodothyronines. Ultimately the monoiodothyronines lose their iodine, and the iodine-free thyronine ring and its metabolites are excreted in the urine. Other metabolites of T_4 and T_3 (deaminated and decarboxylated forms) are excreted in the bile.

Within the blood, T_4 and T_3 circulate bound to protein. The major binding protein is thyroxine-binding globulin (TBG) which carries about 70% of T_4 and T_3 (Hocman, 1981). Thyroxine-binding prealbumin (TBPA) carries about 20% of T_4 and very little if any T_3. Albumin also serves to carry T_4 (10%) and T_3 (30%). Only about 0.03% of T_4 and 0.3% of T_3 are not bound to protein and remain free in the serum.

It was originally believed that only the free hormone was available for entry into tissues. However, the dissociation of T_4 and T_3 from albumin is very rapid (<1 second) and the reaction provides additional "bioavailable" hormone to enter target tissues.

T_3 is the metabolically active thyroid hormone, 20% of which is formed in the thyroid gland and 80% in the periphery from T_4. The latter functions as a prohormone which can be converted to T_3 in a variety of tissues, including the pituitary gland. Actually within the pituitary thyrotroph of the rat there is a different 5′-deiodinase (type II) from that found primarily in liver and kidney (type I 5′-deiodinase). The type II enzyme, for example, is not inhibited by propylthiouracil and has a relatively low Km and Vmax for T_4 (Visser et al, 1983). The nuclear T_3 in the rat pituitary gland is generated locally from T_4 and by a mechanism different from that of liver T_3. A fall in either T_4 or T_3 in the serum leads to a reduction in intracellular T_3 in the pituitary thyrotroph which is the major site for inhibition of TSH secretion (Larsen et al, 1981).

Tests of Thyroid Function

A variety of tests of thyroid function are available to the practicing physician. The interpretation of these tests is not always easy, making the diagnosis of thyroid disease sometimes difficult (Griffen, 1985). For example, critically ill patients often have low levels of T_4 and T_3 in the blood. This condition is often referred to as the euthyroid sick syndrome (Zaloga and O'Brian, 1985). The decrease in circulating thyroid hormones is due, in part, to decreased protein binding, but other factors such as enhanced metabolic clearance rate of T_4 and decreased production and secretion of T_4 are probably involved also. The levels of free T_4 are usually normal and the patient is metabolically euthyroid.

The following tests are frequently performed to assess thyroid status.

SERUM TOTAL T_4

The total concentration of T_4 in the serum is measured by radioimmunoassay (RIA). This value includes both the free and protein-bound T_4. An increase in TBG in the blood will increase total T_4 and a decrease in TBG will decrease serum T_4. A variety of factors will increase or decrease serum TBG (Table 14.5). Normally the serum T_4 ranges between 5 and 12 μg/dl. Because values outside this range may reflect changes in TBG rather than thyroid status it is the usual practice to obtain an estimate of the free fraction as well as the total T_4.

ESTIMATE OF FREE FRACTION OF THYROID HORMONE (IN VITRO UPTAKE TEST)

This test gives an approximation of the amount of T_4 bound to protein. It is performed by incubating the patient's serum with radiolabeled T_4 or T_3. A solid-phase matrix (resin, charcoal) is added, which will bind any labeled T_3 not bound to protein in the patient's serum. After a "standard" interval of time, the proportion of labeled T_4 or T_3 bound by the solid phase is measured. This proportion varies inversely with the

Table 14.5
Causes of Altered Levels of Thyroid-Binding Globulin in Serum

Increased TBG	Decreased TBG
Genetic	Genetic
Hypothyroidism	Androgens
Estrogens	Severe hypoproteinemia
Acute intermittent porphyria	Diphenylhydantoin
	Glucocorticoids (high-dose)
	Nephrosis

overall net binding affinity of the serum proteins. Thus the product of the in vitro uptake value and the serum total T_4 concentration provides a so-called "free T_4 index" or FT_4I, which is analogous to and usually varies with the serum-free T_4. Because of its less intense binding by serum proteins, which leads to higher uptake values and, therefore, reduced counting time and error, labeled T_3 is used more often than is labeled T_4 in these in vitro uptake tests.

In some laboratories, values of the in vitro uptake test are "normalized" by expressing them as a fraction of the uptake value in a standard normal serum. The normalized FT_4I is calculated by multiplying the uptake ratio (patient uptake/pooled normal serum uptake) times the serum total T_4 and has a numerical normal range similar to that of the normal serum total T_4 concentrations.

TBG can be measured directly by RIA. If hereditary defects in TBG production are suspected a direct measurement of serum TBG may be helpful.

SERUM T_3

The total amount of T_3 in serum is measured by RIA and normal values range from 80–180 ng/dl. The concentration of serum T_3 in most patients with hyperthyroidism is elevated even when the serum T_4 value is normal. In hypothyroidism serum T_3 levels may be normal or low. Several factors impair the conversion of T_4 to T_3, resulting in a low serum T_3. Among these are: systemic illness, fasting, surgery, glucocorticoids, radiopaque dyes, and drugs such as propylthiouracil (PTU) and propranolol.

SERUM-FREE T_4 AND T_3

These tests are not available in most laboratories. The measurements are performed by equilibrium dialysis. More recently an RIA for free T_4 has become available. In general, the FT_4I provides sufficient information for most clinical conditions.

SERUM TSH

The amount of TSH in serum is measured by RIA, with normal values ranging from 0.5–4.5 μU/ml. There is a modest diurnal variation. Serum TSH levels are rarely greater than 4 μU/ml in euthyroid individuals. Values are usually <0.5 μU/ml in hyperthyroidism and >10 μU/ml in hypothyroidism. Levels of TSH in serum are decreased by thyroid hormone preparations, corticosteroids, dopamine, and somatostatin. They are also diminished with malnutrition, fever, and stress.

A recently developed immunoradiometric assay for TSH offers greater sensitivity so that the low levels found in euthyroid patients can be measured, whereas the very low levels in hyperthyroidism remain undetectable (Caldwell et al, 1985). In patients with normal TSH values by this sensitive assay and low serum T_4 values pituitary disease should be suspected.

TRH TEST

A dose of 7 μg/kg of TRH is administered intravenously to the patient. A rise in TSH is observed normally 20–30 minutes later and the serum TSH level returns to baseline by 90 minutes. The increment is normally at least 2 μU/ml. In hypothyroidism the response is exaggerated, whereas in hyperthyroidism there is no response.

SERUM rT_3

The level of rT_3 in serum is measured by RIA, with normal values ranging from 10–40 ng/dl. The value is increased in hyperthyroidism, with increased amounts of binding protein, or with decreased activity of 5′-deiodinase. Serum rT_3 levels are decreased in hypothyroidism.

RADIOIODINE UPTAKE

The iodine trapping activity of the thyroid gland can be evaluated by administering ^{123}I (half-life 13 hours) orally to the patient and measuring the level of radioactivity over the thyroid gland at 4 hours and 24 hours after giving the isotope. Normal uptakes are 5–15% at 4 hours and 10–30% at 24 hours. These values are increased in hyperthyroidism and usually decreased in hypothyroidism. It is difficult to distinguish hypothyroidism from euthyroidism because of the large overlap in values. Radioactive iodine uptake is decreased by iodide, corticosteroids, and dopamine.

Technetium (99m-Tc) is a particularly useful radioisotope for children since, in contrast to iodine, it is trapped but not organified by the thyroid and has a half-life of only 6 hours. In addition, the exposure to radioactivity is lower with a technetium scan than with an ^{123}I scan. Imaging is done within 1 hour of administration of the isotope. It may be used for scanning to detect ectopic thyroid tissues or to evaluate thyroid nodules. The disadvantage of technetium is the relatively low uptake by the thyroid and the lack of specificity for thyroid tissue.

SERUM THYROGLOBULIN

This protein can be measured in serum by RIA. It is a helpful test for the presence of thyroid tissue, since in the absence of thyroid cells no thyroglobulin will be detected in the serum.

THYROID FUNCTION DISORDERS

Hypothyroidism

Definition

Hypothyroidism constitutes a clinical state of thyroid hormone insufficiency. Complete or partial lack of thyroid hormone may occur and the condition may be present at birth (congenital) or develop at any time during the individual's life (acquired).

Congenital Hypothyroidism

Epidemiology

Hypothyroidism may be present at birth because of a variety of conditions (Table 14.6). There may be dysgenesis of the thyroid gland or ectopic positioning of the gland. Inborn errors of thyroid hormone synthesis (dyshormonogenesis) and abnormalities of the hypothalamic-pituitary system resulting in decreased TSH production will cause clinical symptoms of thyroid deficiency. Finally iodide deficiency, goitrogens or peripheral resistance to thyroid hormone can cause hypothyroidism.

Developmental defects of the thyroid gland are the most common causes of congenital hypothyroidism (Fisher and Klein, 1981). These occur in about 1/3500–4000 white infants and in about 1/30,000 black infants. One-third of these infants have no thyroid tissue at all on radionuclide scans. The thyroid rudiment, if there is one, is frequently found in an ectopic location anywhere from the base of the tongue to the normal position in the neck. The disorder is usually sporadic, but familial cases have been described. Twice as many females as males are affected.

Most patients with lingual thyroid glands have no functional tissue; however, in about one-quarter of the cases some thyroid tissue is present and responds to TSH by increasing in size. This may produce symptoms of airway obstruction or difficulty in swallowing. There may be enough thyroid hormone produced by the enlarged remnant so that clinical hypothyroidism is not evident at birth, but develops in early childhood.

Hereditary enzyme defects in thyroid hormone synthesis are the second most common cause of congenital hypothyroidism (Fisher and Klein, 1981). In Pendred syndrome goiter due to a peroxidase defect is associated with nerve deafness. The child may be euthyroid or mildly hypothyroid. Other enzyme defects are listed in Table 14.6.

Table 14.6
Causes of Hypothyroidism

Congenital
- Iodide deficiency (cretinism)
- Thyroid dysgenesis (aplasia, hypoplasia, or ectopic gland)
- Inborn errors of thyroid hormone synthesis[1]
- TSH and/or TRH deficiency
- Antithyroid drugs
- Resistance to TSH or thyroid hormone

Acquired
- Thyroiditis
- Ectopic thyroid gland
- TSH and/or TRH deficiency
- Antithyroid drugs (iodide, thiouracil, etc)
- Post-thyroidectomy or ^{131}I
- Infiltrative disease of thyroid: histiocytosis X, cystinosis
- Resistance to TSH or thyroid hormones

[1] Iodide-concentrating defect, peroxidase defect, deficiency of iodotyrosine deiodinase, defect in coupling enzyme (iodotyrosines to iodothyronines), defect in thyroglobulin synthesis.

The above disorders of thyroid development and enzyme function constitute forms of primary hypothyroidism. Disorders of pituitary production of TSH are classified as secondary hypothyroidism, while hypothalamic disorders impairing TRH release are classified as tertiary hypothyroidism.

In certain parts of the world iodine deficiency is endemic and children are born with iodine-deficiency, usually with goiters. Maternal ingestion of goitrogens or administration of radioactive iodine to the mother can result in congenital hypothyroidism.

Natural History

Before neonatal screening programs congenital hypothyroidism was rarely recognized in the newborn except in its most flagrant form (cretinism). Signs and symptoms may not be present at birth or may be insufficient for ready recognition (Klein, 1985). Several clues may be helpful. The hypothyroid newborn tends to be heavier at birth than the normal newborn infant and the physiologic jaundice of the newborn tends to be prolonged (2 weeks) secondary to delayed maturation of hepatic glucuronyl-transferase. Poor peripheral perfusion and mottled skin are early signs. Feeding difficulties are common and the infant is usually sluggish and sleepy. There may be respiratory difficulties secondary to an enlarged tongue. Passage of meconium may be delayed.

On physical examination, older patients will show the classic cretinoid appearance, including puffy myxedematous facies, depressed nasal bridge with pseudohypertelorism, a large protruding tongue with an open mouth, a hoarse cry, large fontanelles (especially the posterior) and wide sutures, umbilical hernia with abdominal distention, cold, mottled or jaundiced skin, hypotonia, and delayed reflex return. It is unusual for a goiter to be palpable, even in infants with enzymatic deficiencies. However, infants exposed to maternal goitrogens in utero may be born with large goiters, which can produce severe airway obstruction.

Infants with secondary or tertiary hypothyroidism often retain the ability to secrete some thyroid hormone so that their symptoms are generally milder and are often associated with symptoms of deficiencies of other pituitary hormones such as ACTH (hypoglycemia), gonadotrophins (small genitalia in males), or vasopressin (DI).

Diagnosis

In 1973, pilot screening programs were begun in Pittsburgh with measurements of TSH in cord blood, in the province of Quebec with T_4 measurements from dried blood on filter paper, and in Belgium with serum TSH determinations. Over the ensuing years more countries and areas joined in the screening program. In general, in North America and Australia T_4 is measured on specimens of dried blood on filter paper obtained at ages 1–5 days of life. In Europe and Japan TSH is measured on dried blood samples.

In the T_4 screening program, infants with low T_4 concentrations undergo further measurement to confirm TSH levels. Such screening programs will detect infants with TBG deficiency as well as those with hypothyroidism. The overall frequency of hypothyroidism in both the T_4 and TSH screening programs is 1:4000, a much higher incidence than had been thought to exist previously.

Once a low T_4 and/or TSH is detected in the serum by the state laboratory the infant's pediatrician is informed of this result. The infant should be examined as quickly as possible, checked for physical evidence of hypothyroidism, and blood should be drawn for additional thyroid hormone analysis. In general, it is wise to obtain: T_4, T_3, FT_4I, and TSH values on the blood sample. For diagnostic purposes a thyroid scan is helpful to look for evidence of thyroid tissue. A bone age should be obtained to assess the duration of the hypothyroidism. Most newborn infants will show ossification of the distal femur, proximal tibia and cuboid bone in the foot. When these centers are not seen the bone age is retarded for a newborn.

The normal values for serum thyroid hormones in the first weeks of life are higher than those found in older infants (Table 14.7). Therefore, values which might seem normal in an older child would be distinctly abnormal in the newborn or premature infant.

The chemical hallmarks of primary hypothyroidism are a low serum T_4 and FT_4I with an elevated serum TSH. The serum T_3 may be in the normal range; if it is decreased the hypothyroidism has probably been longstanding. If the serum T_4 concentration is normal, but the serum TSH level is high, a condition of compensated hypothyroidism exists. This suggests ectopic or hypoplastic thyroid tissue, dyshormonogenesis, or exposure to a goitrogen.

If the T_4 is low and the TSH is normal or low, secondary or tertiary hypothyroidism should be considered. Tests of pituitary function may be appropriate to examine levels of other pituitary hormones and the responsiveness of the pituitary to hypothalamic releasing hormones.

In congenital TBG deficiency the T_4 is low, but the FT_4I is usually normal. The deficiency can be confirmed by obtaining a serum TBG value. This congenital defect is inherited in a sex linked manner so that males are affected; the frequency is about 1:8900.

Treatment

Infants with hypothyroidism should receive L-thyroxine therapy after a blood sample for FT_4I and TSH has been obtained. A thyroid scan should be performed at that time or within a week or so of starting therapy. Therapy should not be delayed for the thyroid scan or additional testing. If the scan is normal, the blood values for thyroid hormones are borderline low normal, and the child is asymptomatic, a period of close observation can be instituted. Any evidence of a rising serum TSH level should suggest a failing thyroid gland. Obviously any evidence of a decline in rate of linear growth and excessive weight gain should alert the physician to the need to institute therapy. If there is any doubt about the presence of hypothyroidism it is safer to place the infant on therapy for the first 2 or 3 years and at that time the thyroid status can be reassessed. A brief interruption of therapy will not be harmful at that time. Since T_3 has a much shorter half-life than does T_4, the following protocol is recommended: 1 month before stopping therapy switch to T_3 (20 μg of T_3 equivalent to 100 μg of T_4) for 1 month, then discontinue therapy for 2 weeks before obtaining a blood sample for T_4, FT_4I, and TSH.

The treatment for each infant must be individualized. In general, a dose of 100 $\mu g/m^2$ of L-thyroxine is recommended, but in all instances the clinical response (growth, physical signs, and symptoms) and thyroid function tests (T_4, FT_4I, TSH) should provide the basis for changes in dose. After the initial evaluation and commencement of therapy, the child should be checked again at 2 weeks, 6 weeks, and 3 months, and every 3 months thereafter for the first 2 years of life. After age 2 years visits every 6 months are sufficient until growth and development are completed. Serum T_4 values should be maintained in the upper half of the normal range for the age of the patient. The TSH values are hard to suppress in early life, but every effort should be made to keep the plasma TSH level under 20 μU/ml in infants.

Table 14.7
Normal Values for Thyroid Hormone Levels in the First Weeks of Life

	Total T_4 (μg/dl)		Total T_3 (ng/dl)		TSH (μU/ml)	
Age	Mean	Range	Mean	Range	Mean	Range
Cord blood	10.2	7.4–13	45	15– 75	9.0	<2.5–17.4
1–3 days	17.2	11.8–22.6	145	32–216	8.0	<2.5–13.3
1–2 wk	13.2	9.8–16.6	250			
2–4 wk	11.0	7.0–15.0	160	160–240	4.0	0.6–10.0
1–4 months	10.3	7.2–14.4	163	117–209	<2.5	<2.5

Sources: Erenberg et al, 1974; Abuid et al, 1974.

Babies who are breast-fed may receive some thyroid hormone from the mother via the breast milk; however, this supply is small and will not protect the infant completely from the effects of hypothyroidism (Franklin et al, 1985).

Prognosis

Recent reviews of results of early therapy in those hypothyroid babies picked up in screening programs are generally encouraging (Barnes, 1985; Klein, 1985). In the New England Collaborative study 146 infants were diagnosed as hypothyroid over a 5-year period from a screening pool of 717,123 newborn infants (Arnold et al, 1984). Those that were adequately treated had IQs on annual psychometric examinations that were not significantly different from those of the control babies. Using somewhat different testing procedures (Griffith's developmental test) the Quebec screening program obtained results suggestive of poorer performance scores by previously diagnosed and treated hypothyroid babies in hearing-speech tests (at 18 and 36 months of age), and in practical reasoning (36 months of age) compared to controls (Glorieux et al, 1983). This group found a significant correlation between initial serum T_4 concentration, BA, and IQ at 36 months. From their results it appears that the duration and severity of fetal hypothyroidism are the most important factors dictating the outcome of mental development in these infants. In agreement with this conclusion is the finding in the New England Collaborative Group Study that 3 of 4 infants with obvious clinical symptoms of hypothyroidism at birth had a significantly impaired IQ when studied later despite early therapy. Nevertheless, all studies agree that early therapy is important in preventing mental retardation.

Acquired Hypothyroidism

Many of the conditions that cause congenital hypothyroidism may also produce symptoms later in life. Hypopituitarism and tumors of the hypothalamic area may appear at any time. Ectopic thyroid tissue or dyshormonogenesis may not produce symptoms of frank hypothyroidism until after infancy. These disorders represent a relatively small percentage of cases of acquired hypothyroidism. Much more frequently seen is acquired hypothyroidism secondary to chronic autoimmune thyroiditis (Hashimoto thyroiditis, chronic lymphocytic thyroiditis).

THYROIDITIS

Definition

This term refers to any inflammation of the thyroid gland that results in injury and damage to thyroidal parenchyma. Three forms of thyroiditis are seen in children: chronic autoimmune thyroiditis, subacute thyroiditis, and acute thyroiditis.

CASE ILLUSTRATION

K.L. was seen by a neurologist at the age of 2 years and 11 months because of slow development. She did not walk until 18 months, was still not toilet-trained, and spoke only a few words with no sentences. She was the product of a pregnancy complicated by ABO incompatability which required an 8-day stay in the nursery for phototherapy for jaundice. Otherwise the delivery and neonatal period were normal.

During infancy she was very quiet, never required any attention, and she seemed uninterested in her environment. She started using single words at 2 years of age. Her weight remained on the 10th centile but length fell off progressively from the 10th centile to a point at the third centile (Fig. 14.9). Her head size was in the 75th centile for age. At the time of her visit to the neurologist skull radiographs and the neurologic examination were normal. A serum T_4 value was 5.9 μg/dl. No TSH was obtained.

At 3 years 2 months she was referred to an endocrinologist. Although there were no overt signs of hypothyroidism, a careful examination of her pharynx revealed an enlarged reddish mass at the base of her tongue. Her serum T_4 was 4.6 μg/dl with a serum TSH of 299 μU/ml. A thyroid scan and uptake showed uptake slightly to the right of the midline in the area of the tongue. There was no uptake in any other area. The 4-hour ^{123}I uptake was 1.7% and the 24-hour value was 1%.

She was diagnosed as having a lingual thyroid and L-thyroxine therapy was started. With this treatment her thyroid chemistries normalized, her linear growth accelerated, and her speech improved. Her parents noted a marked improvement in her personality and the nursery school performance.

The subtlety of the clinical picture of mild thyroid deficiency cannot be overestimated. In any child not growing and developing well, serum values of thyroid hormones should be obtained. TSH is the most critical indicator of a compromised thyroid gland.

Chronic Autoimmune Thyroiditis

Epidemiology

Chronic autoimmune thyroiditis is the most common type of acquired hypothyroidism. Females are affected 6 times as often as males and there is often a family history of hypothyroidism, hyperthyroidism, or goiter. Autoimmune thyroiditis is often associated with chromosomal abnormalities, such as Down syndrome, Turner syndrome, and Klinefelter syndrome. It is also seen more frequently in other diseases with autoimmune components, such as diabetes mellitus (pp. 897), idiopathic adrenal atrophy (pp. 865), and rheumatoid arthritis. The peak incidence of the disease is during early to midpuberty. It is rare to see autoimmune thyroiditis before the age of 4 years.

The thyroid gland is infiltrated with lymphocytes and antithyroid antibodies are present in the circula-

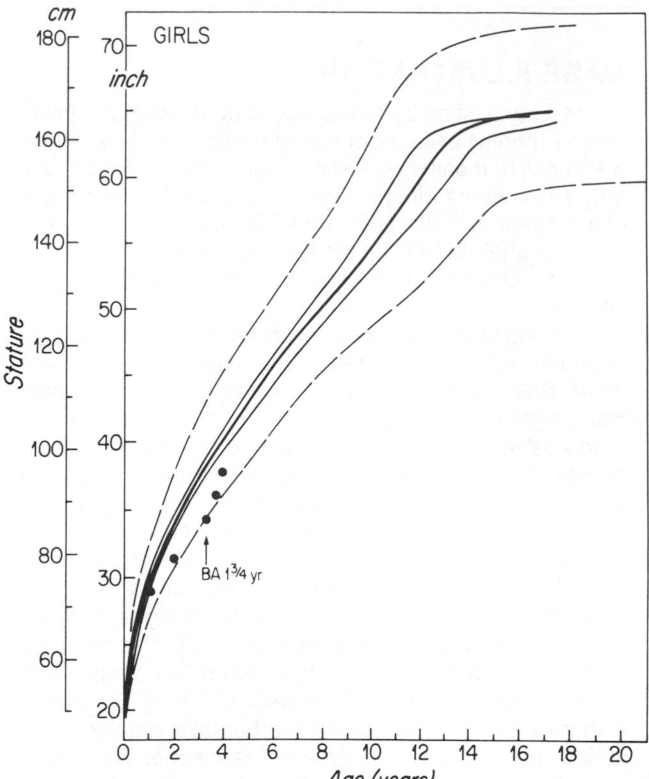

Figure 14.9. Linear growth curve of a patient with a lingual thyroid and hypothyroidism. See Case Illustration for details of diagnosis and treatment.

tion, suggesting that immunologic factors are involved in the pathogenesis of the disorder. The mechanism of the thyroid destruction is unknown; however, there is evidence to support a lymphocyte-mediated cytotoxicity that is targeted and initiated by antithyroid antibodies. The abnormality may reflect a genetically determined deficiency of suppressor cells that allows persistence of a forbidden clone of immunocytes directed against thyroid antigens (Volpe, 1984).

Abnormalities of thyroid hormone biosynthesis and of the release of iodoproteins are observed. Because of the faulty synthesis of thyroid hormone, increased amounts of TSH are secreted and the thyroid gland becomes hyperactive and enlarged.

The degree of fibrosis found in the thyroid gland varies considerably. In the fibrous variety, often seen in adults, fibrous tissue eventually replaces the whole gland. More typical of the condition in children is a minimal fibrosis with hyperplastic thyroid follicular cells surrounded by lymphocyte and plasma cell infiltrates.

Natural History

The onset of signs and symptoms of autoimmune thyroiditis is usually insidious. A nontender goiter appears early and may be noted by the physician on routine physical examination. Clinical symptoms are unusual initially and the thyroid gland is diffusely enlarged, the right lobe often being larger than the left one. The pyramidal lobe may be enlarged also. The consistency of the gland is smooth and soft and the surface often feels granular or pebbly. In later stages the gland feels firm or hard and nodules may be palpable. The nodules show up on thyroid scans as nonradioactive nodules and represent areas of fibrosis.

By far the most common initial symptom of hypothyroidism is a decrease in the growth rate. As with other forms of hypothyroidism the growth deceleration is related to the amount of circulating thyroid hormone. If the thyroid gland has been completely destroyed linear growth will cease completely. Mild obesity (myxedema) is often present as well as delayed development and impaired school performance. In the prepubertal child the body proportions are relatively immature with an increase in the upper/lower body segments.

An early phase of transient thyrotoxicosis may be followed by gradual onset of hypothyroidism. The process develops slowly over several years and it is not uncommon to have a young girl seen for delayed puberty who has not grown in height over 1 or more years and who has autoimmune thyroiditis. The clinical features of hypothyroidism develop slowly also and include: generalized puffiness with altered facial appearance, poor appetite, constipation and lethargy. Features on physical examination in addition to a goiter include: short stature, slow pulse, decreased blood pressure, myxedema, protuberant abdomen, pale thick cool skin, coarse hair, flabby muscles with pseudohypertrophy, delayed deep tendon reflexes, and dull expression.

Although puberty is usually delayed in hypothyroidism, some children exhibit precocious puberty associated with elevated levels of serum gonadotropins. Following treatment with thyroid hormone the previously elevated TSH falls as do the levels of FSH and LH and the changes of precocious puberty regress.

Diagnosis

Early in the stages of autoimmune thyroiditis there are usually no overt signs of hypothyroidism. The gland is enlarged and thyroid function tests show normal concentrations of T_4 and T_3 in the serum but elevated levels of TSH. In those children with clinical symptoms of hyperthyroidism with normal total T_4 and FT_4I, an elevation of serum T_3 may be found.

As the process develops and the thyroid gland can no longer compensate the serum T_4 concentration and, later, the level of T_3 in serum gradually falls and the child becomes clinically hypothyroid. Other associated changes include a decreased basal metabolic rate and an elevated level of serum cholesterol. Linear growth deceleration is one of the first signs of a hypothyroid state in the growing child.

The diagnosis of autoimmune thyroiditis is confirmed by finding antithyroid antibodies, usually of high titer, in the serum. Both antithyroglobulin and antimicrosomal antibodies are usually positive in the patient's serum. Both antibody tests are readily available to the pediatrician. Titers in excess of 1:2000 should be considered strongly suspicious of autoimmune thyroid disease (Hashimoto or Graves disease).

The presence of goiter in a patient with clinical and chemical signs of hypothyroidism and positive thyroid antibodies in the serum does not warrant further investigation such as radioiodine uptake and/or scan or thyroid biopsy. However, in the presence of a single nodule, unexplained regional lymphadenopathy, or expanding thyroid mass during suppressive L-thyroxine therapy, additional tests are required to exclude the presence of thyroid malignancy. These tests should include ultrasonography and radioactive scan of the thyroid gland before thyroid biopsy, when indicated.

Chronic autoimmune thyroiditis can occur as part of a group of disorders known as the autoimmune polyglandular syndromes (Table 14.8).

Treatment

Patients who have thyroid goiter and antibodies but who are clinically euthyroid and whose T_4 and TSH are normal do not necessarily require L-thyroxine therapy (pp. 837). They should continue to be observed at regular intervals, however, since many of these patients may eventually become hypothyroid. Once the diagnosis of hypothyroidism has been established adequate replacement therapy can be achieved by the oral administration of 50–150 μg of L-thyroxine once daily. For the patient who has been hypothyroid for many months or years, therapy should be started with a small dose of L-thyroxine (25–50 μg) which should be increased gradually until the therapeutic dose is reached. Full replacement therapy immediately in such patients may produce symptoms of thyrotoxicosis. The adequacy of the dose of L-thyroxine can be determined by measuring serum levels of TSH and T_4.

Compliance is often a problem in the adolescent. More frequent visits (every 3–6 months) may be necessary during these years of rapid growth and development to monitor the adequacy of therapy and to allow for changes in dose of L-thyroxine should this be required. Once euthyroidism is established and growth is completed, a check of thyroid status can be reviewed at the annual physical check-up.

Patients with transient hyperthyroidism in the early phase of autoimmune thyroiditis do not usually require therapy. Patients at risk for developing autoimmune thyroiditis, such as those with chromosomal abnormalities, diabetes mellitus, and the polyglandular autoimmune syndromes, should have annual determination of serum thyroid antibodies.

Prognosis

The basic autoimmune process will usually bring about destruction of most if not all thyroid function. Replacement thyroid hormone therapy can maintain a euthyroid state in the patient. Compliance may become a problem. In addition, the autoimmune process may eventually involve other endocrine tissues.

Subacute Thyroiditis

Epidemiology

This inflammatory disease of the thyroid gland is rarely seen in children. Only 2–7% of the patients reported in the literature were less than 20 years old; it is most commonly seen in females between the second and fifth decades of life. It probably represents a benign viral infection of the thyroid.

Natural History

The onset of subacute thyroiditis is often preceded by an upper respiratory infection or a prodrome of malaise and fatigue. There is low grade fever and systemic symptoms that resemble viral illness. There is often no leukocytosis.

The thyroid gland is usually swollen and tender, although painless swelling is also seen. There may be symptoms of thyrotoxicosis (pp. 835). Pain in the gland usually involves one side initially, later involving the entire thyroid gland, often radiating to the ear or jaw. The pain is accentuated by extension of the neck and by swallowing. There may be associated dysphagia or hoarseness. Cervical adenopathy is rare.

Most children present with minimal symptoms and signs. There may be no tenderness on palpation of the thyroid gland. The clinical picture in children may be difficult to differentiate from the acute stage of chronic autoimmune thyroiditis.

Table 14.8
Classification of Autoimmune Polyglandular Syndromes[1]

Type	Graves and/or thyroiditis	Gonadal Autoimmune Disease	Hypopara-thyroidism	Addison disease	IDDM	Alopecia	PA
I	10%	12%	[2]	[2]	2%	26%	15%
II	69%	4%	0	100%	52%	1%	1%
III	100%	0	0	0	IIIA	IIIC	IIIB

[1]Abbreviations: IDDM = insulin-dependent diabetes mellitus; PA = pernicious anemia.
[2]At least two of the following three diseases must be present for classification as type I: hypoparathyroidism, Addison disease, and monoliasis.

CASE ILLUSTRATION

A 14-year-old boy was brought to his family physician because of a failure to grow over the previous several years. He had gained excessive weight over the past years but had otherwise been in good health. His school performance had been excellent and he had shown no change in physical activity. There was no family history of thyroid disease. On physical examination he was noted to have pale dry skin and a pulse of 50. His tendon reflexes were somewhat delayed in return. His growth data showed that despite his weight gain his linear growth had ceased completely over the past 4 years (Fig. 14.10). His bone age was 11 years at a chronologic age of 14 years 5 months.

Laboratory values on his serum revealed: T_4 1 μg/dl, FT_4I 1, and TSH > 50 μU/ml. Radioactive iodine uptake was 8%. Thyroid antibodies were positive (both antithyroglobulin and antimicrosomal). A serum cholesterol value was 370 mg/dl. His Hb was 11.

On therapy with L-thyroxine his linear growth rate accelerated (Fig. 14.10) and he lost weight. His physical appearance improved with loss of facial puffiness and general slimming of his body.

COMMENT

This case is typical except for the sex of the patient. The disorder is far more common in females but thyroiditis must be considered in any teenager who is not growing. Unfortunately many years went by without growth in this boy and by the time he received therapy he was at an age when puberty usually occurs. Though he had shown no evidence of pubertal development prior to therapy he underwent a rapid sexual development on therapy. His final height was compromised as a result.

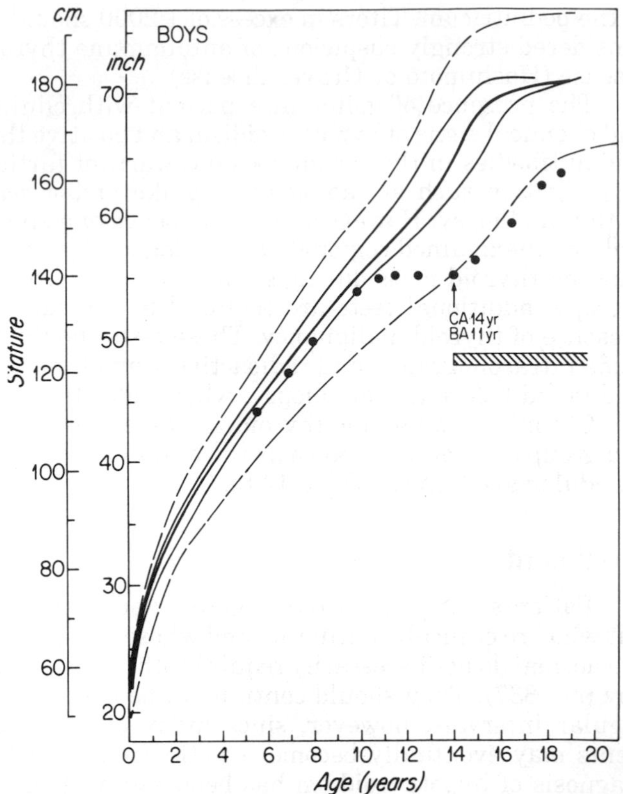

Figure 14.10. Acquired hypothyroidism. Linear growth curve of a young boy with acquired hypothyroidism secondary to autoimmune thyroiditis. See Case Illustration for details. The *shaded bar* represents therapy with L-thyroxine.

Diagnosis

Laboratory findings during the early phase of subacute thyroiditis often suggest mild hyperthyroidism. TSH may be undetectable and the TSH response to TRH administration is absent or impaired.

In contrast to most cases of hyperthyroidism, the 24-hour radioiodine uptake is very low, reflecting the diffuse damage to thyroid follicular cells, resulting in a diminished ability to trap iodine. Thyroid antibodies are absent or show low titers. The erythrocyte sedimentation rate is increased, often to a remarkable extent, during the active phase of the thyroiditis.

Treatment

In mild cases, aspirin is generally adequate to control the symptoms. In more severe cases, glucocorticoids may be needed, but they provide only symptomatic relief and do not alter the underlying disease process. The process eventually resolves.

Acute Thyroiditis

Epidemiology

This form of thyroiditis is rarely seen in children, 61 cases having been reported in the English literature by 1987. *Staphylococcus aureus* and hemolytic streptococci are the major pathogens cultured. In suppurative thyroiditis in children, anaerobic bacteria may be found (Rich and Mendelman, 1987).

Natural History

Acute thyroiditis is often preceded by an upper respiratory infection. There is an abrupt onset of painful, tender swelling in the region of the thyroid gland associated with fever, chills, sore throat, hoarseness, and often severe dysphagia.

The tenderness is usually so severe that the child will not permit an examination of the area. Early in the course of the thyroiditis there may be only an enlarged mass in the region of the thyroid gland, but later there is erythema with regional lymphadenopathy. Either lobe or the entire gland may be affected. In children the left lobe is involved more often than the right lobe.

Diagnosis

Clinical features of high fever with chills, leukocytosis, lymphadenopathy, local erythema, and the reduction of pain on flexion of the neck should suggest the diagnosis of acute bacterial thyroiditis. Aspiration of the affected area for culture in aerobic and anaerobic media and Gram staining of the aspirate are indicated for definitive diagnosis and appropriate therapy. Ultrasonography of the thyroid may demonstrate an abscess, but failure to demonstrate abscess or a definitive organism does not exclude the diagnosis. A barium esophagram is recommended to search for a left pyriform sinus fistula which has been reported in some patients (Rich and Mendelman, 1987).

Treatment

Early therapy with high-dose parenteral antibiotics is essential. Incision and drainage of the area is indicated, however, occasionally complete excision of the abscess by lobectomy may be needed to avoid prolonged drainage from the site.

Prognosis

Thyroid function remains normal in most patients and full recovery is expected.

Hyperthyroidism (Graves Disease)

Definition

Hyperthyroidism constitutes a clinical state of thyroid hormone excess. It is characterized by an accelerated metabolism of virtually all body tissues as a result of increased production of thyroid hormones, which is secondary to an autoimmune process whereby the thyroid gland is stimulated by a TSH-receptor-stimulating immunoglobulin (Volpe, 1984).

Epidemiology and Etiology

Ninety-five percent or more of all cases of hyperthyroidism in children are due to Graves disease. The latter is very rare in infants and young children; the incidence increases with age, and the majority of cases occur during adolescence. It is more common in females than in males with a ratio of between 3 and 5:1, and there is frequently a history of thyroid disease in the family. An increased incidence of Graves disease is observed in Down syndrome, diabetes mellitus, hypoadrenalism and collagen disease.

The etiology of Graves disease involves both genetic and immunologic factors. (Wall, 1987). There is a high familial incidence of the disease with an immunologic relationship to autoimmune thyroiditis. Thyroid-stimulating immunoglobulins, which can interact with the TSH receptor, are found in virtually all patients with Graves disease as well as antibodies against thyroglobulin and microsomal antigens. There is evidence that suppressor cell function is significantly decreased in Graves disease. Aberrant expression of the HLA-DR region of the histocompatibility complex in thyroid tissue from patients with Graves disease has been reported (Hanafusa et al, 1983; Bottazzo et al, 1983).

Infants born of mothers with Graves disease may develop thyrotoxicosis secondary to transplacentally acquired thyroid-stimulating immunoglobulins.

Ophthalmopathy (lid retraction, stare, exophthalmus) occurs in a significant number of children with Graves disease but is rarely as severe as in adults. The cause is unknown but it is thought to have an autoimmune etiology.

Natural History

The onset of thyrotoxicosis in the child is usually insidious, occurring over a period of months and years. Often the disease seems to be precipitated by emotional stress. Common complaints are nervousness, emotional lability, increased appetite but weight loss, school problems, sleep disturbances, and heat intolerance. Fatigue and exhaustion may be prominent, particularly if the child is engaged in physical activities or sports. Amenorrhea or delayed menarche may be noted in adolescent girls.

The most common signs of Graves ophthalmopathy are lid retraction and stare. Mild itching of the eyes and lacrimation may occasionally occur.

In thyroid "storm" the patient has a sudden onset of hyperthermia, severe tachycardia, and restlessness. It is always evoked by a precipitating factor such as acute infection, trauma, or surgical emergency. There can be rapid progression to delirium, coma, and death. This condition is extremely rare in children.

Diagnosis

The thyroid gland is usually symmetrically enlarged, nontender, firm and smooth; however, in some instances the gland is asymmetrical and the consistency may be granular or lobular. Commonly tachycardia and hyperactivity of the precordium are present. A functional murmur is frequently heard. The blood pressure is often elevated with an increased pulse pressure. The skin may be flushed and sweaty with a smooth texture. In some patients thinning of hair may be noted. Associated vitiligo is seen occasionally.

The eyes are often prominent and staring. A lid lag can frequently be demonstrated. Tremor can be demonstrated by having the patient extend the arms and spread the fingers. The linear growth rate is accelerated somewhat. Hyperactive behavior is characteristic.

Laboratory tests of thyroid function reveal increased levels of T_4, free T_4, and T_3 in the blood. Occasionally normal levels of T_4 and increased levels of T_3 are found (T_3 toxicosis). Radioiodine uptake is generally high. Serum TSH is normal or low and the TSH response to TRH is completely abolished in thyrotoxic patients. Titers of antithyroglobulin and antimicrosomal antibodies are elevated in most patients.

Treatment

Three modes of therapy are in use for Graves disease: medical therapy with antithyroid drugs, destruction of the thyroid by ^{123}I, and thyroidectomy (Hamburger, 1985, Wartofsky, 1984).

MEDICAL THERAPY

It is generally recommended that all children under 18 years of age with thyrotoxicosis be treated initially with antithyroid drugs (Dunn, 1984). The major agents used for thyrotoxicosis are drugs of the thionamide class: most commonly, propylthiouracil, methimazole, and carbimazole. These drugs are accumulated by the thyroid gland. Propylthiouracil (PTU), in addition to blocking the intrathyroidal synthesis of thyroxine, blocks the conversion of T_4 to T_3. It is given initially in doses of 300 mg daily, usually 100 mg every 8 hours, although twice daily (150 mg) and even daily (300 mg) regimens have been recommended. Occasionally patients will require a higher (400–600 mg total daily) dose initially. With larger doses it is probably better to increase the frequency of administration of the drug to every 4–6 hours.

Generally some clinical improvement occurs within the first 2 weeks. A normal metabolic state can be restored usually within about 6 weeks. Assessment of the patient at 2- to 3-week intervals is advised at first. Thryoid hormone levels in serum should be determined including a T_3, since the T_4 may fall to normal values but the T_3 may remain elevated. As the thyroid hormone levels fall, the dose of PTU can be reduced gradually to a maintenance dose of 50 mg every 8 hours.

In general, therapy should be continued for at least 1 year. An increase in size of the thyroid gland may suggest noncompliance, too much PTU, or inadequacy of therapy.

If the child is euthyroid after therapy for 1 or more years and if the thyroid gland is of normal size or only very slightly enlarged, treatment should be discontinued. About one-third of patients will have a lasting remission. A recent study suggests that even higher long-term remission rates (about 75%) can be obtained by using doses of drugs several times larger than usual together with replacement doses of T_3 (Romaldini et al, 1983). Side effects are encountered occasionally with the use of antithyroid drugs. Most reactions are mild, such as pruritus, skin rash, urticaria, and arthralgias. It may become necessary to change drugs, although there may be cross-sensitivity from one antithyroid drug to another. Although rare, the most common severe reaction is agranulocytosis, which may occur at any time during the course of therapy but most frequently occurs during the initiation of drug treatment. If the child on antithyroid drugs has fever or sore throat, a white cell count should be obtained immediately. If agranulocytosis is present the antithyroid drug should be discontinued immediately and therapy should be started to combat infection.

If the thyroid gland is very large the likelihood of remission with medical therapy is remote. Medical therapy can be continued until the patient is older and more definitive treatment can be considered.

A β-adrenergic blocking agent such as propranolol is a useful adjunct in the management of the severely toxic patient. Thyroid hormones potentiate the actions of catecholamines, and symptoms such as tachycardia, tremor, and excessive sweating may be relieved with the use of propranolol.

RADIOACTIVE IODINE

Some pediatric endocrinologists and radiotherapists avoid the use of radioactive iodine for the treatment of children with Graves disease. The theoretical risks of such therapy include thyroid carcinoma, leukemia, thyroid nodules, or genetic mutations. Despite these concerns there have been very few documented cases of thyroid carcinoma after ^{131}I therapy for Graves disease and it now seems that there is little likelihood of thyroid cancer occurring with proper radioiodine therapy (Dobyns et al, 1974). From the experience over the past 20 years, a growing number of pediatric endocrinologists believe that radioiodine therapy for Graves disease is safe and effective. Radioiodine should be administered by a specialist in the field. Hypothyroidism occurs eventually in most patients, requiring the administration of thyroid hormone to maintain a euthyroid state.

SURGERY

Surgery is an effective and safe form of therapy for Graves disease in the hands of a highly skilled surgeon under optimal conditions. Complications are low and include transient hypocalcemia, hypoparathyroidism, damage to one or both recurrent laryngeal nerves, wound infections, hemorrhage and keloid formation. Recurrence of hyperthyroidism may occur if all thyroid tissue is not removed. If hypothyroidism occurs, it should be treated with thyroid hormone. Before surgery the child must be treated with antithyroid drugs until a euthyroid state is achieved. About 2 weeks before surgery iodides are administered in the form of Lugol's solution, 5 drops twice daily. The iodide treatment causes the thyroid gland to become less vascular and reduces thyroid function.

Postoperatively the patient must be observed carefully for signs of hypocalcemia (within 24 hours after surgery) or damage to the recurrent laryngeal nerve (hoarseness or stridor).

The decision regarding the mode of therapy for Graves disease in children depends upon many variables, including the availability of a skilled thyroid surgeon and expertise in radiotherapy. Most endocrinologists start with medical therapy but all three modes of therapy should be presented to the patient and/or parents with a thoughtful analysis of the risks and benefits of each method.

THYROID STORM

Thyroid storm requires immediate and vigorous therapy. Intravenous sodium iodide should be started immediately and given in a dose of 1–2 g daily. PTU by nasogastric tube is given in doses of 200–300 mg every 6 hours. Propranolol may be effective in reducing the catecholamine symptoms. Dexamethasone, which reduces the serum level of T_3, is given in doses of 1–2 mg every 6 hours. The temperature can be reduced by placing the patient on a hypothermal mattress. Intravenous fluids and digitalis (if there is evidence of cardiac failure) should be used as required. The mortality is high in this condition but when treated vigorously most patients show improvement within 24 hours.

Prognosis

Remissions of disease can occur spontaneously with or without therapy, but there is no way of predicting which patients will eventually achieve a lasting remission and which will relapse. The condition can recur at any time and lifelong surveillance is essential.

CASE ILLUSTRATION

A 4-year-old girl was seen in clinic with a history of bulging eyes, failure to gain weight, excessive fatigue, and a mass in her neck. On physical examination she was noted to have bilateral exophthalmos, lid lag, and a diffuse enlarged thyroid gland with a loud bruit. Her skin was warm and moist with a velvety texture. Her pulse was 90 and her pulse pressure was increased. She had a moderate tremor of her hands and proximal muscle weakness. Deep tendon reflexes were brisk. Her hair was fine and silky.

At no time had she experienced diarrhea but there was an increased frequency of bowel movements. On close questioning it was apparent that her appetite and caloric intake had increased over the previous year. She was restless in her sleep.

Her laboratory findings included: T_4 13.6 μg/dl, FT_4I 13, TSH <2 μU/ml. ^{123}I uptake at 4 hours was 45% and at 24 hours, 50%. Her bone age was 5 years 9 months and height age was 5 years 5 months.

She was treated with propylthiouracil, starting with a dose of 100 mg three times a day, over a 4-year period before a remission of her Graves disease occurred. She has now been without therapy for 5 years with no evidence of recurrence of her disease.

COMMENT

This case illustrates the value of persisting in medical therapy. On several occasions over the 4-year period a lower dose of PTU was tried, but without success. Eventually she was maintained in a euthyroid state on 50 mg of PTU twice each day and finally she was weaned completely from therapy.

SIMPLE OR COLLOID GOITER

Definition

Any thyroid enlargement in a euthyroid person that does not result from an inflammatory or neoplastic process is defined as simple or colloid goiter.

Epidemiology and Etiology

Next to autoimmune thyroiditis this condition is the most common cause of euthyroid goiters in children (Monteleone et al, 1973). The etiology is unknown but presumably the disorder represents a response to any of several factors that impair the efficiency of the thyroid gland in forming adequate quantities of hormone. The resulting hypersecretion of TSH leads to stimulation of thyroid growth and hormone production. Thus the patient achieves a eumetabolic state at the expense of a large gland. Against this theory is the fact that TSH levels in the serum are usually normal in these patients; however, suppression of TSH with thyroid hormone sometimes causes regression of the goiter.

In most patients with simple goiter no extrinsic goitrogenic factor can be identified. Therefore, many investigators believe that the cause is some intrinsic, probably inborn abnormality in thyroid hormone synthesis. Other postulated causes of simple goiter include both extrinsic (thyroid stimulating immunoglobulins) and intrinsic thyroid growth factors. Iodine deficiency is an uncommon cause of colloid goiter in the United States.

Natural History

Generally these goiters are noted incidentally during a physical examination. Larger goiters may be noticed by the patient and may compress the esophagus or trachea. Long-standing goiters become nodular and are characterized by anatomical and functional heterogeneity and by functional autonomy (Taylor, 1953). This is presumably secondary to prolonged hyperstimulation by TSH or from repeated cycles of hyperstimulation and involution.

Diagnosis

Simple goiter may be difficult to differentiate from early stages of autoimmune thyroiditis. Thyroid antibody titers are negative or very low in patients with simple goiter. Uptake of radioactive iodine on thyroid scintiscanning is symmetrical. Thyroid hormone values are normal, including a normal serum TSH. The patient shows no signs or symptoms of hypo- or hyperthyroidism.

Treatment

Most endocrinologists believe that patients with colloid goiters should be treated with thyroid hormone to prevent later development of multinodular goiter. A similar argument is put forward for hormone treatment of euthyroid patients with goiter secondary to autoimmune thyroiditis.

THYROID NODULES

Definition

A thyroid nodule is a discrete, palpable enlargement of the thyroid gland. Nodules may be single or multiple.

Epidemiology and Etiology

Apparently the propensity to proliferate is not evenly distributed among the follicular cells of the normal thyroid gland, but a growth advantage is a normal feature of some epithelial cells. Therefore, a certain degree of nodularity is present in normal glands. The process is greatly exaggerated whenever a growth-promoting agent, such as TSH, is acting upon the thyroid gland.

Thyroid nodules may be classified as "functioning" (accumulates iodine and synthesizes thyroid hormones) or "nonfunctioning." Functioning nodules show up on thyroid scans as "warm" or "hot" nodules, reflecting the extent of uptake of labeled iodine into the nodule. Hot nodules show intense uptake of isotope with little or no radioactivity appearing in the surrounding gland. Warm nodules take up roughly the same amount of radioactivity as the surrounding thyroid tissue does. Nonfunctioning nodules do not take up labeled iodine and appear on the scan as a "cold" spot (Fig. 14.11).

The presence of a solitary nodule of the thyroid gland in a child or adolescent is uncommon and raises the possibility of malignancy. Of all children with a single nodule in the thyroid gland, about one-third will have neoplasia, most commonly adenoma. The most malignant thyroid tumors do not have the capacity to accumulate and organify significant quantities of radioactive iodine. Their appearance on thyroid scan is that of a cold nonfunctioning nodule. This does not mean, however, that most cold nodules are thyroid carcinomas. Generally about 20% of cold nodules are carcinomas. Papillary carcinomas may show up as "warm" nodules. Adenomas may be functional or nonfunctional. The functional adenomas are autonomous, resulting in suppression of the surrounding thyroid tissue. They may produce hyperthyroidism. The remaining lesions that cause nodularity include: autoimmune thyroiditis, subacute thyroiditis, thyroid abscess, cysts, absence of one lobe and multinodular goiter.

In 1949, Quimby and Werner suggested the possibility of a relationship between radiation and the subsequent development of thyroid carcinoma. This relationship has been verified subsequently. In one study, 76% of patients with thyroid cancer had received neck radiation from 3½ to nearly 14 years before the diagnosis of cancer was made.

Papillary carcinoma is by far the most common type of thyroid cancer in children. These carcinomas often contain follicular elements. They tend to be histologically well differentiated and they usually concentrate iodine. Layered calcium deposits called psammoma bodies are characteristic. The tumor tends to infiltrate surrounding tissue with metastases to regional lymph nodes and lung. Follicular carcinomas may metastasize to lung and bone. A rare carcinoma, medullary carcinoma (see below) involves the calcitonin-secreting cells.

Natural History

Most nodules of the thyroid are identified on routine physical examination. In about three-fourths of patients with carcinoma of the thyroid gland the first sign of disease was one or more firm painless nodules in the neck. Hoarseness, dyspnea, and dysphagia are uncommon initial complaints. Papillary cancers in children are noted for their slow growth. In some cases pulmonary metastases may be the first evidence of thyroid carcinoma. Osseous metastases are uncommon.

Autonomous hyperfunctioning nodules may produce signs of hyperthyroidism.

Diagnosis

In the child with a thyroid nodule a careful history should be taken concerning prior irradiation to the head and neck and family history of thyroid disease. The nodule should be examined for tenderness, which might suggest subacute thyroiditis. Patients with autoimmune thyroiditis may have single or multiple nodules in the thyroid gland. Lymph nodes should be examined for evidence of enlargement and adherence to adjacent tissues.

Both thyroid function tests and assay for thyroid antibodies should be obtained. Radiographs of the chest and neck may reveal pulmonary metastases. Thyroid radio-iodine scan is very important. The finding of a cold nodule when the thyroid appears otherwise normal may indicate adenoma or carcinoma. Ultrasonography is especially helpful in determining whether thyroid nodules are solid or cystic. Finally, a TRH test may be helpful in determining whether or not the nodular cells are responsive to TSH. Hot nodules are usually autonomous and show no response to a tropic stimulus.

Surgical biopsy is essential in cases of suspected malignancy, particularly in a child with prior irradiation to the head and neck.

Treatment

The solitary cold solid nodule should be excised surgically. If the lesion is malignant a total thyroidectomy should be performed. Postoperatively the child should be treated with TSH-suppressive doses of thyroid hormone. Periodic follow-up examinations of the neck region and yearly chest radiographs are instituted. Thyroid function tests may be measured to assure adequacy of the hormone dose and compliance.

Hot nodules producing thyrotoxicosis should be treated with antithyroid therapy or excised. Warm nodules in a euthyroid person may be observed for evidence

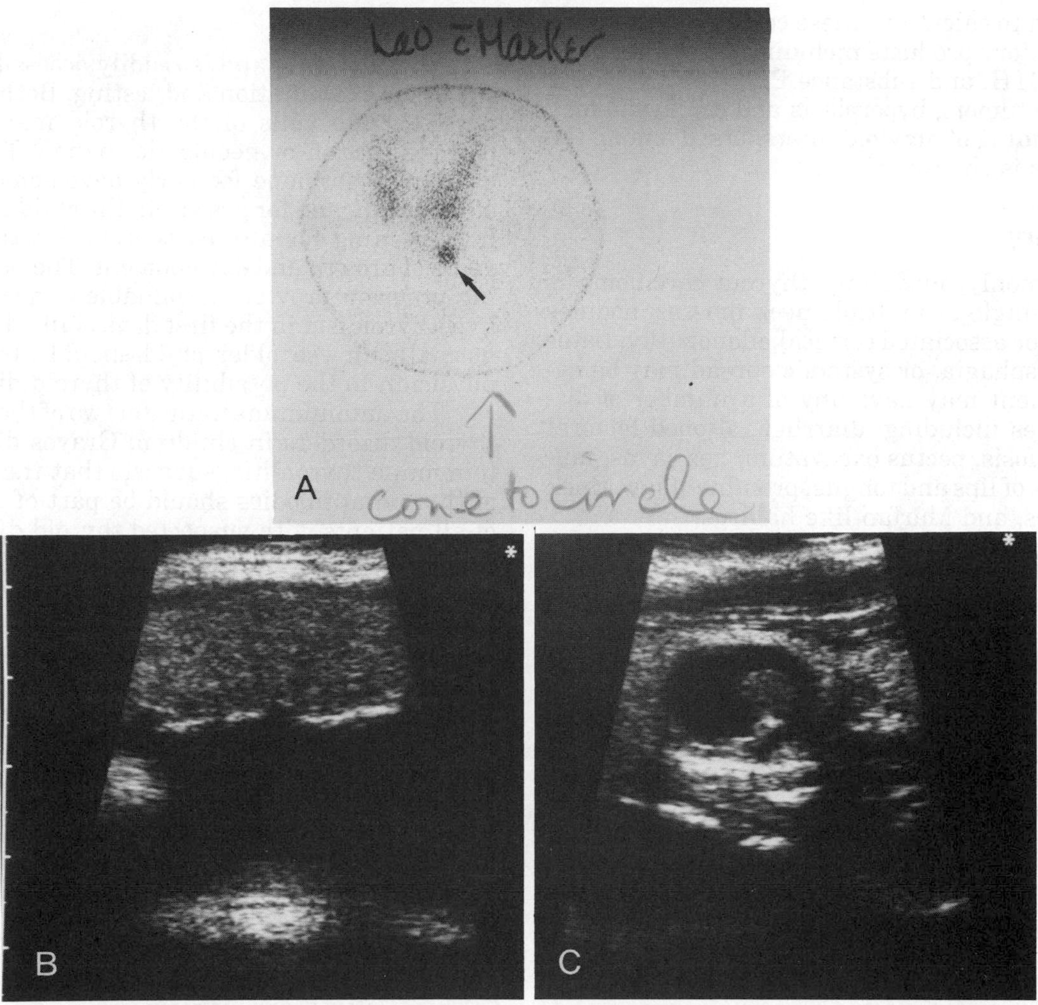

Figure 14.11A and B. This adolescent girl had been seen in endocrine clinic for an asymptomatic nodule in the left lobe of thyroid found by her pediatrician on a thorough physical examination. Radionuclide scan with I^{131} showed a cold area in the left lower pole of the throid gland. (Note: cone to circle on **A**) arrow = marker at lower edge of mass. Ultrasonogram of right lobe showed normal parenchyma **(B)**. A predominantely cystic mass with central solid material was present on the left **(C).** Surgical removal and pathologic examination revealed papillary carcinoma. This was quite an unexpected finding in this patient with no risk factors—specifically no prior irradiation of the area. A cold nodule on radionuclide scans should prompt further examination of the thyroid as malignancy may present in this fashion.

of change in size, consistency, or function. In some instances replacement doses of thyroid hormone cause regression of the nodule. Any increase in size or firmness of a nodule should be investigated surgically.

Multiple cold nodules in a child with autoimmune thyroiditis require close observation. If there is any increase in size or hardening of the nodules a biopsy should be obtained.

Any child with previous history of radiation to the neck area and a thyroid nodule should have a surgical biopsy of the nodule performed.

Prognosis

Because these tumors are slow growing, most children with thyroid carcinoma have an excellent prognosis (Buckwalter et al, 1975).

MEDULLARY CARCINOMA OF THE THYROID

Definition

This tumor represents a carcinoma of the parafollicular "C" cells of the thyroid gland which may occur sporadically or as the result of an autosomal dominant gene in some families.

Epidemiology and Etiology

Medullary thyroid carcinoma accounts for a very small percentage of thyroid carcinomas in children. The tumor may occur alone or in association with other endocrine disorders as part of multiple endocrine neoplasia (MEN type II or III, pp. 840).

In addition to calcitonin these cells may produce a variety of secretory products including serotonin, prostaglandins, ACTH, and substance P.

Within the tumors, hyperplasia and carcinoma may coexist. The finding of amyloid interspersed among the neoplastic cells is characteristic.

Natural History

Most commonly, medullary thyroid carcinoma is first noted as single or multiple neck masses, nodules of the thyroid, or associated cervical adenopathy. Later hoarseness, dysphagia, or systemic spread may be evident. The patient may have any of a number of distinctive features including: diarrhea, slipped femoral epiphyses, scoliosis, pectus excavatum, pes cavus, mucosal neuromas of lips and tongue, prominent jaw, thick eyelids and lips, and Marfan-like habitus.

Diagnosis

Nodules of medullary carcinoma appear cold on thyroid scan. Plasma calcitonin levels are elevated and show enhanced response to calcium infusion or pentagastrin injection. Urinary catecholamines should be checked for evidence of accompanying pheochromocytoma (pp. 867). Parathyroid status should be investigated with measurement of serum calcium and PTH levels. In MEN type II medullary carcinoma, pheochromocytoma and hyperparathyroidism can coexist. In MEN type III medullary carcinoma, pheochromocytoma, and mucosal neuromas coexist.

Treatment

Surgery is the treatment of choice for medullary carcinoma.

Prognosis

Total thyroidectomy is curative if the disease is detected while confined to the thyroid gland. However, metastases to cervical lymph nodes occur during early stages of the disease. The virulence of spread of the tumor varies from patient to patient. Large primary lesions may have distant metastases to lung, liver, and bone.

Prevention

Families of patients with this disorder should be screened with calcium infusion or pentagastrin injection to determine if "C" cell hyperplasia or medullary carcinoma is present. Calcitonin levels greater than normal after stimulation are highly suggestive of increased "C" cell activity. Total thyroidectomy should be carried out in individuals who have "C" cell hyperplasia or tumor.

Postoperatively, calcitonin levels in the serum should be checked periodically. Elevated levels may be the earliest sign of recurrence of tumor.

Summary

The thyroid gland is readily accessible to the physician for examination and testing. Both follicular and parafollicular cells of the thyroid may manifest impaired function or neoplastic change. The importance of thyroid hormone for early development, especially of the brain, and for growth in the child mandates careful screening for altered thyroid function during the years of growth and development. The neonatal screening program provides a valuable service by detecting hypothyroidism in the first days of life. Failure to grow normally in the older child should always alert the physician to the possibility of thyroid disorders.

The autoimmune nature of two of the most common thyroid disorders in children: Graves disease and autoimmune thyroiditis, suggests that the measurement of thyroid antibodies should be part of the evaluation of all patients with suspected thyroid dysfunction.

Solitary nodules of the thyroid gland must receive special screening to rule out the presence of malignancy. Fortunately, thyroid scanning procedures, ultrasound studies, and biopsy as indicated provide valuable information to aid the physician in deciding whether the nodule should be removed surgically.

REFERENCES

Abuid JL, Klein AH, Foley TP Jr, et al: Total and free triiodothyronine and thyroxine in early infancy. *J Clin Endocrinol Metabol* 39:263, 1974.

Arnold MB, Arulanantham K, Bapat V, et al: Characteristics of infantile hypothyroidism discovered on neonatal screening. *J Pediatr* 104:539, 1984.

Barnes ND: Screening for congenital hypothyroidism: The first decade. *Arch Dis Child* 60:587, 1985.

Bottazzo GF, Pujol-Borrell R, Hanafusa T, et al: Role of aberrant HLA-DR expression and antigen presentation in induction of endocrine autoimmunity. *Lancet* 2:1115, 1983.

Buckwalter JA, Thomas CG, Freeman JB: Is childhood thyroid cancer a lethal disease? *Ann Surg* 181:632, 1975.

Caldwell G, Gow SM, Sweeting VM, et al: A new strategy for thyroid function testing. *Lancet* 1:1117, 1985.

Dobyns BM, Sheline GE, Workman JB, et al: Malignant and benign neoplasms of the thyroid in patients treated for hyperthyroidism: A report of the cooperative thyrotoxicosis therapy follow-up study. *J Clin Endocrinol Metabol* 38:976, 1974.

Dunn JT: Choice of therapy in young adults with hyperthyroidism of Graves' disease. *Ann Intern Med* 100:891, 1984.

Erenberg A, Phelps DL, Lam R, et al: Total and free thyroid hormone concentration in the neonatal period. *Pediatrics* 53:211, 1974.

Fisher DA, Klein AH: Thyroid development and disorders of thyroid function in the newborn. *N Engl J Med* 304:702, 1981.

Franklin R, O'Grady C, Carpenter L: Neonatal thyroid function: Comparison between breast fed and bottle fed infants. *J Pediatr* 106:124, 1985.

Glorieux J, Dussault JH, Letarte J, et al: Preliminary results on the mental development of hypothyroid infants detected by the Quebec screening program. *J Pediatr* 102:19, 1983.

Griffin JE: The dilemma of abnormal thyroid function tests—is thyroid disease present or not? *Am J Med Sci* 289:76, 1985.

Hamburger JI: Management of hyperthyroidism in children and adolescents. *J Clin Endocrinol Metabol* 60:1019, 1985.

Hanafusa T, Chiovato L, Doniach D, et al: Aberrant expression of HLA-DR antigen on thyrocytes in Graves' disease: Relevance for autoimmunity. *Lancet* 2:1111, 1983.

Hocman G: Human thyroxine binding globulin (TBG). *Rev Physiol Biochem Pharmacol* 91:45, 1981.

Klein RZ: Infantile hypothyroidism then and now: The results of neonatal screening. *Curr Probl Pediatr* 15:5, 1985.
Lakey T, MacNeil S, Humphries H, et al: Calcium and calmodulin in the regulation of human thyroid adenylate cyclase activity. *Biochem J* 225:581, 1985.
Larsen PR, Silva JE, Kaplan MM: Relationships between circulating and intracellular thyroid hormones: Physiological and clinical implications. *Endocrinol Rev* 2:87, 1981.
Monteleone JA, Danis RK, Tung KSK, et al: Differentiation of chronic lymphocytic thyroiditis and simple goiter in pediatrics. *J Pediatr* 83:381, 1973.
Quimby EH, Werner SC: Late radiation effects in roentgen therapy for hyperthyroidism. *JAMA* 140:1046, 1949.
Rich EJ, Mendelman PM: Acute suppurative thyroiditis in pediatric patients. *Pediatr Infect Dis* 6:936, 1987.
Romaldini JH, Bromberg N, Werner RS, et al: Comparison of effects of high and low dosage regimens of antithyroid drugs in the management of Graves' hyperthyroidism. *J Clin Endocrinol Metabol* 57:563, 1983.
Taylor S: The evolution of nodular goiter. *J Clin Endocrinol Metabol* 13:1232, 1953.
Visser TJ, Kaplan MM, Leonard JL, et al: Evidence for two pathways of iodothyronine 5′-deiodination in rat pituitary that differ in kinetics, propylthiouracil sensitivity, and response to hypothyroidism. *J Clin Invest* 71:992, 1983.
Volpe R: Autoimmune thyroid disease. *Hosp Pract* 19:141, 1984.
Wall JR: Autoimmune thyroid disease. *Endocrinol Metabol Clin North Am* 16:229, 1987.
Wartofsky L: Guidelines for the treatment of hyperthyroidism. *Am Fam Phys* 30:199, 1984.
Zaloga GP, O'Brian JT: Euthyroid sick syndrome. *Am Fam Phys* 31:236, 1985.

Parathyroid Glands 5

Calcium and Phosphorus

Most of the body's calcium and phosphorus is stored in bone. The latter is composed of an organic matrix (collagen, osteocalcin, mucopolysaccharides, sialo proteins, lipids) and calcium phosphate in hydroxyapatite crystals.

Less than 2% of the body content of calcium, magnesium, or phosphate is in the plasma and extracellular fluid, yet the concentration of these minerals outside the cell is kept carefully controlled. Large amounts of Ca^{++}, Mg^{++}, and phosphate continuously enter and leave plasma via intestine, kidney, and bone. Thus, each of these organs participates in the overall regulation of plasma mineral content.

The plasma concentration of calcium (Ca), in particular the ionized Ca, is maintained within narrow limits by a number of regulatory factors, the most important of which are parathyroid hormone (PTH) and vitamin D. The Ca in serum exists in three fractions: (1) a protein-bound fraction (30–50% of total Ca), (2) diffusible nonionized Ca, mostly in complex with phosphate, citrate, bicarbonate, etc (5–15%), and (3) ionized Ca (40–60%). Ca^{++} is the metabolically active form, the concentration of which is regulated tightly. The percentage of Ca bound to protein depends upon the concentration of albumin in serum and the pH. Increases in serum albumin are accompanied by increases in both bound and the total Ca. A decrease in pH results in release of Ca from albumin, leading to an increase in Ca^{++}.

Ca^{++} concentration within the cell varies with changes in calcium fluxes across membranes. Excitation of almost all secretory cells leads to increased permeability of the plasma membrane, allowing calcium to move down its concentration gradient into the cytosol of the cell, thereby activating secretion. The interactions of many hormones with plasma membrane receptors lead to changes in transmembrane calcium flux (pp. 796). Calcium sequestered within organelles of the cell can be mobilized on demand. For example, stores of calcium within the sarcoplasmic reticulum of striated muscles are released into the cytosol when the muscle is excited. In most cells mitochondria contain large amounts of calcium, which can accumulate and be released as conditions indicate.

Several cellular metabolic processes are modulated by alteration of the activity of Ca^{++}-sensitive enzymes. In many cases these effects are mediated by specific "receptor" proteins which first bind Ca^{++} and then interact with enzymes to modify their activity. The most important "calcium receptor" is calmodulin, an ubiquitous protein which forms complexes with calcium. These calmodulin-Ca^{++} complexes function as regulators of many enzymes, including phosphodiesterase, certain adenylate cyclases, phosphorylase kinase, and Ca^{++}-ATPase.

Seventy percent of the phosphate in the circulation is covalently bound in phospholipids and phosphoproteins, while the remaining 30% is inorganic phosphate in serum. In serum, the proportional distribution of magnesium as ionized, protein-bound, and in complex form is similar to that for calcium. Both phosphate and magnesium are found within cells. Magnesium in the cytosol of the cell is largely in complex with phosphate, citrate and other anions such as the adenosine phosphates. Intracellular phosphate is covalently incorporated in many proteins, lipids, and nucleic acids. This phosphorylation of intracellular proteins, especially enzymes, may alter profoundly the biological activity of the molecule.

Ca^{++} reaches the fetus by active transport against a concentration gradient. During gestation there is a gradual increase in fetal serum Ca from about 5.5 mg/dl at the end of the second trimester to about 11 mg/dl at term. After birth total and ionized serum Ca levels fall rapidly (Table 14.9). Serum phosphate also declines in the fetus from values of about 14 mg/dl in the second trimester to about 6 mg/dl at term. After birth there is a brief rise in serum phosphate followed by a fall to adult values (Table 14.9).

Parathyroid Hormone

The hormone produced by the chief cells of the parathyroid gland, PTH, is an 84-amino acid, single chain polypeptide. Usually four parathyroid glands are present, an upper pair located near the junction of the middle thyroid artery and the recurrent laryngeal nerve derived from the fourth branchial pouch and a lower pair usually found lateral to the trachea at the lower pole of the thyroid gland and derived from the third branchial pouch. The chief cells of the parathyroid glands first form a precursor of PTH, called pre-proPTH (Potts et al, 1982), an 115-amino acid polypeptide with a molecular weight of 14,000. Pre-ProPTH is rapidly converted to proPTH which is then converted to PTH, the form stored in and elaborated from secretory granules in the gland. When PTH is released into the circulation it is rapidly cleaved to smaller fragments of molecular weights 4000 and 7000. The latter is biologically inactive but the 4000 molecular weight fragments are potent.

The major target organs of PTH are bone and kidney. Adenylate cyclase activity is stimulated, with production of cyclic AMP; at the same time the intracellular concentration of Ca is increased. In bone, PTH activity requires vitamin D. Both bone resorption and bone formation are regulated by modulation of the activity of osteoclasts and osteoblasts. The activity of osteoclasts is increased by PTH and vitamin D, mobilizing calcium and phosphorus from bone to the extracellular space. In the kidney, PTH causes increased reabsorption of Ca and decreased reabsorption of phosphate by the renal tubules, which results in phosphaturia. Increased renal excretion of sodium, bicarbonate, glucose, and amino acids also occurs. The activity of 1 α-hydroxylase in kidney is increased by PTH, which results in increased formation of 1,25-dihydroxyvitamin D_3 and hence facilitates Ca and phosphate absorption in the intestinal tract.

Several sensitive radioimmunoassays for PTH are available; each assay directed toward measuring various segments of the PTH molecule: the amino-terminus, the carboxy-terminus, and various midsections. Generally all assays recognize the entire molecule as well as specific segments. The problem of multiple circulating fragments of PTH introduces great uncertainties in the interpretation of a particular PTH immunoassay. The bioactive "amino-terminal" fragment of PTH accounts for only 10% of circulating PTH immunoreactivity owing to its short half-life (about 5 minutes) and rapid clearance from the blood. Therefore, the principal fragment(s) present in the peripheral circulation (80%) are derived from the "carboxy-terminal" end of PTH. These fragments have a long half-life (about 1 hour). Although carboxy-terminal fragments are biologically inactive, serum concentrations of these fragments generally reflect the rate of PTH secretion. A decrease in glomerular filtration rate, however, leads to impaired renal clearance of carboxy-terminal fragments from the blood. Thus, in renal insufficiency, radioimmunoassays that measure these fragments may provide misleadingly elevated results for plasma PTH concentration. It is important to ascertain the renal function of the patient before attempting to interpret PTH radioimmunoassays.

The concentration of Ca^{++} in blood is the single most important factor controlling PTH secretion, although the exact mechanism(s) is unknown. Part of the effect of calcium may be mediated by a decrease in cAMP content brought about through calcium stimulation of calmodulin-activated phosphodiesterase. This effect, however, cannot account for most of the calcium-

Table 14.9
Serum Concentrations (mean ± 1 SD) of Calcium, Phosphate and Magnesium at Various Ages (mg/dl)

	Calcium			
	Total	Ionized	Phosphate	Total Magnesium
Cord	10.8 ± 0.7	5.5 ± 0.3	6.2 ± 1.0	1.8 ± 0.1
3–24 hr	9.8 ± 0.8	4.7 ± 0.3	6.6 ± 1.1	1.9 ± 0.2
24–48 hr	9.5 ± 0.9	4.4 ± 0.3	7.5 ± 1.0	1.9 ± 0.2
2–3 days	9.7 ± 0.8	4.5 ± 0.4	8.1 ± 1.2	2.0 ± 0.2
3–4 days	9.8 ± 0.7	4.5 ± 0.4	7.7 ± 1.3	2.0 ± 0.2
4–7 days	10.0 ± 0.9	4.8 ± 0.3	8.2 ± 1.1	2.1 ± 0.2
1 month–15 years	10.0 ± 0.5	4.5 ± 0.3	4.7 ± 0.8	2.1 ± 0.2

Source: David and Anast, 1974.

mediated inhibition of PTH secretion. The principal control exerted by calcium on PTH release may be manifested at the level of fusion of secretory granules within the cell membrane. Low concentrations of calcium cause hyperpolarization of the parathyroid cell concomitantly with increased rates of secretion of PTH.

Other ions can influence PTH secretion. Like calcium, magnesium in increased concentrations inhibits secretion of PTH (Brown, 1982), whereas high concentrations of potassium and lithium stimulate PTH secretion. Since PTH release depends on anion transport across the membrane of the parathyroid cell, the process is inhibited by reducing external chloride.

There is now strong evidence that catecholamines modulate the secretion of PTH. These effects are associated with changes in intracellular levels of cyclic AMP. The catecholamines are not primary regulators, however, and appear to serve as modulators of PTH secretion only when secretion rates are greatly increased. When hormone secretion is suppressed, in the presence of physiologic concentrations of Ca^{++}, epinephrine has little if any effect on rates of secretion of the hormone.

Vitamin D

It is now well established that 1,25-dihydroxyvitamin D_3 (1,25-dihydroxycholecalciferol) is a true steroid hormone (DeLuca, 1988). The biosynthesis of this hormone occurs by a series of steps. Under ultraviolet irradiation, provitamin D_3 (7-dehydrocholesterol) in the skin is converted to previtamin D_3, which isomerizes to vitamin D_3 (cholecalciferol). Blood contains a carrier globulin, vitamin D-binding protein, which transports vitamin D_3 from the skin to the liver. There vitamin D_3 is hydroxylated to 25-hydroxyvitamin D_3 which, in turn, is hydroxylated in the kidney to 1,25-dihydroxyvitamin D_3, the biologically active vitamin D. It acts to increase calcium and phosphate absorption in the gut and to mobilize these components from bone. In addition, receptors for 1,25-dihydroxyvitamin D appear to be widely distributed in various tissues, including kidney, pancreas, parathyroids, skin, placenta, and white blood cells.

Another metabolite of 25-hydroxyvitamin D_3 is 24,25-dihydroxyvitamin D_3, formed also in the kidney. Its mode of action is unknown, but it may be involved in intestinal calcium transport and bone mineralization.

Dietary vitamin D_2 (calciferol) is absorbed primarily from the duodenum and jejunum. This absorption depends upon the presence of bile salts and the capacity to absorb fat. Absorbed vitamin D_2 undergoes the same metabolic transformations to 25-hydroxyvitamin D_2 and 1,25-dihydroxyvitamin D_2 as does vitamin D_3. Radioimmunoassays for vitamin D and its metabolites measure both D_2 and D_3.

Vitamin D, 25-hydroxyvitamin D, and 1,25-dihydroxyvitamin D appear to cross the placenta from mother to fetus. In the neonatal period, serum 25-hydroxyvitamin D concentrations undergo little change; however, values for serum 1,25-dihydroxyvitamin D increase from birth to 24 hours of age in full-term infants (Steichen et al, 1980). The placenta itself also synthesizes 1,25-dihydroxyvitamin D and 24,25-dihydroxyvitamin D from 25-hydroxyvitamin D (Whitsett et al, 1981; Weisman et al, 1979).

Calcitonin

Calcitonin is a hormone produced by the C cells of the thyroid gland. The secretion of calcitonin is increased by hypercalcemia, glucagon, and gastrin and is lowered by hypocalcemia. Calcitonin lowers the concentration of calcium in serum and also inhibits bone formation, decreases intestinal absorption of calcium, and increases urinary excretion of calcium and phosphate. Although calcitonin does play a role in regulating calcium metabolism, other more powerful regulatory factors can maintain a normal serum calcium level even in the presence of marked abnormalities in the secretion of calcitonin.

HYPOCALCEMIA

Definition

Hypocalcemia is a condition of low concentration of Ca^{++} in the serum, often associated with symptoms of neuromuscular irritability, including paresthesias, muscle cramps, and seizures. Decreased concentration of total Ca in serum, with a normal ionized fraction, can exist with hypoproteinemia or acidosis; however, the patient becomes symptomatic only if the concentration of serum Ca^{++} falls below normal. Hypocalcemia often reflects deficient PTH secretion, or deficient generation of active vitamin D metabolites, or both.

Epidemiology

A variety of conditions and diseases can cause hypocalcemia (Table 14.10). Any condition that impairs calcium absorption or enhances its excretion can pro-

Table 14.10
Causes of Hypocalcemia

Neonatal
Early (prematurity, maternal diabetes mellitus, stress)
Late (diet-phosphate load)
Magnesium deficiency
Older Child
Hypoparathyroidism
Pseudohypoparathyroidism
Vitamin D deficiency
Errors in vitamin D synthesis or action
Renal disease
Malabsortion
Magnesium deficiency
Alkalosis
Excess phosphate
Hypoproteinemia

duce hypocalcemia, so that renal failure and malabsorption are common causes. Hypomagnesemia from any cause or any decrease in availability of PTH or vitamin D may produce hypocalcemia.

Some degree of hypoparathyroidism may exist in some neonates. The relatively high level of calcium in serum in utero may suppress the fetal parathyroid glands. Mothers with parathyroid adenomas may produce infants with suppressed parathyroid glands and hypocalcemia.

Neonatal hypocalcemia (within the first 3 days of life) occurs most commonly in premature infants who suffer birth asphyxia or some other neonatal stress and in infants of diabetic mothers. Hypocalcemia of the premature infant may not necessarily be secondary to transient hypoparathyroidism, however, since mean serum PTH levels in these infants at 12–24 hours of age are 3 times greater than the upper limit of normal in older children and adults (Cooper and Anast, 1985).

A diet high in phosphate (cow's milk) may be responsible for hypocalcemia in the infant who has begun oral feedings. Both the ratio of calcium to phosphate and the absolute concentration of phosphate in the diet are important. Increased absorption of phosphate may exceed the renal capacity to excrete this compound, resulting in hyperphosphatemia. The elevated serum phosphate depresses the serum calcium. Cow's milk has a lower calcium to phosphate ratio (1.35:1) than does human milk (2.25:1).

Natural History

Whatever the cause, the clinical manifestations of hypocalcemia are similar. In infants, the usual symptoms are irritability, tremor, twitching, and seizures. Lethargy, poor feeding, and vomiting may occur. In the older child, physical findings include positive Chvostek and Trousseau signs. The Chvostek may be positive in normal infants. It is elicited by tapping the facial nerve just anterior to the ear. A positive response is a twitching of the facial muscles on that side. Trousseau's sign is elicited by inflating a blood pressure cuff to just above systolic pressure for 3 minutes. A positive response is carpospasm. Carpopedal spasm is not usually seen in infants.

In tetany, the extremities, including the wrists are flexed, the thumb is abducted, and the fingers are flexed at the metacarpal phalangeal joint, but extended at other joints. The feet are in the equinovarus position with toes flexed. The Q-T interval of the electrocardiogram is prolonged in hypocalcemia.

Other signs of neonatal hypocalcemia include twitching of the extremities, a high pitched cry and hypotonicity.

Diagnosis

A low concentration of Ca^{++} in serum establishes the diagnosis of hypocalcemia. The serum phosphate levels may be increased, sometimes to 10–12 mg/dl. The clinical and biochemical features in each case depend upon the underlying cause of the hypocalcemia. Renal function (serum creatinine, creatinine clearance) and gastrointestinal function (D-xylose tolerance test, serum carotene, quantitation of stool fat) should be evaluated. Skeletal radiographs should be examined for features of parathyroid disorders or rickets (see below).

Measurements of serum PTH, phosphate, and vitamin D metabolites are essential in defining the category of hypocalcemia (see below).

Treatment

Generally early neonatal hypocalcemia resolves spontaneously within several days. In the asymptomatic hypocalcemic neonate, the serum protein concentration and pH as well as the ionized calcium level should be considered in deciding whether or not to treat. In premature infants who are hypoproteinemic, lower levels of total serum calcium are present normally. All symptomatic infants should be treated. The physician should maintain normal serum calcium levels by intravenous or oral calcium therapy. For acute tetany, a 10% solution of calcium gluconate is given intravenously. The rate of administration should not exceed 1 ml/min and the maximum dose administered at any one time should not exceed 2.0 ml/kg. The intravenous calcium may be repeated three or four times in a 24-hour period as needed to control tetany. After acute symptoms have been controlled, oral calcium may be used to maintain serum calcium levels between 8.0 and 9.0 mg/dl. Neocalglucon (calcium glubionate), which contains 23 mg of calcium/ml, may be given in a dose of 2 ml/kg/day divided into 4–6 doses. In addition, it is recommended that premature infants receive the equivalent of 600–800 IU (international units) of vitamin D daily. Usually treatment can be tapered after 3–4 days.

Hypocalcemia related to diet tends to occur in infants at about 1 week of age. A change in diet will usually correct the condition; however, supplemental calcium may be required initially, with gradual tapering of the dose over several weeks. A 4:1 ratio of calcium to phosphate should be sought once the serum calcium is normal. This can be accomplished by the use of low phosphorus feedings or human milk supplemented with calcium. Serial measurements of serum Ca and phosphate levels are necessary throughout the period of treatment.

In infants with hypomagnesemia, an intramuscular or intravenous dose of 50% $MgSO_4$ is administered in a dose of 0.1–0.2 ml/kg. If given intravenously the rate of infusion must be slow, with electrocardiographic monitoring to detect acute disturbances. It may be necessary to repeat the treatment every 12 or 24 hours, depending upon the clinical response and the serum concentration of magnesium. In many infants with transient hypomagnesemia, one or two injections of magnesium are sufficient, whereas in others, the therapy may be needed for 2–4 days. Those few infants with chronic hypomagnesemia require lifelong treatment with oral magnesium.

Prognosis

The various forms of neonatal hypocalcemia related to prematurity and diet are usually transitory. In cases of maternal hyperparathyroidism with severe suppression of the fetal parathyroid glands the hypocalcemia may be more prolonged. Renal and gastrointestinal disorders carry the prognosis of the underlying disease.

HYPOPARATHYROIDISM

Definition

Hypoparathyroidism is a state of decreased secretion, or peripheral action of PTH. This condition may result from inadequate secretion of PTH, secretion of a biologically inactive PTH, or end organ insensitivity to PTH.

Epidemiology

There are a number of causes of hypoparathyroidism (Table 14.11). Congenital forms of hypoparathyroidism may be familial or sporadic. A rare sex-linked recessive form with early onset in males in the first month of life has been observed, as well as other forms with rare autosomal dominant and autosomal recessive patterns of inheritance. Hypoparathyroidism and thymic aplasia, which result in a severe immunodeficiency and other congenital anomalies, occur together in patients with DiGeorge syndrome. This disorder is due to defective embryological development of the third and fourth branchial pouches, which contain the anlage of the future parathyroid glands and thymus. Hypoparathyroidism has also been reported in association with ring chromosome 16 and 18.

Maternal hyperparathyroidism causes perinatal hypoparathyroidism through chronic suppression of the fetal parathyroid glands by high concentrations of calcium in the fetal plasma.

Deficient secretion of PTH without a known cause is termed "idiopathic hypoparathyroidism"; the most common form occurs as a component of autosomal polyglandular failure (pp. 833). Idiopathic hypoparathyroidism may occur in combination with Addison disease, diabetes mellitus, autoimmune thyroiditis, or gonadal atrophy. Adrenal insufficiency is the most common endocrine abnormality associated with idiopathic hypoparathyroidism. Over one-third of patients with idiopathic hypoparathyroidism have antibodies to parathyroid tissue and 19% have antibodies to adrenal tissue.

Chronic hypomagnesemia may produce a decrease in PTH secretion or a decrease in target tissue responsiveness to PTH.

Damage to the parathyroid glands may occur during thyroid surgery or other surgery in the area of the neck. The incidence of this varies widely in surgical series but is usually less than 2% in experienced hands. The extent of the thyroid resection, the experience of the surgeon, and the diligence in seeking hypocalcemia all contribute to the variation in incidence. The condition may be transient if sufficient viable parathyroid tissue remains.

Table 14.11
Causes of Hypoparathyroidism

Transient hypofunction
Neonatal
Maternal hyperparathyroidism
Congenital aplasia or hypoplasia of parathyroid glands
DiGeorge syndrome
Chromosomal abnormalities
Maternal diabetes mellitus
Familial hypoparathyroidism
X-linked
Autosomal dominant and recessive
Idiopathic hypoparathyroidism
Autoimmune
Congenital hypoplasia
Surgical removal or damage to parathyroid glands
Hemosiderosis
Hypomagnesemia
Ineffective PTH
Unresponsiveness to PTH
Pseudohypoparathyroidism types I and II

Natural History

The most prominent signs and symptoms of hypoparathyroidism are related to the hypocalcemia that results from the deficiency of PTH. Symptoms may range from mild paresthesias to tetany with muscle cramps, carpopedal spasms, laryngeal stridor, and convulsions. Impaired intellectual performance and frank psychoses may occur. Papilledema, presumably related to increased intracranial pressure, may be seen. Metastatic calcification may occur, particularly in the lens, leading to cataract formation.

The skin is often dry and coarse; the hair is brittle with areas of alopecia. The nails are thin and brittle, often with smooth transverse grooves. Monoliasis of the nails and mouth may be present. Dental and enamel hypoplasia may be observed.

The characteristic facies of DiGeorge syndrome are not often missed. The hypertelorism, nasal clefts, low-set notched ear pinnae, shortened lip philtrum, and micrognathia may be associated with aortic arch anomalies, cardiac malformations, and nephrocalcinosis (Kretschmer et al, 1968).

Diagnosis

In hypoparathyroidism, levels of calcium and PTH in serum are low and those of phosphate are high. In addition, concentrations of 1,25-dihydroxyvitamin D in serum are low. When given exogenous PTH, patients with hypoparathyroidism show a prompt rise in urinary cyclic AMP and phosphate and a rise in serum calcium.

Treatment

The main problem at the time of diagnosis is usually tetany or seizures related to hypocalcemia; therefore, the first order of therapy is normalization of serum calcium levels. Once the diagnosis of hypoparathyroidism has been confirmed therapy with vitamin D or one of its metabolites should be started. Administration of 1,25-dihydroxyvitamin D_3 bypasses the defective 1 α-hydroxylation seen in hypoparathyroidism. The initial dose is 0.03–0.08 μg/kg/day up to a maximum of 1–2 μg/day. Large doses of 25-hydroxyvitamin D_3 (3–6 μg/kg/day) or vitamin D (50,000–100,000 units) may be used instead. 1,25-Dihydroxyvitamin D_3 has a rapid onset of action (7–14 days) and a shorter half-life than do the other forms of vitamin D; therefore, the danger of prolonged toxicity is lessened with its use.

Treatment with vitamin D or its metabolites should be initiated slowly with low doses, increasing the dose in a stepwise fashion with careful monitoring of serum calcium values. The dose of vitamin D may need to be increased in patients on anticonvulsant therapy. In general, it is safer to keep serum calcium levels between 8 and 9 mg/dl than at higher normal levels, because of the significant damage to the kidneys (nephrocalcinosis) and central nervous system which may result from hypercalcemia.

Oral calcium supplements are also useful in therapy. Doses of 50 mg of elemental calcium/kg (or 500/mgof calcium gluconate/kg) up to a maximum of 1 g of calcium (10 g calcium gluconate) can be used in three or four divided doses.

If serum magnesium levels fall below 1.5 mg/dl treatment with magnesium salts should be initiated.

Prognosis

The prognosis for hypoparathyroidism is very good, provided that overdosage with vitamin D is avoided. Early diagnosis and treatment should prevent mental retardation.

Patients with polyglandular failure may develop loss of function of other organs and glands. For example, adrenal insufficiency may develop immediately or several years later. Other endocrine glands are involved less often but may develop impaired function as a result of the autoimmune process. Chronic mucocutaneous candidiasis may occur in conjunction with hypoparathyroidism.

PSEUDOHYPOPARATHYROIDISM (Types I and II)

Definition

Pseudohypoparathyroidism is a state of target organ unresponsiveness to PTH. In type I, the defect is presumed to be in the receptor-adenylate cyclase complex. In type II, the defect is apparently in the kidney only, at a site which is after the generation of cAMP, since administration of PTH to such patients results in a rise in urinary concentration of cAMP.

Epidemiology

Pseudohypoparathyroidism type I was first described by Albright in 1942 in three patients with hypocalcemia, hyperphosphatemia, a blunted phosphaturic and calcemic response to exogenous PTH, and a characteristic physical appearance. This syndrome was subsequently termed Albright hereditary osteodystrophy (Albright et al, 1942). The constellation of phenotypic features appears to be expressed independently of the disturbance in calcium metabolism. Family studies suggest variable inheritance. The ratio of involved females to males is 2:1. Recent studies have shown that type I patients have a defect in the G regulatory unit involved in activation of adenylate cyclase (pp. 796). These patients show a high incidence of resistance to other hormones (Levine et al, 1983). In addition to being resistant to PTH many type I patients are hypothyroid, with elevated levels of serum TSH. In some instances, the hypothyroidism was discovered before a diagnosis of pseudohypoparathyroidism was made (Weisman et al, 1985). Patients may also fail to show elevation of serum prolactin in response to TRH. With water deprivation, the urine in type I patients is less concentrated than it is in normal subjects and the patients show much higher concentrations of vasopressin in serum. Some type I patients may be resistant to glucagon and gonadotropins, which suggests a generalized defect that is distal to the receptors for these hormones.

More recently, a separate clinical type, without the physical stigmata of type I, has been reported. These patients (type II) have the biochemical abnormalities of idiopathic hypoparathyroidism but the defect is not in the adenylate cyclase system. It has been suggested that a defective cyclic AMP-dependent protein kinase could be responsible for the observed lack of phosphaturic response to PTH.

Natural History

Type I pseudohypoparathyroidism is associated with short stature, obesity, round facies, shortened metacarpals and metatarsals, subcutaneous calcification, and moderate mental retardation. The fourth digit is most commonly involved and the second digit least commonly. These patients may have impaired smell and taste. As in hypoparathyroidism, cataracts can occur and the skin may be dry and coarse. Hair and nails may be brittle and dental and enamel hypoplasia may occur. Bony changes are prominent: the bones are wide and the calvaria may be thickened.

Some patients have the anatomic features of type I pseudohypoparathyroidism, but no biochemical abnormalities. This condition is sometimes called pseudopseudohypoparathyroidism. Transition from normocalcemia to hypocalcemia has been observed in some of these patients. This disorder is considered to represent an incomplete form of type I pseudohypoparathyroidism.

In type II pseudohypoparathyroidism, none of the above stigmata are present and only the phosphaturic response to PTH is defective.

Diagnosis

Plasma PTH values are high in pseudohypoparathyroidism. In type I pseudohypoparathyroidism, both bone and kidney are unresponsive to PTH. Administration of 200 units of PTH intravenously to children (5–15 units/kg for infants) will normally be followed by a 10-fold rise in urinary cyclic AMP and shortly thereafter by phosphaturia (4- to 6-fold increase). In patients with type I pseudohypoparathyroidism only a slight rise (less than 2-fold) or no rise at all in urinary cyclic AMP and phosphate may occur; however, the phosphaturic response is variable. In type II pseudohypoparathyroidism, the urinary cyclic AMP response to PTH is normal, but phosphaturia does not occur.

Associated endocrine abnormalities may be evident in type I patients with the G unit abnormality. Almost all patients show an elevated basal TSH value and a hyperresponse to TRH. Antithyroid antibody titers are low or absent and a goiter is usually not found.

CASE ILLUSTRATION

The patient was first seen at 6 years of age because of short stature, mental retardation, and chronic otitis media. She was the product of a normal full-term delivery. She was 1 of 10 children and had passed all the usual developmental milestones at the same age as her siblings; however, she was consistently shorter and heavier than her siblings and had to be placed in a special class in school, starting with first grade. She had frequent bouts of otitis media, but was otherwise healthy. There was no family history of mental retardation or endocrine-metabolic disorders.

On physical examination, she was noted to be short and stocky. Her skin was dry and coarse. Her teeth were carious with decreased enamel. Her fourth metacarpals were shortened bilaterally. She had positive Chvostek and Trousseau signs. Her mental status was subnormal.

Laboratory studies showed serum values of calcium of 8.3 mg/dl, magnesium of 2.2 mg/dl, and phosphate of 6.2 mg/dl; serum PTH values were high. Thyroid function tests showed a serum T_4 level of 5.3 μg/dl and an elevated serum TSH (18 μU/ml). Psychometric tests showed her to be in the high-retarded range. Radiologic films of her hands showed shortened fourth metacarpals and some shortening of the first and fifth metacarpals. Skull x-rays showed thickening of the calvaria.

On the basis of her physical appearance, radiologic findings, and laboratory values a diagnosis of pseudohypoparathyroidism was made and she was treated with vitamin D (50,000 u vitamin D per day). She was followed in clinic at 3-month intervals to check serum calcium and phosphate levels as well as urinary excretion of calcium; the dose of vitamin D was adjusted as needed to maintain serum calcium levels between 8 and 9 mg/dl and urinary calcium below 0.25 mg/mg urinary creatinine. On this regimen the patient did well; however, she required special care and supervision because of her mental retardation.

Patients with pseudohypoparathyroidism may have radiological changes compatible with metabolic bone disease, which are similar to those seen in rickets. Irregularity of the epiphyses, with bowing of long bones and pseudofractures may occur.

Treatment

The therapy for pseudohypoparathyroidism is similar to that for hypoparathyroidism. Type I patients with associated endocrinopathies may require appropriate hormone therapy.

HYPERCALCEMIA

Definition

Hypercalcemia is a condition characterized by elevated levels of ionized calcium in serum. Severe hypercalcemia (serum Ca^{++} above 15 mg/dl) is a medical emergency.

Epidemiology

A variety of conditions can cause hypercalcemia (Table 14.12). In general, they can be divided into those conditions associated with excessive production of PTH and those associated with normal or low PTH production and secretion. In the latter group, tumors that secrete an osteoclastic factor or prostaglandins may cause hypercalcemia. Addison disease, because of a lack of the hypocalcemic effect of corticosteroids, is another cause. Ten percent of hyperthyroid patients may be hypercalcemic. Vitamin A and/or vitamin D intoxication, subcutaneous fat necrosis, and immobilization are other causes.

Table 14.12
Causes of Hypercalcemia

Without PTH excess
William's syndrome
Subcutaneous fat necrosis
Familial hypocalciuric hypercalcemia[1]
Vitamin D and/or vitamin A excess
Hyperthyroidism
Prolonged immobilization
Leukemia
Sarcoidosis, Tuberculosis
Addison's disease
PTH excess
Primary hyperparathyroidism
Adenoma
Familial
Hyperplasia
MEA type I
MEA type II
Secondary hyperparathyroidism
Maternal hypoparathyroidism
Renal osteodystrophy

[1] PTH often inappropriately high for degree of hypercalcemia.

Serum Ca^{++} levels are mildly elevated in benign familial hypercalcemia, an autosomal dominant disorder. In idiopathic hypercalcemia of infancy or Williams syndrome the hypercalcemia often resolves spontaneously after the first few years of life.

Hypercalcemia that is caused by hyperfunction of the parathyroid glands will be discussed separately.

Natural History

The clinical manifestations of hypercalcemia include hypotonia, weakness, listlessnes, and irritability. Anorexia, headache, weight loss, constipation, vomiting, polydipsia, and polyuria are other common symptoms. Prolonged or severe hypercalcemia can cause nephrocalcinosis and subsequent hypertension and renal failure.

In infants with extensive subcutaneous fat necrosis, particularly resulting from traumatic delivery, hypercalcemia may develop. The necrosis usually involves the areas subjected to greatest pressure. For example, with forceps delivery the cheeks are affected typically. The signs of hypercalcemia usually occur 1 or several weeks after birth, with vomiting, lethargy, or irritability and fever. As the fat necrosis resolves, serum Ca^{++} levels fall to normal.

In addition to hypercalcemia in infancy, children with Williams syndrome may have aortic stenosis, mental retardation and facial features described as "elfin-like." The features include a broad forehead, hypertelorism, epicanthal folds, prominent pointed ears, large lips, an underdeveloped nasal bridge, and a small mandible. Soft tissue calcification may occur, as well as osteosclerosis secondary to the hypercalcemia. The hypercalcemia may resolve spontaneously.

Patients with familial benign hypercalcemia (hypocalciuric hypercalcemia) have lifelong asymptomatic hypercalcemia; however, in some patients, life-threatening neonatal hypercalcemia has occurred (Gilbert et al, 1985).

Diagnosis

The serum concentration of PTH will be appropriate or low for the level of serum Ca^{++} in these nonparathyroid disorders. The individual diagnoses will depend upon the history, physical examination, and other laboratory data.

The diagnosis of familial hypocalciuric hypercalcemia (FHH) may be confused with that of asymptomatic primary hyperparathyroidism. The parathyroid glands may be hyperplastic in FHH, but only rarely is the concentration of PTH in serum elevated in absolute terms. The PTH levels are, however, elevated for the serum Ca^{++} level. The hypercalcemia begins in infancy and the condition is found in at least one parent. Characteristically the level of Ca^{++} in urine is low relative to that in serum.

Treatment

For mild to moderate hypercalcemia, an infusion of isotonic saline may be given at a rate of 2–4 times that of maintenance. Acutely, cortisone may be useful. The diet should be low in calcium (less than 100 mg/day) and vitamin D should be eliminated.

For severe hypercalcemia, isotonic saline should be infused and furosemide (1 mg/kg intravenously) should be given every 6–8 hours. Cardiac activity and serum and urinary electrolytes should be monitored carefully. Losses of K^{++} and Mg^{++} should be replaced.

HYPERPARATHYROIDISM

Definition

Hyperparathyroidism is defined as a condition associated with long-term increased secretory rate of PTH.

Epidemiology

Hyperparathyroidism is rare in children. It may occur as a discrete entity or in association with other endocrinopathies as part of multiple endocrine neoplasia (MEN) types I and II (pp. 840). It is seen in infants of hypoparathyroid mothers, in vitamin D-deficient rickets (pp. 849), in disorders of vitamin D metabolism, and in renal abnormalities of phosphate excretion. Primary hyperparathyroidism in infancy is exceedingly rare; only 28 cases have been reported in the literature (Ross et al, 1986).

Natural History

Hyperparathyroidism is often asymptomatic and may be diagnosed initially on the basis of hypercalcemia found unexpectedly on biochemical screening of serum.

Infants born with parathyroid hyperplasia and hypercalcemia have symptoms related to the elevated levels of calcium. Respiratory distress, muscular hypotonia and skeletal demineralization occur. Older children may have nausea, constipation, weight loss, headaches, and personality changes. Renal colic and bone pain are less common in children.

Diagnosis

Hyperparathyroidism is usually suspected if the serum calcium level is elevated; however, at times the serum calcium may be normal. There is usually hypophosphatemia, an elevated alkaline phosphatase, and an increased urinary excretion of cyclic AMP. In most patients the carboxy-terminal immunoreactive PTH in serum is elevated, especially when related to the calcium level. The serum level of 1,25-dihydroxyvitamin D has been reported to be raised in primary hyperparathyroidism. Anemia and an increased sedimentation rate may be present. There may be radiologic evidence of bone resorption, cysts, demineralization, and fractures.

Recently, ultrasonography has been found to be useful in locating and sizing the parathyroid glands.

Treatment

With diffuse primary hyperparathyroidism total parathyroidectomy may be necessary. After surgery, such patients require lifelong treatment for hypoparathyroidism. There have been recent attempts at heterotopic autotransplantation in patients undergoing parathyroidectomy for diffuse hyperparathyroidism (Ross et al, 1986). The long-term success of such efforts is not known at this time, although one child is 2 years postsurgery and is doing well without medication (Ross et al, 1986). In children with adenomas, therapy is surgical removal of the tumor.

RICKETS

This deficiency of mineralization seen in growing bones and resulting in bony deformities may be caused by a number of conditions including: vitamin D deficiency, prematurity, defects in hydroxylation of vitamin D, end organ resistance to 1,25-dihydroxyvitamin D and hypophosphatemia. Vitamin D deficiency is discussed in Chapter 00. In this chapter, we shall consider the other causes of rickets.

Rickets in Premature Infants

Epidemiology

Rickets is not uncommon in premature infants. Calcium and phosphate requirements are high in the rapidly growing preterm infant. In a recent study, the fraction of calcium absorbed in premature infants ranged between 65% and 97% and was not influenced by postnatal age, postconceptional age, body weight or intake of various formulae (Ehrenkranz et al, 1985). Thus, the absorption of calcium in premature infants is highly efficient. Rickets has occurred in some premature infants with normal serum levels of 25-hydroxyvitamin D and elevated levels of 1,25-dihydroxyvitamin D (Steichen et al, 1981). These babies improved on formulae with high mineral content, suggesting that in some premature infants rickets may be caused by calcium and phosphate deficiency. Human milk, which has a low phosphate content, may not provide sufficient phosphate in the rapidly growing premature or full-term infant, resulting in rickets associated with phosphate depletion (Sagy et al, 1980; Cosgrove and Dietrich, 1985). Other studies suggest that in some babies a deficiency of vitamin D is the cause of rickets.

Natural History

The patient appears healthy at birth. Symptoms of rickets occur within the first year of life. Hypotonia, weakness, and growth failure are common manifestations of the disorder. There may be a history of convulsions or tetany. Motor retardation may be evident, with poor head control and failure to stand or walk.

Typical signs of rickets include craniotabes, frontal skull bossing, thickening of wrists and ankles, rachitic rosary (enlarged costochondral junctions), and widened ribs. Bowing of long bones may not occur until weight-bearing begins.

Diagnosis

The biochemical abnormalities in premature babies with rickets are similar to those found in older children. Serum concentrations of calcium and inorganic phosphate may be low to low-normal, alkaline phosphatase activity is elevated, and circulating levels of PTH are increased secondary to the hypocalcemia. Radiographs show characteristic bony changes.

Treatment

Vitamin D supplementation and/or high-mineral formulae will usually heal the rickets.

Defects in Hydroxylation of Vitamin D

Epidemiology

Both liver (25-hydroxylation) and kidney (1 α-hydroxylation) are involved in the biosynthesis of biologically active 1,25-dihydroxyvitamin D_3. Cirrhosis of the liver, neonatal hepatitis, biliary atresia, and cholestasis may lead to "hepatic rickets," in which patients the rickets is more likely to be due to impaired fat absorption with associated deficiency of vitamin D rather than to impaired 25-hydroxylation. In some hypocalcemic patients with thalassemia major, 25-hydroxylation in the liver has been found to be impaired, presumably secondary to massive parenchymal hemosiderosis (Zaino et al, 1985).

Phenobarbital and dilantin use can lead to decreased serum concentration of 25-hydroxyvitamin D and rickets. Two mechanisms appear to be involved: (1) a dose-related stimulation of a microsomal enzyme system (hepatic mixed function oxidase), resulting in increased catabolism and excretion of vitamin D and its metabolites, and (2) direct inhibitory effects on intestinal calcium transport and bone metabolism.

An inherited autosomal recessive defect in renal 1 α-hydroxylase has been described. This condition has been termed vitamin D-dependent rickets type I (Table 14.13). The name refers to the fact that large doses of vitamin D are required for treatment in contrast to the physiologic doses required in vitamin D deficient rickets. Small physiologic doses of 1,25-dihydroxyvitamin D are effective, however, since this therapy bypasses the enzyme defect. Production of 1,25-dihydroxyvitamin D also is impaired in renal failure.

Natural History

The signs and symptoms mimic those of vitamin D deficiency rickets: hypotonia, muscle weakness, hypocalcemia, convulsions, and growth failure developing in the first year of life.

Diagnosis

Circulating levels of 1,25-dihydroxyvitamin D are low in association with increased serum PTH and typical rachitic bone changes.

Treatment

Administration of 1,25-dihydroxyvitamin D_3 bypasses the metabolic block. In uremic patients with phosphate retention, oral "phosphate binders" (Am-

Table 14.13
Biochemical Features of Rickets[1]

Type	Plasma Concentration						Urine Concentration		
	Ca	PO4	AP	250HD	1,25D	PTH	Ca	cAMP	PO4
Vitamin D-deficient	↓	↓ or N	↑	↓	↑, N, or ↓	↑	↓	↑	
Vitamin D-dependent									
Type I	↓	↓ or N	↑	↑	↓	↑	↓	↑	
Type II	↓	↓ or N	↑	↑ or N	↑↑	↑	↓	↑	↑
Hypophosphatemic rickets	N	↓	↑	↑	↓	N	↓	N	↑

[1]Abbreviations: AP = alkaline phosphatase, N = normal.

phogel) and a low-phosphate diet help to reduce the degree of hyperphosphatemia and consequent hyperparathyroidism.

End-Organ Resistance to 1,25-Dihydroxyvitamin D (Vitamin D-Dependent Rickets Type II)

Epidemiology

In 1978, Brooks and coworkers described a patient with hypocalcemic rickets who was resistant to the action of 1,25-dihydroxyvitamin D_3. They proposed the term vitamin D-dependent rickets type II to distinguish the disorder from vitamin D-dependent rickets type I. These disorders of end-organ resistance are familial and may be associated with alopecia (Hochberg et al, 1984). Skin fibroblasts from patients can be grown in culture and tested for their ability to bind labeled 1,25-dihydroxyvitamin D_3. Some patients have been shown to have fibroblasts that take up and bind 1,25-dihydroxyvitamin D_3, while others lack these receptors. Fibroblasts from another kindred can bind the hormone, but the affinity of the receptor-hormone complex for nuclear DNA is decreased (Hirst et al, 1985). These disorders are rare.

Natural History

Evidence of rickets and alopecia may manifest at birth or anytime within the first year of life. This is in sharp contrast to babies with vitamin D-dependent rickets type I who appear normal at birth. Those kindreds with vitamin D-dependent rickets type II without alopecia have been diagnosed between 5 and 25 months of age. There is usually a family history of rickets or alopecia. In some kindreds the metabolic defect normalizes and bones heal as the individuals get older, but there is no change in the alopecia.

Diagnosis

Characteristically these patients show evidence of hypocalcemia, hypophosphatemia, increased concentrations of alkaline phosphatase and PTH in the serum, and increased urinary levels of cAMP and phosphate. The serum concentrations of 25-hydroxyvitamin D and 24,25-dihydroxyvitamin D are normal, while the level of 1,25-dihydroxyvitamin D is markedly raised. There is diffuse demineralization of the skeleton with cupping of the epiphyseal-metaphyseal junctions.

Treatment

Megadoses of vitamin D or its metabolites fail to heal the rickets in most patients with alopecia. During childhood, patients without alopecia appeared to respond clinically and radiologically to large doses of vitamin D (17–20 μg of 1,25-dihydroxyvitamin D/day). Spontaneous healing in late childhood has occurred in some cases.

Hereditary X-Linked Hypophosphatemic Rickets

Epidemiology

This condition is the most common form of hereditary rickets. It is most severe in males; females may exhibit only hypophosphatemia. Kindreds have been described with both autosomal dominant and autosomal recessive patterns of inheritance. The renal threshold for phosphate excretion is low and a parallel defect in intestinal phosphate transport may be present. Intestinal absorption of calcium is mildly decreased. In a strain of mice with X-linked hypophosphatemic rickets renal and intestinal transport of phosphate is clearly abnormal; a defect in sodium-dependent phosphate transport has been found in vesicles of brush border membranes from kidneys of affected animals.

Other forms of dysfunction of the proximal renal tubules may result in phosphaturia and rickets (pp. 632). Distal renal tubular acidosis is also associated with hypophosphatemia and rickets.

Diagnosis

These children have a retarded bone age and stature is decreased, with the most severe shortening in the legs. The radiographic features are those of rickets and osteomalacia.

The biochemical features of the disorder include a normal concentration of calcium in serum and a significantly depressed concentration of phosphate appearing at about ages 4–6 months (Table 14.13). Alkaline phosphatase activity in plasma may be high when the rickets is active but is otherwise normal. In general, the serum level of 1,25-dihydroxyvitamin D is low for the degree of hypophosphatemia and the mild secondary hyperparathyroidism.

These children are not usually diagnosed until they have been weight-bearing and have developed bowed legs. Bowing of the legs, medial tibial torsion, and short stature are the major clinical problems.

CASE ILLUSTRATION

A 34-month-old white female was seen for evaluation of bowed legs.

The condition was first noted when the child was about 3 months of age and it was treated by an orthopedic surgeon with leg braces and corrective shoes. The child was on an adequate diet and there were no symptoms of malabsorption or renal disease. She had no skeletal abnormalities other than her bowed legs. She had difficulty running and walking up or down stairs.

Over the first year of life her growth in height and weight fell on the 50th centile line, but over the next 2 years her growth rate declined until her values when first examined in the clinic were on the 3rd centile for weight and below the 3rd centile in height.

The child had a 6-year-old sister with asthma and a brother who had died at 2 months of age of "crib death." There was no family history of renal disease or malabsorption.

On physical examination, prominent bowing of her legs was evident. There were no other abnormalities. Laboratory values revealed: serum BUN 10 mg/dl, creatinine 0.45 mg/dl, Cl 106 mEq/L, pH 7.45, Ca 10.1 mg/dl, phosphate 1.9 mg/dl, and alkaline phosphatase 150 mU/ml. Urinary calcium and amino acid excretion was normal but 24-hour urinary phosphate excretion was elevated at 2.59 g (normal, 0.8–2.0 g). X-rays of hips and legs showed anterolateral bowing of her femur with coarse trabeculation. There was widening and fraying of the distal femur and proximal tibial epiphyses as well as the distal tibial and fibular epiphyses. The growth plate was widened and the bone density was decreased. The changes were considered characteristic of rickets.

On the basis of an adequate vitamin D intake, normal intestinal absorption, low serum phosphate, high urinary phosphate excretion, high serum alkaline phosphatase, and classic radiologic finding of rickets, a diagnosis of hypophosphatemic rickets was made. She was treated with 1,25-dihydroxyvitamin D_3 (Rocaltrol, 0.25 ug twice daily) and phosphorus supplements, seven times a day. On this regimen her serum phosphate levels rose to around 3 mg/dl and her urine calcium/creatine ratios were around 0.3. She improved in linear growth but eventually, at age 9 years, she required bilateral distal femoral osteotomy to correct her severely bowed legs.

Other renal causes of hypophosphatemic rickets such as renal tubular acidosis, Fanconi syndrome, cystinosis, or Lowe syndrome must be considered (pp. 633, 755).

Treatment

Therapy with both inorganic phosphate (1–4 g of elemental phosphorus/day and 1,25-dihydroxyvitamin D_3 have produced good results in these patients. The phosphate must be given by mouth at 4-hour intervals to maintain a nearly normal serum concentration of phosphate. As with any therapy involving vitamin D, serum and urinary calcium levels must be monitored closely in order to avoid hypercalcemia and hypercalcuria, which may lead to permanent kidney damage (Harrison and Finberg, 1981). Vitamin D intoxication is discussed in detail on page 100.

Those patients with severe bone deformities may require surgery.

Summary

Disorders of mineral metabolism may be a result of dietary deficiency or excess or may be secondary to altered PTH and 1,25-dihydroxyvitamin D secretion and/or action. In evaluating the child with abnormal levels of calcium or phosphate a careful dietary and family history must be obtained. Once a dietary deficiency state and known hereditary conditions have been ruled out, the physician should look for evidence of malabsorption or hepatic and renal disorders. In addition, the levels of PTH and vitamin D and its metabolites in blood should be obtained. Evidence of hyper- or hypoparathyroidism must be examined in terms of the known causes of these conditions. End-organ unresponsiveness to PTH and/or vitamin D can be ascertained by appropriate testing.

REFERENCES

Albright F, Burnett C, Smith PH, et al: Pseudo-hypoparathyroidism—an example of "Seabright-Bantam" syndrome. *Endocrinology* 30:922, 1942.

Brooks MH, Bell NH, Love L, et al: Vitamin D-dependent rickets type II. Resistance of target organs to 1,25-dihydroxyvitamin D. *N Engl J Med* 298:996, 1978.

Brown EM: Parathyroid secretion in vivo and in vitro. Regulation by calcium and other secretagogues. *Min Elect Metabol* 8:130, 1982.

Cooper LJ, Anast CS: Circulating immunoreactive parathyroid hormone levels in premature infants and the response to calcium therapy. *Acta Paediatr Scand* 74:669, 1985.

Cosgrove L, Dietrich A: Nutritional rickets in breast fed infants. *J Fam Pract* 21:205, 1985.

David L, Anast CS: Calcium metabolism in newborn infants. The interrelationship of parathyroid function and calcium, magnesium and phosphorus metabolism in normal, "sick", and hypocalcemia newborns. *J Clin Invest* 54:287, 1974.

DeLuca HF: The vitamin D story: A collaborative effort of basic science and clinical medicine. *FASEB J* 2:224, 1988.

Ehrenkranz RA, Ackerman BA, Nelli CM, et al: Absorption of calcium in premature infants as measured with a stable isotope ^{46}Ca extrinsic tag. *Pediatr Res* 19:178, 1985.

Gilbert F, D'Amour P, Gascon-Barre M, et al: Familial hypocalciuric hypercalcemia: Description of a new kindred with emphasis on its difference from primary hyperparathyroidism. *Clin Invest Med* 8:78, 1985.

Harrison HE, Finberg L: Rickets: Primary hypophosphatemic and vitamin D-dependent varieties. *J Pediatr* 99:84:1981.
Hirst MA, Hochman HI, Feldman D: Vitamin D resistance and alopecia: A kindred with normal 1,25-dihydroxyvitamin D binding but decreased receptor affinity for deoxyribonucleic acid. *J Clin Endocrinol Metabol* 60:490, 1985.
Hochberg Z, Benderli A, Levy J, et al: 1,24-dihydroxyvitamin D resistance, rickets, and alopecia. *Am J Med* 77:805, 1984.
Kretschmer R, Say B, Brown D, et al: Congenital aplasia of the thymus gland (DiGeorge syndrome). *N Engl J Med* 279:1295, 1968.
Levine MA, Down RW Jr, Moses AM, et al: Resistance to multiple hormones in patients with pseudohypoparathyroidism. *Am J Med* 74:545, 1983.
Potts JT Jr, Kronenberg HM, Rosenblatt M: Parathyroid hormone: Chemistry, biosynthesis, and mode of action. *Adv Protein Chem* 35:323, 1982.
Ross AJ, Cooper A, Attie MF, et al: Primary hyperparathyroidism in infancy. *J Pediatr Surg* 21:493, 1986.
Sagy M, Birenbaum E, Balin A, et al: Phosphate depletion syndrome in a premature infant fed human milk. *J Pediatr* 96:683, 1980.
Steichen JJ, Tsang RC, Gratton TL, et al: Vitamin D homeostasis in the perinatal period—1,25-dihydroxyvitamin D in maternal, cord, and neonatal blood. *N Engl J Med* 302:315, 1980.
Steichen JJ, Tsang RC, Greer FR, et al: Elevated serum 1,25-dihydroxyvitamin D concentrations in rickets of very low birth weight infants. *J Pediatr* 99:293, 1981.
Weisman Y, Golander A, Spirer Z, et al: Pseudohypoparathyroidism type 1a presenting as congenital hypothyroidism. *J Pediatr* 107:413, 1985.
Weisman Y, Harell A, Edelstein S, et al: 1,25-Dihydroxyvitamin D_3 and 24,25-dihydroxyvitamin D_3: In vitro synthesis by human decidua and placenta. *Nature* 281:317, 1979.
Whitsett JA, Ho M, Tsang RC, et al: Synthesis of 1,25-dihydroxyvitamin D_3 by human placenta in vitro. *J Clin Endocrinol Metabol* 53:484, 1981.
Zaino EC, Yeh JK, Aloia J: Defective vitamin D metabolism in thalassemia major. *Ann NY Acad Sci* 445:127, 1985.

Adrenal Glands 6

Fetal Adrenal

The adrenal gland is one of the earliest endocrine glands to develop in the embryo and it plays a unique role during perinatal life. Several days before there is any indication of a gonadal primordium, cells from the coelomic epithelium on the medial surface of the urogenital ridge, in the dorsomedial angle of the body cavity, begin to proliferate and gradually condense into a discrete mass—the primordium of the adrenal cortex. The proliferation of the cortical cells begins in embryos about 6 mm long (28 days), at a time when all the endocrine primordia except the gonads are visible. By 34 days (10 mm), the cortical anlage is seen as a discrete mass of cells medial to the mesonephros and ventral to the aorta. At about this time primitive cells from the sympathetic primordium begin to invade the adrenal cortex. They will form the future adrenal medulla.

Sometime after 6 weeks' gestation the fetal zone of the adrenal cortex appears and eventually occupies about 80% of the volume of the fetal adrenal. The cells of the fetal zone have decreased activity of 3 β-hydroxysteroid dehydrogenase, an enzyme essential for the biosynthesis of biologically active steroid hormones (Fig. 14.12). This diminished activity exists despite high levels of ACTH and it may be secondary to inhibitory effects of placental steroids, in particular estrogens, which reach the fetus in large quantities (Byrne et al, 1985). These cells are, however, very proficient at sulfurylation of steroids and hydroxylating steroids in the 16 α position. Thus, the products of the fetal zone, and therefore of the fetal adrenal gland, are largely 16 α-hydroxylated-Δ 5-steroids such as 16 α-hydroxydehydroepiandrosterone and its sulfate. Cortisol, aldosterone, and Δ 4-androstenedione are secreted primarily by the adult zone of the fetal adrenal. This zone becomes the definitive adrenal cortex postnatally, whereas the fetal zone disappears within a few weeks or months after birth. It has been postulated that during fetal life the adrenal gland becomes hyperplastic secondary to the relatively high levels of circulating ACTH in the fetus (Byrne et al, 1985). The latter condition represents a response to the relatively low production of glucocorticoids in the fetal adrenal gland in which 3 β-hydroxysteroid dehydrogenase is suppressed by placental estrogens. Once these estrogens disappear after birth, glucocorticoids rise and ACTH levels fall, with resulting regression of that portion of the fetal gland that makes Δ-5-3 β-hydroxysteroids, namely the fetal zone.

The fetal liver is also capable of 16 α-hydroxylating steroids so that estrogens reaching the fetus from the

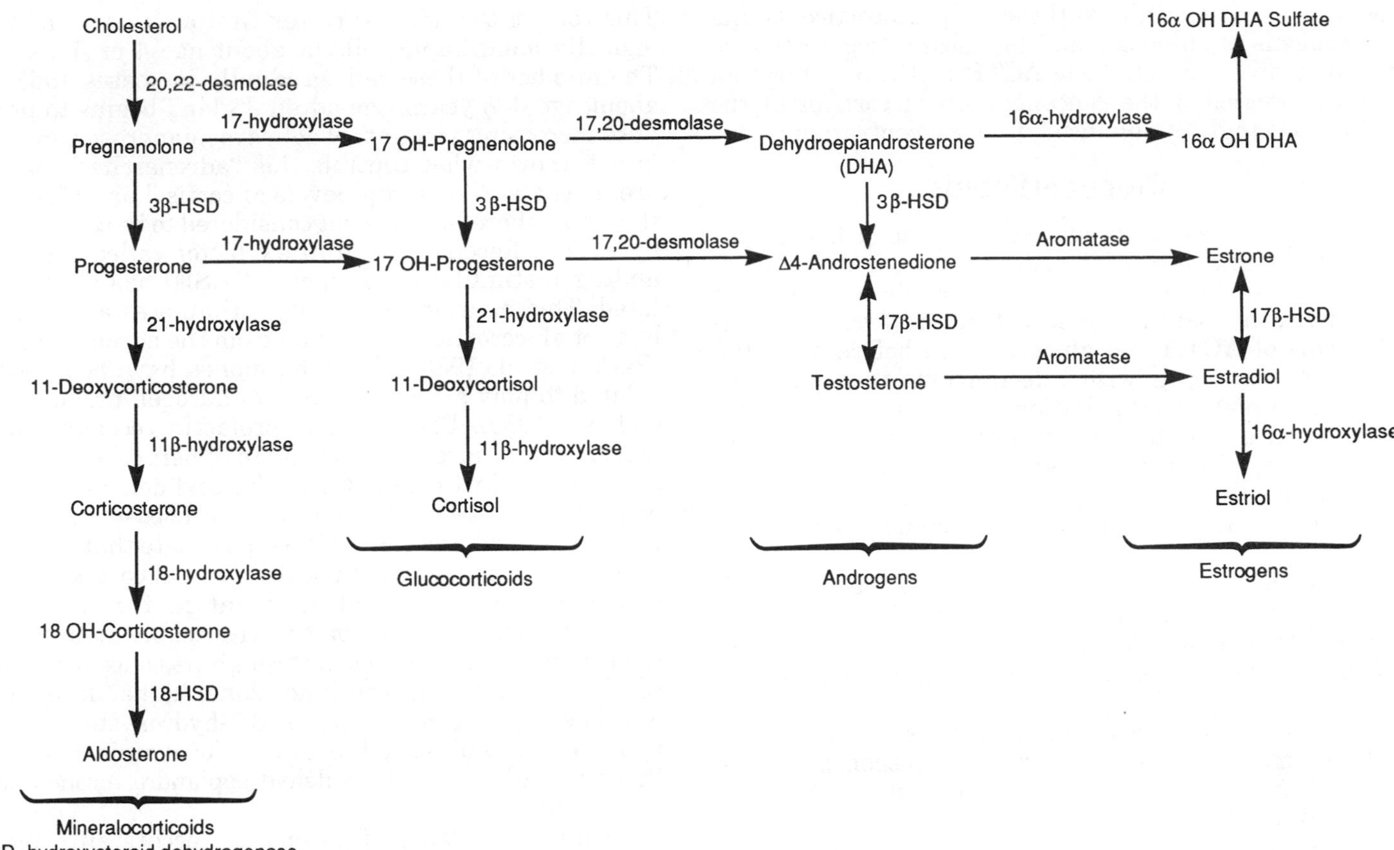

Figure 14.12. Pathways of adrenal steroid biosynthesis.

mother are rapidly converted to estriol (a 16 α-hydroxylated product) and, thus, inactivated.

The human placenta has a very active 3 β-hydroxysteroid dehydrogenase, but lacks 16 α-hydroxylase and 17,20 desmolase (the enzyme that catalyzes the removal of the side chain of the 21-carbon steroids to form androgens, which are the precursors of estrogens). Thus, the human placenta cannot form estrogens de novo but can convert androgens from the maternal and fetal adrenals to estrogens. The fetal zone of the adrenal cannot form cortisol de novo but can convert placental progesterone to cortisol (Fig. 14.12). The attractive complementarity of the enzymes of the fetal adrenal cortex and those of the placenta has encouraged adoption of the concept that the fetus and placenta collaborate in the synthesis of estrogens and glucocorticoids and the term "fetoplacental unit" was coined. It must be remembered, however, that the maternal contributions to steroid metabolism are important also.

The contributions of the fetus to estrogen production are useful in following the condition of the fetus in high-risk pregnancies. A fall in maternal levels of estrogens (especially estriol) may signal a pregnancy in jeopardy. Either hepatic or adrenal insufficiency in the fetus will be reflected by a fall in maternal estriol.

Considerable evidence indicates that glucocorticoids play a major role in the differentiation and maturation of several fetal tissues, including lung, gut, and retina. The circulation of the developing adrenal gland permits blood from the cortex to perfuse the medulla. Exposure of norepinephrine-producing cells in the medulla to high local concentrations of glucocorticoids late in pregnancy and after birth induces N-methyltransferase, an enzyme that catalyzes the conversion of norepinephrine to epinephrine. In the human fetus, epinephrine synthesis rises in pregnancy as the production of glucocorticoids is increased. Since steroids cross the placenta freely, glucocorticoids from the mother are available to the fetus also.

Biosynthesis and Secretion of Adrenocortical Hormones

Three types of hormones are synthesized normally by the adrenal cortex: glucocorticoids, mineralocorticoids, and sex hormones. The production of all three types of hormones is enhanced by ACTH, which interacts with a cell-surface receptor and thereby increases the intracellular concentration of cyclic AMP (see Chapter 1). The actual biosynthesis of the steroid hormones involves a long series of reactions, starting with cholesterol (from the blood) and including sequential side-chain cleavages, hydroxylations, and oxidations of intermediates (Fig. 14.12). The rate-limiting step is the side-chain cleavage of cholesterol, which is stimulated by ACTH. Other steps may be affected by ACTH as well, so that overall synthesis of glucocorticoids and androgens is enhanced and to a lesser degree that of aldosterone. The release of ACTH by the pituitary can be suppressed if the concentration of cortisol in the plasma is high, or enhanced if the concentration is low.

Glucocorticoids

Glucocorticoids, produced in the zona fasciculata and zona reticularis of the adrenal cortex, are secreted episodically, but with an overall circadian pattern. In humans, this pattern is characterized by peak concentrations of ACTH and glucocorticoid before or at the time of awakening, with a decline over the remainder of the 24-hour period. Patients with adrenal insufficiency on adequate replacement therapy continue to have this episodic and rhythmic secretion of ACTH, indicating that this pattern is intrinsic to the hypothalamic control system and independent of feedback control.

The diurnal pattern of ACTH release can be modified by altering the sleep pattern, but only if the change is maintained for several days. The pattern of light and darkness also affects the diurnal rhythm, as does blindness.

Both psychological and physical stress can stimulate ACTH release. Ordinarily the response bears a quantitative relationship to the intensity of the stimulus. When the stress is overwhelming, however, the adrenal may fail and the cortisol level in plasma will fall.

Glucocorticoids in plasma are not in simple solution but are in equilibrium with two plasma proteins: albumin, which has a large capacity but low affinity, and corticosteroid-binding globulin (CBG), a glycoprotein with high affinity but limited capacity. Typically about 90% of plasma cortisol is bound to CBG, 6% is bound to albumin, and 4% is free. It is the free cortisol that is capable of crossing cell membranes and affecting the cellular genome.

Glucocorticoids are metabolized rapidly and excreted in the urine as 17-hydroxycorticosteroids (17-OHCS); however, a small fraction of cortisol is excreted in urine in the free form. Free cortisol as well as other steroid hormones are also found in saliva. Some of the glucocorticoids undergo side-chain cleavage in the liver and the resulting 17-ketosteroids (17-KS) are excreted in the urine.

Sex Hormones

Adrenal androgens such as dehydroepiandrosterone and Δ-4-androstenedione are biologically weak androgens, but they can be converted to biologically active androgens, such as testosterone and dihydrotestosterone, peripherally. The secretion of adrenal androgens occurs episodically and in synchrony with the secretion of cortisol. They are metabolized in the liver to inactive products (reduced ring A) and excreted in the urine as 17-KS.

The zona reticularis, the inner layer of the adrenal cortex, is responsible for the biosynthesis of androgens. This zone of the adrenal cortex first appears as histologically identifiable cells at about age 4 or 5 years. The number of these cells gradually increases and, at about age 6–8 years, the adrenal gland begins to produce increasing amounts of dehydroepiandrosterone. It is not known what controls this "adrenarche." There are no changes in serum levels of cortisol or ACTH at this time; therefore, it is not considered to be controlled by ACTH. Recently, a pituitary factor called cortical androgen stimulating hormone (CASH) has been isolated. This material apparently stimulates androgen, but not glucocorticoid secretion from the adrenal gland (Parker et al, 1983). Other hormones have been postulated to play a role in adrenal androgen production (Adams, 1985). For example, prolactin receptors are present in the adrenal gland and in hyperprolactinemic conditions dehydroepiandrosterone and dehydroepiandrosterone sulfate levels are increased (Lobo et al, 1980). Dickerman and associates (1984) postulate that the apparent functional zonation of the adrenal cortex is imposed by a several-fold gradient in free steroid concentration across the cortex, presumably induced by the centripetal flow of blood through its concentric parenchymal layers. In the inner zone, higher levels of Δ-4-3-ketosteroids may suppress 3 β-hydroxysteroid dehydrogenase and shift the pattern of steroid biosynthesis toward production of dehydroepiandrosterone and its sulfate.

Clinical evidence of adrenarche occurs after biochemical adrenarche with the onset of growth of pubic hair and increased activity of sweat and sebaceous glands. Adrenarche may occur independently of gonadarche.

Thus, secretion of adrenal androgens appears to be controlled by ACTH, by intraadrenal steroidal effects, and probably by hormones such as CASH and prolactin. Under ordinary circumstances pituitary gonadotropins do not influence adrenal androgen production; however, some androgen-producing adrenal carcinomas appear to be responsive to hCG (Wen et al, 1985).

Estrogen production by the normal human adrenal cortex appears to be minimal; however, estrogens may be formed peripherally from adrenal androgens. Both adipose tissue and muscle contribute to the conversion of Δ-4-androstenedione to estrone.

Mineralocorticoids

Aldosterone formation occurs almost entirely in the zona glomerulosa of the adrenal cortex; however, intermediates in the biosynthetic pathway (deoxycorticosterone, corticosterone, and 18-hydroxycorticosterone) are also synthesized by the fasciculata-reticularis cells. Production of these steroids is increased by the administration of ACTH, which enhances the production and release of aldosterone. Nevertheless, the primary regulator of mineralocorticoid synthesis is the renin-angiotensin system. Either renin (the enzyme catalyzing the conversion of angiotensinogen to angiotensin I) or angiotensin II increases both aldosterone secretion and the width of the adrenal zona glomerulosa. Renin is produced in the juxtaglomerular cells of the kidney, which respond to changes in pressure and sodium concentration. Sympathetic nerves of the kidney also modify renin release. Prostaglandins also may be mediators of renin release.

Angiotensin II is formed from angiotensin I by a converting enzyme found in blood and several tissues. Considerable conversion takes place in the lung. Angiotensin II acts directly in the zona glomerulosa, interacting directly with its receptor in these cells without the involvement of cyclic AMP, to stimulate biosynthesis of aldosterone. It also acts on blood vessels to increase peripheral arterial resistance, thus raising blood pressure. Apparently, calcium is required for the stimulation of aldosterone synthesis; the steps involved are increased desmolase activity and enhanced conversion of corticosterone to aldosterone.

In addition to the renin-angiotensin system, potassium can increase aldosterone synthesis by interacting directly with cells of the zona glomerulosa. Minor changes in potassium concentration in the serum can alter aldosterone synthesis and release. Potassium can also modify the release of renin by the juxtaglomerular cells.

An atrial natriuretic peptide (ANP) of 28 amino acids has been isolated from human atria (Kangawa and Matsuo, 1984). Some evidence suggests that this substance is capable of inhibiting aldosterone synthesis in glomerulosa cells in vitro (Atarashi et al, 1984). Increased plasma ANP levels have been found in several clinical conditions including primary aldosteronism. It has been demonstrated in cord blood with higher values in umbilical cord arterial than in cord venous plasma, suggesting that ANP may be secreted by fetal tissue (Yamaji et al, 1986). A glycoprotein formed in the anterior pituitary, aldosterone stimulating factor (ASF), has been found in human urine. This substance has been shown to stimulate aldosterone production by glomerulosa cells in vitro (Sen et al, 1981). The physiologic significance of ANP and ASF in the overall regulation of aldosterone biosynthesis and secretion is unknown.

In plasma, 22% of aldosterone is bound to CBG, 41% to albumin, and 37% is free. A small fraction of secreted aldosterone is excreted unchanged in the urine. A larger fraction (about 15%) is conjugated in both kidney and liver with glucuronic acid at C-18 to form aldosterone glucuronide. A large portion of aldosterone secreted by the adrenal cortex is metabolized in the liver by reduction of ring A of the steroid molecule to form tetrahydroaldosterone conjugated with glucuronic acid at C-3.

Epinephrine

The medullary tissue (chromaffin cells) of adrenal glands contains catecholamines, localized in chromaffin granules. The important catecholamines in the human are dopamine, norepinephrine, and epinephrine. The physiologic stimulus for release of catecholamines from these granules is acetylcholine, which originates in the preganglionic sympathetic nerve endings. Acetylcholine induces changes in the chromaffin cell membrane that result in increased permeability to calcium. Influx of calcium occurs and intracellular calcium rises, triggering extrusion of the soluble contents of the chromaffin granule into the extracellular space (exocytosis).

In addition to catecholamines, the adrenal medulla stores opioid peptides within the chromaffin granules. Both met- and leu-enkephalin have been identified. The human adrenal medulla also contains β-endorphin and other peptides derived from the pro-opiomelanocortin molecule. These opioid peptides are released along with the catecholamines in response to stimulation of the chromaffin cells.

At concentrations normally found in humans, 50–60% of the catecholamines in plasma are loosely bound to protein. Basal levels of epinephrine in plasma range from 20–50 pg/ml, but depending upon the stimulus these values may rise mildly (upright posture), moderately (cigarette smoking, exercise), or markedly (hypoglycemia). Transient rises in plasma levels of epinephrine occur with pain and/or anxiety. The half-life of circulating norepinephrine and epinephrine is less than 1 minute. Norepinephrine released from sympathetic nerve endings is inactivated primarily by reuptake into the sympathetic nerves. The remainder enters the general circulation where, with epinephrine, it is cleared principally by metabolism in the liver, gut, and kidney with formation of metanephrines and 3-methoxy-4-hydroxymandelic acid (VMA), which are excreted in the urine.

The physiologic changes induced by catecholamines are mediated via adrenergic receptors on the surface of effector cells. α-Adrenergic receptors mediate a variety of responses, including vasoconstriction. Many, if not all, β-receptor responses (cardiac stimulation, bronchodilation, and vasodilation) are mediated by cyclic AMP. Norepinephrine is primarily an α-receptor stimulator, whereas epinephrine induces both α- and β-receptor activity. The adrenergic receptors modulate many responses that regulate basic metabolic processes, including glycogenolysis, lipolysis, enzyme secretion, and ion transport. The α-receptor is blocked selectively by phentolamine or phenoxybenzamine, whereas propranolol blocks the β-receptor.

ADRENAL GLAND DISORDERS

Congenital Adrenocortical Hyperplasia

Definition

Congenital adrenocortical hyperplasia (CAH) is a condition associated with inherited enzymatic defects of steroid synthesis that interfere with the biosynthesis of normal amounts of cortisol and, therefore, result in a hyperplastic reaction in the adrenal gland secondary to increased ACTH secretion. In most cases excessive androgens are produced and the female may manifest ambiguous genitalia at birth and/or virilization in later life. A salt-losing syndrome is present in 60–80% of patients with CAH.

Basic Science

Figure 14.12 shows the number of enzymes involved in the conversion of cholesterol to cortisol. Human mutants lacking or deficient in each of these enzymes have been described (Table 14.14). In each instance cortisol production is impaired, resulting in increased secretion of ACTH and hyperplasia of the adrenal gland. It is only at the expense of high levels of circulating ACTH, which result in hyperfunctioning of the adrenal gland and excessive production of androgens, that the plasma concentration of cortisol can be maintained within normal limits in such individuals.

By far the most common of these enzyme deficiencies is lack of 21-hydroxylase, which catalyzes the conversion of 17-hydroxyprogesterone to 11-deoxycortisol (Compound S). The disorder occurs in about 1/5000–15,000 live births, depending upon the population and area involved, and accounts for about 90% of all cases of CAH. It is inherited as an autosomal recessive trait. Close genetic linkage between the genes for human leukocyte antigens (HLA) and the gene for 21-hydroxylase deficiency was first described by Dupont et al (1977). Each parent of a patient with 21-hydroxylase deficiency is an obligate heterozygote carrier and transmits 1 HLA haplotype carrying the gene for 21-hydroxylase deficiency to the patient. Both HLA haplotypes of the patient are linked to the gene for 21-hydroxylase deficiency and therefore any member of the family who shares 1 haplotype with the patient should also carry the gene for the enzyme defect.

Different forms of 21-hydroxylase deficiency are associated with genes for characteristic HLA antigens (Table 14.14). The HLA complex consists of at least four genetic loci which code for HLA-A, HLA-B, HLA-C, and HLA-D/DR. Multiple alleles have been demonstrated for each locus. There are also other loci which have been mapped on chromosome 6 in close linkage with HLA. Apparently the 21-hydroxylase deficiency gene is located between the HLA-A locus and the centromere, but is further away from the centromere than the glyoxalase I locus.

In patients with classical (salt-losing or nonsalt-losing) 21-hydroxylase deficiency the allele HLA-BW47 is found with increased frequency, especially among caucasians throughout Europe and North America. This allele was noted to be most often on one particular haplotype: HLA-A3, BW47, CW6, DR7 (Dupont et al, 1977). There are four complement loci, BF, C2, C4A, and C4B linked to the HLA region on chromosome 6. These loci are very closely linked to one another and are close to HLA-DR (Raum et al, 1981). Fleischnick et al (1983) have found a marked increase in frequency of the rare allele C4B*31 among patients with classical 21-hydroxylase deficiency.

Two "variant" forms of 21-hydroxylase deficiency are associated with HLA-B14; DR1, in which patients have a relatively mild defect in cortisol synthesis and either remain asymptomatic ("cryptic" form) or develop symptoms of virilization in late childhood or at puberty ("late-onset" form).

Evidence suggests that 21-hydroxylase deficiency results from a mutation involving the structural gene for a cytochrome P-450 specific for hydroxylation at carbon 21 of the steroid molecule (White et al, 1984). It is likely that the gene is located near the C4A locus. Apparently two P-450 genes are present, one of which is deleted on the HLA-BW47 haplotype. The authors hypothesize that one gene, under control of ACTH, may be expressed in the zona fasciculata and be responsible for cortisol synthesis, whereas the other gene may be involved in aldosterone synthesis in the zona glomerulosa. Presumably deletions of both genes would cause the salt-wasting form of 21-hydroxylase deficiency. Studies using gene cloning techniques have shown two P-450 (C21) genes each located near the 3′ end of the two C4 genes in a relatively short stretch of human chromosomal DNA. Deletion of one P-450 (C21) gene gives a deficiency of 21-hydroxylation in patients with HLA-BW47 haplotype. The other P-450 (C21) gene is nonfunctional (Higashi et al, 1986).

Table 14.14
Disorders of Adrenal Steroid Biosynthesis[1]

	Ambiguity			Serum		
	M	F	Urine 17-KS	17 OHP	DHA	HLA linkage
21-Hydroxylase						
Classic	0	+	↑↑	↑↑	N or ↑	A3,BW47,DR7
Late onset	0	0	↑	↑↑	N or ↑	B14, DR1
11β-Hydroxylase	0	+	↑↑	↑	N or ↑	
3β-Hydroxysteroid dehydrogenase[2]	+	+	↑[3]	N or ↑	↑↑	
Cholesterol desmolase	+	0	↓↓	↓	↓	
17-Hydroxylase	+	0	↓↓	↓	↓	

[1]N = normal M = male F = female
[2]A late-onset form exists, which is a milder defect not associated with ambiguity of the external genitalia.
[3]Mostly △5–17-KS

Other forms of CAH are much less common. Deficiencies of 11-hydroxylase accounts for 5% of cases and 3 β-hydroxysteroid dehydrogenase, 20,22-desmolase, and 17-hydroxylase deficiencies account for the remainder. These enzyme deficiencies are not genetically linked to the HLA system. Defects in 18-hydroxylase (pp. 865) and 17,20 desmolase (pp. 879) are known; however, these enzymes are involved in aldosterone and androgen synthesis respectively, and do not affect cortisol biosynthesis or result in adrenal hyperplasia.

Natural History

Depending upon the degree and kind of enzyme deficiency the clinical manifestations of CAH may be present at birth or may appear later in childhood or adulthood.

The newborn female with classical 21-hydroxylase deficiency has virilization of the external genitalia, but normal internal genitalia. The clitoris is hypertrophied and there are varying degrees of fusion of the urethral folds and the labioscrotal folds, with formation of a urogenital sinus. In rare instances, masculinization may be so complete that a penile urethra is formed and total fusion of the labioscrotal folds is present. In such cases, it is impossible to differentiate the external genitalia from those of a normal male newborn with bilateral cryptorchidism.

The newborn male with 21-hydroxylase deficiency usually has normal genitalia, but may show genital hyperpigmentation. The diagnosis may not be made until later in childhood when accelerated growth and masculinization of the genitalia are noted. An important difference from true sexual precocity is the presence of prepubertal testes with the markedly enlarged penis and pubic hair. Newborns of both sexes with the salt-losing form of 21-hydroxylase deficiency show evidence of adrenal insufficiency at about 10–14 days of life. There is generally difficulty in feeding, frequent regurgitation, and failure to thrive. Adrenal crisis eventually occurs, with severe dehydration, vomiting (often projectile), pallor, hypotension, and cool clammy skin. Acidosis develops and shock with peripheral collapse may occur. Breast-fed babies may show evidence of salt loss later than do formula-fed babies (Curtis and Bailey, 1983).

Milder forms of 21-hydroxylase deficiency may not be diagnosed until later in life. Most often these patients are females who appear normal at birth and through childhood but at the time of puberty or later develop hirsutism and menstrual irregularities (pp. 888).

Patients with cryptic 21-hydroxylase deficiency are heterozygotes with biochemical evidence of deficiency, but no clinical symptoms of the disorder.

In most patients, deficiency of 11 β-hydroxylase is associated with hypertension as well as virilization. The newborn female is virilized as in 21-hydroxylase deficiency. Salt loss is rarely seen since the enzyme block causes a rise in 11-deoxycorticosterone (DOC), which is a powerful sodium-retaining steroid. However, paradoxical salt loss due to oversuppression of DOC by glucocorticoid therapy has been reported (Hochberg et al, 1984). Excessive production of DOC is thought to produce the hypertension in this syndrome; however, normotensive patients with elevated DOC levels as well as hypertensive patients with normal DOC levels have been reported. A late-onset form has been described in which patients have hirsutism as well as hypertension. As with 21-hydroxylase deficiency, untreated patients show accelerated linear growth and bone maturation.

With 20,22-demolase (cholesterol side-chain cleavage enzyme) deficiency virtually all steroid hormone synthesis is blocked. The condition is often fatal. Affected males have ambiguous or feminine external genitalia. Those patients who survive show evidence of salt loss.

Another early enzyme in steroid hormone synthesis is 3 β-hydroxysteroid dehydrogenase, the deficiency of which affects the biosynthesis of all biologically active steroid hormones. Both salt-losing and nonsalt-losing forms exist (Pang et al, 1983). Salt loss occurs in those patients with enzyme deficiency in the glomerulosa as well as the fasciculata. In the severe form death occurs in infancy owing to salt loss combined with cortisol deficiency. Incomplete masculinization of the newborn male may occur. Mild deficiencies should be included in the differential diagnosis of hirsutism in the pubertal or adult female.

Diagnosis

The diagnosis of CAH should be considered in any newborn child with ambiguous genitalia or in any newborn with male external genitalia plus bilateral cryptorchidism (Fig. 14.13). Such infants may represent incompletely masculinized males or virilized females. It should be remembered at all times that CAH is the most common cause of ambiguous genitalia in the newborn infant. A careful history and physical examination should be followed immediately by buccal smear, karyotyping, and hormone analyses. Depending upon the enzyme deficiency, various cortisol precursors may be produced in excessive amounts (Table 14.14). Many adrenal steroids are elevated in serum of the newborn, a reflection of the activity of the fetal zone of the adrenal cortex which will rapidly involute. For example, the concentration of 17-hydroxprogesterone is normally elevated in umbilical cord blood (mean 1640 ng/dl) but rapidly decreases to 100–200 ng/dl after 24 hours of age. In premature infants it may take longer for this decrease in 17-hydroxyprogesterone and other adrenal steroids to occur. Thus, blood samples for diagnosis of CAH should be obtained after 24 hours of age. Usually the serum cortisol level in patients with CAH is low but within normal limits. Salt losers may have very low cortisol levels.

Males born with salt-losing CAH may be undiagnosed until they are brought in to the hospital in adrenal crisis at 1–2 weeks of age. Serum sodium and chloride levels are low and the serum potassium concentration is elevated. Hyperpigmentation of the genitalia may be evident.

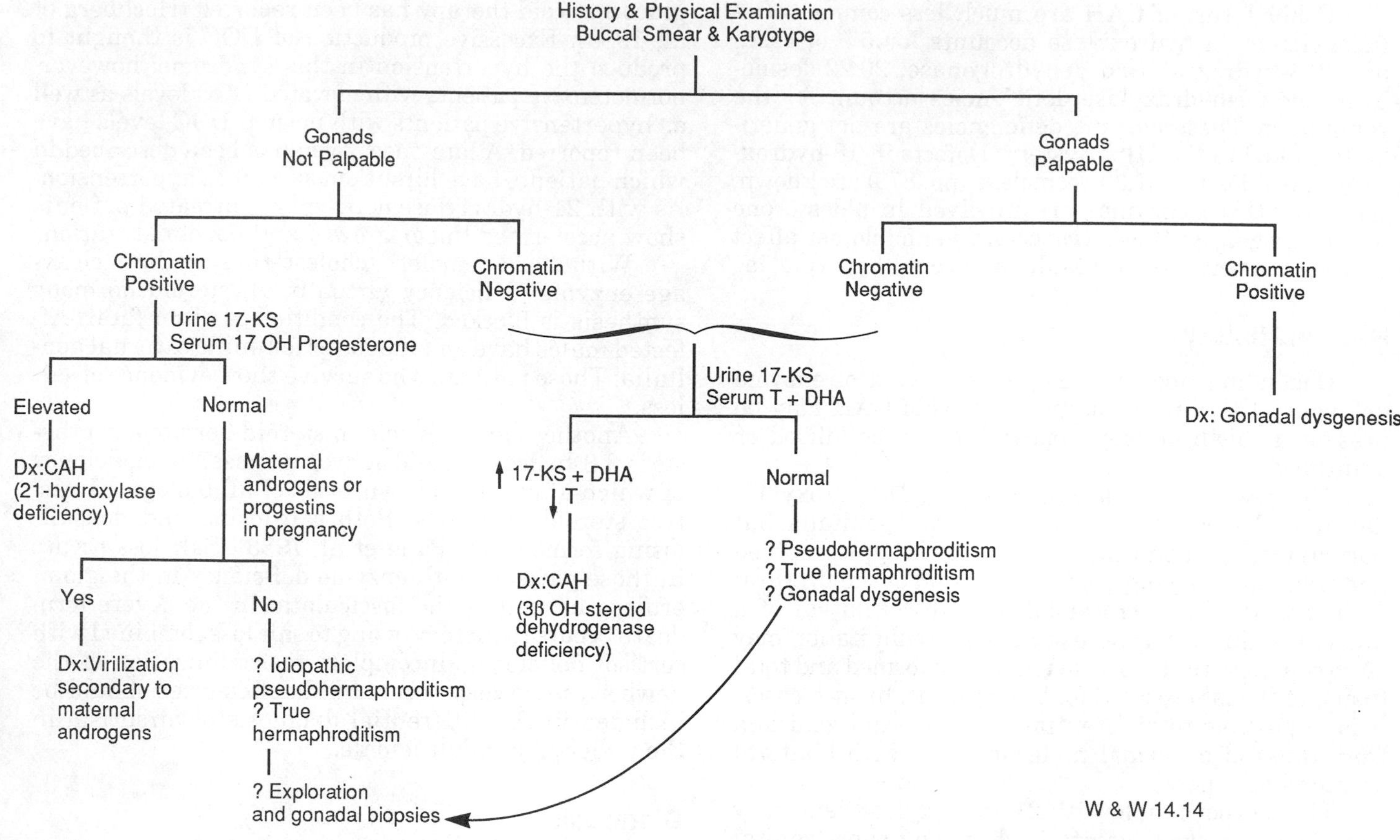

Figure 14.13. Diagnostic evaluation in patients with ambiguous genitalia.

Baseline levels of steroid hormones, particularly a 17-hydroxyprogesterone value well above 1000 ng/dl, obtained in the early morning almost always establish the diagnosis of CAH. If these results are not definitive, an ACTH test can be performed. For this, 1 mg of synthetic ACTH (1-24) is administered intramuscularly after a control blood sample is obtained. Another sample of blood is obtained 1 hour after ACTH administration. Cortisol precursors proximate to the enzyme block will accumulate and their levels in blood and urine will rise disproportionately to that of cortisol. New and associates (1983) have developed nomograms relating the baseline and ACTH-stimulated levels of 17-hydroxyprogesterone, Δ 4-androstenedione, dehydroepiandrosterone and testosterone in 21-hydroxylase deficiency; 17-hydroxyprogesterone is most commonly measured. Those patients with the most severe deficiency of 21-hydroxylase show the greatest rise in these steroids. Patients with the late-onset form of CAH can usually be diagnosed by an ACTH stimulation test (Emans et al, 1983). The differential diagnosis should include polycystic ovarian syndrome.

The patient and members of the family should have blood drawn for HLA haplotypes whenever possible. Parents are obligate heterozygote carriers for the 21-hydroxylase deficiency gene. For example, a child with 21-hydroxylase deficiency may have an HLA haplotype as follows: A3, BW47(W4), CW6, DR7 from one parent and A11, BW35(W6), CW4, DR5 from the other parent. If we find that the father is A3, BW47(W4), CW6,DR7/A3, B7(W6), DR7 and the mother is A11, BW35 (W6), CW4, DR5/A26, BW55(W6), CW3, DRW6, then any child with a haplotype A3, B7(W6), DR7/A26, BW55(W6), CW3, DRW6 does not carry the gene for 21-hydroxylase deficiency. Any offspring of the parents with either A3, BW47(W4), CW6, DR7 or A11, BW35(W6), CW4, DR5 in his HLA haplotype is a carrier of the gene. All offspring of the patient are carriers also. Family members predicted by HLA genotyping to be heterozygous carriers show a higher 17-hydroxyprogesterone response to ACTH stimulation than do family members predicted to be genetically unaffected. Baseline 17-hydroxyprogesterone concentrations in heterozygotes are indistinguishable from those in genetically unaffected subjects; ACTH stimulation is required to unmask the presence of mild 21-hydroxylase deficiency in the heterozygote.

NEW DEVELOPMENTS

Prenatal Diagnosis. Elevated levels of 17-hydroxyprotesterone in the amniotic fluid of fetuses affected with CAH resulting from 21-hydroxylase deficiency have been reported (Pang et al, 1980). In a pregnancy at risk for 21-hydroxylase deficiency, HLA genotyping of amniotic cells provides an additional method for prenatal diagnosis of the defect and can be used also for prediction of a heterozygous carrier fetus (Pollack et al, 1979). There are, however, pitfalls in the prenatal diagnosis of 21-hydroxylase deficiency (Pang et al, 1985). Interpretation of results must be carefully reviewed by knowledgable experts in the field.

Neonatal Screening. A micromethod for measuring 17-hydroxyprogesterone on filter paper has been developed. The hormone is stable on filter paper and the filter paper specimens can be sent to an appropriate laboratory by surface mail. A pilot study screening all infants born in Alaska in a 30-month period showed the method to be feasible and reliable (Pang et al, 1982). Two additional neonatal screening programs have been completed in Italy (Cacciari et al, 1983) and one in Japan (Shimozawa et al, 1984).

Treatment

The immediate medical treatment of the patient in a salt-losing crisis is to administer saline intravenously. As long as adequate amounts of salt are given, mineralocorticoids are not usually necessary; nevertheless, an intravenously injectable preparation (Aldocorten) is available and repeated doses of 0.25 mg may be used as needed to establish a normal blood volume in the patient in shock. Once the acute situation is over, the salt-losing infant will require salt orally, usually added to a bottle containing either formula or mother's milk.

The fundamental aim of endocrine therapy in CAH is to provide replacement of the deficient hormones, thus suppressing ACTH production and preventing further excessive androgen production and virilization. Administration of glucocorticoids both replaces the deficient cortisol and suppresses ACTH overproduction. Several glucocorticoids are available for therapeutic use. Hydrocortisone (cortisol) is used most frequently in infants and young children. It is administered orally at a dose of about 15 mg/m^2/day in three divided doses, generally about one-half in the morning, one-quarter at mid-day, and the final quarter in the evening. Despite the theoretical reasons for using divided doses of hydrocortisone in treating CAH, Winterer et al (1985) have shown that the dose schedule may not be so important. In testing five different schedules for administering the same total dose of hydrocortisone (once, twice, and three times a day, with the major dose in the AM or PM) the authors found no differences in mean 24-hour plasma 17-hydroxyprogesterone levels.

Other steroids besides hydrocortisone may be used for treatment of patients with CAH. Cortisone acetate may be given orally or intramuscularly; however, it has about 80% of the biologic activity of hydrocortisone and the dose must be adjusted accordingly. It is often given intramuscularly at the time of diagnosis, to provide continued sustained levels of glucocorticoids to bring down the markedly high levels of ACTH. Prednisone, prednisolone, and dexamethasone are much more active glucocorticoids per unit weight than is hydrocortisone and are generally used in older children and in adolescents. In small children and infants, dose adjustment with these steroids is difficult and it is easy to overtreat. Excess glucocorticoids can have disastrous effects on linear growth in infancy. Dexamethasone in particular is a long-acting potent glucocorticoid associated with significant suppression of growth. Nevertheless, some clinical studies are being conducted with very small doses of dexamethasone in infants and children, the dose equalling that of the daily hydrocortisone dose of 15 mg/m^2. It is essential to follow both linear growth and bone maturation in these patients in order to avoid a loss in ultimate stature.

Increasing attention has been focused on the role of the renin-angiotensin system in the treatment of CAH. Plasma renin activity is elevated in the simple virilizing as well as in the salt-losing form of CAH. Patients with salt-losing 21-hydroxylase deficiency should receive mineralocorticoid therapy. The question of mineralocorticoid treatment for non-salt losers has been examined. Rosler et al (1977) have shown that the addition of salt-retaining hormone to glucocorticoid therapy in simple virilizing CAH with elevated plasma renin activity improves hormonal control of the disease. Often the dose of glucocorticoid can be reduced in these patients, permitting improved linear growth. As much as 0.15–0.20 mg of fludrohydrocortisone (Florinef) may be needed daily to maintain sodium balance with normal plasma renin activity (Winter, 1980). Hypertension may occur if mineralocorticoid therapy is excessive.

Biochemical monitoring is helpful in adjusting doses of glucocorticoid, but should never supplant evaluation of growth and bone maturation. Measurement of serum steroids has largely replaced 24-hour urinary steroid determinations in many centers; nevertheless, when obtainable, urinary 17-KS represent an integrative function over a 24-hour period and provide different information from the single time value of serum steroids. The most commonly requested values are for serum 17-hydroxyprogesterone and Δ 4-androstenedione. Unfortunately, 17-hydroxyprogesterone levels vary widely depending upon the time of day (marked diurnal variation in patients with CAH) and upon the time since the last dose of cortisol (marked and rapid sensitivity to glucocorticoid suppression). Levels of serum 17-hydroxyprogesterone over 1000 ng/dl are associated with significant elevation of serum androgens and urinary 17-KS. Values less than 200 ng/dl are uniformly associated with low serum concentrations of testosterone, Δ 4-androstenedione and with normal urinary 17-KS (Hughes and Winter, 1978). Therapy should be aimed at maintaining serum 17-hydroxyprogesterone levels between the two extremes of over- and undersuppression. Serum concentrations of 17-hydroxyprogesterone may be high even when clinical and other biochemical criteria of good control are present (Ilondo et al, 1983).

The serum levels of Δ 4-androstenedione have less diurnal variation and correlate better with urinary 17-KS than do any other steroid (Hendricks et al, 1982). It is the serum androgen that best reflects control of

CASE ILLUSTRATION 1

A 3-year- and 7-month-old boy was brought in by his mother because of the appearance of pubic hair over the previous 3 months. The child was the product of a normal pregnancy and delivery and his development was normal in every way. He had a 7-year-old brother who was well developed. The parents were healthy. There was no family history of precocious development. The child had no complaints. There were no headaches, visual problems, nausea or vomiting. He was toilet-trained with no bed-wetting. He was a healthy child except for an occasional ear infection.

On physical examination, the child had a height of 109 cm and a weight of 21 kg. His blood pressure was 90/40. He was a tall, well-developed, muscular boy. Pertinent physical findings included: penis, 10 cm stretch length and 2.9 cm in diameter; testes, 2 cm x 1 cm bilaterally, and stage II pubic hair with 20–25 coarse, dark, curly hairs at the base of the penis.

QUESTIONS AND COMMENTS

What laboratory work-up is in order?

He was diagnosed as a virilized male and the following tests were ordered: 24-hour urine for 17-KS and 17-OHCS, blood for 17-hydroxyprogesterone, cortisol, testosterone, FSH, LH, and radiographs of the skull, hand, and wrist. The results were compatible with CAH, showing elevated 17-KS (11.4 mg/24 hours), elevated plasma 17-hydroxyprogesterone (2400 ng/dl), and advanced bone age (10 years). His serum gonadotropin values were low and the skull films were normal.

How should he be treated? Are mineralocorticoids needed?

He was started on hydrocortisone therapy after initial suppression with decadron 2 mg daily for 6 days. His dose of hydrocortisone was 5 mg, three times daily. His plasma renin activity showed a gradual rise over a period of years and at the age of 9 years he was started on mineralocorticoid therapy (0.05 μg of Florinef daily) in addition to his hydrocortisone. On this combined therapy urinary 17-KS ranged from 1.5 mg/24 hours over the first years to 3.5 mg/24 hours in recent years. Plasma renin activity was reduced from 26.0 to less than 10 on mineralocorticoid therapy. His growth over the years shifted to the 50th centile line, which would bring him to a final height significantly below his genetic potential (M 69 cm, F 78 cm). His bone age at 9 years 2 months is 12 years 1 month, an increment of 2½ years over a period of 5½ years.

The boy is an example of a milder form of classical CAH manifesting itself in early childhood. At no time did he show clinical evidence of salt loss, but his plasma renin activity became elevated eventually and mineralocorticoids were added to his therapeutic regimen. This boy will achieve an acceptable height, but because of his late diagnosis and treatment he will fail to achieve his true genetic target height.

CAH (Korth-Schutz et al, 1978). When there is no significant production of extra-adrenal (testicular) androgens, serum levels of testosterone are useful in monitoring control.

Serum dehydroepiandrosterone values are low in all treated patients with CAH, whether control is good or bad, and, therefore, do not provide a good index of control. Similarly, dehydroepiandrosterone sulfate levels in serum are low. This conjugated steroid has no diurnal variation and is useful as an index of insufficient suppression. Values that are normal for age in a

CASE ILLUSTRATION 2

A 12-day-old infant was admitted to the hospital with a diagnosis of ambiguous genitalia. The infant was the product of a full-term uncomplicated pregnancy. No drugs or hormones were used during the pregnancy. There was no family history of genital anomalies or endocrine disorders.

Shortly after birth the child was noted to have genitalia that were predominantly female but with some ambiguity. A buccal smear at that time showed 5–10% Barr bodies. Blood was drawn for hormone values which subsequently showed a normal serum cortisol value of 13 ug/dl (normal 5–20) and elevated serum values for 17-hydroxyprogesterone and dehydroepiandrosterone. The physical examination of the baby showed an enlarged clitoris (1.5 cm) and partial fusion of the labioscrotal folds. The "labia" were hyperpigmented. No gonads were palpable.

Meanwhile, the child was sent home from the hospital and seemed to do well on Similac feedings; however, there was continued weight loss. The latter plus the steroid values suggested CAH.

In the hospital the child had a serum Na of 137 mEq/L, K of 5.6 mEq/L, Cl of 102 mEq/L, BUN of 4 mg/dl, and a creatinine of 0.5 mg/dl. A karyotype was 46,XX. She showed no clinical signs of salt loss. Her blood pressure was normal.

QUESTION AND COMMENT

What is the diagnosis and how should it be treated?

A diagnosis of CAH 21-hydroxylase deficiency of the nonsalt-losing variety was made and the child was started on 5 mg hydrocortisone three times a day. This dose was tapered after 3 days to 2.5 mg three times a day. On this therapy her serum 17-hydroxyprogesterone value fell to 250 ng/dl. Her electrolytes remained stable; she gained weight and developed normally. She was referred to the surgical service for evaluation of reconstructive genital surgery.

In contrast to the first case of the boy with nonsalt-losing CAH, this condition in girls is detected readily in the newborn period because of the ambiguity of genital development. Barr bodies in the newborn may not be too helpful since they are often low even in normal females. A karyotype should be obtained at all times.

patient with CAH indicate inadequate cortisol therapy. Patients in good control have dehydroepiandrosterone sulfate levels in serum which are below the normal range; however, measurement of this steroid is not useful in detecting patients who are overtreated. Thus, a combination of serum dehydroepiandrosterone, dehydroepiandrosterone sulfate, Δ 4-androstenedione and testosterone (except in male infants and male adolescents) levels can provide information regarding the adequacy of the glucorticoid therapy.

In addition to steroid studies, plasma renin activity should be measured. If elevated, mineralocorticoid therapy should be adjusted. The physician should remember that doses of glucocorticoids that completely suppress androgens also suppress growth. Our knowledge of the pharmacokinetics of glucocorticoid therapy is incomplete; however, some guidelines may be helpful. To prevent overtreatment; urine 17-KS values should be maintained in the low normal range for developmental age (bone age). Serum androgens should be within the normal range. Serum 17-hydroxyprogesterone values should be well under 1000 ng/dl, but values below 300 ng/dl probably indicate oversuppression.

Patients with CAH require extra glucocorticoid coverage during periods of severe stress (high fever, surgery). Generally the dose of glucocorticoid should be doubled or tripled with high fever and preparation for surgery should include a 5- to 10-fold increase in glucocorticoid dose administered intramuscularly the night before and the day of surgery, with intravenous glucocorticoid administered during the operation. Depending on the surgical procedure, high doses of glucocorticoids may be required for 1 or more days postsurgery, but those doses should be tapered as quickly as possible thereafter.

Theoretically it should be possible to administer glucocorticoids to the mother of a fetus at risk for CAH and thus suppress the excessive androgen production during fetal development that causes virilization of the external genitalia of the female fetus. David and Forest (1984) attempted just such therapy in six mothers at risk. Either hydrocortisone or dexamethasone was administered during pregnancy. Two of the offspring, who were subsequently diagnosed as having CAH, showed evidence of adrenal suppression in utero, and in one, normal female genitalia were observed at birth.

Those females born with ambiguous genitalia require surgical evaluation.

Prognosis

Most patients with CAH have an ultimate stature that is somewhat compromised. Children who are adequately treated early in life have a greater final height than do those who are inadequately treated (Kirkland et al, 1978). In males, normal pubertal development and fertility can be expected; however, testicular tumors have occurred in males on inadequate therapy. These tumors probably represent adrenal rest tissue in the testes, which responds to the elevated levels of ACTH.

In females with CAH, sexual development is normal if therapy has been adequate; however, amenorrhea, irregular menses, or oligomenorrhea may occur in 25% or more (Klingensmith et al, 1977; Mulaikal RM et al, 1987).

Money et al (1984) have shown that girls with CAH are more likely to be homosexual and/or bisexual than normal girls or girls with testicular feminization syndrome or Rokitansky syndrome. In a comparable study with boys having CAH, none of the patients was homosexual or bisexual. Other studies by Money have shown that girls with CAH are more likely to indulge in tomboy-like behavior than are other girls. This suggests that masculinizing prenatal hormonal threshold effects can interact with other subsequent environmental factors and contribute to erotosexual differentiation on a hetero/bi/homosexual continuum.

PREMATURE ADRENARCHE

This represents the isolated development of sexual hair at an early age and is presumably due to the early secretion of adrenal androgens. Normally the amount and type of androgen produced at adrenarche is insufficient to produce accelerated physical growth or growth of the penis or clitoris. The genitalia are thus prepubertal and gonadotropin levels are low. Premature adrenarche is benign and requires no treatment. It is, however, essential that all patients showing evidence of virilization (enlargement of penis or clitoris) be investigated for the presence of a virilizing tumor (pp. 864), and attenuated forms of CAH should be excluded.

CUSHING SYNDROME

Definition

Cushing syndrome represents a combination of clinical features including obesity, muscle weakness, hypertension, and skin changes that are secondary to elevated circulating concentrations of glucocorticoids.

Basic Science

Cushing syndrome and disease are rare in children. Cortisol levels in serum may be raised because of exogenous administration or endogenous overproduction of ACTH or cortisol. Those patients with overproduction of pituitary ACTH have Cushing disease. The majority of these patients have pituitary basophilic microadenomas, but some have large invasive pituitary adenomas. Certain pituitary adenomas may be secondary to an initiating hypothalamic stimulus.

Cortisol hypersecretion by adrenal adenomas or carcinomas will produce Cushing syndrome. Adrenal carcinomas in children tend to produce large amounts of androgens, often in excess of cortisol (pp. 864).

During infancy and the first few years of life the basic lesion is usually a tumor of the adrenal gland, either adenoma or carcinoma. After the age of 6 or 7 years the cause is usually excessive pituitary secretion of ACTH with bilateral adrenal hyperplasia. The rare cases of ectopic ACTH production in childhood are seen with such tumors as thymoma and pancreatic neoplasm.

Natural History

The principal clinical features of Cushing syndrome are listed in Table 14.15. The most common features are rapid weight gain and obesity that tends to be centripetal in distribution, involving the trunk (often with a "buffalo hump," a pad of excessive subcutaneous tissue on the back of the neck), abdomen, and facies ("moon face"). The limbs are relatively thin. Weakness is common, largely related to the proximal muscle myopathy. Thigh and shoulder muscle wasting may be evident and the patient may have difficulty rising from a squatting position.

In children, one of the most important signs of Cushing syndrome is the slowing or cessation of linear growth. These children gain weight but do not grow unless the condition is associated with excessive androgen production. Other important features include easy bruising of the skin, plethora, abdominal striae and evidence of mild virilization such as acne and hirsutism. Menstrual abnormalities, hypertension, glucose intolerance, and osteoporosis occur also. Psychiatric changes may be noted.

Diagnosis

All tests for Cushing syndrome rely on the demonstration of sustained, excessive secretion of cortisol and lack of response to normal physiological controls of cortisol production (Table 14.16). The simplest and most reliable test involves attempts to suppress secretion of cortisol by administering the potent glucocorticoid, dexamethasone. The steroid is given orally (20 μg/kg body weight/day) in equal doses every 6 hours for 48 hours. In normal individuals 24-hour urinary 17-OHCS, 17-KS, and free cortisol fall to very low or undetectable levels. Patients with Cushing syndrome show no or only partial suppression at this dose level, but will be suppressed (<1.5 mg 17-OHCS/m^2/day) at higher doses (80 μg/kg body weight/day) of dexamethasone given over a 2-day period.

Table 14.15
Clinical Features of Cushing Syndrome

Weight gain
Impaired linear growth
Centripetal obesity
Hypertension
Skin changes
- Thin skin/bruising
- Acne, greasy skin
- Hirsute
- Plethora
- Abdominal striae
- Pigmentation

Oligo/amenorrhea
Osteoporosis
Glucose intolerance
Muscle weakness

Table 14.16
Tests for the Diagnosis of Cushing Syndrome

Dexamethasone suppression tests
- Low dose—no or partial suppression
- High dose—suppresses with hyperplasia; no suppression with adrenal tumor

Circadian rhythm of plasma cortisol and ACTH
- No diurnal rhythm with hyperplasia or tumor
- Baseline values of ACTH are normal or increased in hyperplasia but decreased with adrenal tumor
- Baseline values of cortisol are normal or increased in hyperplasia and adrenal tumor

Urinary steroids
- 17-OHCS and free cortisol usually elevated in hyperplasia and tumor

Metyrapone test
- Hyperresponse in hyperplasia, decreased or no response with adrenal tumor or ectopic ACTH syndrome

A more rapid test involves the administration of 1 mg of dexamethasone late at night (11:00 or 12:00 PM) and measurement of plasma cortisol concentration the following morning. In normal individuals, cortisol values will be suppressed to less than 5 μg/dl. In general, if a single morning serum cortisol level is only modestly elevated above 15 μg/dl and can be suppressed to below 5 μg/dl after an evening dose of 1.0 mg of dexamethasone, the child probably does not have Cushing disease.

Patients with Cushing syndrome may show a loss of the normal diurnal variation of plasma cortisol and ACTH concentrations; therefore, blood samples drawn early in the morning and late at night may show little difference in hormone values. The 24-hour urinary excretion of 17-OHCS is usually elevated (> 5 mg/m^2/day). The urinary free cortisol level may be elevated (normal <80 μg/m^2/day) and may not be suppressed (<25 μg/m^2/day) on low dose dexamethasone.

The response to the drug metyrapone is useful in differentiating adrenal hyperplasia secondary to pituitary adenoma from adrenal tumors and the ectopic ACTH syndrome. Metyrapone inhibits adrenal 11-hydroxylase, which results in decreased cortisol synthesis, increased ACTH secretion, and increased plasma 11-deoxycortisol, the immediate precursor of cortisol. 11-Deoxycortisol and its metabolites are excreted in the urine as 17-OHCS. Generally, a 24-hour urine and a blood sample are collected before administration of the drug. Metyrapone is then given orally every 4 hours for a total dose of 300 mg/m^2 over 1 day. During metyrapone treatment, 24-hour urine collections are continued as well as for 24 hours after the completion of drug therapy; a blood sample is drawn 4 hours after the last dose of metyrapone. Normally there is a 3-fold increase in urinary 17-OHCS and blood levels of 11 β-deoxycortisol with metyrapone treatment. Pituitary adenomas respond to the metyrapone-induced decrease in plasma cortisol level with enhanced ACTH release and the hyperplastic adrenal glands will produce a greater rise in 11-deoxycortisol production than normal. Thus, plasma 11-deoxycortisol and urinary 17-OHCS levels exceed those found in normal controls. In adrenal tumors and the ectopic ACTH syndrome the chronically suppressed pituitary fails to release ACTH and the metyrapone does not cause an increase in plasma 11-deoxycortisol or urinary 17-OHCS levels.

Striking increases in urinary 17-KS excretion out of proportion to the increased urinary 17-OHCS are characteristic of virilizing adrenal carcinoma. Benign adrenal tumors may produce very little 17-KS. In Cushing disease in children, the 17-KS excretion is usually within normal limits or only slightly elevated.

In summary, the usual criteria for a diagnosis of Cushing syndrome are: (1) absence of diurnal variation of plasma cortisol and ACTH; (2) increased excretion of 17-OHCS in the urine (> 5 mg/m^2/day); (3) failure to suppress urinary 17-OHCS to <1.5 mg/m^2/day by low-dose dexamethasone; (4) suppression of 17-OHCS and usually plasma cortisol and ACTH by high-dose oral dexamethasone; and (5) elevated baseline levels of urinary free cortisol with failure of suppression of free cortisol after dexamethasone.

Cushing syndrome is frequently suspected in obese children, particularly when hypertension and striae are present. Cortisol secretion rates and urinary 17-OHCS are increased in obesity, but when the caloric intake is lowered, these values return to normal. A dexamethasone suppression test may be used to screen obese patients with elevated urinary 17-OHCS values. Both normal and obese individuals will show suppression of urinary 17-OHCS after low-dose dexamethasone, whereas patients with Cushing disease or adrenal tumor will not.

Treatment

Transsphenoidal removal of pituitary adenoma appears to be the best initial approach to treatment of Cushing disease in childhood (Styne et al, 1984). The morbidity of the procedure is low when carried out by an experienced neurosurgeon. The cure rate for microadenomas is high, with minimal loss of pituitary function. Macroadenomas, particularly invasive ones, have a much poorer prognosis.

Other modes of therapy can still be used if surgery fails or if the disease recurs. For example, in some centers, conventional irradiation to the pituitary gland has been found to be a safe and effective therapy for childhood Cushing disease (Jennings et al, 1977), although it has been less successful in others. The potential for damage to vision and the CNS requires that irradiation is only carried out by experienced radiotherapists.

Bilateral adrenalectomy was the treatment most used in the past. Unfortunately, this method requires lifetime steroid replacement therapy and has a high incidence (in 27% of children so treated) of resulting Nelson syndrome, characterized by the development of a pituitary adenoma, hyperpigmentation, and marked elevation of plasma ACTH levels (Hopwood and Kenny, 1977). The tumor of Nelson syndrome can usually be controlled with irradiation to the pituitary.

Long-term medical management for Cushing disease in children has not been popular. Cyproheptadine (a serotonin antagonist) has been successful in some adults, but its use in children with Cushing disease has been disappointing. Ortho, para-DDD [1,1-dichloro-2-(0-chlorophenyl)-2-(p-chloro-phenyl) ethane] and other adrenal suppressive drugs have been used to a limited degree in Cushing disease, but all have potentially undesirable side effects.

The treatment for adrenal tumors is discussed on pages 864.

Prognosis

If therapy for Cushing syndrome is instituted before epiphyseal fusion has occurred some lost growth can be regained. The earlier the age of treatment, the more likely that the deviation from predicted height will be minimal.

Loss of pituitary function may be secondary to surgical or radiation therapy, particularly the latter. Patients may require replacement hormones for life. It is also possible that tumors will recur.

CASE ILLUSTRATION

The patient was a 9-year-old boy with a history of rapid weight gain (42 kg to 52 kg) and failure to grow in height over a 1-year period. His appearance was suggestive of Cushing syndrome, with round face, truncal obesity, prominent interscapular fat pad, and striae. Pubic hair was noted on physical examination but genitalia were normal for age. Urinary levels of 17-OHCS, 17-KS, and free cortisol were elevated and both urinary steroids and serum cortisol were suppressed by high-dose but not by low-dose dexamethasone.

QUESTION AND COMMENT

What is the most likely etiology for this syndrome and how should it be treated?

In this age group, and with the lack of excessive virilization in this patient, the most likely diagnosis is Cushing disease secondary to an ACTH-secreting tumor of the pituitary. The latter was revealed on a CAT scan of the pituitary area.

The patient underwent bilateral adrenalectomy. Subsequently his steroid values returned to normal, his linear growth accelerated, and he sustained a significant loss of weight (back to 40 kg within 6 months). One year after surgery the pubic hair, "moon facies," "buffalo hump," and truncal obesity had disappeared.

With present-day experience this patient would probably have had transphenoidal surgery for removal of the pituitary microadenoma. Because of his adrenalectomy he requires hormonal replacement therapy for life.

ADRENAL TUMORS

Basic Science

The tumors, which are usually unilateral, may be benign, but some are malignant. Adenomas are more likely to produce excess of a single hormone (for example, Cushing syndrome), whereas carcinomas are more likely to show increases in many of the adrenocortical steroids. Carcinomas almost always produce excessive amounts of androgens, especially dehydroepiandrosterone, which results in a clinical picture of virilization. The most common methods of invasion of malignant tumors are contiguous spread into adjoining kidney tissue and metastases to liver, regional nodes, and lung. Histologically differentiation of adenoma versus carcinoma is difficult since pleiomorphism and capsular invasion has been seen in clinically benign tumors.

Epidemiology and Etiology

Adrenocortical tumors are rare in adults and even rarer in children. The majority of tumors seen in children are hormone-secreting tumors, two-thirds being virilizing and one-third producing primarily glucocorticoids. A feminizing tumor of the adrenal gland or an aldosterone-secreting tumor is rarely seen.

Natural History

Adrenal tumors usually occur in infancy or in children under 5 years of age (Lee et al, 1985). Virilizing tumors produce increase in muscle mass, rapid growth, acne, facial and pubic hair, hirsutism, and penile and clitoral enlargement. Axillary hair is uncommon. Boys with virilizing adrenal tumors have prepubertal testes despite penile enlargement.

Less commonly, signs of Cushing syndrome will be the first evidence of an adrenal tumor. The child will show growth arrest, moon facies, and obesity. The growth arrest, however, may be masked if there is a concomitant increase in androgen production with stimulation of growth.

Rarely, signs of feminization or of aldosterone excess may herald an adrenal tumor in a child.

Diagnosis

A tumor may be palpable on abdominal examination. Abdominal sonography and computed tomography are reliable in detecting adrenal tumors.

Hormonal studies are helpful. Urinary 17-KS are characteristically very high in virilizing adrenal tumors, higher than are usually seen in CAH. Urinary 17-OHCS are likely to be elevated in cortisol-producing tumors of the adrenal. Serum dehydroepiandrosterone, dehydroepiandrosterone sulfate, testosterone, and cortisol levels are usually elevated. Steroid production is generally not suppressed by dexamethasone, in contrast to the rapid suppression seen in patients with CAH.

Patients with feminizing adrenal tumors will have high levels of estrogens in blood and urine. The diagnosis of aldosteronomas is discussed on pages 866.

Treatment

The treatment of choice for adrenal tumors is surgical removal. Steroid coverage is essential at the time of surgery since the contralateral adrenal is almost always suppressed. On the day before and on the day of surgery, 50 mg of cortisone acetate can be given intramuscularly. The dose of glucocorticoid should be tapered thereafter.

ADRENOCORTICAL HYPOFUNCTION (Addison Disease)

Definition

Any condition that results in diminished production of steroid hormones will result in a clinical picture of adrenal insufficiency. The term Addison disease is used for those disorders that result in destruction or atrophy of the adrenal cortex associated with both mineralocorticoid and glucocorticoid insufficiency.

Basic Science

Depending upon the cause of the condition, the patient may be deficient in one or more steroid hormones. Disorders of production of CRH and ACTH result in diminished production of glucocorticoids and androgens. The adrenal glands may be hypoplastic at birth either because of pituitary absence or congenital hypoplasia. There are two forms of the latter. The first form is inherited as an autosomal recessive disorder. In these small adrenals the fetal zone is markedly diminished while the adult zone remains well-differentiated. A second form is inherited as an X-linked disorder in males. These adrenals are abnormal in architecture, with persistence of the fetal zone histologic pattern in the cortex. Another inherited form of adrenocortical insufficiency is characterized by an hereditary unresponsiveness of the adrenal cortex to ACTH and is probably autosomal recessive. In contrast to the previous inherited disorders, hereditary adrenocortical unresponsiveness to ACTH is not associated with mineralocorticoid deficiency (Kelch et al, 1972).

Inborn errors of steroid biosynthesis may cause adrenal insufficiency. Deficiencies of enzymes early in the biosynthetic pathway will result in diminished production of all steroid hormones. Those specifically involved in glucocorticoid (pp. 855), androgen (pp. 879), and mineralocorticoid (pp. 865) synthesis are discussed elsewhere.

Destructive lesions of the adrenal cortex, such as infection, hemorrhage, autoimmune disease and adrenoleukodystrophy can cause adrenal insufficiency. Although formerly infections, such as tuberculosis, were the primary cause of Addison disease, today most cases represent the outcome of an autoimmune process (Neufield et al, 1980). Other endocrine glands may be involved in this process also, especially the parathyroid glands, the thyroid glands, and the pancreatic islets (pp. 833).

In the newborn, overwhelming infection or acute hemorrhage (often associated with a traumatic delivery) may result in destruction of the adrenal gland. Fulminating meningococcemia accompanied by adrenal hemorrhage is known as the Waterhouse-Friderichsen syndrome. Septicemia due to other organisms may also cause this syndrome.

Adrenoleukodystrophy is a rare cause of familial adrenal failure (pp. 715). It is an X-linked recessive disorder related to abnormalities of long chain fatty acids in affected tissues (Davis et al, 1979). A related disorder (Wolman disease) is associated with acid lipase deficiency and occurs in infancy.

Adrenal insufficiency may also occur after cessation of long-term glucocorticoid therapy for various diseases.

Natural History

Infants and children with Addison disease may have a variety of clinical complaints including: weakness, fatigue, anorexia, weight loss, dehydration, nausea, vomiting, diarrhea, and hyperpigmentation. The presentation may be gradual or acute. If the more subtle signs of adrenal insufficiency, such as weakness and fatigue, are missed, the child may present later on in adrenal crisis. Convulsions may occur if hypoglycemia is severe.

Diagnosis

On physical examination the most striking finding is hyperpigmentation, particularly of the knuckles, areolae, genitalia, and any existing scars. The buccal mucosa may also show characteristic pigmentation. There may be a history of prolonged tanning.

The laboratory tests may reveal low serum sodium and chloride and the serum potassium may be elevated; however, these findings are variable. In some patients serum concentrations of calcium are elevated. A low fasting blood glucose is frequently present. The early morning plasma cortisol concentration is low, usually less than 5 μg/dl and the serum ACTH will be greater than 200 pg/ml. Plasma renin activity is increased and plasma aldosterone levels are decreased. Urinary 17-OHCS and 17-KS are low. ACTH stimulation (25 u Cortrosyn/m^2) produces little, if any, rise in plasma cortisol (1 hour later), the variable response depending upon the degree of adrenal destruction.

A more prolonged ACTH stimulation test may be indicated in patients suspected of secondary adrenal insufficiency (low ACTH). ACTH may be given intramuscularly every 12 hours for 3 days. In secondary adrenal insufficiency the response will increase with each day of ACTH stimulation. Urinary 17-OHCS as well as plasma cortisol levels may reach normal levels if the test is prolonged to 5 days.

Those patients with autoimmune Addison disease may have antibodies to adrenal antigens in their blood.

Treatment

The treatment for adrenal insufficiency is replacement of those hormones that show defective production. The dose of hydrocortisone is 12–15 mg/m^2/day orally, divided into three doses, plus Florinef (0.05–0.1 mg daily). In older children and adolescents, prednisone may be used instead of hydrocortisone; about one-third the dosage should be administered twice daily. The dose of glucocorticoids should be increased during periods of stress.

Patients in acute adrenal crisis will require appropriate intravenous fluids containing glucose and saline. Volume expansion with saline is absolutely essential and the intravenous fluids should be supplemented with soluble cortisol (hemisuccinate or phosphate) in a dose of about 100 mg/m^2/day (in a continuous infusion). Deoxycorticosterone acetate can be administered intramuscularly in a dosage of 1–2 mg every 24 hours until oral Florinef can be resumed.

Those patients with autoimmune Addison disease should be surveyed carefully for any other signs of polyglandular syndromes.

Before stopping steroids in patients on glucocorticoid therapy for other diseases, the dose of hormone should be reduced to physiologic replacement doses to seek evidence of flare-up of the original disease. Thereafter, the dose can be tapered gradually over a period of 4–5 weeks until complete withdrawal has been achieved. Often glucocorticoids can be administered on an alternate day schedule in controlling certain disease states.

Prognosis

Patients with Addison disease have a life-long loss of adrenal function. Thus, they are vulnerable to periods of stress when normally the adrenal gland would secrete more hormone. The possibility of loss of other endocrine glands must always be considered in the autoimmune form of Addison disease.

HYPOALDOSTERONISM

Definition

Hypoaldosteronism is a condition of decreased aldosterone production or action usually associated with a salt-losing syndrome.

Basic Science

Specific salt-losing syndromes may result from defects in any of the enzymes involved in aldosterone biosynthesis. Those associated with CAH have already been discussed. A selective deficiency of aldosterone may be caused by a defect in 18-hydroxylase, which results in two apparently different forms of this defect. In type I, 18-hydroxycorticosterone production is diminished, and corticosterone and deoxycorticosterone levels are elevated. In type II, there is an increased secretion of 18-hydroxycorticosterone, but this steroid is not converted to the aldehyde derivative to form aldosterone. In both types, levels of aldosterone in plasma are low.

A salt-losing syndrome may also occur in patients with end-organ unresponsiveness to aldosterone (Dillon et al, 1980). This disorder is sometimes called pseudohypoaldosteronism. For those familial cases that have been reported, an autosomal dominant pattern of inheritance with variable expression is suggested.

Natural History

Children with biosynthetic defects in aldosterone synthesis usually present with salt loss, intermittent fever, dehydration, and failure to thrive as early symptoms. These symptoms become less marked with age.

Pseudohypoaldosteronism is associated with repeated episodes of dehydration, vomiting, hyponatremia, hyperkalemia, and failure to thrive during infancy.

Diagnosis

Hyperkalemia and salt loss are common findings in hypoaldosteronism.

Patients with 18-hydroxylase deficiency type I have increased levels of corticosterone and decreased levels of 18-hydroxycorticosterone in plasma. In the type II form, plasma levels of 18-hydroxycorticosterone are elevated. In both types aldosterone levels are low. Depending upon the degree of the defect there may be hyponatremia and hyperkalemia.

Patients with pseudohypoaldosteronism have high levels of plasma renin activity and aldosterone in the presence of hyponatremia and hyperkalemia. Urinary sodium loss is observed, despite otherwise normal renal function.

Treatment

Defects in biosynthesis of aldosterone can be circumvented by the administration of mineralocorticoids.

Therapy in the patient with pseudohypoaldosteronism is with oral sodium chloride supplements. Characteristically, treatment may be discontinued later since the kidneys manage to restore normal amounts of sodium. However, elevated levels of aldosterone and increased plasma renin activity will persist throughout life.

HYPERALDOSTERONISM

Definition

A condition of excess production of aldosterone is designated hyperaldosteronism. The condition may be primary (aldosteronoma or bilateral adrenal hyperplasia) or secondary (excess renin).

Basic Science

Primary hyperaldosteronism is extremely rare in children. The most common cause is bilateral adrenal hyperplasia (Table 14.17). The etiology of the excess aldosterone production is unknown, but in some patients elevated levels of aldosterone-stimulating factor have been found (Carey et al, 1984).

Secondary hyperaldosteronism in children occurs as a result of oversecretion of renin by the juxtaglomerular apparatus, which may be caused by: (1) depletion of extracellular fluid volume, (2) reduction of plasma volume, or (3) sequestration of blood on the venous side of the circulation (cirrhosis). It may also occur in the presence of renovascular abnormalities resulting in unilateral renal ischemia, or, more rarely, in the presence of a renin-producing juxtaglomerular cell tumor (Warshaw et al, 1979) or with hyperplasia of the juxtaglomerular apparatus (Bartter syndrome). The etiology of Bartter syndrome is unknown, but there may be a primary defect in chloride reabsorption.

A rare genetic form of hyperaldosteronism has been described in five separate families in which the aldosterone level is suppressed by dexamethasone. The etiology of this condition, which is transmitted by an autosomal dominant gene is unknown. It has been suggested that aldosterone may be an aberrant product of the ACTH-stimulable zona fasciculata or that ACTH abnormally stimulates glomerulosa secretion of aldosterone. In these patients total mineralocorticoid bioactivity is greater than the radioimmunoassayable activity (deoxycorticosterone, corticosterone, cortisol, plus aldosterone). This suggests the presence of an additional steroid with mineralocorticoid activity that is suppressed by dexamethasone and stimulated by ACTH (Speiser et al, 1985).

Natural History

Systolic and diastolic hypertension are characteristic in all patients. Headaches secondary to hypertension may be present. Other symptoms include fatigue,

Table 14.17
Causes of Hyperaldosteronism

- Primary Hyperaldosteronism
  - Adrenocortical hyperplasia
    - Dexamethasone—suppressible
    - Dexamethasone—nonsuppressible
  - Adrenocortical adenoma
- Secondary Hyperaldosteronism
  - Physiologic
    - Decreased plasma volume (dehydration, hemorrhage)
    - Electrolyte imbalance (K loading, Na depletion)
  - Pathologic
    - With edema (nephrotic syndrome, heart failure)
    - Without edema (renovascular disease)
  - Bartter Syndrome
  - Renal tubular insenstivity to aldosterone

muscle weakness, paresthesias, periodic paralysis, short stature, poor weight gain, polyuria, polydipsia, nocturia, and tetany. Edema may be present in patients with secondary hyperaldosteronism.

In children who develop Bartter syndrome growth may be severely retarded and mental development may be impaired. These children have normal blood pressure. They are brought to medical attention because of weakness, short stature, vomiting, and/or dehydration.

Diagnosis

Hypokalemia (<3.5 mEq/L) is the most consistent biochemical finding. There is also a metabolic alkalosis. Bicarbonate and ammonium excretion is increased. A nephrogenic-type of diabetes insipidus with resistance to vasopressin may be present. Serum calcium and magnesium levels are almost always normal.

Any hypertensive, hypokalemic child who shows renal loss on a normal sodium and potassium intake should be checked for hyperaldosteronism. Primary hyperaldosteronism is established by the presence of elevated plasma or urine aldosterone and concomitant low plasma renin activity (PRA). Unfortunately, PRA in neonates may be difficult to interpret. For example, PRA is significantly higher in neonates than in older infants and children (Siegler et al, 1977). In addition, a series of factors may alter PRA in the neonatal period: hypotension, respiratory distress syndrome, renovascular hypertension, gestational age, postnatal age, and the administration of drugs that stimulate or suppress the release of renin. Therefore, the interpretation of plasma PRA in the neonate should be approached with caution.

The ability to suppress aldosterone levels should be tested. Generally this is performed in the hospital since for these measurements, sodium intake and ambulatory state must be controlled. Plasma aldosterone is measured between 7:00 and 8:00 AM with the patient supine, having been on a high sodium intake (150 mEq daily or more) for the preceding 5 days. Aldosterone levels are not suppressed in primary hyperaldosteronism.

A trial of low-dose dexamethasone (1–2 mg/day) should be given to exclude the diagnosis of dexamethasone-suppressible hyperaldosteronism. Patients with this disorder have no abnormality in cortisol secretion and respond to salt loading and a low-salt diet in a manner similar to patients with primary hyperaldosteronism. Within 48 hours of dexamethasone administration, complete and rapid suppression of urinary and/or plasma aldosterone levels occurs and the PRA increases.

The adrenal lesion in primary hyperaldosteronism may be localized by adrenal venography and/or measurement of aldosterone levels in adrenal veins. A high concentration of aldosterone in adrenal vein blood on one side only suggests tumor; high concentrations in both veins suggest hyperplasia. Computerized tomography and adrenal scanning with labeled cholesterol may be helpful also.

In secondary hyperaldosteronism, serum renin values are high. Bartter syndrome should be considered in any child with hypokalemic alkalosis normal blood pressure, dwarfism, and mental retardation. Aldosterone levels are high as in other forms of secondary hyperaldosteronism and prostaglandin levels in blood and urine also tend to be high.

The causes of hyperaldosteronism are summarized in Table 14.17.

Treatment

Unilateral adrenalectomy is the treatment of choice for a solitary aldosterone-producing tumor. Preoperative correction of hypertension and hypokalemia is necessary. After removal of the tumor, functional hypoaldosteronism may be present for several weeks resulting from prior suppression of the contralateral zona glomerulosa by the tumor. Supplemental salt (6–8 g daily) should be given during this period.

Bilateral adrenal hyperplasia may be treated surgically, but bilateral adrenalectomy improves the hypertension in only a small fraction of patients. Medical therapy with long-term spironolactone may be the treatment of choice.

Dexamethasone-suppressible hyperaldosteronism is treated with glucocorticoids. In most young patients the blood pressure decreases to normal levels within 2 weeks of initiation of glucocorticoid treatment.

The treatment of secondary hyperaldosteronism depends upon the primary cause. For a discussion of renal hypertension and its treatment see page 605. Bartter syndrome can be treated with some success by inhibitors of prostaglandin synthesis, such as indomethacin. Diuretics that conserve potassium or spironolactone may also be useful in conserving potassium and preventing alkalosis.

PHEOCHROMOCYTOMA

Definition

The pheochromocytoma is a rare tumor that arises in chromaffin tissues. In children most of these tumors are located in the adrenal medulla, but they may also be found in aberrant chromaffin tissue.

Epidemiology

Less than 5% of all cases of pheochromocytoma occur in childhood. Boys are affected more often than girls and the peak age of incidence is 9–12 years. Familial cases have been reported either as a single disorder or as part of the multiple endocrine neoplasia (MEN) syndromes (pp. 839). Malignant tumors of chromaffin tissue are rare. In children, pheochromocytoma may be bilateral.

Natural History

The clinical signs and symptoms of pheochromocytoma are related to the overproduction of catecholamines by the tumor. The most significant findings are listed in Table 14.18. The hypertension is usually sustained and systolic pressures may reach levels of 250 mm Hg with corresponding elevations of diastolic pressures. Encephalopathy with convulsions as well as cardiac failure may occur with long-standing hypertension.

The clinical findings are so diverse in this disorder that it is not uncommon to include in the differential diagnosis: essential hypertension, renal disease, thyrotoxicosis, an emotional disorder, or a GI problem.

Diagnosis

The diagnosis of pheochromocytoma depends upon the detection of elevated urinary and blood catecholamines and their metabolites. A 24-hour urine should be collected for norepinephrine, epinephrine, metanephrines, and VMA analyses (Table 14.19). Nearly all patients with tumor will have an abnormally high urinary output of these compounds, although in some patients the high catecholamine production is episodic and may be missed in a single urinalysis. High epinephrine levels suggest that the tumor is intraadrenal or in the organ of Zuckerkandl.

CAT of the abdomen is useful in localizing abdominal tumors over 2 cm in size, as is abdominal ultrasonography. If these techniques fail to demonstrate tumor, selective renal arteriography, aortography, and adrenal venography may be helpful. It is wise to achieve α blockade of the patient before angiography is carried out. Those tumors in the thorax can be detected by chest roentgenography and tomography.

Since pheochromocytoma may be familial, other family members should have urinary catecholamine levels measured. Pheochromocytoma has been associated with medullary thyroid carcinoma (Sipple syndrome); therefore, calcitonin levels should be checked to rule out this possibility. MEA syndromes should be considered in those patients with multiple neural tumors or parathyroid hyperfunction (pp. 848).

Table 14.18
Symptoms and Signs of Pheochromocytoma in Children

Hypertension (sustained or intermittent)
Headache
Sweating
Palpitations, nervousness
Weight loss
Abdominal or chest pain
Polydipsia and polyuria

Treatment

The treatment of choice is surgical excision of the tumor. Adequate preoperative α-adrenergic and/or β-adrenergic blockade should be provided, depending upon the type of catecholamine produced by the tumor. Generally 2–3 weeks of preoperative therapy is required. During surgery, blockade should be continued by the use of intravenous medication.

Continued elevation of blood pressure after 36 hours postoperatively suggests residual tumor or renovascular disease.

Prognosis

The tumor may recur years later. In addition, the patient and family members are at risk for MEA (pp. 839).

Summary

The three different types of steroid hormones produced by the adrenal cortex with their complex, interrelated pathway of biosynthesis, provide a myriad of clinical disorders when adrenal function is disturbed. Excessive production of glucocorticoids (Cushing syndrome), androgens (CAH, virilizing tumor), or mineralocorticoids (hyperplasia, tumor) may occur. Discrete enzymatic deficiencies (CAH, hypoaldosteronism) or destruction of adrenal tissue (Addison disease) can cause specific clinical syndromes. Our present ability to measure levels of steroid hormone in body fluids before and after perturbation with stimulatory (ACTH) and inhibitory (steroids) substances permits the physician to assess adrenal cortical function accurately. These tests provide a framework for diagnostic evaluation of a given clinical picture.

The unique proximity of the adrenal medulla to the adrenal cortex is a necessary condition for normal chromaffin cell function. Only excessive function of these cells with overproduction of catecholamines (pheochromocytoma) produces a distinct clinical syndrome.

REFERENCES

Adams JB: Control of secretion and the function of C_{19}-Δ^5-steroids of the human adrenal gland. *Mol Cell Endocrinol* 41:1, 1985.

Table 14.19
Urinary Values for Catecholamines and 3-methoxy-4-hydroxymandelic Acid in Normal Children[1]

	μg/24 hours Mean ± SD		
Age	Norepinephrine	Epinephrine	3-Methoxy-4-hydroxymandelic Acid
Birth–1 year	10.6 ± 3.4	1.3 ± 1.2	569 ± 309
1–5 years	18.8 ± 7.0	3.2 ± 2.7	1348 ± 443
6–15 years	37.4 ± 16.6	4.8 ± 2.4	2373 ± 698
Over 15 years	50.7 ± 15.7	7.1 ± 3.3	3192 ± 669

[1]From data of Voorhess, 1967.

Atarashi K, Mulrow PJ, Franco-Saenz R, et al: Inhibition of aldosterone production by an atrial extract. *Science* 224:992, 1984.

Byrne GC, Perry YS, Winter JSD: Kinetic analysis of adrenal 3 β-hydroxysteroid dehydrogenase activity during human development. *J Clin Endocrinol Metabol* 60:934, 1985.

Cacciari E, Balsamo A, Cassio A, et al: Neonatal screening for congenital adrenal hyperplasia. *Arch Dis Child* 58:803, 1983.

Carey RM, Sen S, Dolan LM, et al: Idiopathic hyperaldosteronism: A possible role for aldosterone-stimulating factor. *N Engl J Med* 311:94, 1984.

Curtis JA, Bailey JD: Influence of breast feeding on the clinical features of salt-losing congenital adrenal hyperplasia. *Arch Dis Child* 58:71, 1983.

David M, Forest MG: Prenatal treatment of congenital adrenal hyperplasia resulting from 21-hydroxylase deficiency. *J Pediatr* 105:799, 1984.

Davis LE, Snyder RD, Orth DN, et al: Adrenoleukodystrophy and adrenomyeloneuropathy associated with partial adrenal insufficiency in three generations of a kindred. *Am J Med* 66:342, 1979.

Dickerman Z, Grant DR, Faiman C, et al: Intraadrenal steroid concentrations in man: Zonal differences and developmental changes. *J Clin Endocrinol Metabol* 59:1031, 1984.

Dillon MJ, Leonard JV, Buckler JM, et al: Pseudohypoaldosteronism. *Arch Dis Child* 55:427, 1980.

Dupont B, Oberfield SE, Smithwick EM, et al: Close genetic linkage between HLA and congenital adrenal hyperplasia (21-hydroxylase deficiency). *Lancet* 2:1309, 1977.

Emans SJ, Grace E, Fleischnick E, et al: Detection of late-onset 21-hydroxylase deficiency in congenital adrenal hyperplasia in adolescents. *Pediatrics* 72:690, 1983.

Fleischnick E, Raum D, Alosco SM, et al: Extended MHC haplotypes in 21-hydroxylase-deficiency congenital adrenal hyperplasia shared genotypes in unrelated patients. *Lancet* 1:152, 1983.

Hendricks SA, Lippe BM, Kaplan SA, et al: Urinary and serum steroid concentrations in the management of congenital adrenal hyperplasia. *Am J Dis Child* 136:229, 1982.

Higashi Y, Yoshioka H, Yamane M, et al: Complete nucleotide sequence of two steroid 21-hydroxylase genes tandemly arranged in human chromosome: A pseudogene and a genuine gene. *Proc Natl Acad Sci* 83:2841, 1986.

Hochberg Z, Benderly A, Zadik Z: Salt loss in congenital adrenal hyperplasia due to 11β hydroxylase deficiency. *Arch Dis Child* 59:1092, 1984.

Hopwood NJ, Kenny FM: Incidence of Nelson's syndrome after adrenalectomy for Cushing's disease in children. *Am J Dis Child* 131:1353, 1977.

Hughes IA, Winter JSD: The relationship between serum concentrations of 17OH-progesterone and other serum and urinary steroids in patients with congenital adrenal hyperplasia. *J Clin Endocrinol Metabol* 46:98, 1978.

Ilondo MM, Vanderschueren-Lodeweyckx M, Pizarro M, et al: Plasma levels of androgens and 17 α OH-progesterone as an index of the adequacy of treatment in congenital adrenal hyperplasia. *Horm Res* 18:175, 1983.

Irvine WJ: Autoimmunity in endocrine disease. *Rec Progr Horm Res* 36:509, 1980.

Jennings AS, Liddle GW, Orth DN: Results of treating childhood Cushing's disease with pituitary irradiation. *N Engl J Med* 297:957, 1977.

Kangawa K, Matsuo H: Purification and complete amino acid sequence of α-human atrial natriuretic polypeptide (α-hANP). *Biochem Biophys Res Commun* 118:131, 1984.

Kelch RP, Kaplan SL, Biglieri EG, et al: Hereditary adrenocortical unresponsiveness to adrenocorticotropic hormone. *J Pediatr* 81:726, 1972.

Kirkland RT, Keenan BS, Holcombe JH, et al: The effect of therapy on mature height in congenital adrenal hyperplasia. *J Clin Endocrinol Metabol* 47:1320, 1978.

Klingensmith GJ, Garcia SC, Jones HW, et al: Glucocorticoid treatment of girls with congenital adrenal hyperplasia: Effects on height, sexual maturation, and fertility. *J Pediatr* 90:996, 1977.

Korth-Schutz S, Virdis R, Saenger P, et al: Serum androgens as a continuing index of adequacy of treatment of congenital adrenal hyperplasia. *J Clin Endocrinol Metabol* 46:452, 1978.

Lee PDK, Winter RJ, Green OC: Virilizing adrenocortical tumors in childhood: Eight cases and a review of the literature. *Pediatrics* 76:437, 1985.

Lobo RA, Kletzky OA, Kaptein EM, et al: Prolactin modulation of dehydroepiandrosterone sulfate secretion. *Am J Obstet Gynecol* 138:632, 1980.

Money J, Schwartz M, Lewis VG: Adult erotosexual status and fetal hormonal masculinization and demasculinization: 46XX congenital virilizing adrenal hyperplasia and 46XY androgen insensitivity syndrome compared. *Psychoneuroendocrinology* 9:405, 1984.

Mulaikal RM, Migeon CJ, Rock JA: Fertility rates in female patients with congenital adrenal hyperplasia due to 21-hydroxylase deficiency *N Engl J Med* 316:178, 1987.

Neufeld M, MacLaren N, Blizzard R: Autoimmune polyglandular syndromes. *Pediatr Ann* 9:154, 1980.

New MI, Lorenzen F, Lerner AJ, et al: Genotyping steroid 21-hydroxylase deficiency: Hormonal reference data. *J Clin Endocrinol Metabol* 57:320, 1983.

Pang S, Levine LS, Cederqvist L, et al: Amniotic fluid concentrations of Δ^5 and Δ^4 steroids in fetuses with congenital adrenal hyperplasia due to 21-hydroxylase deficiency and in anencephalic fetuses. *J Clin Endocrinol Metabol* 51:223, 1980.

Pang S, Levine LS, Stoner E, et al: Non-salt-losing congenital adrenal hyperplasia due to 3 β-hydroxysteroid dehydrogenase deficiency with normal glomerulosa function. *J Clin Endocrinol Metabol* 56:808, 1983.

Pang S, Murphey W, Levine LS, et al: A pilot newborn screening for congenital adrenal hyperplasia in Alaska. *J Clin Endocrinol Metabol* 55:413, 1982.

Pang S, Pollack MS, Loo M, et al: Pitfalls of prenatal diagnosis of 21-hydroxylase deficiency congenital adrenal hyperplasia. *J Clin Endocrinol Metabol* 61:89, 1985.

Parker LN, Lifrak ET, Odell WD: A 60,000 molecular weight human pituitary glycopeptide stimulates adrenal androgen secretion. *Endocrinology* 113:2092, 1983.

Pollack M, Levine LS, Duchon M, et al: Prenatal diagnosis of CAH due to 21-hydroxylase deficiency by HLA typing of cultured amniotic cells. *Pediatr Res* 13:384, 1979.

Raum DD, Awdeh ZL, Glass D, et al: The location of C2, C4, and BF relative to HLA-B and HLA-D. *Immunogenetics* 12:473, 1981.

Rosler A, Levine LS, Schneider B, et al: The interrelationship of sodium balance, plasma renin activity and ACTH in congenital adrenal hyperplasia. *J Clin Endocrinol Metabol* 45:500, 1977.

Sen S, Shainoff JR, Bravo EL, et al: Isolation of aldosterone-stimulating factor (ASF) and its effect on rat adrenal glomerulosa cells in vitro. *Hypertension* 3:4, 1981.

Shimozawa K, Saisho S, Saito N, et al: A neonatal mass-screening for congenital adrenal hyperplasia in Japan. *Acta Endocrinol* 107:513, 1984.

Siegler RL, Crouch RH, Hackett TN Jr, et al: Potassium-renin-aldosterone relationships during the first year of life. *J Pediatr* 91:52, 1977.

Speiser PW, Martin KO, Kao-Lo G, et al: Excess mineralocorticoid receptor activity in patients with dexamethasone-suppressible hyperaldosteronism is under adrenocorticotropin control. *J Clin Endocrinol Metabol* 61:297, 1985.

Styne DM, Grumbach MM, Kaplan SL, et al: Treatment of Cushing's disease in childhood and adolescence by transphenoidal microadenomectomy. *N Engl J Med* 310:889, 1984.

Vermeulen A, Suy E, Rubens R: Effect of prolactin on plasma DHEA(S) levels. *J Clin Endocrinol Metabol* 44:1222, 1977.

Voorhess ML: Urinary catecholamine excretion by healthy children: Daily excretion of dopamine, norepinephrine, epinephrine, and 3-methoxy-4-hydroxymandelic acid. *Pediatrics* 39:252, 1967.

Warshaw BL, Anand SK, Olson DL, et al: Hypertension secondary to a renin-producing juxtaglomerular cell tumor. *J Pediatr* 94:247, 1979.

Wen X, Villee DB, Ellison P, et al: Effects of adrenocorticotrophic hormone, human chorionic gonadotropin, and insulin on steroid production by human adrenocortical carcinoma cells in culture. *Cancer Res* 45:3974, 1985.

White PC, New MI, Dupont B: HLA-linked congenital adrenal hyperplasia results from a defective gene encoding a cytochrome p-450 specific for steroid 21-hydroxylation. *Proc Natl Acad Sci* 81:7505, 1984.

Winter JSD: Current approaches to the treatment of congenital adrenal hyperplasia. *J Pediatr* 97:81, 1980.

Winterer J, Chrousos GP, Loriaux DL, et al: Effect of hydrocortisone dose schedule on adrenal steroid secretion in congenital adrenal hyperplasia. *J Pediatr* 106:137, 1985.

Yamaji T, Hirai N, Ishibashi M, et al: Atrial natriuretic peptide in umbilical cord blood: Evidence for a circulating hormone in human fetus. *J Clin Endocrinol Metabol* 63:1414, 1986.

Gonads 7

Disordered function of the gonads may result in a variety of clinical syndromes. Both testes and ovaries are capable of producing androgens and estrogens; however, under normal circumstances testes produce predominantly androgens and ovaries produce mostly estrogens. If the appropriate sex hormones are absent or are formed in insufficient or excessive quantities at critical stages in development, abnormal sexual development will occur. Two of the most critical periods are during development in utero and at puberty.

Sexual Differentiation

The gonadal sex of an individual depends upon the chromosomal sex (Fig. 14.14). The Y chromosome is able to direct the bipotential embryonic gonad to differentiate as a testis. The gene for a testis-determining factor, is located on the Y chromosome at the distal portion of the short arm (Simpson et al, 1987). This gene is distinct from the H-Y antigen which had been considered to be the testis—determining factor (TDF) prior to the genetic work of isolating the factor on the distal short arm of the Y chromosome. The H-Y antigen which is a male—specific cell membrane component may be involved in the regulation of spermatogenesis. In the absence of TDF, the indifferent gonad organizes as an ovary.

Once organization of the definitive gonad has occurred, hormone production can begin. The Leydig cells of the testis develop receptors for human chorionic gonadotropin/luteinizing hormone (hCG/LH). The placenta at about 8–10 weeks' gestation forms large amounts of hCG, a small amount of which reaches the fetus. It is the placental hCG that inaugurates testosterone production in the fetal Leydig cells. The fetal pituitary at this stage is not producing significant amounts of gonadotropins.

Both internal and external genitalia are sexually indifferent at 7 weeks' gestation. Secretions from the fetal testis play an important role in male differentiation of these genitalia. Testosterone, elaborated by the Leydig cells of the testis, reaches the wolffian ducts and binds to the androgen receptor there. The ducts are, thus, stimulated to differentiate into epididymis, vas deferens, and seminal vesicles. Local diffusion of testosterone from the testis brings about stabilization and differentiation of wolffian duct structures.

In contrast, male differentiation of the urogenital sinus and external genitalia requires the conversion of testosterone to dihydrotestosterone (DHT) and subsequent interaction of the DHT with androgen receptors in the tissues. The reduction of testosterone is catalyzed by a 5 α-reductase present in these anlage. DHT stimulates growth of the genital tubercle, induces fusion of the urethral and labioscrotal folds, and inhibits the growth of the vesicovaginal septum, thereby preventing the development of the vagina.

Müllerian-inhibiting hormone, which is also produced by the fetal testis (Sertoli cells), induces regression of the müllerian duct (anlage for fallopian tubes, uterus, and upper vagina).

Thus, in the presence of testicular hormones, the wolffian duct differentiates, the müllerian duct regresses, and the urogenital sinus and external genitalia masculinize. In the absence of fetal testicular hormones the müllerian duct differentiates, the wolffian duct regresses, and the urogenital sinus and external genitalia feminize.

In the human, two intact X chromosomes are required for complete development of the ovary. In 45,XO individuals, as well as those with deletions of the X chromosome, ovarian differentiation occurs in utero but oocytes generally fail to survive and folliculogenesis does not occur or is defective. Genes controlling ovarian development are present on both arms of the X chromosome.

During normal fetal development, female germ cells undergo replication and differentiation into oogonia and primary oocytes. By 5 months' gestation, there are 6–7 million germ cells in the two ovaries. Replication of

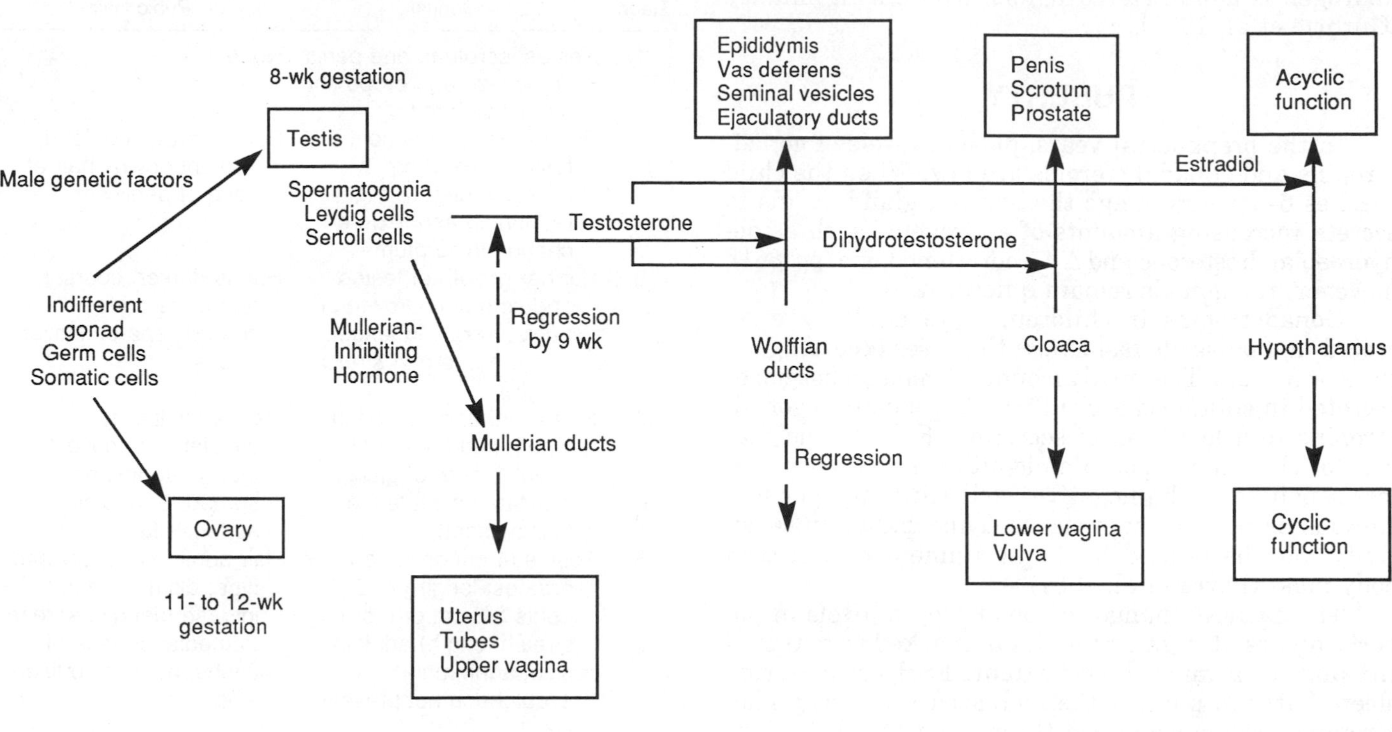

Figure 14.14. Sexual differentiation of reproductive organs. Indifferent organs (in center) will undergo female differentiation in the absence of male genetic factors and testicular hormones.

germ cells ceases by the seventh month of gestation. The oocytes that have formed are arrested in late prophase of the first meiotic division (diplotene state) and remain in this state until ovulation occurs. In contrast to the female, germ cells of the male remain quiescent and do not differentiate until puberty.

In addition to gonadal and genital sexual differentiation, the brain also undergoes differentiation along a male or female pattern, which involves the mode of gonadotropin release by the hypothalamus and differences in behavior patterns. In the male, hypothalamic gonadotropic-releasing hormone (GnRH) and pituitary gonadotropins are released in a pulsatile but relatively constant manner, designated a tonic release. In the female these hormones are released in a cyclic manner that incorporates a preovulatory surge of gonadotropins, which leads to ovulation. Behavioral differences incorporate gender identity and gender role as well as gender orientation. In addition, sexual differences in cognitive function have been described. In the human, sexual differentiation of the brain probably occurs in late intrauterine life. Androgens can masculinize the brain permanently in neonatal animals. The role of androgens versus environmental influences in the sexual differentiation of the human brain has been controversial. It appears that both factors are important and unlike laboratory animals a single exposure of the human female brain to androgen in utero does not cause permanent masculinization of the brain.

Postnatal Gonadal Activity

Beginning about the fifth day of postnatal life levels of gonadotropins in the blood rise. During the first several months the female infant has plasma follicle-stimulating hormone (FSH) levels that are higher than those in comparably aged males and LH levels are higher than those in older female children. The elevation of gonadotropins in both sexes is accompanied by a detectable rise in estradiol in the female and a dramatic increase of testosterone in the male infant. The sex hormones reach a peak at about 3–4 months of age and fall thereafter as the gonadotropin levels decrease.

The precise function of the gonadal secretion in the first year of life is unknown. There is no evidence in the human or monkey that neonatal deprivation or excess of androgen has any permanent effect on hypothalamic pituitary function. Whether neonatal androgens play a specific role in gender identity in humans is uncertain. There is some evidence for a "priming" effect of neonatal androgens on subsequent penile response to androgens. Boys born with micropenis because of androgen deficiency have inadequate androgen-mediated growth of the external genitalia if androgen replacement is started only at the time of normal male puberty, but response may be normal if androgen is administered temporarily during infancy (Guthrie et al, 1973).

PUBERTY

In the prepubertal years, plasma levels of gonadotropins and gonadal steroids are low. When the child reaches 6–7 years of age the adrenal gland begins to secrete increasing amounts of androgens, such as dehydroepiandrosterone and Δ 4-androstenedione (pp. 861); however, the gonads remain quiescent.

Gonadotropins in children, as in adults, are secreted in a pulsatile fashion, with pulses occurring every 2 or 3 hours. The small amounts of gonadal hormones secreted in childhood are sufficient to suppress gonadotropins to a low level of secretion. For reasons that are not clear the hypothalamic-pituitary axis becomes less sensitive to the negative feedback of the gonadal steroids as puberty approaches. This change in sensitivity may be related to the attainment of a critical body mass (Parra et al, 1981).

The earliest change in gonadotropin levels in puberty occurs at night. Episodes of marked secretion of LH and, to a much lesser extent, FSH occur during sleep. Later in puberty the increased levels of gonadotropins become sustained throughout the day, as do the resulting increases in the gonadal sex hormones.

Following the rise in plasma sex hormones, physical signs of sexual development appear. In the male, rising plasma concentrations of FSH bring about increased size of the testes, which occurs before any other physical signs of puberty. The volume or the diameter and length of the testes may be measured as an indicator of the onset of pubertal development. A testicular length of 2.5 cm is indicative of exposure to FSH and the onset of puberty (Table 14.20). Pubic hair often appears after this, followed by increments in linear height and penile length. The staging of puberty is shown in Table 14.20.

A comparable scheme of pubertal development in the female is shown in Table 14.21. The first sign of puberty in the female is the widening and elevation of the areola followed by enlargement of the breast tissue. This breast budding is followed by the appearance of labial and then pubic hair. Complete maturation of breasts takes about 4 years and the time required for full pubic hair development is roughly 3 years. In some girls pubic hair may precede breast budding. The adolescent growth spurt occurs early in girls; 40% of girls reach peak height velocity during the breast-budding stage.

Menarche usually begins during the deceleration phase of the growth spurt, after the breast enlarges. The mean age for menarche for girls in the United States is 12.8 years.

It has been proposed by Frisch (1985) that a particular ratio of fat to lean mass is normally necessary for menarche and the maintenance of regular ovulatory cycles. She suggests that extreme leanness may alter some of the integrating signals from the higher centers of the central nervous system that maintain biologic rhythms.

Table 14.20
Stages of Puberty in the Male

Stage	Genital	Pubic Hair
1	Testes, scrotum, and penis same size and proportion as in childhood	None
2	Beginning enlargement of testes (over 2 cm in greatest length); slight reddening and texture change in scrotum	Sparse growth of long straight downy hair at base of penis
3	Further growth of testes and scrotum. Growth of penis, mostly in length, (7 cm or more in stretch length)	Hair is darker, coarser, and more curled; spreads sparsely over pubes
4	Penis further enlarged in length and breadth; development of glans; prostate palpable (sex hair present)	Hair is adult in type; smaller area covered than in adults; no spread to medial surface of thighs
5	Testes (4 cm or more greatest length) and penis (13 cm or more stretch length) adult in size; adult male escutcheon not present yet	Hair adult in quantity and type; distributed in inverse triangle; spread to medial surface of thighs, but not up linea alba

Menstrual Cycle

Most menstrual cycles are between 25 and 30 days in length. Great variability in cycle frequency and du-

Table 14.21
Stages of Puberty in the Female

Stage	Breasts	Pubic Hair
1	No palpable glandular tissue; areola not pigmented	None
2	Glandular tissue palpable; nipple and breast project as a mound from chest wall	Occasional wispy strands, usually along labia
3	Breast enlarged; areola increased in diameter and more darkly pigmented	Increased dark and coarser hair extending up over pubis
4	Further enlargement with increased areolar pigment; areola and nipple form a secondary mound above level of breast	Dark, coarse, curly hair covering the mons pubis,
5	Areola and nipple no longer project; smooth contour in profile view	Mature including extension of hair to medial aspects of thighs

ration is observed in the first 2 years after menarche. There may be no cycles for several months before a more nearly normal frequency is established. Most of the early cycles are anovulatory. The hormonal changes that occur in the normal menstrual cycle are depicted in Figure 14.15. During follicular development estrogen levels are low, rising about 1 week before the LH peak. Estrogens reach their peak just before or coinciding with the LH surge; they then fall precipituously, before ovulation takes place. Rupture of the follicle occurs about 24–36 hours after the LH peak. Ovulation is followed by the luteal phase, during which large amounts of progesterone are secreted by the granulosa cells. A small rise in estrogen occurs at this time also.

The hormonal regulation of the menstrual cycle is complex. The magnitude and frequency of GnRH pulses are modulated by feedback from ovarian hormones. In addition, ovarian hormones modulate the sensitivity of the pituitary gonadotrophs to GnRH. The negative feedback effect of estrogens on the hypothalamus operates within minutes, whereas positive feedback requires sustained estrogen stimulation, and a significant rise in LH is not seen before 24 hours.

Both FSH and LH are required for estrogen synthesis. FSH induces aromatase, an enzyme complex involved in the conversion of the Δ 4-3 ketone structure of the androgens to the aromatic ring of the estrogens. LH stimulates the synthesis of progesterone plus androgens, which then act as precursors for estrogen synthesis. Thus, the gonadotropins stimulate production of ovarian steroid hormones which, in turn, modulate follicle growth.

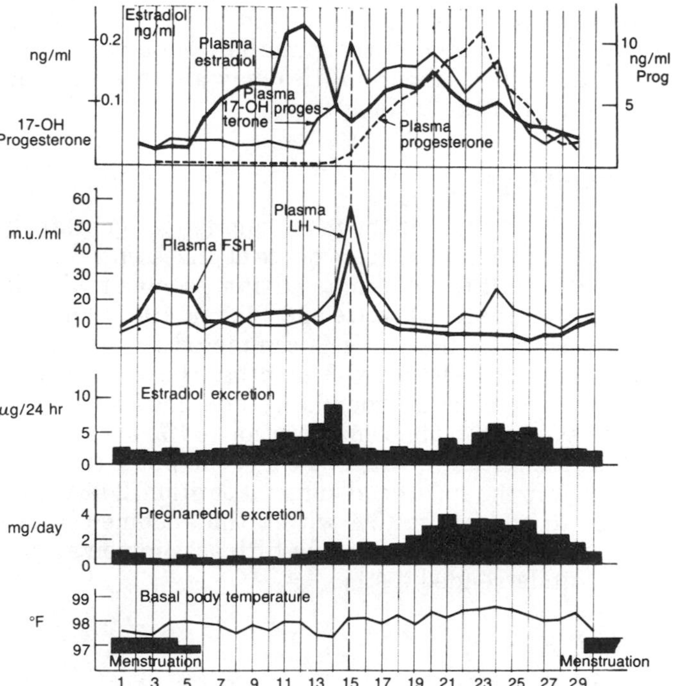

Figure 14.15. Diagram illustrating the concentrations of gonadotropins, estrogens, and progestins in the plasma during a single human menstrual cycle. The urinary excretion of estradiol and pregnanediol and the changes in basal body temperature are also shown. (Reproduced with permission from Villee CA: *Biology*, 7th edition. Philadelphia, WB Saunders, 1977.)

In the early follicular phase of the cycle FSH levels rise initiating follicle growth. As follicles grow the population of cells responding to FSH and synthesizing estradiol increases. The follicle at this stage is a primary follicle in which there are two or more layers of granulosa cells surrounding the oocyte. Under the influence of FSH, a cohort of follicles begins to enlarge, some reaching diameters of 4 mm or more while the rest undergo atresia. As a follicle reaches 8 mm in diameter, the FSH concentration of follicular fluid increases and estradiol secretion by the follicle is enhanced further. The granulosa cells continue to proliferate, eventually forming multilayered concentric cells around the oocyte (secondary follicle). Later, fluid-filled cavities appear within the granulosa layer. The follicular fluid of these antral follicles initially is derived solely from granulosa secretions. In later stages, contributions from capillaries of the surrounding theca cells become significant. The oocyte and its associated cells (cumulus oophorus) are displaced eccentrically and are surrounded by follicular fluid except at the point of attachment to the granulosa layer. Within this fluid are steroid hormones as well as a protein hormone, inhibin, which is a specific inhibitor of FSH. Inhibin activity is found mainly during the follicular phase and its concentration in ovarian venous plasma varies inversely with the concentration of FSH in plasma. Inhibin is produced by the granulosa cells in the ovary and by the Sertoli cells in the testis.

Typically only one follicle reaches preovulatory size (>10–12 mm). It is selected, to the exclusion of all others, by the midfollicular phase (DiZerega and Hodgen, 1981).

As the follicle grows, androgen-producing theca cells proliferate. These androgens may play a role in atresia of follicles as well as provide substrate for estrogen synthesis by granulosa cells. At this stage, the level of estrogen production by the granulosa cells has risen markedly and induces an increase in LH release via a positive feedback effect on the hypothalamus. Apparently the positive feedback effect of estrogens enhances the release of LH more than that of FSH. The effect is one of a predominantly LH surge with subsequent ovulation.

During the follicular phase FSH induces LH receptors in the granulosa cells. These cells now undergo a process of luteinization with enhanced progesterone production under the influence of LH. The granulosa and theca cells together with their surrounding tissues form the corpus luteum. The function of the corpus luteum reaches its peak about 4 days after ovulation and begins to wane about 4 days before menstruation. The sex hormones secreted by the corpus luteum cause a transformation of the endometrium from a proliferative lining (estrogen effect) to a secretory lining (progesterone effect). Spontaneous regression of the corpus luteum occurs if there is no pregnancy. The loss of ovarian hormones brings about a shedding of the uterine lining (menstruation).

Ambiguous Genitalia

Various disorders of development and/or function of the reproductive system in males and females have been described. Perhaps the earliest and most difficult decision for the physician to make is the assignment of sex in the child with ambiguous genitalia (Fig. 14.13, pp. 858). Infants with obviously ambiguous genitalia are candidates for a full evaluation; however, the physician should also be alerted to the possibility of abnormal sexual differentiation in the female with inguinal masses, inguinal herniae, or slight clitoral enlargement as well as in the male with hypospadias, cryptorchidism, or small genitalia and/or gonads. For further discussion of the differential diagnosis of ambiguous genitalia, see pp. 857.

MALE DEVELOPMENT DISORDERS

Hypospadias

Definition

Incomplete fusion of the penile urethra without a urogenital sinus is designated hypospadias.

Epidemiology and Etiology

It is estimated that hypospadias occurs in about 8 of 1000 male births. About 40% of these patients have associated anomalies of the urogenital tract, most of which are mild. The mildest form of hypospadias is coronal, which constitutes 80% of cases.

Theoretically hypospadias represents a state of incomplete masculinization; however, it has been hard to implicate endocrine factors in most cases. Nevertheless, temporary reduction of testosterone production by the fetal testis at the critical stage of urethral fold fusion (before 12–14 weeks' gestation) remains a possible explanation for some of these cases. For example, hypospadias is associated with maternal exposure to progesterone analogues during the first trimester of pregnancy. Progesterone is known to inhibit 3 β-hydroxysteroid dehydrogenase and, thus, block androgen production. A subgroup of males with hypospadias appear to have an abnormality in androgen responsiveness (Keenan et al, 1984; Allen and Griffin, 1984).

There is a 14% recurrence rate of hypospadias for future male siblings. The mode of inheritance in these cases is unknown.

Diagnosis

Careful examination of the newborn male will reveal the presence of even the mildest forms of hypospadias. Extensive endocrine evaluation of the child with a simple coronal hypospadias and otherwise normal genitalia with descended testes is probably unnecessary. For children with more severe degrees of hypospadias or for those with other abnormalities of the external genitalia a full evaluation is indicated (pp. 858).

Treatment

Except in the mildest cases, treatment is surgical correction of the hypospadias.

Cryptorchidism

Definition

The descent of the testes into the scrotum occurs during the last trimester of gestation. Cryptorchidism is defined as the failure of the testes to descend normally through the inguinal canal to their normal position at the bottom of the scrotum by birth. The term ectopic testis is used to describe a testis that has become lodged in the abdominal wall, upper thigh, or within the perineum after passing through the external inguinal ring.

Basic Science

The migration of the testis in the latter part of intrauterine life is dependent upon the normal secretion of LH by the fetal pituitary and of testosterone by the fetal testis. Thus, abnormalities of either the fetal pituitary (hypopituitarism) or the fetal testis can cause cryptorchidism. Concomitant hypopspadias suggests an abnormality of sexual differentiation. Recent studies have shown a significant decline in the early postnatal LH and testosterone surges and diminished responsiveness of LH to GnRH and testosterone to hCG in cryptorchid boys. These same investigators have found antigonadotropic cell antibodies in the serum of cryptorchid children and of their mothers (Pouplard et al, 1985). Structural abnormalities may also prevent normal descent of the testis.

Epidemiology

Cryptorchidism is the most common urogenital abnormality. The estimated incidence of undescended testes is 3.4% in full-term infants, rising to about 30% in premature infants (Schulze and Pfister, 1985). In most boys, descent of the testis is completed in the first 3 months of life. After age 3 months, the incidence of undescended testes is about 0.8%, the same as in adults. The most common abnormal location (44%) is a position high in the scrotum, within 4 cm of the pubic tubercle; 26% occur in the superficial inguinal position, 20% within the canal, and about 10% within the abdomen. Bilateral cryptorchidism is only one-fifth as common as unilateral undescended testis.

Natural History

The histology of the undescended testis is similar to that of the normal testis until about 2 years of age, after which significant differences can be found (Hadziselimovic et al, 1975). The undescended testis has a decreased number of spermatogonia and a decreased tubular diameter compared with the normal descended testis. In addition to changes in tubular morphology, the cryptorchid testis is also more prone to tumor formation. About 10% of all testicular tumors occur in individuals with undescended testes.

Diagnosis

Cryptorchidism must be differentiated from ectopic testes and retractile testes. The parents should be asked if they have ever seen a testis in the scrotum. If so the testis is probably retractile and can usually be "milked" down into the scrotum with the child sitting upright with feet crossed in front of him. Sometimes parents will note a testis in the scrotum when the child is in a warm bath. These testes retract up into the inguinal canal under a variety of conditions, therefore, it is important to conduct the examination in a warm room with warm hands to reduce the cremasteric reflex.

If the testis can be palpated in the inguinal canal but cannot be brought down, ectopic testis is the probable diagnosis. If the testis cannot be felt anywhere it is presumably atrophied or placed within the abdomen. Ultrasonography and/or CAT scan may be helpful in locating the testes in the inguinal canal or abdomen.

Evaluation of serum hormone levels can be helpful. High values for gonadotropins and low testosterone levels would indicate primary gonadal failure. Normal or low values for both gonadotropins and testosterone may suggest the need for a gonadotropin stimulation test. The ability of the testis to descend can be tested by administering hCG (hCG, 3000–4000 IU intramuscularly weekly) or intranasal gonadotropin releasing hormone (GnRH, 200μg every 2 hours, 6 times a day for a total daily dose of 1.2 mg) for 4 weeks. If descent occurs, even though transient, it can be predicted that the testis will descend permanently at puberty. If no testis can be felt, hormone treatment is still beneficial. Analyses of plasma testosterone levels at the beginning and end of the 4-week treatment period will give information regarding the presence of testicular tissue. Leydig cells survive well within the abdomen and can respond to hCG with a rise in testosterone secretion. In those patients receiving GnRH plasma levels of LH and FSH as well as testosterone should rise. An inborn error of testosterone biosynthesis may be present if the testosterone response to hCG is poor. No response suggests absent testes or Leydig cells; however, testes were found in two prepubertal males in whom no response occurred (Bartone et al, 1984).

Cryptorchidism associated with other abnormalities of the external genitalia requires a complete evaluation (pp. 858). The condition is also found in association with various endocrine and chromosomal abnormalities, such as Noonan, Klinefelter, and Kallmann syndromes and trisomy of chromosomes 13, 18, and 21. Since descent of the testis requires abdominal pressure, cryptorchidism is also found in the prune-belly syndrome. Bilateral cryptorchidism with no palpable glands always requires investigation to rule out a condition of female pseudohermaphroditism.

Treatment

Although parenteral hCG has been reported to induce descent into the scrotum in 15–40% of boys with cryptorchidism (Job et al, 1982), the success of hormonal therapy is considerably less in studies where boys with retractile testes have been eliminated from the study group (Rajfer et al, 1986). About 25–50% of the patients who are referred to pediatric surgeons or urologists because of a diagnosis of cryptorchidism will be found to have a retractile testicle when they are examined adequately.

The question of hormonal treatment for true cryptorchidism (high testes) remains unresolved (Colodny, 1986). Hormonal therapy may provide partial descent of these testes and simplify subsequent surgery. Also conversion of gonadocytes to spermatocytes may be under hormonal control. The ultimate answer may be to treat patients with cryptorchidism first with hCG or GnRH for 4–6 weeks and then follow this therapy with orchiopexy for undescended testis in those who do not have complete descent or who have a relapse after a satisfactory initial response. If surgical repair of cryptorchidism is required the present recommendation is for repair to occur before 2 years of age to prevent irreversible damage to the tubular elements of the gland.

Prognosis

There is evidence for malfunction in cryptorchid testes. Androgen production was normal in men who underwent successful unilateral orchiopexy as children (Lipshultz et al, 1976), but prepubertal boys who had bilateral cryptorchidism showed deficient androgen production compared to that of boys with unilateral cyryptorchidism or hypospadias (Walsh et al, 1976). Sperm production may be impaired also in previously cryptorchid testes.

Malignancy may develop in a previously cryptorchid testis many years after apparently successful orchiopexy (Krabbe et al, 1979); therefore, periodic examination of the testis is important in these patients.

Anorchia

Definition

Anorchia is defined as either unilateral or bilateral absence of testicular tissue.

Epidemiology and Etiology

Anorchia is found in 3–5% of boys operated on for cryptorchidism. The internal ducts and external genitalia may be male or there may be ambiguity, depending upon whether testicular tissue was functional at 8–12 weeks' gestation. This condition has been called the "vanishing testis syndrome." One theory for the loss of testes after 12 weeks is that torsion or vascular occlusion occurred at some time during the process of testicular descent.

Occasionally, testes are absent but Leydig cells are present scattered along the genital ducts. This condition has been termed the "Leydig cell only syndrome."

Diagnosis

The absence of a testis can only be diagnosed by a thorough operative search. The vas deferens and epididymis should be sought as well as testicular vessels. These structures may descend into the scrotum without a testis.

Serum gonadotropin levels are elevated in bilateral anorchic boys and the plasma testosterone response to hCG (1000–2000 units intramuscularly every 48 hours for seven doses) is absent. The hCG test is not foolproof, however, and laparotomy is indicated in most cases (Bartone et al, 1984).

Anorchics with ambiguous genitalia require a full investigation.

Treatment

Children with bilateral anorchia require testosterone replacement and prosthetic testes.

Micropenis

Definition

A micropenis is any penis that falls more than 2.5 SD below the mean of normal for stretched length (Table 14.22).

Epidemiology and Etiology

The growth of the penis depends on normal pituitary and testicular production of gonadotropins, testosterone, and growth hormone (Lee et al, 1980). Micropenis may be the only sign of hypopituitarism or disorders of hypothalamic-pituitary function. A variety of syndromes are associated with micropenis (Table 14.23).

Table 14.22
Stretched Penile Length in Normal Males; Values Are Expressed in cm

	Mean	SD	Mean—2.5 SD in cm
Newborn, 30 weeks	2.5	0.4	1.5
Newborn, 34 weeks	3.0	0.4	2.0
Newborn, term	3.5	0.4	2.4
0–5 months	3.9	0.8	1.9
6–12 months	4.3	0.8	2.3
1–2 years	4.7	0.8	2.6
2–3 years	5.1	0.9	2.9
3–4 years	5.5	0.9	3.3
4–5 years	5.7	0.9	3.5
5–6 years	6.0	0.9	3.8
6–7 years	6.1	0.9	3.9
7–8 years	6.2	1.0	3.7
8–9 years	6.3	1.0	3.8
9–10 years	6.3	1.0	3.8
10–11 years	6.4	1.1	3.7
Adult	13.3	1.6	9.3

Diagnosis

All patients with micropenis should be investigated for pituitary function. Specific stigmata of syndromes are helpful in sorting out the possible causes of the condition. Associated hypospadias and/or cryptorchidism suggest the need for an evaluation of ambiguous genitalia.

Patients with micropenis but normal testes should be tested for responsiveness to androgens. Testosterone enanthate, 25–50 mg intramuscularly monthly for three doses should produce lengthening of the penis by 2.0 cm ± 0.6 cm. Alternatively, hCG can be given, with measurement of testosterone levels in serum as well as penile length. This procedure tests the ability of the testis to respond to hCG and the penis to respond to testosterone. Serum testosterone values should be measured 48 hours after the final hCG treatment.

Treatment

If the initial 3-month trial of testosterone or hCG shows a good response in terms of penile length, the patient should be followed carefully for evidence of insufficient growth of the penis later. If the penis again seems small during childhood, an additional 3-month course of treatment is indicated.

In extreme cases (penile length less than 1.9 cm) or in cases showing poor response to hormone treatment, a female sex assignment should be considered.

Prognosis

The responsiveness of the penis to androgen treatment does not necessarily guarantee a penis of normal size at puberty and in adulthood. This is a difficult problem to handle; however, most boys who show good response to androgen will have adequate development of the penis. Unfortunately the suicide rate in these boys is very high and undoubtedly there may be problems with sexual identification and performance. Psychiatric counseling may be extremely important in these patients.

Table 14.23
Disorders Associated with Micropenis

Hypothalamic
Kallman syndrome
Prader-Willi syndrome
Pituitary
Septo-optic dysplasia
GH deficiency
Gonadotropin deficiency
Gonadal
Klinefelter syndrome
Dysgenetic testes
End-Organ
Androgen insensitivity

Gynecomastia

Definition

Gynecomastia is defined as growth of mammary tissue in the male.

Epidemiology and Etiology

Gynecomastia is extremely common in the pubertal boy. Estimates range from 65–80% for incidence of this condition in this age group. Commonly it is bilateral, but it may be asymmetrical or unilateral. It may last for several years. There is some evidence for an increased estrogen to androgen ratio in sera of boys with gynecomastia.

Although puberty is by far the most common "cause" of gynecomastia, palpable breasts are found in boys with a number of conditions including Klinefelter syndrome, androgen receptor defects, thyroid abnormalities, and exposure to certain drugs and hormones (estrogens, meprobamate, phenothiazines, cimetidine, spironolactone, and marijuana). Rarely unilateral enlargement of the breast is the result of neoplasm. If accompanied by galactorrhea, a prolactin-secreting tumor of the pituitary may be present.

Natural History

The gynecomastia of pubertal boys varies from minimal to marked breast development. It persists for about 2 years in 27% of the cases and for 3 years in 7.7%. It is often the cause of extreme embarrassment and emotional turmoil.

Diagnosis

It is important to evaluate all the possible causes of gynecomastia. A careful history may reveal a familial incidence of the condition. Drug ingestion must be reviewed. The physical examination may reveal stigmata of Klinefelter syndrome or hypothyroidism.

Hormonal assays may be very helpful. Serum values for TSH, T4, LH, FSH, prolactin, estradiol, and testosterone should be obtained as well as a 24-hour urine collection for assay of 17-KS.

Skull radiographs and/or CAT scans should be obtained if a pituitary tumor is suspected.

A buccal smear and karyotype will identify Klinefelter syndrome.

Treatment

Specific hormonal disorders should be treated appropriately. Exposure to drugs known to cause gynecomastia should be reduced or eliminated if possible. Unless there is extreme emotional concern, the boy can be reassured that the condition will improve with time.

Until recently, the only therapeutic option was resection. Hormonal intervention had not been uniformly successful. In a report on four nonobese pubertal males, however, dihydrotestosterone heptanoate was given intramuscularly at 2- to 4-week intervals for 16 weeks. Breast size was reduced by 67–68% in all four boys. After a second course of therapy, two boys had a 90% reduction in breast size (Eberle et al, 1986). In a 3-year follow-up of boys treated with percutaneous dihydrotestosterone, 72% responded with no recurrence subsequently (Kuhn et al, 1983). Testolactone, an aromatase inhibitor, has also been used to treat pubertal gynecomastia successfully (Zachmann et al, 1986).

The therapy is too new to permit evaluation of possible late side effects; meanwhile, it is promising and deserves further evaluation.

Delayed Puberty

Definition

Delayed puberty is a term applied to those boys who have an onset of puberty at a chronologic age that is later than the mean age, but within 2 SD of the mean age for the normal male population.

Epidemiology

Delay in onset of puberty is a very common problem in boys and often is associated with a family history of late-onset puberty. Roughly 15% of the normal male population may belong in this group.

Natural History

Typically, these patients are seen in clinic for failure to grow and develop. At age 14 or 15 years these boys show little evidence of sexual development and their linear growth rate may be less than 5 cm per year. They eventually develop sexually and accelerate linear growth rate, but this may not occur for several years and, in some boys, the onset of puberty is delayed until they reach their 20s.

Diagnosis

It is important to distinguish delayed development from other causes of sexual immaturity (pp. 878), particularly hypopituitarism. Careful physical examination may reveal early testicular enlargement (>2.5 cm in length) suggesting that puberty has already begun. Serum levels of gonadotropins may be increased at night, again suggesting an early stage of development.

In the boy with no physical or hormonal evidence of puberty, tests of pituitary function are indicated (pp. 813).

The linear growth pattern of these boys with delayed development will parallel the normal curve without the adolescent growth spurt, whereas in hypopituitarism the curve deviates progressively from the norm. Bone age is appropriate for the degree of sexual development in both conditions.

Treatment

In boys showing early signs of development, reassurance is usually sufficient to allay their anxieties. When psychological problems are evident, a 6-month course of hCG (500 units every 5 days intramuscularly) or testosterone enanthate (100 mg every 3–4 weeks intramuscularly) should be considered. Often when therapy is stopped, the patient will continue to mature on his own. If no progress is made after 6 months without therapy, a second course of hormone therapy may be instituted.

Hormone treatment may shorten ultimate stature and the patient and his parents should be advised of this before therapy is begun.

Male Hypogonadism

Definition

Hypogonadism represents a failure of gonadal function either due to intrinsic defects (hypergonadotropic hypogonadism) or secondary to a lack of gonadotropins (hypogonadotropic hypogonadism).

Hypergonadotropic Hypogonadism

Epidemiology and Etiology

Any condition in which the elaboration of testosterone by the testis is impaired will result in increased production of GnRH by the hypothalamus and greater production and secretion of gonadotropins (Table 14.24).

Klinefelter Syndrome

Definition

This syndrome is characterized by an abnormality of the sex chromosomes and by the presence of small testes with fibrosis and hyalinization of the seminiferous tubules.

Table 14.24
Causes of Hypogonadism in the Male

- Hypergonadotropic
  - Congenital
    - Klinefelter syndrome
    - Gonadal dysgenesis
    - Noonan syndrome
    - Anorchia
    - Abnormalities of testosterone biosynthesis
  - Acquired
    - Castration
    - Leydig cell failure
    - Seminiferous tubule failure
    - Orchitis
- Hypogonadotropic
  - Kallman syndrome
  - Isolated LH deficiency
  - Suprasellar tumors
  - Prader-Willi syndrome
  - Hypopituitarism
  - GH deficiency
  - Pituitary tumors
  - Delayed puberty

Epidemiology and Etiology

The most common cause of primary gonadal failure in boys is Klinefelter syndrome. The prevalence of this disorder as determined by karyotyping of newborn males is about 1/1000. In addition to XXY, the karotype in Klinefelter's syndrome may include up to 4X chromosomes and mosaic patterns (XXXY/XY). An XXY male may result from the fertilization of an XX ovum by a Y sperm or of an X ovum by an XY sperm. The abnormal germ cell results from nondisjunction during meiotic division. Nondisjunction may also occur during mitosis, giving rise in the zygote to an XXY cell line and a nonviable YO line. Studies have shown that both Xs are maternal in 72.5% and one is paternal in 27.5% of cases. The most important etiologic factor is advanced maternal age.

Natural History

Most patients are clinically normal at birth, although a few have been described with abnormalities such as hypospadias and brachyclinodactyly. About 25% of the patients will have delayed speech development and learning disorders.

The classic features of the adolescent boy with Klinefelter syndrome (Table 14.25) include: male phenotype, small, firm testes (usually less than 3 cm and often less than 1.5 cm in length), gynecomastia, azoospermia, and evidence of decreased androgenicity. These patients tend to be taller than average, primarily because of disproportionate growth of the legs. The evidence for increased leg length can be seen at an early age, well before puberty, giving an upper/lower ratio less than normal. Although growth of the legs is increased, that for the arms is not and the arm span of a patient with Klinefelter syndrome is usually less than the height.

Boys with Klinefelter syndrome often have problems in learning and with speech and language development. There may be difficulties in social adjustment, particularly during adolescence.

Diagnosis

The diagnosis of Klinefelter syndrome should be suspected in any male with long legs, small testes,

Table 14.25
Features of Klinefelter Syndrome

Body habitus	Long legs Decreased upper/lower ratio
Genitalia	Testes may be small and firm Penis may be small Hypospadias may be present
Psychosocial	Delay in language development Poorly organized motor function Disturbed body image
Other characteristics	Gynecomastia at puberty

learning disorders, and developmental delay in speech and language.

In addition to the physical features already noted, hormone assays are helpful in diagnosis. Before puberty, these patients have normal plasma concentrations of FSH and LH and the response to GnRH is within the normal range (Ratcliffe, 1982). With the onset of puberty, the concentration of serum testosterone tends to be low and the gonadotropins rise. Response of serum testosterone to administered hCG is subnormal.

The histology of the testis changes with age. There is a progressive reduction in the number of spermatogonia. With the approach of adolescence, pituitary gonadotropins act on the tubules to produce progressive hyalinization. Fibrosis tends to increase with age.

The diagnosis of Klinefelter syndrome is confirmed by the finding of a karyotype of XXY or other variants of multiple X types in cells from blood, skin, or gonads.

Treatment

In patients with androgen deficiency, androgen replacement is indicated. Testosterone enanthate in oil, 200 mg intramuscularly, every 2 or 3 weeks is recommended. Oral androgen preparations are less effective and their use includes the risk of hepatic tumors and abnormalities of liver function.

Gynecomastia may require surgery.

Prognosis

Early diagnosis and treatment with testosterone may be effective in containing ultimate stature and decreasing the degree of gynecomastia. Once hyalinization of the tubules has occurred, sperm disappear and infertility is the rule.

Noonan Syndrome

Definition

This syndrome is characterized by hypogonadism, webbed neck, ptosis, congenital heart disease, and short stature.

Epidemiology

The incidence of this syndrome is about 1/8000, most new cases arising by spontaneous mutation. It is familial and is usually transmitted by the affected female mainly because of reduced fertility in the male. It occurs equally in males and females. The chromosomal constitution is normal and the gonadal differentiation is appropriate for the chromosomal sex.

Natural History

Males with this syndrome are usually cryptorchid with hypoplastic testes. Androgen deficiency is common. These patients have characteristic triangular facies with narrow maxilla, micrognathia, and high-arched palate. The most common cardiac malformations are pulmonic stenosis and atrial septal defect. Other clinical features are similar to those found in patients with Turner syndrome: low-set ears and posterior hairline, cubitus valgus, lymphedema of hands and feet, clinodactyly, shield chest, and widely spaced hypoplastic nipples. Pectus excavatum, renal anomalies, and varying degrees of impaired mental development are frequently seen.

Diagnosis

This syndrome should not be called "male Turner syndrome," although many of the somatic characteristics are similar to those found in Turner syndrome. The two syndromes are quite different. There are no chromosomal abnormalities in Noonan syndrome. Those male patients manifesting the somatic features of Turner syndrome plus chromosomal abnormalities, such as 45,XO/46,XY mosaicism, might more appropriately be labeled as having male Turner syndrome.

Treatment

Those patients showing evidence of androgen deficiency should receive replacement hormone therapy.

Gonadal Dysgenesis

For a complete discussion of this disorder, see page 882.

Enzymatic Defects in Testosterone and/or DHT Biosynthesis

Definition

Disorders of testosterone biosynthesis include any defect in one or more of the enzymes involved in the conversion of cholesterol to testosterone and DHT.

Epidemiology

Defects in enzymes involved in the early steps of testosterone biosynthesis have been discussed in Chapter 6. Those specific for androgen biosynthesis include: (1) 17, 20-desmolase deficiency (conversion of 17-hydroxypregnenolone to dehydroepiandrosterone and 17-hydroxyprogesterone to Δ 4-androstenedione) and (2) 17-hydroxysteroid dehydrogenase deficiency (conversion of Δ 4-androstenedione to testosterone). In addition, a defect in 5 α-reductase severely impairs conversion of testosterone to DHT, which is necessary for masculinization of the external genitalia.

These conditions have an autosomal recessive inheritance and are very rare.

Natural History

Clinically these patients show incomplete masculinization. The defect may be so severe that a female sex assignment is given at birth. Males with 17-β-hydroxysteroid dehydrogenase deficiency or 5-α-reductase deficiency may have a gender change at puberty from female to male. The features of each enzyme defect are shown in Table 14.26.

Table 14.26
Biochemical and Clinical Features of Enzymatic Defects in Androgen Biosynthesis

Defect	17,20-desmolase	17β-hydroxysteroid dehydrogenase[1]	5α-reductase
External genitalia	Female → Ambiguous → Hypoplastic male	Female → Ambiguous	Ambiguous
Müllerian ducts	Absent	Absent	Absent
Wolffian ducts	Development dependent upon degree of enzymatic defect		Normal
Puberty:			
Virilization	Possible	Common	Common
Breasts	Possible	Variable	None
Elevated plasma steroids	17-hydroxy-progesterone	Δ4-androstenedione estrone	↑ testosterone: DHT ratio

[1] Also termed 17-ketosteroid reductase.

Diagnosis

Hormonal analyses will reveal an accumulation of steroids proximal to the enzymatic defect (Table 14.26).

Treatment

Androgen replacement therapy is usually necessary in those patients reared as males. Gonadectomy is recommended with estrogen replacement at puberty in those 46XY patients reared as females.

Hypogonadotropic Hypogonadism

A deficiency of gonadotropins may be due to pituitary failure (hypopituitarism, pituitary tumors) or to hypothalamic dysfunction (Kallmann syndrome, suprasellar tumors, Prader-Willi syndrome).

Hypopituitarism

Deficiencies of LH and FSH can occur as part of idiopathic hypopituitarism (pp. 811) or secondary to pituitary or hypothalamic tumors (pp. 813). In particular, prolactinomas may impair gonadotropin secretion (pp. 890). The latter are rare in males. See page 811 for a complete discussion of hypopituitarism.

Kallmann Syndrome

Definition

Kallman syndrome is a disorder of isolated gonadotropin deficiency characteristically associated with anosmia or hyposmia.

Epidemiology and Etiology

The prevalence of Kallmann syndrome is not known, but it probably ranks second to Klinefelter syndrome as a cause of hypogonadism in man. Although it does occur in women it is far more common in men. The pattern of inheritance in most families is compatible with X-linked or autosomal transmission. In certain kinships, the disorder is associated with midline abnormalities. New mutations occur commonly.

The underlying defect is apparently hypothalamic since repeated GnRH treatments will cause a rise in serum gonadotropins in virtually all patients. The histologic findings at autopsy have been aplasia of the olfactory bulb, normal pituitary glands, and hypoplasia of the hypothalamus.

Natural History

Individuals with Kallmann syndrome may be diagnosed in childhood because of the presence of micropenis and/or cryptorchidism. Midline defects may also be noted early in life. These children grow normally, but fail to undergo puberty.

Less severely affected individuals with partial defects in FSH and/or LH ("fertile eunuch syndrome") are difficult to differentiate from normal boys with delayed development.

Diagnosis

The differential diagnosis between delayed development and Kallmann syndrome may be difficult, particularly if anosmia or other characteristic defects are not present. Observation for a period of time for signs of puberty is indicated. Hormone studies, including 24-hour serum gonadotropin levels and gonadotropin response to GnRH, may be helpful. A nocturnal rise in LH and a significant rise in plasma LH after administration of 100 μg of GnRH intravenously are indicators of impending sexual maturation.

Treatment

Androgen therapy may be used for treatment of micropenis (pp. 876) or to instigate pubertal development in patients with Kallmann syndrome. In adulthood, these patients are usually infertile unless provided with appropriate doses of gonadotropins. With the present availability of GnRH, pulsatile administration of this hormone has been effective in inducing fertility in men with Kallmann syndrome (Crowley et al, 1980).

Prognosis

The present use of GnRH administered in pulses, mimicking the normal biologic rhythm of gonadotropin release, has paved the way for effective treatment of patients with hypogonadotropic hypogonadism. Previously infertile patients have successfully become fathers under this therapy.

Precocious Puberty

Definition

Precocious puberty is a condition of advanced sexual maturation. Boys showing evidence of stage 2 sexual development before 9 years of age are considered precocious. Penile enlargement without evidence of significant increased testicular growth suggests early androgen secretion and does not constitute true central precocity.

Epidemiology and Etiology

Although in some cases early maturation of the hypothalamic-pituitary reproductive axis is the cause, in 64% of sexually precocious boys an organic cause is found. Central precocity may stem from disturbances of hypothalamic function secondary to head trauma, CNS infections or tumors. In the CNS, some tumors act by blocking inhibitory pathways for GnRH regulation (gliomas, astrocytomas) and others act by secreting hCG (germinomas, teratomas) or GnRH (hamartomas).

Virilization in boys, unaccompanied by evidence of hypothalamic-pituitary activation of gonadotropin secretion, may be caused by certain forms of adrenal hyperplasia (pp. 855) or by tumors of the adrenal cortex or the testis. The incidence of testicular neoplasms for the total male population is only 0.002%. Testicular neoplasms tend to occur in the first year of life, although Leydig cell tumors tend to occur after 2 years of age. Precocity is rarely associated with primary hypothyroidism.

Natural History

The first sign of true precocity in boys is the enlargement of the testes followed by penile growth, accelerated linear growth, and development of pubic hair. In patients with virilization alone, the testes will show some enlargement but disproportionately less than expected for the degree of penile growth. Depending upon the amount of androgen exposure the patient will show accelerated linear growth, pubic hair, and muscular development. Deepening of the voice and appearance of facial hair occur late in puberty or with exposure to large amounts of androgen.

If the precocity is secondary to tumor or infection in the CNS, symptoms suggestive of the condition may be evident, although often the first sign of tumor in the hypothalamic region may be the development of precocity.

Diagnosis

Levels of androgens (testosterone, dehydroepiandrosterone, and its sulfate, and Δ 4-androstenedione) and gonadotropins (FSH, LH) should be measured in serum and urine. Radiographs of the hand and wrist for bone age and of the head are indicated. Abdominal ultrasonography and/or CAT scan may be helpful if adrenal tumor is suspected. Patients with central precocity will show hormone values appropriate for the stage of pubertal development. In contrast, patients with androgen-secreting tumors will have low levels of serum gonadotropins, but elevated values for androgens. If the primary androgen secreted is testosterone (some adrenal and testicular tumors), the urinary excretion of 17-KS will not be increased significantly. Adrenal androgens produced by adrenal tumors will be secreted as 17-KS and raise the level of urinary 17-KS.

If the serum concentrations of LH are elevated in a precocious boy, a serum analysis for the β subunit of hCG should be obtained to look for an hCG-producing tumor.

Treatment

Tumors should be treated surgically or with radiation whenever possible. Chemotherapy is sometimes helpful in adrenal carcinoma. In the past, hormone therapy for central precocity utilized medroxyprogesterone acetate with some success; however, the side effects can be a problem. More recently, the use of analogues of GnRH has proved satisfactory for the treatment of sexual precocity (pp. 886). The long-term effects of these analogues, however, are unknown.

FEMALE DEVELOPMENT DISORDERS

Delayed Onset of Puberty

Definition

Delay in the onset of puberty is present if secondary sexual characteristics have not begun to appear by 15 years of age.

Epidemiology and Etiology

It is estimated that delayed puberty occurs in 2–3% of adolescent girls. It is a less common complaint among girls than among boys. Constitutional delay in growth and pubertal development is the result of a physiologic delay in the maturation of the hypothalamic-pituitary-gonadal axis. Frequently, there is a family history of delayed development.

Although most cases of female delayed development are constitutional, other causes of delayed puberty must be considered (Table 14.27). Tumors or inflammatory disorders in the region of the hypothalamus may alter the release of GnRH. Various forms of hypopituitarism, including those secondary to operative or radiation therapy for pituitary tumors may involve the gonadotropes (pp. 812). Kallmann syndrome may occur in females as well as males (pp. 880). Laurence-Moon-Biedl and Prader-Willi syndromes are discussed on page 764. Both anorexia nervosa and bulimia occur primarily in young women and represent syndromes of bizarre eating patterns, which result in severe restriction of caloric intake and functional hypogonadotropic hypogonadism. These conditions are being seen in increasing numbers of girls and, at present, anorexia nervosa is one of the most common causes of hypogonadotropic hypogonadism in pediatric practice.

Natural History

Those patients with constitutional delayed puberty are seen for failure to grow and develop normally. They are otherwise normal and in time they will undergo pubertal development.

Diagnosis

In most cases the diagnosis of constitutional delayed puberty can be made from the family history, the record of the patient's growth, the physical examination, bone age, and serum assays of gonadotropins. The growth pattern as the girl approaches the age of puberty is likely to deviate further from her genetic centile. The bone age is delayed and is usually equal to the height age. The serum levels of gonadotropins are appropriate for the stage of pubertal development and are therefore less than expected for the patient's chronologic age. A radiograph (or CAT scan) of the hypothalamic-pituitary area for evidence of tumor should be included.

A GnRH response test is often helpful in differentiating constitutional delayed puberty (normal response) from pituitary deficiency (poor response) and gonadal failure (enhanced response).

Table 14.27
Causes of Delayed Puberty in Girls

Constitutional Delayed Puberty
Hypogonadotropic Hypogonadism
Hypothalamus and/or pituitary
Trauma
Congenital anomalies
Tumors
Infection or inflammation
Idiopathic hypopituitarism
Kallman syndrome
Laurence-Moon-Biedl syndrome
Prader-Willi syndrome
Functional gonadotropin deficiency
Chronic disease
Anorexia nervosa
Bulimia
Hypergonadotropic Hypogonadism
Gonadal dysgenesis
Other forms of primary ovarian failure
Autoimmune
Postoophorectomy
Resistant ovary syndrome
17-Hydroxylase deficiency

Treatment

Reassurance is the treatment of choice. Hormonal therapy for constitutional delay of puberty should be considered in those girls who have marked psychological disability resulting from the delay in sexual maturation. Premature hormone therapy may compromise adult stature. These patients should be re-evaluated periodically for other causes of delayed puberty.

Gonadal Dysgenesis (Turner Syndrome)

Definition

Various forms of abnormal gonadal development exist and belong under the general category of gonadal dysgenesis. One form is Turner syndrome, characterized by abnormality of X chromosomal karyotype associated with short stature, characteristic phenotypic stigmata, and ovarian failure. The designation of "pure gonadal dysgenesis" has been applied to phenotypic females with 46,XX or 46,XY karyotype who have rudimentary streak gonads and remain sexually infantile, but who are of normal or tall stature and lack the somatic stigmata of Turner syndrome.

Epidemiology and Etiology

Abnormalities of the sex chromosomes resulting in the loss of all or part of an X chromosome occur in 1 of 2000–5000 liveborn phenotypic females. The most common karyotype is 45,X (50–60% of all cases). Considering that most 45,X conceptuses do not survive beyond 28 weeks' gestation, the actual occurrence of this karyotype in the early embryo is higher, probably about 0.8%. Studies of abortuses have shown that the 45,X karyotype occurs in about 10% of spontaneous abortions. This is probably the most common chromosomal anomaly in humans.

The chromosomal anomaly may be a consequence of nondisjunction or chromosome loss during meiosis in either parent or the result of anaphase lag or nondisjunction in the early cleavage divisions after fertilization. Family studies of X-linked traits such as color blindness and the Xg blood group indicate that loss of the paternally derived sex chromosome occurs more commonly: about 75% of 45,X individuals lose the paternal X chromosome and 25% lose the maternal X chromosome.

Patients with Turner syndrome have an increased likelihood of developing autoimmune disorders. The most common is autoimmune (Hashimoto) thyroiditis; rheumatoid arthritis, inflammatory bowel disease, and diabetes mellitus occur also. Parents of patients with Turner syndrome have an increased incidence of thyroid autoimmunity. It is possible that a genetic predisposition to develop autoantibodies increases the prevalence of a 45,X constitution in the offspring.

Other forms of gonadal dysgenesis include both chromatin-positive and chromatin-negative variants. The most common finding in chromatin-positive gonadal dysgenesis is 45,X/46,XX mosaicism. Patients with this form of mosaicism generally have fewer of the somatic anomalies found in classic Turner syndrome. Depending upon the number of gonadal cells with a 46,XX karyotype, functional ovarian tissue may be present. Structural anomalies of the X chromosome include isochromosome for the long arm of the X chromosome, a ring chromosome (loss of both ends of a chromosome with union of the proximal breaks), and deletions of the short or long arm. The presence of a Y chromosome (chromatin-negative gonadal dysgenesis) modifies the female Turner phenotype leading to various degrees of masculine differentiation, from bilateral streaks in the phenotypic female to bilateral dysgenetic testes. In mixed gonadal dysgenesis, development is asymmetrical with a streak gonad on one side and a rudimentary testis on the other side. There is an increased propensity for patients with 45,X/46,XY mosaicism to develop gonadal tumors.

The poor growth in patients with Turner syndrome is not secondary to hormone insufficiency. Generally growth hormone (GH) and T4 are secreted in normal amounts and somatomedin C (SmC) levels are normal during childhood. During pubertal development SmC levels rise in normal girls but remain prepubertal in girls with gonadal failure.

Natural History

The features of the typical patient with Turner syndrome are listed in Table 14.28. The diagnosis may be suspected at birth if puffiness of the dorsum of the hands and/or feet is present. More commonly, unless a karyotype is performed, the first indication of a problem may be poor growth. The growth deficit is more pronounced in the legs than in the upper body, resulting in an abnormal upper to lower segment ratio. Usually by 5 years of age these girls are 2.5 SD below the mean for age. The mean height at 11 years of age is 124 cm and no pubertal growth spurt occurs. A mean adult height of 142.5 cm has been reported in these patients. The poor growth is the result of a combination of events: (1) intrauterine growth retardation (1 SD below the normal mean for length and weight at birth), (2) a gradual decline in velocity of growth in height during childhood, and (3) the absence of a pubertal growth spurt. There is, however, a strong positive correlation between ultimate height attained and midparental height, as is found in normal children.

Table 14.28
Features of Turner Syndrome in Order of Frequency

Short stature
Gonadal failure
Abnormal upper/lower ratio
Otitis media
Characteristic facies
Cardiovascular anomalies
Cubitus valgus
Low posterior hair line
Renal anomalies
Shortened metacarpals
High-arched palate
Autoimmune thyroiditis
Webbed neck
Edema of hands and feet

The disturbance in growth involves other bones also and contributes to many of the somatic features of Turner syndrome. Developmental abnormalities of the trochlear head lead to an increase in the carrying angle, resulting in cubitus valgus. Hypoplasia of one or more cervical vertebrae results in a short neck which contributes to the low hairline. Poor growth of the metacarpals and metatarsals (particularly the fourth metacarpal) may produce shortening of one or more of these bones. Facial characteristics of Turner syndrome probably reflect abnormal development of many bones.

Other developmental abnormalities result in lymphatic malformation and obstruction. Generalized edema may be present in the 45,X abortus. Resolution of the edema in the neck region leaves redundant skin forming a webbed neck, although patients who never had significant distention in the neck region may not show this characteristic and, indeed, only 25% have any webbing at all. Residual edema of hands and feet may persist after birth or occur intermittently during childhood and adolescence.

Patients with Turner syndrome may have an abnormal structural relationship of the middle ear to the eustachian tube. This, coupled with abnormalities in the shape of the palate (high-arched), creates a situation which predisposes to fluid collection and secondary infection. Bilateral otitis media is commonly seen with as many as 68% of patients having significant middle ear infection. Such infections may contribute to the conductive hearing loss reported in patients with Turner syndrome; however, a sensorineural hearing loss also exists and appears to develop with age, representing a degenerative rather than a congenital abnormality.

Additional congenital anomalies of development may include coarctation of the aorta, aortic stenosis, renal abnormalities (horseshoe kidney, duplication of the renal pelvis and ureter, and hydronephrosis), pigmented nevi, and abnormal nail development.

Girls with Turner syndrome show little or no sexual development. The genital ducts and external genitalia are female but immature. The gonads are replaced by fibrous streaks of connective tissue. It is not uncommon for these girls to be brought to the clinic initially with the problems of short stature and delayed development. Those girls who are mosaics may show some gonadal function. Even individuals with only 45,X cell lines in multiple tissues have been fertile (Kohn et al, 1980), but this is unusual and presumably some XX cells were present in the gonads.

Patients with Turner syndrome may have difficulties in school, especially in those subjects dealing with spatial relationships, such as mathematics. Verbal ability is not affected. These girls have a tendency to seek careers in fields involving caretaking, such as nursing and teaching.

Patients with chromatin-negative gonadal dysgenesis may be phenotypic males, females, or ambiguous. The extent of gonadal function will depend upon the number of gonadal cells with XX or XY karyotype.

Diagnosis

Any newborn with lymphedema of the hands and/or feet should have a buccal smear performed on cells from the buccal mucosa and karyotype analysis of white blood cells. Any female who is short and has delayed development also requires chromosomal analysis. Many girls with Turner syndrome will have classic stigmata, but some will not; therefore, these features, although helpful if present, do not rule out the disorder if absent. In particular, those girls who have a mosaic karyotype may not have all (or indeed any) of the classic physical features of Turner syndrome.

Measurement of serum levels of gonadotropins is extremely helpful. Even during childhood (ages 4–10 years), gonadotropin values in girls with ovarian failure will be above the very low-normal levels seen at this age. In the immediate postnatal years and during the adolescent years, gonadotropin secretion is markedly increased over normal values. Response of gonadotropins to administered GnRH is exaggerated in affected compared to normal girls. Estrogen levels in serum are very low in 45,X individuals, but some estrogen secretion and breast development may occur in mosaic individuals.

Thyroid function and antibodies should be checked and an intravenous pyelogram may be indicated because of the increased incidence of renal anomalies in these patients.

In patients with chromatin-negative gonadal dysgenesis complete investigation of the reproductive system is required, especially if there is any ambiguity of the external genitalia.

Treatment

Therapy should be directed toward augmenting stature and inducing adolescent development. Both androgens and estrogens in small doses have been recommended for enhancing growth. Oxandrolone, an anabolic androgen, has been reported to augment height in some patients. Physiologically small doses of estrogen also show promise (Ross et al, 1983), but long-term studies have not been completed. Cuttler et al (1985) have shown that on low-dose estrogen treatment (90–220 ng/kg/day of ethinyl estradiol) for 2–12 months, patients with Turner syndrome (mean age 13 years) have a rise in mean serum SmC concentration from 0.72 ± 0.06 U/ml before treatment to 1.17 ± 0.17 U/ml during estrogen treatment. At high doses (250 μg/day of ethinyl estradiol), estrogen apparently suppresses SmC levels. Presumably, estrogens may increase SmC concentrations in serum by augmenting GH secretion.

GH therapy for Turner syndrome is currently being evaluated. The combination of hGH and low-dose estrogen or androgen therapy may prove to be desirable in achieving better growth in these girls but, as yet, not enough studies have been performed to warrant recommending their use.

Full replacement estrogen treatment should be deferred as long as possible to achieve better linear growth.

CASE ILLUSTRATION

The patient was seen by her physician at 13 years 10 months of age because of short stature and lack of sexual development. Her mother had started menses at age 13 years and two older sisters had achieved menses by ages 13 and 11 years. Their respective adult heights were 157 cm and 160 cm. Another sister, age 9 years, already was showing early breast development. Both parents were tall.

The patient was 2.4 kg in weight at birth and 49.5 cm in length. She was always considered small in comparison to her siblings at the same age. Her growth had always been well below the third centile. She had repeated ear infections in infancy with a tonsillectomy and adenoidectomy being performed at age 4 years.

At the age of 13 years 10 months, she was 130.5 cm tall and weighed 35.2 kg. Her physical examination revealed a very short girl with a wide chest and increased internipple distance. She had no webbing of the neck, but the hair line was low in the back of the neck. Her palate was high-arched and she had an increased carrying angle. There was some shortening of the fourth metacarpals.

A buccal smear revealed absence of Barr bodies. A karyotype was 45,X. Serum values of both FSH and LH were elevated and estrogens were not detectable.

A diagnosis of Turner syndrome was made and the patient was started on estrogen therapy, followed 6 months later by cyclic estrogen-progesterone therapy. On this regimen she showed modest growth and breast development. Her final adult height was 139 cm.

All too often, patients with Turner syndrome are not identified until adolescence when they fail to develop. Despite her extremely short stature, particularly as compared to the family growth pattern, no investigation of this patient's growth occurred during childhood. Any girl growing below the third percentile should have a karyotype performed. The final height in this patient was typical of that achieved by patient's with Turner syndrome. Present attempts to use small doses of estrogens or androgens, starting at a younger age, may permit better growth of these patients.

Low-dose estrogen (Ross et al, 1983) or androgen may be useful in the early years (12–15 years). Later, larger doses of estrogen (0.3 mg conjugated) by mouth can be given daily for the first 21 days of the month. Over the next 2 or 3 years, the estrogen dose can be gradually increased as needed for full physiological effect. The minimal dose of estrogen should be used (usually 0.6–1.25 mg of conjugated estrogen or 10 μg of ethinyl estradiol). Progestins should be given on days 17–21 of the month to induce menstruation.

These girls and their families need much guidance from the physician. Frank discussion of the reproductive facts at the appropriate age as well as organized support groups including other patients with Turner syndrome and their parents are helpful. These girls are very maternal and frequently express the wish for children. With new techniques of in vitro fertilization and embryo transplantation, the possibility of bearing a child exists.

Medical follow-up to monitor evidence of autoimmune disease and cardiac or renal anomalies is important.

Patients with chromatin-negative gonadal dysgenesis may require a sex assignment at birth. In patients assigned a female gender, the gonads should be removed and the external genitalia repaired as needed. In infants receiving a male gender assignment, all gonadal tissue except that which appears histiologically normal and is in the scrotum should be removed and prosthetic testes should be inserted into the scrotal sacs. Removal of müllerian remnants must be performed also. Hypospadias should be repaired.

Acquired Ovarian Failure

Definition

A condition of hypergonadotropic hypogonadism in a normal female with a normal karyotype should suggest an acquired form of ovarian failure.

Epidemiology and Etiology

Any injury to the ovary, whether it be autoimmune, chemical, or secondary to radiation, can result in ovarian failure. The autoimmune disorders may involve failure of one or more endocrine glands including the gonads. In addition to injury to the ovary, hypogonadism can also reflect an end-organ insensitivity to pituitary gonadotropins.

Natural History

The patient with autoimmune oophoritis is likely to have evidence of other autoimmune diseases, such as thyroiditis, Addison disease, and monoliasias; however, in some cases lack of pubertal development may be the only manifestation of autoimmune disease. A history of prior abdominal radiation therapy or chemotherapy for malignancy should alert the physician to the possibility of ovarian failure.

Patients with end-organ insensitivity may show evidence of a more generalized defect such as pseudohypoparathyroidism.

Those patients who develop ovarian failure after pubertal development will have secondary amenorrhea.

Diagnosis

Ovarian antibodies should be measured for evidence of autoimmune disease. Gonadotropin values will be found to be high with low levels of serum estrogens.

Treatment

Replacement estrogen and progestin therapy is indicated.

Precocious Puberty

Definition

Girls whose pubertal development begins before age 8 years are considered to have precocious puberty. True precocious puberty involves development of both pubic hair and breasts and an acceleration of linear growth. Vaginal bleeding may occur cyclically.

Epidemiology and Etiology

In 80% of females with accelerated sexual development the precocity is constitutional. No lesions of the CNS are found, but the frequent finding of abnormal EEGs suggests that undetected abnormalities may be present.

The various causes of precocious puberty in girls are listed in Table 14.29. Gonadotropin-dependent or independent mechanisms may be involved. Intracranial lesions are responsible for precocity in 4% of girls. These lesions characteristically involve the tuber cinereum, the mammillary bodies, or the floor of the third ventricle. Ovarian neoplasms account for 1–2% of cases of female precocity. The other causes are far less commonly observed.

Table 14.29
Causes of Sexual Precocity in Girls

Hypothalamic-pituitary
- Tumor of central nervous system
- Congenital anomalies of central nervous system
- Trauma
- Postinfectious
- McCune-Albright syndrome
- Neurofibromatosis
- Hypothyroidism

Other Causes
- Ovarian tumors
  - Granulosa—theca cell tumor
  - Granulosa—luteal and follicular cysts
- Adrenal feminizing tumors
- Iatrogenic

Natural History

In constitutional precocious puberty, development follows a normal pattern but begins at an earlier age. As a result of this early development, bone maturation is accelerated and the patient's ultimate stature is compromised. If the onset of sexual development occurs before age 6 years, the final height is likely to be under 5 feet.

Intracranial lesions (neoplasms, infections, developmental defects, trauma) may manifest themselves by causing headaches or visual disturbances; however, often the only sign of these lesions is precocity.

Diagnosis

The diagnosis of constitutional precocious puberty is made by the process of exclusion. The differential diagnosis of sexual precocity in girls is summarized in Figure 14.16. There are several conditions to be considered.

NEUROGENIC PRECOCITY

Skull films and/or CAT scan may reveal an intracranial lesion responsible for the precocity. Some tumors actually secrete gonadotropins: hypothalamic hamartomas may be a source of GnRH and some pineal teratomas secrete hCG. Assays for gonadotropins and for the β-subunit of hCG should be performed on blood specimens of patients suspected of an intracranial lesion.

NEUROCUTANEOUS SYNDROMES (pp. 741)

A careful family history may reveal the presence of this condition in relatives. Brownish, irregular cafe au lait spots may be present on the skin, especially on the trunk. Neurofibromas may be visible on any part of the body.

MCCUNE-ALBRIGHT SYNDROME

This form of precocity is associated with cafe au lait pigmentation occurring in nevi that have an irregular (coast of Maine) border, and polyostotic fibrous dysplasia. Occasionally, hyperthyroidism, Cushing syndrome, gigantism-acromegaly, and ovarian cysts are present. Not all patients have all features. Pigmentation may be absent, and not all patients with fibrous dysplasia and pigmentation have sexual precocity.

The cause of this syndrome is unknown. Pituitary adenomas capable of secreting LH and FSH and/or GH have been reported, and in those patients with Cushing's syndrome and hyperthyroidism, nodular hyperplasia that is independent of pituitary control may be observed. Some luteinized follicular cysts in the ovary are believed to function autonomously.

HYPOTHYROIDISM

Thyroid function tests (serum T4, resin T3, and TSH) should be performed in all girls with precocious puberty, retarded growth, and a delayed bone age. Clinical signs of hypothyroidism may or may not be present. Often the patient will have mild galactorrhea and milky fluid can be expressed from the breasts by careful manipulation. Serum prolactin levels are usually elevated as are estrogens. Ultrasonography of the pelvis may show multicystic ovaries.

Gonadotropin levels in serum are elevated based on immunoassays, but biological activity is not usually detectable (Beitins and Bode, 1980). The common α subunit of the gonadotropins and TSH and an overlap in the negative feedback regulation of pituitary hormone secretion may result in overproduction of gonadotropins, as well as TSH and prolactin, in response to the thyroid deficiency. Prolactin may enhance ovarian responsiveness to gonadotropins, resulting in increased estrogen production and breast development.

ADRENAL OR OVARIAN NEOPLASMS

Careful abdominal and pelvic examinations are extremely important to detect feminizing adrenal tumors (extremely rare) or ovarian tumors or cysts. Estrogen levels in girls with granulosa cell tumors of the ovary may be markedly elevated; however, in many of these patients, estrogen levels do not exceed those of the normal adult female. Nevertheless, a very high serum estradiol value should suggest an ovarian neoplasm.

INCOMPLETE SEXUAL PRECOCITY

Both premature thelarche and premature adrenarche are conditions quite separable from true precocious puberty. Premature adrenarche is discussed on pp. 861. Premature thelarche is the appearance of breast development before the age of 8 years, unaccompanied by other signs of pubertal development. This condition is not unusual in infants and very young children. The pathogenesis of the condition is unclear. There may be a slight increase in estrogen production or enhanced sensitivity of breast tissue to the normal low levels of estrogen in childhood. Vaginal smears do show slight estrogenization as compared to smears in normal girls. Normal or slightly increased plasma concentrations of estradiol, LH, and FSH are present. No accelerated linear growth or advancement of bone age is evident in these girls. The breast development usually ceases or tissue regresses over a period of months or years. Normal puberty occurs at an appropriate age.

Treatment

Intracranial lesions must be treated by appropriate measures (surgery, radiation). Tumors of the ovary or adrenal require surgical exploration and removal when possible. Chemotherapy or radiation therapy may be indicated.

Every attempt should be made to control the progress of sexual precocity. At present, long-acting GnRH agonists offer the best mode of therapy (Crowley et al, 1981; Mansfield et al, 1983). Chronic administration of these analogues causes regression in secondary sexual

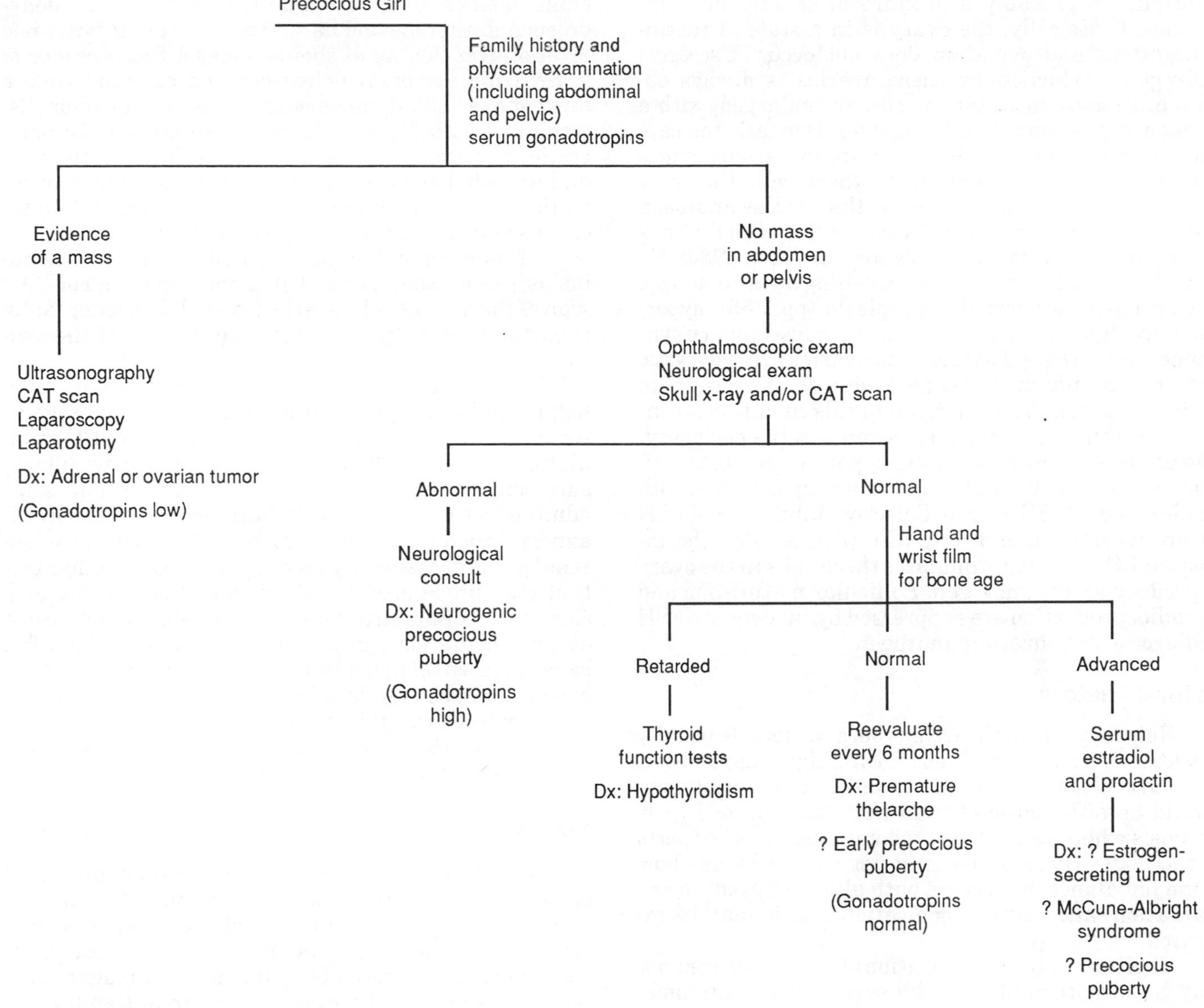

Figure 14.16. Evaluation of girls with evidence of sexual precocity.

changes and stops the rapid progression in bone maturation. Long-range effects of these analogues are still unknown.

Thyroid replacement treatment will cause regression of premature sexual maturation associated with hypothyroidism.

No treatment other than careful follow-up is required for precocious thelarche.

Girls who mature precociously physically are still immature psychologically. Considerable effort should be made to "talk things out" with these girls. It should be made clear to the parents that pregnancy is possible unless treatment is instituted. These children are often considered older than they are because of their development and friends or relatives may treat them accordingly.

Hyperandrogenism

Definition

Any condition resulting in excessive production of androgens may produce clinical signs of masculinization and a hyperandrogen state.

Epidemiology and Etiology

Only two organs produce androgens in the female: the adrenal gland and the ovary. Disorders of the adrenal gland are discussed on page 855. The ovary is the most common source of excess androgens in the peripubertal period. Although tumors of the ovary may cause masculinization, more commonly excess ovarian androgens are due to polycystic ovary syndrome. This syndrome is probably a mixture of several different entities. Classically, the ovary is in a state of continuous estrus and ovulation does not occur. Excessive androgen production by these ovaries is always observed. In most cases the ovaries are enlarged, with a thickened glistening white capsule. Beneath the capsule are many small follicular cysts in various stages of atresia, often with prominent theca cells that may be luteinized. It is now apparent that excess androgen from any source can lead to the constellation of findings observed in polycystic ovary syndrome (Yen, 1980). Included are such disorders as Cushing syndrome (pp. 861), congenital adrenal hyperplasia (pp. 855), hyper- and hypothyroidism, obesity, and polycystic ovary syndrome. In all these disorders the ovaries are polycystic and the chronic anovulation is due to inappropriate feedback signals. The androgen in this condition is converted to estrogen, primarily estrone, in the periphery. The estrogen feeds back on the hypothalamic-pituitary axis to induce inappropriate gonadotropin secretion with an elevated LH/FSH ratio. Selective inhibition of FSH by an ovarian inhibin may also play a role. The increased LH secretion stimulates theca cells in the ovary to produce excess androgen. Follicular maturation and estradiol production are suppressed by inadequate FSH and excess intraovarian androgen.

Natural History

Hair may appear in areas where the female usually has little hair: face, chest, abdomen, thighs, upper arms, and back. This form of excess hair, called hirsutism, should be differentiated from the condition of hypertrichosis where vellus hair predominates on other parts of the body. Hypertrichosis is not caused by sex hormone imbalance, but occurs with glucocorticoid excess, starvation, and certain medications, or it may be inherited.

Virilization (masculinization) is characterized not only by hirsutism but also by severe acne, clitoromegaly, deepening of the voice, and male muscular development. The extent of hirsutism and/or virilization will depend upon the amount and biological activity of circulating androgens.

In polycystic ovarian syndrome, hirsutism is common, but virilization is not often seen. The hirsutism increases with time and becomes less amenable to therapy. The disorder is usually observed in patients in their late teenage years. Most of the patients have a normal menarche and secondary sexual development, but have progressive development of hirsutism and obesity. Occasionally, these patients have dysfunctional uterine bleeding (pp. 666) at menarche. More often, secondary amenorrhea (pp. 890) or oligomenorrhea is seen later.

Diagnosis

Any condition with severe virilization should suggest an adrenal or ovarian tumor and appropriate measures should be used to investigate the possibility. Measurement of serum levels of androgen should include testosterone, Δ 4-androstenedione, and dehydroepiandrosterone and its sulfate. A serum testosterone level of over 200 ng/dl should suggest the presence of a virilizing tumor. A dehydroepiandrosterone sulfate level of over 800 μg/dl suggests an adrenal tumor. Estrone and estradiol should be measured also. In polycystic ovarian syndrome, estrone levels are elevated and estradiol is normal. Serum gonadotropin concentrations may provide evidence of the LH preponderance often seen in polycystic ovarian syndrome.

Often a tumor can be palpated on careful abdominal or pelvic examination. Ultrasonography and/or CAT scan of the area may locate the lesion. Ultrasonography is particularly helpful in assessing the size of the ovaries.

Tests of adrenal and ovarian function are often helpful in locating the source of the excess androgens. An ACTH stimulation test (pp. 858) and an hCG stimulation test (2000–3000 IU daily for 2 days), with measurements of appropriate hormones before and after administration of the tropic hormone, may aid in diagnosis. Such tests are not foolproof, however; the adrenal gland occasionally responds to hCG. Another test that may prove useful is the dexamethasone suppression test. Administration of 0.5 mg of dexamethasone every 6 hours for 4 days is usually followed by a fall in serum cortisol and adrenal androgens. Failure of the plasma androgen levels to fall suggests an ovarian source of the androgens; again, these results can be misleading at times since ovarian sources of excess androgens may be suppressed by dexamethasone.

Treatment

Disorders of adrenal androgen excess are discussed on page 855. Polycystic ovarian syndrome is best treated by establishing normal menstrual cycles and cosmetic attention to the hirsutism. In general, an estrogen-dominant oral contraceptive pill is used. Hirsutism may require electrolysis for control. Certain antiandrogens (spironolactone or cimetidine) may be effective in ameliorating hirsutism.

Patients who are overweight should be placed on a weight reduction program. Weight loss alone occasionally results in a normalization of menstrual cycles.

In those rare patients with a virilizing tumor of the ovary, surgical removal and/or radiation therapy and/or chemotherapy is indicated.

Prognosis

The prognosis of patients with ovarian virilizing tumors depends on the cell type of the tumor and the ease of surgical removal. Patients with polycystic ovarian syndrome can be reassured concerning fertility. Ovulation can be induced with a variety of agents (clomiphene, gonadotropins, GnRH) and wedge resection. For reasons not clearly understood, removal of a wedge of ovarian tissue will often stimulate normal ovulatory cycles. In young adults, however, hormonal treatment is usually successful.

MENSTRUAL DISORDERS

Menstrual problems in the adolescent girl are very common. Abnormal bleeding (dysfunctional) may occur or the menstrual cycles may occur infrequently (oligomenorrhea) or not at all (amenorrhea). In all cases of menstrual irregularities, a careful pelvic and/or rectal examination should precede all other studies. For a discussion of dysfunctional uterine bleeding, see page 666.

Amenorrhea

The failure of menstrual periods to occur may be primary or secondary. In either case it is important to investigate the possibility of pregnancy. Teen pregnancies are being seen in increasing numbers in pediatric practice and with the office urine test for hCG a diagnosis can be made quickly from a random urine sample. Once pregnancy has been eliminated as a possibility, the various causes of amenorrea should be considered (Table 14.30).

Primary Amenorrhea

Definition

Primary amenorrhea is a failure of menarche to occur by 16 years of age.

Epidemiology and Etiology

Primary amenorrhea can be caused by a variety of factors including severe malnutrition, vigorous physical training, or chronic disease. In many cases of primary amenorrhea there has been some error in embryonic sexual differentiation. Of these, about one-half are due to the syndrome of gonadal dysgenesis (pp. 882), one-third to müllerian dysgenesis, and one-sixth to errors in genital development.

Table 14.30
Causes of Amenorrhea

- Physiologic
  - Delayed puberty
  - Pregnancy
- Anatomic
  - Congenital absence of uterus
  - Imperforate hymen
- Hypothalamic-pituitary dysfunction
  - Organic disease in area of hypothalamus/pituitary
  - Psychogenic
  - Nutritional
  - Sustained vigorous exercise
  - Systemic causes
    - Chronic illness
    - Metabolic or endocrine disorders
- Gonadal dysfunction
  - Gonadal dysgenesis
  - Premature ovarian failure
  - Resistant ovary syndrome
  - Testicular feminization syndrome
  - Virilizing tumor of ovary or adrenal
  - Polycystic ovarian disease
  - True hermaphroditism

Most of the factors giving rise to delayed puberty also cause primary amenorrhea. Those patients with no secondary sexual characteristics either have primary ovarian failure or lack gonadotropin stimulation of normal ovaries. These conditions have been discussed previously and will not be reviewed here.

Those patients with normal female secondary sex characteristics but no menses may have an anatomic abnormality (absent uterus) or a chromosomal abnormality (46,XY).

Patients with heterosexual development have excessive androgen production which may be secondary to a virilizing tumor or adrenal hyperplasia.

These disorders are summarized in Table 14.30 and those not previously discussed will be considered individually.

Anatomical Abnormality

Diagnosis and Treatment

Careful examination to determine the presence and patency of the vagina should be undertaken. The hymen may be imperforate and a lower abdominal swelling may be felt. Rectal examination may reveal a distended vagina. The hymen should be perforated to allow menstrual fluid to escape.

If the vagina is patent, a careful examination to search for a uterine cervix should be performed. Absence of a cervix (and, therefore, uterus) suggests the possibility of a chromosomal abnormality. Buccal smear and a karyotype of the patient should identify presence of a Y chromosome. The patient with a Y chromosome and no evidence of masculinization is most likely to have androgen insensitivity or complete testicular feminization syndrome. If a chromatin-positive buccal smear is present, the most likely diagnosis is congenital absence of the uterus.

Ultrasonography is very helpful in locating internal genital structures. Surgical removal of tissue inappropriate to the sex of the individual (for example, testes in testicular feminization syndrome) should be performed.

Testicular Feminization Syndrome

Definition

An X-linked disorder in which affected genotypic males are phenotypic females is designated testicular feminization syndrome.

Epidemiology and Etiology

In the complete form of this syndrome either androgen receptors are absent in target cells or postreceptor activity is defective. Ineffective androgen action during embryogenesis results in lack of male differentiation of the wolffian ducts and the external genitalia. Since testes are present in these patients, mullerian-inhibiting factor is secreted normally and the mullerian ducts regress. Thus, these patients lack fallopian tubes, uterus, and the upper portion of the vagina. The external genitalia and the urogenital sinus are female in development.

Natural History

Since these individuals appear as normal females the diagnosis is not suspected unless another member of the family has already been diagnosed as having testicular feminization syndrome. Occasionally inguinal hernias are present at birth and testicular tissue is found. More often, however, no problem is suspected until pubertal development occurs, but no menses follow.

Diagnosis

On physical examination, the vagina is found to be short and the uterine cervix is absent. These girls have a paucity of sexual hair which may provide a clue to the disorder. A chromosomal analysis will show a 46,XY karyotype. Incomplete forms of androgen insensitivity may result in patients with various degrees of masculinization. Plasma levels of LH are high, but FSH values may be normal or only slightly elevated. Both testosterone and estradiol concentrations in plasma are increased in these patients.

Treatment

Gonadectomy should be performed. Vaginal dilatation by the patient or her sexual partner is usually sufficient so that surgery of the vagina is not necessary. After gonadectomy, estrogen therapy is required.

Secondary Amenorrhea

Definition

Secondary amenorrhea is defined as the absence of menses for at least 6 months after menarche has occurred.

Epidemiology and Etiology

The most common causes of secondary amenorrhea in young girls are those affecting hypothalamic pituitary function. Some patients with secondary amenorrhea have elevated values for plasma prolactin (Pepperell, 1983). Since prolactin secretion is episodic, a single determination may not reveal hyperprolactinemia and measurement should be repeated if the condition is suspected. A significant number of patients with high prolactin values do not have galactorrhea, and vice versa.

Amenorrhea may be the result of nutritional and/or psychogenic factors. Anorexia nervosa may be associated with primary or secondary amenorrhea (pp. 000). Weight reduction associated with loss of 30% of body fat or more will result in amenorrhea (Wentz, 1980). Women who undertake vigorous exercise programs, such as long distance running, have a high incidence of amenorrhea (Dale et al, 1979) as do ballet dancers (Frisch et al, 1980).

In addition to hypothalamic-pituitary dysfunction, ovarian failure may be a cause of either primary or secondary amenorrhea. Destruction of the ovary may be secondary to (1) an autoimmune oophoritis (pp. 885), (2) irradiation or chemotherapy, or (3) systemic disease, such as galactosemia (pp. 915) and cerebellar ataxia. Other causes of amenorrhea are listed in Table 14.30.

Diagnosis and Treatment

Figure 14.17 summarizes the diagnostic procedures recommended for patients with primary or secondary amenorrhea. Treatment is individualized for each disorder.

Galactorrhea-Amenorrhea Syndrome

Definition

Galactorrhea is defined as any persistent discharge of milk or milk-like secretions from the breast in the absence of parturition or beyond 6 months postpartum in a non-nursing mother. When accompanied by amenorrhea and hyperprolactinemia, a condition of chronic anovulation exists.

Epidemiology and Etiology

Galactorrhea occurs in a wide variety of disorders, most commonly in patients with normal menstrual periods and no associated endocrine disease. Often the galactorrhea represents a residuum of postpartum lactation. Prolactin levels in these cases are usually within the normal range. In all probability these women have breast tissue that is extremely sensitive to the normal levels of prolactin.

Galactorrhea is accompanied by amenorrhea in a large percentage of cases. Galactorrhea-amenorrhea is classically associated with elevated levels of plasma prolactin which are often secondary to prolactin-secreting adenomata (prolactinomas) of the pituitary gland. There is much evidence now that the hypersecretion of prolactin in patients with prolactinomas is a result of hypothalamic dysfunction. Such patients have been noted to have loss of the sleep-entrained increase in prolactin, a decrease in pulsatile release of gonadotropin, and diminished responsiveness to chlorpromazine and arginine. When GnRH is administered to women with hyperprolactinemia from prolactinomas, there is a prompt secretion of LH and FSH; therefore, the functional defect lies in the hypothalamus. Dopamine functions as an inhibitor of both LH and prolactin release. It is postulated that a dysfunction of the hypothalamic dopaminergic mechanism might be the pathophysiologic basis for both the development of prolactinomas and the loss of cyclic gonadotropin secretion. It has been observed that LH pulses occurred infrequently in women with hyperprolactinemia and amenorrhea (Moult et al, 1982; Sauder et al, 1984).

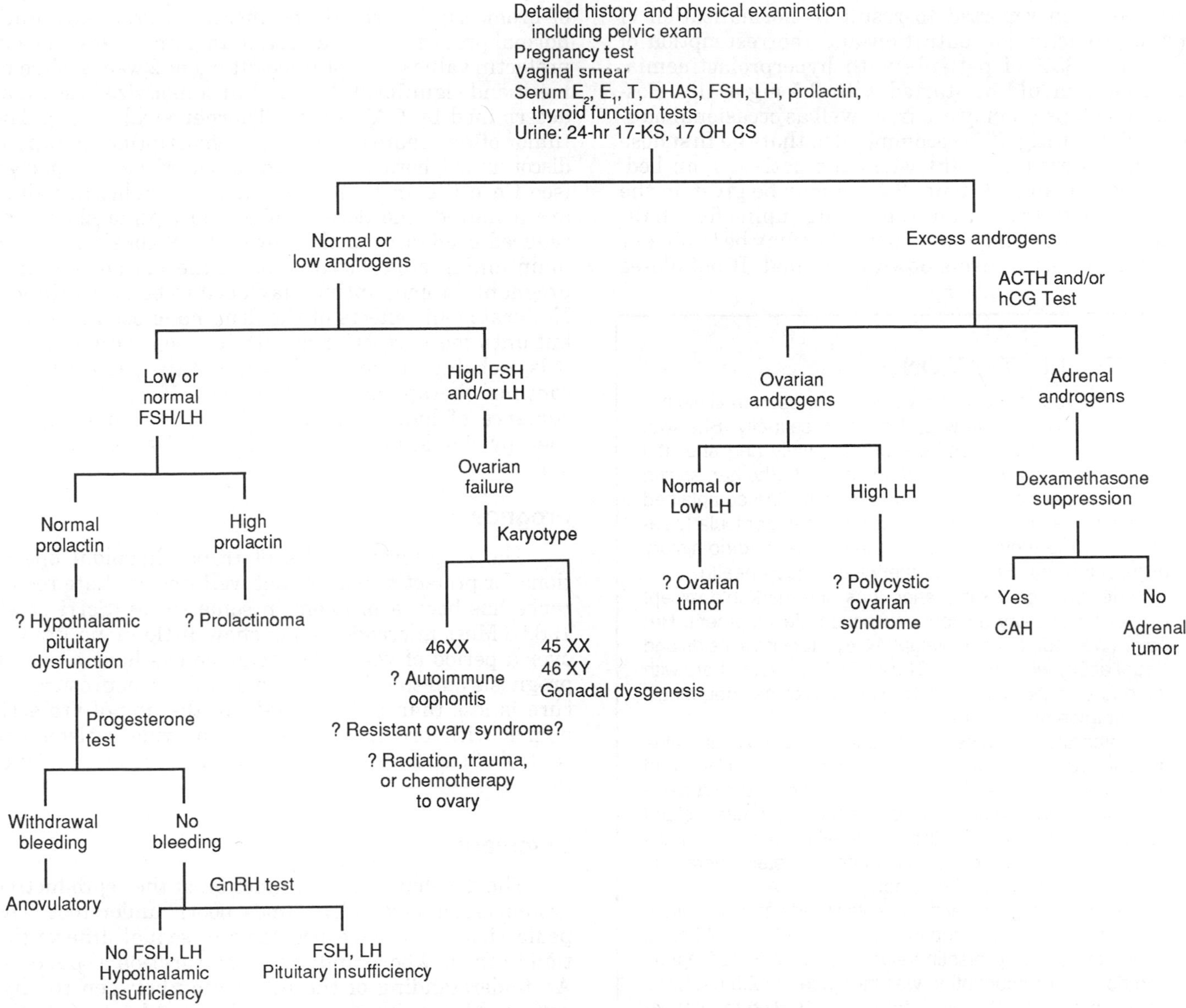

Figure 14.17. Evaluation of the patient with amenorrhea.

Diagnosis

The diagnosis of a prolactin-secreting tumor rests upon the demonstration of persistent hyperprolactinemia and typical radiographic changes in the sella turcica. The serum prolactin values may be moderately or markedly elevated. Normal values for serum prolactin concentration are less than 25 ng/ml. Radiographic changes suggestive of a pituitary tumor include thinning of sella surfaces, bulging of the floor of the sella, enlargement of the sella, or local destruction or erosion of the floor of the sella. These changes are found in only about half the patients with hyperprolactinemia and amenorrhea. High-resolution CAT scans or magnetic resonance imagining of the pituitary area may show evidence of tumor. Visual field abnormalities and/or diminished visual acuity are rare findings.

Basal serum gonadotropin and estrogen concentrations are low or normal in women with prolactinomas. Many of these patients will show impaired GH response to provocative stimuli.

Treatment

Transsphenoidal surgery has been widely used in the United States for the treatment of prolactinomas. It is associated with greater than 80% cures in experienced hands (Randall et al, 1983), although late recurrence of hyperprolactinemia has been reported (Serri et al, 1983).

In general, patients with large tumors (macroadenomas) do less well with surgery and recent use of the dopamine agonist, bromocriptine, suggests this mode of therapy may be better for such patients. Bromocriptine has been reported to result in normalization of serum prolactin concentration and the resumption of menses in 85% of patients with hyperprolactinemia. Treatment should be started with 2.5 mg orally. Postural hypotension may occur, as well as occasional nausea and vomiting. It is recommended that the first dose be administered at night when the patient is in bed. As tolerated, an additional 2.5 mg may be given in the morning, with the patient remaining supine for a half-hour afterward. The total of 5 mg/day may be sufficient to bring prolactin levels down to normal. If not, doses of bromocriptine should be increased gradually until normal prolactins are achieved. In many cases, normal prolactin values are obtained after 1 or 2 weeks of treatment and significant decrease in tumor size is seen, as determined by CAT scans (Thorner et al, 1981). The tumor often regains its size if bromocriptine therapy is discontinued; however, presumed "cures" have been seen (see Case Illustration). Once normal prolactin values are achieved, the dosage of bromocriptine should be reduced gradually to the lowest level consistent with maintaining euprolactinemia. If the patient becomes pregnant, bromocriptine may need to be discontinued. No teratogenic effects of the drug have been reported, but until more experience with its use is accumulated, it is probably in the best interest of the patient to discontinue therapy during pregnancy. If any signs of recurrence of hyperprolactinemia occur, bromocriptine therapy should be reinstituted at the lowest dose possible.

CASE ILLUSTRATION

A 19-year-old college student was seen in clinic because of failure to grow and develop sexually. She was shorter than other members of her family and she had apparently not grown since grade school. She had shown no breast development and no menses. She complained of occasional headaches, which had been particularly severe over the previous 4 or 5 months. She had no history of galactorrhea. She was otherwise in good health.

Her physical examination was unremarkable except for her lack of any evidence of sexual development. Her height was 152 cm and weight 44 kg. Her visual fields and visual acuity were normal. The optic discs were sharp with venous pulsations bilaterally. The rest of her neurologic examination was normal.

Laboratory studies revealed a serum prolactin value of over 900 ng/ml. Lateral radiographs of her skull showed a large sella turcica. CAT scan of the sella turcica demonstrated a symmetrical enlargement of the pituitary gland which protruded toward the suprasellar area. The mass measured about 1.5 cm in maximum diameter. There was no calcification within the tumor.

A diagnosis of prolactinoma was made and the patient was started on bromocriptine, 2.5 mg, at night. Within 2 weeks the serum prolactin value had fallen to 136 ng/ml. The dose of bromocriptine was increased to 2.5 mg twice daily and the prolactin value dropped to 10.2 ng/ml. Repeat CAT scan of the tumor area revealed a decrease in size of the mass so that it was no longer visible. Her headaches had disappeared and serum estrogen values which had been less than 30 pg/ml pretreatment rose to 62 pg/ml. The patient now showed breast development and linear growth.

The bromocriptine dose was gradually tapered over a period of 1 year. During that time the patient had her first menstrual period. Prolactin levels remained in the normal range after discontinuance of bromocriptine.

The patient has continued to do well and after 2½years without bromocriptine she continues to have normal prolactin levels, normal menses, and no radiologic or clinical evidence of tumor.

This case points out several interesting aspects of prolactinomas. Onset of hyperprolactinemia before pubertal development can prevent sexual development and retard growth. Although this patient may represent a medical "cure" of prolactinoma, most patients require continuous treatment with bromocriptine treatment and/or surgery.

Prognosis

The long-term results of transsphenoidal operations for prolactinoma are not well known. Late recurrence has been a problem in some series (Serri et al, 1983). Most microadenomas show little or no growth over a period of years. Macroadenomas have a poorer prognosis and the chance for a definitive neurosurgical cure is less than 50%. Long-term therapy of prolactinomas with bromocriptine may provide satisfactory control of tumor growth and normal reproductive function.

Summary

The development and function of the reproductive system is complex and, at times, poorly understood. The pediatrician may face problems of sexual differentiation in the newborn and sexual maturation at puberty. An understanding of the interaction between the hypothalamic-pituitary axis and the gonads provides the basic knowledge for diagnosing errors in development of reproductive function. The psychologic trauma of inadequate or delayed sexual development can far outweigh that associated with other more life-threatening disorders. The physician must be prepared to reassure the patient and/or parents concerning problems of sexual identity or function.

REFERENCES

Allen TD, Griffin JE: Endocrine studies in patients with advanced hypospadias. *J Urol* 131:310, 1984.

Bartone FF, Huseman CA, Maizels M, et al: Pitfalls in using human chorionic gonadotropin stimulation test to diagnose anorchia. *J Urol* 132:563, 1984.

Beitins IZ, Bode HH: Hypothyroidism with elevated gonadotropin secretion. *Pediatr Res* 14:475, 1980.

Colodny AH: Undescended testes—is surgery necessary? *N Engl J Med* 314:510, 1986.

Crowley WF Jr, Beitins IZ, Vale W, et al: The biologic activity of a potent analogue of gonadotropin-releasing hormone in normal and hypogonadotropic men. *N Engl J Med* 302:1052, 1980.

Crowley WF Jr, Comite F, Vale W, et al: Therapeutic use of pituitary desensitation with a long-acting LHRH agonist: A potential new treatment for idiopathic precocious puberty. *J Clin Endocrinol Metabol* 52:370, 1981.

Cuttler L, Van Vliet G, Conte FA, et al: Somatomedin C levels in children and adolescents with gonadal dysgenesis: Differences from age-matched normal females and effect of chronic estrogen replacement therapy. *J Clin Endocrinol Metabol* 60:1087, 1985.

Dale E, Gerlach DH, Wilhite AL: Menstrual dysfunction in distance runners. *Obstet Gynecol* 54:47, 1979.

DiZerega GS, Hodgen GD: Folliculogenesis in the primate ovarian cycle. *Endocrinol Rev* 2:27, 1981.

Eberle AJ, Sparrow JT, Keenan B: Treatment of persistent pubertal gynecomastia with dihydrotestosterone heptanoate. *J Pediatr* 109:144, 1986.

Frisch RE: Fatness, menarche and female fertility. *Perspect Biol Med* 28:611, 1985.

Frisch RE, Wyshak G, Vincent L: Delayed menarche and amenorrhea of ballet dancers. *N Engl J Med* 303:17, 1980.

Guthrie RD, Smith DW, Graham CB: Testosterone treatment for micropenis during early childhoold. *J Pediatr* 83:247, 1973.

Hadziselimovic F, Herzog B, Seguchi H: Surgical correction of cryptorchidism at two years: Electron microscopic and morphometric investigations. *J Pediatr Surg* 10:19, 1975.

Job JC, Canlorbe P, Garagorri JM, et al: Hormonal therapy of cryptorchidism with human chorionic gonadotropin (hCG). *Urol Clin North Am* 9:405, 1982.

Keenan BS, McNeel RL, Gonzales ET: Abnormality of intracellular 5 α-dihydrotestosterone binding in simple hypospadias: Studies on equillibrium steroid binding in sonicates of genital skin fibroblasts. *Pediatr Res* 18:216, 1984.

Kohn G, Yarkoni S, Cohen MM: Two conceptions in a 45,X woman. *Am J Med Genet* 5:339, 1980.

Krabbe S, Berthelsen JG, Volsted P, et al: High incidence of undetected neoplasia in maldescended testes. *Lancet* 1:999, 1979.

Kuhn JM, Roca R, Laudat MH, et al: Studies in the treatment of idiopathic gynecomastia with percutaneous dihydrotestosterone. *Clin Endocrinol* 19:513, 1983.

Lee PA, Mazur T, Danish R, et al: Micropenis I. Criteria, etiologies, and classification. *Johns Hopkins Med J* 146:156, 1980.

Lipshultz LI, Caminos-Torres R, Greenspan CS, et al: Testicular function after orchiopexy for unilaterally undescended testis. *N Engl J Med* 295:15, 1976.

Mansfield MJ, Beardsworth DE, Loughlin JS, et al: Long-term treatment of central precocious puberty with a long-acting analogue of luteinizing hormone-releasing hormone. *N Engl J Med* 309:1286, 1983.

Moult PJA, Rees LH, Besser GM: Pulsatile gonadotropin secretion in hyperprolactinemic amenorrhea and the response to bromocriptine therapy. *Clin Endocrinol* 16:153, 1982.

Parra A, Cervantes C, Sanchez M, et al: The relationship of plasma gonadotropins and androgen concentrations to body growth in boys. *Acta Endocrinol* 98:137, 1981.

Pepperell RJ: A rational approach to ovulation induction. *Fertil Steril* 40:1, 1983.

Pouplard A, Job JC, Luxembourger I, et al: Antigonadotropic cell antibodies in the serum of cryptorchid children and infants and of their mothers. *J Pediatr* 107:26, 1985.

Rajfer J, Handelsman DJ, Swerdloff RS, et al: Hormonal therapy of cryptorchidism: A randomized double-blind study comparing human chorionic gonadotropin and gonadotropin releasing hormone. *N Engl J Med* 314:466, 1986.

Randall RV, Laws ER Jr, Abboud CF, et al: Transsphenoidal microsurgical treatment of prolactin-producing pituitary adenomas: Results in 100 patients. *Mayo Clin Proc* 58:108, 1983.

Ratcliffe SG: The sexual development of boys with the chromosome constitution 47,XXY (Klinefelter's syndrome). *Clin Endocrinol Metabol* 11:703, 1982.

Ross JL, Cassorla FG, Skerda MC, et al: A preliminary study of the effect of estrogen dose on growth in Turner's syndrome. *N Engl J Med* 309:1104, 1983.

Sauder SE, Frager M, Case GD, et al: Abnormal patterns of pulsatile lutenizing hormone secretion in women with hyperprolactinemia and amenorrhea: Responses to bromocriptine. *J Clin Endocrinol Metabol* 59:941, 1984.

Schulze KA, Pfister RR: Evaluating the undescended testis. *Am Family Phys* 31:133, 1985.

Serri O, Rasio E, Beauregard H, et al: Recurrence of hyperprolactinemia after selective transphenoidal adenomectomy in women with prolactinoma. *N Engl J Med* 309:280, 1983.

Simpson E, Chandler P, Goulmy E, et al: Separation of the genetic loci for the H-Y antigen and for testis determination on human Y chromosome. *Nature* 326:876, 1987.

Thorner MO, Perryman RL, Rogol AD, et al: Rapid changes of prolactinoma volume after withdrawal and reinstitution of bromocriptine. *J Clin Endocrinol Metabol* 53:480, 1981.

Walsh PC, Curry N, Mills RC, et al: Plasma androgen response to hCG stimulation in prepubertal boys with hypospadias and crytorchidism. *J Clin Endocrinol Metabol* 42:52, 1976.

Wentz AC: Body weight and amenorrhea. *Obstet Gynecol* 56:482, 1980.

Yen SSC: The polycystic ovary. *Clin Endocrinol* 12:177, 1980.

Zacharias L, Wurtman RJ, Schatzoff M: Sexual maturation in contemporary American girls. *Am J Obstet Gynecol* 108:833, 1970.

Zachmann M, Eiholzer U, Muritano M, et al: Treatment of pubertal gynaecomastia with testolactone. *Acta Endocrinol* 113(Suppl 279):218, 1986.

Pancreas

8

The pancreas consists of an exocrine portion and an endocrine portion. The latter, the islets of Langerhans, contains at least four endocrine cell types: the α, β, Δ, and PP cells, which produce, respectively, the peptides glucagon, insulin, somatostatin, and pancreatic polypeptide. β Cells form a central core of the islet which is surrounded by either Δ and α cells (tail and body of the pancreas) or Δ and PP cells (head of the pancreas). Normally glucagon secretion is suppressed by insulin. Conversely, insulin secretion is directly stimulated by glucagon. Minute amounts of somatostatin suppress both insulin and glucagon secretion. The relation of the islet cells to the blood vascular system exposes α cells to the highest circulating concentrations of insulin in the body and, thus, facilitates the role of insulin as an inhibitor of glucagon release. It has been suggested that the three hormones insulin, glucagon, and somatostatin influence neighboring islet cells in a paracrine fashion. Thus, the cells of the islets undoubtedly form a complex micro-organ in which both systemic and paracrine influences coordinate and integrate function for the overall regulation of the metabolism of glucose and other fuel molecules.

HORMONES OF THE PANCREATIC ISLETS

Insulin

The human insulin gene, which is located in band p15 of the short arm of chromosome 11, consists of a coding sequence for a 1430-nucleotide mRNA precursor which is interrupted by two intervening sequences (introns) of 179 and 786 nucleotides. After excision of the two introns, the mRNA molecule for preproinsulin is formed. The latter is synthesized on the rough endoplasmic reticulum of the β cell. The signal sequence is then removed to form proinsulin, which is transferred to the Golgi apparatus. Proinsulin is converted to insulin by cleavage of a 33-amino acid connecting C-peptide. The released insulin is stored in cytoplasmic granules available for secretion by exocytosis. As the contents of the granules are discharged into the circulation, both insulin and C-peptide are released. The measurement of C-peptide levels in blood can serve as a sensitive index of endogenous insulin secretion, for unlike insulin, C-peptide is metabolized very little by the liver.

The concentration of glucose in serum is the principal regulator of insulin secretion in the human; however, other factors, such as amino acids, fatty acids, ketones and hormones, as well as the autonomic nervous system may also modulate insulin secretion. The gastrointestinal hormones (secretin, gastrointestinal polypeptide [GIP], pancreozymin, gastrin, and gut glucagon) increase insulin secretion and may account for the greater rise in serum insulin after oral as compared to intravenous glucose. Other hormones such as pancreatic glucagon, growth hormone (GH), and cortisol stimulate insulin secretion under certain conditions, whereas catecholamines and somatostatin inhibit insulin release.

The mechanism of insulin release involves a flux of Ca^{++} into the β cell. Thus, Ca^{++} is the primary trigger of insulin release, whereas cyclic adenosine monophosphate (AMP) acts as an amplifier of the secretory signal. During a constant stimulation, the rate of insulin release is biphasic. For example, glucose initiates acute secretion of insulin, which is followed shortly thereafter by a state of refractoriness to glucose in the β cell, so that the rate of insulin secretion is decreased, despite ongoing stimulation. This inhibitory action persists for several minutes, even after glucose withdrawal. The third phase involves an amplification of the insulin response with time so that a late increase in secretion rate is seen.

The overall effects of insulin are both metabolic and growth-promoting. In general, the metabolic effects are observed at low concentrations of hormone and occur rapidly after exposure of cells to insulin. Growth-promoting effects are seen usually with high concentrations of insulin and require hours or days to be manifested. The latter effects are important in fetal growth and organogenesis and in tissue repair and regeneration. Insulin promotes glucose storage (as glycogen and fat) and protein synthesis and decreases the utilization of fat for energy. The principal target tissues for insulin action are muscle, liver, and adipose tissue. In muscle, insulin stimulates the uptake of glucose and its oxidation and storage as glycogen, and increases the uptake of amino acids and protein synthesis. Insulin does not have a direct effect on glucose transport in liver; however, it does increase both glucose oxidation and glycogen synthesis and inhibits glycogen breakdown and gluconeogenesis. In adipose tissue, insulin increases the transport of glucose across the cell membrane and increases both glucose oxidation and conversion into triglycerides.

The exact mechanism of insulin action is uncertain (Kahn, 1985). The insulin receptor is a symmetrical peptide consisting of two α and two β subunits. It is known that insulin binds to the 135,000 dalton α subunit of the insulin receptor, resulting in activation of the tyrosine-specific protein kinase that is intrinsic to the 95,000 dalton β subunit. Both subunits of the insulin receptor are glycoproteins with complex carbohydrate side chains. The insulin receptor is synthesized from a single chain proreceptor of molecular weight 190,000, containing both subunits. The synthesis occurs in the rough endoplasmic reticulum, followed by glycosylation of the receptor in the Golgi apparatus, and final cleavage to yield α and β subunits inserted into the plasma membranes. The insulin-receptor complex is internalized. Some of the receptor is degraded but most of the molecules are recycled back to the membrane.

The insulin-mediated activation of the tyrosine-specific protein kinase of the receptor initiates a phosphorylation cascade that regulates metabolic pathways. Insulin not only activates the receptor kinase but it also causes: (1) conformational change in the receptor, (2) aggregation of receptors, (3) rapid changes in Na^+ and K^+ flux, (4) internalization of the hormone-receptor complex, and (5) generation of possible soluble intracellular second messengers. These events occur within seconds or minutes (Fig. 14.18). Later actions of insulin involve stimulation of synthesis of protein, lipid, RNA, and DNA.

Many of the insulin effects involve anticyclic AMP actions mediated by insulin-stimulated phosphoprotein phosphatases. Other effects of insulin are similar to those generated by cyclic AMP. For example, glucagon and insulin act on hepatocytes to stimulate the same amino acid transport system. Insulin also activates serine-specific protein kinases that phosphorylate enzymes and other cellular components. Finally, insulin stimulates the translocation of membrane-bound proteins from intracellular sites to the plasma membrane, a process occurring in glucose transport. Like the insulin receptor, glucose transporters are present in many cell types. In cells in which insulin has little or no effect on glucose transport, there appears to be a smaller intracellular pool of transporters.

Glucagon

Like the preproinsulin gene, the preproglucagon gene consists of both coding sequences or exons (six) and introns (five). The five introns are removed to form preproglucagon mRNA. As with insulin, the signal sequence of preproglucagon is removed to form proglucagon which is subsequently processed to glucagon.

The mechanism whereby glucagon works at the molecular level is better understood than is the case with insulin. Glucagon binds to the regulatory unit of the glucagon receptor, which is somehow coupled to the catalytic subunit of adenylate cyclase by an inhibitory guanine nucleotide-binding regulatory protein (pp. 796). The latter activates adenylate cyclase. Cyclic AMP concentrations in liver rise within seconds after the administration of glucagon. Cytosolic cyclic AMP binds to the inactive dimeric form of the cyclic AMP-dependent protein kinase; activation of this kinase initiates all the known actions of glucagon.

In the liver, glucagon causes increased glycogenolysis, gluconeogenesis, and ketogenesis and decreased glycogen synthesis, glycolysis, and lipogenesis (Fig. 14.18). Insulin opposes these actions of glucagon largely by decreasing intracellular levels of cyclic AMP and the activity of the cyclic AMP-dependent protein kinase. When insulin is not present the unopposed action of glucagon greatly increases hepatic cyclic AMP and protein kinase activity, initiating the catabolic cascade.

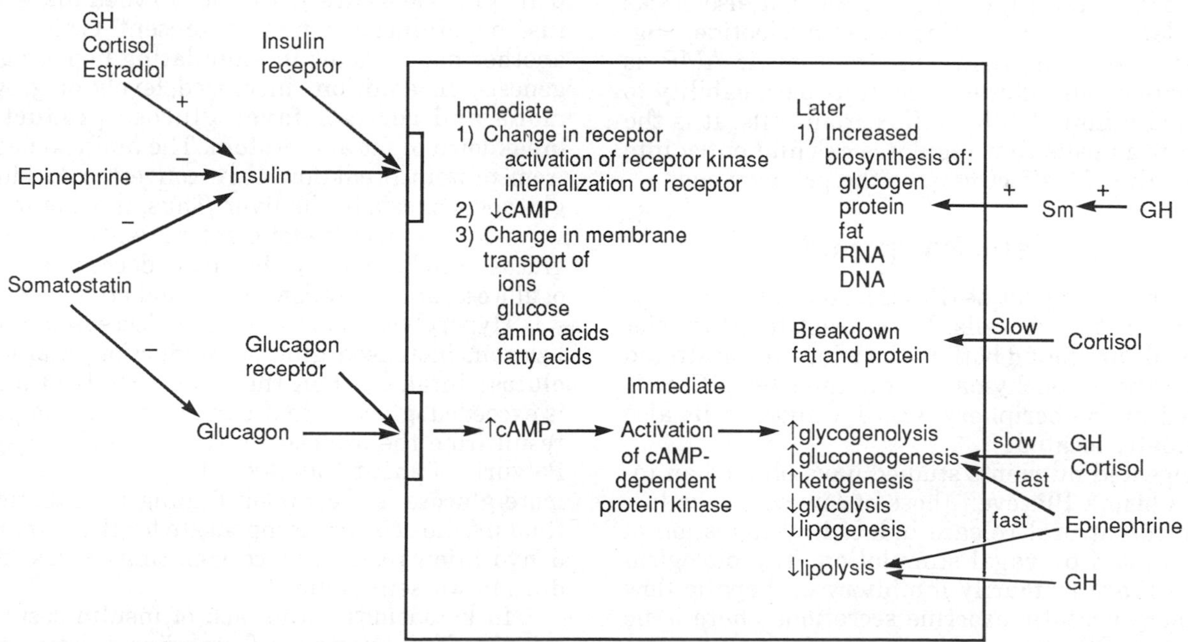

Figure 14.18. Hormonal control of metabolism within the cell. + = stimulation of production; − = suppression of production. Both cortisol and GH produce an insulin-resistant state.

The overriding signal to both α and β cells is the ambient glucose concentration. The α cells that synthesize glucagon are probably under the constant restraining influence of insulin within the islet microcirculation. Apparently glucagon release by α cells can be suppressed by a rise in blood glucose, however, independently of the β cells and insulin. Glucopenia stimulates glucagon secretion largely via an intrapancreatic α-adrenergic mechanism.

A molecule similar to glucagon is also synthesized in the gastrointestinal tract.

Somatostatin

This hormone is distributed widely in cells throughout the nervous system and is present in many extraneural tissues, including the gut and the pancreas. As a pituitary regulator (inhibits secretion of GH and thyroid-stimulating hormone [TSH] and, under certain conditions, of prolactin and corticotropin [ACTH] also) it is a true neurohormone. Somatostatin also acts as a neurotransmitter in other areas of the CNS. In the gut and pancreas somatostatin influences the function of adjacent cells and, thus, has paracrine characteristics. It also can influence its own secretion (an autocrine role).

Somatostatin is a cyclic peptide containing 14 amino acids. It is synthesized as a preprohormone and processed in a manner similar to that of insulin and glucagon. The action of somatostatin in gut and pancreas is inhibitory, decreasing secretions of many tissues, including salivary glands, pancreas, and gut mucosa. In the pancreatic islets, somatostatin inhibits the secretion of both insulin and glucagon.

Somatostatin acts by first binding to specific receptors on plasma membranes of target cells. Although it reduces the concentration of cyclic AMP, it also blocks the stimulatory effects of this cyclic nucleotide, suggesting an action "downstream" from cyclic AMP as well. Somatostatin reduces membrane permeability to calcium and stimulates K^+ efflux from cells. It is the K^+ efflux from cells that regulates calcium entry into cells; thus, the K^+ effect may be the primary one.

Pancreatic Polypeptide

Pancreatic polypeptide (PP) is a 36-amino acid peptide formed in the PP cells. In contrast to other islet cells, PP cells are found both in the islets and scattered in the exocrine parenchyma. Within the islets, PP cells are located in the periphery where α and Δ cells also are principally located.

All ingested nutrients studied have elicited an increase in plasma PP, even those of low caloric value. The most potent oral release induced by ingestion of food is mediated by vagal stimulation. The biological effects of PP are primarily inhibitory on hepatic flow of bile and pancreatic exocrine secretion. There is no evidence that PP affects secretion by islet α, β, or Δ cells.

HYPERGLYCEMIA

Insulin-Dependent Diabetes Mellitus (Type I, Juvenile Onset)

Definition

This form of diabetes mellitus has its onset most commonly in childhood and adolescence. The disorder is caused by a deficiency of insulin, resulting in alterations in carbohydrate, lipid, and protein metabolism.

Basic Science

The symptoms and signs of diabetes result from hyperglycemia and glucosuria due to a lack of insulin. In addition to deficient insulin secretion, it is now clear that acquired deficiencies of the secretion of some counterregulatory hormones occur commonly in patients with IDDM (Cryer et al, 1986). For example, secretion of glucagon in response to decreased levels of plasma glucose become deficient early in the course of IDDM in the vast majority of patients. This is a selective defect; glucagon responses to other stimuli are intact. Secretion of epinephrine in response to plasma glucose decrements may also be deficient in some patients with IDDM, particularly later in the course of the disease (Bolli et al, 1983). Defects in the responses of glucagon and epinephrine to lower plasma glucose levels increase the risk of severe hypoglycemia in diabetic patients.

The failure of the diabetic patient to secrete insulin results in an inability to transport glucose and amino acids into muscle and adipose tissue. As a result these tissues are unable to utilize normal amounts of these substances for energy production and protein synthesis. Insulin deficiency is a major cause of unrestrained hepatic gluconeogenesis. In uncontrolled diabetes mellitus, hyperglucagonemia is present typically and is another major factor in stimulating hepatic gluconeogenesis. In addition, increased levels of growth hormone and cortisol favor glucose production and breakdown of fat and protein. The amino acids derived from protein breakdown are converted to glucose via gluconeogenesis in the liver. Thus, the metabolic pathways in the insulin-deficient patient favor increased glucose production by the liver, decreased utilization of glucose, and breakdown of fat and protein (Fig. 14.18).

Hyperglycemia results from decreased glucose utilization, increased glucose production, and continued glucose intake. When the renal threshold for glucose is exceeded, glycosuria occurs. Polyuria and polydipsia result from the osmotic diuresis caused by glycosuria. Polyuria of about 100–300 ml/kg/day containing 5% or more glucose is a common finding in diabetics. When fluid intake does not compensate for the urinary losses, dehydration results. Once vomiting occurs, the dehydration worsens rapidly.

In ketoacidosis, the lack of insulin results in the release of free fatty acids from adipose tissue. Normally fatty acids are oxidized in the liver to provide energy for gluconeogenesis; however, in diabetes mellitus this oxidation is incomplete, resulting in the accumulation of ketone bodies (acetoacetate, β-hydroxybutyrate, acetone). At physiologic pH, the ketoacids dissociate, releasing hydrogen ions and ketone anions. The latter are excreted as sodium or potassium salts. The hydrogen ion remaining plus the loss of basic ions required for anion excretion results in acidosis. Total body depletion of both sodium and potassium occurs in ketoacidosis, although serum levels of both cations may be normal.

Epidemiology

Diabetes mellitus (both insulin-dependent and insulin-independent types) occurs in about 2–10% of the entire population. About 5% of diabetics are diagnosed in childhood. A Michigan study gives a prevalence of 1.6 diabetics per 1000 school-age children (Gorwitz et al, 1976).

Insulin-dependent diabetes mellitus (IDDM) is caused by a lack of insulin secondary to destruction of pancreatic cells. The latter may be secondary to a disease process (for example, see Cystic Fibrosis; however, extensive evidence now suggests that cell destruction in most cases of IDDM is the result of a chronic progressive autoimmune process (Eisenbarth, 1986). There are reasons to believe that T-lymphocytes and not islet cell antibodies are the major determinants of β cell destruction. In pancreatic transplants between identical twins, in which the pancreas from one twin without diabetes is transplanted to the other identical twin with diabetes, islet cell destruction in association with massive T-cell infiltration occurred within weeks (Sutherland et al, 1984). The actual destruction of the β cells may be mediated by lymphokines (Mandrup-Poulsen et al, 1985). The process is slow except in transplanted pancreases and total destruction of the β cells may take up to 9 years in some adults. Although basal insulin levels may be normal in newly diagnosed cases, insulin production in response to a variety of secretagogues is blunted and usually disappears completely over a period of months to years. A limited capacity for insulin secretion may remain for a period of time, usually not exceeding 5 years in children.

Other autoimmune diseases such as Addison disease, Hashimoto thyroiditis, and pernicious anemia occur with increased frequency in diabetics with type I disease. All of these autoimmune diseases including type I diabetes mellitus are associated with an increased frequency of finding certain histocompatibility antigens, in particular, HLA-B8, HLA-BW15, DW3, and DW4 (Deschamps et al, 1980). In type I diabetes the inheritance of HLA-B8 or BW15 appears to confer a 2- to 3-fold relative risk for development of the disease. When both B8 and BW15 are inherited together the relative risk increases to 7- to 10-fold.

The mechanism of inheritance of predisposition for type I diabetes mellitus is unknown. The observed risk to individuals with one sibling with diabetes is about 5–10%. The risk to offspring of one juvenile diabetic is about 2%. The results are not compatible with either a simple recessive or dominant inheritance. Offspring of diabetic fathers are at greater risk than those of mothers (Warram et al, 1984). The concordance rate among identical twins in whom one has insulin-dependent diabetes is only 50%, suggesting environmental triggering factors. In animals, a number of viruses can cause a diabetes-like syndrome. In man, epidemics of mumps, rubella, and coxsackievirus have been associated with subsequent increases in frequency of type I diabetes, and the occurrence of acute diabetes mellitus induced by a coxsackie B4 virus has been documented (Yoon et al, 1979).

In summary, present evidence suggests that a virus (or other environmental factors) may trigger an autoimmune reaction to β cells in patients who have inherited a diabetogenic gene(s) linked to the HLA locus.

Natural History

Most children with diabetes mellitus have a history of polyuria, polydipsia, polyphagia, and weight loss. Generally, the symptoms have been present for days or weeks, but usually less than a month. The onset of enuresis in a previously toilet-trained child may be an early sign.

It is less common (30% or less) for a child to present with frank diabetic ketoacidosis, air hunger, Kussmaul breathing, acetone on the breath, obtundation of consciousness or coma, vomiting, dehydration, ketonemia, hyperglycemia, glucosuria, and ketonuria. Leukocytosis and abdominal pain that mimic appendicitis are common in children and may be associated with elevated serum amylase that does not necessarily indicate the existence of pancreatitis. Abdominal pain is most commonly seen with ketoacidosis.

Although symptoms of diabetes usually begin abruptly, not uncommonly the child may experience a more insidious onset with lethargy, weakness, and weight loss developing over days or weeks.

After the initial control of hyperglycemia with insulin therapy almost all patients show a decline in insulin requirement. Of these patients, 65% achieve a "partial remission" characterized by remarkably good metabolic control and an insulin requirement of less than 0.5 U/kg/day. A small group (3%) will have a "total remission" characterized by normal metabolism for a minimum of 3 months without the need for insulin therapy (Drash et al, 1980). This period of partial or complete remission (often referred to as the "honeymoon period") may last for several months and, in some cases, as long as 1–2 years. Inevitably, however, insulin requirements increase slowly, leading to complete absence of β-cell function in most patients by 1–2 years after diagnosis. Occasionally, there may be an abrupt loss of remission, usually associated with intercurrent infection, emotional stress, or physical or emotional trauma.

Complete remission is very uncommon in children diagnosed under 5 years of age, but the chance of remission increases commonly in older children and adolescents. Partial remission, however, can occasionally occur in young children.

Diagnosis

With the classical symptoms and signs of glycosuria, ketonuria, and hyperglycemia, a random blood glucose level over 200 mg/dl establishes the diagnosis of diabetes mellitus. Glycosuria without hyperglycemia may reflect impaired glucose reabsorption in the kidney tubules. Hyperglycemia from other causes generally is accompanied by specific signs and symptoms unlikely to be confused with those of diabetes mellitus.

A glucose tolerance test is not necessary to make the diagnosis if glycosuria, ketonuria, and hyperglycemia are present. In patients with asymptomatic glycosuria, a fasting and 2-hour postprandial blood glucose value should be obtained. If the results are equivocal a glucose tolerance test is recommended. The amount of glycosylated hemoglobin also should be measured.

Oral Glucose Tolerance Test

Preparation

The patient should be on a high carbohydrate diet for 3 days before the test; with a minimum of 50–60% of calories as carbohydrate. No food should be taken after midnight before the day of the test.

Medication

Glucose is given orally (1.75 g/kg body weight, with a maximum dose of 75 g) after a baseline sample of blood is drawn.

Sampling

Sample times are 0, 60, 120, and 180 minutes. Each blood sample should be analyzed for levels of glucose and insulin.

Interpretation

In the normal fasting individual, the concentration of glucose in plasma should be less than 110 mg/dl; values before 2 hours should not exceed 180 mg/dl, and the glucose concentration at 2 hours after an oral glucose challenge should be 140 mg/dl or less (Table 14.31). In diabetics, the 2-hour value is usually over 200 mg/dl. Insulin response to a glucose challenge in diabetics is usually subnormal.

Glycosylated Hemoglobin or Hemoglobin A1c (HbA1c)

Total glycosylated hemoglobin represents a combination of HbA1a, HbA1b, and HbA1c. The last-mentioned is a minor fraction of adult hemoglobin, which is formed by the postsynthetic linkage of glucose to the N-terminal of the β chain of the globin molecule (Bunn, 1981). Since HbA1c is formed throughout the lifespan of the red cell, the quantity of HbA1c in the blood reflects the average level of blood glucose throughout the lifespan of the red cell. Thus, in diabetics HbA1c is usually elevated, reflecting the integrated "time-averaged" blood glucose concentration over the preceding 2–3 months. In some laboratories total glycosylated hemoglobin is measured rather than HbA1c. There are two portions of HbA1c, a labile and a stable portion. The labile portion, which is affected by acute changes in blood glucose, accounts for up to 10–25% of HbA1c and can spuriously elevate HbA1c levels. Only changes of 20–25% or more are significant. The upper limit of normal for HbA1c in most laboratories is about 4–6% and that for total glycosylated hemoglobin is about 5.6–7.6%.

Table 14.31
Normal Glucose and Insulin Values for Glucose Tolerance Test

Time	Glucose (plasma mg/dl)	Mean Insulin 1.5–6 years	(μU/m) 6–11 years
0	≤110	8	15
1 hour	≤160	40	60
2 hour	≤140	35	55
3 hour	≤130	18	20

Either of the following are considered diagnostic of diabetes mellitus:

1. Presence of classical symptoms plus random plasma glucose over 200 mg/dl.
2. In asymptomatic individuals, both fasting venous plasma glucose > 140 mg/dl on at least two occasions and a 2-hour postprandial and one other value (between meal or glucose dose and 2-hour value) > 200 mg/dl.

A patient is considered to have impaired glucose tolerance if the glucose concentration 2 hours after oral glucose is over 140 mg/dl and > 200 mg/dl between 0 and 2 hours of the oral glucose test. The fasting glucose concentration must be below the value that is diagnostic of diabetes.

Diabetic Ketoacidosis

Diagnosis

Diabetic ketoacidosis (DKA) should be suspected in an acutely ill, dehydrated child who is breathing rapidly. The plasma pH is less than 7.3 and the plasma bicarbonate level is less than 20 mEq/L in DKA. Ketoacidosis is the leading cause of death in young patients with IDDM (Krane et al, 1985).

Serum Na^+ levels are often normal; however, hypo- or hypernatremia may be present, depending upon the balance between water and sodium loss. Hyperglycemia will reduce the "normal" serum sodium. For each 100 mg/dl increase in blood glucose, serum sodium is decreased 1.6 mEq/L. Thus, a "normal" serum sodium in a patient with a blood glucose of 1100 mg/dl would be 140 mEq/L minus 1.6 times 10 or 124 mEq/L. Hyperlipidemia, which is seen in some patients in ketoacidosis, spuriously decreases serum sodium because the volume of the serum occupied by lipid does not contain electrolytes.

The serum K^+ level should be monitored since it may fall precipitously with treatment.

Laboratory studies should include serum glucose, ketones, electrolytes, bicarbonate, and osmolarity. In severe DKA, the ketone bodies may be mainly in the form of β-hydroxybutyrate, which is not detected by the nitroprusside reaction (Acetest tablets) that routinely measures "ketones." During the recovery process, β-hydroxybutyrate is converted to acetoacetate which is detectable with Acetest tablets and may cause a rise in the ketone titer early in recovery before a fall is demonstrated. Both glucose and osmolarity will be elevated, the extent depending upon the degree of hyperglycemia.

Treatment

The first objective in therapy is the elimination of overt clinical symptoms.

Patients with severe ketoacidosis require rehydration and correction of the acidosis. Intravenous fluid therapy should be started immediately after the initial assessment and blood samples are obtained. Over the first 60 minutes of normal saline infusion, 10–20 ml/kg should be given. This can be repeated if necessary to expand the blood volume and raise the blood pressure. Once the circulation is stabilized, a switch to half-normal saline should be made to replace fluid deficits and to provide maintenance fluids.

Dehydration can be assumed to be about 10%. The rate of fluid replacement is adjusted so that only one-half of the calculated deficit is replaced over the first 8 hours, with the remainder of the deficit being replaced over the next 16–20 hours.

Glucose replacement is begun with a 5% solution when the glucose level approaches 300 mg/dl. Potassium is considerably depleted in ketoacidosis; therefore, K^+ should be started early even if the serum K^+ is normal or elevated. In practical terms, the first hour or so of fluid should be K^+-free; thereafter replacement potassium should be added to subsequent infusates. Phosphate is also significantly depleted in DKA, so that phosphate should be included in the intravenous fluid. Serum Ca^{++} should be monitored to avoid hypocalcemia secondary to the phosphate therapy and correction of the acidosis.

There is considerable disagreement about the use of bicarbonate in treating DKA. In general, bicarbonate is used only in patients with severe metabolic acidosis as indicated by an arterial pH of 7.0–7.1 or a bicarbonate value of less than 5 mEq/L. When used, sodium bicarbonate should be given by slow intravenous infusion over several hours and should be discontinued when the pH reaches 7.2.

Traditionally, DKA is treated with intravenous and subcutaneous insulin injections, the dose depending upon the extent of hyperglycemia and ketonemia (Table 14.32). Injections are repeated every 2–4 hours while blood glucose levels and acid-base status continue to be monitored. When blood glucose has fallen to about 300 mg/dl, subsequent insulin injections (0.25–0.5 u/kg body weight) may be given subcutaneously every 6–8 hours while infusion of 5% glucose is maintained until the child can tolerate solid food. Once food intake is established, half the previous day's total insulin dose is given in an intermediate-acting form (NPH or Lente). Adjustment in insulin dose by using a combination of intermediate- and short-acting forms twice daily is made on a daily basis.

An alternative means of regular insulin therapy, routinely used in major centers, utilizes a continuous low-dose infusion with a priming dose of 0.1 u/kg followed by 0.1 u/kg/hr until blood glucose levels approach 300 mg/dl. At that time, subcutaneous injections of insulin at a dose of 0.25–0.5 u/kg may be given every 6–8 hours while the glucose infusion is continued until the child can fully tolerate food.

Complications during or as a result of treatment for diabetic ketoacidosis include: inadequate fluid replacement, unrecognized hypokalemia, overuse of bicarbonate, overzealous phosphate replacement with resultant hypocalcemia, unrecognized cerebral edema, and peripheral or pulmonary edema (insulin edema as fluid overload). CT scans are helpful in detecting subclinical brain swelling (Krane et al, 1985).

ROUTINE MANAGEMENT

Insulin Regimens. At the onset of diabetes, or after recovery from acidosis, the total daily dose of insulin is roughly 0.5–1.0 u/kg of body weight. Various

Table 14.32
Insulin Regimen for Diabetic Ketoacidosis[1]

Blood Glucose	Total Insulin Dose (given every 2–4 hours)	Intravenous Dose (every 2–4 hours)	Intramuscular or Subcutaneous Dose (every 2–4 hours)
>900 mg/dl	2 u/kg	1 u/kg	1 u/kg
600–900 mg/dl	1 u/kg	0.5 u/kg	0.5 u/kg
300–600 mg/dl	0.5 u/kg	0.25 u/kg	0.25 u/kg

If ketones are only modestly elevated, the total dose of insulin may be halved.
[1]See text for continuous low-dose infusion regimen for insulin treatment of diabetic ketoacidosis.

insulin preparations provide short, medium, or long action (Table 14.33). Long-acting insulins are not usually used in children at the outset; rather a combination of intermediate- and short-acting insulins is the mainstay of therapy. Although some children can be managed with a single daily injection of a mixture of intermediate- and short-acting insulin, most children eventually require injections twice daily. Therapy must be individualized, but in general, roughly two-thirds of the daily dose of insulin is given 30 minutes before breakfast and roughly one-third is given 30 minutes before the evening meal. Each injection consists of intermediate- and short-acting insulins in the proportion of 2:1 or 3:1, mixed in the same syringe. Injection sites should be rotated among arms, thighs, buttocks and abdomen. When children are sufficiently mature and responsible they can be taught to administer their own insulin injections and to monitor their own diabetic control, but always with parental supervision.

Continuous subcutaneous insulin infusion systems are used by a minority of pediatricians to treat a small number of highly selected children with diabetes mellitus. The infusion pumps are small and externally located, usually attached to the patient's belt. Insulin is delivered subcutaneously via a catheter with its attached needle placed under the skin of the abdomen. The available pumps have variable speeds for delivery of insulin; a basal rate is used continuously (basal mode), and a prandial rate applied just before and during meals (bolus mode), thus, mimicking the dynamics of insulin release of the human pancreas. Although use of the insulin pump in teenaged and young adult populations has been successful (Tamborlane et al, 1984), there is no question that effective use of the pump requires extraordinary effort on the part of the patient, the physician, and the therapeutic team; which is far more demanding than standard insulin therapy. Thus, patients selected for a pump must be highly motivated, mature, and intelligent. Brink and Stewart (1986) found that use of the insulin pump in an office setting with a prolonged period of follow-up improved but did not normalize blood glucose and HbA1c levels. They found that 30% of their patients discontinued using the pump for various reasons.

Many investigators believe that comparable metabolic control can also be achieved by multiple-dose (3–4/day) regular insulin ± basal ultralente therapy, tight nutritional management, and home glucose monitoring.

Table 14.33
Insulin Preparations

Type	Peak Action (hour)	Duration of Action (hour)
Regular	2–4	4–6
NPH	6–8	18–24
Semilente	2–4	12–16
Ultralente	12–18	24–36
Lente	6–12	24–28

Diet

The diet of the diabetic child should include three well-balanced meals and snacks at midmorning, in the afternoon, and at bedtime. In general, in planning dietary recommendations for diabetic patients, foods with a low glycemic response should be favored. The physician or dietician should emphasize day-to-day constancy of both timing of meals and snacks, and the composition and amounts of foods, especially those high in carbohydrate. Many physicians use a food exchange system to keep the content as well as the amount of food relatively constant.

Although concentrated sweets have generally been prohibited except on special occasions, many physicians are reevaluating dietary recommendations for patients with diabetes. It has become clear that specific foods differ in their ability to raise blood glucose (glycemic index). For example, glucose, potatoes, and honey elicit similar postprandial glycemic responses, whereas rice, beans, and fructose yield a much flatter glycemic-response curve (Jenkins et al, 1981). The glycemic response to a single food may differ depending upon differences in preparation of the food. Ingestion of whole rice results in a much flatter blood glucose curve than does ingestion of rice flour (O'Dea et al, 1980). Wheat in pasta elicits a lower blood glucose peak than does wheat in bread (Jenkins et al, 1983). Interestingly, fructose elicits a considerably lower postprandial glycemic response than those produced by glucose, sucrose, and some starches (Bantle et al, 1983).

Other factors influence glycemic response also. Fat slows down gastric emptying reducing the glycemic response. Protein stimulates insulin release and will affect glycemic response in normal individuals.

Special adjustments in meal planning and insulin must be made during the adolescent growth spurt and with vigorous exercise. Exercise usually lowers the blood glucose by increasing (a) glucose consumption, (b) mobilization of insulin from the injection site (especially during leg exercise with subcutaneous insulin given in the thigh), and (c) insulin receptors. Simply eating an additional snack or adding to a regular snack before unusual exercise is usually sufficient to avoid hypoglycemia. Concomitant reduction of insulin dose is usually necessary for planned vigorous exercise and when exercise is prolonged or repetitive. Vigorous exercise may produce a delayed hypoglycemia late at night or early in the morning. Thus, the athlete may need to take a larger evening snack to avoid hypoglycemia.

Home Monitoring of Diabetic Control

Glucose-oxidase-impregnated strips for measuring glucose concentrations in blood and urine have been available for several years. Spot tests of urine can be made, but generally it is better to collect urine "blocks" over specific time intervals. Daytime blocks collected from 8:00 AM to noon, from noon to 4:00 PM, and from 4:00 PM to 8:00 PM, and an overnight collection (8:00 PM to 8:00 AM) of urine can be analyzed for glucose content and provide an overall evaluation of glucosuria.

Unfortunately day to day variations in urine blocks or in glucose analyses of individual voidings make urine testing less helpful than home blood glucose monitoring in evaluating diabetic control.

Home blood glucose monitoring techniques have improved so that measurements provide accurate and reproducible results (Skyler, 1981). The physician should emphasize to the patient that to obtain accurate and reliable data good technique is essential. Adjustments of insulin dosage can be made according to well-established algorithms (Skyler et al, 1981).

Ketones in the urine can be tested with appropriate test materials (Acetest tablets). Ketonuria should alert the patient to adjustment of the insulin dosage so that diabetic ketoacidosis can be avoided. Urinary ketones should be tested routinely in the patient who has a blood glucose level over 240 mg/dl, or urinary glucose level of 5% or more; such ketones should always be measured if the patient is sick.

Education

A very important member of the therapeutic team is the nurse-clinician educator responsible for overall education of the patient and family so that all may have an understanding of all aspects of diabetes mellitus and its management. This aspect of diabetes care cannot be overemphasized. It is only with a firm grasp of the fundamental biology of the diabetic condition that the patient will be motivated to perform daily monitoring and to follow suggested dietary guidelines. It is important that the patient and family understand the long-term complications of diabetes (see Prognosis) and how careful diabetic control may prevent some of these problems.

Long-Term Observations

Growth of the child with diabetes is an important indication of control. At the time of diagnosis most diabetics are of normal height, but underweight. Poorly controlled diabetes will impair growth severely (Mauriac syndrome).

Periodic measurements of serum triglyceride and cholesterol levels in blood are helpful in ascertaining the degree of overall diabetic control. Hypercholesterolemia is an important risk factor for ischemic heart disease and should be treated by modification of the diet and drugs if necessary. Urine protein determinations should be obtained periodically, to follow renal function. Periodic fundoscopic examinations are also recommended; and the recognition of diabetic retinopathy early is of especial importance because therapy with photocoagulation can alter the course of this complication.

Because of the increased incidence of autoimmune endocrine disease in diabetics, the patient should be checked for goiter or other evidence of endocrine dysfunction. Antibodies for thyroid, gonadal, or parathyroid gland tissue can be measured as indicated by the clinical condition of the patient.

COMPLICATIONS OF INSULIN THERAPY

Hypoglycemia

The symptoms of hypoglycemia are secondary to (1) adrenergic activation of the sympathetic nervous system and (2) insufficient glucose for normal neural function. The former elicits perspiration, tachycardia, tremor, pallor, anxiety, and uneasiness; the latter may cause behavioral changes, confusion, obtundation, convulsions, or coma. If the patient is conscious, ingestion of sugar tablets, table sugar, or orange juice may be sufficient treatment. In the home, an intramuscular injection of 1 mg of glucagon should be used until the patient can be brought to the hospital. In the unconscious patient, intravenous glucose is required.

In those patients with autonomic neuropathy and epinephrine deficiency the usual adrenergic warning symptoms are lacking and neuroglycopenia is the sole manifestation of hypoglycemia. These patients are unaware of hypoglycemia until neurological symptoms occur. This condition is uncommon in children.

After an episode of hypoglycemia (often undetected) rebound hyperglycemia (Somogyi phenomenon) may occur. The pathogenesis of this phenomenon in diabetics involves the activation of counterregulatory systems by the hypoglycemia. In nondiabetic persons, increased secretion of counterregulatory hormones (epinephrine, glucagon, GH, cortisol) would be offset by a compensatory increase in insulin secretion, so that hyperglycemia would not occur. The diabetic with defective β cells is unable to respond appropriately to the hyperglycemia. To prevent the Somogyi phenomenon the initial hypoglycemia must be avoided. This is best accomplished by an overall reduction in insulin dose. The Somogyi effect is frequently seen in children with IDDM.

Hypoglycemia often occurs during the night in patients with IDDM. Morning hyperglycemia may be the result of activation of counterregulatory systems by nocturnal hypoglycemia. However, early morning increases in plasma glucose concentrations (or insulin requirements) may be observed without prior hypoglycemia (dawn phenomenon). Since suppression of nocturnal GH secretion by infusion of somatostatin attenuates or prevents this phenomenon, and administration of GH exacerbates it, GH appears to play a prominent role in the etiology of the dawn phenomenon (Campbell et al, 1985). It is important to distinguish among the Somogyi phenomenon, the dawn phenomenon and simple waning of previously injected insulin as a cause of early morning hyperglycemia, because the treatment of each is different. For the dawn phenomenon and insulin waning, adjustment of the evening dose of intermediate-acting insulin to provide additional coverage between 4:00 AM and 7:00 AM is needed. This frequently means giving intermediate acting insulin at bedtime (about 10:00 PM) instead of before supper; i.e., three shots/day. Management of the Somogyi phenomenon consists of reducing the evening insulin dose or providing late-evening carbohydrate (or both) to avoid nocturnal hypoglycemia. Testing blood glucose levels at bedtime, 2:00–4:00 AM, and 7:00 AM for several days may be necessary to determine which of these three causes is most likely in a given patient.

Hypertrophy and Lipoatrophy

Atrophy of subcutaneous tissue at the site of insulin injection is probably an allergic response to impurities in the insulin preparation. Switching to pure pork or human insulin and injecting this pure insulin into or around the atrophic area may be beneficial.

Hypertrophy at sites of insulin injection is due to repeated injections into the same site. The involved site should be avoided and new sites used for subsequent injections.

Insulin Allergy

Allergic reactions may develop during insulin therapy or later. Local reactions are characterized by erythema, pruritus, and induration at the injection site. Systemic allergy may be manifested by generalized urticaria, angioneurotic edema, or anaphylaxis. Local reactions may be reduced by the use of purified pork or biosynthetic human insulin with an antihistamine. Sometimes switching to a different type of insulin (NPH from Lente or vice versa) will reduce the allergic response. If there is no improvement with antihistamines, dexamethasone injected with the insulin may reduce allergic response. Desensitization is required for systemic reactions.

Insulin Resistance

Anti-insulin antibodies may develop during insulin therapy. Insulin requirements may be extremely high in patients with very high antibody titers and with high insulin-binding capacity. The use of a less antigenic form of insulin, such as purified pork or human insulin, decreases the requirement for insulin in about half the patients. There is cross-reactivity, however, among the different insulins. Sulfated insulin, a chemically modified form of beef or pork insulin that contains an average of six sulfate groups per molecule, combines less avidly with antibodies to beef and pork insulin. Patients with insulin resistance, when switched to sulfated insulin, will require only about 15% of their former insulin dose, and even less as the antigenic stimulus is removed and the antibody titer falls. In the patient who does not respond to less antigenic insulins, steroids may be required. Glucocorticoid therapy will result in a rapid reduction in insulin requirement in most patients. Because of the known insulin resistance effect of glucocorticoids, the dose of steroid should be tapered as quickly as possible (usually 2–3 weeks) and discontinued when the patient is no longer resistant to insulin.

Prognosis

The prognosis for patients with IDDM is largely dependent upon the degenerative complications of the disease. Microvascular complications include retinopathy, neuropathy, and nephropathy. Atherosclerosis and its sequelae (stroke, myocardial infarction, gangrene) are considered macrovascular complications. These complications begin to appear 10–15 years after the onset of diabetes.

Whether diabetic complications can be prevented or delayed by meticulous control is under study. Some evidence suggests that tight diabetic control may be able to delay or even prevent some of the degenerative changes. The process of protein cross-linking which may cause structural changes and which is caused by glycosylation end-products is inhibited by aminoguanidine (Brownlee et al, 1988). Such therapy in the future may prevent certain complications of diabetes. In the young patient with many years of life ahead, the hope of a prophylactic advantage makes careful diabetic control a reasonable goal. Meticulous control, however, is rarely achieved unless the patient is highly motivated.

New developments for treatment of diabetes mellitus are being tested. The so-called "artificial pancreas," a closed loop system which adjusts the insulin infusions to changes in concentration of blood glucose, may be useful for bedside treatment of ketoacidosis and management of patients during surgery. Islet cell and pancreatic transplants are presently being evaluated. The role of the immune system in the etiology of β cell destruction suggests that drugs that affect this process might be useful. Cyclosporin is under study for this purpose in 1988.

Noninsulin-Dependent Diabetes Mellitus (Type II, Adult Onset)

Definition

This form of diabetes is characterized by a nonketosis-prone glucose intolerance that is relatively stable over years. Sufficient insulin is produced by the β cell to prevent diabetic ketoacidosis.

Epidemiology

Often associated with obesity, noninsulin-dependent diabetes mellitus (NIDDM) is the most common of the hyperglycemic states; the incidence is higher in older obese subjects than in the young. Nevertheless, impaired glucose tolerance has been found in about 15–25% of grossly obese preadolescents and in about 40% of obese adolescents. Subsequently some of these children may develop overt diabetes.

The inheritance of NIDDM is probably multifactorial. Familial aggregation of this form of diabetes is more common than is the case with IDDM. Concordance of identical twins for NIDDM is 90–100%, compared to about 50% in IDDM (Barnett et al, 1981). A form of maturity-onset diabetes of the young (MODY) appears to have an autosomal dominant inheritance. In 85% of the cases of MODY there is a strong family history of NIDDM. Thus, MODY may be a separate, genetically determined form of NIDDM.

Natural History

The etiology of NIDDM is unknown. Unlike IDDM, there is no evidence of an autoimmune etiology. It is clear that both an "insulin-insufficient" state and an "insulin-resistant" state coexist in most patients. Obesity itself can lead to the development of insulin resistance, and, since the great majority of patients with NIDDM (80%) are overweight, obesity-induced insulin resistance frequently contributes to hyperglycemia in these patients. However, the insulin resistance is greater than that which can be accounted for on the basis of obesity alone. Furthermore, many nonobese patients with NIDDM are also insulin-resistant.

Some but not all children with impaired glucose tolerance subsequently develop clinical diabetes. In those who do, signs of hyperglycemia occur (polyuria, polydipsia), but ketosis does not usually develop.

The clinical picture in MODY is usually mild and many affected individuals are asymptomatic. These patients are usually adolescents who are of normal weight or only slightly obese.

Diagnosis

Children with close relatives who are diabetic and those with evidence of stress glucosuria or reactive postprandial hypoglycemia should be considered at greater risk than normal for developing diabetes mellitus. Currently, the best test to evaluate β cell secretory reserve is an intravenous glucose tolerance test with measurement of the first phase insulin secretion (1- and 3-minute values). A low insulin response to intravenous glucose and the presence of islet cell antibodies in the blood are highly predictive of diabetes mellitus. Since insulin responses to a glucose challenge tend to increase with growth from the age of 3 years through a mean age of 15 years, normal insulin values must be adjusted for age (Table 14.31).

Treatment

Caloric restriction and increased physical activity in obese children with NIDDM may normalize blood glucose levels. Those children with hyperglycemia who fail to respond to dietary restriction and exercise may require insulin therapy. Some children will respond to oral hypoglycemic agents.

OTHER DIABETIC SYNDROMES

A number of specific syndromes are associated with glucose intolerance. IDDM secondary to cystic fibrosis is the most common, with hemochromatosis, chronic pancreatitis, or steroid therapy less common.

A far less common syndrome is lipotrophic diabetes, characterized by severe insulin resistance and generalized atrophy of adipose tissue (Senior and Gellis, 1964).

A syndrome of insulin resistance plus acanthosis nigricans (type B) has been described in which antibodies to the insulin receptor have been found in the sera of patients (Kahn et al, 1976). In virtually all of these patients there are features of a more generalized autoimmune disease. The insulin resistance in these patients is often severe, requiring large doses of insulin to normalize blood glucose concentrations. The course of the diabetes is variable and several patients have had spontaneous remissions.

Another form of insulin resistance and acanthosis nigricans (type A) can be associated with hypogonadism. In this disorder, there is a decrease in receptor number with normal receptor affinity and no antireceptor antibodies.

Hypoglycemia

Definition

Hypoglycemia represents a condition in which the blood glucose level is below the norm for age. The lower limit of normal blood glucose values is 40 mg/dl.

Basic Science

Blood glucose is obtained from the diet directly or via production by the liver (glycogenolysis and gluconeogenesis) and kidney (gluconeogenesis). Glucose is used by all tissues but certain tissues such as red cell and brain derive all or almost all of their energy from metabolism of glucose. Insulin is the primary glucoregulatory hormone via its effects on hepatic production and utilization of glucose. Other hormones (epinephrine, GH, glucagon, cortisol) also play a role by enhancing glucose production.

Persistent hypoglycemia secondary to decreased production and overutilization of glucose usually is due to excess insulin. Excess production of insulin may be due to diffuse β cell hyperplasia, nesidioblastosis (a disorder of regulation of insulin secretion), or a β cell adenoma (insulinoma). In the infant with hyperinsulinism there is usually a disordered secretion of insulin, whereas in the older child hyperinsulinism is almost always caused by an insulinoma. Some patients with hyperinsulinemia develop severe hypoglycemia when given leucine.

Persistent hypoglycemia secondary to decreased production of glucose is most commonly due to (1) inborn errors of metabolism involving the gluconeogenic enzymes, (2) deficiency of one or more counterregulatory hormones (see appropriate chapters), or (3) decreased substrates such as alanine (ketotic hypoglycemia).

Persistent hypoglycemia in the infant is likely to be caused by hyperinsulinism, or by enzyme or hormone deficiencies. In the older child, the most likely causes of hypoglycemia include ketotic hypoglycemia, islet cell adenoma, GH deficiency, or glucocorticoid deficiency.

Epidemiology

Hypoglycemia is a relatively common problem of infancy and childhood. Since the level of circulating glucose depends upon the balance between production

Table 14.34
Causes of Hypoglycemia in Childhood

Transient Neonatal
Decreased production (small-for-dates, premature)
Increased utilization (hyperinsulinism)
Infants of diabetic mothers
Erythroblastosis
Beckwith-Wiedemann syndrome
Persistent Neonatal and Early Infancy
Decreased production
Enzyme deficiencies[1]
Metabolic abnormalities[2]
Hormone deficiencies
Increased utilization (hyperinsulinism)
Nesidioblastosis, β-cell hyperplasia, adenoma
Older Children
Decreased production
Enzyme deficiencies[1]
Hormone deficiencies
Ketotic hypoglycemia
Increased utilization (hyperinsulinism)
Islet cell adenome

[1]Glucose-6-phosphatase, debrancher enzyme, phosphorylase, phosphorylase kinase, glycogen synthetase, fructose 1,6-diphosphatase, phosphoenolpyruvate carboxykinase, pyruvate carboxylase.
[2]Galactosemia, fructose intolerance, maple syrup urine disease.
In addition, salicylates, alcohol or fulminant hepatitis can cause hypoglycemia.

and utilization, a variety of disorders may cause the condition (Table 14.34).

The incidence of transient hypoglycemia is increased in preterm infants, infants with intrauterine growth retardation, and in infants who suffer stress. This is partly due to the reduced hepatic glycogen stores in the premature and small-for-dates babies. In infants of diabetic mothers (IDM) and infants with erythroblastosis or Beckwith-Wiedemann syndrome, a state of hyperinsulinism exists and hypoglycemia occurs commonly in these babies after birth.

Natural History

The normal infant born at term shows an immediate fall in blood glucose concentration during the first 4–6 hours after birth. The fall in blood glucose coincides with an increase in plasma glucagon levels, perhaps due in part to stimulation by the release of catecholamines after cutting the umbilical cord. These adaptive hormonal changes trigger an immediate release of glucose from hepatic glycogen stores. In addition, circulating levels of GH are high at birth favoring lipolysis and the release of fatty acids as a source of energy. Maintenance of normoglycemia during the neonatal period depends upon adequate reserves of glycogen and fat and effective glycogenolysis and gluconeogenesis.

IDM have a characteristic appearance. They are overweight for gestational age, with increased body fat and increased length. Many babies with nesidioblastosis have a similar physical appearance. Infants with Beckwith-Wiedemann syndrome are characterized by exomphalos, macroglossia, visceromegaly, and gigantism, in addition to hyperinsulinemic hypoglycemia. In such infants, there is a high prevalence of ear lobe anomalies.

The hypoglycemia is more severe in infants with hyperinsulinemia and enzymatic defects, symptoms usually developing within the first 6 months of life. Many become hypoglycemic even after a very short fast. Hepatomegaly in these children should suggest a form of glycogen storage disease (pp. 911). Infants with documented nesidioblastosis develop severe intractable hyperinsulinemic hypoglycemia, usually within the first 3 days of life.

Hormone deficiencies (GH, cortisol) generally cause a less severe form of hypoglycemia which manifests in late infancy and early childhood.

The typical patient with ketotic hypoglycemia is a boy between 2 and 7 years of age who is underweight, and born small-for-gestational age or after a difficult delivery. During caloric restriction, often during intercurrent infection or after a burst of intense physical activity, the child develops symptomatic hypoglycemia which may progress to convulsions. The episodes may be recurrent, but are finally outgrown.

Diagnosis

A careful history is the cornerstone of diagnosing hypoglycemia in the child. Details of the pregnancy and delivery, the birthweight of the infant, the presence of fetal distress or birth asphyxia should be ascertained. The family history should be checked for previous infant deaths or metabolic acidosis (genetic enzyme abnormalities). In the differential diagnosis, the following points are important: (1) age of onset of symptoms; (2) temporal relationship of symptoms to meals, specific foodstuffs, and fasting; and (3) the child's growth and neurologic development. Short stature and small genitalia (in boys) may indicate hypopituitarism (pp. 811). The physical examination may reveal an enlarged liver, suggesting abnormal glycogen metabolism, defects in gluconeogenesis or galactosemia (pp. 915). Abnormal pigmentation may suggest Addison disease (pp. 864).

A blood sample drawn while the child is hypoglycemic is of crucial importance in diagnosing the type of hypoglycemia. Since most affected infants and children give a history of symptomatic hypoglycemia after a fast, an early morning blood sample after an overnight fast in the hospital may show a glucose level below 40 mg/dl. Alternatively, a briefer period of fast during the day, when hospital personnel are available to observe the child, may be indicated. Blood levels of glucose, insulin, free fatty acids, and ketones should be obtained every 2 or 3 hours during the fast. If the overnight fasting is not associated with an abnormally low plasma glucose, a more prolonged fast may be indicated.

A urine sample should be obtained when the child is hypoglycemic and analyzed for ketone bodies ("ketotic" vs "nonketotic" hypoglycemia), positive reducing sugars (galactosemia, fructose intolerance), catecholamines, and organic acids (fatty acid metabolic disorders, pp. 951).

The diagnosis of hyperinsulinemia depends upon the demonstration of a high value for plasma insulin in relation to the value for blood glucose during a hypoglycemic episode. The latter may be induced by fasting. In the presence of organic hyperinsulinism, fasting hypoglycemia is accompanied by low plasma levels of free fatty acids and ketones because of inhibition of lipolysis and ketogenesis by insulin. Conversely, if hypoglycemia is due to noninsulin-mediated reduction in glucose production (defect in glycogenolysis or in gluconeogenesis), there will be an associated elevation of plasma free fatty acids and ketones. In normal children, the plasma insulin value is less than 10 μU/ml in the presence of hypoglycemia. With a plasma glucose concentration of less than 45 mg/dl and a plasma insulin concentration of greater than 10 μU/ml, a diagnosis of endogenous hyperinsulinism is likely. A number of simultaneous blood insulin and glucose values should be obtained to verify the diagnosis. Hyperinsulinemia is often associated with increased insulin sensitivity to leucine or a high protein meal; therefore, in children in whom this diagnosis is suspected, a leucine tolerance test may be performed. Leucine (150 mg/kg body weight orally) is given and glucose and insulin in the blood are measured at 0, 15, 30, 45, 60, 90, and 120 minutes. This test should only be performed in infants who can maintain a normal blood glucose during a 4- to 5-hour fast.

In laboratories that perform C-peptide assays, blood can be checked for this byproduct of insulin production. A plasma C-peptide concentration greater than 1.5 ng/ml in the presence of hypoglycemia indicates endogenous hyperinsulinism. In theory, measurement of plasma C-peptide should be more sensitive for diagnosis than that of insulin, since, in contrast to insulin, C-peptide is degraded little if at all by the liver.

CAT scan of the upper abdomen may be helpful in locating a pancreatic tumor, although insulinomas are often small and may not be detected. Ultrasonography and arteriography may be useful in localizing insulinomas.

In children with ketotic hypoglycemia, ketonuria and symptomatic hypoglycemia will develop after 8–16 hours of fasting. Normal children can sustain a fast of 24–36 hours without symptoms. During the test, periodic blood samples should be analyzed for insulin, GH, cortisol, alanine, lactate, and β-hydroxybutyrate. If the child becomes symptomatic, a blood sample should be obtained for the above tests and the test terminated with intravenous glucose. Typically the blood tests will show no evidence of hyperinsulinism, lactic acidosis, or hormone deficiency. In children with ketotic hypoglycemia, serum levels of alanine are significantly lower after a fast than they are in normal fasted children. β-Hydroxybutyrate in blood and ketones in urine are elevated in affected children on fasting. Very often, ketotic hypoglycemia is a diagnosis of exclusion, once inborn errors of metabolism and hormone deficiencies have been eliminated as possible causes of the hypoglycemia.

Treatment

With the decreased likelihood of adenoma in infants with hypersinulinemia, medical therapy may be tried. Diazoxide (8–12 mg/kg body weight) should be administered along with a low protein diet if the child is sensitive to leucine. If this does not maintain the blood glucose in the normal range, a higher dose (up to 15–20 mg/kg) of diazoxide may be tried before subjecting the child to a laparotomy. If on surgery no adenoma is detected, a 50–80% pancreatectomy should be performed. Diazoxide and a low protein diet may be continued after surgery if necessary. If the blood glucose still cannot be kept in the normal range, total pancreatectomy is indicated.

In the older child with hyperinsulinism, adenoma is by far the most common cause of the condition. Therapy consists of surgical removal.

The therapy of hypoglycemia secondary to enzyme or hormone deficiencies is discussed elsewhere (see Section 15).

Children with ketotic hypoglycemia should have frequent feedings. During intercurrent illnesses the child's urine should be tested for ketones, and if positive, liquids rich in carbohydrate should be given. Usually after age 8 or 9 years, these measures are no longer necessary.

Prognosis

Infants less than 1 year of age with recurrent hypoglycemia have a high incidence of acquired irreversible brain damage. Rapid diagnosis and therapy of the hypoglycemia can help protect the brain from such damage.

REFERENCES

Bantle JP, Laine DC, Castle GW, et al: Postprandial glucose and insulin responses to meals containing different carbohydrates in normal and diabetic subjects. *N Engl J Med* 309:7, 1983.

Barnett AH, Eff C, Leslie RDG, et al: Diabetes in identical twins. A study of 200 pairs. *Diabetologia* 20:87, 1981.

Bolli G, De Feo P, Compagnucci P, et al: Abnormal glucose counterregulation in insulin dependent diabetes mellitus. *Diabetes* 32:134, 1983.

Brink SJ, Stewart C: Insulin pump treatment in insulin dependent diabetes mellitus. *JAMA* 255:617, 1986.

Brownlee M, Cerami A, Vlassara H: Advanced glycosylation end products in tissue and the biochemical basis of diabetic complications. *N Engl J Med* 318:1315, 1988.

Bunn HF: Non-enzymatic glycosylation of protein: Relevance to diabetes. *Am J Med* 70:325, 1981.

Campbell PJ, Bolli GB, Cryer PE, et al: Pathogenesis of the dawn phenomenon in patients with insulin-dependent diabetes mellitus: Accelerated glucose production and impaired glucose utilization due to nocturnal surges in growth hormone secretion. *N Engl J Med* 312:1473, 1985.

Cryer PE, White NH, Santiago JV: The relevance of glucose counterregulatory systems to patients with insulin-dependent diabetes mellitus. *Endocrinol Rev* 7:131, 1986.

Deschamps I, Lestradet H, Bonaiti C, et al: HLA genotype studies in juvenile insulin-dependent diabetes. *Diabetologia* 19:189, 1980.

Drash A, LaPorte R, Becker D, et al: The natural history of diabetes mellitus in children: Insulin requirements during the initial two years. *Acta Pediatr Belg* 33:66, 1980.

Eisenbarth GS: Type I diabetes mellitus: A chronic autoimmune disease. *N Engl J Med* 314:1360, 1986.

Gorwitz K, Howen GG, Thompson T: Prevalence of diabetes in Michigan school-age children. *Diabetes* 25:122, 1976.

Jenkins DJA, Wolever TMS, Jenkins AL, et al: Glycemic response to wheat products: Reduced response to pasta but no effect of fiber. *Diabet Care* 6:155, 1983.

Jenkins DJA, Wolever TMS, Taylor RH, et al: Glycemic index of foods: A physiological basis for carbohydrate exchange. *Am J Clin Nutr* 34:362, 1981.

Kahn CR: The moelcular mechanism of insulin action. *Ann Rev Med* 36:429, 1985.

Kahn CR, Flier JS, Bar RS, et al: The syndromes of insulin resistance and acanthosis nigricans: Insulin-receptor disorders in man. *N Engl J Med* 294:739, 1976.

Krane EJ, Rockoff MA, Wallman JK, et al: Subclinical brain swelling in children during treatment of diabetic ketoacidosis. *N Engl J Med* 312:1147, 1985.

Mandrup-Poulsen T, Bendtzen K, Nielsen JH, et al: Cytokines cause functional and structural damage to isolated islets of Langerhans. *Allergy* 40:424, 1985.

O'Dea K, Nestel PJ, Antonoff L: Physical factors influencing post-prandial glucose and insulin responses to starch. *Am J Clin Nutr* 33:760, 1980.

Senior B, Gellis SS: The syndromes of total lipodystrophy and of partial lipodystrophy. *Pediatrics* 33:593, 1964.

Skyler J (ed): Symposium on home glucose self-monitoring. *Diabet Care* 4:392, 1981.

Skyler JS, Skyler DL, Seigler DE, et al: Algorithms for adjustment of insulin dosage by patients who monitor blood glucose. *Diabet Care* 4:311, 1981.

Sutherland DER, Sibley R, Chinn P, et al: Twin-to-twin pancreas transplantation: Reversal and reenactment of the pathogenesis of Type I diabetes. *Clin Res* 32:561A, 1984.

Tamborlane WV, Press CM: Insulin infusion pump treatment of Type I diabetes. *Pediatr Clin North Am* 31:721, 1984.

Warram JH, Krolewski AS, Gottlieb MS, et al: Differences in risk of insulin-dependent diabetes in offspring of diabetic mothers and diabetic fathers. *N Engl J Med* 311:149, 1984.

Yoon JW, Austin M, Onodera T, et al: Virus-induced diabetes mellitus: Isolation of a virus from the pancreas of a child with diabetic ketoacidosis. *N Engl J Med* 300:1173, 1979.

DOROTHY B. VILLEE

The author acknowledges John Crigler, Joseph Wolfsdorf, Reid Larsen, Craig Rudlin, and Thomas Carpenter for their help in reviewing this section.

Section 15

Hereditary Metabolic Diseases

The pediatrician is unlikely to be in practice for very long or to serve for any length of time as attending physician on a pediatric ward before encountering at least one patient with an inborn error of metabolism. At least 58 disorders have been recognized in newborn infants (Burton, 1987) and well over 200 have been catalogued (McKusick, 1987). In fact, as more inborn errors are recognized this area of pediatrics is assuming an increasing role in both private practice and medical center referral. Hence, it is important for the pediatrician to develop a system for identifying the patient who might have an inborn error, for assessing whether an inborn error is indeed the cause of the problem, and perhaps even determining the general category of the putative error.

A metabolic diagnosis is important for several reasons. First, and certainly of paramount importance, it can lead to therapy that might reverse the acute symptoms and prevent chronic damage. Second, it may lead to treatment that will ameliorate some of the features of the disease even if some degree of damage is already irreversible. Third, even if treatment is not possible or would be of no benefit, diagnosis may provide genetic information that can be valuable for future family planning or prenatal diagnosis. Finally, even if therapy is not possible and genetic information has little or no value to the family, a metabolic diagnosis is very often important by providing the family and health providers with the satisfaction of a name and an explanation for disability in the child.

Many physicians tend to avoid the subject of metabolic diagnosis because it appears to be complicated and to require extensive knowledge of biochemistry. Suspicion of a metabolic disorder and subsequent diagnosis, however, is neither very complicated nor does it require the skill of a biochemist. A systematic approach that recognizes certain clinical presentations and utilizes generally available laboratory tests is required. This introduction is an attempt to provide such an approach—to take the mystery out of the diagnosis of inborn errors of metabolism.

SYSTEM FOR METABOLIC DIAGNOSIS

The symptoms of an inborn error may best be considered according to the age of the patient since certain inborn errors tend to present clinically in the newborn or early infancy periods while others present later in childhood. The system below includes the most prominent clinical and laboratory features of the inborn errors according to category of age (Table 15.1).

Newborn

Acute Presentations

Three main classes of acute presentation exist.

Class 1 disorders are characterized by lethargy, coma, hypotonia, tachypnea, poor feeding, excessive weight loss, hepatomegaly, and, possibly, seizures and/or vomiting. Laboratory tests should include bacterial cultures, blood gases or serum electrolytes, blood glucose, blood ammonia, blood lactate, complete blood count, and urinalysis.

Class 2 presentation is characterized primarily by signs of liver disease, including jaundice, hepatomegaly, and, occasionally, increased bleeding tendency. Signs of CNS involvement such as lethargy, poor feeding, and hypotonia may be present. Laboratory tests should include bacterial cultures, liver function tests (including PT and PTT), blood glucose, and urinalysis with test for reducing substance (not simply a dipstick for glucose).

The presence or absence of coagulopathy is important. In liver disease with a metabolic cause, coagulopathy (increased PT and PTT) is usually present, whereas in conditions with nonmetabolic liver disease (biliary atresia, hepatitis, etc) coagulopathy is often absent until the stage of liver failure.

Class 3 encompasses presentation of the neonate with nonketotic hyperglycinemia. Lethargy develops in the first or second day of life, progressing to unresponsiveness with marked hypotonia and, often seizures. All laboratory tests are normal including blood gases, serum electrolytes, blood glucose, blood ammonia and lactate, complete blood counts, and urinalysis.

Newborn Screening

Certain tests are included in newborn screening as listed in Table 15.2. Newborn screening may provide a diagnosis before the disorder presents clinically. The process begins with a telephone call or letter from the

Table 15.1
Characteristics of Acute Presentations of Metabolic Disorders in the Newborn (details are described in the text)

Observation	Possible Cause	Test Requested
Class 1 Metabolic acidosis Hypoglycemia Hyperammonemia Ketonuria Leukopenia (occasionally)	Organic acid disorder	Urinary organic acids; blood and urine amino acids
Same as above but urinary ketones negative or no greater than trace to 1+	Fatty acid oxidation defect	Same as above
Metabolic acidosis Ketonuria Increased blood lactate	Pyruvic acidemia	Same as above
Hyperammonemia (without metabolic acidosis)	Urea cycle disorder	Blood and urine amino acids; urinary orotic acid
Class 2 History of milk ingestion Urine reducing substance positive, but glucose negative	Galactosemia	Blood galactose, galactose 1-phosphate, and galactose enzymes
Hypoglycemia	Hereditary tyrosinemia	Blood and urine amino acids, urinary organic acids
History of soy-based formula ingestion Urine glucose-positive Hypoglycemia	Hereditary fructose intolerance	Blood and urine amino acids
Class 3 Lethargy Marked hypotonia Possible seizures Standard laboratory tests normal	Nonketotic hyperglycinemia	Blood and urine amino acids; urinary organic acids

newborn screening laboratory. The neonate is usually well, although in disorders such as galactosemia or maple syrup urine disease, the infant may already have developed early symptoms of disease that are unrecognized as medically important.

Infant

Acute Presentations

These are virtually identical to the acute presentations described for the neonate, except that the neonatal course is normal and episodic acute presentations usually occur beginning at 3–4 months of age when protein intake begins to increase. The disorders that should be considered are identical to those in the neonate. Whether the disorder presents in the newborn or later in infancy seems to depend upon the degree of metabolic block. When there is almost no residual activity of the affected enzyme producing an essentially complete metabolic block, the clinical symptoms occur within the first few days after birth. When there is some residual enzyme activity and an incomplete metabolic block, presentation is later.

Table 15.2
Metabolic Disorders for which Newborn Screening is Conducted and the Likely Clinical State of the Newborn

Disorder	Frequency of Screening	Clinical State of Newborn	Positive Cases Detected in Massachusetts July 1985–June 1986 (84,846 screened)
Phenylketonuria	All programs	Normal	4
Congenital hypothyroidism	All programs	Normal	11
Galactosemia	Many programs	I ll	1
Maple syrup urine disease	Some programs	I ll	1
Homocystinuria	Some programs	Normal	0
Biotinidase deficiency	Some programs	Normal	—[1]

[1]Not screened in Massachusetts program.

The most frequent type of acute clinical presentation of an organic acid disorder or urea cycle defect in the infant is similar to that of *Reye syndrome* with lethargy or coma, hepatomegaly, and hyperammonemia. Metabolic acidosis usually signifies a disorder of organic acids, whereas in the absence of metabolic acidosis, a urea cycle defect is likely.

The presentation of metabolic liver disease described for the neonate also applies to the older infant, except that α-1-antitrypsin deficiency should be considered in the infant, whereas this disorder does not produce neonatal liver disease. A serum α-1-antitrypsin assay is indicated for all infants with metabolic liver disease.

Nonketotic hyperglycinemia also may present in the older infant; rather the later onset form of this disease with developmental delay and myoclonic seizures presents in the older infant.

Chronic Presentations

Any infant with *developmental delay* or *failure to thrive* should be considered for a metabolic diagnosis. Evaluation should include blood and urine amino acids, urine organic acids, blood glucose, gases, ammonia, and lactate, and urinalysis that includes tests for reducing substance and ketones.

Child

Acute Presentations

Acute presentation in the child is identical to that described for the infant, with the same exceptions as those for the neonate. In the child, the "Reye syndrome" presentation of an organic acid disorder or a urea cycle defect may be even more characteristic of classic Reye syndrome than in the infant.

Chronic Presentations

Mental retardation is the most frequent characteristic of the chronic metabolic disorders in the child. Some of these, such as phenylketonuria and congenital hypothyroidism should be identified by routine screening, and repeat testing for them should be considered in any child who shows signs of mental retardation. Most other metabolic disorders that cause mental retardation are not screened in the newborn. Consequently, any child with mental retardation or with any degree of reduced mentality or unusual behavior should receive assays of amino acids in blood and urine and urinary organic acid analysis.

REFERENCES

Burton BK: Inborn errors of metabolism: The clinical diagnosis in early infancy. *Pediatrics* 79:359, 1987.

McKusick VA: Molecular defects in mendelian disorders. In Scriver CR, et al (eds): *The Metabolic Basis of Inherited Disease*, Sixth Edition. New York, McGraw-Hill, 1987.

Carbohydrate Metabolism Disorders 1

GLYCOGEN STORAGE DISEASES

There exists a series of inherited defects involving glycogen metabolism in liver, muscle, and other tissues. These defects are secondary to specific enzyme deficiencies resulting in the accumulation of normal or structurally abnormal glycogen.

Basic Science

The pathways of synthesis and degradation of glycogen are depicted in Figure 15.1. The first enzyme deficiency of glycogen metabolism to be demonstrated was that of glucose-6-phosphatase (von Gierke disease) by Cori in 1952. Since then individuals with deficient or absent activity for each of the other enzymes have been described and a system of numbering these diseases sequentially was set up.

Epidemiology and Genetics

These disorders are very rare and are inherited as autosomal recessive traits with the exception of phosphorylase b kinase deficiency which is inherited in an X-linked recessive manner.

In debranching enzyme deficiency, there is widespread variability in tissue enzyme activity even with single affected families. In Israel, this disease accounts for 73% of the glycogen storage disease disorders. There was a minimal prevalence of 1:5420 in a non-Ashkenazi Jewish community which originated in North Africa. No debrancher deficiency has been seen in the Ashkenazi Jews.

GSD Type I—Glucose-6-Phosphatase (von Gierke disease)

Definition

This disorder represents a genetic deficiency in glucose-6-phosphatase (type I) or in the transport of glucose-6-phosphate across the hepatic microsomal membrane (type Ib). As a consequence, glycogen accumulates in the liver, kidney, and intestine.

Basic Science

Glucose-6-phosphatase catalyzes the conversion of glucose-6-phosphate (G-6-P) to glucose (Fig. 15.1). The enzyme is located on the microsomes and is characteristically totally absent in vitro in these patients. Treating the hepatic microsomes of some patients with detergent (which opens up microsomal vesicles) restores enzyme activity to normal. A defect in G-6-P transport across hepatic microsomes has been postulated for these patients (Narisawa et al, 1983).

Natural History

Affected children show rapid enlargement of the liver during infancy. Growth is impaired and the musculature is flabby and poorly developed. Hepatomegaly is accompanied by enlargement of the kidney (seen on roentgenographic examination) but rarely is the spleen involved.

Hypoglycemia may be severe and result in convulsions, especially in early life. The hypoglycemia is unresponsive to epinephrine and glucagon. Because of the enzyme block, metabolism in the liver is funneled toward glycolysis with accumulation of lactate and pyruvate producing a chronic metabolic acidosis. Other pathways in the liver are overwhelmed also with the accumulation of triglycerides, phospholipids, cholesterol, and uric acid. The patients are resistant to ketosis, which is attributed to the high pyruvate providing adequate oxaloacetate and thereby preventing acetyl coenzyme A accumulation.

Excess triglycerides appear as xanthomas over the extensor surfaces of the extremities. Gouty tophi from the hyperuricemia may have similar distribution later in life.

Platelet function is abnormal resulting in frequent bleeding episodes such as nosebleeds. Intermittent bouts of diarrhea have also been reported. A Fanconi-like syndrome (aminoaciduria, glycosuria, and phosphaturia) occurs in patients with glucose-6-phosphatase deficiency. In addition, osteoporosis is usually present, possibly secondary to a negative calcium balance related to the chronic acidosis. Clinically, these patients improve with age and are less difficult to manage.

As individuals with type I glycogen storage disease grow older, they may manifest impaired renal function. Three deaths from renal failure were reported by Chen et al (1988).

Diagnosis

In any child with enlarged liver, hypoglycemia, and failure to grow the diagnosis of glucose-6-phosphatase deficiency should be considered. A glucagon or epinephrine test will show a greatly diminished rise in blood glucose and increase in blood lactate. The individual responses, however, are variable; therefore, specific assay of enzymes performed in vitro on liver biopsy material is necessary. The glycogen content of the liver tissue will be elevated in addition to the deficiency of glucose-6-phosphatase. In some patients with glucose-6-phosphatase deficiency, the morphology of liver tissue or a CAT scan of the liver may show evidence of adenomatous nodules. More rarely, hepatocellular carcinoma is found on liver biopsy.

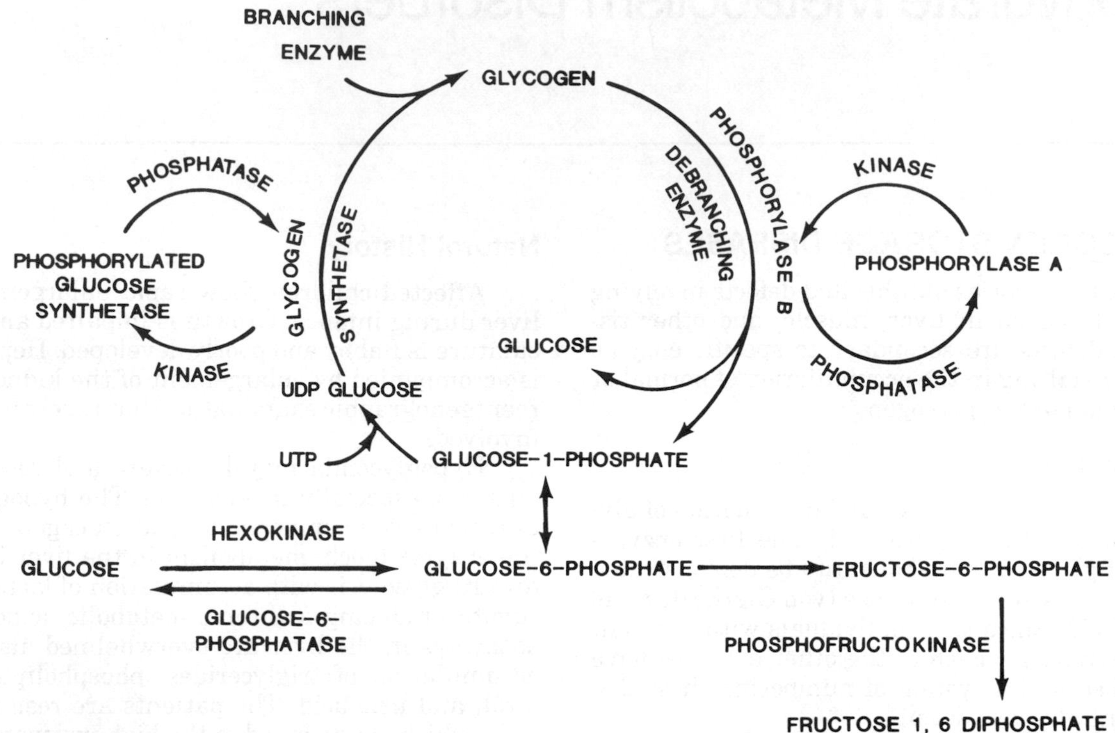

Figure 15.1. Pathways of glycogen metabolism.

Treatment

Restoration of normal blood glucose levels restores the biochemical abnormalities to normal and the child improves. The liver defect is bypassed by providing a steady input of glucose to the child (Folk and Greene, 1984). This is achieved by frequent feedings during the day coupled with continuous nasogastric feeding at night. Children on this regimen grow normally and manifest no biochemical abnormalities in the blood (Slonim et al, 1979).

As children grow older, oral feedings of uncooked corn starch made up in a slurry every 4–6 hours plus their regular diet maintains normal blood glucose and reversal of the biochemical abnormalities (Chen et al, 1984). The total glucose intake must be carefully calculated to avoid swings in blood glucose and insulin levels. This is a disorder that requires careful management of caloric and glucose intake in order to avoid triggering gluconeogenic responses in the liver, which may bring about a host of metabolic and hormonal changes. It is the latter that are responsible for the clinical syndrome of von Gierke disease.

In the past, patients with this disease have had portocaval shunting in order to have ingested substrates bypass the liver. Although growth afterward is improved, fasting hypoglycemia remains troublesome and the procedure is no longer recommended.

Prognosis

With continuous feeding regimens, these patients do very well. Growth is normal and all evidence of clinical von Gierke disease gradually disappears. As these children grow older, management may be more flexible, particularly with corn starch feedings to help maintain a more even glycemic response throughout a 24-hour day (Smit et al, 1984).

GSD Type II—α-1,4-Glucosidase (Acid Maltase Deficiency, Pompe Disease)

Definition

This disorder is characterized by a deficiency of the lysosomal enzyme α-1,4-glucosidase (acid α-glucosidase) with either a severe, fatal infantile form (Pompe disease) or a milder form starting in either childhood or adulthood.

Basic Science

This enzyme is responsible for breaking the α-1,4-linkages in glycogen in the process of its degradation within lysosomes. As a result of deficiency of this enzyme, glycogen accumulates in lysosomes of liver, muscle, heart, and in most other tissues. The gene for the enzyme is located on chromosome 17. A cDNA for human acid α-glucosidase has been used to investigate the defect (Martiniuk et al, 1986). The authors found absent mRNA for the enzyme in one patient with the infantile form of the disease and decreased size and amount of mRNA in an adult onset cell line. No major deletions were found in genomic DNA in patients with this disease, suggesting that a point mutation or a small deletion (or insertion) in the gene could be the origin of the defect.

Natural History

In the infantile form of this disease the patient presents with profound hypotonia, muscle weakness, and congestive heart failure during the first year of life. The heart is strikingly enlarged, but the liver is usually of normal size prior to the onset of cardiac decompensation. There are no abnormalities of glucose homeostasis, and blood lactate, uric acid, and lipid levels are normal. Most patients are dead by 1 year of age; the cause of death is cardiorespiratory failure, pneumonia, or aspiration.

In the slower form of the deficiency, the symptoms are primarily muscle weakness and hypotonia without clinical heart disease. Death (generally before 19 years of age) usually results from pneumonia and respiratory failure.

If the disorder starts in adulthood, the primary complaint is muscle weakness. The disease is slowly progressive and mimics other chronic myopathies.

Diagnosis

The diagnosis is established by the demonstration of an increased tissue (usually muscle biopsy) concentration of glycogen (seen on electron microscopy within the lysosomes) and an acid α-1,4-glucosidase deficiency. Properly prepared leukocytes may be used for diagnosis also (Broadhead et al, 1978). Fibroblasts cultured from amniotic fluid are reliable for prenatal diagnosis (Butterworth and Broadhead, 1977).

Treatment

There is no specific treatment as yet for this disorder.

Type III—Amylo-1,6-glucosidase (Debrancher) Deficiency

Definition

This enzyme deficiency results in (1) an accumulation of an abnormal glycogen with short outer branches and (2) a clinical picture similar to that of a mild von Gierke disease.

Basic Science

Only the outer residues of glycogen can be removed by phosphorylase. Debrancher enzyme catalyzes two successive reactions. It first transfers three glucosyl residues from a branch containing four residues onto another glycogen chain so as to lengthen it. This permits action of phosphorylase on the lengthened chain. The amylo-1,6-glucosidase then catalyzes the hydrolysis of the single residue remaining at the branch to yield free glucose. Starvation in GSD type III induces the degradation of glycogen to within four units of the branch point. Glycogen with such short outer chains is called a limit dextrin; the term limit dextrinosis is sometimes used for GSD type III.

Natural History

When limited to the liver, the clinical course of this GSD is milder than that of glucose-6-phosphatase deficiency. Hypoglycemia and growth defects are much milder and the serum concentrations of lactate, lipids and uric acid are generally normal. There is no renal enlargement in GSD type III in contrast to glucose-6-phosphatase deficiency. Hepatomegaly occurs in young patients but disappears at puberty in some. Moderate cardiomegaly is usually found.

In those patients lacking both liver and muscle debrancher enzymes, muscle weakness and short stature occur during childhood.

Galactose and fructose are readily converted to glucose in these patients in contrast to GSD type I where severe metabolic acidosis can be produced by administering these sugars.

The rise in blood glucose level after administration of epinephrine or glucagon is variable in these patients. A normal response to glucagon 2 hours after feeding, but not after a 14-hour fast has been reported.

In the older patients, muscle wasting and weakness may occur. Occasionally, the disorder presents in adulthood as a progressive muscle weakness.

Diagnosis

In addition to decreased or absent debrancher activity the glycogen content in liver is usually increased and is found to have short outer branches. Some patients have normal muscle glycogen content; in others it is elevated. Van Hoff and Hers (1967) have described a series of biochemical subtypes of debrancher deficiency.

Treatment

Frequent feedings are indicated for the child with symptoms of debrancher deficiency. Nocturnal nasogastric feedings have been very beneficial. High-protein feedings may be helpful in those patients with myopathy (Slonim et al, 1984).

Prognosis

The outlook for a long life is good. The development of myopathy and cardiac hypertrophy remains a concern.

GSD Type IV—α-1,4-Glucan:α-1,4-Glucan-6-α-glucosyltransferase (Brancher) Deficiency

Definition

This rare enzyme deficiency results in the synthesis of abnormal glycogen with reduced branching. The glycogen resembles amylopectin which is not normally present in liver and causes progressive fibrosis and cirrhosis.

Basic Science

This enzyme catalyzes the transfer of a segment of 1,4-residues from a chain of at least 11 residues in length to another segment at a point four residues removed from the nearest branch. In patients with clinical evidence of brancher deficiency, studies have shown a deficiency of brancher enzyme in liver and leukocytes.

Natural History

These patients appear normal at birth but soon fail to thrive. Hepatomegaly is seen early. The weight gain is poor and the liver and spleen increase progressively in size. There is actually a reduced amount of glycogen in the liver, the hepatomegaly being due to progressive fibrosis and cirrhosis. Neurologic dysfunction may include poor development, hypotonia, muscular atrophy, and decreased deep tendon reflexes. The neurologic findings correlate with autopsy data on the accumulation of amylopectin in the nervous system.

Diagnosis

A deficiency of brancher enzyme can be demonstrated in leukocytes and in fibroblasts as well as in liver tissue.

Treatment

These infants should be treated for the liver failure and ascites which develops.

Prognosis

Death in childhood, generally by the second year of life, is the rule.

GSD Type V—Muscle Phosphorylase Deficiency (McArdle Syndrome)

Definition

The lack of the enzyme in muscle which breaks the 1,6-linkages of glycogen to release glucose-1-phosphate causes muscular dysfunction. The latter is characterized by painful cramps on strenuous exercise, at a time when the stored glycogen in the muscle cell would ordinarily be used to provide energy.

Basic Science

The enzyme glycogen phosphorylase exists in three isoenzymatic forms: liver, muscle, and brain. The muscle form is the only isozyme expressed in skeletal muscle. Two patients with McArdle disease had a lack of mRNA for muscle phosphorylase (Daegelen et al, 1983). The gene which is located on chromosome 11 is small (13 kb). No major deletions or gene rearrangements have been described in patients with McArdle disease. For a more complete discussion see Gautron et al, 1987.

Natural History

Patients with muscle phosphorylase deficiency are clinically normal and have no abnormalities at rest. Liver phosphorylase is presumably normal. The patients are not hypoglycemic and have a normal response to glucagon.

Even in childhood, exercise is often tolerated well but with prolonged or severe exercise in adolescence or adulthood, the patient develops muscle cramps. If exercise is continued, myoglobinuria results. Characteristically, the patient with McArdle disease shows fewer symptoms after age 40 years but more wasting and weakness of muscles. Renal failure may occur secondary to the myoglobinuria.

Diagnosis

These patients demonstrate an absence of the rise in venous lactate which follows anaerobic exercise. A specific diagnosis is made on muscle biopsy tissue which shows an increased concentration of normal glycogen and a deficiency of glycogen phosphorylase. The activity of the enzyme in liver and smooth muscle is normal.

Treatment

Avoidance of extreme exercise is the best treatment. In some cases, isoproterenol, which increases (1) the concentration of fatty acids in serum and (2) the blood flow to muscle, has been successful in treating these patients. A high-protein diet will increase muscle endurance in these patients (Slonim and Goans, 1985).

Prognosis

The prognosis varies with the patient. Those patients with more severe symptoms may develop renal failure in late life. Most do well with restriction in exercise.

GSD Type VI—Liver Phosphorylase Deficiency (Hers Disease)

Definition

This is a disorder of diminished phosphorylase activity in liver and leukocytes.

Basic Science

The enzyme deficiency is difficult to differentiate from phosphorylase b kinase deficiency. Since there is about 25% of normal phosphorylase activity present in the liver, the patient is generally asymptomatic or has very mild symptoms.

Natural History

Affected children may have hepatomegaly early in life but they are usually asymptomatic. Hypoglycemia does not occur.

Diagnosis

The demonstration of low activity of the hepatic phosphorylase system is consistent with but not diagnostic of GSD type VI. The liver phosphorylase must be separated and assayed specifically for a definitive diagnosis.

Leukocytes may also show defective activity of glycogen phosphorylase; however, the enzyme may be inactivated to varying degrees by the isolation process itself. Thus, leukocyte assays are not always reliable.

Phosporylase activity in muscle is normal.

Treatment

There is no treatment.

Prognosis

The outlook is good.

GSD Type VII—Muscle Phosphofructokinase Deficiency

Definition

This disorder is characterized by a deficiency (1–3% of normal) of phosphofructokinase in muscle and erythrocytes but not in liver.

Basic Science

Phosphofructokinase is a tetrameric protein under the control of three structural genetic loci that code for muscle (M), liver (L), and platelet (P) subunits (DiMauro et al, 1986). Mature muscle expresses only M and, therefore, contains the tetramer M4. Erythrocytes express both M and L; therefore, the enzyme may be in the form M4 or L4 or as any one of three hybrids. In patients with GSD type VII, there is usually a 50% reduction in erythrocyte phosphofructokinase activity. Liver and kidney (which express L and P) are not affected. Heart and brain express all three subunits; therefore, these two tissues have a partial enzyme deficiency. Clinically, there is no evidence of cardiopathy or brain disease. The gene for the M subunit is on chromosome one, while the genes for L and P are on chromosomes 21 and 10, respectively.

Natural History

These patients appear clinically identical to patients with an absence of muscle phosphorylase activity.

Diagnosis

The diagnosis is established by the presence of painful cramps after exercise, the demonstration of no rise in venous lactate after anaerobic exercise, and muscle biopsy showing increased glycogen content and absence of phosphofructokinase activity. Hyperuricemia can be found after exercise; normal levels return after 48 hours of bed rest (Mineo et al, 1987).

Treatment

The avoidance of strenuous exercise is the only treatment suggested.

GSD VIII—Hepatic Phosphorylase b Kinase Deficiency

Definition

Glycogen phosphorylase requires specific enzymes for both activation and inactivation. In vitro studies showing reduced phosphorylase activity might arise from phosphorylase deficiency per se or from deficiency of the kinase which activates phosphorylase. Patients with the kinase deficiency show an X-linked inheritance of the disorder in most cases.

Natural History

Females who carry this gene (heterozygotes) may have modest hepatomegaly. Affected males (hemizygotes) have substantial hepatomegaly but no hypoglycemia or hyperlipidemia.

The response to epinephrine and glucagon is variable. Liver enzymes are elevated in plasma. The kinase may be assayed in liver biopsy and in fibroblasts or leukocytes. The content of glycogen in affected tissues is increased and the phosphorylase as well as kinase activities are reduced.

Treatment

There is no treatment.

Prognosis

The outlook is good.

Prenatal Diagnosis of the Glycogen Storage Diseases

Type I glycogen storage disease cannot be diagnosed prenatally because glucose-6-phosphatase is not present in normal cultured human fibroblasts. Techniques of molecular genetics should permit prenatal diagnosis in the near future.

Pompe disease and brancher deficiency can be reliably diagnosed in utero using fibroblasts grown from amniotic fluid (Butterworth and Broadhead, 1977).

Widespread tissue variability of debrancher deficiency makes prenatal diagnosis difficult. Other glycogen storage diseases are of such mild course that prenatal diagnosis is unwarranted.

GALACTOSE METABOLIC DEFECTS

Definition

Three inborn errors of galactose metabolism are known, each due to an inherited deficiency of one of the three enzymes of the galactose metabolic pathway whereby glucose 1-phosphate is formed (Fig. 15.2).

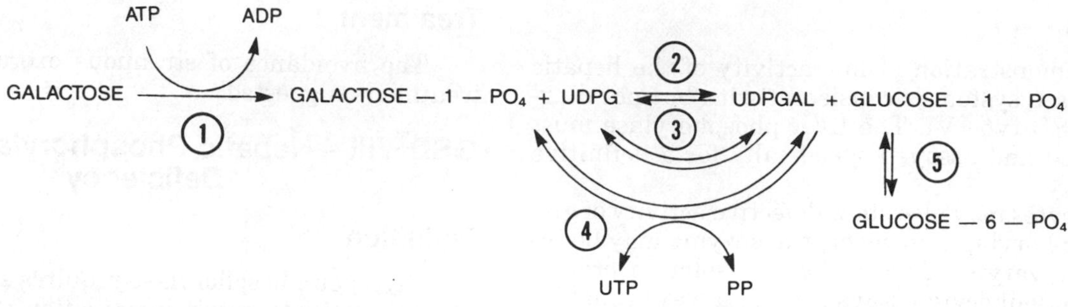

(1) GALACTOKINASE

(2) GALACTOSE — 1 — PHOSPHATE URIDYLTRANSFERASE

(3) URIDINE DIPHOSPHATE GALACTOSE — 4 — EPIMERASE

(4) URIDINE DIPHOSPHATE GALACTOSE (OR GLUCOSE) PYROPHOSPHORYLASE

(5) PHOSPHOGLUCOMUTASE

Figure 15.2. Pathway of galactose metabolism. The enzyme defects associated with disorders of galactose metabolism are: (*1*) galactokinase deficiency; (*2*) galactose-1-phosphate uridyl transferase deficiency; (*3*) uridine diphosphate galactose-4-epimerase deficiency.

Classical galactosemia, the best known and most frequent of these inborn errors, is due to a deficiency of galactose 1-phosphate uridyltransferase (transferase), a key enzyme in the pathway responsible for the transfer of galactose 1-phosphate to UDP-glucose, releasing glucose 1-phosphate and forming UDP-galactose. Galactokinase deficiency is due to a defect in galactokinase, the first enzyme in the pathway, which is responsible for the conversion of galactose to galactose 1-phosphate. The most recently described inborn error, UDP-galactose-4-epimerase (epimerase) deficiency, is due to deficiency of the enzyme that catalyzes the interconversion of UDP-galactose and UDP-glucose. All three disorders are inherited in an autosomal recessive fashion. (Komrower, 1982)

Basic Science

The sugar of milk is lactose, a glucose-galactose disaccharide. After ingestion, lactose is hydrolyzed by intestinal lactase releasing free glucose and galactose. These monosaccharides are absorbed into the portal system and enter the liver, where galactose is catabolized. A deficiency in galactose 1-phosphate uridyltransferase, characteristic of galactosemia, results in the accumulation of both galactose 1-phosphate and galactose, the latter due to product inhibition of galactokinase by the excess galactose 1-phosphate. In galactokinase deficiency, only galactose accumulates since the metabolic block prevents the phosphorylation of galactose to galactose 1-phosphate. In UDP-galactose-4-epimerase deficiency both galactose 1-phosphate and galactose accumulate, since this defect prevents the regeneration of UDP-glucose, thereby limiting the amounts of this cosubstrate for the transferase reaction. UDP-galactose also accumulates in epimerase deficiency.

Epidemiology

The prevalence of galactosemia is about 1/40,000 live births, that of galactokinase deficiency is of the order of 1/1 million live births, and that of epimerase deficiency is unknown at this time. It may be as rare as galactokinase deficiency.

Natural History

Neonates with galactosemia who are fed milk, either from the breast or formula, can present with a fulminant illness characterized by lethargy, feeding intolerance, weight loss, hyperbilirubinemia, and liver dysfunction with coagulopathy. About 25% of these infants develop sepsis, usually by the end of the first or second week of life, most often due to *Escherichia coli*. Physical examination discloses a lethargic, hypotonic infant with hepatomegaly and jaundice. Ophthalmologic examination often reveals the presence of "water droplet" cataracts. If milk is not withdrawn, and the infant spontaneously survives the neonatal illness, the disease produces mental retardation, cirrhosis, and cataracts. These features usually develop during the first year of life. Females also develop ovarian failure with streak ovaries in adolescence or young adult years. Most of the clinical features of galactosemia seem to be due to the accumulation of galactose 1-phosphate, since galactokinase deficient patients who accumulate galactose but not galactose 1-phosphate only develop cataracts.

Several variant transferase deficiency states exist in which patients have 10–35% of normal transferase activity, the most frequent of which is Duarte-galactosemia. Patients with these variants are usually asymptomatic but, on rare occasions, they can present with any of the clinical manifestations of galactosemia, depending on the degree of residual enzyme activity.

Patients with galactokinase deficiency develop cataracts as the sole manifestation of the disorder. The cataracts are due to the accumulation of galactitol, a metabolite of galactose which forms in the lens of the eye and is trapped there. This is also the origin of the cataracts in galactosemia.

Patients with the epimerase deficiency have only been recently described and little is known about the natural history of this disorder. It appears that those with an enzyme deficiency limited to the erythrocytes are asymptomatic, while those with a more generalized deficiency may have a phenotype similar to that seen in galactosemia, viz. failure to thrive, jaundice, hepatomegaly, and liver dysfunction.

Diagnosis

Since newborn screening for galactosemia is performed routinely in many states in the United States and in many countries of Europe and Asia, patients with galactosemia and sometimes other galactose metabolic defects are often identified by newborn screening before they become seriously ill. Screening identifies galactose and galactose 1-phosphate in the newborn blood specimen or transferase activity by a specific spot enzyme assay. The metabolite assay can lead to the diagnosis of any of the galactose metabolic defects: infants with galactosemia or epimerase deficiency will have increased levels of galactose and galactose 1-phosphate, while those with galactokinase deficiency will have only increased levels of galactose. The spot assay for transferase activity identifies infants with galactosemia or other transferase variants but will not identify infants with galactokinase and epimerase deficiencies.

In the absence of newborn screening, the diagnosis is suspected on the basis of clinical symptoms. A urine test for reducing substance ("Clinitest") should be performed. The presence of reducing substance that is not glucose ("Clinistix" negative) provides a presumptive diagnosis of galactosemia or other defect in galactose metabolism.

Once an infant has been identified by any of these methods, the diagnosis can be confirmed by assay of the appropriate enzyme in red blood cells, cultured fibroblasts, or liver. Patients who have received blood transfusions obviously will not be distinguished accurately by measurement of the enzymes in blood. Hence, at least 4 months should be allowed for the disappearance of donor erythrocytes before the enzyme is measured in these patients.

Blood should be collected for culture, liver function studies (including coagulation times), and measurements of galactose, galactose 1-phosphate, and galactose metabolic enzymes. Blood glucose also should be determined because of the frequency of hypoglycemia in galactosemia. Serum electrolyte levels should be obtained because symptomatic infants with galactosemia are often dehydrated. Since sepsis and bacterial meningitis represent such a dire threat to the neonate with galactosemia, cultures of urine and CSF are indicated.

Treatment

The infant should be admitted to the hospital, milk feedings discontinued, and intravenous glucose and electrolytes given. Intravenous antibiotics with coverage for Gram-negative organisms should be initiated. If a coagulopathy is present, fresh-frozen plasma and vitamin K may be required before lumbar puncture. Milk withdrawal will usually lead to clearing of galactose from the blood and urine within 24–48 hours. Galactose 1-phosphate also decreases markedly in the blood but will remain in the erythrocytes at a low level (1–3 mg/dl). Signs of liver disease usually disappear in 3–4 days. If the cultures are negative, antibiotics can be discontinued. After 1–2 days, feedings of a soy-based formula or other milk-free formula may begin.

Older children with galactosemia should remain on a milk-free diet with the addition of vitamins and calcium. The guidance of a nutritionist should be sought since milk solids are common additives in foods and lactose is used as a filler in many medications. Close attention to product labels and education of the parents and eventually the child are required. Compliance with the diet can be monitored by measuring galactose 1-phosphate in red blood cell or whole blood or urinary galactose. Nevertheless, even well-treated galactosemic patients may accumulate small amounts of galactose 1-phosphate in the blood. This is believed to be formed endogenously from UDP-glucose and may have a role in some of the complications of this disorder discussed below.

Patients with galactokinase deficiency are also put on a milk-free diet, which eliminates the galactose and prevents the development of cataracts.

Patients with epimerase deficiency who are symptomatic should be treated in the same way as those with galactosemia. Milk restriction has modified the clinical and biochemical abnormalities. These patients may require a small amount of galactose to promote the synthesis of galactosides, including the brain gangliosides.

Prognosis

Children with galactosemia in whom treatment begins early in life do not develop the classical triad of mental retardation, cirrhosis, and cataracts. It has been recognized, however, that even well-treated patients may develop learning disabilities, speech and language difficulties, neurologic disease, and behavioral problems (Fishler et al, 1972; Lo et al, 1984; Waisbren et al, 1983). In addition, girls with galactosemia develop gonadal (ovarian) failure (Kaufman et al, 1981; Kaufman et al, 1986). This is hypergonadotrophic in nature and seems to be independent of early treatment or dietary compliance. The problems associated with ovarian failure include not only amenorrhea or oligomenorrhea and infertility, but also poor secondary sexual development and osteoporosis due to estrogen deficiency. Hormones may be required at puberty to produce pubertal changes. Current research is underway in various laboratories to determine the cause of these complications.

Milk restriction seems to prevent cataracts in children with galactokinase deficiency. Little is known about the eventual outcome of symptomatic children with epimerase deficiency.

Prevention

Prenatal diagnosis of galactosemia is available through amniocentesis and subsequent measurement of transferase activity in cultured amniocytes. The first trimester diagnosis of galactosemia by chorionic villus sampling and transferase assay has also been reported (Kleijer et al, 1986).

Mothers at risk for having galactosemic children are often placed on a milk-restricted diet with calcium supplementation during pregnancy on the premise that this may decrease the galactose load to the fetus and thereby eliminate the complications of the disease.

CASE ILLUSTRATION

The newborn screening blood specimen collected at 36 hours of age from a 4-day-old female infant and tested in the Newborn Screening Program at the State Laboratory Institute contained markedly increased galactose and galactose 1-phosphate. No galactose 1-phosphate uridyltransferase activity was detected by the Beutler spot test. The pediatrician was informed of these findings and told that galactosemia was the suspected diagnosis. The infant had been clinically normal. The pediatrician saw the infant that day and found that the urine was strongly positive for reducing substance. He referred the infant to the Children's Hospital, Boston, where she was seen that evening in the Emergency Room by a metabolic specialist.

History revealed normal, full-term pregnancy, labor, and delivery. Birth weight was 3100 g. The infant was formula-fed, did well in the nursery, and was discharged at 36 hours of age. At home she had been well until the day she was seen when she appeared somewhat lethargic and began feeding less vigorously than before. On physical examination in the Emergency Room she weighed 2900 g (200 grams less than birth weight), was mildly jaundiced, had slightly reduced activity, and was mildly hypotonic. There were no other abnormal findings. In particular, she did not have hepatosplenomegaly and her eyes appeared normal with no gross evidence of cataract.

Venipuncture was performed to obtain blood for studies. During and following venipuncture it was noted that multiple bruises appeared on her arm and that bleeding at the site of the venipuncture continued for 15 minutes despite vigorous pressure to control bleeding. Coagulopathy was suspected and was confirmed by a prothrombin time 51.0/12.8 seconds and partial thromboplastin time $>$ 100/33 seconds. Other laboratory results included SGOT 600 U, SGPT 500 U, LDH 750 U, alkaline phosphatase 355 U, bilirubin 5.5 total/1.7 mg/dl direct, blood glucose 50 mg/dl, and urine positive for reducing substance but negative for glucose.

It was clear that this 4-day-old infant had galactosemia and that the disorder had already caused severe liver dysfunction despite the absence of hepatomegaly and other clinical findings that would have pointed to liver disease. Her lethargy and poor feeding with weight loss also indicated the beginning of a CNS effect from the galactosemia.

Cultures of blood, urine, and CSF were obtained and, because of the high frequency of sepsis among galactosemic neonates, intravenous antibiotic therapy was begun. Attention was given to coverage for Gram-negative sepsis, particularly *E. coli,* since this organism accounts for at least 80% of the sepsis in galactosemia. The intravenous fluid also contained glucose and maintenance electrolytes. Formula feeding was discontinued. Additional blood was collected for quantitative assay of galactose 1-phosphate uridyltransferase which later was reported to be undetectable, consistent with classic galactosemia.

During the next 4 days of hospitalization, the infant improved. Urine was examined daily; reducing substance had disappeared by the end of the first hospital day. Examination of blood for galactose and galactose 1-phosphate by daily filter paper blood collection and testing at the State Laboratory disclosed disappearance of these metabolites by the end of the second hospital day. Serum bilirubin rose to 10 total/4.0 direct mg/dl on the second hospital day, but by the fourth day had declined to 3.5 total/1.6 direct mg/dl. Her coagulopathy also began to resolve and by the fourth hospital day her PT was 39/12.5 seconds and PTT 74/33 seconds. Other tests of liver function returned to normal. Cultures remained negative and antibiotics were discontinued on the fourth day. Ophthalmologic examination by direct ophthalmoscopy and slit-lamp revealed "water droplet" cataracts without opacity in both lenses. She was begun on a soy-based formula. By the fifth hospital day when she was discharged, she weighed 3200 g (gain of 300 g from admission), was active, and had normal muscle tone.

At outpatient follow-up 1 week later, she was clinically normal. Her coagulopathy had cleared as evidenced by PT 11.5/12.5 seconds and PTT 29.3/33 seconds. She continued with the soy-based formula and has followed a milk-free diet since beginning solid foods. At 2 years of age she is a healthy girl with normal growth and development. Her urine has consistently been free of reducing substance and her blood has had no detectable galactose and only a trace of galactose-1-phosphate. Nevertheless, she has early signs of an expressive language defect and of hypergonadotrophic hypogonadism, complications often observed despite early diagnosis and treatment.

Nevertheless, galactose 1-phosphate has been elevated in cord blood even in galactosemic infants of mothers who strictly adhered to the diet. Therefore, it appears that the galactosemic fetus can produce galactose 1-phosphate endogenously (Irons et al, 1985).

HEREDITARY FRUCTOSE INTOLERANCE

Definition

Hereditary fructose intolerance is an autosomal recessive inborn error of metabolism due to a deficiency of fructose 1-phosphate aldolase, one of the enzymes of the fructose catabolic pathway. This deficiency results in loss of the ability to metabolize fructose 1-phosphate. Affected infants have recurrent vomiting, fail to grow, and may develop severe liver disease following the introduction of fructose in the diet.

Basic Science

Affected individuals have a deficiency of the enzyme fructose 1-phosphate aldolase B which can be demonstrated in the liver, kidney cortex, and small intestine. After ingestion of fructose, patients with hereditary fructose intolerance accumulate fructose 1-phosphate and become hypoglycemic due to inhibition of gluconeogenesis. Intracellular phosphate is depleted and inorganic phosphate in serum is decreased. Increased serum magnesium may reflect reduced ATP in fructose-metabolizing tissues, with release of cellular magnesium, since ATP is a strong chelator of magnesium.

Epidemiology

The prevelence of this disorder is about 1/20,000 in Switzerland. This may be an underestimate since many affected children and adults may remain undiagnosed (Gitzelmann et al, 1983). It is diagnosed much less frequently in the United States.

Natural History

The ingestion of fructose or sucrose (a fructose containing disaccharide) initiates symptoms in patients with this disorder. Conversely, affected children and adults may remain healthy as long as they do not ingest fructose or sucrose. Accordingly, breast-fed infants remain normal until they are weaned and fruits and vegetables are introduced. The most common reason for clinical presentation in the neonate or young infant is the ingestion of a soybean-based formula containing sucrose.

Symptomatic infants and young children have feeding intolerance, fail to thrive and often vomit. Less frequent symptoms at this age include hypoglycemia (which may be short-lived), metabolic acidosis, lethargy, hepatic dysfunction with coagulopathy, shock, seizures, renal tubular acidosis, hypoproteinemia, rickets, or seizures. The diagnosis is difficult when the young infant presents only with failure to thrive and acidosis.

When undiagnosed during infancy, the disease process continues with exacerbations and remissions depending on the dietary intake of fructose. As they grow older, most children develop an aversion to sweets and, through this self-restriction, remain in "remission." The most prominent symptoms in older children include hepatomegaly and poor growth; acute episodes of illness are rare. Some patients may be diagnosed in childhood during evaluation for hepatomegaly while adults may be discovered only by chance or after the diagnosis in a relative.

Diagnosis

The diagnosis of hereditary fructose intolerance should be suspected from the clinical signs and symp-

CASE ILLUSTRATION

This youngster was first seen at The Children's Hospital at 19 months of age for evaluation of poor growth and recurrent vomiting and diarrhea. He was below the fifth percentile for both height and weight, length 74 cm, weight 7.14 kg.

He weighed 4 lb 13 oz at term (by dates) and was observed for 15 days after birth in hospital of birth because of a nuchal cord and fetal bradycardia. He had an initial serum glucose of 23 mg/dl but no further hypoglycemia in the newborn period.

At 3 months of age he weighed 9 lb 2 oz but had sufficient recurrent vomiting that he was admitted to another hospital for evaluation of either pyloric stenosis or chalasia. His hematocrit at the time was 32%. Otherwise, all studies, including sweat test, stool fat, and immunoglobulins were normal.

He was described by his mother as a finicky eater, which was also noted during the hospitalization.

During the admission to The Children's Hospital, a diet assistant noted that the mother reported the child refused all sweets. The infant was observed to refuse Isomil in the hospital but took glucose solutions. Extensive psychiatric and social service evaluations were undertaken as well as observations by the "feeding" team. The conclusion was that he had the ability to eat but had a very variable appetite. A referral was made to an early intervention program and no specific medical reason for his persistent vomiting and poor appetite was ascertained.

At age 2 years, he was re-evaluated and found to have hepatosplenomegaly. This resulted in a subsequent admission, where hypoglycemia was documented and intolerance to an oral fructose load was established by increased lactate levels and gastrointestinal symptoms. Hereditary fructose intolerance was diagnosed.

In retrospect, the history of aversion to all sweets made sense. The fact that this was overlooked by innumerable doctors, even though his mother was quick to make the observation, is a lesson not to be forgotten. The child subsequently did very well on a diet that was fructose- and sucrose-free. The mother's reaction to all of this was: "you mean I'm not crazy."

toms, as well as from a careful history, particularly a nutritional history. Reducing substance in the urine (fructose and/or glucose), hyperaminoaciduria, and increased blood methionine and tyrosine (usually secondary to liver involvement) are common. The beneficial effect of fructose withdrawal either by discontinuation of dietary fructose or by the administration of intravenous fluids with glucose favors the diagnosis.

The diagnosis can be confirmed either by assay of the enzyme in a liver biopsy specimen or by an intravenous fructose loading test. This loading test should be performed only after several weeks of abstinence from fructose. The moderate challenge dose of 200 mg/kg should be used since higher doses can precipitate fatal metabolic consequences (Steinmann and Gitzelmann, 1981). Affected individuals will develop hypoglycemia, reduced serum phosphate and increased serum magnesium and uric acid in response to the fructose load.

Treatment

Treatment of an acute episode includes the elimination of sucrose and fructose from the diet and the administration of intravenous fluids containing glucose. Correction of the coagulopathy might require the administration of fresh-frozen plasma. Liver and kidney symptoms may not resolve for several days.

Chronic treatment includes the avoidance of sucrose or fructose in the diet. Patients should inform health providers of their diagnosis since many intravenous fluid solutions contain fructose or sorbitol which may be life-threatening to affected individuals.

Prognosis

After recovery from an acute episode and with continued restriction of fructose, patients experience catch-up growth and develop normally. Intellectual function is said to be normal in treated patients. Small children may continue to have hepatomegaly despite adequate dietary therapy (Odievre et al, 1978).

Fructose-1,6-Diphosphatase Deficiency

Definition

Fructose-1,6-diphosphatase deficiency is an inborn error of the gluconeogenic pathway. It appears to be an autosomal recessive disorder. The clinical phenotype includes neonatal ketoacidosis, lethargy, and hepatic disease.

Basic Science

The enzyme defect, fructose-1,6-diphosphatase, is demonstrable in liver, jejunum, kidney, and leukocytes. Gluconeogenesis is severely impaired since this is a key gluconeogenic enzyme.

Epidemiology

The exact incidence of this disorder is not known. As of 1983, 38 cases were reported in the literature (Gitzelmann et al, 1983).

Natural History

This is a severe and life-threatening disorder. About half of the patients present in the first 4 days of life, with hyperventilation, ketoacidosis, lethargy, hypotonia, hepatomegaly, and hypoglycemia (Baerlocher et al, 1971). Episodes in older children usually occur during periods of febrile illness or infection and are precipitated by fasting and/or vomiting. Affected children who have fasted can very quickly develop ketoacidosis and hypoglycemia with hyperventilation, lethargy, seizures, hepatomegaly, and muscle weakness. In contrast to hereditary fructose intolerance, hepatic dysfunction, renal tubular acidosis, and a history of aversion to sweets are usually absent.

Since fructose-1,6-diphosphatase is so important for gluconeogenesis, patients become dependent on dietary glucose. They also have a reduced tolerance to fructose and sorbitol, which can cause reactive hypoglycemia. Prolonged fasting results in hypoglycemia when the liver shifts from glycogenolysis to gluconeogenesis for energy production.

Diagnosis

The diagnosis is confirmed by demonstration of the enzyme deficiency in liver or leukocytes (Alexander et al, 1985). Fasting and tolerance tests should not be performed until several weeks after an acute illness, and then only with caution. As in hereditary fructose intolerance, an intravenous fructose tolerance test with a moderate dose of 200 mg/kg of fructose is recommended (Gitzelmann et al, 1983). This will result in reduced blood glucose and phosphate and increased lactate, uric acid, magnesium, and alanine in affected individuals.

Acute episodes are treated by correction of the hypoglycemia and acidosis with intravenous solutions of glucose and sodium bicarbonate.

Chronic treatment includes avoidance of fasting and the elimination of fructose and sucrose in the diet. Acute exacerbations of the disease with illness can usually be treated by avoiding fasting, and administering glucose and/or sodium bicarbonate.

Prognosis

The prognosis after prompt diagnosis and with institution of adequate therapy may be good.

Prevention

Heterozygote detection has been reported by assay of the enzyme in leukocytes (Alexander et al, 1985). Hence, prenatal diagnosis from fetal blood samples is potentially possible.

PYRUVIC ACIDEMIAS

Pyruvate Dehydrogenase (PDH) Complex Deficiency

Definition

Pyruvate dehydrogenase deficiency leads to pyruvate accumulation and lactic acidosis, defined as a blood lactate level greater than 2 mMol/L.

Basic Science

Anaerobic glycolysis leads to the production of pyruvate. Much of the pyruvate is reduced to lactate, producing a lactate to pyruvate ratio of approximately 10:1. Pyruvate is also aerobically degraded to acetyl-CoA or to form oxaloacetate (Fig. 15.3). Disorders of pyruvate degradation produce lactic acid accumulation (lactic acidosis) as well as increased blood pyruvate. In lactic acidosis secondary to hypoxia, the lactate to pyruvate ratio is increased because of a shift from aerobic to anaerobic glycolysis and an increased intracellular ratio of NADH to NAD, which drives pyruvate reduction to lactate. Common causes of secondary lactic acidosis include those leading to tissue hypoxia such as shock, sepsis, congenital heart disease, some of the organic acid metabolic disorders, malignancies, and severe illness. Primary lactic acidosis is either idiopathic or due to a defect in pyruvate catabolism.

Mammalian PDH complex is located in the inner mitochondrial membrane. Its primary function is to control the supply and oxidative metabolism of two-carbon fragments derived from carbohydrates and amino acids (Stansbie, 1986),

The complex is under tight metabolic control. It consists of three catalytic enzymes arranged in a cubic cluster (E_1-pyruvate dehydrogenase, E_2-dihydrolipoyl transacetylase, E_3-dihydrolipoyl dehydrogenase), two regulatory enzymes (Mg^{++}-ATP-dependent protein kinase and phosphoprotein phosphatase) which, respectively, inhibit or activate the E_1 component of the complex, and five cofactors (thiamine pyrophosphate, lipoic acid, coenzyme A, flavin adenine dinucleotide, and NAD^+). Clearly, there are numerous potential sites for mutations, any one of which could result in deficient PDH activity. This complexity also leads to difficulties in measuring activities of the different components.

The main function of the PDH complex is to catalyze the oxidative decarboxylation of pyruvate to form acetyl-CoA, CO_2, and reduced NAD^+ (Fig. 15.3). Since acetyl-CoA is a central intermediate in oxidative and biosynthetic pathways and is critical for the production of citrate, the major metabolic problem seen in affected individuals is the energy deficit that results from deficient production of acetyl-CoA. This energy deficit becomes especially critical during illness, starvation, and other causes of metabolic stress.

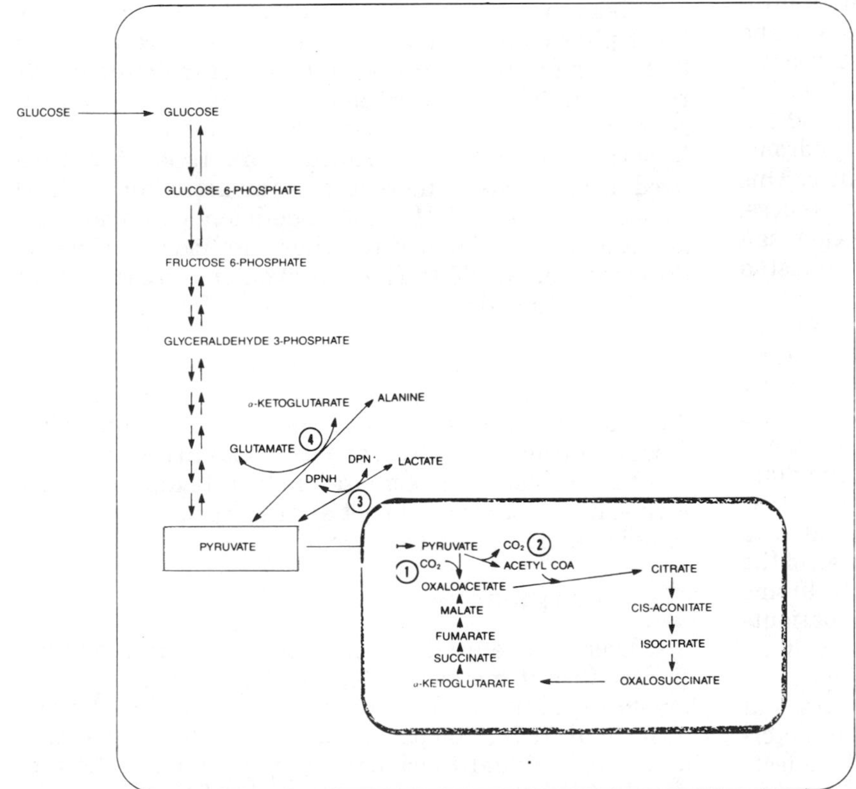

Figure 15.3. Pathway for pyruvate production and metabolism. (*1*) Pyruvate carboxylase. (2) Pyruvate dehydrogenase complex.

Epidemiology

The incidence of this disorder is unknown. Primary lactic acidosis is inherited in an autosomal recessive manner.

Natural History

The majority of reported cases have had a defect attributed to the E_1 component of the complex, although because of the aforementioned difficulties in measurement of activities of the components of the complex, some may have been misclassified. Thus, the natural history of the various disorders is not known with certainty (Stansbie 1986).

Patients with deficiencies of the E_1 component appear to fall into two clinical groups: those who are generally in the second decade of life and present with attacks of intermittent cerebellar ataxia and weakness, usually following a febrile illness; and those in the second group who typically present in the first few hours to few months of life with severe metabolic acidosis and hypotonia. These infants usually die during the first years of life. Psychomotor retardation, seizures (often myoclonic), ophthalmoplegia, optic atrophy, microcephaly, and facial dysmorphisms have been reported in both groups of patients.

Patients with deficiency of the E_2 component present with severe neurologic disease, usually from birth, leading to profound psychomotor retardation. Optic atrophy and microcephaly also have been reported.

Like patients in the second group with E_1 deficiency, those with deficiency of the E_3 component present as neonates with severe metabolic acidosis and hypotonia. They usually die within the first 2 years.

There has also been one reported patient with a pyruvate dehydrogenase complex activity of 10–30% of normal who had a central hypoventilation syndrome and who required chronic ventilatory assistance. This patient also had intermittent ataxia and weakness, psychomotor retardation, seizures, ophthalmoplegia, and changes in pigment in the retinal epithelium (Johnston et al, 1984).

There is some confusion whether patients with Leigh disease, or subacute necrotizing encephalomyelopathy, have pyruvate metabolic defects. There have been many reports of children with ataxia, hypotonia, seizures, and developmental retardation who had increased blood levels of lactate and pyruvate, and in whom the diagnosis of subacute necrotizing encephalomyelopathy was made at autopsy. Patients have been documented to show deficiency of total pyruvate dehydrogenase, of the E_1 component, of pyruvate carboxylase, or cytochrome oxidase. To add to the confusion, many other patients with subacute necrotizing encephalomyopathy diagnosed at autopsy have had no abnormalities of pyruvate metabolism. For the moment at least, it appears that Leigh disease is a clinically and biochemically heterogeneous group of disorders that may include defects in pyruvate metabolism.

Diagnosis

The common biochemical abnormalities seen in patients with PDH complex deficiencies include increased levels of lactate and pyruvate in blood, with preservation of the normal lactate to pyruvate ratio and increased levels of alanine and/or proline in the blood and urine. Patients with E_3 deficiency also have increased levels of the branched-chain amino acids and 2-oxo glutamate in blood and urine. Some patients also have increased blood ammonia levels. Acutely ill patients can present with severe metabolic acidosis and lactic aciduria.

Definitive diagnosis requires demonstration of the specific enzyme deficiency. Measurement of the different components is possible in fibroblasts, leukocytes, platelets, and liver, muscle, brain, or other tissue.

Of 40 cases with lactic acidosis, a specific diagnosis was made by biochemical study of cultured skin fibroblasts in 14. Eight had a deficiency of the PDH complex, five had pyruvate carboxylase deficiency, and one had phosphoenolpyruvate carboxylase deficiency (Robinson et al, 1980). Therefore, the majority of patients with lactic acidosis are still without a specific metabolic diagnosis even with use of current assay systems.

Treatment

Treatment of acute metabolic acidosis in these patients may require large doses of intravenous bicarbonate or acetate (often 1 mEq/kg/hour). If this therapy is not effective, hemodialysis may be necessary. Large concentrations of glucose should *not* be given as this may lead to even higher levels of pyruvate and lactate. Most physicians caring for these patients recommend 3–4 mg/kg/min of glucose, unless metabolic demands require higher concentrations of glucose. Sodium benzoate has also been used successfully for treatment of hyperammonemia (McCormick et al, 1985). We have used intravenous dichloroacetate (an activator of PDH) in one child with PDH complex deficiency in whom the acidosis was refractory to other methods of therapy (Stacpoole et al, 1983). The improvement occurred more slowly than would have been expected from a dichloroacetate effect.

Chronic treatment of these patients, involving the use of thiamine, lactogenic (high fat, low carbohydrate) diets, and/or bicarbonate or citrate, has been somewhat disappointing. These therapeutic modalities may control the acidosis and decrease the lactate and pyruvate levels, but apparently do not alter the progressive neurologic deterioration that occurs.

CONTROVERSY

Dichloroacetate has been used orally in a few patients since it has been successful in lowering lactate levels in adults with secondary lactic acidosis (Stacpoole et al, 1978; Stacpoole et al, 1983). Dichloroacetate activates residual PDH activity by inhibiting the protein kinase, the regulatory inhibitor of the E_1 component of the complex. In one child with PDH complex deficiency, oral dichloroacetate lowered the lactate and pyruvate levels, but it did not alter the clinical course of the disease (McCormick et al, 1985). There is concern about the chronic use of dichloroacetate since it can cause paralysis in dogs and has been implicated in polyneuropathy in an adult (Stacpoole et al, 1979).

Prognosis

The prognosis for most of these patients is poor. Current treatment modalities only appear to stabilize the biochemical abnormalities and do not alter the chronic course of the illness.

Prevention

Prenatal diagnosis is theoretically possible by means of assay of the enzyme in cultured amniotic fluid cells. This may be considered in families where deficiencies of total PDH or one of the components have been demonstrated in cultured fibroblasts.

Pyruvate Carboxylase Deficiency

Definition

Pyruvate carboxylase deficiency can occur as one component of multiple carboxylase deficiency or as an isolated deficiency. It is one cause of primary lactic acidosis.

Basic Science

Pyruvate carboxylase catalyzes the conversion of pyruvate to oxaloacetate, the first reaction of gluconeogenesis (Fig. 15.3). This reaction also provides the 4-carbon intermediate for the Krebs cycle.

Epidemiology

The incidence of this defect is not known. It is inherited as an autosomal recessive trait.

Natural History

Several different clinical presentations have been reported in pyruvate carboxylase deficiency (Blass, 1983). One group of patients presented in early childhood with seizures, psychomotor retardation, hypotonia, acidosis, and chronic neurologic deterioration. Others presented with a severe ataxic encephalopathy or with findings consistent with a diagnosis of Leigh disease (see discussion of PDH complex deficiency in previous section). Patients have also presented in the neonatal period, often on the first day of life, with severe acidosis and hypoglycemia.

Diagnosis

Affected individuals have increased levels of lactate and pyruvate in blood and of alanine and/or proline in blood and urine. Hypoglycemia and ketosis also may be present.

Definitive diagnosis requires the demonstration of the enzyme deficiency in cultured skin fibroblasts, lymphocytes, liver, brain, or other tissue.

Treatment

Treatment of an acute episode may require large amounts of intravenous bicarbonate for correction of the acidosis. Chronic treatment has included the use of thiamine, which has led to decreased lactate levels in some cases.

Prognosis

Although treatment may lead to decrease in lactate levels, the chronic progression of the disorder appears not to be altered.

Prevention

Heterozygote detection is possible by the demonstration of intermediate levels of enzyme activities in fibroblasts and lymphocytes.

Prenatal diagnosis has been performed by assay of the enzyme in cultured amniotic fluid cells obtained at 17 weeks gestation (Marsac et al, 1982).

REFERENCES

Alexander D, Assaf M, Khudr A, et al: Fructose-1-6-diphosphatase deficiency: Diagnosis using leukocytes and detection of heterozygotes with radiochemical and spectrophotometric methods. *J Inher Metabol Dis* 8:174, 1985.

Baerlocher K, Gitzelmann R, Nussli R, et al: Infantile lactic acidosis due to hereditary fructose 1,6-diphosphatase deficiency. *Helv Paediatr Acta* 26:489, 1971.

Baker L, Wingrad AI: Fasting hypoglycaemia and metabolic acidosis associated with deficiency of hepatic fructose-1,6-diphosphatase activity. *Lancet* 2:13, 1970.

Blass JP: Inborn errors of pyruvate metabolism. In Stanbury JB, et al (eds): *The Metabolic Bases of Inherited Disease.* New York, McGraw-Hill, 1983, p. 193.

Broadhead DM, Butterworth J: Alpha-glucosidase in Pompe's disease. *J Inher Metabol Dis* 1:153, 1978.

Butterworth J, Broadhead DM: Diagnosis of Pompe's disease in cultured skin fibroblasts and primary amniotic fluid cells using 4-methylumbelliferyl-alpha-D-glucopyranoside as substrate. *Clin Chim Acta* 78:335, 1977.

Chen YT, Cornblath M, Sidbury JB: Cornstarch therapy in Type I glycogen storage disease. *N Engl J Med* 310:171, 1984.

Chen YT, Coleman RA, Scheinman JI, et al: Renal disease in type I glycogen storage disease. *N Engl J Med* 318:7, 1988.

Daegelen D, Munnich A, Levin MJ, et al: Absence of functional messenger RNA for glycogen phosphorylase in the muscle of two patients with McArdle's disease. *Ann Hum Genet* 47:107, 1983.

DiMauro S, Miranda AF, Sakoda S, et al: Metabolic myopathies. *Am J Med Gen* 25:635, 1986.

Fishler K, Donnell GN, Bergren WR, et al: Intellectual and personality development in children with galactosemia. *Pediatrics* 50:412, 1972.

Folk CC, Greene HL: Dietary management of Type I glycogen storage disease. *J Am Diet Assoc* 84:293, 1984.

Gautron S, Daegelen D, Mennecier F, et al: Molecular mechanisms of McArdle's disease. *J Clin Invest* 79:275, 1987.

Gitzelmann R, Steinmann B, Van Den Berghe G: Essential fructosuria, hereditary fructose intolerance, and fructose-1,6, diphosphatase deficiency. In Stanbury JB, et al (eds): *The Metabolic Basis of Inherited Disease.* New York, McGraw-Hill, 1983, pp. 118–140.

Irons M, Levy HL, Pueschel S, et al: The accumulation of galactose-1-phosphate in the galactosemic fetus despite milk avoidance. *J Pediatr* 107:261, 1985.

Johnston K, Newth CJL, Sheu K-FR, et al: Central hypoventilation syndrome in pyruvate dehydrogenase complex deficiency. *Pediatrics* 74:1034, 1984.

Kaufman FR, Kogut MD, Donnell GN, et al: Hypergonadotrophic hypogonadism in female patients with galactosemia. *N Engl J Med* 304:994, 1981.

Kaufman FR, Donnell GN, Roe TF, et al: Gonadal function in patients with galactosaemia. *J Inher Metabol Dis* 9:140, 1986.

Kleijer WJ, Janse HC, Van Diggelsen OP, et al: First-trimester diagnosis of galactosemia. *Lancet* 1:748, 1986.

Komrower GM: Galactosaemia thirty years on: The experience of a generation. *J Inher Metabol Dis* 5(suppl): 96, 1982.

Lo W, Packman S, Nash S, et al: Curious neurologic sequelae in galactosemia. *Pediatrics* 73:309, 1984.

Marsac C, Augereau C, Feldman G, et al: Prenatal diagnosis of pyruvate carboxylase deficiency. *Clin Chem Acta* 119:121, 1982.

Martiniuk F, Mehler M, Pellicer A, et al: Isolation of a cDNA for human acid alpha-glucosidase and detection of genetic heterogeneity for mRNA in three alpha-glucosidase deficient patients. *Proc Natl Acad Sci* 83:9641, 1986.

McCormick K, Viscardi RM, Robinson B, Heininger J: Partial pyruvate decarboxylase deficiency with profound lactic acidosis and hyperammonemia: Responses to dichloroacetate and benzoate. *Am J Med Genet* 22:291, 1985.

Mineo I, Kono N, Hara N, et al: Myogenic hyperuricemia a common pathophysiological feature of glycogenosis types III, V and VII. *N Engl J Med* 317:75, 1987.

Narisawa K, Otomo H, Igarashi Y, et al: Glycogen storage disease Type Ib: Microsomal glucose-6-phosphatase system in two patients with different clinical findings. *Pediatr Res* 17:545, 1983.

Odievre M, Gentil C, Gautier M, Alagille D: Hereditary fructose intolerance in childhood. *Am J Dis Child* 132:605, 1978.

Robinson BH, Taylor J, Sherwood WG: The genetic heterogeneity of lactic acidosis: occurrence of recognizable inborn errors of metabolism in a pediatric population with lactic acidosis. *Pediatr Res* 14:956, 1980.

Slonim AE, Coleman RA, Moses WS: Myopathy and growth failure in debrancher enzyme deficiency: Improvement with high-protein nocturnal enteral therapy. *J Pediatr* 105:906, 1984.

Slonim AE, Goans PJ: Myopathy in McArdle's syndrome: Improvement with a high protein diet. *N Engl J Med* 312:355, 1985.

Slonim AE, Lacy WW, Terry A, et al: Nocturnal intragastric therapy in type I glycogen storage disease: Effect on hormonal and amino acid metabolism. *Metabolism* 28:707, 1979.

Smit GPA, Berger R, Potasnick R, et al: The dietary treatment of children with Type I glycogen storage disease with slow release carbohydrate. *Pediatr Res* 18:879, 1984.

Stacpoole PW, Moore GW, Kornhauser DM: Metabolic effects of dichloroacetate in patients with diabetes mellitus and hyperlipoproteinemia. *N Engl J Med* 298:526, 1978.

Stacpoole PW, Moore GW, Kornhauser DM: Toxicity of chronic dichloroacetate. *N Engl J Med* 300:372, 1979.

Stacpoole PW, Harman EM, Curry SH, et al: Treatment of lactic acidosis with dichloroacetate. *N Engl J Med* 309:390, 1983.

Stansbie D, Wallace SJ, Marsac C: Disorders of the pyruvate dehydrogenase complex. *J Inher Metabol Dis* 9:105, 1986.

Steinmann B, Gitzelmann R: The diagnosis of hereditary fructose intolerance. *Helv Paediatr Acta* 36:297, 1981.

Van Hoff F, Hers HG: The subgroups of type III glycogenosis. *Eur J Biochem* 2:265, 1967.

Waisbren SE, Normal TR, Schnell RR, et al: Speech and language deficits in early-treated children with galactosemia. *J Pediatr* 102:75, 1983.

Inborn Errors of Amino Acid Metabolism 2

Evaluation for metabolic disease in children with developmental delay, clinical illness, or positive results from routine newborn screening usually includes the measurement of amino acids in the blood, urine, or both, since amino acid disorders are among the most frequently identified inborn errors of metabolism. Although many of these disorders are extremely rare, others are more frequent and are likely to be encountered because of their clinical presentation in infancy or from routine newborn screening. Therapy may prevent irreversible damage or even death in many of these disorders; for optimal benefit treatment must be initiated as soon as possible, often within the first few days or weeks of life.

PHENYLKETONURIA

Definition

Phenylketonuria (PKU) is an inborn error of metabolism involving the major degradative pathway of the amino acid phenylalanine. The salient biochemical feature is an increased level of phenylalanine in the blood (hyperphenylalaninemia). PKU should always be identified by routine newborn screening as will infants with incomplete blocks in phenylalanine metabolism such as atypical PKU and mild persistent hyperphenylalaninemia.

Basic Science

PKU results from deficient activity of phenylalanine hydroxylase, the enzyme responsible for conversion of phenylalanine to tyrosine (Fig. 15.4). This enzyme is encoded by a gene located on chromosome 12. In PKU, this gene is mutant on both homologous chromosomes. Phenylalanine hydroxylase deficiency results in the accumulation of phenylalanine in the blood, urine, CSF, and tissues when the diet is normal. Phenylalanine metabolites such as phenylpyruvic acid, phenyllactic acid, phenylacetic acid, phenylacetylglutamine, and hydroxyphenylacetic acid are also present in the urine. The name "phenylketonuria" is derived from the presence in the urine of phenylpyruvic acid, a phenylketone. If some residual phenylalanine hydroxylase activity is present, mild persistent hyperphenylalaninemia results.

Epidemiology

PKU is an autosomal recessive disorder. The general prevalence of PKU in the United States and in many other countries is about 1/12,000 live births. There are ethnic variations in the frequency, however, so that among different countries and even among different states in the United States the prevalence may vary between 1/6000–1/25,000. The highest frequencies are reported among the Irish, those of Irish descent, and in Poland; the lowest national frequency reported is 1/100,000 in Japan. PKU is extremely rare among blacks and Ashkenazi Jews but relatively frequent among Yemenite Jews in Israel. The prevalence of "atypical PKU" and MPH are both less than that of PKU, each approximating 1/40,000.

Natural History

Untreated PKU causes developmental delay and mental retardation, often severe. The delay is usually suspected by 6 months of age and is quite evident by the end of the first year. Autistic behavior with seizures (minor motor and myoclonic) and hyperactivity often occur in early childhood. Later, aggressive behavior becomes evident and may be so difficult to control that the family is disrupted. Some untreated individuals

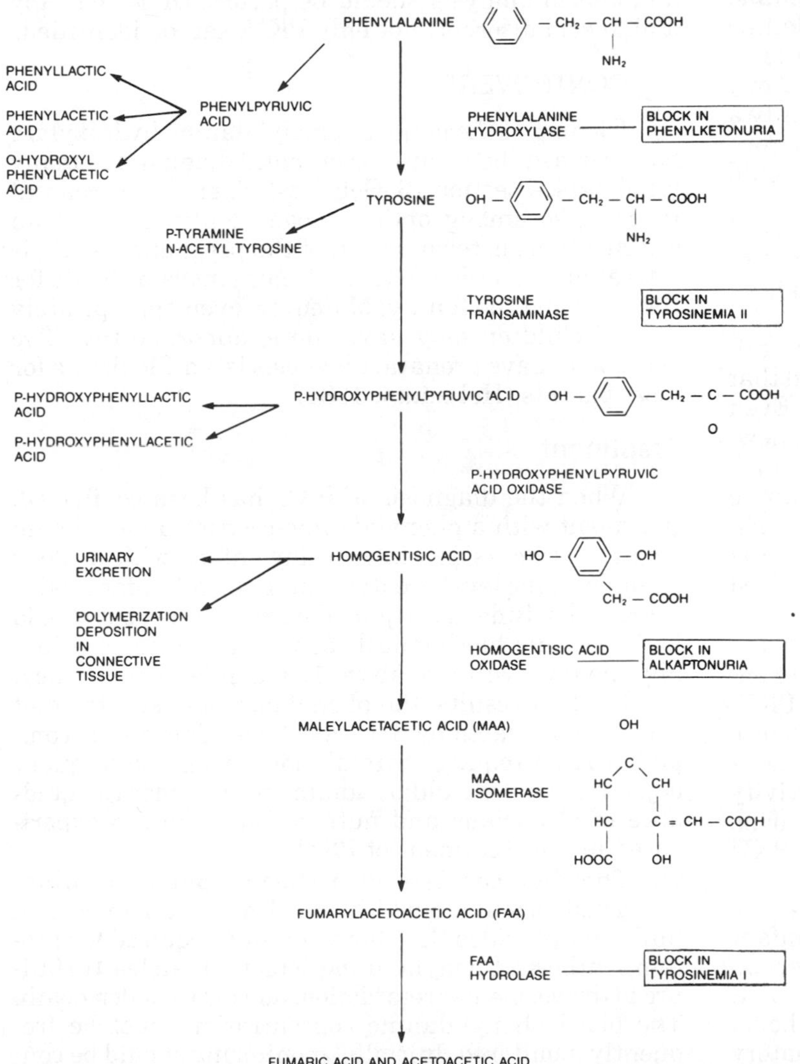

Figure 15.4. Pathway of phenylalanine and tyrosine metabolism. The metabolic disorders in this pathway are indicated adjacent to the corresponding enzymes that are involved.

have a "musty" or "mousy" odor believed to be due to the accumulation of phenylacetic acid. Eczema, scleroderma-like skin changes, and dilution of hair and skin color have also been features of untreated PKU (Jervis, 1937).

The precise cause of the brain toxicity and damage is not known, but these appear to result from the accumulation of phenylalanine and/or its metabolites. The strongest evidence for this is that dietary restriction of phenylalanine instituted early in infancy prevents the mental retardation and other signs of neurologic damage.

Diagnosis

PKU should always be identified in the neonatal period by newborn screening. Such screening for PKU is routine in the United States, Canada, and many other countries. Neonates with PKU are clinically normal; thus, PKU cannot be diagnosed on the basis of symptoms or clinical findings until neurologic damage has progressed to an irreversible state.

Identification of the neonate with PKU is based on finding an increased concentration of phenylalanine in the blood specimen collected for newborn screening. Most infants with PKU will have a blood phenylalanine concentration at least 4 mg/dl or greater. This is at least a two-fold increase over the normal level of 2 mg/dl. Occasionally, an infant with PKU will have only a slightly increased phenylalanine level in the newborn screening specimen; therefore, repeat specimens should be obtained in any infant whose blood phenylalanine concentration is above 2 mg/dl. The filter paper blood specimen for routine screening is usually collected at 2–3 days of age when most infants are discharged from the newborn nursery. The recent trend toward earlier nursery discharge, however, has complicated the collection process since it is often incorrectly assumed that PKU cannot be identified in an early specimen. Even if discharge occurs during the first day of life, the newborn blood specimen should be obtained at that time. In most infants with PKU, the blood phenylalanine level is increased as early as the first few hours of life. When the newborn blood specimen is obtained during the first 24 hours of life a second filter paper blood specimen should be collected at 1–2 weeks of age to be certain that PKU or other disorders are not missed.

The urine ferric chloride test that detects phenylpyruvic acid is usually negative in neonates with PKU, since the formation of this phenylalanine metabolite requires the activity of phenylalanine transaminase, a slowly maturing enzyme that may have low activity until the infant is several months old. Thus, the urine ferric chloride test is effective only in identifying PKU in older infants and children.

When an increased concentration of phenylalanine in blood is identified by newborn screening, the infant should be referred to a pediatric metabolic center experienced in the diagnosis and treatment of PKU. If referral is not possible, contact with such a center should be established quickly so that the proper confirmatory tests are performed and the appropriate treatment initiated without delay.

For the confirmation of PKU, all amino acids should be measured in the blood by an accurate quantitative technique (e.g., amino acid analyzer). A blood phenylalanine concentration of 20 mg/dl or greater with a normal or reduced concentration of tyrosine is evidence of classic PKU. Hyperphenylalaninemia less than 20 mg/dl is indicative of either "atypical PKU" (blood level that is consistently greater than 12 mg/dl but less than 20 mg/dl) or mild persistent hyperphenylalaninemia (blood level that is greater than 2 mg/dl but less than 12 mg/dl). Infants with a pterin defect can have any degree of hyperphenylalaninemia and must be differentiated from those with PKU and mild persistent hyperphenylalaninemia (see section on Pterin Defects).

Despite routine screening programs, PKU can be missed in the newborn period and, hence, this disorder should be considered in any infant with developmental delay or a child with mental subnormality (Levy, 1986). The absence of eczema or the presence of dark hair and normal complexion should not be considered incompatible with PKU; not all children with PKU have blond hair and fair skin. In fact, a complete blood and urine amino acid analysis should be performed so that any amino acid disorder, not only PKU, can be identified.

CONTROVERSY

Cloning of the gene for phenylalanine hydroxylase has provided the means for prenatal diagnosis in many families (see Section 13, Genetics). There is no prenatal therapy, so among options upon identification of an affected fetus is termination of the pregnancy. PKU is a treatable disorder, but the treatment is difficult for the child and the family. Moreover, even appropriately treated children may have subtle abnormalities. The decision to have prenatal diagnosis is a difficult one for most parents (Holtzman, 1984).

Treatment

When the diagnosis of PKU has been confirmed, treatment with a phenylalanine-restricted diet should begin as soon as possible in any infant with a blood phenylalanine level greater than 12 mg/dl. Infants with MPH probably do not require dietary therapy, but should have periodic biochemical monitoring since occasionally the level will rise above 12 mg/dl later in infancy.

For best results, the phenylalanine-restricted diet should be initiated by 3 weeks of age. This diet is complicated and requires careful monitoring and frequent adjustments; it should be administered under the guidance of physicians and nutritionists who are experienced in the treatment of PKU.

The diet consists of a special phenylalanine-restricted formula to which is added a small amount of milk that provides the phenylalanine required for protein synthesis. Phenylalanine depletion can lead to failure to thrive, mental retardation, and even sudden death. The blood phenylalanine concentration must be frequently monitored. Initially, monitoring should be conducted at least weekly or even semiweekly, since infants with PKU will vary considerably in their tolerance for phenylalanine. Later in infancy and childhood, monitoring may be less frequent. The blood phenylalanine level should be maintained between 4 and 10 mg/dl.

It is possible to continue breast-feeding infants with PKU. Only 2 or 3 breast feedings per day are allowed; a specially formulated phenylalanine-free formula without added milk is used for the other feedings. As in formula-fed infants, the blood phenylalanine level must be monitored frequently, and changes in the ratio of breast feedings to special formula feedings made accordingly.

As the infant grows, low protein foods such as fruits and vegetables in measured amounts are added to the diet. Since the artificial sweetener aspartame (Nutrasweet) contains phenylalanine, individuals on dietary treatment for PKU should be careful to avoid the many foods, drinks, and medications that contain this substance. Whether those not on dietary treatment should restrict aspartame intake is not known as of 1987.

Children with PKU may benefit from dietary treatment even when the diagnosis is delayed. Improvement is almost always noted when the diet is initiated before 3 years of age. For instance, we have seen substantial developmental progress in a girl who was quite delayed when treatment began at 2 years of age. In general, however, the sooner the diet begins, the better the outcome.

CONTROVERSY

Most centers treating children with PKU now recommend continuation of the phenylalanine-restricted diet indefinitely. Previously, many centers recommended discontinuing the diet at 5 or 6 years of age, but decreased IQ scores in many children who discontinued the diet has prompted this change. Some adolescents with PKU who discontinued the diet have also had changes in behavior and emotional status. Some centers also recommend that girls with PKU remain on the diet so that treatment is continued even at conception and the complications of maternal PKU avoided (see below) (Kaufman, 1986).

Prognosis

The prognosis for patients with PKU who have been on a phenylalanine-restricted diet since early infancy is quite good (Koch et al, 1984). Mental retardation and other signs of neurologic damage such as seizures and autistic behavior are prevented as well as somatic features, such as eczema. Nevertheless, learn-

CASE ILLUSTRATION

The *first* of these two histories illustrates the child with PKU who was identified by newborn screening and treated with diet from early infancy. This girl came to attention when on newborn screening her blood specimen contained an increased concentration of phenylalanine. She was referred by her pediatrician to a metabolic center where PKU was confirmed on the basis of a phenylalanine level of 41 mg/dl (normal less than 2 mg/dl) and normal concentration of other amino acids in her blood. She began the phenylalanine-restricted diet at 8 days of age. Excellent metabolic control was achieved with blood phenylalanine levels consistently within the range of 2–10 mg/dl and normal growth and development was maintained. When she was 5 years old, the diet was discontinued in accordance with center policy at that time. Her intelligence has remained within normal range and she completed high school with a "C" average. However, her IQ decreased from 132 at 5 years of age to 85 at age 16 years, and psychologic assessments disclosed deficits in fine motor performance. These changes are probably at least partially related to discontinuation of the diet.

The *second* history illustrates the child in whom PKU was missed by newborn screening and who did not begin treatment until later in childhood. This 4-year-old boy was referred for assessment of mental retardation, autism, and hyperactivity. He did not talk and was not toilet-trained. His hyperactive behavior tended to be aggressive, presenting a formidable problem to his family. Neurologic assessment revealed hyperactive deep tendon reflexes and hypertonia in addition to mental retardation. His autistic-type behavior included sitting in a corner and rocking back and forth for long periods of time. EEG was abnormal, with a sharp wave focus and slow spike waves. A blood amino acid analysis obtained for evaluation of mental retardation with unknown etiology disclosed a phenylalanine level of 40 mg/dl. Urine was positive for phenylketones on ferric chloride testing. These findings established the diagnosis of PKU.

Past history revealed that a newborn blood specimen had been collected when the infant was 4 days of age and was submitted for PKU screening, but was interpreted as normal by the screening laboratory. During his first few months of life he was irritable and thought to have colic. By age 9 months developmental delay was evident in that he could not yet sit unsupported and was socially unresponsive. At age 18 months, he began to exhibit autistic behavior and received his first developmental evaluation. Testing for PKU and hypothyroidism was recommended but was not performed. As he became older the mental retardation became more noticeable and the hyperactivity more difficult to control.

Dietary therapy for PKU began at 4 years of age soon after the diagnosis of PKU became known. He and his family complied with dietary recommendations and excellent metabolic control was achieved. His autistic behavior disappeared soon after the diet began and his development and behavior substantially improved. Nevertheless, he remains mentally retarded.

ing difficulties may be experienced by even the most carefully treated individual (Koch et al, 1984).

Prevention

Prevention of the complications of PKU can be accomplished by early diagnosis through newborn screening and by early institution of a phenylalanine-restricted diet.

The detection of carriers for the PKU genetic mutation is possible by measurement of the blood phenylalanine: tyrosine ratio in the fasted state. However, misleading results can occur with this approach. Molecular genetic techniques recently developed may soon become widely available and provide highly reliable carrier detection for most families with PKU.

Since phenylalanine hydroxylase activity is expressed only in the liver, prenatal diagnosis of PKU through amniocentesis and enzyme analysis has not been possible. Analysis of the phenylalanine hydroxylase gene by recombinant DNA techniques, however, has made prenatal diagnosis available to about 90% of couples known to be at risk. The fetal DNA required can be obtained from amniotic fluid cells or from chorionic villi. A more detailed discussion of the newer application of prenatal diagnosis by DNA analysis is provided in Section 13, Genetics.

Gene transfer therapy may be available in the future but remains experimental in 1987 (Ledley, 1987).

Maternal Phenylketonuria

This is another complication of PKU that may be preventable by dietary therapy. Women with PKU have children who are mentally retarded and microcephalic and who also may have congenital heart disease and low birth weight. These abnormalities are most likely secondary to fetal damage resulting from the maternal abnormally elevated substances that cross the placenta since nonphenylketonuric as well as phenylketonuric offspring are affected. The women at highest risk for having damaged offspring are those with blood phenylalanine levels greater than 20 mg/dl when untreated. (Lenke and Levy, 1980). Some women with atypical PKU also may be at high risk. Treatment with a phenylalanine-restricted diet during pregnancy, however, especially when begun before conception, may prevent the fetal damage in maternal PKU. Several normal offspring from such treated mothers have been reported. Maternal PKU will become more important in the future, as more girls with PKU who were identified by newborn screening, and hence, were treated early enter their child-bearing years. It has become increasingly important to locate adolescent girls and young women with PKU who have been lost to follow-up, and together with those who are still being followed in the PKU clinics, inform them about maternal PKU and the importance of dietary treatment before and during pregnancy (Rohr et al, 1987; Drogari et al, 1987).

TETRAHYDROBIOPTERIN DEFICIENCY

Definition

Persistent hyperphenylalaninemia may result not only from a defect in phenylalanine hydroxylase as in PKU but also from a deficiency of tetrahydrobiopterin (BH_4), the cofactor which activates phenylalanine hydroxylase. There are at least three genetically distinct enzymatic defects that can cause a deficiency of BH_4; collectively, they are known as the pterin defects.

Basic Science

BH_4 is the cofactor necessary for aromatic amino acid hydroxylation. Therefore, it is not only required for the hydroxylation of phenylalanine to tyrosine, but it is also necessary for the hydroxylation of tyrosine and of tryptophan (Fig. 15.5). Thus individuals with BH_4 deficiency have reduced amounts of monoamine neurotransmitters such as dopamine and norepinephrine (derived from tyrosine hydroxylation) and serotonin (derived from tryptophan hydroxylation) as well as hyperphenylalaninemia.

The three known metabolic defects that produce a deficiency of BH_4 are inherited as distinct autosomal recessive traits. The first to be described, dihydropteridine reductase deficiency, results in lack of BH_4 regeneration from quinonoid-BH_2. The other two, 6-pyruvoyl-tetrahydropterin synthase deficiency and GTP cyclohydrolase deficiency, lead to a defect in the synthesis of BH_4.

Epidemiology

About 0.5–1% of infants with persistent hyperphenylalaninemia detected by newborn screening have one of the pterin defects. The frequency is probably no greater than 1/1,000,000 in the population or about three affected children born in the United States each year.

Natural History

Infants with pterin defects almost always have come to medical attention because of persistent hyperphenylalaninemia identified by newborn screening. They have usually been mistakenly diagnosed as having PKU and have been treated with a phenylalanine-restricted diet. Unlike children with PKU, however, they have become neurologically damaged despite early dietary intervention. The symptoms usually appear by 4 months of age and include feeding difficulty, hypotonia, slow motor development, lethargy, and seizures. Later, mental retardation and profound neurologic complications develop. The neurotransmitter deficiencies may play a major role in the neurologic damage.

Diagnosis

A newborn infant with persistent hyperphenylalaninemia should be tested for biochemical evidence of a pterin defect. Diagnosis is possible by measurement

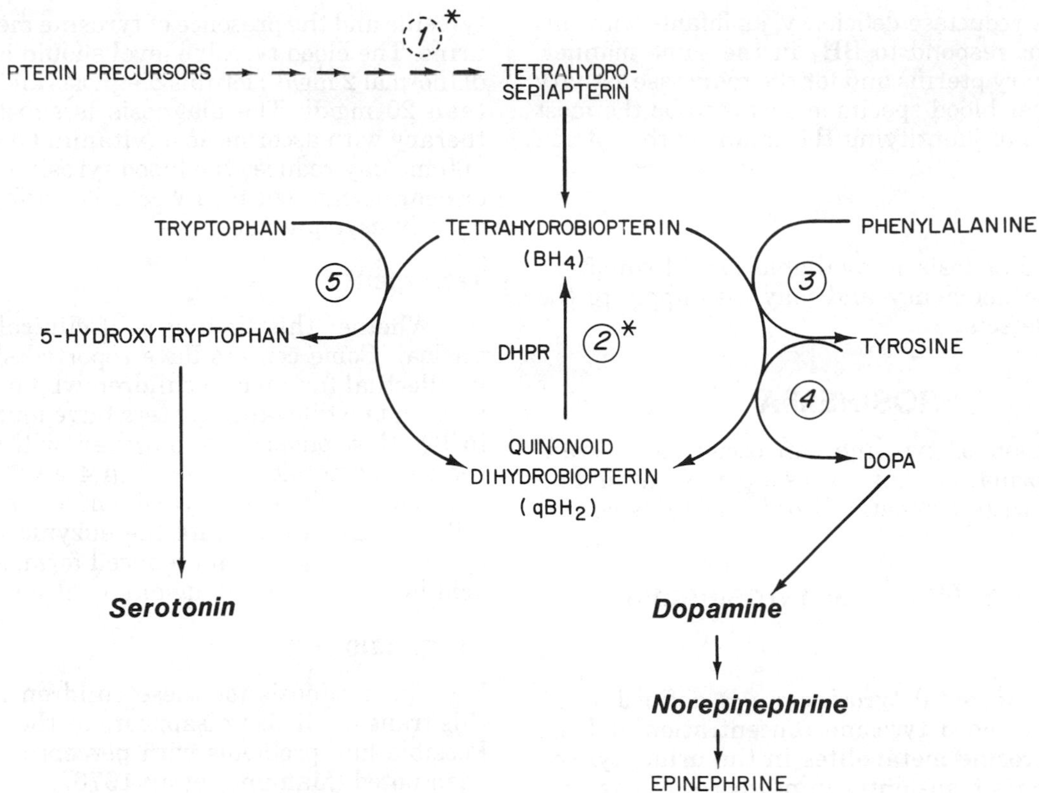

Figure 15.5. Pterin pathway. (*1*) BH_4 synthetic enzymes. (*2*) Dihydropteridine reductase. (*3*) Phenylalanine hydroxylase. (*4*) Tyrosine hydroxylase. (*5*) Tryptophan hydroxylase.

of neopterin and biopterin in the urine, which can be performed on a filter paper specimen of urine.[1] In GTP cyclohydrolase deficiency both biopterin and neopterin are markedly reduced. In the 6-pyruvoyl-tetrahydropterin synthetase defect urinary biopterin is very low but neopterin is normal; this is expressed as a low biopterin percentage. In dihydropteridine reductase deficiency, urinary biopterin is normal or more often, increased, but neopterin is low, resulting in an increased biopterin percentage. In PKU, the percentage of urinary biopterin is essentially the same as in normal infants. Dihydropteridine reductase activity can also be measured in blood specimens on filter paper. All three pterin defects can be identified by enzyme assay in cultured skin fibroblasts. Several infants with urinary pterin abnormalities have had an isolated peripheral defect in biopterin synthesis without involvement of the central nervous system. This seems to be a benign condition and can be differentiated from a serious defect in biopterin synthesis by measuring monoamine neurotransmitter metabolites in the CSF. The levels of these metabolites will be normal in a peripheral defect but reduced when the defect also involves the CNS. Accordingly, any infant suspected of having a pterin defect should have a lumbar puncture with examination of neurotransmitter metabolites in the CSF.

[1] The test is offered by Dr. Edwin Naylor, Western Pennsylvania Hospital, 4800 Friendship Avenue, Pittsburgh, PA 15224.

Treatment and Prognosis

Treatment for infants and children with pterin defects includes administration of the neurotransmitter precursors L-dopa and 5-hydroxytryptophan, which are distal to the hydroxylation reactions in the neurotransmitter biosynthetic pathways. In addition, the phenylalanine-restricted diet is necessary since the hyperphenylalaninemia should be controlled. BH_4 is also effective in the treatment of 6-pyruvoyl-tetrahydropterin synthase and GTP cyclohydrolase deficiency. Folinic acid (citrovorum factor; 5-formyltetrahydrofolate) has been added to the regimen in several patients with dihydropteridine reductase deficiency and has resulted in sufficient clinical improvement to suggest that this is an important therapy in this disorder (Irons et al, 1987). There are indications that initiation of therapy early in infancy may prevent the irreversible neurologic damage that is seen in these patients.

CONTROVERSY

A challenge test with BH_4 has been used to differentiate hyperphenylalaninemic infants with the pterin defects from those with PKU. The basis of this test is that BH_4 administered orally or intravenously will result in a marked decline of the blood phenylalanine level within 2–4 hours if the infant has a pterin defect, but little or no reduction if the infant has PKU. This therapeutic test seems to be reliable in the diagnosis of biopterin synthesis defects but may not diagnose dihydropteridine reductase deficiency, as infants with this defect may not respond to BH_4 in the same manner. Assay for urinary pterins and for the reductase activity in a filter paper blood specimen seems to be the most reliable means of identifying the infant with a pterin defect.

Prevention

Prenatal diagnosis is available for dihydropteridine reductase deficiency and may also apply to the other pterin defects.

TYROSINEMIA

An elevation of tyrosine can occur either transiently in a normal newborn or as a persistent finding in the infant with a genetic disorder of tyrosine metabolism.

Transient Neonatal Tyrosinemia

Definition

Transient neonatal tyrosinemia is defined as an increase in the blood tyrosine concentration and the presence of tyrosine metabolites in the urine (tyrosyluria) that occurs transiently in newborn infants (Avery et al, 1967).

Basic Science

Transient neonatal tyrosinemia is due to the delayed maturation of p-hydroxyphenylpyruvic acid oxidase, the enzyme responsible for the degradation of p-hydroxyphenylpyruvic acid, a product of tyrosine oxidation (Fig. 15.4). Hence tyrosine, p-hydroxyphenylpyruvic acid, and metabolites derived from the latter accumulate.

Epidemiology

This formerly occurred in as many as 5–10% of newborn infants, predominantly premature infants fed formulas containing half skimmed milk. Reduction in protein intake through the greater use of breast-feeding, however, and formulas with lower protein concentrations has substantially decreased the frequency.

Natural History

Transient tyrosinemia usually appears after the first or second week of life, and reaches a peak at 2 or 3 months of age when the protein intake has substantially increased. It is much more frequent among premature infants than among full-term infants. This is probably related to the general immaturity of enzyme systems in premature infants.

Diagnosis

The diagnosis is suspected when an infant, particularly a premature one, is found to have an increased concentration of tyrosine in the blood and increased tyrosine and the presence of tyrosine metabolites in the urine. The blood tyrosine level should be at least 4 mg/dl (normal 2 mg/dl) for this diagnosis and is often greater than 20 mg/dl. The diagnosis is substantiated when therapy with ascorbic acid (vitamin C) in a dose of 50–100 mg/day reduces the blood tyrosine level to normal or near normal within 1 week. The affected infants are usually asymptomatic.

Treatment

Whether this finding is of clinical importance is unclear. Some centers have reported slightly reduced intellectual function in children who had transient tyrosinemia while other centers have found no reduction in IQ. Most physicians, however, will advise limiting the protein intake to less than 4 g/kg/day in children who had had transient tyrosinemia. Since ascorbic acid (vitamin C) will activate the enzyme in most infants by maintaining it in its reduced form, a daily ascorbic acid intake of 50–100 mg/day is also recommended.

Prognosis

The prognosis for these children is very good as this transient defect disappears as the infants mature. Possible late problems with perceptual function have been noted (Mamunes et al, 1976).

Hereditary Tyrosinemia (Tyrosinemia I)

Definition

Hereditary tyrosinemia is an inherited disorder of tyrosine metabolism that causes severe liver disease in infancy.

Basic Science

The enzyme defect in hereditary tyrosinemia seems to be a deficiency in fumarylacetoacetase (fumarylacetoacetate hydrolase), the enzyme that degrades fumarylacetoacetate to fumarate and acetoacetate (Fig. 15.4). Deficient activities of p-hydroxyphenylpyruvic oxidase and tyrosine transaminase have also been found in the livers of these patients, but these seem to be secondary enzyme defects. The most prominent amino acid findings are increased tyrosine and methionine in the blood and increased tyrosine and tyrosine metabolites in the urine (tyrosyluria). Notably, succinylacetone is found in the urine. This organic acid is the excretory product of fumarylacetoacetate, which is unstable, and its presence seems to be specific for this disease. Serum α-fetoprotein is also markedly elevated, apparently as a consequence of the type of liver disease that occurs in hereditary tyrosinemia; an enormous elevation is a major characteristic of the disorder (Hostetter et al, 1983).

Epidemiology

This is a very rare genetic disorder. The highest known frequency is in the French-Canadian population where the carrier frequency has been estimated in some regions to be as high as 1/14 persons. The pattern of inheritance is autosomal recessive.

Natural History

There are two clinical presentations of hereditary tyrosinemia. The most dramatic or early onset, occurs in the first week or two of life. These infants develop hepatomegaly, jaundice, coagulopathy, and other signs of severe liver disease. Liver function continues to deteriorate rapidly and death usually occurs by 2–3 months of age.

More often, the second, or later onset, type of clinical presentation is encountered. Affected infants develop jaundice and hepatomegaly at the end of the first or second month of life. At that time, liver function tests are abnormal, with evidence of coagulopathy. They may also have the renal Fanconi syndrome with glucosuria, hyperphosphaturia, proteinuria, and generalized aminoaciduria. The disease is progressive during the next few months, with development of cirrhosis and hypophosphatemic rickets. The CNS is spared. Further complications are associated with liver disease, including esophageal varices, bleeding diatheses, and eventually, hepatic failure (Fig. 15.6).

Diagnosis

The diagnosis of hereditary tyrosinemia may be difficult. Increased tyrosine and methionine in the blood and the presence of tyrosyluria can be associated with liver disease from many different causes. Therefore, these findings are not specific for hereditary tyrosinemia. The diagnosis can be established, however, by the presence of succinylacetone in the urine. In addition, activity of erythrocyte Δ-amino levulinic acid dehydratase is reduced, presumably due to inhibition by succinylacetone. A markedly increased level of serum α-fetoprotein is also highly suggestive of the diagnosis. The diagnosis is confirmed by the demonstration of reduced or absent fumarylacetoacetase activity in cultured skin fibroblasts or liver.

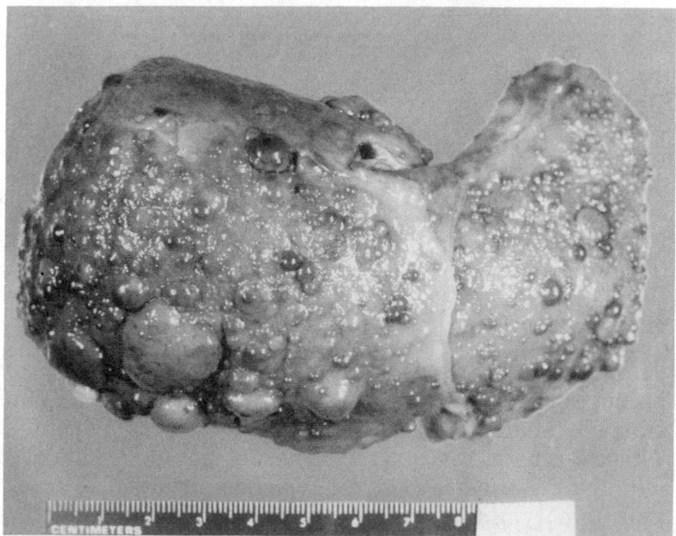

Figure 15.6. Postmortem appearance of liver in an infant who died at 8 months of age while awaiting a liver transplant.

Treatment

Treatment for this condition has included a special diet restricted in tyrosine and phenylalanine, the precursor amino acid to tyrosine, as well as therapy for the complications of the liver disease. The diet is successful in reversing the renal abnormalities and the rickets, but has only rarely halted progression of the liver disease.

Liver transplantation has been performed in a number of children with hereditary tyrosinemia. Most are living and have had no evidence of disease in the donor liver. Thus, this may be the treatment of choice for severely affected infants (Starzl et al, 1985).

Prognosis

Most infants with hereditary tyrosinemia have progressive liver disease and die with liver failure during infancy or early childhood. Those who live into later childhood almost always develop fatal hepatocellular carcinoma. Rare individuals with hereditary tyrosinemia, probably those with a milder variant of the disorder, have lived into adulthood and, in rare instances, have even recovered from any evidence of liver disease.

CONTROVERSY

Several patients who received liver transplants have continued to excrete succinylacetone. This is believed to result from enzyme deficiency in extrahepatic sites. Nevertheless, it is not yet certain that the transplanted liver will remain free of liver disease. The occurrence of hepatocellular carcinoma has been reported in the transplanted liver of one patient (Starzl et al, 1985).

Prevention

Prenatal diagnosis is available. Amniotic fluid obtained at midtrimester contains increased succinylacetone when the fetus is affected. Cultured amniocytes contain little or no fumarylacetoacetase.

Tyrosinosis (Tyrosinemia II)

Definition

Tyrosinosis is a very rare inborn error that affects the skin and eyes as well as the CNS, but not the liver or kidney. It is also known as the Richner-Hanhart syndrome.

Basic Science

Tyrosinosis is an autosomal recessive disorder in which the enzymatic defect is a deficiency of cytosolic tyrosine aminotransferase with normal mitochondrial aspartate (tyrosine) aminotransferase (Fig. 15.4). Deficiency of the cytosolic enzyme, which is responsible for most of the conversion of tyrosine to p-hydroxyphenylpyruvate, results in accumulation of tyrosine in the blood. The increased tyrosine enters the mitochondria of nonhepatic cells which lack p-hydroxyphenylpyruvate oxidase activity, resulting in an accumulation of p-hydroxyphenylpyruvate and other tyrosine metabolites. The increased tyrosine and tyrosine metabolites appear in the urine.

The hypertyrosinemia leads to the deposition of tyrosine crystals. It is believed that this deposition disrupts lyosomes leading to the release of proteolytic enzymes which in turn leads to the inflammatory changes seen in the skin and eyes of these patients. Unlike hereditary tyrosinemia (tyrosinemia I), patients with tyrosinosis do not have liver, bone, or kidney disease.

Epidemiology

Only a few patients with this disorder have been described.

Natural History

Patients with tyrosinosis have eye, skin, and neurologic findings. Ophthalmologic symptoms usually develop within the first few months of life, often before the skin lesions, and include increased lacrimation, photophobia, and ocular pain. Long-term effects include corneal scarring, nystagmus, and glaucoma. Neurologic manifestations include developmental delay in early childhood with later manifestations of mild to moderate mental retardation.

Hyperkeratotic skin lesions of the hands and feet are often the most striking clinical feature of the disorder (Fig. 15.7). These lesions are limited to the palms and the soles and are painful and tender. The skin lesions have a predilection for the tips of the digits and thenar and hypothenar eminences.

Diagnosis

The diagnosis may be suspected on the basis of the clinical features, which in their aggregate are not seen in any other disorder. The biochemical findings of increased tyrosine in the blood and increased tyrosine and its metabolites in the urine (tyrosyluria) in association with the clinical syndrome establishes the diagnosis.

Treatment and Prognosis

The skin and eye lesions can be controlled by a diet that is restricted in tyrosine and phenylalanine. It appears that, analogous to PKU, the mental retardation may be prevented if the diet is initiated early in infancy. Dietary therapy must be monitored by periodic determinations of blood tyrosine and urinary tyrosine metabolites.

Prevention

Newborn screening for blood tyrosine elevations could identify infants with tyrosinosis and lead to early treatment that might prevent the clinical expression of this disorder. Most newborn screening programs do not include tyrosine screening, however, and those few that do have not yet reported an identified case.

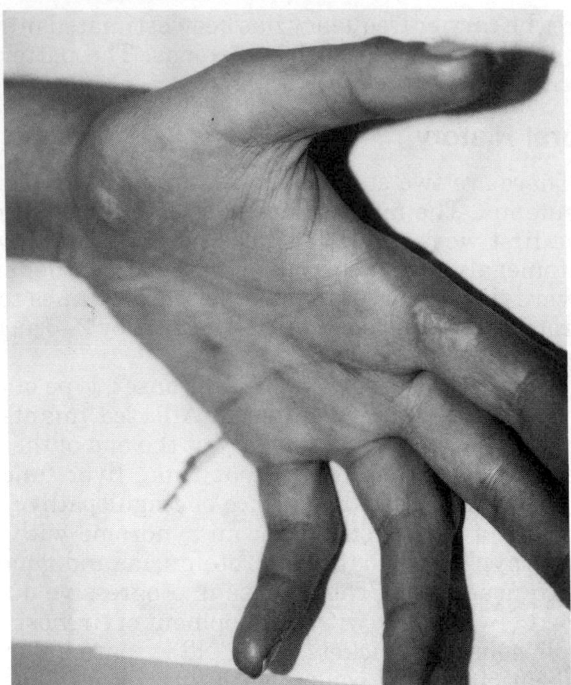

Figure 15.7. Keratotic skin lesions that are pathognomonic of the rare type II tyrosinosis. These lesions were present in infancy, and come and go with the level of serum tyrosine. The young man is now a 30-year-old mildly retarded adult.

Prenatal Diagnosis

This is not yet possible for tyrosinosis.

ALKAPTONURIA

Definition

Alkaptonuria is due to an inborn error in the degradation of homogentisic acid, an intermediate in tyrosine metabolism. It produces osteoarthritis and pigmentation of connective tissue known as ochronosis (Srsen, 1979).

Basic Science

The basic defect in this condition is a deficiency of homogentisic acid oxidase, an enzyme that is responsible for the degradation of homogentisic acid (Fig. 15.4). This results in the accumulation of homogentisic acid which, in tissues, is oxidized to benzoquinoneacetic acid and its polymers. These compounds bind to connective tissue macromolecules and produce ochronosis. Homogentisic acid is also excreted in large quantities, imparting a dark color to the urine.

Epidemiology

The prevalence of alkaptonuria has been reported to be 1/25,000 in Slovakia. It is probably much less frequent in other areas of the world. Only two cases have been identified among 800,000 infants who have received urine screening in Massachusetts.

Natural History

The first sign of alkaptonuria is dark staining of the diapers. Later in childhood, the axillary regions become pigmented. Increased pigmentation of ear cerumen (dark brown to black) may also occur in childhood. Pigmentation of the eyes, usually beginning after 20 years of age, is most striking in the sclerae, but also occurs in the cornea, bulbar conjunctiva, tarsus, and skin of the eyelid (Srsen and Srsnova, 1979).

The systemic complications of alkaptonuria chiefly relate to the deposition of ochronotic pigment in the joints, the genitourinary system, and the heart. Males are more frequently affected with genitourinary complications, which include the formation of prostatic calculi and renal stones. Males also have more severe joint disease, and may be incapacitated by it.

Diagnosis

The characteristic clinical findings and the identification of homogentisic acid in the urine establish the diagnosis. Urine from patients with alkaptonuria is also positive on testing for reducing substance and will darken upon standing or with alkalinization.

Treatment

There is no known effective treatment for this disorder, although some have advocated a diet low in phenylalanine and tyrosine.

ALBINISM

Definition

Albinism comprises a heterogeneous group of disorders caused by inherited metabolic defects of the pigment cells of the eye, skin, and hair. There are three major categories of albinism: oculocutaneous albinism, ocular albinism, and oculocutaneous and ocular albinoidism.

Basic Science

Extensive reviews of albinism and other disorders of pigment metabolism are available (Witkop, 1983; Witkop et al, 1983). The basic defect in this group of disorders occurs in the melanocyte system of the eye, skin, and hair. The symptoms and signs seen in the various forms of albinism are determined by the specific defect(s) of the melanocyte in the various organ systems that occur in the particular disorder.

Natural History

Oculocutaneous albinism exists in 10 distinct forms. Nine are inherited in an autosomal recessive manner, while one is an autosomal dominant trait. These patients have in common decreased or abnormal pigmentation of the skin, hair, and eyes. Ophthalmologic abnormalities also include decreased visual acuity with hypoplasia of the fovea, varying degrees of nystagmus, and photophobia. In the classic form of oculocutaneous albinism, there is no detectable pigment in skin, hair or eyes and no activity of tyrosinase, the enzyme that catalyzes the first step of tyrosine conversion to melanin. The other forms of oculocutaneous albinism are tyrosinase-positive, and patients with any of these forms may develop increasing pigmentation of skin, hair, and eyes and increasing visual acuity with age.

The Chédiak-Higashi syndrome, the Hermansky-Pudlak syndrome, and the Cross syndrome are three oculocutaneous albinism syndromes that include abnormalities in addition to those mentioned above. Recurrent infections, neutropenia, and development of lymphoreticular malignancy are characteristic of the Chédiak-Higashi syndrome in which severe chemotactic abnormalities are a major feature. Patients with the Hermansky-Pudlak syndrome present with a history of easy bruisability and bleeding owing to a defect in platelet aggregation. Accumulation of a ceroid-like material and lipids in the reticuloendothelial tissue, urine, oral and gastrointestinal mucosa, and the lung are also features of this syndrome. These accumulations can result in restrictive lung disease and ulcerative colitis. In the Cross syndrome, additional findings include microphthalmia, corneal clouding, and retardation of physical and mental development.

Patients with ocular albinism present with primary ocular involvement and usually have normal hair and skin pigmentation, although they may be less pigmented than their siblings. This is inherited as an X-linked or autosomal recessive disorder.

Oculocutaneous and ocular albinoidism can be distinguished from the other types of albinism by the absence of hypoplasia of the fovea, lack of nystagmus or photophobia, and usually by the lack of visual impairment. These patients have reduced pigmentation of the hair, skin, and irides. Autosomal dominant and recessive inheritance has been reported for the various forms of albinoidism.

Diagnosis

The various forms of albinism are diagnosed on the basis of characteristic clinical findings, which include reduced or absent skin and hair pigmentation, and upon the classic ophthalmologic findings noted on careful eye examination. The ophthalmologic findings are the most important in diagnosing any form of albinism. These include hypoplasia of the fovea, nystagmus, transillumination of the irides, photophobia, depigmentation of the fundi, and decreased visual acuity.

The hair bulb tyrosine incubation test will distinguish tyrosinase-negative oculocutaneous albinism from tyrosinase-positive types. Pigment formation in the hair bulbs of patients with the tyrosinase-positive forms of the disorder can be seen after incubation of the hair with tyrosine.

Treatment

Treatment is aimed at the three major problems encountered by these patients. Sensitivity of their skin to sunlight and their susceptibility to skin neoplasia are treated by avoidance of sunlight and the use of protective clothing and sunscreens. Their visual defect is treated with corrective lenses, tinted to reduce photophobia.

Prevention

Prenatal diagnosis of albinism has been reported in one case. Electron microscopic examination of fetal skin samples collected by means of fetoscopy at 20 weeks of gestation revealed arrest of melanosome development in the hair bulb melanocytes.

HYPERMETHIONINEMIA

Definition

This disorder is characterized by an increased level of methionine in the absence of homocystine, in contrast to homocystinuria (see next disorder), which features both increased methionine and the presence of homocystine. Its mode of inheritance is unknown since, so far, only isolated cases have been described.

Basic Science

The first patient with isolated hypermethioninemia was found to have a deficiency in liver methionine adenosyltransferase, the first enzyme in methionine degradation which is responsible for the synthesis of S-adenosylmethionine, an important methyl donor (Fig. 15.8). It is evident that deficient activity of the transferase would result in hypermethioninemia and several cases with deficiency of hepatic methionine adenosyltransferase have been described. Still other cases of isolated hypermethioninemia, however, have had normal liver transferase activity. The origin of the hypermethioninemia in these cases has not been identified.

Epidemiology

We have identified only one infant with isolated hypermethioninemia among almost 2 million neonates who have received newborn blood screening for elevation of methionine. In Japan, the frequency from routine newborn screening has been about 1 per million.

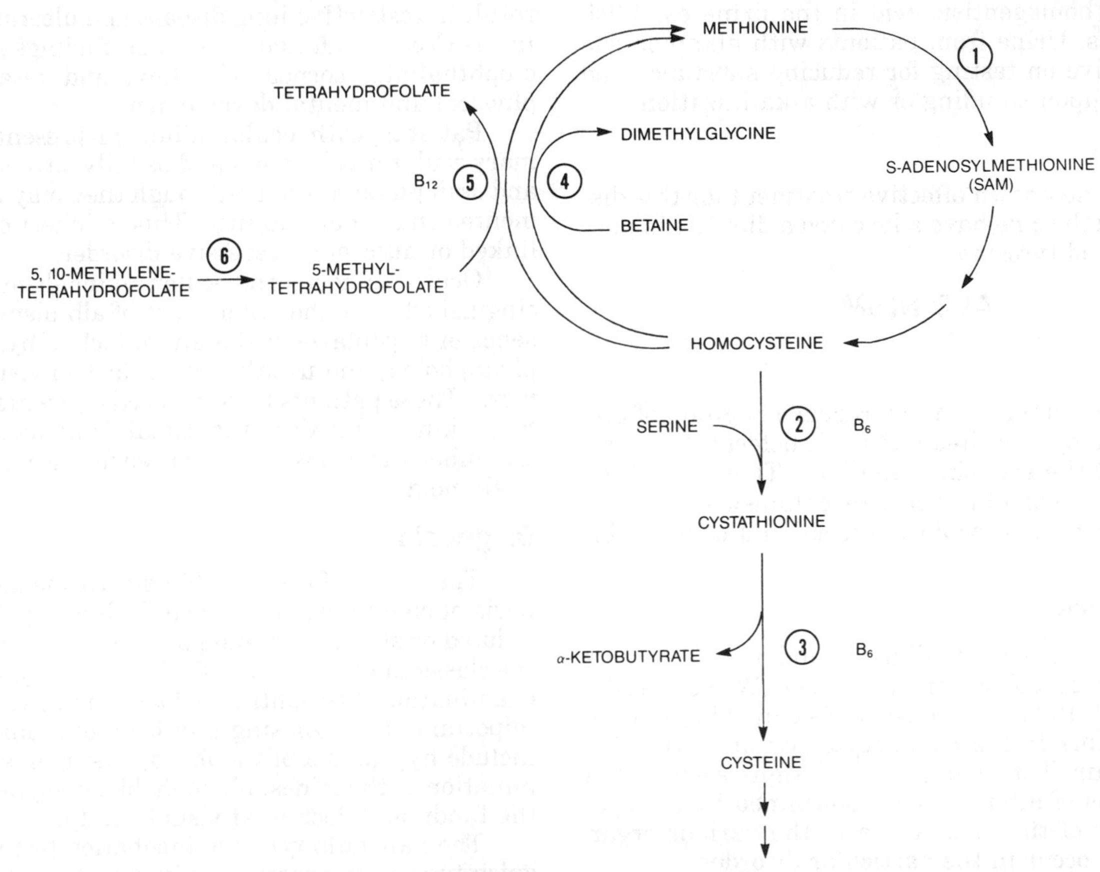

Figure 15.8. Pathway of methionine metabolism. (*1*) Methionine adenosyltransferase. (*2*) Cystathionine β-synthase. (*3*) Cystathionase. (*4*) Betaine-homocysteine methyltransferase. (*5*) 5-methyltetrahydrofolate-homocysteine methyltransferase. (*6*) 5,10-methylene-tetrahydrofolate reductase.

Natural History

Patients with hypermethioninemia and liver methionine adenosyltransferase deficiency have been clinically normal. This includes a 31-year-old man who was studied because of an unusual breath odor that resulted from large amounts of a methionine metabolite. On the other hand, children without deficiency of adenosyltransferase have had clinical abnormalities ranging from mental retardation and proximal muscle disease to fatty degeneration of the liver (Gaull et al, 1981).

Diagnosis

This is based on the presence of persistently increased levels of blood and urine methionine without other amino acid changes, particularly the absence of homocystinuria. Diagnosis of the form of hypermethioninemia associated with methionine adenosyltransferase deficiency can be confirmed by assay of its activity in liver obtained by biopsy. Diagnosis of the form associated with normal liver adenosyltransferase activity also is supported by studies of activity in biopsied liver, although the metabolic block in this form cannot be determined by this assay alone. Increased serum folate concentrations have been reported in most, but not all, patients who do not have methionine adenosyltransferase deficiency.

Treatment

The increased level of methionine in blood can be reduced by a methionine-restricted diet, although this does not seem necessary for patients who are asymptomatic. Reducing the methionine level may be helpful in reversing fatty degeneration of the liver in some patients without the transferase deficiency. Whether other symptoms associated with hypermethioninemia would also benefit from the diet is not known.

Prognosis

Prognosis seems to be good for those patients with methionine adenosyltransferase deficiency, but as yet unknown for others.

Prevention

Prenatal diagnosis is not yet possible.

HOMOCYSTINURIA

Definition

This autosomal recessive disorder is characterized by the presence of homocystine, most markedly demonstrated in urine. It is among the best known of the amino acid disorders because of its striking phenotype which includes not only mental retardation but also dislocation of the ocular lenses, long and thin extremities similar to the appearance in the Marfan syndrome, and a predisposition to arterial changes that lead to thromboembolic disease.

Basic Science

The metabolic block is in the conversion of homocysteine to cystathionine. This step is normally catalyzed by cystathionine β-synthase, an enzyme that requires pyridoxine (vitamin B_6) for activity (Fig. 15.8). In homocystinuria, cystathionine β-synthase activity is deficient. As a result of this block, homocysteine accumulates and is measured in blood and urine as homocystine, its oxidized disulfide form. Methionine is usually increased since the homocysteine blocked in its pathway of transsulfuration (i.e., to cystathionine) is methylated back to methionine (Fig. 15.8). Cystine is decreased or absent, not only because of reduced synthesis of cystathionine, the precursor of cysteine, but primarily because one of its major synthetic enzymes, cysteine sulfhydrase, is the same protein as cystathionine β-synthase.

The pathogenetic agent in homocystinuria is unknown. Comparing isolated hypermethioninemia with homocystinuria, however, provides a clue. In both types of disorders, methionine is increased, but only in homocystinuria does homocysteine accumulate, and only homocystinuria is characterized by mental retardation, dislocated ocular lenses, skeletal defects, and vascular changes. Accordingly, most investigators believe that homocysteine or a closely related metabolite is most likely the toxic compound.

Epidemiology

Although the frequency of identification from routine newborn screening for increased blood methionine is about 1/335,000, this is clearly an underestimate since it is known that newborn screening misses up to one-half of affected infants. Hence, the most likely frequency is probably between 1:100,000 and 1:200,000.

Natural History

The infant with homocystinuria is usually normal, although thromboembolic complications of the CNS during the first year of life have been described. During the second or third year, developmental delay is noted. Dislocated ocular lenses (ectopia lentis) follows, usually between 4 and 10 years of age. Severe myopia is the first sign of ectopia lentis and may precede the actual dislocation by several months to a year or longer. The characteristic long, thin extremities (dolichostenomelia) may not appear until later in childhood or during adolescence, but osteoporosis, especially of the spine, may already have been present for some time. Thromboembolic events such as cerebrovascular occlusions or pulmonary emboli usually do not occur until adult years, but have been reported in children and even infants with homocystinuria.

The phenotype of homocystinuria is quite variable. About 50% of affected individuals are not mentally retarded and some are quite intelligent. The external skeletal features are minor or absent in many patients, although most have some degree of osteoporosis. The vascular complications may not occur during early and even middle adult years and may not occur at all in some patients. On the other hand, almost all homocystinuric individuals will have ectopia lentis. Those patients responsive to pyridoxine (see below) tend to have later onset of the clinical complications and less severe complications than do those nonresponsive to pyridoxine.

Diagnosis

The presence of homocystine in urine as detected by amino acid screening is the most characteristic biochemical marker for homocystinuria and is usually the first indication of the disease in children and adults. Further amino acid studies disclose the presence of homocystine also in blood, usually increased methionine but little or no cystine. Other amino acid findings are normal. The diagnosis can be confirmed by assay of cystathionine β-synthase activity in cultured skin fibroblasts or liver, but this is usually not necessary for clinical purposes when the biochemical and clinical features of homocystinuria are present.

Treatment

About 50% of affected individuals are biochemically responsive to pyridoxine and can be treated with supplements of pyridoxine hydrochloride varying from 25–1000 mg/day. Most of these patients also require some degree of protein or methionine restriction in the diet in order to maintain normal or near normal amino acid values. Patients who are not responsive to pyridoxine require a methionine-restricted diet for metabolic control, similar to that used for the treatment of PKU. It consists of a special formula containing little or no methionine but the other amino acids and is supplemented with cystine. The solid foods allowed are those low in, or free of, protein.

Children who are nonresponsive to pyridoxine and will not accept the diet may be treated with betaine, a methyl donor that stimulates homocysteine methylation via betaine-homocysteine methyltransferase (Fig. 15.8). This therapy reduces or eliminates homocysteine but raises the level of methionine. Nevertheless, betaine may be beneficial since homocysteine, not methionine, seems to produce the clinical complications. The dose of betaine varies from 6–9 g/day.

Surgical procedures may be necessary for complications from dislocated lens or for fractures secondary to osteoporosis. Thromboembolic events may occur more readily postoperatively in homocystinurics than in normal individuals. Thus, surgery should only be performed when absolutely necessary. The amount of intravenous fluid provided before and after surgery should be greater than usual so that the patient is maintained in a somewhat hypervolemic state and the tendency for coagulation is thereby lessened.

Prognosis

This must remain guarded. Thromboembolic events are a threat to any individual with homocystinuria. Complications from dislocated lenses may occur at any time. Osteoporosis may worsen and complications such as pathologic fractures may occur. On the other hand, some patients have very few complications even into adult years.

Prevention

Prenatal diagnosis is possible by measurement of cystathionine β-synthase activity in cultured aminocytes. Heterozygote detection is also possible by measurement of total homocysteine in blood after methionine loading (Boers et al, 1986).

CYSTATHIONINEMIA

Definition

This is an autosomal recessive disorder of cystathionine degradation characterized by accumulations of cystathionine in urine and blood. It is probably benign.

Basic Science

The enzyme defect is in cystathionase which normally cleaves cystathionine to cysteine and α-ketobutyrate (Fig. 15.8); hence, cystathionine accumulates. The enzyme requires vitamin B_6 for its activity.

Epidemiology

Based on newborn urine screening in Massachusetts the frequency of this disorder is about 1/70,000.

Natural History

A variety of clinical abnormalities have been described with cystathioninuria, including seizures, hypoplastic genitalia, thrombocytopenia, renal calculi, diabetes insipidus and diabetes mellitus. Nevertheless, most children with cystathioninuria, including those identified by routine newborn urine screening, have been normal. On balance, therefore, cystathioninemia seems to be a benign disorder. Our experience in Massachusetts supports this, although a few of the children whom we have followed from the newborn period have had hyperactive behavior.

Diagnosis

Increased cystathionine in urine and blood without other amino acid abnormalities suggests the presence of this disorder. Cystathioninuria may also be secondary to liver disease, neuroblastoma, ganglioblastoma, hepatoblastoma or vitamin B_6 deficiency and is often transient in the newborn period. Small amounts of cystathionine may be excreted by heterozygotes for the disorder. Thus, to diagnose cystathioninemia associated with cystathionase deficiency, the cystathionine accumulation must be persistent, other causes of cystathioninuria must be eliminated and the cystathioninuria should be in excess of 1000 μMole/g creatinine. The diagnosis can be confirmed by assay of cystathionase activity in liver or cultured lymphoid cell lines, but the likelihood that the disorder is benign would militate against liver biopsy or even the labor involved in culturing cells.

Treatment

Most individuals with cystathioninemia are responsive to pyridoxine. Usually 100–200 mg of pyridoxine hydrochloride per day will greatly reduce or eradicate the cystathionine accumulation. An occasional affected individual is nonresponsive to pyridoxine but they have been clinically normal.

Prognosis

Prognosis is good for this benign disorder.

Prevention

Prenatal diagnosis is not available. Heterozygote detection is possible on the basis of urinary measurement of cystathionine.

HOMOCYSTEINE METHYLATION DEFECTS

Definition

These defects comprise a group of inborn errors that limit the capacity of homocysteine to be methylated to methionine (Fig. 15.8). They are often also referred to as methionine remethylation defects. All produce developmental delay and other features of neurologic damage.

Basic Science

Two pathways are capable of methylating homocysteine. The major methylation pathway utilizes the methyl group from 5-methyltetrahydrofolate and is mediated by 5-methyltetrahydrofolate-homocysteine methyltransferase (Fig. 15.8). This pathway requires vitamin B_{12} or, more precisely, methylcobalamin (Mecbl), one of the two coenzymatically active forms of B_{12}. The minor of these involves betaine and is mediated by betaine-homocysteine methyltransferase (Fig. 15.8).

Two of the three inborn errors of homocysteine methylation involve defect in the synthesis of methylcobalamin from the precursor B_{12}. One of these is cobalamin C (D) mutation, a defect in the synthesis of adenosylcobalamin, the other B_{12} coenzyme, as well as methylcobalamin while cobalamin E mutation is a defect in methylcobalamine synthesis alone. The reduced amounts of available methylcobalamin result in reduced activity of 5-methyltetrahydrofolate homocysteine methyltransferase. The third inborn error is a defect in 5,10-methylene-tetrahydrofolate reductase, the enzyme which produces the 5-methyltetrahydrofolate necessary for homocysteine methylation (Fig. 15.8).

Metabolic blocks in homocysteine methylation result in homocysteine accumulation (i.e., homocystinuria) and a reduced methionine level (hypomethioninemia). Cystathionine accumulation (cystathioninuria) will also sometimes appear.

Epidemiology

These defects are very rare; fewer than 30 cases of cobalamin C mutation have been described and perhaps fewer than 15 cases of cobalamin E mutation are known. Similarly, only 70 or 80 cases of 5, 10-methylenetetrahydrofolate reductase deficiency have come to attention.

Natural History

The cobalamin defects produce the unusual pediatric combination of neurologic disease and megaloblastic anemia. In the cobalamin C mutation, there is often evidence of intrauterine growth retardation, with low birth weight and microcephaly at birth. Growth delay continues postnatally and may result in severe failure to thrive, leading to death in early infancy. Those infants who survive manifest developmental delay by 2 or 3 months of age. Megaloblastic anemia also appears at this time as does evidence of visual impairment. Ophthalmologic examination reveals retinal degeneration (Robb et al, 1984). Seizures and other features of neurologic disease, including moderate to severe mental retardation, develop as the child becomes older.

5,10-Methylenetetrahydrofolate reductase deficiency is also characterized by failure to thrive and neurologic disease, but is notably different from the cobalamin defects in that megaloblastic anemia is absent. The neurologic disease is often severe, with microcephaly and seizures in addition to mental retardation.

Diagnosis

The key to the diagnosis of a cobalamin defect is the combination of neurologic disease and megaloblastic anemia. This combination should trigger amino acid studies of blood and urine and organic acid analysis of urine. The amino acid studies will disclose the presence of homocystine and perhaps cystathionine, usually with a reduced level of methionine in blood. In cobalamin C (D) mutation methylmalonic acid is detected in urine on organic acid analysis but in cobalamin E mutation urine organic acids are normal. Despite the megaloblastic anemia, serum vitamin B_{12} and folate levels are normal or even elevated, eliminating vitamin B_{12} or folate deficiency as the cause of the megaloblastic changes. The diagnosis of cobalamin C (D) mutation can be confirmed by genetic complementation analysis using cultured skin fibroblasts. Cobalamin E mutation may be confirmed by studies of 5-methyltetrahydrofolate-homocysteine methyltransferase activity in cultured skin fibroblasts as well as by complementation analysis.

5,10-Methylenetetrahydrofolate reductase deficiency is diagnosed by the presence of homocystine and a normal or low level of blood methionine. Confirmation of the diagnosis requires the demonstration of reduced enzyme activity in cultured skin fibroblasts.

Treatment

Large doses of intramuscular vitamin B_{12} result in rapid reversal of the megaloblastic anemia in the cobalamin defects. The doses used vary from 0.5–1.0 mg weekly or biweekly to 1.0 mg every other day. Growth and development may not improve although the progressive downhill course may be halted by therapy. The retinal degeneration, however, has not responded to therapy. Specific administration of methylcobalamin may be the treatment of choice for the cobalamin E mutation since this is a singular deficiency of this B_{12} coenzyme. 5,10-Methylene-tetrahydrofolate reductase deficiency has not consistently responded to therapy but at least one case has partially benefited from folate supplements, vitamin B_{12}, methionine, and folinic acid (Harpey et al, 1981). Betaine has also been used in the treatment of this disorder.

Prognosis

Prognosis is guarded for all of these defects. The neurologic disease usually progresses, although a continued downhill course often ending in death may be halted by therapy.

Prevention

Prenatal diagnosis and prenatal therapy with vitamin B_{12} administration to the mother has been successful in one case of cobalamin E mutation (Rosenblatt et al, 1985). The prenatal diagnosis of the other cobalamin defects has not been reported but presumably can be made. Whether prenatal therapy for the cobalamin C (D) mutation would be successful as it has been in the cobalamin E mutation is unknown, but the similarity between the two disorders suggests that it might be. Prenatal diagnosis has also been successful for 5,10-Methylenetetrahydrofolate reductase deficiency by measuring the enzyme and detecting deficient activity in cultured amniocytes and chorionic villi.

HISTIDINEMIA

Definition

Histidinemia is an inborn error of histidine metabolism inherited in an autosomal recessive pattern. It was formerly believed to cause speech defects and mental retardation, but more recent studies indicate that it is benign.

Basic Science

The first step in metabolic degradation of histidine is nonoxidative deamination to urocanic acid. This step is catalyzed by histidase, a zinc-requiring enzyme. In histidinemia, histidase activity is markedly deficient. As a consequence, histidine and its metabolites such as imidazolepyruvate, imidazolelactate, imidazoleacetate, and imidazoleacetic acid riboside accumulate when a normal diet is ingested. In contrast, urocanic acid, which is produced by histidase activity, and is usually found in large quantities in skin and sweat, is absent (Fig. 15.9).

Epidemiology

The results of newborn screening indicate that histidinemia occurs in 1/15,000 to 1/20,000 newborns in the United States and Europe. It seems to be unusually frequent in Canada and Japan, however, occurring in 1/8000 newborns.

Natural History

The first report of histidinemia described a child who had poor speech but normal intelligence. The poor speech was ascribed to the histidinemia. Family screening, however, disclosed a sister who had histidinemia but who was clinically normal. In subsequent studies, histidinemia was occasionally discovered in children who received amino acid screening for evaluation of

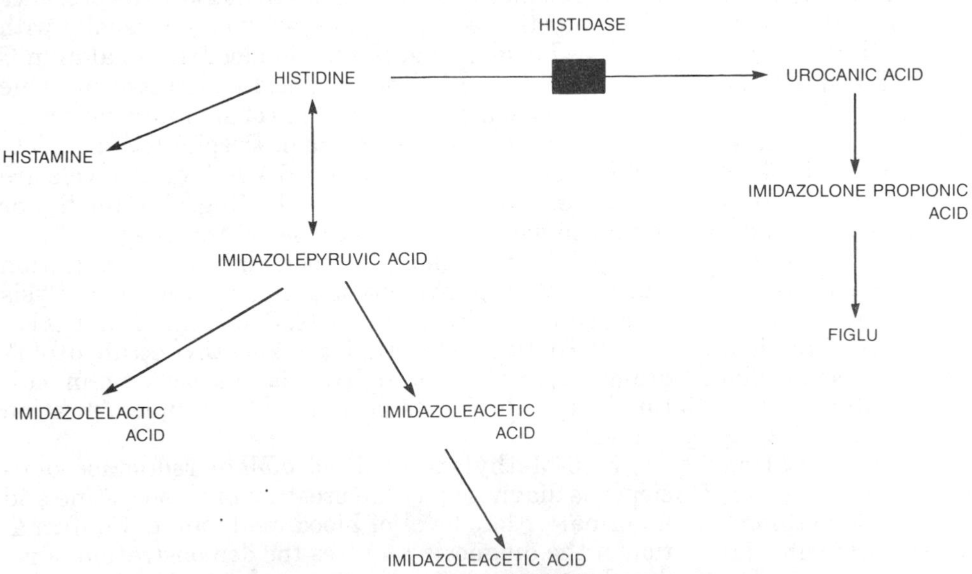

Figure 15.9. Pathway of histidine metabolism. Histidinemia is due to a defect in histidase, the enzyme responsible for the conversion of histidine to urocanic acid.

mental retardation. Many of these children also had poor speech. As in the original report, however, normal children with histidinemia also were identified in family screening.

Follow-up studies of histidinemic infants discovered through routine newborn screening disclosed that most of these infants have not been treated for histidinemia and almost all have had normal growth and development. They have not had speech difficulties and, as older children, have had IQ scores and school performances comparable with their unaffected siblings. Therefore, histidinemia appears to be a benign metabolic disorder, although perinatal hypoxia might predispose an occasional histidinemic infant to CNS deficits.

Diagnosis

The diagnosis is made either through routine newborn screening or amino acid screening for the evaluation of clinical disease. The former consists of screening for increased histidine in the newborn blood specimen or by identifying increased histidine and its metabolites in filter paper specimens of urine collected at 3–4 weeks of age. The blood histidine level in histidinemia is usually 8–14 mg/dl, several times greater than the normal level of less than 2 mg/dl. Urinary histidine is often 50-fold greater than normal.

The diagnosis may be confirmed by the direct measurement of histidase activity in clippings of cuticular skin which in histidinemia is less than 5% of normal. A simpler method of confirmation is the demonstration of absence of urocanic acid in an homogenate of cuticular skin or in sweat. As described under "Basic Science," the absence of urocanic acid reflects little or no histidase activity.

Treatment

Histidine is an essential amino acid or, at least, a semi-essential one. Thus, its level in the body can be controlled by the dietary intake of histidine. A histidine-restricted diet, including special histidine-free formulas, has been developed for the treatment of histidinemia. Proper administration of this diet with frequent monitoring of histidine and other amino acids in blood will control the histidine level in histidinemia and will maintain normal growth and development. Nevertheless, dietary treatment is probably not necessary.

Prognosis

The outcome is good even without therapy.

Prevention

Prenatal diagnosis for histidinemia is not available as histidase activity is not expressed in cultured amniocytes, so the diagnosis of histidinemia through amniocentesis and enzyme analysis is not possible. The gene that encodes histidase has been cloned in the rat, so DNA analysis for histidinemia may soon be possible.

Maternal Histidinemia

Fertility is not impaired in histidinemia. Women with histidinemia have had normal pregnancies and their offspring have usually been normal.

CYSTINOSIS

Definition

Cystinosis is a disorder of cystine metabolism that results in the intracellular accumulation of free, nonprotein cystine crystals in the reticuloendothelial system, as well as kidneys, bone marrow, and cornea. The infantile form is nephropathic while intermediate or late onset forms do not have nephropathy.

Basic Science

The basic defect is not known. However, the efflux of cystine from lysosomes is absent or nonfunctional (Gahl et al, 1982).

Epidemiology

The disorder is a rare autosomal recessive disease.

Natural History

The most severe infantile form may present with growth failure and repeated episodes of dehydration after 6 months of age. Anemia, photophobia, and vitamin D-resistant rickets result from renal tubular damage (Toni-Debre-Fanconi syndrome). Variations in the course occur between families, but the severity tends to be similar within families. In the absence of treatment, death occurs from renal failure in childhood.

Hypothyroidism develops in many patients from cystic accumulation in the gland.

Diagnosis

Cystine crystals may be seen in bone marrow. Leukocyte cystine content can be measured to monitor the effects of therapy (da Silva et al, 1985).

Treatment

Cysteamine, 50 mg/kg/day divided into three equal doses by mouth has been effective in depleting intracellular stores of cystine and, if started before the tissues are damaged, is compatible with normal life (Thoene and Lemons, 1980). Adverse side effects of fever, seizures, hepatotoxicity, and portal hypertension have been reported. The long-term outcome of treated patients is not known as of 1987.

Prevention

Heterozygotes have elevated free cystine in peripheral blood leukocytes. Fibroblasts grown in tissue culture permits prenatal diagnosis.

PROLINE AND HYDROXYPROLINE DISORDERS

Proline and hydroxyproline, while usually included among the amino acids, are more accurately classified as imino acids. Unlike amino acids, in which the nitrogen is in a primary amino group, the nitrogen of the imino acids is bound within a ring.

This subsection includes the disorders of proline and hydroxyproline metabolism as well as prolidase deficiency, a disorder in which proline and hydroxyproline-containing imidodipeptides are not cleaved.

Hyperprolinemia

Definition

Two inborn errors are associated with increased levels of proline. Hyperprolinemia type I is due to a defect in proline oxidase, the first degradative enzyme in the proline pathway. Hyperprolinemia type II is due to a defect in the second enzyme, Δ-1-pyrroline-5-carboxylic acid (PCA) dehydrogenase. The inheritance pattern of each disorder is autosomal recessive.

Basic Science

Proline is a nonessential compound which can be synthesized from glutamic acid or ornithine. It is found predominantly in collagen. The first step in proline degradation, catalyzed by proline oxidase, results in the formation of PCA. A block in this step produces hyperprolinemia type I, with increased proline in blood and urine. Pyrroline-5-carboxylic acid is then converted to glutamic acid by pyrroline-5-carboxylic acid dehydrogenase. This enzyme is defective in hyperprolinemia type II and results in the urinary excretion of pyrroline-5-carboxylic acid in addition to the accumulation of proline.

Proline shares a renal tubular transport system with hydroxyproline and glycine (the iminoglycine system). Accordingly, when this system is saturated by the excess proline to which it is exposed in hyperprolinemia, renal transport of hydroxyproline and glycine is impaired, and they along with proline are increased in urine. This accounts for the iminoglycinuria that is frequently present in hyperprolinemia.

Epidemiology

We have identified four infants with hyperprolinemia type I and two infants with hyperprolinemia type II among 800,000 who have received routine newborn urine screening in Massachusetts. This is a frequency of 1/200,000 for hyperprolinemia type I and 1/400,000 for hyperprolinemia type II.

Natural History

Hyperprolinemia type I appears to be benign. Although a few reported patients have had renal anomalies, deafness and mental retardation, most of the recognized cases have been normal. The four infants we identified by urine screening have remained clinically normal through childhood while continuing normal diets.

Hyperprolinemia type II, on the other hand, produces CNS dysfunction in at least some affected individuals. The two infants we identified by routine screening, now teenagers, have learning disorders. In addition, one has a markedly abnormal electroencephalogram although she has not had overt seizures. This has been reported in other patients with hyperprolinemia type II. We have also diagnosed hyperprolinemia type II in two adolescents who were screened because of mental retardation. Both have had generalized seizures. Asymptomatic individuals with hyperprolinemia type II have also been described.

Diagnosis

Hyperprolinemia of either type is identified by finding an increased level of proline in blood when amino acids are measured for evaluation of a clinical problem or after iminoglycinuria is found by urine amino acid testing. In hyperprolinemia type I, the blood proline level is usually 7–15 mg/dl (normal 2–5 mg/dl). In hyperprolinemia type II, the blood proline level is considerably higher, often exceeding 30 mg/dl. In addition, PCA (and Δ-1-pyrroline-3-hydroxy-5-carboxylic acid) are present in the urine in hyperprolinemia type II but are absent in hyperprolinemia type I.

The diagnosis of hyperprolinemia type I can be confirmed by assay of proline oxidase in liver. Hyperprolinemia type II can be confirmed by the absence of PCA dehydrogenase activity in cultured skin fibroblasts or leukocytes.

Treatment

There is no proven treatment available. Dietary restrictions of proline and amino acids such as ornithine and glutamic acid that can be used to synthesize proline have been attempted in hyperprolinemia type II but have resulted in little or no reduction in blood proline.

Prognosis

Hyperprolinemia type I is most likely benign and is probably compatible with normal growth and development. The prognosis for hyperprolinemia type II is unknown. The mental retardation and seizure disorder seen in some patients do not seem to be progressive.

Prevention

Prenatal diagnosis of hyperprolinemia type II can probably be made by assay of PCA dehydrogenase in cultured amniocytes (or chorionic villi), although this has not yet been reported.

Maternal Hyperprolinemia

Pregnancies have occurred in women with hyperprolinemia type I. No complications were noted during these pregnancies and the offspring were normal.

Hydroxyprolinemia

Definition

This is an inborn error of hydroxyproline degradation. Levels of hydroxyproline are increased in blood and urine.

Basic Science

Hydroxyproline is a constituent of connective tissue, primarily collagen. It is synthesized by the hydroxylation of collagen proline. Although synthesis can occur nonenzymatically in the presence of ascorbic acid (vitamin C), it is largely mediated by the enzyme prolyl hydroxylase. Free hydroxyproline and hydroxyproline released by cleavage of imino acid-containing dipeptides are generated during collagen turnover. The hydroxyproline is degraded to Δ-1-pyrroline-3-hydroxy-5-carboxylic acid by the enzyme hydroxyproline oxidase, which is presumably defective.

Epidemiology

Hydroxyprolinemia has been reported very rarely. We have identified only one case in screening 800,000 newborn infants.

Natural History

The original patient with hydroxyprolinemia and several others have been mentally retarded, but were, in fact, screened because of mental retardation. Other individuals identified through family studies or by routine screening have been normal. The child we have followed, now 3 years old, is growing and developing at a faster rate than her biochemically normal dizygotic twin sister. Thus, hydroxyprolinemia seems to be a benign disorder.

Diagnosis

Individuals with hydroxyprolinemia have a 10- to 20-fold increase in the plasma hydroxyproline level. All other plasma amino acid values are normal, including that of proline. Urine hydroxyproline concentration is also markedly increased. In contrast to hyperprolinemia, however, patients with hydroxyprolinemia do not have iminoglycinuria, presumably because the concentration of hydroxyproline rarely, if ever, is elevated to the level necessary for saturation of the iminoglycine renal transport system, and displacement of glycine and proline from that system.

Treatment

No treatment is available.

Prognosis

Hydroxyprolinemia seems to be benign and compatible with normal growth and development.

Prevention

Prenatal diagnosis for hydroxyprolinemia has not been developed.

Maternal Hydroxyprolinemia

One woman with hydroxyprolinemia is known to have had a normal pregnancy with the birth of a normal child.

PROLIDASE DEFICIENCY

Definition

Prolidase deficiency is an autosomal recessive inborn error in which prolidase, an imidodipeptidase that cleaves certain proline- and hydroxyproline-containing imidodipeptides, is deficient. The disorder results in a striking tendency for development of severe and intractable ulcerative cutaneous lesions of the lower extremities.

Basic Science

The C-terminal imino acid-containing dipeptides that are released during collagen turnover are cleaved by prolidase, a manganese-activated enzyme. When prolidase activity is deficient, these dipeptides (imidodipeptides) accumulate in the body and can be readily identified in blood and urine. The clinical disease that results, primarily ulcerative skin lesions, has not yet been satisfactorily explained on the basis of the biochemical abnormalities. A plausible explanation, however, is that proline released intracellularly from imidodipeptides is necessary for recycling into collagen and that, in the absence of this release, the equilibrium of collagen metabolism is altered.

Epidemiology

Very few cases have been reported. It is possible that this reflects, to some extent, the lack of suspicion of inborn errors by dermatologists and internal medicine specialists who are more likely to see these patients than are pediatricians, as the skin lesions often do not appear until adolescence. We have identified one infant among 800,000 who received routine urine screening in the newborn period. Two siblings of this infant also have prolidase deficiency but had not been screened. Thus, the frequency might be about 1:300,000.

Natural History

The major feature of prolidase deficiency is the presence of chronic ulcers of the legs. The lesions may appear in childhood but more often do not become evident until adolescence. They are often accompanied and may be preceded by a chronic dermatitis consisting of crusting erythematous lesions on the face, soles, and palms. About 50% of patients have been mentally retarded or had only borderline intelligence. Several have also had splenomegaly. Facial dysmorphism, including ptosis, ocular proptosis, and prominent cranial sutures, have also been reported.

Diagnosis

The disorder is usually discovered by the presence of glycylproline in an amino acid screen of urine. Further study of urine will disclose the excretion of several other imidodipeptides including aspartylproline, leucylproline, alanylproline, and prolylproline. The blood contains identifiable glycylproline, which is not detectable in normal blood. The diagnosis is confirmed by the demonstration of markedly deficient or absent prolidase activity but normal prolinase activity (the enzyme that cleaves N-terminal imidodipeptides) in erythrocytes or leukocytes.

Treatment

No satisfactory treatment has yet been devised for prolidase deficiency. Prolidase requires manganese for optimal activity and manganese supplementation has been used in the treatment of several patients, but has not produced a clear biochemical or clinical response (Charpentier et al, 1981).

Prognosis

The leg ulcers improve with nonspecific treatment that includes antibiotics and leg elevation. However, they tend to reappear. Other features of the disorder also continue. No long-term follow-up studies have yet been reported.

Prevention

Prolidase activity is deficient in erythrocytes from umbilical cord blood (Naughten et al, 1984). Thus, the disorder is expressed in the fetus and probably can be identified by enzyme assay of cultured amniocytes, although prenatal diagnosis has not yet been reported. No treatment is known that will prevent development of the clinical abnormalities.

HYPERORNITHINEMIAS

Ornithine is a nonprotein amino acid that plays an important role in the urea cycle and in the metabolism of proline, creatine, and the polyamines. The major source of ornithine is the arginine from dietary protein.

Hyperornithinemia is the major biochemical feature of two distinct inborn errors of metabolism, gyrate atrophy of the choroid and retina, and the HHH (hyperornithinemia-hyperammonemia-homocitrullinuria) syndrome.

Gyrate Atrophy of the Choroid and Retina

Definition

Gyrate atrophy of the choroid and retina is an autosomal recessive inborn error of metabolism due to a deficiency of the enzyme ornithine-Δ-aminotransferase (OAT). Poor vision with night blindness is the major clinical feature.

Basic Science

The inherited deficiency of ornithine-Δ-amino transferase, which has been demonstrated in cultured skin fibroblasts, phytohemagglutinin stimulated lymphocytes, muscle, liver, and hair roots of affected individuals results in hyperornithinemia and explains the biochemical abnormalities that are seen in this disorder. OAT is a pyridoxine (B_6) requiring enzyme. Several pyridoxine responsive patients have been described (Berson et al, 1981). How hyperornithinemia leads to chorioretinal degeneration and cataracts is not known.

Epidemiology

Gyrate atrophy of the choroid and retina has been reported in over 90 patients, half of whom are Finnish.

Natural History

Affected individuals present with myopia, night blindness, and loss of peripheral vision, usually beginning in the first decade of life. Untreated, these symptoms progress to tunnel vision and finally to total blindness by the third or fourth decade. All of the patients also have posterior subcapsular cataracts. Examination of the ocular fundus characteristically reveals sharply demarcated areas of chorioretinal degeneration.

Diagnosis

The diagnosis is suggested by the history and clinical examination. Electroretinography reveals decreased amplitude. Mitochondrial abnormalities in liver and skeletal muscle, and the existence of "tubular aggregates" in type 2 skeletal muscle fibers have also been described.

Plasma ornithine values are characteristically 10- to 20-fold greater than normal; increased urinary excretion of ornithine is also seen.

Confirmation of the diagnosis depends upon demonstration of decreased OAT activity in cultured cells and/or tissues of the patient.

Treatment

A low protein, arginine-restricted diet decreases the plasma ornithine level and has been reported to decrease the progression of symptoms in several patients. Pyridoxine supplementation decreases ornithine in patients with a pyridoxine responsive form of this disorder (Berson et al, 1981). Some treated patients reported improvement in visual function.

Creatine administration has led to improvement of the histologic abnormalities in the muscle of affected individuals.

Prevention

Prenatal diagnosis of this disorder is theoretically possible by measurement of ornithine Δ-amino transferase activity in cultured amniotic cells. Carrier detection is possible since obligate heterozygotes have been shown to have about 50% of normal transferase activity in cultured skin fibroblasts.

The gene for ornithine Δ-transferase has been cloned and assigned to chromosome number 10 (Mitchell et al, 1986a; Ramesh et al, 1986).

Hyperornithinemia-Hyperammonemia-Homocitrullinuria (HHH Syndrome)

Definition

The HHH syndrome is an autosomal recessive inborn error of metabolism that results in hyperornithinemia, hyperammonemia, and homocitrullinuria.

Basic Science

The primary defect in this disorder is unknown, but is believed to be an impairment of ornithine transport from the cytoplasm across the inner mitochondrial membrane into the mitochondrion (Hommes et al, 1986). This would produce a block in the urea cycle at the level of ornithine transcarbamylase (Fig. 15.10), and would result in hyperammonemia. The origin of homocitrullinuria is unknown.

Epidemiology

Twelve patients have been reported with this rare inborn error of metabolism.

Natural History

Affected individuals present with seizures, mental retardation, and symptoms related to hyperammonemia, including episodic vomiting, lethargy, and coma. There is usually a history of growth retardation, developmental delay, and self-induced protein restriction.

Diagnosis

The diagnosis is suggested by the clinical history in a patient with hyperammonemia, and confirmed by the demonstration of increased levels of plasma ornithine and urinary homocitrulline. Most patients also have increased levels of glutamine and alanine in the blood, and increased urinary orotic acid.

Treatment

Protein restriction to less than 1.2 g/kg/day has resulted in a decrease in plasma ornithine concentration and in postprandial hyperammonemia. In one patient, arginine supplementation led to decreased blood ammonia levels. Ornithine supplementation has also been reported to decrease ammonia levels, but ornithine loading in a patient with the HHH syndrome did not protect the patient from hyperammonemia induced by amino-nitrogen loading.

Prevention

Since the primary defect in this disorder is not known, there is no available method of prenatal diagnosis.

UREA CYCLE DISORDERS

Definition

The urea cycle comprises six enzymes that operate in a cyclic fashion devoted to the production of urea. An inborn error of metabolism has been identified for each of the enzymes in the cycle. Those disorders are inherited in an autosomal recessive fashion, except for ornithine transcarbamylase deficiency, which is inherited as an X-linked recessive.

Basic Science

One molecule of urea is synthesized by each revolution of the urea cycle. Two nitrogen atoms enter the cycle. The first is derived from ammonia, which is produced continuously from amino acids and purines, while the second nitrogen is derived from aspartate which enters the cycle at another point. The liver is the major site for urea synthesis.

The first three enzymes of the cycle, N-acetylglutamate synthetase, carbamylphosphate synthetase I (CPS I), and ornithine transcarbamylase (OTC), are intramitochondrial. The last three enzymes, argininosuccinate synthetase, argininosuccinate lyase, and arginase, function in the cytosol. These enzymes and the reactions in the cycle that they catalyze are shown in Figure 15.10. An enzymatic defect at any step results in accumulation of metabolites proximal to that step and a reduction or absence of metabolites distal to the step. The most proximal metabolite is ammonia, which accumulates in the presence of any of the defects. CPS and OTC deficiencies cause reduced citrulline and arginine. Argininosuccinate synthetase deficiency produces increased citrulline (citrullinemia), argininosuccinate lyase deficiency produces argininosuccinate (argininosuccinic acidemia) and arginase deficiency results in increased arginine (hyperargininemia). In addition to these amino acid abnormalities, orotic acid, an organic acid derived from carbamyl phosphate (Fig. 15.10), is increased in the urine in all of the urea cycle defects except for CPS deficiency, in which the production of carbamyl phosphate is limited. A comprehensive review of hyperammonemia by Batshaw et al (1982) should be consulted for further details.

Epidemiology

The exact prevalence of inborn errors of metabolism of the urea cycle is not known, but has been estimated at about 1/10,000.

Natural History

The main clinical features of the urea cycle disorders include protein intolerance with hyperammonemia and episodic lethargy, leading to developmental delay or mental retardation, and hepatomegaly.

One patient with N-acetylglutamate synthetase deficiency has been described (Bachmann et al, 1981). This patient presented on the third day of life with

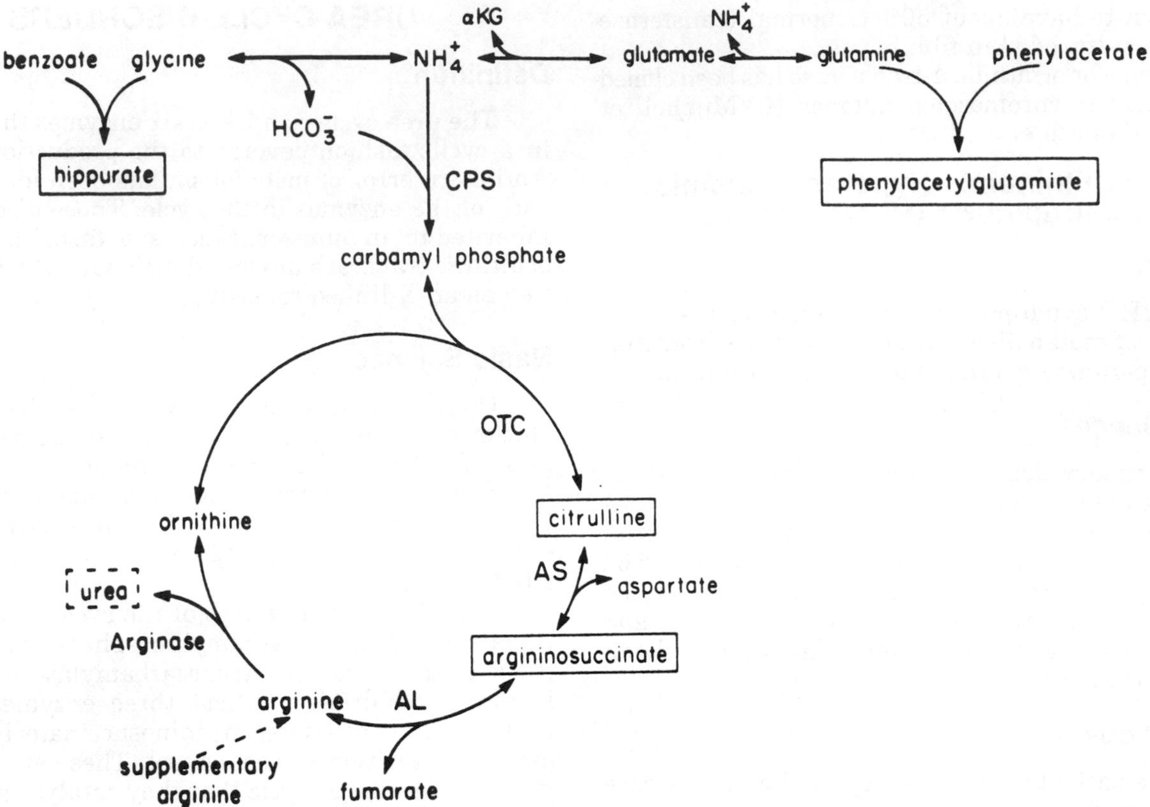

Figure 15.10. Pathways in the urea cycle.

hyperammonemia in the absence of orotic aciduria and a nonspecific hyperaminoaciduria.

CPS I deficiency is of two types: In the neonatal form, characteristic signs of hyperammonemia appear in the first 3 days of life. These include vomiting, lethargy, seizures, respiratory distress, and coma. Severe cerebral edema and pulmonary and gastrointestinal hemorrhages develop as the disease progresses. These patients are severely ill and often do not survive the neonatal illness. In the later onset forms, patients present later during the first or second year of life, with a picture that may be indistinguishable from Reye syndrome, with lethargy or coma, hyperammonemia, and hepatomegaly. These children often have a chronic episodic history of feeding intolerance, irritability, lethargy, vomiting, or seizures. The neonatal form is associated with an absence of CPS I activity, while late onset patients may have a partial deficiency of this enzyme. In both forms, patients often have recurrent hyperammonemic crises precipitated by febrile illnesses, increased protein intake, or even constipation despite treatment for the urea cycle disorder.

OTC deficiency also has a neonatal and a late onset form. In this X-linked disorder, there is often a history of deaths in the neonatal period among males on the mother's side of the family. Hemizygous males usually present with severe neonatal hyperammonemia, with signs and symptoms similar to those in the neonatal form of CPS I deficiency. Heterozygous females generally present with recurrent hyperammonemia later in life similar to the "Reye" phenotype of late onset CPS I deficiency, although severe neonatal hyperammonemia may also be encountered in females. The severity of illness in the female depends on the pattern of X-chromosome inactivation (lyonization) in the liver cells and, hence, the residual enzyme activity. If the X-chromosome that carries the mutant OTC gene has been inactivated in most of the cells, the residual OTC activity will be higher than if the X-chromosome carrying the normal OTC gene has been preferentially inactivated. In the former instance, the female is likely to be asymptomatic or only mildly symptomatic, while in the latter case the female might have severe recurrent hyperammonemia. Although OTC-deficient patients who present with the later onset form of the disorder are usually females, recently several males have been described who initially presented as older children or adults. Presumably they have a different mutation of the OTC locus from that which produces neonatal disease. As in CPS I deficiency, any affected individual can become hyperammonemic during an acute febrile illness or with increased protein intake.

Citrullinemia, due to argininosuccinate synthetase deficiency, and argininosuccinic acidemia, due to argininosuccinate lyase deficiency, can also present with severe neonatal hyperammonemia or with later onset forms. As in CPS I and OTC deficiencies, the later onset forms of argininosuccinate synthetase and lyase deficiencies typically involve a history of recurrent hyperammonemic crises or mental retardation and seizures. In addition to hyperammonemia, argininosuccinate lyase deficiency is also associated with dry, brittle hair and with microscopic nodular protrusions along the shaft of the hair.

The clinical picture in patients with a deficiency of arginase, the last enzyme of the urea cycle, is different from that seen in other disorders. Children with arginase deficiency do not have neonatal illness and rarely have the "Reye" phenotype of later onset. Their most characteristic feature is a "scissoring gait" due to spasticity of the lower extremities which usually progresses to spastic diplegia. Ataxia, choreoathetosis, seizures, hepatomegaly, dysphagia, and vomiting have also been reported in these patients. Recurrent episodes of hyperammonemia may occur but are usually not as severe as in the other urea cycle disorders. As in the other disorders, there is considerable heterogeneity of expression. Some patients show mild impairment of intellectual function as the only manifestation of illness.

Diagnosis

Any patient with lethargy, coma, or other signs that suggest a urea cycle disorder should have a blood ammonia level determined immediately. In a urea cycle disorder, the blood ammonia level is typically 5–30 times normal. Respiratory alkalosis due to stimulation of respiratory drive by the hyperammonemia may also be observed, as well as increased serum transaminases of liver origin, a nonspecific hyperaminoaciduria, and an increase in the blood alanine and glutamine levels. Glucose and electrolyte concentrations are usually normal. Urine should be examined for organic acids since organic acid disorders are often accompanied by hyperammonemia, although usually in a setting of severe metabolic acidosis and hypoglycemia.

The most important laboratory tests in establishing the specific enzyme deficiency in the urea cycle are analyses of amino acids in blood and urine and of orotic acid in urine. Metabolite accumulation proximal to the blocked enzyme step and reduced product distal to the block provides each urea cycle disorder with a characteristic pattern. Low or undetectable blood citrulline levels are seen in patients with CPS I and OTC deficiency. The urine orotic acid analysis (discussed below) will distinguish between these two. Patients with citrullinemia (argininosuccinate synthetase deficiency) typically have marked elevations of citrulline in blood and urine. Those with argininosuccinic acidemia (argininosuccinate lyase deficiency) have increased levels of argininosuccinic acid in the blood and urine (more readily identifiable in urine), and those with arginase deficiency have 4- to 20-fold elevations of arginine in the blood. Patients with arginase deficiency also have been reported to have a curious vitamin K-resistant clotting abnormality.

The urine orotic acid analysis can help distinguish between some of the urea cycle disorders. Patients with OTC deficiency typically present with a striking orotic aciduria, whereas in CPS I deficiency urinary orotic acid is normal or reduced. Increased orotic acid levels also are present in patients with enzyme defects distal to the OTC step, although the elevation is less striking than is that in OTC deficiency. The increased orotic acid is derived from carbamyl phosphate, a co-substrate with ornithine for OTC, which accumulates in the mitochondria when OTC activity or enzyme activities distal to OTC are deficient. The accumulated carbamyl phosphate enters the cytosol where it becomes available for conversion to pyrimidines such as orotic acid, uridine, and uracil.

A definitive diagnosis of the enzyme deficiency requires measurement of tissue enzyme activity. This is readily available in patients with deficiencies of the last three enzymes of the cycle since these cytosolic enzymes can be measured in a variety of tissues, including cultured skin fibroblasts, lymphocytes, and/or erythrocytes. Enzyme diagnosis is somewhat more difficult for the first three disorders of the cycle, for which the enzymes are intramitochondrial, as these enzymes can only be measured in liver specimens obtained by percutaneous or open liver biopsy. There have been reports of patients who have more than one urea cycle enzyme deficiency, which may complicate the interpretation of data obtained by standard methods of diagnosis described above.

Treatment

Until recently, the treatment of patients with urea cycle disorders consisted only of a protein-restricted diet and, for acute episodes, high caloric intravenous fluids. This therapy was of very limited effectiveness and did little to reduce very high morbidity and mortality in these disorders. With the recent introduction of medications such as sodium benzoate and sodium phenylacetate to activate alternate pathways of waste nitrogen disposal (Fig. 15.10) and advances in hemodialysis and peritoneal dialysis, many of these infants and children are surviving. The hallmarks of this therapy for acute hyperammonemia episodes include the prompt introduction of protein restriction, intravenous sodium benzoate, sodium phenylacetate, and arginine, and peritoneal dialysis or, if available, hemodialysis. Hemodialysis has been shown to be much more efficient in controlling hyperammonemia than is either exchange transfusion or peritoneal dialysis, and is the method of choice. Sodium benzoate and sodium phenylacetate conjugate glycine and glutamine, which are readily excreted as hippurate and phenylacetylglutamine, respectively (Fig. 15.10). A specific protocol for this therapy has been published by the group at the Johns Hopkins Hospital (Brusilow et al, 1984; Batshaw et al, 1982). Intravenous glucose (10–20%) and lipids also should be given to spare amino acids and reduce endogenous proteolysis. The neurologic status should be observed carefully since hyperammonemia may produce severe cerebral edema, with increased intracranial pressure sufficient to cause herniation of the brain stem and death. Patients with argininosuccinic acidemia (argininosuccinate lyase deficiency) may respond dramatically to intravenous arginine alone, which warrants the use of higher doses of arginine in patients suspected of having this disorder.

The chronic treatment of these patients includes the use of various combinations of sodium benzoate, sodium phenylacetate or phenylbutyrate, and citrulline or arginine, in addition to a high-calorie, protein-restricted diet and close monitoring of clinical status and blood ammonia levels. Particular attention should be given to blood ammonia concentrations during episodes of febrile illness as these children are extremely susceptible to recurrent episodes of severe hyperammonemia throughout life.

Bartholomew and colleagues have reported the benefit of prospective treatment of neonates at risk for a urea cycle disorder (Bartholomew et al, 1986). With protein restriction and the organic acid medications provided, a number of affected infants have remained clinically normal and maintained normal blood ammonia levels throughout the neonatal and early infancy periods.

Prognosis

Although the morbidity and mortality associated with urea cycle disorders have been improved by advances in intensive care, dialysis, and use of sodium benzoate and sodium phenylacetate, affected patients still experience many problems. Some infants die in the neonatal period despite therapy, and those that survive are often neurologically impaired (Msall et al, 1984). The prognoses for patients with CPS I deficiency as well as citrullinemia and argininosuccinic acidemia appear to be better than that for males with OTC deficiency, while the prognosis for females heterozygous for OTC deficiency depends to some extent on their residual enzyme activity.

Prevention

Prevention involves genetic counseling and prenatal diagnosis. Since neither CPS I nor OTC activity is expressed in cultured amniocytes, until recently the only method of prenatal diagnosis possible was by means of fetal liver biopsy and measurement of these enzymes in liver. Now, the cloned genes for both CPS I and OTC are available, making prenatal diagnosis by means of fetal DNA analysis possible in some families at risk for having infants with these disorders. Prenatal diagnosis of citrullinemia and argininosuccinic acidemia is possible by measurement of ASAS and ASAL activities in cultured amniocytes, respectively. In addition, increased levels of citrulline and argininosuccinic acid have been reported in the amniotic fluid of an affected fetus. Prenatal diagnosis of arginase deficiency requires the measurement of arginase in fetal red blood cells obtained by means of fetoscopy.

Carrier detection of females for OTC deficiency can be accomplished by demonstration of increased urinary ammonia and/or orotic acid after oral protein loading. A preliminary report describes a new method of carrier detection that relies on an exaggerated urine orotic acid response to allopurinol (Brusilow and Valle, 1986). Heterozygotes for arginase deficiency have been reported to have increased concentrations of arginine in leukocytes.

Transient Hyperammonemia of the Neonate

Definition

Transient hyperammonemia of the neonate (see pp. 140, Neonatology) was first recognized in premature infants or those who were small for gestational age, but has also been recognized in term infants. It is not believed to be an inherited disorder.

Basic Science

The cause of this phenomenon is unknown. The activities of urea cycle enzymes in several patients were found to be normal and in other patients amino acid and orotic acid studies have not indicated a urea cycle defect. The disorder may be due to the relative inability of an immature urea cycle to handle the increased ammonia production that can occur in neonates in a hypercatabolic state.

Epidemiology

The prevalence of this disorder is not known.

CASE ILLUSTRATION

A 4-kg full-term male was born after an uneventful pregnancy and normal vaginal delivery. He seemed normal at birth, but by the third day of life was tachypneic, obtunded, and had a seizure. On evaluation at the hospital, he was found to have a respiratory alkalosis and blood ammonia level of 2000 μg/dl. Blood urea nitrogen was 4 mg/dl. Further studies revealed deficiency of ornithine transcarbamylase (OTC).

Therapy included immediate hemodialysis to lower the ammonia level, since the length of time that the serum ammonia is over 300 μg/dl is thought to be a critical factor in neuronal damage. Exogenous protein was restricted, and excess calories were provided by intravenous dextrose and lipids to minimize proteolysis. Intravenous sodium benzoate and sodium phenylacetate were given to bind endogenous ammonia before it entered the urea cycle. The resulting hippurate and phenylacetylglutamine were excreted in the urine.

The infant was subsequently given sodium benzoate, sodium phenylacetate, and arginine, and his serum ammonia was maintained within a normal range. He continues to do well.

Natural History

Affected infants present with hyperammonemia that in general develops earlier than that seen in disorders of the urea cycle, often during the first 24 hours of life. Symptoms and signs of hyperammonemia, which include lethargy, seizures, coma, and respiratory alkalosis, occur. Patients have significantly lower birth weights and gestational ages, and plasma ammonia concentrations are higher at an earlier age than are those seen in patients with urea cycle disorders.

Diagnosis

As noted above, blood ammonia concentrations are increased (often greater than 1000 μg/dl) and blood gas analysis reveals respiratory alkalosis. Orotic aciduria is not present and blood and urine amino acid concentrations are essentially normal. In particular, citrulline levels are normal or slightly increased.

Treatment

Since the hyperammonemia is reversible and rarely recurs, treatment to control the hyperammonemia should be aggressive, and instituted promptly. The treatment is that for acute hyperammonemic episodes as described under Treatment for the urea cycle disorders.

Prognosis

Without prompt and appropriate therapy, many of these infants will die in the neonatal period. With therapy, however, the prognosis for these infants is very good. They do not develop recurrent hyperammonemic episodes and appear to recover from their initial episode without neurologic sequelae.

Lysinuric Protein Intolerance

Definition

First described in Finland, lysinuric protein intolerance (also known as "hyperdibasic amino aciduria") is an autosomal recessive disorder, which is due to defective transport of dibasic amino acids.

Basic Science

The underlying defect is believed to be impaired transport of the dibasic amino acids in the kidneys, intestinal tract, and liver. This leads to increased urinary excretion of the dibasic amino acids and decreased circulating levels of these amino acids. It is the impaired transport of ornithine across the hepatocyte membrane, however, that appears to cause the clinical complications. This results in insufficient intracellular and intramitochondrial ornithine to support the activity of ornithine transcarbamylase (OTC), an important intramitochondrial enzyme of the urea cycle (Fig. 15.10).Thus, there is reduced carbamylase activity in the presence of a normal enzyme. Hyperammonemia with protein intolerance follows.

Epidemiology

The reported prevalence of this disorder is 1/60,000–80,000 births in Finland, but cases have been reported in many other countries around the world.

Natural History

Growth retardation, protein intolerance, and signs of hyperammonemia are the earliest manifestations of this disorder. The protein intolerance usually begins in infancy and is marked by feeding difficulties, vomiting, diarrhea, and failure to thrive. As the children become older, overt signs of protein aversion develop. Developmental delay and mental retardation also have been reported.

Other signs and symptoms include osteoporosis and short stature, hepatosplenomegaly, opacities of the lens of the eye, sparse and brittle hair, hyperelastic skin, and loose joints. Some patients also have signs of bone marrow depression.

Diagnosis

The diagnosis of this disorder may be suspected by the clinical features. Osteoporosis may be striking and this as well as short stature has brought attention to a number of these children. The diagnosis is further suspected when the patient has hyperammonemia, decreased levels of lysine, arginine, and ornithine, with increased levels of alanine and glutamine in blood, increased levels of the dibasic amino acids in urine, and, often, increased concentrations of orotic acid in urine. The dibasic aminoaciduria might suggest the diagnosis of cystinuria, although cystine is not prominent in urine in lysinuric protein intolerance. Nevertheless, this disorder should be considered in any child with "cystinuria," especially if short stature is present.

Treatment

The administration of citrulline in large doses has produced major improvements in the clinical features of lysinuric protein intolerance (Carpenter et al, 1985). Citrulline can enter the hepatocyte and lead to the intracellular formation of ornithine via the urea cycle. The cytosolic ornithine formed then enters the mitochondria and acts as substrate for the OTC-mediated reaction, thus alleviating the urea cycle block. Measurement of orotic acid excretion is useful in monitoring therapy and determining adequate citrulline dosages.

Prognosis

Oral citrulline therapy has been very effective in increasing protein tolerance and bone mass, and in improving linear growth in affected patients.

NONKETOTIC HYPERGLYCINEMIA

Definition

Nonketotic hyperglycinemia is defined as a persistent increase in glycine without ketoacidosis. The

CASE ILLUSTRATION (Abstracted from *N Engl J Med* 312:290, 1985)

This 23-month-old infant of Italian descent was referred because she had a compressed fracture of the wrist after a minor fall, and the radiograph showed severe osteopenia. She weighed 3.9 kg at birth, and was well until about 1 year of age, when regurgitation and diarrhea were noted with the introduction of solid foods. These subsided, but her weight fell from the 30th percentile to the 15th percentile and her height moved from the 20th percentile to below the 3rd percentile between 16 and 26 months of age. Her developmental milestones were normal. On examination, she was fair-skinned and red-haired unlike her darker complexioned parents and brother. No ocular or dental abnormalities were present. She had a Cushingoid appearance, with reduced muscle mass and a puffy facies. Laboratory studies showed normal calcium, phosphorus, magnesium, copper, alkaline phosphatase, vitamin D metabolites, and serum cortisol. The fasting ammonia was normal but urinary excretion of lysine and glutamine were elevated. Dibasic amino acids (ornithine, lysine, and arginine) were reduced in the serum.

Further studies showed a four-fold elevation in plasma ammonia after an intravenous infusion of alanine, showing an impaired urea cycle function. Oral protein loading led to an increase in orotic acid excretion. The administration of citrulline with an identical protein load lowered orotic acid excretion.

After 7 months of oral citrulline supplementation, her appearance improved dramatically. Her previously red hair became dark brown and her linear growth accelerated. Radiographic studies showed an increase in bone density. By 2 months of therapy, her plasma amino acids were nearly normal, as was the ammonia level.

entity was named to differentiate it from ketotic hyperglycinemia. We now know that "ketotic hyperglycinemia" is not a specific disorder but is ketoacidosis and hyperglycinemia secondary to any one of several organic acidopathies, notably propionic acidemia and methylmalonic acidemia (see section on organic acid disorders). Consequently, the term "ketotic hyperglycinemia" has disappeared, replaced by the names of the specific organic acid disorders. Nonketotic hyperglycinemia, however, persists in metabolic nomenclature since it designates what is believed to be a specific autosomal recessive disorder of glycine degradation.

Basic Science

Glycine is involved in many synthetic reactions, including the formations of serine, porphyrins, purines, glutathione, bile acids, and glyoxylate. The most important of these for glycine degradation is the synthesis of serine. The defect in nonketotic hyperglycinemia is in glycine conversion to serine, normally mediated by the glycine cleavage reaction. In this reaction, glycine is decarboxylated to yield carbon dioxide and the methyl group for hydroxymethyltetrahydrofolate. The latter compound is used to form serine. Although hydroxymethyltetrahydrofolate is derived from many sources other than glycine, the lack of glycine cleavage sufficiently limits its availability so that serine synthesis is impaired. Perhaps of much greater importance in nonketotic hyperglycinemia is the increased glycine that results from the defect in glycine cleavage.

The major problem in nonketotic hyperglycinemia may be the accumulation of glycine in the brain. The glycine cleavage reaction is present in normal brain but absent in brain from patients with nonketotic hyperglycinemia. Brain glycine as well as CSF glycine is markedly increased in these patients. Since glycine is a postsynaptic inhibitory neurotransmitter, it is possible that excessive glycine so inhibits neurotransmission as to produce the clinical disease.

Epidemiology

We are aware of six infants with nonketotic hyperglycinemia identified in New England during the past 15 years. This is an incidence of about 1:350,000. It is likely that this is an underestimation, however, since some infants with nonketotic hyperglycinemia may die without diagnosis.

Natural History

We have observed three clinical phenotypes associated with nonketotic hyperglycinemia. The neonatal form is the most dramatic and may be the most frequent. Typically an infant is born after a normal pregnancy with normal labor and delivery who seemed to be normal during the first day of life but becomes markedly lethargic and hypotonic by the second or third day. Before the end of the first week the infant becomes unresponsive and extremely floppy. Many of these infants will have seizures, either myoclonic or generalized. The usual laboratory results are normal, including cultures, electrolytes, liver function studies, blood gases, ammonia, and others.

The second phenotype, "late onset," is represented by the infant who has had a normal neonatal course but at 3–6 months of age is noted to be developmentally delayed and, often, to have myoclonic seizures. The seizures disappear but the child becomes mentally retarded, usually moderate in degree.

The third phenotype is represented by the child who is clinically normal but who has persistent elevation of glycine in urine. We have observed one such case identified by routine newborn urine screening. In contrast to clinically abnormal children who have markedly increased CSF glycine levels, this child had only a slightly increased level suggesting that his defect is peripheral and excludes the CNS.

Diagnosis

Increased concentrations of glycine in blood and urine in an infant with the acute clinical characteristics of nonketotic hyperglycinemia or in a mentally retarded child are the initial findings in this disorder. Careful attention should be given to whether metabolic acidosis or ketonuria are evident, in which case the hyperglycinemia may be secondary to an organic acid disorder ("ketotic hyperglycinemia"). Regardless, any infant or child with increased glycine should have a urine organic acid screen, which will be normal in nonketotic hyperglycinemia. CSF should be examined for amino acids. The CSF glycine value is usually 15- to 25-fold greater than normal while the blood glycine concentration is 3- to 5-fold increased. Thus, the plasma-CSF glycine ratio, usually about 30, is reduced to 4–8 in nonketotic hyperglycinemia.

Treatment

There is no effective treatment for nonketotic hyperglycinemia. Sodium benzoate has been used in attempts to reduce the amount of glycine via formation of hippuric acid, but this has not been accompanied by clinical benefit, perhaps because benzoate does not readily enter the CNS. Strychnine has been given because it competes with glycine for postsynaptic neurotransmitter receptor sites. Some neonates treated with strychnine have developed better muscle tone and older infants are reported to have better development than otherwise expected, but strychnine has not been beneficial for most patients. Diazepam has been reported to improve seizure control and increase responsiveness to stimuli but we have not seen improvement in the two patients we have treated with this drug.

Prognosis

Infants with the neonatal phenotype often die within the first month of life. Those that survive are usually left with profound brain damage, exhibiting severe developmental delay and generalized seizures that are often intractable. Late onset disease is much milder, and symptoms may not appear until adolescence.

Prevention

Successful prenatal diagnosis on the basis of increased glycine:serine ratio in second trimester amniotic fluid has been reported (Applegarth et al, 1986). Whether this is a reliable method for the prenatal diagnosis of nonketotic hyperglycinemia remains to be determined. The enzyme defect has been found in the placenta from an affected pregnancy, which suggests that prenatal diagnosis by chorionic villus testing may be possible (Hayasaka et al, 1987).

REFERENCES

Adcock MW, O'Brien WE: Molecular cloning of cDNA for rat and human carbamyl phosphate synthetase I. *J Biol Chem* 259:13471, 1984.

Applegarth DA, Ingram P, Hingston J, et al: Hyperprolinemia type II. *Clin Biochem* 7:14, 1974.

Applegarth DA, Levy HL, Shih VE, et al: Prenatal diagnosis of nonketotic hyperglycinemia. *Prenat Diag* 6:257, 1986.

Avery ME, Clow CL, Menkes JH, et al: Transient tyrosinemia of the newborn. Dietary and clinical aspects. *Pediatrics* 39:160, 1967.

Bachmann C, Drahenbuhl S, Colombo JP, et al: N-Acetylglutamate synthetase deficiency: A disorder of ammonia detoxication. *N Engl J Med* 304:543, 1981.

Ballard RA, Vinocur B, Reynolds JW, et al: Transient hyperammonemia of the preterm infant. *N Engl J Med* 299:920, 1978.

Bartholomew D, Reichel R, Brusilow S: Prospective diagnosis and treatment of urea cycle defects. *Am J Hum Genet* 39 (Suppl):A4, 1986.

Batshaw ML, Brusilow S, Waber L, et al: Treatment of inborn errors of urea synthesis. *N Engl J Med* 306:1387, 1982.

Beaudet AL, O'Brien WE, Bock HGO, et al: The human argininosuccinate synthetase locus and citrullinemia. In Harris H, Hirschhorn K (eds): *Advances in Human Genetics,* Vol 15. Plenum Publishing Corp, 1986, p 161.

Bernar J, Hanson RA, Kern R, et al: Arginase deficiency in a 12-year-old boy with mild impairment of intellectual function. *J Pediatr* 108:432, 1986.

Berson EL, Shih VE, Sullivan PL: Ocular findings in patients with gyrate atrophy on pyridoxine, and low-protein, low arginine diets. *Ophthalmology* 88:311, 1981.

Bienfang DC, Kuwabara T, Pueschel SM: The Richner-Hanhart syndrome-report of a case with associated tyrosinemia. *Arch Ophthalmol* 94:1133, 1976.

Boers G, Smals A, Kloppenbong P, et al: Heterozygosity for homocystinuria in premature arterial disease. *N Engl J Med* 314:850, 1986.

Brusilow S, Valle D: Allopurinol induced orotic aciduria: A test for heterozygosity for ornithine transcarbamylase deficiency. *Am J Hum Genet* 39:(Suppl):A6, 1986.

Bursilow SW, Danney M, Waber LJ, et al: Treatment of episodic hyperammonemia in children with inborn errors of urea synthesis. *N Engl J Med* 310:1630, 1984.

Carpenter TO, Levy HL, Holtrop ME, et al: Lysinuric protein intolerance presenting as childhood osteoporosis. *N Engl J Med* 312:290, 1985.

Charpentier C, Dagbovie K, Lemonnier A, et al: Prolidase deficiency with iminodipeptiduria therapy. *J Inher Metabol Dis* 4:77, 1981.

Coulombe JT, Kammerer BL, Levy HL, et al: Histidinaemia. Part III: Impact; a prospective study. *J Inher Metabol Dis* 6:58, 1983.

da Silva VA, Zurbrugg RP, Lavanchy P, et al: Long-term treatment of infantile nephropathic cystinosis with cysteamine. *N Engl J Med* 313:1460, 1985.

Donn SM, Swartz RD, Thoene JG: Comparison of exchange transfusion, peritoneal dialysis, and hemodialysis for the treatment of hyperammonemia in an anuric newborn infant. *J Pediatr* 95:67, 1979.

Drogari E, Beasley M, Smith I, et al: Timing of strict diet in relation to fetal damage in maternal phenylketonuria: An international collaborative study by the MRC/DHSS phenylketonuria register. *Lancet* 2:8565, 1987.

Eady RAJ, Gunner DB, Garner A, et al: Prenatal diagnosis of oculocutaneous albinism by electron microscopy of fetal skin. *J Invest Dermatol* 80:210, 1983.

Freij, BJ, Levy HL, Dudin G, et al: Clinical and biochemical characteristics of prolidase deficiency in siblings. *Am J Med Genet* 19:561, 1984.

Gahl WA, Bashan N, Tietze F, et al: Cystine transport is defective in isolated leukocyte lysosomes from patients with cystinosis. *Science* 217:1263, 1982.

Gahl WA, Finkelstein JKD, Mullen KD, et al: Hepatic methionine adenosyltransferase deficiency in a 31-year-old man. *Am J Hum Genet* 40:39, 1987.

Gaull GE, Tallan HH, Lonsdale D, et al: Hypermethioninemia associated with methionine adenosyltransferase deficiency: Clinical, morphological and biochemical observations on patients. *J Pediatr* 98:734, 1981.

Goldsmith LA, Kang E, Bienfang DC, et al: Tyrosinemia with plantar and palmar keratosis and keratitis. *J Pediatr* 83:798, 1973.

Goldsmith LA, Reed J: Tyrosine-induced eye and skin lesions. A treatable genetic disease. *JAMA* 236:382, 1976.

Guttler F: Phenylketonuria: 50 years since Folling's discovery and still expanding on clinical and biochemical knowledge. *Acta Paediatr Scand* 73:705, 1984.

Harpey JP, Rosenblatt DS, Cooper BA, et al: Homocystinuria caused by 5,10-methylenetetrahydrofolate reductase deficiency: A case in an infant responding to methionine, folinic acid, pyridoxine and vitamin B_{12} therapy. *J Pediatr* 98:275, 1981.

Hayasaka K, Tada K, Fueki N, et al: Feasibility of prenatal diagnosis of non-ketotic hyperglycinemia: Existence of the glycine cleavage system in placenta. *J Pediatr* 110:124, 1987.

Holtzman NA: Ethical issues in the prenatal diagnosis of phenylketonuria. *Pediatrics* 74:424, 1984.

Holzgreve W, Golbus MS: Prenatal diagnosis of ornithine transcarbamylase deficiency utilizing fetal liver biopsy. *Am J Hum Genet* 36:320, 1984.

Hommes FA, Roesel RA, Metoki K, et al: Studies on a case of HHH-syndrome (hyperammonemia, hyperornithinemia, homocitrullinuria). *Neuropediatrics* 17:48, 1986.

Horwich AL, Fenton WA, Williams KR, et al: Structure and expression of a complementary DNA for the nuclear coded precursor of human mitochondrial ornithine transcarbamylase. *Science* 224:1068, 1984.

Hostetter MK, Levy HL, Winter HS, et al: Evidence for liver disease preceding amino acid abnormalities in hereditary tyrosinemia. *N Engl J Med* 308:1265, 1983.

Hudak ML, Jones MD, Brusilow SW: Differentiation of transient hyperammonemia of the newborn and urea cycle enzyme defects by clinical presentation. *J Pediatr* 107:712, 1985.

Irons M, Levy HL: Metabolic syndromes with dermatologic manifestations. *Clin Rev Allerg* 4:101, 1986.

Irons M, Levy HL, O'Flynn et al: Folinic acid therapy in treatment of dihydropteridine reductase deficiency. *J Pediatr* 110:61, 1987.

Jervis GA: Phenylpyruvic oligophrenia. *Arch Neurol Psychiatry* 38:944, 1937.

Kaufman S: Problems in diagnosis and therapy of hyperphenylalaninemia. *J Pediatr* 109:572, 1986.

Koch R, Azen C, Friedman EG, et al: Paired comparisons between early treated PKU children and their matched sibling controls on intelligence and school achievement test results at eight years of age. *J Inher Metabol Dis* 7:86, 1984.

Kolvraa S, Brandt NJ, Christensen E: Nonketotic hyperglycinemia. *Acta Paediatr Scand* 68:629, 1979.

Ledley F: Somatic gene therapy for human disease. Background and prospects. *J Pediatr* 110:1, 1987.

Lenke RR, Levy HL: Maternal phenylketonuria and hyperphenylalaninemia: An international survey of the outcome of treated and untreated pregnancies. *N Engl J Med* 303:1202, 1980.

Levy HL: Maternal phenylketonuria. Review with emphasis on pathogenesis. *Enzyme* 38:312, 1987.

Levy HL: Phenylketonuria-1986. *Pediatr Rev* 7:269, 1986.

Levy HL, Waisbren SE: Effects of untreated maternal phenylketonuria and hyperphenylalaninemia on the fetus. *N Engl J Med* 309:1269, 1983.

Lombeck I. Wendel U, Versieck J, et al: Increased manganese content and reduced arginase activity in erythrocytes of a patient with prolidase deficiency (iminodipeptiduria). *Eur J Pediatr* 144:571, 1986.

Mamunes P: Intellectual deficits after transient tyrosinemia in the term neonate. *Pediatrics* 57:675, 1976.

Marescau B, Pintens J, Lowenthal A, et al: Arginase and free amino acids in hyperargininemia: Leukocyte arginine as a diagnostic parameter for heterozygotes. *J Clin Chem Clin Biochem* 17:211, 1979.

Mitchell G, Valle D, Willard H, et al: Human ornithine-delta-aminotransferase (OAT): Cross-hybridizing fragments mapped to chromosome 10 and Xp11.1-21. *Am J Hum Genet* 39 (Suppl):A163, 1986a.

Mitchell GA, Watkins D, Melancon SB, et al: Clinical heterogeneity in cobalamin C variant of combined homocystinuria and methylmalonic aciduria. *J Pediatr* 108:410, 1986b.

Mollica F, Pavone L, Antener I: Pure familial hyperprolinemia: Isolated inborn error of amino acid metabolism without other anomalies in a Sicilian family. *Pediatrics* 48:225, 1971.

Msall M, Batshaw ML, Suss R, et al: Neurologic outcome in children with inborn errors of urea synthesis. *N Engl J Med* 310:1500, 1984.

Mudd SH, Levy HL, Skovby F: Disorders of transsulfuration. In Scriver CR, et al, (eds): *The Metabolic Basis of Inherited Disease*. New York, McGraw Hill, in press.

Naughten ER, Proctor SP, Levy HL, et al: Congenital expression of prolidase defect in prolidase deficiency. *Pediatr Res* 18:259, 1984.

Old JM, Purvis-Smith S, Wilcken B, et al: Prenatal exclusion of ornithine transcarbamylase deficiency by direct gene analysis. *Lancet* 1:73, 1985.

Perheentupa J, Visakorpi JK: Protein intolerance with deficient transport of basic amino acids. *Lancet* 2:813, 1965.

Potter JL, Timmons GD, Silvidi AA: Argininosuccinic aciduria: The hair abnormality revisited. *Am J Dis Child* 134:1095, 1980.

Raijman L: Double deficiencies of urea cycle enzymes in human liver. *Biochem Med* 21:226, 1979.

Ramesh V, Eddy R, Shows TB, et al: Chromosomal assignment of human ornithine aminotransferase. *Am J Hum Genet* 39 (Suppl):A166, 1986.

Robb RM, Dowton SB, Fulton AB, et al: Retinal degeneration in vitamin B_{12} disorder associated with methylmalonic aciduria and sulfur amino acid abnormalities. *Am J Ophthalmol* 97:691, 1984.

Robinson MJ, Menzies IS, Sloan I: Hydroxyprolinemia with normal development. *Arch Dis Child* 55:484, 1980.

Rohr FJ, Doherty LB, Waisbren SE, et al: New England maternal PKU project: Prospective study of untreated and treated pregnancies and their outcomes. *J Pediatr* 110:391, 1987.

Rosenblatt DS, Cooper BA, Schmutz SM, et al: Prenatal vitamin B_{12} therapy of a fetus with methylcobalamin deficiency (cobalamin E disease). *Lancet* 1:1127, 1985.

Rowe PC, Newman SL, Brusilow SW: Natural history of symptomatic partial ornithine transcarbamylase deficiency. *N Engl J Med* 314:541, 1986.

Rozen R, Fox J, Fenton WA, et al: Gene deletion and restriction fragment length polymorphisms at the human ornithine transcarbamylase locus. *Nature* 313:815, 1985.

Schuh S, Rosenblatt DS, Cooper BA, et al: Homocystinuria and megaloblastic anemia responsive to vitamin B_{12} therapy. *N Engl J Med* 310:686, 1984.

Schutgens RBH, Ket JL, Hayasaka K, et al: Nonketotic hyperglycinaemia due to a deficiency of T-protein in the glycine cleavage system in liver and brain. *J Inher Metabol Dis* 9:208, 1986.

Scriver CR, Levy HL: Histidinaemia. Part I; Reconciling retrospective and prospective findings. *J Inher Metabol Dis* 6:51, 1983.

Sellcoe DJ: Familial hyperprolinemia and mental retardation. *Neurology* 19:494, 1969.

Simell O, Mackenzie S, Clow CL, et al: Ornithine loading did not prevent induced hyperammonemia in a patient with hyperornithinemia-hyperammonemia-homocitrullinuria syndrome. *Pediatr Res* 19:1283, 1985.

Simell O, Perheentupa J, Rapola J, et al: Lysinuric protein intolerance. *Am J Med* 59:229, 1975.

Srsen S: Alkaptonuria. *Johns Hopkins Med* J 145:217, 1979.

Srsen S, Srsnova K: Diagnosis of alkaptonuria in children. *Padiatrie und Padologie* 14:163, 1979.

Starzl TE, Zitelli BJ, Shaw BW, et al: Changing concepts: Liver replacement for hereditary tyrosinemia and hepatoma. *J Pediatr* 106:604, 1985.

Thoene JG, Lemons R: Cystine depletion of cystinotic tissues by phosphocysteamine (WR638). *J Pediatr* 96:1043, 1980.

Trauner DA, Page T, Greco C, et al: Progressive neurodegenerative disorder in a patient with nonketotic hyperglycinemia. *J Pediatr* 98:272, 1981.

Tsujii T, Morita T, Matsuyama Y, et al: Sibling cases of chronic recurrent hepatocerebral disease with hypercitrullinemia. *Gastroenterologia Japonica* 11:328, 1976.

Valle D, Goodman SI, Applegarth DA, et al: Type II hyperprolinemia. Delta-pyrroline-5-carboxylic acid dehydrogenase deficiency in cultured skin fibroblasts and circulating lymphocytes. *J Clin Invest* 58:598, 1976.

Valle D, Simell O: The Hyperornithinemias. In Stanbury JB, et al (eds): *The Metabolic Basis of Inherited Disease*. New York, McGraw-Hill, 1983, pp. 382-401.

Witkop CJ: Abnormalities of pigmentation. In Emery AEH, Rimoin DL (eds): *Principles and Practice of Medical Genetics*. London, Churchill Livingston, 1983, pp. 622-652.

Witkop CJ, Quevedo WC, Fitzpatrick TB: Albinism and other disorders of pigment metabolism. In Stanbury JB, et al (eds): *The Metabolic Basis of Inherited Disease*. New York, McGraw-Hill, 1983, pp. 301-346.

Woo SLC, Lidsky AS, Guttler F, et al: Cloned human phenylalanine hydroxylase gene allows prenatal diagnosis and carrier detection of classical phenylketonuria. *Nature* 306:151, 1983.

Organic Acid Metabolism Disorders 3

Each of the inborn errors of metabolism in this section is characterized by a block in the degradation of an organic acid intermediate in an amino acid catabolic pathway. Most of these are pathways of branched-chain amino acids (leucine, isoleucine, and valine) and result in either accumulations of both amino acids and organic acid metabolites, such as in maple syrup urine disease, or in an intermediary organic acid(s) alone. A few organic acid disorders occur in the degradative pathway of other amino acids. All of the disorders have specific organic acid accumulations that can be identified by appropriate organic acid analysis of urine.

MAPLE SYRUP URINE DISEASE

Definition

Maple syrup urine disease also known as branched-chain ketonuria, is an autosomal recessive disorder that affects the catabolism of the branched-chain amino acids.

Basic Science

The defect in maple syrup urine disease is a deficiency of the branched-chain ketoacid dehydrogenase, a complex mitochondrial enzyme that normally converts the branched-chain ketoacids to their acyl-CoA esters. The enzyme deficiency results in accumulations of the branched-chain amino acids leucine, isoleucine, and valine, their respective ketoacids 2-ketoisocaproic acid, 2-keto-3-methylvaleric acid, and 2-ketoisovaleric acid, and the corresponding hydroxy acids. The 2-keto- and hydroxy acids of isoleucine and leucine are believed to be responsible for the characteristic odor that is much like maple syrup and the ketoacid of leucine has been implicated in the CNS dysfunction that may be profound in the disorder.

The severity of the disease depends on the residual activity of the branched-chain ketoacid dehydrogenase. With little or no residual activity, the classic or most severe form occurs, with 3–5% of residual activity, the intermediate form occurs, and with 5–8% of residual activity, the intermittent form occurs.

Epidemiology

The prevalence has been about 1/200,000 live births in newborn screening programs. It has been reported in all racial and ethnic groups.

Natural History

In the classical form of the disease, infants develop feeding intolerance, vomiting, and lethargy by the end of the first week of life. Severe ketoacidosis rapidly progresses with the development of coma. Delay in treatment leads to death or, if the infant survives, to severe neurologic impairment with mental retardation. Other symptoms and signs include hyper- or hypotonia, nystagmus, and the characteristic odor of maple syrup or curry which is best recognized in the urine or on the diaper.

In milder degrees of the disorder, which include the intermittent, intermediate, and thiamine-responsive forms, the presentation is later in infancy, or perhaps not until early childhood, with episodic and milder clinical manifestations. The symptoms in these children include neurologic abnormalities, ataxia, seizures, vomiting, recurrent episodes of ketoacidosis, and the abnormal odor. The ketoacidosis, which is usually milder than that seen in the classical form, usually occurs during febrile illness or increased protein intake. In the intermittent form, however, the ketoacidotic episodes may be as severe as those seen in classic disease and can result in death or irreversible brain damage. Children with the intermittent form are clinically normal during remission but can die during an acute episode. Those with the intermediate form are mentally retarded unless treated from early infancy.

Although all affected members of a kinship usually have the same form of maple syrup urine disease, different forms may occur in the same family. A report from France documented a family in which the proband had the classic form with neonatal presentation and had 1.9% of normal dehydrogenase activity, while the father and two siblings were found to have a milder form, with 5–10% of normal dehydrogenase activity. It was postulated that the father and siblings were compound heterozygotes for the classical mutant gene and a "variant" allele (Frezal et al, 1985).

Diagnosis

During an acute episode, patients present with severe metabolic acidosis, hypoglycemia, and ketonuria. The urine is also strongly positive for ketoacids by the DNPH test.

The diagnosis is suspected by the characteristic clinical presentation and the maple syrup odor. The odor is not always evident, however, especially early in infancy. The diagnosis is confirmed by the presence of markedly increased levels of branched-chain amino acids, including alloisoleucine, in the blood and urine and by the demonstration of branched-chain ketoacids in blood and urine. The intermediate and intermittent forms are differentiated by the presence of amino acid and organic acid elevations even during remission in the former, but normal amino acid levels during remission in the latter.

Confirmation of the diagnosis depends upon the demonstration of the enzyme defect in cultured skin fibroblasts or leukocytes from the patient.

Treatment

During acute illness, treatment must be immediate. The infant requires an intensive care setting and close neurologic monitoring. Peritoneal dialysis or hemodialysis is effective in clearing the abnormally accumulated metabolites and should be performed as soon as possible. Intravenous glucose and bicarbonate must be given, the former to provide adequate calories to decrease the high catabolic rate and the latter to control the acidosis. Anticonvulsant medications may be required for seizures. All protein intake is discontinued until the branched-chain amino acid concentrations return to normal.

Chronic treatment of the classic and intermediate forms of the disorder includes the use of a special diet restricted in the branched-chain amino acids, but allowing sufficient protein to support growth. Careful monitoring of the child's biochemical status, especially during febrile illnesses, is necessary to prevent acute exacerbations of the disease.

Patients with the milder variants that are thiamine-responsive usually require thiamine in doses of 10–150 mg/day, generally in conjunction with a diet restricted in the branched-chain amino acids and/or protein. The intermittent form does not require dietary treatment, but the child must be monitored with appropriate acute therapy during febrile illnesses or trauma.

Prognosis

If treatment of the neonatal form of the disorder is initiated within the first week of life, normal mental and physical development can be seen. Newborn screening programs for maple syrup urine disease have greatly improved the prognosis for infants with this disorder by identifying infants during the first week of life, often before life-threatening symptoms appear. Untreated, or late treated, the disorder can be fatal or the child may be left with severe psychomotor and neurologic dysfunction.

Patients with the intermediate or intermittent form of the disorder who are responsive to thiamine have had a decrease in the number of ketoacidotic episodes while receiving thiamine therapy with or without a restricted diet.

Prevention

Prenatal diagnosis is available by measurement of enzyme activity in cultured amniotic fluid cells. There is considerable overlap in activity between carriers and noncarriers, which makes carrier detection unreliable.

ISOVALERIC ACIDEMIA

Definition

Isovaleric acidemia is an autosomal recessive disorder in the intermediary metabolism of leucine, resulting from deficiency of the enzyme isovaleryl-CoA dehydrogenase. It is often associated with an odor similar to that of sweat, which has given isovaleric acidemia the appellation "sweaty foot syndrome."

Basic Science

Isovaleryl-CoA dehydrogenase catalyzes the conversion of isovaleryl-CoA, a metabolite of leucine, to 3-methylcrotonyl-CoA. Deficiency of this enzyme leads to an accumulation of isovaleryl-CoA which can conjugate with glycine to form isovalerylglycine. If the conjugation capacity is exceeded by either too rapid formation of isovaleryl-CoA, or the glycine stores are limited, or both, the excess isovaleryl-CoA is cleaved to the free acid or to 3-hydroxyisovaleric acid.

Epidemiology

The incidence of this disorder is not known.

Natural History

Isovaleric acidemia can present as an acute or a chronic disorder. In the acute form of the disease, affected neonates present with feeding intolerance, lethargy, seizures, metabolic acidosis, ketonuria, hyperammonemia, and a characteristic odor of "sweaty feet." The disease can progress quickly to coma and death if treatment is not initiated promptly. Survivors of this acute phase develop a chronic form of the illness, which is characterized by recurrent episodes of ataxia, vomiting, lethargy, ketoacidosis, and the "sweaty foot" odor, usually precipitated by febrile illness or increased protein intake. The symptoms subside after therapy is instituted. Patients often give a history of aversion to dietary protein. The frequency of these recurrent episodes has been found to diminish with increasing age. Patients with either form are often mentally retarded.

Diagnosis

The acute phase of the disorder is associated with hypoglycemia, severe metabolic acidosis, ketonuria, and hyperammonemia. Patients may also develop bone marrow depression with leukopenia, thrombocytopenia, and anemia during these episodes.

The diagnosis is suggested by the clinical history and characteristic odor and substantiated by finding increased levels of isovaleric acid in the blood and isovalerylglycine, isovaleric acid, and 3-hydroxyisovaleric acid in the urine.

Confirmation of the diagnosis depends upon the demonstration of decreased enzyme activity in cultured skin fibroblasts.

Treatment

Treatment of the acute disorder often requires an intensive care setting. Intravenous glucose in large amounts and bicarbonate should be given. Anticonvulsant therapy may be necessary for seizure control. Protein intake is discontinued during acute therapy.

Chronic therapy includes a diet restricted in leucine, with close monitoring of biochemical status, especially during febrile illnesses. Several investigators have found that addition of glycine to the diet increases the conjugation of isovaleryl-CoA to isovalerylglycine, thus reducing the accumulation of isovaleric acid and preventing acute exacerbations of the disorder. Carnitine supplementation may act in a similar fashion.

Prognosis

Early treatment of the acute neonatal form of the illness and effective subsequent control of the chronic phase can lead to normal mental and physical development. Untreated, the disease can be rapidly fatal or lead to severe neurologic deficits.

Prevention

Prenatal diagnosis is theoretically possible by measurement of enzyme activity in cultured amniotic fluid cells or by the demonstration of isovalerylglycine in the amniotic fluid.

3-HYDROXY-3-METHYLGLUTARYL-CoA LYASE DEFICIENCY

Definition

3-Hydroxy-3-methylglutaryl-CoA lyase deficiency is an autosomal recessive disorder in the intermediary metabolism of leucine.

Basic Science

3-Hydroxy-3-methylglutaryl-CoA lyase is a mitochondrial enzyme that catalyzes the final step of leucine degradation, the intramitochondrial cleavage of 3-hydroxy-3-methylglutaryl-CoA to acetoacetic acid and acyl-CoA. Therefore, this enzyme is involved in both leucine catabolism and ketone body formation. Lack of this enzyme results in the inability to form ketone bodies, an especially important function during fasting or times of acute illness when increased energy requirements are needed.

Epidemiology

The incidence of this rare disorder is not known.

Natural History

This disorder may present in the early neonatal period with symptoms of vomiting, hypotonia, lethargy, metabolic acidosis, severe hypoglycemia, and coma. Some patients present with similar signs and symptoms later in infancy or within the first years of life. These later episodes are usually associated with febrile illness, fasting, or increased protein intake.

Diagnosis

Severe hypoglycemia, metabolic acidosis, and the inability to form ketones are hallmarks of the disorder. Urine organic acid analysis is diagnostic and reveals the presence of 3-hydroxy-3-methylglutaric, 3-methylglutaconic, 3-hydroxyisovaleric, and 3-methylglutaric acids in large amounts.

Confirmation of the diagnosis depends upon the demonstration of enzyme deficiency in leukocytes or cultured fibroblasts.

Treatment

Treatment of the acute episodes requires correction of the hypoglycemia and acidosis with intravenous glucose and bicarbonate. Chronic treatment of the disorder includes the use of a leucine-restricted diet and avoidance of prolonged fasting.

Prognosis

Inadequate treatment of acute exacerbations can result in neurologic sequelae. Leucine restriction, avoidance of fasting, and prompt treatment of acute exacerbations can result in normal mental and physical development.

Prevention

Prenatal diagnosis of this disorder has been reported by demonstration of increased levels of hydroxymethylglutaric acid and 3-methylglutaconic acid in maternal urine at 23 weeks of gestation. Prenatal diagnosis is also theoretically possible by measurement of enzyme activity in cultured amniotic fluid cells, or by organic acid analysis of amniotic fluid.

3-KETOTHIOLASE DEFICIENCY

Definition

3-Ketothiolase deficiency is an autosomal recessive inborn error in the intermediary metabolism of isoleucine.

Basic Science

3-Ketothiolase is the enzyme responsible for the conversion of 2-methylacetoacetyl-CoA to propionyl-CoA and acetyl-CoA in the last step of isoleucine catabolism. Deficiency of this enzyme results in the accumulation of 2-methylacetoacetyl-CoA and its metabolites.

Epidemiology

The incidence of this rare disorder is not known.

Natural History

Affected patients can present in either infancy or early/late childhood with episodic ketoacidosis and accompanying symptoms which include vomiting, tachypnea, and lethargy. There may also be a history of protein aversion. Untreated, the acute episodes can be fatal or lead to neurologic sequelae. Acute episodes may occur during times of febrile illness or increased protein intake.

Diagnosis

During acute exacerbations, patients present with metabolic acidosis and ketonuria. Examination of urine organic acids reveals 2-methyl-3-hydroxybutyric acid, tiglylglycine, and, occasionally, 2-methylacetoacetic acid.

Confirmation of the diagnosis depends upon the demonstration of deficient enzyme activity in cultured skin fibroblasts.

Treatment

Treatment of the acute phase requires the use of intravenous glucose and bicarbonate. Chronic treatment includes a protein-restricted diet, and close monitoring of biochemical status, especially during episodes of febrile illness.

Prognosis

Effective management of acute episodes and protein restriction can lead to normal growth and development.

PROPIONIC ACIDEMIA

Definition

Propionic acidemia, formerly known as ketotic hyperglycinemia, is an autosomal recessive disorder due to deficiency of propionyl-CoA carboxylase (Wolf et al, 1981).

Basic Science

Propionyl-CoA carboxylase is the enzyme responsible for the conversion of propionyl-CoA to methylmalonyl-CoA (Fig. 15.11). Propionyl-CoA is an intermediate in the catabolism of isoleucine, valine, threonine, and methionine as well as of odd-chain fatty acids and cholesterol.

Deficiency of the enzyme leads to the accumulation of propionic acid in the blood and urine, as well as in the accumulation of its various metabolites, including 3-hydroxypropionate, propionylglycine, methylcitrate, tiglylglycine, and tiglic acid. The accompanying ketoacidosis is believed to be due to the accumulation of these metabolites. Inhibition of the glycine cleavage pathway is also believed to cause hyperglycinemia, hyperglycinuria and hyperammonemia.

Epidemiology

The exact incidence of this disorder is not known.

Natural History

Affected infants present in the first few days of life with vomiting, tachypnea, respiratory distress, feeding intolerance, lethargy, severe ketoacidosis, and hyperammonemia. Seizures and hepatomegaly also may occur, and coma and death can rapidly ensue if aggressive treatment is not instituted immediately. Bone marrow suppression of all cell lines may be present, and cerebellar hemorrhage has been reported. Infants who survive the neonatal period are subject to recurrent acute ketoacidotic episodes throughout life, usually associated with febrile illness or increased protein intake. Feeding intolerance and the refusal to accept food by mouth is frequent and many patients have required gastrostomy to maintain adequate nutrition.

A few patients have presented later in infancy with failure to thrive, seizures, and developmental delay. Some of these patients have been found to be responsive

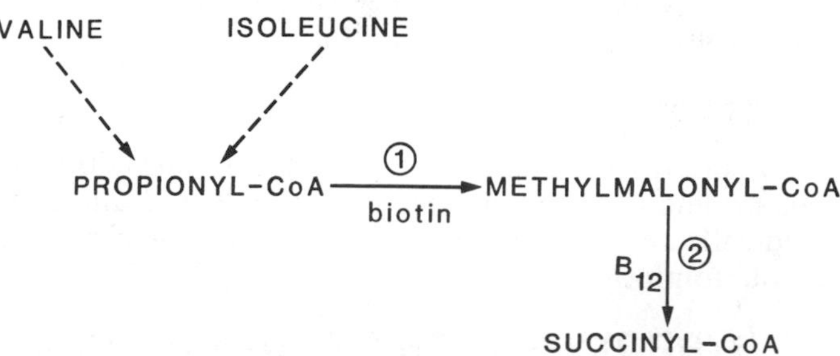

Figure 15.11. Conversion of propionyl-CoA to methylmalonyl-CoA.

to biotin, and most may be found to have multiple carboxylase deficiency rather than specific propionic acidemia (see multiple carboxylase deficiency further in this section).

Diagnosis

During an acute episode, patients present with profound ketoacidosis, hypoglycemia, and hyperammonemia.

Amino acid analysis reveals an increased concentration of glycine in the blood and urine. Short-chain fatty acid analysis discloses increased levels of propionate in the blood and urine. Organic acid analysis of the urine characteristically reveals the presence of methylcitrate and 3-hydroxypropionate, as well as propionylglycine, tiglylglycine, tiglic acid, acetoacetic acid, and 3-hydroxybutyrate. Medium-chain ketones such as butanone, pentanone, and hexanone also are present in the urine.

Confirmation of the diagnosis depends upon the demonstration of deficient enzyme activity in liver, leukocytes, or cultured skin fibroblasts.

Treatment

Aggressive and intensive treatment is required for acute episodes at any stage. Peritoneal dialysis and/or hemodialysis may be required for elimination of the abnormal metabolites. High concentrations of intravenous glucose are necessary to provide enough calories to reduce the increased catabolic rate. Intravenous bicarbonate in large quantities, often up to 1 mEq/kg/hour, is required to neutralize the large quantities of acids being produced. All protein should be discontinued.

For patients who survive the neonatal episode, chronic treatment includes the use of a special diet restricted in the four offending amino acids, but with sufficient protein and other amino acids to permit adequate growth and nutrition. Calories must be plentiful to meet the energy requirements of a growing child. Close monitoring of biochemical status is required, especially during times of febrile illness. Oral bicarbonate or citrate therapy also may be required chronically to treat acidosis. Carnitine therapy may also be indicated.

Prognosis

The acute neonatal episode is commonly fatal or may result in severe neurologic sequelae. If the infant survives the neonatal period, the chronic disorder is difficult to manage and requires close supervision of diet and biochemical status. Some patients do relatively well on chronic therapy, especially as they grow older, while others have problems with growth, osteoporosis, or recurrent acute exacerbations of the disorder.

Prevention

Carrier detection for this disorder has been found to be unreliable because of overlap of enzyme activity between carriers and noncarriers.

Prenatal diagnosis is available by measurement of propionyl-CoA carboxylase activity in cultured amniotic fluid cells or by the demonstration of excess methylcitrate in the amniotic fluid.

METHYLMALONIC ACIDEMIA

Definition

Methylmalonic acidemia is an autosomal recessive inborn error of metabolism due to a defect in methylmalonyl-CoA mutase or a defect in the production of adenosylcobalamin, the vitamin B_{12} cofactor for the enzyme.

Basic Science

Methylmalonyl-CoA mutase is responsible for the conversion of methylmalonyl-CoA to succinyl-CoA in the catabolic pathways of isoleucine, valine, methionine, and threonine (Fig. 15.11). Decreased activity of this enzyme leads to the accumulation of methylmalonyl-CoA. The defect may occur in the mutase itself, or in the biosynthesis or availability of adenosylcobalamin, the mutase coenzyme.

About half the patients with methylmalonic acidemia are responsive to vitamin B_{12}, while the other half are unresponsive. Many of those who are unresponsive to vitamin B_{12} develop symptoms in the newborn period and have an intrinsic mutase defect.

One patient has been described with minimal methylmalonic aciduria (50 mg/dl) responsive to vitamin B_{12}. The defect was in the transport of cobalamin from lysosome to cytoplasm (Rosenblatt et al, 1985).

Epidemiology

This is a rare disorder. Between 1968 and 1974, only 17 infants with methylmalonic aciduria were detected by routine urine screening of most newborn infants in Massachusetts.

Natural History

Methylmalonic acidemia can present in the neonatal period with a course identical to that of propionic acidemia. Affected infants develop tachypnea, vomiting, lethargy, and ketoacidosis, often progressing rapidly to coma and death during the first few days of life, if not aggressively treated. Cerebellar hemorrhage, which complicates the acute episode has also been reported.

Those surviving the neonatal period often develop recurrent episodes of ketoacidosis, usually in association with febrile illness.

Many of the cobalamin (B_{12})-responsive patients present later in infancy or during the first year. Symptoms include failure to thrive, vomiting, lethargy, and developmental delay. Patients may also present with an acute ketoacidotic episode and, later, recurrent episodes of ketoacidosis.

A benign variant of methylmalonic acidemia apparently unresponsive to B_{12} may be one of the more frequent forms of this disorder and has been identified by newborn urine screening. These children have low levels of methylmalonic acid in blood and urine, but have normal growth and development, and do not require dietary or vitamin therapy (Ledley et al, 1984).

Diagnosis

During an acute episode, patients present with hypoglycemia, ketoacidosis, thrombocytopenia, and neutropenia. The presence of large amounts of methylmalonic acid in urine is diagnostic. Methylcitrate and 3-hydroxypropionate may also be seen, as well as increased levels of glycine in the blood and urine.

Confirmation of diagnosis depends upon the demonstration of deficient enzyme activity in cultured skin fibroblasts.

Treatment

Treatment of the acute episode requires the administration of intravenous glucose in high concentrations, along with intravenous bicarbonate to treat the acidosis. Large doses (1–2 mg/day) of cyanocobalamin or hydroxycobalamin should also be administered. Peritoneal dialysis or hemodialysis may be necessary in profoundly ill neonates.

Chronic treatment of those with the vitamin B_{12}-responsive form of the disorder includes long-term therapy with vitamin B_{12}. Chronic treatment of those with the vitamin B_{12}-unresponsive form of the disorder involves the use of a protein-restricted diet low in the four amino acids that are precursors of propionate. The degree of protein restriction should permit adequate growth while minimizing the accumulation of methylmalonic acid. Carnitine therapy is also indicated.

Continuous ambulatory peritoneal dialysis has been used in a vitamin B_{12}-unresponsive patient to increase the excretion of methylmalonic acid. The dialysis allowed increased protein intake and accelerated the growth in the child, but was not without the complications inherent in peritoneal dialysis.

Prognosis

Patients with the vitamin B_{12}-unresponsive form may be difficult to manage, but careful monitoring of biochemical status and aggressive treatment of acute illness can lead to normal mental and physical development. Those with the vitamin B_{12}-responsive form have been shown to have decreased levels of methylmalonic acid in blood and urine on therapy, decreased numbers of ketoacidotic episodes, and often normal growth and development.

Prevention

Prenatal diagnosis of this disorder is available by measurement of the enzyme activity in cultured amniotic fluid cells, or of methylmalonic acid in amniotic fluid or maternal urine during pregnancy (Ampola et al, 1975).

Prenatal therapy has been used to protect a fetus with the vitamin B_{12}-responsive form of the disorder diagnosed in utero. The mother was treated with cyanocobalamin during the last 2 months of her pregnancy and the infant had only very low levels of methylmalonic acid at birth.

MULTIPLE CARBOXYLASE DEFICIENCIES: HOLOCARBOXYLASE SYNTHETASE DEFICIENCY AND BIOTINIDASE DEFICIENCY

Definition

Multiple carboxylase deficiency describes a group of inborn errors of metabolism that are characterized by deficiencies in the biotin-dependent carboxylases. Two categories exist within this group, one due to holocarboxylase synthetase deficiency and the other due to biotinidase deficiency. Both are inherited as autosomal recessive traits.

Basic Science

The 4 mitochondrial biotin-dependent carboxylases in mammalian tissues are propionyl-CoA carboxylase, pyruvate carboxylase, 3-methylcrotonyl-CoA carboxylase, and acetyl-CoA carboxylase. Biotin activates these carboxylases by covalently binding with the enzyme. The binding process is mediated by an enzyme known as holocarboxylase synthetase. A deficiency of this enzyme produces markedly deficient carboxylase activity with symptoms occuring during the first days of life (Fig. 15.12).

A second enzyme known as biotinidase is necessary for the recycling of biotin so that it can be used again to activate the carboxylases (Fig. 15.12). Specifically, following its activity function, each carboxylase with attached biotin (holocarboxylase) is degraded in the lysosome by a protease. The biotin is released not as free biotin but still covalently bound to a lysine residue from the degraded enzyme. This bound biotin (called biocytin) must be cleaved and free biotin released if the biotin is to be available for another cycle of carboxylase stimulation. The enzyme that cleaves biocytin is called biotinidase. Biotinidase deficiency produces a later onset form of multiple carboxylase deficiency.

Isolated deficiency of 3-methylcrotonyl CoA carboxylase has been reported in two patients but it is unclear whether these patients might indeed have multiple carboxylase deficiency.

Acquired biotin deficiency can produce biochemical and clinical findings similar to those in multiple carboxylase deficiency.

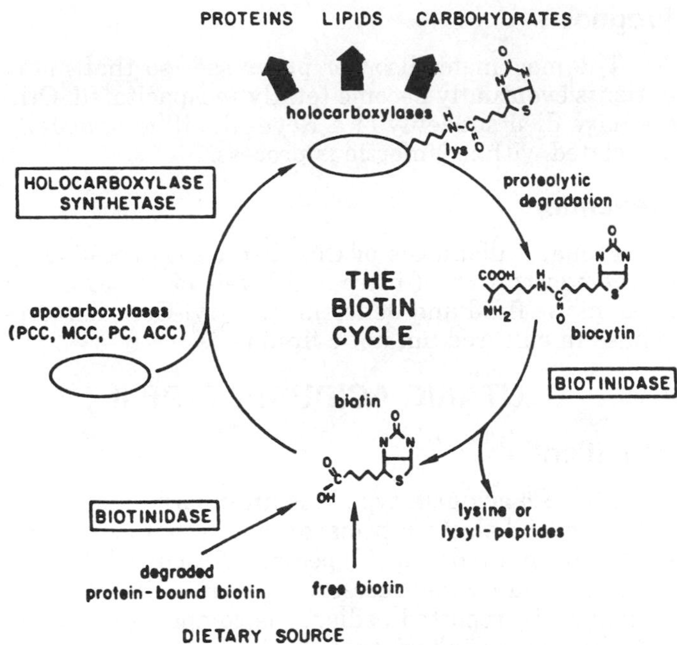

Figure 15.12. The biotin cycle.

Epidemiology

The incidence of holocarboxylase synthetase deficiency is not known. The prevalence of biotinidase deficiency has been estimated to be about 1/40,000 from a pilot newborn screening study (Wolf et al, 1985). In New England it is 1:30,000.

Natural History

Patients with the early onset form of multiple carboxylase deficiency (holocarboxylase synthetase deficiency) often present in the newborn period with vomiting, lethargy, metabolic acidosis, hypoglycemia, ketonuria and hyperammonemia. If they survive the neonatal illness, they are subject to acute exacerbations later in life.

Patients with the later onset form of the disorder (biotinidase deficiency) may present from 3 months to 2–3 years of age. The symptoms include alopecia, a skin rash which may have monilial superinfection, seizures, developmental delay, hypotonia, ataxia, and hearing loss. Several infants identified through newborn screening have been found to have subtle neurologic signs in the first few months of life. Organic aciduria and ketoacidosis may appear late in the course of the disease. Recent research reveals that the skin changes seen may be associated with abnormalities in fatty acid composition.

Diagnosis

Organic acid analysis of urine in both forms of multiple carboxylase deficiency reveals the presence of 3-methylcrotonylglycine, 3-hydroxyisovaleric acid, 3-hydroxypropionate, and methylcitrate.

The specific diagnosis depends upon the measurement of carboxylase activities in leukocytes or fibroblasts. If these are deficient, biotinidase activity and holocarboxylase synthetase activity are then measured to determine which form of the disorder the child has. A rapid and easier method of confirmation is to measure biotinidase activity in serum, whole blood, or erythrocytes in any child with the findings of multiple carboxylase deficiency. This is done as a single screening procedure in a number of routine newborn screening programs. If biotinidase activity is deficient, the diagnosis of biotinidase deficiency is confirmed. If biotinidase activity is normal, more elaborate enzyme studies for holocarboxylase synthetase deficiency should then be performed.

Treatment

The treatment of the acute form of multiple carboxylase deficiency requires the prompt use of intravenous glucose and bicarbonate to correct the biochemical abnormalities seen. Patients with this form of the disorder also respond to biotin in doses of 10–80 mg/day.

Patients with biotinidase deficiency have been found to respond to 10–20 mg/day of biotin, although there is some evidence to suggest that even lower doses may be adequate for treatment of this disorder.

Prognosis

Since patients with both forms of the disorder respond to biotin, the prognosis for most patients is good, provided that acute episodes are treated quickly and aggressively.

Prevention

Prenatal diagnosis of holocarboxylase synthetase deficiency is available by measurement of the activities of the three carboxylase activities in cultured amniotic fluid cells and by organic acid analysis of the amniotic fluid. Prenatal diagnosis of biotinidase deficiency is also possible by measurement of biotinidase activity in cultured amniotic fluid cells. Prenatal therapy of an affected fetus, diagnosed in utero, with biotin has also been reported.

GLUTARIC ACIDURIA TYPE I

Definition

Glutaric aciduria type I is an autosomal recessive inborn error of metabolism due to deficiency of glutaryl-CoA dehydrogenase. It produces neurologic deficits as well as mental retardation.

Basic Science

The deficiency of glutaryl-CoA dehydrogenase in affected individuals results in deficient oxidation of glutaryl-CoA, an intermediate in the metabolism of lysine, hydroxylysine, and tryptophan. As a result, glutaric acid accumulates in blood, urine, and CSF as well as in the brain and other tissues.

Decreased activity of the enzyme has been demonstrated in liver, leukocytes, and cultured fibroblasts of affected individuals.

Postmortem examination of a patient has revealed neuronal loss and fibrous gliosis in the caudate and putamen, as well as slight atrophy of the cerebellar cortex. In addition, fatty changes were seen in the liver, kidney, and myocardium. These pathologic changes correlate well with the symptoms seen.

Epidemiology

The incidence of this rare disorder is not known.

Natural History

Affected individuals present in either infancy or childhood with a progressive movement disorder consisting primarily of choreoathetosis and dystonia, with or without spasticity. Dysarthria and megacephaly can also be seen. In addition, some patients have been reported as having intermittent or chronic metabolic acidosis associated with episodic irritability, lethargy, vomiting, and hypoglycemia. Seizures, mental retardation, and death from a Reye-like illness also have been reported.

Diagnosis

Laboratory findings in affected patients may reveal metabolic acidosis with ketonuria, hypoglycemia, and abnormal liver function tests. CT scan of the head discloses a characteristic enlargement of the aqueduct of Sylvius and bilateral areas of reduced density often misinterpreted as subdural effusions.

Organic acid elevations in the urine (glutaric acid, β-hydroxyglutaric acid, and glutaconic acid) are diagnostic. Increased levels of lactic, β-hydroxybutyric, β-hydroxyisovaleric, adipic, and suberic acids may also be present in urine.

Confirmation of the diagnosis depends upon the demonstration of deficient activity of glutaryl-CoA dehydrogenase in cultured skin fibroblasts or leukocytes.

Treatment

At least one patient had improved tone and some increase in motor activity when treated with a diet restricted in lysine and tryptophan. Another approach to therapy includes the use of riboflavin and lioresal (4-amino-3-(4-chlorophenyl)butyric acid), a GABA analog, in conjunction with a low-protein diet. This prevented progressive neurologic deterioration in one patient.

Prognosis

The movement disorder progresses so that many patients eventually become totally incapacitated. Others have died suddenly of a Reye-like illness, usually associated with an infectious process.

Prevention

Prenatal diagnosis of this disorder is possible by the demonstration of increased levels of glutaric acid in amniotic fluid and deficient glutaryl-CoA dehydrogenase in cultured amniotic fluid cells.

GLUTARIC ACIDURIA TYPE II

Definition

Glutaric aciduria type II is an inborn error of the mitochondrial electron transport chain that usually results in neonatal death. All pedigrees reported thus far suggest an autosomal recessive pattern of inheritance, although one reported pedigree is compatible with X-linked recessive inheritance.

Basic Science

Glutaric aciduria type II, also known as multiple acyl-CoA dehydrogenase deficiency, is due to a defect in the electron transfer flavoprotein (ETF) or to ETF dehydrogenase deficiency. Both of these mitochondrial flavoproteins function in the respiratory chain to move electrons from the flavin adenine dinucleotide (FAD) of several dehydrogenases to coenzyme Q. Some of the dehydrogenases are involved in amino acid metabolism, while others are involved in the β-oxidation of fatty acids, accounting for the multiplicity of symptoms and biochemical abnormalities seen in affected infants (Goodman et al, 1977; 1986).

Epidemiology

The incidence of this disorder is not yet known. From the paucity of reported cases it appears to be quite rare. Since death usually occurs within the first few days of life, however, many cases may have been unrecognized.

Natural History

The disorder has three modes of presentation. These are neonatal onset with congenital anomalies, neonatal onset without congenital anomalies, and a later onset form which in some (or all) cases may be synonymous with ethylmalonic-adipic aciduria (Goodman et al, 1977; Sweetman et al, 1979). Symptoms are primarily due to the defect in fatty acid oxidation which is important for ketone body formation and in supplying energy for skeletal and cardiac muscle function and for gluconeogenesis.

Onset of disease in the neonatal period is characterized by profound metabolic acidosis and hypoglycemia, often present on the first day of life. Hyperammonemia and hypotonia may also be present and hepatomegaly and cardiomyopathy often appear. Among the congenital anomalies reported are polycystic kidneys, defects of the abdominal wall (omphalocele), and anomalies of the external genitalia. Potter-type facies, perhaps secondary to the severe renal malformations, has been described in several infants. All affected infants have died within the first few weeks of life.

Patients with the "late onset" form of the disorder present during infancy or childhood with intermittent vomiting, hypoglycemia, and metabolic acidosis. Several have also had cardiomyopathy, and hepatomegaly.

Diagnosis

As with the other disorders of fatty acid metabolism, the hallmarks of glutaric aciduria type II are metabolic acidosis and nonketotic hypoglycemia, the latter due to the defect in fatty acid oxidation. A "sweaty feet" odor has been noted in several of the patients.

The diagnosis of this inborn error is based on the demonstration of the typical organic aciduria in a patient with nonketotic hypoglycemia. The organic acids present in the urine, predominantly glutaric and lactic acids, are derivatives of the substrates of the flavoprotein dehydrogenases. In addition, dicarboxylic acids such as adipic acid, suberic acid, and sebacic acid and hydroxyacids such as hydroxybutyric acid, p-hydroxyphenyllactic acid, hydroxyisovaleric acid, and hydroxyisocaproic acid are also found. Sarcosine is intermittently present.

Treatment

There is no effective treatment for this disorder. Some patients have shown a temporary response to large doses of riboflavin. Carnitine may be indicated.

Prognosis

Most infants with the neonatal form of the disorder die during the first few weeks of life.

Prevention

Prenatal diagnosis of glutaric aciduria type II has been accomplished by demonstration of markedly increased amounts of glutaric acid in the amniotic fluid (Goodman et al, 1977).

REFERENCES

Ampola MG, Mahoney MJ, Nakamura E, et al: Prenatal therapy of a patient with vitamin B_{12}-responsive methylmalonic acidemia. *N Engl J Med* 293:313, 1975.

Bartlett K, Ghneim HK, Stirk HJ, et al: Enzyme studies in biotin-responsive disorders. *J Inher Metabol Dis* 8 (Suppl 1):46, 1985.

Buchanan PD, Kahler SG, Sweetman L, et al: Pitfalls in the prenatal diagnosis of propionic acidemia. *Clin Genet* 18:177, 1980.

Cohn RM, Yudkoff M, Rothman R, et al: Isovaleric acidemia: Use of glycine therapy in neonates. *N Engl J Med* 299:996, 1978.

Dave P, Curless RG, Steinman L: Cerebellar hemorrhage complicating methylmalonic and propionic acidemia. *Arch Neurol* 41:1293, 1984.

Dunger DB, Snodgrass GJAI: Glutaric aciduria Type I presenting with hypoglycaemia. *J Inher Metabol Dis* 7:122, 1984.

Duran M, Shutgens RBH, Ketel A, et al: 3-hydroxy-3-methylglytaryl coenzyme A lyase deficiency: Postnatal management following prenatal diagnosis by analysis of maternal urine. *J Pediatr* 95:1004, 1979.

Duran M, Wadman SK: Thiamine-responsive inborn errors of metabolism. *J Inher Metabol Dis* 8 (Suppl 1):70, 1985.

Frezal J, Amedee-Manesme O, Mitchell G, et al: Maple syrup urine disease: Two different forms within a single family. *Hum Genet* 71:89, 1985.

Goodman SI: Inherited metabolic disease in the newborn: Approach to diagnosis and treatment. *Adv Pediatr* 33:197, 1986.

Goodman SI, Norenberg MD, Shikes RH, et al: Glutaric aciduria: Biochemical and morphologic considerations. *J Pediatr* 90:746, 1977.

Hyman DB, Tanaka K: Specific glutaryl-CoA dehydrogenating activity is deficient in cultured fibroblasts from glutaric aciduria patients. *J Clin Invest* 73:778, 1984.

Ledley FD, Levy HL, Shih VE, et al: Benign methylmalonic aciduria. *N Engl J Med* 311:1015, 1984.

Leibel RL, Shih VE, Goodman SI, et al: Glutaric acidemia: A metabolic disorder causing progressive choreoathetosis. *Neurology* 30:1163, 1980.

Matsui SM, Mahoney MJ, Rosenberg LE: The natural history of the inherited methylmalonic acidemias. *N Engl J Med* 308:857, 1983.

Middleton B, Bartlett K, Romanos A, et al: 3-ketothiolase deficiency. *Eur J Pediatr* 144:586, 1986.

Moreno-Vega, Govantes JM: Methylmalonic acidemia treated by continuous peritoneal dialysis. *N Engl J Med* 312:1641, 1985.

Ney D, Bay C, Saudubray JM, et al: An evaluation of protein requirements in methylmalonic acidaemia. *J Inher Metabol Dis* 8: (Suppl 1):132, 1985.

Packman S, Golbus MS, Cowan MJ, et al: Prenatal treatment of biotin-responsive multiple carboxylase deficiency. *Lancet* 1:1435, 1982.

Packman S, Sweetman L, Baker H, et al: The neonatal form of biotin-responsive multiple carboxylase deficiency. *J Pediatr* 99:418, 1981.

Proud VK, Patterson J, Rizzo WB, et al: Skin abnormalities in biotinidase deficiency may be associated with alterations in fatty acid composition. *Am J Hum Genet* 39 (Suppl):A18, 1986.

Roe CR, Bohan TP: L-carnitine therapy in propionic acidaemia. *Lancet* 1:1411, 1982.

Rosenblatt DS, Hosack A, and Matiaszuk NV: Defect in vitamin B_{12} release from lysosomes: Newly described inborn error of vitamin B_{12} metabolism. *Science* 228:1319, 1985.

Seccombe DW, Snyder F, Parsons HG: L-carnitine for methylmalonicaciduria. *Lancet* 2:1401, 1982.

Sweetman L, Weyler N, Shafai T, et al: Prenatal diagnosis of propionic acidemia. *JAMA* 242:1048, 1979.

Tada K, Hayasaka K: Nonketotic hyperglycinaemia: Clinical and biochemical aspects. *Eur J Pediatr* 146:221, 1987.

Tanaka K, Rosenberg LE: Disorders of branched chain amino acid and organic acid metabolism. In Stanbury JB, et al (eds): *The Metabolic Basis of Inherited Disease*. New York, McGraw-Hill, 1983, pp. 440-473.

Wolf B, Sweetman L, Gravel R, et al: Propionic acidemias: A clinical update. *J Pediatr* 99:835, 1981.

Wolf B, Grier RE, Secor McVoy JR, et al: Biotinidase deficiency: A novel vitamine recycling defect. *J Inher Metabol Dis* 8 (Suppl 1):53, 1985.

Yudkoff M, Cohn RM, Puschak R, et al: Glycine therapy in isovaleric acidemia. *J Pediatr* 92:813, 1978.

Fatty Acid Oxidation Defects

4

Fatty acid oxidation plays a major role in energy metabolism (Saudubray et al, 1982). It provides the main source of energy during fasting in peripheral tissues, and is necessary for gluconeogenesis and ketone body formation in the liver. Several inborn errors of metabolism in which there is defective oxidation of fatty acids have been described. These include the "dicarboxylic acidurias" which are due to inherited disorders of the acyl-CoA dehydrogenases; ethylmalonic aciduria and glutaric aciduria type II which are due to a defect in a common electron transfer flavoprotein (ETF) or a defect in ETF dehydrogenase; and reduced transport of long-chain fatty acids into the mitochondria as can be seen in either carnitine deficiency or carnitine palmitoyl transferase deficiency. The clinical presentations of these disorders vary, but a common feature of all is hypoketotic hypoglycemia with dicarboxylic aciduria, indicating a defect in the β-oxidation of fatty acids.

ACYL-CoA DEHYDROGENASE DEFICIENCIES—"DICARBOXYLIC ACIDURIAS"

Definition

Inherited disorders of the short-, medium-, and long-chain acyl-CoA dehydrogenases have been described (Divry et al, 1983; Stanley et al, 1983; Bougneres et al, 1985; Hale et al, 1985). All appear to be inherited in an autosomal recessive pattern.

Basic Science

During fasting, or other periods of catabolic stress, oxidation of fatty acids to ketones in the liver provides energy for gluconeogenesis; utilization of fatty acids also helps conserve glucose for brain metabolism. The fatty acid is transported into the mitochondrion by carnitine (Fig. 15.13). Three acyl-CoA dehydrogenases mediate intramitochondrial fatty acid oxidation. Each is active with a particular range of fatty-acid chain length; viz. long-chain, medium-chain, and short-chain. Two other dehydrogenases, isovaleryl-CoA and isobutyryl-CoA, act on intermediates of branched-chain amino acid oxidation. All of these enzymes require electron transfer flavoprotein as an electron acceptor. Absence of any acyl-CoA dehydrogenase blocks oxidation of fatty acids with the characteristic chain length. The medium-chain dehydrogenase, however, also has some activity against short-chain fatty acids, so that absence of the medium-chain dehydrogenase blocks the oxidation of medium-chain fatty acids and partially blocks short-chain fatty acid oxidation as well. During conditions that require increased energy production, such as prolonged fasting or illness, an inherited acyl-CoA dehydrogenase deficiency leads to metabolic derangements produced by decreased oxidation of fatty acids and, therefore, decreased metabolites in the Krebs cycle and the gluconeogenic pathway.

Epidemiology

The incidence is not yet known. Our recent experience suggests that the frequency may be similar to that of other organic acid disorders, perhaps 1:200,000. The medium-chain dehydrogenase deficiency seems to be the most frequent of these defects.

Natural History

Patients can present at any age, although most do so during early childhood. The common mode of presentation for medium-chain dehydrogenase deficiency

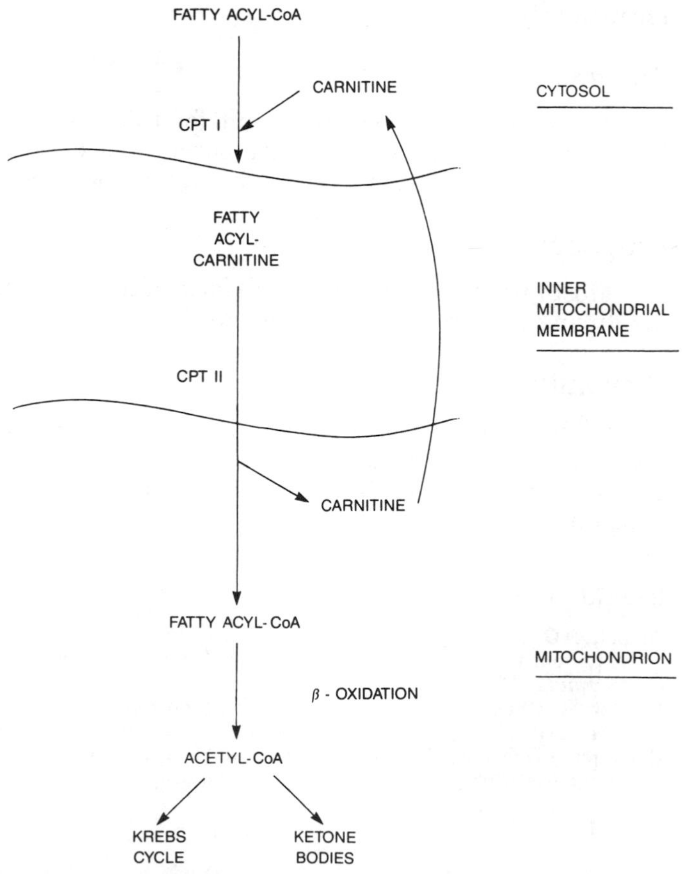

Figure 15.13. Role of carnitine in transport of fatty acyl-CoA.

is recurrent life-threatening episodes of hypoglycemia, coma, hyperammonemia, and metabolic acidosis, often associated with fasting or illness and resembling Reye syndrome. The key biochemical feature in these patients is the lack of ketone production during fasting and in the presence of hypoglycemia, indicating a defect in fatty acid oxidation. Significant hepatomegaly and hypotonia occurs during the acute episodes. Death may occur secondary to cardiorespiratory arrest and/or cerebral edema.

Short-chain and long-chain acyl-CoA dehydrogenase deficiencies may have more chronic presentations than does medium-chain deficiency. The short-chain defect results in failure to thrive, muscle weakness, hypotonia, and developmental delay during the first year of life. The long-chain disorder causes a striking skeletal and cardiac myopathy with hepatic dysfunction and developmental delay noted during the first or second year of life. These defects may also rarely cause the acute Reye-like picture observed with the medium-chain disorder.

Diagnosis

Any child who presents with a Reye-like illness characterized by hypoglycemia, hyperammonemia, acidosis, coma, and lack of ketosis should be investigated for a disorder of fatty acid oxidation. Some investigators believe that "Reye syndrome" in any child less than 2 years of age is most likely to be due to medium-chain ACD deficiency.

During the acute episode the presumptive diagnosis of a fatty acid oxidation defect secondary to acyl-CoA dehydrogenase deficiency can be made by the absence of ketosis and ketonuria and by analysis of the urine for organic acids by gas chromatographic and/or mass spectroscopic techniques. The presence of urinary dicarboxylic acids and related metabolites, including suberylglycine is pathognomonic. These patients also may have elevated levels of free fatty acids in plasma and decreased levels of free carnitine in plasma and muscle. The specific diagnosis can be then confirmed by assay of acyl-CoA dehydrogenase activity in liver, white blood cells, or cultured skin fibroblasts from the patient (Coates et al, 1985).

The diagnosis of medium-chain deficiency can also be made by obtaining an acylcarnitine profile after an oral carnitine load. The deficiency of medium-chain acyl-CoA dehydrogenase results in the accumulation of medium-chain acyl-CoA compounds which bind to free carnitine, forming particular acylcarnitines, especially octanoylcarnitine. These can be identified in urine by a specific gas chromatographic/mass spectroscopic method. This test permits the diagnosis of medium-chain deficiency without the risk of fasting or a dietary fat challenge which can precipitate an acute episode.

Treatment

Treatment of an acute episode is an emergency and whenever possible should be given in a center experienced in the care of acute metabolic disorders. Blood should be obtained for measurement of amino acids, carnitine, and other relevant tests and urine should be collected for organic acid and amino acid analysis. Intravenous glucose-containing fluids should be administered immediately for correction of the hypoglycemia and to decrease the catabolic state. Acidosis should be treated with intravenous sodium bicarbonate. Intravenous carnitine should also be administered to provide the free carnitine as it mediates the transfer of long-chain fatty acids into mitochondria and that binds potentially toxic fatty acid acyl-CoA derivatives and removes them from the mitochondria. Careful monitoring of electrolytes, glucose, blood gases, blood ammonia, and cardiorespiratory and neurologic function is also necessary.

Chronic treatment of patients includes the administration of oral carnitine and adjustment of the diet to contain decreased amounts of the specific fatty acids that cannot be metabolized by the patient. Because of the high concentration of carnitine in breast milk, breast-feeding may be protective for infants with these disorders, particularly those with medium-chain dehydrogenase deficiency. Some investigators also have reported improvement in the cardiomyopathy seen in patients with long-chain dehydrogenase deficiency after treatment with carnitine and a specific diet.

Prognosis

With prompt treatment of intercurrent infections and acute episodes by immediate hospitalization and specific therapies, the prognosis for patients with these disorders is good. Recent reports of sudden infant and child death in siblings of asymptomatic children found to have medium-chain acyl-CoA dehydrogenase deficiency raise the possibility of sudden death as one of the complications of this disorder (Duran et al, 1986; Roe et al, 1986).

Prevention

These disorders can be diagnosed at birth by enzyme assay of lymphocytes derived from cord blood. The diagnosis of medium-chain dehydrogenase deficiency can be made by 1 week of age on the basis of the urine acylcarnitine profile after 5–6 days of breast-feeding. Prenatal diagnosis of these disorders is possible by measurement of the specific enzymes in cultured amniotic fluid cells.

CARNITINE DEFICIENCY

Definition

Carnitine is an amine that transports long-chain fatty acids into the mitochondria for subsequent β-oxidation. There are two main forms of primary carnitine deficiency, myopathic and systemic, each believed to be inherited in an autosomal recessive manner. In addition, there are numerous causes of secondary carnitine deficiency.

Basic Science

Carnitine is synthesized endogenously from lysine and methionine. The major source of carnitine, however, is dietary, particularly breast milk, meat, and dairy products. In addition, many infant formulas have been supplemented with carnitine.

Long-chain fatty acids are transported across the inner mitochondrial membrane as acylcarnitines. The fatty acid then uncouples from the carnitine yielding fatty acyl-CoA, which undergoes β-oxidation, and free carnitine, which returns to the cytosol (Fig. 15.13). Other functions of carnitine may include the facilitation of oxidation of branched chain α-ketoacids, the shuttling of acyl moieties shortened by β-oxidation out of hepatic peroxisomes, and the modulation of the acyl-CoA/CoA-sulfhydryl ratio in mammalian cells (Engel and Rebouche, 1984).

Ninety-eight percent of total body carnitine is in the muscle, with the remainder in the liver and extracellular fluid. In tissues and physiologic fluids, L-carnitine is present in both free and esterified forms. The latter includes short-chain and long-chain fatty acyl-carnitine esters. Many of the symptoms and signs of carnitine deficiency are due to defective fatty acid oxidation and to deficiency of free carnitine in muscle.

Epidemiology

The incidence of primary carnitine deficiency is not known; secondary carnitine deficiency, however, is quite frequent. It is usually due to reduced carnitine intake, such as occurs in special diets for metabolic disorders that restrict meats and dairy products and when organic acids accumulate and esterify free carnitine.

Natural History

Primary carnitine deficiencies, myopathic and systemic, each present with a characteristic clinical picture (Engel and Rebouche, 1984; Rebouche and Engel, 1983).

Primary myopathic carnitine deficiency may be due to defective transport of carnitine into muscle. Onset of symptoms may occur from early childhood to adulthood. Patients present with mild to severe muscle weakness (both at rest and upon exertion), symptoms of cardiomyopathy and cardiac compromise, and myoglobinuria. Pregnancy may lead to worsening of symptoms.

Primary systemic carnitine deficiency is generally diagnosed early in childhood, although patients can present any time from infancy to adult years. Presenting symptoms include muscle weakness (often progressive), hepatomegaly and hepatic dysfunction, cardiomyopathy and cardiac compromise, hypoglycemia, and recurrent episodes of acute encephalopathy with vomiting which may be fatal. The acute attacks are usually triggered by illness and fasting. Fasting leads to increased mobilization of fatty acids the utilization of which is limited by the primary carnitine deficiency. These signs and symptoms may be mistakenly diagnosed as Reye syndrome or an organic acid disorder. Sudden death has also been reported with systemic carnitine deficiency that followed a prolonged illness (Legge, 1985). A distinct form may present as familial cardiomyopathy associated with skeletal weakness (Waber et al, 1982).

Secondary carnitine deficiency may produce any or all of the features of primary systemic carnitine deficiency.

Diagnosis

The diagnosis of primary muscle carnitine deficiency depends on the demonstration of reduced free carnitine in muscle tissue. Serum and liver carnitine levels may be normal. Pathologic examination reveals increased lipid in skeletal muscle. This lipid excess may also be seen in leukocytes and Schwann cells.

The diagnosis of primary systemic carnitine deficiency depends on the demonstration of decreased free carnitine levels in muscle, liver, and serum. Again, there is increased deposition of lipid in skeletal muscle, as well as in heart muscle, liver, and other tissues. Patients with an acute exacerbation of the disorder can present with hypoglycemia, hyperammonemia, increased muscle and liver serum enzymes, a coagulopathy, and dicarboxylic aciduria identified by urine organic acid analysis.

Treatment

Replacement therapy with oral L-carnitine has led to improvement in muscle strength and cardiac function in patients with either the myopathic or systemic forms of carnitine deficiency (Waber et al, 1982; Prockop et al, 1983). In addition, dietary manipulations, which include maintenance of caloric input (particularly with carbohydrate) and the addition of medium-chain triglycerides to the diet, have been beneficial (Angelini et al, 1976).

Treatment of acute attacks of systemic carnitine deficiency includes the administration of intravenous glucose and carnitine.

Prognosis

As noted above, treatment of patients with the myopathic or systemic forms of carnitine deficiency has been successful. Whether the severe cardiomyopathy seen in some patients can be successfully treated depends upon the degree of cardiac compromise at the time of presentation.

CARNITINE PALMITOYLTRANSFERASE DEFICIENCY

Definition

Carnitine palmitoyltransferase deficiency is an inborn error of fatty acid metabolism that affects muscle and the kidneys. Most cases are believed to be due to autosomal recessive inheritance, but several sporadic cases have also been described.

Basic Science

The two forms of carnitine palmitoyltransferase (known as I and II) are located on the external and matrix surfaces of the inner mitochondrial membrane, respectively (Fig. 15.13). Both function in the transport of fatty acids into the mitochondria (Engel and Rebouche, 1984). Carnitine palmitoyltransferase I couples carnitine to the fatty acid for transport across the mitochondrial membrane; whereas type II uncouples the acylcarnitine, releasing free carnitine and the fatty acid.

Epidemiology

The incidence of this inborn error is not known.

Natural History

The clinical presentation of patients with carnitine palmitoyltransferase deficiency is varied. Symptoms may begin at any time, from childhood to adult years. They usually consist of episodes of muscle cramps and rhabdomyolysis in association with myoglobinuria. Respiratory insufficiency has also occurred during acute episodes (DiDonato et al, 1981).

Patients differ with regard to the stimulation or trigger for the rhabdomyolysis. Exercise, fever, and illness have precipitated the symptoms in many patients, while in others, the symptoms may begin spontaneously.

Diagnosis

During an acute episode, affected individuals present with myoglobinuria, azotemia, and increased levels of liver and muscle enzymes in serum. Increased baseline and fasting levels of triglycerides, cholesterol, and free fatty acids due to defective utilization of free fatty acids may also be seen in the disorder. The muscle does not contain excess lipid based on pathologic examination. Patients differ in their ability to make ketones while fasting; some patients form ketone bodies while others do not.

Carnitine palmitoyltransferase activity can be measured in muscle, liver, platelets, and cultured fibroblasts. Patients have had a wide range of enzyme activity, demonstrating the biochemical heterogeneity in this disorder. Patients have shown specific deficiencies of either carnitine palmitoyltransferase I or II; a few patients have decreased activities of both forms.

Treatment

Treatment of an acute episode includes the administration of intravenous glucose solutions. Renal insufficiency may require renal dialysis.

Prognosis

The prognosis depends to a large extent on the degree of renal compromise that has occurred.

Prevention

Detection of heterozygotes by demonstration of intermediate levels of enzyme activity in platelets has been reported in one family (Angelini et al, 1981).

REFERENCES

Angelini C, Lucke S, Cantarutti F: Carnitine deficiency of skeletal muscle: Report of a treated case. *Neurology* 26:633, 1976.

Angelini C, Freddo L, Battistella P, et al: Carnitine palmitoyltransferase deficiency: Clinical variability, carrier detection, and autosomal recessive inheritance. *Neurology* 31:883, 1981.

Bank WJ, DiMauro S, Bonilla E, et al: A disorder of muscle lipid metabolism and myoglobinuria. *N Engl J Med* 292:443, 1975.

Bougneres PF, Rocchiccioli F, Kolvraa S, et al: Medium-chain acyl-CoA dehydrogenase deficiency in two siblings with a Reye-like syndrome. *J Pediatr* 106:918, 1985.

Coates PM, Hale DE, Stanley CA, et al: Genetic deficiency of medium-chain acyl coenzyme A dehydrogenase: Studies in cultured skin fibroblasts and peripheral mononuclear leukocytes. *Pediatr Res* 19:671, 1985.

DiDonato S, Castiglione A, Rimoldi M, et al: Heterogeneity of carnitine-palmitoyltransferase deficiency. *J Neurol Sci* 50:207, 1981.

Divry P, David M, Gregersen N, et al: Dicarboxylic aciduria due to medium chain acyl CoA dehydrogenase defect. *Acta Paediatr Scand* 72:943, 1983.

Duran M, Hofkamp M, Rhead WJ, et al: Sudden child death and "healthy" affected family members with medium-chain-acyl-coenzyme A dehydrogenase deficiency. *Pediatrics* 78:1052, 1986.

Engel AG, Rebouche CJ: Carnitine metabolism and inborn errors. *J Inher Metabol Dis* 7 (Suppl 1):38, 1984.

Goodman SI, Frerman FE: Glutaric acidaemia type II (Multiple acyl-CoA dehydrogenation deficiency). *J Inher Metabol Dis* 7(Suppl 1):33, 1984.

Hale DE, Batshaw ML, Coates PM, et al: Long-chain acyl coenzyme A dehydrogenase deficiency: An inherited cause of nonketotic hypoglycemia. *Pediatr Res* 19:666, 1985.

Legge M: Systemic carnitine deficiency as the cause of a prolonged illness and sudden death in a six-year-old child. *J Inher Metabol Dis* 8:159, 1985.

Niederwieser A, Steinmann B, Exner U, et al: Multiple acyl-CoA dehydrogenation deficiency (MADD) in a boy with nonketotic hypoglycemia, hepatomegaly, muscle hypotonia and cardiomyopathy. *Helv Paediatr Acta* 38:9, 1983.

Prockop LD, Engel WK, Shug AL: Nearly fatal muscle carnitine deficiency with full recovery after replacement therapy. *Neurology* 33:1628, 1983.

Rebouche CJ, Engel AG: Carnitine metabolism and deficiency syndromes. *Mayo Clin Proc* 58:533, 1983.

Roe CR, Millington DS, Maltby DA, et al: Recognition of medium-chain acyl-CoA dehydrogenase deficiency in asymptomatic siblings of children dying of sudden infant death of Reye-like syndromes. *J Pediatr* 108:13, 1986.

Saudubray JM, Coude FX, Demaugre F, et al: Oxidation of fatty acids in cultured fibroblasts: A model system for the detection and study of defects in oxidation. *Pediatr Res* 16:877, 1982.

Stanley CA, Hale DE, Coates PM, et al: Medium-chain acyl-CoA dehydrogenase deficiency in children with non-ketonic hypoglycemia and low carnitine levels. *Pediatr Res* 17:877, 1983.

Sweetman L, Nyhan WL, Trauner DA, et al: Glutaric aciduria Type II. *J Pediatr* 96:1020, 1980.

Treem WR, Witzleben CA, Piccol DA, et al: Medium-chain and long-chain acyl CoA dehydrogenase deficiency: Clinical, pathologic and ultrastructural differentiation from Reye's syndrome. *Hepatology* 6:1270, 1976.

Waber LJ, Valle D, Neill C, et al: Carnitine deficiency presenting as familial cardiomyopathy: A treatable defect in carnitine transport. *J Pediatr* 101:700, 1982.

Peroxismal Disorders

5

In these disorders the defect is in the peroxisome, a small subcellular organelle in which a number of reactions occur, including that of catalase, the β-oxidation of very-long-chain fatty acids, the oxidation of phytanic acid, and the degradation of pipecolic acid. The disorders show accumulation of bile acid precursors and very-long-chain fatty acids with impaired synthesis of plasmalogens. Minor congenital anomalies are associated with these disorders (Moser, 1987).

For a discussion of adrenoleukoclystrophy see page 715.

REFSUM DISEASE

Definition

Refsum disease, also known as phytanic acid storage disease, is an autosomal recessive inborn error of phytanic acid degradation.

Basic Science

The enzyme defect in Refsum disease is a deficiency of phytanic acid α-oxidase, an enzyme that normally catalyzes the conversion of phytanic acid to α-hydroxyphytanic acid. Deficiency of this enzyme results in large accumulations of phytanic acid in blood and other body tissues and organs.

Epidemiology

The incidence of this disorder is unknown.

Natural History

The tetrad of retinitis pigmentosa, peripheral neuropathy, cerebellar ataxia, and a high CSF protein in the absence of pleocytosis has been found in virtually all reported patients. The symptoms may begin in childhood, but some patients have presented as late as the fifth decade. The earliest symptom reported appears to be night blindness. Other symptoms include failing vision, extremity weakness, and gait abnormalities. Among other features are nerve deafness, anosmia, nystagmus, nonspecific ECG abnormalities, and skin lesions, which include icthyosis-like changes ranging from mild hyperkeratosis of the palms and soles to florid icthyosis of the trunk.

Diagnosis

Increased serum phytanic acid levels are found in all affected patients. Definitive diagnosis depends upon demonstration of a decreased rate of phytanic acid oxidation in cultured skin fibroblasts. In some cases, abnormal peroxisomes are visible with electron microscopy.

Treatment

Since phytanic acid is exclusively exogenous in origin, attempts at treatment have concentrated on decreasing phytanic acid in the diet. The use of plasmapheresis has also been reported with promising results. Some improvement in peripheral neuropathy has followed reduction in serum phytanate.

Prognosis

The disease usually runs a protracted course with progressive deterioration, although more than half of the reported patients have had long periods of remission.

Prevention

Heterozygote detection is possible by measurement of phytanic acid oxidation in cultured skin fibroblasts.

ZELLWEGER DISEASE

Definition

Zellweger disease, also known as the cerebrohepatorenal syndrome, is an autosomal recessive disorder characterized by the absence of peroxisomes and peroxisomal function. It is a lethal disorder of infancy.

Basic Science

The basic defect in this disorder is not known, but is believed to be due to an abnormality in peroxisomal formation or maintenance leading to the diminished function of all peroxisomal enzymes. Infants have significant elevations of unbranched long chain fatty acids, especially those of 26 carbon chain length.

Epidemiology

The prevalence of this disorder is estimated to be about 1/100,000 live births.

Natural History

Affected infants present in the newborn period with a characteristic facies, severe hypotonia, and hepatomegaly. The liver disease progresses to cirrhosis and death usually occurs by 1 year of age. The abnormal facial features include a high narrow forehead, hypertelorism, epicanthal folds, shallow supraorbital ridges, a broad nasal bridge, abnormal helices, and a high arched palate. Stippled irregular calcification of the patella or greater trochanter are highly characteristic of this disorder. Other features include the lack of mental or motor development, ocular abnormalities (cataracts, corneal opacities, glaucoma), seizures, and renal cortical cysts.

Diagnosis

The diagnosis is suggested by the clinical features of the disorder and the demonstration of increased levels of very-long-chain fatty acids and pipecolic acid in the serum or cultured fibroblasts. Electron microscopy of various tissues reveals the absence of peroxisomes.

Treatment

There is no known therapy for this disorder.

Prognosis

As noted above, death usually occurs in the first year of life.

Prevention

Prenatal diagnosis is possible by demonstrating increased very-long-chain fatty acids and decreased plasmalogens in cultured amniotic fluid cells.

INFANTILE REFSUM DISEASE

Definition

Infantile Refsum disease is an autosomal recessive disorder that shares features of both Refsum disease and Zellweger disease.

Basic Science

Infants with this inborn error have a disturbance in phytanic acid metabolism, probably in phytanic acid oxidation. They accumulate very-long-chain fatty acids in plasma and fibroblasts, have elevated plasma pipecolic acid, abnormal bile metabolites in plasma, and impaired de novo plasmologen biosynthesis in fibroblasts. All of these aberrations suggest multiple peroxisomal dysfunction and tend to make this disorder more like a variant of Zellweger disease then an early presenting form of Refsum disease, in which only phytanic acid oxidation is disturbed. Patients also exhibit decreased activity of acyl-CoA:dihydroxyacetone phosphate acyltransferase, a membrane-bound peroxisomal enzyme, which strengthens the case for multiple peroxisomal dysfunction.

Epidemiology

Only a few cases of this disorder have been reported as of 1987.

Natural History

Clinical features include dysmorphic facies, retinitis pigmentosa, neurosensory hearing loss, hepatomegaly, osteopenia, delayed growth, and delayed psychomotor development. These features are present from infancy.

Diagnosis

Affected children have increased plasma phytanic acid, increased pipecolic acid in plasma, urine, and CSF, abnormal bile metabolites in plasma, and the accumulation of very-long-chain fatty acids in plasma and fibroblasts. The diagnosis is confirmed by the demonstration of a deficiency of phytanic acid oxidase in cultured skin fibroblasts.

Treatment

Studies are currently being performed to determine the efficacy of a diet restricted in long-chain fatty acids and phytanic acid.

Prognosis

The prognosis for children with this disorder treated with the restricted diet is not yet known.

CONRADI-HUNERMANN FORM OF CHONDRODYSPLASIA PUNCTATA

Definition

This disorder is characterized by focal calcification in cartilagenous tissues associated with a deficiency of erythrocyte plasmalogens and the enzyme dihydroxyacetone phosphate acyltransferase.

Epidemiology

This rare disorder is an autosomal dominant. Milder related forms are autosomal recessive or X-linked.

Natural History

Short stature, punctate calcifications in spine, sternum and lower extremities, cataracts, icthyosis, and a shallow nasal bridge are found in this disorder. The lower limbs are asymmetrical.

Diagnosis

The diagnosis is suggested by the constellation of findings.

Treatment

Supportive care is all that is available in 1988.

Lipoprotein Metabolism Disorders

6

The importance of identification of children with disorders of lipid metabolism was long appreciated since some are at risk of premature atherosclerosis and myocardial infarction. The 1984 Lipid Research Clinics Coronary Primary Prevention trial in adult men treated for 7 years reinforced the importance of early detection by finding a 24% reduction in incidence of myocardial infarction deaths when plasma cholesterol was reduced by cholestyramine therapy.

Basic Science

Cholesterol and triglycerides are transported in the blood with associated apoproteins; the complexes are called lipoproteins (Breslow, 1985). Dietary lipids, together with apolipoproteins form chylomicrons that are hydrolyzed by lipoprotein lipase in the capillary endothelium. The lipoprotein particles (or remnants) are bound and internalized into the hepatocyte by membrane receptors specific for the apoE on the particles (Mahley, 1988). The dietary cholesterol partially regulates hepatic cholesterol metabolism.

The liver secretes very low density lipoproteins (VLDL) and apoproteins which then undergo conversion to low density lipoproteins (LDL). Another specific receptor on most cell membranes allows the LDL to be recognized, bound and internalized for membrane synthesis.

The liver also secretes high density lipoproteins that accept cholesterol from VLDL and LDL as well as tissues. The cholesterol is esterified by lecithin: cholesterol acyltransferase (LCAT).

Hypercholesterolemia is defined as a fasting cholesterol greater than 200 mg/dl for both sexes in the first 2 decades. Hypertriglyceridemia is defined as a fasting triglyceride level over 100 mg/dl in the first decade and over 130 mg/dl in the second decade.

If a family history of premature heart attacks is present, LDL and HDL cholesterol should be ascertained. Elevation of LDL over about 130 mg/dl is indication for treatment.

Low levels of HDL cholesterol are associated with an increased risk of atherosclerosis. If levels are extremely low, the condition is known as Tangier disease. High levels may be protective as in familial hyperalphalipoproteinemia, which is associated with low apoA-I and apoA-II levels. In other words, high levels of HDL are good and low levels of LDL are good.

Epidemiology

In a Danish study of 1407 children and young adults whose fathers had died from myocardial infarctions before age 45 years, 15% had hypercholesterolemia and 8% had hypertriglyceridemia (Andersen et al, 1982).

FAMILIAL HYPERCHOLESTEROLEMIA

See Table 15.3 for other hyperlipoproteinemias.

Definition

This is a disorder of lipid metabolism that is characterized by a variety of mutations at the LDL-receptor locus on the short arm of chromosome 19. The result

Table 15.3
Types of Hyperlipoproteinemias

Primary Genetic Defects	Frequency	Defect	Manifestations
Familial hypercholesterolemia	1/500	LDL receptor deficiency	Xanthomas, atherosclerosis
Familial combined hyperlipidemia	1/100	Possible excess VLDL	Hyperinsulinism
Familial hypertriglyceridemia	2–3/1000	Unknown	Obesity, hyperinsulinemia, hyperuricemia
Lipoprotein lipase deficiency (chylomicronemia)	1/6000		Chylomicronemia, xanthomas, pancreatitis
Secondary Hyperlipidemias			
Tangier disease	Rare	Low levels HDL and apoA I and II	Atherosclerosis, yellow tonsils, splenomegaly, neuropathy, corneal lesions
Abetalipoproteinemia	Rare autosomal dominant (may be recessive)	No VLDL or LDL, low cholesterol and triglycerides	Fat malabsorption, cerebellar ataxia, retinitis pigmentosa, acanthocytosis
Lecithin-cholesterol acyltransferase (LCAT) deficiency	Very rare	Reduced levels of all plasma apoproteins	Anemia, proteinuria, corneal opacities

is a marked increase in plasma LDL cholesterol. In a well-studied group of French Canadians with a mutation that led to a diminished number of receptors, the clinical outcome varied dramatically even among homozygous individuals (Hobbs et al, 1987).

Epidemiology

This disorder is an autosomal dominant that occurs in 1/500 individuals. It has been found in higher frequency among some Lebanese and among Afrikaners in South Africa.

Natural History

Homozygous individuals (about 1 per million) have elevated plasma cholesterols (over 500 mg/dl) from birth. At birth or in the first years of life, they develop cutaneous xanthomas over tendons of knees, ankles, and elbows. Coronary atherosclerosis may be present in childhood. Untreated, most die of myocardial infarction before age 30 years.

Heterozygotes may also have developed xanthomas over tendons, and soft tissue deposits of cholesterol esters in eyelids and arcus corneae. Achilles tendonitis may be an early sign.

Diagnosis

Heterozygotes have plasma cholesterol levels of above 250 mg/dl.

Treatment

Dietary restriction of cholesterol is advised. Cholestyramine or colestipol resin will reduce LDL cholesterol. Since both drugs interfere with the absorption of fat-soluble vitamins, plasma vitamin A and prothrombin levels should be measured, and supplements provided if needed.

Homozygous individuals require regular plasmapheresis, or ileal bypass surgery and portocaval shunt. Liver transplantation has a potential role (Bilheimer et al, 1984).

Prognosis

The prognosis, even within families with the same gene deletion, is extremely variable.

HDL DEFICIENCY STATES (TANGIER DISEASE)

Tangier disease is a rare familial disorder of lipoprotein metabolism.

Individuals with Tangier disease synthesize a defective apo A-I that does not associate normally with lipoproteins. Since it is catabolized rapidly, the plasma levels fall to about 1% of normal. The disorder is characterized by very low levels of HDL and cholesterol, and elevated serum triglycerides (Bojanovski et al, 1987).

The clinical manifestation may present in childhood and result from deposition of cholesteryl esters in reticuloendothelial tissues including tonsils, which may appear enlarged and yellow, the spleen, peripheral nerves, liver, lymph nodes, skin, and cornea. Coronary artery disease may appear in either the homozygotes or heterozygotes in middle age. Cardiac valvular involvement has also been recognized in adults.

WOLMAN DISEASE

Definition

Wolman disease is a disorder of lipid metabolism characterized by an accumulation of cholesterol and triglycerides that produces poor growth, hepatosplenomegaly, and calcification of the adrenals.

Basic Science

The defect is a deficiency of lysosomal acid lipase caused by allelic recessive genes at the same locus on chromosome 10. Consanguinity has been found in several reported families. Chemical analyses of liver and spleen reveal increased cholesteryl ester and triglycerides up to 100 times normal values. The enzyme defect is demonstrable in leukocytes and cultured fibroblasts (Coates et al, 1979).

Epidemiology

The frequency of this rare disorder is not known.

Natural History

The onset of failure to grow, diarrhea, and vomiting is usually within the first weeks of life. Soon hepatosplenomegaly is apparent and the abdomen becomes greatly distended. The diagnosis is often first considered when plain radiographs of the abdomen show punctate or stippled calcification of the adrenals.

Death from progressive inanition is usual before 6 months of age, and rarely do affected children live over 1 year.

Diagnosis

The diagnosis may be made at laparotomy from the finding of enlarged yellow liver, spleen, and mesenteric nodes. Biopsy confirms lipid storage and chemical analysis reveals an increase in cholesteryl esters and triglycerides. Demonstration of a deficiency of lysomal acid lipase is confirmatory. A deficiency of the same enzyme is found in a more chronic disorder known as cholesteryl ester storage disease.

Treatment

No specific treatment has been found effective.

Prevention

Heterozygotes can be detected by assay of acid lipase in leukocytes. Prenatal diagnosis is possible.

GAUCHER DISEASE (GLUCOSYL CEREBROSIDE LIPIDOSIS)

Definition

Gaucher disease is an inborn error of lipid metabolism that results in an accumulation of glucocerebrosides throughout the reticuloendothelial system in the skin, the bone marrow, and in some forms of the disease (neuronopathic) in the brain. Chronic Gaucher disease is a slowly progressive disorder without nervous system involvement. Infantile Gaucher disease has marked cerebral involvement and is rapidly fatal (Table 15.4).

Basic Science

Glucocerebroside levels have been measured postmortem in the brains of patients with the neuronopathic forms of Gaucher disease (types 2 [onset in infancy] and 3 [onset in childhood or adolescence]). The greatest concentrations were found in the occipital cortex with lesser amounts elsewhere in the brain. Brain stem structures are relatively spared. The enzymatic defect is inactivity of a lysosomal ceramide glucoside cleaving enzyme, glycosyl ceramide β-glucosidase (Brady et al, 1966). A genetic marker for at least some individuals with neuronopathic disease was reported by Tsuji et al (1987).

The typical Gaucher cell is 20–80 μ in diameter, round, oval, or spindle-shaped with a fibrillar cytoplasm that represents stored glucocerebroside. The cells are found in liver, spleen, lymph nodes, and bone marrow.

Epidemiology

The type 1 (adult) form of Gaucher disease is most common in Ashkenazi Jews (frequency 1/2500) but has appeared in all ethnic groups. The inheritance of all forms of Gaucher disease is recessive. A few dominant-transmission pedigrees have been described.

Natural History

The onset of the rare infantile form of the disease may be in the first few months of life with slow development and hepatosplenomegaly. In the most severely affected infants, swallowing difficulties lead to aspiration and chronic bronchopneumonia. Death usually occurs before 2 years of age.

The more chronic form of the disease or the adult type, is about 20 times as common as the infantile form. It is characterized by hypersplenism; anemia and thrombocytopenia, bone pain, and joint swelling are common and pathologic fractures as well as osteomyelitis have been reported. Other findings may include yellow-brown pigmentation in exposed areas of the body.

Diagnosis

The Gaucher cells are almost pathognomonic and bone marrow biopsy is essential to the diagnosis. The spleen or liver can be extracted for lipids and the glyco lipids can be separated by thin layer chromotography. The most diagnostic test is measurement of the enzyme, glucosyl ceramide β-glucosidase in leukocytes or cultured skin fibroblasts. Patients have less than 20% of normal activity.

Table 15.4
Lipid Storage Diseases[1]

Condition	Defect	Clinical Features
Disorders with visceromegaly		
Infantile generalized gangliosidosis (pseudo Hurler)	β-galactosidase	Somewhat resembles Hurler, about half have retinal cherry-red spots
Gaucher	Glucocerebrosidase	Bulbar signs early, occasional cherry-red spots
Niemann-Pick (type A)	Sphingomyelinase	Intellectual deterioration, anemia
Juvenile onset		
Niemann-Pick (types C and D)	Unknown	Onset 2–4 years, neurologic symptoms dominate, hepatosplenomegaly
Gaucher	Glucocerebrosidase	Ataxia, myoclonus, anemia
Disorders without visceromegaly		
Tay Sachs	Hexosaminidase A	Cherry red spot; early onset neurologic deterioration
Infantile neuronal ceroid lipofuscinosis[2]	Unknown	Onset between 1 and 2 years; progressive neurologic deterioration
Late infantile amaurotic idiocy	Unknown	Onset 2–6 years, retinal degeneration, seizures, neurologic deterioration
Farber disease	Ceramidase	Early onset deformed and painful joints with numerous subcutaneous nodules and plaques, death is usual before 2 years, prenatal diagnosis is possible.

[1]Modified from Menkes JH: *Textbook of Child Neurology*, 3rd edition. Philadelphia, Lea & Febiger, 1985, p. 61.

[2]Neuronal ceroid-lipofuscinoses include Batten disease, Spielmeyer-Vogt disease, Jansky-Bielschowsky disease, Kufs disease and amaurotic familial idiocy. Diagnosis can be made by finding abnormal inclusions in neurons in a rectal biopsy.

Treatment

In individuals who have evidence of hypersplenisms, splenectomy can provide relief, although in some patients the bone lesions may be exacerbated within a few months of surgery. Partial splenectomy may be preferable (Rubin et al, 1986). The orthopedic problems require the supervision of an orthopedist. General supportive care is necessary for these patients who may have considerable pain.

Attempts at bone marrow transplantation have been undertaken in some of the severely affected children with normalization of their enzyme levels, but no improvement in the condition of tissues in which the abnormal cerebrosides have been accumulated (Rappeport and Ginns, 1984).

Prevention

Prenatal diagnosis is available for all types of Gaucher disease. Affected infants will have less than 20% of normal activity of the enzyme and carriers will have about 60% of normal activity.

TAY-SACHS DISEASE

Definition

This gangliosidosis is the most fulminant of all cerebroretinal degenerative diseases. The neurons are distended with lipid-soluble GM_2 ganglioside. Liver, spleen, and serum also contain excess gangliosides. The biochemical defect is an abnormality of hexosaminidase.

Natural History

Ganglioside accumulation starts in fetal life, affected infants appear normal at birth. By ages 3–10 months, listlessness, irritability, and developmental regression are noted. Hypotonia is characteristic. A cherry-red spot in the macula is found in Tay-Sachs disease (see also Section 13, Genetics) and, in some instances of Niemann-Pick disease.

Neurologic symptoms progress to loss of all voluntary movements, spasticity, and convulsions. Death usually comes by the second or third year, but some survive to ages 5 or 6 years.

Diagnosis

The presence of progressive neurologic findings, a cherry red macula, and lack of visceromegaly are characteristic. Hexosaminidase levels on serum are diagnostic.

Treatment

Only supportive treatment is available.

Prevention

Serum hexosaminidase levels can detect heterozygotes. Prenatal diagnosis is possible from amniotic fluid fibroblast cultures.

NIEMANN-PICK DISEASE

Definition

This gangliosidosis exists in at least six major forms. It is characterized by the accumulation of sphingomyelin and nonesterified cholesterol in the reticuloendothelial system. The clinical picture is diverse, with some families having the disease present in infancy and be rapidly fatal, and others with onset at ages 2–4 years. Other entities may occur in adults as visceromegaly without neurologic involvement.

Basic Science

The pathologic findings are large lipid-laden cells in the reticuloendothelial system in liver, spleen, bone marrow, lungs, and lymph nodes. Sphingomyelin accumulates in ganglion cells of cerebrum, cerebellum, brain stem, spinal cord, and in the choroid plexus. A lysosomal sphingomyelin-cleaving enzyme, sphingomyelinase is deficient in the reticuloendothelial system in groups A and B disease. The metabolic lesion in group C disease is faulty regulation of low density lipoprotein uptake (Pentchev et al, 1987).

Epidemiology

Group A disease is inherited in an autosomal recessive manner, with a predilection for Ashkenazi Jews (Crocker and Farber, 1958). Groups A and B disease are primary mutations.

Natural History

Features that most commonly occur in the various types of Niemann-Pick disease include hepatosplenomegaly, anemia, poor growth, in association with progressive neurologic dysfunction. Impaired upward gaze, dementia, and seizures are characteristic.

Type A disease has its onset in the first year of life with hepatosplenomegaly and poor growth and development. Persistent neonatal jaundice, diarrhea, and lymphadenopathy may be the earliest symptoms. CNS involvement includes seizures and spasticity. Retinal cherry red spots are found in about 50% of patients.

Type B disease is characterized by the absence of neurologic manifestations, but has other features in common with type A disease.

Type C disease is probably a group of metabolic disorders characterized by sphingomyelin storage with normal sphingomyelinase levels. The clinical features are diverse, with onset between 2 and 4 years. Neurologic symptoms predominate, and hepatosplenomegaly is usually less marked than in type A disease.

Occasionally disorders of sphinyomyelin storage are found in adults. The metabolic defect in these variants is not known.

Diagnosis

The abnormal cells may be found in bone marrow or lymph node biopsy. A deficiency of sphingomyelinase in leukocytes or skin fibroblasts is pathognomonic for A and B.

Treatment

Only supportive therapy is available.

Prevention

Sphingomyelinase deficiency can be demonstrated in cultured amniotic fluid fibroblasts (Beaudet and Manschrek, 1982). Detection of individuals at risk of developing neurologic symptoms is about 80% accurate with molecular probes. This finding opens the way to bone marrow transplantation before neuronal destruction occurs.

FABRY DISEASE (α-GALACTOSIDASE A DEFICIENCY)

Definition

Fabry disease (storage of trihexosylceramide) is noted for a punctate angiectatic skin rash with progression to renal involvement, corneal opacities, and a progressive neuropathy. The condition is the result of a heterogeneous group of mutations that affect synthesis, processing, and stability of α-galactoside A (Lemansky et al, 1987).

Epidemiology and Natural History

This is a condition whose prevalence is about 1:40,000. It is transmitted as a sex-linked condition with occasional expression in heterozygous females. The onset is usually in childhood, but may be in the second or third decades. Storage of lipids in skin and small blood vessels leads to the early dermatologic findings, especially around hips and genitalia. A rash with a butterfly distribution can occur on the face. The peripheral neuropathy may present as intermittent burning pain in feet and fingertips.

Diagnosis

A biopsy of peripheral nerve may show swelling and disruption of unmyelinated axons. A deficiency of α-galactoside A in plasma or skin fibroblasts confirms the diagnosis.

Treatment

Phenytoin sufficient to bring the plasma level to 4 μg/ml may provide relief of pain in the extremities. Treatment of renal failure by dialysis and eventually kidney transplantation has had some success.

Prognosis

The disorder is progressive, and death is usually from hypertension and renal failure.

FARBER DISEASE (DISSEMINATED LIPOGRANULOMATOSIS)

Definition

This rare disorder of infancy is characterized by widely distributed periarticular granulomas that present as large, firm subcutaneous nodules, marked capsular distention of all joints with contractures, hoarseness, poor growth, and slow development. Hepatosplenomegaly may be present.

Basic Science

Foam cells within the granulomas contain periodic acid Schiff (PAS)-positive material. Ultrastructural examination reveals concentric lamellar bodies in cytoplasm (Abenoza and Sibley, 1987). Free ceramide accumulates in lymph nodes, liver, kidneys, and lungs. The neurons may be involved, and spinal fluid protein is elevated. The basic defect is lysosomal acid ceramidase deficiency (Jameson et al, 1987).

Epidemiology and Natural History

The disorder is a sex-linked recessive condition. Affected males may die in infancy or live to adulthood. Most signs and symptoms relate to the abnormal accumulation of lipids that may be present at birth. The material deposits in smooth muscle and endothelium of blood vessels. The hoarse cry results from involvement of laryngeal cartilage by granulomas.

Diagnosis

Biopsy of a granuloma will show PAS-positive foam cells. A deficiency of acid ceramidase has been found in kidney and cultured skin fibroblasts.

Treatment

Physiotherapy is appropriate to lessen the disability from the arthropathy. No specific therapy is known, although eventually enzyme replacement therapy deserves consideration.

Prognosis and Prevention

The disorder is progressive. Prenatal diagnosis has been made with cultured amniotic fluid fibroblasts.

REFERENCES

Abenoza P, Sibley RK: Farber's disease: A fine structural study. *Ultrastruct Pathol* 11:397, 1987.

Andersen GE, Hejl M, Christensen NC et al: Frequency of hyperlipaemia in 1407 children and young adults whose father had died from ischaemic heart disease prior to the age of 45 years. *Ugeskr Laeger* 144:926, 1982.

Beaudet AL, Manschrek AA: Metabolism of sphingomyelin by intact cultured fibroblasts: Differentiation of Niemann-Pick disease types A and B. *Biochem Biophys Res Commum* 105:14, 1982.

Bilheimer DW, Goldstein JL, Grundy SM, et al: Liver transplantation to provide low-density-lipoprotein receptors and lower plasma

cholesterol in a child with homozygous familial hypercholesterolemia. *N Engl J Med* 311:1658, 1984.
Bojanovski D, Gregg RE, Zech LA, et al: In vivo metabolism of proapolipoprotein A-I in Tangier disease. *J Clin Invest* 80:1742, 1987.
Brady RO, et al: Demonstration of a deficiency of glucocerebroside-cleaving enzyme in Gaucher's disease. *J Clin Invest* 45:1112, 1966.
Breslow JL: Human apolipoprotein molecular biology and genetic variation. *Ann Rev Biochem* 54:699, 1985.
Coates PM, Cortner JA, Hoffman GM, et al: Acid lipase activity of human lymphocytes. *Biochem Biophys Acta* 572:225, 1979.
Crocker AC, Farber S: Niemann-Pick disease: A review of 18 patients. *Medicine* 37:1, 1958.
Gibberd FB, Page NGR, Billimoria JD, et al: Heredopathia atactica polyneuritiformis (Refsum's disease) treated by diet and plasma exchange. *Lancet* 1:575, 1979.
Goldfischer S, Collins J, Rapin I, et al: Pseudo-Zellweger syndrome: deficiencies in several peroxisomal oxidative activities. *J Pediatr* 108:25, 1986.
Goldstein JL, Brown MS: The low density lipoprotein pathway and its relation to atherosclerosis. *Ann Rev Biochem* 46:897, 1977.
Hobbs HH, Brown MS, Russell DW, et al: Deletion in the gene for the low-density lipoprotein receptor in a majority of French Canadians with familial hypercholesterolemia. *N Engl J Med* 317:734, 1987.
Holmes RD, Wilson GN, Hajra AK: Peroxisomal enzyme deficiency in the Conradi-Hunerman form of chondrodysplasia punctata (letter). *N Engl J Med* 316:1608, 1987.
Jameson RA, Holt PJ, Keen JH: Farber's disease (lysosomal acid ceramidase deficiency). *Ann Rheum Dis* 46:559, 1987.
Lemansky P, Bishop DF, Desnick RJ, et al: Synthesis and processing of the human lysosomal enzyme alpha galactosidase A in human fibroblasts. Evidence for different mutations in Fabry disease. *J Biol Chem* 262:2062, 1987.
Lipid Research Clinics Program: The Lipid Research Clinics Coronary Primary Prevential Trial Results I and II. *JAMA* 251:351, 365, 1984.
Mahley RW: Apolipoprotein E: Cholesterol transport protein with expanding role in cell biology. *Science* 240:622, 1988.
Moser HW: New approaches in peroxisomal disorders. *Dev Neurosci* 9:1, 1987.
Moser HW: Peroxisomal disorders. *J Pediatr* 108:89, 1986.
Nyhan WL, Sakati NA: *Diagnostic Recognition of Genetic Disease.* Philadelphia, Lea & Febiger, 1987.
Pentchev PG, Comly ME, Kruth HS, et al: Group C Niemann-Pick disease: Faulty regulation of low-density lipoprotein uptake and cholesterol storage in cultured fibroblasts. *FASEB J* 1:40, 1987.
Poll-The BT, Saudubray JM, Ogier H, et al: Infantile Refsum's disease: Biochemical findings suggesting multiple peroxisomal dysfunction. *J Inher Metabol Dis* 9:169, 1986.
Rappeport JM, Ginns EI: Bone marrow transplantation in severe Gaucher's disease. *N Engl J Med* 311:84, 1984.
Rubin M, Yampolski I, Lambrozo R, et al: Partial splenectomy in Gaucher's disease. *J Pediatr Surg* 21:125, 1986.
Tsuji S, Choudary PV, Martin BM, et al: A mutation in the human glucocerebrosidase gene in neuronopathic Gaucher's disease. *N Engl J Med* 316:570, 1987.
Van Crugten JT, Paton B, Poulos A: Partial deficiency of dihydroxyacetone phosphate acyltransferase activity in both classical and infantile Refsum's diseases. *J Inher Metabol Dis* 9:163, 1986.
Wolman M, Sterk VV, Gatt S, et al: Primary family xanthomatosis with involvement and calcification of the adrenals. Report of two more cases in siblings of a previously described infant. *Pediatrics* 28:742, 1961.

Purine/Pyrimidine Metabolism Disorders 7

HGPRT DEFICIENCY—LESCH-NYHAN SYNDROME

Definition

The Lesch-Nyhan syndrome is an X-linked recessive inborn error of metabolism due to the deficiency of hypoxanthine-guanine phosphoribosyltransferase (HGPRT).

Basic Science

Hypoxanthine-guanine phosphoribosyltransferase is an enzyme that normally catalyzes the transfer of the phosphoribosyl moiety of 5-phosphoribosyl 1-pyrophosphate to the 9 position of hypoxanthine to form inosine monophosphate or of guanine to form guanosine monophosphate. These are part of a recycling or salvage pathway which is more efficient than the synthesis of purines de novo.

Deficiency of HGPRT results in a 200-fold increase in the rate of uric acid synthesis. The resulting hyperuricemia leads to nephrolithiasis and explains the renal aspects of the disorder. The relation between the biochemical findings and the profound CNS disease in this disorder, however, is not understood.

Absent or decreased activity of HGPRT has been demonstrated in fibroblasts, leukocytes, and erythrocytes. Several variants of the disorder have been reported, either with altered residual activities or altered properties of the enzyme. Patients with residual enzyme activity often do not have the full complement of clinical symptoms.

Epidemiology

The prevalence of this disorder has been estimated to be about 1/300,000.

Natural History

Hemizygote males have hyperuricemia, mental retardation, and neurologic findings that include spasticity, hyperreflexia, choreoathetosis, and self-mutilatory behavior. They often exhibit aggressive behavior toward others. Interestingly, they seem to be aware of their inability to prevent themselves from self-mutilation and often show a desire to be restrained, becoming extremely agitated when the restraints are removed. The hyperuricemia can lead to nephrolithiasis and eventually to renal failure if not controlled. Other symptoms include anemia, growth retardation, immunologic dysfunction, and arthritis.

Diagnosis

The diagnosis is suggested by the characteristic clinical phenotype and confirmed by the demonstration of HGPRT deficiency in erythrocytes or cultured skin fibroblasts. Patients also exhibit increased serum uric acid, increased 24-hour excretion of uric acid, and an increased ratio of uric acid to creatinine in a random urine sample.

Treatment

Most treatment modalities have been unsuccessful in arresting the clinical progression of the disorder. Control of hyperuricemia, however, can be achieved with allopurinol. Behavior modification techniques may also be helpful in decreasing the aggressiveness and self-mutilatory behavior. Patients should have adequate restraints, helmets, and mouth guards to protect themselves from injury.

Prognosis

The prognosis appears to depend upon the severity of the renal disease, as most deaths occur secondary to renal failure. The disorder is a candidate for gene transfer, but at least one attempt was unsuccessful.

Prevention

Heterozygote detection is possible by measurement of HGPRT in cultured skin fibroblasts. Prenatal diagnosis is possible by means of amniocentesis and measurement of HGPRT activity in cultured amniotic fluid cells. About one-half of patients can be diagnosed at the nucleic acid level with RNase A cleavage analysis (Gibbs and Caskey, 1987).

HEREDITARY XANTHINURIA

Definition

Hereditary xanthinuria is an autosomal recessive inborn error of metabolism due to deficiency of xanthine oxidase.

Basic Science

Xanthine oxidase, a molybdenum-requiring enzyme, is responsible for the successive oxidation of hypoxanthine to xanthine, and of xanthine to uric acid. Therefore, affected individuals present with a large excess of urinary xanthine and hypoxanthine in conjunction with decreased uric acid in the urine.

Epidemiology and Natural History

The incidence of this rare disorder is not known. Affected individuals usually present in the third decade, but the disorder can appear in childhood. Patients present most commonly with urinary stones and hematuria due to the complications of nephrolithiasis. Muscle pain due to deposition of xanthine and hypoxanthine crystals and recurrent polyarthritis can also be seen.

A combined deficiency of xanthine oxidase and sulfite oxidase as a result of defects in molybdenum metabolism has been described. The neurologic symptoms of sulfite oxidase deficiency overshadow the symptoms of xanthine oxidase deficiency in these patients.

Diagnosis

Decreased uric acid levels in urine and serum as well as increased urinary xanthine and hypoxanthine levels are found in these patients. Confirmation of the diagnosis depends upon the demonstration of xanthine oxidase deficiency in jejunal, hepatic, or renal tissue.

Treatment

Treatment is difficult and consists of alkalinization of the urine with oral alkalinizing agents and a large fluid intake to dilute the urine. When xanthine stones are present, allopurinol is also used to inhibit residual xanthine oxidase activity and, thereby, decrease the conversion of hypoxanthine to xanthine, as hypoxanthine is more soluble.

Patients with the combined deficiency of xanthine and sulfite oxidase may respond to treatment with molybdenum.

Prognosis and Prevention

The prognosis depends upon the severity of the renal disease. Heterozygotes are asymptomatic but may excrete excessive quantities of urinary oxypurines.

HEREDITARY OROTIC ACIDURIA

Definition

Orotic aciduria is an autosomal recessive disorder of pyrimidine metabolism and a rare cause of vitamin B_{12}-unresponsive megaloblastic anemia.

Basic Science

The basic metabolic defect in this disorder is that of pyrimidine nucleotide deficiency due to reduced activity of two enzymes acting sequentially in the pathway of de novo pyrimidine synthesis; orotate phosphoribosyltransferase and orotidylic acid decarboxylase (ODC) deficiency is seen in type I orotic aciduria, while an isolated deficiency of ODC is seen in type II orotic aciduria. The loss of two adjacent enzymes is most easily explained by a defect in a genetic control mechanism. The clinical manifestations probably result from a deficiency of compounds necessary for the synthesis of nucleic acids and certain critical cofactors.

Epidemiology

The incidence of this disorder is not known.

Natural History

About one-half of the affected individuals have presented in the first year of life, while the remainder have usually presented by 5 years of age. Clinical symptoms include failure to thrive, lethargy, moderate developmental delay, and severe hypochromic anemia with leukopenia. Increased crystalluria associated with orotic acid excretion can cause hematuria and ureteral and urethral obstruction. Some patients have had normal growth and development.

Diagnosis

Affected individuals have 1000- to 2000-fold increases in orotic acid excretion in the urine. Increased excretion of orotidine is also seen. Bone marrow examination reveals megaloblastic changes. Confirmation of the diagnosis depends upon the demonstration of decreased orotate phosphoribosyltransferase and ODC activity in liver or cultured skin fibroblasts.

Treatment

The anemia in these patients does not respond to therapy with iron, vitamin B_{12}, folic, or folinic acid. Oral uridine administered in doses of 100–150 mg/kg/day has produced marked improvement in the hematologic abnormalities, and an improvement in growth and development, but a lesser effect upon the mental deficits that may be seen in this disorder.

Prevention

Heterozygotes demonstrate partial deficiency of the two orotic enzymes and increased orotic acid levels in the urine, but remain asymptomatic. Prenatal diagnosis is theoretically possible by demonstration of each enzyme deficiency in cultured amniotic fluid cells.

REFERENCES

Duran M, Beemer FA, Heiden CVD, et al: Combined deficiency of xanthine oxidase and sulfite oxidase: A defect of molybdenum metabolism or transport. *J Inher Metabol Dis* 1:175, 1978.

Fox RM, Wood MH, Royse-Smith D, et al: Hereditary orotic aciduria. *Am J Med* 55:791, 1973.

Gibbs RA, Caskey CT: Identification and localization of mutations at the Lesch-Nyhan locus by ribonuclease A cleavage. *Science* 236:303, 1987.

Kelley WN: Hereditary orotic aciduria. In Stanbury JB, et al (eds): *The Metabolic Basis of Inherited Disease.* New York, McGraw-Hill, 1983, p. 1202.

Seegmiller JE: Inherited deficiency of hypoxanthine-guanine phosphoribosyltransferase in X-linked uric aciduria (the Lesch-Nyhan syndrome and its variants). In Harris H, Hirschorn K (eds): *Advances in Human Genetics.* Vol 6. New York, Plenum Press, 1976, p. 5.

Tubergan DG, Krooth RS, Heyn RM: Hereditary orotic aciduria with normal growth and development. *Am J Dis Child* 118:864, 1969.

Van Heeswijk PJ, Blank CH, Seegmiller JE, et al: Preventive control of the Lesch-Nyhan syndrome. *Obstet Gynecol* 40:109, 1972.

Metal Metabolism Disorders

8

MENKES DISEASE

Definition

Menkes disease, also known as Menkes steely-hair or kinky-hair disease, is an X-linked disorder due to defective absorption of copper by the intestine and other body cells (Menkes et al, 1962).

Basic Science

The basic defect is unknown but it seems to be related to decreased intestinal absorption of copper. This results in a deficiency of copper in serum and tissues as well as a deficiency in ceruloplasmin, the copper-binding proteins. The clinical manifestations of this disorder may be secondary to deficient synthesis of the copper-containing enzymes.

Epidemiology

The prevalence of this disorder in Australia is estimated at 1/50,000–1/100,000 births.

Natural History

Males present in infancy with abnormal hair, characteristic facies, hypotonia, hypothermia, developmental delay, seizures, osteoporosis, and metaphyseal fractures. Later, arterial degeneration due to defective elastin synthesis, and failure to grow become evident. Recurrent gastrointestinal and respiratory infections also occur and hydronephrosis has been noted.

The characteristic facial features include pudgy cheeks, a cupid's bow upper lip, pallor, and abnormal eyebrows which are horizontal and tangled.

The hair is normal at birth, but then becomes sparse, tangled, dull, and, with secondary growth, depigmented. The hair strands break easily, resulting in a short stubble with a steel-like texture. On microscopic examination, pili torti are seen.

An affected female with an X-autosome translocation and the clinical and biochemical features of Menkes disease has been reported (Kapur et al, 1986).

Diagnosis

Characteristic laboratory findings include decreased serum copper and ceruloplasmin, decreased content of copper in the liver and brain.

Confirmation of the diagnosis requires the demonstration of a disturbance in copper transport resulting in increased copper and metallothionein content in cultured skin fibroblasts and lymphocytes.

Radiographs of long bones show metaphyseal spurs and a diaphyseal periosteal reaction.

Treatment

There is no effective treatment for this disorder. Therapy with oral or parenteral copper has resulted in increased serum copper and ceruloplasmin levels but has not resulted in clinical improvement. Menkes recommends that copper therapy be instituted as soon as the diagnosis is made and continued until it is evident that cerebral degeneration cannot be arrested (Menkes, 1985).

Prognosis and Prevention

Death usually occurs between 3 months and 3 years of age. Prenatal diagnosis is possible by demonstration of disturbed copper handling in cultured fibroblasts from amniotic fluid.

REFERENCES

Danks DM, Campbell PE, Walker-Smith J, et al: Menkes kinky-hair syndrome. *Lancet* 2:1100, 1972.

Kapur S, Higgins JV, Delp K, et al: Menkes syndrome in a female with X-autosome translocation. *Am J Human Genet* 39(Suppl):A67, 1986.

Menkes JH: *Textbook of Child Neurology,* 3rd edition. Philadelphia, Lea & Febiger, 1985, p. 94.

Menkes JH, Alter M, Steigleder GK, et al: A sex-linked recessive disorder with retardation of growth, peculial hair, and focal cerebral and cerebellar degeneration. *Pediatrics 29:764, 1962.*

Inborn Errors of Transport

9

In contrast to the inborn errors of metabolism in which the proximal defect is an enzyme responsible for the conversion of one metabolite to another, the inborn errors of transport are due to a defect in a transport protein or carrier that moves the amino acid across a cell membrane against a concentration gradient. These disorders involve the kidney and the small intestine. Unlike the metabolic disorders which produce an increased blood level of the involved amino acid(s), in the transport disorders, blood amino acids are normal or may even be slightly reduced while the concentration of certain urinary amino acids is greatly increased.

Primarily from the study of inborn errors of transport it is now known that certain carrier proteins in the kidney are responsible for the transport of certain *groups* of amino acids. For instance, specific carriers have been identified for the transport of the following: cystine and the dibasic amino acids; the neutral amino acids; and the imino acids, proline and hydroxyproline and glycine. Other amino acid transport systems in the kidney are also known.

This section will focus on the three best known amino acid transport disorders. One, cystinuria, is a prominent cause of urinary stones. Another, Hartnup disorder (defective transport of neutral amino acids) is benign except under certain conditions of clinical stress. The third, iminoglycinuria, seems always benign.

CYSTINURIA

Definition

Cystinuria is an autosomal recessive disorder of renal and intestinal transport that results in markedly increased quantities of cystine and dibasic amino acids in urine. It is an important cause of urinary stones, especially in children and adolescents.

Basic Science

A specific transport system in the renal tubule transports cystine and the dibasic amino acids (ornithine, lysine, and arginine). Presumably, it is this system that is defective in cystinuria. Studies of kidney slices from individuals with cystinuria have shown a defect in dibasic amino acid transport but not in cystine transport. Thus, the precise basis for all of the biochemical features of cystinuria in the urine has not yet been demonstrated. Nevertheless, the huge quantities of cystine and the dibasic amino acids in the urine indicate that the defect involves all four of these amino acids. Of these, only cystine causes clinical difficulty as it is poorly soluble especially in acidic environments such as urine and in large quantities precipitates out of the urine to form stones.

The transport defect is also expressed in the intestinal mucosa. Studies in vitro have demonstrated different patterns of impairment in cystine and dibasic amino acid uptake: in type I there is no transport of cystine or the dibasic amino acids; in type II, cystine transport is reduced and there is no transport of lysine; in type III, cystine transport may be normal or reduced and the reduction in lysine transport is variable.

Epidemiology

Cystinuria accounts for about 5–10% of adults who have urinary stones, but perhaps as many as 15–20% of children and adolescents who form stones. Routine newborn urine screening in Massachusetts has disclosed a frequency of about 1:12,000. In Australia, the frequency among newborns is somewhat lower, at 1:17,000, while in Quebec, it is only 1:40,000. Cystinuria is very rare among blacks.

Natural History

Cystinuria tends to be asymptomatic until adolescence or young adult years when urinary calculi begin to develop. In our follow-up of over 60 cystinuric children identified by routine newborn screening only one or two developed stones before adolescence but at least five adolescents have had stones. Since most of the screened children are only now reaching adolescent years, this suggests a fairly high frequency of stone formers among adolescent cystinurics. The stones tend to form more readily during prolonged recumbency when there is urinary stasis. For instance, one of the children we have followed formed stones when he was confined to bed with a femoral fracture. Stones may also form during periods of physical exertion if this is accompanied by dehydration that produces excessively concentrated urine. This occurred in one of our patients during late summer football practice. Localization of the calculi is not very different from noncystinuric stone formation, i.e., most often in the kidney, somewhat less often in the ureter, and infrequently in the bladder (Pavanello et al, 1981). Cystinuric stones, however, are much more frequently bilateral and recurrent than are noncystinuric stones.

Diagnosis

In the absence of routine newborn urine screening for amino acid disorders, cystinuria in childhood is almost always diagnosed during evaluation for urinary calculi. In fact, any child with a urinary stone should have a urine amino acid analysis that includes a nitroprusside screening test for cystine. The characteristic amino acid findings of markedly increased cystine and the dibasic amino acids are very striking and definitive. Although other metabolic disorders may produce some features of this urinary amino acid pattern (e.g., lysinuric protein intolerance), only cystinuria includes the full pattern.

Treatment

There is no single or entirely satisfactory therapy for cystinuria. It is preferable if urinary stones can be passed without surgery, especially in cystinuria when ureteral stones in particular tend to recur at the site of the operative lesion. Encouragement of water intake is the safest therapy, but it is difficult to induce the child to drink sufficient quantities for maintenance of a dilute urine. Compliance with waking during the night to drink water is particularly difficult, although this is an important element of water therapy since cystine stones tend to develop at night when the urine becomes relatively concentrated. Alkalinization of urine is effective in preventing the formation of stones since cystine is much more soluble in an alkaline than in an acidic environment, but extraordinarily large amounts of a base such as baking soda must be ingested and this is almost impossible for most children. Chelating therapies such as penicillamine and mercaptopropionylglycine (MPG; Thiola) which bind cysteine in a soluble disulfide and reduce the amount of the much less soluble cystine that is excreted, have been used with some success. These drugs are quite toxic, however, and must be used with caution since they may produce the nephrotic syndrome and other complications.

Prognosis

Without therapy, the prognosis in cystinuria for someone who has formed a stone is for continued development of urinary stones with attendant complications that include urinary tract obstruction and infection. This leads to loss of kidney tissue and eventually to renal failure. Prompt treatment that leads to removal or evacuation of the stone(s) is the first line of treatment. Truly effective therapy, however, lies in preventing stone formation. This can sometimes be achieved with increased water intake or alkalinization of urine. If these measures fail, therapy with penicillamine or mercaptopropionylglycine may be in order.

Prevention

Prenatal diagnosis has not yet been reported in cystinuria. We and others have found that amniotic fluid at delivery or during the third trimester contains increased amounts of cystine and the dibasic amino acids when the fetus has cystinuria. This suggests that prenatal diagnosis for cystinuria might be possible during the second trimester, by measuring amino acids in amniotic fluid obtained by amniocentesis.

HARTNUP DISORDER

Definition

This is an autosomal recessive hyperaminoaciduria that at first resembles a generalized hyperaminoaciduria but on closer examination is recognized as involving only the neutral amino acids.

Basic Science

The defect is in the renal and intestinal carrier system for the neutral amino acids. Hence, these amino acids appear in much higher concentrations than normal in the urine. Clinical consequences of this transport defect may be related to impaired uptake of the neutral amino acid tryptophan in the intestine, which might limit the amount of niacin (a tryptophan product) that can be formed and produce a state of niacin deficiency.

Epidemiology

The frequency of Hartnup disorder as determined by routine newborn urine screening is 1:18,000 in Massachusetts, 1:25,000 in Australia, and 1:40,000 in Quebec.

Natural History

Most individuals with the Hartnup urinary findings are asymptomatic as shown by the follow-up of children identified by newborn screening in both Massachusetts and Australia. Nevertheless, a photosensitive skin rash as well as intermittent ataxia and mental retardation have been described in association with Hartnup disorder. The differences in clinical features may be explained by a tendency for lower plasma amino acids, perhaps genetically determined but independent of the Hartnup genotype, among the few symptomatic patients (Scriver et al, 1987). Hence, the availability of tryptophan for the synthesis of niacin might be limited both by impaired intestinal transport of tryptophan due to the Hartnup defect and further reduction of the blood tryptophan level by another mechanism.

Diagnosis

The urinary amino acid profile is characteristic for Hartnup disorder. Neutral amino acid levels are markedly increased while amino acids in the dibasic, acidic, and iminoglycine groups are absent or present in normal quantities. Also present in the urine are organic acid metabolites of tryptophan such as indolepyruvate, indolelactate, and indoleacetate. These urinary findings are due to bacterial decomposition of the unabsorbed tryptophan in the intestine with the formation and absorption of tryptophan metabolites. Fecal free amino acid levels are usually increased in a pattern similar to that noted in the urine, although the intestinal defect in amino acid transport may not be present in all individuals with the renal defect. The diagnosis may be supported by intestinal biopsy with the demonstration in vitro of reduced transport of neutral but not other amino acids.

Treatment

Most individuals with the Hartnup disorder are asymptomatic and do not require therapy. For those who develop symptoms, nicotinic acid or nicotinamide may be helpful. Amounts of nicotinamide from 50–300 mg/day have been administered orally. In some reported cases, this has resulted in clearing of a rash or amelioration of ataxia.

Prognosis

Hartnup disorder seems to be benign in most individuals. With therapy, the prognosis for those who develop symptoms seems to be good.

Prevention

Prenatal diagnosis has not yet been reported. Carrier detection is not yet possible.

IMINOGLYCINURIA

Definition

This is an autosomal recessive disorder in the renal transport of the iminoglycine group, which includes the two imino acids, proline and hydroxyproline, and the amino acid glycine. It is often referred to as renal iminoglycinuria to differentiate this entity from the secondary iminoglycinuria associated with the hyperprolinemia.

Basic Science

There are at least three carrier systems in the renal tubule that are involved in transport of the imino acids and glycine. One is characterized by high capacity and low affinity for the imino acids, glycine, and the neutral amino acids. Of the other two, one has low capacity and high affinity for transport of the imino acids and the other is specific for glycine with similar functional characteristics. Renal iminoglycinuria is due to a defect in the first of these three systems. The consequence of this defect is reduced renal tubular transport of the imino acids and glycine with corresponding increased urinary excretion of these compounds. The excess imino acids and glycine cannot be adequately transported by the low capacity second and third systems. A defect in the intestinal transport of proline occurs in some but not all individuals with renal iminoglycinuria.

Epidemiology

The prevalence of renal iminoglycinuria detected by routine newborn urine screening is 1:12,000 in Massachusetts and 1:10,000 in Australia. The relatively large number of case reports from Israel and the high percentage of Jewish infants among those identified in Massachusetts suggest that the gene frequency for renal iminoglycinuria is particularly high among Jews.

Natural History

Renal iminoglycinuria seems to be a benign disorder. Virtually all affected infants and children followed after newborn screening identification in Massachusetts have been asymptomatic. The occasional symptoms reported in children and adults with iminoglycinuria have been variable without a pattern that would indicate a relationship to the disorder.

Diagnosis

Markedly increased urinary concentrations of proline, hydroxyproline, and glycine with normal concentrations of other urinary amino acids and normal plasma amino acid concentrations is the hallmark of renal iminoglycinuria. Because iminoglycinuria is a normal transient finding in many newborn infants and may persist until several months of age, only when iminoglycinuria persists beyond the age of 6 months should the diagnosis of renal iminoglycinuria be accepted. The transient iminoglycinuria of early infancy is usually much less striking than the iminoglycinuria of the infant with renal iminoglycinuria as a disorder.

Treatment

No treatment known will reduce the degree of iminoglycinuria and none is necessary for this benign disorder.

Prognosis

This is a benign disorder with no implications for health or longevity.

Prevention

Prenatal diagnosis has not been made. Carriers of this recessive gene have isolated hyperglycinuria and are usually readily identifiable.

REFERENCES

Levy HL: Hartnup disease. In Goldensohn ES, Appel SH (eds): *Scientific Approaches to Clinical Neurology*. Vol. 1. Philadelphia, Lea & Febiger, 1977, pp. 75-84.

Pavanello L, Rizzoni G, Dussini N, et al: Cystinuria in children. *Eur Urol* 7:139, 1981.

Scriver CR, Mahon B, Levy HL, et al: Hartnup phenotype: Mendelian transport disorder, multifactorial disease. *Am J Hum Genet* 40:401, 1987.

Statten M, Ben-Zvi A, Shina A, et al: Familial iminoglycinuria with normal intestinal absorption of glycine and imino acids in association with profound mental retardation, a possible "cerebral phenotype." *Helv Paediatr Acta* 31:173, 1976.

Wilcken B, Yu JS, Brown DA: Natural history of Hartnup disease. *Arch Dis Child* 52:38, 1977.

Mucopolysaccharide (MPS) Metabolism Disorders

10

A group of inherited disorders of mucopolysaccharide metabolism are characterized by the accumulation of glycosamino glycans in various organs. Specific lysosomal enzymes are required for the degradation of mucopolysaccharides; specific deficiencies of these enzymes result in a particular constellation of abnormalities.

The nomenclature of the disorders follows the name of the individuals who described the clinical features (Hunter, Hurler, Pfaundler, Sanfilippo, Morquio, Scheie, Maroteau, and Lamy). Alternately, they are known as MPS I (Hurler), MPS II (Hunter), MPS III (Sanfilippo), MPS IV (Morquio), MPS V (Scheie), MPS VI (Maroteau-Lamy), and MPS VII (Sly) (Table 15.5).

A very rare group of disorders are called mucolipidoses. The best known is I-cell disease (for inclusion cell) or mucolipidosis II.

These conditions should be suspected in the context of a positive family history since they are autosomal recessives, except for Hunter syndrome, which is X-linked. They are not often recognized at birth, but affected infants show developmental delays, hepatosplenomegaly, and later multiple bony changes diagnosed radiographically. Corneal clouding is present in types I, V, and VI. Neurologic abnormalities are found in types I, II, and III but not in IV, V, or VI.

Throughout this section, we refer to treatment as "supportive only" for most of these conditions, to indicate the absence of any treatment directed toward the underlying problem. This brief notation fails to define the extent of supportive treatment required and its impact on the life of the affected child and family. A multidisciplinary team with experience with children with progressive storage disorders, demyelinating diseases, or other chronic handicapping conditions can be of great help in maintaining the best possible function. The pediatrician has a major role in coordinating the many medical services that will be required and in mobilizing special education. Genetic counseling is of great importance to make certain prenatal diagnosis is used if possible.

HURLER DISEASE (MPS I)

Definition

This is the most severe of the group of mucopolysaccharidoses. Most all tissues accumulate dermatan and heparan sulfates so that brain, viscera, and bones become progressively involved.

Basic Science

See Table 15.5 for biochemical defect.

Natural History

Normal at birth, in the first year of life affected infants show hepatosplenomegaly and developmental delay. After the first year, the facies becomes "coarse" with frontal bossing and a large head. Obstructive hy-

Table 15.5
Biochemical Abnormalities in Mucopolysaccharidoses

Name	Urinary MPS HS[1]	Urinary MPS DS[1]	Neurologic Signs	Defect
Hurler	+	+	Severe	α-L-iduronidase
Hunter	+	+	Severe	Iduronosulfate sulfatase
Sanfilippo	+		Moderate mental retardation (becomes severe)	Heparan N sulfate α-N-acetylglucosaminidase acetyl CoA: α-glucosaminide N acetyl transferase N-acetyl-α-glucosaminide 6-sulfatase
Morquio	–	–	Rare	Galactase-6-sulfatase
Scheie	+	+	None	α-L-iduronidase
Maroteaux Lamy		+	None	N-acetylgalactosaminase-4-sulfatase (arylsulfatase B)
Sly	+	+	Variable	β-glucuronidase

[1]HS = heparan sulfate, DS = dermatan sulfate.

drocephalus may develop. The bridge of the nose may be depressed. Clouding of the corneas progresses and is usually noticed about 1 year of age. Bone, joints, and CNS involvement lead to eventual immobility.

Diagnosis

Urinary excretion of heparan sulfate is increased. Definitive diagnosis depends on measurement of a deficiency of α-L-iduronidase in white blood cells, serum, or cultured skin fibroblasts.

Radiographic changes include shortening of radius and ulna, wide metaphyses and irregular epiphyses (Dysostosis multiplex). The metacarpals and phalanges are thickened and irregular. Kyphosis is prominent in most patients. The vertebral bodies are ovoid with beaked projections in lower thoracic and upper lumbar regions. Hair is profuse and coarse.

Treatment

The only treatment available is bone marrow transplantation, which has been reported to result in arrest of mental deterioration and clearing of the corneas.

Prognosis

In the absence of bone marrow transplantation, the course is progressive and death from bronchopneumonia is usual in early to middle childhood.

Prevention

Antenatal diagnosis is possible from identification of the enzyme defect in fibroblasts cultured from amniotic fluid.

HUNTER DISEASE (MPS II)

Definition

This is a rare disorder with variable severity from mild abnormality in facial structure to dwarfism and cardiovascular disease. Joint involvement is invariable. Corneal clouding is unusual.

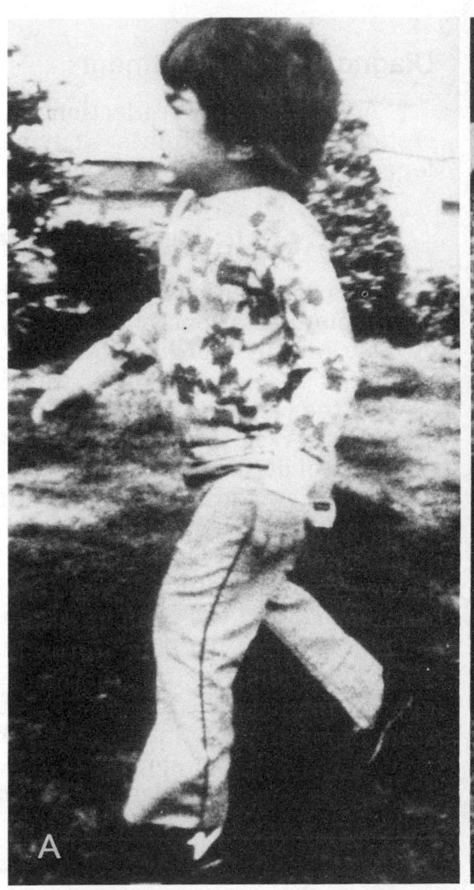

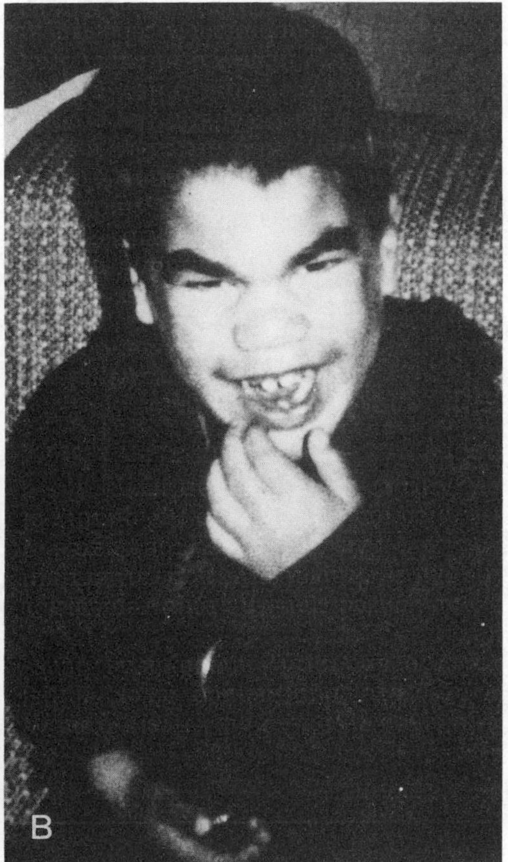

Figure 15.14. This youngster with Hunter disease was born after a normal pregnancy and had an uneventful infancy. He walked by 18 months, said words at the same time, and was in the 90th percentile for height. **A.** By age 2 years he had an unusual appearance and decelerated development. Studies included urine sulfatase activity which was unmeasurable. The subsequent course was regressive with decreased mobility by age 6 years, and essentially immobile at 9 years, loss of language by age 9 years, and (**B**) difficulty feeding. Both liver and spleen were palpable at 3 cm below the costal margins. The corneas remained clear (courtesy of Dr. Allen Crocker).

Natural History

In its most severe form, involvement of the CNS leads to mental retardation, seizures, persistent diarrhea, and death by age 12 years. Some individuals are less affected and live into their 20s (Figs. 15.14 and 15.15).

Diagnosis and Treatment

Cultured fibroblasts are deficient in iduronate sulfatase. Treatment is supportive only.

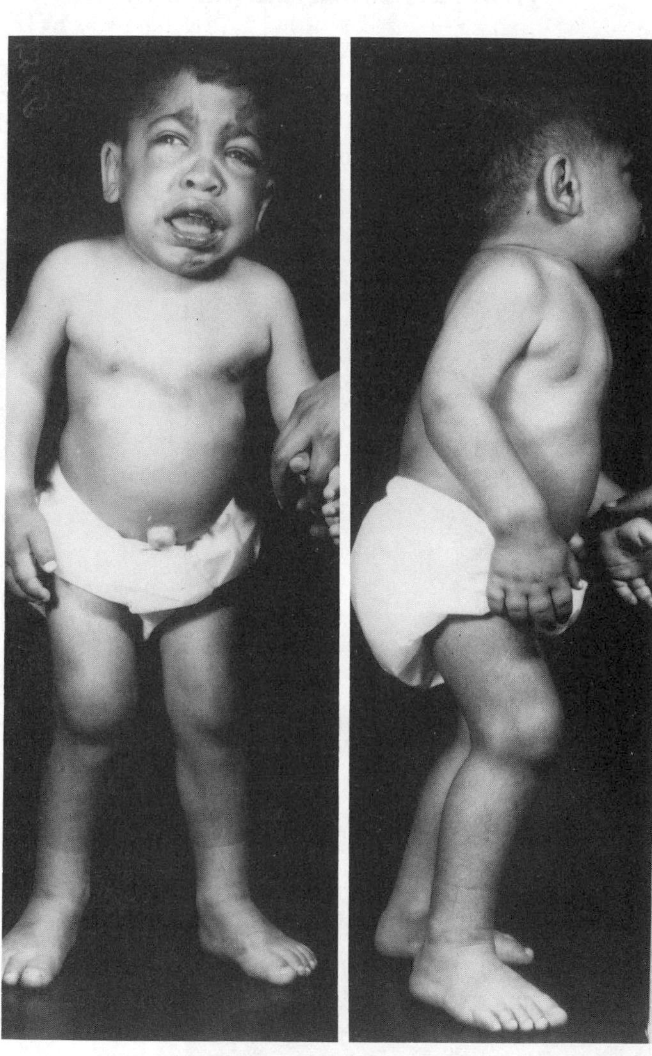

Figure 15.15. This patient presented at age 2 years for evaluation of a chronic nasal discharge and a peculiar facies. He was of Portuguese ancestry with no known consanguinity. This photograph was taken at age 6 years and shows his major skeletal problems and coarse features. His intelligence was normal, a point that distinguishes Maroteau-Lamy syndrome (MPS VI) from Hurler disease, which it resembles closely in other respects. He was blind and partially deaf. He succumbed at age 9 years with his cardiomyopathy and unexplained massive gastrointestinal hemorrhage (courtesy of Dr. Allen Crocker).

Prevention

Prenatal diagnosis from amniotic fluid fibroblasts is possible.

SANFILIPPO DISEASE (MPS III)

Definition

At least four biochemically distinguishable forms of Sanfilippo syndromes are known. The clinical features are similar with an onset of deceleration of development, followed by regression between 2 and 5 years. Facial features are coarse, but less so than in other mucopolysaccharidoses.

Natural History

Since there is no growth retardation or corneal clouding, recognition of this disorder is not usual before age 2 years. Diarrhea may be an early sign. Loss of extension of interphalangeal joints is a common observation late in the course of disease. Neurologic findings include mental retardation, ataxia, tremor, and eventually bulbar dysfunction. Most individuals die by age 20 years.

Diagnosis and Treatment

A 24-hour urine collection will show elevated excretion of heparan sulfate. Enzymes assays are needed for a definitive diagnosis. Treatment is supportive only.

SCHEIE DISEASE (MPS V)

This disorder is characterized by corneal clouding. Other manifestations of MPS may be absent or may develop late in life. Involvement of connective tissue may lead to compression of the median nerves as it crosses the carpal tunnel of the wrist.

Hurler-Scheie complex is characterized by excess secretion of dermatan sulfate and heparan sulfate from a deficiency of iduronosulfate sulfatase. The mucopdysaccharides are stored in liver and spleen. Patients may present with skeletal deformities and short stature. Corneal clouding occurs. Mental function is usually normal and the condition is compatible with long life.

Radiological features include enlargement of the sella, sclerosis of the base of the skull, irregularities of acromial joints, and flat femurs with short metaphyses. Skeletal changes of spine and hands are minimal, in contrast to Hurler disease (Schmidt et al, 1987).

I-CELL DISEASE (MUCOLIPIDOSIS II)

This rare disorder is sometimes confused with Hurler disease, since it has many of the same features. It is distinguished by a more rapid deterioration and early death. Gingival hyperplasia is common; corneal clouding is mild or absent. Cardiovalvular disease is frequent. There is no excess excretion of heparan.

KNIEST SYNDROME

This disorder is not apparent until after 1 year of age, when the relatively short trunk and limbs are evident. The head is larger with a depressed nasal bridge. Joints are stiff. Other features are lordosis, kyphoscoliosis, and osteoporosis. Retinal detachment and deafness occur. The diagnosis is confirmed by excess keratan sulfate in the urine.

MUCOLIPIDOSIS IV

This lysosomal storage disease, first described in 1974, is characterized by profound psychomotor retardation. The condition is found mainly in Ashkenazic Jews and has an autosomal recessive pattern of inheritance. The natural history is onset in the first months of life of motor delay and visual disturbances. Vision may be severely reduced from corneal opacities and retinal degeneration. The course may be protracted over years. Comprehension of language is severely limited and expressive language is usually nonexistent. Most children are growth retarded, but some are normal. The diagnosis depends on observation of typical storage organelles seen by electron microscopy of conjuctivae on skin. Abnormal gangliosides can be identified in cultured fibroblasts (Amir et al, 1987).

REFERENCES

Amir N, Zlotogora J, Bach G: Mucolipidosis type IV: Clinical spectrum and natural history. *Pediatrics* 79:953, 1987.

Dorfman A, Matalon R: The mucopolysaccharidoses (a review). *Proc Natl Acad Sci* (USA) 73:630, 1976.

McKusick VA, Neufeld EF: The mucopolysaccharide storage diseases. In Stanbury JB, Wyngaarden JB, Fredrickson DS, et al (eds): *The Metabolic Basis of Inherited Disease,* 5th edition. New York, McGraw-Hill, 1983.

Menkes J: *Textbook of Child Neurology,* 3rd edition. Philadelphia, Lea & Febiger, 1985, pp. 41-50.

Muenzer J: Mucopolysaccharidoses. A review. *Adv Pediatr* 33:269, 1986.

Schmidt H, Ullrich HJ, von Lengerke J, et al: Radiological findings in patients with mucopolysaccharidosis I (H/S) Hurler-Scheie syndrome. *Pediatr Radiol* 17:409, 1987.

Other Disorders 11

RHABDOMYOLYSIS: MALIGNANT HYPERTHERMIA

Definition

Rhabdomyolysis in association with hyperthermia refers to the destruction of muscle. It may be an inherited condition that is triggered by fever and especially by certain anesthetics.

Basic Science

This is an autosomal dominant condition that can be identified by elevated levels of creatine phosphokinase in serum. The underlying pathophysiology is unknown. Defects in phosphorylase or carnitine palmitoyl transferase may occur in some patients.

Natural History

This myopathy should be considered in families with a history of hyperthermia and sudden death following general anesthesia. Occasionally, rhabdomyolysis occurs in association with minor infections or after extreme physical exertion.

Diagnosis

The hereditary disorder is associated with elevations in serum CPK and during an attack it may reach greater than 40,000 units. The urine contains myoglobin. Acute renal failure is the major complication.

Treatment

The metabolic disturbances demand immediate intervention. If the temperature is elevated, anesthetics must be discontinued, and the patient must be actively cooled with ice blankets and intravenous iced saline. Dantrolene is given in doses of 1–3 mg/kg as a bolus intravenously and sodium bicarbonate is infused in 1–2 mEq/kg increments as needed to combat acidemia and hyperkalemia. In extreme cases, extracorporeal circulation may be needed for heat exchange.

CASE ILLUSTRATION

A 7-month-old female was admitted to our hospital with apparent sepsis. She was in good health until 2 weeks before admission when she developed upper respiratory infection symptoms, which resolved. Two days before admission she developed vomiting, diarrhea, and low grade fever. On the day of admission she appeared lethargic, prompting a septic work-up. The white blood count was 18,000/mm^3, with 80% polys and 12% bands, hematocrit of 34.7%, platelet count 300,000/mm^3; urinalysis was notable for 3+ protein, positive heme test, 1–2 white blood cells and 4+ bacteria per high powered field on a bag specimen. Spinal tap was normal. An SGOT was 336 U. Because of the vomiting and the elevated SGOT, a serum ammonia was measured and found to be normal. The physical examination showed a well-nourished white female with normal vital signs. She was afebrile. There was impressive generalized hypertonia but no other discernible abnormalities.

QUESTIONS AND COMMENTS

How should this patient be managed?

This 7-month-old previously healthy infant demonstrated marked hypertonia, diarrhea, an elevated SGOT, and heme-positive urine, suggestive of either myoglobin or hemoglobin. Since there was no evidence of hemolysis, presence of myoglobin was suspected. A repeat SGOT was 4310 U, with a CPK greater than 40,000 U, thus, consistent with rhabdomyolysis.

Initial management requires that the extent of metabolic damage be documented and treated and that acute renal failure be avoided. Since the muscle is a storehouse for potassium, phosphate, uric acid, and creatinine, one must monitor these particular metabolites during the presence of rhabdomyolysis, since serum levels may markedly increase these metabolites, often to dangerously high levels. For example, a low BUN to creatinine ratio is an important clue for rhabdomyolysis. The serum calcium may be decreased either because it coprecipitates with phosphate or because it is sequestered by injured muscle. All these aberrations must be quickly recognized and treated appropriately.

While acute renal failure is a major cause of mortality, the exact mechanism underlying the phenomenon is unclear. Avoidance can be accomplished by high urine flow and by alkalinizing the urine since at or below a pH of 5.6 myoglobin precipitates along with urate in the urine. High fluid intake and forced diuresis will prevent this from happening.

In this patient, the potassium was slightly above 5.0 mEq/L but other electrolytes were essentially normal. The creatinine rose to a maximal level of 1.3 mg/dl. Urine output was maintained at 2–3 cc/kg/hour with IV fluids and furosemide. Several days after admission, the enzymes dropped markedly and the child's muscle strength improved.

What are the causes of rhabdomyolysis?

Rhabdomyolysis can be categorized as traumatic, exertional, metabolic, hereditary, inflammatory, and idiopathic. There was certainly no evidence of trauma in this patient. Metabolic defects and carbohydrate and fat metabolism may be playing a role. While a defect such as phosphorylase deficiency as seen in McArdle disease is not seen until later childhood during exertion, cartinine palmityl transferase deficiency can present in infancy, which may have been the case in this infant. Other possibilities, although not relevant in this child, would include anesthetic-induced myolysis causing the malignant hyperthermia syndrome, a toxin-induced myopathy, and rhabdomyolysis in the setting of inflammatory myopathies due to systemic lupus or dermatomyositis. A definitive diagnosis can often be very difficult to obtain. A muscle biopsy with electron microscopic inspection and assays for specific enzymes could be useful in elucidating the underlying metabolic defect. This was not performed in this patient due to parental refusal of the procedure.

REFERENCES

Flewellon EH, Nelson TE, Jones WP, et al: Dantrolene dose response in awake man: Implications for management of malignant hyperthermia. *Anesthesiology* 59:275, 1983.

Menkes JH: Metabolic diseases of the nervous system. In: *A Textbook of Child Neurology,* 3rd edition. Philadelphia, Lea & Febiger, 1985.

Sandhoff K, Conzelmann E: The biochemical basis of gangliosidoses. *Neuropediatrics* 15(Suppl):85, 1984.

HARVEY LEVY
MIRA IRONS
DOROTHY VILLEE
MARY ELLEN AVERY

Section 16

Immunology

The mechanisms by which our bodies defend themselves against invasion by foreign agents are remarkable. A variety of cells (lymphocytes, phagocytes) and of proteins (antibodies and complement) are marshalled to fight infection. In this section on Immunology, we discuss diseases characterized by recurrent infections because of the failure of one or several of the immunologic mechanisms involved in the protection against and the elimination of foreign organisms. (For a general review of molecules of the immune system, see Tonegawa S: *Sci Am* 253:122, 1985.)

Compartments of the Immune System

1

The immune system can be divided into four compartments: the B-lymphocyte or antibody system; the T-lymphocyte system; the complement system; and the phagocytic system. Abnormalities may occur in one or more compartments and result in predisposition to recurrent infections.

A list of the immune deficiency diseases according to the last WHO classification is shown in Table 16.1.

B-CELL COMPARTMENT

Definition

B cells are a class of lymphocytes characterized by the presence of surface immunoglobulins, and by the ability to differentiate into plasma cells that secrete abundant quantities of immunoglobulin. The activation, proliferation, and differentiation of B cells is aided by signals or factors provided by T cells. Immunoglobulins specifically bind and opsonize the stimulating antigen or organisms. Upon binding antigen, antibodies can activate the complement cascade, causing cytolysis of the organisms (by fixing C1–C9) and/or facilitating their phagocytosis by neutrophils and monocytes, which carry surface receptors for the Fc portion of IgG and for C3 (Metzger and Kinet, 1988).

Immunoglobulins can be divided into five major classes or isotypes based on their structure and function: IgG, IgM, IgA, IgD, and IgE. All the immunoglobulins consist of two major polypeptide chains, heavy chains and light chains. The five isotypes are distinguished by antigenic determinants on the constant regions of the heavy chain. The special properties of each of the isotypes are summarized in Table 16.2.

The IgG group is the major antibody in blood and tissues and comprises the major antibody response to antigenic stimulation. It is the only class of antibody that can cross the placenta. IgG antibodies can be further subdivided into four subclasses, again based on minor antigenic determinants of the heavy chain (Table 16.2).

IgM antibody consists of five immunoglobulin units linked by disulfide bonds. Primary antibody responses usually begin with the secretion of IgM antibody. The IgM-producing B cells later switch to the production of heavy chain constant regions of other isotypes to produce antibody of the IgG, IgA, or IgE isotype. Since the variable regions used in the construction of the heavy chain remain the same, the antigenic specificity of the secreted antibody is unchanged (Fig. 16.1).

IgA is the predominant antibody in secretions. IgA exists mostly as a dimer consisting of two units joined by a small, 15,000-dalton polypeptide, the J chain. Secretory IgA is synthesized by plasma cells in the lamina propria and transported through the lining epithelium via the attachment of a 60,000-dalton secretory piece. Two subclasses of IgA, IgA1 and IgA2, are recognized. Normal serum IgA is about 90% IgA1 and 10% IgA2. In secretions, the amounts of IgA2 and IgA1 are almost equal.

IgD is present in very small quantities in serum. Its role is not well understood. The majority of B cells bear IgD on their surface together with other surface isotypes.

IgE antibodies are unique in that they have the capacity to bind to high affinity receptors on mast cells and basophils. When allergen binds and cross-links two or more allergen-specific IgE antibodies on the surface of the mast cell, degranulation of these cells occurs. Degranulation releases preformed mediators such as histamine, eosinophil chemotactic factors of anaphylaxis, and platelet-activating factor, and also triggers the synthesis and release of leukotrienes (Talbot et al, 1985). These mediators cause allergic reactions by increasing vascular permeability and smooth muscle contraction, and by producing a local inflammatory reaction that is thought to play an important role in the pathogenesis of chronic allergic disorders (Kaliner, 1984).

Normal Development and Maturation of B Cells

B cells pass through a complex series of stages before their development into antibody-producing plasma cells (Fig. 16.2). Just as the thymus provides an inductive microenvironment in which lymphoid progenitor cells undergo T cell differentiation and clonal expansion, the fetal liver and later the bone marrow are the sites in mammals where lymphoid cells undergo commitment to differentiate along B-cell lines.

B cells are marked by a diverse assortment of cell-surface components, the expression of which varies as a function of differentiation. These include the membrane-bound immunoglobulins, Fc receptors for IgG and other immunoglobulin isotypes, HLA-DR determinants, receptors for Epstein-Barr virus, for mitogens (e.g., lipopolysaccharides), for growth and differentiation factors produced by T cells, and for the complement components C3b and C3d.

The first recognizable cell of B-cell lineage makes its appearance in the fetal liver during the seventh week of gestation in man. These cells, called pre-B cells, are large, rapidly dividing cells, which contain small amounts of intracytoplasmic IgM, and lack both surface immunoglobulin and functional surface receptors for antigens and C3. Immature B lymphocytes bearing sur-

Table 16.1
Classification of Primary Immunodeficiency Diseases[1]

A. Predominant antibody defects
 1. X-linked agammaglobulinemia
 2. X-linked hypogammaglobulinemia with growth hormone deficiency
 3. Autosomal recessive agammaglobulinemia
 4. Immunoglobulin deficiency with increased IgM (and IgG)
 5. IgA deficiency
 6. Selective deficiency of other immunoglobulin isotypes
 7. κ-Chain deficiency
 8. Antibody deficiency with normal γ-globulin levels or hypergammaglobulinemia
 9. Immunodeficiency with thymoma
 10. Transient hypogammaglobulinemia of infancy
 11. Common variable immunodeficiency with predominant B-cell defect
  a. Nearly normal B-cell number with $\mu^+ \delta^+$, without $\mu^+ \delta^-$, $\mu^+ \gamma^+$, γ^+, or α^+ cells
  b. Very low B-cell number
  c. $\mu^+ \gamma^+$ or γ^+ "nonsecretory" B cells with plasma cells
  d. Normal or increased B-cell number with $\mu^+ \delta^+ \gamma^+$, $\mu^+ \alpha^+$, γ^+, and α^+ B cells
 12. Common variable immunodeficiency with predominant immuno-regulatory T-cell disorder
  a. Deficiency of helper T cells
  b. Presence of activated suppressor T cells
 13. Common variable immunodeficiency with autoantibodies to B or T cells
B. Predominant defects of cell-mediated immunity
 14. Combined immunodeficiency with predominant T-cell defect
 15. Purine-nucleoside phosphorylase deficiency
 16. Severe combined immunodeficiency with adenosine deaminase deficiency
 17. Severe combined immunodeficiency
  a. Reticular dysgenesis
  b. Low T- and B-cell numbers
  c. Low T-cell and normal B-cell numbers (Swiss)
  d. "Bare-lymphocyte syndrome"
 18. Immunodeficiency with unusual response to Epstein-Barr virus
C. Immunodeficiency associated with other defects
 19. Transcobalamin 2 deficiency
 20. Wiskott-Aldrich syndrome
 21. Ataxia telangiectasia
 22. Third- and fourth-pouch/arch (DiGeorge) syndrome

[1]Reproduced with permission from Rosen FS, Cooper WD, Wedgewood RJP: *N Engl J Med* 311:235, 1984.

face IgM first appear in the human fetal liver around the eighth week of gestation. These cells are similar to mature B cells in that they can interact with antigen, but their development is easily aborted by antibodies to IgM determinants and they are highly susceptible to clonal abortion by multivalent antigens. Furthermore, they display a paucity or absence of Fc and C3 receptors. These cells migrate from fetal liver and bone marrow to the spleen.

During the final stages of B-cell development, immature B lymphocytes become mature B lymphocytes expressing all of the surface determinants needed for collaboration with helper T cells and macrophages, including multiple immunoglobulin isotypes, Ia or HLA-DR determinants, and Fc and C3 receptors. Soon after B cells are formed in fetal liver or bone marrow, they enter the circulation and migrate to form lymphoid follicles in special areas of the spleen, lymph nodes, Peyer's patches, and other secondary lymphoid tissues. They accompany T cells in recirculating through lymphatic and vascular channels, but travel the circuit less often than do T cells. Throughout life, millions of B cells are generated each day in the bone marrow, but most probably live for only a few days after migration to the spleen.

The genetically polymorphic HLA-DR molecules serve as recognition elements in the interaction with T cells—a basic requirement for antigen activation of the resting B cell. On antigen interaction with surface antibody molecules and on autologous helper T-cell interaction with HLA-DR and antigen (processed by the B cell), the resting B cell is induced to enlarge and to express receptors for nonantigen-specific T-cell factors that deliver signals for proliferation and for differentiation into plasma cells. Activated B cells may undergo a reciprocal loss of other cell-surface molecules, such as IgD and C3 receptors.

Some members of the activated B-cell clone do not undergo terminal plasma-cell differentiation. These long-lived cells serve as memory B cells, which are triggered relatively easily by antigen. The final step in B-cell differentiation is the plasma cell. The progression from activated B lymphocyte is marked by a gradual loss of HLA-DR and surface immunoglobulin along with conversion from synthesis of membrane-type to secretory immunoglobulin molecules with their hydrophilic tails. Plasma cells rarely divide and usually live for only a few days.

T cells have an important regulatory influence on the terminal differentiation of mature B cells into plasma

Table 16.2
Properties of Immunoglobulins

Property	IgG				IgA	IgM	IgD	IgF
	IgG1	IgG2	IgG3	IgG4				
Molecular weight ($\times 10^{-3}$)	150	150	150	150	150	150–600	900	190
Present in secretions					++	−		
Crosses placenta	+	±	+	+	−	−	−	−
Fixes complement	++	+	++	−	−	++		−
Binds to mast cells	−	−	−	+	−	−	−	++
Binds to macrophages	++	+	++	±		−		

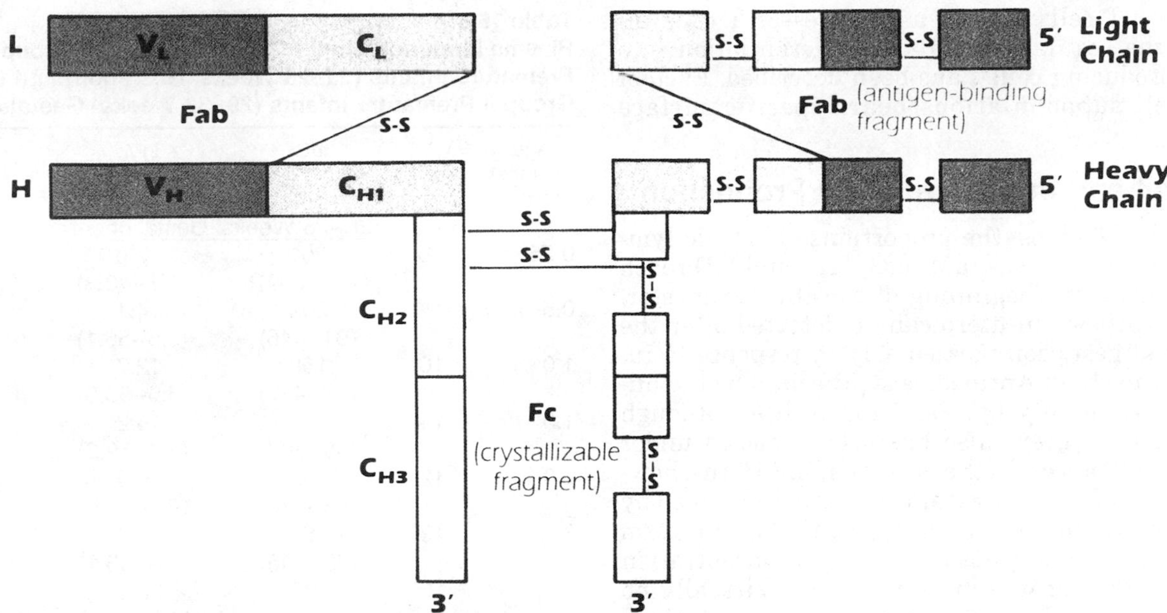

Figure 16.1. An immunoglobulin is composed of two identical heavy chains and two identical light chains with constant and variable regions that are called domains. Immunoglobulins belong to five different classes based on differences in the amino acid sequences of their constant (C) domain. The order of synthesis of antibodies is as follows: The B-cell recognizes an antigen, becomes a plasma cell, and makes an IgM antibody. After 7–10 days, an IgG molecule is formed. At sites on mucosal cells, secretory IgA is formed. Abbreviations: L = light chain; H = heavy chain; Fab = antigen-binding fragment; Fc = crystallizable fragment; C = constant domain; V = variable domain; V_L and V_H = bind antigen; S-S = disulfide bonds between chains and within each domain (shown in one-half of molecule) C_{H1} = usually links to C_L; C_{H2} = binds complement; C_{H3} = attaches to cell receptors; 5′ = amino terminal; 3′ = carboxy terminal. Reproduced with permission from Henley WL: *Pediatr Ann* 16:465, 1987.

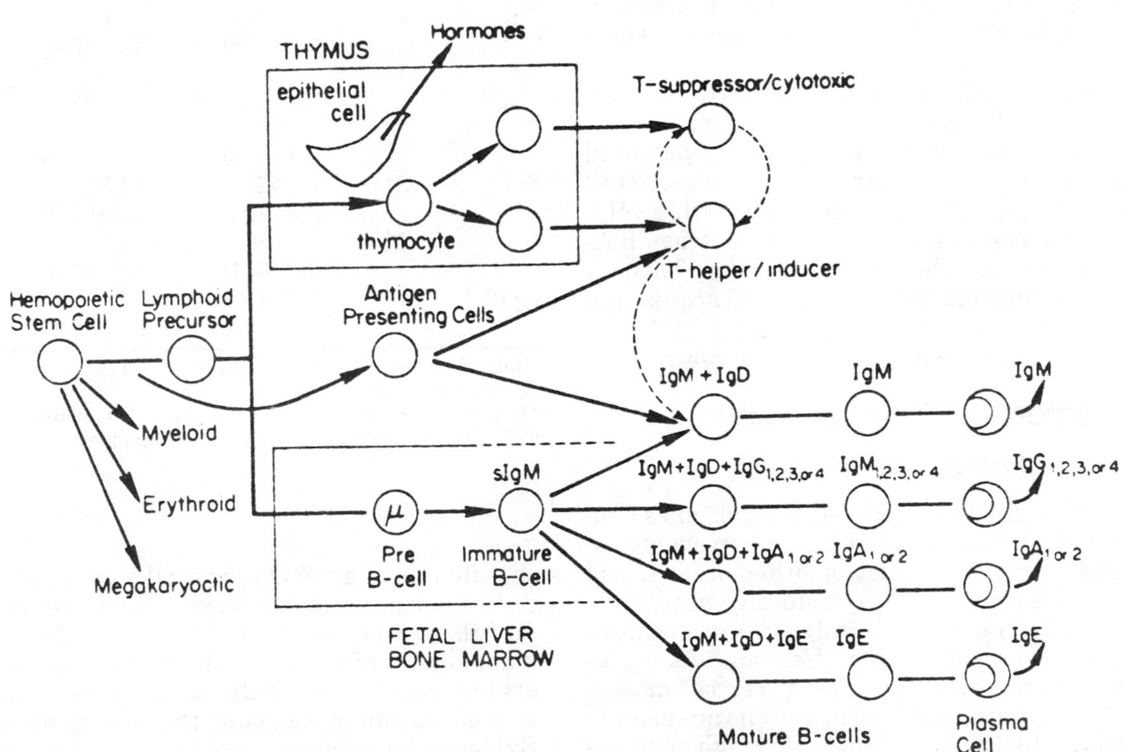

Figure 16.2. Schematic representation of T- and B-cell ontogeny. Reproduced with permission Rosen FS, et al: *N Engl J Med* 311:235, 1984. Originally published in Meeting Report, Primary Immunodeficiency Diseases. WHO Scientific Group on Immunology in *Clin Immunol Immunopathol* 28:450, 1983. Academic Press, Inc.

cells. Helper T cells as well as suppressor T cells involved in the regulation of B-cell differentiation into antibody-producing cells have been described. Each of these T-cell subpopulations bears specific surface markers.

Neonatal and Infant Antibody Production

In human fetuses, the proportions of splenic lymphocytes bearing surface IgM, IgG, IgA, and IgD reach adult values by the beginning of the third trimester. Antibody synthesis in utero can be detected after the 20th week of gestation particularly in response to intrauterine infection. Antibodies synthesized by the human fetus are mainly IgM, and rarely IgA, although IgG synthesis in utero also has been detected under special circumstances. In the normal human fetus, however, the bulk of circulating antibodies are obtained by transfer of maternal IgG via the placenta. The full-term human newborn infant has a serum IgG concentration slightly higher than the maternal level. Virtually no maternal IgA and IgM cross the placenta and, thus, cord blood contains less than 1% of IgA and about 10% of IgM found in maternal serum.

Maternal IgG is slowly catabolized, with a half-life of up to 1 month, and by the third month of life 87% of maternal IgG has been degraded. Because of the delayed onset of IgG synthesis in the normal human infant, a physiologic hypogammaglobulinemia is observed between 4 and 9 months, but levels of serum IgG rapidly start rising toward normal adult values by the end of the first year of age. Premature infants may suffer recurrent infections associated with severe hypogammaglobulinemia due to birth before completion of transplacental transfer of maternal γ-globulin (Table 16.3).

The functional maturation of the B cell is an orderly process. For example, the ability to make antibodies to polysaccharide antigens is usually acquired relatively late in infancy. Immunization results first in the formation of IgM-antibody responses, with a relatively slow progression to IgG-antibody production. IgA-antibody responses are the last to mature. This response pattern is reflected by the sequential acquisition of adult levels of serum immunoglobulins: IgM at 1 year, IgG at 5–7 years, and IgA at 10–14 years.

Table 16.3
Plasma Immunoglobulin Concentrations in Group I Premature Infants (25–28 Weeks' Gestation) and In Group II Premature Infants (29–32 Weeks' Gestation)[1]

Age (months)	*n*	IgG[2] (mg/dl)	IgM[2] (mg/dl)	IgA[2] (mg/dl)
		25–28 Weeks' Gestation		
0.25	18	251 (114–552)[3]	7.6 (1.3–43.3)	1.2 (0.07–20.8)
0.5	14	202 (91–446)	14.1 (3.5–56.1)	3.1 (0.09–10.7)
1.0	10	158 (57–437)	12.7 (3.0–53.3)	4.5 (0.65–30.9)
1.5	14	134 (59–307)	16.2 (4.4–59.2)	4.3 (0.9–20.9)
2.0	12	89 (58–136)	16.0 (5.3–48.9)	4.1 (1.5–11.1)
3	13	60 (23–156)	13.8 (5.3–36.1)	3.0 (0.6–15.6)
4	10	82 (32–210)	22.2 (11.2–43.9)	6.8 (1.0–47.8)
6	11	159 (56–455)	41.3 (8.3–205)	9.7 (3.0–31.2)
8–10	6	273 (94–794)	41.8 (31.1–56.1)	9.5 (0.9–98.6)
		29–32 Weeks' Gestation		
0.25	42	368 (186–728)[3]	9.1 (2.1–39.4)	0.6 (0.04–1.0)
0.5	35	275 (119–637)	13.9 (4.7–41)	0.9 (0.01–7.5)
1.0	26	209 (97–452)	14.4 (6.3–33)	1.9 (0.3–12.0)
1.5	22	156 (69–352)	15.4 (5.5–43.2)	2.2 (0.7–6.5)
2.0	11	123 (64–237)	15.2 (4.9–46.7)	3.0 (1.1–8.3)
3	14	104 (41–268)	16.3 (7.1–37.2)	3.6 (0.8–15.4)
4	21	128 (39–425)	26.5 (7.7–91.2)	9.8 (2.5–39.3)
6	21	179 (51–634)	29.3 (10.5–81.5)	12.3 (2.7–57.1)
8–10	16	280 (140–561)	34.7 (17–70.8)	20.9 (8.3–53)

[1]Data of Ballow et al: *Pediatr Res* 20:899, 1986.
[2]Geometric mean.
[3]The normal ranges in parentheses were determined by taking the antilog of (mean logarithm ± 2 SD of the logarithms).

Assessment of Humoral Immunity

Clinical Findings

Patients with antibody deficiency syndromes usually present with a history of recurrent pyogenic infections of the respiratory tract or other organs, and chronic gastrointestinal disease including giardiasis. The bacterial infections are mainly due to encapsulated, pyogenic organisms such as *Haemophilus influenzae, Streptococcus pneumoniae, Staphylococcus aureus,* and *Neisseria meningitidis*. Viral infections are usually cleared normally by these patients, although they are prone to recurrent infections with the same virus since they cannot produce a protective antibody level against the offending agent. On physical examination, the presence or absence of lymphoid tissue should be sought. Tonsils are absent in patients with X-linked agammaglobulinemia. Radiologic studies may be helpful in evaluating the size of the adenoid tissue and the thymus gland and in assessing the sinuses and lung fields. Evidence for recurrent infections such as scars from previous abscesses or chronic otitis media also should be noted.

Immunologic Findings

The measurement of serum immunoglobulins is an important screening test in the diagnosis of deficiencies in immunity. Measurements of IgG subclasses can be performed by single radial immunodiffusion, but such determinations are limited to a few laboratories because antisera to IgG subclasses are scarce.

Other screening tests for antibody production in vivo include the assessment of specific antibody formation. Isohemagglutinin should be present in all normal individuals except those with group AB red cells. Titers should be greater than 1:8 in normal subjects over the age of 3 years. Antibodies to streptolysin O and other streptococcal antigens are found in the serum of most individuals after infancy. The determination of serum antibody titers after tetanus or diphtheria immunizations or immunization with *H. influenzae* and pneumococcal vaccines provides valuable information about the ability of an individual to mount specific antibody responses. Most of the antibody response to tetanus and diphtheria resides in the IgG 1 subclass (with some IgG 3), whereas the antibody response to carbohydrate antigens resides almost exclusively in the IgG 2 subclass.

When a patient is found to have low immunoglobulin levels, additional in vitro tests are warranted to characterize the site of the B-cell defect. Enumeration of circulating B lymphocytes is based on the presence of several surface receptors not found on T cells. These include immunoglobulins on the B-cell surface, C3 and Fc receptors, and B-cell-specific antigens, such as B1 and B2 (Nadler et al, 1981).

HUMORAL IMMUNITY DISORDERS

Transient Hypogammaglobulinemia of Infancy

Definition

Transient hypogammaglobulinemia of infancy is characterized by an abnormal prolongation and accentuation of the physiologic hypogammaglobulinemia resulting from a delay in the onset of immunoglobulin synthesis in these infants (Tiller and Buckley, 1978; Rieger et al, 1980).

Basic Science

The normal full-term newborn infant has a serum IgG level that is the same or sometimes slightly higher than that of the mother, reflecting an active transport of IgG across the placenta during the last trimester of pregnancy. Although the human fetus is capable of forming antibodies in utero after the 20th week of gestation when adequately stimulated, the normal infant usually does not begin significant synthesis of IgG until age 2–3 months. The maternal IgG is slowly catabolized with the usual half-life of 25–30 days. Hence, between 4 and 9 months of age, a physiologic hypogammaglobulinemia occurs.

Epidemiology

This condition affects both male and female infants. In some cases, there is a familial occurrence.

Natural History

Affected infants usually present after 6 months of age with recurrent viral and pyogenic infections of the upper and lower respiratory tract and rarely the skin or meninges. Recurrent otitis and bronchitis are the most common infections observed in these patients. Nevertheless, many infants with transient hypogammaglobulinemia are free of significant infection, and have been found incidentally among relatives of immunodeficient persons. Such infants usually have no specific physical findings, usually thrive, and have normal peripheral lymphoid tissue.

Patients with transient hypogammaglobulinemia of infancy have been found to be capable of synthesizing specific antibodies to human type A and B erythrocytes, and to diphtheria and tetanus toxoid well before immunoglobulin concentrations become normal. Lymphocyte studies in vitro show neither abnormalities in numbers of circulating B or T cells, nor in response to mitogen stimulation. In some cases the disorder is associated with food allergy (Fineman et al, 1979).

Lymph nodes from these patients display very small or no germinal centers, with marked reduction in the number of plasma cells. Since these patients have a normal number of circulating B cells, the defect presumably involves terminal differentiation of B cells into antibody-producing plasma cells. A defect in the number and function of helper T cells has been found to underlie transient hypogammaglobulinemia of infancy. No evidence has been presented for increased suppressor cell activity in these patients.

Treatment

The majority of patients with transient hypogammaglobulinemia do not require γ-globulin replacement therapy. These patients usually thrive, do not have significant life-threatening infections, and their serum IgG level is usually above 200 mg/dl. Immunoglobulin levels should be measured every 3–4 months. In those patients with severe recurrent infections, γ-globulin replacement therapy is indicated, usually for 12–36 months. It is discontinued when there is evidence for in vivo IgG synthesis. These patients should be investigated thoroughly and followed carefully to distinguish this condition from other permanent immunodeficiencies.

Prognosis

Patients with transient hypogammaglobulinemia of infancy usually recover spontaneously around 4 years of age when immunoglobulin production becomes normal. After the onset of normal IgG synthesis, their prognosis is excellent.

X-linked Agammaglobulinemia

Definition

This disorder, also called congenital agammaglobulinemia or Bruton disease, is characterized by the early onset of recurrent pyogenic infections. These patients have low serum concentrations of all immunoglobulin classes, no circulating B cells, and the absence of plasma cells in all lymphoid tissues. T cells, however, are normal in number and function.

Basic Science

The selective B-cell defect in congenital agammaglobulinemia is probably the result of a maturational block in early B-cell development in the transition of pre-B cells to B cells. The proposed mechanism is the failure of the variable gene of the heavy chain to join the constant μ chain gene (Conley et al, 1986; Kwan et al, 1986).

Epidemiology

This disease is transmitted in an X-linked recessive pattern with lateral male relatives being affected.

Natural History

Male infants with X-linked agammaglobulinemia are usually asymptomatic during the first several months of life, presumably because of the passive protection afforded by placentally transferred maternal γ-globulin. After 6 months of age, when maternal γ-globulin has been catabolized, the affected infants manifest recurrent infections, many with encapsulated pyogenic organisms such as staphylococci, pneumococci, streptococci, and influenzae. Depending on the environment of the child, the presence of older siblings and other circumstances, however, the onset of recurrent infections may be as late as 2 years of age. The most common sites of infection involve the upper and lower respiratory tract causing pneumonia, otitis, purulent sinusitis, and bronchiectasis as well as meningitis, sepsis, pyoderma, and osteomyelitis. These infections usually can be controlled with appropriate antibiotics, but they recur persistently until prophylactic γ-globulin therapy is instituted. Without early replacement of γ-globulin, many of these children acquire chronic progressive bronchiectasis and ultimately die of pulmonary complications. The gastrointestinal tract is usually free of disease, unless intestinal malabsorption due to giardiasis occurs (Ochs et al, 1972).

Children with X-linked agammaglobulinemia have an increased susceptibility to infection with hepatitis virus, and enteroviruses such as ECHO and polio virus. Patients with persistent and potentially fatal CNS ECHO virus infections, as well as paralytic polio resulting from administration of live polio vaccine, have responded to treatment with high doses of iv γ-globulin (with or without intrathecal γ-globulin) containing antibodies to the culprit strain of the virus (Mease et al, 1981). Chronic inflammation and swelling of the large joints, which resembles rheumatoid arthritis, develop in one-third to one-half of these children before the diagnosis is established. This complication resolves with the institution of γ-globulin replacement.

Several patients with X-linked agammaglobulinemia have also developed syndromes resembling dermatomyositis in conjunction with disseminated ECHO virus infection. This complication of the disease is generally fatal, despite use of steroids or antimetabolites (Gotoff et al, 1972).

Diagnosis

The serum of children with X-linked agammaglobulinemia is marked by severe deficiency of all major immunoglobulin classes. The IgG levels are usually less than 100 mg/100 ml. Serum IgA and IgM are usually present in concentrations less than 1% of adult values. Cellular immunity is intact, with normal delayed hypersensitivity, normal T-cell number, normal in vitro response to mitogens, antigens, and allogeneic cells and occurrence of florid poison ivy dermatitis and ampicillin rashes. With very few exceptions, patients with X-linked agammaglobulinemia lack circulating lymphocytes bearing surface immunoglobulin.

Treatment

Replacement therapy with immune serum globulin has been effective in preventing the severe recurrent pyogenic infections in these patients (Cunningham-Rundles et al, 1984). Antibiotics are unnecessary for those patients on maintenance γ-globulin therapy except when specific infections supervene.

Common Variable Agammaglobulinemia

Definition

This immunodeficiency has also been termed acquired agammaglobulinemia or common variable immunodeficiency. As its name suggests, this syndrome represents a heterogeneous group of disorders united by hypogammaglobulinemia. These disorders were originally grouped together because they could not be classified unequivocally. Included are cases previously classified as non-X-linked (or sporadic) hypogammaglobulinemia, and 'acquired' primary hypogammaglobulinemia. Patients in this category have immunodeficiency that varies in time of onset as well as clinical and immunologic pattern.

Basic Science

The etiology of common variable agammaglobulinemia is unknown. Although there is no clear genetic influence on the occurrence of this disease, common variable agammaglobulinemia has occurred in siblings, and family members of patients with this disease have a higher incidence of hypogammaglobulinemia, selective IgA deficiency, and autoimmune disease. The development of infectious mononucleosis has also been associated with common variable agammaglobulinemia.

Epidemiology

Both sexes are affected equally, and in some cases, familial occurrence has been reported.

Natural History

In this disease, symptoms rarely occur before the age of 6 years, and in most patients the disease begins in the second or third decade of life. Recurrent and chronic respiratory tract infections, particularly paranasal sinusitis, bronchitis, and pneumonia are prominent features. Any patient with chronic progressive bronchiectasis should be suspected of having this disease (Hausser et al, 1983).

A frequent complication of common variable agammaglobulinemia rarely seen in the congenital disease is a sprue-like syndrome with diarrhea, malabsorption, steatorrhea, and protein-losing enteropathy occurring in up to 60% of the patients. These gastrointestinal abnormalities may be associated with heavy bacterial overgrowth, jejunal villous atrophy or intestinal nodular lymphoid hyperplasia, but frequently the intestinal biopsy is perfectly normal. *Giardia lamblia* infection is common and appears to be responsible for many of the gastrointestinal complications seen in these patients. In such cases, treatment with metronidazole (Flagyl) has been beneficial.

Patients with common variable agammaglobulinemia frequently have associated hematologic disorders, including pernicious anemia, hemolytic anemia (including Coombs test-positive hemolytic anemia), anemia from folate or vitamin B_{12} malabsorption, leukopenia, and/or thrombocytopenia.

The nondeforming polyarthritis and/or polyarthralgias responsive to γ-globulin replacement seen in congenital agammaglobulinemia may also be seen in the acquired disease. Furthermore, autoimmune disorders such as rheumatoid arthritis, systemic lupus erythematosus, and idiopathic thrombocytopenic purpura are seen in patients with acquired agammaglobulinemia and in their relatives at a much higher incidence than in the normal population.

Another distinguishing feature of common variable agammaglobulinemia is the frequent occurrence of noncaseating granulomas of the lungs, spleen, liver, and skin. An infectious etiology for these lesions has not been identified, but steroids have been reported to be helpful in their treatment. Amyloidosis, hemolytic-uremic syndrome, and an increased incidence of malignancy, particularly reticuloendothelial tumors, have also been reported in these patients.

Diagnosis

IgG levels are usually less than 500 mg/100 ml, and IgA and IgM levels less than 50 mg/100 ml. Although most patients have normal or increased numbers of circulating B cells, plasma cells are rarely found in lymph nodes, bone marrow and spleen, but may be found in the intestinal lamina propria.

Patients with common variable agammaglobulinemia usually have low isohemagglutinin titers, and a markedly reduced antibody response on challenge with a variety of antigens. Despite the immunoglobulin deficiency, auto-antibodies such as rheumatoid factor or anti-red blood cell antibody resulting in Coombs test positive hemolytic anemia have been reported frequently.

In addition to the B-cell deficiency, many of these patients have or eventually develop T-cell abnormalities. Over 50% of patients eventually exhibit cutaneous anergy.

Several investigators have demonstrated that patients with common variable agammaglobulinemia are heterogeneous in terms of the site at which differentiation of B cells into antibody-secreting cells is blocked. About 25% of patients have an extreme reduction or absence of immunoglobulin-bearing lymphocytes in the circulation. The remaining patients have a normal or increased number of circulating B cells. These patients have defects involving the terminal differentiation of B lymphocytes into immunoglobulin-secreting plasma cells. Most patients with common variable agammaglobulinemia probably have an intrinsic defect in B-cell differentiation (Geha et al, 1974; Waldmann et al, 1974). (For discussion of treatment, see pp. 993.)

Selective IgG Subclass Deficiency

Definition

Patients with selective IgG subclass deficiency frequently have normal or slightly decreased levels of total IgG, because, with the exception of IgG1, the other subclasses make up a minor portion of total IgG. Nevertheless, the disproportionate synthesis of certain IgG subclasses is of clinical significance because the biologic properties of immunoglobulins in the various IgG subclasses differ. A deficiency of a quantitatively less important subclass conceivably could lead to disease if a specific antibody activity was found exclusively within that specific subclass. The relative distribution of the four IgG subclasses among serum in normal adults is 65–70%, 23–28%, 4–7%, and 3–4% for IgG1, IgG2, IgG3, and IgG4, respectively.

The most common subclass deficiency is IgG2. Deficiency of IgG3 alone or in combination with IgG1 can also cause recurrent infection.

Basic Science

Schur et al (1979) and Oxelius (1974) reported deficiency of specific subclasses in patients with recurrent infections, particularly bronchopneumonia and otitis media. *H. influenzae* and pneumococci were implicated more frequently in these infections since the antibody response to the capsular antigens of these bacteria resides almost exclusively in the IgG2 subclass (Siber et al, 1980). Although the total serum IgG was normal, on immunoelectrophoresis IgG showed restricted heterogeneity.

The important role that IgG2 plays in the antibody response against bacterial polysaccharides has been further substantiated by several observations. First, children under the age of 2 years respond poorly to most polysaccharide antigens, including pneumococcal, meningococcal, and *H. influenzae* type b capsular polysaccharides. This correlates with the fact that IgG2 levels are particularly low in infants under the age of 2 years and that adult levels of IgG2 are not attained as quickly as in other subclasses.

Selective Antibody Deficiency Syndrome

An important and newly discovered antibody deficiency syndrome is a selective deficiency in the ability to respond to certain antigens. Individuals with this syndrome have normal total levels of IgG, absence of IgG^2 and have recurrent sinopulmonary infections. Many of these patients, however, completely fail to respond to immunization with carbohydrate antigens such as those of *H. influenzae* type b (Umetsu et al, 1985). Absence of IgG antibody response to polysaccharide antigens has been described in individuals with normal IgG subclasses (Ambrosino et al, 1987; 1988).

Selective IgA Deficiency

Definition and Epidemiology

This condition is defined by the presence of reduced levels of serum IgA (< 10 mg/100 ml) associated with normal or even elevated levels of IgG or IgM. Selective IgA deficiency is the most common form of immunodeficiency; the incidence is reported to be between 1/500 and 1/700. Controversy exists as to the clinical significance of IgA deficiency since some patients remain healthy throughout their life, while others have significant disease. IgA deficiency with recurrent infections has been associated with IgG2 subclass deficiency. Most cases of IgA deficiency occur sporadically, although numerous instances of familial occurrence have been reported. The mode of inheritance of this defect within such families has been variable and, thus, is not clearly established. Increased incidence of selective IgA deficiency is observed in families with hypogammaglobulinemia (Underdown and Schiff, 1986).

Basic Science

IgA in bone marrow plasma cells and serum is predominantly (90%) IgA1. In contrast, IgA in secretions and intestinal plasma cells contains equal amounts of IgA1 and IgA2. The B cells capable of producing IgA2 found in peripheral blood are, thus, possibly "in transit." In some persons with serum IgA deficiency, IgA2-producing plasma cells may be plentiful in the gut, and the apparent defect of serum IgA may reflect the lack of serum IgA1 only. Most IgA-deficient persons, however, lack both serum and secretory IgA1 and IgA2.

IgG2 and IgG4 deficiencies may be associated with selective IgA deficiencies. Nearly half of patients with selective IgA deficiency are also deficient in IgE. Thus, the disorder may not be an isolated or selective defect in IgA, particularly in symptomatic patients; instead, it may reflect a more general abnormality in the terminal differentiation of the B cell.

Natural History

In a recent survey of reported cases of immunodeficiency, over half the patients with selective IgA deficiency had frequent infections and a quarter had autoimmune or collagen vascular disease. Symptomatic IgA deficiency accounts for 10–15% of cases involving clinically serious immunodeficiency.

The deficiency of IgA may not be primary, or isolated. It may occur after the administration of drugs, such as phenytoin. Under these circumstances, the deficiency may be the result of the induction of suppressor T cells that interfere with B-cell maturation.

Certain autoimmune diseases occur with greater frequency in patients with IgA deficiency than would be expected in the normal population. Rheumatoid arthritis and systemic lupus erythematosus appear to be most frequent, but dermatomyositis, pernicious anemia, thyroiditis, idiopathic Addison disease, Sjogren syndrome, pulmonary hemosiderosis, chronic active hepatitis, and autoimmune hemolytic anemia also have been reported.

Diagnosis

In the disorder, serum and secretory IgA levels are undetectable by radial immunodiffusion (< 5 mg/dl). With more sensitive techniques, however, trace amounts of IgA can be found in most patients with selective IgA deficiency. In rare cases, patients with normal secretory IgA, but decreased serum IgA, have been reported. By definition, normal levels of the other major immunoglobulin classes are found.

Patients with selective IgA deficiency have an increased number of autoantibodies directed to human immunoglobulins (antihuman IgA, antihuman IgM, and antihuman IgG), thyroid antigens, DNA, muscle tissue, gastric parietal cells, mitochondria, and basement membranes. As many as half of the patients with IgA deficiency have anti-IgA antibodies. Patients with anti-IgA antibodies are at high risk for anaphylactoid reactions after administration of blood products, such as plasma or immune serum globulin that contains IgA.

The majority of patients with selective IgA deficiency have antibodies against milk; 40% of the patients have, in addition, IgA antibodies directed against normal serum from cow, goat, and sheep (anti-bovidae antibody). These antibodies cross-react with milk, and may obscure the diagnosis of IgA deficiency by producing precipitation spurious lines when IgA quantitation is performed using radial immunodiffusion plates. In such patients, horse or rabbit antihuman IgA should be used for the immunoprecipitation.

Absence or markedly reduced amounts of serum IgA cannot be considered as diagnostic of a selective IgA immunodeficiency. Symptomatic patients with diminished levels of serum IgA require further examination to determine definitively the actual nature of their problem. The evaluation should include quantitation of IgG and IgA subclasses, and determination in secretions of IgA and its associated secretory piece, as well as studies of B- and T-cell function. Such an evaluation has clinical relevance, since patients with associated IgG-subclass defects may benefit from immunoglobulin replacement therapy.

Treatment

Treatment is symptomatic for patients with IgA deficiency, focusing on conditions that may occur in association with this immunodeficiency, such as recurrent infections, celiac disease, collagen-vascular disease, etc. Use of IgA-free γ-globulin preparations is indicated only in cases with severe recurrent infections.

Immunodeficiency with Increased IgM

Definition

This form of dysgammaglobulinemia is characterized by a deficiency of IgA and IgG associated with normal or elevated serum IgM levels.

Epidemiology

This disease occurs in an X-linked form, sporadically in families without an X-linked inheritance, and in association with the congenital rubella syndrome.

Natural History

Males with the X-linked form of the disease present in the first or second year of life with recurrent pyogenic infection including otitis media, pneumonia, and septicemia. In addition to their increased susceptibility to infection, many of these patients develop cyclic or persistent neutropenia, thrombocytopenia, renal lesions, and aplastic and hemolytic anemia, presumably as manifestations of autoimmune disease induced by IgM antibodies. Enlarged cervical lymph nodes and hepatosplenomegaly are frequent findings. Malignant IgM-producing B-cell lymphomas of the intestinal tract have been reported in several cases.

Diagnosis

Patients with hyper-IgM immunodeficiency have been shown to have IgM-bearing B cells in the circulation, but not IgG- or IgA-bearing B cells. When peripheral blood lymphocytes from these patients are stimulated in vitro with pokeweed mitogen, they synthesize IgM but not IgG (Geha et al, 1979), which suggests that the development of B cells may be arrested at the IgM synthesizing stage. The cause of this block is unknown. In some cases, T-cell factors can overcome the defect in vitro, suggesting the lack of adequate production of B-cell maturation factors (Levitt et al, 1983).

Treatment of Children with Antibody Deficiency Syndrome

Overall Treatment—Summary

Prophylactic antibiotics are usually given during the winter months for the less severe cases. In children who have IgA deficiency, it is important to make sure that anti-IgA antibodies are absent. If they are present, a preparation free of IgA should be instituted.

Intravenous γ-globulin is started at 400 mg/kg initially and then maintained at 200 mg/kg every 2 weeks

CASE ILLUSTRATION

R.W. is a 4-year-old boy who had a history of recurrent upper respiratory and ear infections starting at age 8 months. These infections occurred predominantly between October and May and their incidence was decreased after the insertion of tubes. Twice he was diagnosed as having bronchitis because of cough, fever, and a noisy chest. Wheezing has occurred intermittently during the course of several episodes of upper respiratory infection. For the past 4 months, he had been tired and had a persistent cough and foul-smelling breath.

Physical examination revealed a child of normal height and weight. Positive findings included tenderness over the right maxillary area, and crusty mucus in both nostrils.

A chest radiograph was normal. Radiographs of sinuses revealed total opacification of the right maxillary sinus and extensive thickening of the mucosa of the left maxillary sinus.

QUESTION AND COMMENT

What immune defect is suggested and how should it be evaluated and treated?

Serum immunoglobulins of IgG 580 mg/dl, IgM 20 mg/dl, and IgA 100 mg/dl were all normal for his age. Serum IgG subclasses were IgG1 400 mg/dl, IgG2 10 mg/dl, IgG3 80 mg/dl and IgG4 60 mg/dl. IgG2 level was under 2 SDs below the mean of age. The anti-*Haemophilis influenzae* capsular antigen (HIBCP) titer in this child was 100 ng/ml before HIBCP immunization and rose to only 300 ng/ml after immunization. The protective level is 300 ng/ml, and the expected postimmunization level for this age is >1200 ng/ml.

The diagnosis of IgG2 subclass deficiency was made and the child was started on prophylactic trimethoprim-sulfa, 5 cc daily. After he was given a 4-week course of amoxicillin (250 mg tid) and of pseudoephedrine, which resulted in the clearing of his sinuses, the frequency of his ear infections markedly decreased and his "energy level" returned to normal. In the coming summer, prophylaxis was discontinued. The following September he had two episodes of otitis, after which prophylactic antibiotics were reinstituted successfully.

R.W. has a cousin, who had a similar problem. When she failed to improve on prophylactic antibiotics, she was started on replacement therapy with iv γ-globulin. This resolved her problems with infections.

or a higher dose every 3 weeks. Side effects from γ-globulin therapy are rare, but include fever, chills, muscle cramps, urticaria, and rarely, anaphylaxis (Burks et al, 1986).

It should be emphasized that the requirement for γ-globulin depends on the clinical situation rather than the serum level of IgG. This is because the degree of protection against infection is related to the quality of the circulating IgG rather than the quantity.

T-CELL COMPARTMENT

Definition

The T cells constitute another major class of lymphocytes that is involved in several immune mechanisms. Several subsets of T cells exist, each with specific effector mechanisms. T cells in one subset, characterized by the presence of the cell determinant-4 membrane (CD4) antigens (OKT4, or Leu3), are called helper/inducer cells, because they help B cells in the process of differentiation to antibody-secreting cells. In addition, helper/inducer T cells are involved in expanding another subset of cytotoxic and suppressor T cells, which are characterized by the presence of CD8 antigens (OKT8 or Leu2). The function of cytotoxic cells is to bind to and destroy target cells, such as tumor cells or virus infected cells. The function of suppressor cells is to down-regulate immune responses by directly affecting the responding cell (e.g., antibody production by the B cell), or by affecting the helper T cell (e.g., the helper T cell necessary for B-cell differentiation into an antibody-producing cell).

T cells are responsible for contact sensitivity (e.g., poison ivy dermatitis), delayed hypersensitivity reactions (e.g., tuberculin test reactivity), immunity to intracellular organisms (viruses, tuberculosis, brucella), immunity, fungal organisms, and graft-versus-host diseases.

Development of T Cells

Thymic Development

Precursors of both B and T lymphocytes arise from pluripotential stem cells that appear first in the blood islets of the embryo and yolk sac at about the fourth week of gestation. Such cells later migrate to the fetal liver and then to the bone marrow, when these tissues become hematopoietic. At 9 weeks of gestation, bone marrow precursor cells start to migrate to the thymus where they are induced to become lymphoid cells. The exact nature of the thymic differentiation signal as well as the stem cell receptor for the signal remain undefined.

T-cell Differentiation Within the Thymus

About 90% of the thymocytes are located in the thymic cortex, and only 5–10% are in the thymic medulla. Outer cortical thymocytes are the most immature lymphoid T cells, many of which die within the cortex, while others migrate from cortex to medulla as they undergo further differentiation.

During migration to the medulla, maturing thymocytes become resistant to the lytic effects of corticosteroids and acquire immunocompetence. Medullary thymocytes can recognize and respond with proliferation to alloantigens in a mixed lymphocyte culture and to the polyclonal T-cell mitogens concanavalin A and phytohemagglutinin. Cortical thymocytes lack these capabilities.

Thymic epithelial cells produce soluble factors that may influence the growth and maturation of T cells even after they migrate to the periphery. Several biologically active peptides, or thymic hormones, have been identified—e.g., thymosin, thymopoietin, and thymic facteur serique. Thymic hormones are produced at higher rates in young persons, and a sharp drop in blood levels is usually seen in the third decade of life.

Additional information regarding the differentiation of human thymocytes has been provided by monoclonal antibodies directed against specific T-cell surface antigens (Reinherz et al, 1980a). Immature thymocytes, which account for about 10% of the thymocyte population, bear both OKT9 and OKT10. The OKT6 marker appears later in development and is present on about 70% of thymocytes. At this stage, cells additionally and concurrently express OKT4 and OKT8. As maturation proceeds, the OKT6 marker is lost, and OKT3 is acquired. It is at the mature thymocyte stage that T cells segregate into OKT4 (helper) and or OKT8 (suppressor) cytotoxic subpopulations. As the thymocyte becomes a circulating T cell, the OKT10 antigen is lost.

T-Cell Circulation

Mature T cells leave the thymus by passing through the walls of medullary venules into the peripheral circulation. Lymphocytes can be detected in the peripheral circulation at 7–8 weeks of gestation. By the 10th week, these cells constitute over 50% of the circulating white cells. Circulating T cells exit from the blood via high cuboidal endothelial cells lining the venules of the paracortical areas of the lymph nodes and Peyer patches. After a period of residence in lymph nodes, lymphocytes enter the lymphatic system via the afferent channel and travel to the thoracic duct, from which they reenter the peripheral circulation.

Lymph nodes can be found in the human embryo as early as 11 weeks and are well populated with lymphoid cells by birth. B and T cells have distinct areas of residence within the node; B cells occupy primary and secondary follicles located in the lymph node cortex, whereas T cells accumulate in the paracortical areas (Fig. 16.2).

T-Cell Subpopulations

The standard method for identification of human T cells has utilized their ability to form rosettes with sheep erythrocytes. Recently, monoclonal antibodies have characterized T-cell subsets as follows. The monoclonal antibody designated OKT3 reacts with 95% of peripheral blood T cells. OKT4 antibodies detect a subclass comprising 55–60% of the total peripheral blood T-cell population, which has T-helper function. OKT8 detect a separate and distinct subset of T cells, which has suppressor activity.

Helper T cells are induced to undergo blast transformation and cell division when they interact with antigen presented by monocytes and HLA-DR determinants on antigen-presenting cells. In addition, the plant lectins, phytohemagglutinin, concanavalin A, and pokeweed mitogen which bind to a variety of cell-surface glycoproteins, are capable of polyclonal T-cell activation. In each case, macrophages or other accessory cells are required for activation. They produce a factor, interleukin-1 which, in turn, induces the helper T cell to produce a T-cell growth factor, interleukin-2, and to express cell surface receptors for interleukin-2 molecules. Acquisition of HLA-DR and release of soluble factors by activated T cells are important in the immune response. These lymphokines include macrophage chemotactic and activation factors, B-cell growth and differentiation factors, and γ-interferon.

Cytotoxic T-cell precursors can be preactivated by contact with the appropriate antigen, such as a budding virus, and HLA-A, -B, and -C molecules present on all nucleated cells, but they require interleukin-2 and other factors from helper T cells for their conversion into active cytotoxic cells. Suppressor T cells also depend on helper T cells for their activation. Activated suppressor T cells, in turn, release soluble factors that suppress helper T cells, dampening the immune response.

T-Cell Immunodeficiency Diseases

Definition

T cells are important for the elimination of viruses, the response to fungi, foreign cells, tumor surveillance, and for providing help for B cells to differentiate into autoantibody-producing cells. Thus, T-cell immunodeficiency can result in severe fungal and viral infections as well as bacterial infections and in failure to thrive. T-cell deficiencies cover a wide spectrum which ranges from total failure of T-cell development as is seen in severe combined immunodeficiency to more selective and subtle defects, such as those seen in chronic mucocutaneous candidiasis.

Since T cells pass through multiple stages in thymic development and since T-cell activation is a multistage process that involves sequential steps, it is not surprising to find distinct defects in T-cell maturation and/or activation which would all result in functional T-cell deficiencies.

Laboratory Investigation of T-Cell Function

A complete blood count and differential is important because lymphopenia is often seen in severe combined immunodeficiency. Chest radiographs are helpful; observation of a thymic shadow rules out classical severe combined immunodeficiency.

A delayed hypersensitivity skin test is very useful in assessing T-cell function. Tetanus toxoid (1:10, dilution of fluid T1 injected intradermally) is very useful, as all children have been immunized with the toxoid (Borut et al, 1980). At 1 year of age up to 80% of children will have a positive 48-hour skin test to this toxoid. Monilia, mumps, and others can be added.

Total T-cell and T-cell subset distribution can be readily measured in vitro by use of monoclonal antibodies specific to T-cell surface antigens, T3 for total T cells, T4 for helper T cells, and T8 for suppressor T cells. The most important in vitro test, however, is the assessment of T-cell function, as in many situations T cells are present in normal numbers but do not function. The test measures T-cellular proliferation after stimulation with plant lectins (e.g., phytohemagglutinin concanavalin A) and, more important, after stimulation with antigens to which the child has been exposed (e.g., tetanus toxoid, diphtheria toxoid, or *Candida*). Earlier events of T-cell activation, such as IL2 receptor expression can also be measured.

Primary T-Cell Deficiency (Severe Combined Immunodeficiency)

Definition

Because T cells play a central role in the immune system, abnormalities in the T-cell compartment may be responsible for a diverse spectrum of immune deficiencies. When T-cell deficiency is severe, both the T- and B-cell compartments are paralyzed, resulting in severe combined T-/B-cell immunodeficiency.

Epidemiology

Severe combined immunodeficiency can be inherited as an autosomal recessive or an X-linked recessive trait. Consequently, 75% of patients with the disorder are male; half the autosomal recessive cases involve a deficiency of the enzyme adenosine deaminase. A handful of autosomal recessive cases are characterized by purine nucleoside phosphorylase deficiency. Some patients may have an intrathymic defect that causes the disease. In some cases, the T cells that are present do not express HLA-A and HLA-B antigens; this is termed the "bare-lymphocyte syndrome." These "bare" lymphocytes are not functionally competent.

Natural History

Patients with T-cell deficiency usually present with recurrent infections with fungi, viruses, or *Pneumocystis carinii*. The thymus is often absent on chest radiograph, and lymphopenia may be observed. Diarrhea is often present, accompanied by growth retardation, and wasting. These children are susceptible to graft-versus-host disease from T cells from a variety of sources, including blood products, or transplacentally derived maternal T cells.

Diagnosis

Examination usually reveals absence of tonsils and lymph nodes, abnormal lung examination with rales, and rhonchi, evidence of wasting, and oral thrush. Chest radiographs show absence of a thymic shadow. Circulating lymphocytes may be decreased, and serum immunoglobulins are markedly decreased. Neutropenia, anemia, monocytosis, thrombocytosis, and eosinophilia may be present. Delayed skin tests are always negative. T cells are generally absent and often B cells may be absent as well. Proliferative responses to both mitogens and antigens are absent. AIDS must be ruled out.

The number of mature T cells is consistently low, although some patients have B lymphocytes in their circulation that behave normally in vitro when mixed with normal T cells. Some patients have normal numbers of circulating lymphocytes that are immature. When mature T cells are present, they are frequently of maternal origin. Although immunoglobulins are very low in most cases, IgM components may be present in the blood.

The clinical syndrome in purine-nucleoside phosphorylase deficiency has a remarkable resemblance to the acquired immunodeficiency syndrome, except that deficiency of the phosphorylase results in orotic acidemia. Most patients have undue susceptibility to opportunistic infections. The number of T cells is extremely low, but the number of B cells is normal. Although in vitro T-cell responses to mitogens and antigens are virtually absent, antibody formation is normal, and immunoglobulin levels are within the normal range (Gelfand et al, 1978). The gene for purine nucleoside phosphorylase has been localized to chromosome 14. The enzyme has been usually undetectable in the reported cases.

Treatment

Whenever severe combined immunodeficiency is suspected, great care must be taken to limit exposure to infection, and to avoid use of any nonirradiated blood to prevent graft-versus-host disease. Zoster-immune globulin is indicated if exposure to varicella has occurred. The disease is cured by bone marrow transplantation. For the 60% of patients with no suitable sibling donors, a moderate degree of success has been achieved with transplants of fetal liver (Keightley et al, 1975), and implants of fetal thymus or thymic epithelium (Hong et al, 1976). None of these procedures has proved as satisfactory as bone marrow grafts in establishing lymphoid chimerism. It is now possible to use parental marrow with success after depletion of T cells, which could cause fatal acute graft-versus-host disease. T cells can be removed with monoclonal antibodies or lectin columns (Reisner et al, 1983).

Prognosis

Unless bone marrow transplantation is performed death usually occurs within the first weeks.

DiGeorge Syndrome (Thymic Hypoplasia, Third and Fourth Pouch Syndrome)

Definition

This syndrome is probably a developmental rather than an inherited disease, due to dysmorphogenesis of the third and fourth pharyngeal pouches, which results in hypoplasia or aplasia of the thymus and of the parathyroid glands. It is associated with abnormalities of the great vessels (right-sided aortic arch, transposition, etc), atrial and ventricular septal defects, esophageal atresia, bifid uvula, short philtrum, mandibular hypoplasia, hypertelorism, and low-set notched ears. These children often present for cardiac evaluation in the neonatal period, and develop hypocalcemic seizures. Cardiac defects are the most common cause of death.

Basic Science

Experimental elimination of limited areas of the cephalic neural crest early in embryonic development can result in a cluster of developmental defects similar to the multiple organ defects in the DiGeorge syndrome. Thus, DiGeorge syndrome could result from failure of neural-crest mesenchymal derivatives to migrate and interact properly with pharyngeal epithelium. A similar syndrome has been described in the women who ingest large doses of retinoic acid (Lammer et al, 1985).

Diagnosis

The severity of thymic hypoplasia is extremely variable. Although complete thymic aplasia does occur, with the resulting immunodeficiency resembling that of severe combined immunodeficiency, most patients have partial T-cell function which appears to improve with time. Mature T cells are decreased in peripheral blood, while immature T cells (OKT 9+ and OKT 6+) are found in increased number. Proliferative responses to mitogens and antigens may be decreased or normal. Serum immunoglobulins are often normal for age, although IgA may be diminished and IgE may be elevated.

Treatment

Because of the considerable variability in the severity of immune deficiency, which also improves with time, it is difficult to evaluate the benefit of various treatment modalities. Treatment must, therefore, be individualized. Aggressive therapy of infections with antibiotics may be sufficient. The immunologic defect can be corrected by fetal thymic implants (Cleveland et al, 1968).

Graft-versus-Host Disease

Definition

Graft-versus-host disease is a manifestation of severely impaired cellular immunity and is characterized by multisystem disease that may remit or be fatal.

Basic Science

When a T-cell deficient host receives a transfusion of HLA-incompatible immunocompetent T cells, necrosis of skin, liver, and gastrointestinal tract can result. This event can occur with intrauterine transfusions in preterm infants with erythroblastosis fetalis and in children with severe combined immunodeficiency who receive blood transfusions. It is more commonly seen after bone marrow transplantation.

Epidemiology

Some degree of graft-versus-host disease occurs in about 60% of allogeneic transplants.

Natural History

The acute disease begins 7–14 days after grafting, and starts with a maculopapular skin eruption, or even a "scalded skin" syndrome and alopecia. The epidermis shows coagulation necrosis. Liver changes include periportal necrosis, which may result in liver failure. Chronic diarrhea and malabsorption are serious manifestations. Latent viral infections may become manifest, and opportunistic infections may be lethal.

Diagnosis

The clinical findings are so characteristic in immunocompromised individuals who have received incompatible T cells by any route (even transfusions) that the diagnosis is obvious. A Coombs test-positive anemia, thrombocytopenia, and leukopenia are common in the severe form. A skin biopsy is diagnostic, but rarely needed.

Treatment

In some instances, glucocorticoids or antilymphocyte globulins are helpful (Tsoi, 1982). Cyclosporin A is effective. Recent approaches used to prevent acute graft-versus-host disease associated with bone marrow transplant have consisted of depleting the donor bone marrow of T cells by use of monoclonal antibodies and complement or by absorption on lectin columns.

Prognosis

In some patients, the only manifestation is a fleeting skin rash. In others, a chronic debilitating illness results. Even in those who recover, autoimmune disorders such as dermatofibrosis, progressive hepatitis, or Sjogren syndrome may develop weeks or years later.

Chronic Mucocutaneous Candidiasis

Candida constitute part of the normal flora of the oral mucosa, the gastrointestinal tract, and the skin. Clinical candidal disease is often seen when the ecologic balance is upset by intrinsic or extrinsic manipulations. Thus, antibacterial chemotherapy frequently results in candidal proliferation and disease. Such infections are transient, in contrast to the persistent and recurrent infections of the skin, mucous membrane, and/or nails with *Candida*. Chronic mucocutaneous candidiasis (see pp. 1118) is not a single clinical entity, but is a collection of related syndromes, and it, therefore, includes both patients who have limited local disease and those with extensive cutaneous (*Candida* granuloma) or mucous involvement. Patients with the disorder do not generally suffer from invasive candidiasis.

Diagnosis

Numerous immunologic defects have been noted in patients with chronic mucocutaneous candidiasis. Cell-mediated immunity is most frequently impaired, with patients failing to show delayed skin test hypersensitivity reactions to *Candida* antigens. In addition, peripheral blood leukocytes from such patients show impaired proliferative responses and lymphokine production when they are exposed to *Candida* antigen in vitro. Other immunologic abnormalities seen in some patients include deficient secretory IgA, abnormal complement system, and impaired macrophage/monocyte function.

Natural History

Certain patients need close observation, particularly children, in whom special attention should be paid to the development of concomitant polyendocrine failure—including hypofunction of the adrenal, thyroid, and parathyroid glands—ovarian failure, and pernicious anemia. Children from a family with a history of chronic mucocutaneous candidiasis and polyendocrinopathy are at special risk. Also, those patients in whom one endocrine deficiency has been identified must be monitored for the development of other endocrine failures.

Treatment

Treatment is directed toward correcting the underlying endocrine or immunologic problem and eradicating or controlling the infection. Many antifungal compounds are now available, including ketoconazole, clotrimazole, miconazole, amphotericin B, nystatin, and flucytosine.

Wiskott-Aldrich Syndrome

Definition

This X-linked syndrome which presents in infancy is characterized by a triad of eczema, thrombocytopenia, and recurrent infections.

Basic Science

The basic defect in Wiskott-Aldrich syndrome is unknown. The relationship of a decrease in a cell surface membrane glycoprotein (gp 115) on lymphocytes and platelets to disease pathogenesis is not yet clear.

Natural History

Initially, patients develop otitis, sinopulmonary bacterial infections, sepsis, and meningitis, but later, when T-cell function diminishes, infections with fungi, viruses, and *Pneumocystis carinii* occur. Death can occur secondary to infection, or from hemorrhage, or from a reticuloendothelial malignancy.

Diagnosis

The diagnosis is confirmed by the presence of platelets that are half the normal size. IgG levels are normal or slightly low, IgM is usually low, and IgA and IgE are elevated (Bruce and Blaese, 1974). Isohemagglutinins and responses to polysaccharide antigens are markedly diminished. In vitro mitogen responses are often normal, although responses to antigens are usually absent.

In patients with this syndrome, the T cells progressively decline in number and function, so that profound lymphopenia does not usually become apparent until 6 years of age. The mixed lymphocyte responses are depressed more than is the response to nonspecific mitogens. Platelets turn over rapidly, and there is decreased thrombopoiesis.

Treatment

Treatment is directed mainly at control of bleeding and at control of infection with antibiotics. Splenectomy has been useful in increasing the platelet content. Bone marrow transplantation has been shown to be highly successful in reversing all the defects in Wiskott-Aldrich syndrome.

Ataxia Telangiectasia

Definition and Natural History

This autosomal recessive syndrome is a progressive disorder characterized by progressive cerebellar ataxia beginning in early childhood, associated with increasing telangiectasia beginning inconspicuously in the bulbar conjunctivae and later spreading to the skin. The immune deficiency is variable, although progressive bacterial sinopulmonary infection occurs in most patients. Tumors, particularly of the lymphoreticular system, are the most common cause of death.

Basic Science

Numerous chromosomal breaks and translocations have been reported, the majority of which were clustered at chromosome 14q12 with translocations to chromosome 6, 7, and X. The immunologic defect in ataxia-telangiectasia is complex. The thymus gland has a fetal appearance microscopically. T cell function is variably depressed. Half the patients have low IgG levels, and three-quarters have low IgE levels. IgA is undetectable in half the patients and very low in 30%. Autoantibodies, particularly to IgA, are commonly found. Those who lack IgG2 as well as IgA appear to be at higher risk of infection (Oxelius et al, 1982).

Treatment

There is no satisfactory therapy for this fatal disease.

Hyper-IgE Syndrome

Definition

The hyper-IgE syndrome is a primary immunodeficiency characterized by recurrent staphylococcal abscesses and markedly elevated levels of serum IgE (Buckley et al, 1972).

Natural History

These patients have a lifelong history of severe recurrent staphylococcal abscesses involving the skin, lungs, joints, and other sites. Pruritic dermatitis is usually present, which differs from typical atopic dermatitis, and respiratory allergic symptoms are usually absent. Laboratory features include exceptionally high serum levels of IgE, near-normal levels of IgG, IgA,

CASE ILLUSTRATION

A.J., a boy who was the product of a first cousin marriage, presented at age 4 months with two episodes of otitis and with thrush and pneumonia. Chest radiograph revealed hyperinflation and linear infiltrates and absent thymus. Shortly after admission, he developed diarrhea. White cell count was 6000/mm^3 with 10% lymphocytes (< 1000/mm^3 lymphocytes is indicative of lymphopenia). Lymphocyte phenotyping showed 17% T3+ cells, 10% T4+ cells, 5% T8 cells, 8% surface immunoglobulin cells (B cells) and that 58% of the cells had the Leu 11 antigen characteristic of natural killer cells. Proliferation in vitro to phytohemagglutinin gave 20,000 counts per minute with a control of 300,000 cpm. Phenotyping revealed cells exclusively of the XX karyotype, i.e., maternal cells. Adenosine deaminase was normal in the child. HLA typing revealed no histocompatibility with either parent. Bone marrow was obtained from the mother, after she was depleted of T cell by in vitro treatment with a pan T-cell antibody and complement, and given to the child.

A few days before the transplant, the child was given cyclophosphamide and rabbit antilymphocyte serum for 5 days to remove any immunocompetent cells capable of rejecting the graft. Two weeks later, a mild graft-versus-host disease appeared, characterized by a measles-like skin rash, fever, diarrhea, and eosinophilia. This subsided in 1 week, after which lymphocyte counts steadily rose to normal and the phytohemagglutinin response became normal. The child was discharged in excellent condition. Six months later his cells proliferated to tetanus toxoid after immunization with the toxoid and his serum IgG levels started to increase steadily. Eighteen months later, this child is immunologically normal and thriving.

and IgM, pronounced blood and sputum eosinophilia, abnormally low anamnestic antibody responses to booster immunizations, poor antibody- and cell-mediated responses to neoantigens, abnormal mixed leukocyte culture responsiveness to genetically disparate family members, and variable presence of chemotactic defects.

Diagnosis

Serum IgE is very high (usually >10,000 IU/ml). Delayed cutaneous anergy to ubiquitous antigens, such as *Candida* and streptokinase-streptodornase is found in about one-half of the patients. In vitro studies of cell-mediated immunity have revealed normal lymphocyte, proliferative responses to the phytohemagglutinin, concanavalin A, and pokeweed mitogen in all but two patients. By contrast, lymphocyte-proliferative responses to the antigens *Candida albicans* and tetanus toxoid were absent or very low in all tested. Serum hemolytic complement and phagocytic function were normal. A variable defect in neutrophil chemotaxis has been described (Fontan et al, 1976).

AIDS in Children

Transplacental acquisition of the AIDS-causing virus (HIV) results in a syndrome which, in infants, involves infections that are usually seen with B-cell dysfunction. The children grow poorly, have lymphadenopathy, often parotid hypertrophy and suffer from bacterial infections (otitis, sepsis, pneumonia) as well as pneumonias due to Epstein-Barr virus and cytomegalovirus. Hypergammaglobulinemia and a positive HIV antibody test are present (Ammann et al, 1985). A few children show hypogammaglobulinemia. Treatment is palliative. Intravenous γ-globulin decreases the frequency of infections without appearing to affect the ultimate fatal outcome (Clavelli and Rubinstein, 1986) (see pp. 1039).

Immunodeficiency with Unusual Response to Epstein-Barr Virus

Patients, both male and female, have been described in whom Epstein-Barr virus infection had an untoward outcome in the form of B-cell lymphomas, marrow aplasia, fatal infectious mononucleosis, or agammaglobulinemia (see pp. 1033). Initially these patients appeared immunologically normal. After the infection, their B cells and immunoglobulins were decreased, however, and the predominant T cells in the circulation were natural killer cells.

Complement System 2

Definition

The complement system is a network of protein components that interact in an orderly sequential fashion. This interaction has been referred to as a 'cascade' in analogy with the coagulation system, and in both systems the activity of one component depends on the activation of the prior component(s) in the sequence. The interaction occurs along the classical pathway or the alternative pathway, or both. The early components (1–3) become activated when they are enzymatically cleaved. The later components (5–9) interact nonenzymatically.

Basic Science

A few basic principles of the biochemistry of complement require description. The enzymatic cleavage of C3 occurs by either of two mechanisms: (1) activation of the early classical complement components, C1, C4, and C2 to form an enzyme designated the classical pathway C3 convertase; or (2) activation of the proteins of the alternative pathway to form another enzyme, the alternative pathway C3 convertase. These enzymes cleave C3, and with the cleavage of C3, C5 is cleaved and the terminal components are added in the order C6–C9, allowing lysis of the target (Fig. 16.3). Func-

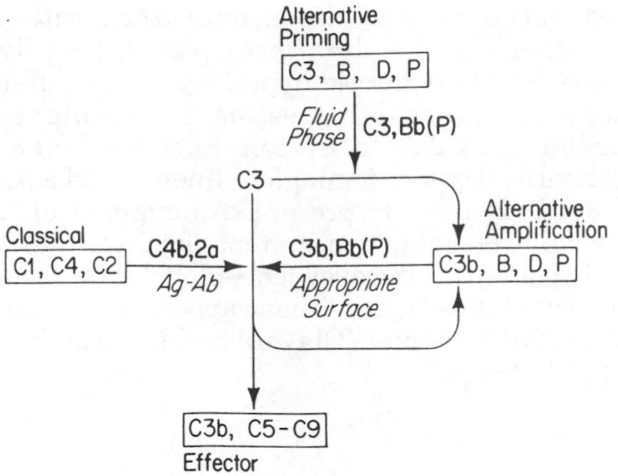

Figure 16.3. Relation of the classical and alternative pathways of complement activation to C3 and the effector sequence. Reproduced with permission from Fearon DT, Austen KF: *N Engl J Med* 303:259, 1980.

tional activities relevant to host defense that are generated as a consequence of complement activation are summarized in Table 16.4.

In the presence of convertase activity, C3 is cleaved and two products are formed: C3a, an anaphylatoxin, which is released, and C3b which covalently binds to cell surfaces. The presence of C3b on a surface permits recognition by cells with C3b receptors, namely, B lymphocytes and phagocytic cells (neutrophils, monocytes, and macrophages). Under most circumstances, in the absence of C3b, phagocytosis is inefficient. It is not surprising, therefore, that patients with a deficiency of C3 often present with severe pyogenic infections. B lymphocytes also bind to C3d, the large cleavage product of C3, through a C3d receptor, that serves also as an attachment receptor for Epstein-Barr virus (Mold et al, 1986).

In the presence of C3b both the classical and alternative C3 convertases acquire the ability to cleave C5. A small fragment, C5a, is released. This peptide is a potent anaphylatoxin and chemoattractant (Eliasson et al, 1977). The larger cleavage fragment (C5b) attaches to the convertase and allows the binding, without cleavage, of C6. This stabilized complex (C5b6) then disassociates from the enzyme and reacts with C7. The activated C5b67 complex then binds C8 and C9. This assembled complex (C5b6789) inserts into the cell, and lysis occurs.

The similarities between the early classical pathway components and those of the alternative pathway are quite striking. Activity of both pathways requires a surface-bound protein, C4b and C3b, respectively. When covalently bound to an appropriate surface, the proteins act as membrane binding sites for C2 and factor B, respectively. C2 and factor B are comparable in many respects. They are of similar size and structure and both are heat-labile. In the presence of Mg^{++} both are cleaved by serine proteases (C1 and factor D, respectively) to the catalytic subunits of convertase activity. Each component hydrolyzes the same arginine-linked peptide bond in its natural substrates C3 or C5. Finally, the structural genes for C2 and factor B are closely linked with the major histocompatibility complex (MHC) on the short arm of human chromosome 6. Both loci are situated close to each other outside the MHC (Raum et al, 1979).

The similarities between the control mechanisms of the classical and alternative pathways are also extensive. Both C2a and Bb are labile and spontaneously dissociate from the membrane binding site to form inactive species. Both compete for binding with control proteins (C4bp and factor H, respectively) that potentiate inactivation of the membrane binding proteins by the same enzyme, factor I (C4b/C3b INA). The ability to cleave C5 is acquired by both C3 convertases upon the further binding of C3b.

PRIMARY DEFICIENCIES OF THE COMPLEMENT SYSTEM

Deficiencies of each component of the classical pathway have been described, as have deficiencies of the control proteins, C1 INH and factors I, H, and D, and propendin. In addition to the primary inherited protein deficiencies, certain functionally deficient complement proteins have been identified. These deficiencies and the associated clinical findings are summarized in Table 16.4. A defect in complement function should be suspected in any patient with collagen vascular disease, with recurrent pyogenic infection, or with neisserial infections.

C1q Deficiency

A primary selective deficiency of C1q was first described in a 10-year-old boy who suffered from an episode of meningitis, recurrent septicemia, recurrent otitis media, and persistent moniliasis of his oral cavity and nails. In this and other patients, C1q has been lacking in the serum by both hemolytic and immunochemical assays (Berkel et al, 1979). Transfusion of fresh-frozen plasma resulted in clinical improvement lasting about 10 days in one case. Although C1q activity rose after the infusion, it returned to undetectable levels by 24 hours after infusion. Complement levels from the patients' parents and siblings have been normal, and it has not appeared that the probands' deficiency has had an inherited basis.

C1r Deficiency

Complete deficiency of C1r has been reported in fewer than a dozen patients who showed manifestation of autoimmune disease at the time of the initial description. Some patients have had low levels of C1s, which may be an associated primary defect or may be secondary to the absence of C1r (Rick et al, 1979).

Table 16.4
Inherited Deficiencies in Complement and Complement-Related Protein[1]

Deficient Protein	Observed Pattern of Inheritance at Clinical Level	Reported Major Clinical Correlates[2]
C1q	Autosomal recessive	Glomerulonephritis, systemic lupus erythematosus
C1r	Probably autosomal recessive	Syndrome resembling systemic lupus erythematosus
C1s	Found in combination with C1r deficiency	Systemic lupus erythematosus
C4	Probably autosomal recessive (two separate loci, C4A and C4B)[3]	Syndromes resembling systemic lupus erythematosus
C2	Autosomal recessive, HLA-Linked	Systemic lupus erythematosus, discoid lupus erythematosus, juvenile rheumatoid arthritis, glomerulonephritis
C3	Autosomal recessive	Recurrent pyogenic infections, glomerulonephritis
C5	Autosomal recessive	Recurrent disseminated neisserial infections, systemic lupus erythematosus
C6	Autosomal recessive	Recurrent disseminated neisserial infections
C7	Autosomal recessive	Recurrent disseminated neisserial infections, Raynaud phenomenon
C8 β chain or C8 $\alpha-\gamma$ chains	Autosomal recessive	Recurrent disseminated neisserial infections
C9	Autosomal recessive	None identified
Properdin	X-linked recessive	Recurrent pyogenic infections, fulminant meningococcemia
Factor $\overline{D}$	?	Recurrent pyogenic infections
C1 inhibitor	Autosomal dominant	Hereditary angioedema, increased incidence of several autoimmune diseases[4]
Factor H	Autosomal recessive	Glomerulonephritis
Factor I	Autosomal recessive	Recurrent pyogenic infections
CR1	Autosomal recessive[5]	Association between low numbers of erythrocyte CR1 and systemic lupus erythematosus
CR3	Autosomal recessive[6]	Leukocytosis, recurrent pyogenic infections, delayed umbilical-cord separation

[1]Reproduced with permission from Frank MM: *N Engl J Med* 316:1528, 1987.
[2]Note that many people with complement deficiencies, especially of C2 and the terminal components, are clinically well. A substantial number of patients with defects in C5 through C9 have had autoimmune disease.
[3]The deficiency in persons lacking C4A or C4B is referred to as "q0," for quantity zero. Thus, such a deficiency can be designated C4Aq0 or C4bq0. Persons with such deficiencies are reported to have a higher than normal incidence of autoimmune diseases. Similarly, heterozygous C2-deficient persons are reported to have an increased incidence of autoimmune disease.
[4]Approximately 85% of cases involve silent alleles, and 15% involve alleles encoding for dysfunctional variant C1-inhibitor protein.
[5]Homozygosity for a low (not absent) numerical expression of CR1 on erythrocytes is detectable in vitro and appears to be associated with systemic lupus erythematosus. An acquired defect in the number of CR1 receptors may also be operative.
[6]Low but not absent levels of leukocyte CR3 are detectable in both parents of most CR3-deficient children.

C4 and C2 Deficiency

C4 deficiency has been described in association with systemic lupus erythematosus. C2 deficiency appears to be the most common complement component deficiency of man, with an estimated prevalence of 1 in 10,000 and a gene frequency of 1–2%. Many of these individuals have been detected either because their serum was used for laboratory tests or population studies, or because they are related to a symptomatic C2-deficient patient. Thus, the true prevalence of this disorder in the general population may be underestimated. Whether these individuals remain in good health is yet to be determined.

The association of C2 deficiency with collagen-vascular disease was first described by Agnello and colleagues (1972), and since then many similar cases have been identified.

It is, thus, apparent that complement deficiencies are associated with autoimmune disease states and that this association is quite striking in deficiencies of the early classical pathway components C1, C4, and C2. The reasons for this are obscure at present.

Most of the patients with isolated C2 deficiency described to date have not had serious infections. Thus, defective classical pathway opsonization may be compensated for by a functioning alternative pathway. There have been few reports, however, of C2 deficiency associated with bacteremic illnesses.

C3 Deficiency

The major complement deficiencies that give rise to recurrent infections are those that severely affect C3 levels. This is because of the important role of C3 in opsonization. The clinical manifestations are recurrent severe bacterial infections. C3 deficiency is a rare autosomal recessive C5 disorder.

C5 Deficiency

Of 10 C5-deficient patients described, seven had increased susceptibility to infection, especially *Neisseria* infections, either recurrent meningococcal meningitis or gonococcal arthritis.

C6, C7, and C8 Deficiency

Patients with C6, C7, or C8 deficiency have increased susceptibility to neisserial infections (Lee et al, 1979).

C9 Deficiency

C9 deficiency has been reported in the absence of association with infections (Lint et al, 1978) or with meningococcal meningitis.

C1 INH Deficiency (Hereditary Angioneurotic Edema)

Definition

C1 INH deficiency leads to hereditary angioneurotic edema (HANE), a condition characterized by intermittent episodes of edema.

Basic Science

While most patients (85%) have markedly reduced levels (5–30%) of the inhibitor protein, some patients synthesized a nonfunctioning but antigenically similar protein. These patients cannot be distinguished clinically and the inheritance pattern is identical. Absence of C1 INH allows the unchecked activation of C2 and C4 by C1, and during acute episodes, C2 and C4 are characteristically depressed. The activity of all other components, including C1, is usually normal. When the level of C1 is depressed, it is usually no lower than 50% of normal, and the degree of C1 depression correlates roughly with the level of C4. With activation of the classical complement pathway, the concomitant release of vasoactive complement fragments occurs, resulting in increased permeability of the vascular bed, followed by the extravasation of fluid and protein.

Natural History

Edema is typically located peripherally and is nonpitting and nonpruritic. Episodes may occur spontaneously or after trauma, anxiety, or stress and usually last for 24–72 hours. While many patients have little or no serious difficulty, others present with swelling of submucosal surfaces severe enough to occlude the upper airway and threaten life. The association of HANE and systemic lupus erythematosus has been reported, and it appears that the prevalence of lupus-like illnesses is much greater in patients with hereditary angioneurotic edema than in the general population.

In addition to the inherited forms of this disease, C1 INH deficiency may be acquired in adult life in association with an underlying malignancy, usually a lymphoproliferative disorder. C1q levels are characteristically normal in hereditary angioneurotic edema but reduced in acquired C1 INH deficiency.

Treatment

The treatment of hereditary angioneurotic edema consists primarily of avoiding precipitating factors, usually trauma. Fresh plasma transfusions have been used prophylactically when trauma is unavoidable, e.g., with surgery or dental work, but this carries the potential risk from infusion of the substrate (C4, C2) of the uncontrolled, activated enzyme. The infusion of purified C1 INH has been effective in aborting acute attacks (Gadek et al, 1980). Androgens have been used successfully in the treatment of the disorder; in particular the semi-synthetic androgen Danazol, which has minimal virilizing activity, has proved useful in preventing acute episodes (Gelfand et al, 1976). The clinical improvement noted with Danazol is related to increased serum levels of C1 INH by a currently unknown mechanism. Danazol cannot be used in children. The treatment of acquired angioedema is directed toward the underlying disorder.

C3b Factor I INA Deficiency

Definition

To date, the patients described with a deficiency of factor I INA illustrate the role of this enzyme in regulating the function of the alternative complement pathway. In the absence of factor I, C3b persists longer, causing the activation of factor B and the unchecked activation of the alternate pathway. This results in unchecked consumption of C3.

Natural History

Because of persistent low C3 levels, patients with factor I C3b suffer from recurrent episodes of meningitis, otitis, and septicemia. The continuous generation of the mast cell anaphylotoxin C3a from C3 leads to a tendency for recurrent hives.

Diagnosis

Tests for the presence of a specific complement component are of two types:

1. Immunochemical: This uses purified antibody to a specific complement component, usually in a single radial immunodiffusion technique.
2. Hemolytic: In this test all necessary components are added to antibody-coated red cells except the component being measured. The ability of the test serum to supply the missing component, and therefore allow lysis of the red cells, is quantitated. This is a very sensitive assay in which dysfunctional components, by definition, cannot participate. Thus, either absolute or functional deficiency of a complement component will be detected.

Phagocytic System

3

The phagocytic cell system comprises neutrophils and monocytes/macrophages. The primary function of the phagocytic system is engulfment and killing of microbial organisms. The reticuloendothelial system, especially the spleen, also plays a vital role in filtering pathogenic organisms from the blood. Phagocytosis is greatly enhanced by opsonization of the organisms with antibody and complement.

Phagocytic cell disorders can be classified into (1) disorders of numbers, i.e., quantitative disorders, or (2) disorders of function. These could affect leukocyte movement, the capacity of the leukocyte to engulf particles, or its ability to generate intracellular killing activity.

QUANTITATIVE DISORDERS

Adequate numbers of neutrophils are required for normal host defenses. When the absolute neutrophil count falls below 500/mm^3, susceptibility to infection increases greatly (Bodey et al, 1966). This fall can occur secondary to antimetabolite therapy, or to autoimmune disease with antineutrophil antibodies or T cells that inhibit granulocyte maturation. Neutropenia may be congenital (Kostman syndrome, Shwachman syndrome) or may occur in cycles of every 15–35 days (cyclic neutropenia). Bone marrow transplantation has been successful in children with congenital neutropenia (see pp. 528).

QUALITATIVE DISORDERS

Defects in Chemotaxis

Basic Science

In the absence of specific antibody or in response to antibody of certain subclass specificity, microorganisms can generate C3a and C5a from C3 and C5 in serum by activating the incompletely defined alternate complement pathway or properdin system. Nonspecific proteases released from bacteria or damaged tissue can attack C3 and C5 directly to yield C3a and C5a. Aggregating platelets also release a protein that generates a chemotactic factor from C5. Since both the classic and alternate complement pathways and the nonspecific proteases act on C3 and C5, these proteins are absolutely required for the chemotactic activity of complement.

Neutrophils rapidly enter inflammatory foci, whereas monocytes enter more slowly. Greater mobility underlies the prompt response of neutrophils to chemotactic stimulation relative to monocytes.

Natural History and Diagnosis

Defective chemotaxis results in superficial infections of skin and mucous membranes. Once bacteria invade the blood stream they are efficiently cleared by resident phagocytic cells. The diagnosis of defective chemotaxis can be made easily by the bedside Rebuck skin window which involves scraping the skin, placing a coverslip on the area and looking 4 hours and 24 hours later for the presence of exuded neutrophils and macrophages, respectively.

A rare condition has been described in children with neutropenia, depressed neutrophil mobility, and recurrent infection; this constellation of findings was termed the "lazy leukocyte syndrome." Abnormal chemotactic responsiveness was found in two children with mannosidosis (Desnick et al, 1976).

Disorders of chemotaxis can be secondary, as a consequence of circulating inhibitors. Inhibitors of granulocyte chemotactic responsiveness have been identified in patients with Hodgkin disease and with hepatic cirrhosis. Abnormal granulocyte chemotaxis also has been identified in patients with "immotile cilia syndrome" and with Shwachman syndrome.

Defects in Phagocytosis

Basic Science

The prototype of these diseases is deficiency of a family of three leukocyte cell adhesion molecules (LeuCAM). Three cell surface molecules have been described. MO1 (on monocytes), LFA1 (lymphocyte functional antigen on T cells and B cells), and P150/90 (on monocytes). These molecules are dimers with a shared beta chain. They are all involved in cell-cell adhesion. MO1 has been shown to be the receptor for the fragment of the third component of complement (C3bi) and its expression is essential for bacterial phagocytosis, chemotaxis and adherence. LFA1 is important for T cell-monocyte interaction. The function of P150/95 is unknown.

Natural History

A syndrome has been discussed in which the common B chain of these three adhesion molecules is not expressed. Patients with this syndrome have severe recurrent pyogenic infections. Delayed separation of the umbilical cord was noted in some of these patients.

Diagnosis

The diagnosis is made by demonstrating absence of MO1 antigen by fluorescence technique and by the failure of the neutrophils to ingest opsonized bacteria efficiently.

Treatment

Treatment consists of chronic administration of antibiotics and in severe cases, of bone marrow transplantation.

Prognosis

The severity of the defect is variable. Cases with the lowest expression (<1% of normal) of Leu-CAM suffer the most severe, recurrent, potentially fatal, infections.

Defects in Intracellular Killing: Chronic Granulomatous Disease

Definition

The prototype of these defects is chronic granulomatous disease. Opsonized bacteria undergo phagocytosis but the mechanism for producing superoxide, which is needed for intracellular killing, is defective. This results in deep-seated bacterial infections, pneumonias, and abscesses.

Basic Science

The gene that is abnormal in the X-linked form of the phagocytic chronic granulomatous disease has been cloned without reference to a specific protein by relying on its chromosomal map position (Royer-Pokora et al, 1986). The transcript of the gene is expressed in the phagocytic lineage of hematopoietic cells and is absent or structurally abnormal in four patients with the disorder. The nucleotide sequence of complementary DNA clones predicts a polypeptide of at least 468 amino acids with no homology to proteins described previously. The protein has an estimated molecular mass of, at a minimum, 54 kilodaltons, is probably basic, and must play an important role in the respiratory burst of neutrophils.

Epidemiology

About 500 children with this condition have been described in the medical literature. Although it is clearly underreported, the condition is still extremely rare. It is usually inherited in an X-linked recessive manner. Sporadic cases can occur from deletions of a segment of the X-chromosome.

Natural History

The organisms that pose the greatest problems are those that do not produce hydrogen peroxide and/or produce the enzyme catalase, which converts hydrogen peroxide to water and oxygen. Such organisms include staphylococci, *Klebsiella, Serratia, Salmonella,* and certain fungi, like *Aspergillus* and *Candida.* Organisms that produce their own hydrogen peroxide, including streptococci, pneumococci, *Haemophilus influenzae,* and meningococci do not cause problems. When the offending organism is not killed in the neutrophil, more neutrophils and macrophages are summoned to the scene and form a granuloma, hence the name of the disease. Histologically, the granulomas are full of pigmented, lipid-filled histiocytes. When they achieve sufficient size, they can cause obstruction in and around various lumens.

Patients with chronic granulomatous disease have severe infections accompanied by generalized granulomatous processes and hypergammaglobulinemia. The earliest lesions are staphylococcal infections of skin around the ears and nose. Hepatosplenomegaly is a constant finding, suggesting spread of bacteria to the reticuloendothelial system. Pulmonary disorders occur in nearly all children with the disease and include hilar lymphadenopathy, bronchopneumonia, empyema, and lung abscess.

Gastrointestinal disorders are frequent in patients with chronic granulomatous disease and include obstruction, perianal fistula, vitamin B_{12} malabsorption, and steatorrhea. Rectal and jejunal biopsies may reveal characteristic histiocytes. Osteomyelitis, particularly of the small bones of the hands or feet, occurs frequently. Patients are especially susceptible to fungal infections. *Aspergillus* is encountered most frequently in these patients and is associated with pneumonia, osteomyelitis and soft tissue lesions.

Diagnosis

Chronic granulomatous disease is distinguished by an inability of leukocytes to change nitroblue tetrazolium (NBT) from colorless to deep blue during phagocytosis (NBT test).

Treatment

The management of patients with chronic granulomatous disease includes appropriate antibiotic therapy to treat bacterial infection and surgical drainage of suppurative lesions. Prophylactic treatment with antibiotics helps decrease the number of infections. Bone marrow transplantation has been successful in correcting the defect (see also pp. 532).

Chediak-Higashi Syndrome

This syndrome is inherited in an autosomal recessive manner (see pp. 531). It consists of partial albinism, hypopigmentation, recurrent fever and infection (most often with *S. aureus),* and abnormal leukocyte morphology. Phagocytosis is normal but bactericidal killing of *S. aureus, Streptococcus,* and *Pneumococcus* is decreased, more so in polymorphonuclear cells than in monocytes.

Natural History

There is anemia, hypersplenism, and abnormal platelet function. An accelerated lymphomatous phase is observed, with hepatosplenomegaly, lymphadenopathy, neutropenia, anemia, and perivascular infiltra-

CASE ILLUSTRATION

A 17-month-old boy had been diagnosed with chronic granulomatous disease as a newborn, since an older brother had died at 8 years of generalized aspergillosis from that disorder. The patient was admitted because of being profoundly underweight, pale, and wasted.

The patient had been treated with prophylactic antibiotics, and during the first year of life experienced very few problems.

At about 11 months of age he was noted to have intermittent episodes of vomiting, which were neither bilious nor bloody, and unassociated with fever. Nevertheless, from that time he failed to gain weight and was admitted for evaluation of that problem.

On physical examination his weight was less than the fifth percentile. He appeared wasted, irritable, and chronically ill. The liver was palpable at the right costal margin, but there was no splenomegaly. No abdominal masses were felt. Laboratory studies revealed hematocrit of 34%, reticulocyte count of 4%, white blood count of 19,100 mm^3, 43% polys, 43% lymphs, 4% monos, 5% eos, and 4% atypical lymphs. Platelets were normal, sedimentation rate was 22 mm/hr. The rest of the examination and laboratory studies were unrewarding, except to document that indeed enough calories had been provided, but there were significant losses because of the postprandial vomiting.

QUESTION AND COMMENT

What is the etiology of this patient's vomiting? How would you further evaluate the symptoms?

An upper gastrointestinal series was performed and showed severe gastric antral narrowing, a fairly common complication of chronic granulomatous disease. Granulomas form in an annular manner around the antrum of the stomach and set up a significant inflammatory reaction.

The youngster was treated with liquid enteral feedings through a nasogastric tube and intravenous antibiotics. Gradually his vomiting subsided and he was able to absorb enough nutrients to begin to gain weight.

It was of concern whether the degree of malnutrition could be explained on the basis of chronic infection or whether additional possible causes should be pursued vigorously. Although it was unlikely that chronic infection itself would have been responsible for severe inanition, it was responsible for producing obstruction of the antrum of the stomach which, in turn, by causing vomiting, led to the extreme weight loss. In the absence of a previously established diagnosis of chronic granulomatous disease, the differential would have included gastric ulcer, Crohn disease, even leukemic infiltration, lymphosarcoma, tuberculosis, and granulomas.

Some patients with chronic granulomatous disease have malnutrition attributable to a persistent diarrhea with associated malabsorption. Fungal and bacterial overgrowth may be present in the intestinal tract, with microabscesses throughout the large and small bowel. Sometimes the diarrhea can be ascribed to *Clostridium difficile* infection associated with the chronic use of oral antibiotics. None of the latter were seen in this patient.

tion. Death occurs as a result of infection (65%), bleeding (15%), both (15%), or respiratory failure due to the lymphohistiocytic and reticular cell infiltrates. In some cases, cyclic AMP levels in leukocytes are low.

Treatment

Ascorbic acid and agents that increase cyclic AMP have been reported to be beneficial in some patients. Bone marrow transplantation after ablative therapy results in correction of the defects.

MANAGEMENT OF THE CHILD WITH RECURRENT INFECTIONS

The diagnostic evaluation of the child with recurrent infections depends to a great extent on the severity and frequency of infections, on what types of infections are occurring, and on what diagnostic categories are being considered. For example, in patients with severe and recurrent disease, one proceeds with testing including sophisticated procedures until a diagnosis can be made. On the other hand, in patients with recurrent infection with limited morbidity, initial screening tests are sufficient. Normal tests are reassuring suggesting that immune dysfunction is not present. Nonspecific tests such as a complete blood count, differential, and erythrocyte sedimentation rate are helpful as first steps. Nonimmunologic diseases should not be overlooked and tests such as sweat electrolytes should be performed.

Clinical Features Associated with Immunodeficiency

Because of the similarities of each isolated infection in normal and in immune deficient children, how does one identify the patient likely to have real disease?

First, the patient with immune deficiency differs from a normal child in that when the former develops a viral upper respiratory infection, complications from that infection invariably occur, i.e., a secondary bacterial otitis media or sinusitis occurs. This secondary infection may occur in normal hosts, but with a much lower frequency. The immunologically normal child recovers completely from these infections within several days, whereas the immune compromised child has symptoms which often persist for weeks or months.

Second, in children with true immunodeficiency, there is accrual of morbidity from the repetitive infections. For example, scarring of tympanic membranes may occur with repeated otitis media. Perforation of the tympanic membrane, chronic ear drainage, hearing loss, pulmonary scarring and restrictive lung disease, clubbing, chronic recurrent conjunctivitis may also occur. The patient may appear chronically ill, irritable, lethargic, with chronic purulent nasal discharge, chronic cough, or with chronic rales or rhonchi.

Third, the patient with immune deficiency may present with severe infection, which may be recurrent. Normal children may develop one episode of severe infection; however, recurrence is very suggestive of immunodeficiency.

Fourth, the patient with immune deficiency may present unusually, for example, with recurrent meningitis, recurrent sepsis, or osteomyelitis, or with unusual reactions to live vaccines.

Fifth, uncommonly encountered agents may cause infection, such as fungi, protozoa, viruses, mycobacteria, or Gram-negative bacteria, or bacteria that are ordinarily not pathogens.

Other diagnostic features include other family members who may have had recurrent infections or a family history that may include childhood death. Chronic diarrhea and malabsorption are common in immunodeficiency. Hepatosplenomegaly and arthritis may be present. Ataxia may be present suggesting ataxia telangiectasia, neonatal tetany, and cardiac disease may have occurred suggesting DiGeorge syndrome, petechiae may be present suggesting Wiskott-Aldrich syndrome, chromosomal trisomy 21 may be present suggesting Down syndrome in which a subtle T-cell deficiency is often present. Any persistent rash that is unusual often is the presenting symptom in immunodeficiency.

Diagnosis

If the frequency or severity of infections are significant, then the following laboratory tests are useful (Table 16.5).

Tests for B-cell Function

Indications

Recurrent sinopulmonary infections occur with B-cell deficiency. The extent of disease should be confirmed, e.g., with sinus or chest radiographs. If parents belong to high risk group for AIDS, HIV antibody should be checked.

Immunoglobulin Levels

Total protein/albumin levels are useful in interpreting low immunoglobulin levels. Low albumin suggests low synthetic rate for all proteins or increased loss of proteins, e.g., protein losing enteropathy or loss through skin disease. High levels of immunoglobulin suggests intact immunity, e.g., CGD, or immotile cilia syndrome, and very high levels suggest AIDS.

Specific antibody levels

Antibody levels to tetanus, diphtheria, ASLO, isohemagglutinins are measured. High titers to antigens such as tetanus or diphtheria (after immunization) indicate the ability to make antibody and rule out severe B cell dysfunction which is seen in diseases such as X-linked agammaglobulinemia, and acquired aggammaglobulinemia. Patients with transient hypogammaglobulemia and IgG subclass deficiency have normal titers to potent protein antigens, such as tetanus or diphtheria toxoids. However, patients with IgG subclass deficiency have impaired responses to bacterial polysaccharide antigens.

IgG Subclass Levels

Few laboratories can give reliable results. In the face of normal total IgG levels and significant recurrent sinopulmonary infection, IgG subclass deficiency should be ruled out.

Table 16.5
Evaluation of Immunodeficiency

Suspected Abnormality	Diagnostic Studies: Initial	Diagnostic Studies: Confirmatory or Addition
Humoral defect		
Antibody deficiency	Serum immunoglobulins	IgG subclones Antibody levels and response to immunization with tetanus, Hib B cell number, in vitro synthesis of immunoglobulins
Defect of cell-mediated immunity	Delayed-hypersensitivity skin tests, lymphocyte counts, chest film for thymic shadow	Lymphocyte response to mitogens and antigens, Total T cells and T-cell subsets IL2 receptor expression and IL2 synthesis
Complement deficiency	Complement hemolytic titer (CH_{50})	Individual component determinations
Phagocyte defect		
Neutropenia	White cell and differential counts	Examination of marrow, hematologic studies
Abnormal chemotaxis	Leukocyte migration	Inflammatory Rebuck skin window, blood smear
Cellular defect of phagocytosis	Phagocytosis assay	Phagocyte bacterial killing, MO1 profile
Intracellular killing (CGD)	Nitroblue tetrazolium test Phagocyte bacterial killing	Phagocyte bacterial killing, blood smear (Chediak-Higashi)

Enumeration of Peripheral Blood B Cells

Absence of lymphocytes expressing surface antibody suggests severe immune deficiency such as X-linked agammaglobulinemia.

Test for T-Cell Function

Indications

Recurrent fungal infections, recurrent sinopulmonary infections, severe infections, opportunistic infections, or ataxia-telangiectasia are indications for T-cell function testing.

Complete Blood Count, Differential

Lymphopenia is suggestive of T-cell disorder. Thrombocytopenia and platelets with small size suggest Wiskott-Aldrich syndrome.

Chest Radiographs

Absence of a thymic shadow may indicate T-cell disease.

Delayed Skin Tests—Tetanus Toxoid, Monilia

These tests are often misinterpreted. The site should be observed 48–72 hours after placement for induration. Erythema may be present but is not sufficient for a positive result. Induration at 12–24 hours is also not sufficient since this is usually the result of an Arthus reaction and does not reflect T cell function. Negative tests are seen in 10–30% of normals, and in patients on daily steroids. In such cases, the patient may be boosted with tetanus toxoid, and the skin test can be repeated 7 days later. A positive skin test when read properly rules out serious T-cell deficiency.

Enumeration of T-Cell Numbers with Monoclonal Antibody and Flow Cytometry (T-cell Subsets)

T-cell numbers are decreased in many T-cell deficiencies. T-helper/suppressor cell numbers are abnormal in transient hypogammaglobulinemia, in AIDS, and in many disorders of immunoregulation.

Functional T-Cell Studies

Proliferation to mitogens (phytohemagglutinin [PHA], pokeweed mitogen [PWM], concanavalin A), and to antigens (tetanus toxoid [TT], diphtheria toxoid, monilia), or to alloantigens (MLR) indicates intact T-cell function. Responses to TT require prior immunization. Loss of the response to PHA invariably indicates severe T cell deficiency, e.g., SCID. The PWM response is often the first mitogen response lost in AIDS. Poor responses to TT are occasionally seen in normal individuals.

Tests for Complement

Indications

Recurrent Bacterial Infection

A C3 level is often sufficient to rule out complement deficiency as a cause of recurrent infection. In the case of recurrent *Neisseria* infection, test for total hemolytic activity is helpful (CH50), to rule out deficiency of C5, C6, C7, or C8. If the CH50 is low, deter-

CASE ILLUSTRATION

The patient is an 11-month-old male with recurrent episodes of otitis media, persistent nasal symptoms and cough. At 2 months of age, he developed bronchiolitis with cough, wheezing, associated with otitis media. Symptoms resolved after several days on antibiotics. At 3 months of age, symptoms of cough and wheezing returned. Purulent ocular discharge began, accompanied with purulent nasal discharge, and irritability. These symptoms improved slowly over several weeks but recurred at 4 months of age. Otitis media was then diagnosed and was treated with 10 days of antibiotics. Since then, he has had recurrent episodes of otitis, occurring as often as every 2–3 weeks, associated with cough, nasal discharge, occasionally with mild fever.

COMMENT

This history may or may not be that of an immunologically abnormal child. The series of episodes of otitis beginning at 4 months of age may be a single persistent infection treated for an inadequate period of time. This patient should be treated with a long course of antibiotics until the infection is completely eradicated.

Nonimmunologic reasons for recurrent infection should also be sought. For example, are the parents heavy smokers, is there evidence of allergic disease, is anatomic disease likely?

With regard to immunologic disease, the degree to which such a diagnosis is pursued with diagnostic studies depends on whether the patient has accrued morbidity from recurrent infection: Is he growing? Is his development normal? Are his tympanic membranes scarred or perforated? Is the chest radiograph abnormal? If the morbidity is minimal, the following *screening* tests can be performed to rule out immunologic disease:

1. Complete blood count, differential, erythrocyte sedimentation rate
2. Quantitative immunoglobulins
3. Measurement of a specific antibody response (e.g., to tetanus toxoid)
4. Delayed type skin test (e.g., to tetanus toxoid, monilia).

Further testing will depend on the results of the screening tests and on whether or not infections/and or morbidity continue to occur, despite prophylactic antibiotics. In this case, no evidence of immunodeficiency was found on screening.

mination of levels of specific complement components is indicated.

Angioedema

C4 levels are invariably reduced in hereditary angioneurotic edema, and this can be used as a screening test. C2 levels are reduced in acute attacks of HANE. The diagnosis is confirmed by determination of C1 INH levels.

Tests for Phagocytic Function

Indications

Patients with chronic, recurrent bacterial infections, e.g., perianal abscesses, especially if normal B and T cell function have been documented, should have tests for phagocytic function.

Nitroblue Tetrazolium Test

This test is abnormal in chronic granulomatous disease. The normal increase in metabolic activity of granulocytes following phagocytosis reduces NBT to purple formazan. Leukocytes from patients with CGD cannot reduce NBT in the normal fashion.

Leukocyte Mobility

A rebuck skin window is performed by abraiding the skin and placing a coverslip on the skin. After several hours, the coverslip is examined for infiltrating neutrophils. Absence of neutrophils indicates failure of neutrophil chemotaxis.

Other

Complete blood count may reveal neutropenia, bone marrow is useful to evaluate neutropenia, examination of neutrophils and monocytes for expression of Mo-1/LFA-1 antigen to rule out Mo-1/LFA-1 deficiency.

Principles of Treatment of Immunocompromised Children 4

The following points should be kept in mind in managing patients with immune deficiency.

1. Avoid transfusion with blood products, since donor lymphocytes may cause lethal graft-versus-host disease in immunocompromised hosts. When blood products are required, they should be irradiated before use to prevent graft-versus-host disease.
2. Avoid live virus vaccines (polio virus, measles, mumps, rubella, BCG) especially in patients with T-cell deficiencies, and avoid live polio virus vaccine in patients with severe agammaglobulinemia.
3. Prophylactic antibiotics. In children with antibody deficiency syndrome and sinopulmonary infections of mild-to-moderate severity, a trial of prophylactic antibiotics is often used. Single daily doses of amoxicillin trimethoprim/sulfamethoxazole, are used. The prophylactic antibiotics usually are needed from October to May in the United States.
4. Chronic diarrhea in children with immunodeficiency is often due to *Giardia* and/or to subsequent lactase deficiency, which can be diagnosed by a lactase breath test. Examination of stools for bacteria and parasites, especially *Giardia*, is useful. Dietary restriction and appropriate antimicrobials and γ-globulin are effective.
5. Replacement γ-globulin. Human γ-globulin is derived from pooled human plasma and, therefore, contains all the antibodies normally occurring in the donor population. γ-Globulin may be administered by the intramuscular or by the intravenous route. Preparations are not interchangeable, however; those intended for intramuscular use cannot be given intravenously since they contain aggregates of IgG that can cause anaphylaxis.

   Intramuscular γ-globulin contains little IgA or IgM. It is administered at a dose of 0.6–0.7 ml/kg (100 mg/kg every 3–4 weeks), with a loading dose of three times the maintenance dose. The administration of intramuscular γ-globulin may be associated with adverse reactions (fever, chills). Rarely, anaphylactic reactions may occur, especially in patients with IgA deficiency.

   Intravenous γ-globulin has several advantages over intramuscular γ-globulin. Higher doses can be given, therefore achieving higher serum levels and better protection against infection. Also, it is relatively painless. On the other hand, it is time-consuming (3–4 hours). The loading dose is 400 mg/kg, and the maintenance dose is 200–300 mg/kg, which is given every 3–4 weeks. Reactions to intravenous γ-globulin are generally mild, with fever, chills, and rarely a drop in blood pressure. These reactions usually can be avoided by slower infusion (6–8 hours) and pretreatment with diphenhydramine and aspirin.

6. Bone marrow transplantation. Immunodeficiency syndromes in which the T cells are defective (e.g., severe combined immunodeficiency, Wiskott-Aldrich syndrome), or in which the phagocytic cells are affected (e.g., chronic granulomatous disease) are treated with bone marrow transplantation. Bone marrow is harvested from a histocompatible donor and infused into the patient. Residual immune function in the recipient must be ablated before transplant to allow engraftment. Complications of bone marrow transplantation include infection and graft-versus-host disease. Bone marrow transplants from haploidentical donors have been used successfully when the marrow has been rigorously depleted of mature T cells, which can cause fatal graft-versus-host disease (Table 16.6).

Table 16.6
Estimated Experience from Bone Marrow Transplants for Correction of Primary Immune Deficiency 1968–1986 (Worldwide)[1]

Defect	HLA Identical Total	HLA Identical Surviving	%	HLA Mismatched Total	HLA Mismatched Surviving	%
Severe T-cell deficiency	132	105	80	167	97	58
Wiskott-Aldrich syndrome	41	33	80	13	3	23
Leu-CAM	2	1	50	2	2	100
Chediak-Higashi	5	4	80	2	0	0
Chronic granulomatous disease	6	1	17	0	0	0
Total	186	144	77%	184	102	55%

[1]Modified from Buckley RH: *Pediatr Ann* 16:420, 1987.

Hypersensitivity Reactions 5

Hypersensitivity reactions represent tissue injury on the basis of an immune response. There are four basic types. Type 1 is the immediate or anaphylactic type, type 2 the cytotoxic type, type 3 the immune complex or arthus type, and type 4 a delayed hypersensitivity reaction. Each of these types of hypersensitivity reactions is dealt with briefly below.

TYPE 1 HYPERSENSITIVITY

Basic Science

Type 1 hypersensitivity is mediated by IgE, an immunoglobulin that is cell-bound to the basophil or mast cell. When an antigen is encountered by these cells, the molecules of IgE cross-link and, in doing so, stimulate mediator release with the assistance of intracellular calcium in the basophil, or matachromatic granules in the mast cell. These mediators result in smooth muscle contraction, vasodilation, edema, mucous secretion, vascular leakage, and pruritus (Serafin and Austen, 1987).

Some of the mediators during an anaphylactic or immediate hypersensitivity response include histamine and other chemotactic factors that will draw eosinophils or polymorphonuclear neutrophils to the site of an antigen antibody reaction, thus producing the tissue inflammation. In addition, these immediate mediators are responsible for the formation of prostaglandin-generating and platelet-activating mediators, which subsequently cause rapid platelet aggregation with sequestration of platelets in involved tissues, especially the lung with subsequent vaso- and bronchoconstriction. The formation of prostaglandins leads to smooth muscle contraction and increased vascular permeability along with increased infiltration by polymorphonuclear neutrophils. Leukotrienes can also be formed in a later phase along with the prostaglandin and platelet activating factors of the type 1 hypersensitivity reaction. These too will lead to smooth muscle contraction in pulmonary airways and are responsible for what was once termed the slow-reacting substance of anaphylaxis.

Epidemiology

Type 1 hypersensitivity reactions are clinically manifest as allergic disease including rhinitis, asthma, and drug allergy. Systemic anaphylaxis is the most serious consequence of type 1 hypersensitivity reactions. The most common causes for anaphylaxis include some antibiotics, in particular, the penicillins and the cephalosporins. Contrast media used for radiologic studies may also result in an anaphylactoid response. The food groups that have the highest incidence of causing anaphylaxis include fish and shell fish in particular, nuts, milk, and eggs. Exercise and aspirin have also been associated with increased risk of an immediate hypersensitivity reaction.

Natural History

The immediate clinical manifestations of anaphylactic or type 1 hypersensitivity reaction can involve the cutaneous manifestations of diffuse flushing and generalized urticaria with angioedema. Respiratory manifestions include allergic rhinitis, laryngeal edema, bronchospasm, and even respiratory arrest. Cardiovascular changes (in particular, hypotension and tachycardia) and gastrointestinal signs and symptoms including nausea, vomiting, abdominal pain, and diarrhea are also associated with type 1 hypersensitivity.

The delayed phenomenon of a hypersensitivity reaction usually occurs 2–48 hours following the initial antigen antibody exposure and manifests itself as giant hives and angioedema as well as continued generalized anaphylaxis as described above. These late phase reactions differ from the immediate response by a lack of production of some prostaglandins and generation of smaller amounts of kinins.

Treatment

Respiration and circulation must be attended to in any child experiencing anaphylaxis. If there is compromise of the airway, epinephrine at a dose of .01 ml/kg of a 1:1000 solution can be administered subcutaneously, while oxygen is simultaneously being administered. If an insect bite has caused an anaphylactic reaction, a tourniquet applied proximal to a bite on an extremity may result in delayed release of the allergic substance. Once improvement has been noted, other antihistimine agents such as diphenhydramine given at a dose of 1–2 ml/kg every 6 hours for 48 hours can be useful to suppress any further flare-up of the hypersensitivity. Hypotension may require treatment with intravenous fluids in order to stabilize blood pressure. Bronchospasm may benefit from the use of aminophyllin and, if anaphylaxis is severe, tracheal intubation and intravenous vasopressors may also be useful.

Prevention and Prognosis

It is very important that every attempt be made to determine the specific allergen that is responsible for the anaphylactic episode so that further re-exposure can be avoided. Some specific allergens can be evaluated by RAST testing or by specific skin testing to allergens. If penicillin is suspected as the cause for anaphylaxis then skin testing can confirm sensitivity. Patients who are allergic to penicillin may be able to undergo desensitization to the allergen although this procedure is usually done by an experienced immunologist or allergist. If an insect sting has resulted in anaphylaxis then it is important that these children be given an anaphylaxis kit and wear medical alert identification. These kits allow immediate administration of epinephrine should a repeat episode occur. Patients allergic to contrast dye may benefit from pretreatment with diphenhydramine and corticosteroids to avoid an anaphylactic reaction.

TYPE 2 HYPERSENSITIVITY

Type 2 hypersensitivity reactions are cytotoxic ones that result in the death of a target cell carrying the antigen responsible for the reaction. It is usually a result of the linkage of an IgG molecule (and occasionally an IgM) to the antigen with subsequent binding of the Fc fragment of the immunoglobulin by a receptor on an "effector" cell, which can be either a polymorphonuclear phagocyte (requiring the assistance of complement) or a mononuclear phagocyte with subsequent phagocytosis and lysis of the target cell. There is also a subpopulation of lymphoid cells called killer cells which can also interact with IgM antibody which can also serve as an effector cell for a type 2 hypersensitivity reaction.

A classic example of a type 2 hypersensitivity reaction is hemolysis on the basis of ABO incompatibility or Rh incompatibility. In addition, this type of reaction may lead to destruction of skin cells of the dermal epidermal junction otherwise known as pemphigus or may result in nephrotoxicity with reactions of both pulmonary and glomerular basement membrane (as seen in Goodpasture syndrome).

TYPE 3 HYPERSENSITIVITY

Type 3 hypersensitivity is an immune complex hypersensitivity in which circulating antigen antibody complexes are formed through the help of IgG1 or IgG3, subsequently resulting in complement fixation and then deposition of the total immune complex into the endothelium of blood vessels. The complement system acts as a chemotactic mediator and draws polymorphonuclear neutrophils to the area of the immune complex deposition, which then phagocytose these complexes and release lysosomal enzymes; these enzymes go on to damage endothelial surfaces as well as platelets resulting in increased vascular permeability and further vascular endothelial injury.

The characteristic type 3 hypersensitivity reaction is the vasculitis and arthus phenomenon in which a previously sensitized individual is re-exposed to an antigen that leads to antibody production and subsequent vasculitis, localized edema and swelling within 1–2 hours of exposure to the antigen, with maximum reaction seen 3–6 hours and then diminishing after 10–12 hours.

Endogenous antigens may include such molecules as DNA which can result in an autoimmune disorder like systemic lupus erythematosus. Exogenous antigens may include infectious agents such as viruses, bacteria, fungi or drugs. One common immune complex disorder is poststreptococcal glomerulonephritis which results from streptococcal antigen exposure and immune complex deposition in the glomerular membrane.

TYPE 4 SENSITIVITY

Type 4 sensitivity is cell-mediated immunity. It results when certain types of T cells become sensitized to antigens resulting in the release of lymphokines, which are mitogenic or lymphocyte transforming factors that lead to blast transformation and lymphocyte proliferation. Response usually requires 48–72 hours and, hence, the type 4 is referred to as a delayed hypersensitivity reaction. The cell-mediated hypersensitivity reaction is usually mediated by sensitized lymphocytes from the T8 or suppressor subset.

Examples of type 4 hypersensitivity reactions include the Mantoux tuberculin test which turns positive after 48 hours if there is sensitivity to the purified protein derivative. Poison ivy also develops on the basis of a delayed hypersensitivity reaction. Transplantation rejection and graft rejection also result from cell-mediated immunity.

REFERENCES

Agnello V, DeBracco MME, Kunkel HG: Hereditary C2 deficiency with some manifestations of systemic lupus erythematosus. *J Immunol* 108:837, 1972.

Ambrosino DM, Siber GR, Chilmonczyk BA, et al: An immunodeficiency characterized by impaired antibody responses to polysaccharides. *N Engl J Med* 316:790, 1987.

Ambrosino DM, Umetsu DT, Siber GR, et al: Selective defect in the antibody response to *Haemophilus influenzae* type B in children with recurrent infections and normal IgG subclass groups. *J Allergy Clin Immunol* June, 1988.

Ballow M, Cates KL, Rowe JC, et al: Development of the immune system in very low birth weight (less than 1500 g) premature infants: Concentrations of plasma immunoglobulins and patterns of infections. *Pediatr Res* 20:899, 1986.

Berkel AI, Loos M, Sanal O, et al: Clinical and immunological studies in a case of selective complete Clq deficiency. *Clin Exp Immunol* 38:52, 1979.

Bodey GB, Buckley M, Sathe YS, et al: Quantitative relationships between circulating leukocytes and infection in patients with acute leukemia. *Ann Intern Med* 64:328, 1966.

Borut TC, Ank BJ, Gard SE, et al: Tetanus toxoid skin test in children: Correlation with in vitro lymphocyte stimulation and monocyte chemotaxis. *J Pediatr* 97:567, 1980.

Bruce RM, Blaese RM: Monoclonal gammopathy in the Wiskott-Aldrich syndrome. *J Pediatr* 85:204, 1974.

Buckley RH, Wray BB, Belmaker EZ: Extreme hyperimmunoglobulinemia E and undue susceptibility to infection. *Pediatrics* 49:59, 1972.

Burks AW, Sampson HA, Buckley RH: Anaphylactic reactions after gamma globulin administration in patients with hypogammaglobulinemia. *N Engl J Med* 314:560, 1986.

Clavelli TA, Rubinstein A: Intravenous gamma-globulin in infant acquired immunodeficiency syndrome. *Pediatr Infect Dis* 5:S207, 1986.

Cleveland WW, Fogel BJ, Brown WT, et al: Foetal thymic transplant in a case of DiGeorge's syndrome. *Lancet* 2:1211, 1968.

Conley ME, Brown P, Pickard AR, et al: Expression of the gene defect in X-linked agammaglobulinemia. *N Engl J Med* 315:564, 1986.

Cooper MD: Pre-B cells: Normal and abnormal development. *J Clin Immunol* 1:81, 1981.

Cunningham-Rundles, et al: Efficacy of intravenous immunoglobulin in primary humoral immunodeficiency disease. *Ann Intern Med* 101:435, 1984.

Desnick RJ, Sharp HL, Grabowski GA, et al: Mannosidosis: Clinical, morphologic, immunologic, and biochemical studies. *Pediatr Res* 10:985, 1976.

Eliasson R, Mossberg B, Camner P, et al: The immobile cilia syndrome: A congenital ciliary abnormality as an etiologic factor in chronic airway infections and male sterility. *N Engl J Med* 297:1, 1977.

Fineman SM, Rosen FS, Geha RS: Transient hypogammaglobulinemia, elevated immunoglobulin E levels, and food allergy. *J Allergy Clin Immunol* 64:216, 1979.

Fontan G, Lorente F, Rodriguez MCG, et al: Defective neutrophil chemotaxis and hyperimmunoglobulinemia E—a reversible defect? *Acta Paediatr Scand* 65:509, 1976.

Frank MM: Complement in the pathophysiology of human disease. *N Engl J Med* 316:1525, 1987.

Gadek JE, Hosea SW, Gelfand JA, et al: Replacement therapy in hereditary angioedema. *N Engl J Med* 302:542, 1980.

Geha RS, Alami S, Farah F, et al: The B cell defect in hyper IgM immunodeficiency. *J Clin Invest* 64:385, 1979.

Geha RS, Schneeberger E, Merler E, et al: Heterogeneity of "acquired" or common variable agammaglobulinemia. *N Engl J Med* 291:1, 1974.

Gelfand EW, Dosch HM, Biggar WD, et al: Partial purine nucleoside phosphorylase deficiency: Studies of lymphocyte function. *J Clin Invest* 61:1071, 1978.

Gelfand JA, Shlerins RD, Alling DW, et al: Treatment of hereditary angioedema with Danazol. *N Engl J Med* 295:1444, 1976.

Gotoff SP, Smith RD, Sugar O: Dermatomyositis with cerebral vasculitis in a patient with agammaglobulinemia. *Am J Dis Child* 123:53, 1972.

Hausser C, Virelizier JL, Buriot D, et al: Common variable hypogammaglobulinemia in children. *Am J Dis Child* 137:833, 1983.

Henley WL: Hypersensitivity reaction in tissue injury. *Pediatr Ann* 16:422, 1987.

Hong R, Santosham M, Schulte-Wisserman H, et al: Reconstitution of B and T lymphocyte function in severe combined immunodeficiency disease after transplantation with thymic epithelium. *Lancet* 2:1270, 1976.

Johnston RB: Recurrent bacterial infections in children. *N Engl J Med* 310:1237, 1984.

Kaliner M: Hypotheses on the contribution of late-phase allergic responses to the understanding and treatment of allergic diseases. *J Allergy Clin Immunol* 73:311, 1984.

Keightley RG, Lawton AR, Cooper MD, et al: Successful fetal liver transplantation in a child with severe combined immunodeficiency. *Lancet* 2:850, 1975.

Kwan SP, Kunkel L, Bruns G, et al: Mapping of the X-linked agammaglobulinemia locus by use of restriction fragment length polymorphism. *J Clin Invest* 77:649, 1986.

Lammer EJ, Chen DT, Hoar RM, et al: Retinoic acid embryopathy. *N Engl J Med* 313:837, 1985.

Lee TJ, Snyderman R, Patterson J, et al: *Neisseria meningitidis* bacteremia in association with deficiency of the sixth component of complement. *Infect Immunol* 24:656, 1979.

Levitt D, Haber P, Rich K, et al: Hyper IgM immunodeficiency: A primary dysfunction of B lymphocyte isotype switching. *J Clin Invest* 72:1650, 1983.

Lint TF, Zeitz HJ, Scott D, et al: Hereditary deficiency of the ninth component of complement (C) in man. *Clin Res* 26:714A, 1978.

Mease PJ, Ochs HD, Wedgwood RJ: Successful treatment of echovirus meningoencephalitis and myositis-fasciitis with intravenous immune globulin therapy in a patient with X-linked agammaglobulinemia. *N Engl J Med* 304:1278, 1981.

Metzger H: Antibodies as effector molecules. *Harvey Lect* 80:49, 1986.

Metzger H, Kinet J-P: How antibodies work: Focus on F_c receptors. *Fed Am Soc Exp Biol J* 2:3, 1988.

Mold C, Cooper NR, Nemerow GR: Incorporation of the purified Epstein-Barr virus/C3d receptor (CR2) into liposomes and demonstration of its dual ligand binding functions. *J Immunol* 136:4140, 1986.

Nadler LM, Stashenko P, Hardy R, et al: Characterization of a human B cell-specific antigen (B2) distinct from B1. *J Immunol* 126:1941, 1981.

Ochs HD, Ament ME, Davis SD: Giardiasis with malabsorption in X-linked agammaglobulinemia. *N Engl J Med* 287:341, 1972.

Oxelius VA: Chronic infections in a family with hereditary deficiency of IgG2 and IgG4. *Clin Exp Immunol* 17:19, 1974.

Oxelius VA, Berkel AI, Hanson LA: IgG2 deficiency in ataxia-telangiectasia. *N Engl J Med* 306:515, 1982.

Paterson MC, Smith PJ: Ataxia telangiectasia: An inherited human disorder involving hypersensitivity to ionizing radiation and related DNA-damaging chemicals. *Annu Rev Genet* 13:291, 1979.

Raum D, Glass D, Carpenter CB, et al: Mapping of the structural gene for the second component of complement with respect to the human major histocompatibility complex. *Am J Human Genet* 31:35, 1979.

Reinherz EL, Kung PC, Goldstein, et al: Discrete stages of human intrathymic differentiation: Analysis of normal thymocytes and leukemic lymphoblasts of T cell lineage. *J Proc Natl Acad Sci USA* 77:1588, 1980a.

Reinherz EL, Schlossman SF: Current concepts in immunology. *N Engl J Med* 303:370, 1980b.

Reisner Y, Kapoor N, Kirkpatrick D, et al: Transplantation for severe combined immunodeficiency with HLA-A.B.D.Dr incompatible parental marrow cells fractionated by soybean agglutinin and sheep red blood cells. *Blood* 61:341, 1983.

Rick KC Jr, Hurley J, Gewurz H: Inborn Clr deficiency with a mild lupus-like syndrome. *Clin Immunol Immunopathol* 13:77, 1979.

Rieger CHL, Nelson LA, Peri BA, et al: Transient hypogammaglobulinemia of infancy. *J Pediatr* 91:601, 1980.

Rosen FS, Wedgwood RJ, Aiuti F, et al: Primary immunodeficiency diseases: Report prepared for the WHO by a Scientific Group on Immunodeficiency. *Clin Immunol Immunopathol* 28:450, 1983.

Royer-Pokora B, Kunkel LM, Monaco AP, et al: Cloning the gene for an inherited human disorder—chronic granulomatous disease—on the basis of its chromosomal location. *Nature* 322:32, 1986.

Samuelson B: Leukotrienes mediators of immediate hypersensitivity reactions and inflammation. Science 220:568, 1983.

Schur PH, Rosen F, Norman ME: Immunoglobulin subclasses in normal children. *Pediatr Res* 13:181, 1979.

Serafin WE, Austen KF: Mediators of immediate hypersensitivity reactions *N Engl J Med* 317:30, 1987.

Siber GR, Schur PH, Aisenberg AC, et al: Correlation between serum IgG2 concentrations and the antibody response to bacterial polysaccharide antigens. *N Engl J Med* 303:178, 1980.

Sullivan TJ: Pathogenesis and management of allergic reactions to penicillin and other beta-lactan antibiotics. *Pediatr Infect Dis* 1:644, 1982.

Talbot SF, Atkins PC, Goetzl, et al: Accumulation of leukotriene C4 and histamine in human allergic skin reactions. *J Clin Invest* 76:650, 1985.

Tiller TL Jr, Buckley RH: Transient hypogammaglobulinemia of infancy: Review of the literature, clinical and immunologic features of 11 new cases, and long-term follow-up. *J Pediatr* 92:347, 1978.

Tonegawa S: The molecules of the immune system. *Sci Am* 253:122, 1985.

Tsoi MS: Immunological mechanisms of graft-versus-host disease in man. *Transplantation* 33:459, 1982.

Umetsu DT, Ambrosino DM, Quinti I, et al: Recurrent sinopulmonary infection and impaired antibody response to bacterial capsular polysaccharide antigen in children with selective IgG-subclass deficiency. *N Engl J Med* 313:1247, 1985.

Underdown BJ, Schiff JM: Immunoglobulin A: Strategic defense initiative at the mucosal surface. *Ann Rev Immunol* 4:389, 1986.

Waldmann TA, Durm M, Broder S, et al: Role of suppressor T cells in pathogenesis of common variable hypogammaglobulinemia. *Lancet* 2:609, 1974.

Wilson M: Immunology of the fetus and newborn: Lymphocyte phenotype and function. *Clin Immunol Allergy* 5:271, 1985.

Wykoff RF, Pearl ER, Saulsbury FT: Immunologic dysfunction in infants infected through transfusion with HTLV III. *N Engl J Med* 312:294, 1985.

RAIF GEHA
LEWIS FIRST
DALE UMETSU

Consultants
Richard Johnston
Fred Rosen

Portions of the section are taken directly with permission from Chapter 5 by Leung DYM, Rosen FS, and Geha RS; and Chapter 9 by Altenburger KM and Johnston RBJ in Chandra RK (ed): *Primary and Secondary Immunodeficiency Disorders*. New York, Churchill Livingstone, 1983.

Section 17

Infectious Diseases

Infections are such an important cause of illness in children that discussion of aspects of them appear throughout this book, particularly in Neonatology, Pulmonology, Immunology, and Well Child Care. In this section, we have selected some general topics, and a brief review of the principal organisms and illnesses they produce, alphabetically by class (virus, bacteria, fungi, parasite).

Worldwide, the death toll from potentially preventable infectious diseases is staggering. The National Research Council survey of diseases in the third world reported on estimated rates of infectious diseases and assigned a priority for accelerated vaccine development in the following order

Organism	Deaths/year
Streptococcus pneumoniae	10,000,000
Rotavirus diarrhea	900,000
Malaria	2,000,000
Typhoid fever	500,000
Shigella	500,000
Hepatitis B	800,000
Haemophilus influenzae type b	145,000

The field of microbiology has been revolutionized by new concepts in molecular biology, which are beginning to illuminate some aspects of infectious disease and carry promise of producing genetically engineered vaccines. Meanwhile, clinical infectious disease has emerged as an important new subspecialty, as internists and pediatricians are faced with patients who continue to encounter new pathogens, or old pathogens in new suits, or have altered responses to infection. Ever more chemotherapeutic agents are discovered and await clinical trials for efficacy and safety. It is hardly surprising that entire textbooks are now devoted to infectious diseases of infants, or infants and children. A relatively new journal, *Pediatric Infectious Disease* by McCracken and Nelson and published by Williams & Wilkins, has been a help to clinicians who try to keep abreast of new developments, and to this writer who is doing the same. Three textbooks have been particularly helpful: Hanshaw, Dudgeon, and Marshall: *Viral Disease of the Fetus and Newborn,* 2nd edition, Philadelphia, WB Saunders, 1985; Feigin and Cherry: *Textbook of Pediatric Infectious Diseases*. Philadelphia, WB Saunders, 1987; and Marks: *Pediatric Infectious Diseases for the Practitioner*. New York, Springer-Verlag, 1985. The Report of the Committee on Infectious Diseases of the American Academy of Pediatrics, 20th edition 1986, known as the "red book," is an invaluable guide to diagnosis and treatment of infectious diseases.

REFERENCE

Leeper P: Vaccines for the third world. *News Report National Research Council* 36:4, 1986.

General Considerations

1

FEVER

Definition

Fever is an increase in the body temperature because of an elevation in the "set point" above 37.1°C in the hypothalamic thermoregulatory center. Fever can originate from CNS pathology, deficiency in peripheral cooling mechanisms, overproduction of heat as in extreme exercise, or in association with infectious disease.

Basic Science

Fever associated with infection is the response of the CNS to an inflammation. The key mediator in the response is interleukin 1, formerly known as "endogenous pyrogen" or "leukocyte endogenous mediator." The change in name distinguishes it as a monokine derived principally from phagocytic monocytes in contrast to interleukin 2 which is a lymphokine that is released by activated helper T cells (Dinarello, 1984).

Interleukin 1 is released when monocytes come in contact with microorganisms or their products such as endotoxins and exotoxins. In addition to its effect on the hypothalamic temperature regulating centers, it is responsible at least in part for changes in white cell counts and acute phase reactants. A specific inhibitor of interleukin 1 has been identified in urine of febrile patients which suggests the presence of a biofeedback mechanism for regulation of interleukin 1.

Interleukin 1 is thought to act on cell membranes to release arachidonic acid, the precursor of prostaglandins and leukotrienes which are responsible for fever production. Aspirin and cortisone are believed to interfere with prostaglandin synthesis in the hypothalamus itself.

Natural History

When the hypothalamic set point is elevated, the body senses a need to conserve heat and mechanical thermogenesis is accomplished by chills. Peripheral vasoconstriction is evident from cold hands and feet until body temperature reaches the new set point, at which time the patient is comfortable. When the stimulus for fever is withdrawn, peripheral cooling mechanisms come into action. Flushing represents peripheral vasodilation and sweating enhances cooling by evaporation. These reactions have been described as the "crisis" that heralds recovery.

Newborns do not develop as high fevers as older children, and they do not have the capacity for mechanical thermogenesis. When chilled, or when the "set point" for temperature is elevated, they release epinephrine and norepinephrine that stimulates peripheral vasoconstriction and promotes breakdown of triglycerides into fatty acids in brown fat. These responses are termed chemical thermogenesis. One explanation for the relative inability of infants to mount a febrile response is suggested by the decreased ability of monocytes from cord blood to produce interleukin 1 (Dinarello et al, 1981).

Diagnosis

Measurement of body temperature requires assurance that the thermometer is calibrated to read correctly. The best available site to approximate core temperature is the rectum with the lubricated thermometer inserted at least 3 cm above the anal sphincter and left in place until the reading stabilizes which averages 3 minutes. The normal values are 37.8 ±0.5°C with higher values in the evening and lower ones in the morning. Oral temperatures are unreliable unless the patient can cooperate and keep the thermometer under the tongue with mouth closed. In general, oral temperatures are 0.5–1.5°C below rectal values. The axilla is useful for monitoring temperatures in infants, and approximates oral values.

Treatment

The decision to attempt to lower body temperature rests on whether the elevation is thought to be a useful host defense, or the source of discomfort and at high levels a possible cause of brain damage.

In general, elevations of temperature up to 40°C are probably more beneficial than harmful. Some host defenses such as phagocyte mobility and bacteriocidal activity are increased by temperature elevation. When body temperature is over 40°C, about 5% of children will have seizures, and all will be irritable and clearly uncomfortable. For these reasons, gentle interventions to lower temperature are usually undertaken. Simply undressing the child in temperate climates and leaving him naked, or nearly so at ambient temperatures of 23–25°C will ensure a fall in temperature. Tepid water sponging is widely used, but probably has little advantage over undressing. Cold water is to be avoided except in extreme hyperthermia (above 42°C) since it makes the child miserable, and crying and vasoconstriction are counterproductive.

If the temperature is over 40°C, antipyretic drugs are usually prescribed. Acetaminophen is the best tolerated and most effective one available. Aspirin is not recommended for children and adolescents because of the association of Reye syndrome after its use.

General Considerations in a Child with Fever

Fever is the most common manifestation of infection and its presence should bring that possibility to mind at any age. In general, in the first few months of life temperature elevations with infection are low grade. Thereafter young infants can develop very high fevers, often very suddenly. Elevations to 40°C are commonly found with minor respiratory infections, otitis, or infectious diarrhea. Temperatures over 40°C are more commonly associated with more severe illness such as pneumonia or meningitis.

In older children, recurrent high fevers may be associated with rheumatoid arthritis, lupus, or malignancies such as leukemia. Osteomyelitis, Crohn disease or systemic infections such as tuberculosis need to be considered when fever persists or recurs in the absence of obvious explanations.

Not all temperature elevations are the result of disease. Small infants in particular have a reduced capacity to defend themselves from extremes of environmental temperatures and may present on a hot day, wrapped in blankets, with a high fever which promptly falls when the infant is undressed. Vigorous exercise can lead to hyperthermia, sometimes of extreme and dangerous degree as seen in marathoners on a hot day. Further evaluation would depend on a search for specific abnormalities.

Yet another situation in which body temperatures can rise rapidly to lethal levels is known as malignant hyperthermia. Inherited as an autosomal dominant trait, this rare disorder presents after inhalational anesthesia. An abnormal release of calcium from muscle cells activates adenosine triphosphatase and releases heat by uncoupling of oxidative phosphorylation. Mild elevations of creatinine phosphokinase may be found in affected individuals. Treatment is rapid cooling, intravenous fluids to maintain urine output in face of myoglobinuria, and the muscle relaxant dantrolene given intravenously. Prevention is possible with oral dantrolene 4–7 mg/kg the day before anesthesia.

Acute Phase Reactants

Clinicians have come to depend on two readily measured indicators of an inflammatory response, the erythrocyte sedimentation rate (ESR) and the C-reactive protein (CRP). Both measurements depend on the production of a heterogeneous group of proteins that are synthesized primarily in the liver, in response to cellular injury, inflammation, or pregnancy.

The ESR depends primarily on levels of serum fibrinogen. This asymmetric molecule affects erythrocyte aggregation by dampening the repulsive charges on the red cell surface; red cells can then form stacks or rouleaux which sediment in plasma at an increased rate. Abnormalities in size and shape of red cells, as in sickle cells, acanthocytosis, and poikilocytosis interfere with aggregation and prevent an appropriate rise in ESR. Anemia, on the other hand, is associated with a disproportionately elevated ESR. The same events that increase the ESR cause a much greater increase in CRP levels.

Named for the original observation that serum from acutely ill patients contained a substance that precipitated with the C fraction of the capsular polysaccharide of the pneumococcus, CRP has been extensively studied in a number of conditions characterized by injury or inflammation. The low basal blood level of CRP is about 600 ng/ml. The level can double in about 8 hours and rise a thousand-fold within 2 days, as can be demonstrated after surgery.

Elevation of CRP is, at least in part, mediated by interleukin 1 production by macrophages, and to some extent by prostaglandins (Gewurz et al, 1982). Anti-inflammatory drugs such as cortisone and indomethacin diminish CRP levels. The protein itself has many different binding capacities, some of which are calcium dependent, such as phosphocholines that are widely distributed among microbes. Apparently, CRP and its ligand modulate the inflammatory response in a manner analogous to antibodies. Its main function is thought to be the recruitment of complement by the classic, but not alternative pathway. Complexes of CRP and some of its ligands are also platelet activators, stimulating the release of thromboxane A_2.

Formerly, measurement of CRP was time-consuming, and thus, this assay was less applicable to clinical decision making than the ESR. Sensitive immunologic assays are now available, including enzyme-linked immunosorbent assays (ELISA) which should make this indicator of inflammation of much greater clinical usefulness.

Epidemiology

DAY CARE CENTERS

At the present time, about 11 million children in the United States are enrolled in day care centers. Poor hygiene where groups are in close contact allows epidemic spread. Certain organisms thrive under these conditions, particularly those that can survive for extended periods (from hours to weeks) on environmental surfaces. These include rotavirus, hepatitis A virus, and *Giardia lamblia*. Campylobacter has also caused outbreaks of diarrhea. Overall, however, the incidence of infection in most centers is no greater than that found in large families or by exposure to adults who smoke.

Other organisms are particularly important in younger children and immunocompromised hosts. For example, *Haemophilus influenzae* can cause serious disease in infants under 18 months. Cytomegalovirus may be spread by asymptomatic children who shed the virus in their urine and infect others. Infection is usually benign, but may cause illness in the immunocompromised host. Chickenpox is highly communicable and is spread by respiratory droplets or direct contact with secretions. Since about one-third of cases (more than 1 million each year) occur in children under age 5 years, it is important for parents to prevent spread by keeping their children at home until 1 week after the rash first appears. Immunosuppressed individuals should receive varicella zoster immune globulin within 96 hours of exposure. In fact, it is incumbent upon parents to ensure that their children are fully immunized and do not attend the center if they have any sign of illness. Center directors also have the responsibility of ensuring that all the staff members are immunized and that proper hygiene (hand-washing, etc) is practiced. State health officials should be notified promptly if a significant pathogen is isolated from a child who attends the center (see also pp. 51–52).

GENERAL ASPECTS OF ANTIMICROBIAL THERAPY

The use of antimicrobial drugs is so common in pediatrics that it seems pertinent to review some of the general principles in this section. The mechanism of action can be summarized briefly in Table 17.1. The reader is referred to textbooks on pharmacology for more detailed information on mechanism of action and to Koren G, Prober CG, Gold R (eds): *Antimicrobial Therapy in Infants and Children.* New York, Marcel Dekker, Inc., 1988 for an excellent review of this topic.

Antimicrobial drugs are capable of either killing (bacteriocidal), or inhibiting (bacteriostatic) microorganisms. Antibiotics are defined as chemical substances that are produced by certain species of microorganism.

The aim of therapy is to achieve a sufficient concentration of drug to kill the organism without harming the host. The definition of resistance of an organism to an antimicrobial agent is defined by the concentration of the drug required to inhibit or kill the organism that exceeds the concentration that can be tolerated by the host.

Susceptibility of a microbe to a drug depends on a number of factors including the ability of the drug to reach the organism. For intracellular organisms, drugs such as rifampin, chloramphenicol, and trimethoprim are the most active. Common drugs that are excluded from cells are penicillins, cephlosporins, and aminoglycosides. With respect to the environment of the host, sometimes purulent material can bind antibiotics and reduce the effective concentration at the desired site. Furthermore both pH and oxygen tension of the local environment can also influence antimicrobial activity. Anaerobic situations found in some relatively avascular environments of abscesses may lessen the effectiveness of aminoglycosides.

The rate of bacterial killing is dependent not only on the number of bacteria present and the concentration of the drug in the tissue, but also other host defense mechanisms including blood flow to the tissue site and mobilization of monocytes or leukocytes.

Table 17.1
Mechanisms of Action for Antimicrobial Agents

Effect on Microbial Cells	Representative Drug(s)
Inhibition of cell wall synthesis or activation of host enzymes that disrupt cell walls to cause loss of viability	Penicillins, cephalosporins, vancomycin
Increase in cell membrane permeability, resulting in loss of intracellular constituents	Amphotericin B
Altered function of ribosomes, causing disruption of protein synthesis (reversible inhibition)	Chloramphenicol, tetracyclines, erythromycin, lincomycin, clindamycin
Binding of drug to ribosomes, causing misreading of mRNA code and production of abnormal polypeptides	Aminoglycosides
Disruption of nucleic acid metabolism	Rifampin, metronidazole
Blocking of essential metabolism events critical to microorganism (antimetabolites)	Trimethoprim, sulfonamides, metronidazole

Testing of microbial sensitivity involves ascertainment of the lowest concentration of the antimicrobial agent that prevents visible growth of microorganisms after 18–24 hours of incubation (the minimum inhibitory concentration or MIC). The lowest drug concentration that results in nearly total killing of bacteria is known as minimum bacteriocidal concentration (MBC).

The choice of an antimicrobial agent requires knowledge of how the agent is metabolized. Most drugs are detoxified in the liver and/or depend on the kidney for excretion. Under certain conditions such as age or illness, those organs responsible for metabolism and subsequent detoxification of the drugs may be impaired. Agents that are dependent on the integrity of the liver for detoxification include most of the penicillins, chloramphenicol, clindamycin, erythromycin, isoniacid, and metronidazole. Drugs that have as their major route of excretion the kidney include all of the aminoglycosides and most of the cephalosporins.

Since individual responses to given antibiotics can vary significantly, it is useful to follow blood levels when possible. This is mandatory in the case of the use of chloramphenicol in infants in whom liver conjugation may or may not be effective, and blood levels can accumulate to significant and potentially harmful values (Gray Baby syndrome).

The choice of antimicrobial therapy is complicated for the physician by the number of new drugs and the zeal of their manufacturers in advertising them. The cephalosporins come as first generation, second generation, and third generation drugs as of mid-1986 (Yogev, 1986). The generations are distinguished by their in vitro activity against Gram-negative bacteria. First generation drugs, such as cephazolin, are active against *Escherichia coli, Proteus mirabilis,* and *Klebsiella pneumoniae.* Second generation agents such as cefuroxime are, in addition, effective against *H. influenzae, Neisseria,* and *Enterobacter* species, although resistance is common. Third generation cephalosporins have the widest spectrum of activity and are most useful for Gram-negative infections. Ceftriaxone is one of the most widely used drugs in treatment of meningitis. It is usually combined with ampicillin when given to newborn infants to provide coverage for *Listeria monocytogenes.* The long half-life in low birth weight infants, and the potential to displace bilirubin from albumin-binding sites make ceftriaxone inappropriate in preterm infants. Cefotaxime is preferable for treatment of proven susceptible Gram-negative enteric bacilli (Fink et al, 1987). The third generation cephalosporins are ineffective against *L. monocytogenes, Enterococcus,* and some *Pseudomonas* species. Ceftazidime is the best of the cephalosporins against *P. aeruginosa.*

Considerations in the choice of drug include knowledge of minimal concentrations needed to inhibit 90% (MIC_{90}) of bacteria tested, levels achieved in blood and other body fluids and time to achieve half-initial concentration.

Other considerations include side effects and costs. The cephalosporins have few side effects. Diarrhea has been reported in 0.3–6% of children, and superinfection with resistant bacteria in 1–3%. Cost depends in part on half-life, since a drug with a long half-life needs to be administered less often. Once daily administration of ceftriaxone is effective for most indications.

Illustrations of the role of cephalosporins include:

(a) Documented penicillin allergy (other than a rash only)—cefazolin is useful against *S. aureus,* and has only about 5% cross-reactivity with penicillin.
(b) When chloramphenicol is associated with neutropenia, a second or third generation cephalosporin can be substituted.
(c) When resistant *Pseudomonas* infections are present, ceftazidime in combination with tobramycin has a role.

In general, cephalosporin use should be undertaken with knowledge that wide use will undoubtedly lead to resistance to these valuable antimicrobials.

Antibacterial Combinations

The simultaneous use of more than a single antimicrobial agent has evolved because, in some circumstances, one cannot be sure initially of the sensitivity of the organism to a single agent. Moreover, some antibiotics appear to be synergistic. For example, ampicillin and gentamicin are synergistic against some enterococci. In other circumstances, some combinations of drugs can be antagonistic. For example, ototoxicity may be enhanced when two drugs (such as kanamycin and furosemide) with this potential are administered simultaneously (Brummett et al, 1975). In general, antimicrobial combinations are not usually recommended (except in severe illness) since the potential for adverse effects or the possibility of benefit is unpredictable in a given individual.

Antiviral Drugs

Now that it is possible to identify the specific viruses associated with the large number of infectious diseases of childhood, it would seem optimal to have a number of agents from which to choose that might be either virustatic or virucidal. Alas, that is not often the case, probably because of the enormous difficulty in finding drugs that will damage the intracellular replicative cycle of the virus without destroying the host cell. Nevertheless, better understanding of the mechanisms of viral action lends promise to the development of effective drugs (Hirsch and Kaplan, 1987).

One of the first agents to be developed was amantadine (1-adamantanamine hydrochloride) which is able to inhibit influenza A virus replication. Clinical studies with this agent in diverse settings has demonstrated that prophylaxis can be accomplished with 55–80% protection against influenza illness during outbreaks of influenza A. Apparently it is less effective in the prevention of infection than in the prevention of illness but that can be an advantage if subclinical infection can confer immunity. Some side effects such as anxiety, jitteriness, and insomnia have been noted but they seem to clear rapidly.

Amantadine is effective in the treatment of influenza A disease, primarily in young adults with uncomplicated disease. Ordinarily this disease is short-lived and self-limited so the benefit of treatment is only modest.

Its principal use would be in prophylaxis of individuals at risk of serious infection during an epidemic. This would include immune suppressed individuals, as well as those with chronic pulmonary disease, and other chronic illness that could be exacebated by even mild infection.

Much interest has been focused on interferons that are produced by human cells and are thought to be one of the natural ways of defense against viral infections. Although interferons are now available through recombinant DNA technology, their clinical efficacy as antiviral agents has not been established.

Another group of agents have been evolved for treatment of herpesvirus infections. Herpesvirus can cause minor infections such as cold sores or can cause chronic genital disease or sometimes destructive and fatal CNS disease. When acquired by the newborn, it can be fatal. It has also been lethal for immunocompromised individuals. Thus, development of antiherpes compounds has been most welcome. The first one to be found effective was vidarabine (ara-A). Vidarabine is a purine nucleoside analogue with activity against herpes simplex. The compound inhibits viral nucleic acid synthesis. It has been evaluated against all sorts of herpes infections. A limitation in its use is that it is poorly soluble so that it has to be given in large quantities of liquid which is a hazard for patients with encephalitis.

Acyclovir is a more widely used inhibitor of certain herpes viruses. It is active against herpes simplex 1 and 2 as well as varicella zoster virus. It can be administered intravenously in smaller amounts of fluid and a topical form is also available.

The most extensive use of acyclovir will be in the therapy of genital herpes where it has been shown to be moderately effective when administered locally and very effective when given intravenously. The optimal duration of treatment is under investigation currently.

Fortunately, acyclovir has been well-tolerated with no significant toxicity but the drug has not been around long enough to be certain of long-term hazards.

Ribavirin is a nucleoside analogue of guanosine and is active against replication of respiratory syncytial virus in vitro. The only studies to date of its use in human infants involved administration by aerosol in which the amount delivered is problematic. Nevertheless, in several clinical trials a shortening of the duration of shedding of virus was found as well as some reduction of severity of illness (Hall et al, 1983; Taber et al, 1983). It seems possible that the deposition of the drug in the lower respiratory tract acted directly to interfere with the growth of the virus. However, a critical review of published studies concluded that clinically significant benefits from ribavirin in treatment of RSV infection were limited (Wald et al, 1988).

REFERENCES

Bart KJ (ed): Child Day Care Infectious Disease Study Group. Considerations of infectious diseases in day care centers. *Pediatr Infect Dis* 4:124, 1985.

Brummett RE, Traynor J, Brown R, et al: Cochlear damage resulting from kamamycin and furosemide. *Acta Otolaryngol* 80:86, 1975.

Caldwell BM (ed): *Group Care for Young Children. A Supplement to Parental Care*. Lexington, MA, Lexington Books, DC Heath and Co., 1987.

Dinarello CA: Interleukin-1. *Rev Infect Dis* 6:51, 1984.

Dinarello CA, Shparbar M, Kent EF, et al: Production of leukocytic pyrogen from phagocytes of neonates. *J Infect Dis* 144:337, 1981.

Dolin R: Antiviral chemotherapy and chemoprophylaxis. *Science* 12:96, 1985.

Eichenwald HF: Antimicrobial therapy in infants and children: update, 1976–1985. Part I. *J Pediatr* 107:161, 1985; Part II. *J Pediatr* 107:337, 1985.

Fink S, Karp W, Robertson, A: Ceftriaxone effect on bilirubin-albumin binding. *Pediatrics* 80:873, 1987.

Florman AL: Interleukin 1 and monitoring of acute infections. *Pediatr Infect Dis* 4:450, 1985.

Gewurz H, Mold C, Siegel J, et al: C-reactive protein and the acute phase response. *Adv Int Med* 27:345 1982.

Hall CB, McBride JT, Walsh EE, et al: Aerosolized ribavirin treatment of infants with respiratory syncytial viral infection. *N Engl J Med* 308:1443, 1983.

Hirsch MS, Kaplan JC: Antiviral therapy. *Sci Am* 256:76, 1987.

Liu C: Antiviral drugs. *Med Clin North Am* 66:235, 1982.

Mitchell D, Laburn HP: Pathophysiology of temperature regulation. *Physiologist* 28:507, 1985.

Roberts RJ: *Drug Therapy in Infants*. Chapter 4. Philadelphia, WB Saunders, 1984 pp. 39–93.

Scarr S: *Mother Care Other Care*. New York, Warner Books, 1985, p. 205.

Taber LH, Knight V, Gilbert BE, et al: Ribavirin aerosol treatment of bronchiolitis associated with respiratory syncytial virus in infants. *Pediatrics* 72:613, 1983.

Wald ER, Dashefsky B, Green M: *In re* ribavirin: A case of premature adjudication? *J Pediatr* 112:154, 1988.

Yogev R: A strategy for evaluating which of the new cephalosporins to use. *Pediatr Ann* 15:470, 1986.

Meningitis

2

Definition

Meningitis is a generalized term for inflammation of the meninges due to both infectious and noninfectious etiologies. Infectious organisms can include bacteria, viruses, fungi, mycoplasma, protozoa, and rickettsia. Noninfectious etiologies can be due to exposure to chemicals or some antineoplastic agents as well as due simply to a sympathetic reaction to localized pathology. Although the natural course, treatment, and prognosis usually depend on the etiologic agent, some generalizations are possible to help distinguish bacterial from nonbacterial causes.

Basic Science

The most common mechanism for meningitis is for bacteria to reach the meninges by the hematogenous route after dissemination from a primary focus elsewhere. Studies on infant rats and monkeys suggest that the nasopharynx may be the most common focus for transient bacteremia and subsequent meningitis. Another route of spread is from contiguous foci such as infections in the mastoids and sinuses with extension into the meninges. Patients with otitis media are felt to develop meningitis more often from hematogenous spread than from direct invasion of the meninges from the middle ear. A rare mechanism is when an anatomic, traumatic, or postsurgical abnormality such as a neurenteric or dermal fistula at the base of the brain or in the sacrococcygeal area allows a direct portal of entry for organisms into the spinal fluid. Once an organism has gained access to the cerebrospinal fluid (CSF), host defenses appear less capable of controlling rapid growth of organisms as well as they would in the blood stream. Occasionally, if sampled early, spinal fluid will reveal organisms only, and it may be as long as 24 hours after initial infection that white blood cells suggestive of the inflammatory reaction appear.

The inflammatory reaction causes many of the complications of meningitis including cranial nerve palsies, or thrombosis of penetrating cerebral vessels. Analysis of an inflamed spinal fluid may show elevated protein, believed to be secondary to the opening of tight junctions of cerebral capillaries during the inflammatory process. Complement and antibody enter the CSF with other serum proteins. This elevation in CSF proteins is detected 16–18 hours after invasion by a bacterial organism. In addition, bacteria may result in diminished CSF glucose levels. This hypoglycorrhachia results, in part, from impaired glucose transport and also from increased glucose use by the brain during the tissue hypoxia produced by the inflammatory response. The inflammatory exudate can further interfere with the normal circulation of spinal fluid and lead to a low pressure hydrocephalus. In general, the longer the disease goes undiagnosed, the greater the chances of complications.

Seizures occur in 20–30% of cases of meningitis and may be the only presenting sign of the disease along with fever. Most seizures associated with meningitis are brief febrile seizures, although they may be prolonged and associated with electrolyte imbalance, increased intracranial pressure, or if occurring late in the course, may represent a cortical vein thrombosis, arteritis, cerebral infarction, a subdural effusion, empyema, or even a brain abscess.

Epidemiology

It is estimated that 30,000 infants and children under the age of 15 years will contract bacterial meningitis in a given year in the United States, and that 3000 will die of this disease, and 10,000 have some permanent neurologic sequelae. About 100,000 children will develop the usually milder viral meningitis in a given year (Fig. 17.1). Regardless of etiology, 90% of all cases of meningitis occur within the first 5 years of life, and the peak incidence occurs in the 6- to 12-month age range. Genetic factors appear to have some role in susceptibility in that males are more susceptible than females (Ward et al, 1981).

Natural History

The earliest signs and symptoms of meningitis regardless of etiology are subtle and nonspecific and can include fever, lethargy, vomiting, irritability, and, in older children, a headache. Because of the subtlety of these symptoms, in younger children in particular, clinicians will often proceed to do a lumbar puncture as part of a "rule out sepsis" work-up with the intent of diagnosing the disease at an early stage. Twenty-four hours into the illness more dramatic symptoms will occur including irritability with high-pitched cry, respiratory distress secondary to a metabolic acidosis, interference with the midbrain's respiratory control mechanism, and seizures. Physical examination at this later stage will be notable for bulging fontanelle, nuchal rigidity, hypo- or hyperthermia, or cranial nerve palsy. Neonates with meningitis may demonstrate jaundice, an abnormal Moro reflex, opisthotonus, apnea, in addition to cranial nerve palsies, convulsions, poor feeding, fever, and possibly coma. Late onset complications of meningitis include subdural effusions,

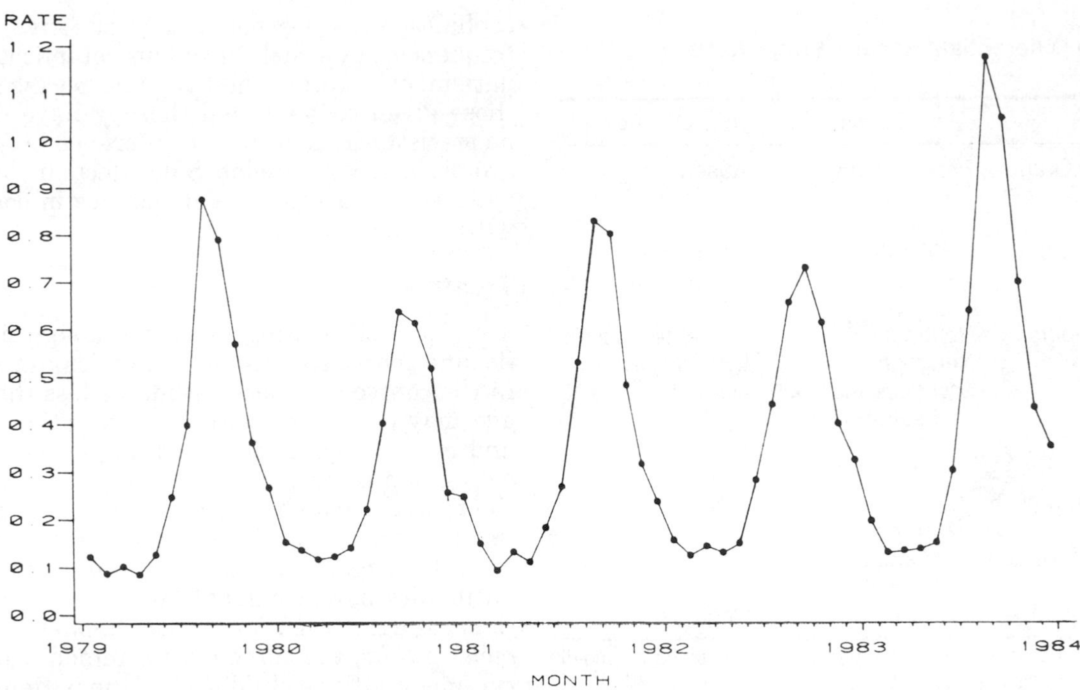

Figure 17.1. Reported cases of aseptic meningitis per 100,000 population, by month, in the United States 1979–1983. Yearly peak incidences occur in the same months as enterovirus infections. From CDC: *MMWR*, Annual Summary 32:15, 1984.

subdural empyema, cortical vein thrombosis, abscess, and significant neurologic disability.

Diagnosis

In the early stages of meningeal infection, the signs and symptoms may be subtle. Two physical findings that can help to confirm the diagnosis of nuchal rigidity are the Brudzinski sign, which is the flexion of the hip and knee joints when the neck is flexed, and Kernig sign in which there is resistance to knee extension when the thigh is flexed to 90°. In infants less than 1 year of age, a full fontanelle should suggest meningitis; nuchal rigidity or a positive Brudzinski or Kernig sign is less apt to be present.

If the diagnosis of meningitis is entertained and the patient does not demonstrate papilledema on physical examination or have a focal neurologic deficit, a lumbar puncture should be performed which should not be delayed by waiting for a CT scan or other tests. If the progression of the signs and symptoms is such that they are present and progressively worse over a period of less than 24 hours, a bacterial etiology is most likely.

Appropriate cultures include blood, urine, and CSF, the latter being necessary to make the diagnosis. If papilledema is present or Reye syndrome, lead encephalopathy, brain abscess, or tumor are diagnostic possibilities, a CT scan should be obtained before performing the lumbar puncture, since it is contraindicated with increased intracranial pressure. Antibiotics, however, need not be withheld before performing a CT scan if suspicion of meningitis is raised in a toxic-appearing child.

Examination of CSF should focus on a cell count, Gram stain and culture, and a protein and glucose. A CSF Gram stain will demonstrate organisms 80% of the time if they are present. A single CSF culture will be positive in over 90% and a blood culture positive in 50% of infected patients. Meningococcal and *Listeria* organisms are the most apt to be missed in Gram stain. A CSF cell count can be estimated by staining the CSF fluid with methylene blue to identify white cells or by treating the fluid with glacial acetic acid to hemolyze red cells. The more definitive count, however, should be determined by centrifuging spinal fluid at 1500 g for 15 minutes, and then performing a differential cell count on the spun sediment (see Table 17.2).

Serum electrolytes and osmolarity, blood urea nitrogen, glucose, liver function tests, clotting studies, and latex agglutination for *Haemophilus influenzae, N. meningitides,* and group B streptococci, and CSF from blood and urine are important baseline measurements. Urine for electrolytes and osmolarity, and routine urinalysis should also be obtained.

RECENT DEVELOPMENTS

New diagnostic techniques include detection of bacterial capsular antigens in CSF, serum, or urine. Latex particle agglutination, enzyme linked immunosorbent assay (ELISA), and counter immunoelectropheresis (CIE) assays are all used for this purpose. The simplest test is the latex particle agglutination which has been found to be more sensitive than CIE (Ward, 1978; Daum et al, 1982).

Table 17.2
Guidelines to Differentiate Bacterial from Aseptic Meningitis

CSF Findings	Bacterial	Aseptic
Organisms on Gram stain	Present early	Absent
Cell count[1]		
Early (6–8 hours)	>200/mm³	<200/mm³
Late		<2000/mm³
Differential		
Early (6–8 hours)	Neutrophils	Some neutrophils
Late	Neutrophils	Lymphocytes
Glucose	Low (less than 50% of serum level)	Normal
Protein		
Under 1 month of age	>200 mg/dl	
After 1 month of age	> 40 mg/dl Up to 1500 mg/dl	
Latex agglutination	Positive	Negative

[1]Correction for red cells in spinal fluid, protein increases about 1 mg/dl for every 1000 red cells.

To distinguish a bacterial from a viral meningitis, the use of quantitative C-reactive protein (CRP) is useful, but not definitive. Bacterial meningitis has been found to have high serum CRP levels (greater than 50 mg/L), whereas viral meningitis has low (less than 50 mg/L) CRP levels. Moreover, an elevated CRP or a subsequent increase in serum CRP may indicate a complication of a bacterial meningitis such as a subdural abscess, or a concurrent bacterial infection superimposed on a viral meningitis (Corrall et al, 1981). It is hypothesized that the CRP interacts with bacteria in the CSF and as an opsonin is then rapidly cleared from the CSF by the bacteria. Therefore, serum CRP determinations are currently recommended over CSF-CRP determinations (Peltola et al, 1984).

Treatment

NEW DEVELOPMENTS

A new approach to assist in the choice of the most effective antibiotic in treating bacterial meningitis with a cephalosporin is to combine in vitro data obtained from minimal inhibitory concentrations (MICs) and in vivo data (the CSF level) achieved, to produce an index that reflects the degree to which achievable CSF levels exceed the MICs for various bacteria. This number is called the "inhibitory quotient" and normally should exceed 10 if possible. Thus, the greater the inhibitory quotient the more effective the antibiotic is expected to be.

Inhibitory quotients and MICs for the traditionally recommended antibiotics (ampicillin, chloramphenicol, and gentamicin) demonstrate lower activity than the new cephalosporins against most of the bacterial pathogens as demonstrated, suggestive that the more active cephalosporins are potentially effective in vivo. The frequencies by which infectious complications occur in patients who receive new cephalosporins as opposed to those given conventional therapy have demonstrated no statistically significant difference between the two groups in gross sequelae. Side effects include increased episodes of neutropenia and diarrhea in patients treated with the new cephalosporins.

Treatment

Bacterial meningitis carries a significant morbidity and mortality unless antibiotics are started early in the course of illness. Neonates less than 28 days of age may be treated with a combination of ampicillin and an aminoglycoside such as gentamicin, since *E. coli,* group B streptococcus, and *L. monocytogenes* are the most common bacterial etiologies for meningitis in the newborn in the United States. For children beyond 1 month of age, ampicillin and chloramphenicol are the antibiotics most commonly used because of the effectiveness against *H. influenzae, S. pneumoniae,* and *N. meningitidis,* the three most common causes of bacterial meningitis in childhood. If the patient is clinically deteriorating with progressive lethargy, seizures, and cranial nerve findings, or if petechiae or purpura are present and meningococcemia is probable, antibiotics should be given immediately with blood and spinal fluid cultures obtained subsequent to providing therapy. All antibiotics used must be capable of penetrating the CSF in adequate enough concentration to kill bacteria. Although gentamicin has poor CSF penetration it is felt that penetration is somewhat improved in an inflammatory state where more of the antibiotic can diffuse across the blood brain barrier. Intravenous therapy is continued usually for at least a week to 10 days and sometimes longer if signs or symptoms persist.

Because of reports that *H. influenzae* might not be sufficiently treated by ampicillin and gentamicin in infants 2–8 weeks of age, increasing attention has been given to the use of new cephalosporins that can cover for *H. influenzae,* provide good CSF penetration, and treat the other normal pathogens of neonatal meningitis. None of the cephalosporins can be used as single drug therapy if *Listeria* is prevalent, so penicillin or ampicillin should certainly be added to a cephalosporin regimen, if that organism is under consideration.

If the patient appears in septic shock, respiratory and cardiovascular support should be provided at once. Inappropriate antidiuretic hormone (SIADH), may occur in meningitis and is characterized by a decrease in the serum sodium and serum osmolarity in the presence of an elevation of urine sodium and urine osmolarity. Treatment is performed by providing fluids at two-thirds to three-quarters maintenance, taking into account increased maintenance requirements if the patient has a fever, and monitoring fluid restriction by following serum osmolarity and urine sodium excretion.

The management of increased intracranial pressure in meningitis is also of concern in the course of therapy. In an infant, the presence of increased intracranial pressure is monitored by following daily head circumferences. This problem can be treated by (1) reducing CSF volume via placement of a ventricular catheter for external drainage (although this is rarely applied to the routine bacterial cases of meningitis); (2) by reduction of cerebral blood volume via induction of hypocarbia by hyperventilation until the intracranial pressure decreases to 20 mm Hg or less; or (3) by reduction of cerebral mass using either fluid restriction, mannitol or glycerol infusions, diuretics, or corticosteroids. Unfortunately, while the latter measures are helpful for increasing intracranial pressure secondary to trauma, or a malignancy, their role in a bacterial meningitis has yet to be proven (see pp. 1324).

The use of mannitol or glycerol is contraindicated in the setting of renal failure or in the setting of a poor systemic blood pressure. Seizures can occur in 20–30% of cases, most often in infants and need to be managed with appropriate airway support and anticonvulsants.

Serial head circumference measurements are important in infants to ascertain presence of a subdural effusion as well as for evidence of increased intracranial pressure. Only 10% of subdural effusions will have symptoms such as persistent or recurrent fever, persistent lethargy or coma, an elevation in head circumference, persistent focal seizures, or positive transillumination of the skull. CT scans can help make the diagnosis. Only if symptoms progress or persist should the effusion be tapped.

CONTROVERSY

Although antibiotics are standard therapy for bacterial meningitis, therapeutic dilemmas still exist.

When is it appropriate to treat a presumptive viral meningitis when a bacterial etiology can not be totally ruled out? While the criteria for distinguishing bacterial from viral meningitis in untreated patients will suggest a bacterial etiology, a clinical gray zone exists in which bacterial and viral meningitis can both appear. In fact, two-thirds of early viral meningitis can have a predominance of neutrophils. Therefore, the therapeutic approach should depend on clinical suspicion until better studies or better diagnostic tests are available. There are two therapeutic choices. First, treat all patients with antibiotics pending results of cultures and then discontinue antibiotics if cultures are negative at 48 hours. Second, monitor the patient closely under observation in the hospital without antibiotic treatment and then repeat the lumbar puncture at 8–12 hours. If the child has a viral meningitis a greater than 75% chance exists that the CSF will shift from a predominance of neutrophils to a predominant lymphocytosis over this period of time (Feigin and Shackelford, 1973).

What is appropriate in the case of a partially treated meningitis, i.e., a patient who is diagnosed as having white cells in the CSF after receiving antibiotics for a previously diagnosed infection? Unfortunately partial treatment with an antibiotic will produce cell counts that will mimic a viral meningitis, although the glucose and protein and the differential cell counts are not altered by earlier treatment if a bacterial etiology is present. Cultures are not reliable since they can be negative after antibiotic treatment has begun with a drug that can penetrate the CSF, such as amoxicillin or a cephalosporin. Given this uncertainty, children with partially treated meningitis are admitted to hospital and treated for the full 10-day course.

Who needs a repeat lumbar puncture and how long should you treat? In general, 5 successive afebrile days, in combination with a CSF cell count less than 50 and a CSF glucose greater than 45 mg/dl on a repeat lumbar puncture at the end of the afebrile days and a negative culture usually indicate sterilization of spinal fluid. Unfortunately, some patients have cell counts below 50 or CSF glucose higher than 45 mg/dl at the end of 5 afebrile days and still demonstrate relapse in symptoms at the end of 10–14 days of therapy. Thus, routine repeat puncture is not recommended. If no clinical improvement occurs or focal neurologic signs or a seizure appears after a period of clinical improvement, or prolonged or recurrent fever is present, or the child is under 12 weeks of age, a repeat lumbar puncture is warranted at a much earlier point in the therapy to ensure appropriate therapeutic success with the antibiotics chosen. The rate of sterilization of CSF after the start of adequate antibiotic therapy will correlate inversely with the concentration of bacteria in the CSF at the time of diagnosis of bacteria. Sterilization is usually accomplished within 1 hour if the initial bacterial count in CSF is less than 100,000 bacteria/ml but can last longer if the count is larger than 10 million bacteria/ml with the common pathogens. In neonatal meningitis with coliform organisms, sterilization of the CSF may not occur for 3 or more days. Patients who sterilize rapidly are less apt to demonstrate permanent neurologic abnormalities following treatment (Feigin and Shackelford, 1973).

What is the best response to a prolonged fever during appropriate treatment of bacterial meningitis? About 13% of cases of bacterial meningitis demonstrate fever lasting longer than 10 days. *H. influenzae* meningitis tends to cause fever longer than meningococcal or pneumococcal meningitis. If fever occurs in excess of 5 days, in addition to the possibility of recurrence or resistance of the infecting organism, consider subdural effusions, phlebitis, drug fever, or a nosocomially acquired infection as possible etiologies. If fever persists at the end of 10–14 days of therapy, a repeat lumbar puncture should certainly be performed.

Prognosis and Follow-up

Most of the studies demonstrating evidence of permanent neurologic damage secondary to meningitis have involved patients who have had *H. influenzae* as an etiology for the disease. In these circumstances, mortality has ranged 1–2% of all cases. Risk factors that can predict permanent neurologic damage include a delayed sterilization of CSF, the presence of focal neurologic deficits at the time of diagnosis, and/or an increased antigen burden (greater than 1 million colony-forming units of bacteria per ml of CSF). Other poor prognostic factors include seizures for a period of greater than 4 days, CSF protein over 1000 ml/dl, CSF leukocytes greater than 10,000/mm^3, and a CSF glucose of less than 10 mg/dl. Serial CRP determinations correlate with the risk of complications, in that a secondary rise in serum CRP concentrations has been associated with increased incidence of complications. As soon as a hearing deficit can be detected corrective measures such as hearing aids and speech therapy are indicated (Sell, 1983).

Since hearing impairment is the most common neurologic sequel to bacterial meningitis in children (Dodge et al, 1984), it is mandatory that all children have their hearing tested about 1 month after resolution of the disease, since transient deafness may occur during the course of the illness. In younger infants who will not cooperate for a routine hearing evaluation, auditory-evoked potentials are useful to help detect sensory neural deafness (Kotagal et al, 1981).

Prevention

H. influenzae vaccine is the best form of prevention in infants over age 18 months. Greater efforts must still be made to prevent even more cases due to other organisms or to prevent *Haemophilus* disease in the very young who can not mount an adequate immune response (Claesson et al, 1988).

REFERENCES

Bolan G, Barza M: Acute bacterial meningitis in children and adults: A perspective. *Med Clin North Am* 60:233, 1985.

Claesson BA, Trollfors B, Lagergard T, et al: Clinical and immunologic response to the capsular polysaccharide of *Haemophilus influenzae* type b alone or conjugated to tetanus toxoid in 18- to 23-month-old children. *J Pediatr* 112:695, 1988.

Corrall CJ, Pepple JM, Moxon ER, et al: C-reactive protein in spinal fluid of children with meningitis. *J Pediatr* 99:365, 1981.

Daum RS, Siber GR, Kamon JS, et al: The evaluation of a commercial latex particle agglutination test for rapid diagnosis of *Haemophilus influenzae* type B infection. *Pediatrics* 69:466, 1982.

Dodge PR, Davis H, Feigin RD, et al: Prospective evaluation of hearing impairment of the sequelae of acute bacterial meningitis. *N Engl J Med* 311:869, 1984.

Feigin RD, Shackelford PG: Value of repeat lumbar puncture in the differential diagnosis of meningitis. *N Engl J Med* 289:571, 1973.

Kotagal S, Rosenberg C, Rudd D, et al: Auditory evoked potentials in bacterial meningitis. *Arch Neurol* 38:693, 1981.

Nelson JD: Management problems in bacterial meningitis. *Pediatr Infect Dis* 4:S41, 1985.

Peltola H, Luhtala K, Valmari P: C-reactive protein as detector of organic complications during recovery from childhood purulent meningitis. *J Pediatr* 104:869, 1984.

Sell SH: Long term sequelae of bacterial meningitis in children. *Pediatr Infect Dis* 2:90, 1983.

Teele DW, Dashefsky B, Rakusan, T, et al: Meningitis after lumbar puncture in children with bacteremia. *N Engl J Med* 305:1079, 1981.

Ward JI: Rapid diagnosis of *Haemophilus influenzae* type B infections by latex particle agglutination NCIE. *J Pediatr* 93:37, 1978.

Ward JI, Lum MKW, Bender TR, et al: *Haemophilus influenzae* disease in Alaskan Eskimos: Characteristics of a population with an unusual incidence of invasive disease. *Lancet* 1:1281, 1981.

Yogev R: Advances in diagnosis and treatment of childhood meningitis. *Pediatr Infect Dis* 4:321, 1985.

Pneumonia 3

Pneumonia is an infection of lung parenchyma. Bacteria, viruses, fungi, rickettsia, and parasites are all capable of producing pneumonia and are discussed individually later in this section.

Most lower respiratory tract infections in infants and children are preceded by upper respiratory infections that are usually viral. Injury to the epithelial surfaces and alteration of the usual bacterial flora invite secondary bacterial infection. Presumably aspiration of infected secretions sets up lobar or lobular infection which is characteristic of bacterial pneumonias. Beyond the first few months of life, most pneumonias are viral. School-age children may be infected with *Mycoplasma pneumoniae*.

In infants under 3 months of age in the United States, group B streptococcal pneumonia, *Chlamydia, Staphylococcus aureus,* and some Gram-negative organisms are the most likely organisms that can cause pneumonia. Group B streptococcal pneumonia and *Chlamydia* infections are acquired from an infected vagina during delivery. The onset of symptoms may be in the first hours of life in the case of group B streptococcal pneumonia or up to 4 months of age in the case of *Chlamydia*. If the infant has not received erythromycin ophthalmic ointment as prophylaxis in the delivery room, conjunctivitis may appear approximately 1–3 weeks after birth. The symptoms are mild and easily overlooked. Pneumonia is associated with low-grade fever, occasional paroxysmal coughing, mild tachypnea and rales (Stagno et al, 1981).

Staphylococcal pneumonia is most commonly acquired as a nosocomial nursery infection. It is characterized by mild prodromata, fever, upper respiratory infection, and sometimes vomiting and diarrhea. An abrupt onset of severe respiratory distress or a pneumothorax is characteristic. Radiographs may show pleural thickening or effusion, and loculated air in the subpleural surfaces (pneumatococles). Untreated staphylococcal pneumonia is usually fatal.

Beyond the first 3 months of life, *S. pneumoniae* (pneumococcus) is the most common organism and accounts for nearly 90% of acute bacterial pneumonias in children who are not immunocompromised or with underlying disease such as cystic fibrosis.

Viral pneumonias occur at all ages, from congenital infections with rubella and cytomegalovirus to early onset systemic herpes infection acquired during delivery. The most common cause of lower respiratory tract infection in the first year of life is respiratory syncytial virus-associated bronchiolitis.

In many instances, several pathogens may coexist in a sick infant. *Chlamydia* and *Cytomegalovirus* were most commonly found in mixed infections by Stagno et al, 1981.

In developing countries, bacterial infection in the wake of the immune suppression of measles remains a major problem. In studies in which lung aspirate and viral cultures or serology were conducted, adenovirus, herpes virus, or enteroviruses were identified, but not shown to be causative in about one-third of patients. Bacteria were present in more than half the patients, with *Haemophilus influenzae, S. pneumoniae,* and *S. aureus* most prominent. Other studies report less morbidity when penicillin is given to children admitted to a hospital with cough and fever than in an untreated control group (Shann, 1986).

Most pneumonias in infants and children cannot be distinguished by clinical or radiographic findings, but require laboratory identification. The presence of pneumonia, however, is a clinical diagnosis based on some or all of the following findings (in order of increasing severity):

Fever
Tachypnea
Retractions
Nasal flaring
Expiratory grunt
Shortness of breath
Anxiety
Cyanosis
Respiratory failure

In infants, chest percussion is unrewarding in most pneumonias. A flat percussion note indicates effusion and hyperresonance indicates pneumothorax, but infiltrates can rarely be detected by percussion. A mediastinal shift can be readily palpated. Auscultation is useful to assesss the presence of air exchange, rales, and rhonchi. Wheezes may be heard with prolonged expirations, but they can also be felt by palpation of the chest wall.

In older children, percussion and auscultation help localize the involved areas, and allow assessment of progression of disease (or recovery). In the event of a probable viral etiology (deduced by knowledge of likely organisms in a given setting, and a white blood count usually less than 15,000 cells), in a child who is not clinically very ill, the presence of rales will establish the diagnosis of pneumonia and radiographs are not indicated. If the condition worsens, or the course is prolonged, chest radiographs can be of help in identifying effusions, hilar nodes, or abscesses that can occur with secondary infection and cannot be identified on physical examination.

Sputum is usually swallowed by infants and young children. Deep suction may produce some mucus and sputum and should be stained and cultured if pneumonia is suspected. However, contamination with oral organisms makes interpretation difficult in the presence of mixed flora. Nasopharyngeal washings are useful for rapid identification of respiratory syncytial virus, influenza, and parainfluenza.

Microbial diagnosis can sometimes be made by a positive blood culture during the acute phase of the disease. Culture of lung aspirate or lung biopsy is necessary to determine the etiology in individuals with negative blood cultures. Nasopharyngeal and throat cultures are not reliable sources of microbes in the lung.

The treatment of acute-onset pneumonia in a previously well child is usually with oral penicillin or amoxicillin, pending results of a blood culture which is positive in one-third of patients with *S. pneumonia* or *H. influenzae* infection. Lung aspirate is rarely undertaken in such situations. Sputum is examined if available, but in young children it cannot often be obtained. If the chest radiograph shows a diffuse infiltrate, and cold agglutinins are positive and suggest the diagnosis of mycoplasma, erythromycin is the drug of choice. If a pleural effusion is present, a thoracentesis is appropriate to withdraw fluid for examination and culture.

In immunocompromised individuals, persistent pneumonias or pulmonary infiltrates that do not respond to penicillin require an etiologic diagnosis. Lung aspirate of involved areas is the least invasive approach. Aspiration of bronchial secretions through a fiberoptic bronchoscope is sometimes recommended. Lung biopsy may be necessary if pneumocystis or fungal infections are suspected. Treatment is dictated by the nature of the pulmonary pathogen.

Since pneumonia is such a common and serious condition in developing countries, and an etiologic diagnosis is often unobtainable, WHO guidelines propose the use of procaine penicillin if injections are feasible.

If not, either amoxicillin or cotrimoxazole orally are recommended for severe cases (Pio, 1986).

REFERENCES

Pio A: Acute respiratory infections in children in developing countries: An international point of view. *Pediatr Infect Dis* 20:179, 1986.

Shann F: Etiology of severe pneumonia in children in developing countries. *Pediatr Infect Dis* 5:247, 1986.

Stagno S, Pifer LL, Hughes, WT, et al: Infant pneumonitis associated with cytomegalovirus, *Chlamydia, Pneumocystis* and *Ureaplasma*: A prospective study. *Pediatrics* 68:322, 1981.

Viruses 4

Viruses cause a disproportionate amount of illness in childhood. Not only do they include some of the most prevalent pathogens, but some of the most lethal as well. They can cause significant disease in their own right, and also trigger exacerbation of other chronic illnesses such as nephrosis or cystic fibrosis. Viral respiratory tract infections are a major source of morbidity and are the most common diseases experienced among individuals in the United States.

PERSPECTIVES IN VIROLOGY

Alice S. Huang, Ph.D.

The major challenge in virology lies in understanding pathogenesis. Only when mechanisms of the virus-host interactions are known, will there be a rational basis for the control of viral diseases. An important aspect of understanding pathogenesis for many viruses is their ability to convert to a persistent or latent state. We now know that many viruses infect their hosts mainly during the first few years after birth and continue to reside in the host for many years, if not for life. What do we know of these mechanisms of persistence? This perspective will present three such mechanisms and discuss their implications for viral pathogenesis.

The mechanisms are: (1) genetic changes leading to persistence; (2) phenotypic changes leading to altered surface antigens; and (3) latency in differentiated cells. Before describing these mechanisms, let us first review the current state of the science in virology (Evans, 1982; Fields, 1985).

Viruses have been with us for a long time. They are, of course, most noticeable when they cause disease, particularly lethal ones, or very disfiguring ones. Historically there are many examples. An Egyptian relief from the early days of the pharoahs shows a shrunken leg resulting from asymmetric paralytic poliomyelitis. Socrates described "dog days" when humans bitten by dogs go mad or rabid. Chinese literature during the Middle Ages described variolation, or passive transfer of material from human pox lesions, to protect others from small pox. However, it is only over the past 20 years that most viruses have been characterized and related to the diseases that they cause. There are at least 25 different virus groups that cause human disease. They have been characterized as separate groups by their different biochemical strategies of replication. When negatively stained each group has a different morphology by electronmicroscopy.

The nucleic acid sequences of many prototypical viruses are known. Their gene products are characterized as individual protein species. Computerized protein conformational analyses, as well as some biophysical data, in particular, X-ray crystallographic results, are now known about these gene products. Even human viral pathogens, which reproduce poorly in the laboratory or not at all, are being studied by the cloning of their nucleic acid genomes. Albeit descriptive, such data are essential for studying agents which cause disease.

The future lies in understanding the function(s) of these genes and the interactions of their products with nucleic acids during the regulation of viral gene expression.

Together with the advances in molecular virology, dramatic advances are being made in understanding the immune system. A large number of ongoing investigations are on the response of the host immune system to viral infections. Viral proteins, particularly their surface antigens, are extraordinarily immunogenic. Studies with T- and B-cell clones from the immune system as well as mixed lymphocyte-macrophage cultures are providing information as to which specific parts, or epitopes, of the viral proteins are seen by the immune system. This, together with sequence data, has led to a whole generation of subunit, peptide, or vaccinia-vectored vaccines which may offer protection against viral infections.

Such studies on the host immune response point to that part of the immune system which protects us from viral disease. As we uncover the details of these mechanisms, there will be manipulations of the immune system so that protection against certain viral diseases can be enchanced and damage from the immune response itself reduced. On the other hand, viruses themselves appear to manipulate the immune system to their own advantage. Examples abound where viruses utilize antibodies to attach to *fc* receptors and therefore, enter cells and spread more effectively. Also, viruses produce excess soluble antigens which react with antibodies and prevent their ability to neutralize viruses. Virus-infected cells can evade host immune surveillance by limiting the expression of new viral antigens or removing them completely from the surface of cells by immune modulation. Lastly, viruses can directly attack cells of the immune system, resulting in their death.

Although viruses are best studied in their lytic phase, where 10–100,000 progeny are generated per cell, it has become increasingly evident that the virus lifestyle is far from being so simple. As an obligate intracellular parasite, the virus has evolved a variety of mechanisms to avoid damaging the host cell and to coexist. What mechanisms do viruses use to remain hidden? What can we do to coax them out? The ability of viruses to persist or remain latent and our understanding of these host cell interactions lie at the fundamental basis of pathogenesis. Herein lies the challenge.

The first example of a mechanism for persistence lies in mutational flexibility (Holland et al, 1982; Parvin et al, 1986). Viruses have an intrinsic rapid rate of mutation. Although they can be cloned by plaque isolations so that the population is genetically homogenous, after several cycles of growth the population becomes heterogenous again, harboring many mutations. This rate of mutation can be as high as 3% of the progeny, greater than a million times the rate of mutations in bacteria. After infection with influenza virus, isolations on successive days from the same patient will show mutational changes. This selection of genetically mutated virus explains why our antibodies to one strain of influenza virus may not be as protective against a similar strain next year. This is known as antigenic drift.

One of these naturally occurring genetic mutations among viruses is due to deletions and rearrangements of nucleic acid pieces (Huang, 1986). The effects of such changes on the virus are more subtle than simply antigenic alterations. It has been known for some time that in animal virus preparations, not all virus particles are infectious. Many of these noninfectious virus particles contain deletions which play a significant role in the biology of the virus host interaction. Deletions, as much as two-thirds of the genome or more, may occur. These, in turn, alter the virulence of the virus preparation itself.

How such effects are brought about depends on how infections are initiated. Rather than a single infectious unit or virion initiating the disease process, recent evidence indicates that successful transmission usually requires more than one virus particle. The presence of deletion mutants in a population can result in an inhibition of the growth of the normal infectious virus and enhance the growth of the deleted virus. On a population level, a cyclic pattern of production is established, very similar to what population biologists call predator-prey relationships. Studies on this cyclic pattern show that the response of the host cell varies considerably depending on the ratio of infectious virus to deleted virus that infect a given cell as well as on the total amount of virus present. Such cyclic patterns in vitro can be initiated with identical amounts of standard virus but result in different patterns if different amounts of deleted virus are mixed in. With a preparation containing excess deleted virus, growth of the virus will be initially inhibited; whereas, a preparation with fewer such particles will result in an opposite cyclic pattern. At a given time thereafter, very different amounts of infectious standard virus may be present. Similarly, if deleted virus is inhibited in its ability to interfere, a high titer of infectious virus is maintained throughout the time course. Therefore, population heterogeneity may contribute to the self-limiting nature of viral diseases. Interference may explain why viruses persist in a subclinical form. Although our immune system is known to play a major role in determining the outcome of an infection, viruses themselves, through an interactive population effect, may also be very important. These interactions among virus particles as they progress from the initial site of inoculation to their target organ are postulated to be a major determinant in whether virus infections remain silent or cause disease (Cave et al, 1985).

The second example of viral persistence is not at the genetic level but at a phenotypic level. Viruses can hide from our host immune defenses either by passing directly from cell to cell or by the incorporation of other proteins on their surfaces. This latter phenomenon is particularly interesting and is called phenotypic mixing or "wolves in sheep's clothing" (Zavada, 1982). Unrelated RNA, as well as DNA viruses, can coinfect cells and produce a variety of progeny. Some resemble the parents and are neutralized by antiserum made against each parent. Others carry mixed antigens and are neutralized by either antisera. And finally, the wolves in sheep's clothing, where the surface antigens have been totally exchanged, escape from antibodies directed against the parent, but are neutralized by antibodies against the donor virus. In addition, the new surface coat extends the host range of the virus to include the host range of the other parent.

Phenotypic mixing probably occurs more commonly, since we now know many viruses can coexist in a single host. What are the possible consequences of such mixing? Could viruses hide by failing to make their own coats? Could one virus rescue another by providing new coats, and could the new coats cause viruses to attach to cells which they normally do not enter and cause disease?

The last mechanism in this perspective on persistence is the latency of viruses in differentiated cells (Roizman, 1982; Weiss et al, 1982). Many of the DNA viruses, as well as the RNA retroviruses, have two very distinctive lifestyles. Some behave like killers, resulting in the death of the cell. Others stably associate with the host genetic information indefinitely. Viral latency occurs often in differentiated tissues. Only when the cells are coaxed to proliferate rapidly, by some mitogenic challenge to the host immune system or by special culture conditions in vitro, will the virus reproduce itself and exit from the cell. DNA viruses, as well as retroviruses, require cellular DNA synthesis during their replication cycle. Specialized differentiated cells do not divide unless stimulated by a mitogen. As we know more about growing these cells in the laboratory we will be uncovering a whole host of occult viruses. Already by the use of interleukin-2 and mitogens on T lymphocytes, several human lymphotropic viruses have been isolated.

Therefore, by giving examples of how viruses might persist, we have uncovered mechanisms of how viruses hide. The details of such viral interactions with host cells as well as interactions with each other will form the future of animal virology research. These sophisticated intracellular parasites pose great challenges. They offer excitement for the infectious disease researcher and hope to the clinician.

REFERENCES

Cave DR, Hendrickson FM, Huang AS: Defective interfering particles modulate virulence. *J Virol* 55:366, 1985.

Evans AS: *Viral Infections of Humans,* 2nd edition. New York, Plenum Medical Book Co., 1982, pp. 1–720.

Fields BN: *Virology*. New York, Raven Press, 1985, pp. 1–1614.

Holland JJ, Spindler K, Horodyski I, et al: Rapid evolution of RNA genomes. *Science* 215:1577, 1982.

Huang AS: Modulation of viral disease processes by defective interfering particles. In Ahlquist P, Domingo E, Holland JJ (eds): *RNA Genetics: Variability*. New York, CRC Press, 1986.

Parvin JD, Moscona A, Pan WT, et al: Measurement of the mutation rates of animal viruses: Influenza A virus and poliovirus type 1. *J Virol* 59:377, 1986.

Roizman B. *The Herpesviruses*. New York, Plenum Press, Vol. 1 and 2. 1982–1983, pp. 1–445 and 1–439.

Weiss R, Teich N, Varmus H, et al: *RNA Tumor Viruses*. Cold Spring Harbor Monograph Series. 1982, pp. 1–1396.

Zavada J: The pseudotypic paradox. *J Gen Virol* 63:15, 1982.

ADENOVIRUSES

Definition

Adenoviruses are most frequently associated with prolonged high fever, tonsillitis, otitis, pneumonia, and gastroenteritis. Disseminated, sometimes fatal infections with adenovirus 7 have been reported. Adenoviruses have long been known to produce epidemic illnesses, such as pharyngeal-conjunctival fever and atypical pneumonias among military recruits. The name was suggested in 1956 for the group of viruses with characteristic involvement of lymphadenoid tissue (Enders et al, 1956). More than 40 types cause human infection.

Basic Science

The viruses are DNA viruses without envelopes. The virion is an icosahedron (20 sides) with a central core. They are classified according to their guanine-cytosine content and DNA homology as well as by serotypes.

The initial infection is often in the upper respiratory tract, but it may progress to the lower tract or to the gastrointestinal tract. Blood stream invasion can occur, with a morbilliform or petechial rash. Prolonged carrier states can exist in young children in nasopharynx and stool.

Epidemiology

In a controlled prospective study, Brandt et al (1969) reported that by conservative estimate 7% of respiratory disease in children was caused by adenoviruses types 2, 1, 5, and 3 in that order. Illness is most common between 6 months and 5 years of age, but may occur at any age.

Only about half of those in whom the virus is recovered will have respiratory illness (Fox et al, 1977). No seasonal variation has been reported.

Natural History

In a prospective study from Finland, Ruuskanen et al (1985) used a radioimmunassay to detect adenovirus hexon antigen in hospitalized febrile children. They found that in the 105 children with adenovirus infection, tonsillitis was present in 41%, gastroenteritis in 12%, pneumonia in 9%, otitis media in 9%, and febrile convulsions in 9%. Fever lasted 2–13 days; the highest value was 39.4° C. Diarrhea and vomiting were common; conjunctivitis was present in 12%. Seventeen percent of patients had no identifiable source of infection.

Tonsillitis is often exudative and hard to distinguish from streptococcal disease except for a younger average age group and lack of response to antibiotics.

Gastroenteritis has been associated with diarrhea in hospitalized children, many of whom also had upper respiratory tract symptoms.

A late complication from adenovirus types 7 and 21 is bronchiolitis obliterans. This infection can cause a severe necrotizing bronchiolitis or angitis (unilateral hyperlucent lung; Wohl and Chernick, 1978).

Diagnosis

The white blood count is variable, as is the sedimentation rate. Immunoassay on tissue permits identification of the antigen in 24–30 hours (Ruuskanen et al, 1984).

Treatment

No antiviral agents have been found to be very effective, although a few studies with ribavirin have been encouraging. However, only two strains of adenovirus caused 80% of illness in a Nashville study which suggests the possibility of development of an effective vaccine (Edwards et al, 1985).

Prevention

No vaccine is available for routine use.

CORONAVIRUS

Definition

Coronaviruses are a family of RNA viruses that cause respiratory infections in humans and more severe diseases in a number of animals.

Basic Science

First isolated from individuals with upper respiratory infections in 1965, coronaviruses are large (80–160 nm) RNA viruses with a lipid-soluble coat. They are transmitted by the fecal-oral route or by droplet spread. Although prevalent in animals, animals are not thought to be a reservoir for human infection.

Epidemiology

Outbreaks occur in temperate zones between December and April, in contrast to rhinovirus outbreaks that occur mostly in the fall. Some evidence suggests they cycle every 2–4 years. In some studies, coronaviruses have been found to cause 8–15% of upper respiratory infections. Immunity is not lasting, and reinfection is common.

Natural History

Experimental infection in volunteers has shown a 3-day incubation period, with a 6- to 7-day duration of illness. Sore throat, cough, nasal discharge and fever characterize the illness. The virus can persist for months in stools of asymptomatic individuals, but it has not been shown to cause gastroenteritis.

Diagnosis

Complement fixation tests are used in epidemiologic studies. The virus is difficult to isolate, and it is not sought routinely in mild upper respiratory illness. It can be seen by electron microscopy.

Treatment

Only supportive treatment is available.

Prevention

Handwashing is the best prevention. No vaccines are available.

CYTOMEGALOVIRUS

Cytomegalic Inclusion Disease

Definition

Cytomegalovirus (CMV), a DNA virus member of the herpes virus group that is often present in a latent form, can cause serious multisystem disease in susceptible hosts. Increasingly, cytomegalic virus inclusion disease (CID) has come to be an important problem not only in the perinatal period but in immunocompromised individuals of any age. CMV-induced mononucleosis occurs in previously healthy young adults.

Basic Science

The suggestion that the congenital syndrome we now call CID had a viral etiology dates from the 1920s, but it was not until the 1950s that several groups at the same time reported independently the isolation of the human CMV. CMV is one of five known herpes viruses of humans. Many species can be infected with this virus, including dogs, hamsters, sheep, and chimpanzees. Hanshaw et al (1985) provided evidence that CMV, Epstein-Barr virus, and varicella-zoster viruses are antigenically related.

The most striking morphologic feature of a CMV-infected cell is a large intranuclear inclusion of 8–10 μ in diameter with an overall enlargement of the cell of 25–40 μ. The nuclear inclusion is usually located centrally and is composed of aggragates of chromoten and virus particles.

The human infection primarily involves epithelial cells, but curiously human fibroblasts are required for in vitro growth. It is thought that the infection spreads from cell to cell producing foci of enlarged cells with inclusions.

Antigenic heterogeneity exists. No complement fixing cross-reactivity has been identified between human and nonhuman CMV strains. Strains can be distinguished by use of restriction endonuclease analysis of purified DNA (Huang et al, 1980).

Rapid diagnosis is possible with electron microscopic examination of cells in the urine. Stagno and colleagues (1980) found the electron microscopic examination positive in less than 1 hour in 92 specimens later found to contain the virus. Rapid detection of CMV in urine through DNA hybridization has also been described by Chou and Merrigan (1983).

Epidemiology

The condition varies widely in incidence as a function of the prevalence of the virus in women of childbearing age. The prevalence of the virus in pregnant women has been studied by Reynolds et al (1973) who found the virus excreted from urine or cervix in 12% of such women. In their study, 40% of infants born to mothers who were excreting the virus became infected, but none of the infants were ill. (Overall, about 10% of infected infants are symptomatic.) Acquisition and initial replication of virus occurred despite appreciable levels of maternal antibody. The later rise in antibody titers documented the fact that the infections were recent. In the United States as a whole, CMV infection is found in 50–60% of pregnant women.

Acquired CMV infection can be monitored by use of restriction enzyme analysis of CMV DNA that permits identification of different strains. In studies in day care centers, more than 50% of adults are seropositive and 5% of teachers are excretors of virus. Transmission of infection is unusual from adult to adult; children, however, can acquire infection from other children, most commonly in those under 28 months of age. They can also be a source of adult infection (Pass et al, 1987).

Infection that comes from transfusions occurs 3–12 weeks later; after tissue transplantation it appears between 6 weeks and 4 months later.

Natural History

The importance of CMV as a cause of major birth defects, particularly mental retardation, has been documented by several surveys. About 1% of all infants are infected with CMV at birth. The percentage varies with socioeconomic status reaching about 2% in individuals of low socioeconomic groups. Most of these infants have inapparent infections that can be detected only because they are excreting the virus in the urine or are making antibodies to it. About 10% of the infected group have serious disseminated infection with hepatosplenomegaly, thrombocytopenia, jaundice, and sometimes cerebral calcifications and microcephaly. Transient neutropenia is commonly seen. Chorioretinitis and deafness have been associated with the disseminated disease which is occasionally fatal. Even children with inapparent infection in the newborn period can have later sequelae, including hearing loss and depressed IQ scores.

Diagnosis

Most infected infants are not diagnosed in the newborn period unless they have an overwhelming disseminated infection and blood is drawn for TORCH titers. Most infants with acquired CMV infection become ill after they leave the nursery. Some of the infection acquired postnatally apparently comes from maternal virus shed in breast milk. When exposed to the virus in the genital tract during delivery, the rate of infection of young infants is about 58%.

The manifestations of the acquired illness are principally hepatosplenomegaly and anemia. Severe pneumonias have been reported principally in infants delivered through an infected vagina. Notably infections acquired during birth or from breast milk were not prevented by substantial levels of maternally derived neutralizing antibody. The acquired infection, however, produced minimal morbidity.

Acquisition of infection from blood transfusion in infants of seronegative mothers can result in severe and sometimes fatal generalized disease (Yeager et al, 1981). Only seronegative (<1:8) individuals should be donors of blood for newborn infants. Irradiation of donor blood is not adequate.

LABORATORY DIAGNOSIS

Indirect fluorescent CMV IgM antibody is usually elevated. Cord serum IgM is usually elevated, atypical lymphocytosis is present, thrombocytopenia of less than 100,000, platelets occurs in more than half the infants, as does conjugated hyperbilirubinemia. Increased spinal fluid protein may be present (Pass et al, 1980). The diagnosis can be confirmed by culture of the organism from a fresh urine specimen or throat swab. Rapid culture methods based on immunofluorescent detection of early viral proteins with monoclonal antibodies now allow detection in 2 days.

CONTROVERSY

There is some question about the wisdom of allowing a mother known to be shedding CMV in her breast milk to continue nursing her infant. Presumably her infant would have acquired antibodies transplacentally, so that it is unlikely that the infant will suffer any adverse consequences, although he may acquire infection and spread the virus. Certainly it is a warning not to bank breast milk so that infants who are seronegative or prematurely born might receive CMV-infected milk (Rawls et al, 1984; Dworsky et al, 1983).

Treatment

Treatment is supportive only.

Prognosis

The majority of infants with CMV infection are asymptomatic. Neurologic sequelae are more common when virus excretion is found soon after birth. If excretion occurs after 8 weeks of age, sequelae are rare

> **CASE ILLUSTRATION**
>
> A 2-month-old male infant was admitted for tachypnea, low-grade fever, and a cyanotic spell at home. His birth history was entirely unremarkable, with excellent weight gain and normal activity until 1 day before admission when his respiratory symptoms developed. Examination on arrival showed tachypnea, grunting and mild cyanosis, and an infant who appeared uncomfortable. Chest radiograph was notable for a right middle lobe infiltrate. He received intravenous antibiotics until cultures were negative and improved rapidly. On the day of planned discharge, CMV was isolated from the posterior nasopharyngeal secretions.
>
> **QUESTION AND COMMENT**
>
> **Can the symptoms be attributable to CMV?**
>
> Because of acute onset and prompt response to antibiotics, it is improbable that CMV caused the illness.
>
> While we usually recommend a broad spectrum antibiotic for bacterial pneumonias in this age group, nonbacterial pathogens are probably much more common. With maximal effort to identify by culture or immunochemical technique in the infant 1–3 months of age with pneumonia, up to 63% recovery of a pathogen has been achieved.

(Paryani et al, 1985). The worst prognosis is for infants with microcephaly at birth, and neurologic and ocular signs at 1 year (Conboy et al, 1986).

Prevention

Acquired infection is best prevented by hand washing after exposure to an infected infant. Blood provided for infants should be from CMV-negative donors or frozen in glycerol.

Cytomegalovirus-Induced Mononucleosis

Definition

CMV-induced mononucleosis is a febrile illness that is difficult to distinguish from Epstein-Barr (EB) virus-induced mononucleosis. It is characterized by lymphadenopathy, splenomegaly, and a peripheral monocytosis with a negative heterophil antibody test.

Epidemiology

The disorder was first recognized in 1965 and is probably underdiagnosed. However, when appropriate serologic studies are done, it is evident the disease is fairly common. Jordan et al (1973) described nine cases seen over a 10-month period, and Horwitz et al (1986) discussed 82 patients seen over a 15-year period. The youngest patient in their series was 6 years old.

Natural History

Young, previously well adults may acquire CMV infection in the absence of transfusions or other recognized sources. The illness presents with fever that lasts several days to weeks, myalgias, lymphadenopathy, and splenomegaly. About one-third of the patients have a sore throat, but exudative tonsillitis is rare. Other findings include headache, abdominal pain, or diarrhea.

Diagnosis

Blood smears are indistinguishable from those of EB virus infection. Atypical lymphocytes are prominent from a few to 40/100 white cells. Thrombocytopenia and hemolysis may occur. The heterophil antibody test is negative. A CMV-IgM test is sensitive but may cross-react with EB virus. It is seldom indicated in patients whose blood smears in the first few weeks of illness are normal.

Treatment

Treatment is supportive, limited experiences with cortisone or acyclovir have been unimpressive.

ENTEROVIRUS

Coxsackievirus

Definition

Coxsackieviruses have been associated with a wide variety of illnesses including the common cold. Coxsackie B virus was recognized as a pathogen for neonates in the mid-1950s when it was identified as the cause of an acute myocarditis and meningoencephalitis in newborn infants in a nursery. The virus was originally isolated in the town of Coxsackie in New York state by Dalldorf and Sickles (1948). Congenital coxsackie B virus infection has been described as a cause of hepatitis and encephalomyocarditis. It is not known to be a teratogen, although the association of coxsackie B6 with congenital CNS malformations is suggestive. Coxsackie A16 is the major cause of hand, foot, and mouth syndrome.

Basic Science

Coxsackieviruses, echoviruses, and poliomyelitis viruses are the three main groups of RNA viruses that constitute enteroviruses. All three groups of enteroviruses are antigenically distinct and each has several serologic subtypes.

Epidemiology

Epidemic outbreaks of enteroviruses usually occur in the warmer months. Epidemics of coxsackie B5 have resulted in aseptic meningitis in newborn infants as well as in older children. The illness acquired in utero may present as early as 48 hours of age with hepatitis, encephalitis, and myocarditis. Occasionally, however, an infected infant may be asymptomatic.

Natural History

The incubation period is usually 3–6 days. Infants who acquire the illness may have a mild temperature elevation, nonspecific upper respiratory symptoms, and diarrhea. Later in the illness there may be an excessive tachycardia, tachypnea, cyanosis, and circulatory collapse in association with myocarditis.

In an older age group (young adults), epidemic pleurodynia (Bornholm disease) is most commonly caused by group B coxsackieviruses. The illness is most common among children 5–15 years of age. It is characterized by the abrupt onset of pain over the lower rib cage or upper abdomen with moderate fever, sometimes associated with sore throat, headache, and general malaise but cough is notably absent. Some individuals only experience a mild ache, but others have severe pain along the costal margin, aggravated by breathing. Pleurodynia should be considered whenever a child has a febrile illness with periumbilical pain. Pain may last for several hours during which time nothing is heard on auscultation. Pleural friction rubs are unusual. The illness usually last for 4–7 days. In the newborn, coxsackieviruses have been associated with myopericarditis. In older children the disorder usually follows an upper respiratory infection by about 2 weeks. The symptoms are those of myocarditis and include chest pain, shortness of breath, fever, and malaise, which has sometimes been confused with angina. A pericardial friction rub has been noted in more than half the patients during the course of illness. Enlargement of the cardiac silhouette may be the result of myocardial weakness and dilatation or a pericardial effusion. ECG abnormalities of ST segment elevations are usually present and severe myocardial disease may lead to the development of Q waves and arrhythmias.

Hand, foot, and mouth syndrome, most common in children less than 5 years old, has a short incubation period of less than a week, and presents as mild fever, malaise, and complaint of a sore mouth. After a few days an enanthem appears especially within the mouth. The lesions are 4–8 mm in diameter and frequently ulcerate. The hands, more commonly than feet, are the site of vesicular lesions 3–7 mm which clear in about a week. Trunk, thighs, and buttocks may be involved. Aseptic meningitis may be associated with this disorder.

The condition is most commonly due to coxsackie A16, but has been reported with other serotypes and enteroviruses.

Diagnosis

Attempts should be made to recover the virus in tissue culture or suckling mice. Serologic tests have a limited value in diagnosis. The identification of neutralizing antibody in ventricular fluid from infants with severe anatomic defect of the CNS is provocative and deserves further evaluation.

Treatment

Treatment is supportive only. No antiviral agent has been shown to be effective against coxsackie A or B virus. Immune globulin may be of benefit in immunocompromised patients.

Prognosis

Neonatally acquired myocarditis is said to have a mortality of about 50%, with death occurring within 1 week of onset. Older children and adults have a better prognosis, but may have recurrences of their myopericarditis. Chronic constrictive pericarditis has been reported with onset from 5 weeks to 1 year after the acute illness.

ECHO VIRUSES

Definition

ECHO viruses are normal inhabitants of the human gastrointestinal tract. They can cause neurologic illness. Apart from epidemics in newborn infants in which hepatic necrosis can occur, they rarely are associated with fatal illness.

Basic Science

The five most prevalent types are types 9, 4, 6, 11, and 30 (Cherry, 1981a). The virus is acquired through the oral or respiratory routes, and extends to regional lymph nodes. Viremia occurs about the third day, and illness depends on viral multiplication in secondary sites and later viremia from seeding. Approximately 90–95% of infections are asymptomatic.

Epidemiology

Enteroviruses have a worldwide distribution. Outbreaks of illness depend on clusters of susceptible individuals in a population. In temperate climates, illness is most common in August, September, and October.

Natural History

ECHO viruses produce nonspecific febrile illnesses of about 3 days' duration. Pharyngitis may be present. Vomiting and diarrhea are usually mild. Abdominal pain is often present, but is poorly localized. Mesenteric adenitis and peritonitis may occur. In newborns, the disease is much more serious and can be fatal (Carolane et al, 1985). Hepatitis, and even hepatic necrosis have been reported (Modlin, 1980).

A variety of skin manifestations have accompanied ECHO virus infection. The rash is usually erythematous and macular, but may be petechial. Conjunctivitis is frequent.

Epidemic aseptic meningitis is most commonly seen in ECHO 4, 9, and 30 infections. The simultaneous occurrence of an exanthem and fever should suggest the diagnosis. The duration of illness is 3–5 days. The virus has been associated with Guillain-Barré syndrome.

Hemangioma-like lesions have been seen in ECHO 25 and 32 infections.

Diagnosis

Virus isolation in association with symptoms is highly suggestive.

Treatment

No specific treatment for any enteroviral infection is available.

Prevention

In nursery outbreaks, passive protection with pooled human globulin (0.2 ml/kg im) may be useful. General good hygiene to lessen fecal-oral spread is the best known prevention.

EPSTEIN-BARR VIRUS

Infectious Mononucleosis

Definition

Infection with the Epstein-Barr virus (EBV, one of the herpes group) induces infectious mononucleosis. The disease occurs in children and young adults, and is characterized by fever and lymphoid hyperplasia. It is usually self-limited but can be associated with a chronic histiocytic response that may be fatal in immunocompromised hosts.

Basic Science

Infectious mononucleosis is invariably associated with EBV, as shown by seroconversion and by reaction to EBV-specific IgM antibody. The virus has been recovered from throat washings of individuals with clinical illness.

The virus belongs to the herpes group, with a capsid surrounded by a lipid-containing coat and a core of DNA. It is relatively large (110–120 nm) and easily inactivated. Transmission requires close contact, usually of the mucous membranes, between individuals.

The EBV was first isolated from cultured cells derived from African Burkitt lymphoma. The wide variety of host responses to this virus probably relate more to host differences than to any property of the virus. The common response to infection is a proliferation of lymphoid tissue. Atypical lymphocytes in peripheral blood are probably activated T cells. The EBV genome is in B cells.

Epidemiology

Infectious mononucleosis can be seen in children in the first year of life, although it is more commonly recognized in older children and in adolescents in whom contact of mucous membranes may occur, hence the name "the kissing disease." The incidence of infection is not known since much of it is subclinical, although it is clear that it can occur in epidemics in institutions. Presumably most humans have had asymptomatic infections at some stage. About one-third of infected adolescents develop symptoms. No seasonal predilection is found. Males are more commonly symptomatic than are females.

Natural History

The incubation period is 10–60 days. The most common single manifestation, and frequently the first, is low-grade fever, which may reach a height of 40–41°C during the peak of the disease. Lymphadenopathy occurs in more than 90% of the patients, and is frequently generalized. Prominence of the posterior cervical chain and axillary nodes, in addition to the anterior cervical chain from inflamed tonsils, suggests the widespread distribution of the infection. The virus persists for life in salivary glands and B lymphocytes. The ability of the virus to reactivate depends on the integrity of the cellular immune system.

The rashes are predominantly maculopapular, but can be petechial and in some resemble erythema multiforme. Complications include splenic rupture, hemolytic anemia, Bell palsy, transverse myelitis, and pneumonia.

Diagnosis

In general, there is a moderate elevation of white count to 10,000–15,000 cells with a predominance of lymphocytes. Atypical lymphocytes range from a few to as many as 40/100 white cells. A severe neutropenia occurs during the course of disease in 5–10% of children. Thrombocytopenia has been identified in a few of these patients. The complications of infectious mononucleosis can be very severe, particularly if the individual has an underlying impairment of host defenses. Pneumonia, meningitis, encephalitis, Guillain-Barré syndrome, hemolytic anemia, elevated liver transaminases, glomerulonephritis, and orchitis have all been reported. Superimposed bacterial infections are relatively rare.

LABORATORY DIAGNOSIS

The virus cannot be isolated directly. The rapid slide test to determine the presence of antibodies is widely used as a screening test. Quantitation of antibodies is done with the Paul-Bunnell-Davidsohn test which utilizes sheep and horse erythrocytes as agglutination indicator cells. These tests detect the heterophil antibodies in about 80% of children over age 4 years, but are less reliable in younger children. More specific serologic tests are possible with the measurement of IgM antibodies to EBV-capsid antigen. IgG antibodies to that antigen can also be measured. The EBV nuclear antigen can be determined late in the illness by techniques described by Henle and associates

(1974). Virus identification was first reported by Chang et al (1973) from material in the oropharynx of infected children. He found the virus could transform lymphocytes from cord blood of normal infants. Prolonged oral excretion has been observed (Miller et al, 1973).

Treatment

There is no specific treatment for EBV-infectious mononucleosis. Prednisone relieves some of the discomfort from cervical adenopathy and tonsillar enlargement within 24–48 hours, without adverse effects. In chronic malignant forms of the disease, more drastic chemotherapy is in order (see pp. 584).

Prevention

EBV infection confers lasting immunity. No vaccine is available in part because of the association of this virus with malignant lymphoproliferative disease.

CONTROVERSY

Chronic Mononucleosis-like Syndrome. EBV infection has been thought to be responsible for a syndrome of "recurrent mononucleosis" characterized by fatigue, myalgias, arthralgias, pharyngitis, headache, lymphadenopathy, and moderate hepatosplenomegaly. The symptoms and findings usually present for 2–4 months. The condition is seen mostly in female adolescents and young adults. Serology is not helpful in diagnosis of an individual, although as a group they tend to have elevated antibody titers against EBV antigens, especially VCA-IgG and EA-Ab.

The nonspecific nature of the symptoms and the lack of any diagnostic test make it possible that this syndrome could be caused by any number of agents. The diagnosis should be considered provisional and other causes of chronic fatigue considered (Holmes et al, 1987).

ROSEOLA (EXANTHEM SUBITUM)

Definition

Roseola (exanthem subitum) is one of the classic exanthems of childhood. It has a characteristic clinical course but no identified etiologic agent. (It was once known as "sixth" disease, when the common exanthems were numbered.) The course is that of a viral illness, hence its inclusion in this section.

Epidemiology

Roseola is an acute febrile illness that occurs commonly during the summer and early fall but can occur at any time of year. It is rare in infants before 3 months of age, and also rare after 4 years of age. One attack confers lasting immunity. It usually occurs sporadically but when it does occur in epidemics, the incubation period is between 5 and 15 days.

Natural History

Roseola should always be suspected in the presence of the acute onset of a high fever in a previously well child, without severe systemic signs and defervescence 3–5 days later at which time an erythematous maculopapular rash appears most prominently on the neck and trunk but involves the face and proximal extremities as well. It is not particularly itchy and desquamation is not present. The rash persists for 24–48 hours and then disappears.

Diagnosis

The diagnosis can be very complicated during the period of high fever and before the rash appears. These children have been worked up for sepsis and meningitis, and treated for pharyngitis and otitis. The pediatrician may attribute the rash to some of the drugs used during the febrile illness and the diagnosis may be missed altogether. An important distinguishing feature is that most rashes in association with drugs have fever concurrent with the rash. In roseola, the fever has subsided by the time the rash appears.

No laboratory tests are of particular value, except that the white blood count is usually low normal. The percentage of lymphocytes may increase to 80% and then return to normal after the rash disappears.

Complications

There have been neurologic complications from roseola although they are uncommon. Since no specific virus has been incriminated as the cause of roseola it is difficult to know what agents were responsible for the encephalitis and occasional residual hemoplasia.

Treatment

There is no specific treatment for roseola. When the temperature is over 40°C, acetaminophen is appropriate.

HERPES SIMPLEX

Definition

Herpes simplex (HSV) infections are among the most common in human infections. Infected individuals are usually asymptomatic. However, infections in newborns due to both type 1 and type 2 virus can be lethal. (Type 1 virus is primarily nongenital, and type 2 is often genital although these are not clear distinctions).

Basic Science

HSV replicates within cell nuclei; it is easily isolated in many tissue culture systems and produces typical cytopathic changes within 24–48 hours after inoculation. Types 1 and 2 share 50% sequence homology in their genome, but have unique biologic properties (Corey and Spear, 1986).

Serological tests are of less value since they are not completely reliable and, in infants at least, the disease is so fulminant that it is inappropriate to wait for serologic evidence of infection when the virus can usually be isolated from the lesions.

Epidemiology

The virus is found worldwide. The annual incidence of new cases of adult genital herpes is estimated to be as high as 4 million per year in the United States, with about 100 million episodes of recurrent labial herpes. The prevalence of genital infection in pregnant women is under 1%. HSV antibodies were found in 63% of adults in the Framingham Massachusetts Heart Study, 47% of whom had episodes of cold sores (Blackwelder et al, 1982).

Neonatal herpes, most commonly caused by type 2 virus, is not reported to the Centers for Disease Control so its incidence can only be estimated between 1/3500 and 1/30,000 live births (Frau and Alexander, 1985). The risk of infection in the infant whose mother has primary herpes is about 50%. The risk of infection in the infant born vaginally to a mother with recurrent infections is very low since neutralizing antibody crosses the placenta (Prober et al, 1987).

Natural History

CONGENITAL HERPES

Transmission of the virus in utero may occur through transplacental spread or ascending infection through the cervix. The organism can be spread venereally or by any direct contact with mucous membranes. During vaginal birth there is contamination of the infant's scalp, eyes, skin, umbilical cord, and upper respiratory tract. Vesicular lesions may be present on the day of birth, presumably from intrauterine infection. When the infection is acquired during delivery, illness may appear at 1–4 weeks of age. The vesicular lesions may appear first on the exposed skin, especially the scalp, and conjunctivitis is common. The predominant symptoms are lethargy, temperature instability, hepatomegaly, and CNS signs. Some infants will have keratitis in addition to conjunctivitis and coreoretinitis. Before the advent of chemotherapy, about 75% of infants in whom congenital herpes infection was diagnosed died.

Involvement of the CNS may be the dominant clinical feature and is the most serious. Congenital herpes is one of the causes of frank seizures and increased intracranial pressure with a bulging fontanelle. The signs may progress rapidly and lead to coma and eventually death. Several spinal fluid proteins are usually elevated by the time the child is symptomatic, and surprisingly the cell count is usually less than 400/mm^3. Nonspecific changes may be evident on the EEG. Hepatic involvement is common and as in the case of the CNS, may be fulminant. Some infants proceed to develop disseminated intravascular coagulation. Not all these infants are jaundiced, but an elevated bilirubin level usually includes both the direct and indirect components.

OTHER HERPETIC INFECTIONS

The cycle of infection is primary mucocutaneous infection, spread to neural ganglia, latency, reactivation, and recurrent infection. Although understanding of this cycle is rudimentary, it is recognized that latency can be lifelong. Presumably host immune responses maintain latency, but can be overcome under a number of stresses that must deregulate the immune surveillance mechanisms.

Diagnosis

The diagnosis is usually made on clinical grounds. Clusters of vesicular lesions on the scalp and trunk in particular are characteristic. The systemic manifestations of malaise, CNS, and hepatic involvement are most characteristic. Some infants have respiratory distress as well and widespread involvement of the lung is a recognized complication. Disseminated herpetic disease may be indistinguishable from enterovirus infection or bacterial sepsis.

Treatment

Fortunately there are now somewhat effective drugs to treat genital herpes simplex infection. Vidarabine has been effective. Acyclovir, which is an acyclic analogue of nucleoside guanine, specifically enters herpes virus-infected cells and inhibits the viral DNA polymerase that is needed for viral replication. The drug is available in topical, oral, and intravenous preparations. Acyclovir is effective in treatment of initial genital herpes, and also in the treatment of immunosuppressed patients who have been at risk of systemic herpes simplex infection (Meyers et al, 1982). The oral preparation is best; topical preparations only reduce virus shedding.

Experience with acyclovir in treating neonatal HSV infections is limited, although some reports have been very encouraging (Whitley et al, 1980a).

Unfortunately, there are some adverse effects, such as nephrotoxicity, which is presumably reversible. The long-term safety of the drug is not known, and it is not recommended for pregnant women or nursing mothers. Some organisms have developed resistance to acyclovir.

Prognosis

With disseminated infection or CNS disease, the outlook is very poor even with treatment. The case fatality rate is about 50% (Straus et al, 1985). In older children, subclinical infection can be present and the cause of later neurologic sequelae. If the involvement is localized to the skin, or eye, or mucous membranes, treatment with topical acyclovir may be effective and complete recovery is possible.

If the mother has vaginal lesions within 6 weeks of term, delivery should be by cesarean section within 4–6 hours of membrane rupture. If infection is primary, some obstetricians would deliver by section even if membranes were ruptured more than 6 hours, since the risk of the infant having the disease is 40–50%.

Contact isolation is essential for the duration of illness.

No effective vaccines are available as of 1988.

CONTROVERSY

What is the pediatrician's responsibility to an infant born vaginally to a mother with vaginal lesions? In general, if the infection is primary, the infant will be cultured and treated soon after birth. If the lesions are a recurrence, we culture and observe since the risk is 3–5%. Infants should receive local ophthalmic drugs as well as parenteral antiviral therapy.

CASE ILLUSTRATION

A 7-year-old male presented with lethargy, headache, and vomiting over 1–2 days. His examination was initially notable for visual hallucinations, disorientation to time and place, and a unilateral upgoing toe. CSF results revealed 41 white cells with 9% polys, 47% lymphs, 44% monos, and 6 red blood cells, a protein of 10, and a glucose of 70. EEG showed spikes in the right temporal area with spread to frontal area of the brain. The patient's mental status cleared significantly over his first 6 hours of hospitalization. Despite high suspicion of his having an enterovirus, the focal findings on physical examination and an EEG could not be ignored and a herpes encephalitis was considered in the differential.

QUESTION AND COMMENT

Is a brain biopsy indicated, or should an antiviral agent be started empirically?

While brain biopsy at present remains the definitive method of diagnosis, it is difficult to subject a fully alert patient to this procedure before beginning empiric treatment with an antiviral agent such as acyclovir, since the side effects upon proper administration are minimal. If treatment is witheld until the patient's neurologic status deteriorates, antiviral therapy may not be effective. On the other hand, empirical treatment with an antiviral agent may exclude identification of other possibly treatable etiologies (that a brain biopsy could diagnose). In short, the clinical likelihood of this patient having herpes simplex encephalitis versus the risks and benefits of biopsy in the treatment must be carefully considered.

A review of the literature on this subject is complicated and confusing. One study supports the idea of brain biopsy before treating, while another will be equally convincing in promoting empirical treatment, particularly if the examination shows focal or suspicious EEG findings. The team taking care of this patient weighed all the variables, observed the patient's general clinical improvement, and elected to treat him with acyclovir without brain biopsy. He subsequently did well and his neurologic examination which was already near baseline before starting treatment, returned to normal. We hope future noninvasive tests will obviate the need for brain biopsy in making the diagnosis of herpes encephalitis.

VARICELLA ZOSTER

Definition

Chickenpox and herpes zoster (shingles) are caused by a virus that persists throughout life in the sensory ganglia. Chickenpox, the first infection, usually occurs during childhood and presents initially on the trunk as discrete pruritic vesicular lesions. Zoster or shingles represents a reappearance of the virus in a distribution of from 1 to 3 sensory dermatomes as a cluster of vesicular lesions (Weller, 1953; Weller, 1983).

Basic Science

Herpes varicellae or V-Z virus is one of the herpes virus group in the category of a DNA virus. Giant cells induced by the viruses can be recovered from the base of vesicles from a cutaneous lesion and can be identified rapidly by a Tzanck preparation. The virus can be distinguished from HSV by immunofluorescence with suitable monoclonal antibodies.

Complement-fixing antibodies can be identified and persist for many years. With the emergence of zoster infections there is a rise in CF antibody.

Congenital varicella is a rare condition partly because most women have had varicella before pregnancy. The prevalence in the collaborative project of some 30,000 pregnancies was 0.7/1000. Confirmatory laboratory diagnosis depends on detection of the antibody by complement fixation. Infection of mother 5 days before birth or 1 day after is especially dangerous for the fetus who may have viremia and no passive antibodies from mother. Intrauterine infection is more common with maternal varicella than with maternal herpes zoster (Paryani and Arvin, 1986; Alkalay et al, 1987).

Epidemiology

Varicella occurs in 90/100,000 individuals each year in the United States. Sixty percent of cases occur between 5 and 9 years of age, and 80% in children less than 10 years old (Preblud, 1981). Outbreaks occur beginning in early autumn and peak in the spring (Fig. 17.2).

Natural History

Man is the only reservoir of infection for the varicella zoster virus. Thus, the disease depends on direct contact or airborne droplet infection. Introduction of the virus into the household usually results in infection in nearly all susceptible persons. Individuals are believed to be contagious for 1–2 days before, and 5–6 days after the onset of the rash until crusted. The incubation period is 14–16 days but may be as early as 11 days or as late as 21 days after contact.

There are few systemic symptoms with the first attack. Complications, however, can occur including

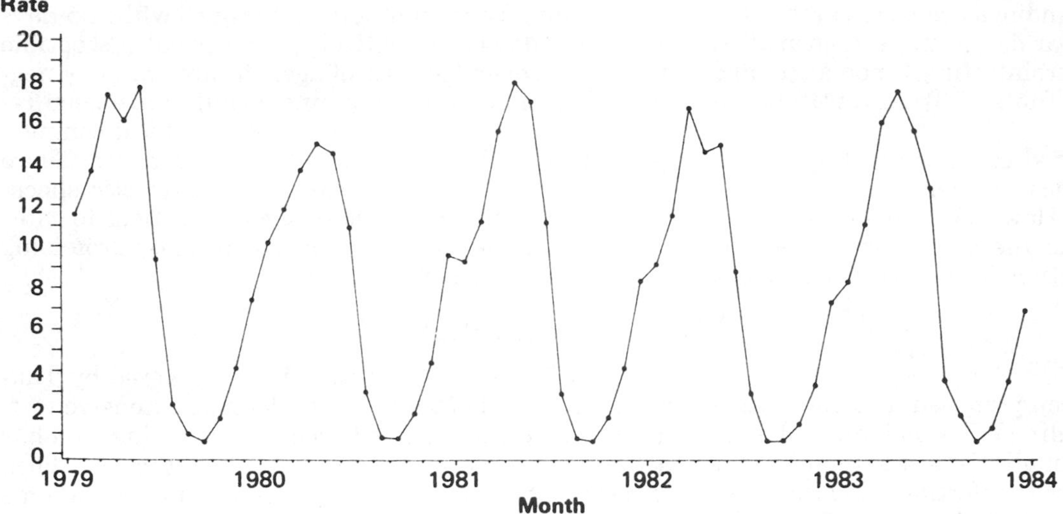

Figure 17.2. Reported cases of varicella per 100,000 cases, by month, United States 1979–1983. Varicella was the second most frequently reported infectious disease (gonorrhea was first) in the United States in 1983. Note the peak incidence is between March and May. From CDC: *MMWR* 32:71, 1984.

those related to bacterial superinfection, thrombocytopenia, hepatitis, arthritis, and sometimes encephalitis or meningitis. Reports of Reye syndrome have been noted after some instances of chickenpox. In the immune deficient patient, chickenpox can be most severe and characterized by high fever and continuing new lesions into the second week of the illness.

The lesions of varicella appear as small clusters of red papules which very shortly develop a clear teardrop-shaped vesicle on an erythematous base. The contents become cloudy after 24 hours and the vesicles are easily broken with the formation of small scabs. The lesions first appear on the trunk, spread later onto the face and scalp, but rarely involve the distal extremities. Most individuals have some degree of malaise and fever. Pruritis can sometimes be severe. Mucous membrane involvement is common in the mouth, but unusual in the genital areas. When individuals have an associated thrombocytopenia, the rash can be hemorrhagic. Purpura fulminans has been described at the end of the first week in individuals with varicella infection.

Diagnosis

The virus can be isolated during the first 3–4 days of the skin eruption. It can be identified by a Tzanck preparation or direct electron microscopy and by immunofluorescence. Infection is best confirmed by testing acute and convalescent sera.

Complications

Bacterial superinfections, particularly in children less than 5 years of age, remain the most common complication of chickenpox. Usually, these are minor superficial infections, but they may be more extensive and require hospitalization.

Treatment

No treatment for varicella is usually required except for general supportive care. Usually the fever is low grade and aspirin should be avoided because of the reported association with Reye syndrome. Strict isolation of these patients is indicated when they require hospitalization. In fact, it would be appropriate to avoid hospitalization of children with varicella since the immunosuppressed population in the hospital would be so susceptible to infection. In severe cases, acyclovir is effective.

VARICELLA IN PREGNANCY

The risk of serious illness in the mother is probably no higher than in the general population, although deaths from varicella pneumonia have been reported. The virus can infect the placenta and, in turn, the fetuses who may have skin lesions, pneumonia, hepatitis, among other lesions. No increase in fetal death or premature births has been noted in maternal varicella. If the maternal rash is within 5 days of delivery, the infant is at greatest risk of serious disease, since there would be inadequate time for maternal antibodies to develop and cross the placenta. An infant infected just before or after birth should be given v. zoster immune globulin (VZIG) as soon as possible.

Overall transmission of virus to infant occurs in 26% of cases. Usually the infant has skin lesions that appear between 5 and 10 days of life and require isolation from other infants. Systemic infection is rare, but accounts for a 5% case fatality rate, hence the recommendation for VZIG. If the infant becomes tachypneic or develops a fever or rash, systemic varicella may become apparent even after ZIG. Acyclovir may be useful.

FETAL VARICELLA SYNDROME

Varicella infection between 8 and 20 weeks of pregnancy may be associated with a wide variety of abnormalities. The virus apparently causes necrosis of nerve cells which, in turn, leads to malformations. The condition should be suspected in any infant of a mother who had chickenpox between 8 and 20 weeks, and who is born with skin lesions in the distribution of a dermatome. Other common findings are limb paresis, hydrocephalus, seizures, bulbar dysphagia, eye anomalies, skeletal hypoplasias, gastrointestinal anomalies, and genitourinary anomalies (Table 17.3) (Arvin, 1986; Alkalay et al, 1987).

The number of reported cases is small (30 as of 1987) probably because most women of child-bearing age have had chickenpox. However, under-recognition may be a factor because of the many conditions that can result from fetal infection. The mortality is about 30%.

Prevention

In certain immune-compromised patients, varicella zoster immune globulin (VZIG) is indicated after exposure. This immunoglobulin is of maximal benefit within 96 hours of exposure to infection and it may not be beneficial after that time. It is not useful in the treatment of clinical infection. It is probable that the duration of immunity will equal the half-life of the immunoglobulin (approximately 3–4 weeks). The recommended dose is 125–625 units/kg given im. Recipients of the immunoglobulin should include all immunocompromised children: those with neoplastic disease who have been exposed to the disease, all newborn infants whose mothers had lesions within 5 days before or 2 days after delivery, and normal susceptible adolescents over 15 years of age who are antibody negative. Reactions to the immunoglobulin have been reported but appear to be infrequent. The most common reaction is local discomfort at the injection site. There has been a rare reported case of anaphylactic shock, but otherwise no other serious adverse reactions to date.

A vaccine is under evaluation and looks promising (Lawrence et al, 1988).

CONTROVERSY

An effective vaccine was first discovered by Takahashi et al in 1974 and has undergone extensive testing ever since. It is a live herpes virus vaccine, and has not been licensed for fear of increasing the likelihood of zoster infections in adults or in others who become immune-suppressed. It has been administered safely to individuals with leukemia in remission. A review of the pros and cons of this controversial subject appeared as a supplement to *Pediatrics* 78:1986 under the title "Current status of varicella vaccine."

Table 17.3
Summary of Details in 18 Cases of Congenital V-Z[1]

Illness or Defect	No.
Maternal varicella in pregnancy	14
Maternal zoster in pregnancy	3
Maternal zoster varicellosus in pregnancy	1
Gestational age at maternal illness	8–20 weeks
Infants born "small for gestational age"	8
Cutaneous scars	13
Hypoplasia of a limb	10
Muscular atrophy	9
Rudimentary digits	5
Psychomotor retardation	7
Seizures	3
Muscular paralysis	4
Other CNS signs or symptoms Cortical atrophy Microcephaly Horner syndrome	7
Microphthalmus	8
Chorioretinitis	4
Cataracts and nystagmus	8
Facial asymmetry	3
Recurrent chest infections	4
Delayed development in infancy	7
Deaths	7
Survivors	11

[1] Reproduced with permission from Hanshaw DB, Dudgeon JA, Marshall WC: *Viral Diseases of the Fetus and Newborn*. Philadelphia, WB Saunders, 1985.

Shingles

Definition

Herpes zoster is a reactivation of latent infection with varicella zoster virus which starts with neuralgic pain in the area of the dermatome and is followed by an outcropping of vesicles.

Epidemiology

The incidence of this condition (shingles), which always occurs in patients who have had a history of varicella infection, increases with each decade. Second attacks are very rare. The disease is particularly threatening in individuals with malignancies and those who are receiving immunosuppressive drugs.

Natural History

Typically the illness presents as a neuralgia, sometimes accompanied with malaise and fever. After a few days red papules appear, usually unilaterally and are distributed in the area of the dermatome. The most commonly involved segments are those of the second dorsal to the second lumbar nerves, but can occur with other nerves including the trigeminal. When the seventh nerve is involved it is called the Ramsay Hunt syndrome which represents paralysis of the facial nerve and vesicles in and around the external ear canal.

The course of the illness is for the lesions to become vesicular then pustular and finally scab over a period of 5–10 days. Successive crops may appear, but always in clusters and along a dermatome. Fever, pain, and tenderness are likely to persist during the several weeks that the vesicles are present and regional lymph nodes are enlarged.

Diagnosis

The diagnosis depends on thc the characteristic cluster of lesions in a dermatome. In the first few days of the rash it is possible to isolate the virus from scrapings of the bases of the vesicles or from vesicular fluid. A Tzanck preparation will show multinucleated giant cells. Occasionally, the spinal fluid will have a mild lymphocytosis. A rise in varicella zoster virus antibody titer occurs during the 2 weeks following the illness.

CASE ILLUSTRATION

A 6-year-old female was brought to the emergency room with a 2-day history of a red raised slightly tender rash in the groin and buttocks. She had been well previously with an exposure to chickenpox at 2 months of age, but no apparent disease afterward, and no other episodes of rashes. On examination, she was afebrile, and had an erythematous, papulovesicular rash, in a dermatomal distribution over the left thigh and groin, without fever, organomegaly, or altered mental status. She was sent home with a diagnosis of varicella zoster, presumably reactivated from her primary asymptomatic infection in infancy, but returned the next day with scattered vesicular lesions over all parts of the body in addition to her dermatomal zoster, as well as with vomiting and mild dehydration. Again she had no mental status changes, or organomegaly. Her liver function tests were normal and she was admitted for observation and rehydration.

QUESTIONS AND COMMENTS

What conditions predispose to the appearance of zoster in a previously well child?

In adults, zoster has been associated with immunosuppressed states such as extreme old age, leukemia, lymphoma, and chemotherapy. The appearance of zoster in childhood is especially prevalent after primary infection in utero or within the first 6 months of life, and may be the first symptomatic manifestation of varicella zoster virus infection since the primary infection may have had an attenuated or asymptomatic course. Disseminated infection occurring with zoster has been related to lower levels of antivaricella zoster virus antibody and is a hallmark of the viremia that occurs in some episodes of zoster.

How should such a case be treated?

Prevailing opinion suggests that systemic chemotherapy with ara A or acyclovir be reserved for patients with systemic manifestations of disseminated disease—i.e., hepatitis or encephalitis—or with underlying risk factors for the development of systemic illness—i.e., malignancy, chemotherapy, or immunodeficiency. Such therapy has been shown to reduce the severity and incidence of systemic manifestations in these settings. In our patient, the disseminated pox were not associated with systemic signs and an uneventful recovery followed without antiviral systemic therapy.

Treatment

The treatment is symptomatic. Aspirin should be avoided, particularly in children because of the possible risk of Reye syndrome. In immunocompromised patients, acyclovir is appropriate. The prognosis is usually good.

Prevention

Varicella zoster can spread rapidly among household contacts, usually within about 2 weeks of exposure. The incubation period is between 8 and 21 days. Patients with zoster who require hospitalization should be treated as if they had chickenpox. Zoster infection is a reason to stay home from school until all blisters have dried, which is normally 1–2 weeks.

HUMAN IMMUNODEFICIENCY VIRUS (HIV) AIDS (Acquired Immunodeficiency Syndrome)

Definition

AIDS was first recognized as a clinical entity in 1981, and later recognized as the end-stage of infection with human immunodeficiency virus. The underlying problem is immunosuppression from loss of T4 lymphocytes, which predisposes to overwhelming opportunistic infections. In the early stages, before opportunistic infection occurs, the disorder is referred to as AIDS-related complex (ARC).

A summary definition of HIV infection in children under 13 years is shown in Table 17.4 published by The Centers for Disease Control (1987). A classification is proposed in Table 17.5.

Basic Science

The causative agent of AIDS is human immunodeficiency virus (HIV) formerly known as HTLV III, lymphadenopathy AIDS virus (LAV), and AIDS-associated retrovirus (ARV). The virus is a member of the lentivirus, or slow virus, subgroup of retroviruses and is closely related to a number of viruses that cause chronic degenerative neurologic and immunologic diseases of animals.

Table 17.4
Summary of the Definition of HIV Infection in Children

Infants and children under 15 months of age with perinatal infection
- Virus in blood or tissues or
- HIV antibody and evidence of both cellular and humoral immune deficiency and one or more categories in class P-2 or
- Symptoms meeting CDC case definition for AIDS

Older children with perinatal infection and children with HIV infection acquired through other modes of transmission
- Virus in blood or tissues or
- HIV antibody or
- Symptoms meeting CDC case definition for AIDS

Table 17.5
Summary of the Classification of HIV Infection in Children under 13 Years of Age

Class P-O. Indeterminate infection

Class P-1. Asymptomatic infection
- Subclass A. Normal immune function
- Subclass B. Abnormal immune function
- Subclass C. Immune function not tested

Class P-2. Symptomatic infection
- Subclass A. Nonspecific findings
- Subclass B. Progressive neurologic disease
- Subclass C. Lymphoid interstitial pneumonitis
- Subclass D. Secondary infectious diseases
  - Category D-1. Specified secondary infectious diseases listed in the CDC surveillance definition for AIDS
  - Category D-2. Recurrent serious bacterial infections
  - Category D-3. Other specified secondary infectious diseases
- Subclass E. Secondary cancers
  - Category E-1. Specified secondary cancers listed in the CDC surveillance definition for AIDS
  - Category E-2. Other cancers possibly secondary to HIV infection
- Subclass F. Other diseases possibly due to HIV infection

The AIDS virus causes immunosuppression by infecting the T4 lymphocytes. The loss of these inducer and helper cells takes place gradually from blood, lymph nodes, spleen, and other tissues. The virus selectively inhibits the growth of T4 lymphocytes and eventually destroys them, although it probably remains latent in a few cells.

In children, the earliest consequence of loss of T4 lymphocytes is usually a lack of direction to B cells, which produce large amounts of nonspecific (and ineffective) immunoglobulins. Somewhat later in the course of the disease, T-cell deficiency results in susceptibility to fungal infections, *Pneumocystis carinii* pneumonia, and chronic diarrhea (Pifer et al, 1988). The virus apparently can invade the CNS and produce psychosis and brain atrophy (Laurence, 1985; Belman et al, 1988). The virus can invade intestinal mucosa and neurons. Chronic diarrhea and cerebral atrophy may be the consequence.

Epidemiology

Groups at risk of acquiring AIDS are homosexuals (24–68% positive), their heterosexual contacts, iv drug users with contaminated needles (2–72%), hemophiliacs (40–88% positive), and other transfusion recipients. The problem has been particularly serious among Haitians and in Zaire. The total number of children reported to the Communicable Disease Center in the United States as of July 1987 was 520. Seventy-five percent were from mothers with AIDS, 14% received blood or blood products before antibody screening in blood banks, 5% were hemophiliacs, and in 6%, no risk factors were identified. Sixty-four percent died by 1987.

Among United States military recruits, the prevalence of confirmed positive antibody tests for HIV was 1.5/1000 in 1985–1986 (Burke et al, 1987). The rate of infections is highest in Central and East Africa where the annual incidence is 0.75% (Quinn et al, 1986). Worldwide, a total of 73,747 cases were reported to WHO as of 9 December 1987 (Piot et al, 1988).

Natural History

The time from initial infection with HIV to onset of symptoms is variable, but probably on average is several years. In homosexual men infected with HIV, only 5–20% have developed disease within the first 2–5 years after becoming infected (Curran, 1985). The infants of infected adults, who presumably were infected in utero, may fail to gain weight or grow appropriately in the first year of life. Chronic diarrhea and sustained fever are major manifestations. Their initial contact with a physician may be for a severe infection, which in association with lymphadenopathy, cardiomyopathy, and hepatosplenomegaly should arouse suspicion. The course of illness depends in part on the chance encounter with pathogens such as *Candida*, herpes, cytomegalovirus, or *Pneumocystis*. A lymphocytic interstitial pneumonia results from EB virus infection. The disorder is probably uniformly fatal. The course may extend over months or a few years. The oldest child with congenital infection we know of is 9 years old (as of 1988) (Ammann, 1985). (See Section 12 for neurologic findings.)

Diagnosis

A positive titer to HIV antibody beyond 15 months of age when maternal antibody has disappeared is strong evidence of disease. Before 15 months of age, definite diagnosis is more difficult since one-half of infants born to infected mothers (and carrying transplacentally transmitted HIV antibody) are not infected. The most significant other finding is evidence of a depression in T-suppressor lymphocytes, with polyclonal elevation of immunoglobulins (up to six to eight times normal). It is important to exclude primary immunodeficiency disorders where clinical features may resemble AIDS, by a negative antibody test in the child and parents.

Infants can acquire infection in utero, during delivery, from close contact with an infected mother, and from breast milk. The diagnosis of infection in the infant depends on detection of an anti-HIV antibody of the IgM isotype. The absence of the antibody at birth, and its peak level at 8 weeks suggests a primary perinatal infection. Confirmation of infection in infants requires identification of the virus by culture or the presence of antigen.

Some infants with congenital HIV infection have been noted to have a prominent forehead, greater than normal palpebral fissure length, hypertelorism, flattened nasal bridge, and occasionally hydrocephalus.

These features may or may not represent an HIV embryopathy (Marion et al, 1987; Qazi et al, 1988).

Treatment

No treatment is known for underlying immunodeficiency, although several drugs are being evaluated in 1987. If *P. carinii* pneumonia is present, trimethoprim sulfa should be given indefinitely. Intravenous γ-globulin is under study as a mode of treatment. (Calvelli and Rubenstein, 1986). Newer antiviral drugs are under investigation (Oleske et al, 1988).

Prevention

Unfortunately, no vaccine is available, and hence, the best precaution is to modify lifestyle by less promiscuity and avoidance of intravenous drug abuse (Fineberg, 1988). An advance was made with the ability to detect antibodies in blood donors, so that, at present in the United States, the blood supply is almost completely safe. The kinds of precautions taken with patients with hepatitis are appropriate for patients hospitalized with AIDS. Immunization of infants with AIDS with attenuated vaccines is not advised (measles, rubella, mumps, polio). Inactivated poliovaccine may be given (CDC, 1986b). Family contacts should *not* be given live polio vaccine.

NEW DEVELOPMENTS

During the first 6 years of awareness of AIDS in the United States, about 55,000 cases are known. The estimate for the next 5 years is about 235,000 new cases (Barnes, 1986). Nearly 18,000 people have died from AIDS by December 1986. The problem is staggering in the absence of a vaccine to prevent it or effective treatment. Only education is available to break the chain of transmission from sexual contact, contaminated blood or needles, and birth from an infected mother.

CASE ILLUSTRATION

A 13-month-old male infant of a mother who was a drug abuser presented with a history of lethargy, irritability, and rapid breathing. The mother had had several hospitalizations for pneumonia and was known to be chronically neutropenic. The infant had had no well child visits and no immunizations. The pregnancy was said to have been uneventful and the birth weight was 3.2 kg. However, the infant never gained weight appropriately, and at 13 months weighed only 7.2 kg, with a length of 72 cm, and a head circumference of 44 cm. All measurements are less than the third percentile.

On examination, it was evident that he had generalized lymphadenopathy, anemia, and hepatosplenomegaly. The liver was 4 cm down, the spleen 5 cm down. He was febrile and irritable and, for that reason, a lumbar puncture was performed. The spinal fluid showed 23 white blood cells, all lymphocytes with a protein of 18, and a glucose of 16. The hemogram revealed a hematocrit of 21, blood count of 16,400 with normal differential. The sedimentation rate was 33. On hospitalization it was evident that he had persistent elevations in temperature reaching 41°C at one point. A chest radiograph showed patchy infiltrates bilaterally. He was treated with ampicillin for 10 days because of the inability to rule out a bacterial cause of his pneumonia. There was no improvement. While in the hospital, he developed profuse diarrhea and abdominal distention. Stool cultures were negative, as were blood cultures and spinal fluid culture. Serology for toxoplasmosis, rubella, cytomegalovirus, and herpes were all negative. Immunoglobulins were all elevated. A *Candida* skin test was negative, T cells were depressed with T4 being approximately half the predicted normal number. It was ascertained later that blood from both the mother and the infant was positive for HIV antibody.

The infant remained in the hospital for 3 months without significant change in clinical course. A volunteer grandmother, appropriately dressed in gown and gloves, visits the child daily and provides some substitute mothering. The infant remains withdrawn and continues to fail to gain weight.

QUESTIONS AND COMMENTS

What questions are most appropriate when taking the history of an infant who has failed to thrive?

After the usual family and past histories have been recorded, it is essential to explore the social history. In our patient, the fact that the mother was a drug abuser and had been hospitalized for pneumonia was not learned at the time of admission. Concern was aroused early, however, about her capacity as a caregiver since the infant had had no immunizations.

Should a child with AIDS be placed in a foster home, if parents have AIDS?

Parents with AIDS who are well enough and competent as parents can care for the child. If not, a foster home seems plausible if foster parents are willing to enforce the same kind of precautions they would in caring for a child with hepatitis. The virus has been identified in saliva and tears, but transmission by contact with those secretions alone has not been documented (as of mid-1988). The patient should be protected from individuals with infections such as chickenpox, measles, herpes simplex, and tuberculosis. AIDS children should not receive live virus vaccines that are mandated for school attendance such as measles, rubella, and mumps. They should receive inactivated polio vaccine, and DPT, and *H. influenzae* vaccines.

Adolescents with AIDS should be aware of the risk of sexual transmission, and spread through shared needles and syringes.

If a mother with AIDS becomes pregnant, what is the risk to the fetus?

Although the data are limited, in a study of 20 women who had previously delivered a baby with AIDS, 65% of the next pregnancies resulted in another infected infant. Among infected primiparas, 35% had infected infants (Rubenstein, 1986).

INFLUENZA

Definition

Influenza is a respiratory illness caused by many different strains of influenza virus.

Epidemiology

Influenza comes in epidemics every few years, with the peak attack rate in January through March (Fig. 17.3). Types A and B viruses prevail in different areas. Other types may appear during worldwide outbreaks. Influenza accounts for between 4% and 8% of all deaths signed out as pneumonia. Individuals with underlying chronic lung disease or other debilitating illness are most at risk. Outbreaks with influenza A (H3N2) were reported in nursing homes in the United States in 1984–1985. The incidence of influenza infections is not known since many cases are not reported.

Basic Science

Influenza viruses, classified as orthomyxoviruses, are negative strand RNA viruses of three major antigenic types, A, B, and C. The current nomenclature specifies type and subtype. Thus, in January 1986 in the United States, influenza was reported as the result of infection with type A (H3N2) virus. H stands for hemagglutinin and N for neuraminidase subtypes. Occasionally, the viruses are identified by the country or region in which they were first isolated. Thus, epidemics result from Asian flu or Hong Kong flu.

The biologic and antigenic diversity of influenza viruses, called antigenic drift, results from point mutations. Mutant viruses emerge with the capacity to grow in the presence of antibodies from previous infections. Thus the need to anticipate the most likely strains of influenza in time to make a vaccine to protect in an epidemic.

Influenza viruses can affect individuals of any age particularly during epidemics. They characteristically involve the alveolar lining cells, and may disrupt surfactant synthesis. In its most severe form, influenza pneumonia resembles acute respiratory distress syndrome. The lungs become atelectatic, and edema and hemorrhage occur. With continued breathing of oxygen-enriched mixtures, the lesions of oxygen toxicity are superimposed with hyaline membrane formation.

Natural History

The virus is spread by inhalation of droplets aerosolized by a coughing patient. It may also spread by direct contact. The incubation period is 1–7 days. Influenza begins with sudden onset of high fever, headache, and myalgia. After several days, the chest film may show diffuse infiltrates reminiscent of adult respiratory distress syndrome. The clinical spectrum is wide and includes pleural effusion. With severe fulminant disease, hypoxemia may be present.

Diagnosis

Virus may be recovered from respiratory secretions just before and during the period of symptoms. Routine laboratory studies are not helpful. The white count may be normal or elevated.

Treatment

Most attacks of influenza last 2–5 days and are self-limited. If fever is high, acetaminophen may be used, but aspirin should be avoided because of its possible role in postinfluenza Reye syndrome.

Mechanical ventilation may be required for influenza pneumonia. Added oxygen may be needed, but since it can aggravate already inflammed alveolar tissues, it should not be given in excess of the amount needed to keep arterial oxygen over 80 mm Hg.

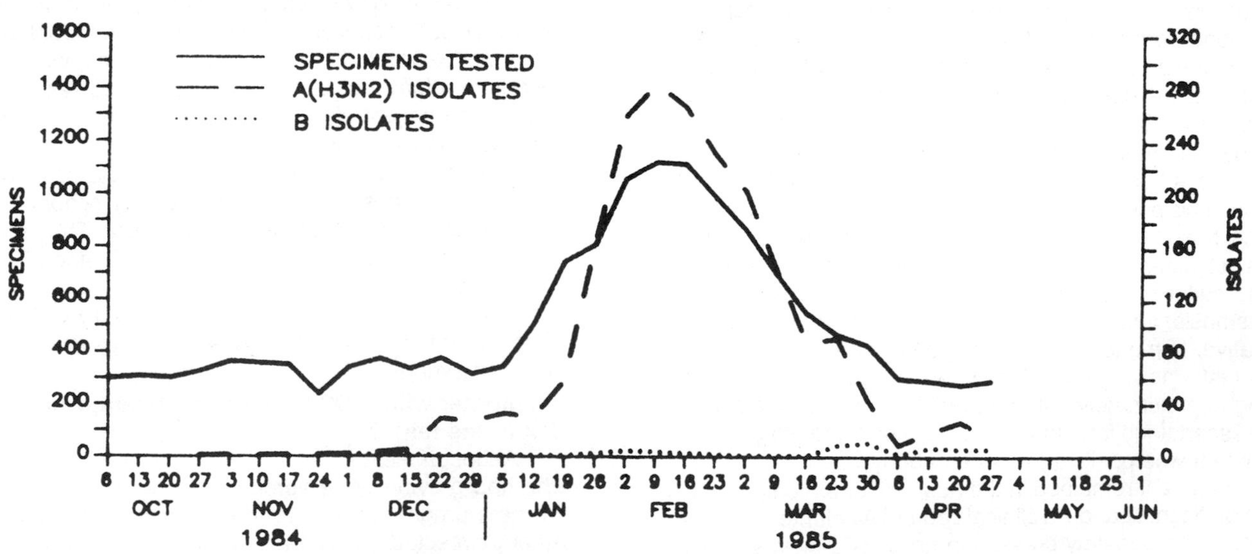

Figure 17.3. Laboratory diagnosis of influenza reported to Centers for Disease Control by WHO Collaborating Laboratories. From CDC: *MMWR* 34:442, 1985.

The drug of choice in 1988 is oral amantadine, 5–8 mg/kg/day, maximum 200 mg/day given every 12 hours. (Adult doses are up to 550 mg/day.)

CONTROVERSY

Ribavirin has in vitro activity against influenza, but it has not been evaluated in terms of efficacy as an aerosol.

Corticosteroids, advocated by some physicians, appear to enhance pulmonary oxygen toxicity in animals. Their use is not justified on the basis of current information.

Prevention

Influenza vaccine is updated annually on knowledge of strains of virus most likely to produce illness in a given region. The vaccine contains highly purified, inactivated, egg-grown viral particles that produce a type-specific hemagglutinin antibody in about 2 weeks. Some local redness and swelling occur in about one-third of individuals immunized, and 5% have some mild fever and myalgia. A split product preparation is sometimes used in children to reduce symptoms. Anaphylaxis from eggs is a contraindication.

Children for whom annual immunization against influenza is recommended include those with chronic asthma, cystic fibrosis, or other chronic lung disease such as bronchopulmonary dysplasia. Children undergoing chemotherapy for cancer and those with congenital heart disease are also at risk. It is important for medical personnel in close contact with patients to be immunized to avoid becoming ill in an epidemic, or be themselves carriers of infection.

Since there is overlap of groups at risk for pneumococcal disease and influenza, the vaccines can be given at different sites at the same time. (Pneumococcal vaccine is given only once; influenza vaccine is given annually.)

Amantadine is effective in preventing illness caused by type A influenza (not type B). When given within 24–48 hours of onset of symptoms, the course is shorter and less severe.

LASSA FEVER

Definition

This viral illness seen most commonly in tropical West Africa and Central Africa causes an acute febrile illness which may be very mild or progressively fatal. It was first recognized in 1969 among missionary nurses in Lassa, Nigeria. The viruses are small RNA viruses of the arenavirus group, related to lymphocytic choriomeningitis.

Epidemiology and Natural History

The incidence is unknown, although it is quite common in endemic areas. The incubation is 3–16 days, with the insidious onset of fever and malaise, with headache. Bradycardia, hypotension, pharyngitis, and lymphadenopathy are common, as is facial and neck swelling, and occasionally, conjunctival injection and a macular rash. In the more severe cases there is an altered sensorium, and pulmonary edema and ascites are common. Convalescence may be prolonged with generalized weakness, loss of hair, and irreversible hearing impairment.

Diagnosis

The laboratory findings include leukopenia in about half the patients and, frequently, massive proteinuria. Patchy infiltrates may be evident on chest radiographs. Definitive diagnosis depends on isolation of the lassa virus from serum or urine or other body fluids. Serologic diagnosis is possible with IgM and IgG specific indirect immunofluorescent antibodies. A serum asparate aminotransferase level of > 150 IU/L is associated with a case fatality rate of over 50% (McCormick et al, 1986).

Treatment

Until 1986, treatment was supportive only. An encouraging report on the efficacy of ribavirin, given orally or intravenously in an epidemic in Sierra Leone, makes it the drug of choice. It can be given at any time during the illness, as well as for postexposure prophylaxis (McCormick et al, 1986).

Prognosis

The case fatality rate in epidemics has been 36–76%.

Prevention

The virus is spread person to person, thus, full isolation precautions are appropriate, including gloves, gowns, and masks. Attention should be given to decontamination of bed linen and all objects with which the patient has had contact.

The virus has been identified in rats. Lessening human exposure to rats could reduce the risk of disease.

MUMPS VIRUS

Definition

The mumps virus belongs to the group of paramyxoviruses and has only one known serotype that is pathogenic for humans. The disease is mainly associated with parotid involvement, orchitis, or CNS manifestations.

Epidemiology

The mumps virus is endemic worldwide (now rare in the U.S.) and its only known host is the human. In unimmunized populations epidemics tended to occur every 2–5 years throughout the year, but often with a peak in late winter or early spring. During the summer months it has been associated with aseptic meningitis.

Since the introduction of the live attenuated mumps vaccine, a dramatic decrease in reported cases has been observed in those states that have intensive immunization programs (Fig. 17.4).

Natural History

The mumps virus is transmitted in affected saliva or is airborne through droplets. The infection rates in susceptible populations have been as high as 80%. The period of communicability extends from several days before the onset of symptoms to several days thereafter, but the virus has been isolated as late as 9 days after the onset of parotitis. Infection with the virus or immunization is thought to confer immunity for life.

The virus proliferates in the upper respiratory tract epithelium and then enters the circulation. It then localizes in glandular and neural tissue.

The onset of symptoms is usually that of an acute generalized disease with fever, malaise, and headache. Most patients develop parotitis which may appear in one or both parotid glands. Earache, jaw tenderness with chewing, and dry mouth are among the presenting complaints which worsen over the next several days. Sucking a sour stimulus produces significant worsening of the pain. The swelling is at the angle of the jaw, and obliterates the angle, often extending to the lower portion of the ear which may be displaced up and out. Defervescence and resolution of parotid tenderness takes about a week.

Infection can also be established in the testes and epididymis, particularly in adolescents or adults. Orchitis usually occurs 1–2 weeks after parotitis, but it may occur without parotitis. Symptoms begin abruptly with testicular swelling and tenderness and associated nausea, vomiting, and headache. The testicle may enlarge three or four times and become very tender. Later, some degree of atrophy develops in nearly half the affected organs.

Oophoritis has been reported in as many as 5% of postpubertal females with mumps. If the right ovary is involved, it can resemble appendicitis.

CNS involvement is characterized by an aseptic meningitis which occurs in 1–10% of patients with parotitis. Meningeal symptoms develop any time between a week before or several weeks after the parotitis. Lymphocytic dominance with fewer than 500 cells is usual, but white cell counts may rise to over 2000 in the spinal fluid. The spinal fluid glucose is usually normal, and the protein is normal or slightly elevated. These findings revert to normal after about a week and sequelae are uncommon. Encephalitis is very rare with an estimated frequency of 3/1000 cases. It can be very serious with seizures and cortical blindness. High fevers are common. Recovery is usually complete, but fatalities have been reported.

Pancreatitis is another manifestation of mumps and occurs in approximately 5% of the patients. Infection with mumps virus has been implicated as a possible cause of juvenile onset diabetes. There has been documentation of onset of diabetes within a few weeks following clinically diagnosed mumps. An association has been found between mumps infection and endocardial fibroelastosis (St. Geme et al, 1972).

Diagnosis

The clinical features are diagnostic. Laboratory findings are of little value, except that the serum amylase is elevated in 90% of the patients with parotitis and serum lipase levels are normal distinguishing mumps from pancreatitis. Serologic tests are rarely done but it is possible to evaluate the S antigen by complement fixation antibody titers which rise in the first week of illness and V antigen by complement fixation antibody titers that follow with a rise several weeks later and may persist at low levels for years. If the titer

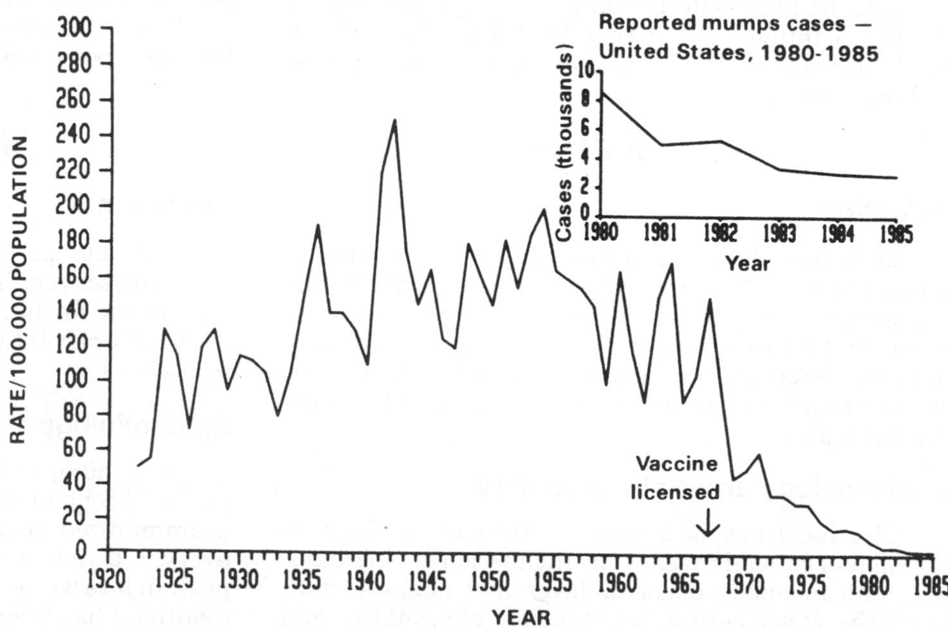

Figure 17.4. Mumps incidence rates showing the sustained fall after the vaccine was licensed. The school-age population accounted for the majority of cases in 1984. From CDC: *MMWR* 35:216, 1986.

rises during convalescence it is diagnostic. Neutralizing antibodies appear during convalescence.

Treatment

There is no specific therapy for mumps.

Prevention

The live attenuated mumps vaccine which is prepared in chick embryo cell cultures has been found to be 95% effective. Immunization is usually given at about 15 months of age, in combination with measles and rubella vaccination. It is particularly important to ensure that all pregnant women have been immunized against mumps, although not during pregnancy (Aase et al, 1972). Although mumps virus is not a recognized teratogen, there is evidence that it can infect the placenta and has been associated with abortion. The risk of endocardial fibroelastosis in the offspring of a mother who has had mumps during pregnancy is about 2% which is significantly higher than the risk in the general population. It has been suggested that the virus causes interstitial myocarditis in the fetus which may produce persistent left ventricular dilatation and mitral valve insufficiency (Hutchins and Vie, 1972).

PARVOVIRUS INFECTION (ERYTHEMA INFECTIOSUM)

Definition

Parvoviruses are associated with a number of acute febrile illnesses, with and without rashes. Erythema infectiosum, the "fifth disease," is associated with human parvovirus (B19). It derives its name from its place as the fifth classic exanthem of childhood: measles, scarlet fever, rubella, roseola infantum, and erythema infectiosum. The B19 parvovirus also can cause aplastic crises in hemolytic diseases, and a polyarthralgia in normal adults (Ozawa et al, 1986).

Epidemiology

Erythema infectiosum has been most common in Japan where it appears in outbreaks about every 10 years. The association of the virus with erythema infectiosum was first made by Anderson et al in 1983. Presumably many patients before then were thought to have rubella or other viral illness. In sero epidemiologic surveys, prevalence of antihuman parvovirus antibodies increases with age. Apparently many attacks are asymptomatic. Acquisition of antibodies indicative of infection occurs usually between ages 4 and 10 years (Anderson, 1982).

Natural History

This mild febrile illness sometimes has a typical rash characterized by a "slapped check appearance," and later a lace-like rash mostly over the extremities, but not on palms or soles. In epidemics, some individuals are ill without a rash. Arthralgias are common. Some children have transient red cell aplasia in association with hemolytic anemia.

A wider spectrum of pathology from human parvovirus continues to emerge as more investigators search for it (Plummer et al, 1985). An example is an association with fetal hydrops reported during an epidemic of erythema infectiosum.

Diagnosis

The diagnosis is not difficult in the midst of an epidemic since the prominence of the rash on the cheeks distinguishes it from most other acute exanthems. Serologic diagnosis can be made by countercurrent immunoelectrophoresis (CIE) and radioimmunoassay. During one epidemic reported from Japan, 97% of the patients, but only 15% of control children, had CIE-reactive antibody. An anti-HPV IgM was present in all patients tested. The peripheral white count is usually normal with a relative lymphocytosis.

Treatment

The treatment is supportive only.

Prognosis

The prognosis is excellent.

POLIOMYELITIS

Definition

Poliomyelitis is a paralytic disease that can occur in epidemics and has a range of severity from subclinical to fatal bulbar disease.

Basic Science

Polioviruses, coxsackie, and echoviruses, (collectively enteroviruses) are grouped together because of shared physical and chemical properties, as well as a shared habitat, the human gastrointestinal tract.

They are single-stranded RNA viruses of the Picornavirus family, consisting of 20–30 nm particles of naked protein capsids with a dense central core as seen by electron microscopy. High resolution crystallography has made possible three-dimensional analysis of poliovirus. Each of the three major capsid proteins contains a core reminiscent of the pattern seen in icosahedral viruses. Differences in orientation of proteins probably account for the high degree of specificity with respect to the cells that can be infected by the different picornaviruses (Hogle et al, 1985; Baltimore, 1985).

Enteroviruses each have multiple serologic types. Polioviruses have three serotypes, type I being most likely to produce paralysis. Humans are the only natural host. Enteroviruses are transmitted from person to person usually by the fecal-oral route, with the oropharynx being the portal of entry. Only 1–2% of infections result in paralytic polio even in epidemic areas. The milder aseptic meningitis syndrome occurs in only 4–8% of infected individuals (Horstmann, 1981).

Epidemiology

Worldwide poliomyelitis continues to occur among unimmunized individuals. Wild strain polio is very rare in the United States (only three cases in 1980–1984). More than 274,000,000 doses of oral vaccine have been given between 1973 and 1984. Vaccine-related polio occurred in 104 instances or 1 case per 2.64 million doses. Thirteen of these cases were in immunocompromised patients.

Natural History

The initial infection is either in the lymphoid tissue of the pharynx or the intestinal tract. Careful studies have demonstrated that the virus enters the lymphatics and regional lymph nodes where it replicates. The virus can penetrate the CNS from the regional lymph nodes or there may be an associated viremia. The virus has tropism for anterior horn cells and establishes an inflammation with mononuclear cells.

Poliomyelitis may present in several forms: nonparalytic polio, aseptic meningitis, paralytic polio, and bulbar disease.

Differences in virulence are assumed on the basis of widely differing attack rates in epidemics. Predisposing factors for paralysis include: strenuous exercise, recent trauma, and evidence exists that tonsillectomy, even in the past, increases the likelihood of bulbar poliomyelitis. There is some evidence that genetic factors predispose to paralysis since histocompatibility antigen HLA 3 and HLA 7 have been associated with an increased risk of paralysis.

Diagnosis

During an incubation period of 9–12 days there may be variable manifestations: fever, headache, sore throat, and muscular pains, may be transient and subside in a few days. Nonparalytic polio is well-known during epidemics.

In other patients, there may be an aseptic meningitis presenting as stiffness of the neck and back with headache and somewhat more fever than in the subclinical infection. It is assumed that paralysis occurs in only 1/10 of a percent of all polio virus infections in children.

Muscle pain is characteristic of severe illness. The paralysis may follow several days after the onset of pain and tends to be asymmetric and involve proximal muscles of the extremities, and legs more than arms. The paralysis is likely to progress over 2–3 days but ceases when the patient becomes afebrile. There is no sensory loss in paralytic poliomyelitis.

The bulbar involvement is most serious and often is first noted by a nasal voice from involvement of the muscles of the soft palate. Encephalitis may be present and lead to seizures and loss of consciousness. Respiratory failure is not uncommon and prolonged dependence on mechanical ventilation is a well-known outcome of the more serious infections.

LABORATORY FINDINGS

Polio viruses can be isolated from throat secretions during the first week of illness, and may be present in the feces for several weeks longer. The virus is rarely isolated from the spinal fluid. The peripheral white blood count is normal or slightly elevated. CSF findings may show pleocytosis with modest elevations of the proteins.

Treatment

There is no specific antibody treatment and, therefore, only supportive measures are available.

Prognosis

During epidemics the overall mortality was between 5% and 10%, although much higher in immunodeficient individuals, and those with bulbar poliomyelitis. Some estimate of the long-range outcome can be made about 1 month after the initial illness. It is said that no additional return of function can be expected beyond 9 months, but careful physical therapy and bracing in growing children can provide continuing support.

Recently, there has been a disturbing recurrence of muscle weakness in individuals who had their acute attacks of poliomyelitis many years earlier. The pathogenesis of this is not understood.

Prevention

Oral polio vaccine is usually given at 2, 4, 6, and either 15 or 18 months and again at 4–6 years of age in normal children. If an immunodeficient state is suspected, killed polio vaccine should be substituted for live vaccine.

RABIES

Definition

Rabies is an RNA virus that is transmitted from animals to humans by bites, and travels by nerves to brain to cause a fatal encephalitis.

Basic Science

Known from ancient times, the feared consequences of animal bites are now reasonably well-understood and preventable (Kaplan et al, 1986). The virus can infect all species of mammals. It is a member of the rhabdovirus group and apparently exists in only one antigenic type. Skunks and racoons are the principal transmitters of disease to humans, although foxes, vampire bats, cats, dogs, and farm animals have inflicted disease on humans.

Epidemiology

Vaccination of dogs and cats has reduced the number of cases in the United States drastically in recent years. No human cases were reported in the U.S. in 1986. It is estimated that worldwide 4,000,000 people per year are given postexposure vaccination.

Natural History

Most human infections follow a bite by a rabid animal. Saliva from the animal is inoculated into subcutaneous or muscular tissue and the virus enters peripheral nerves. It moves passively by axoplasmic flow to neurons, and is not exposed to the immune system. Once in the spinal cord, it moves rapidly to the brain. Extreme irritability and excitement precede depression. The incubation period is variable, but usually 20–90 days after exposure. The incubation period is shorter in children than adults; bites on the face have shorter periods than bites on extremities. Itching and pain may occur at the site of the bite.

Diagnosis

The acute CNS finding lasts about 2–10 days before death. Only rare recoveries have been reported with optimal intensive care.

The pathognomonic sign is hydrophobia. Attempts to swallow result in painful spasms of laryngeal and pharangeal muscles. Meningismus is common. Flaccid paralysis of the bitten limb may occur.

Spinal fluid may show a mononuclear pleocytosis. The white count in peripheral blood has increased polymorphonuclear cells.

Treatment

Immediate treatment is mandatory. Local: Thorough cleansing of the wound as soon as possible is imperative. Ethyl alcohol (43%) should be applied. Rabies hyperimmune globulin (RIG) should be given as soon as possible (20 IU/kg), followed by the first dose of vaccine. Human diploid cell vaccine (HDCV) has replaced duck embyro vaccine. Usually, five doses are given in a 4-week period (immediately, days 3, 7, 14, and 28). Adverse effects are uncommon, although allergic responses can occur with a booster. Protection lasts about 4 years (Fayaz et al, 1981).

Prevention

Vaccination of domestic animals, and avoidance of wild animals is the best prevention. Individuals such as veterinarians or other animal handlers, or those exposed to bats should receive vaccination before exposure. If exposure is continuous, and infection likely, boosters are recommended every 4 years. For definitive guidelines to prevention and treatment, the reader is referred to the Report of the Committee on Infectious Diseases, American Academy of Pediatrics (20th edition, 1986).

QUESTION AND COMMENT

How do you decide when to immunize a youngster who was bitten by an unknown and untraceable dog?

There are no clear answers to this question. If the bite was unprovoked, or drew blood, immunization is appropriate. Any lesion on head or neck would be more serious than an abrasion on an extremity. In general, superficial wounds inflicted through clothing are not associated with infection.

Knowledge of prevalence of rabies in the environment is helpful. In the United States in 1983, 5878 cases were reported in animals, only 132 of which were from dog bites. Skunks and racoons are the major sources of human infection. The situation is different in many other parts of the world. Children at greatest risk are those in India, Iran, Philippines, Thailand, and North Africa where immunization should be considered.

RESPIRATORY SYNCYTIAL VIRUS

Definition

Respiratory syncytial virus (RSV) is associated with bronchiolitis in infants and bronchitis and upper respiratory infections in older children and adults. It has a high attack rate and does not produce lasting immunity. It is the most important respiratory pathogen of infancy (see also bronchiolitis).

Basic Science

RSV belongs to the family Paramyxoviridae. It is medium sized (120–300 nm) with a lipid envelope surrounding RNA.

Epidemiology

The virus is widely distributed throughout the world and produces seasonal outbreaks in the temperate climates usually during November to March. The severity of illness may vary from year to year, but in almost all instances it is the infant under 2 years of age or immunocompromised children who are most severely affected (Hall et al, 1986).

Prevalence

RSV has been implicated in 5–40% of pneumonias of young children, and up to 90% of the cases of bronchiolitis. The organism is rarely recovered from individuals who do not have respiratory symptoms.

Spread of infection is largely through contamination of objects with respiratory secretions. Hand-to-hand spread has been shown to be an important mode of transmission. Particle aerosols are unstable at low humidity, but have some stability at higher relative humidities. Apparently, touching contaminated secretions and then the eyes or nasal mucosa is sufficient to inoculate a susceptible person.

Natural History

The signs of infection with RSV include fever, cough, rhinitis, pharyngitis, and evidence of lower tract disease characterized by retractions, wheezing, occasional rales, and rhonchi. Some infants become severely short of breath, hypoxic, and hypercapnic, although that is unusual. Hypoxia can readily be corrected by increasing inspired oxygen modestly (25–30%). The duration of illness is usually at least 7 days and sometimes up 2–3 weeks. Evidence of airway hyperreactivity persists for many months and even years in individuals who had bronchiolitis in infancy.

Clinical symptomatology is quite characteristic and diagnosis is rarely a problem. The only condition with which it could be confused would be asthma in infancy unassociated with RSV infection. Radiographic findings are usually characterized by a diffuse interstitial pneumonitis and hyperinflation of the lung. The peripheral blood count is unrevealing.

Some infants shed virus for long periods suggesting that they may have an abnormal immune response. Infants are born with some maternal antibody which tends to disappear in the first months of life. Specific IgA antibody can be detected in nasal secretion of infants of all ages but the antibody is not neutralizing and its role remains to be delineated.

Diagnosis

Diagnosis can usually be made by recovery of the virus from the anterior nasal wash, and rapid identification is possible by immunofluorescent techniques. Serologic diagnosis is rarely of help in management of these patients.

Treatment

An antiviral agent, ribavirin has been shown to have some benefit when administered by aerosol (Hall et al, 1983). Its use is currently restricted to hospitalized children with severe disease or those with conditions that put them at risk of severe illness such as immunocompromised infants, low birth weight infants, and those with bronchopulmonary dysplasia.

The mainstay of treatment is humidified oxygen, since arterial oxygen tensions may be dangerously low (see bronchiolitis). Mist is not indicated since it can be irritating to reactive airways.

Prevention

Nosocomial infection is common among hospitalized children during epidemics. Strict attention to handwashing, and avoidance of contact between infants and adults who may have RSV infection of the upper airway seems reasonable. No vaccine is available (Chanock et al, 1977).

RHINOVIRUSES

Definition

The 113 known serologically distinct rhinoviruses are the most common cause of colds. Infection is usually restricted to the upper respiratory tract.

Basic Science

Members of the picornaviruses, rhinoviruses are small, nonenveloped, icosahedral (20-sided, hexagonal in cross-section), single stranded RNA viruses. The virus attaches to a respiratory epithelial cell, invades it, and rapidly replicates. It is estimated that each infected cell may produce up to 1000 infectious particles in 15 hours. Man is the major host, although subclinical infections have been established in chimpanzees and gibbons. Because of their serologic diversity, attempts at vaccine production to rhinoviruses have been futile. As many as half of individuals from whom rhinoviruses have been isolated may not develop four-fold or greater increases in serum antibodies. Transmission is usually person-to-person by hand spread of nasal secretions.

Epidemiology

In temperate climates in the northern hemishpere, illness predominates between October and April. No figures for incidence are available, but the common cold is indeed common. The virus is most prevalent in infants and young children.

Natural History

The incubation period is 2 days, with virus detectable on the third day. Serum antibodies to different serotypes develop and increase so adults may be protected from nearly half of the viruses. Nasal antibodies confer some protection. About 24 hours after experimental infection, nasal IgA secretion increases. Rhinorrhea begins about 48 hours later, with a transudate that contains IgG. Serum IgG appears at 1 week and reaches a peak at 1 month. The illness lasts about 8–10 days.

Although usually associated with colds, rhinoviruses have been associated with exacerbations of wheezing in asthmatics (Empey et al, 1976). The relation to more serious illness including sudden infant death syndrome has been suggested but not proven.

Diagnosis

Specific viral diagnosis is not possible on the basis of clinical symptoms. Recovery of the virus in epidemics is suggestive, but not diagnostic. Serologic diagnosis is possible, but not usually worthwhile for a brief self-limited illness.

Treatment

Treatment is supportive only.

Prevention

The many antigenically distinct types of rhinoviruses make the development of suitable vaccines improbable. No effective chemoprophylactic agents have been found. The efficacy of vitamin C in excess of normal requirements remains controversial because of inconsistent results of clinical trials.

Control for spread of infection by hand-washing with dilute solutions of elemental iodine is the only proven effective method (Hall, 1977).

ROTAVIRUS

Definition

First associated with diarrhea in infants in Australia in 1975, rotavirus is now recognized as one of the major pathogens associated with diarrheal episodes, found in about 22% of outpatients and 39% of inpatients in The Children's Hospital, Washington, DC (Brandt et al, 1979).

Basic Science

Rotavirus is a member of a family that includes reoviruses and orbiviruses and is distinguished by being associated with diarrheal disease in newborn or young humans, calves, mice, piglets, lambs, rabbits, primates, goats, kittens, and other animals.

The viruses are double-shelled surrounding double-stranded RNA and exist in at least two serotypes capable of infecting humans (type 1 and type 2).

The organism is transmitted by the fecal-oral route. The organism can be seen in biopsy specimens from the duodenum. It is associated with severe mucosal changes, including shortened and blunted villi as well as mononuclear cell infiltrations of the lamina propria.

Apparently, illness with type 1 virus does not protect against illness from type 2 virus.

Epidemiology

Rotavirus is one of the most commonly associated agents in severe diarrhea of infancy. The incidence of disease caused by it is unknown, since excretion of rotavirus occurs in children with and without diarrhea (Burke et al, 1985).

Natural History

There are no pathognomonic clinical features of diarrhea associated with rotavirus. Affected individuals are likely to have vomiting, watery stools, and quickly become dehydrated. Vomiting usually lasts about 2 days and diarrhea lasts about 5 days. In some individuals, prolonged diarrhea with mucosal damage can result in disaccharidase deficiency.

Diagnosis

The most practical tests for diagnosis are antigen detection through counter immune electrophoresis or an ELISA. The virus can be readily isolated from feces.

Treatment

No specific treatment for the virus is indicated. The patient needs general supportive care for the dehydration associated with the diarrhea. Agents that alter the mobility of the gastrointestinal tract are not indicated.

Prevention

Rotavirus infection is highly contagious through direct person-to-person contact. Effective hand-washing and disinfection of contaminated objects can control the spread.

Several vaccines are under investigation and have been promising when given before the epidemic season. They may be useful in high risk groups, but are not available or recommended for routine immunization (Vesikari et al, 1985).

RUBEOLA (MEASLES)

Definition

Measles virus causes an exanthem and a pathognomonic enanthem (Koplik spots) in epidemics among susceptibles. It is capable of severe and sometimes fatal complications, especially among malnourished children.

Basic Science

Measles virus is pleomorphic, 150–300 nm in diameter with an outer lipoprotein envelope and a nucleocapsid of about 5% RNA. It is distributed worldwide. Transmission of this highly contagious virus is by droplet nuclei, inhaled by susceptible individuals.

Following infection, hemagglutination inhibiting and neutralizing antibodies appear about 2 weeks after exposure, and reach a peak at 4–6 weeks. The titer decreases slowly but persists for life. Cell-mediated immunity is important in resistance to infection. Immunocompromised patients frequently die from progessive measles infection. During infection, T, B, and null lymphocytes are suppressed for about a week, which accounts for postmeasles anergy (Coovadia et al, 1977).

The most significant histologic feature is the wide distribution of multinucleated giant cells. They appear on the respiratory surface, lymph nodes, spleen, and thymus and may have 100 or more nuclei. The pulmonary epithelium may contain many giant cells and slough into the airway (giant cell pneumonia).

Epidemiology

Outbreaks of measles used to be predictable whenever groups of susceptible children were crowded in relatively close quarters, such as schoolrooms. The epidemics started when windows were shut, first in northern parts of the United States in the fall, and progressively farther south (Wells, 1944).

The severity of illness among groups of individuals with no previous exposure, mode of transmission and lifelong immunity was described in a classic study on

CASE ILLUSTRATION (from CDC: *MMWR* November 29, 1985)

A 17-year-old girl had been infected with measles while traveling in California during the 2 weeks before going to a Christian Science camp in Colorado on July 24, 1985. She developed measles and exposed 110 campers and 25 counselors, none of whom had been immunized. Even though the camp was closed on July 27, and all exposed individuals were quarantined, a total of 50 associated cases occurred, 34 in the second generation, and 16 in the third. No serious complications were reported.

COMMENT

This episode illustrates dramatically the high attack rate of measles in a susceptible population. It also raises the question of whether religious beliefs should be acceptable as an exemption from immunization. The risk of spread in the community is small if most individuals are immunized. If individuals refuse immunization, they must accept quarantine in epidemic settings to protect themselves and lessen the likelihood of transmission of the virus.

the Faroe islands in 1846 by Panum. Before measles vaccine was available, about 400,000 cases were reported in the United States each year (population about 200 million).

In the 1980s in the United States, one of the largest groups of susceptibles comprises individuals who grew up in the 1960s and were not immunized as infants. The decline in natural infection decreased their exposure until they traveled to parts of the world where the disease is endemic, such as Central America and Africa. In 1985, 18.5% of the 1802 cases of measles reported to the Centers for Disease Control in the United States were among college students.

Natural History

The primary site of infection is the respiratory epithelium, with spread of the virus to regional lymph nodes, and then a primary viremia. Virus multiplication persists in the respiratory epithelium for about 2 weeks. During the fifth to seventh day of infection, secondary viremia leads to the early manifestations of disease that include conjunctivitis, generalized transitory rash, fever, and Koplik spots (± 1-mm papules on an erythematous base) on the oral mucosa opposite the lower molars. About 4 days later, the typical exanthem occurs at the peak of the respiratory symptoms. It starts at the hairline and spreads from head to feet. It initially is maculopapular, but becomes confluent with microvesicles on top of a generalized erythematous base. With healing after 6–7 days, a fine desquamation occurs.

Pharyngitis, cough, and lymph node enlargement are common features. In malnourished populations, tracheitis and pneumonia can be lethal complications.

Neurologic involvement can be detected by electroencephalography in about half the patients. Clinical encephalitis occurs in about 1/1000 cases. Symptoms occur during the exanthem or earlier. Headache, involuntary movements, disorientation, and coma may occur; long-term sequelae include selective brain damage, deafness, and hemiplegia. Cerebrospinal fluid abnormalities include mild mononuclear pleocytosis, mild protein elevation, and normal glucose.

Other complications of measles include a hemorrhagic form probably from disseminated intramuscular coagulation. Thrombocytopenic purpura can occur. Measles in pregnancy may be associated with spontaneous abortion. Death from complications of measles occurs in 1/3000 reported cases in the United States.

A serious late complication of measles is subacute sclerosing panencephalitis. It follows natural measles in about 1/100,000 infections. The mean incubation pe-

CASE ILLUSTRATION

A 10-year-old from El Salvador now living in Boston (March 1986) visited his grandparents in Central America and, while there, developed fever, nausea, vomiting, and weakness. Two days later, he had green watery stools and was assumed to have acquired gastroenteritis. The next day he complained of headache, photophobia, and developed a cough and coryza. After 1 week of illness, he returned to Boston and came to Children's Hospital for evaluation.

He looked tired and ill, and had a temperature of 39°C, pulse 20, respiratory rate 20. He had a rash that had started 8–12 hours earlier behind the ears and on the face, then spread down the body. The rash was erythematous with fine macules and papules. Conjunctivitis was prominent. The diagnosis was suspected when 1-mm white papules were seen on the buccal mucosa opposite the second molars. The rest of the physical examination was unremarkable. A white blood count was 4900 with 70% bands, and 15% polys.

The Koplik spots disappeared 2 days later but the leukopenia persisted. Palms and soles were involved in the erythematous rash. Desquamation occurred first on the face and later on the body.

COMMENT

In retrospect, this youngster had been immunized at 13 months, an age at which vaccine failure can occur. The recommended age of measles, mumps, and rubella immunization is 15 months. Once again, suspicion of measles should be heightened by a history of exposure in a region where it is endemic. Given the rarity of it, the diagnosis may be delayed and other immunocompromised children put at risk if a child with measles is hospitalized. A search for Koplik spots in children with fever, conjunctivitis, and an exanthem is well worthwhile.

riod is 7 years. The risk after live measles vaccine is less with mean incubation period of 3.3 years. The symptoms are insidious behavioral and intellectual deterioration, leading to seizures, difficulties with speech, dementia, decorticate rigidity, and death in 6–9 months (see pp. 727).

Diagnosis

Smears of the buccal mucosa will show clusters of multinucleated giant cells. Paired sera will demonstrate a rise in titer of specific antibodies. The virus can be recovered from nasal swabs.

Usually the clinical features and course of illness are so typical that laboratory confirmation is unnecessary. If the patient is seen at the early stages of illness and Koplik spots are present, the diagnosis is clear. Later, in the presence of pneumonia or other complictions, the diagnosis may depend on laboratory confirmation.

Treatment

Treatment is supportive only.

Prevention

In 1963, an inactivated (killed) vaccine and a live attenuated vaccine (Edmonston B strain) were licensed in the United States. The killed vaccine was used until 1967, and the Edmonston strain until 1972. In 1968, another attenuated vaccine (Moraten strain) was licensed and is currently in use in the United States (1987).

Active immunization with live attenuated measles virus vaccine induces immunity in 95% of susceptible persons. Vaccine-induced antibodies persist for years; only time will tell if they persist for life. In the United States, live measles vaccination is recommended at 15 months of age; in societies where the attack rate is high among younger infants, administration should be considered as early as 6 months of age. Unimmunized individuals or those born between 1963 and 1967 who may have received killed vaccine should be immunized if they attend college, or expect to travel in the developing world.

In areas of high prevalence of tuberculosis, a tuberculin test should be given before measles immunization, since the vaccine can suppress cellular immune responses.

Measles immunization is contraindicated in pregnancy or in an individual on immune suppressant therapy. It is dangerous in any individual with primary immunologic disorders, AIDS, or generalized malignancies.

If an unimmunized individual has been exposed to measles, live measles vaccine can be effective if given within 72 hours and less than 6 days earlier, γ-globulin is recommended (0.25 mg/kg, maximum dose 15 ml). For immunocompromised hosts, the dose is 0.5–15 ml/kg.

A personal or family history of convulsions is not a contraindication to immunization (CDC: *MMWR* July 10, 1987).

The duration of immunity after immunization with Schwarz strain live measles vaccine is at least 21 years (Miller, 1987).

Atypical Measles

Some individuals who received a killed measles vaccine in the 1960s develop a characteristic giant cell pneumonia on exposure to natural measles 4–6 years after immunization. The vaccine was removed from the United States market in 1968, and the disease is now very uncommon. It can occur (rarely) among individuals immunized with live vaccine.

Basic Science

The clinical syndrome appears to be an arrest in the natural evolution of illness. Annunziato et al (1982) proposed that the killed vaccine did not induce adequate antibody response to prevent cell-to-cell spread of the virus; rather it produced hemagglutinin antibody capable of a hypersensitivity reaction to wild virus infection.

Natural History

The incubation period is 7–14 days, with sudden onset of high fever and headache. Abdominal pain, dry nonproductive cough, pleuritic chest pain, and weakness are common; Koplik spots are rare.

The rash differs from measles by first appearing on distal extremities with cephalad spread. It is prominent on palms and soles and wrists and ankles. It may be vesicular and petechial. Numbness, paresthesias, and hepatosplenomegaly may occur. Some individuals have persistent nodular pulmonary lesions.

Diagnosis

Marked elevations in antibody titers occur by the 10th day of illness.

Treatment

Treatment is supportive only.

Prevention

Avoidance of killed measles vaccine is the only method of prevention.

SMALLPOX (VARIOLA)

Definition

The last case of smallpox known to occur in the world was in 1978 as a result of a laboratory accident in England. The last cases known to occur in an epidemic were in Somalia in 1977. Since then, through an extensive international effort coordinated by the World Health Organization, smallpox has been eradicated and the virus is now confined to a few designated laboratories (Henderson, 1984).

Since the disease is of such historic importance, and since there is a remote possibility of its reappearance, it seems appropriate to include some information pertinent to the disease and its eradication in a textbook of pediatrics in the 1980s. For a comprehensive report, see "The Global Eradication of Smallpox" Geneva, 1980, WHO publication.

Basic Science

Smallpox (variola) virus depends on a human host or cells of a human host for its survival. In 1967, a negative staining technique was introduced so that electronmicroscopy became a rapid and accurate method of diagnosis. The virus particles were large and brick-shaped and could be identified in scrapings from macular or pustular lesions or even in suspensions prepared from crust. Variola can be distinguished from other pox viruses by the distinctive lesions it produces in the chick chorioallantois. Serologic tests involving demonstration of complement fixation, hemagglutination, and neutralizing antibody are all available. Of all these methods, electronmicroscopy was found to have the greatest sensitivity.

Natural History

Smallpox has occurred worldwide in individuals of all ages and races. Four recognizable clinical types of smallpox have been described. First, the ordinary or most frequent form, corresponds to the classical description of the disease. The incubation period is 10–12 days from exposure to the onset of a febrile illness. The actual range of the incubation period may be somewhat greater (suggested to be 7–17 days). The pre-eruptive stage of the illness starts with fever, headache, prostration, muscle aching, and often nausea and vomiting which persists for 2–3 days before the rash develops. The earliest lesions are small macules which after about a week form vesicles and then pustules. During the second week scabs form and over the subsequent 1–2 weeks fall off leaving deep pigmented areas. After many weeks, these develop into facial pock marks. The eruption usually shows a centrifugal distribution.

The modified form of the disease occurs in vaccinated individuals and resembles the ordinary form, but is less severe. A third type is called the flat form which is frequently fatal. The pre-eruptive illness is severe and the lesions are slow to mature. The vesicles tend to be flat, soft, and velvety to touch. They do not become pustules. Some progress to a fourth form of the disease, the hemorrhagic small pox which is almost invariably fatal. The pre-eruptive illness is severe with much facial pallor and extreme prostration. In the fulminating form, lesions develop bleeding around them in addition to subconjunctival bleeding, and bleeding from the mouth and gums. Death is likely to occur between the fifth and seventh days of the illness when only a few cutaneous lesions are present.

Reported case fatality rates varied tremendously from year to year and region to region. It seems probable that there were viruses of differing pathogenicity and there were certainly hosts of greater or lesser susceptibility. The case fatality rates were highest in the early years of life, particularly infancy and had been as high as 26% among some unvaccinated individuals and as low as 0.2% in other outbreaks. In the last recorded outbreak of 3229 cases in Somalia in 1977 there were 12 fatalities.

Treatment

Since there was no known treatment for this extraordinarily serious disease, it became evident that the goals should be elimination of the virus first proposed by the World Health Assembly in 1958. The following characteristics made it conceivable that smallpox could be eradicated:

1. The recognition of cases is comparatively simple.
2. It was transmitted solely person to person. There were no known animal reservoirs.
3. The transmissibility of infection is low and epidemics were slow to develop. Between each generation of cases there was an interval of 2–3 weeks which made it possible to immunize some of the exposed individuals.
4. Transmission requires close contact, so susceptible persons were readily identified.
5. Within any one epidemic, the chances of transmission were relatively few.
6. A surveillance system could be mounted that would identify all outbreaks promptly and containment of the affected individual was feasible by mobilizing local health workers.

Clearly, the eradication of smallpox must stand as one of the most notable achievements in the history of preventive medicine.

Vaccination

The essential method of breaking the transmission chain of smallpox was mass vaccination. It had, of course, been demonstrated in Europe and North America that the disease could be eliminated by obtaining high levels of immunity. It became evident that coverage of about 80% of the population by vaccination was sufficient for eradication. This was achieved in most of the countries of the world with the freeze-dried vaccine that was stable in tropical climates and did not require refrigeration. It was given by a bifurcated needle with results comparable to those achieved with multiple pressure or scarification methods. The dose used was only .0025 ml.

COMPLICATIONS OF VACCINATION

The requirement for universal vaccination was dropped in the United States some years before the disease was eliminated from the world, because the incidence of complications, particularly, postvaccinal encephalitis exceeded the chances that an individual who did not leave the United States would acquire the illness. Another complication was in individuals with eczema who had a spread of the virus to multiple sites on the skin. It was estimated that there was about 1 death per million vaccinated individuals resulting from complications of primary vaccination and 1 death per 4 million following revaccination.

COST OF ERADICATION

It was estimated that the WHO and participating countries spent $313,000,000 between 1967 and 1979. It is conservatively estimated that quarantine programs and the maintenance of routine vaccination for international travelers plus the cost of complications of vaccination amounted to $1 billion per year. These rough calculations underscore the cost-effectiveness of preventive programs.

The problem of preventable infectious diseases worldwide must remain in focus by those of us who reside in societies where immunization is nearly universal. Approximately 4 million children die each year from preventable infections. Estimates for 1983 are that over 2.5 million died of measles and its complications, over 1 million died of neonatal tetanus, 735,000 died of pertussis, and about 350,000 died of polio (Henderson, 1984). These startling numbers remind us of the need for continuing vigilance in assuring that our children are immunized, and stimulate our participation in programs such as UNICEF to try to eliminate forever at least measles and polio, since they share with smallpox only a human host and the availability of effective means of immunization. Since both measles and polio vaccines must be hept cold to be effective, the problem is a significant one, but surely not beyond our means to solve.

ARTHROPOD-BORNE ENCEPHALIDITES

Definition

Arthropod-borne viruses are the most common agents in epidemics of encephalitis. Encephalitis is to be distinguished from aseptic meningitis, which is most commonly caused by enteroviruses, although they can also cause encephalitis. Many arthropod-borne viruses are named for the region where they first caused epidemics, and include Eastern equine, Western equine, Venezuelan equine, St. Louis, California, and La Crosse.

Epidemiology

Encephalitis of all causes resulted in 1500–1800 cases being reported each year in the United States. Eastern equine virus is more common in the very young, and St. Louis virus disease is seen in older individuals.

Natural History

These viruses all require an arthropod vector to introduce the virus through the human skin. Animal reservoirs include a wide variety of wild animals in-

CASE ILLUSTRATION

A 6-year-old female presented to the hospital in coma with irregular breathing, decorticate posturing, and bilateral upgoing toes. She had been well until 4 days before admission when she developed headache, chills, vomiting and fever to 101.5°F, unresponsive to acteominophin. Three days before admission she became lethargic, complained of a stiff neck, and continued to vomit. She was admitted to a local hospital where physical examination was notable for fever, photophobia, and meningismus. White count at that time was 21,500, with 77% polys and 8% bands. Lumbar puncture showed slightly cloudy CSF, with 10 red cells, 1384 white cells, with 97% polys, 3 mononuclear cells, a glucose of 70 with a serum glucose of 128, and a protein of 46, with a negative Gram stain. Ampicillin and chloramphenicol were started. Two days before hospital admission she had a generalized seizure, multiple episodes of confusion with lip smacking behavior. An EEG showed generalized slowing without an epileptic focus. On the day before admission, she was responsive only to painful stimuli. A head CT showed small ventricles and a repeat lumbar puncture showed 6 red cells, 318 white cells, with 54% polys, 46% mononuclear cells, a protein of 62, and a glucose of 87 with serum glucose of 142. For further management of her meningoencephalitis she was transferred to our hospital.

QUESTION AND COMMENT

What further diagnostic work-up is indicated?

From a diagnostic standpoint, the most likely etiologies for this patient's symptoms were that of a viral meningoencephalitis, with herpes simplex and Eastern equine encephalitis, heading the list. A more careful history showed that the patient was living in an endemic area south of Boston where Eastern equine encephalitis had been reported. Acyclovir was started to cover the possibility of herpes simplex as the causative organism and measurements to lower intracranial pressure were instituted. These included pentobarbitol coma and muscular paralysis. On the third hospital day, serologic titers for Eastern equine encephalitis were positive and all antibiotics including acyclovir were discontinued. Intracranial pressure control measures were continued during the first week of hospitalization and she was weaned over the following week, during which time she was extubated. She was initially left with a severe neurologic deficit, although progressed to a slow recovery of purposeful activity during the following year. Repeat brain stem-evoked potentials showed normal brain stem conduction time and she was subsequently left with a mild bilateral hearing loss, and special educational needs.

This patient's course is unusual in that the prognosis is generally poor with a high immediate mortality and predominance of major neurologic deficits in the survivors. No antiviral agent has been found effective and, at present, supportive measures for intracranial hypertension provide the best treatment.

cluding rodents, and birds such as sparrows and pheasants. Despite the name equine, horses, like humans are end-stage hosts for these viruses and are not involved in their transmission cycle. Outbreaks are more likely after wet weather that creates swamps in which mosquitoes breed. Symptoms are headache, vomiting, fever, irritability, lethargy, and altered consciousness. Focal neurologic signs and seizures are common in the more serious cases. These diseases may be mild and self-limited, but can be fulminant and fatal, especially Eastern equine encephalitis.

Diagnosis

EEGs show focal or generalized dysrhythmias. CSF may be normal or show moderate lymphocytosis (usually under 1000 cells/mm^3). Polymorphonuclear cells may be present. Glucose concentration is normal. CSF IgM may be elevated and specific antibodies should be sought in serum and spinal fluid.

CT scans are useful to rule out abscess, tumor or other conditions that could produce similar symptoms.

For discussion of brain biopsy, see herpes encephalitis.

Treatment

See Section 12 (Neurology) for relief of increased intracranial pressure. No specific antiviral therapy is available.

Prognosis

In epidemics, outcome depends on virus type and host factors. Mortality ranges from rare (Colorado tick fever) up to 60% (Eastern equine encephalitis). Residual neurologic damage frequently occurs.

DENGUE

Definition

Dengue fever, an influenza-like illness, is a viral disease of man caused by any one of four related flavivirus serotypes transmitted by Aedes mosquitoes. Epidemics of dengue occur in many tropical and subtropical countries around the world. A more severe form, known as dengue hemorrhagic fever/dengue shock syndrome, has been a major pediatric health problem in Southeast Asia and recently in the Caribbean.

Basic Science

Dengue viruses belong to the flavivirus group along with yellow fever and St. Louis encephalitis viruses. Flavivirus virions are enveloped and have a single stranded positive RNA genome. Dengue virus grows well in macrophages in vitro but the identity of the permissive cell in vivo remains obscure. Dengue hemorrhagic fever may have an immune mediated pathogenesis. Non-neutralizing antibody can enhance the binding and internalization of infectious dengue virus to macrophages. Precisely how this abnormal antibody-mediated infection might lead to the release of vascular permeability and complement activating factors, which may be the mediators of hemorrhage and shock, is not clear (Halstead, 1988).

Epidemiology

Outbreaks occur in urban areas especially in Asia in monsoon season and in Africa. Hemorrhagic fever is most common in the Philippines, Thailand, and Malaysia. Outbreaks of dengue have been reported with increasing frequency in Central American and Caribbean countries. In 1984 over 27,000 cases were reported from Mexico (CDC, 1986c).

Natural History

The incubation period is 2–7 days, followed by fever up to 41°C and severe headache and myalgias. A transient macular rash may coexist with the fever. Nausea, vomiting, lymphadenopathy, and taste aberrations may occur. After defervescence, a morbiliform rash appears and spares palms and soles and later may desquamate. Fever may recur. The hemorrhagic form also known as dengue shock syndrome may evolve from the milder one with rapid clinical deterioration, shock and multiple petechiae, and ecchymoses in association with thrombocytopenia and hemoconcentration.

Laboratory Diagnosis

Pancytopenia may occur on the third and fourth day and persist or recur. Isolation of the virus and/or serology establish the diagnosis.

In the severe form, hemoconcentration, thrombocytopenia, and hyponatremia occur. Fibrinogen levels are low and fibrin split products are present.

Treatment

No specific antiviral therapy exists.

The dengue shock syndrome is managed as hypovolemia shock by rapid intravenous infusion of saline or colloid. Prophylaxis is by insect repellants or avoidance of endemic areas. No effective vaccine is currently available.

FLAVIVIRUS (YELLOW FEVER)

Definition

Yellow fever is caused by a flavivirus and transmitted by Aedes Aegypti and other mosquitoes in tropical climates. The illness is of sudden onset, involves many systems, and is often fatal.

Basic Science

The virus is a member of the flavivirus family that includes dengue, and St. Louis and Japanese encephalitis. It is an RNA virus, which is endemic in tropical America and Africa. Unvaccinated humans, especially children in locations where vaccination programs have been curtailed, are susceptible. Some evidence suggests individuals of blood group O are most susceptible for unknown reasons.

A live attenuated 17D vaccine developed in the 1930s and modified later has been safe and effective. It is not advised in infants under 4 months of age because of risk of vaccine-induced encephalitis.

Recently, major advances in understanding flavivirus organization at the molecular level have been reported (Rice et al, 1985). Knowledge of the molecular structure and the location of the genes for the structural polypeptides should allow preparation, through recombinant DNA technology, of specific and active immunogens not only for yellow fever, but also dengue and St. Louis and Japanese encephalitis.

Epidemiology

Yellow fever has been a major killer and was the first virus incriminated as a cause of human disease. The havoc wrought by yellow fever has been described poignantly in histories of the Spanish American war (1898) and the building of the Panama Canal. Yellow fever is preventable by immunization and mosquito control, so that it is rare in most urban areas except in wartime when immunization programs have been abandoned. It is seen in forest workers and others who may be in geographic isolates in endemic areas.

Natural History

The incubation period is usually 3–6 days. The illness has a wide spectrum from mild febrile episodes to fatal disease with the classic triad of icterus, hemorrhages and albuminuria. The abrupt onset is characterized by fever up to 40°C, headache, myalgia, vomiting, and epigastric pain. Prostration, and severe epistaxis, melena, ecchymoses and gingival bleeding occur before death in the seventh to tenth day of illness. Renal and hepatic failure occur.

Diagnosis

Leukopenia occurs in the first week. Albuminuria begins on the fourth or fifth day. Specific diagnosis depends on virus isolation from the blood obtained during the first 4 days. Serologic diagnosis can be made on paired acute and convalescent specimens.

Treatment

No specific treatment exists. Supportive care is all that is available.

Prognosis

The case fatality rate in South American outbreaks in the 1960s was 22%.

Prevention

Mosquito control is essential, including mosquito-proof rooms and netting. Vaccination provides long-lasting protection beginning 10 days after inoculation with the 17D vaccine.

RUBELLA (GERMAN MEASLES)

Definition

Rubella is a highly contagious virus that causes a relatively mild exanthem in children, but can be devastating to the fetus if acquired just before or during the first 8 weeks of pregnancy. Man is the only reservoir of infection.

Basic Science

Rubella virus resembles measles in that it apparently has a single antigenic strain. No subtypes have been identified. Nevertheless, the organism may vary in virulence from time to time. Extensive epidemics in the 1940s and 1960s are hard to explain on any other basis.

The antigens consist of an HA antigen located at the cell surface and identified by hemadsorption. Two complement fixing antigens have been identified and two precipitating antigens have been found. The virus, first isolated in 1962, can be cultivated in a large number of cells that are suitable for diagnostic purposes.

Virus isolation is the preferred method of diagnosis in the newborn period as it can be recovered from the urine nasopharynx or other tissues. The cord blood serology is usually positive for the hemagglutination-inhibition (HI) test. Diagnosis of postnatal rubella usually is made by the appropriate serology.

Epidemiology

In regions where immunization is practiced, rubella should be of very low incidence. In 1984, in the United States the incidence was 0.3/100,000 population. Before immunization, the peak age was 5–14 years with an annual incidence of 26/100,000 population. In closed communities such as institutions, or even some classrooms, nearly all susceptible individuals become infected, particularly in the spring (Fig. 17.5).

Recent outbreaks have occurred on college campuses and among office workers who have never been immunized (mean age 25 years).

Natural History

The incubation period is usually 14–21 days. The disease is infective 7 days before the rash, and up to 12 months later in infants who acquired the infection in gestation. Virus is spread to other individuals via contact.

Diagnosis

The illness is usually mild, with low-grade fever, and usually with a rash that is characterized by discrete maculopapular eruptions and flushing, particularly on the face. Mild itching is present; the rash disappears by the third day with minimal desquamation. The most characteristic feature is postauricular or posterior cervical lymphadenopathy which appears before the rash and may last a week or more. The pha-

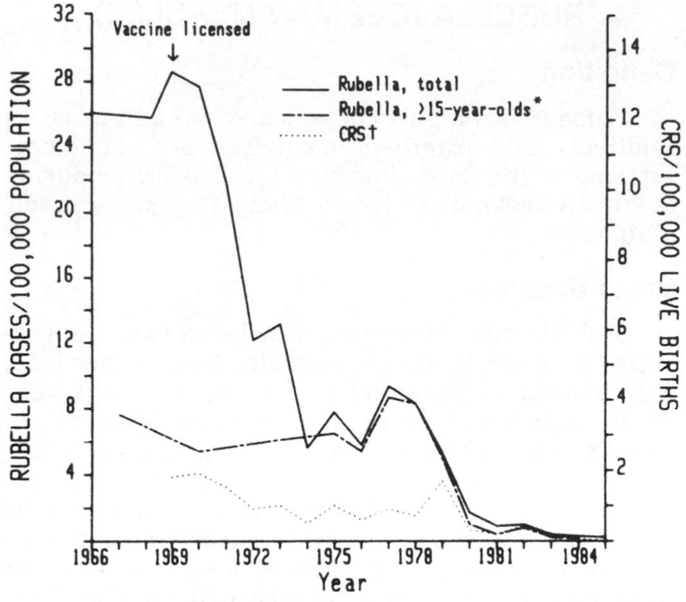

Figure 17.5. Reported incidence of rubella and congenital rubella syndrome in the United States 1966–1985. From CDC: *MMWR* 35:130, 1986.

ryngeal mucosa is inflamed. Mild enlargement of the spleen is common, and white cell count is lowered. Polyarthritis may be present, and may last for several days to 2 weeks.

Differential diagnosis from roseola infantum may be difficult. In general, roseola is characterized by a high fever which resolves with appearance of the rash. Low-grade fever and lymphadenopathy are more characteristic of rubella.

A single attack confers lifelong immunity. Serologic surveys showed that nearly 80% of adults had antibody.

Congenital rubella is the most feared form of infection. It can be acquired transplacentally during the first trimester, or later with different manifestations. Maternal infection within a month before conception or through the second trimester can affect the fetus. The manifestations depend on the time of infection. Cataracts occur when infection occurs before the 60th day after the last menstrual period; heart disease can occur with infection any time in the first trimester, and deafness from infection anytime in the first two trimesters.

Epidemiology

The fetus can be affected about 15–25% of the time with first trimester disease in the mother, 5–7% in the fourth month, and 1–2% in the fifth month. The infant can excrete the virus in nasopharyngeal secretions and urine for many months after birth and be a threat to other susceptible individuals.

Diagnosis

The infants are often undersized for gestational age. Lesions evident at birth may be glaucoma, cataracts, purpura (blueberry muffin syndrome) hepatosplenomegaly, pneumonia, and meningoencephalitis. Osseous lesions include a large anterior fontanelle and lesions in the long bones. Provisional zones of calcification are irregular (Rudolph et al, 1965). Cardiac lesions include patent ductus, septal defects, and peripheral stenosis of pulmonary arteries. Myocardial necrosis has been reported. Hearing loss from involvement of the organ of Corti is common. Immunologic abnormalities with elevated IgG and depressed IgM make the infants prone to infection or histiocytosis.

Now that rubella infection is so rare in the United States, it is possible that infants with congenital rubella will not be diagnosed. A useful set of criteria for diagnosis has been proposed by The Centers for Disease Control in Atlanta (Table 17.6).

Table 17.6
Criteria for Classifying Congenital Rubella Syndrome (CRS) Cases[1]

CRS confirmed. Defects present and one or more of the following:

A. Rubella virus isolated.
B. Rubella-specific IgM present.
C. Rubella hemagglutination-inhibition (HI) titer in the infant persisting above and beyond that expected from passive transfer of maternal antibody (i.e., rubella HI titer in the infant which does not fall off at the expected rate of one twofold dilution/month).

CRS compatible. Laboratory data insufficient for confirmation and any two complications listed in A or one from A and one from B:

A. Cataracts/congenital glaucoma (either or both count as one), congenital heart disease, loss of hearing, pigmentary retinopathy.
B. Purpura, splenomegaly, jaundice, microcephaly, mental retardation, meningoencephalitis, radiolucent bone disease.

CRS possible. Some compatible clinical findings which do not fulfill the criteria for a compatible case.

Congenital rubella infection only. No defects present but laboratory evidence of infection.

Stillbirths. Stillbirths which are thought to be secondary to maternal rubella infection.

Not CRS. One or more of any of the following inconsistent laboratory findings in a child without evidence of an immunodeficiency disease:

A. Rubella HI titer absent in a child 24 months of age or younger.
B. Rubella HI titer absent in mother.
C. Rubella HI titer decline in an infant consistent with the normal decline of passively transferred maternal antibody after birth (the expected rate of decline of maternal antibodies is one twofold dilution/month).

[1] Reproduced from *MMWR*, 35:132, 1986.

LABORATORY FINDINGS

Latex agglutination, fluorescence immunoassay, and enzyme immunoassay tests are used to detect infection. Virus isolation is slow and not generally available.

Treatment

No specific treatment is available. If a susceptible individual is exposed to rubella, intramuscular immune serum globulin is indicated within the first 7–8 days after exposure. There is little indication for this approach except in nonimmune pregnant women who do not want an abortion.

Prognosis

The rubella virus may be isolated from peripheral mononuclear cells years after an acute attack. The association of persistent viruses and chronic arthritis in children was confirmed by Chantler et al (1985) on the basis of recovery of virus from mononuclear lymphoreticular cells in peripheral blood and synovial fluid. The virus has also been isolated from children with Still disease, and adults with seronegative spondyloarthritis, some of whom had no history of rubella, but most of whom had received rubella vaccine.

When vaccinated individuals fail to show seroconversion (by hemagglutination inhibition), they may have rubella-specific antibody detectable by ELISA. These individuals are most likely to have persistence of rubella virus. After congenital infection, another possible site for viral persistence is in chondrocytes in developing cartilage and perhaps other tissues as well.

Prevention

Rubella vaccine is recommended for all children at about 15 months of age. Serologic status of all women of child-bearing age and individuals who work with young mothers and children should be known, and if negative, they should be immunized. Health care personnel likewise should be screened and immunized if they do not have antibodies.

There is a finite risk of fetal infection from the RA 27/3 vaccine currently used in the United States. About 5% of infants of mothers immunized in the first trimester were infected. Thus, pregnant women should not be immunized and others should not become pregnant for 3 months after immunization (Sever, 1984). There has never been a bad fetal outcome in this situation, so that if vaccine is given inadvertently, abortion is not recommended.

Prenatal diagnosis can be carried out on fetal blood obtained by fetoscopy at 20–25 weeks. Unfortunately, first trimester infection can probably not be identified before 22 weeks (Morgan-Capner et al, 1984)

Theoretically, rubella can be eliminated if all susceptible individuals are immunized since there is no known animal host. Significant progress toward that end has been achieved, with the rate of reported cases between 1964 and 1968 at 24.3/100,000 population, down to 0.3/100,000 in 1984 (*MMWR* 35:130, 1986; Bart et al, 1985).

CONTROVERSY

As of 1986 in the United States, a number of women of child-bearing age have not been immunized and are at risk of having the disease during pregnancy. Proof of rubella immunity by serologic testing is a part of prenatal care and family counseling. Postpartum immunization is appropriate in seronegative individuals. Should rubella vaccine be offered to all women when they have contact with the health care system for any reason? Should all college students be required to provide proof of immunity as a part of college entry? Should all health care workers be required to do the same? The answer to these questions from our perspective is yes. The tragedy of the congenital rubella syndrome is so great, and the means of prevention so safe and inexpensive that efforts should continue to protect women who were above the age at which routine immunization was offered when the vaccine was licensed in 1969.

UNCONVENTIONAL VIRUSES

Definition

This relatively new group of viruses are infectious agents with unusual physical and chemical properties as well as biological behavior. Two are known to cause disease in man, Kuru and Creutzfeldt-Jakob disease (CJD) (Gadjusek, 1977).

Basic Science

Characteristic of these viruses is their long incubation period, their unusual resistence to chemical and physical agents, including ionizing radiation, the absence of an inflammatory response, and a chronic slowly progressive disease without remissions or any reported recovery. The pathology is "degenerative" with amyloid plaques, gliosis with no inclusion bodies, no antigenicity, and no alteration in pathogenesis by immunosuppression. The immune B-cell and T-cell functions are intact in vivo and in vitro and there is no cytopathic effect in infected cells in vitro.

Epidemiology

In one of the exciting chapters of medical history, the high incidence of Kuru among tribes in the highlands of New Guinea was discovered by Gadjusek whose extensive studies have been outlined in his book as well as his acceptance speech for the Nobel Prize (1977). Once it became apparent that the mode of transmission of the virus was through the ingestion of infected brain, with the abandonment of that practice, the disease has nearly disappeared. On the other hand, Creutzfeldt-Jakob disease appears to be increasing, partly through medical interventions. Man-to-man transmission has been reported in the recipient of corneal grafts from a donor who, retrospectively, had the disease. It is probable that some children who received growth hormone made from material from human pituitaries have acquired the same disease months or even years later. No transmission of CJD has been reported through blood transfusions or other direct contact. Neurosurgeons, however, have acquired the disease.

Natural History

Both Kuru and CJD are related to scrapie which is widely distributed among sheep, goats, mice, and monkeys.

The incubation period for CJD or Kuru is more than 2 years and sometimes more than 2 decades (Prusiner et al, 1982). The basic lesion is a progressive vacuolation in the dendritic and axonal processes of neurons. An extensive proliferation of glial cells is characteristic; and, finally, the gray matter becomes spongiform. There is usually no evidence of cells or alterations of protein in CSF throughout the course of the infection. There is also no evidence of an immune response to the causative virus. Kuru presents with a cerebellar ataxia and tremors that are episodic and shivering-like. There is a reasonably rapid progression to motor incapacity, and death follows in less than a year from the onset of symptoms. The word Kuru means shivering or trembling in the FORE language of New Guinea. Before the cause of the disease was elucidated, it was found in about 1% of the population. It affected male and female children and adult females, but was rare in adult males. In retrospect, this was a clue to the mode of acquisition of the infection since it was the females who participated in the ritual cannibalism.

CJD is rare and has a familial pattern of inheritance in about 10% of the patients. The affected adults demonstrate myoclonus and characteristic paroxysmal bursts of high voltage and slow waves on the EEG. That disease is regularly transmissible to chimpanzees and even the domestic cat with pathology that is similar to that of Kuru.

It is not clear as to the range of illness associated with CJD virus but possibility of its involvement in Alzheimer disease and amyotrophic lateral sclerosis is of great interest.

Diagnosis

There are no laboratory studies that help in the diagnosis of these conditions except by exclusion. Knowledge of the pertinent epidemiology and likelihood of exposure is crucial to making the diagnosis. It should be suspected any time there is the possibility of direct infection by ingestion or injection of infected nervous tissue including pituitaries.

Treatment

No treatment is known other than supportive.

Prevention

Avoidance of human exposure to infected nervous tissue is the best means of prevention.

REFERENCES

Aase JM, Noren GR, et al: Mumps-virus infection in pregnant women and immunologic response of their offspring. *N Engl J Med* 286:1379, 1972.

Alkalay AL, Pomerance JJ, Rimoin DL: Fetal varicella syndrome. *J Pediatr* 111:320, 1987.

Ammann AJ: The acquired immunodeficiency syndrome in infants and children. *Ann Intern Med* 103:734, 1985.

Anand A, Gray ES, Brown T, et al: Human parvovirus infection in pregnancy and hydrops fetalis. *N Engl J Med* 316:183, 1987.

Anderson LJ: Role of parvovirus B19 in human disease. *Pediatr Infect Dis* 6:711, 1987.

Anderson MJ, Jones SE, Fisher-Hoch SP, et al: Human parvovirus: The cause of erythema infectiosum (fifth disease)? *Lancet* 1:1378, 1983.

Anderson MJ: The emerging story of a human parvovirus-like agent. *J Hyg (London)* 89:1, 1982.

Annunziato D, Kaplan MH, Hall WW, et al: Atypical measles syndrome pathologic and serologic findings. *Pediatrics* 70:203, 1982.

Ayres JC, et al: The sequelae of eastern equine encephalomyelitis. *N Engl J Med* 240:960, 1949.

Baltimore D: Picornaviruses are no longer black boxes. *Science* 229:1366, 1985.

Barnes DM: Grim projections for AIDS epidemic. *Science* 232:1589, 1986.

Bart KJ, Orenstein WA, Preblud S, et al: Elimination of rubella and congenital rubella from the United States. *Pediatr Infect Dis* 4:14, 1985.

Belman AL, Diamond G, Dickson D, et al: Pediatric acquired immunodeficiency syndrome. Neurologic syndromes. *Am J Dis Child* 142:29, 1988.

Blackwelder WC, Dolin R, Mittal KK, et al: A population study of herpes virus infections and HLA antigens. *Am J Epidemiol* 115:569, 1982.

Borsky M: Herpes zoster in infancy. *Am J Dis Child* 134:618, 1980.

Brandt CD, Kim HW, Vargosko AJ, et al: Infections in 18,000 infants and children in a controlled study of respiratory tract disease. 1. Adenovirus pathogenicity in relation to serologic type and illness syndrome. *Am J Epidemiol* 90:484, 1969.

Brandt CD, Kim HW, Yolken RH, et al: Comparative epidemiology of two rotavirus serotypes and other viral agents associated with pediatric gastroenteritis. *Pediatr J Epidemiol* 110:243, 1979.

Braun P: The clinical management of suspected herpes virus encephalitis: A decision analytic view. *Am J Med* 69:895, 1980.

Brunell PA: Varicella-zoster infections. In Feigin R, Cherry J: *Textbook of Pediatric Infectious Diseases*. Philadelphia, WB Saunders, 1981, p. 1206.

Brunell PA, Kotchmar GS: Zoster in infancy: Failure to maintain virus latency following intrauterine infection. *J Pediatr* 98:71, 1981.

Burke DS, Brundage JF, Herbold JR, et al: Human immunodeficiency virus infections among civilian applicants for United States military service, October 1985 to March 1986. *N Engl J Med* 317:131, 1987.

Burke V, Gracey M, Masters P: Rotavirus in children. *J Infect Dis* 152:646, 1985.

Calvelli TA, Rubenstein A: Intravenous gamma globulin in infant acquired immunodeficiency syndrome. *Pediatr Infect Dis* 5:5207, 1986.

Carolane DJ, Long AM, McKeever PA, et al: Prevention of spread of echovirus 6 in a special baby unit. *Arch Dis Child* 60:674, 1985.

CDC: Classification system for human immunodeficiency virus (HIV) infection in children under 13 years of age. *MMWR* 36:225, 1987.

CDC: Dengue—the Americas. *MMWR* 35:51, 1986.

CDC: Human T-lymphotropic virus type III/lymphadenopathy-associated virus antibody prevalence in U.S. military recruit applicants. *MMWR* 35:421, 1986a.

CDC: Imported dengue fever—United States 1984. *MMWR* 34:488, 1985.

CDC: Influenza—United States 1983–1984 season. *MMWR* 33:417, 1984.

CDC: Measles in a population with religious exemption to vaccination—Colorado. *MMWR* 34:718, 1985.

CDC: Measles on colleges campuses—United States, 1985. *MMWR* 34:445, 1985.
CDC: Measles prevention. *MMWR* 36:409, 1987.
CDC: Poliomyelitis—United States 1975–1984. *MMWR* 35:180, 1986.
CDC: Postexposure prophylaxis of hepatitis B. *MMWR* 33:285, 1984.
CDC: Prevention and control of influenza. *MMWR* 34:261, 1985.
CDC: Recommendations for initial management of suspected or confirmed cases of Lassa fever. *MMWR* 28:3S–12S, 1980.
CDC: Recommendations for protection against viral hepatitis. *MMWR* 34:313, 1985.
CDC: Recommendations of immigration practices advisory committee. *MMWR* 35:595, 1986b.
CDC: Revision of the case definition of acquired immunodeficiency syndrome for national reporting—United States. *MMWR* 34:373, June 28, 1985.
CDC: Rubella vaccination during pregnancy—United States 1971–1982. *MMWR* 32:429, 1983.
CDC: Update: Acquired immunodeficiency syndrome—United States. *MMWR* 34:245, May 10, 1985.
CDC: Update: Influenza activity—United States. *MMWR* 34:140, 1985.
Chang RS, Lewis JP, Abildgaard CF: Prevalence of oropharyngeal excreters of leukocyte-transforming agents among human population. *N Engl J Med* 289:1325, 1973.
Chanock RM, Richardson LS, Belshe RB, et al: Prospects for prevention of bronchiolitis caused by respiratory syncytial virus. *Pediatr Res* 11:264, 1977.
Chantler JK, Tingle AJ, Petty RE: Persistent rubella virus infection associated with chronic arthritis in children. *N Engl J Med* 313:1117, 1985.
Cherry JD: Measles. In Feigin RD, Cherry JD (eds): *Textbook of Pediatric Infectious Diseases*. Philadelphia, WB Saunders, 1981b.
Cherry JD: Non-polio enteroviruses. In Feigin RD, Cherry JD (eds): *Textbook of Pediatric Infectious Diseases*. Philadelphia, WB Saunders, 1981a.
Chesney PJ, Dick EC: Coronaviruses. In Feigin RD, Cherry JD (eds): *Textbook of Pediatric Infectious Diseases*. Philadelphia, WB Saunders, 1981, pp. 1160–1167.
Chou S, Merigan TC: Rapid detection and quantification of human cytomegalovirus in urine through DNA hybridization. *N Engl J Med* 308:921, 1983.
Conboy TJ, Pass RF, Myers GJ, et al: Symptomatic congenital cytomegalovirus infection and mental retardation. *Pediatr Res* 20:160A, 1986.
Cooper LZ, Ziring PR, Ockerse AR, et al: Rubella: Clinical manifestations and management. *Am J Dis Child* 118:18, 1969.
Coovadia HM, Brain P, Hallett AF, et al: Immunoparesis and outcome in measles. *Lancet* 1:619, 1977.
Corey L, Spear PG: Infections with herpes simplex virus. *N Engl J Med* 314:686, 1986.
Curran JW: The epidemiology and prevention of the acquired immunodeficiency syndrome. *Ann Intern Med* 103:657, 1985.
Dalldorf G, Sickles GM: An unidentified filterable agent isolated from feces of children with paralysis. *Science* 108:61, 1948.
Dick EC, Chesney PJ: In Feigin RD, Cherry JD (eds): *Textbook of Pediatric Infectious Diseases*. Philadelphia, WB Saunders, 1981, pp. 1167–1186.
Douglas RG Jr: In Stein JH (ed): *Picornaviruses. Internal Medicine*. Boston, Little Brown & Co., 1983, p.1252.
Dworsky M, Yow M, Stagni S, et al: Cytomegalovirus infection of breast milk and transmission in infancy. *Pediatrics* 72:295, 1983.
Edwards KM, Thompson J, Paolini BS, Wright PI: Adenovirus infections in young children. *Pediatrics* 76:420, 1985.
Elliot DL, Tolle SW, Goldberg L, et al: Pet-associated illness. *N Engl J Med* 313:985, 1985.
Empey DW, Laitinen LA, Jacobs, L, et al: Mechanisms of bronchial hyperactivity in normal subjects after upper respiratory tract infection. *Am Rev Respir Dis* 113:131, 1976.
Enders JF, Bell JA, Dingle JH, et al: "Adenoviruses": Group name proposed for new respiratory tract viruses. *Science* 124:119, 1956.
Farquhar J, Gadjusek DC: *Kuru Early Letters and Field Notes from the Collection of D. Carleton Gadjusek*. New York, Raven Press, 1981.
Fayaz A, Simani S, Nour-Salehii S, et al: Booster effect of human diploid cell antirabies vaccine in previously treated persons. *JAMA* 246:2334, 1981.
Fineberg HV: Education to prevent AIDS: Prospects and obstacles. *Science* 239:592, 1988.
Fox JP, Hall CE, Cooney MK: The Seattle virus watch VII: observations of adenovirus infections. *Am J Epidemiol* 105:362, 1977.
Frau LM, Alexander ER: Public health implications of sexually transmitted diseases in pediatric practice. *Pediatr Infect Dis* 4:453, 1985.
Gadjusek DC: Unconventional viruses in the origin and disappearance of Kuru. *Science* 197:943, 1977.
Gallo RC: The AIDS virus. *Sci Am* 256:47, 1987.
Gear JHS, Bowen GS, Kemp GE: Yellow fever. In Feigin RD, Cherry JD (eds): *Textbook of Pediatric Infectious Diseases*. Philadelphia, WB Saunders, 1981.
Glezen WP: Pathogenesis of bronchiolitis: Epidemiologic considerations. *Pediatr Res* 11:239, 1977.
Glezen WP, Paredes A, Taber LH: Influenza in children. *JAMA* 243:1345, 1980.
Guess HA, Broughton DD, Melton LJ, et al: Chicken pox hospitalizations among residents of Olmstead County, Minnesota 1962–1981. *Am J Dis Child* 138:1055, 1984.
Hall CB: The shedding and spreading of respiratory syncytial virus. *Pediatr Res* 11:236, 1977.
Hall CB, McBride JT, Walsh EE, et al: Aerosolized ribavirin in the treatment of respiratory syncytial viral infection: A randomized double-blind study. *N Engl J Med* 308:1443, 1983.
Hall CB, Powell KR, MacDonald NE, et al: Respiratory syncytial viral infection in children with compromised immune function. *N Engl J Med* 315:77, 1986.
Halstead SB: In Feigin RD, Cherry JD (eds): *Textbook of Pediatric Infectious Diseases*. Philadelphia, WB Saunders, 1981, pp. 1140–1149.
Halstead SB: Pathogenesis of dengue: Challenges to molecular biology. *Science* 239:476, 1988.
Hanshaw B, Dudgeon JA, Marshall WC: *Viral Diseases of the Fetus and Newborn*. Philadelphia, WB Saunders, 1985.
Hayden FG, Halperin SA: In Stein JH (ed): *Internal Medicine*. Boston, Little Brown & Co., 1983.
Henderson RH: Vaccine preventable diseases of children. The problem is protecting the world's children's vaccines and immunization within primary health care. New York, Rockefeller Foundation, p.1–17, 1984.
Henle W, Henle G, Horwitz CA: Epstein-Barr virus-specific diagnostic test in infectious mononucleosis. *Hum Pathol* 5:551, 1974.
Hogle JM, Chow M, Filman DJ: Three-dimensional structure of poliovirus at 2.9 A resolution. *Science* 229:1358, 1985.
Holmes GP, Kaplan JE Stewart JA, et al: A cluster of patients with a chronic mononucleosis-like syndrome. *JAMA* 297:2297, 1987.
Horstmann DM: In Feigin RD, Cherry RD (eds): *Textbook of Pediatric Infectious Diseases*. Philadelphia, WB Saunders, 1981.
Horwitz CA, Henle W, Henle G, et al: Clinical and laboratory evaluation of cytomegalovirus-induced mononucleosis in previously healthy individuals. Report of 82 cases. *Medicine* 65:124, 1986.
Huang ES, Alford CA, Reynolds DW, et al: Molecular epidemiology of cytamegalo infections in women and their infants. *N Engl J Med* 303:958, 1980.
Hutchins GM, Vie SA: The progression of interstitial myocarditis to idiopathic endocardial fibroelastosis. *Am J Pathol* 66:483, 1972.
Jarrat M: Herpes simplex infections. *Arch Dermatol* 119:99, 1983.
Jespersen CS, Littauer J, Sagild U: Measles as a cause of fetal defects. A retrospective study of ten measles epidemics in Greenland. *Acta Paediatr Scand* 66:367, 1977.
Jordan MC, Roussenau WE, Stewart JA, et al: Spontaneous cytomegalovirus mononucleosis. *Ann Intern Med* 79:153, 1973.
Juretic M: Natural history of herpetic infection. *Helv Paediatr Acta* 21:356, 1966.
Kaplan, Turuer GS, Warrell DA: *Rabies: The Facts*. New York, Oxford University Press, 1986.
Kline JO (ed): *Report of the Committee on Infectious Diseases, American Academy of Pediatrics,* 19th edition, 1982, Evanston, IL, 1982.
Laurence J: The immune system in AIDS. *Sci Am* 253:84, 1985.
Lawrence R, Gershon AA, Holzman R, et al: The risk of zoster after

varicella vaccination in children with leukemia. *N Engl J Med* 318:543, 1988.

Marion RW, Wiznia AA, Hutcheon G, et al: Fetal AIDS syndrome score: Correlation between severity of dysmorphism and age at diagnosis of immunodeficiency. *Am J Dis Child* 141:429, 1987.

McCormick JB, King IJ, Webb PA, et al: Lassa fever. Effective therapy with ribavirin. *N Engl J Med* 314:20, 1986.

Meyers JD, Wade JC, Mitchell CD, et al: Multicenter collaborative trial of intravenous acyclovir for treatment of mucocutaneous herpes simplex virus infection in the immunocompromised host. *Am J Med* 73:229, 1982.

Miller C: Live measles vaccine: A 21 year follow up. *Br Med J* 295:22, 1987.

Miller G, Niederman JC, Andrews LL: Prolonged oropharyngeal excretion of Epstein-Barr virus after infectious mononucleosis. *N Engl J Med* 288:229, 1973.

Modlin JF: Fatal echovirus II disease in premature neonates. *Pediatrics* 66:775, 1980.

Monath TP: Arboviruses of Central and South America. In Feigin RD, Cherry JD (eds): *Textbook of Pediatric Infectious Diseases*. Philadelphia, WB Saunders, 1981.

Morgan-Capner P, Roderick CH, et al: Prenatal diagnosis of rubella. *Lancet* 2:343, 1984.

Oleske JM, Connor EM, Grebenau MD, et al: Treatment of HIV infected infants and children. *Pediatr Ann* 17:332, 1988.

Ozawa K, Kurtzman G, Young N: Replication of the B19 parvovirus in human bone marrow cell cultures. *Science* 233:883, 1986.

Panum PL: Observations made during the epidemic of measles in the Faroe Islands in the year 1846. *Med Class* 3:829, 1939.

Paryani SG, Arvin AA: Intrauterine infection with varicella-zoster virus after maternal varicella. *N Engl J Med* 314:1542, 1986.

Paryani SG, Yeager AS, et al: Sequelae of acquired cytomegalovirus infection in premature and sick term infants. *J Pediatr* 107:451, 1985.

Pass RF, Little EA, Stagno S, et al: Young children as a probable source of maternal and congenital cytomegalovirus infection. *N Engl J Med* 316:1366, 1987.

Pass RF, Stagno S, Myers, GJ, et al: Outcome of symptomatic congenital cytomegalovirus infection: Results of long term longitudinal followup. *Pediatrics* 66:758, 1980.

Piot P, Plummer FA, Mhala FS, et al: AIDS: An international perspective. *Science* 239:573, 1988.

Plotkin SA, Clark HF: Rabies. In Feigin RD, Cherry JD (eds): *Textbook of Pediatric Infectious Diseases*. Philadelphia, WB Saunders, 1981, pp. 1267–1275.

Plummer FA, Hammond GW, Forward K, et al: An erythema infectiosum-like illness caused by human parvovirus infection. *N Engl J Med* 313:74, 1985.

Preblud SR: Age specific risks of varicella complications. *Pediatrics* 68:14, 1981.

Prober CG, Sullender WM, Yasukawa LL, et al: Low risk of herpes simplex virus infections in neonates exposed to the virus at the time of vaginal delivery to mothers with recurrent genital herpes simplex infections. *N Engl J Med* 316:240, 1987.

Prusiner SB, Gadjusek DC, Alpers MP: Kuru with incubation periods exceeding two decades. *Ann Neurol* 12:1, 1982.

Qazi QH, Sheikh TM, Fikrig S, et al: Lack of evidence for craniofacial dysmorphism in perinatal human immunodeficiency virus infection. *J Pediatr* 112:7, 1988.

Quinn TC, Mann JM, et al: AIDS in Africa: An epidemiologic paradigm. *Science* 234:955, 1986.

Ragozzino MW: Risk of cancer after herpes zoster. *N Engl J Med* 307:393, 1982.

Rawls WE, Wong CL, Blajchman M, et al: Neonatal cytomegalovirus infections: The relative role of neonatal blood transfusion and maternal exposure. *Clin Invest Med* 7:13, 1984.

Reeves WC, et al: Risk of recurrence after first episodes of genital herpes: Relation to HSV-type antibody response. *N Engl J Med* 305:315, 1981.

Report of the National Advisory Committee on Immunization: *The Canada Disease Weekly Report*. Vol 10, April 21, 1984.

Reynolds DW, Stagno S, Myers GJ, et al: Maternal cytomegalovirus excretion and perinatal infection. *N Engl J Med* 289:1, 1973.

Rhodes AR: Herpes zoster in neoplastic disease. *JAMA* 36:2174, 1976.

Rice CM, Lenches EM, Eddy SR, et al: Nucleotide sequence of yellow fever virus: Implications for Flavivirus gene expression and evolution. *Science* 229:726, 1985.

Rubenstein A: Pediatric AIDS. In *Current Problems in Pediatrics* XVI, 366, 1986.

Rudolph AJ, Singleton EB, et al: Osseous manifestations of congenital rubella syndrome. *Am J Dis Child* 110:428, 1965.

Ruuskanen O, Meurman O, Sarkkinen H: Adenoviral diseases in children: A study of 105 hospital cases. *Pediatrics* 76:79, 1985.

Ruuskanen O, Sarkkinen H, Meurman O, et al: Rapid diagnosis of adenoviral tonsillitis: A prospective clinical study. *J Pediatr* 104:725, 1984.

Southern P, Oldstone MBA: Medical consequences of persistent viral infection. *N Engl J Med* 314:359, 1985.

Spencer MJ, Cherry JD: Adenoviral infections. In Feigin R, Cherry JD (eds): *Pediatric Infectious Diseases*. Philadelphia, WB Saunders, 1981, p. 1279.

Stagno S, Brasfield DM, Brown MB: Infant pneumonitis associated with cytomegalovirus, chlamydia, pneumocystis and ureaplasma: A prospective study. *Pediatrics* 68:322, 1981.

Stagno S, Pass RF, Reynolds DW, et al: Comparative studies of diagnostic procedure for congenital cytomegalovirus infection. *Pediatrics* 62:251, 1980.

Stagno S, Whitley RJ: Herpes virus infections of pregnancy Part II Herpes simplex virus and varicella zoster virus infections. *N Engl J Med* 313:1327, 1985.

St. Geme JW, Noren GR, Adams P: Proposed embryopathic relation between mumps virus and primary endocardial fibroelastosis. *N Engl J Med* 286:1379, 1972.

Straus SE, et al: Herpes simplex virus infection: biology, treatment and prevention. NIH Conference Report. *Ann Intern Med* 103:404, 1985.

Sumaya CV, Ench Y: Epstein-Barr virus infectious mononucleosis in children. 1. Clinical and general laboratory findings. *Pediatrics* 75:1003, 1985.

Sumaya CV, Ench Y: Epstein-Barr virus infectious mononucleosis in children. 2. Heterophil antibody and viral-specific responses. *Pediatrics* 75:1011, 1985.

Takahashi M, Otsuka T, Okuno Y: Live vaccine used to prevent the spread of varicella in children in hospital. *Lancet* 2:1288, 1974.

Takahashi M: Clinical overview of varicella vaccine: Development and early studies. *Pediatrics* 78:736, 1986.

The Global Eradication of Smallpox, Final report of the Global Commission for the Certification of Smallpox Eradication, Geneva, 1980, Publication of the World Health Organization.

The Medical Letter. Oral acyclovir for genital herpes simplex infection. 27:41, 1985.

Vesikari T, Isolauri E, et al: Clinical efficacy of the RIT 4237 live attenuated bovine rotavirus vaccine in infants vaccinated before a rotavirus epidemic. *J Pediatr* 107:189, 1985.

Wald ER, Dashefsky B, Green M: *In re* ribavirin: A case of premature adjudication? *J Pediatr* 112:154, 1988.

Weller TH: Serial propagation in vitro of agents producing inclusion bodies derived from varicella and herpes zoster. *Proc Soc Exp Biol Med* 83:340, 1953.

Weller TH: Varicella and herpes zoster. *N Engl J Med* 309:1434, 1983.

Wells MW: The seasonal patterns of measles and chicken pox. *Am J Hyg* 40:279, 1944.

Whitley RJ, Nahmias AJ, Soong S, et al: Vidarabine therapy of neonatal herpes simplex virus infection. *Pediatrics* 66:495, 1980.

Whitley RJ, et al: Herpes simplex encephalitis, clinical assessment. *JAMA* 247:17, 1982.

Whitley RJ, et al: Natural history of herpes simplex virus infection of mother and newborn. *Pediatrics* 66:49, 1980.

Winter WD: Eastern equine encephalomyelitis in Massachusetts in 1955. *N Engl J Med* 255:262, 1956.

Wohl MEB, Chernick V: Bronchiolitis. *Am Rev Respir Dis* 118:759, 1978.

Yeager AS, Itafleigh MT, Arvin AM, et al: Prevention of transfusion acquired cytomegalovirus infections in new born infants. *J Pediatr* 98:281, 1981.

Yolken RH, Kim, HW, Clem T, et al: Enzyme-linked immunoabsorbent assay (ELISA) for detection of human reovirus-like agent of infantile gastroenteritis. *Lancet* 2:263, 1977.

Bacteria 5

ACTINOMYCOSIS

Definition

Actinomycosis is a rare disorder in children characterized by suppurative skin lesions, draining sinuses, and even more rarely, systemic infection.

Basic Science

The organisms are Gram-positive slow-growing anaerobic bacilli with branching hyphae. Human illness is mostly from *Actinomyces israelii*. The organisms are normal inhabitants of nasopharynx and gastrointestinal tract, and cause illness when they infect damaged tissue. "Sulfur granules" may appear in the secretions that are about 2 mm diameter, light yellow, and are clumps of calcified mycelia (they have been reported in other infections as well).

Epidemiology

The incidence is unknown, although it is uncommon in the United States.

Natural History

The most common infection is cervicofacial actinomycosis. The organism enters subcutaneous tissues after trauma or a tooth infection, and produces a painless swelling along the mandible. Eventually it becomes fluctuant and surrounding tissue is discolored and indurated. Draining fistulas are characteristic. Pulmonary lesions are associated with persistent empyema. Abdominal infections occur after appendicitis or penetrating wounds.

Diagnosis

Histologic findings are sulfur granules and Gram-positive filamentous bacilli are characteristic. The organism can be grown from infected tissue.

Treatment

Surgical drainage of abscesses and excision of infection tissue are indicated. Intravenous penicillin for 6–8 weeks followed by oral penicillin for 6–12 months may be required for healing of deep infections.

BRUCELLOSIS

Definition

Brucellosis is a febrile illness caused by several species of *Brucella* including *B. melitensis, B. abortus, B. suis,* and *B. canis*. It is primarily a disease of animals and is acquired by people in contact with infected animals.

Basic Science

The major reservoirs of brucellosis are goats, sheep, cows, swine, and kennel-raised dogs. Other animals may be infected but are not commonly a source for human infection.

The microorganisms are small, Gram-negative, nonmotile bacilli. They can remain viable in water or fomites for many days and also may be found in improperly pasteurized or unpasteurized milk and cheese products.

Transmission from animals to humans occurs mostly through the ingestion of infected milk or meat. Workers in meat-processing plants and veterinarians are at particular risk.

Epidemiology

Only about 10% of the reported cases of brucellosis each year involve children. The disease is reportable, and in 1987, 116 cases were reported in the United States.

Natural History

The organisms enter the body through eye, skin abrasions or oral pharyngeal membranes. They enter the lymphatic system and are localized in the regional lymph nodes where they multiply before invading the bloodstream. In the blood stream they are engulfed by phagocytes and monocytes and transported to the reticuloendothelial system (spleen, liver, bone marrow, lymph nodes, and kidney). Brucellae remain viable in the macrophages for long periods of time, and stimulate the production of multiple, minute granulomas composed of epithelial cells, lymphocytes, monocytes, plasma cells, and giant cells. Sometimes there is central necrosis but the granulomas do not typically undergo caseation. Infections with *B. suis* in particular can form abscesses.

After general dissemination there is apparently production of endotoxin which provides a stimulus to humoral and cellular immune responses. The organism provokes delayed hypersensitivity of the tuberculin type. Infection produces a moderate degree of immunity so reinfection is infrequent.

The chief symptoms are chills, fever, headache, weakness, myalgias, and arthralgias. Multiple other symptoms including anorexia, weight loss, dizziness, tinnitus, epistaxis, and hematuria may occur. The most notable clinical finding is generalized lymphadenopathy and splenomegaly.

The chronic form of brucellosis has many nonspecific symptoms and may be masked as a fever of unknown origin.

Complications are rare but can include meningoencephalitis, pneumonitis, abscesses, and osteomyelitis, as well as diffuse interstitial nephritis. Subacute bacterial endocarditis also has been reported.

Diagnosis

Since the clinical picture is nonspecific, diagnosis depends upon laboratory confirmation. A standard agglutination test is the best generally available. Serial samples of sera should be obtained to demonstrate a rising titer. The agglutination test remains positive, but with reduced titers for many months or even years. Blood cultures and specimens from infected tissues should be taken during active infection since the organism can be recovered in about half the cases. The laboratory should be notified that *Brucella* may be the offending organism so that incubation is done in an elevated CO_2 atmosphere.

The formerly widely used *Brucella* skin test is no longer recommended; not only are the results unreliable but the test may cause a rise in titer in the agglutination test.

Treatment

In older children the tetracyclines administered orally in doses of 25–40 mg/kg/day divided into three or four doses for 3 weeks are usually adequate, although relapses may occur. For patients who do not tolerate tetracycline, trimethoprim-sulfamethoxazole is effective. Sometimes the rapid destruction of the organisms leads to a Herxheimer reaction which can be alleviated with short courses of hydrocortisone.

Prevention

Efforts to eliminate brucellosis from cattle have been underway for many years with significant success. Vaccines are currently available for cattle, goats, and sheep. Unfortunately, control programs have been less effective in swine and no vaccine is available, hence there is a continuing exposure of the population to brucellosis.

CAMPYLOBACTER

Definition

Formerly known as *Vibrio fetus, Campylobacter* is a frequent cause of gastroenteritis in children (Karmali and Fleming, 1979). Improved isolation techniques developed in recent years have clarified the role of this organism, first isolated from an infant by Eden in 1962.

Basic Science

The organism has three known species, *C.fetus, C. intestinalis,* and *C. jejuni,* and is a thin Gram-negative motile rod with a single flagellum at one or both poles. Visible growth of the bacteria may require 5–14 days after inoculation, but growth can be observed in 72 hours if the organisms are incubated on sheep blood and chocolate agar in 5–10% CO_2. *C. jejuni* requires selective medium and incubation at 42°C.

Epidemiology

The incidence is not known, but the organisms are frequently found in stools of children with gastroenteritis and very rarely in neonates with meningitis (Lee, et al, 1985). It can be spread venereally, or through contaminated food or water. Household pets have also been implicated as reservoirs of infection.

Natural History

Oral ingestion is thought to be followed in 2–11 days by an enterotoxin-induced watery diarrhea, and vomiting. It is not ordinarily invasive, although either transient or persistent and fatal bacteremia may be present, especially in neonates. Most commonly in older children the illness is enteric and can resemble ulcerative colitis or intussusception, with blood and mucus present in stools 2–4 days after onset of symptoms. Fever, malaise, abdominal pain and distention, and myalgia have been reported (Feigin, 1981). Venereal transmission has been documented in homosexual relationships, and is thought to occur in heterosexual ones.

Diagnosis

The diagnosis depends on recovery of the organism from stool. Direct phase microscopy of feces is sometimes helpful. The possibility of infection with *Campylobacter* should be considered whenever *Salmonella* or *Shigella* are suspected.

Treatment

The organism is usually sensitive to gentamicin, kanamycin, and chloramphenicol. When septicemia is present, gentamicin is considered the drug of choice. Milder illnesses with *C. jejuni* have been successfully treated with erythromycin 40 mg/kg/day for 1 week.

Prognosis

The outlook is poorest in newborns and immunocompromised hosts infected with *C. intestinalis.* Most other patients, especially those infected with *C. jejuni,* recover completely.

CLOSTRIDIA

Botulism

Definition

Botulism is a severe form of food poisoning caused by a neurotoxin from *Clostridium botulinum.*

Epidemiology

An increasing number of outbreaks have been reported in recent years, mostly from home-processed foods, especially vegetables and fruits. Cases have been reported from Scandinavia, Japan, and Canada, but true incidence is not known in this epidemic disorder which is characterized by sporadic outbreaks.

Natural History

Spores of *C. botulinum* are ubiquitous in soil and can contaminate fresh foods. They can survive boiling for several hours, and thrive on food previously cooked and left at ambient temperature for at least 16 hours. Boiling for 5 minutes before serving inactivates the toxin. Honey is another source of food poisoning from botulinum.

The onset of symptoms is usually abrupt, as early as 6 hours, more likely about 36 hours after ingestion of contaminated food, but it can be delayed for 3 weeks. Early onset illness has a poor prognosis. Nausea, vomiting, abdominal pain, and diarrhea may occur early in the course. Diplopia, ptosis, facial weakness, and thick speech can progress rapidly to respiratory failure and quadriplegia. The patient remains alert and has no sensory deficit. Maximal weakness more commonly develops 7–10 days after onset of symptoms. In contrast to Guillain Barré syndrome, the weakness is descending. In infants, the signs are poor sucking or swallowing, ptosis, ophthalmoplegia, and constipation. Affected individuals are afebrile and have normal spinal fluid (Arnon and Chin, 1979; Polin and Brown, 1979).

Diagnosis

Diagnosis depends on identification of the toxin or the organism in the patient or the suspected food. Specimens of feces (at least 50 g), vomitus and serum should be refrigerated and examined as soon as possible. They must be in sealed containers labeled "hazardous" since small amounts of toxin can be highly toxic. An ELISA permits identification of the toxin in feces within 24 hours (Dezfulian et al, 1985).

Treatment

If the patient is seen within a few hours of exposure, vomiting should be induced and gastric lavage with ipecac is appropriate. Enemas have been recommended to eliminate unabsorbed toxin. Fast-acting laxatives such as magnesium sulfate may be useful.

Prompt administration of trivalent botulinum antitoxin gives rapid relief, and full recovery is the rule in treated patients. The recovery in children may be very gradual, over weeks or months. Ventilatory support is often required.

Prognosis

The mortality rate is about 20–25%. Relapses can occur after a period of steady improvement, for reasons that are obscure. Presumably the spores persist and excrete more neurotoxin in some individuals.

CASE ILLUSTRATION

A 5-month-old white male presented after 3 weeks of constipation, progressive weakness, and failure to gain weight. He had had a benign perinatal history and was well until the onset of an upper respiratory infection 3 weeks before his admission. Constipation followed and no stools were noted for 10 days. Superimposed on this constellation of symptoms was a regression in developmental milestones, decreased activity with muscle weakness, and a poor suck over 3–4 days, that resulted in poor oral intake and dehydration. The baby had been breast-fed since birth, with canned baby foods introduced at age 3 months, but no honey or Karo syrup.

Initial examination revealed a weak, irritable but alert male infant with height, weight, and head circumference in the 50th percentile. Chest movement was shallow. Cardiac and abdominal examination were benign. Rectal examination was notable for stool in the ampulla with diminished sphincter tone. Neurologic examination showed an expressionless face, poor gag and suck, with flaccid tongue and generalized diffuse muscle weakness, although reflexes were 2+ and symmetrical.

Baseline laboratory values were entirely normal, except for some mild hypoxia noted on arterial blood gas.

QUESTIONS AND COMMENTS

Is this case consistent with the diagnosis of infantile botulism?

Despite the lack of a clear dietary etiology and the presence of reflexes, EMG studies done shortly after admission were found to be pathognomonic for infantile botulism. In fact, review of the literature on infantile botulism indicates that only in a few cases can a source be identified and in more than one-third reflexes were present at the initial time of diagnosis, and constipation was present often as long as 3 weeks before the muscle weakness was noted. Without the EMG findings, diagnosis would have awaited growth of the organism or identification of the toxin in the stool, although stools are only rarely positive for toxin in infants, in contrast to the situation in adult food-borne botulism.

How should this infant be treated?

Treatment for infantile botulism is essentially supportive (respiratory and/or nutritional); antitoxins, antibiotics, or drugs that alter the release of acetylcholine have not been helpful in children. This patient was treated with stool purgatives and gavage feeds, and over the subsequent weeks showed improvement in respiratory mechanics and muscle tone. It took several months, however, for the baby to achieve a full recovery.

Clostridium difficile

Definition

C. difficile (see also pp. 444) is a widespread potential pathogen capable of causing a mild exudative enteropathy, or an antibiotic-associated pseudomembranous colitis.

Basic Science

The organism is an obligate anaerobe that produces at least two potent toxins. It is so often associated with other pathogens, it has been difficult to assign a pathogenic role to *C. difficile*. Frequently it may be present in stools of asymptomatic individuals. The toxins are cytopathic, and capable of producing death in infant monkeys (Arnon et al, 1984).

Epidemiology

The organism is most commonly found in the stools of infants fed formula. It is rarely associated with infection in infancy, but is associated with membranous colitis in older children and adults. Nosocomial spread has been well-documented in nurseries.

Natural History

Studies on infant monkeys show that intraperitoneal or intravenous injection of toxins cause an illness characterized by progressive hypothermia and loss of muscle tone after a few hours. Respiratory failure precedes a flat EEG. This quiet death has been compared to that of infants with sudden infant death syndrome.

Diarrhea associated with *C. difficile* is usually bloody and mucousy. It may be present and associated with membranous colitis especially in children who have been on long-term antibiotic therapy. Symptoms can resemble appendicitis.

Diagnosis

Recovery of the organism in stools and identification of cytopathogenic effects in tissue culture is suggestive but not confirmatory of its role in illness. It is more significant in the absence of other pathogens. Sigmoidoscopy is a good immediate diagnostic test and is very suggestive when the findings are flagrant.

Treatment

Vancomycin 50 mg/kg/day every 6 hours orally for 7–17 days is usually very effective. Metronidazole, (Flagyl) is also effective. If relapse occurs, retreatment is indicated and sometimes effective.

CONTROVERSY

The data are not adequate to define the role of this toxin-producing organism in disease other than in antibiotic-associated pseudomembranous colitis where the response to vancomycin is so effective.

The possible association with sudden infant death syndrome, discussed by Cooperstock et al, 1982 and Arnon et al, 1984, is of interest, since it seems possible that *C. difficile* may cause no symptoms as long as it is in the colon of normal individuals, but can produce illness when antibiotics eliminate competing enteric flora, or when its toxins can enter the circulation for whatever reason. Why the latter event would occur in the otherwise asymptomatic infants in the first year of life who become victims of sudden death is unexplained.

Clostridia perfringens

Definition

C. perfringens is a spore-forming anerobic bacterium associated with a wide variety of infections, most notably gas gangrene secondary to wound infection. The organism is commonly found in the colon of asymptomatic carriers.

Basic Science

Clostridia produces a number of toxins that explain its toxicity. The most important is a lecithinase which destroys tissue and produces hemolysis. Collagenase, hyaluronidase, fibrinolysins, and others contribute to tissue necrosis thrombosis and gas gangrene.

Epidemiology

The organism is often found among other flora and isolated in 5–10% of anaerobic wound infections.

Natural History

Gas gangrene is heralded by pain in the region of a wound, then edema and hemorrhage. The surrounding skin may be tense, blanched, and later has a bronze coloration. Systemic toxemia and tachycardia are common. Crepitus may be felt under the involved skin. Hemolysis with rapid onset of jaundice may occur and may lead to toxic delirium and later shock.

Enteric infection is much less severe. It is a common form of food poisoning starting 6–12 hours after ingestion of contaminated meat. The illness is usually over in 24 hours although the organism may be recovered in stools for long periods (carrier state).

The organism has been associated with more severe bowel problems, including (rarely) neonatal necrotizing enterocolitis or toxic megacolon.

Diagnosis

Gas gangrene can be diagnosed by observation of gas formation and necrosis in the presence of severe pain and toxemia. Specimens from wound exudate should be refrigerated and sent to a suitable laboratory to search for the organism.

Recovery of the enterotoxin-producing organism in stools of individuals with food poisoning, of the same serotype as food in the contaminated food, establishes the association.

Treatment

If only cellulitis is present, incision and drainage and antimicrobials are effective. If gas gangrene is present, radical surgical debridement of the wound with drainage is imperative. Penicillin G or cephalosporins in penicillin-sensitive individuals are the antibiotics of choice. Chloramphenicol is also effective. Food poisoning from *C. perfringens* does not require antibiotic therapy.

Prognosis

Wound infection carries a 15–35% mortality rate, dependent on size of wound and duration of infection before initiating treatment. In individuals at high risk, a type C toxoid may be helpful.

Clostridium tetani

Definition

C. tetani is the spore-forming anerobic bacillus that causes tetanus, by producing a neurotoxin that causes tonic spasms of skeletal muscles. The disease is completely preventable with immunization.

Basic Science

This Gram-positive organism is present in soil and human feces. Developing spores give the organism its drumstick shape. After extrusion, spores are resistant to boiling, but are killed by heating at 120°C for 15–20 minutes, or exposure to sunlight. In shady or dark areas, they can survive in soil for months and they are carried in the intestines of many animals and humans.

The spores multiply in tissues, but do not produce inflammation. Illness is caused by two exotoxins. One, tetanospasmin, is a highly potent toxin; it is thought to be transported in nerves, with initial penetration close to the site of inoculation. It exerts its effects at the motor end plates of skeletal muscle, the spinal cord, the brain and the autonomic nervous system. The toxin inhibits release of acetylcholine from nerve terminals. Within the CNS it suppresses inhibitory influences on motor neurons which explains spasms and seizures.

Epidemiology

The incidence is highest in unimmunized individuals exposed to dung. In the United States in 1985–1986, 147 cases were reported for a rate of 0.3/100,000 (CDC, 1987). Contamination of the umbilicus is the most common route of infection in infants in underdeveloped areas of the world. Infants of immunized mothers are protected by passive transfer of antibodies across the placenta.

Natural History

The usual incubation period is 3–21 days, but it may be shorter or as long as several months. The median incubation period is 7 days. The greater the distance from site of infection to the CNS, the longer is the incubation period.

The most common form of illness follows introduction of the bacteria through a penetrating wound or burn. It has followed septic abortions.

In over half the patients, trismus is the first symptom. Irritability, meningismus, dysphagia, and muscle rigidity follow. Groups of muscles are involved, including chest, abdomen, and back which results in opisthotonus, and generalized tonic seizures are common. Glottic and laryngeal spasms are life-threatening. Temperature elevation, profuse sweating, cardiac arrhythmias, and tachycardia are sometimes present.

Sometimes the disease may be localized to muscles in the region of infection. Persistent painful spasm of muscles close to the lesion is characteristic.

Diagnosis

The most pathognomonic sign is trismus. The diagnosis depends on the typical clinical features and although recovery of the organism from the wound may be possible, it is not necessary to establish the diagnosis.

Treatment

Human hyperimmune globulin, 5 units intramuscularly, is the treatment of choice for neonatal tetanus. Tetanus toxoid should also be given to stimulate active immunity. For wound infection in older individuals, 3000–6000 units intramuscularly is recommended. Penicillin is recommended in all cases since it kills the vegetative form of the organism. Seizures are best controlled with secobarbital or pentobarbital, 10 mg/kg/day. Intravenous diazepam has been found to be effective in doses of 0.1–0.2 mg/kg every 2–8 hours. Severe forms of tetanus may require muscle relaxants and mechanical ventilation.

Meticulous nursing care in a subdued environment can be life-saving. Frequent suctioning and reassurance may obviate need for a tracheostomy or endotracheal intubation, although these may be required if laryngospasm is a problem. Adequate caloric intake should be maintained by gavage. Pyridoxine, 100 mg/day, has been reported to decrease morbidity in an uncontrolled study (Godel, 1983).

Prognosis

If untreated, the disease is usually fatal. Nevertheless, early debridement, administration of hyperimmune globulin, and meticulous nursing care can promote recovery. The case-fatality rate among unimmunized and inadequately immunized adults in the United States 1985–1986 was 31%.

Prevention

Immunization should be universal. Active immunization with tetanus toxoid is very effective. After the four injections given in the first year of life, a booster is given on school entry, and every 10 years thereafter. Serum antitoxin levels of 0.01 unit/ml indicate adequate protection. An attack of tetanus does not confer immunity.

Immunization of pregnant women is safe. Two doses of toxoid a month apart, with the second dose 2 weeks before delivery will protect the infant who will receive antibodies across the placenta. The mother's third dose can be given postpartum to protect future pregnancies.

DIPHTHERIA (*Corynebacterium diphtheriae*)

Definition

Diphtheria is an acute infectious disease from the toxin of *Corynebacterium diphtheriae,* a Gram-positive pleomorphic bacillus. Its clinical importance in the United States largely ended with world use of immunization in the late 1920s and 1930s (English, 1985).

Basic Science

C. diphtheria is most frequently identified with toxigenic strains. Pappenheimer and Murphy (1983) examined the DNA from toxigenic and nontoxigenic strains and found close similarity. Since immunization has been widespread, carrier rates of nontoxigenic strains have remained nearly constant. Both carriers and patients with toxigenic strains are observed sporadically, usually after contact with cases in developing countries.

Epidemiology

The organism is distributed worldwide, but rarely causes diseases in the United States where at least 80% of the population have been immunized in infancy. The disorder reaches a peak in autumn and winter months. Only one case was reported to the Centers for Disease Control in the United States for the first 6 months of 1985 and three cases in all of 1987.

Natural History

The incubation period is 2–4 days. Bacilli localize in the mucosa of the upper respiratory tract, but may also involve skin or eyes. A toxin is absorbed to the cell membrane and causes tissue necrosis with a localized inflammation, which widens and deepens and forms a tough adherent gray membrane. Serosanguinous nasal discharge and membranous involvement of tonsils and adenoids are characteristic.

The circulating toxin can cause myocarditis 10–14 days after onset and peripheral neuritis may appear after 3–7 weeks.

SYMPTOMS

The clinical picture of diphtheria is one which presents wide variations, depending upon the principal location of the disease (cutaneous, conjunctival, vulvovaginal, and aural infection can occur), its severity, and its complications. For practical purposes the following groups may be considered.

1. Mild cases, in which there is either no membrane, or the amount of membrane is small and limited to the tonsils or to the nose, with few or none of the constitutional symptoms that follow absorption of the diphtheria toxin. These cases have the characteristics of a local disease.
2. Severe cases of pharyngeal disease can be divided into two types: those in which there is marked evidence of constitutional poisoning from diphtheria toxins; and, those with laryngeal stenosis. In the former there is usually an extensive formation of membrane in the pharynx and sometimes in the nose. The larynx may be involved secondarily to disease in the pharynx or nose, or it may be primarily affected.
3. Cases of mixed infection (septic cases). In many of the cases of the two preceding groups, streptococci are found in the throat, but there are neither sufficient numbers nor are they virulent enough to modify the course of the disease. In those cases designated mixed infection, the constitutional and local symptoms of diphtheritic toxemia are accompanied by significant general septicemia, usually streptococcal. In these cases inflammation is especially prominent, not only in the pharynx but sometimes in the lymph glands and cellular tissue of the neck, this may be followed by suppuration or sloughing. This form is frequently complicated by bronchopneumonia even without laryngeal disease, and sometimes by severe nephritis.

Diagnosis

The diagnosis must be made on clinical criteria in order to initiate prompt treatment. Direct smears of material from diphtheritic lesions are unreliable. Specimens of the membrane, or material beneath it should be obtained and placed on Loeffler, tellurite, or blood agar medium. For determining toxigenicity, two guinea pigs must be inoculated with a broth suspension of the organism; one is given diphtheria antitoxin before intracutaneous inoculation. An inflammatory reaction will appear in 24 hours in the control animal, but not in the one given antitoxin. The Schick test, diphtheria toxin injected intracutaneously, will produce a local inflammatory response that peaks at 5 days in the absence of antitoxin. Ten millimeters of induration indicates susceptibility to diphtheria. The test is useful in determining the immune status of an individual, but takes too long to be helpful in diagnosis.

An electrocardiogram may reveal arrhythmias or ST segment changes if myocarditis is present. Other laboratory tests are of little value. The white blood count can be elevated or normal. Anemia from hemolysis is unusual.

Treatment

Diphtheria antitoxin must be given intravenously when the condition is serious, or intramuscularly for less serious cases: 20,000–50,000 units on 2 or 3 successive days is effective. Penicillin has a bactericidal effect, and should be given intravenously if the child cannot swallow. After the first few days, 600,000 units of procaine penicillin G twice daily intramuscularly for 10 days is recommended.

Preliminary testing for sensitivity to horse serum is essential, as is the availability of 1:1000 aqueous epinephrine in case of anaphylaxis.

Prognosis

Mortality rates vary, mostly as a function of time to make the diagnosis and the presence of early onset myocarditis. The case fatality rate is 3–25%.

Prevention

Prevention should be universal with the series of DPT immunizations in the first year of life. If these have not been given, primary immunization of children over 6 years may be carried out with absorbed diphtheria and tetanus toxoids (Td). Two doses are required intramuscularly or subcutaneously 4 weeks apart, with a booster 1 year later. Immunization is not always effective; in the event of an epidemic, a booster injection of toxoid is recommended. The Shick test is not useful for diagnosis, but can be used to determine the immune status of contacts. Carriers of diphtheria require erythromycin 40 mg/kg/24 hours for 7–10 days. If a contact has symptoms, treatment with antitoxin and penicillin (as in a case of diphtheria) is indicated.

Escherichia coli

Definition

E. coli species (see also pp. 430) are the most common organisms in the normal intestinal flora, but the organisms can produce purulent meningitis in newborns, pyelonephritis and occasionally, a dysentery-like illness in populations throughout the world (see pp. 611 for pyelonephritis).

Basic Science

The somewhat paradoxical situation that *E. coli* organisms inhabit healthy normal intestines where they have an important physiologic function, but also are capable of producing purulent meningitis in infants and pyelonephritis in girls and young women, has been explained, at least partially, by the knowledge that there are different strains of *E. coli* responsible for each of the diseases they cause. Their names indicate their site of injury: meningitic, pyelonephritogenic, enteroinvasive (*Shigella*-like), and enterohemorrhagic, enterotoxigenic, and enteroadherent.

The mechanism of virulence depends on surface proteins that promote or adhere to different epithelial surfaces. They can be seen as fimbriae or pili on the surface of the bacillus. Gene probes for some species are now available to detect the pili or adherence factors on the different strains. Once adherent, the bacteria produce exotoxins that can affect protein synthesis and cause cell death.

Epidemiology

The organisms are distributed worldwide, and illness associated with them is common, although true incidence is unknown.

Natural History

Toxin-producing pathogenic *E. coli* organisms are found in many foodstuffs. Infection by pathogenic strains can produce symptoms in the intestine, the urinary tract, or systemically. Person-to-person transmission is the major problem in nursery epidemics. Nothing distinguishes *E. coli*-induced diarrhea from that of many other Gram-negative organisms including *Shigella* species. Explosive "rice water" diarrhea, or bloody diarrhea can produce profound dehydration within hours of onset. Mortality rates above 50% have been reported in nursery outbreaks, the "summer diarrhea" of the past. More recently, traveler's diarrhea has been attributed to pathogenic strains of *E. coli* among nonimmune visitors.

Diagnosis

Most of the specific etiologic agents (e.g., enterotoxic strains, hemorrhagic strains, adherent strains, invasive strains) are not readily identifiable by routine clinical laboratories. Similar illnesses are caused by rotavirus, *Vibrio cholerae, Salmonella, Shigella,* and *Yersinia* species, as well as the more recently identified *Campylobacter*. The disease is usually self-limited within a few days or a week.

Treatment

Replacement of fluid and electrolyte losses remains the mainstay of treatment. No evidence supports the use of antimicrobial or antiperistaltic agents. For *E. coli* meningitis, ampicillin and an aminoglycoside, or third generation cephalosporins are the agents of choice.

Prognosis

With early and appropriate oral rehydration, the prognosis is excellent.

Prevention

Although no vaccines are available in 1985, the use of molecular biologic techniques holds promise for the near future (Levine, 1985).

GONOCOCCUS

Definition

Strains of *Neisseria gonorrhoeae* are the cause of a highly contagious and widespread venereal disease, which can produce serious infection in the eyes of infants born to mothers with a contaminated vaginal canal, and can present with urethritis, vaginitis, and systemic complications in older individuals. Sequelae include sterility and ectopic pregnancy.

Basic Science

Gonorrheal infection in adults is limited to sites with columnar or transitional epithelium such as the mucous membranes of the urethra, the cervix, the rectum, and the pharynx. Once the organism has penetrated the mucous barrier, it can affect other areas such as synovial fluid and endocardium.

The organism produces an extracellular IgA_1 protease that cleaves secretory IgA and allows the establishment of infection. Virulence depends on extracellular surface pili which apparently facilitate attachment of the microbe to human epithelial cells (Britigan et al, 1985).

In recent years there has been an increase in the development of penicillin-resistant organisms so that higher and higher doses of penicillin have been required for treatment. Resistance may be plasmid-mediated and may be the result of induction of β-lactamase production in some strains that inactivate penicillin. In parts of southeast Asia and Africa, 30–60% of gonococcal isolates produce β-lactamase. Strains that produce disseminated infection, however, are highly sensitive to penicillin.

Epidemiology

Gonorrhea is the most prevalent reportable venereal disease in the United States with approximately 900,000 cases/year during 1980-1984.

Natural History

Asymptomatic carriers are considered a major source of new gonococcal infections. It is much more likely to be asymptomatic in females, although genital infection often is associated with dysuria, urinary frequency, and an increase in vaginal discharge. Because these findings may mimic cystitis, many gonococcal infections in females are unrecognized. In adolescent girls, fever and abdominal pain may indicate salpingitis and peritonitis from ascending infection.

In males, the gonococcus is the most common cause of urethritis which produces significant dysuria. The clinical disease follows a 2- to 7-day incubation period and presents as urethral discharge which is usually purulent but may be clear. If untreated, the discharge may persist an average of 8 weeks but then remit spontaneously.

Very few gonococcal infections lead to disseminated disease. In fact, some individuals with disseminated disease are unaware of the existence of urogenital gonorrhea. The skeletal system is involved mainly with arthralgia and both sterile and purulent arthritis. In gonococcemia, a skin rash, characterized by pustules with erythematous bases, is present, most commonly on the extremities; some pustules can become bullous and necrotic. Endocarditis and meningitis are very rare.

Individuals with inherited deficiencies of C5, C6, C7, or C8 (components of complement), are unusually susceptible to systemic infection with the gonococcus. They lack bactericidal activity in their serum and hence are susceptible to serious disease.

Diagnosis

Diagnosis requires the demonstration of Gram-negative intracellular diplococci in smears of urethral discharge in men and cervical secretions in women, and is confirmed by culture of the organism. Pharyngeal and rectal swabs should be examined in the investigation of sexual contacts of children with suspected gonorrhea. Blood or fluid from swollen joints should be examined as well.

The organism is usually cultured on chocolate-blood agar in an enriched CO_2 atmosphere. Selective media are essential for rectal, cervical, and pharyngeal cultures. Accurate speciation of all *Neisseria* organisms cultured from children is necessary if there is any question of sexual abuse.

Treatment

For infants with any form of gonococcal disease intravenous administration of 75,000–100,000 units daily of aqueous penicillin G should be instituted as soon as possible (four divided doses for 7 days). Once drug sensitivities are known (minimal inhibitory concentrations), the appropriate drug can be substituted for penicillin if needed. A single intramuscular dose of 125 mg ceftriaxone has been proven effective (Laga et al, 1986). Older children with disseminated infection should be treated with up to 10 million units of aqueous penicillin G intravenously for at least 3 days, followed by amoxicillin, 500 mg by mouth four times daily to complete at least 7 days of therapy. Uncomplicated urethritis or cervicitis in adolescents is treated with amoxicillin, 3.0 g, or ampicillin 3.5 g, by mouth or aqueous procaine penicillin G, 4.8 million units intramuscularly, and probenecid, 1.0 g by mouth. (For patients sensitive to penicillin, ceftriaxone, 250 mg intramuscularly, is effective.) After the single dose of any of the above, oral tetracycline, 500 mg four times daily for 7 days, or doxycycline, 100 mg twice daily for 7 days, is recommended to treat possible coexisting *C. trachomatis* infection.

The changing patterns of resistance to antimicrobials require up-to-date information on the most effective agents in a given place at a given time. In 1985, strains resistant to penicillin were most sensitive to cefuroxime and cefotaxime (CDC surveillance summaries, 1984).

Prevention

Humans are the only known reservoir for gonococci which are sexually transmitted. Thus, prevention depends on early recognition and treatment of infected individuals and their sexual contacts. Despite much research toward production of an appropriate vaccine, in 1985 the problems remain insurmountable. (For a review of vaccine development, see Britigan et al, 1985).

Gonorrhea Ophthalmia

Vaginal delivery from an infected mother can place the infant at risk of acquiring gonorrhea in the conjunctivae and the pharynx, as well as the anal canal. Gonococcal ophthalmia, however, is of special concern because it can lead to blindness (see Section 20). Fortunately, it is now largely prevented by screening for gonorrhea during pregnancy, treating of infected women, and by routine administration of antimicrobial drops in the eyes of all newborn infants (1% silver nitrate instilled in both eyes in the immediate neonatal period). Although over 90% effective, silver nitrate produces a chemical conjunctivitis in 90% of infants. Ophthalmic ointments containing other agents such as tetracycline (1.0%) or erythromycin (0.5%) are also effective. Many pediatricians advocate erythromycin, which has the advantages of being less irritating to the conjunctivae. Early reports that it was also effective against *Chlamydia* have not been confirmed.

CASE ILLUSTRATION

A 14-year-old sexually active black male developed pain in the right eye 2 weeks before presenting at the hospital. Examination revealed he had a severe anterior uveitis which was treated with steroid and atropine drops.

Two days later he complained of pain in the left ankle and on complete examination, a urethral discharge was noted. Treatment with high-dose procaine penicillin, probenecid, and doxycycline was started on the assumption of gonococcal or chlamydial infection.

Shortly thereafter his left knee became warm and swollen, leading to the possibility that he had a purulent arthritis or an immunologic response to antigens, as in Reiter syndrome. Aspiration of the joint produced 25,000 white cells, 95% polys, but a negative Gram stain and subsequent negative culture. Culture of the urethral exudate revealed gonorrhea. Further laboratory studies that were important included a negative PPD, and negative tests for rheumatoid factor, and antinuclear antibody. His tissue type was HLA-B27 which is observed in 60–80% of patients with Reiter syndrome.

Four days after onset of treatment, most of the symptoms except the uveitis had improved. Systemic steroids and antiflammatory doses of aspirin were then instituted, with further subsidence of all manifestations.

QUESTIONS AND COMMENTS

Reiter syndrome consists of the triad of urethritis, conjunctivitis, and arthritis, but usually the urethritis is nonbacterial. In this case, the gonococcus was cultured from the urethral discharge.

Reiter syndrome in young children sometimes follows infection with *Shigella* and *Yersinia* as well as *Chlamydia*. The designation is usually restricted to those situations in which infectious urethritis and gonococcal disease have been excluded. In this instance the child apparently had the appropriate tissue type for susceptibility to Reiter disease and probably the gonococcus was the initiating organism.

This youngster had pain in the left ankle as well as the left knee. Would this be typical of gonococcal arthritis?

The most common manifestation of gonococcal arthritis is confined to a single joint, often the knee, with evidence of effusion and the ability to recover the organism from the joint fluid. Occasionally in disseminated disease from hematogenous spread, arthritis may be present in multiple joints as well as tenosynovitis, dermatitis, carditis, and even meningitis. This patient probably did not have hematogenous spread, but more likely an immune response to the organism causing the urethritis inasmuch as several joints were involved (with sterile effusion in the knee), and he also had uveitis, which is not the characteristic eye lesion in gonorrhea, but is seen in Reiter syndrome.

Treatment

Infants whose mothers have gonorrhea at the time of delivery should receive a single dose of 50,000 U of penicillin G (20,000 U for low birth weight infants) intramuscularly. Infants with gonococcal ophthalmia or other gonococcal infections should receive intravenous penicillin for at least 7 days or until all signs of infection are gone. The eyes should be irrigated with saline at least hourly. If the organism is resistant to penicillin, cefotaxime or gentamicin may be used.

CONTROVERSY

Gonorrhea remains so prevalent worldwide that most pediatricians recommend routine prophylaxis. The most widely used preparation is 1% silver nitrate in ampules since it is effective and no resistant strains or hypersensitivity reactions have been observed. The chemical conjunctivitis is mild and self-limited.

The argument for use of erythromycin or tetracycline ointments rests on the observation that they are effective against gonococcal infection and less irritating, but alas, they are more expensive than silver nitrate (Hammerschlag, 1988).

The choice is up to the physician except in those regions that mandate the use of silver nitrate (see also pp. 1220, Section 20).

Haemophilus influenzae

Definition

H. influenzae is the most serious pathogen in young children in industrialized countries. It is the leading cause of bacterial meningitis in children, and accounts for most epiglottitis, cellulitis, septic arthritis, and some cases of pneumonia and occult bacteremia in young children.

Basic Science

H. influenzae are Gram-negative pleomorphic coccobacilli. Most of the invasive infections in children are due to an encapsulated strain classified as type B on the basis of the capsular polysaccharide, polyribose phosphate. Of the organisms identified with otitis media, 85–90% are not encapsulated and, hence, are nontypable strains.

Antibody to polyribophosphate (PRP) is opsonic in serum and is protective.

The ability to mount an antibody response to *H. influenzae* is age-dependent. Serum concentrations sufficient to prevent infection are rarely seen after immunization with pure polysaccharide vaccine before 24 months. The conjugated vaccine provides sufficient protection after 18 months to warrant its routine administration.

Epidemiology

About 12,000 cases of meningitis are reported annually in the United States, primarily among children under 4 years of age, for a rate of 40/100,000 children under age 4 years. The mortality rate is 5% and neurologic sequelae are observed in as many as 25–35% of survivors.

Serious *H. influenzae* infections spread among family members and occasionally in day care centers. Whether 2–6% of susceptible children will acquire infection, or fewer, remains controversial. The highest prevalence of systemic disease occurs among the native Inuit population of Alaska where the rate is 491 cases/100,000 children under 5 years of age. Caucasian children with Hib infections other than epiglottitis were significantly more likely to lack the G 2m(n) allotype than controls (Ambrosino et al, 1985).

Natural History

The period of highest susceptibility is among individuals under 2 years of age, but cellulitis, epiglottitis, and arthritis are commonly seen in children under 5 years, and rarely may be seen later, even in adults.

Septicemia precedes invasion of organs. *H. influenzae* has a predilection for the meninges (pp. 1021), synovial membranes (pp. 1288) pericardium, and other serous surfaces such as the middle ear, epiglottis (pp. 1197), or trachea (pp. 1197). Cellulitis, particularly of the cheek or periorbital region, may appear in association with an upper respiratory infection. The onset is acute, and is usually without a history of injury. The lesion is indurated, dusky red, and tender. Blood cultures as well as an aspirate from the edge of the lesion are usually positive for *H. influenzae* type b.

Type b infection is overwhelmingly the most common after the first month of life. In a review of 88 cases of culture-proven sepsis in newborns, from *H. influenzae* only 20% were type B and more than half were non-typeable. The condition was most common in infants under 30 weeks gestational age, in whom the mortality was 90% (Friesen and Cho, 1986). The onset of symptoms is usually in the first day with respiratory distress with rapid evolution of circulatory collapse. Prompt diagnosis and appropriate antibiotics can produce prompt improvement. The mortality rate in infants is about 12%.

Anemia accompanies *H. influenzae* type B infections in nearly 90% of children. Many are moderately anemic on admission, and nearly all become anemic during the illness. Since reticulocyte counts are low, decreased red cell production probably contributes to the anemia. Elevated carboxyhemoglobin levels, consistent with hemolysis were reported in 75% of children with *H. influenzae* meningitis (O'Brien et al, 1981). The mechanism of the anemia, elucidated by Shurin et al (1986) is hemolysis when the capsular polysaccharide of *H. influenzae* type B binds to erythrocytes in the presence of complement. The anemia is self-limited, and full recovery occurs within 21 days.

Diagnosis

The organism can be cultured from blood early in the illness, and from cerebrospinal fluid even before a cellular response. Needle aspiration at the leading edge of cellulitis can also reveal organisms that can be identified by Gram stain or culture. Rapid diagnosis by latex particle agglutination facilitates diagnosis, but false-positive findings in serum and urine reduce the value of this test. False-negative values are rare. Arthritis associated with *H. influenzae* meningitis may be septic or reactive. Thus, aspiration and culture are necessary to ascertain whether prolonged antibiotics or anti-inflammatory agents are appropriate.

Treatment

Treatment with intravenous antibiotics should begin immediately; the choice of antibiotic depends on knowledge of recent local experience with sensitivities. Resistance to *H. influenzae* correlates mainly with production of a plasmid-mediated β-lactamase enzyme. If β-lactamase is produced, the organism is resistant to ampicillin, but should respond to chloramphenicol. The therapeutic range of chloramphenicol is 10–20 μg/ml, and serum levels should be measured. Cefuroxime in high dosage is an effective second generation cephalosporin and cefotaxime or ceftriaxone are the preferred third generation agents (Barson et al, 1985; Higham et al, 1985). Third generation cephalosporins may be useful if the organism is resistant to chloramphenicol or the drug is contraindicated in a given patient. After chloramphenicol is discontinued, rifampin should be given for 4 days (20 mg/kg/day) in a single daily dose to eliminate the carrier state and possible recurrence in infants under age 2 years.

Prognosis

Neurologic and learning disabilities are present in nearly half of the children who survive *H. influenzae* meningitis. About 20% have significant hearing deficits; spastic hemiparesis, quadriplegia, poor coordination, lowered I.Q., and impaired vision from chorioretinitis are found alone or in combination in about 10% of survivors. It is well to note, however, that 50% of survivors are normal in all respects (Sell, 1987).

Prevention

Concerns have been expressed that the 90% effectiveness of the *Haemophilus* b polysaccharide vaccine will prove disappointing and may undermine public confidence in other more effective vaccines (see also pp. 18, Section 1). On balance, the vaccine is expected to prevent more than 2500 cases of meningitis each year in the United States, but surely some immunized children will develop the disease.

CASE ILLUSTRATION

The fulminant nature of *H. influenzae* infection in a 3-year-old is illustrated by the following case. This previously well child suddenly became drowsy and was found to have a temperature of 40°C. There were no specific complaints, but the fever persisted and then over the next several hours there was a rapid progression of respiratory difficulty. Excessive salivation was noted and the youngster rejected all fluids.

On presentation about 6 hours after fever was first noted, the child was markedly distressed with labored respirations. She held her head in a slightly forward position but was not drooling at the time of initial examination. Other aspects of the physical examination were within normal limits.

She was taken immediately to the operating room where under direct laryngoscopy moderate swelling and erythema of the epiglottis was noted and she was intubated with a no. 4 catheter. Blood cultures were drawn and she was started immediately on ampicillin and chloramphenicol in doses of 200 mg/kg/day and 75 mg/kg/day, respectively. Her white blood count was 29,900 with 68 polys, 18 bands, and 8 lymphs. *H. influenzae* latex fixation was positive on both blood and urine samples.

Over the subsequent hours it was apparent that she was not appropriately responsive. She made withdrawal responses to painful stimuli but did not respond to verbal commands. She gradually became more obtunded and was hypoventilating with a pH of 7.14, P_{CO_2} of 66 and a P_{O_2} of 70, with bicarbonate 22. About 12 hours after the onset of the illness it was evident that she had a dilated right pupil that did not react to light and deviated to the right. She was hyporeflexic and had a Babinski bilaterally. A CT scan of the brain revealed diffuse brain stem and thalamic edema. Vigorous efforts to lower intracranial pressure by mannitol and hyperventilation to produce hypocarbia were carried out, but no improvement was noted. Despite mechanical ventilation and measures to maintain blood pressure and reduce intracranial pressure, she died within 24 hours of the onset of symptoms, and after more than 15 hours of intravenous ampicillin and chloramphenicol.

Subsequently *H. influenzae* were cultured from her blood and spinal fluid, which clearly explains the major and catastrophic neurologic collapse. It is unusual for meningitis to be present in a child with epiglottitis.

QUESTIONS AND COMMENTS

Who should receive the vaccine?

A major recent advance has been the availability of a polysaccharide vaccine for prevention of *H. influenzae* type B disease (*MMWR*, April 19, 1985). The new vaccine was developed by Smith and colleagues who demonstrated its effectiveness in children over 2 years of age (1973). Some improved responses have been observed in infants 18 months of age, but in general, those 18–23 months do not respond as reliably as those 2 years or older. Thus, this vaccine, while very welcome, does not provide protection from *H. influenzae* infection in infancy where attack rates are highest. Only 35–40% of disease occurs among children 18 months or older, and only 25% occurs in children over 2 years of age (Peltola et al, 1984).

In 1988, an improved conjugate vaccine is available and recommended for all infants at 18 months of age (see pp. 18).

Is prophylaxis of close family, friend, or professional contacts warranted?

In general, we advise prophylaxis against *H. influenzae* Type B with rifampin, for children 20 mg/kg/once daily for 4 days and for adults, 600 mg/kg/single dose for 4 days. Rifampin prophylaxis is not recommended for households in which all contacts are 48 months old or older.

The risk of invasive disease acquired from contacts in day care centers is considered too small to justify rifampin prophylaxis for all contacts. Individual discretion in use of prophylaxis is in order (Osterholm et al, 1987).

Vaccine failures are possibly related to genetic factors since the Gm immunoglobulin phenotype is associated with an increased risk of vaccine failure (Granoff et al, 1986).

Moxon (1986), in presenting the reasons why most European countries are not recommending routine immunization at age 2 years with the vaccine, cites expense and failure to achieve high immunization rates with other more effective vaccines. (He noted that in the United Kingdom only 60% of preschool children have been immunized against measles.) He also noted the "virtual certainty" that an improved conjugated *H. influenzae* type B vaccine will be available within a few years. In 1988, the improved conjugated vaccine was licensed and recommended for all children at 18 months of age (CDC, 1988; Claesson et al, 1988).

KLEBSIELLA

Definition

Klebsiella is a widely distributed potential pathogen which is found in 5% of normal individuals, but is capable of producing septicemia, pneumonia, and meningitis in newborn infants and others with impaired host defenses. It is a common cause of urinary tract infection.

Basic Science

This Gram-negative intestinal bacterium exists in at least 70 serotypes, but types 1 and 2 are most commonly pathogenic. *Klebsiella,* like *Enterobacter* and *Pseudonomas* are common causes of nosocomial infection. They can persist for long periods on moist surfaces, such as incubators, and are pathogens when the inoculum is large and host defenses are suppressed.

Natural History

Spread of the organism is usually by hand after contact with surfaces contaminated by infected stools, or by aerosol in respiratory therapy equipment. The illness most commonly manifests as pneumonia and onset may be insidious. In severe infections, pneumatoceles and abscess formation occur. Before antibiotics became available, the mortality was 80%.

Diagnosis

The organism can be isolated from purulent tracheal exudate, blood and lung aspirates, and stool.

Treatment

The organism may respond to an aminoglycoside or cephalosporins pending sensitivities.

LEGIONELLA (LEGIONNAIRE DISEASE)

Definition

Legionella pneumophila was identified as a pathogen only when it was responsible for an acute febrile respiratory illness that afflicted members of the American Legion at a convention in a Philadelphia hotel in 1976. Hence, the name of the organism. In retrospect, outbreaks of respiratory illness in Washington, DC in 1965, and Pontiac, Michigan in 1968 were attributed to the same organism by analysis of stored serum and tissue samples from exposed guinea pigs. Subsequently other species of *Legionella* have been incriminated in outbreaks of nosocomial infection, principally among individuals who are immunosuppressed.

Legionella pneumophila has 39 serogroups, 14 of which have been implicated in infections in humans.

Basic Science

The organism is a Gram-negative bacillus, whose spread is airborne. It has been recovered from environmental water sources, including ultrasonic nebulizers and shower heads; air conditioners have been shown to serve as sources of the organism. The organism survives for many months in tap water at room temperature. It grows best on agar at 35°C. The pulmonary infiltrate of macrophages and polymorphonuclear cells surrounds respiratory bronchioles, but not the major bronchi. Bacteremia has been demonstrated in some cases.

Epidemiology

Legionnaire disease tends to appear in clusters often associated with specific buildings, such as hospitals or hotels. Since legionellosis is probably underdiagnosed in sporadic cases, the 833 cases reported in the United States in 1986 is an underestimate of prevalence.

Natural History

The usual incubation period is from 2–10 days with outbreaks occurring most often in summer or fall. Although the disease tends to afflict middle-aged patients with chronic underlying diseases, such as diabetes or immunosuppression, it can occur at any age. For unknown reasons, renal transplant recipients seem to be at particular risks.

One form of *Legionella* infection (Legionnaire disease) is characterized by high fever with a relative bradycardia. The temperature tends to be sustained at levels over 39°C. Pneumonia is fulminant with rales and consolidation. Cough is almost universally present, but there is minimal sputum. Diarrhea often begins early in the illness and may be watery, but without blood or mucus. Headache, confusion, nausea, myalgia, generalized malaise, and pleuritic pain are characteristic.

The chest radiograph shows patchy, alveolar infiltrates, but is nonspecific (Evans et al, 1981). Leukocytosis and elevated sedimentation rates are the rule, although leukopenia may develop and carry with it a poor prognosis. Disseminated intravascular coagulation has been seen in some of the fatal cases. Proteinuria is common and hematuria and renal failure have been described.

Legionella infections have been the cause of endocarditis in some patients with prosthetic valves. All patients had a long history of postoperative fatigue, night sweats, and weight loss (Tompkins et al, 1988).

A second form of the disease known as Pontiac fever begins 1–2 days after inhalation of *L. pneumophila*. It is characterized by high fever, headache, and extreme prostration for 2–7 days, but notably does not involve the lungs. In all reported cases, the patients survived.

Diagnosis

Diagnosis depends on the recovery of the organism or a direct fluorescent antibody test, preferably on transtracheal or other uncontaminated specimens. Alternatively, the diagnosis can be made by demonstrating an appropriate increase in antibody titers. A fourfold increase to 1:128 or greater is considered diagnostic, and a single high titer is suggestive. Sera should be obtained early in the illness and 3–6 weeks after symptoms subside to establish a diagnostic change.

Treatment

The standard treatment is with oral erythromycin 40 mg/kg/24 hours in four divided doses which often gives a prompt clinical response. Therapy is advised for at least 3 weeks, or until symptoms have disappeared. When oral medication cannot be tolerated, intravenous erythromycin is available.

Prognosis

The mortality rate depends on the underlying condition of the patient. In immunosuppressed patients in whom the diagnosis is made retrospectively, the mortality may be as high as 80%. Some individuals fail to respond to antibiotic therapy and proceed to develop bronchiolitis obliterans. If there is a deterioration in lung function after an initial improvement, it is appropriate to consider this complication and treat with high doses of glucocorticoids orally.

LISTERIOSIS

Definition

Listeria monocytogenes, is a widely distributed organism capable of mild or fatal infections in fetus, newborn, and immunocompromised individuals.

Basic Science

This Gram-positive motile rod was first associated with infection in 1917, and characterized in 1927. Not until 1940 did it acquire the name *L. monocytogenes.* Its virulence may depend on the fact that it is an intracellular parasite and, thus, avoids bactericidal activity by phagocytes. It can withstand pasteurization of milk.

Infected infants fail to have a specific antibody response or a cell-mediated immune response to *L. monocytogenes.* Infected mothers have a significantly greater lymphoblastogenic proliferative response than do control mothers. The microagglutination titer and opsonizing activity of infected mothers was also elevated (Issekutz et al, 1984).

The nature of the natural immunity of term infants and older individuals has not been defined. The reasons for susceptibility to infection in pregnancy likewise are unknown, but are clearly of great importance.

Epidemiology and Natural History

Among newborn infants, *L. monocytogenes* is among the bacteria known to cause an uncommon disease, neonatal meningitis (group B streptococci, enterococci, and *E. coli* K1 are the most common organisms in The Children's Hospital, Boston). Pregnant women may have a flu-like episode preceding abortion which is the result of *Listeria* infection.

L. monocytogenes is a common animal infection, with outbreaks identified among rabbits, cattle, chickens, goats, and others. In humans, the disease may be sporadic or epidemic. In a major epidemic in the Canadian Maritime provinces, the route of infection was consumption of raw cabbage grown in soil contaminated by manure from a flock of infected sheep (Schlech, 1984). In a Massachusetts epidemic, pasteurized milk from infected cows was the vehicle of infection (Fleming et al, 1985).

Diagnosis

Early onset disease is acquired by the infant either from transplacental or ascending infection. Chorioamnionitis can be found in association with abortion or preterm birth. The onset and course are similar to group B streptococcal disease. The infant may appear well at delivery, but within hours may be in a septic shock. The overall mortality is about 30%.

Late onset disease usually occurs at about 1 week of age (but may occur as late as the fourth or fifth week) and presents as meningitis. The spinal fluid contains multiple cells including large numbers of polys and monos, and glucose is depressed. The organism is almost always type IV B. The mortality is about 10%.

The diagnosis depends on culture of the organism since no satisfactory serological test is available. IgM is not elevated in infected infants.

Treatment

Ampicillin or penicillin and an aminoglycoside are effective. The optimal regimen is unknown, but usually penicillin and gentamicin for 1 week followed by penicillin for 1–2 weeks are effective. The organism is not sensitive to cephalosporins.

Prevention

Prompt treatment of maternal listeriosis seems appropriate, although its effectiveness is unknown.

Infants may be colonized and asymptomatic. It is not known whether treatment will prevent late onset disease. Isolation is important; treatment is optional, but is probably worthwhile.

Delivery by cesarean section will not prevent the disease.

Prognosis

The harmful effects of infection are greatest among preterm infants. Survivors of early onset disease do well. Meningitis may have more complications such as hydrocephalus or neurological developmental delay (Evans et al, 1984).

MENINGOCOCCUS

Definition

Neisseria meningitidis is a Gram-negative nonmotile encapsulated coccus whose only reservoir is humans. It is a common cause of meningitis and septicemia.

Basic Science

N. meningitidis has been shown by DNA hybridization to be closely related to *N. gonorrhoeae,* but causes a very different kind of disease. *N. meningitidis* may be encapsulated or fimbriated, and has pili in about 80% of isolates. The relationship of fimbria or pili to virulence is unclear. Isolates are grouped on the basis of capsular polysaccharides or cell wall-associated protein antigens. Protein antigen identification is useful in tracking epidemics. Unlike *N. gonorrhoeae*, antibiotic susceptibility has been constant in recent years.

Epidemiology

N. meningitidis is the most common cause of meningitis and septicemia in children beyond 2–3 years of age, although it can occur in infants (Clegg et al, 1980). Outbreaks occur in crowded conditions, wartime and in institutions, with epidemics occurring mostly in winter in 7- to 10-year intervals in the United States. In nonepidemic years the nasopharyngeal carrier rate is 5–15%. About 75% of organisms isolated in the United States are group B or C meningococci, although outbreaks with group A have been reported.

Natural History

Invasive disease is thought to occur within days of acquiring a new strain of *N. meningitidis* before the 7- to 10-day interval required for appearance of specific serologic responses. The importance of host factors is illustrated by recurrent infections in individuals with congenital deficiency of terminal components of complement C5-C9.

Once the organism is in the blood, it can replicate very rapidly and produce an illness that can be lethal within a few hours after the first symptoms, usually headache and fever. Approximately 15% of children with meningococcal disease develop "fulminant meningococcemia." Alternatively, the infection can be transient and benign.

The organism shows marked preference for the meninges, but also attacks synovial membranes and adrenal glands. Endotoxin (lipopolysaccharide) is thought to be involved in the fulminant form. Extensive endothelial damage occurs, so that petechiae rapidly merge into ecchymoses, and sometimes purpura fulminans and gangrene. Adrenal involvement is common, and, when associated with profound shock, is called Waterhouse-Friderichsen syndrome. Serum cortisol levels are often elevated during the illness.

Symptoms include a macular rash which may become papular or petechial. Headache, stiff neck, confusion, and coma can ensue very quickly. Disseminated intravascular coagulation with a consumptive coagulopathy aggravates the condition and heralds death. Meningitis may be the only manifestation of the disease; similarly, suppurative complications such as pericarditis, eye infections, and arthritis can occur without meningitis.

Diagnosis

The clinical syndrome is often so characteristic that penicillin should be given immediately, after which blood cultures (on chocolate agar), Gram stains of petechial aspirates, lumbar puncture, and blood counts, can be obtained. Other laboratory data are of little value.

Treatment

Once meningococcemia is suspected, prompt initiation of intravenous penicillin is the ideal treatment. If that is not feasible, a stat intramuscular injection should be given pending availability of an intravenous line. A dose of 300,000 unit/kg/day is recommended. If the individual is allergic to penicillin, chloramphenicol or third generation cephalosporins are effective.

N. meningitidis may persist in the upper respiratory tract after treatment for meningitis (Abramson et al, 1985). Consequently, treatment with rifampin at the time of discharge has been recommended.

Prevention

Chemoprophylaxis is recommended for family members and personnel in close contact with a child subsequently found to have meningococcemia. The risk of illness is about 0.5%. If the child has been in day care, or in close proximity with playmates, they are also candidates for prophylaxis. Rifampin, 10 mg/kg/dose for four doses (twice daily) is recommended for children, and 600 mg twice daily for four doses in adults. It should not be given to pregnant women in the first trimester.

CASE ILLUSTRATION

A 2-week-old female presented to the emergency room with a 2-day history of fever, diarrhea, and poor oral intake. Her perinatal course was entirely unremarkable. Her initial physical examination was notable for a temperature of 103°F rectally, blood pressure of 80 systolic, irritability, and a few petechial lesions scattered throughout her trunk. Initial laboratory values were notable for a white count of 6.7, with 34% polys and 10 bands, and a sedimentation rate of 10, cerebrospinal fluid (CSF) contained 172,600 white cells (50% polys), and 6550 red cells. CSF protein was 165, CSF glucose 45, with a peripheral serum glucose of 69 and a Gram stain positive for Gram-negative intracellular diplococci. CSF and blood cultures subsequently grew out meningococcus group B. The patient initially responded to penicillin, her only complication of disease being a coagulopathy, which was easily corrected. The family received rifampin prophylaxis before carrier status could be obtained and, hence, etiology for the exposure could not be ascertained.

QUESTION AND COMMENT

What is the etiology of meningococcal disease in the neonate?

Previous case reports have documented meningococcal disease in the neonate (in less than 1% of meningitis cases) with exposure thought to be secondary to respiratory and/or maternal genitourinary colonization. Absence of bacterial antibodies to *N. meningitidis* appears to correlate well with the onset of disease.

CASE ILLUSTRATION

A 5-month-old black male presented with 1 day of fever and irritability. His perinatal history was essentially noncontributory, and except for an upper respiratory infection and otitis 1 month before his current illness, he was in good health. In the emergency room he was found to have a temperature of 40.3°C rectally, and otitis media in the right ear. Blood count was 10,400 mm^3 with 59% polys and 7 bands, and CSF findings revealed 1 red cell, 8 white cells, with 76% polys, 15 lymphs, 12% monos, a protein of less than 10, and a glucose of 72. Cultures of blood, urine, and cerebrospinal fluid were obtained and the patient was sent home on amoxicillin. Over the next 2 days the patient's temperature returned to normal and except for diminished appetite he was apparently his usual active self. A blood culture at 48 hours was positive for *N. meningococcus*, and the patient was called back in for re-evaluation. Repeat examination at that time revealed an afebrile, playful, well-hydrated infant with a retracted, slightly mobile right tympanic membrane. Repeat blood count was notable for a white count of 9600 mm^3, 24% polys, 63% lymphs, 19% monos, and a repeat lumbar puncture was notable for 2200 red cells and 20 white cells, with 45% polys, 47% lymphs.

QUESTIONS AND COMMENTS

How should this child be subsequently evaluated and treated for his meningococcal disease?

Since a partially treated meningitis could not be ruled out, the patient was admitted for a parenteral antibiotic therapy of presumptive meningococcal meningitis and bacteremia. We mention this case because of the mild way that meningococcal disease presented and to cite the possible benefit that oral antibiotic therapy provided. A review of the fever and bacteremia literature suggests a 5% incidence of meningococcus accounts for all bacteremias in children between 2 and 24 months, with approximately half of these cases being unsuspected. All patients had fever greater than 38.8°C, but none had a rash or signs of shock. White blood count usually ranged between 5000 and 15,000 mm^3 instead of the usual leukocytosis previously reported for pneumococcal or *H. influenzae* bacteremia. Initial lumbar punctures were normal. At initial presentation, those children diagnosed as having an otitis or pneumonia received oral antibiotics for home use and anecdotally these children did well in handling their meningococcal infection, although almost all subsequently received parenteral penicillin when the blood culture turned positive. Two patients in whom oral antibiotics were not given initially died despite subsequent therapy after a positive blood culture was reported.

Since oral levels of penicillin can exceed the minimal inhibitory concentration needed for treatment for meningococcus, it seems reasonable to believe that an oral antibiotic can be useful as an initial treatment for this often unsuspected bacteremia. However, there has been no evidence other than a few case reports that show that a full course of oral therapy is as good as parenteral antibiotics for the treatment of bacteremia (in regard to outcome and sequelae) and no report shows oral therapy is beneficial in the treatment of meningococcal meningitis. Moreover, there are cases of meningitis that have been reported, despite initial usage of oral amoxicillin in unsuspected meningococcal disease.

In retrospect, this child with a temperature over 40°C and with blood cells in his spinal fluid should have been admitted for parenteral antibiotics when first seen.

Should all children under 2 years of age with fever and no obvious focus or leukocytosis receive oral antibiotics to avoid the risk of meningococcal disease?

Unfortunately, the data currently available do not yet permit such a conclusion. Nor is it even clear that antibiotics used at first encounter will avert a fatal outcome if a patient has more fulminant meningococcal disease. Of note, this patient was placed on intravenous penicillin for 10 days and subsequently did well.

Purified polysaccharide vaccines are available for serogroups A/C/Y/W-135. High risk individuals, such as military recruits, deserve immunization. Routine immunization is not recommended. The safety of the vaccine in pregnant women has not been established. γ-Globulin is ineffective.

Mycobacterium Tuberculosis

Worldwide, tuberculosis remains a leading cause of death and disability. In North America improved living standards, surveillance programs, and effective chemotherapy have resulted in a greatly reduced incidence of the disease, and the closing of sanitoria for its treatment. Nonetheless, the disease persists, and physicians should be alert to its manifestations and current approaches to therapy.[1]

Definition

Tuberculosis is caused by infection with *Mycobacterium tuberculosis*. Bovine tuberculosis is now unknown in the United States, but continues to be a problem in developing countries. Mycobacterium avian intracellulare is an opportunistic infection whose importance as a pathogen has come into focus in immunodeficient individuals.

[1]For a fascinating discussion of tuberculosis in history, the reader is referred to Dubos R, Dubos J: *The White Plague Tuberculosis, Man and Society*; Boston, Little, Brown, and Co., 1952.

Basic Science

The tubercle bacillus is rod-shaped, 1–4 μ long and 0.3–0.6 μ in diameter. The bacilli are difficult to stain (acid fast) but can be made to fluoresce after staining with auramine or rhodamine. The bacilli grow slowly and are obligate aerobes which also require CO_2. Their oxygen and carbon dioxide requirements are best met by alveolar gases in the relatively underperfused apices of upright adults (This observation is thought to explain the apical localization of adult tuberculosis, and the random localization of the primary complex in children in whom hydrostatic effects on the pulmonary circulation are less evident when the child is upright.)

The pathogenesis of primary pulmonary tuberculosis in children is the result of inhalation and deposition of organisms in the peripheral lung. Histiocytes carry some of the organisms via lymphatics to the regional lymph nodes which subsequently become enlarged. The peripheral lesion, which is often invisible until it calcifies, and the enlarged mediastinal nodes constitute the Ghon tubercle (in the periphery) and the primary complex (tubercle plus nodes).

Hypersensitivity to tuberculin requires 3–8 weeks from initial infection. Invasion of the infected area by lymphocytes, and nodal enlargement induce transformation of mononuclear cells to epithelial cells which cluster to form tubercles. The primary forms may dissolve, or become necrotic or caseous. If the area of caseation is extensive, it may rupture into a bronchus, be aspirated and induce tuberculous pneumonia. Alternatively, granulomas may appear in the bronchial lumen (endobronchial tuberculosis).

If many bacilli are inhaled, and/or host defenses are impaired, bacillemia follows. Hematogenous tuberculosis can deposit organisms in many different sites producing miliary lesions usually 3–6 months after the primary infection.

Tubercle bacilli synthesize proteins that can produce a delayed-type hypersensitivity response. Some of the manifestations of the disease, such as pleural effusions, are a response to a peripheral lesion which sensitizes the pleura, much as an intradermal injection of the proteins induces a positive tuberculin test (see below).

The relationship between this allergic response and immunity has been the subject of intense study, since Arnold Rich first discussed the issues in his classic text, *Pathogenesis of Tuberculosis*. Probably immunity depends on other factors thought to be mediated by phagocytes and mononuclear cells. Immunity is not complete, however, inasmuch as reactivation and reinfection are well known.

Newborn infants have some immunity conferred by transplacental transfer. Keller et al (1987) reported immunity in infants of tuberculin-positive mothers at 4–6 weeks of age, but found less at 3 months. They did not find evidence of transfer by human milk.

Epidemiology

Tuberculosis is most common in urban slums where crowding enhances the likelihood of infection. Epidemics have been found in shelters for the homeless. Malnutrition depresses host defenses and further increases risk of infection. In the United States, control programs lessen the number of active cases, but the continued flow of illegal immigrants perpetuates the risk in areas where they settle. In 1986, 22,768 cases of tuberculosis (all ages) were reported in the United States, for a rate of about 1/1000 population. About 1200 cases were in children under 15 years. Worldwide, an estimated 8 million cases appear each year.

Almost all cases of tuberculosis are acquired from close contact. Congenital tuberculosis can occur, with widespread involvement of liver, spleen, and peritoneal surfaces from bacillemia via the umbilical vein. Prompt diagnosis and treatment are compatible with recovery; delayed diagnosis can be disastrous (Nemir and O'Hare, 1985).

Natural History

The disease is spread mostly by aerosolized droplets from an infected individual who is coughing. Repeated contact increases the likelihood of infection, so that children are most likely to acquire the disease from a parent or other adult in the household, a teacher, or school bus driver. Congenital tuberculosis is very uncommon, but can be acquired when the placenta is seeded during maternal bacteremia.

Bovine tuberculosis is acquired by ingestion of raw milk from infected cows, and is most likely to present as cervical adenitis or intestinal tuberculosis.

The severity of infection is related to the size of the inoculum, the virulence of the organism, and hypersensitivity to it. Protection depends on host resistance that can be native or acquired. It seems probable that certain racial groups are at greater risk, namely blacks, American Indians, and Inuit, whereas other groups, such as Jews, are less susceptible. Age is a factor, not only with respect to susceptibility, but also by its influence on the natural history and manifestations of disease. Disseminated disease occurs more often in the first 2 years of life and again at puberty. Women of menstrual age are at greater risk than men of similar age. Older men have more serious disease than older women, which may be cultural rather than biologic.

The severity of tuberculosis is enhanced by underlying disease, such as after measles when T-cell function is depressed, in diabetes, lymphoma, or other malignancies. When host defenses are suppressed by cortisol chemotherapeutic agents, tuberculosis that has been asymptomatic and latent for years, may become manifest.

The initial contact is often difficult to pinpoint, except in the instances of newborn infants exposed to infected medical personnel during brief stays in a hospital nursery (Light et al, 1974).

Presenting findings may be low-grade fever, anorexia, or cough. Children may never cough unless endobronchial disease or irritation is present, and they rarely produce sputum. Tubercle bacilli may be found in swallowed pulmonary mucus and can be recovered by gastric aspiration done first thing in the morning, before breakfast. Most cases of childhood tuberculous infection are not diagnosed on the basis of symptoms, but more commonly by routine tuberculin tests, or testing done because of exposure.

Discussion of the systemic manifestation of tuberculosis will be found under the relevant organ systems.

Diagnosis

The tuberculin test is the principal screening and diagnostic tool. Two antigens are available: purified protein derivative (PPD) and old tuberculin (OT). PPD is dispensed in a vial that should be kept refrigerated. OT can be kept refrigerated for up to a month), but it varies in potency and gives more nonspecific reactions. It may be deposited on tines and is available in a disposable unit. The four prongs can be pushed through skin quickly and relatively painlessly. One or more 2-mm papules is doubtful-positive, and confluence of the four papules is positive. With PPD or OT used with multiple puncture devices, a high false-positive rate (about 20%) limits their usefulness.

PPD is administered with syringe and 25-gauge needle. Exactly 0.1 ml of intermediate strength (5 tuberculin units) is injected into the volar surface of the forearm. A wheal should follow the injection. The test is read 24–72 hours later. Induration of less than 5 mm is negative; 5–9 mm is doubtful; and 10 mm or greater is positive. This test, called a Mantoux, may produce a severe local reaction in some individuals. If ocular tuberculosis is suspected, or there is reason to expect a strongly positive test, it may be wise to omit the test and search for the organism. Dilute solutions of OT may be preferable. If a local reaction is severe, application of hydrocortisone ointment is helpful.

Interpretation of the multiple puncture or intradermal (Mantoux) tests must be made with attention to the many factors that can affect the tests. There is no gold standard, or totally dependable test. The Mantoux (5Tu PPD) comes closest, and is the test with which others are compared. It is the preferred test even for mass screening. However, if the goal of screening is to identify every infected person, a 1- to 2-mm induration for the multiple puncture (TINE host) with PPD provides a very sensitive, but not very specific test. If the tests are being used to determine who needs chemoprophylaxis, a high degree of specificity is desired and the Mantoux is preferred.

Since false-negative tests may occur in overwhelming disease, possibly in malnutrition, or for up to 9 months after measles or some other viral illnesses (Kipps, 1966) or immunizations, it may be necessary to test for anergy with another antigen such as *Candida* or tetanus on the opposite arm. Almost all persons have had contact with *Candida* (after the first few months of life) and will give a positive response if T-cell mediated delayed hypersensitivity is intact.

Previous immunization with BCG is not a contraindication to tuberculin testing since the 5 TU of PPD rarely produces induration over 9 mm in immunized individuals, nor does previous infection with atypical mycobacteria that can cross-react with tuberculosis.

Definitive diagnosis depends on culture of the bacilli. Sputum, or swallowed organisms obtained from early morning gastric aspirates may be seen on smear for rapid presumptive diagnosis, or grown on suitable media for positive identification. Unfortunately, growth is slow so results may not be evident for 3–6 weeks. Biopsy specimens should be cultured and examined for characteristic histology of granulomas, necrosis, and giant cells.

An enzyme-linked immunosorbent assay (ELISA) for serodiagnosis has been evaluated in field studies and compared with sputum examinations. The ELISA has a sensitivity of 69% specific. In combination, the results were a highly satisfactory 92% sensitive and 88% specific (Daniel et al, 1986).

Treatment

Current concepts of the treatment of tuberculosis have evolved as a result of clinical trials to establish efficacy and toxicity of a number of drugs. It has been suggested that distinct populations of organisms exist in human infection, and their susceptibilities to antituberculosis drugs differ. Group 1 organisms are rapidly growing and metabolically active. They respond to bactericidal doses of isoniazid, rifampin, and streptomycin. Group 2 organisms have spurts of activity and respond best to rifampin. Group 3 organisms are within macrophages and respond best to pyrazinamide. Group 4 organisms are dormant, relatively unresponsive and require prolonged therapy.

Since clinical trials are often not applicable to all populations, it has been difficult to provide definitive recommendations based on sound scientific data. For that reason, consensus achieved by experienced individuals comes closest to providing guidelines for the physician, who must individualize treatment on the basis of drug sensitivities and patients' responses.

A "consensus conference" report, published in 1986, provides the basis for current recommendations (Table 17.7).

The daily dosage of antituberculosis drugs in children are shown in Table 17.8.

Other Issues Related to Therapy

If the diagnosis of tuberculosis as a cause of illness is made while a child is in the hospital, the question of isolation and duration of hospitalization arises. If the patient is coughing, isolation is necessary until che-

Table 17.7
Treatment of Tuberculosis[1]

1. A 6-month regimen consisting of isoniazid, rifampin, and pyrazinamide given for 2 months followed by isoniazid and rifampin for 4 months is effective treatment in patients with fully susceptible organisms who comply with the treatment regimen. It may be advisable to include ethambutol in the initial phase when isoniazid resistance is suspected.
2. A 9-month regimen consisting of isoniazid and rifampin is also highly successful. The need for an additional drug in the initial phase is not certain unless isoniazid resistance is suspected, in which case ethambutol should be included until susceptibility tests have been reported.
3. In the presence of documented resistance to isoniazid, rifampin and ethambutol, perhaps supplemented initially by pyrazinamide, should be given for a minimum of 12 months.
4. Children should be treated in essentially the same ways as adults using appropriately adjusted doses of the drugs. However, consideration must be given to the important differences in the approach to management in children.
5. Extrapulmonary tuberculosis should be managed according to the principles and with the drug regimens outlined for pulmonary tuberculosis.
6. The major determinant of the outcome of treatment is patient compliance. Careful attention should be paid to measures designed to foster compliance and to ensure that patients take the drugs as prescribed.

Treatment of tuberculous infection:

1. Preventive therapy with isoniazid given for 6–12 months is effective in decreasing the risk of future tuberculosis.
2. Persons for whom preventive therapy is indicated include: household members and other close contacts of potentially infectious persons; newly infected persons; persons with past tuberculosis or with a significant tuberculin reaction and abnormal chest films in whom current tuberculosis has been excluded; infected persons in special clinical situations such as silicosis, diabetes mellitus, adrenocorticosteroid therapy, immunosuppressive therapy or diseases, AIDS or positive tests for antibodies to AIDS virus, hematologic and reticuloendothelial malignancies, end-stage renal disease, and clinical conditions associated with rapid weight loss or chronic undernutrition; tuberculin skin test reactors younger than 35 years of age.
3. In persons younger than 35 years of age, routine monitoring for adverse effects of isoniazid should consist of a monthly symptom review. For persons 35 years and older, in addition to monthly symptom reviews, hepatic enzymes should be measured prior to starting isoniazid and periodically throughout treatment.
4. Persons at high risk of developing severe forms of tuberculosis, if infected due to contact with a patient having isoniazid-resistant organisms, should be treated with rifampin rather than isoniazid. Lower-risk contacts can be treated with isoniazid and observed carefully.
5. As with treatment of tuberculosis, the key to success of preventive therapy is patient compliance.

[1]Reproduced with permission from *Am Rev Respir Dis* 134:355, 1986.

motherapy is well established (perhaps 3–4 weeks) and gastric aspirates are negative. Otherwise, isolation is not required.

The length of hospitalization should depend on the severity of illness, and not be dictated by the identification of organisms. That is, children with tuberculous meningitis require care for the meningitis, whether or not it is tuberculous. Sometimes an adverse social situation will make hospitalization necessary to ensure delivery of medication.

Most children with positive tuberculin tests and a primary complex can be treated as outpatients. If they are asymptomatic, they can attend school and participate in normal activity. Bed rest is not needed. Close follow-up and home visits are essential to ensure that the primary source is identified and under treatment, and that prescribed drugs are being taken and tolerated.

CONTROVERSY

Controversy continues to exist about the duration of chemotherapy, largely because there are few long-term studies with currently used drugs. In one evaluation of short-course treatment for children, Abernathy et al (1983) concluded that their regimen of 10–20 mg/kg rifampin and 20–40 mg/kg isoniazid twice a week for 8 months was safe, effective, inexpensive, and facilitated compliance.

Prevention

Contacts of newly discovered cases who have a tuberculin reaction of 5-mm induration or greater are at risk of tuberculosis and should receive chemoprophylaxis. Some controversy exists about chemotherapy for tuberculin-negative contacts who may have been infected but not yet converted their skin tests. Preventive therapy is recommended for 3 months, when a repeat tuberculin test is given. If positive, with a negative chest radiograph, therapy should be continued for a total of 12 months. If the reaction is negative and exposure has ended, therapy may be discontinued.

Isoniazid is the only drug widely studied as preventive therapy. Side effects include hepatitis, which is extremely rare in individuals under 20 years of age, and peripheral neuropathy, mood changes, and hypersensitive reactions, which are also very rare. Toxicity is reduced if the drug is taken at bedtime in a dose of 10 mg/kg/day (maximum, 300 mg).

If the contact is with an organism completely resistant to isoniazid, rifampin is recommended. If the organism is only partially resistant, isoniazid and rifampin are recommended.

BCG

BCG is the generic term for a number of live attenuated vaccines derived from *M. bovis*. The name stands for bacillus of Calmette and Guerin, who developed the original strain. Much controversy has surrounded recommendations for use of BCG, in part because studies have been conducted on different pop-

Table 17.8
Daily Dosage of Antituberculosis Drugs in Children[1]

Child's Weight		Isoniazid (tablets, 100 and 300 mg) Dosage: 10–20 mg/kg/day		Rifampin (capsules, 150 and 300 mg) Dosage: 10–20 mg/kg/day		Pyrazinamide (tablets, 250 mg) Dosage: 15–30 mg/kg/day		Ethambutol (tablets, 100 and 400 mg) Dosage: 15–25 mg/kg/day		Ethionamide (tablets, 250 mg) Dosage: 15–20 mg/kg/day		Streptomycin (vials, 1 and 4 mg) Dosage: 20–40 mg/kg/day[2]	
lbs	kg	mg	mg/kg	mg	mg/kg	mg	mg/kg	mg	mg/kg	mg	mg/kg	mg	mg/kg
15–21	6–9.5	100	17–10	150	25–16	125	20–13	100	17–10	125	20–13	120–200	20–25
22–29	10–13	150	15–11	150	15–11	250	25–19	150	15–11	250	25–19	200–250	20–19
30–40	14–18	200	14–11	300	21–16	375	26–21	200	14–11	250	18–14	300–350	21–19
41–51	19–23	250	13–11	300	15–13	500	26–21	250	13–11	500	26–21	400–450	21–19
52–62	23.5–28	300	12–11	300	13–10	500	21–18	300	12–11	500	21–18	450–600	19–21
63–78	28.5–35	350	12–10	450	14–13	750	26–21	350	12–10	750	26–21	600–700	21–20
79–89	35.5–40	400	11–10	450	13–11	1,000	28–25	400	11–10	750	21–19	700–800	20
90–100	40.5–45	450	10	600	15–13	1,250	30–28	450	10	1,000	24–22	800–900	19–20
100+	46+	500	11	600	13	1,250	27	500	10	1,000	22	1,000	20

[1]Modified from *Am Rev Respir Dis* 134:356, 1986.
[2]Intramuscularly.

ulations with different results, and because not all vaccines have similar potency. Efficacy has been greatest in areas of high prevalence, and has lasted up to 20 years. In areas where atypical mycobacterial infections are endemic, efficacy has not been proven, probably because atypical organisms have some of the same beneficial effect in enhancing immunity.

Freeze-dried vaccines are currently recommended for infants who are tuberculin-negative but are in a household where adults are sputum-positive, or are not complying with therapy. The dose is usually 0.05 ml for newborns and 0.1 ml for older individuals, injected intradermally. On occasion, a local abscess with axillary lymphadenopathy occurs, which resolves over a few months. No treatment is indicated. In developing countries, BCG immunization has to be dictated by prevalence rates and feasibility of administering the vaccine. In general, high prevalence is an infection rate of more than 1% per year.

BCG is contraindicated in immunosuppressed individuals.

Recommendations for BCG administration:

1. The age of immunization should be 3–9 months. If it is to be given earlier, the dose should be reduced by about half. (Earlier administration, that is, after birth, may be appropriate if follow-up at 3 months is uncertain.)
2. It is customary to use the outer side of upper left arm at insertion of deltoid.
3. The multiple puncture technique is preferred.

MYCOBACTERIA (Nontuberculous, Atypical)

Definition

Some species of atypical mycobacteria are capable of causing disease that mimics in every respect that caused by *M. tuberculosis*. For the most part, however, infections are subclinical or disease is localized, particularly in children, to the cervical lymph nodes.

Basic Science

In the United States the most frequently identified myocbacteria are *M. avium-intracellulare, M. scrofulaceum,* and *M. kansasii,* with *M. fortuitum* and *M. chelonis* being found especially in hospitalized or immunocompromised patients. These organisms are identified on the basis of their staining properties, colony appearance on specialized media, and their pigment production without being exposed to light. More than 300 strains of mycobacteria exist with diverse cell surface components. (Most laboratories depend on regional or reference laboratories, or the Centers for Disease Control, Atlanta, Georgia for identification.)

Epidemiology

The incidence of infections with atypical mycobacteria is not known. It is clear, however, that many of the organisms are endemic in the southeastern United States, and have been reported from most regions in the States. Although the organisms are widespread the incidence of clinical disease is much less than that due to *M. tuberculosis*. It does not appear that any animal serves as an important reservoir for human disease.

Natural History

The striking difference between atypical mycobacterial disease and tuberculosis is the tendency for atypical disease to be localized. The absence of many constitutional symptoms with these organisms is usual.

The incubation period is not known and the natural course of disease is variable, with spontaneous recovery usually the rule. Consequently, drug therapy alone is not indicated for atypical infection of the cervical lymph nodes.

In individuals with impaired host defenses such as those with AIDS, atypical mycobacteria can become disseminated and behave much like miliary tuberculosis. The mortality in these individuals is high (see American Thoracic Society position paper: Mycobacterioses and the acquired immunodeficiency syndrome. *Am Rev Respir Dis* 136:492, 1987).

Another route of infection is through a skin lesion, which may become the site of infection with *M. marinum,* acquired in swimming pools or fish tanks. The lesion is a chronic granuloma which is self-limited.

Diagnosis

Although skin tests to specific antigens are not always helpful, most individuals with active atypical mycobacteria infection have a modest response to intermediate PPD (less than 10 mm of induration).

The affected cervical nodes are most commonly close to the mandible, but may be at other locations. They are initially firm and painless, but may progress to caseation and spontaneous rupture. More often they remain firm for some months then regress. The differential diagnosis includes *M. tuberculosis* or *M. bovis,* cat scratch disease, or lymphoma. The only certain way to distinguish adenitis from atypical mycobacteria is by aspiration of a node, followed by smear and culture. Some physicians advocate initiating antituberculous therapy before aspiration and continuing for the 2–3 months required for identification of a positive culture. Chemotherapy alone is probably not appropriate in an otherwise healthy child. Total excision of node is favored to avoid continued suppuration and scarring.

Treatment

Localized disease may require surgical excision. Antituberculous drugs are rarely indicated. In disseminated disease, rifampin is the drug of choice, in combination with ethionamide and other drugs based on sensitivity testing. Treatment of some strains requires multiple drugs based on sensitivities. Rapidly growing organisms require entirely different drugs, such as amikacin and cefoxitin (see American Thoracic Society position paper: Mycobacterioses and the acquired immunodeficiency syndrome. *Am Rev Respir Dis* 136:492, 1987).

Mycobacterium Leprae (LEPROSY)

Definition

Infection with *Mycobacterium leprae* includes a wide variety of responses stemming from initial infection of peripheral nerves. Skin ulcerations may be present and eyes, mucosa, the respiratory tract, and muscles may be involved. The infection, which has a long incubation period, is chronic and progressive.

Basic Science

M. leprae is an acid-fast organism with an unusual epidemic pattern. It is not highly contagious but clearly can be transmitted by personal contact. The initial lesion is usually in the skin and it is possible that the organism reaches the peripheral nerves via this route.

Epidemiology

Although rare in the United States (206 cases reported during 1987), it is estimated that worldwide there are about 15 million individuals with leprosy. Most of them are in Africa, Southeast Asia, and South America. Some 4 million reside in India.

The disease can occur at any age and young children are at risk, although it is uncommon in infants. About 20% of new cases occur in children of families with no known infected individuals.

Natural History

Illness is a manifestation of the host response to the organism. Like tuberculosis it is thought that many individuals are infected but never develop symptoms. What host factors predispose to illness is not clear, but males are more commonly infected than are females.

The range of findings can be from tuberculoid lesions in the skin, characterized by hypopigmented anesthetic macules which persist for many months, to the more severe form of the disease, which is disseminated through the blood stream, and is designated lepromatous leprosy. Nervous system involvement occurs with enlargement of peripheral nerves especially the ulnar nerve, but others overlying bony prominences. Tenderness and paralysis are characteristic in the area innervated by the affected nerve. Trigeminal lesions may result in anesthesia of the cornea, with major eye complications. Tuberculoid leprosy is more common in children; lepromatous disease is rare in childhood.

Lepromatous leprosy is characterized by multiple papular skin lesions which in the early stages are not associated with decreased sensation or sweating. Later, however, peripheral nerves are destroyed and anesthesia can become extensive. As the disease progresses the skin becomes thickened and waxen to produce the characteristic "leonine" facies. The peripheral anesthesia is responsible for the recurrent trauma and eventual amputation of digits and extremities.

Diagnosis

The diagnosis should be suspected whenever there are palpable thickened peripheral nerves and/or skin lesions with localized anesthesia. Bacteriologic diagnosis can be made from biopsy of the skin lesions.

The drug of choice in treatment is dapsone (2 mg/kg/24 hours). Individuals with lepromatous leprosy may require life-long treatment, but other forms of the disease are usually cured in 3–10 years. A number of antimycobacterial drugs exist and any physician who has a patient with leprosy is well advised to consult the CDC for the most appropriate current therapy (Felice and Fraser, 1978).

General supportive care includes measures to eliminate or lessen the likelihood of trauma to insensitive extremities. Reconstructive surgery may be helpful under certain circumstances.

Prognosis

Untreated systemic leprosy is usually progressive and lethal in 10–20 years. The milder tuberculoid leprosy may be self-limiting in 1–3 years, but can lead to some deformities.

NOCARDIA

Definition

Nocardia asteroides is a Gram-positive, acid fast, aerobic bacterium that resides in soil and is distributed worldwide. It is most commonly identified as a cause of chronic pulmonary infection in immunocompromised hosts.

Epidemiology

The organism may be associated with other "opportunistic" bacteria in causing illness in immunocompromised hosts. Three-quarters of the infections are pulmonary. It is estimated that 500–1000 individuals annually have nocardiasis in the United States (Frazier et al, 1977).

Natural History

Exposure to *Nocardia* is especially likely in situations where dust is inhaled (as at major construction sites or in dust storms). Pulmonary lesions may be focal and chronic. In advanced disease, abscesses form and empyema is likely. Metastatic disease may occur in brain and kidney, but rarely bone (Curry, 1980).

Diagnosis

The organism may be recovered from skin abscesses, or from aspiration of pulmonary infiltrates. It is rarely found in the blood. No serologic tests are available.

Treatment

Sulfonamides are effective: sulfadiazine or trimethoprim-sulfamethoxazole for months or even years may be required to eradicate the organism. Optimal blood levels are 12–20 μg/dl. For severe infection, additional antibiotics may be needed.

Prognosis

The mortality in untreated disease among immunologically normal people is about 20%. Overall mortality is close to 50%.

PERTUSSIS

Definition

Pertussis is an acute disease of the respiratory tract caused by *Bordetella pertussis*.

Epidemiology

In immunized populations pertussis is rare. In the United States, 2493 cases were reported in 1983. Individuals most at risk are infants who have not had a full course of immunization inasmuch as at least three doses of DTP are believed to be necessary for protection. Moreover, in recent outbreaks, some children who had been appropriately immunized have acquired the disease.

Natural History

The incubation period is 7–14 days, before a mild upper respiratory infection ensues. This catarrhal stage may last for 1–3 weeks during which the disorder is most contagious. Later a paryoxysmal cough (followed by an inspiratory "whoop") develops, which may persist for weeks. Much viscid white mucus may be produced. Vomiting is not unusual after a paroxysm. The coughing may lead to inadequate food intake and exhaustion, especially in small infants. Cyanosis, vomiting, and apneic spells are common in young infants, who may not have the "whoop."

Intercurrent infections are common and may prolong morbidity or be lethal. Complications include secondary infection, atelectasis, and residual bronchiectasis. Apnea and sudden death have occurred after paroxysms of coughing. Convulsions may occur in association with an encephalopathy that may be of hypoxic etiology.

Diagnosis

Laboratory findings may include an absolute and relative lymphocytosis to levels of 20,000–30,000. The peripheral smear may resemble leukemia. Culture of *B. pertussis* is difficult, but possible with culture of nasopharyngeal swabs on Bordet-Gengou agar or Regan-Lowe transport media inoculated at the bedside. Fluorescent antibody tests are available, but are not always reliable. Cultures and fluorescent antibodies are negative after 4–5 weeks.

DIFFERENTIAL DIAGNOSIS

Difficulty in culture and fluorescent antibody identification of *B. pertussis* has been confirmed in many situations in which the clinical syndrome resembles pertussis, but tests for the organism are negative. In such situations, adenovirus has been recovered, but not in excess of that found in individuals with positive cultures of *B. pertussis*. Keller et al (1980) found *B. pertussis* or *B. parapertussis* in 36 of 100 patients with clinical pertussis and in 78% of patients and immediate family groups. Adenovirus was isolated from 33% of those with positive cultures, and 14% of those with negative cultures.

Treatment

Erythromycin estolate eliminates *B. pertussis* but does not shorten the course of illness. Nonetheless, we treat with 50 mg/kg/24 hours orally in four divided doses for 2 weeks. Pertussis immune globulin is of no benefit.

General supportive measures include hospitalization of infants under 1 year of age to ensure adequate hydration and oxygenation. Mist therapy is contraindicated because of further local irritation to the airways. Sedation is also contraindicated. Isolation should be enforced for 5 days after initiation of erythromycin or 3 weeks after the onset of coughing.

Prognosis

The mortality is less than 1% with good supportive care. Postpertussis bronchiectasis can occur, but it is rare.

Prevention

The currently available vaccine is recommended with the caution that it is only 60–85% effective. Moreover, side effects of fever and seizures may occur. The estimated incidence of temperature over 40°C is 1:333 and the rate of convulsion with hyporesponsiveness is 1:1750. Either of these reactions contraindicates further doses of pertussis vaccine. The risk of encephalopathy with permanent neurologic damage is between 1 in 110,000 and 1 in 310,000.

New acellular vaccines are currently being evaluated; meanwhile the risk of serious illness from immunization is less than the risk of death from pertussis (0.5%; Brunnell, 1985).

Antibiotic prophylaxis of close contacts of a pertussis patient is recommended. Erythromycin, 250 mg orally four times a day for 10–14 days, is appropriate for adults. Children require 40 mg/kg/day orally four times a day for 10–14 days. Contacts under 7 years of age who have been immunized should receive a booster.

PSEUDOMONAS

Definition

The most prevalent pathogenic species of *Pseudomonas* is *P. aeruginosa,* although *P. cepacia* has been isolated with increasing frequency in the 1980s. Individuals most at risk of infection with these ubiquitous organisms are those with cystic fibrosis (see pp. 248) and those who are immune suppressed for any reason, including congenital and acquired immunodeficiencies, malignancies, malnutrition, or immunosuppressant chemotherapy.

Basic Science

Pseudomonas aeruginosa is an aerobic motile Gram-negative rod with a single flagellum and pili. It is found in soil and water, and most environments such as sinks, incubators, and respiratory therapy equipment. The organism produces a weak endotoxin that may cause diarrhea, and several proteolytic enzymes that are thought to be responsible for the necrosis in some burns and wound infections. The organism resists phagocytosis, and once having invaded the lung, for example, is very hard to eradicate.

Pseudomonas cepacia, first recognized as a major pathogen in cystic fibrosis patients in 1984, is a distant relative of *P. aeruginosa* and is more closely related to *Alcaligenes fecalis* and *Aquaspirillum serpens.* The organism can use penicillin as a sole carbon source, and survive in some iodophors and chlorhexidine. (Preparations with ethyl alcohol are bacteriocidal.) It is resistant to most antibiotics. The organism is of low virulence, and the reasons for its pathogenicity in cystic fibrosis patients are unknown (Prince, 1986).

Epidemiology

Human infection is unusual except in the conditions noted above.

Natural History

The organism is ubiquitous and may be found in any break in the skin, especially in deep wounds and burns. It is one of the organisms associated with prolonged use of intravenous or urinary catheters. Septicemia may occur, with macular skin lesions that characteristically have central necrosis.

Almost all individuals with cystic fibrosis eventually develop chronic pulmonary disease and their sputum contains mucoid colonies of *P. aeruginosa* or *P. cepacia.* Colonization can occur in infants, and be present at the time of diagnosis, before antibiotics or respiratory therapy equipment are used, although both have been suggested as reasons for colonization.

Diagnosis

The organism is readily grown on standard laboratory media.

Treatment

Recommendations for treatment of patients with cystic fibrosis colonized with *Pseudomonas* can be found on page 252. Septicemia with *P. cepacia* should be treated with drugs to which the organism is sensitive. Sensitivity changes frequently, so recommendations in one geographical location may not be appropriate in another. Trimethoprim-sulfamethoxazole or ceftazidime are sometimes effective.

Prevention

Because the spread of infection is from contaminated equipment, including respiratory therapy equipment, standing basins of water, and humidity chambers in incubators, careful attention to proper cleaning procedures is of utmost importance.

SALMONELLA

Definition

Salmonella organisms are capable of causing gastrointestinal infections that may be mild or severe, and enteric or typhoid fever. They may also produce a carrier state that can be lifelong. *Salmonella* organisms can localize to one site during bacteremia.

Basic Science

These Gram-negative organisms have three main antigens in the envelope of the bacillus: flagella (H);

cell wall (O); and an (O)-blocking antigen (V_i). Nearly 1400 serotypes have been recognized by bacteriophage typing, and most are capable of causing diseasc in humans. *S. enteriditis* organisms are usually ingested from contaminated food or water, and may be killed by acid gastric contents. If the inoculum is large, however, they can enter the intestine and invade the mucous lining, but they do not destroy the epithelial cells. Septicemia occurs, but is usually transient in most infections.

Some serotypes enter the lymphatics and the systemic circulation and reach cells in the reticuloendothelial system, where multiplication occurs. *S. typhi,* one of the causes of typhoid fever, evokes a mononuclear response in the intestine, and commonly produces ileus rather than diarrhea.

The carrier state occurs when organisms are sequestered in the liver and biliary tract. They may be shed in large numbers into the intestine without causing disease and are excreted in the stools. The carrier site of nontyphi *Salmonella* is not clear, but possibly is in the intestine.

Some individuals are at increased risk of *Salmonella* infections. Those with achlorhydria or gastrectomy can be explained by the deficiency of gastric acids. Predisposition of children with sickle cell disease to *Salmonella* osteomyelitis may be the result of injury from old bone infarcts favoring localization of the organism, coupled with deficient opsonization in these functionally splenectomized individuals. Disorders that compromise the immune system, such as leukemia and lymphomas and other malignancies, predispose to *Salmonella* septicemia.

Epidemiology

Outbreaks of *Salmonella* infection can occur whenever contaminated food or drink is consumed, most commonly in the summer months in this country, but at any time in warmer climates. Over 44,000 cases were reported in 1983. *S. typhimurium* is the most common serotype associated with infection in man. *S. typhi* causes 300–500 cases of typhoid fever annually in the United States. The disease is rare and milder in children than in adults.

Most salmonellae are common in foodstuffs and animals but the only reservoir of *S. typhi* is human.

Natural History

TYPHOID FEVER

The incubation period for *S. typhi* is 6–14 days or longer. The disease usually presents with fever, headache, and increasing abdominal pain, and ileus, but no diarrhea. The fever tends to persist and increase with an associated bradycardia. The spleen may be enlarged, and there is generalized lymphadenopathy.

Only 10–20% of patients will have discrete papular "rose spots" at the end of the first week. They are most commonly seen over the anterior chest and abdomen.

If untreated, temperatures of 39–41°C are sustained, and a number of complications may ensue, including pneumonia, encephalopathy, and perforation of the intestine followed by a green-watery (pea soup) diarrhea. Osteomyelitis, carditis, and liver abscesses have occurred.

About 3% of patients who recover will become asymptomatic carriers, with women three times more likely to be carriers than men. Antibiotics are ineffective in treating carriers.

GASTROENTERITIS

Acute gastroenteritis from *Salmonella* species is often associated with fever and occurs from 12–48 hours after ingestion of organisms. The symptoms may be mild or severe. Stools are loose, but usually are not bloody. Occasionally overwhelming illness can result from salmonellosis. Gastroenteritis accounts for about 70% of *Salmonella* infections. Symptoms subside in 2–5 days in normal individuals.

EXTRAINTESTINAL INFECTIONS

Although uncommon, *Salmonella* pyelonephritis and cystitis can occur in typhoid fever. Pericarditis, endocarditis, pneumonia, and infections of the biliary tract are all described. Cholecystitis is the frequent intraabdominal infection. The biliary tree is a sanctuary for *Salmonella* and may be responsible for the chronic carrier state (Cohen et al, 1987). Children may have a reactive arthritis several weeks after the diarrhea subsides.

Diagnosis

TYPHOID FEVER

The diagnosis of typhoid fever may be difficult in the early stages. Blood cultures will be positive in about 80% of patients for about 2 weeks. Urine and stool cultures may be positive following septicemia. Rose spots are the classic lesions; if biopsied, bacilli may be cultured from them. Leukopenia (less than 5000) with a relative granulocytosis (average 65–95%) are characteristic in childhood (Caglar et al, 1983). Elevated serum glutamic-oxaloacetic transaminase (SGOT) and reversed albumin: globulin ratios result from damage to liver cells. Serologic tests are helpful. The Widal reaction detects increases in O and H agglutinating antibodies.

GASTROENTERITIS

Isolation of the organism from stools is usually possible. Smears of stools may show polys.

Treatment

GASTROENTERITIS

Antibiotics are not indicated in this self-limited illness, since they have been shown to prolong the time of bacterial shedding, except in infants less than 1 year old who have a high rate of bacteremia. Oral electrolyte solutions are usually adequate to maintain hydration. No antidiarrheal agents are recommended for children.

TYPHOID FEVER

This should be treated with chloramphenicol unless the patient has had marrow suppression or has a resistant strain. Trimethoprim sulfamethoxazole or intravenous ampicillin is effective in divided doses for at least 14 days.

Prognosis

Gastroenteritis in otherwise healthy individuals is self-limited. *Salmonella* infections of any sort in debilitated or malnourished children can be serious. *Salmonella* meningitis has about 40% mortality. Reinfection can occur, but repeated infections are unusual.

CASE ILLUSTRATION

A 3-month-old female presented to the emergency room in shock apparently from acute lower gastrointestinal bleeding. She was born at term to a healthy mother after an uneventful pregnancy, labor, and delivery, and went home feeding on Similac. She was well until 2 months of age when she had the onset of mild diarrhea with blood streaks but she had no systemic signs. Examination at that time revealed a healthy-appearing infant with normal abdomen, loose stools with moderate blood streaks, hematocrit 33%, reticulocyte count of 1%, and a stool Gram stain that was culture negative. She was thought to have milk protein allergy and the formula was changed to a soy-based formula. Over the next week she was seen three more times with improvement of her loose stools, which were heme-negative. Repeat laboratory tests continued to show a stable hematocrit, normal white count, but elevated partial thromboplastic time (PTT) thought to be consistent with laboratory error, given her complete clinical recovery.

She remained well until 3 days before admission, when she began to produce loose stools mixed with blood and mucus. Although she developed a low-grade temperature and mild vomiting she continued to be normally active and hungry. On the morning of admission her temperature was 41°C, she stopped eating, began vomiting, and had voluminous bright red bloody stools per rectum. She was referred to the hospital for evaluation.

She had received her immunizations on time, had been growing well, and had no other medical problems.

On arrival she was pale, listless, and slightly cyanotic with very poor perfusion. Temperature was 41°C, heart rate 180, respiratory rate 55, blood pressure 70 systolic. There was no rash, cutaneous or mucosal bleeding or bruising, or adenopathy. Her peripheral pulses were decreased but the cardiac examination was otherwise unrevealing. Abdomen was slightly distended with decreased bowel sounds, diffuse peritoneal signs and guarding, but no mass effect was felt. There was grossly bloody stool in the diaper, Gram stain of which showed moderate amounts of polys. Neurologically she was listless, but had no focal signs.

Within a half-hour of arrival, she had a hypotensive episode requiring massive volume support, systemic vasopressors, and intubation. Nasogastric tube revealed coffee-ground stomach contents. Her initial hematocrit was 36, white count 5600, with 18% polys, 24% bands, and platelet count 54,000. Prothrombin time was 53/12 (PT), PTT was greater than 100. An arterial blood gas evaluation was notable for a serum bicarbonate of 10, and an incomplete respiratory compensation to a metabolic acidosis. A radiograph of the abdomen revealed multiple dilated loops, but no free peritoneal air.

QUESTION AND COMMENT

What are the diagnostic possibilities in this child and how should she be managed?

The initial diagnostic possibilities included a volvulus or malrotation with intestinal ischemia, generalized septicemia with a consumptive coagulopathy, an enteric infection, hemolytic uremic syndrome, or chronic appendicitis. Based on clinical criteria, the infant appeared to have perforated her bowel and antibiotics including ampicillin, gentamicin, and clindamycin were administered. An upper gastrointestinal series showed a normal stomach and esophagus, and normal placement of the ligament of Treitz; a barium enema showed normal filling of the appendix without striking abnormalities of the colonic mucosa.

Over the initial 24 hours the infant required platelet and plasma transfusions, and vasopressor support for ongoing blood loss, fever, pulmonary capillary leak, and probable disseminated intravascular coagulation suggestive of endotoxemia. While she appeared to be gravely ill, suggesting some undiagnosed intestinal ischemia, she did not have the typical hyperkalemia and refractory metabolic acidosis typically seen with ongoing tissue death.

On the second day of hospitalization her stool and blood cultures grew out Gram-negative rods which were serologically typed *Salmonella* group B. In retrospect, the fever, bloody diarrhea, colitis, and bandemia all pointed to an enteric pathogen, but the presentation in shock made gastrointestinal bleeding the most striking feature. The presentation of *Salmonella* infections (both typhoid and nontyphoid) with gastrointestinal hemorrhage, peritonitis, or microperforation is well known, with a disturbing incidence of poor outcome such that surgical intervention (to remove the most severely infected bowel segments and reduce endotoxemia) has been required. Whether or not the earlier report of abnormal clotting and rectal bleeding in this patient represented an initial infection with *Salmonella* remains speculative; it clearly argues for the aggressive treatment of symptomatically trivial *Salmonella* infections in this young age group. This patient's *Salmonella* group B was found to be sensitive to chloramphenicol but intermediate to ampicillin, and despite addition of high doses of chloramphenicol, disseminated intravascular coagulation, progressive hepatitis, cardiovascular and respiratory compromise persisted, resulting in the necessity for mechanical ventilation and maximal supportive efforts. Nevertheless she went on to show a progressive bulging fontanelle and brain edema on CT, suggestive of *Salmonella* meningitis. Despite maximal supportive efforts, the patient died after a week of hospitalization. Autopsy confirmed the diagnosis of *Salmonella* meningitis in addition to bacteremia and gastroenteritis.

CASE ILLUSTRATION

A 5-year-old male presented with a 1-week history of fever and pallor. He had been well except for an episode of prolonged fever that resolved spontaneously 17 months before admission. He had been well since that time and had spent a month in rural Portugal, returning 10 days before admission. One week before admission he developed an unremitting fever (to 40°C) not responsive to antipyretics, and detailed review of systems was essentially negative except for anorexia and lethargy. After 6 days of high fever his physician reported a normal physical examination and urinalysis, and a blood count notable for hematocrit of 31, white blood cell count of 6.4 (65% polys, 3% bands), an MCV of 88, and an ESR of 65. Of note, a 2-year-old sibling began to experience vomiting and low grade fever several days before admission, although parents and another younger sibling remained well.

Because of the persistent fever he was admitted to hospital and he appeared tired but in no distress. Temperature was 39.9°C, heart rate 120, respiratory rate 30, and blood pressure 100/70. Height and weight were in the 50th percentile. His examination was notable for some small anterior cervical nodes bilaterally; a 2–3 over 6 systolic murmur heard best at the left upper sternal border radiating out to the axilla; a benign abdomen without hepatosplenomegaly; guaiac-negative stools; no meningismus; and a normal neurological examination. There was no obvious localized infection. Initial laboratory values continued to show hematocrit ranging between 27 and 30 with an MCV of 88, a white count of 8600 (54% polys and 9% bands), adequate platelets, a reticulocyte count of 2.6%, and an ESR of 69. Blood smear showed slight hypochromia without visible evidence of hemolysis. Chemistries were normal except for a lactic dehydrogenase (LDH) of 304 (but with normal SGOT and bilirubin). Chest radiograph and ECG were within normal limits.

QUESTION AND COMMENT

Should any further tests be obtained, should the child be treated, and if so, for what?

The diagnostic possibilities for this child were many. Initially, the question of subacute bacterial endocarditis was raised since the patient had presented with fever and a new murmur. The medical team managing this patient admitted the child to observe fever spikes, and to obtain blood cultures concurrent with them. Within the first 48 hours, five blood cultures were obtained, and on the third day of admission all blood cultures were positive for Gram-negative rods identified as *Salmonella* typhi. This result was somewhat surprising in light of the absence of other often associated signs and symptoms—e.g., headache, abdominal pain with paralytic ileus, rose spots, bradycardia, and/or splenomegaly. Of note, *S. typhi* was subsequently cultured from stools. The patient was treated with chloramphenicol to which the organism was sensitive, with good clinical response and he continues to do well. His anemia was thought to be secondary to a mild hemolytic picture that has been described in patients with typhoid fever.

It is of interest that the 2-year-old sibling who had been well at the onset of the patient's illness, subsequently developed vomiting, mild diarrhea, and high fever. His stool and blood cultures were also positive for *S. typhi* and treatment with chloramphenicol was also started. The other family members were cultured, but not treated in the absence of bacterial growth and they remain asymptomatic. It is hypothesized that the exposure came from contaminated food or water while visiting rural Portugal, 2 weeks before the onset of symptoms.

Prevention

Vaccines are available for *S. typhi,* but are not effective with heavy exposures. No parenteral vaccine is recommended for routine use. A new live attenuated oral vaccine for typhoid is recommended.

SHIGELLA

Definition

Infections with shigellae cause a diarrheal syndrome with watery, mucus-containing, and sometimes bloody stools. Shigellosis is one of the most common causes of acute bacillary dysentery.

Basic Science

The nonmotile Gram-negative rods are classified into four groups (*S. dysenteriae, S. flexneri, S. boydii,* and *S. sonnei*) and 39 serotypes. *S. sonnei* is most common in the United States. The bacilli have cell wall (O) antigens, but lack the flagellar antigens found in *Salmonella* and *E. coli.* Virulence of the organisms varies, and is thought to depend on side-chain sugars of the O antigen. Isolation from stools is often difficult.

The organisms invade intestinal epithelial cells, multiply within them and promote an intense inflammatory reaction. Toxins are thought to produce most of the symptoms by promoting transudation of fluid into the intestinal lumen.

Epidemiology

Transmission is by the fecal-oral route. Epidemics occur wherever diarrheal disease is prevalent, and especially in institutions. Children 1–4 years of age are most susceptible, and many are asymptomatic carriers. Very small numbers of organisms (as few as 10) can produce illness in susceptible populations. Nearly 20,000 cases were reported in the United States in 1983, and nearly half were in children under 9 years of age.

Natural History

The incubation period is short, usually 2–7 days. The onset is acute, with fever and crampy abdominal pain, tenesmus, soon followed by watery or pasty stools which persist for several days. The lesion is an acute colitis with blood and mucus often present in the stools. Systemic effects include convulsions which may be associated with the high fever, but do occur without fever, presumably from a neurotoxin. Rarely, bacteremic chronic urinary tract infection may occur from *Shigella* infection.

Diagnosis

Examination of the stool reveals sheets of polys. The organism can be isolated from fresh specimens. Leukocytosis is characteristic. The symptoms are similar to those with other enteric infections including *Campylobacter, Yersina enterocolitica, Salmonella,* amebiasis, and invasive *E. coli.* Only bacterial diagnosis culture can distinguish the causative agent. Fresh stool specimens should be delivered promptly to the laboratory for isolation of shigellae.

Treatment

Since the natural course is only 2–3 days, no antibiotics are required. In severe illness, seen early, trimethorprim-sulfamethoxazole for 5 days can shorten the duration of diarrhea and eradicate the organism. Antidiarrheal drugs should be avoided since they prolong excretion of the organism. Oral electrolyte solutions are usually adequate to maintain hydration.

Prognosis

Prognosis is excellent, except among malnourished or otherwise host defense compromised children.

Prevention

Experimental oral vaccines have been effective in institutions, but are not available for routine use. Strains resistant to most antibiotics develop. Hand-washing remains the most effective way to reduce fecal-oral spread.

STAPHYLOCOCCUS

Definition

Staphylococci are the most common causes of pyogenic skin infections and may be associated with systemic disease including pneumonia, empyema, endocarditis, osteomyelitis, and meningitis. Certain strains are also common causes of food poisoning.

Basic Science

Staphylococci are nonmotile Gram-positive members of the family of *Micrococcaceae.* They grow aerobically in clusters and are classified on the basis of being coagulase-positive or -negative, and subclassified into strains by bacteriophage typing. *S. aureus* strains are coagulase-positive and usually produce a yellow pigment. *S. epidermidis* strains are coagulase-negative and produce a white pigment.

The various strains produce a variety of toxins and enzymes that permit the organism to invade tissues. Some of the toxins are hemolysins, which can cause tissue necrosis and injure leukocytes as well as hemolyze red cells. Another toxin, leukocidin, which is produced by most strains of *S. aureus,* also has the capacity to destroy leukocytes (hence its name), and interacts with the phospholipids of cell membranes to increase their permeability. An exfoliative toxin associated with phage group II staphylococci is the cause of the "scalded skin syndrome" or Ritter disease. It is also associated with a scarlatiniform eruption. Enterotoxins are elaborated by many strains of *S. aureus* and can produce vomiting and diarrhea and sometimes profound hypotension, including toxic shock syndrome (see pp. 1088).

Among the enzymes that may be released by certain strains are coagulase, staphylokinase, penicillinase, or β-lactamase, (an inactivator of penicillin), and hyaluronidase (a spreading factor).

Coagulase-negative staphylococci, once thought to be nonpathogenic normal flora, have been identified as a potential source of bacteremia in newborns and immunocompromised hosts.

Epidemiology

Staphylococcal infections are widespread, but their true incidence is unknown. It is estimated that 20–30% of normal individuals carry *S. aureus* in their anterior nares, and the organism is widely distributed on the skin. Transmission is usually by direct contact. The newborn infant is particularly susceptible, with the common sites of colonization being the nasopharynx, the skin, and the umbilicus. Rapid spread among infants through handling by nursery personnel is especially serious with some virulent strains such as phage type 80/81.

Disease occurs when the skin is penetrated, particularly by foreign bodies, or indwelling catheters, or prosthetic valves. Skin injury or disease, as in acne, provides a fertile site for growth of the omnipresent staphylococci. The ability to produce disease is thought to be related to the capacity of the virulent strains to inhibit chemotaxis.

Natural History

Pyogenic skin infections, especially bullous impetigo, are the most frequent forms of staphylococcal disease. Multiple staphylococcal abscesses may occur in individuals with deficient granulocyte function and with hyperimmunoglobin E. Infants in particular are prone to respiratory tract disease. Pneumonia may be primary or follow a viral infection. In infants under 1 year of age who are most susceptible, the onset can be sudden and severe, with widespread necrotizing pneumonitis and development of pneumatoceles, pneumothorax, and empyema. In some adolescents, staphylococcal infections can be very severe.

Sepsis is less common but can occur with localized infection appearing in bones, joints, kidneys, heart, or brain. High fever and either leukopenia or leukocytosis are common.

Meningitis may follow bacteremia or be a complication of *Staphylococcus* otitis media, periorbital cellulitis, or osteomyelitis of the skull.

Nosocomially acquired infection with *S. epidermis* is an increasing problem, particularly in intensive care nurseries. It has replaced group B streptococci as the pathogen most commonly isolated from blood cultures in newborn infants.

Diagnosis

Diagnosis depends on the isolation of the organism from the site of infection. The organism is readily grown and identified on the basis of Gram stain and coagulase. Patterns of sensitivity should always be assessed since degree of antibiotic resistance in different strains is extremely variable.

Treatment

Because staphylococcal infection may cause suppuration, antibiotic therapy alone is often not adequate. Abscesses require draining particularly in the case of empyema or osteomyelitis. If a foreign body has served as the focus of infection it should be removed.

Since in some areas more than 90% of staphylococci are resistant to penicillin, initiation of therapy should be with a penicillinase-resistant agent such as methicillin, oxacillin, or nafcillin (200 mg/kg/24 hours intravenously in six divided doses). The response of the patient to treatment as well as reports from the laboratory on the sensitivity of the organism dictate subsequent treatment. After the patient becomes afebrile, oral administration of these drugs is usually satisfactory. For meningitis and other serious illnesses, intravenous administration remains preferable. For acute osteomyelitis, an initial intravenous course can be followed by oral regimens if compliance can be assured, and serum killing power of the antibiotic against the organism is known. If individuals are sensitive to penicillin, a first generation cephalosporin or clindamycin may be effective.

S. epidermidis is a coagulase-negative organism that may be resistant to most drugs. Vancomycin may be required. Blood levels should be monitored since the renal excretion varies in small infants (Reed et al, 1987). Methicillin-resistant staphylococci can be killed by vancomycin.

Prognosis

Staphylococcal septicemia is a very serious condition and carries a mortality rate of 80% or more if untreated. Staphylococcal pneumonia in infancy is fatal unless it is recognized promptly and treated with high doses of antibiotics intravenously. A white count depressed below 5000 is a grave prognostic sign.

Prevention

During epidemics, such as occurred in the mid-1950s and early 1960s in the United States, hexachlorophene bathing of infants was widely used to establish a barrier at the site of initial colonization. This approach is no longer recommended, since transcutaneous absorption, particularly in premature infants, can produce toxic blood levels. Hexachlorophene solutions or organic iodide compounds are appropriate for hand-washing of adult caretakers. Deliberate colonization of infants with avirulent strains such as 502A was once practiced to establish competition with more virulent ones. This approach is now used very selectively since fatal septicemia was reported from an "avirulent" strain.

Staphylococcal Pneumonia

A 3-month-old female presented to the hospital with cough and fever. Four days before admission she had had a low-grade temperature, cough, and coryza. Two days later she developed a fever to 39°C, with irritability and poor feeding; she was diagnosed as having tonsillitis by her pediatrician and was sent home on amoxicillin. On the day of admission she demonstrated increased tachypnea and was admitted to the hospital. On physical examination she was an alert, irritable infant with nasal flaring and occasional grunting. Her temperature was 39.4°C, heart rate 160/min, respirations were 66/min and labored. Her pulmonary examination was notable for coryza and coarse upper airway breath sounds with coarse rhonchi at bases and in the right anterior lung field. Her hematocrit was 32, white blood cell count 21,800, with 49% polys and 19% bands; urinalysis and CSF findings were within the normal limits. Chest radiograph showed a rounded density in the lateral segment of the right middle lobe consistent with pneumonia. An arterial blood gas on 30% O_2 showed a PO_2 of 148 mm Hg, PCO_2 of 26 mm Hg, and a pH of 7.51.

QUESTION AND COMMENT

What are the most likely diagnostic possibilities in this child, and how should she be managed?

The lack of response to ampicillin should come as no surprise: not only would a viral etiology explain this patient's symptoms (including cytomegalovirus, respiratory syncytial virus, parainfluenza, and adenovirus) but bacterial etiologies would have included *Staphylococcus, Mycoplasma,* and *Pertussis,* before *Haemophilus influenzae* and *Pneumococcus.* Ampicillin would not provide adequate coverage for most of these bacterial pathogens. A chest radiograph 12 hours later showed increased extension of pneumonia in the right lower and middle lobes with new small pleural effusions. A thoracentesis was performed for the effusion and 37,200 white blood cells were obtained with 85% polys, 1% bands, and a Gram stain that showed polys and Gram-positive cocci in clusters. Cultures subsequently grew out *S. aureus;* the patient was promptly changed to oxacillin to which she had a good clinical response.

Toxic Shock Syndrome

Definition

Toxic shock syndrome is a multisystem disease of acute onset with fever, hypotension, a characteristic rash with subsequent desquamation, mainly in menstruating young women between 15 and 24 years of age. This syndrome was first described by Todd et al (1978).

Basic Science

The offending agent in toxic shock syndrome is a toxin secreted by *S. aureus*. The puzzling question has been why this toxin is more likely to cause disease in women who insert absorbent materials into the vagina during menses. One product in particular, Rely tampons, was the most strongly assoicated product in the 1980 epidemic. All tampons with polyester foam were withdrawn from the market and the number of cases of toxic shock syndrome fell. It was apparent that the introduction of polyester foam and polyacrylate rayon in the late 1970s corresponded with the first reports of the syndrome.

Studies in vitro show that staphylococci multiply and produce toxin at an elevated rate when in an environment with low magnesium. Mills et al (1985) proposed that the offending fibers could absorb magnesium ions and the resulting environment promoted toxin production. Restoration of magnesium ions in vitro reduced toxin production. These findings are consistent with the observation that the symptoms are most common when menstrual flow lessens, about the fourth day of the period. Since tampons with polyester fibers were removed from the market, the number of cases has decreased, but the disorder has not disappeared.

Only a small percentage of users of Rely tampons developed toxic shock. One probable explanation is that the toxin, TSST-1 is so widespread that most people have antibodies to it by 20 years of age. Alternatively, some individuals may have a genetically determined susceptibility to shock from the toxin.

Epidemiology

As of April 16, 1984 cases reported to the Centers for Disease Control included 2385 in females, and only 124 (5%) in males. Cases have been reported from all 50 states, and many other countries. The peak incidence was in 1980, and the disorder has declined progressively ever since (Fig. 17.6). Although reported in newborn infants and in older persons, almost 60% of menstruating cases were aged 15–24 years, and 25% were 25–34 years old. The association with extravaginal staphylococcal infections is well-known, although the incidence is not (Buchdahl et al, 1985; Davis, 1980).

Natural History

Toxic shock syndrome is associated with vaginal *S. aureus* (usually phage-group-1) infections in menstruating women who use tampons. Other cases have followed cesarean section wound infections, mastitis, and nasal surgery with nasal packing. Sporadic cases with other *S. aureus* infections such as furuncles and insect bites have occurred. The case fatality rate has dropped consistently from 5% in 1980 to 2.6% in 1983.

Diagnosis

The syndrome is defined by symptoms of high fever, low blood pressure, and a diffuse erythematous "sunburn-like" rash which characteristically begins on

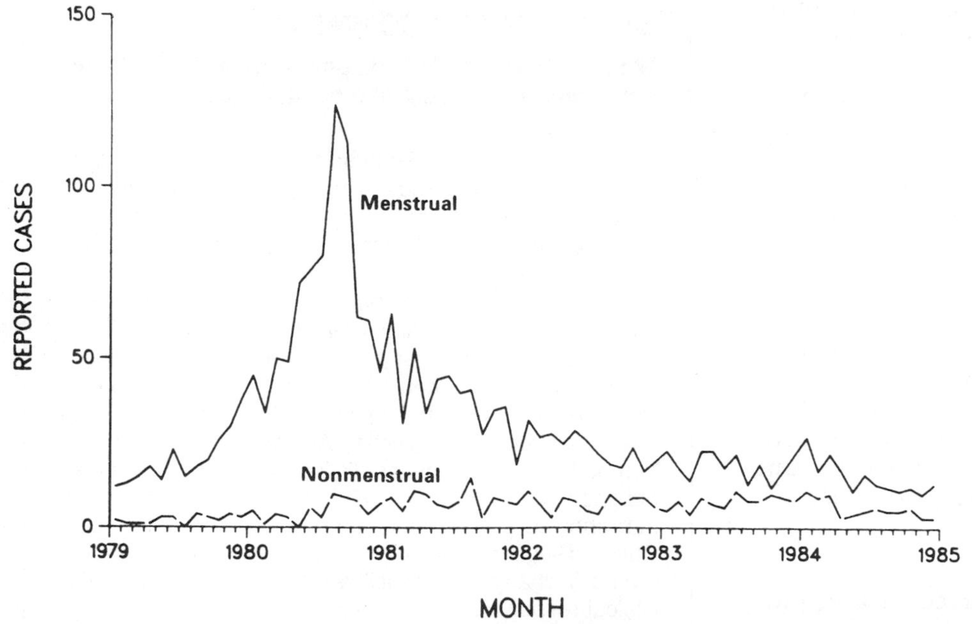

Figure 17.6. Toxic shock syndrome by month of onset 1976–1984. Of the total cases, 2669 were in females and 146 were in males. Cases in nonmenstrual women accounted for 27% of the total reported in 1984. From CDC: *MMWR*, Annual Summary 1984, 33:63, 1986.

CASE ILLUSTRATION

A 15-year-old white female had the onset of fever (39.5°C) and myalgia during the second day of her menses. She had been in good health until this illness and regularly used tampons during periods.

This illness was noted for dizziness, sore throat, and nausea, followed the next day by watery diarrhea, mild abdominal pain, and a diffuse urticarial erythema. An episode of syncope led to her seeking medical care, at which time her blood pressure was 80/60. Laboratory examinations revealed normal hematocrit, white count and platelets. She had elevated fibrin split products and mild elevation of liver function. She was given intravenous fluids and improved over the next few days. *S. aureus* phage group I was isolated from her vagina. Desquamation of areas of skin accompanied lessening of systemic signs.

COMMENT

The diagnosis in a menstruating woman who uses polyester-containing materials that can be inserted into the vagina is not difficult. Much greater diagnostic perplexity results when males or other individuals exhibit similar symptoms.

QUESTIONS AND COMMENTS

What were the likely reasons for the rarity of this condition before 1978, and the peak prevalence in 1980?

The introduction of synthetic fibers into certain brands of tampons corresponded to the initial outbreak and the withdrawal of the products was associated with fewer cases.

Why are the symptoms most likely to occur toward the end of the menstrual period?

The occurrence of symptoms late in the period may be the result of reduced menstrual flow, and more opportunity for the organisms to produce high concentrations of toxin.

Why might this condition be inaccurately reported?

The condition is not usually considered in males or in nonmenstruating females. The origin of the toxin in such circumstances is unclear. It may be that some cases of Kawasaki disease are falsely labeled toxic shock since there are no pathognomonic signs or symptoms or diagnostic tests.

palms and soles. It resembles scarlet fever, but has also been confused with Kawasaki disease and leptospirosis. In severe cases, liver and renal failure can lead to death. Severe vomiting and diarrhea are common. There is no specific diagnostic test. Culture of strains of staphylococci that produce a toxin known as TSST-1 is possible in most cases. Muscle creatine kinase levels may be elevated.

Treatment

Early treatment includes intravenous fluids and colloid to restore volume, ventilatory support if needed, and cardiovascular support with dopamine if the blood pressure remains low. Removal of tampons and contraceptive devices and vaginal irrigation to eliminate the offending toxins is mandatory. Intravenous antistaphylococcal drugs such as oxacillin or nafcillin should be given for 10 days to prevent recurrences.

Prevention

The best prevention of toxic shock syndrome is to avoid inappropriate (prolonged) use of tampons.

STREPTOCOCCUS

Group A

Definition

Streptococci are among the most common pathogens capable of mild or serious disease, with or without sequelae in infancy and childhood.

Basic Science

Streptococci are Gram-positive spherical cocci, of the family lactobacillaceae. Lancefield in the 1930s separated these organisms into groups on the basis of the carbohydrate components in the cell wall. The outer portion of the cell wall contains proteins some of which are related to the virulence of the organism. The M protein is an antiphagocytic antigen. Other proteins (T and R) are not clearly related to virulence.

Disease is produced by the toxins. Group A hemolytic streptococci produce more than 20, including erythrogenic toxins (A, B and C), streptolysins (O and S), streptokinases (A and B), deoxyribonucleases (A, B, C, and D), hyaluronidase, and others.

Epidemiology

Group A streptococci are present in 15–20% of children and, thus, are components of normal flora. The incidence of disease is not known. They are most often associated with disease in January to May and also in the fall when school opens. Pharyngitis associated with streptococci occurs most often between 4 and 11 years of age (see sections on rheumatic fever and nephritis for incidence of nonsuppurative complications).

Natural History

The organism is spread from person to person by direct contact or by droplets. It can be spread in contaminated milk or occasionally in water. The organism can initiate an acute inflammatory response. The erythrogenic toxin is responsible for the rash in scarlet fever, from hyperemia and a polymorphonuclear invasion in the corium of the skin.

Pharyngitis results from deposition of large numbers of organisms on the pharyngeal mucosa. The M protein prevents phagocytosis and permits multiplication of the organism. Streptolysin O has a toxic effect on leukocytes; their lysis promotes the inflammatory reaction.

The incubation period is 1–3 days. Manifestations in infants are a clear nasal discharge, nonspecific irritability, and a low-grade fever. If the illness persists for 4–6 weeks, the condition is called streptococcosis, which is most common between 6 months and 3 years. Otitis media and lymphadenopathy are common.

In older children, tonsillitis and pharyngitis predominate. The tonsils may be covered with purulent yellow exudate, and the pharynx and palate will be infected. Petechial and edema of the palate are characteristic. In untreated cases retropharyngeal abscesses may develop. If pain is present, the child may have trismus.

Scarlet fever has a 1- to 7-day incubation period. The onset is acute with fever of 39–40°C or higher, pharyngitis, headache, and often vomiting. Early in the course the tongue is white with red edematous papillae (white strawberry tongue). The white coat is sloughed, and the tongue is bright red (red strawberry tongue). The rash starts in axillae, groin, and neck, but then becomes generalized. After 5–7 days fever and rash subside, but desquamation of skin on the face, trunks, and finally hands and feet may continue for 4–6 weeks.

Impetigo is a superficial pyoderma caused by group A β-hemolytic streptococci. (Staphylococci may be present, but are thought to be secondary invaders. They are responsible for bullous impetigo.) The organisms may invade a superficial abrasion, mosquito bite, poison ivy, or any wound. The lesions are characterized as pustular, and usually cluster. Regional lymphadenitis may occur, but bacteremia is rare.

Deep skin infections with group A streptococci are designated cellulitis or erysipelas. The skin is swollen, indurated, with a raised margin. Fever and vomiting are common. Bacteremia and metastatic spread may occur. Osteomyelitis, pneumonitis, arthritis, meningitis and pyelonephritis can result; rarely bacterial endocarditis occurs.

Diagnosis

The organisms can be grown on a 5% sheep blood agar plate, and are readily presumptively identified by bacitracin sensitivity, or fluorescent antibody staining.

Serologic responses to antistreptolysin O can be measured. An increase to greater than 166 Todd units occurs in most untreated children.

Kits are now available for rapid tests, which are fairly sensitive and highly specific. Specific antibody tests (e.g., antihyaluronidase) are helpful in certain clinical situations. Results are known in about 1 hour or less. The high costs and false-positives as well as false-negative results have prevented wide use of the test kits (Medical Letter, 1985).

Treatment

BASICS

Penicillin is the drug of choice. Almost all strains of group A streptococci are sensitive to bacteriocidal concentrations. Blood and tissue levels should be maintained for 10 days. Oral penicillin (200,000 units) given three times a day for 10 days is satisfactory if compliance is assured. Otherwise children are given intramuscular benzathine penicillin in a single dose of 600,000 units which provides appropriate blood levels for about 1 month. For serious illness, intravenous administration is needed. Erythromycin, 50 mg/kg/day or clindamycin 30 mg/kg/day are effective for individuals who are allergic to penicillin, provided that they are given for 10 days.

CONTROVERSY

Since a carrier state is common, what is the criterion for determining when pharyngitis is caused by streptococci? A discussion of this question in 1985 discloses continuing differences of opinion (Breese et al, 1985). In general, we treat if there is marked tonsillar and pharyngeal redness, anterior cervical adenopathy and redness of the soft palate, and a positive culture. It could be argued that the culture is superfluous in the presence of the characteristic findings, and treatment with penicillin is both safe and effective. Other conditions, such as infectious mononucleosis and some viral infections are indistinguishable from streptococcal pharyngitis. Although they will not be made worse by penicillin, clearly they will not respond to it. Conversely, a positive culture in the presence of mild upper respiratory tract disease does not require treatment. A quantitative measure after second streaking of a colony may be helpful in borderline cases (10–50 colonies are indication for treatment). We do not recommend culture of children under 4 years of age with upper respiratory infections since streptococci are unlikely to be the cause, and rheumatic fever and glomerulonephritis are rare in that age group in the United States. Rheumatic fever occurs at a rate of 0.64/100,000 population. (This is not true in underdeveloped countries where both infection and complications can occur in malnourished children in particular; Massell et al, 1988.)

Reculture after 10 days of therapy is not widely recommended, nor do we practice it unless symptoms persist. Some children have repeated illness at close intervals from group A streptococci. Cultures of family members, and treatment with penicillin prophylaxis has been proposed during seasons of high incidence, or in closed communities such as prisons, military establishments, or other institutions. Alternatively, treatment of the individual with another antibiotic may be more practical and sometimes effective.

Prevention

Children with a history of rheumatic fever require continuous prophylaxis with oral penicillin (see Section 6, pp. 386.) Recurrent episodes of streptococcal infection may also be prevented with oral prophylaxis during the months of high prevalence of infection. Individuals with recurrent streptococcal pharyngitis may respond after a course of rifampin (20 mg/kg/dose every day for 4 days; Chaudhary et al, 1985).

Prognosis

The main concern about acute streptococcal disease is the risk of rheumatic fever and glomerulonephritis. Indeed, the reason for cultures, and a 10-day course of penicillin for acute streptococcal disease is the belief that the late complications (including suppurative ones) will be reduced.

Group B Streptococcus

The emergence of serious disease from type III group B streptococcal infections (see also Section 4, pp. 195) since the early 1970s has been puzzling and disturbing inasmuch as treatment of infected infants even within the first hour of infection has not been effective. (Before the 1970s, the organism was known mostly as a cause of udder infection in cows.)

Basic Science

Improved survival of infants with group B streptoccal disease will depend on better insight into pathogenesis. Conventional treatment with antibiotics and pressors usually fails to reverse shock. Extensive studies in animal models support the hypothesis that a toxin produces myocardial dysfunction. Peevy et al (1985) in a rabbit model, produced shock with heat-killed group B streptococci, and prevented the hemodynamic changes with prior treatment with indomethacin (a prostaglandin synthetase inhibitor). These observations suggest the shock is the result of myocardial dysfunction that is mediated by prostaglandins. The clinical relevance of these observations awaits further study.

Epidemiology

Epidemiologic studies show 5–30% of pregnant women are colonized with group B streptococci in the vagina, the rectum or both. About one-half of their infants will be colonized on the skin, nasopharynx, or rectum, but only 1% of colonized infants will develop disease (Siegel et al, 1982). In many nurseries in Europe and America (at least) group B streptococcus is the leading cause of neonatal septicemia. Early onset infection, before 5–7 days of age, affects 2–3 babies per 1000 live births in the United States.

QUESTION AND COMMENT

Why is 10 days of treatment recommended?

The recommendation dates from the 1950s, when 10 days was more effective in eradicating group A streptococci from the pharynx of asymptomatic carriers. In a study by Schwartz et al (1981), children with streptococcal pharyngitis had fewer clinical and bacteriologic recurrences when treated with oral penicillin V for 10 days than did those on 7 days of treatment.

It is only an assumption that 10 days of penicillin reduces the risk of rheumatic fever in the 1980s (Gerber and Markowitz, 1985).

CASE ILLUSTRATION

A 5½-year-old male presented to the emergency room in marked respiratory distress. Five days before admission he developed a barking cough. Three days before admission he began to complain of right upper quadrant abdominal pain. On the day of admission he was seen by his pediatrician who noted a temperature of 39°C and a clear chest on physical examination. He was sent home only to return 6 hours later with a temperature of 41°C and a respiratory rate of 52, looking cyanotic, and in severe respiratory distress. A white blood cell count was 19,000 with 35% polys and 50% bands, and a chest radiograph revealed right upper lobe and right lower lobe infiltrates. Ampicillin and oxacillin were instituted for treatment of a presumptive bacterial pneumonia.

Over the next 24 hours the patient's respiratory status further deteriorated and he became increasingly hypoxic and hypercarbic. A repeat chest radiograph showed complete opacification of the right lung field with fluid layering out on the lateral view. He was intubated and a chest tube was placed with initial drainage of 600 ml of purulent fluid. Concurrent with this was profound hypotension and clotting abnormalities consistent with a picture of septic shock and disseminated intravascular coagulation. Cultures of pleural fluid and throat were both positive for group A β-hemolytic streptococcus.

QUESTION AND COMMENT

How common is streptococcus as a cause of childhood empyema and pneumonia?

While group A streptococcus represents less than 10% of bacterial isolates of childhood pneumonia, this case is typical in the rapidity (i.e., hours versus days) and severity of its clinical course once it invades the lung of a presumed normal host. Moreover, empyema has been reported in 100% of cases of streptococcal pneumonia, and this one is no exception. It is thought that viral or other bacterial superinfections may predispose to a streptococcal pneumonia, although in this patient no second organism was found. That blood cultures remained negative is not unusual since previous studies have shown that only 55% of cases have a positive blood culture (Molteni, 1977). Other studies suggest that from 33–66% of patients with streptococcal pneumonia can have a positive throat culture as did our patient. The natural course of streptococcal pneumonia is a slow resolution with patients remaining febrile with pleuritic chest pains for at least a week. Such was the case with our patient who had a slow but steady improvement after initiation of penicillin and after a brief course of intubation and vasopressor support.

CASE ILLUSTRATION

An 8-year-old male presented to the emergency room with polyarthralgias, left elbow effusion, and fever. He had been in excellent health until 10 days before admission when he had a sore throat and impetigo of both elbows, which had been treated with erythromycin. Eight days before admission he fell on his left knee, sustaining a superficial cut which healed uneventfully. Six days before admission he had nausea, vomiting, and diarrhea lasting 2 days and the onset of fever (to 103°F) and chills, which persisted until the day of admission. He began limping because of right heel pain without erythema, effusion, or radiographic findings. Later the right heel became erythematous and warm, and the left elbow became erythematous, tender, warm, and swollen. On the day of admission he had diffuse tenderness along the spine and the left shoulder as well. He had no rash, chest pain, chorea, insect bites, urinary changes, trauma, or recent dental work or travel. He had no known allergies and no family history of collagen vascular disease. Physical examination revealed a well-nourished male in significant pain. His temperature was 38.2°C orally, heart rate was 100, respiratory rate was 28, blood pressure was 100/70. His cheeks were flushed but there were no petechiae. The impetigo had healed. There was no meningismus, adenopathy, or pharyngitis. Chest was clear. Cardiac examination was normal except for a 2/6 flow murmur at the left lower substernal border without radiation. Abdomen was soft without organomegaly, stool was guaiac-negative. He had marked tenderness of the left shoulder, both heels, and thoracic spine without bony tenderness or effusion. The right heel was slightly red and markedly warm. The left elbow was warm, tender, and swollen. He could not walk because of heel tenderness. Knees and hips were apparently not involved. The neurological examination was entirely normal. Laboratory studies included a hematocrit of 32, white count of 12,700, with 55 polys and 5 bands, platelets of 290,000 and a sedimentation rate of 59. Chest radiograph and ECG were normal. Urinalysis revealed 2–3 white cells, but was otherwise negative. Shoulder and ankle films were normal. A left elbow film revealed effusion without bony changes. The elbow effusion was tapped.

QUESTION AND COMMENT

What are some diagnostic possibilities and how should this child be managed?

While rheumatic fever, serum sickness, juvenile rheumatoid arthritis (JRA), Lyme arthritis, staphylococcal and gonococcal septic arthritis were all considered, aspiration of the joint fluid provided a definitive diagnosis. The joint fluid was straw-colored with 14,000 white cells (mostly polys), a protein of 500 mg/dl, glucose of 12 mg%, and Gram-positive cocci in pairs and chains. Shortly after the joint aspiration the patient had an episode of shaking chills, cyanosis, and hypotension; penicillin and chloramphenicol were administered pending the results of cultures. Blood cultures and the joint fluid grew out group A *Streptococcus* at 12 hours into his hospital course. Serum fibrinogen and fibrin split products were elevated consistent with disseminated intravascular coagulation. A bone scan was recommended to rule out osteomyelitis and showed changes consistent with septic arthritis of the left elbow only. Operative drainage of the effusion was subsequently performed. On high dose penicillin (400,000 units kg/day divided every 4 hours), symptoms resolved and there was improvement in the elbow and right ankle.

Group A streptococcal sepsis and arthritis are not very common. Groups D and B have been isolated in patients with multiple septic joints and endocarditis, but this patient had no other evidence of endocarditis. Throat cultures grew group A *Streptococcus* resistant to erythromycin with which this patient had been treated for his primary diagnosis of impetigo. The possibility of a rheumatic component cannot be excluded since this patient met the Jones criteria (for acute rheumatic fever) having polyarthritis, arthralgia, fever, and elevated sedimentation rate, white count, antistreptolysin O (ASLO) titer, and a positive throat culture, but the persistent findings in the elbow and ankle despite negative bone scan make a disseminated septic process most likely. He received 2 weeks of high-dose intravenous penicillin and then 2 more weeks of oral penicillin to maintain serum-cidal levels.

Natural History

Infants at risk of infection are those who lack antibody to type B III, the type most often associated with late onset meningitis in the United States. (In Finland it is type Ib or Ic) (Vesikari et al, 1985). The organism is spread by vertical transmission, either through ruptured membranes and amnionitis, or during passage through the birth canal. The reasons for early onset versus late onset (up to 6 months of age) presentation are not clear. Presumably the late onset illness is acquired from mother or other individuals, or in nursery.

Diagnosis

The early onset form presents within hours or rarely days after birth with sudden onset of peripheral vascular collapse, apnea, tachypnea, hypoxia, and often a diffuse pulmonary infiltrate which may be difficult to distinguish from hyaline membrane disease. Infection may have begun in utero and precipitated premature labor. About one-third of the infants also develop meningitis.

Late onset disease occurs mostly in term infants. It usually presents 1–12 weeks after birth, and cannot be distinguished clinically from other fulminant bacterial meningitides. It can present with adenitis, septic arthritis, and osteomyelitis. In some instances the organism (type III) can be recovered from the maternal vagina.

Laboratory diagnosis depends on demonstration of Gram-positive cocci in nasal swab, gastric aspirate, which establishes exposure, and positive culture of blood or spinal fluid for evidence of infection. Rapid diagnosis is possible with latex agglutination or counterimmunoelectrophoresis (CIE) in which antisera from immunized rabbits can detect the capsular antigens of the bacteria in body fluids. The test can be completed within 30 minutes, although it is relatively insensitive. The neutrophil count may be depressed, although fatal disease has been reported with normal levels (Christensen et al, 1985).

Treatment

Intravenous penicillin is the treatment of choice; 250,000–400,000 u/kg/day, given in divided doses every 8 hours intravenously is recommended. An aminoglycoside is usually given in addition for the first week. (Swingle et al, 1985).

Prognosis

Even with early administration of drug, early onset disease is about 50% fatal; late onset disease has a mortality of 20–40%. About one-third to one-half of the survivors of group B streptococcal meningitis have neurologic sequelae. Careful follow-up and counseling of parents is essential to maximize the potential of these infants. Risk factors are coma at time of hospitalization, CSF protein over 300 mg/dl, and neutrophil counts below 1000/mm^3 (Edwards et al, 1985).

Prevention

As prophylaxis against group B streptococcus, penicillin, given within an hour of birth may reduce but does not eradicate early onset disease (0.2 case/1000 live births versus 1.2 cases/1000 controls). It had no effect on late onset disease, 0.5/1000 treated versus 0.4/1000 controls) (Siegel et al, 1982).

The most effective prevention of infection in the infant is treatment of the mother at the onset of labor with intravenous ampicillin (2 g) followed by 1 g every 4 hours until delivery. The mothers selected for treatment were those with positive culture, premature onset of labor, or more than 12 hours of ruptured membranes (Boyer and Gotoff, 1986).

The possibility of immunization of mothers in the third trimester with streptococcal polysaccharide was explored by Baker et al (1985). Results are promising but preliminary. The use of intravenous immune globulin has been encouraging in several studies (Christensen et al, 1985).

CASE ILLUSTRATION

A 1-month-old black female presented with increasing left hip pain for 1–2 weeks. Her perinatal history was entirely benign. The mother had a full-term gestation without complications, and a normal spontaneous vaginal delivery with the baby being sent home on day 3 of life. She appeared well at a 2-week visit, but shortly thereafter began to have pain on both active and passive movements of the left hip and knee, without fever, rash, or erythema. When swelling of the hip was noted, she was brought to the emergency room where examination revealed an afebrile infant with the left hip flexed and externally rotated with decreased range of motion. Her blood count was 14,500 with 66 polys, 1 band, ESR 49. A complete septic work-up was performed with blood and CSF culture subsequently showing no growth. A hip radiograph showed lateral displacement of the left femoral head. Because of the high suspicion of a joint effusion, the baby underwent exploration and drainage of the left hip joint. Pus was noted over the left hip capsule, which subsequently grew B *Streptococcus*.

QUESTIONS AND COMMENTS

How common is a group B *Streptococcus* septic arthritis, and how should it be treated?

Although *Staphylococcus aureus* previously has been thought to be the major cause of perinatal septic arthritis, there has been an increasing incidence of group B streptococcal joint and bone infections over the past 10 years. In fact, group B streptococcal osteomyelitis and/or septic arthritis is believed to be the second most common localizing site of late onset group B streptococcal disease (the first being meningitis). Previous case reports confirm a lack of maternal perinatal complications predisposing to infection, and most cases appear without other systemic signs, as did this one. Although osteomyelitis is often seen accompanying the arthritis (believed to be secondary to vascular perforation of epiphyseal growth plates and joint capsule), no bone involvement was noted by radiographic studies or direct observation in this patient. Duration of therapy is 3 weeks with intravenous aqueous penicillin at a dose of 100,000–200,000 units kg/day, divided every 4 hours.

Streptococcus Pneumoniae (Pneumococcus)

Definition

Streptococcus pneumoniae is a widespread normal inhabitant of the upper respiratory tract which can become pathogenic and be responsible for both upper and lower respiratory tract infections.

Basic Science

The organism is a Gram-positive encapsulated diplococcus. More than 80 serotypes have been identified on the basis of the type-specific capsular polysaccharide. Only the smooth encapsulated strains are pathogenic for humans. Virulence appears to be related in part to the size of the capsule and to the capsular material that impedes phagocytosis.

Somatic antigens also have been isolated. C substance is a cell wall antigen that is not related to specific serotypes.

CASE ILLUSTRATION—MENINGITIS

A 29-day-old white female was brought to the hospital with a 1-week history of coryza. Two days before admission she was sleepier than usual. On the evening before admission she was irritable and fed poorly. Perinatal history was completely unremarkable. A 2-year-old sibling had had symptoms of an upper respiratory infection.

On physical examination the infant was irritable and alert with a temperature of 39.6°C, heart rate of 148, respirations of 44, and blood pressure of 90 systolic. The examination was otherwise entirely unremarkable. Laboratory investigation revealed a hematocrit of 35.7, white count of 7400, with 45% polys and 5% bands. The CSF had 745 white cells, with 89% polys, 4% lymphs, 7% monos, and 8 red cells, with a glucose of 27 mg/dl and a serum glucose of 77 mg/dl, and a protein of 98 mg/100 dl. The Gram stain revealed many polys but no organisms despite very careful search. Urinalysis was normal as was a chest radiograph. Other laboratory results were remarkable for a mild hyponatremia. Cultures of blood and CSF were sent as well as latex agglutination for group B *Streptococcus* and *H. influenzae* on urine, blood, and CSF.

QUESTIONS AND COMMENTS

What is the role of the new cephalosporins in the treatment of meningitis in such a young infant?

The findings in this infant were thought to be most consistent with bacterial meningitis, given the high CSF cell count, predominance of polys, and low CSF glucose. The choice of antibiotics is complicated by the fact that this child was at an age of transition between the neonatal and infancy period; Gram-negative infection in babies without neonatal complications is very unusual after 1 month of age. On the other hand, *H. influenzae* becomes a leading pathogen after this time, with group B *Streptococcus* and *Pneumococcus* straddling both periods.

To cover these organisms either regimen of the old standby antibiotics, i.e., ampicillin and an aminoglycoside and chloramphenicol, or a new third-generation cephalosporin, such as ceftriaxone in combination with ampicillin may be used. There is now reasonable evidence that cefuroxime and ceftriaxone are effective therapy for *H. influenzae* meningitis and that moxalactam is as effective as ampicillin and amikacin in the treatment of neonatal Gram-negative meningitis. The choice involves balancing efficacy and familiarity against the known or unknown side-effects of these drugs. This child was initially treated with ampicillin, gentamicin, and chloramphenicol although the cephalosporins would probably have been just as efficacious. Before the organism was identified, we would have included ampicillin since *Listeria* are not covered by cephalosporins.

Twenty-four hours after starting the antibiotics, Gram-positive cocci and pairs and chains grew from the first blood culture and CSF, subsequently identified as group B streptococcus and the treatment with ampicillin and gentamicin was continued for 2 weeks. Her recovery was complete.

What is the role of latex agglutination tests in the diagnosis of bacterial disease?

Of interest is the fact that the group B streptococcal latex agglutination test on CSF and urine was negative. This test has been shown to be moderately sensitive and very specific for group B streptococci. However, it is often negative if only a small inoculum of bacteria is available. Thus, specimens such as urine are best concentrated in order to maximize the sensitivity of the test. In this case, there were insufficient fluids to concentrate. When the latex test remains positive, inadequate therapy is a possibility.

Epidemiology

Pneumococcus is the most common cause of acute otitis media in children and a frequent cause of pneumonia, sinusitis, and bacteremia with meningitis (Austrian et al, 1977). Most infections with *Pneumococcus* occur before 2 years of age, after which significant immunity is acquired. Only about 15% of pneumococcal acquisitions result in disease, however, which is most common within 1 month of infection (Gray et al, 1980).

Natural History

Pneumococci are commonly found in the naso- and oral pharynx in the absence of infection. The production of disease necessitates invasion of the respiratory mucosa. The pathogenesis of pneumonia may well be aspiration of contaminated secretions from the upper airway. Alternatively, it could possibly follow bacteremia.

As in most infectious disease, the likelihood of an individual succumbing to disease is a function of the number of bacteria, their virulence, and inversely proportional to resistance which can be both native and acquired.

A predisposition to bacteremia from pneumococcal infection exists among individuals who are immunodeficient, especially those who are homozygous with respect to C3 deficiency and are subject to severe and recurrent infections. One of the mechanisms for removal of the organism is opsonization which is deficient in these individuals. Previous splenectomy or congenital asplenia is also an increased risk factor. The functional asplenia in patients with sickle cell anemia predisposes them to fulminant pneumococcal infection for similar reasons.

Clinical manifestations depend on site of infection. Infection in the middle ear may spread locally to mastoids and even meninges. Empyema, septic arthritis, and pericarditis may complicate the course.

Pneumococcal bacteremia may exist in the absence of any localized sign or symptom, and is called "occult bacteremia." It is most common in children 6–24 months of age who have a body temperature of 39°C or higher and a white blood count greater than 15,000/ml^3. In spite of the high fever, many of these children do not appear ill and often the bacteremia is self-limited. In others these findings herald the development of pneumonia or meningitis.

Primary peritonitis is also associated with pneumococcal infection. Although the route of entry of organisms is not known it presumably follows from the transient bacteremias. The clinical findings include the sudden onset of abdominal pain, nausea and vomiting, usually with fever. The condition is particularly common in children with the nephrotic syndrome.

Diagnosis

The diagnosis of pneumococcal infection depends on the recovery of the organism, either from the nose, throat, blood stream, or spinal fluid. Rapid diagnosis can be made with a direct quellung test utilizing pneumococcal serum that contains antibodies to 82 different types. A latex fixation test is useful for CSF but not serum or urine.

Peripheral blood is characterized by a pronounced leukocytosis, often with white cells in excess of 30,000. A Gram stain of the buffy coat of a centrifuged specimen may reveal Gram-positive diplococci.

Treatment

Penicillin remains the most effective drug against pneumococci. Children with uncomplicated otitis or pneumonia respond to 50,000 u/kg/day in four divided oral doses for 7–10 days. For meningitis, 400,000 u/kg/day aqueous penicillin G iv is required until the child is afebrile for 5 days, or a minimal course of 10 days. The reason for the high dose is suboptimal penetration of penicillin into CSF. Tube dilution studies should be carried out on pneumococci isolated from CSF.

For patients allergic to penicillin, erythromycin, chloramphenicol, and cephalosporins are effective alternatives.

In regions where strains of penicillin-resistant pneumococci are prevalent, such as South Africa, intravenous vancomycin is the drug of choice (Oppenheim and Koornhof, 1986).

Prevention

A new 23-valent pneumococcal vaccine was licensed in 1983 and is composed of capsular polysaccharide antigens from many of the most common serotypes.

A previously available 14-valent vaccine included only 71% of the types that cause bacteremia and meningitis in adults. Now the new 23-valent vaccine covers 97% of the types of pneumococci that cause bacteremia and meningitis in children and in 65% of the types associated with acute otitis media.

Children younger than 5 years of age have relatively poor antibody response to some of the polysaccharide antigens but can respond to others. In one study, vaccination of healthy infants at 6 months stimulated an increase in serum antibody against only 1 of 8 vaccine antigens, and that stimulation did not persist. A better response takes place in children immunized between ages 2 and 6 years, but the best response is in those over 6 years. For detailed guidelines, see Report of Committee on Infectious Diseases, American Academy of Pediatrics, 20th edition, 1986, Elk Grove Village, IL 60007.

TULAREMIA

Definition

Tularemia is an acute febrile illness caused by *Francisella tularensis* usually acquired after contact with wild rabbits. The ulceroglandular syndrome is the most common manifestation.

Basic Science

The organism is a coccobacillary Gram-negative nonmotile, nonencapsulated organism.

Epidemiology

The disease is very rare, and under 300 cases were reported to the Centers for Disease Control during 1985. Evans et al (1985) described an experience gained over 30 years with 88 cases. Seventy-five percent were ulceroglandular in type, and 25% were typhoidal with two deaths.

The disease has been found in most parts of the northern hemisphere. It is most common in southeastern and north central states during the summer months when ticks, which are vectors, and rabbit hunting are most prevalent. Dogs can disseminate ticks, and cats can be infected.

Natural History

The organism can gain access to the body through the bite of a tick or an infected animal and occasionally through the respiratory or gastrointestinal tract. It then enters the lymphatics and bacteremia persists for about the first week. An overwhelming inoculation can result in an extreme toxemia in association with septicemia characterized by shock, renal failure, and death. More commonly at any time between 1 and 21 days after exposure, there is the onset of chills and fever, headache and photophobia, with enlarged lymph nodes, liver and spleen, and a variety of skin rashes including erythema nodosum, which may appear during the second week of the illness. The different types of tularemia have been described under the headings of ulceroglandular, glandular, oculoglandular, typhoidal, or pharyngeal and pneumonic, each of which focuses on the predominant symptoms from this widespread granulomatus illness (Jacobs et al, 1985).

Diagnosis

A history of exposure is of central importance. No pathognomonic clinical features of the disease exist, although cutaneous ulcers occur in over half the patients. An agglutination test is usually employed for diagnosis. Paired samples with a demonstration of a rise in titer are considered diagnostic (peak titers are between the 11th and 16th day). Culturing should not be carried out in routine hospital laboratories because of the danger to the personnel. Special laboratories are available and information can be obtained from local state health department or the Centers for Disease Control.

Treatment

Streptomycin is the drug of choice for the treatment of tularemia in doses of 30–40 mg/kg/day for 10 days. Although tetracyclines and chlorampenicol are also effective, relapse may occur after they have been discontinued.

Prevention

Children should be aware of handling sick or dead rabbits or rodents. No effective vaccine is available; the disease is so rare that immunization of the general population is not warranted. Nevertheless, if individuals are at risk because of the nature of their work for example, they should contact the Centers for Disease Control for access to unlicensed vaccine.

VIBRIO CHOLERAE

Definition

Cholera, caused by *Vibrio cholerae,* is characterized by a fulminant secretory diarrhea, which is fatal without fluid replacement.

Basic Science

Vibrio cholerae is a Gram-negative motile bacillus with a single flagellum. The name comes from the apparent "vibrations" of the organism in wet preparations. The organism synthesizes a protein enterotoxin, which produces the diarrhea, and a neuraminidase and a mucinase which hydrolyze intestinal mucus. The toxins activate ATP to form 3'5'-cyclic adenosine monophosphate (cAMP), which in turn stimulates a secretory mechanism in the intestinal mucosa that moves liquid and electrolytes from the extracellular space into the intestinal lumen. Agglutinating antibodies reach a peak 1–2 weeks after onset of disease, but wane after a few months, which accounts for the frequency of reinfection.

Epidemiology

Cholera has been, and in some regions continues to be, one of the most devastating pandemics of history. It is seen mostly in Bangladesh, India, and other regions of Asia. Only a few cases are reported each year in the United States. It is one of the few causes of death from acute gastroenteritis in adults.

Natural History

V. cholerae are ingested by mouth and colonize in the small intestine. Watery diarrhea of gradual or sudden onset characterizes the illness. Vomiting may precede the diarrhea. The stools are described as like rice water. Progressive dehydration is the most severe threat to life. Children may be febrile, lethargic, and prone to seizures. Hypovolemia and potassium losses lead to renal failure. Rehydration without added potassium promotes fluid shifts from extracellular to intracellular spaces with profound hypokalemia.

Diagnosis

The extensive water losses from diarrhea in endemic areas suggest the diagnosis. Confirmation depends on identification of the organism in the stool.

The watery stool is isotonic with serum and contains about 50 mMol of bicarbonate per liter. The loss of bicarbonate contributes to a profound metabolic acidosis, which is made even worse by lactic acidemia and renal failure from hypovolemia and shock. The acidosis is normochloremic in part because the rapid development of dehydration does not permit sufficient time for the kidneys to retain chloride (Wang et al, 1986).

Treatment

Treatment requires replacement of lost fluid, which can be done with adequate amounts of WHO oral electrolyte solutions. Even in individuals who are vomiting, this solution is tolerated and is life-saving (Pierce and Hirschhorn, 1977).

Antibiotics can shorten the course of illness. Tetracycline, 30 mg/kg/day for 2–3 days is effective in children. Trimethoprim-sulfamethoxazole is also effective. Nevertheless, antibiotics are of less importance than early institution of oral fluid replacement and may not be necessary.

YERSINIA ENTEROCOLITICA

Definition

Yersinia is a widely distributed Gram-negative coccobacillary pathogen of the small intestine that produces acute and chronic diarrheal disease in young children, and a variety of systemic symptoms in older individuals.

Basic Science

This organism has been known since 1939, but its role in disease was not widely appreciated until the work of Carlsson et al in 1964. Now that most laboratory personnel recognize its characteristics, it is more commonly identified as an important cause of enteric and systemic infections.

Organisms invade Peyer patches and regional lymph nodes in the distal ileum. Systemic spread with microabscess production can occur. The terminal ileitis can include the appendix.

Epidemiology

The organism has been identified in outbreaks of diarrheal disease in institutions, as well as in sporadic cases from contaminated water and food. Many animals harbor the organism, which appears to thrive in colder climates and may persist for prolonged periods in fresh water. The incidence of infection is not known, since reporting is not required.

Natural History

The incubation period is not known. Infection in children results in abdominal pain, often mimicking appendicitis, but is from mesenteric adenitis. Matted lymph nodes are found in the region of the terminal ileum at operation. In older children and young adults the disease is more commonly restricted to the bowel, and produces a watery diarrhea which may persist for several weeks. An acute polyarthritis can occur weeks after the onset of diarrhea and persist for several months.

Sometimes a full-blown Reiter syndrome with uveitis, conjunctivitis, erythema nodosum, and myocarditis follows Yersinia infection. Septicemia, usually in host-compromised adults, has about 40% mortality. Individuals with iron-overload states are at high risk.

Diagnosis

If the laboratory is alerted that Yersinia may be present, the organism can be identified in fresh stool specimens. Acute and convalescent sera are necessary to identify serotypes. Peripheral leukocytosis is common.

Treatment

Most strains are sensitive to tetracyclines, chloramphenicol, and sulfonamides. No evidence supports their use in shortening the course of disease, however, and the resemblance of late manifestations to some drug reactions gives caution to use of antimicrobials. Only if the organism is recovered from the blood or in immunodeficient individuals would most experts advise their use.

Prognosis

Most infections in previously healthy children are acute and self-limited. Individuals with immune-deficiency disorders have a serious prognosis and require early antimicrobial therapy.

Prevention

Only avoidance of the organism (by not drinking water in streams and lakes, for example) is effective prevention. No vaccines are available.

CASE ILLUSTRATION

A 5-month-old male was admitted with fever and bloody diarrhea. He was well until 10 days before admission when loose stools developed. For 1 week before admission, there were intermittent fevers (38.7°C). Three days before admission, a bilateral otitis was diagnosed and he was treated with amoxicillin. Because he continued to remain febrile and irritable he was brought to the emergency room where initial examination showed a temperature of 38.7°C with evidence of a resolving bilateral otitis and an otherwise unremarkable physical examination. Rectal examination was notable for guaiac-negative stool and many polys on Gram stain. Because of his young age, fever, and irritability, a septic work-up was performed with a white count of 18,200 thousand with 9% polys and 28% bands, hematocrit of 32, and a normal platelet count. CSF and urinalysis were unremarkable. Cultures of blood, urine, CSF, and stool were obtained.

QUESTIONS AND COMMENTS

What are the diagnostic possibilities, and how should this child be treated?

This child was admitted with the working diagnosis of bacterial colitis, and possible complicating sepsis. *Salmonella* and *Shigella* were considered most likely etiologies. Pneumococcal or *H. influenzae* bacteremia were also possible, given the presence of the otitis. The infant was given intravenous trimethoprim-sulfamethoxazole while cultures were pending. After 2 days, all cultures were negative and the baby was discharged without antibiotics because diarrhea was resolving. Two days after discharge a stool culture grew out Gram-negative bacteria that were later identified as *Yersinia enterocolitica.*

Given the finding of *Yersinia*, does this child need further treatment?

Treatment remains controversial. Whereas the bacteria are usually sensitive to trimethoprim-sulfamethoxazole in vitro, there are no data which show that antibiotics shorten the duration of the diarrhea or provide a bacteriologic cure. Nor is it known whether earlier therapy can provide better results. This patient was followed carefully but further antibiotics were withheld. He recovered fully.

YERSINIA PESTIS (formerly *Pasteurella pestis*)

Definition

Yersinia pestis is a Gram-negative nonmotile, pleomorphic bacillus that causes bubonic plague. It is endemic in rodents and spreads among them by fleas. The organism is endemic in the American West.

Epidemiology

The infection is very rare in the western world. Only 10 cases were reported in the United States in

1986. Apparently only certain rodent populations are reservoirs of the bacillus and spread of infection to humans requires close contact with infected rats and the vector fleas. Once the bacillus is in the human population, it can spread directly from inhalation of respiratory droplets. However, persistence of the disease depends on continuing contact with infected rodents and their fleas.

Plague has had an important effect in human history. Epidemics of The Black Death have killed millions of people in Europe and Asia. From 1346–1352 it is estimated that about 20 million people died from the plague in Europe alone. About 75% of those infected in the 14th century died from it.

Natural History

Bacilli are transmitted into humans through flea bites. The organisms enter lymphatics and multiply in regional lymph nodes. The enlarged, tender nodes are called buboes, hence, the name bubonic plague. If the bacilli enter the blood stream, meningitis, pneumonia, and intravascular coagulation may occur. The incubation period is 2–6 days, except after human-to-human spread, when it can be a matter of hours.

The victim has fever, tachycardia, myalgia, and eventually delirium and shock. Vomiting and bloody diarrhea may occur.

Diagnosis

The diagnosis should be considered in individuals in contact with rodents. Smears of purulent exudates or sputum, stained with Giemsa or Wayson stain, may reveal the organism.

Treatment

Streptomycin is bactericidal for *Yersinia pestis*. It can be given intramuscularly for 10 days. Tetracycline is also effective and can be given orally if the individual is not severely ill or vomiting. Chloramphenicol can be used if the organism is resistant to other drugs with early treatment. The mortality is under 10%. The septicemic form, however, has a higher case fatality rate (about 70%) (Mann et al, 1980).

Prevention

Prevention consists of elimination of infected rodents or, at least, avoidance of contact with them. If the latter is not feasible, a heat-killed vaccine is available. Chemoprophylaxis is indicated after known exposure.

REFERENCES

Abernathy RS, Dutt AK, Stead WW, et al: Short-course chemotherapy for tuberculosis in children. *Pediatrics* 72:801, 1983.

Abramson JS, Spika JS: Persistence of *Neisseria meningitidis* in the upper respiratory tract after intravenous antibiotic therapy for systemic meningococcal disease. *J Infect Dis* 151:370, 1985.

Ambrosino D: Correlation between G2M(N) immunoglobulin allotype and human antibody response and susceptibility to polysaccharide encapsulated bacteria. *J Clin Invest* 75:1935, 1985.

American Thoracic Society: Treatment of tuberculosis and tuberculosis infection in adults and children. *Am Rev Respir Dis* 134:355, 1986.

Arnon SS, Chin J: The clinical spectrum of infant botulism. *Rev Infect Dis* 1:614, 1979.

Arnon SS, Mills DC, Day PA: Rapid death of infant rhesus monkeys injected with *Clostridium difficile* toxins A and B: Physiologic and pathologic basis. *J Pediatr* 104:34, 1984.

Austrian R, Howie VM, Ploussard JH: The bacteriology of pneumococcal otitis media. *Johns Hopkins Med J* 141:104, 1977.

Baker RD, Edwards MS, et al: Neonatal immunity to Type III group B streptococcal (III GBS) polysaccharide from maternal third trimester vaccination. *Pediatr Res* 19:287A, 1985.

Barson WJ, Miller MA, Brady MT, et al: Prospective comparative trial of ceftriaxone vs conventional therpay for treatment of bacterial meningitis in children. *Pediatr Infect Dis* 4:362, 1985.

Beem MO, Saxon EM: Respiratory tract colonization and a distinctive pneumonia syndrome in infants infected with *Chlamydia trachomatis*. *N Engl J Med* 296:306, 1977.

Borgado F, et al: Hemolytic anemia, splenic abscess and pleural effusion caused by *Salmonella typhi*. *J Infect Dis* 142:945, 1980.

Boyer KM, Gotoff SP: Prevention of early-onset neonatal group B streptococcal disease with selective intravenous chemoprophylaxis. *N Engl J Med* 314:1665, 1986.

Breese B, Denny FW, Dillon H, et al: Consensus: Difficult management problems in children with streptococcal pharyngitis. *Pediatr Infect Dis* 4:10, 1985.

Britigan BE, Cohen MS, Sparling PF: Gonococcal infection: A model of molecular pathogenesis. *N Engl J Med* 312:1683, 1985.

Brunnell PA: Prevention of pertussis, *Haemophilus* and varicella infections. *Pediatr Infect Dis* 4:439, 1985.

Buchanan GR: The mild anemia of acute infection. *Pediatr Infect Dis* 4:225, 1985.

Buchdahl R, Levine M, Wilkins B, et al: Toxic shock syndrome. *Arch Dis Child* 60:563, 1985.

Caglar MK, Ozsoylu MD, Kaura G: Relative granulocytosis in childhood typhoid fever. *J Pediatr* 102:603, 1983.

CDC: Annual Summary 1983. *MMWR* 32:3, 1984; CPC of Massachusetts General Hospital. *N Engl J Med* 311:172, 1984.

CDC: Botulism from fresh foods—California. *MMWR* 34:156, 1985.

CDC: Changing trends in gonococcal antibiotic resistance in the United States, 1983-84 in CDC surveillance summaries. 33:11SS, 1984.

CDC: *Chlamydia trachomatis* infections. *MMWR* (Suppl) 34:35, 1985.

CDC: Drug-resistant tuberculosis among the homeless—Boston. *MMWR* 34:429, 1985.

CDC: *MMWR* 34:111, 1985.

CDC: *MMWR* 34:299, 1985.

CDC: Pertussis—Washington 1984. *MMWR* 34:390, 1985.

CDC: Polysaccharide vaccine for prevention of *Haemophilus influenzae* type B disease. *MMWR* 34:201, 1985.

CDC: Sexually transmitted diseases treatment guidelines 1985. *MMWR* 34(Suppl 4S):815, 1985.

CDC: Tetanus—United States 1985–1986. *MMWR* 36:477, 1987.

CDC: Update: Prevention of *Haemophilus influenzae* type B disease. *MMWR* 37:13, 1988.

Chaudhary S, Bilinsky SA, Hennessy JL, et al: Penicillin V and rifampin for the treatment of group A streptococcal pharyngitis: A randomized trial of 10 days penicillin vs 10 days penicillin with rifampin during the final 4 days of therapy. *J Pediatr* 106:481, 1985.

Christensen RD, Hill HR, et al: Intravenous human immune globulin prevents neutropenia, neutrophil supply exhaustion and death in experimental group B streptococcal sepsis. *Pediatr Res* 19:289A, 1985.

Claesson BA, Trollfors B, Lagergard T, et al: Clinical and immunologic responses to the capsular polysaccharide of *Haemophilus influenzaė* type B alone or conjugated to tetanus toxoid in 18- to 23-month-old children. *J Pediatr* 112:695, 1988.

Clegg HW, et al: Fulminant neonatal meningococcemia. *Am J Dis Child* 134:354, 1980.

Cochi S, Broome CV, Hightower AW: Immunization of US children with *Hemophilus influenzae* type b polysaccharide vaccine. *JAMA* 253:521, 1985.

Cohen JI, Bartlett JA, Corey GR: Extra-intestinal manifestations of *Salmonella* infections. *Medicine* 66:349, 1987.

Committee on Infectious Diseases: *Haemophilus* type b polysaccharide vaccine. *Pediatrics* 76:322, 1985.

Cooperstock MS, Steffen E, Yolken R, et al: *Clostridium difficile* in normal infants and sudden infant death syndrome: A relationship with infant formula feeding. *Pediatrics* 70:91, 1982.

Curry WA: Human nocardiasis. *Arch Intern Med* 140:818, 1980.

Daniel TM, DeMurillo GL, Sawyer JA,et al: Field evaluation of enzyme-linked immunosorbent assay for the serodiagnosis of tuberculosis. *Am Rev Respir Dis* 134:662, 1986.

Davis JP: Toxic shock syndrome: Epidemiologic features, recurrence, risk factors and prevention. *N Engl J Med* 303:1429, 1980.

Dezfulian M, Yolken R, Bartlett J: Rapid diagnosis of a case of infant botulism by enzyme immunoassay. *Pediatr Infect Dis* 4:399, 1985.

Dubos R, Dubos J: *The White Plague*. Boston, Little, Brown and Co., 1952.

Eden AN: Vibrio fetus meningitis in a newborn infant. *J Pediatr* 61:33, 1962.

Edmonson RS, Flowers WW: Intensive care in tetanus. Management, complications and mortality in 100 cases. *Br Med J* 1:1401, 1979.

Edwards MD, Rench, MA, Haffar AAM, et al: Long-term sequelae of group B streptococcal meningitis in infants. *Pediatrics* 106:717, 1985.

English PC: Diphtheria and theories of infectious disease: Centennial application of the critical role of diphtheria in the history of medicine. *Pediatrics* 76:1, 1985.

Escola J, Peltola H, Takala AK, et al: Efficacy of *Haemophilus influenzae* type b polysaccharide-diphtheria toxoid conjugate vaccine in infancy. *N Engl J Med* 317:717, 1987.

Evans JR, Allen AC, Bortolussi R, et al: Follow-up study of survivors of fetal and early onset neonatal listerosis. *Clin Invest Med* 7:329, 1984.

Evans ME, Gregory DW, Schaffner W, et al: Tularemia: A 30-year experience with 88 cases. *Medicine* 64:251, 1985.

Evans AF, Oakley RH, Whitehouse GH: Analysis of chest radiographs in Legionnaires' disease. *Clin Radiol* 32:361, 1981.

Feigin RD: Campylobacter fetus infections. In Feigin RD, Cherry J (eds): *Textbook of Pediatric Infectious Diseases*. Philadelphia, WB Saunders, 1981, p. 833.

Felice GA, Fraser DW: Management of household contacts of leprosy patients. *Ann Intern Med* 88:538, 1978.

Finegold SM: Clostridial intoxication and infection. In Feigin RD, Cherry JM (eds): *Textbook of Pediatric Infectious Diseases*. Philadelphia, WB Saunders, 1981, p. 837.

Fleming DW, Cochi SL, MacDonald KL: Pasteurized milk as a vehicle of infection in an outbreak of listerosis. *N Engl J Med* 312:404, 1985.

Frazier AR, Rosenow EC, Roberts GD. Nocardiasis: A review of 25 occurring during 24 months. *Mayo Clin Proc* 50:657, 1977.

Friedman AD, Fleischer GR: Unsuspected meningococcemia treated with orally administered amoxicillin. *Pediatr Infect Dis* 1:38, 1982.

Friesen CA, Cho CT: Characteristic features of neonatal sepsis due to *Haemophilus influenzae*. *Rev Infect Dis* 8:777, 1986.

Frost WH: Diphtheria in Baltimore: A comparative study of morbidity, carrier prevalence and antitoxic immunity in 1921-24 and 1933-36. In Maxcy KF (ed): *Papers of Wade Hampton Frost MD, A Contribution to Epidemiological Method*. New York, Commonwealth Fund, 1941.

Geiseler PJ, Nelson KE, Reddi KT: Unusual aspects of salmonella meningitis. *Clin Pediatr* 19:699, 1980.

Gerber MA, Markowitz M: Management of streptococcal pharyngitis reconsidered. *Pediatr Infect Dis* 4:578, 1985.

Godel JC: Trial of pyridoxine therapy for tetanus neonatorum. *J Infect Dis* 145:547, 1982.

Good AE: Streptococcal endocarditis initially seen as septic arthritis. *NY Arch Intern Med* 138:805, 1978.

Granoff DM, Shackelford PG, Suarez BK, et al: *Hemophilus influenzae* type B disease in children vaccinated with type B polysaccharide vaccine. *N Engl J Med* 315:1584, 1986.

Gray BM, Converse GM III, Dillon HC Jr: Epidemiologic studies of *Streptococcus pneumoniae* in infants: Acquisition, carriage, and infection during the first 24 months of life. *J Infect Dis* 142:923, 1980.

Grayston JT, Kuo CC, Wang SP, et al: A new *Chlamydia psittaci* strain. TWAR, isolated in acute respiratory tract infections. *N Engl J Med* 315:161, 1986.

Hammerschlag MR: Chlamydial infections. *Pediatr Rev* 3:77, 1981.

Hammerschlag MR: Neonatal ocular prophylaxis, *Pediatr Infect Dis* 7:81, 1988.

Hendren WH, Haggerty RJ: Staphylococcal pneumonia in infancy and childhood: Analysis of 75 cases. *JAMA* 68:6, 1958.

Higham M, Cunningham FM, Teele DW: Ceftriaxone administered once or twice a day for treatment of bacterial infections of childhood. *Pediatr Infect Dis* 4:22, 1985.

Hornick RB: Salmonella infections. Shigella infections. In Feigin RD, Cherry JD eds: *Textbook of Pediatric Infections*. Vol I, Philadelphia, WB Saunders, 1981, pp. 455–464; 464–469.

Hyams JS, et al: Salmonella bacteremia in the first year of life. *J Pediatr* 96:57, 1980.

Iosub S, Bamji M, Stone RK, et al: More on human immunodeficiency virus embryopathy. *Pediatrics* 80:512, 1987.

Issekutz TB, Evans J, Bortolussi R: The immune response of human neonates to *Listeria monocytogenes* infection. *Clin Invest Med* 7:281, 1984.

Jacobs RF, Condrey YM, Yamauchi T: Tularemia in adults and children: A changing presentation. *Pediatrics* 76:818, 1985.

Johnson RO, et al: Diagnosis and management of infantile botulism. *Am J Dis Child* 133:586, 1979.

Kaplan EL: Acute rheumatic fever. *Pediatr Clin North Am* 25:817, 1978.

Karmali MA, Fleming PC: *Campylobacter* enteritis in children. *J Pediatr* 94:527, 1979.

Keller MA, Aftandelians R, Connor JD: Etiology of pertussis syndrome. *Pediatrics* 66:50, 1980.

Keller MA, Rodriguez AL, Alvarez S, et al: Transfer of tubercular immunity from mother to infant. *Pediatr Res* 22:227, 1987.

Keusch GT: *Yersinia enterocolitica* infections. In Feigin RD, Cherry JD (eds): *Textbook of Pediatric Infections*. Vol I. Philadelphia, WB Saunders, 1981, pp. 470–475.

Kipps A: The duration and possible significance of the depression of tuberculin sensitivity following measles. *S Afr Med J* 40:104, 1966.

Kirby BD, Snyder KM, Meyer RD, et al: Legionnaires' disease: Report of 65 nosocomially acquired cases and review of the literature. *Medicine* 59:188, 1980.

Laga M, Naamara W, Brunham RC, et al: Single dose therapy of gonococcal ophthalmia neonatorum with ceftriaxone. *N Engl J Med* 315:1382, 1986.

Lee MM, Welliver RC, LaScolea LJ: Campylobacter meningitis in childhood. *Pediatr Infect Dis* 4:544, 1985.

Lenoir AA, Granoff PD, Granoff DM: Immunogenicity of *Haemophilus influenzae* type b polysaccharide-*Neisseria meningitidis* outer membrane protein conjugate vaccine in 2- to 6-month old infants. *Pediatrics* 80:283, 1987.

Levine MM: *Escherichia coli* infections. *N Engl J Med* 313:445, 1985.

Light I, Saidleman M, Sutherland JM: Management of newborns after nursery exposure to tuberculosis. *Am Rev Respir Dis* 109:415, 1974.

Lincoln EM, Sewell EM: *Tuberculosis in Children*. New York, McGraw Hill, 1963.

Mangenello FP, et al: Neonatal meningococcal meningitis and meningococcemia. *Am J Dis Child* 133:651, 1979.

Mann JM, Shandler L, Cushing AH: Pediatric plague. *Pediatrics* 69:762, 1982.

Markowitz M, Gordis L: *Rheumatic Fever—Diagnosis, Management and Prevention*. 2nd edition. Philadelphia, WB Saunders Co, 1972.

Massell BF, Chute CG, Walker AM, et al: Penicillin and the marked decrease in morbidity and mortality from rheumatic fever in the United States. *N Engl J Med* 318:280, 1988.

McEvedy C: The bubonic plague. *Sci Am* 258:118, 1988.

Medical Letter: Rapid office diagnostic tests for streptococcal pharyngitis. 27:49, 1985.

Melish ME, Glasgow LA: Staphylococcal scalded skin syndrome. *J Pediatr* 78:958, 1971.

Melish ME: Staphylococcal infections. In Feigin R, Cherry J (eds): *Pediatric Infectious Diseases*. Philadelphia, WB Saunders, 1981.

Memon IA, et al: Group B streptococcal osteomyelitis and septic arthritis: Its occurrence in infants less than 2 months old. *Am J Dis Child* 133:921, 1979.

Mills JT, Parsonnet J, Hickman RK, et al: Control of production of toxic shock syndrome toxin-1 (TSST-1) by magnesium ion. *J Infect Dis* 151:1158, 1985.

Mofenson LM: Lyme disease: Recognition, treatment and prevention. Report of State Laboratory Institute. Department of Public Health, Commonwealth of Massachusetts, June 3, 1985.

Molteni RA: Group A Beta hemolytic streptococcal pneumonia clinical course and complications of management. *Am J Dis Child* 131:1366, 1977.

Moseley SL, Echeverria P, Seriwatana J, et al: Identification of enterotoxigenic *Escherichia coli* by colony hybridization among three enterotoxin gene probes. *J Infect Dis* 145:863, 1982.

Moxon ER: *Haemophilus influenzae* vaccine. *Pediatrics* 77:258, 1986.

National ACCP Consensus Conference on Tuberculosis. Iseman MD, Sbarbaro JA (eds): *Chest* 87:(Suppl)115S-149S, 1985.

Nelson SJ, Granoff D: Salmonella gastroenteritis in the first 3 months of life. A review of management and complications. *Clin Pediatr* 21:709, 1982.

Nemir RL, O'Hare D: Congenital tuberculosis. Review and diagnostic guidelines. *Am J Dis Child* 139:284, 1985.

O'Brien RT, Santos JI, Glasgow L, et al: Pathophysiologic basis of anemia associated with *Haemophilus influenzae* meningitis. *J Pediatr* 98:928, 1981.

O'Hanley P, Low D, Romero I, et al: Gal-Gal binding and hemolysis phenotypes and genotypes associated with uropathogenic *Escherichia coli. N Engl J Med* 313:414, 1985.

Oppenheim B, Koornhof, HJ: Antibiotic-resistant pneumococcal disease in children at Baragwanath Hospital, Johannesburg. *Pediatr Infect Dis* 5:520, 1986.

Osterholm MT, Pierson LM, White KE, et al: The risk of subsequent transmission of *Hemophilus influenzae* type B disease among children in day care. *N Engl J Med* 316:1, 1987.

Pai CH, Gillis F, Tuomanen E, et al: Placebo-controlled double-blind evaluation of *Yersina enterocolitica* gastroenteritis. *J Pediatr* 104:308, 1984.

Pappenheimer AM Jr, Murphy JR: Studies on the molecular epidemiology of diphtheria. *Lancet* 2:923, 1983.

Peevy KJ, Chartrand SA, Wiseman HJ, et al: Myocardial dysfunction in group B streptococcal shock. *Pediatr Res* 19:511, 1985.

Peltola H, Kayhty H, Virtanen M, et al: Prevention of *Hemophilus influenzae* type B bacteremic infections with the capsular polysaccharide vaccine. *N Engl J Med* 310:1561, 1984.

Pickett J, Berg B, Chaplin E, et al: Syndrome of botulism in infancy. Clinical and electrophysiologic study. *N Engl J Med* 295:770, 1976.

Pierce NF, Hirschhorn N: Oral fluid—a simple weapon against dehydration in diarrhoea: How it works and how to use it. *WHO Chron* 31:87, 1977.

Pifer LLW, Woods DR, Edwards CC, et al: *Pneumocystis carinii* serologic study in pediatric acquired immunodeficiency syndrome. *Am J Dis Child* 142:36, 1988.

Polin RA, Brown LW: Infant botulism. *Pediatr Clin North Am* 26:345, 1979.

Prince A: *Pseudomonas cepacia* in cystic fibrosis patients. *Am Rev Respir Dis* 134:644, 1986.

Pyati SP, Pildes RS, Jacobs NM, et al: Penicillin in infants weighing two kilograms or less with early-onset group B streptococcal disease. *N Engl J Med* 308:1383, 1983.

Reed MD, Kliegman RM, Weiner JS, et al: The clinical pharmacology of vancomycin in seriously ill preterm infants. *Pediatr Res* 22:360, 1987.

Reingold AL, et al: Age specific differences in duration of clinical protection after vaccination with meningococcal polysaccharide A vaccine. *Lancet* 2:114, 1985.

Reingold AL: Epidemiology of toxic-shock syndrome: United States, 1960-1984. *MMWR* 33:1955, 1985.

Rettig PJ: *Chlamydia* infections in pediatrics: Not for babies only. *J Pediatr* 104:82, 1984.

Sato P, Madtes DK, Thorning D, et al: Bronchiolitis obliterans caused by *Legionella pneumophila. Chest* 6:87, 1985.

Schachter J, Sweet RL, Grossman M, et al: Experience with the routine use of erythromycin for Chlamydial infections in pregnancy. *N Engl J Med* 314:276, 1986.

Schachter J, Grossman M, Sweet RL, et al: Prospective study of perinatal transmission of *Chlamydia trachomatis. JAMA* 255:3374, 1986.

Schlech WF: New perspectives in the gastrointestinal mode of transmission in invasive *Listeria monocytogenes* infection. *Clin Invest Med* 7:321, 1984.

Schlesinger PA, Duray PH, Burke BA, et al: Maternal-fetal transmission of the Lyme disease spirochete, Borrelia bargdorferi. *Ann Intern Med* 103:67, 1985.

Schwartz RH, Wientzen RL, Pedrira F, et al: Penicillin V for group A streptococcal pharyngitis. *JAMA* 246:1790, 1981.

Sell SH: *Haemophilus influenzae* type B meningitis: Manifestations and long term sequelae. *Pediatr Infect Dis* 6:775, 1987.

Sewell EM, O'Hare D, Kendig EL: The tuberculin test. *Pediatrics* 54:650, 1974.

Shulman ST (ed): Management of Pharyngitis in an Era of Declining Rheumatic Fever. Report of 86th Ross Conference on Pediatric Research. Columbus OH, Ross Laboratories, 1984.

Shurin SB, Anderson P, Zollinger J, et al: Pathophysiology of hemolysis in infections with *Haemophilus influenzae* type B. *J Clin Invest* 77:1340, 1986.

Siegel JD, McCracken GH Jr, Threlkeld N, et al: Single dose penicillin prophylaxis of neonatal group B streptococcal disease. Conclusion of a 41 month controlled trial. *Lancet* 1:1426, 1982.

Smith DH, Peter G, Ingram DL, et al: Responses of children immunized with the capsular polysaccharide of *Haemophilus influenzae* type B. *Pediatrics* 52:637, 1973.

Smith MHD, Marquis JR: Tuberculosis and other mycobacterial infections. In Feigin R, Cherry J (eds): *Textbook of Pediatric Infectious Diseases.* Philadelphia, WB Saunders, 1981, pp. 1051–1054.

Steere AC, et al: The spirochetal etiology of Lyme disease. *N Engl J Med* 308:733, 1983.

Steere AC, et al: Successful parenteral penicillin therapy of established Lyme arthritis. *N Engl J Med* 312:869, 1985.

Street L, Grant WW, Alva JD: Brucellosis in childhood. *Pediatrics* 55:416, 1975.

Swingle HM, Bucciarelli RL, Ayouh EM: Synergy between penicillins and low concentrations of gentamicin in the killing of Group B streptococci. *J Infect Dis* 152:515, 1985.

Tait KA, Lawrenchuk DW, et al: Legionellosis-Staffordshire England and Wayne County Michigan. *MMWR* 34:344, 1985.

Teele DW, Marshall R, Klein JO: Unsuspected bacteremia in young children. *Pediatr Clin North Am* 26:773, 1979.

Todd S, Fishaut M, Kapral F, Welch T: Toxic shock syndrome associated with phage group I staphylococci. *Lancet* 2:116, 1978.

Tompkins LS, Roessler BJ, Redd SC, et al: Legionella prosthetic-valve endocarditis. *N Engl J Med* 318:530, 1988.

Turner TB, Stafford ES, Goldman L: Studies on the duration of protection afforded by active immunization against tetanus. *Bull Johns Hopkins Hosp* 94:204, 1954.

Vesikari T, Janas M, Gronroos P, et al: Neonatal septicaema. *Arch Dis Child* 60:542, 1985.

Victoria MS, Shah BR: Bacillus Calmette-Guerin lymphadenitis: A case report and review of literature. *Pediatr Infect Dis* 4:295, 1985.

Viscide RP, Bartlett JG: Antibiotic-associated pseudomembraneous colitis in children. *Pediatrics* 67:381, 1981.

Wang F, Butler T, Rabbani GH, et al: The acidosis of cholera. *N Engl J Med* 315:1591, 1986.

Ward J, Lum MKW, Bender TR: Influenza disease in Alaska. In: Sell SH, Wright PF(eds): *Haemophilus Influenzae.* New York, Elsevier, 1982.

Weinstein L: Tetanus. *N Engl J Med* 289:1293, 1973.

Welch DF, Marks MI: Is *Clostridium difficile* pathogenic in infants? *J Pediatr* 100:393, 1982.

Wilson R, et al: Clinical characteristics of infant botulism in the United States: A study of the 9 California cases. *Pediatr Infect Dis* 277:148, 1982.

Wise MB, Beaudry PH, Bates DV: Long-term followup of staphylococcal pneumonia. *Pediatrics* 38:398, 1966.
Wolinsky E: Nontuberculus mycobacteria and associated diseases. *Am Rev Respir Dis* 119:107, 1979.
Yow MD: Brucellosis. In Feigin R, Cherry J (eds): *Textbook of Pediatric Infectious Diseases*. Philadelphia, WB Saunders, 1981, pp. 828-833.

Treponemes 6

SYPHILIS

Definition

Infection with *Treponema pallidum,* a flagellated highly mobile spirochete, acquired by transplacental transmission beyond the fourth month of gestation, can result in stillbirth or the manifestations of disease in liveborn infants.

Epidemiology

Once one of the most common congenital infections, syphilis is now rare, but staging a modest comeback. Approximately 30,000 cases of syphilis in adults are reported each year in the United States (12.2 cases/100,000 population in 1984). The incidence of congenital syphilis is about 1 in 10,000 live births in the United States, 244 cases were reported in 1984, and 365 were reported in 1986. Texas, California, Florida, and metropolitan New York City accounted for 80% of all reported cases of congenital syphilis.

Natural History

The organism enters the fetal circulation and reaches its first target, the liver; it may involve skin, mucous membranes, lips and anus, bones, and CNS. The lungs may be involved in an extensive pneumonia, called pneumonia alba, most commonly seen in stillbirths which occur in the third trimester in 20–30% of cases of early maternal syphilis. The risk of transmission to the fetus approaches 100% in untreated primary or secondary syphilis.

Some infected infants are asymptomatic for the first few weeks. The majority may have persistent snuffles, with a serosanguinous discharge. Cutaneous lesions are copper-colored, and desquamative, especially over the perioral or perinasal and diaper regions. Palms and soles may be involved. In heavily infected infants, the rash can be generalized. Radial cracks appear at mucocutaneous junctions which may persist for years as rhagades.

More than 90% of infants have osteochondritis and periostitis, with thickening of the periosteum. The lesions resemble those of scurvy, but appear within the first 3 months, which is earlier than scurvy.

Hepatomegaly, lymphadenopathy, anemia from bone marrow involvement may be severe, and cause hydrops. Congenital nephrosis may result from syphilitic infection (Oppenheimer and Hardy, 1971).

Signs of CNS involvement may not be evident in the newborn, but may be manifested by an elevated protein and mononuclear cells up to 300/ml CSF. Dental changes (Hutchinson teeth or notched upper central incisors, abnormal enamel and excessive cusps on first lower molars) appear with permanent teeth eruption. Fetal or perinatal death occurs in 40% of affected infants (CDC, 1988).

Diagnosis

Dark-field examination of any nasal discharge is advised; the placenta and umbilical cord are good sites for collection of specimens. The best laboratory test is identification of a specific IgM antibody (IgM-FTA, ABS) (fluorescent-labeled antihuman immunoglobulin), although it may not be positive at birth if infection was acquired late in gestation. Unfortunately this test is only available in specialized research laboratories. The most widely used test is the FTA-ABS test (fluorescent treponemal antibody-absorption), but it is time-consuming and is not recommended for general screening because of false-positive and false-negative reactions.

If the mother has positive serology (VDRL or other flocculation test), the infant will have a similar positive test on cord blood. If the mother has not been treated, the positive value could mean infection, and the infant should be treated. If mother was adequately treated, the infant need not be treated if asymptomatic, but repeat serology should be done at 1 month. A falling titer indicates the infant's antibodies were acquired by passive transfer of antibody from mother (Srinivasan et al, 1983).

Treatment

All infants should have an examination of CSF as a baseline before starting therapy. Infants without CNS involvement require a dose of 50,000 u of aqueous procaine penicillin per kg/day in two divided doses administered im or iv for 10 days. With nervous system findings, crystalline penicillin G 50,000 u/kg/day for a minimum of 2 weeks is recommended. Despite intensive therapy, the organism may persist in ocular fluid for months (Hardy et al, 1970). Continuation of treatment should be considered until spinal fluid has cleared. Retreatment is indicated if signs or symptoms recur (Srinivasan et al, 1983).

Prevention

Serologic tests for syphilis in the first trimester should identify mothers who need treatment. In high-risk mothers, such as drug addicts and promiscuous women, tests in the second or third trimesters are indicated.

LYME DISEASE

Definition

Lyme arthritis (named for Old Lyme, Connecticut where it was first recognized in 1975) is caused by a

CASE ILLUSTRATION

A 17-year-old woman arrived at The Children's Hospital, Boston emergency room complaining of perivaginal lumps and dysuria of 2 days' duration. She was sexually active but denied any unusual discharge, pain, fever, arthralgias, rash, or nausea. Her last menstrual period was 2 weeks before her visit and of usual duration. She used no contraception, was otherwise well, and had no previous pregnancies. On examination she appeared well. Pharynx, chest, heart, abdomen, and lymph nodes were normal. The skin was clear except for slightly tender, erythematous, flat, lesions on the labia and vulva. A copious white vaginal discharge was present. The cervix, uterus, and adnexae were normal. Neurologic examination was also normal. Microscopic examination of the discharge revealed live *Trichomonas* and probable Gram-negative intracellular diplococci. Urinalysis revealed pyuria, hematuria, and bacteria. Gonorrhea cultures and RPR (rapid plasma reagin) and β-HCG were sent. She was thought to have probable condyloma accuminata, gonococcal cervicitis, a urinary tract infection, and *Trichomonas* vaginitis. She was to be treated with ampicillin alone pending diagnosis of possible pregnancy, but walked out of the emergency room. The following day her HCG (pregnancy test) was negative but the RPR (for syphilis) was floridly positive.

QUESTION AND COMMENT

What diagnostic and therapeutic work-up is advised?

Repeated phone calls were unsuccessful in bringing this woman to our emergency room until a life-threatening illness was mentioned. She finally returned for further serologic testing and definitive treatment. An FTA-ABS obtained at that time was positive at 1:512 confirming the diagnosis of syphilis. While evaluation for sexually transmitted disease in adolescents is a routine procedure in an emergency room, serologic screening for syphilis in this population is often regarded as superfluous. Nonetheless, more than 25,000 cases of syphilis are reported each year in the United States with actual cases at least twice that frequent. Prevalence estimates suggest that there are 0.6% cases in indigent adolescent mothers, 1% in nulliparous females less than 16 years of age at a teenage health clinic, and 2–3% in the total maternity population (Ginsburg, 1983). In retrospect, this mother's condylomalata were initially diagnosed as being accuminata but were probably manifestations of spirochetal rather than viral disease.

Generalized lymphadenopathy, papular or erythematous rashes, and warts in the prepubertal child should raise the suspicion of syphilis. In children, congenital acquisition is often assumed but sexual abuse should be the most pressing concern for an emergency room physician. An RPR or VDRL will become positive between 2 and 6 weeks after exposure. Since false-positives can ocur in many inflammatory states, a specific antitreponemal antibody test should be performed. The titer of a specific FTA-ABS study reflects the state of disease—it rises through the secondary stage of syphilis and falls gradually over 2 years after effective treatment.

During the incubation period, syphilis is probably eradicated by single high dose penicillin or amoxicillin used to treat gonococcus, and thus, it is probably more common than usually estimated because it is undiagnosable at this stage. Effective therapy for primary, secondary, or latent syphilis requires prolonged blood levels of penicillin. For disease of less than 1 year of duration, intramuscular benzathine penicillin G is the treatment of choice; follow-up quantitative serologic tests should confirm efficacy of therapy. This follow-up is of obvious importance in pregnancy. While seropositivity in the newborn may reflect maternal antibody, prompt treatment is recommended before waiting the 3–6 months necessary to see a falling titer in the child.

Treatment failures are related to reinfection after treatment, or treatment only in the third trimester in established infection. Even some mothers treated at an appropriate stage of infection have had infants with congenital syphilis, which highlights the need for prevention (CDC, 1986; 1988).

spirochete transmitted by the "deer tick" Ixodes dammini, and other ticks as well.

Epidemiology

The disease occurs in endemic regions, especially the Northern coastal area of New England in late spring and summer. During one summer in a town of 5000, 39 children and 12 adults were infected. The illness has been seen on four continents. From 1984–1986, approximately 1500 cases of Lyme disease were reported annually in the United States (CDC, 1988).

Natural History

The etiologic agent is a spirochete, *Borrelia burgdorferi* which is found in a variety of hosts including the white-footed mouse, deer, and probably many other animals. The juvenile ticks feed on the infected animal and acquire the spirochete. The ticks which are very small, attach to vegetation in grassy or wooded environment, then reach human skin by direct contact.

The first symptom, a skin rash, begins 3–32 days after the bite as an erythematous macule or papule, expands, and has a clearing region, which may be indurated or later, necrotic (Fig. 17.7). The rash extends over the trunk and proximal extremities. Periorbital edema, conjunctivitis, and urticaria may follow. A flu-like syndrome follows with fever, myalgia, and arthralgia. Meningismus and lymphadenopathy are common. If untreated, the symptoms resolve in several weeks, but may recur with arthritis (in up to 60%) as soon as 1 week or as late as 22 months after the tick bite. Neurologic involvement includes meningitis, facial palsies, and nerve root pain. As many as 6–10% of infected individuals have myopericarditis, and fluctuating atrioventricular block. No long-term cardiac sequelae have been reported.

Maternal-fetal transmission in the first trimester led to death in one infant with congenital heart disease and spirochetes in spleen and bone marrow.

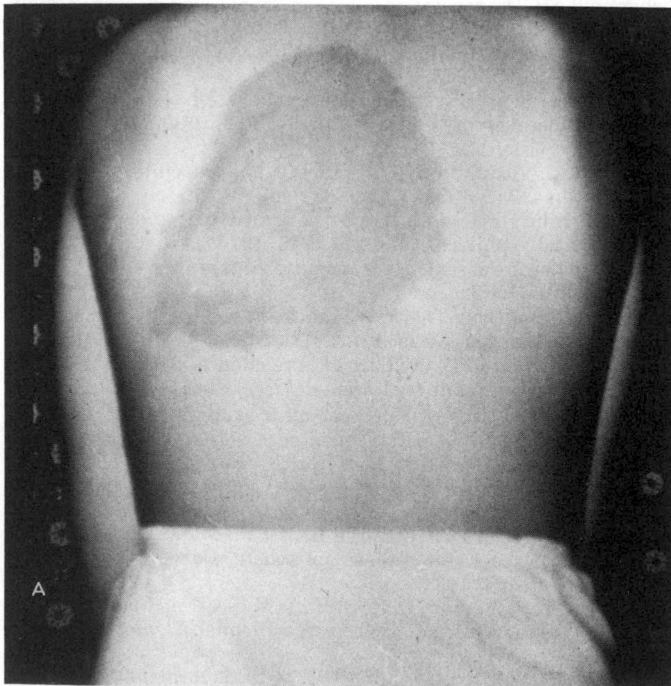

Figure 17.7. Skin lesion in Lyme disease, erythema chronicum migrans began as a papule, then expanded with a clearing region in the center. Reproduced with permission of Dr. Allen Steere and *Ann Intern Med* 86:685, 1977.

Diagnosis

No simple test is diagnostic. The history of exposure in an endemic area, with the characteristic rash is enough to warrant the presumed diagnosis and initiate therapy. Serologic techniques to identify the disease are now available, although they are not well standardized.

Treatment

Oral antibiotic treatment with penicillin V, 50 mg/kg/day in divided doses is effective. Erythromycin is an acceptable alternative. If the child presents with complications, high-dose intravenous penicillin for at least 10 days is recommended. Ceftriaxone is a possible alternative.

Prevention

The best prevention is avoidance of the tick, or prompt removal although the ticks are small and may be hard to find.

LEPTOSPIROSIS

Definition

Infection with many species of the spirochete *Leptospira* causes protean manifestations with fever and multiorgan involvement.

Epidemiology

Leptospira infect almost all mammals, including dogs and rats. It is estimated that 5% of household dogs and 40% of stray dogs are seropositive (Elliot et al, 1985). The incidence of human infection is low; only 34 cases were reported in the United States in 1985.

Natural History

Ingestion or direct exposure of mucous membranes to organisms in urine, blood, or tissues of infected animals is followed by about a 10-day incubation period, then a septicemic illness. The initial phase of anicteric illness which lasts about a week, and is marked by pulmonary involvement, fever, malaise, headache, and conjunctival effusions, is followed by an immune phase which may lead to fever, rash, meningitis, or uveitis. Lumbar puncture may reveal elevated CSF pressure and pleocytosis, first with polys, then monos up to 500/mm^3.

CASE ILLUSTRATION (from Rennels M, DeJarnette J, *University Pediatrics*, 1984 University of Maryland, Baltimore)

A 4-year-old white female was bitten by a tick behind her right ear. Five days later, redness and swelling were noted at the site. One day later her temperature reached 40°C, and she was lethargic. Sneezing, coughing, and coryza developed and lasted 5 days, after which a preauricular exanthem was noted, which had a sharp border and a clearing center. It was not pruritic. A few days later a right facial palsy developed.

Her general physical examination was in other respects normal. Her white blood count was 12,700, 53% polys, 37% lymps, 7% monos, 1% eos, and 2% atypical lymphs. Hematocrit was 38 and ESR 42. She had 106 white cells in her spinal fluid (9% polys, 50% lymphs, 41% monos). Protein was 25 and glucose was 68. Immunoglobulins were normal, as was a CT scan of the brain and an EEG. An ELISA titer of IgM directed against the spirochete of Lyme disease was 1:400 (significant). No organisms were recovered from spinal fluid.

She received intravenous penicillin 55,000 u/kg/day for 10 days and prednisone 1 mg/kg/day for 7 days, with resolution of her symptoms and her facial weakness.

QUESTIONS AND COMMENTS

What is the most characteristic part of the clinical syndrome? What complications should be looked for?

The rash is most characteristic. It progresses as an expanding erythematous ring with the bite in the center. Later many areas of erythema may appear and fade, then recur.

Half the patients will have arthritis of one or more large joints, which may persist. High-dose intravenous penicillin can reverse even established arthritis (Steere et al, 1983).

Days or even months later, cardiac arrythmias or myocarditis may occur. Meningoencephalitis and peripheral neuritis have been seen.

What treatment would you have used if the child had been allergic to penicillin?

A 14-day course of ceftriaxone (50 mg/kg/day) is an effective alternative.

The icteric form of leptospirosis, known as the Weil syndrome, is far more serious, and involves impaired renal and hepatic function. Fever may persist throughout the septicemic and immune phases of the illness. Jaundice, sometimes intense, may result from an elevation of both indirect and direct reacting bilirubin. The peak concentration, which may reach 80 mg/dl, usually occurs within the first 7 days. Liver function tests are abnormal, but stools are rarely acholic. Renal dysfunction is marked by proteinuria, with casts and red and white blood cells in the urinary sediment. In some patients, azotemia is present, and impaired renal function is marked by oliguria and signs of acute tubular necrosis. Hyponatremia is a consistent finding in severe cases.

Diagnosis

Laboratory diagnosis is difficult and culture requires special media, and incubation for several weeks. A four-fold rise in agglutination titer over 2 weeks is confirmatory. A single titer of greater than 1/100 with an appropriate clinical picture is diagnostic. Fluorescent antibody techniques are available. Specimens of serum, urine, or spinal fluid may be sent to the National Leptospirosis Laboratory at the Centers for Disease Control in Atlanta, Georgia.

Treatment

High doses of intravenous penicillin or doxycycline are indicated for about 10 days, although their benefit is not clear. Careful attention to supportive care is required but even so mortality from the icteric form of the disease is about 5–10%.

Prevention

Canine vaccines are available, which prevent illness in dogs, but do not prevent dogs from shedding organisms and transmitting the infection to humans. Avoidance of contaminated soil or water is the best prevention.

REFERENCES

CDC: Congenital syphilis—United States 1983–1985. *MMWR* 35:625, 1986.

CDC: Guidelines for the prevention and control of congenital syphilis. *MMWR* 37 (No. S-1):1, 1988.

Eichenfield AH: Diagnosis and management of Lyme disease. *Pediatr Ann* 15:583, 1986.

Elliot DL, Tolle SW, Goldberg L, et al: Pet-associated illness. *N Engl J Med* 313:985, 1985.

Frau LM, Alexander ER: Public health implication of sexually transmitted diseases in pediatric practice. *Pediatr Infect Dis* 4:453, 1985.

Ginsburg CM: Acquired syphilis in prepubertal children. *Pediatr Infect Dis* 2:232, 1983.

Hardy JB, Hardy PH, et al: Failure of penicillin in a newborn with congenital syphilis. *JAMA* 212:1345, 1970.

Lynch PJ: Therapy of sexually transmitted diseases. *Med Clin North Am* 66:915, 1982.

Medical Letter of Drug Therapy: Treatment of sexually transmitted diseases. *Med Lett* 24:29, 1982.

Mumford DM, Smith PB, Goldfarb JL: Prevalence of venereal disease in indigent pregnant adolescents. *J Reproduc Med* 19:83, 1982.

Oppenheimer EH, Hardy JB: Congenital syphilis in the newborn infant: Clinical and pathological observations in recent cases. *Johns Hopkins Med J* 129:63, 1971.

Rennels M, DeJarnette J: Lyme Disease. *University Pediatrics* 3:3, 1984.

Schlesinger PA, Duray PH, Burke BA, et al: Maternal-fetal transmission of the Lyme disease spirochete, *Borrelia burgdorferi*. *Ann Intern Med* 103:67, 1985.

Srinivasan G, Ramamurthy RS, Bharathi S, et al: Congenital syphilis: A diagnostic and therapeutic dilemma. *Pediatr Infect Dis* 2:436, 1983.

Steere AC, Hutchinson GJ, Rahn DW, et al: Treatment of the early manifestations of Lyme disease. *Ann Intern Med* 99:22, 1983.

Taber LH, Feigin RD: Spirochetal infections. In Speck WJ (ed): Symposium on Unusual Infections. *Pediatr Clin North Am* 26:377, 1979.

White ST, Lota FA, Ingram DL: Sexually transmitted diseases in sexually abused children. *Pediatrics* 72:16, 1983.

Other Infections

7

CAT SCRATCH DISEASE

Definition

Cat scratch disease which may be caused by a recently identified bacillus, depends on history of contact or scratch from a cat or dog, and negative studies for other forms of lymphadenopathy. Biopsy of a lymph node gives characteristic histopathology and special staining techniques can allow identification of Gram-variable bacilli, best seen with specific silver stains (Wear et al, 1983).

Basic Science

For many years, cat scratch disease was recognized as a benign, self-limited form of regional lymphadenopathy following a cat scratch or, occasionally, other kinds of skin abrasions. Traditional cultures for bacteria were always negative, since organisms fail to grow on blood agar, chocolate agar, or thioglycollate medium. Bacilli were first identified in 1983 in 34 of 39 lymph nodes examined by a silver impregnation stain. They have been identified in the walls of capillaries and sometimes within macrophages that line the sinuses in or near the germinal centers of the lymph node. They can exist as single organisms, in chains, or in clumps. Bacilli were also identified in histiocytes and in necrotic foci (Wear et al, 1983). An unusual bacteria has been isolated (English et al, 1988).

Epidemiology

The incidence of this condition is unknown since probably many times it is not brought to the attention of a physician. It has been recognized worldwide, and appears to be more common in the fall and winter. One group practice in Florida reported 1200 cases seen over a 30-year period (Carithers, 1985).

Clinical Findings

A papule or pustule often develops at the site of the scratch or infected skin lesion. Most commonly, the extremities are involved but occasionally the inoculation can be on the trunk or neck. Regional lymphadenitis and mild systemic signs including fever, occur 10–30 days after the cat scratch. Nodes that drain the area become enlarged, often tender, and about 25% of them suppurate. The regional lymphadenopathy may persist for 2 weeks to 8 months (average about 2 months).

Other manifestations that have been reported are rare but include a generalized maculopapular rash, erythema multiforme, or nodosum, conjunctivitis, mesenteric adenitis, peripheral neuritis; rarely, 1–6 weeks after the onset of adenopathy, an encephalopathy may develop. The encephalitis can be severe but is usually completely reversible (Torres et al, 1978).

Diagnosis

A skin test was formerly used since it was about all that was available to confirm the diagnosis. However, the antigens are poorly standardized and there is a 5% false-positive reaction. Furthermore, it has not been made commercially available. Diagnosis in this era depends on exclusion of other causes of lymphadenopathy and, if needed, biopsy and appropriate staining to identify the bacilli in tissue.

It is important to distinguish this disease from other forms of localized adenopathy including atypical tuberculosis, rat bite fever, Hodgkins disease, and some other bacterial and fungal infections.

No treatment has been fully evaluated. The disease is eventually self-limited. Aspiration of flocculant nodes may be necessary if they appear likely to rupture but this is rarely needed.

CHLAMYDIA TRACHOMATIS

Definition

Chlamydia trachomatis infection is a widespread venereal disease that can infect infants during the course of delivery. It is the most prevalent of all sexually transmitted diseases in the United States today (CDC, 1985).

Basic Science

Chlamydiae are bacteria that share some properties with viruses. They resemble bacteria in that they have cell walls, divide by binary fission, and contain both DNA and RNA. Like viruses they grow only intracellularly and require cell culture for growth in the laboratory.

Epidemiology

It has been estimated that there are between 15,000 and 30,000 infants each year who have pneumonia caused by *C. trachomatis*. In a study of women in city hospitals, the organism was found in the vagina of 2–13% of women (Hammerschlag, 1978), and a study of asymptomatic women college students revealed that 4.6% were found to be infected with this organism. Of infants born to infected mothers, 18–50% will develop

CASE ILLUSTRATION

A 2½-year-old was in good health until found unresponsive with his eyes deviated. Tonic clonic movements of the limbs were noted, and he assumed an opisthotonic position. On examination he was afebrile, pale, and had persistent generalized seizures. The only abnormality was a firm, red lymph node in the right axilla. Laboratory studies revealed a normal blood count, electrolytes, urea nitrogen, calcium, and glucose. CSF was normal. A CT scan of the brain was normal. The seizures lasted for about an hour despite intravenous diazepam (Valium), diphenylhydantoin (Dilantin), and phenobarbital. After seizures were controlled, the child was arousable but disoriented.

Further questioning revealed that he had been scratched on the right arm by a cat. The node had been present for 1 week before the onset of seizures. He was markedly improved the day after admission, and discharged on diphenylhydantoin and phenobarbital. The lymph node did not suppurate, and gradually diminished in size over the subsequent week.

QUESTIONS AND COMMENTS

How long should he be kept on anticonvulsants?

We do not know, but in the absence of a recurrence, we discontinued them when the axillary node was no longer palpable.

Is it unusual to be afebrile with cat scratch fever, as it is often called?

The majority of children have no constitutional symptoms. Some temperature elevation is found in about 30% of patients with the disease.

Was the lymph node biopsied?

We did not biopsy or excise the node. The history of a cat scratch with regional adenopathy and encephalopathy, and prompt recovery made any other diagnosis improbable. The histology is nonspecific, and the putative organism very difficult to stain or grow.

Why was a skin test not performed?

He was tested with PPD (tuberculin test) and found to be negative. The antigens for cat scratch disease are no longer available.

How common is encephalopathy?

We have no figures for incidence, but in Carithers series (1985), only 1/1200 patients developed it. It can occur from 3 days to 6 weeks after adenopathy appears, but is most common 1–2 weeks later.

conjunctivitis between 1 and 3 weeks after birth unless prophylaxis with erythromycin ophthalmic ointment is provided. Approximately 1 of 6 exposed infants will develop pneumonia (Schachter et al, 1986).

Natural History

The clinical spectrum of *C. trachomatis* infections is very wide. Although most infections in women are asymptomatic, the organism can cause mucopurulent cervicitis and pelvic inflammatory disease. Infection in pregnancy can cause postpartum endometritis.

Infants delivered via the vaginal route from infected mothers are very likely to have conjunctivitis beginning 5–14 days after delivery, too late to be the result of chemical irritation caused by silver nitrate or other ophthalmic solutions. Pneumonia is most often seen between 4 weeks and 3 months of age, with or without antecedent conjunctivitis.

Diagnosis

The most prominent symptom is a cough that frequently is paroxysmal and interferes with feeding. Sometimes fine rales may be present. Radiographs may be disproportionately severe in the presence of mild symptoms, but the only distinguishing radiographic features are widespread infiltrates. Most of the affected infants are afebrile.

The chlamydiae are shed from the respiratory tract and can be isolated from nasopharyngeal aspirates; conjunctival shedding has also been noted.

According to Beem and Saxon (1977), infants with pneumonia had high immunofluorescent antibody titers to lymphogranuloma venereum type I.

The organism can be seen as an iodine-staining cytoplasmic inclusion obtained from the conjunctival or nasopharyngeal aspirates. Antigen tests are available; a rise in serum antibodies detected by immunofluorescence confirms the infection. IgG and IgM are elevated. An absolute eosinophilia of $>400/mm^3$ is usual.

The diagnosis of *C. trachomatis* cervicitis in adolescents is suggested by a yellow mucopurulent discharge. A Gram stain that shows more than 10 polys per oil immersion field (1000 X) suggests *C. trachomatis* infection. Culture of material from the endocervix is the "gold standard" of diagnosis, but it is not widely available. Antigen detection tests are available, and improving each year.

Treatment

The organisms are sensitive to a number of antimicrobial agents, including erythromycin, tetracycline, and sulfonamides. Erythromycin is preferred treatment for children in four divided doses for 2–3 weeks. The mother and father also should receive erythromycin (*The Medical Letter* 30:5, 1988).

Prevention

Maternal screening at the first prenatal visit of all women under age 20 years, all unwed women, and married women with multiple sex partners or a history of other sexually transmitted disease, allows identification and treatment of infected mothers-to-be. Erythromycin ethylsuccinate (400 mg four times a day for 7 days) given at 36 weeks' gestation was 92% successful in treating maternal illness, and reduced the rate of illness in infants (Schachter et al, 1986).

Increased use of barrier contraceptives can reduce the likelihood of infection.

CASE ILLUSTRATION

An 18-year-old female presented with a 3-day history of sharp right upper quadrant abdominal pain. She was well until 2 weeks before admission, when she began to experience sharp intermittent suprapubic pain without dysuria, vaginal discharge, fever, nausea, or vomiting. Evaluation at that time was notable for bilateral lower quadrant tenderness but no adnexal or cervical motion tenderness and no vaginal discharge. CBC, sedimentation rate, and urinalysis were normal. Cervical cultures and a urine pregnancy test were also negative. No specific etiology for the pain was determined. Two days later she had the onset of menstrual flow, heavier and 5 days earlier than usual, lasting 5 days. During this time she continued to complain of suprapubic crampy pain.

Three days following her menses she developed the onset of pulling sharp pain in the right upper quadrant. It intensifed in quality such that on the night before admission she could not sleep and developed headache and low-grade fever. The patient was sexually active and used oral contraception. She continued to have no vaginal discharge after her menses, nor did she have sore throat, tenderness, nausea, cough, sputum production, or shortness of breath. She had had alternating constipation and diarrhea for the last few weeks.

Physical examination revealed a well-appearing but uncomfortable young woman with normal vital signs and an otherwise benign physical examination, except for the abdomen. Abdominal examination was notable for involuntary guarding and much tenderness over the liver, without generalized peritoneal signs, masses, costovertebral angle tenderness, or abnormal breath sounds. Pelvic examination revealed a scant cervical discharge, but again no cervical or adnexal tenderness; rectal examination was normal with guaiac-negative stool. A Gram stain of the cervical smear was notable for 5–10 white cells, but no organisms were seen. White blood count was 9100, with 68% polys, 3% bands, 5% lymphs, 12% monos, 1% eos, and 1% atypical lymphs. Sedimentation rate was 58 mm/hour, and urinalysis and liver function tests were normal. Pregnancy test was negative, as was a chest radiograph. She was admitted with the suspicion of having Fitz-Hugh-Curtis syndrome, although an appendiceal or liver abscess, Crohn's disease, or cholecystitis could not be ruled out.

QUESTION AND COMMENT

What was the next step in the diagnostic work-up, and how could the diagnosis of Fitz-Hugh-Curtis syndrome be confirmed?

Shortly after admission, an abdominal ultrasonographic examination was performed, which did reveal fluid in the cul-de-sac with a normal liver and gall bladder. A laparoscopy followed and showed pus around the Fallopian tubes, adnexa, and around the liver with a normal gall baldder and appendix visualized, thus confirming the diagnosis of Fitz-Hugh-Curtis syndrome.

Fitz-Hugh-Curtis syndrome is a late complication of pelvic inflammatory disease. It has been reported in up to 13% of females with acute pelvic inflammatory disease, about half of whom have been asymptomatic. The mechanism is felt to be essentially a lower genital tract infection during the menses. While this case did not demonstrate the presence of tenderness on cervical motion, presence of low-grade fever, some peritoneal signs, and an ESR, were consistent with the diagnosis. Usual organisms include *Gonococcus, Chlamydia,* and mixed anerobes. Cultures obtained at laporoscopy on this patient were negative for gonococci, but a rise in serum antibodies by immunofluorescence suggested a chlamydial infection, with a subsequent rise from acute to convalescent serum. The patient was treated initially with cefoxitin, and doxycycline, since the latter is effective for the treatment of *Chlamydia.*

TRACHOMA

Definition

Repeated exposure of conjunctivae to *C. trachomatis* causes trachoma, which is the major cause of preventable blindness in the world in 1985.

Epidemiology

Approximately 500 million people are estimated to have trachoma.

Natural History

Eye infection occurs in endemic regions, including the Middle East, North Africa, and India. In the United States, it is seen in Indian reservations and among the Mexican-American population of California. Transmission by contact occurs in poor hygienic surroundings.

In nonendemic areas, inclusion conjunctivitis (blenorrhea) can be acquired by newborns who are exposed during delivery through an infected vagina.

Recurrent infections in endemic areas often begin in childhood, with a chronic follicular conjunctivitis. Follicles (which are germinal centers of B lymphocytes) appear first on the upper tarsal plate and upper limbus. Photophobia and lacrimation are common. As the disorder progresses, neovascularization of the cornea occurs, with development of a pannus. Chronic recurrences lead to conjunctival scarring.

Diagnosis

Immunotyping has identified types A, B, and C as predominant in endemic trachoma. Types D, E, G, and F are the ones commonly found in the genital tract in nonendemic areas.

Treatment

Topical application of erythromycin is not protective in newborns. Infants with conjunctivitis require oral or intravenous erythromycin. Control of recurrent infection involves improved hygiene. Mass chemotherapy is not feasible with current antibiotics. Repeated topical applications to infected children suppress infection and reduce transmission (Taylor, 1985).

Prevention

Improved living conditions and less crowding have been associated with a reduction in trachoma. No effective vaccine is available.

CHLAMYDIA PSITTACI (PSITTACOSIS)

Definition

Psittacosis usually presents as a type of pneumonia from inhalation of *Chlamydia psittaci*. Systemic manifestations may occur.

Epidemiology

Psittacosis is usually seen only among individuals in contact with birds, including poultry workers, veterinarians, and pet-store personnel. (Parrots, parakeets, and other birds may be infected.) There were 142 cases reported in the United States in 1983. In 1986, a new organism, possibly a strain of *C. psittaci,* TWAR, was identified as the cause of pneumonia, and is spread human-to-human with no known bird reservoir. TWAR antibody has been found in 25–45% of adults (Grayston et al, 1986).

Natural History

Infected birds aerosolize organisms with cough or spread infection via feathers or dust, and inhalation of infected particles by humans leads after 1–3 weeks to an abrupt onset of fever, toxicity, cough, and bradycardia. The white blood count may be depressed. The disease can spread rapidly and, if untreated, has a 20–30% mortality rate. Occasionally psittacosis lacks respiratory involvement and is characterized by severe headache, chills, fever, and a protracted course. Hepatitis, myocarditis, endocarditis, and meningitis have been observed. Erythema multiform or nodosum may occur.

The recently described diseases caused by the TWAR strain (named after the laboratory designation of the first isolates) produce upper and lower respiratory tract disease. Severe sore throat followed by chronic bronchitis with production of yellow mucoid sputum have been noted. Diffuse or lobar pneumonia indistinguishable from that caused by mycoplasma may persist for weeks. Prompt recovery has followed treatment with tetracyclines or erythromycin. White blood counts have been normal in these patients (Grayston et al, 1986).

The TWAR strain illness differs from bird-associated psittacosis in the absence of severe headache and myalgias, and the presence of severe pharyngitis. Neither organism has produced conjunctivitis, which is common with *C. trachomatis*.

Diagnosis

The organism may be recovered from throat swabs or in sputum. Serologic complement fixation tests are available for both strains of *C. psittaci*.

Treatment

Tetracyclines or chloramphenicol are effective when given in divided doses every 6 hours for at least 10 days.

Prognosis

If untreated, the disease associated with bird reservoirs can spread rapidly and may be fatal. After the introduction of tetracyclines, the mortality fell to less than 1%. The TWAR strain illness is not known to be fatal.

KAWASAKI SYNDROME (MUCOCUTANEOUS LYMPH NODE SYNDROME)

Definition

Kawasaki syndrome is a clinical syndrome of unknown etiology characterized by a panvasculitis. High fever, conjunctivitis, dermatitis, arthritis, and later, aneurysms of coronary vessels are characteristic. The Centers for Disease Control (CDC) case definition is fever for 5 days or more without other more reasonable explanation and at least four of the following criteria:

1. bilateral conjunctival infection;
2. at least one of the following mucous membrane changes: injected or fissured lips, injected pharynx, or "strawberry" tongue;
3. at least one of the following extremity changes: erythema of palms or soles, edema of the hands or feet, or generalized or periungual desquamation;
4. rash; and
5. cervical lymphadenopathy (at least one lymph node 1.5 cm or greater in diameter) (Rauch and Hurwitz, 1985).

Basic Science

The syndrome is a reaction to something, perhaps the toxin of a yet to be identified microorganism or a lymphotropic virus. Polymerase activity and reverse transcriptase activity has been found in the supernatants of cultures from infected patients (Burns et al, 1986). An unusual constellation of immunologic responses has been described. An activation of IgA positive T cells of the T4-helper subset occurs, followed by a large number of IgG and IgM plaguing cells in peripheral blood. Later, hypergammaglobulinemia from polyclonal B-cell activation reflects a polyclonal B-cell activation. Suppressor T cells are depressed. By the third week of illness these findings revert to normal (Leung et al, 1983).

Despite extensive epidemiologic studies, no evidence of person to person transmission has been reported. Antecedent respiratory illness has occurred in more affected infants than controls, but no etiologic agent has been identified.

Epidemiology

First described in Japan in 1967, the syndrome has affected over 50,000 children in Japan, and has been recognized in many other parts of the world. Although usually sporadic, outbreaks have been reported in New York and Massachusetts (Bell et al, 1981), and multiple other sites since. In the temperate climates, outbreaks are most likely in spring and fall.

Natural History

The syndrome occurs mostly in infants and children under 5 years of age from upper socioeconomic groups. It is characterized by sudden onset of high fever and a generalized skin rash which may resemble scarlet fever or a drug reaction, and sometimes involves

CASE ILLUSTRATION
(courtesy of Dr. Jane Newburger)

A 3-year-old white male, previously in excellent health, had an attack of pharyngitis and cervical adenitis with high fever. Throat culture at the time was negative. He was treated with amoxicillin with some improvement, but then the fever recurred. He was placed on cefaclor for 24 hours but with persisting fever and increase in the swelling of the cervical nodes. He was seen in the emergency room. The white count was 13,600 with 62 polys, 27 bands, 9 lymphs, 1 basophil, 1 atypical lymph. A repeat throat culture was uninformative. His erythrocyte sedimentation rate was 51.

Physical examination on admission showed swelling of the left cervical lymph nodes. He appeared ill with a temperature of 40°C and had a diffuse erythematous rash over his chest and abdomen, with large confluent regions over his neck and back. The rash also involved hands and soles of the feet. Examination of his eyes revealed inflamed conjunctivae and photophobia. His tonsils were mildly enlarged but there was no exudate, and his neck was supple. He was alert, oriented, but very irritable. There were no other abnormalities on examination. Negative throat cultures, blood cultures, and urine cultures, with persisting symptoms made it increasingly clear that his illness was consistent with Kawasaki syndrome. He was treated with 80 mg/kg/day of aspirin throughout his 9-day hospital course and for 2 weeks after his discharge home; all of the acute manifestations had subsided but hydrops of his gall bladder was diagnosed by ultrasonography 2 days before discharge. Liver function studies remained normal.

Six days later while still on aspirin he was seen in follow-up and noted to have residual arthralgias and mouth sores, with photophobia and some peeling of hands and feet. He had been observed at home to have one episode where he suddenly felt short of breath and said his stomach hurt. This lasted about a minute with pallor but then resolved. Later when he was blowing bubbles he suddenly held his chest, shivered, and became pale. His mother noted that his heart was pounding and he was brought to the clinic where an echocardiogram revealed tubular dilatation of the left main and proximal left circumflex coronary arteries with discrete aneurysms. Because of concern that these could be attacks of myocardial ischemia, he was readmitted to the hospital. A chest radiograph was normal, as was an ECG. LDH isoenzymes and CPK (MB bands) were determined and within normal limits. After 6 days of careful monitoring he had no further symptoms, and was discharged a second time. On follow-up 6 weeks later, he was found to be asymptomatic and there was clear evidence of regression of his coronary artery aneurysms, such that they were no longer visible. He continues on aspirin. The long term function of seriously involved coronary vessels is not known. He receives periodic exercise tests to look for possible exercise-induced myocardial ischemia. He continues well, on full activity.

QUESTIONS AND COMMENTS

With what conditions can Kawasaki disease be confused?

Clearly the initial symptoms were indistinguishable from a streptococcal sore throat or a viral pharyngitis with cervical adenitis. It was the persistent fever and lack of response to antibiotics that provoked suspicion of Kawasaki disease and the appearance of the rash made the diagnosis highly probable. The subsequent evolution of the rash to desquamation is typical of Kawasaki syndrome but not restricted to it. The observation of hydrops of the gall bladder by ultrasonography is very consistent and the development of coronary artery aneurysms establishes the diagnosis in the 15% who have them.

What further laboratory studies might have been helpful?

T-cell enumeration shows a characteristic depression in supressor cells. In this patient, 41% were helper-inducer cells (normal 35–50), and only 7% were supressor-cytotoxic cells (normal 18–30).

The platelet count may become elevated late in the disease.

Uveitis is found in 80% of children with Kawasaki disease, which may be detectable only on slit-lamp examination (Burns et al, 1985).

What other form of therapy might have been offered this child?

Currently, we use intravenous γ-globulin in combination with salicylates during the active state of disease (see Treatment). This patient's complete recovery and reversal of his aneurysms was spontaneous.

palms and soles. Desquamation of skin of digits is common during recovery. Boys may have desquamation in inguinal areas as well. Edema of the extremities may be marked. Lips and mucous membranes are inflamed, and the tongue has a strawberry appearance. Cervical lymphadenopathy is prominent in about half the patients. Spiking fevers may be present for a few weeks. Later in the course of the disease, about day 12 or several weeks therefter, coronary artery aneurysms appear in about 15–20% of the infants. Carditis occurs in about 40% of patients in the acute stage of illness; mitral regurgitation is seen in 8–11%, and aortic regurgitation in 5%. Most of the valvular lesions disappear after the acute illness. Death occurs in about 0.5–2% of all cases, usually from cardiac complications.

Diagnosis

The syndrome should be considered in children with prolonged fever, conjunctival infection, oropharyngeal inflammation, diffuse rash, and lymphadenopathy. Edema of peripheral extremities is characteristic. Anterior uveitis occurs in over 80% of children in the first week of illness. No single laboratory test is diagnostic. About the ninth day of illness, the platelet count may be elevated. Acute phase reactants are elevated and the pattern of immunologic response is characteristic. Reversible hydrops of the gallbladder has been described, as has sterile pyuria, aseptic meningitis, and arthritis.

Treatment

The recommended treatment in 1988 is aspirin, 100 mg/kg/day through the 14th day of illness, then 3–5 mg/kg/day until all symptoms have resolved. In the acute stage, intravenous γ-globulin, 400 mg/kg/day for 4 consecutive days is given. In a prospective randomized clinical trial of intravenous γ-globulin with aspirin, compared to aspirin alone, the results favored the combined therapy with a reduction in the prevalence of coronary artery abnormalities (Newburger et al, 1986; Nagashima et al, 1987).

Prevention

There is no known method of prevention.

MEDITERRANEAN FEVER

Definition

Mediterranean fever is a familial amyloidosis that mimics infectious diseases, and is characterized by amyloid protein deposits primarily in kidney, liver, spleen, and adrenals.

Epidemiology

Mediterranean fever is found predominantly in individuals of sephardic Jewish origin, but also in Armenians and Arabs.

Natural History

This rare disorder may present in childhood or adolescence with episodes of fever and sterile peritonitis. The fevers have an abrupt onset and short duration (24–48 hours) associated with severe abdominal pain, polyserositis, and rashes. They occur as often as weekly, or as infrequent as yearly.

Renal amyloidosis may present with proteinuria and eventual nephrotic syndrome. Recurrent atelectasis has been noted.

Treatment

Colchicine reduces the frequency of the febrile attacks, but its effect on amyloid deposition is unknown. The usual dose is 0.6 mg orally tid.

Mycoplasma/Ureaplasma

Definition

Mycoplasma and *Ureaplasma* are two genera of the same family. Although over 50 species have been identified, only nine *Mycoplasma* and *Ureaplasma* species infect humans. They are small organisms without a cell wall, and are widely distributed in nature. Pneumonia is one of the major causes of respiratory infections in school-age children and young adults. Genital *Mycoplasma* or *Ureaplasma* infection is very common, and may be associated with premature onset of labor.

Epidemiology

The peak age incidence for pneumonia from this organism is 10–15 years, with epidemics occuring among college students and military personnel. It is responsible for 40–60% of pneumonia cases in that age group. Between 50 and 80% of pregnant women carry other *Mycoplasma* organisms in their genital tracts.

Natural History

The lung is the primary site of involvement with *M. pneumoniae*. The incubation period is variable, but on the average between 2 and 3 weeks. The onset of illness is gradual and there are no diagnostic signs or symptoms. Sore throat is frequent and cough is a major symptom.

Humans with antibodies are protected from subsequent infection. Cell-mediated immunity has a role as well since reactive lymphocytes appear in peripheral blood following both natural and experimental infection. Denny and colleagues (1971) have made the interesting observation that small children are commonly infected with *M. pneumonia* but rarely become ill. It is not until their lymphocytes can be stimulated by the antigen that they develop disease. Thus, it is the immunologic response of the host that is responsible for much clinical illness.

The organism can establish infection in the CNS, heart, and joints. Although rare, meningitis can occur with a predominance of mononuclear cells in the spinal fluid. *Mycoplasma* is one of the causes of so-called aseptic meningitis, since the organism does not grow on ordinary media. Encephalitis and transverse myelitis have been described. Skin lesions include maculopapular rashes and erythema nodosum. A few patients have had a Stevens-Johnson syndrome in association with *Mycoplasma* infection.

Intrauterine infection with *U. urealyticum* can be manifest as respiratory distress at birth, with a prolonged and sometimes fatal course. The possibility should be suspected in any infant with persistent respiratory distress from birth (Quinn et al, 1985).

Genital *Mycoplasma* infection is associated with low birth weight. Erythromycin, 1 g/day/6 weeks in the last trimester seemed to reduce the number of low birth weight infants in a small study reported by Kass and Platt (1984). It is not clear whether the benefit was from reduction in *U. urealyticum, M. hominis, C. trachomatis,* or other sexually transmitted infections.

Diagnosis

Radiographic findings are variable, but often include bilateral, diffuse infiltrates. Occasionally, a lobar infiltrate is present. Pleural effusions are evident in 10–15% of patients. Laboratory findings are nonspecific. A number of serologic responses follow *M. pneumoniae* infection. Cold hemagglutinins are common but nonspecific. More specific immunologic responses can be demonstrated by complement fixation and radio-immuno precipitation. Acute phase serum should be obtained at the time of diagnosis and convalescent serum in 10 days to 3 weeks to demonstrate a specific antibody rise. The organism can be grown on artificial media supplemented with yeast extract and horse serum, but this is not widely available.

Treatment

Erythromycin is the drug of choice in children, because it has minimal untoward side effects. Treatment should be continued for 7–10 days. For children under 25 kg the dose is 50 mg/kg/day in four divided doses. For those over 25 kg, the dose is 250 mg every 6 hours.

Prevention

No effective vaccine exists. It is possible that none will be available since the clinical manifestations of *M. pneumoniae* are immunologically mediated. Thus, the use of any vaccine in children would seem inappropriate.

Prognosis

In general, most patients with *M. pneumoniae* infection recover fully; only when infection becomes systemic or is superimposed on chronic lung disease it may be fatal. Pneumonia acquired by the fetus before birth can result in stillbirth or neonatal death.

CASE ILLUSTRATION

A 13-year-old white female presented with 1 day of lethargy and ataxia following 1–2 weeks of upper respiratory infection symptoms. She had been afebrile throughout this time and, on arrival to our hospital, had a physical examination notable for mild papilledema, a supple neck, and nonfocal neurologic examination that revealed obtundation with purposeful response to painful stimulation but no response to verbal command, hypotonia, symmetrical reflexes, and bilateral upgoing toes. CBC showed a hematocrit of 39, white blood count of 5000, with 77% polys, 12% bands, and normal platelets with sedimentation rate of 28. A CT scan showed no evidence of cerebral edema and a lumbar puncture was notable for 40 white cells, (50% lymphs), 0 red cells, a protein of 40, and a gluocse of 97. Of note, a chest radiograph showed a question of right middle lobe infiltrate or atelectasis, and cold agglutinins at the bedside were weakly positive.

QUESTION AND COMMENT

Can this whole spectrum of symptoms be attributable to *Mycoplasma*?

It was thought that this patient's clinical presentation was consistent with a meningoencephalitis. Although many possible causes including other various viral, bacterial, and fungal etiologies as well as toxin exposure were considered, given the light coma, nonfocal examination, lack of fever, and absence of red cells in the CSF and an EEG showing diffuse slowing throughout without a discrete temporal focus, *Mycoplasma* infection seemed most likely. Therefore, we did not perform a brain biopsy or start empiric antiviral therapy. Instead the patient was begun on erythromycin, which has been shown to reduce the duration of respiratory symptoms, although it does not cross the blood-brain barrier. Over the initial week of hospitalization, she became fully oriented, although she was still intermittently lethargic. Of most interest was her antimycoplasmal antibody titer in serum drawn on admission and reported as positive at 1–32,000 at the end of the first week of hospitalization. Thus, the diagnosis was confirmed.

A review of the literature on *Mycoplasma pneumoniae* encephalitis suggests that our patient's clinical presentation including LP and EEG was consistent with the several hundred cases that have been reported to date in which the cerebrum, cerebellum, spinal cord, and/or nerve routes have been affected (Lerer and Kalavsky, 1973). The mechanism for the CNS involvement is unknown, but may involve a neurotoxin, immunocomplexes, or direct exposure to the organism, since the organism has recently been cultivated from CSF for the first time. Studies looking at prognosis in these patients suggested focal neurologic findings, CSF white blood cell counts over 100, and a CSF protein over 100 mg% have a worse outlook for neurologic recovery. Our patient met none of these criteria and subsequently went on to regain full neurologic function.

REFERENCES

Beem MO, Saxon EM: Respiratory tract colonization and a distinctive pneumonia syndrome in infants infected with *Chlamydia trachomatis*. *N Engl J Med* 296:306, 1977.

Bell DM, Brink EW, et al: Kawasaki syndrome: Description of two outbreaks in the United States. *N Engl J Med* 304:1568, 1981.

Burns JC, Joffe L, Sargent RA, Glode MP: Anterior uveitis associated with Kawasaki syndrome. *Pediatr Infect Dis* 4:258, 1985.

Burns JC, Geha RS, Newburger JW: Polymerase activity of lymphocyte culture supernatants from patients with Kawasaki disease. *Nature* 323:814, 1986.

Carithers HA: Cat-scratch disease. An overview based on a study of 1200 patients. *Am J Dis Child* 139:1124, 1985.

Cassell GH, Cole BC: Mycoplasma as agents of human disease. *N Engl J Med* 304:80, 1981.

CDC: *Chlamydia trachomatis* infections. *MMWR* 34:535, 1985.

CDC: Lyme disease—Connecticut *MMWR* 37:1, 1988.

Clyde WA Jr: Neurological syndromes and *Mycoplasma infection*. *Arch Neurol* 37:65, 1980.

Denny FW, Clyde WA, Glezen WP: *Mycoplasma pneumoniae* disease: Clinical spectrum, pathophysiology, epidemiology, and control. *J Infect Dis* 123:74, 1971.

English CK, Wear DJ, et al: Cat-scratch disease. *JAMA* 259:9, 1988.

Fernald GW: Role of host response in *Mycoplasma pneumoniae* disease. *J Infect Dis* 127:S55, 1973.

Fernald GW, Collier AM, Clyde WA: Respiratory infections due to *Mycoplasma pneumoniae* in infants and children. *Pediatrics* 55:327, 1975.

Furusho K, Nakano H, Shinomiya K, et al: (Letter). *Lancet* 2:1055, 1984.

Grayston JT, Kuo CC, Wang FT, et al: A new *Chlamydia psittaci* strain, TWAR, isolated in acute respiratory tract infection. *N Engl J Med* 315:161, 1986.

Hammerschlag MR: *Chlamydia pneumonia* in infants. *N Engl J Med* 298:1083, 1978.

Kass EH, Platt R: Urinary tract and genital mycoplasmal infection. In Wald NJ (ed): *Antenatal and Neonatal Screening*. New York, Oxford University Press, 1984, p 345.

Kato H, Kioke S, Yamanoto M, et al: Coronary aneurysms in infants and young children with acute febrile MCLNS. *J Pediatr* 86:892, 1975.

Lake AM, Oski FA: Peripheral lymphadenopathy in children: 10 year experience with excisional biopsy. *Am J Dis Child* 132:357, 1978.

Lerer RJ, Kalavsky SM: Central nervous system diseases associated with *Mycoplasma pneumoniae* infection. *Pediatrics* 52:658, 1973.

Leung DYM, Chu ET, Wood N, et al: Immunoregulatory T cell abnormalities in MCLNS. *J Immunol* 130:2002, 1983.

McCormack WM, Alpert S, McComb DE, et al: Fifteen month followup study of women infected with *Chlamydia trachomatis*. *N Engl J Med* 300:123, 1979.

Medical Letter: Treatment of sexually transmitted diseases. 30:5, 1988.

Nagashima M, Matsushima M, Matsuoka H, et al: High-dose gammaglobulin therapy for Kawasaki disease. *J Pediatr* 110:710, 1987.

Newburger JW, Takahashi M, Burns JC, et al: The treatment of Kawasaki syndrome with intravenous gamma globulin. *N Engl J Med* 315:341, 1986.

Quinn PA, Gillan JE, et al: Intrauterine infection with *Ureaplasma urealyticum* as a cause of fatal neonatal pneumonia. *Pediatr Infect Dis* 4:538, 1985.

Rauch AM, Hurwitz ES: Centers for Disease Control (CDC) case definition of Kawasaki syndrome. *Pediatr Infect Dis* 4:702, 1985.

Schachter J, Sweet RL, Grossman M, et al: Experience with the routine use of erythromycin for chlamydial infections in pregnancy. *N Engl J Med* 314:276, 1986.

Taylor HR: Report of a workshop: Research priorities for the control of trachoma. *J Infect Dis* 152:383, 1985.

Thompson SE, Washington AE: Epidemiology of sexually transmitted *Chlamydia trachomatis* infections. *Epidemiol Rev* 5:95, 1983.

Torres JR, et al: Cat scratch disease causing reversible encephalopathy. *JAMA* 240:1628, 1978.

Wear DJ, Margileth AM, Hadfield TL, et al: Cat scratch disease: A bacterial infection. *Science* 221:1403, 1983.

Rickettsia 8

RICKETTSIAL DISEASE

Rickettsia are obligate intracellular parasites, maintained in nature by an animal reservoir and transmitted to humans by an insect vector. The illnesses are usually characterized by sudden onset, high fever of 1 or more weeks, headache, malaise, prostration, characteristic rash in most of them, and an underlying vasculitis. During convalescence they induce serum agglutinins against specific *Proteus* strains (OX 19, OX 2, and OX K). The latter is identified with scrub typhus. The test is called Weil-Felix reaction, and is positive with epidemic murine typhus and Rocky Mountain Spotted Fever (RMSF). It is not positive in patients with rickettsial pox, or Q fever. A convalescent serum titer of 1:160 or higher is usually diagnostic; antibiotics may blunt the serological response. More sensitive and specific tests are complement fixation reactions to group specific soluble rickettsial antigens. Complement fixation antibodies usually appear during the second and third week of illness, and even later if antibiotics were begun in the first 3–5 days.

Isolation of the organism from the blood is difficult and it involves intraperitoneal injection into male guinea pigs. The organism can be identified in skin biopsy material with immunofluorescent techniques, although such methods are not widely available. The organism can be seen as early as the fourth day of illness or as late as the tenth day.

Differential Diagnosis

The rickettsial diseases are closely related to each other and can be distinguished partly on epidemiologic grounds. Epidemic typhus is transmitted to man in the feces of the human body louse, *Pediculus humanus*. Murine typhus is transmitted by rat feces, and scrub typhus is mite-borne. RMSF is transmitted by ticks. Rickettsial pox is carried by a small colorless mite.

The rash resembles that of meningococcemia but differs in that the meningococcal rash develops early during the onset of the illness, and the rickettsial rashes usually appear about the fourth day of fever, and only gradually become petechial. Sometimes the rash of RMSF is confused with rubella, or rubeola, or that of Kawasaki disease. It is very difficult to distinguish RMSF from epidemic louse-born typhus, since both can be very severe with peripheral vascular collapse, ecchymotic skin lesions, renal failure, and delirium. The major difference is that the rash of RMSF appears first in the cooler distal extremities (*R. rickettsii* grows at 25°C) whereas in epidemic typhus, the rash usually appears first over the axillary folds and trunk, and rarely involves palms, soles, face (*R. prowazekii* grows at 32° C). Murine typhus is a much milder disease and may be distinguished mostly by specific serologic reactions.

Therapeutic Considerations

Early diagnosis and early treatment carry a good prognosis. If the disease is strongly suspected, treatment should be initiated since definitive serologic data may not be available until after the patient has died. Chloramphenicol is the drug of choice in children, with an initial oral dose of 50 mg/kg/day given in divided doses every 6–8 hours until the patient has been afebrile for 4–6 days. Sometimes in acutely ill patients intravenous loading dose would be recommended. The response to treatment is usually prompt when initiated early in the illness before the vasculitis is well-established. Improvement usually is evident within 36–48 hours with defervescence in 2–3 days.

RICKETTSIALPOX

Definition

Rickettsialpox is a mild febrile illness following infection by *R. akari* transmitted from mice by mites.

Epidemiology

The disease is rarely diagnosed, and since it is not reportable in the United States, no indication of prevalence is available.

Natural History

The site of the bite usually develops into a small papule, later with an ulcer and a dark crust that heals leaving a scar. There may be regional lymphadenopathy and intermittent fever for a week or so. Headache, photophobia, and myalgia are common. During the febrile period, there can be a generalized maculopapular rash which spares the palms and soles. The disease is self-limited and no deaths have been reported.

Diagnosis

A rising titer of specific complement fixation antibodies confirms the diagnosis.

Treatment

No treatment is indicated for mild illness. Tetracycline is effective for more severe illness (Brettman et al, 1981).

Prognosis

The prognosis is excellent.

ROCKY MOUNTAIN SPOTTED FEVER

Definition

Rocky Mountain Spotted Fever (RMSF) is a rickettsial disease transmitted by tick bite. It is reported most frequently from Oklahoma, North Carolina, and other states in the west-south-central regions.

Basic Science

RMSF and other rickettsial diseases are characterized by an exanthem that involves the small blood vessels of the skin, subcutaneous tissue, lungs, and CNS. Endothelial swelling leads to thrombosis and necrosis of skin. Occluded vessels are surrounded by mononuclear cells, plasma cells and macrophages.

The organism is *Rickettsia rickettsii* and is found in many rodents who do not become ill. The transmission to man is via the wood tick, *Dermacentor andersoni*, or the dog tick *Dermacentor variabilis*.

Sporadic clusters of cases have been reported from unlikely areas such as New York City (Salgo et al, 1988).

Epidemiology

Reported cases in the United States have risen from about 0.10/100,000 population in 1960 to about 0.50/100,000 population in 1983. This apparent increase may represent improved reporting. Only Maine and Vermont reported no cases in the most recent 3-year period. (The disease is not reportable in Alaska or Hawaii.)

Natural History

The incubation period in children is variable, between 1 and 8 days before the onset of headache, myalgia, and fever. Only half the patients have a history of tick bite, and local reaction at the site of the bite is uncommon. The disease is most prevalent between April 1 and August 31 in the United States. Individuals under 19 years of age account for about half of the cases, with the highest incidence in 5- to 9-year-olds. The incidence is higher for males than females, and higher for whites than blacks. The overall case-fatality ratio in 1981–1983 was 4% (Fishbein et al, 1985).

Diagnosis

Almost all patients have fever and myalgia, headache, and rash. The rash may appear a few days after the onset of fever and myalgia. It starts on the ankles, wrists, and lower legs, then spreads to the whole body, including hands and soles. At the beginning it is maculopapular, but later petechial and purpuric. Splenomegaly is common, as are other systemic signs including facial edema, CNS symptoms, myocarditis, and pneumonitis. Nearly half the patients have thrombocytopenia, and in severe forms, disseminated intravascular coagulation. In uncomplicated cases, recovery occurs in the third week of illness.

Cases of RMSF can be confirmed by a complement fixation titer of equal to or greater than 16, or a single indirect fluorescent antibody titer of over 64, or with paired serum specimens a four fold rise in titer. Isolation of the organism by skin biopsy confirms the diagnosis. Four-fold increases in the Weil-Felix assay (proteus OX 19 or OX 2), or positive latex agglutination provide evidence of probable infection (Fishbein et al, 1985).

Treatment

Chloramphenicol is the drug of choice in children, but it is not always effective; 50–75 mg/kg/day intravenously is recommended to be continued until the patient is afebrile for 48 hours. Tetracyclines in the same dose may be useful in older children or adolescents. Vigorous supportive therapy in the event of shock may be required.

CONTROVERSY

Glucocorticoids have been advocated, but no critical evaluation has been undertaken.

Prognosis

For those patients who report having been bitten by a tick, prompt treatment at the onset of symptoms with chloramphenicol or tetracyclines is usually effective. Thus, in retrospect, those patients who died were less likely to have reported a tick bite within 2 weeks of onset of illness, and less likely to have been treated with chloramphenicol or tetracyclines.

CASE ILLUSTRATION

An 8-year-old white child was admitted in July with a complaint of rash and fever. One week before admission a tick was found in her hair. Six days before admission she developed a stiff neck and a temperature of 40°C. Her pediatrician diagnosed otitis and treated her with amoxicillin and erythromycin. The following day she had an erythematous rash on the ankles, wrists, palms, and soles and a worsening of symptoms with stiff neck and continuing fever. Amoxicillin was discontinued on the assumption that some of the symptoms could be related to the drug. However, she continued to be febrile and had significant nausea and vomiting.

When admitted she appeared very sick, with a temperature of 40°C, and a heart rate of 150. She had an erythematous macular and papular rash on the distal extremities, including palms and soles. Some lesions would blanche, but others were petechial, several millimeters in diameter. She had slight conjunctivitis and a stiff neck. There was no significant lymphadenopathy. Her chest was clear. The abdomen was diffusely slightly tender without palpable organs. Neurologic examination was within normal limits. Her white blood count was 15,200, 88% polys, 7 lymphs, 5 monos, hematocrit 44, sedimentation rate 33. Her spinal fluid showed 17 white blood cells, 28% polys, 67% lymphs, 5% monos, protein 18, glucose 68, and Gram stain negative. Blood cultures were subsequently negative. The Weil-Felix agglutination was positive and complement fixation studies were later returned as positive, confirming the diagnosis of RMSF. The differential included the possibility of meningococcemia, gonococcemia, or syphilis, but previous treatment with amoxicillin had not produced any response. She was treated with chloramphenicol on admission on the assumption of the diagnosis before the serologic tests confirmed it. On that regimen she became asymptomatic promptly, and was discharged after 3 days with advice to continue oral chloramphenicol another 4–6 days.

QUESTIONS AND COMMENTS

With what condition could RMSF be confused?

In this instance, when it was recognized there was a fever, a rash with involvment of palms and soles, and aseptic meningitis, after treatment with amoxicillin, the most likely possibilities included RMSF and enteroviral infection. The history of a tick having been removed 1 week before admission and the prompt response to chloramphenicol made RMSF most likely. It was only later that the serology was returned and confirmed the diagnosis.

Why was a skin biopsy not done?

It is clear that rickettsia can be demonstrated as early as 3–4 days in macular lesions. On the other hand, the sensitivity of this test is low and the presumptive diagnosis was so strong that it was felt inappropriate to subject the patient to biopsy. Confirmation came from serologic studies later.

Prevention

No vaccine is available.

Q FEVER

Definition

Q fever due to *Coxiella burnetii* infection first described in adults in 1937, is a febrile illness which is usually characterized by fever, headache, and pneumonia.

Epidemiology

This condition is not usually considered by pediatricians because of the rarity of reports among children even in endemic areas. A recent report from the Netherlands describes the illness in 18 children younger than 3 years of age seen during a 16-month period. The authors suggest that the condition may be underdiagnosed. Its incidence in this country is not known (Richardus et al, 1985). Individuals at risk are those who work with sheep (including researchers) and in textile mills that process wool. Contact with an infected parturient cat was responsible for an outbreak of Q fever in Nova Scotia (Marrie et al, 1988).

Natural History

Q fever differs from most rickettsial diseases in that it is usually transmitted by inhalation of dust rather than through the bite of an insect. The incubation period is 9–20 days. The condition is characterized by relapsing episodes of fever, often considered fever of unknown origin. Over half of the patients have pneumonia and, less often, febrile convulsions, meningeal irritation, hepatitis, or an exacerbation of asthma. A wide variety of nonspecific symptoms including anorexia, myalgia, nausea, vomiting, and headache were seen in the infants in the Netherlands. A few of the children had an erythematous skin rash which persisted for several days. Only one child had purpuric lesions on the face and legs that occurred during the course of the *C. burnetii* infection.

Diagnosis

Leukocytosis persists with a mean value of 25,000 and a shift to immature cells. Complement fixing antibodies show a more than four-fold rise. The diagnosis can be confirmed by the demonstration of a specific IgM antibody in serum diluted to more than 1:16 by an indirect immunofluorescence test. The Weil-Felix test is not positive in Q fever.

Treatment

Chloramphenicol is the drug of choice and it is usually recommended that treatment be continued until the patient has been afebrile for about 5 days. Some advocate adding tetracyclines in the case of adults with Q fever, but this is not appropriate in young children.

Prognosis

Most patients recover in a month or two.

Prevention

Most infected individuals have had contact with animals, and/or have ingested unpasteurized milk. The organism apparently persists in feces of infected animals. It may also exist in an animal tick cycle and has been recognized in individuals bitten by *Dermacentor andersoni*. Avoidance of fomites associated with infected animals is the best prevention. Nonimmune individuals who are exposed to sheep can be immunized.

TYPHUS

Definition

Typhus is the name of a group of rickettsial diseases which can be epidemic (*R. prowazekii*) or endemic (*R. mooseri*). Both forms are characterized by flu-like symptoms of fever, headache, weakness, followed in 4–7 days by a rash. Epidemic typhus has not been reported in the United States in recent years. Scrub typhus is caused by *R. tsutsugamushi* and is seen only in Asia.

Natural History

Epidemic typhus has no animal host, but is spread by lice or by lice-contaminated clothing, bedding, or furniture that aerosolizes lice feces; thus, organisms can be transmitted to human hosts through inhalation, ingestion, or skin abrasions. The incubation period is less than 2 weeks and the illness lasts about a week.

Endemic typhus (murine) has a rat reservoir and may be transmitted by rat fleas or lice. It is found worldwide; 25 cases were reported in the United States in 1985.

Human infection can occur from the excreta of an infected flea entering at the site of a bite, or from inhalation of infected flea feces. The illness is usually mild and is distinguished from epidemic typhus by serology. The incubation period is 6–14 days, with flu-like symptoms of headache, arthralgia, and fever lasting 9–14 days. The rash begins on the trunk and has a peripheral spread. Unlike RMSF, it rarely involves palms, soles, or face. The lesion is maculopapular with ill-defined borders and is rarely purpuric.

Scrub typhus (Tsutsugamushi disease) is seen exclusively in a region bounded by Japan, the Solomon Islands, and Pakistan. It is transmitted by mites that are both reservoirs and vectors, and humans are infected by a bite. The site of the bite becomes necrotic in over half the cases. Regional lymphadenopathy precedes an acute febrile illness by 1–2 weeks. Headache, macular rash on the trunk which later extends to the limbs, generalized lymphadenopathy, and hepatosplenomegaly are common.

Diagnosis

The Weil-Felix reaction is positive in louse-borne and flea-borne typhus. The reaction depends on the antigenic similarity of strains of *Proteus vulgaris* and rickettsiae. The antibody titers rise during the illness but do not persist more than several months.

Treatment

As with other rickettsial diseases, chloramphenicol, 50 mg/kg/day in four divided doses orally or intravenously, is effective. Mild illness is probably often mistaken for a viral exanthem and does not require treatment.

Prognosis

Mortality from epidemic typhus can be high in situations of crowding and poverty, expecially among adults. Case fatality rates for endemic typhus in children are less than 1%.

Prevention

Control of rat reservoir and use of insecticides to kill lice will control spread of typhus.

REFERENCES

Bernard KW, Helmick CG, Kaplan JE, et al: Surveillance of Rocky Mountain Spotted Fever in the United States 1978–1980. *J Infect Dis* 146:297, 1982.

Brettman LR, Lewin S, Holzman RS, et al: Rickettsialpox: report of an outbreak and a contemporary review. *Medicine* 60:363, 1981.

Fishbein DB, Kaplan JE, Bernard KW, et al: Surveillance of Rocky Mountain Spotted Fever, United States 1981–1983. *MMWR* 33:1555, 1985.

Marrie TJ, MacDonald A, Durant H et al: An outbreak of Q fever probably due to contact with a parturient cat. *Chest* 93:98, 1988.

Richardus JH, Dumas AM, Huisman J, et al: Q fever in infancy: A review of 18 cases. *Pediatr Infect Dis* 4:369, 1985.

Salgo MP, Telzak EE, Currie B, et al: A focus of rocky mountain spotted fever within New York City. *N Engl J Med* 318:1345, 1988.

Woodward TE: Rocky Mountain spotted fever: Epidemiological and early clinical signs are keys to treatment and reduced mortality. *J Infect Dis* 150:465, 1984.

Fungi 9

ASPERGILLOSIS

Definition

Infection with *Aspergillus fumigatis* can cause granulomatous lesions of the skin, vagina, and invasive disease of nasal sinuses, bones, lungs, and meninges, especially in immunocompromised patients. A diffuse allergic response may occur, known as allergic bronchopulmonary aspergillosis.

Epidemiology

Some asthmatic patients hospitalized with chronic pulmonary disability have allergic bronchopulmonary aspergillosis (Henderson et al, 1968). As more individuals undergo chemotherapy for leukemia and other malignancies, the presence of symptomatic and even fatal invasive aspergillosis has become an increasing problem.

Natural History

The organism is saphrophytic and grows in masses of matted mycelia in bronchiectatic, tuberculous, or histoplasmotic cavities. "Fungus balls" may be evident without invasion.

Aspergillus is an ubiquitous organism with airborne spores. Outbreaks have occurred during construction where dust can carry spores. Sometimes air conditioning or heating ducts have been incriminated (Mahoney et al, 1979).

Endogenous routes of transmission include spread from the nasopharynx and gastrointestinal tract (Krick and Remington, 1976).

Allergic bronchopulmonary aspergillosis, a disease superimposed on chronic pulmonary disease, was first recognized in 1952. In immunosuppressed patients, a rapidly invasive infection can produce a necrotizing pneumonia. Some individuals become sensitized to the organism and develop wheezing, fever, sputum with characteristic brown plugs, and eosinophilia.

Diagnosis

Bronchopulmonary aspergillosis is usually considered when the blood eosinophil count rises to more than 1000/mm^3. The diagnosis is probable when immediate skin reactivity to the antigen is positive, precipitating antibodies are present, serum IgE concentration exceeds 1000 ng/ml, pulmonary infiltrates and proximal bronchiectasis are evident. Pulmonary blebs and bullae occur in advanced stages (Mendelson et al, 1985). Hyphae may be seen in the sputum of individuals with invasive disease.

Migratory pulmonary infiltrates, and areas of atelectasis are commonly seen on chest radiographs.

Treatment

Aspergillomas (fungus balls) in the lung are sometimes resected. Allergic bronchopulmonary aspergillosis responds to corticosteroids. Systemic aspergillosis, almost exclusively seen in immunosuppressed patients, requires intravenous amphotericin B. The duration of therapy will depend on the individual's response. Since the drug is nephrotoxic, BUN and creatinine should be followed.

Prognosis

Individuals can be asymptomatic with localized infection. Disseminated disease, particularly in leukemia, is almost always fatal.

Prevention

It is difficult to avoid contact with this ubiquitous organism. However, it behooves those who care for immunosuppressed patients to be sure air is filtered to remove spores in rooms where such patients are under care. The occurrence of hospital-acquired infection should stimulate immediate environmental investigation.

CASE ILLUSTRATION

A previously healthy 14-year-old black male was admitted in severe respiratory distress. About 3 weeks earlier, he had a low-grade fever, headache, and vomiting with a persistent mild cough. The cough became more severe and productive of yellow sputum. His pediatrician diagnosed pneumonia and prescribed erythromycin and theophylline, but there was no significant improvement.

On admission his temperature was 38°C, respiratory rate 80, and he was severely ill. On 70% inspired oxygen, his arterial oxygen tension was 53, and P_{CO_2} 41, with a pH of 7.42. He had a marked leukocytosis of 36,000, with a 75% polys. A chest radiograph showed a diffuse infiltrative process with a reticular nodular pattern. A tracheal aspirate was negative for bacteria and acid-fast bacilli, and a tuberculin test and a test for infectious mononucleosis were negative. Because of the extent and seriousness of the process, open lung biopsy was carried out which revealed extensive involvement with *A. fumigatus.* No other organisms were identified.

After this surprising observation, a more detailed history revealed he had been spreading woodchips around his garden. He had not traveled and there was no close exposure to animals. The rarity of invasive aspergillus in immunocompetent hosts triggered an investigation into this patient's host defense mechanisms. It was subsequently ascertained that he had chronic granulomatous disease, unknown to himself or members of his family. This had been his first serious infection. He recovered completely after treatment with amphotericin, and was advised to lead a normal life but to wear a mask when he is working in his garden or spreading woodchips.

BLASTOMYCOSIS

Definition

Blastomycosis, caused by *Blastomyces dermatitidis,* starts as a pulmonary infection but can disseminate to other organs particularly the skin and bones.

Natural History

The organism is widely distributed in the United States and Canada, particularly in the midwest and central south. The natural habitat of the organism is still unclear, but soil near a beaver pond was incriminated in the epidemic (Klein et al, 1986). It is thought that humans acquire infection by inhalation of oval conidia. The incubation period can range 3–15 weeks (mean about 6 weeks). Although the illness is widely recognized in adults, very few instances of infection in children have been reported until recently (Klein et al, 1986).

The clinical manifestations are usually described as predominantly pulmonary with the possibility of dissemination to other organs and a chronic cutaneous form. The initial pulmonary infection may be mild or may progress to pneumonia with pleuritis. Occasionally, cavities can occur in the lung, but more commonly the pulmonary infection heals without scarring or calcification.

In the disseminated disease, which can be fatal, the skin was involved in more than half of the patients. One-third of the patients had liver, bone, CNS, or splenic involvement.

The chronic cutaneous disease occurs as one or more subcutaneous nodules most commonly on exposed surfaces. The lesions eventually ulcerate and if untreated form elevated granulomatous lesions. The organisms can be found in the microabscesses within the lesion. Long bone involvement is a complication of disseminated blastomycosis.

Diagnosis

The organism has a characteristic morphology which permits a presumptive diagnosis on examination of body fluids or tissue obtained by biopsy. Definitive diagnosis depends on culture. The blastomycin skin test is not reliable, nor are serologic tests (immunodiffusion and complement fixation). An assay of in vitro transformation of lymphocytes from patients in the presence of an antigen from blastomyces is promising (Bradsher, 1984).

Treatment

Since the untreated disease has a high case fatality rate, it is important to identify the organism and initiate treatment. Amphotericin B, given intravenously is effective. Ketoconazole, an oral imidazole, may be effective and preferable in milder cases.

CANDIDA ALBICANS INFECTION (MONILIASIS)

Definition

Congenital, disseminated, or acquired superficial infections with species of *Candida* may occur, especially in newborn infants and immunocompromised patients, and in individuals who receive intravenous alimentation. The omnipresent yeast, *C. albicans,* infects nearly all individuals at some time during life, so that a positive skin test is used as a test of T-cell function. Unless the inoculum is very large, or the individual's defenses are compromised, most infections are superficial or subclinical. Other *Candida* species can cause infection. *C. parapsilosis* has been reported as a cause of meningitis.

Epidemiology

One longitudinal study of infants showed that by 4 weeks of age, 82% of infants were found to have *Candida* in the mouth (Russell and Lay, 1973). Fungal colonization, predominantly *Candida,* was found in 26.7% of very low birth weight infants. Two-thirds were colonized at 1 week of age (Bayley et al, 1986). Disseminated candidiasis, once rare, is currently more common because of the use of intravenous alimentation and immunosuppressive chemotherapy. Chronic mucocutaneous candidiasis may occur alone or in patients with hypoparathyroidism or Addison disease.

Natural History

CONGENITAL INFECTION

Intrauterine infection can occur with maternal disease and involvement of the placenta. Ascending infection from the vaginal flora has been reported to contribute to spontaneous abortion. Some infants have been born with a diffuse macular rash and pneumonia from *Candida* infection. Cord lesions of 1- to 3-mm yellowish white plaques have been described in intrauterine infection (Schirar et al, 1974).

Colonization with *C. albicans, C. tropicalis,* and *T. pullulens* appears early in infants. *C. parapsilosis* appears at 2–3 weeks of age. The most common sites are rectal, oral, endotracheal, and groin in that order in low birth weight infants (Bayley et al, 1986).

THRUSH

The most common infection in infants is oral thrush, usually presenting in the second week. The lesions are plaques of white, friable, pseudomembranous material on a red base over the tongue and buccal mucosa. The diagnosis can be confirmed by a KOH preparation of scrapings from a typical lesion, and by culture.

CUTANEOUS LESIONS

Localized involvement of skin creases and diaper area are also common. Multiple tiny vesicopustules merge to form brightened scaly plaques. Satellite lesions are characteristic. Localized disease will respond to nystatin applied locally. Usually ointments are tolerated best.

DISSEMINATED CANDIDIASIS

Invasive disease occurs in about 7–8% of colonized infants. It can also occur as the consequence of contaminated intravenous solutions. Infants of less than 28 weeks' gestation or on intravenous alimentation are at greatest risk. In all intensive care units, and among immunocompromised hosts, *Candida* is an ever-present threat. Contamination of urinary and vascular catheters, and any indwelling devices may be portals of entry.

OPHTHALMITIS

Ophthalmitis is an occasional complication and justifies fundoscopic examination whenever the condition is suspected. Osteomyelitis, endocarditis, and meningitis have been reported in addition to the more common pneumonia.

Diagnosis

No characteristic radiographic or serologic tests are diagnostic. Occasionally, the organism can be found in the buffy coat of a centrifuged blood specimen. Culture of the organism from a nonpermissive site is diagnostic, albeit rarely accomplished. Demonstration of the organism may depend on lung biopsy or marrow aspiration. Rarely a budding yeast form has been found in spinal fluid.

Treatment

Nystatin suspension, 100,000–200,000 units by mouth four times a day for 10–14 days usually cures oral thrush. Failure of the lesions to resolve requires an investigation for an immune deficiency state.

Disseminated candidiasis should be treated vigorously. Amphotericin B is the drug of choice. Ketoconazole and miconazole may be used for milder disease or if response is inadequate to the first drugs (Smith and Congdon, 1985). Only flucytosine was effective in the one case of meningitis from *C. parapsilosis.*

Prevention

Candida is widely distributed and can be considered normal flora in healthy individuals. Overgrowth occurs after antibiotic therapy or in immunocompromised individuals.

Candida may be acquired in hospitals from contaminated equipment. Clearly the need for indwelling tubes should be strictly monitored and they should be used for a minimal period.

COCCIDIOIDOMYCOSIS

Definition

Coccidioides immitis is a fungus which infects by aspiration into the respiratory tract. Very rarely it can infect the skin.

Epidemiology

The spores of this fungus are widely distributed throughout the western and southwestern parts of the United States, as well as Central and South America. Occasional cases have been reported in Australia and other areas of the world. The spores are airborne as a result of windstorms or digging, and archaeologists are at special risk. It is estimated that there are probably 100,000 new cases each year in the United States.

Natural History

The fungus grows in pulmonary tissue and establishes an acute inflammatory reaction. Polys predominate early in the process and, later, granulomas are formed. Large cavitary lesions can occur similar to those found in tuberculosis. Hilar lymph nodes enlarge and may rupture in a manner similar to that of tuberculous infection. Very rarely, perhaps in 1% of all symptomatic cases, there can be hematogenous spread, particularly to the meninges. Individuals of darker races and pregnant women of all races are at greatest risk.

Diagnosis

Many individuals are infected as evidenced by positive skin tests, but never become ill. The incubation period is thought to be 10–20 days, with the onset then of fever, muscle aches, headaches, and a nonproductive cough. A skin rash is present in about half of the patients, either as a maculopapular or urticarial lesion on the lower trunk or thighs. Later, a more typical erythema nodosum with painful subcutaneous nodules, especially over the anterior tibial surfaces can be seen.

The acute pulmonary infection may be mild and transient or fulminating and lethal. Spontaneous recovery comes in about 95% of patients with symptomatic disease.

The radiographic changes mimic tuberculosis, histoplasmosis, or blastomycosis. Pleural effusion and pleural thickening is common. There may be areas of cavity and even honeycombing within the lungs.

CASE ILLUSTRATION

A 23-year-old white male archaeology student was digging for dinosaur bones in southern California when he experienced a low-grade fever, an intensely itchy rash, chest pain, myalgia, and arthralgias. Gradually the rash became a toxic erythema present over the trunk and limbs. He became short of breath and a few fine inspiratory crackles were heard. The chest roentgenograms revealed patchy areas of consolidation and his sputum was positive for *C. immitis*. His blood gases revealed a Pao_2 of 40 mm Hg.

Pulmonary consolidation increased and pulmonary failure was evident about 1 week into the course of the illness. He was intubated and maintained with 10 cm H_2O of water continuous positive airway pressure in an inspired oxygen of 0.6. He was started on intravenous amphotericin B and oral ketoconazole with gradual improvement. However, he had not returned to his usual state of health for at least 9 months after discharge from the hospital (patient cited by Larson et al, 1985).

Serologic tests can substantiate the diagnosis. Confirmation comes from direct microscopic examination of sputum or biopsy material which reveals the distinctive sporangia. Antibodies to *C. immitis* in CSF can be demonstrated by either complement-fixation tests or by immunodiffusion (Drutz et al, 1978).

Treatment

The disease is usually self-limited, but when symptoms occur the drug of choice is amphotericin B. Other newer antifungal agents have activity against the organism in vitro and in vivo but their superiority to amphotericin B has not been demonstrated to date.

CRYPTOCOCCUS NEOFORMANS

Definition

Cryptococcus causes infections primarily in the lungs but also skin and CNS, particularly in individuals who are immunocompromised.

Basic Science

C. neoformans is a widely distributed yeast, found particularly in soil contaminated by pigeon droppings. Humans are infected principally by inhalation of aerosolized organisms that can enter air conditioning systems, or be stirred up at building sites. The organism is spherical or ellipsoid and is surrounded by a distinctive thick-walled gelatinous capsule that is composed of a polysaccharide. At least four serotypes are known, and only serotype A is found commonly in eastern and central United States.

Epidemiology

This opportunistic infection is most likely to be found in situations where a number of individuals are immunocompromised. Normal individuals may develop the disease if heavily exposed to the organism. The disease is one of the problems encountered by patients with AIDS.

Natural History

Most of the initial infections are in the form of asymptomatic pulmonary foci which may be found on routine chest radiograph. It is possible to have hematogenous dissemination and meningoencephalitis as a consequence of cryptococcosis. Individuals infected with cryptococci have general constitutional symptoms such as malaise, low-grade fever, and often a chronic dry cough.

Cutaneous lesions may appear as painless erythematous papules and occasionally pustules and nodules that gradually enlarge and ulcerate and may be purulent.

Diagnosis

If the lungs are the only site of cryptococcal disease, the diagnosis will require transbronchial or open lung biopsy. With fiberoptic bronchoscopy it is often possible to obtain by brushings enough material to demonstrate the organism. Transbronchial biopsy is necessary to know if the organism has invaded tissue. Occasionally, it can be found in asymptomatic individuals. The organism can be grown on media such as Sabouraud glucose agar, but it rarely grows well and may require up to 6 weeks.

In meningoencephalitis, a latex agglutination test for the polysaccharide capsular antigen can provide rapid diagnosis (Snow and Dismukes, 1975).

Treatment

The most common form of cryptococcosis is an isolated pulmonary lesion which, if asymptomatic, may not require treatment. If the individual is immunosuppressed, however, it is appropriate to use amphotericin B. If hematogenous spread is a possibility then amphotericin combined with flucytosine is recommended. The duration of therapy is dependent on the individual's response.

Prognosis

The outlook is good if the individuals have been treated with amphotericin B before serious meningoencephalitis develops. Most of the pulmonary forms of the disease are reversible with treatment and solitary lesions may regress without treatment.

HISTOPLASMOSIS

Definition

Histoplasma capsulatum is a ubiquitous fungus that is found free in certain soils. If inhaled it can be the source of pulmonary disease, and is capable of causing disseminated disease.

Epidemiology

This is the most prevalent systemic fungus infection, especially in the western Appalachian slopes bordering on the tributaries of the Ohio, Missouri, and Mississippi Rivers. About 80–90% of young adults have positive skin tests to the fungal antigen. The organism has been found in many other areas of Europe and North America, including Montreal, Canada.

Natural History

H. capsulatum is found in chicken dung and even in feathers. Sites of old farms exposed by construction can be the source of the organisms which have become aerosolized and infect individuals. One of the most severe epidemics occurred in Arkansas, when coal dust from a strip mine was shovelled into bins near classrooms with open windows. After the 10- to 14-day incubation period, 36 pupils became febrile, had a cough, and prostration. Later, 146 children showed positive serology for histoplasmosis. (The tale of solving this puzzling epidemic was told by Berton Roueche in the *New Yorker*, September 17, 1960.)

Usually there is a primary focus in the lung with regional lymphatic spread and some local inflammation. Mononuclear cells are literally filled with phagocytized yeast cells. There is relatively little inflammation around each focus. In most respects, the disorder resembles tuberculosis, including having a tendency for hematogenous spread. Hypersensitivity can occur, which can be determined by histoplasmin skin tests. The interval from the primary inoculation to positivity of the skin test is 3–6 weeks. Skin tests can produce positive serology, hence they are not widely used.

Most infected individuals are asymptomatic. Symptomatic illness begins 7–21 days after exposure with chills, fever, headache, malaise, and myalgia. A nonproductive cough and pleural pain may occur. Chest radiographs may show patchy pneumonitis and enlarged hilar nodes. Healing may occur with calcification around the sites of infection.

Progressive disseminated disease is more common in young infants and in those individuals who are immunosuppressed. Hepatosplenomegaly and anemia result from widespread involvement of the reticuloendothelial system. Dissemination to all organs of the body has been reported. Nodules and ulceration of the skin or mucous membranes have been described.

Diagnosis

Organisms may be seen in infected secretions and tissues. Gastric washings are not usually very helpful. The chest radiograph may be quite characteristic with multiple areas of radiodensity, although it can be normal. Complement fixation test may be positive. A radioimmunoassay for detection of *H. capsulatum* antigen in serum, urine, or CSF is a useful new method for diagnosis of disseminated disease (Wheat et al, 1986).

Treatment

The benign forms of the disease are self-limited and no treatment is indicated. Rapidly progressive disease may be treated with amphotericin B intravenously. The dose and duration of therapy must be individualized.

REFERENCES

Bayley JE, Kliegman RM, Fanaroff AA: Disseminated fungal infections in very low birth weight infants: Clinical manifestations in epidemiology. *Pediatrics* 73:144, 1984.

Bayley JE, Kliegman RM, et al: Fungal colonization in the very low birth weight infant. *Pediatrics* 78:225, 1986.

Bodey GP, Fainstein V (eds): *Candidiasis*. New York, Raven Press, 1985.

Bradsher RW: Development of specific immunity in patients with pulmonary or extrapulmonary blastomycosis. *Am Rev Respir Dis* 129:430, 1984.

Brueton NJ: Allergic bronchopulmonary aspergillosis complicating cystic fibrosis in childhood. *Arch Dis Child* 55:348, 1980.

Christie A: Histoplasmosis. In Kendig E, Chernick V (eds): *Disorders of the Respiratory Tract of Children*. Philadelphia, WB Saunders, 1983, p. 721.

Drutz DJ, Catanzaro A: Coccidiomycosis. *Am Rev Respir Dis* 117:559 and 727, 1978.

Faix RG: *Candida parapsilosis* meningitis in a premature infant. *J Pediatr Infect Dis* 2:462, 1983.

Hammerman KJ, et al: Pulmonary cryptococcosis clinical forms and treatment. *Am Rev Respir Dis* 108:1116, 1973.

Henderson AH, English MP, Vecht RJ: Pulmonary aspergillosis: A survey of its occurrence in patients with chronic lung disease and a discussion of the significance of diagnostic tests. *Thorax* 23:513, 1968.

Johnson DE, Thompson TR, Green TP: Systemic candidiasis in very low birth weight infants (under 1500 grams). *Pediatrics* 73:138, 1984.

Klein BS, Vergeront JM, Weeks RJ, et al: Isolation of *Blastomyces dermatiditis* in soil associated with a large outbreak of blastomycosis in Wisconsin. *N Engl J Med* 314:529, 1986.

Krick JA, Remington JS: Opportunistic invasive fungal infections in patients with leukemia and lymphoma. *Clin Hematol* 5:245, 1976.

Larson RA, Jacobson JA, Morris AH: Acute respiratory failure caused by primary pulmonary coccidioidomycosis. *Am Rev Respir Dis* 131:739, 1985.

Mahoney DH, Steuber P, Starling KA, et al: An outbreak of aspergillosis in children with acute leukemia. *J Pediatr* 95:70, 1979.

Medoff G, Kobayashi GS: Fungal diseases. In: Feigin RD, Cherry JD (eds): *Textbook of Pediatric Infectious Diseases*. Philadelphia, WB Saunders, 1981.

Mendelson EB, Fisher MR, Mintzer RA, et al: Roentgenographic and clinical staging of allergic bronchopulmonary aspergillosis. *Chest* 87:334, 1985.

Reynolds RJ, Penn RL, Grafton WD, et al: Tissue morphology of *Histoplasma* capsulation in acute histoplasmosis. *Am Rev Respir Dis* 130:317, 1984.

Russell C, Lay KM: Natural history of *Candida* species and yeasts in oral cavities of infants. *Arch Oral Biol* 18:957, 1973.

Sathapatayavongs B, Batteiger BE, Wheat LJ, et al: Clinical and laboratory features of disseminated histoplasmosis during two large urban outbreaks. *Medicine* 62:263, 1983.

Schirar A, Rendu C, Viehl JP, et al: Congenital mycosis (*Candida albicans*). *Biol Neonate* 24:273, 1974.

Smith H, Congdon P: Neonatal systemic candidiasis. *Arch Dis Child* 60:365, 1985.

Snow RM, Dismukes WE: Cryptococcal meningitis: Diagnostic value of cryptococcal antigen in cerebrospinal fluid. *Arch Intern Med* 135:1155, 1975.

Stone HH: Studies in the pathogenesis, diagnosis, and treatment of *Candida* sepsis in children. *J Pediatr Surg* 9:127, 1974.

Wheat LJ, Kohler RB, Tewari RP: Diagnosis of disseminated histoplasmosis by detection of *Histoplasma capsulatum* antigen in serum and urine specimens. *N Engl J Med* 314:83, 1986.

Wientzen RL, Utz JP: Coccidioidomycosis. In: Kendig E, Chernick V (eds): *Disorders of the Respiratory Tract of Children*. Philadelphia, WB Saunders, 1983, p. 744.

Parasitic Infections 10

Rapid air travel and increased mobility of people throughout the world expose populations and individuals to a wide variety of unfamiliar organisms. Consideration of the possibility of parasitic infection is the responsibility of all clinicians. Although many parasites are endemic in certain regions of the world, sporadic cases of unusual infections can occur in almost any setting especially among travelers.

Parasitic infection is enhanced when groups of individuals are in a situation where fecal-oral spread can occur. In this country, some day care centers or wards for retarded are foci of epidemics of parasitic infection.

Some of the more common organisms and the disorders they produce will be discussed here. For more details the reader is referred to other sources, such as Beaver PC, Jung RC, Cupp EW: *Clinical Parasitology*,

9th edition. Philadelphia, Lea & Febiger, 1984; or Brown and Neva: *Basic Clinical Parasitology,* 5th edition. New York, Appleton-Century-Crofts, 1983. Recommendations and doses of drugs for treatment of parasitic infections are listed in *The Medical Letter* 30:15, 1988.

Definition

A parasite lives on or in a host, which is usually larger and provides protection and nutrition. A single host, or several intermediates may be involved. Individual life cycles vary, and provide the basis for understanding diagnosis and infection. Hosts that transmit parasites to man are called vectors. When a parasite is located within the body, the relationship is termed an infection, when the organism is restricted to skin it is an infestation.

Epidemiology

Worldwide, parasitic infections are among the most common disorders, contributing immensely to morbidity and, in the case of malaria in particular, to death. It is estimated that 200 million people have malaria, 200 million have schistosomiasis, and nearly 2 billion have some form of intestinal parasite.

Diagnosis

Details of laboratory diagnosis are beyond the scope of this book. They are critically important to accurate diagnosis. Any physician who suspects a parasitic infection should consult an experienced laboratory technician for proper methods of preparation of specimens.

MUCORMYCOSIS

Exposure to *Rhizopus, Absidia,* and *Mucor* is common but disease is unusual. The dimorphic fungi are distributed worldwide and are commonly found in fruit or bread mold.

Natural History

Infection is limited to children with diabetes mellitus, and individuals who are immunocompromised, such as those with leukemias, and individuals in severe malnutrition.

The spores are inhaled and invade the nasal, tracheal, or gastrointestinal mucosa. Extension can involve the bones of the face and extend into sinuses and meninges. Pulmonary infection can have an acute febrile onset with invasion of pulmonary vessels and hematogenous extension to other organs. Lung abscess can develop and include a mycetoma.

Diagnosis

Biopsy can demonstrate the hyphae that are characteristic of the organism. Culture of bronchial washes can reveal the organism.

Treatment

Treatment of the underlying disease is essential to control spread of infection. Intravenous amphotericin B is indicated for systemic infection. Local debridement is advised for cutaneous or local infection.

AMEBIASIS

Definition

Amebiasis is caused by *Entameba histolytica,* one of the intestinal protozoa.

Epidemiology

Prevalence of infection may be 50% in densely crowded poverty-stricken areas of the world. It is estimated to be 15% of the population of India (Nanda et al, 1984). In contrast, it is probably close to zero in well-sanitized locales. Infection is most common in warm climates.

Natural History

The infection is spread by infective cysts in stools which can contaminate food and drinking water. Cockroaches and house flies can spread the cysts.

Trophozoites penetrate the mucous membrane of the bowel in regions of relative stasis such as cecum, appendix, and colon. A small abscess forms and may ulcerate. Amebae can enter the portal vein and lodge in one or more areas of the liver, or travel to lungs and pleura.

Diagnosis

Most infected individuals are asymptomatic. Symptoms occur when tissue is invaded and results in a regional ulcerative colitis. The onset is insidious, and systemic symptoms are unusual. The stools lack odor and are accompanied by a clear mucus or blood. Repeated fresh stool examinations may be required to identify the protozoa.

Liver abscess should be considered in the presence of upper quadrant tenderness or mass, with fever and leukocytosis. The organism may be difficult to identify in aspirates of the abscess.

Treatment

Treatment depends on the nature of the process. See current texts for available information.

CONTROVERSY

The question of treatment of asymptomatic individuals has been the subject of debate. Nanda et al (1984) added valuable information from a study in India that followed individuals with infection confirmed by rectal biopsy and stool culture. They documented spontaneous eradication without treatment, and recommended treatment only in persons working as food handlers or in contact with immunocompromised individuals, including premature infants.

ANCYLOSTOMA DUODENALE (HOOKWORM)

Definition

This common infection in tropical and subtropical areas is caused by *Ancylostoma duodenale* or *Necator americanus,* nematodes that live in the human intestine and produce chronic blood loss and anemia.

Natural History

The adult worms reside in the jejunum and feed on blood. They expel ova into the feces. The eggs hatch in damp shady soil and become infective larvae in about 2 weeks. They can then penetrate the skin of bare feet, enter the blood stream, go to lungs, exit through alveolar walls, migrate up the tracheobronchial tree and are swallowed. With heavy infection, pulmonary lesions may be evident, and cough and dyspnea may occur. Itching of the soles of feet and between toes may indicate entrance of the larvae. Otherwise, the affected individuals are usually asymptomatic until anemia develops.

Diagnosis

Ova can be seen in fecal smears. Occult blood in stools is common, as are hypoalbuminemia and moderate eosinophilia. It is important to quantify the worm burden by doing fecal egg counts and correlate it with hemoglobin levels and iron intake.

Treatment

Mebendazole (100 mg bid for 3 days for children over 2 years) is effective not only for hookworms, but also for ascariasis, enterobiasis, and trichuriasis. It is contraindicated in pregnancy.

Pyrantel pamoate in a single oral dose of 11 mg/kg is a possible alternative.

Prevention

Hookworm disease is prevalent in crowded communities where individuals walk barefoot. Inadequate sanitation is often the central problem. Vigorous control programs can eradicate the disease.

ASCARIS LUMBRICOIDES

Definition

Infection with the nematode *Ascaris lumbricoides* is a cause of gastrointestinal symptoms and pneumonia with eosinophilia when the larvae migrate.

Epidemiology

This large round worm is distributed worldwide, but is more common in moist, warm climates. The rate of infection is as high as 95% in parts of Africa, and it is estimated that about 1 billion people are infected in the world.

Natural History

The worm is normally located in the small intestine. Its life cycle depends on the gravid female depositing 200,000 eggs daily, which require 3–4 weeks to become infective. On ingestion, the larva hatches in the small intestine, penetrates the intestinal wall and enters the portal circulation (Fig. 17.8). It is carried to the heart, then the lungs, where it breaks through the capillaries and becomes a fourth stage larva. It then moves up the tracheobronchial tree and enters the esophagus. When it reaches the intestine it becomes sexually mature and the cycle is repeated.

Diagnosis

The infected individual is usually asymptomatic. When numbers of larvae are migrating, it is possible

CASE ILLUSTRATION

A 3-year-old boy was sent from Puerto Rico to the United States by his uncle to be evaluated for wheezing. Asthma was apparently diagnosed in infancy, necessitating multiple subsequent hospitalizations in San Juan, one for as long as 6 months and another for 3 months. Five siblings in the family also had asthma. On arrival at our hospital, the youngster was acyanotic but tachypneic with a respiratory rate of 80, retracting and tachycardic with heart rate 130. He was slightly febrile with a temperature of 38.5°C, and was noted to be small for 3 years of age, with a weight of 11.8 kg. Rales and expiratory wheezes were heard in both lower lung fields. The rest of the examination was entirely benign. Despite usage of short-acting β agents and phosphodiesterase inhibitors in the emergency room, the wheezing failed to clear sufficiently to allow the child to be discharged, and he was admitted for further evaluation of his persistent reactive airway disease.

QUESTION AND COMMENT

Given this patient's history, what further diagnostic work-up is indicated to determine an etiology for his wheezing?

A more careful history was obtained and it was determined that there had been "white worms" appearing in the child's stools. In fact, all five siblings with "asthma" also had such worms in their stools. A CBC was obtained and showed a white blood count of 16,200 with 12% polys, 1% bands, 43% lymphocytes, and 41% eosinophils. Inspection of this child's stool revealed mucousy, grossly bloody stool with multiple long 6- to 12-inch pink worms. A chest film showed basilar infiltrates. The combination of pulmonary infiltrate, esosinophilia, wheezing, and worms suggested that the patient had Loeffler syndrome.

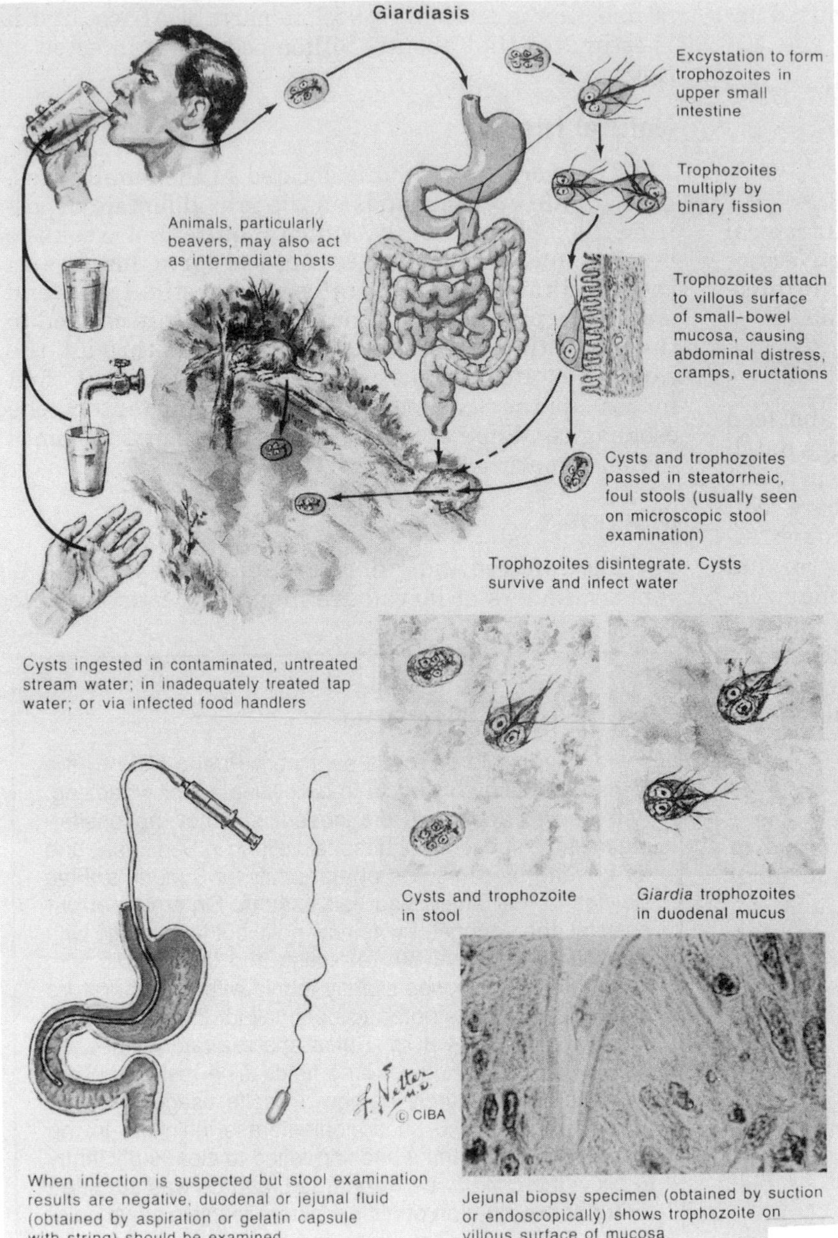
Giardiasis
Excystation to form trophozoites in upper small intestine
Trophozoites multiply by binary fission
Trophozoites attach to villous surface of small-bowel mucosa, causing abdominal distress, cramps, eructations
Animals, particularly beavers, may also act as intermediate hosts
Cysts and trophozoites passed in steatorrheic, foul stools (usually seen on microscopic stool examination)
Trophozoites disintegrate. Cysts survive and infect water
Cysts ingested in contaminated, untreated stream water; in inadequately treated tap water; or via infected food handlers
Cysts and trophozoite in stool
Giardia trophozoites in duodenal mucus
When infection is suspected but stool examination results are negative, duodenal or jejunal fluid (obtained by aspiration or gelatin capsule with string) should be examined
Jejunal biopsy specimen (obtained by suction or endoscopically) shows trophozoite on villous surface of mucosa
© CIBA

Figure 17.8. *Giardia lamblia*. © 1984 Copyright CIBA Pharmaceutical Company, Division CIBA-GEIGY Corporation. Reprinted with permission from *Clinical Symposia*, illustrated by Frank H. Netter, M.D. All rights reserved.

to see a constellation of symptoms such as fever, malaise, nausea, vomiting, diarrhea, and even CNS disorders. Migration through the lungs may produce bronchospasm or pneumonitis (Loeffler syndrome.) A high eosinophil count will suggest that stage of infection, which usually subsides in 7–10 days.

Large numbers of adult worms may become entangled and produce intestinal obstruction. Migrating worms may enter the biliary tree or even the pancreatic duct. Rarely, a worm enters the appendix.

The adult worm may be passed in feces or even through the nose.

Treatment

A number of antihelmintic agents are effective. Mebendazole, 100 mg twice daily for 3 days, for children over 2 years has been useful. Piperazine citrate elixir in a dose of 75 mg/kg po for 2 days is an alternative.

Prevention

Improved sanitation is the essential method of control. When human feces are used as fertilizer, avoidance of green vegetables and salads is advised.

BABESIOSIS

Definition

Infection from *Babesia microti,* a tick-borne intraerythrocytic parasite is designated babesiosis.

Epidemiology

This increasingly common (but still rare) infection has been found in the temperate climates. The incidence of illness in humans is not known but the infection is common among domestic animals throughout the world and depends on transmission by an infected tick. Human to human transmission has not been observed. Infection in the United States is often in association with deer herds. It was first described on Nantucket Island in 1977 (Ruebush et al) and is endemic in Martha's Vineyard and Long Island and Shelter Island in New York.

Natural History

The symptoms include fever, anorexia, sweating, general myalgia, often diagnosed as flu. The disease can be very serious in splenectomized individuals. Mild splenomegaly and hepatomegaly often accompany the acute infection. The incubation period is thought to be 1–3 weeks. The duration of illness is several weeks, with a prolonged carrier state.

Diagnosis

The diagnosis is based on examination of the blood which shows the parasites in the erythrocytes. They resemble the ring form of *Plasmodium,* but unlike malarial parasites, there is no pigment. Antibodies to *B. microti* can be detected in serum by an indirect immunofluorescent method.

Treatment

There is no need for therapy in the milder forms of the disease. Clindamycin and quinine in combination have been effective in an animal model. In the event of a severe episode of babesiosis, the reader is advised to contact the Centers for Disease Control for information on the latest possibly effective drugs.

Prevention

Avoidance of ticks in endemic areas is the only known prevention. Like malaria, the disease has a carrier state and can be transmitted by blood transfusion.

CRYPTOSPORIDIOSIS

Definition

Cryptosporidium is an intestinal parasite, of the same family as toxoplasma, that was first recognized in 1976 as an important cause of self-limited diarrhea in infants and older individuals as well.

Basic Science

Cryptosporidium is a protozoan, of which 11 species have been identified. The life cycle is completed within one host who ingests oocysts. The organisms undergo an asexual stage of development followed by a sexual stage, and are found attached to the surface of the bowel epithelium. The life cycle is completed in about 12 days with the passage of more infected oocysts. The organism is found mostly in the small and large bowel.

The illness is more common and more serious in immunocompromised patients, such as those with AIDS, in whom it can produce a voluminus, watery stool. When it occurs in immunocompetent individuals, infection can lead to watery diarrhea for several weeks, but is self-limited.

Epidemiology

Outbreaks of watery diarrhea associated with cryptosporidiosis have been reported from several centers. The true incidence is unknown, but reports from Australia, Finland, England, and New England find that about 2% of stool samples from patients with diarrhea are positive for this parasite. In a study in Costa Rica, *Cryptosporidium* has been found in 4% of cases of diarrhea, making it the fifth most common cause of illness (Mata et al, 1984; after rotavirus, enterotoxigenic *E. coli, Campylobacter,* and *Shigella*). In immunocompromised hosts, it can produce a cholera-like illness. Individuals with asymptomatic infection have been found to excrete oocyts 7 days after exposure.

What proportion of otherwise unknown causes of diarrhea will be ascribed to this agent remains to be determined. In New England, it is most common in summer and autumn (Case records of the Massachusetts General Hospital, 1985).

Natural History

The organism is widely distributed among the young of animals such as calves, lambs, goats, rabbits, cats, dogs, and rodents. It is associated with watery diarrhea in young children who have been in good health. Low-grade fever may be present and abdominal pain is prominent, symptoms persist for 1–10 days, but may last for 4 weeks.

Diagnosis

An immunofluorescence test may show seroconversion. A modified acid-fast stain of the stool smear may reveal the organism. Identification of the organism in the stool does not necessarily indicate an etiologic relationship, since it may coexist with other pathogenic organisms (Campbell and Current, 1983). In biopsy specimens the organism may be visible adherent to the intestinal mucosa when examined by light or electron microscopy.

Treatment

Treatment is supportive only. Spiramycin has been recommended but its efficacy is not established.

Prognosis

The prognosis is excellent unless the host is immunocompromised.

CASE ILLUSTRATION

A previously well 6-year-old girl had the sudden onset of vomiting with low grade fever, abdominal cramps, and dark brown watery stools that did not contain blood or mucus.

Two weeks before admission the child and her mother visited an animal clinic where they noted that several horses and other animals appeared to have a diarrheal illness. They lived on a horse farm with dogs, cats, gerbils in the home, and bats in the vicinity.

Physical examination was remarkable only for a pale, sick-looking irritable youngster with abdominal pain and some diffuse tenderness over the lower quadrants. The urine and blood counts were normal as were all blood chemistries. Abdominal radiographs revealed multiple air-fluid levels with minimally dilated loops of small bowel. Routine examination of the stool revealed no neutrophils, ova, or parasites and the culture was negative for all pathogens. A test for occult blood was negative.

A modified acid-fast stain of a stool smear was carried out to search for *Cryptosporidium* oocysts and they were identified. Confirmation by a sugar flotation method followed.

(Case history abstracted from case records from the Massachusetts General Hospital. *N Engl J Med* 313:805, 1985)

QUESTIONS AND COMMENTS

What would be the likely causes of an acute noninflammatory diarrhea?

Certainly the illness was consistent with a viral gastroenteritis and probably rotavirus, Norwalk virus, and enteric adenovirus would be the most likely pathogens. Rotavirus is thought to be associated with half of all hospital admissions worldwide for infectious diarrhea. Norwalk virus is more common in older children and adults and can produce an illness similar to this one, but usually vomiting is prominent. It tends to occur in epidemics and is not likely to be as serious as the illness in our patient.

Two parasitic protozoa, *Giardia* and *Cryptosporidium* are both capable of illnesses of this sort. *Giardia* is frequently water-borne in settings where animals can contaminate the water. Commonly, the organism is not seen on microscopic examination of the stool. It also produces a noninflammatory severe diarrhea, but characteristically giardiasis is associated with foul-smelling stools, which were not present in this patient.

How should such a child be treated?

The most immediate need was for rehydration, which was accomplished initially intravenously but soon oral intake was reestablished. The diarrhea decreased by the third day of hospitalization, and she was discharged asymptomatic on the fourth day. No medications were given.

Prevention

Hand-washing is the best means of preventing the spread of infection.

ECHINOCOCCOSIS (HYDATID DISEASE)

Definition

Echinococcus infection is caused by larvae of *Echinococcus granulosa* which have a tendency to develop one or more cysts.

Epidemiology

Hydatid disease is common only in endemic areas such as ranches in Australia, South America, and Mediterranean countries. It is also endemic in Alaska and Canada. Children are most commonly infected.

Natural History

Dogs, wolves, and other carnivores are the hosts, who pass infective ova in their feces. Ingested eggs hatch in the human intestine, and larvae enter the portal circulation and spread throughout other tissues. Multiple organ involvement occurs in more than 20% of patients with liver, lung, muscle, bone, kidney, and brain spread in that order. In children, the lung is most commonly involved (Rausch, 1986).

Most patients have a single cyst, but 15–30% will have multiple cysts in one or more organs. The symptoms depend on the site of the cyst. Many are silent, until they become secondarily infected or rupture. Up to one third of pulmonary cysts rupture and produce fever, cough, hemoptysis or "coughing up grape skins." Hepatic cysts may present as a mass, or right upper quadrant pain. Bone cysts may be the site of a pathologic fracture.

Diagnosis

Hydatid disease is most commonly identified by radiographs. Before rupture, the pulmonary cyst has a sharply delineated border and may be surrounded by areas of atelectasis. Once ruptured, it has a crescent appearance. Calcification is rarely seen in children.

Eosinophilia is not prominent, although IgE levels are elevated. Serological testing is available in the United States through Centers for Disease Control. False-negative tests occur in 10–30% of infected individuals. Definitive diagnosis is made by identification of the organism in resected lesions.

Treatment

A densely calcified cyst usually indicates death of the organism, and it rarely expands. If found as an incidental lesion, excision may be optional. Expanding lesions, all pulmonary lesions, and symptomatic ones require surgical excision; great care should be taken not to rupture cysts, inasmuch as the contents can produce anaphylaxis. Aspiration is contraindicated. Prolonged high doses of praziquantel or mebendazole have been reported to be effective in individuals with inoperable echinococcosis.

Prevention

In endemic areas dogs should be kept from raw meat. Individuals acquire the disease only by ingesting eggs in material contaminated with feces. Once again, handwashing can break the chain of infection.

ENTEROBIUS VERMICULARIS (PINWORM)

Definition

Pinworm infection (enterobiasis) involves the intestine and produces symptoms from eggs deposited in the perianal area.

Epidemiology

Pinworms are widespread worldwide, especially in crowded indoor living. It is the most common of all human nematode infections.

Natural History

These light yellow worms with a pointed tail inhabit the cecum and adjacent parts of large and small intestine. The gravid female migrates to the anus to deposit eggs, which are infective and may survive several weeks outside the body. Reinfection by hand contamination is common.

Diagnosis

Most infected individuals are asymptomatic. The major symptom is pruritis ani, which can cause restlessness, interfere with sleep, and occasionally is associated with enuresis. A cellophane tape should be pressed against the perianal skin (adhesive side down) when the child awakens. Eggs fasten to the underside of tape and can be seen under a microscope.

Treatment

Pyrantel pamoate is the drug of choice, 11 mg/kg po for the first dose, with a second dose in 2 weeks, if necessary. A single dose of 100 mg of mebendazole is also efficacious.

Prevention

In the days before effective medication, it was customary to advise that sheets and night clothes should be changed daily, and the bedroom floor kept clean. Good hygiene and housekeeping are a good idea, but vigorous laundering is probably not necessary. Inasmuch as the ova are likely to infect other members of the household, the whole family should be tested, and treated if necessary. Careful hand-washing will break the chain of reinfection.

GIARDIA LAMBLIA

Definition

Giardiasis is a noninflammatory infection of small bowel which produces a protracted diarrhea.

Epidemiology

Widely distributed in drinking water, this organism has been responsible for major outbreaks of gastrointestinal symptoms, especially diarrhea in children (Meyer and Jarroll, 1980). The parasite is a particular problem in some day-care centers (Pickering et al, 1984). During an epidemic in Rome, New York in 1975 a survey found 10.6% of the population had a giardia-like illness (Shaw, 1977).

Natural History

Transmission can be from infected animals to human, and human to human. Infection with *Giardia* is usually asymptomatic in children. When present, the symptoms range from mild foul-smelling diarrhea, flatulence, and anorexia, to crampy abdominal pain, epigastric tenderness, and a celiac-like syndrome.

Diagnosis

The organism is pear-shaped, with two oval nuclei and four pairs of flagella. Cysts have a thick wall around four small nuclei. The cysts may be found in the stools, but more often in duodenal aspirates (string test; Rosenthal et al, 1980). Duodenal or jejunal biopsy will sometimes reveal the organism when aspirates are negative (Fig. 17.8, pp.1124).

Diagnosis has been greatly simplified by detection of *Giardia* antigen in the feces by counterimmunoelectrophoresis. Examination of stools within a few hours of collection revealed the antigen in 94% of infected patients. No false-positives were found. Further confirmation of the specificity of the test was disappearance of the antigen 1–2 weeks after eradication of infection with antigiardial therapy (Vinayak et al, 1985). The test is not commercially available as of 1988.

Treatment

Quinacrine hydrochloride in a dose of 5 mg/kg/day, three times daily for 1 week is effective. Furazolidone in suspension has been useful in children. Metronidazole (Flagyl) has been widely used, but is not approved for children in the United States except for amebiasis. The dose is 40 mg/kg for two doses a week apart.

CONTROVERSY

The treatment is safe and side effects rare. When the symptoms have persisted for some weeks and other etiologies seem unlikely, a therapeutic trial with quinacrine may be less toxic than repeated duodenal aspirates.

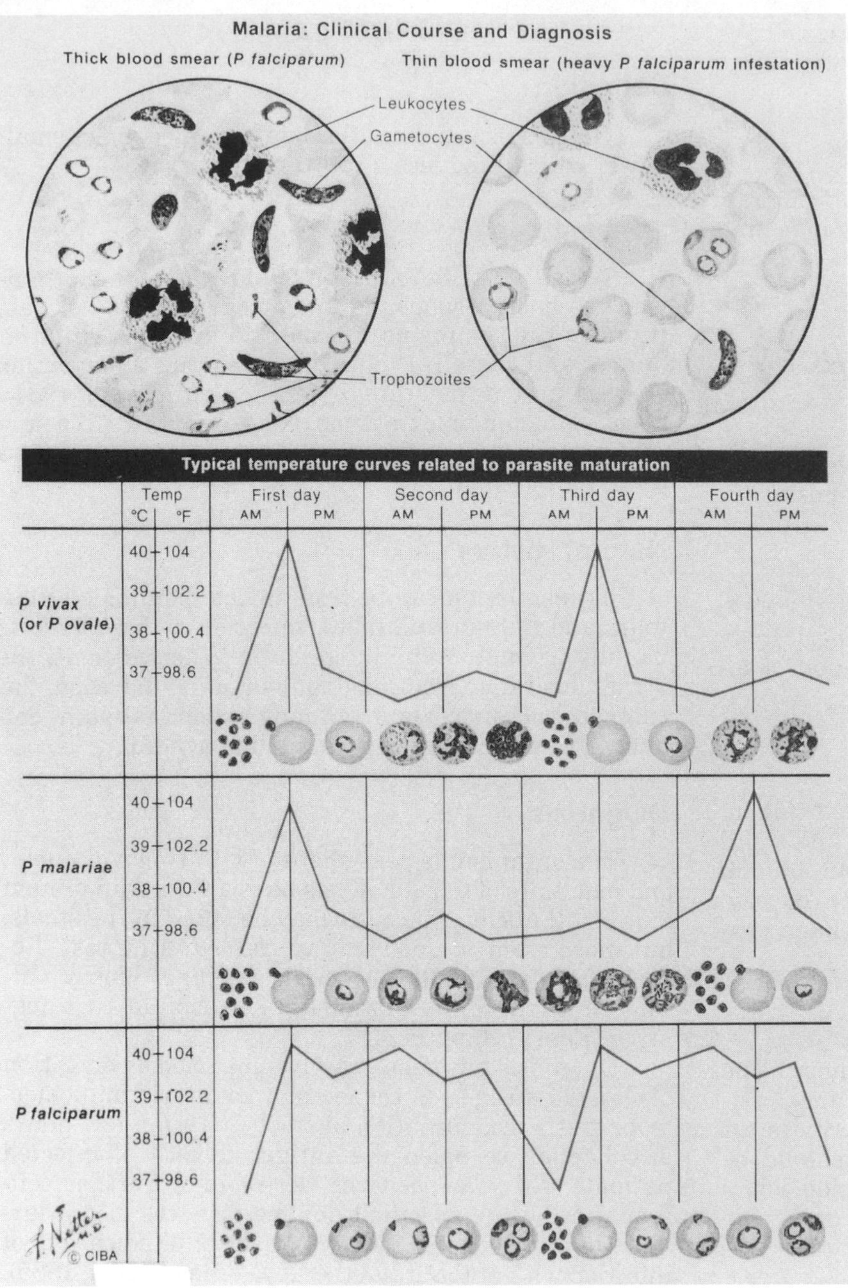

Figure 17.9. Blood smears and temperature course in malaria.

Should asymptomatic children in day care centers be treated? We do not think so, since reinfection is so likely. Only if anemia, diarrhea, or growth delay occur would chemotherapy be indicated.

LEISHMANIASIS

Definition

Leishmaniasis is a group of diseases caused by species of *Leishmania*. Visceral leishmaniasis, also known as Kala-azar, cutaneous leishmaniasis (old world and American), and mucocutaneous leishmaniasis are caused by morphologically and serologically identical organisms but are different clinically and occur in a defined geographical distribution.

Basic Science

Leishmaniasis is transmitted by sandflies and the organism infects many wild and domesticated animals, as well as man. The sandfly ingests infected blood, incubates the amastigotes, which transform to flagellates that divide by binary fission and migrate to the insect oral cavity. In the human, the organisms enter the reticuloendothelial system of the spleen and liver, and later bone marrow and lymph nodes. They are engulfed

CASE ILLUSTRATION

Two siblings both with juvenile onset diabetes mellitus from 2 years of age presented for evaluation of diarrhea. The oldest, a 13-year-old female, complained of sporadic, watery diarrhea for 4 weeks, vomiting for 2 weeks, and abdominal pain for 7 days' duration. Stool cultures were negative. Her examination was remarkable for right and left lower quadrant tenderness to palpation and guaiac-negative stool. CBC and urinalysis were also unremarkable. Her brother, a 10-year-old, complained of loose brown stools 3 times a day for weeks, as well as a decrease in appetite and similar abdominal pain. His examination showed upper epigastric tenderness and guaiac-negative stool. His CBC and urinalysis were likewise normal. The family had recently moved to a rural area of New Hampshire and were drinking well water.

QUESTION AND COMMENT

How should the diagnostic and therapeutic work-up proceed?

It was thought that the leading diagnosis was an infectious diarrhea and, given the history of the well water, *Giardia lamblia* was considered likely. Diagnosis of giardiasis by stool examination alone may be disappointing. The excretion of cysts is unpredictable and the identification of trophozoites requires a fresh sample amount of stool. If the symptoms are severe enough to demand a clinical diagnosis, repeat examination of stools or a duodenal aspirate is likely to be more helpful. This was done in the older sibling where examination of intestinal duodenal secretions was positive for parasites.

Three drugs are recommended for eradicating the infection. These are: metronidazole, quinacrine, or furazolidone. The first is highly efficacious but is not as yet supplied as a liquid. Quinacrine is also unavailable as a liquid, transiently stains the skin yellow, and is associated with gastrointestinal upset in young children. Furazolidone is not as efficacious as its two competitors, but works well in some patients. These children were treated with metronidazole and had a complete resolution of symptoms (Vinayak et al, 1985).

by macrophages and can be found in the duodenum, jejunum, and kidneys. The latent period from insect bite to manifestation of disease is variable, reported as early as 10 days and as late as 10 years.

Epidemiology

The diseases are prevalent in South and Central America, and from the Mediterranean countries to China, as well as in the Sudan, Kenya, and Nile valley.

Natural History

Infant Kala-azar is described as having a sudden or insidious onset of high fever, vomiting, diarrhea, and anemia. The spleen becomes greatly enlarged, a bleeding diathesis develops and without treatment, death ensues. In older children, the disease is more chronic and produces emaciation and hepatosplenomegaly. Intercurrent infections aggravate the course and may prove fatal.

Cutaneous leishmaniasis is restricted to the site of the bite and is a reaction to the parasite which produces a chronic ulcer that can be mistaken for carcinoma. Healing occurs over 3–18 months, but leaves a hyperpigmented depressed scar.

Diagnosis

Visceral disease can be diagnosed by finding the organism in stained smears of peripheral blood, or from culture on specialized media. Splenic puncture is widely practiced in endemic areas to obtain macrophages that contain the organism. (The procedure is hazardous if a bleeding diathesis is present.) Serum globulins are markedly elevated. A fluorescent antibody test is highly specific.

Treatment

Kala-azar responds to pentavalent antimonials, and pentamidine isethionate or amphotericin B. Cutaneous disease can be diagnosed by examination of tissue from non-necrotic areas of the ulcer. Treatment may be local with injections of quinacrine into the area of the ulcer.

Prognosis

Untreated, the visceral disease is fatal in 75–85% of cases; treated, the cure rate is 85–95%.

Prevention

Sandflies have been controlled in some areas by insect sprays, but they are so widespread that their elimination is improbable. The best prevention is protective clothing and insect repellants applied to exposed skin.

MALARIA

Worldwide, malaria is a major cause of death. The ubiquitous *Anopheles* mosquito is the vector for *Plasmodium*, the malarial parasite, and man may be a long-term host. Only about 60 of the 200 known species of *Anopheles* are considered vectors (Wyler, 1983).

Definition

The disease has been recognized for centuries by the quotidian, tertian, and quartan fever cycles that are now understood in terms of the life cycle of the *Plasmodium* species of malaria: *P. falciparum, P. vivax, P. malariae,* and *P. ovale*. The parasites can be seen in red cells best in between the peaks of fever.

Basic Science

The life cycle of this parasite is best depicted in the Figure 17.10 (pp. 1130).

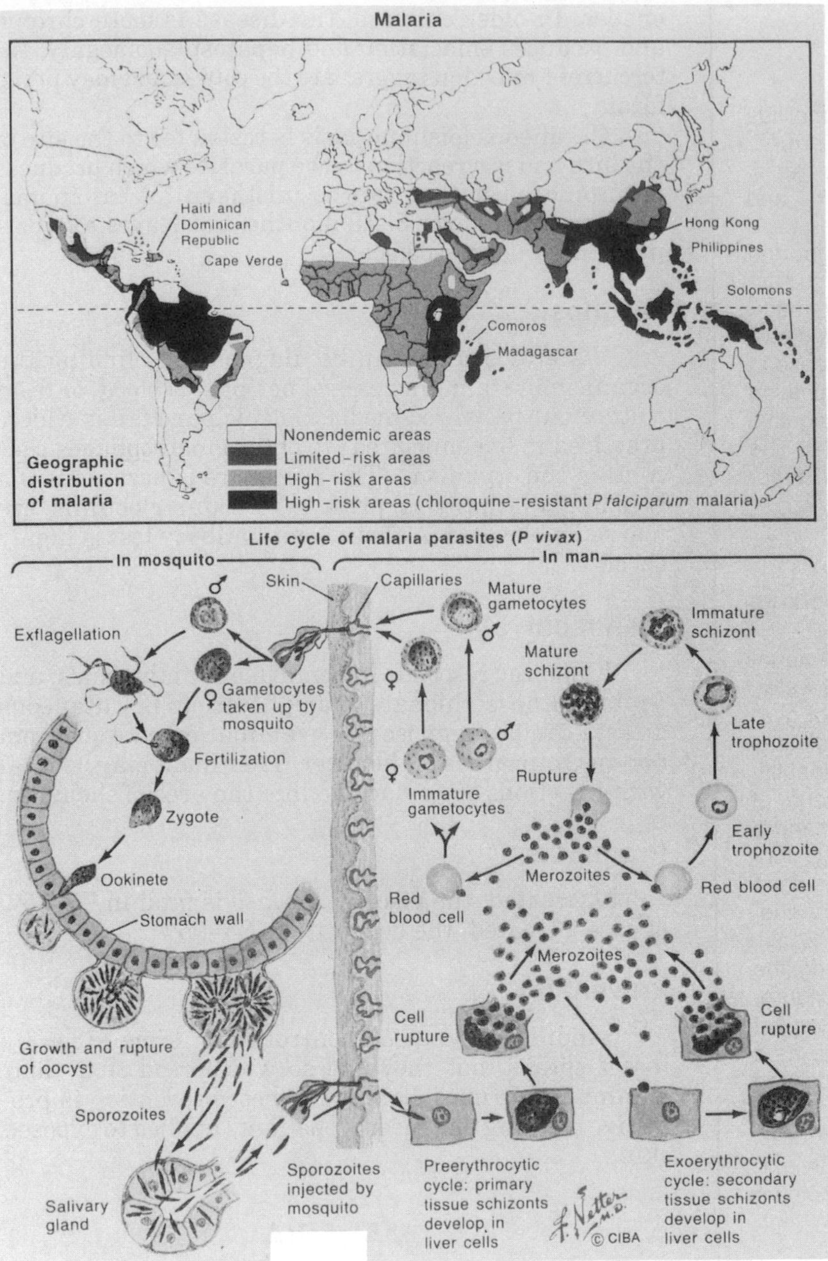

Figure 17.10. Life cycle of *Plasmodium* parasite.

Epidemiology

P. falciparum is most prevalent in tropical areas of the world. *P. vivax,* the most common form, has a wider distribution and has been prevalent in temperate zones of North America, Europe, and Asia. *P. malariae* and *P. ovale* are much less common, and are mainly found in Africa. The disease afflicts between 200 and 400 million individuals of all ages. In Africa, it kills about 10% of its victims. It is estimated that about one-third of the world's population is exposed to malaria.

Natural History

The natural history of disease and protean manifestations can also be shown schematically. An incubation period of 10–150 days, depending on the parasite, precedes evidence of infection. If suppressive therapy has been given the incubation period is prolonged.

The outstanding clinical features are paroxysms of fever (>40°C) which appear at regular intervals. However, this periodicity may be absent early in the infection. Initially, the victim experiences chills for up to an hour or two, then fever for 1–4 hours. Sweating follows for another few hours and the patient feels better. Fever is the response to merozoites liberated into the blood stream. Associated symptoms include headache, muscular pains, abdominal pain, and even hallucinations. In the more serious infection with *P. falciparum* in particular, cerebral malaria is a dreaded complication. Massive hemoglobinuria (Blackwater Fever) results in anemia and jaundice. Acute respiratory distress may be a feature and shock and renal failure can be lethal.

The signs may be more subtle in the infant. Fever may be less pronounced. Jaundice and splenomegaly, with anemia, may be the most prominent signs.

In those areas where malaria is uncommon, the diagnosis is often not entertained until a laboratory technician calls attention to the parasite seen in a peripheral blood smear. As indicated in Fig. 17.9 (pp. 1128) thick films aid in detection of the parasite.

CONGENITAL MALARIA

At least 150 cases of this rare form of malaria have been described. The mother may or may not have been symptomatic during pregnancy and may have acquired her disease from residence in an endemic area or by transfusion. The child is usually normal at birth but becomes symptomatic at 3–12 weeks of age. Fever, hepatosplenomegaly, listlessness, loss of appetite, and a progressive hemolytic anemia should arouse suspicion.

Diagnosis

The differential diagnosis is similar to that for most congenital or perinatally acquired infections, and the diagnosis can be overlooked unless someone examines the peripheral blood smear with care. This method is both sensitive and specific, but is time consuming. Serologic studies can confirm the diagnosis, although they do not accurately discriminate between past and current infections. If intrauterine transmission has occurred, IgM antibody may be present in cord blood (Thomas and Chit, 1980; Hindi and Azimi, 1980).

The future will doubtless see routine use of specific DNA probes for epidemiologic surveys (Barker et al, 1986).

Treatment

Identification of the parasite together with knowledge of the country of residence provide the necessary information to select the drug or combination of drugs most suitable for treatment. Chloroquine and quinine remain useful drugs. If the organism is likely to be chloroquine resistant, quinine is recommended. Since sensitivities change, the best advice for North American pediatricians is to call the Centers for Disease Control in Atlanta for current recommendations.

Prevention

Travelers to endemic areas are advised to use chloroquine for prophylaxis. The dose for children is 5 mg base/kg po once weekly, beginning 1 week before arrival and continuing for 6 weeks after last exposure. Mosquito control remains the most important means of prevention of spread of malaria. Work on vaccines is underway and clinical trials with sporozoite vaccines are in progress. No vaccines for general use are available as of 1987 (Miller et al, 1986).

CASE ILLUSTRATION

A 16-year-old male from El Salvador, who had been in the United States for only 4 months, was admitted to the emergency room with a 7-day history of daily fevers and chills, occurring once and sometimes twice a day. He described having had an episode in El Salvador with red urine for which he took an unknown medicine which turned his urine green. Otherwise his past medical history was unremarkable. On physical examination he looked toxic and had a temperature of 39.7°C. Physical examination was entirely normal including no hepatosplenomegaly, no altered mental status, and no focal neurologic signs. The hematocrit was 40, the white blood count was 4900 mm^3, with 66% polys and 6% bands. The ESO was 40. Bilirubin was 1.2 total over 0.3 direct. SGOT was 5, and SGPT 14. Twelve hours after admission the patient was afebrile and looking well.

QUESTIONS AND COMMENTS

What further diagnostic and therapeutic work-up is indicated?

Diagnosis on this patient was made by observation of the peripheral blood smear. While scanning the Wright stain, large ring forms were noted consistent with the diagnosis of malaria. The peripheral smear will not necessarily show the ring forms and a thick smear is necessary. The waxing and waning fever pattern in this patient is highly suggestive of malaria and prompted physicians to search for the ring forms.

What type of *Plasmodium* species is most consistent with this patient's presentation and how should he be treated?

Based on the specific morphology of the parasites on the patient's smear, including large amebial forms and developing schizonts, the likelihood of a diagnosis of vivax malaria was small. This was incompatible with a history of probable relapses; and with the nature of the malaria in that endemic area (86% of malaria in El Salvador being *P. vivax*). Since *P. vivax* is not resistant to chloroquine the patient was started on an oral regimen of that drug, 10 mg po stat, followed by 5 mg/kg po q 6 hours later and then daily thereafter for 2 days to which he had a gratifying symptomatic response. He was discharged to receive a subsequent "radical cure" with primaquine—i.e., elimination of the persistent extraerythrocytic phase in the liver, characteristic of *P. vivax* although not of *P. falciparum*.

CONTROVERSY

In areas where resistant *P. falciparum* exists, the question is whether to use pyrimethamine-sulfadoxine in addition to chloroquine. Since it was first recommended by the CDC in 1982, some severe cutaneous reactions have been reported, six of which were fatal. The reactions resemble Stevens-Johnson syndrome and toxic epidermal necrolysis. For this reason, in 1985, the CDC revised its recommendation since the risk, although small, is too great to justify routine prophylaxis for travelers (*MMWR* 34, April 12, 1985).

ONCHOCERCIASIS (FILARIASIS)

Definition

Infection with *Onchocerea volvulus* is acquired through the bite of a fly and involves primarily skin and eyes.

Epidemiology

Worldwide, 20–50 million are infected, especially in W. Africa and C. America (river blindness). In some tropical villages, as many as 30% of people are blind.

Natural History

The infecting fly deposits larvae in the subcutaneous tissue where they mature into adult worms. When surrounded by fibrous tissue they form a nodule within which they reproduce. The microfilariae invade the eye and may infect all layers from conjunctiva to optic nerve.

Diagnosis

Microfilaria may be seen in skin shavings. They are also visible within the anterior chamber and cornea of the eye as seen through an ophthalmoscope.

Treatment

Ivermectin and other new drugs are promising (White et al, 1987).

Prevention

Control of flies which breed along rivers and streams is difficult but desirable.

PNEUMOCYSTIS CARINII

Definition

Pneumonia, caused by *Pneumocystis carinii* infection, is usually associated with immune suppression. It is commonly found in individuals with immune deficiency disorders or who are immune suppressed by chemotherapy. After total body irradiation it is so common that prophylaxis with trimethoprim-sulfamethoxazole is often prescribed, but remains controversial. Immunocompetent infants are also at risk in the first weeks of life.

Epidemiology and Natural History

The occurrence of *Pneumocystis* infection depends on the number of individuals at risk and precautions taken to prevent infection. It has been found in about 60% of AIDS patients (Hughes, 1984). In 1986, the number of deaths from *P. carinii* exceeded the number of deaths from all types of tuberculosis in the United States.

Onset in preterm infants occurs between 2 and 12 weeks, with the major findings cough and tachypnea. The course is 10–50 days when treated. Coinfection with pathogenic viruses is common.

Diagnosis

Patients are usually afebrile. Rales and wheezing may or may not be present. The chest radiograph sometimes looks worse than the patient; overdistention is the rule with discrete nodules or extensive alveolar opacification.

Laboratory findings include elevated IgM, with mild leukocytosis and occasionally a moderate eosinophilia. Two to five months after onset, IgG antibodies to *P. carinii* are present.

Lung lavage or lung aspirate may yield the organism (Leigh et al, 1985). It can be seen with suitable stains such as methenamine silver. In some patients, open lung biopsy may be preferred. In severely ill patients, tracheal brushings or lung lavage may be preferred (Leigh et al, 1985).

Treatment

Trimethoprim-sulfamethoxazole, adjusted to 20 mg/kg/day of trimethoprim oral or iv in four doses for 14 days has been found effective. If the response is poor after 3–5 days, or if adverse side effects are present, pentamidine isethionate, 4 mg/kg/day intravenously, is recommended for 10–21 days. Trimetrexate with leucoviron is an alternative therapy (Allegra et al, 1987).

Prognosis

Mortality approaches 100% in untreated patients. With treatment, it remains between 25 and 50% as long as the host is immunocompromised. Complete recovery is possible within about 6 months after treatment.

Prevention

Trimethoprim and sulfamethoxazole are effective prophylaxis. Pentamidine by aerosol is also effective.

SCHISTOSOMIASIS

Definition

Schistosomiasis is a chronic trematode infection in which adult blood flukes reside in veins of liver, intestine, and bladder, and produce eggs whose antigens cause chronic inflammation and illness.

Basic Science

Schistosoma mansoni (occurs in Africa and South America), *S. japonicum* (occurs in Asia), and *S. haematobium* (occurs in Africa and the middle East). They are three closely related parasites. Mated pairs produce eggs which reach the lumens of intestine and bladder and are passed into fresh water. The eggs hatch, releasing a free swimming larva which penetrate the tissues of certain snails and sporocysts from which in turn develop free swimming cercariae. The cercariae attach to human skin and penetrate within seconds to minutes after contact. They then move to lungs via lymphatics, then migrate to the liver where they mature in the portal venous system and its tributaries. Adult worms can live as long as 20 years in a human host. They do not replicate in the human, however. Eggs appear in human feces and urine 5–12 weeks after exposure, depending on species of trematode. Immunity is incomplete and repeated infections occur.

Epidemiology

Estimates are that about 200 million people who live in the endemic areas of Asia, Africa, and South America are infected.

Natural History

Clinical manifestations appear in relation to parasite development. Entry into the skin produces pruritic papular lesions in water-exposed areas. When the schistosomules enter the lung and lymphatics, a serum sickness-like illness may occur. The chronic phase evolves as the eggs lead to inflammation and fibrosis of liver and portal hypertension. *S. haematobium* infection involves the bladder and ureters and can lead to an obstructive uropathy.

Secondary exposure of sensitized individuals produces more intense reactions, including urticaria, especially in areas of skin that are exposed to water. Fever, abdominal pain, diarrhea, cough, and weight loss follow. Eosinophilia may exceed 90%.

Intestinal schistosomiasis produces granulomatous inflammation, which results in diarrhea and anorexia. Papillomas may develop in the colon. Later, hepatosplenic involvement can lead to esophageal varices. Proteinuria is a complication of immune complex nephritis in some patients. Central nervous system involvement from focal granulomas in the cerebrum may cause convulsions, and granulomas in the spinal cord can cause transverse myelitis.

Diagnosis

Given the multiorgan system involvement, diagnosis can be difficult, particularly in nonendemic areas. Inquiry into possible exposure, as with travel and skin exposure to possibly infected bodies of water should raise suspicion. A definitive diagnosis depends on identification of viable eggs in feces or urine. A rectal biopsy is a useful procedure in a patient with diarrhea. Proctoscopy, colonoscopy, cystoscopy, and intravenous pyelography may delineate the extent of disease.

Treatment

New drugs given by mouth have revolutionized the treatment of schistosomiasis. Praziquantel, 40 mg/kg once orally is currently the treatment of choice for all types.

Prognosis

Some infected individuals do not experience severe symptoms. On the other hand complications of hepatic and renal involvement may have a fatal outcome.

Prevention

Control focuses on elimination of the human-to-snail life cycle by case identification and sewage management. Anti-schistosomal drugs that can be given orally are being used in mass campaigns.

NEW DEVELOPMENTS

Although no vaccine is available as of 1988, several schistosome proteins have been found immunogenic in human and protective in baboons (Capron et al, 1987).

STRONGYLOIDES STERCORALIS

Definition

Strongyloides stercoralis is a nematode that is capable of causing chronic abdominal discomfort, diarrhea, and malabsorption.

Epidemiology

The distribution is worldwide and an estimated 40 million people are infected. Infection is most prominent in the tropics and is considered for the most part to be a human infection although it has been found in dogs.

Natural History

Infection is acquired by invasion of the skin by a larva where it enters the lymphatics and then the venous system. The larvae are carried to the heart and lungs, migrate up the trachea to the glottis where they are swallowed and then establish themselves in the duodenum and proximal jejunum. They do not attach to the mucosa but become buried in the folds and can lay up to 40 eggs a day.

It is felt that at least half of the infected individuals are asymptomatic. Those with heavy invasion, however, can have repeated reinfection and disseminated disease produced by the migrating larvae.

Symptoms can vary from anorexia, nausea, and vomiting to constipation or chronic diarrhea. In the chronic stage, malabsorption with a protein-losing enteropathy may ensue.

The inflammatory response is an eosinophilia which may reach 10–12%.

Diagnosis

The condition is most prominent in individuals who are debilitated or on immunosuppressive therapy. Eosinophilia is an important clue, but the diagnosis depends on demonstration of the filariform larvae in the stool or duodenal aspirate. Frequently, stool examinations are negative, so if the infection is suspected repeat examinations are indicated.

Treatment

Thiabendazole, 25mg/kg twice daily, administered orally for 2 successive days is usually effective in bringing about a cure. The drug is detoxified in the liver and the dose should be reduced in individuals with liver disease.

Prognosis

With repeated infection, the "hyper infection" syndrome and disseminated strongyloidiasis may lead to a fatal outcome. Presumably the bowel wall can become permeable to Gram-negative organisms, and Gram-negative bacteremia and even meningitis have been reported.

TAENIA SOLIUM (CYSTICERCOSIS)

Definition

T. solium is the pork tapeworm. Infection with the larvae cause cerebral cysticercosis. Man serves as a host for adult worms and also for the larval stage, i.e., cysticerci.

Epidemiology

Frequent infections are found in Asia, eastern Europe, and Latin America. Infection in United States is rare, except among immigrants from Latin America. The frequency of cysticercosis in routine autopsies in Mexican children is 0.1–0.6% (Norman and Kapadia, 1986).

Natural History

Infection with the adult worm is acquired by ingesting pork containing cysticerci; it may survive for years in the human intestine producing an average of 50,000 eggs per day. Cysticercosis is acquired by ingestion of eggs in water contaminated with raw sewage or vegetables fertilized with soil containing eggs. Hogs are the intermediate host.

The eggs hatch in the small intestine and the embryos penetrate the intestinal wall and may be widely distributed to subcutaneous tissue, muscle, viscera, and central nervous system. Only heavy infection produces symptoms of muscle pain and weakness, fever, meningoencephalitis, or seizures.

Diagnosis

Segments of the adult worm may be found in stools or around the perianal area. The proglottids or scolex must be recovered to distinguish the organism from *T. saginata*. Calcified lesions may be seen on radiographs. In the brain, a cyst containing low-density fluid with a calcified dead larva is characteristic. The cerebrospinal fluid may have a lymphocytosis, but protein and glucose are usually normal. A radioimmunoassay is available for anticysticerci IgG in serum and spinal fluid (Miller et al, 1984).

Treatment

Praziquantel has been successful in the treatment of cysticercosis in adults, and in at least one child reported by Norman (1986). If cerebral edema is present, dexamethasone and phenobarbital are appropriate. Resection of isolated brain cysts may be appropriate if the lesion is superficial or if a biopsy is needed for diagnosis. Nidosamide or praziquantel will kill the adult tapeworms.

Prevention

Cooking pork prevents the infection with adult worms. Since person-to-person spread of eggs can occur, screening contacts in households is appropriate.

Prognosis

Mortality in children treated symptomatically is 3–5%; serious morbidity is 67—80% of children reported from Mexico and South Africa (cited by Norman et al, 1986).

TOXOCARIASIS: VISCERAL LARVA MIGRANS

Definition

Visceral larva migrans is a syndrome caused chiefly by the migrating larvae of the helminth *Toxocara canis* or *catti*. It is widespread wherever there is a significant dog or cat population. Occasionally other parasitic helminths such as *Baylisascaris procyonis* can cause a similar disease (Fox et al, 1985).

Natural History

Human infection takes place when embryonated eggs derived from dog or cat feces are ingested. Toddlers and young children who tend to eat soil and dirt are most likely to be infected. The eggs hatch in the small intestine and the larvae migrate to various organs of the body, principally liver, lungs, eye (ocular larva migrans), and brain. In time, a granuloma forms around the larvae. During the migration stage a high eosinophil count is characteristic. Man is an abnormal host and the larvae do not become adult worms. Toxocara may coexist with other soil-transmitted infections such as *Ascaris* or *Trichuris*.

Prevalence

Serologic surveys show past exposure in about 10% of the population in the United States.

Diagnosis

Many of the infections are subclinical with the only evidence being an elevated eosinophil count and positive flourescent antibody test. An ELISA is also available; titers of 1:32 or above has good specificity. Elevated anti-A or anti-B isoagglutinin titers are common. Biopsy of the liver may show the presence of the parasite, but is rarely indicated. The diagnosis should be considered whenever a toddler has muscular pains and urticarial rashes with hepatomegaly. More extensive involvement can be present, such as ocular toxocariasis, which may lead to blindness. On funduscopic examination, the ocular lesion, chorioretinitis, is usually unilateral and often painless. Migration of the larva to the central nervous system may produce epilepsy.

Treatment

The lesions often subside on their own in 6–18 months and the prognosis is usually good. Fatal meningoencephalitis is rare. Treatment is often unsatisfactory. Diethylcarbamazine has some effect on the larva stage. Thiabendazole, 50 mg/kg/day po divided every 12 hours for 5 days or longer is recommended by Nelson (1985). Corticosteroids may be indicated for severe symptoms and for eye involvement.

Prevention

Periodic treatment of dogs and cats with antihelmintics is a wise precaution, particularly in households with toddlers.

TOXOPLASMOSIS

Definition

Toxoplasmosis is a generalized granulomatous disease caused by *Toxoplasma gondii,* an intracellular protozoan parasite.

Epidemiology

Inapparent infection is widespread, throughout the world, especially among individuals who consume raw meat. The domestic cat can be a reservoir of infective oocysts. Sever reported on serum from 23,000 pregnant women seen in the collaborative perinatal research project in the United States in the 1960s. Thirty-eight percent had evidence of past infection, but only 5 infants in the group had proven congenital toxoplasmosis. Estimates of frequency of congenital infection are from 1–4/1000 live births. In Paris in the 1970s, Desmonts reported 84% of women of child-bearing age with antibodies. Fetal infections were present in one-third of the newly infected mothers. Clinical disease was present in 11% of infants.

Natural History

Few instances of congenital infection have been found among mothers who became infected before pregnancy. Severe involvement of the fetus occurred only in mothers who acquired infection in the first and second trimesters. Later infection resulted in mild or subclinical involvement in the newborn.

A strong correlation exists between positive placental involvement and infection in the fetus. Treatment of maternal infection with spiramycin reduced by more than half the expected number of congenital infections (Desmonts and Couveur, 1974).

The most likely source of infection, at least in the French experience, was ingestion of raw meat. This was supported by the observation that children in a tuberculosis hospital became seropositive at a rate of 9% per month when provided with two extra feedings of undercooked mutton per week. Raw or rare meat was presumed to have therapeutic effects (Feldman, 1974).

The majority of infants have no symptoms at birth, but in the following weeks may have fever, hepatosplenomegaly, and persistent jaundice. Chorioretinitis is usually the first clinical finding, but it may not be evident until several weeks or even months after birth. Rashes and pneumonia have been reported. Anemia, thrombocytopenia, and eosinophilia are occasionally present. The classic triad of chorioretinitis, hydrocephalus, and intracranial calcifications is present in only a small proportion of cases, although chorioretinitis was found in 86% of Eichenwald's series of 150 cases (1957).

Convulsions and mental retardation are late findings.

Diagnosis

The major concern of the pediatrician is the diagnosis of congenital toxoplasmosis, acquired by invasion of the fetal blood during maternal parasitemia. It is thought that the fetus can be infected only during the initial maternal infection (which is usually asymptomatic) inasmuch as mothers with chronic infection do not transmit disease to subsequent fetuses.

The diagnosis depends on serologic tests, particularly an indirect fluorescent antibody and an ELISA. Both can be adapted to measure specific IgM antibody. At birth, the titer in the infant may be the same or higher than that in the mother even in the absence of congenital infection. If the infant is infected, the titer will rise to peak at about 1 year. A negative antibody titer usually excludes the diagnosis, although seronegative cases have been seen.

Eye examination, skull radiographs, and CSF examination are helpful in diagnosis.

Treatment

Since evidence of ongoing disease may be lacking at birth, it seems appropriate to treat all infants with positive and rising IgM titers.

The recommended drugs are pyrimethamine (with supplemental folinic acid) and trisulfapyrimidine and sulfadiazine. The combinations and duration depend on the infant's response, but in general treatment for 1 year is advised. Bone marrow depression may occur from pyrimethamine.

Prognosis

Most symptomatic infants develop severe ocular and neurological disease. Even with treatment, congenital toxoplasmosis can become active years after birth. Exacerbations of chorioretinitis with loss of vision are the main findings (Koppe et al, 1986).

Prevention

Prenatal diagnosis by culture of fetal blood and amniotic fluid, tests of fetal blood for specific IgM, and ultrasonography of fetal brain have been reported by Daffos et al in 1988. Treatment of mothers of infected fetuses with spiramycin and pyrimethamine and sulfadiazine reduced the severity of infection.

TRICHINOSIS

Definition

This infection, first described in 1835, is caused by *Trichinella spiralis,* a parasite that is widely distributed in pork, bears and walrus. Thus, it appears worldwide, even in the Arctic. Its manifestations depend on migration of larval stages derived from adult females in the intestine (where they produce abdominal pain, nausea, and diarrhea) with systemic signs of antigenemia (which include fever and periorbital edema), to the muscles where they encyst (muscular tenderness), and myocardial failure.

Basic Science

Study of the reaction of host to parasite is essential to the production of vaccines and therapeutic agents. Antigens extracted from infective larvae have been shown to produce strong resistance to a subsequent challenge in mice. Immunized mice are able to expel adult worms from the intestine at an accelerated rate, as well as inhibit their multiplication. The target antigens are expressed only on the developing larvae, suggesting that they produce defective adults (Silberstein and Despommier, 1985).

Epidemiology and Natural History

No accurate information on amount of clinical disease is available. In the United States, 60 cases were reported to the CDC in 1984. It is estimated that 4% of Americans harbor *Trichinella* worms, but most have never been diagnosed. Infection is most common among those who ingest raw meat, since organisms are sometimes present in beef prepared in the same grinder used in preparation of sausages. After ingestion, the larvae are liberated in the small intestine to become adult nematodes 1–2 mm long. The female deposits larvae that enter the circulation and deposit in striated muscle, especially, the diaphragm, tongue, and abdominal muscles, but also peripheral muscles. The larvae become encysted in the muscle and may remain viable for years. They migrate through the myocardium and produce myocarditis.

Diagnosis

In the invasion stage, mild gastrointestinal symptoms may occur within 48 hours of ingestion. In the migration stage, fever and hypereosinophilia are present. The migrating larvae produce periorbital edema, muscle tenderness, fever, and tachycardia and may affect the central nervous system 8–10 days later. By the third week of infection, encystment has occurred, and serologic tests become positive.

Laboratory tests include an ELISA which is specific. A skin test of antigen gives an immediate type hypersensitivity response. Serum enzymes such as glutamic and pyruvic transaminases are elevated. The diagnosis may require muscle biopsy which is positive in 90% of clinically suspected cases. Most cases are probably diagnosed as flu and few persisting symptoms are present.

CASE ILLUSTRATION

The first case, described in 1859, was of a young servant girl in Germany who was preparing meat for the Christmas holiday. She was described as tired, dizzy, had a fever, and excruciating muscle pain. When admitted to a hospital, she was diagnosed as having typhoid. Fifteen days after admission she died and the pathologist, Zenker, removed a sliver of muscle from her arm and examined it under a microscope. He saw dozens of tiny worms wriggling in the muscle.

COMMENT

This story, related by Gina Kolata (1985) surely describes an overwhelming infection by *Trichinella spiralis,* and is hardly typical of the usual case. Nonetheless, it brings home the problem of diagnosis of nonspecific symptoms that mimic acute viral illness, and makes us wonder how often the diagnosis is missed. A great increase in eosinophils in peripheral blood should alert us to the possible diagnosis. It is estimated that only 1/1000 to 1/3000 cases are ever diagnosed.

Treatment

Oral prednisone for 3–5 days plus thiabendazole brings relief of life-threatening CNS involvement. No other treatment is indicated at this time. Consultation with CDC in Atlanta is appropriate.

Prevention

The United States does not require testing of pork for *Trichinella,* even though the Common Market countries do. An ELISA is now available, and may be used by pork producers who would like to certify their meat as *Trichinella*-safe.

Meanwhile, consumers should continue to be sure all pork products are thoroughly cooked. Those individuals who like raw ground beef need to be assured their beef is not put through a grinder in which pork has been ground. A consultation with the butcher is in order.

TRICHURIASIS (HUMAN WHIPWORM)

Epidemiology and Natural History

Trichuris trichiura is widespread in warm moist regions of the world, including southern United States. It is the most common parasite recovered from the Puerto Rican population in Boston.

Man is the only natural host and spread of infection is the fecal-oral route. Infection is most common among the poor, among institutionalized children, and in day care centers.

The organism threads its entire body in the epithelium of the colon. As it matures, the posterior portion is extruded and copulation and deposition of eggs occurs.

Diagnosis

Heavy infection can result in dysentery. Anal sphincter tone may be lost, and rectal prolapse may occur. Hypochromic anemia is common from chronic blood loss. Peripheral eosinophilia may be present but seldom is over 15%.

Treatment

Mebendazole, 100 mg po twice a day for 3 days, is standard treatment for all patients regardless of weight.

Prevention

Sanitary disposal of feces would reduce infection. No method has been found to destroy infective eggs in soil.

TRYPANOSOMIASIS (AFRICAN SLEEPING SICKNESS)

Definition

Sleeping sickness is the result of infection by certain trypanosomes. In equatorial Africa, the tsetse fly is the vector of *T. gambiense* and *T. rhodesiense* parasites that, when transmitted to animals and humans, cause this lethal disease.

Basic Science

These parasites, currently the topic of intense investigation, have evolved a remarkable way of surviving in their hosts. They enter the blood stream and multiply there. The immune system produces antibodies which kill the organism, except that a few change their surface coats, survive, and multiply again until finally the immune system is overwhelmed. Eventually they invade the central nervous system and cause fatal sleeping sickness. For a review of current research, see Kolata (1984) and Donelson and Turner (1985).

Epidemiology

It is estimated that 1 million people in sub-Sahara, central and east Africa are infected. Some 20,000 new cases are reported each year. It is of serious concern because livestock too are infected, and the reservoir of infection is enormous. The trypanosome and the tsetse fly together are responsible for making about 4 million square miles of Africa uninhabitable for cattle.

Natural History

These flagellates multiply in the tsetse fly and migrate to the salivary glands. The infective fly inoculates a wound bite, and the organisms multiply in the animal or human blood, lymph, and extracellular spaces. A massive immune response occurs after 14–21 days in Rhodesian infection, or after weeks or years in Gambian-type infections. Recurrent bouts of fever, erythema multiforme-type rashes, and lymphadenopathy ensue. Invasion of the central nervous system is heralded by headache, followed by mental deterioration, tremors, seizures, and finally coma and death.

Diagnosis

Identification of trypanosomes in blood, bone marrow, lymph node aspirates, or cerebrospinal fluid by smear or culture and animal inoculation establishes the diagnosis. Elevated levels of IgM-specific antibody are diagnostic.

Treatment

In the early phases of the disease, suramin (20 mg/kg) intravenously on days 1, 3, 7, 14, and 21 has been effective. Pentamidine, 4 mg/kg daily for 10 days has also been advocated. For treatment of late stages of this disorder no drug has been very effective. Consultation with parasitologists or the Centers for Disease Control in Atlanta is mandatory for the latest information in this rapidly changing area.

Prevention

The pecularity of the organism, namely the ability to change its surface antigens, complicates any hope of an effective vaccine. Elimination of the tsetse fly also seems unlikely. The best current prevention is to wear protective clothing when in an endemic area.

TRYPANOSOMIASIS (CHAGAS DISEASE)

Definition

Chagas disease is a potentially fatal disease caused by a flagellated protozoa, *Trypanosoma cruzi*.

Epidemiology

An estimated 25,000 transfusion-induced cases occur annually in Brazil alone. Infants and children are frequently infected in endemic areas. The incidence of infection is high in poverty areas of South and Central America.

Natural History

The organism is found in the feces of the reduviid bug, which lives in the walls of mud and thatch houses. If it is rubbed into a skin wound it will produce a painful red nodule. The incubation period is 2–3 weeks. Soon there is local lymphadenopathy, facial edema, unilateral conjunctivitis with intermittent or continuous fever. During the systemic phase, the organism may involve myocardium, liver, or produce a meningoencephalitis. Invasion of adipose cells produces tender subcutaneous nodules. The acute stage lasts 20–30 days.

Chronic Chagas disease is more commonly diagnosed than the acute form, and may follow an undiagnosed acute illness. The symptoms depend on the affected organ, and include cardiac, meningoencephalitic, myxedematous, or adrenal dysfunction. Megaesophagus or megacolon may be present. Dysphagia is the chief symptom of megaesophagus; gastroesophageal reflux is common.

Diagnosis

An elevated mononuclear response is often present. The organism may be found in peripheral blood, bone marrow, or aspirates of lymph nodes or spleen.

Treatment

A nitrofuran derivative (Nifurtimox) in a dose of 5–15 mg/kg/day for 120 days has been of benefit, but has not been shown to cure the chronic disease. It is highly toxic and should not be used without confirmation of the diagnosis. A consultation with the Centers for Disease Control in Atlanta, Georgia is advisable.

Prognosis

The disease is more serious in children than adults, and death may occur within the first month, or later from complications such as cardiac failure.

REFERENCES

Allegra CJ, Chabner BA, Tuazon CU, et al: Trimetrexate for the treatment of *Pneumocystis carinii* pneumonia in patients with the acquired immune deficiency syndrome. *N Engl J Med* 317:978, 1987.

Barker RH, Suebsaeng L, Rooney W, et al: Specific DNA probe for the diagnosis of *Plasmodium falciparum* malaria. *Science* 231:1434, 1986.

Beaver PC, Jung JC, Cupp EW: *Clinical Parasitology,* 9th edition. Chapter 11. Philadelphia, Lea Febiger, 1984.

Black RE, Dykes AC, Sinclair SF, et al: Giardiasis in day-care centers: Evidence of person to person transmission. *Pediatrics* 60:486, 1977.

Campbell PN, Current WL: Demonstration of serum antibodies to *Cryptosporidium* sp. in normal and immunodeficient humans with confirmed infections. *J Clin Microbiol* 18:165, 1983.

Capron A, Dessaint M, Capron M, et al: Immunity to Schistosomes; Progress toward vaccine. *Science* 238:1065, 1987.

Case records of the Massachusetts General Hospital. (Case 48-1984). *N Engl J Med* 311:1425, 1984.

Case records of the Massachusetts General Hospital. (Case 39-1985). (cryptosporidiosis) *N Engl J Med* 313:805, 1985.

Case records of the Massachusetts General Hospital. (Case 11-1986). Cerebral cysticercosis. *N Engl J Med* 314:767, 1986.

Case records of the Massachusetts General Hospital. (Case 47–1987) *Strongyloides* infection. N Engl J Med 317:1332, 1987.

CDC: Revised recommendations for preventing malaria in travelers to areas with chloroquine-resistant *Plasmodium falciparum. MMWR* 34:April 12, 1985.

Daffos, F, Forestier F, Capella-Pavlovsky M, et al: Prenatal management of 746 pregnancies at risk for congenital toxoplasmosis. *N Engl J Med* 318:271, 1988.

Desmonts G, Couvreur J: Congenital toxoplasmosis: A prospective study of 378 pregnancies. *N Engl J Med* 290:1110, 1974.

Donelson JE, Turner MJ: How the trypanosome changes its coat. *Sci Am* 252:44, 1985.

Dupont HL: Cryptosporidiosis and the healthy host. *N Engl J Med* 312:1319, 1985.

Eberson F: Eradication of hookworm disease in Florida. *J Fla Med Assoc* 67:736, 1980.

Eichenwald H: Congenital toxoplasmosis; A study of 150 cases. *Am J Dis Child* 94:411, 1957.

Feldman HA: Congenital toxoplasmosis, at long last . . . Editorial, *N Engl J Med* 290:1138, 1974.

Fox AS, Kazacos KR, Gould NS, et al: Fatal eosinophilic meningoencephalitis and visceral larva migrans caused by the racoon ascarid Baylisascaris procyonis. *N Engl J Med* 312:1619, 1985.

Glickman LT, Schantz PM: Epidemiology and pathogenesis of zoonotic toxocariasis. *Epidemiol Rev* 3:320, 1981.

Godson CN: Molecular approaches to malaria vaccines. *Sci Am* 252:52, 1985.

Hindi RD, Azimi PH: Congenital malaria due to *Plasmodium falciparum. Pediatrics* 66:977, 1980.

Hughes WT: *Pneumocystis carinii* pneumonitis. *Chest* 85:810, 1984.

Hughes WT: *Pneumocystic carinii* pneumonitis (editorial). *N Engl J Med* 317:1021, 1987.

Isaacs D: Cryptosporidium and diarrhoea. *Arch Dis Child* 60:608, 1985.

Johnson GM, Baldwin JJ: Pulmonary mucormycosis and juvenile diabetes mellitus. *Am J Dis Child* 135:567, 1981.

Katz M, Despommier DD, Deckelbaum RJ: Cryptosporidiosis or an Aesop fable for modern times. *Pediatr Infect Dis* 6:619, 1987.

Keating JP: In Feigin RD, Cherry JD: *Textbook of Pediatric Infectious Diseases*. Philadelphia, WB Saunders, 1981.

Kline MW: Mucormycosis in children: Review of the literature and report of cases. *Pediatr Infect Dis* 4:672, 1985.

Kolata G: Testing for trichinosis. *Science* 227:621, 1985.

Kolata G: Scrutinizing sleeping sickness. *Science* 226:956, 1984.

Koppe JG, Loewer-Sieger H, de Roever-Bonnet H: Congenital toxoplasmosis: Long-term followup of 20 years. *Lancet* 1:254, 1986.

Leigh M, Henshaw NG, Wood RE: Diagnosis of Pneumocystic carinii pneumonia in pediatric patients using bronchoscopic bronchoalveolar lavage. *Pediatr Infect Dis* 4:408, 1985.

Markell EK, Voge M: In *Medical Parasitology*. Philadelphia, WB Saunders, 1971, p.86.

Mata L, Bolanos H, Pizzaro D, et al: Cryptosporidiosis in children from Highland Costa Rican rural and urban areas. *Am J Trop Med Hyg* 33:24, 1984.

Meyer EA, Jarroll ELO: Giardiasis. *Am J Epidemiol* 111:1, 1980.

Miller B, Goldberg MA, Heiner D, et al: A new immunologic test for CNS cysticercosis. *Neurology* 34:695, 1984.

Miller LH, Howard RJ, Carter R, et al: Research toward malaria vaccines. *Science* 234:1349, 1986.

Nanda R, Baveja U, Anaud RS: Entomoeba histolytica cyst passers: clinical features and outcome in untreated subjects. *Lancet* 2:301, 1984.

Nash TE, Neva FA: Recent advances in the diagnosis and treatment of cerebral cysticercosis. *N Engl J Med* 311:1492, 1984.

Nelson JD: *Pocketbook of Pediatric Antimicrobial Therapy*, 6th edition, Baltimore, Williams & Wilkins, 1985.

Nime FA, Burek JF, Page DL, et al: Acute enterocolitis in a human being infected with protozoan *Cryptosporidium. Gastroenterology* 70:592, 1976.

Norman RM, Kapadia C: Cerebral cysticercosis: treatment with praziquantel. *Pediatrics* 78:291, 1986.

Pickering LK, Woodward WE, DuPont HI, et al: Occurrence of *Giardia lamblia* in children in day-care centers. *J Pediatr* 104:522, 1984.

Pifer LL, Hughes WT, Stagno S, et al: *Pneumocystis carinii* infection: Evidence for high prevalence in normal and immunocompromised children. *Pediatrics* 61:35, 1978.

Rausch RL: Life cycle patterns and geographic distribution of Echinococcus species. In: Thompson RCA (ed): *The Biology of Echinococcus and Hydatid Disease*. London, Allen and Unwin, 1986.

Rosenthal T, Liebman WM: Compariative study of stool examinations, duodenal aspiration and pediatric entero-test for giardiasis in children. *Pediatrics* 96:278, 1980.

Ruebush TK, Juranek DD, et al: Human babesiosis on Nantucket Island. *N Engl J Med* 297:825, 1977.

Sever JL: Perinatal Infections. In Prevention of Mental Retardation. Proc of Conference June 9-11, 1966. Public Health Service, 1972.

Shaw PK, Brodsky RE, Lyman DO, et al: A community outbreak of giardiasis with evidence of transmission by a municipal water supply. *Ann Intern Med* 87:426, 1977.

Silberstein DS, Despommier DD: Effects on *Trichinella spiralis* of host responses to purified antigens. *Science* 227:948, 1985.

Smith MA, Clegg JA: Vaccination against *Schistosoma mansoni* with purified surface antigens. *Science* 227:535, 1985.

Stagno S, Pifer LL, Hughes WT, et al: *Pneumocystis carinii* pneumonitis in young immunocompetent infants. *Pediatrics* 66:56, 1980.

Sutton DL, Kamoth KR: Giardiasis with protein-losing enteropathy. *J Pediatr Gastro Nutr* 4:56, 1985.

Tasker WG, Plotkin SA: Cerebral cysticercosis. *Pediatrics* 63:761, 1979.

Thomas V, Chit CV: A case of congenital malaria in Malaysia with IgM malaria antibodies. *Trans R Soc Trop Med Hyg* 74:73, 1980.

Vinayak VK, Kum K, Chandna R, et al: Detection of *Giardia lamblia* antigen in the feces by counterimmunoelectrophoresis. *Pediatr Infect Dis* 4:383, 1985.

White AT, Newland HS, Taylor HR, et al: Controlled trial and close-finding study of ivermectin for treatment of onchocerciasis. *J Infect Dis* 156:463, 1987.

Wiedermann BL, Kaplan SL, Marino B: Prevalence and significance of cryptosporidiosis in children. *Pediatr Infect Dis* 4:292, 1985.

Wilson CB, Remington JS, Stagno S, et al: Development of adverse sequelae in children born with sublinical toxoplasma infection. *Pediatrics* 66:767, 1980.

Wilson JF, Diddams AC, Ralisch RL: Cystic hydatid disease in Alaska. *Am Rev Respir Dis* 98:1, 1968.

Woldorf J, Mark EJ: Case records of the Massachusetts General Hospital (Diabetes and pulmonary mucormycosis). *N Engl J Med* 317:614, 1987.

Wolfson JS, Richter JM, Waldron MA, et al: Cryptosporidiosis in immunocompetent patients. *N Engl J Med* 312:1278, 1985.

Wyler DJ: Malaria-resurgence, resistance and research. *N Engl J Med* 308:875, 935, 1983.

Zaman V, Keong LA: *Handbook of Medical Parasitology*. New York, ADIS Health Science Press, p 38, 1982.

MARY ELLEN AVERY
LEWIS R. FIRST
ALICE HUANG

Consultants
Donald Goldmann
Melvin Marks
Kenneth McIntosh
Edward O'Rourke
Thomas Weller
Donna Ambrosino

Section 18

Dermatology

Essential to any physical examination is the careful observation of the color, texture, and condition of the skin and identification of any abnormalities of skin or appendages, such as nails or hair. The skin mirrors health or disease and gives important evidence of age and lifestyle.

Although a variety of disorders affect only the skin, in other conditions lesions of the skin may be manifestations of more serious underlying illness and, indeed, may provide important clues to the diagnosis of these diseases. This section describes the more common disorders that primarily affect the skin and have little significance for general well-being, such as minor disorders of the newborn and neonate, as well as those serious conditions, such as bullous lesions, which may even be life-threatening. Those skin lesions that may be important clues to underlying disorders, such as purpuric lesions in meningococcemia, Henoch-Schönlein purpura, or leukemia, or the viral exanthems which, indeed, may herald the infection, are touched upon in this section for differential diagnosis, but are discussed in the context of underlying disease (see sections on Infectious Diseases, Neurology, Rheumatology). All the figures in this section were kindly provided by Dr. Arthur Rhodes.

For a more thorough discussion of cutaneous manifestations of systemic illness, the reader is referred to Hurwitz S: *The Skin and Systemic Disease in Children*. Chicago, Year Book Medical Publishers, 1985.

Minor Lesions of the Newborn

1

This chapter includes a number of mild, generally self-limited disorders that occur in newborns and infants. Most require no, or only minimal, treatment, but diaper dermatitis is considered in some detail because it is so common and carries some risk of concomitant infection.

ERYTHEMA TOXICUM

This common, self-limited inflammatory reaction occurs only in the first days of life, mostly in term infants. Lesions may be present at birth, but more commonly appear between 24 and 48 hours, or even later. About half of all infants are affected with this disorder of unknown etiology.

The lesions are 1- to 2-mm papules that evolve into a sterile pustulo-vesicle surrounded by erythema, and edema that may be extensive (up to 3 cm). The lesions are most prominent on the trunk, but can involve the whole body. The eruption resolves spontaneously after 3–6 days.

Diagnosis is usually obvious on inspection but, if in doubt, a Wright stain of a smear of the contents of a vesicle will reveal large numbers of eosinophils. Recurrence is rare if, indeed, it does occur (Fig. 18.1).

MILIARIA

Miliaria results from a disturbance of sweat secretion. It is aggravated by heat and humidity, and appears frequently in infants under phototherapy.

A mild form of miliaria results from sweat retention in the epidermis and presents as clear vesicles without inflammation. If the obstruction results in rupture of the intradermal part of the sweat duct, the vesicle may be surrounded by inflammatory cells. The distribution is most commonly in intertriginous areas, but all parts of the body may be involved.

The disorder is self-limited when the infant is in a cooler environment.

MILIA

Milia, multiple 1- to 2-mm keratin-filled white papules, occur on the face of about 40% of term infants. It is a minor and usually temporary defect that produces an invagination of epidermis that becomes filled with keratin. The lesions disappear spontaneously within a few weeks (Fig. 18.2).

SEBORRHEA

Seborrhea is a common scaling disorder of the scalp which occurs in the first week or two of life, and is sometimes called cradle cap. The lesions result from excessive oil gland excretion (seborrhea) and have no or minimal evidence of inflammation. A much less common but more severe form of seborrhea is known as seborrheic dermatitis. The lesions are yellow, greasy, scaly, and have an erythematous base. Usually they involve scalp, postauricular areas, and the face, most commonly at 1–3 months of age (Fig. 18.3).

If seborrhea becomes extensive or persists, it may be much more serious. An intractable form is associated with a functional defect of the fifth component of complement and is called Leiner disease. In addition, scaling, greasy, often hemorrhagic papules manifesting in early or late infancy may be the result of histiocytic infiltration and signify Letterer-Siwe disease (histiocytosis X).

If seborrheic lesions are present in older infants, they may be manifestations of tinea capitis infection, or psoriasis. The latter lesions are "fixed" plaques that appear red and scaly. Biopsy may be required to distinguish these lesions.

Treatment

Cradle cap, which usually is improved by frequent shampooing, is self-limited. If scaling persists, 1% hydrocortisone cream is helpful. Alternatively, 1% salicylic acid and/or 3% sulfur in cold cream may be applied after washing.

SCLEREMA

Sclerema neonatorum is now a very rare condition characterized by widespread, noninflammatory, nonpitting induration of the skin in debilitated and often hypothermic infants. Attention to fluid balance and thermal environment has resulted in elimination of this severe derangement in modern nurseries.

SUBCUTANEOUS FAT NECROSIS

Subcutaneous fat necrosis is a rare condition appearing at 1–6 weeks of age in otherwise healthy infants. It is characterized by single or multiple circumscribed erythematous nodules or plaques that appear most commonly on the buttocks or thighs. Trauma and anoxemia may be factors in pathogenesis. The fat pads of the cheeks can be affected if pinched by overenthusiastic caretakers. When the condition is extensive, calcification can occur within the lesions. Rarely, the lesions liquefy and drain. Hypercalcemia has been described in some infants. Skin biopsy may result in nonhealing ulceration. Intact lesions usually heal spontaneously in 2–12 weeks, while ulcerating lesions take

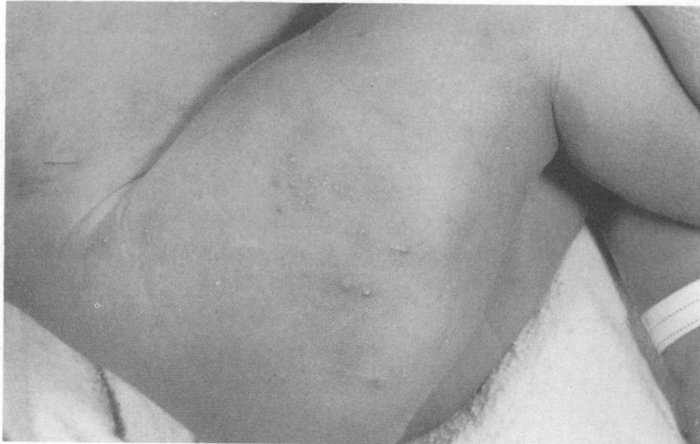

Figure 18.1. Erythema toxicum in a 3-day-old infant.

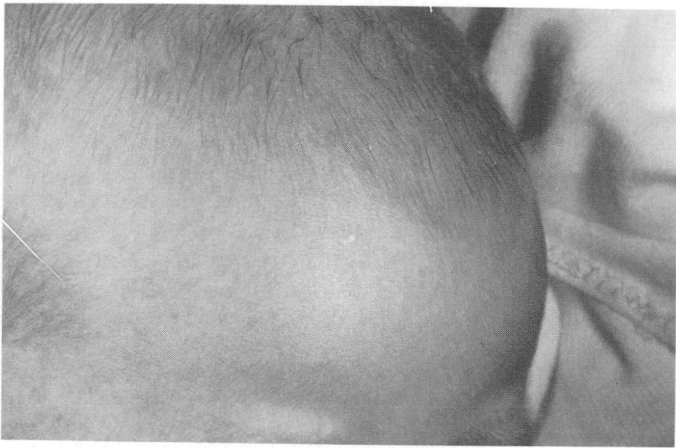

Figure 18.2. Milium on the forehead of a newborn.

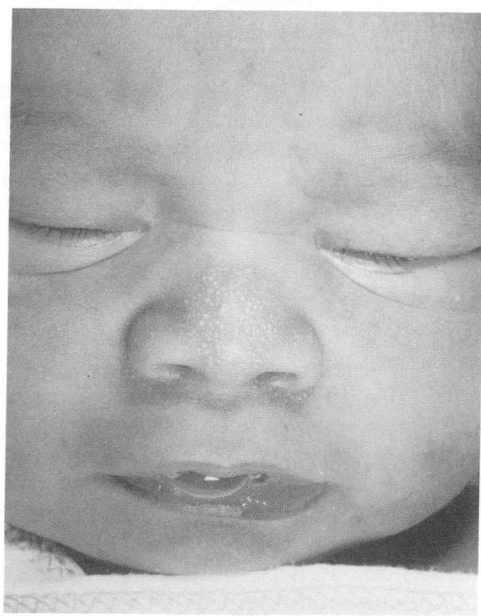

Figure 18.3. Sebaceous hyperplasia of the nose in a newborn. These common pinpoint yellow lesions regress in the first weeks of life.

longer to heal, usually leaving prominent scars. It is doubtful that systemic corticosteroids influence the course of disease.

SUCKING BLISTERS

Isolated blisters on an extremity or central upper lip occur in about 1/100 otherwise healthy infants. They are presumed to occur in utero from infant sucking. The hypothesis is strengthened by their prompt resolution and the failure to develop new ones after birth. No treatment is needed (Fig. 18.4).

HARLEQUIN COLOR CHANGES

This occurs on the 3rd or 4th day of life in otherwise normal infants. It is a remarkable finding of reddening of one side of the body and blanching of the other, with a sharp line of demarcation nearly in the midline. The phenomenon may last for a few minutes or a few hours. The cause is unknown, but it seems likely to be a manifestation of autonomic immaturity. It is self-limited and has no known prognostic importance.

TRANSIENT NEONATAL PUSTULAR MELANOSIS

Pustular melanosis is a transient, self-limited inflammatory disorder occurring in less than 1% of newborns, more readily appreciated in black infants. The small superficial pustules are present at birth, espe-

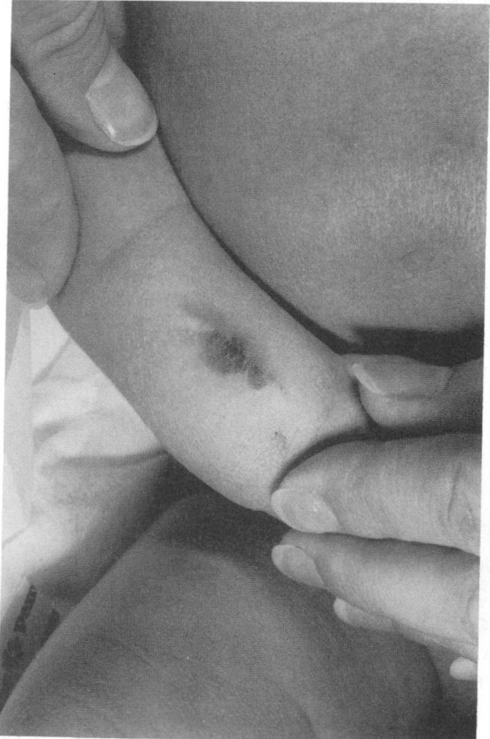

Figure 18.4. Hemorrhagic sucking blister on the forearm of a 3-day-old newborn. The frequency of this finding appears to be less than 1/500 newborns.

cially around the neck, forehead, and back, although they can be elsewhere. Wright stains reveal polys but rare eosinophils. Gram stains fail to reveal pathogens. The lesions may become macular and hyperpigmented but resolve after a few months.

DIAPER DERMATITIS

This inclusive term designates a wide variety of inflammatory processes in the diaper area. They are likely to be initiated by contact irritation and aggravated by infection. Sometimes, other dermatologic conditions, such as psoriasis and histiocytosis X may involve the diaper area.

Epidemiology and Natural History

Nearly every infant, at some time or another, has some inflammation in the diaper region. This is aggravated by prolonged exposure to urine and feces, and in infants who may sit in one place for prolonged periods, such as in a car seat. The natural course of inflammation depends on the likelihood of infection, which can result from bacteria and yeast. One of the most common organisms associated with diaper dermatitis is *Candida albicans,* which has been recovered from as many as 70% of cases of diaper dermatitis. This organism may be a primary offender in some instances because it is capable of penetrating the stratum corneum of the skin if it is sufficiently warm and moist. Leyden and Kligman (1978) showed a correlation between the number of *Candida* organisms recovered from the stool and the severity of the diaper dermatitis (Figs. 18.5 and 18.6).

Diagnosis

There is little difficulty in diagnosing diaper dermatitis, although there is somewhat more difficulty in identifying the cause. The skin is frequently colonized by *Staphylococcus aureus* and pustules may be evident in the inflamed area, due to *Candida* or *S. aureus.*

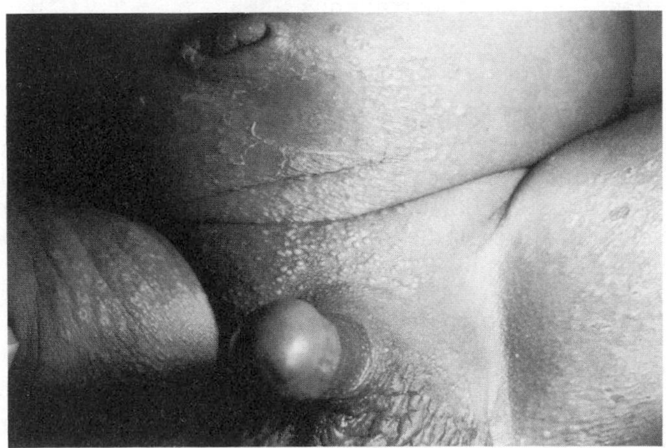

Figure 18.5. *Candida* diaper dermatitis. Note the pustules and fine scaling.

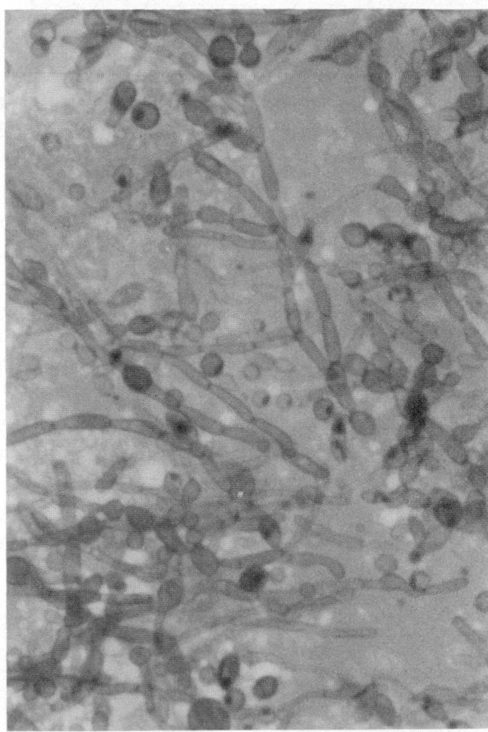

Figure 18.6. *Candida* diaper dermatitis, positive potassium hydroxide preparation showing pseudohyphae and budding spores.

The most common cause of diaper dermatitis is irritation and chafing, aggravated by occluded wetness. The problem of a diagnosis of an underlying disorder, such as seborrheic dermatitis or psoriasis, is more complicated. Eczema is not likely to be limited to the diaper area, but it certainly may be present in this location after the first 8–12 months of life. Seborrheic dermatitis may be present and is usually associated with erythema and fine scaling in the scalp and axillary area, as well as the diaper area. Histiocytosis X is characterized by discrete or confluent pink to hemorrhagic papules with a greasy scale.

Psoriasis may be localized in the diaper area and can be distinguished by "fixed" circumscribed plaques of erythema. The thick, silvery scale, typical of psoriasis in the older age group, is unlikely to be present in moist occluded areas. A family history of psoriasis occurs in about 50% of cases, but a positive family history is less likely for younger individuals.

Treatment

In all instances the mainstays of treatment are avoidance of occlusion of the inflamed area by plastic or rubber and attention to appropriate cleansing. Gentle washing with warm water is usually all that is required. Sometimes a very mild soap may be used to remove feces, but its use should always be followed by thorough rinsing. Harsh rubbing with a towel should be avoided. Rather, the area should be patted dry and then covered by a thick layer of petrolatum. There is little rationale to cover the diaper area with powders of any type particularly because the chance of aspiration of powders may outweigh benefits to be gained. Cautious application of small amounts of cornstarch is helpful if the area is not grossly inflamed (Leyden, 1984).

If significant inflammation is present, 1% hydrocortisone ointment is usually effective. Once the inflammation has subsided, a protective ointment such as petrolatum USP, or a paste containing zinc oxide may be useful. If *Candida* is suspected, an antifungal ointment is useful. Nystatin after each diaper change will usually result in reduction of the rash in 5–7 days. If the gastrointestinal tract is involved, oral nystatin may be indicated.

Because mothers often feel embarrassed by a diaper dermatitis and feel that perhaps they have been negligent, the pediatrician should provide the appropriate steps for prevention, while assuring the mother that almost every child has this condition at some time. Avoidance of wetness and occlusion by frequent diaper changes, daily warm water baths, and early diagnosis and treatment of *Candida* can reduce the problem to a minimum.

REFERENCES

Leyden JJ: Cornstarch, *Candida albicans* and diaper rash. *Pediatr Dermatol* 1:322, 1984.

Leyden JJ, Kligman AM: The role of microorganisms in diaper dermatitis. *Arch Dermatol* 114:56, 1978.

Solomon LM, Esterly NB: Miscellaneous skin disorders. In: Avery ME, Taeusch HW (eds): *Diseases of the Newborn*. Philadelphia, WB Saunders, 1984.

GENERAL REFERENCES

Solomon LM, Esterly NB: *Neonatal Dermatology*. Philadelphia, WB Saunders, 1973.

Solomon LM, Esterly NB, Loeffel ED: *Adolescent Dermatology*. Philadelphia, WB Saunders, 1978.

Developmental Defects 2

ABSENCE

Congenital absence of skin can occur as a 1- to 2-cm circular or oval patch usually in the midline of the posterior scalp. The lesions are readily recognizable by their punched-out appearance. The surface is covered by a smooth membrane. Gradually epithelialization from surrounding tissue occurs, leaving a scar (Figs. 18.7 and 18.8).

The lesion may be inherited as an autosomal dominant with variable penetrance (Deeken and Caplan, 1970). More extensive congenital defects of skin have been described, but are very rare (Solomon and Esterly, 1973). Underlying skull defects and associated cardiac malformations occur rarely.

CONGENITAL DERMAL SINUSES

Dermal sinuses may be located at any level along the dorsal midline and appear as dimples or as tracts that connect skin with CNS. They may be overlooked unless a careful search is made. Sometimes they are associated with hypertrichosis or a vascular nevus (Fig. 18.9).

Diagnosis can sometimes be established by injection of radiopaque material. If a tract exists to CNS, meningitis may occur (Fig. 18.10).

Treatment is surgical excision as soon as the diagnosis is made. A search for other sinuses or anomalies should be undertaken.

ECTODERMAL DYSPLASIAS

Ectodermal dysplasia is a diffuse congenital disorder of epidermis and at least one of its appendages. By definition, it is not progressive (Solomon et al, 1987). The two rare inherited ectodermal dysplasias described below are distinguished by whether sweating is abnormal or normal.

Anhidrotic Dysplasia

Definition

Anhidrotic ectodermal dysplasia is characterized by the absence of sweating and usually is accompanied by defective dentition. Hair is usually present, but may be sparse.

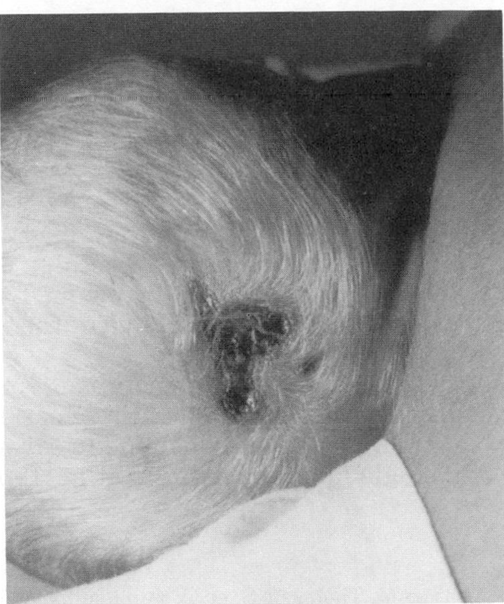

Figure 18.7. Aplasia cutis congenita in a 1-day-old white male, presenting as a hemorrhagic plaque. These lesions are rare, occurring in an estimated 1/5000 to 1/10,000 newborns.

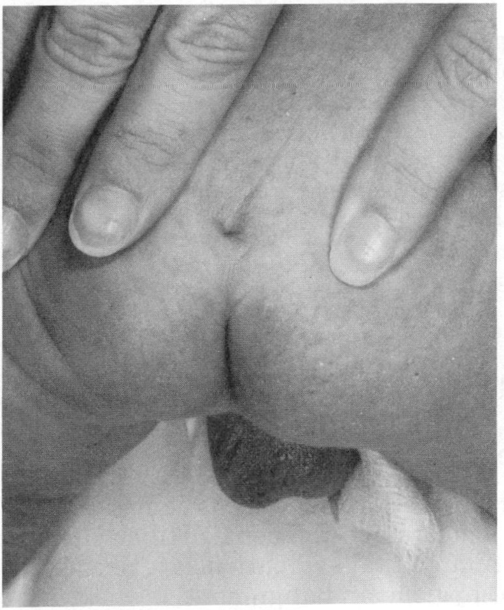

Figure 18.9. Sacral dimple in a newborn. This finding may be associated with malformation of the vertebrae and/or spinal cord.

Epidemiology

This is a rare disease that is usually inherited in an X-linked recessive manner. Carrier females may have minor signs such as a patchy decrease in sweating, but the full phenotypic expression may appear in affected females (Clarke et al, 1987).

Natural History

The most serious manifestation of the condition is the reduction or absence of sweating, which produces significant heat intolerance. In undiagnosed infants the febrile episodes may lead to hospitalization for evaluation of a fever of unknown origin. When it is shown, however, that the infant's temperature rises concomitantly with the temperature of the environment, the diagnosis is clear.

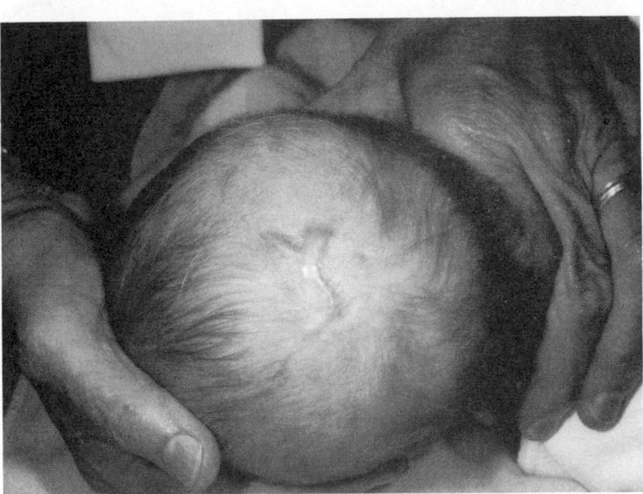

Figure 18.8. Aplasia cutis congenita. Same patient as shown in Figure 18.7, at age 6 weeks. The lesion has healed, forming a hairless scar.

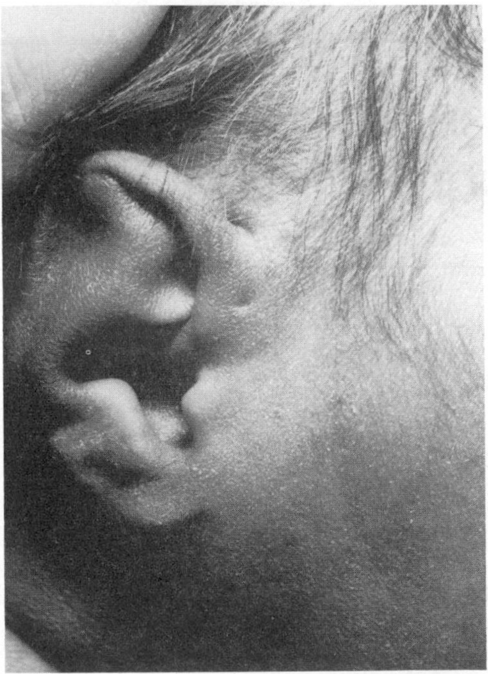

Figure 18.10. Preauricular sinus in a newborn. These lesions may be associated with fistulous middle ear connections.

The facies are characteristic, with frontal bossing and a depression of the central facial area which results in a "dish-face" profile. Eyebrows are sparse and eyelashes are likely to be absent or very delicate. The skin around the eyes can be wrinkled and sometimes hyperpigmented. Dental abnormalities may range from total absence of the teeth to defective peg-shaped incisors, which are prone to caries (see pp. 1231).

Diagnosis

If the diagnosis is in doubt, a skin biopsy will not have any eccrine glands. Eccrine sweat glands will be noticeably absent on examination of fingertips.

Treatment

Avoidance of overheating is imperative for these patients. If tears are deficient, artificial tears can be used. Regular dental evaluations are needed to optimize dental hygiene and alignment.

Hidrotic Ectodermal Dysplasia

Definition

This form of ectodermal dysplasia is characterized by sparse hair and hypoplasia or absence of nails, but sweating is normal in this form of the disease.

Epidemiology

This is a rare condition, inherited as an autosomal dominant trait.

Natural History

The nails may appear to be thickened and discolored, with longitudinal ridges or they may be thin, brittle, and hypoplastic. Hair on the scalp, which is usually very fine, is sparse and slow growing. Eyebrows and lashes are often absent. In this form the facies is normal.

Sensorineural deafness, polydactylism, and other abnormalities have been reported in these patients. Elevated sweat chlorides have been found in several generations of a single family (Robinson et al, 1962).

REFERENCES

Clarke A, Sarfarazi M, Thomas NS, et al: x-linked hypohidrotic ectodermal dyplasia: DNA probe linkage analysis and gene localization. *Hum Genet* 75:378, 1987.

Deeken JH, Caplan RM: Aplasia cutis congenita. *Arch Dermatol* 102:386, 1970.

Robinson GC, Miller JR, Bensimon JR: Familial ectodermal dysplasia with sensorineural deafness and other anomalies. *Pediatrics* 30:797, 1962.

Solomon LM, Cook B, Klipfel W: The ectodermal dysplasias. *Dermatol Clin* 5:231, 1987.

Solomon LM, Esterly NB: *Neonatal Dermatology*. Philadelphia, WB Saunders, 1973.

Vascular Lesions and Disorders of Pigmentation 3

HEMANGIOMAS AND VASCULAR MALFORMATIONS

Definition

Hemangiomas are localized vascular tumors of proliferating endothelium that may be superficial, subcutaneous, or mixed. Those in which there is a proliferation of capillaries are designated "capillary" hemangiomas, while others are venous and/or lymphatic malformations and contain large, irregular spaces that are lined by a single layer of endothelial cells. For any given hemangioma, the parenchymal pattern is uniform, but it changes with age. (Mulliken and Young, 1988).

STRAWBERRY HEMANGIOMAS

Natural History

These flat or raised red hemangiomas may be single or multiple, superficial or deep. The superficial lesions are red and lobulated, resembling strawberries. The deeper lesions may not involve the skin, but present as a subcutaneous, vascular, or lymphatic mass.

Some lesions appear as very small, raised hemangiomas at birth, but are often overlooked until they start to enlarge during the subsequent weeks and continue to grow for 3–6 months. Others appear in the first weeks of life and follow a similar growth cycle. They then become stationary and usually involute slowly over the next few years. The strawberry lesions turn gray and become fibrotic, and eventually disappear with minimal residua.

In some cases, the hemangiomas are extensive, sufficiently large to occlude an eye or interfere with nasal passages and larynx, or even to cause destruction of portions of the external ear.

Multiple hemangiomas that can involve many organs (disseminated hemangiomatosis) but especially the liver, are rare, and often fatal. The rapidly expanding multiple hemangiomas can lead to platelet consumption and a depletion of circulating clotting factors known as Kasabach-Merritt syndrome. Fibrin split products are elevated.

Treatment

Prednisone in doses of 2 mg/kg/day for 6–12 weeks is worth a trial for all hemangiomas with complications such as obstruction of a vital structure, unusually rapid growth frequent trauma, hemorrhage, infection, or platelet consumption. Some hemangiomas begin to regress within a few weeks of treatment and may regrow as steroids are tapered. Other hemangiomas do not respond.

Many proliferating hemangiomas also respond to irradiation, but it is not recommended because of the risk of hypoplasia of underlying tissues and skin atrophy. The late cosmetic result is poorer after radiation than with natural regression. The same is true of argon laser therapy. Nevertheless, if the hemangioma obstructs the larynx and does not respond to prednisone, lasers can be helpful. Surgery has a role, mainly in reconstruction after the lesions have regressed.

Prognosis

Hemangiomas usually involute during the first years of life. Complete resolution occurs in 50% of children by age 5 years and in over 90% by age 7 years. Only a few fail to regress completely. Acceleration of the natural course of regression by prednisone occurs in about half the treated patients (Mulliken, 1984).

VASCULAR MALFORMATIONS

Telangiectatic nevi, sometimes called stork bites or salmon patches, are present at birth, and their growth parallels the child's growth. They do not have proliferating endothelium, nor do they invade adjacent tissue. The lesions are pale, irregular red areas found around the eyelids, glabella, forehead, or back of neck which become less prominent with age. Such nevi are present in about one-third of newborn infants. The typical lesion is bright to dark red, flat, with a sharp outline (Fig. 18.11).

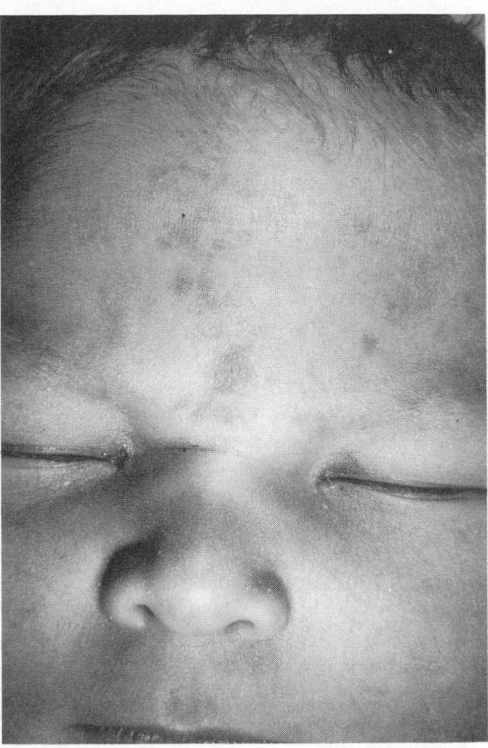

Figure 18.11. Salmon patches (nevus flammeus) on the forehead and glabella in a newborn. This fixed erythema fades by 6–12 months of age.

PORT WINE STAINS

When a vascular malformation involves the cheek or upper lip, it is more likely to persist as a "port wine stain." Port wine stains are much less common than are nuchal lesions. When they are in the region of the ophthalmic branch of the trigeminal nerve, glaucoma may be present. A port wine stain that affects one side of the face may also involve the ocular orbit and the meninges, as well as mouth, tongue, and buccal mucosa. This combination of vascular malformations is called Sturge-Weber syndrome. The best treatment is masking make-up. If the lesion is nodular, excision and grafting are possible. Careful neurologic and ophthalmologic evaluation is essential.

Treatment

Most of the nevus flammeus group of skin hemangiomas and port wine stains do not respond to treatment. Patients use masking ointments if the lesions are on the face.

CAFÉ-AU-LAIT SPOTS

A light brown or tan sharply demarcated flat mark is called a café-au-lait spot. Such marks are present from birth in about 1% of white babies and 12% of blacks, in whom the spots are darker than the surrounding skin. They can range in size from about 1 cm to lesions that cover a significant part of the body. In general the presence of large lesions or six or more small ones indicates an underlying condition, such as neurofibromatosis (see p. 741) or McCune-Albright syndrome (see p. 886). The McCune-Albright syndrome frequently has one large café-au-lait spot. The lesions have skin markings identical to normal skin, remain lifelong, and are histologically without nevus cells or melanocyte proliferation.

MONGOLIAN SPOTS (BLUE NEVI)

Mongolian spots (Fig. 18.12) are brown to slate gray macular areas of varying size located mainly over the lumbosacral area. Multiple lesions on limbs, flanks, and shoulders can occur. The discoloration of the skin is from collections of melanin-producing spindle-shaped melanocytes deep in the dermis. They are thought to be due to an arrest in the migration of a collection of melanin-producing cells that normally move through the dermis to their epidermal destinations. The spots are found in 96% of black and 90% of Asian infants but in fewer than 10% of white children. Most of the spots fade during the first few years of life, but some remain throughout life. They are of no clinical significance, except that they should not be mistaken for bruises.

FRECKLES

Sun-induced, small brown spots are called solar lentigines, or freckles. These flat spots are restricted to sun-exposed skin. Histologically, they are characterized by a proliferation of melanocytes. Freckles tend to fade after withdrawal of ultraviolet exposure, and are not known to have malignant potential.

CONGENITAL NEVOMELANOTIC NEVI

Most nevi (Fig. 18.13) are slightly raised dark brown lesions found in about 1% of newborns and 62% of white adults (fewer in blacks). Fewer than 10% of these nevi are larger than 3–4 cm in diameter. Those that are over 10 cm in diameter are called large and occur in 1/20,000 newborns. Those that cover very large areas, as in a "bathing suit" distribution are called giant nevi and occur in about 1/500,000 newborns.

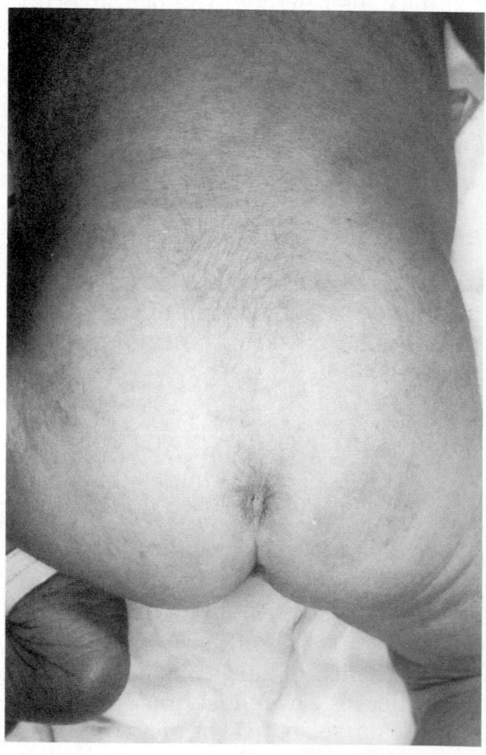

Figure 18.12. Mongolian spots on the buttocks and sacrum of a black newborn.

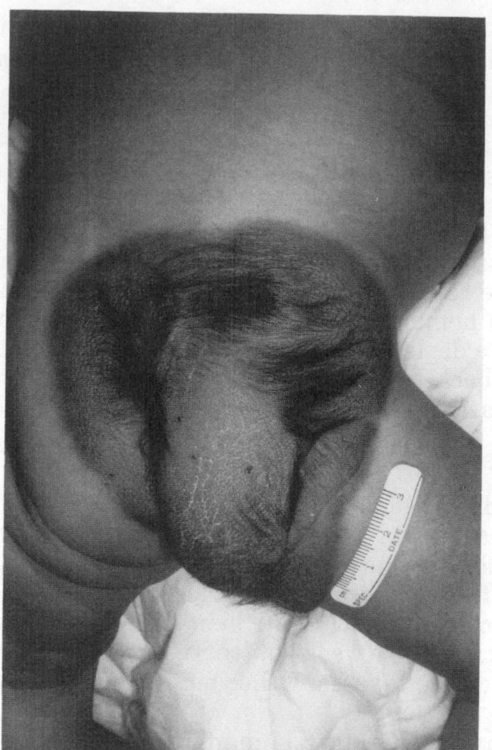

Figure 18.13. Giant congenital nevus covering the buttocks of a 3-week-old white male. The lifetime risk of melanoma for individuals with giant congenital nevi is at least 6.3%; 50% are diagnosed in the first 3–5 years of life.

Giant nevi are obvious at birth, and are of concern not only because they are unsightly, but because they have at least a 6% chance of giving rise to malignant melanoma. The brown or black lesions are raised and have a fleshy feel and a leathery look. Coarse hairs sometimes grow from the nevus, but they may not be present at birth.

Treatment

Evaluation for possible excision of giant nevi in the first months of life is recommended if the infant's general condition would permit toleration of the multiple procedures. Dermabrasion has its advocates, but does not remove all nevus cells which may be in the deep dermis or subcutaneous fat and may give rise to melanomas (Rhodes, 1983).

Treatment of smaller congenital nevocellular nevi is controversial. Such nevi may account for some cases of melanoma, which argues for early primary excision. Nevertheless, melanoma before puberty is very rare, and some dermatologists recommend waiting until the child is old enough to have the lesions excised under local anesthesia. Any atypical appearance or recent growth may warrant early excision (Fig. 18.14).

Any lesion with very dark or irregular pigmentation or an uneven surface should be evaluated for possible excision at any age because of the possibility of malignancy (Figs. 18.15–18.17).

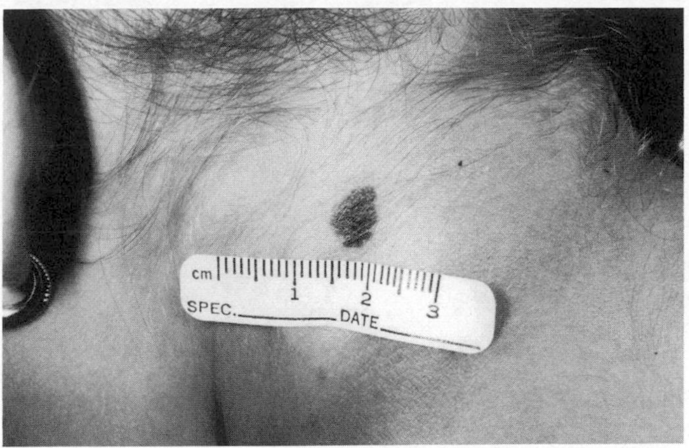

Figure 18.14. Small congenital nevus on the neck of a 3½-year-old white female child. The risk of melanoma for persons with small congenital nevi may be as high as 5% by age 60 years; melanoma is rare before age 12 years, but increases sharply thereafter.

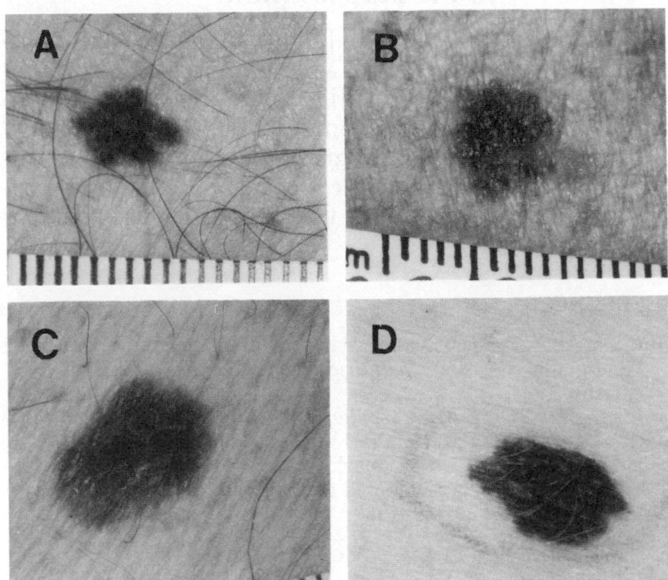

Figure 18.15. Dysplastic melanocytic nevi **(A-D).** Dysplastic nevi are irregularly and/or darkly pigmented nevi that have a relatively large size (>5 mm) and an irregular and/or fuzzy border. Dysplastic nevi occur in 2% of white individuals, first seeming apparent at the end of the first decade of life. Dysplastic nevi confer an estimated 25- to 43-fold increased melanoma risk for individuals who have them, as well as being formal histogenic precursors of cutaneous melanoma. In the familial melanoma setting, dysplastic nevi are an autosomal dominant trait conferring a lifetime melanoma risk of 56% by age 59 years (Rhodes AR: Pigmented birthmarks and precursor melanocytic lesions of cutaneous melanoma identifiable in childhood. *Pediatr Clin North Am* 30:435, 1983).

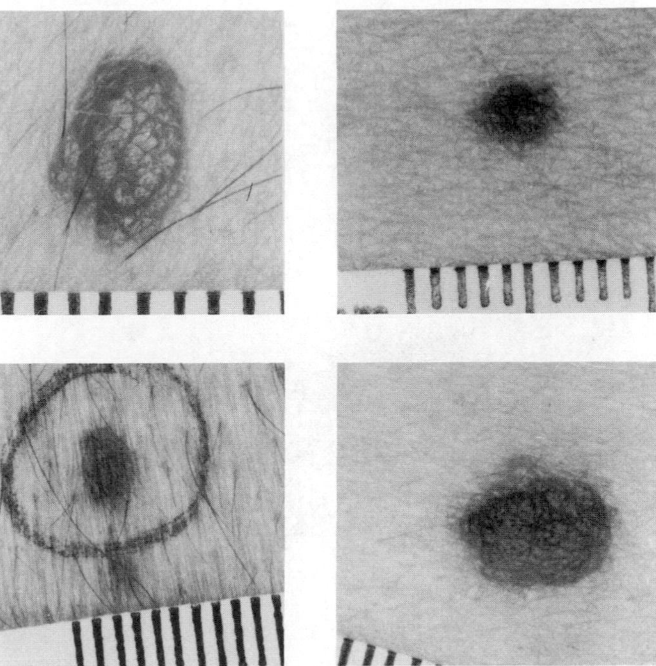

Figure 18.16. Typical acquired nevi. Approximately 70% of white adults have one or more typical acquired pigmented nevi. Typical acquired nevi are small (usually less than 5 mm), with a uniform speckled pigment pattern distributed symmetrically, and relatively smooth and well-demarcated borders.

TUBEROUS SCLEROSIS

The initial lesion of this multisystem dominantly inherited disorder is a 1- to 3-cm diameter "white leaf" macule which is sharply demarcated and is best seen under a Wood lamp. Single or multiple lesions most commonly appear on the trunk. Later, adenoma sebaceum develops as red or brownish nodules in a butterfly distribution on the nose and cheeks. They first appear at 2–5 years of age and, by adolescence, are present in about 80% of patients.

Tuberous sclerosis also is characterized by seizures from sclerotic patches in the cortical gray matter, and multiple benign tumors of fibrous tissue in kidneys, heart, liver, and lungs. Nearly half the patients have retinal lesions appearing as white or yellow raised areas near the optic disc.

Diagnosis depends on a constellation of findings. The white leaf macule is pathognomonic, although not always present.

ALBINISM

Albinism can present as a congenital defect in pigmentation that affects skin, hair, and eyes, with photophobia, nystagmus, and reduction in visual acuity. Oculocutaneous albinism is usually inherited as an autosomal recessive disorder. The basic defect is an interference with melanin production stemming from a deficiency or functional defect in tyrosinase. Affected individuals of all races should be protected from ex-

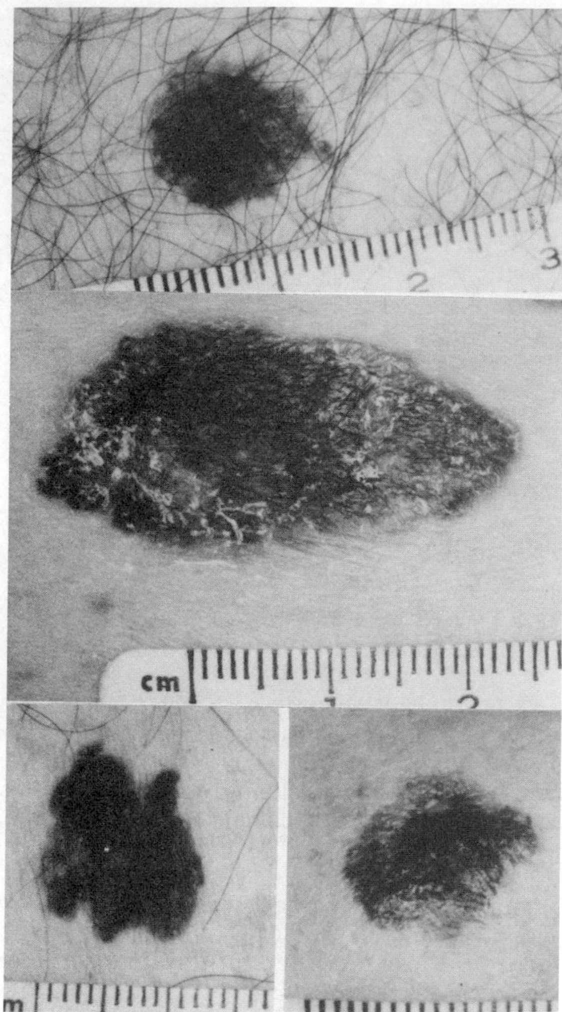

Figure 18.17. Cutaneous melanomas of the superficial spreading type. Cutaneous melanomas are characterized by their relatively large size (>5 mm in 99% of cases), are very dark, and/or show haphazard displays of color (black, brown, pink, blue, and gray), often with irregular borders and uneven surfaces. The 5-year survival for persons with cutaneous melanoma (all stages) diagnosed between 1972 and 1982 was 83%. The best indication of prognosis for persons with melanoma is microscopic tumor thickness: the 7-year survival for thin lesions (<0.76 mm) is 99%, whereas that for thick lesions (4 mm or more) is 39%.

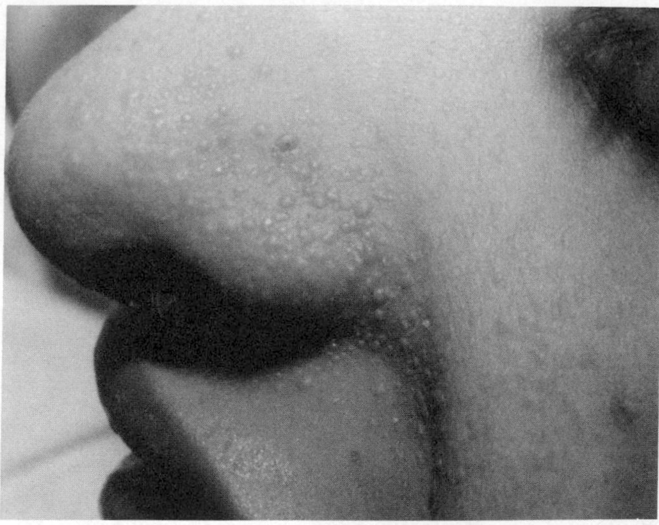

Figure 18.18. Brownish-red elevated nodes (adenoma sebaceum) appeared in a butterfly distribution in this 14-year-old boy with tuberous sclerosis.

cessive sun exposure because they are prone to sun-induced skin cancers. No other treatment is available.

Partial Albinism

Partial albinism (piebaldism) is an uncommon autosomal dominant disorder with regions of absent melanocytes, identical to vitiligo. The affected areas are mostly on the head and ventral surfaces, and involve skin and hair. It is not progressive. Vitiligo has a similar appearance, but is not congenital and is often progressive. The only available treatment is to use masking substances.

REFERENCES

Mulliken JB: Cutaneous vascular lesions of children. In: Serafin D, Georgiade NG (eds): *Pediatric Plastic Surgery*. St. Louis, CV Mosby, 1984.

Mulliken JB:, Young AE: *Vascular Birthmarks: Hemangiomas and Malformations*. Philadelphia, WB Saunders, 1988.

Rhodes AR: Pigmented birthmarks and precursor melanocytic lesions of cutaneous melanoma identifiable in childhood. *Pediatr Clin North Am* 30:435, 1983.

Bullous Lesions

4

Common to all bullous disorders is an impairment in coherence of certain layers of skin. Disease can affect the desmosomes that hold epidermal cells together, or the basement membrane that separates epidermis from the dermis. Biopsy is usually necessary to ascertain the site of involvement.

ALLERGIC CONTACT DERMATITIS

Definition

Allergic contact dermatitis is a hypersensitivity reaction to an antigen applied to the skin. It is T-cell-mediated and initially requires several days to develop. Subsequent contact with the same antigen provokes an inflammatory response in 8–12 hours.

The clinical manifestations are intense pruritus, eczematous lesions that may be edematous, and even vesiculobullous. Lichenification, scaling, and pigmentation may follow rupture of bullae and secondary infection (Fig. 18.19).

One familiar form of contact dermatitis is poison ivy (oak or sumac), called rhus dermatitis. It is typically vesiculobullous and is a local response to the antigens. Spread to other regions of the body can occur by hand or contaminated clothing.

Other common forms of contact dermatitis are reactions to metals such as nickel used in jewelry, cosmetics, and many industrial agents.

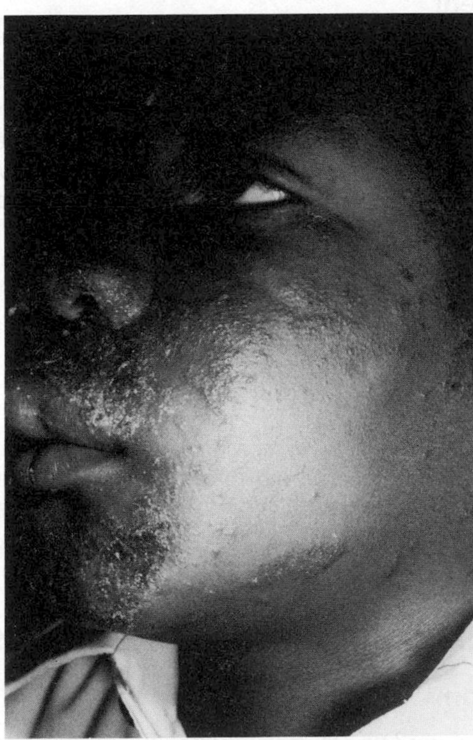

Figure 18.19. Poison ivy contact dermatitis. Note the edema, crusting, papules, and plaques.

Diagnosis

The diagnosis should be made from a careful history of possible contact with a sensitizing substance. If this is unrewarding, patch tests with selected groups of possible antigens can be helpful, although they are never definitive without a history of exposure.

Treatment

In the acute phase when bullous lesions are present, wet cloths applied to the lesions can be soothing. In severe cases oral prednisone, 1 mg/kg/day in divided doses for 1–2 weeks may be necessary. Topical hydrocortisone ointment is not helpful in the blister stage, but provides relief if the dermatitis is dry.

Prevention

The best prevention is to avoid contact with sensitizing allergen.

ERYTHEMA MULTIFORME EXUDATIVUM (STEVENS-JOHNSON SYNDROME)

Definition

Bullous lesions of skin and mucous membranes in association with fever and prostration occur in erythema multiforme exudativum (Stevens-Johnson syndrome).

Basic Science

The cause of this presumed hypersensitivity reaction is not known. It often follows infection, including Herpes simplex and *Mycoplasma pneumoniae*. Some instances are thought to be drug-related. Lupus erythematosus has rarely been associated with the syndrome.

Epidemiology

The relatively rare disorder can occur at all ages, and is 3–4 times more common in males than in females.

Natural History

The initial lesions are erythematous and papular, expanding with a dusky center which leads to blister formation. Lesions can appear almost anywhere, but usually spare the scalp. They can be scattered or confluent. High fever and prostration accompany the severe form of this illness, which has a 10% mortality rate. The course is usually 1–4 weeks, although mucous membrane involvement can last longer and the disease can recur. Scarring of the cornea may lead to blindness.

Treatment

Maintenance of hydration and prevention of secondary infection are goals of treatment. Prednisone, 1–2 mg/kg/24 hours, is often used, but its efficacy is unproven. If widespread herpetic infection is present, particularly ocular involvement, corticosteroid administration is contraindicated. Acyclovir has been used to prevent recurrent erythema multiforme associated with herpes simplex infection.

STAPHYLOCOCCAL SCALDED SKIN SYNDROME (RITTER DISEASE)

Definition

The staphylococcal scalded skin syndrome (SSSS; Fig. 18.20) is a response of the skin to certain strains of staphylococci that produce an epidermolytic toxin. The severe form is characterized by blisters, bullae, and exfoliation with some resemblances to heat injury, hence the name.

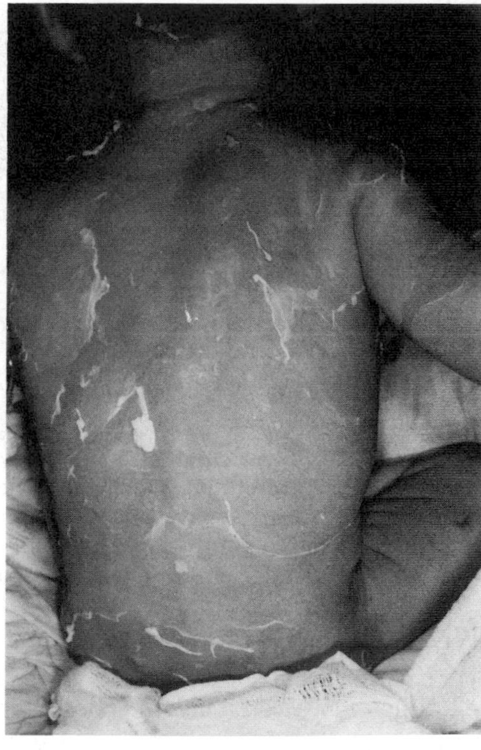

Figure 18.20. Staphylococcal scalded skin syndrome (SSSS). This 16-month-old infant developed purulent staphylococcal conjunctivitis, followed in 4 days by the development of red skin and blistering. The blistering is the result of the systemic dissemination of the staphylococcal exfoliative toxin, which is produced at the site of purulent conjunctivitis.

Natural History

The onset is usually sudden and progression rapid in an otherwise well child. A staphylococcal infection may or may not be identified as a local area of impetigo, conjunctivitis, or, in newborns, as an infected umbilical or circumcision site. Initially the skin is red and tender. Within a few days, the epidermis will separate from the dermis under very light pressure (Nikolsky sign). Blisters and bullae may form and rupture. Sheets of epidermis separate, leaving moist red surfaces, which heal within a few days, then undergo flaky desquamation. The process is usually self-limited, resolving in about 2 weeks. The skin heals without scars.

Diagnosis

Staphylococci are not present in intact bullae, but are usually found in distant foci, such as nares, conjunctiva, sinuses, or throat. Organisms isolated from patients produce an exfoliative toxin that induces epidermolysis in newborn mice. They are usually phage group II organisms, types 3A, 3B, 3C, 55 and 71. Staphylococcal sepsis may also result in SSSS (Lillibridge et al, 1972).

The diagnosis is made on clinical grounds and biopsy is not usually necessary, unless toxic epidermal necrolysis (TEN) is being considered. The cleavage plane of SSSS is high in the epidermis, and no inflammation is present unless the skin is infected secondarily. If desquamated skin is examined, only the cornified layer is seen in contrast to TEN, where the whole epidermis is necrotic, with a subepidermal cleavage plane.

Treatment

The children are miserable and should be handled as little as possible. They are best treated with warm water baths to debride the desquamating epidermis and reduce bacterial colonization. Oral antibiotics effective against staphylococci (oxacillin or nafcillin), or, if the patient is sensitive to penicillin, erythromycin, 30–50 mg/kg/day in four doses, is required.

Systemic and local corticosteroids have been tried and, rather than being beneficial, may enhance susceptibility to secondary infection (Melish and Glasgow, 1971; Rudolph et al, 1974).

Prevention

Because staphylococci are ubiquitous, it is unlikely that all infections can be prevented. Hospital personnel can be warned to avoid working with patients if they have paronychias. Meticulous hand-washing can reduce hospital-spread infection.

TOXIC EPIDERMAL NECROLYSIS

Definition

Toxic epidermal necrolysis (TEN) is a drug-induced injury to skin characterized by a generalized erythematous rash that rapidly evolves into bullae and peeling.

Basic Science

Clinically, the erythema, blisters, and peeling are the same as seen in SSSS. In TEN, mucous membranes are more often involved. The distinguishing feature is the histology, which shows a line of cleavage at the dermal-epidermal junction and an infiltrate of leukocytes. In SSSS, the cleavage plane is intraepidermal, and the outlook for recovery without scar formation is much better.

Epidemiology

TEN is much less common in children than is SSSS. Frequent offending drugs are phenobarbital, phenytoin, allopurinol, sulfonamides, and penicillin (Manzella et al, 1980).

Natural History

Systemic toxicity may be marked in individuals with TEN. Loss of epidermis is associated with egress of fluids and many of the problems encountered with burns. The disease can be protracted and has at least a 25–50% mortality, usually related to electrolyte disturbances and infection.

Diagnosis

A skin biopsy is essential to distinguish the self-limited SSSS from the more serious TEN.

Staphylococci may be cultured from either disorder, and conversely, may not always be identified in SSSS.

Treatment

Withdrawal of the offending drug is of first importance. Early administration of a β-lactamase-resistant penicillin is essential in SSSS, but may aggravate TEN. Steroids are not helpful.

CASE ILLUSTRATION

A 7-year-old female noted oral cold sores 4 days before she experienced an erythematous rash around the lips and separately on the trunk. She was placed on dicloxacillin for the presumed diagnosis of impetigo. However, it was obvious the next day that her skin had become very red and was noted to peel off with rubbing. Blisters appeared below the neck and both ears.

She had been on oxacillin for an upper respiratory infection 2 weeks before this episode.

On admission, the patient was anxious but nontoxic and afebrile. She had marked erythema of face, trunk, and vulva with sheets of desquamating skin. Large bullae were present on the lips and behind the right ear. The palms, soles, and fingers were not involved. The mucous membrane was slightly red, but no blisters were seen. The peripheral blood count and urinalysis were normal. A punch biopsy of the skin was performed.

COMMENT

At this juncture, the major question was whether this was SSSS or a reaction to the previous dicloxacillin, i.e., drug-induced TEN. Pending results of the biopsy, therefore, antibiotics were initially withheld. However, the report of the biopsy showed intraepidermal cleavage consistent with SSSS and oxacillin was then administered with prompt healing of the lesions. No staphylococci of phage types known to be associated with SSSS were isolated from this child, but she recovered completely and, in retrospect, it appears that SSSS was the correct diagnosis, despite the negative cultures.

EPIDERMOLYSIS BULLOSA

Definition

Epidermolysis bullosa (EB) comprises a group of inborn errors that result in bullous lesions in response to minimal trauma or shearing forces.

Basic Science

The group consists of about 20 disorders defined by the site of separation of skin layers. EB simplex arises from a blister in the basal layer of the epidermis, especially at pressure points. Other forms of the disease may involve the dermis and are associated with diminished or absent anchoring fibrils and degeneration of collagen. An altered form of collagenase capable of accelerating the breakdown of collagen has been found to be elevated in infants with recessive dystrophic EB. Recent studies with monoclonal antbodies permit delineation of the specific membrane antigen defect in the dystrophic forms of EB (Fine et al, 1984; Bello, 1985; Figs. 18.21 and 18.22).

Epidemiology

It is estimated that between 25,000 and 50,000 individuals in the United States have one or another form of EB. All but one of the types is hereditary, presumably based on defects in a single gene that initiate the fragile attachments of layers of epidermis and dermis. The most common form is EB simplex, an autosomal dominant disorder that is present at birth or in infancy. A less common dominant form of epidermal disease is Weber-Cockayne disease.

Natural History

EB simplex appears in infancy and usually improves by puberty. Lesions are most common over feet, hands, elbows and knees, and may involve nails. The level of cleavage is restricted to the epidermis, so that no scarring occurs. In contrast, Weber-Cockayne disease does not appear in the neonatal period, mostly involves hands and feet, and after marked shearing trauma, results in blisters that do not leave scars.

Recessive dystrophic EB disease often results from consanguineous matings. The lesions, which are present at birth, are usually extensive, involving mucous membranes as well as skin. The split is in the papillary dermis and, hence, results in scarring, with inevitable deformities of hands and feet. Esophageal and duodenal

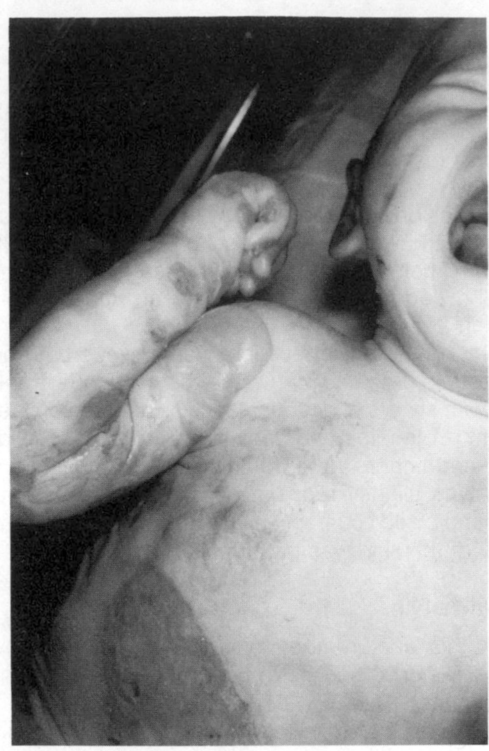

Figure 18.21. Junctional epidermolysis bullosa. This 3-week-old female infant developed progressive blistering at sites of shearing trauma from simple handling, with progressive denudation of skin at sites of blister formation. She died of *Candida* sepsis at age 6 weeks.

strictures may arise. Oral and laryngeal lesions may occur. Blisters in the dystrophic disease form easily and are slow to heal, usually rapidly resulting in widespread disease, infection, and death.

Treatment

Clinical trials with phenytoin, which inhibits some types of collagenase, have been promising in some cases of EB dystrophia. Evaluation is difficult because of the heterogeneous nature of the disorders so that there are relatively few patients in some groups. For information on current research write to Dystrophic Epidermolysis Bullosa Research Association of America (DEBRA), Kings County Hospital Center, 451 Clarkson Avenue, Brooklyn, NY 11203.

Meticulous attention to prevention of trauma and infection of skin is the keystone of therapy. All objects with which the infant or child comes in contact should be padded, and only soft toys left within reach. Hot water and adhesive tape should not be used. Petrolatum can be applied to crusted areas to prevent adherence to sheets or clothes. Rubber gloves and incubators (promoting steam and moist warmth, respectively) aggravate all forms of epidermolysis bullosa in the newborn period.

Prevention

Genetic counseling is appropriate. Prenatal diagnosis by in utero skin biopsy is currently experimental.

ACRODERMATIS ENTEROPATHICA

Definition

This is a rare autosomal recessive disorder characterized by bullous and eczematous skin lesions which are widely and symmetrically distributed. Transient zinc deficiency states that occur during the first year of life are identical in presentation to acrodermatis enteropathica, except that the acquired form of disease resolves with zinc therapy and zinc may then be discontinued. In acrodermatis enteropathica, zinc must be continued for life.

Natural History

The onset is usually during the first year of life after weaning from breast milk to cow's milk. The hair assumes a peculiar red tint and becomes sparse. Conjunctivitis, photophobia, and even corneal dystrophy may be present. In the advanced stages of this disease

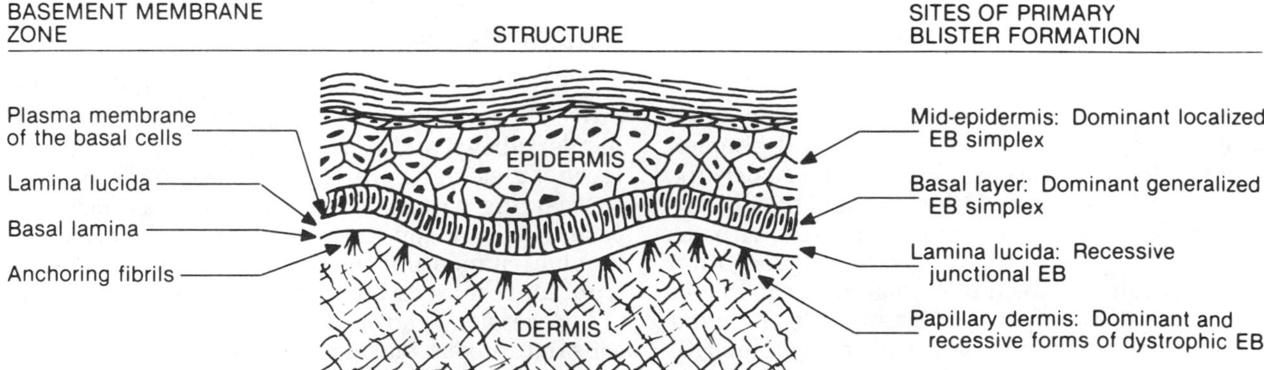

Figure 18.22. Diagram of blistering. Illustration courtesy of National Institute of Arthritis, Musculoskeletal and Skin Diseases, National Institutes of Health.

the infants are miserable, with chronic diarrhea, stomatitis, nail dystrophy, and growth retardation. They frequently have intercurrent bacterial infections. Without treatment, the infants become marasmic and eventually die.

Diagnosis

Diagnosis depends on the clinical findings and evidence of a low concentration of plasma zinc and alkaline phosphatase, a zinc-dependent enzyme. The basic metabolic defect appears to relate to intestinal absorption of zinc.

Treatment

Oral therapy with zinc is curative, although it must be continued throughout life. Optimal doses range from 50 mg zinc sulfate or acetate to 150 mg for older children. Blood zinc levels should be monitored.

PEMPHIGUS

Definition

Pemphigus vulgaris is a serious bullous disease which can have its onset in childhood, although this is rare.

Natural History

Initial symptoms may be painful oral ulcers which persist for weeks or months and subsequently large bullae appear on nonerythematous skin, mostly on the head and trunk. When they rupture, the surface is painful, raw, and tends to heal slowly. The avulsion of epidermis on gentle pressure (Nikolsky sign) is positive.

The blisters arise in crops and can be confused with bullous pemphigoid, Stevens-Johnson syndrome, chronic bullous disease of childhood, and dermatitis herpetiformis. In bullous pemphigoid, the lesions are on an erythematous base and are pruritic. The diagnosis of bullous pemphigus can be made on histologic examination with demonstration of immunoglobulin G (IgG) and C3 in the basement membrane zone.

Treatment

In pemphigus vulgaris, IgG is usually demonstrable between epidermal cells on a direct or indirect assay. These diseases can be suppressed with corticosteroid therapy. The course can be rapid and fatal or spontaneous resolution may occur.

DERMATITIS HERPETIFORMIS

Definition

Dermatitis herpetiformis is a chronic subepidermal blistering disorder characterized by pruritic papules, clusters of which become vesicular, usually over the back and buttocks. The base is pruritic and the condition is characterized by microabscesses that become encrusted and persist for weeks.

Natural History

The condition, which is most common in adults, appears to be associated with gluten-sensitive enteropathy, although celiac symptoms are not usually present. A gluten-free diet, nonetheless, can lead to resolution of the skin lesions or reduction in the need for drug therapy. Diagnosis is best made with biopsy and demonstration of IgA in the dermal papillae by direct immunofluorescence.

Treatment

Prolonged treatment (6–12 months) on a gluten-free diet is helpful in some cases. Oral sulfapyridine or dapsone provides relief from the itching but, because they have potentially serious side effects, they should not be used unless symptoms need to be suppressed.

MAST CELL DISEASES (URTICARIA PIGMENTOSA)

Definition

Mast cell infiltrates may be solitary or manifest as disseminated nodular or bullous eruption.

Natural History

This disorder of unknown etiology of infancy is characterized by collections of mast cells in the dermis, and rarely, other organs. The lesions may be present at birth, but are more common in infancy. The lesions, which vary in size from a few millimeters to a few centimeters, are usually oval and have a pink-yellow to tan pigmentation. They may be solitary or generalized.

Periodic release of histamine may cause pruritus or flushing. Even hypotension, wheezing, and diarrhea can ensue. Mast cells may infiltrate other organ systems, including liver and bone.

Diagnosis

Stroking the lesions may produce urticaria or even blistering. Dermatographia is common in these infants. The diagnosis is confirmed by biopsy and examination for mast cells with Giemsa or toluidine blue.

Treatment

Treatment is directed at avoiding irritation of the skin by mechanical means or by reducing induction of release of mast cells. Thus, vigorous rubbing should be avoided as well as administration of medications such as aspirin, alcohol, morphine compounds,and curare that may induce release of histamine from mast cells. Exposure to heat, cold, and trauma should also be avoided. Antihistamines may relieve pruritus.

Prognosis

Spontaneous resolution of symptomatic disease usually occurs by puberty, although pigmentation may persist. Mast cell leukemia, rarely present in the infantile and childhood disease, is more common when disease develops after puberty.

REFERENCES

Bello M: Researchers seek causes of enigmatic blistering disorders. Res Resources Reporter IX: 9:1, US Department Health and Human Services, 1985.

Briggaman RA: Hereditary epidermolysis bullosa with special emphasis on newly recognized syndromes and complications. *Dermatol Clin* 1:263, 1983.

Fine JD, Breathnach SM, Hintner H, et al: KFI monoclonal antibody defines a specific basement membrane antigen defect in dystrophic forms of epidermolysis bullosa. *J Invest Dermatol* 82:35, 1984.

Lillibridge CB, Melish ME, Glasgow LA: Site of action of exfoliative toxin in the staphylococcal scalded-skin syndrome. *Pediatrics* 50:728, 1972.

Manzella JP, Hall CB, Green JL, et al: Toxic epidermal necrolysis in childhood: Differentiation from staphylococcal scalded skin syndrome. *Pediatrics* 66:291, 1980.

Melish ME, Glasgow LA: The staphylococcal scalded skin syndrome—the expanded clinical syndrome. *J Pediatr* 78:959, 1971.

Rudolph RD, Schwartz W, Leyden JJ: Treatment of staphylococcal toxic epidermal necrolysis. *Arch Dermatol* 110:559, 1974

Hypersensitivity Lesions 5

ATOPIC DERMATITIS (ECZEMA)

Definition

This pruritic inflammatory skin disorder, most common in young children, is characterized by chronic exacerbations and remissions of superficial erythematous, papular, and sometimes weeping lesions, which may be confined to areas of flexion or may be generalized. The combination of clinical findings, a family history of asthma, allergic rhinitis, atopic eczema and, often, an elevated IgE level, support the diagnosis (Table 18.1).

Basic Science

It is generally agreed that recurrent exposure to allergens of many sorts may aggravate a potential disorder, i.e., both the T-lymphocyte system and adenyl cyclase systems. The role of allergy in atopic dermatitis is debated.

As many as 80% of patients with atopic dermatitis have increased susceptibility to severe skin infections, not only to *Staphylococcus aureus,* but also herpes simplex and vaccinia. They also have an increased susceptibility to dermatophytoses. All of these findings support the likelihood that there is a fundamental abnormality in cell-mediated immunity. Some authors have described a decrease in the number of circulating T lymphocytes in patients with atopic dermatitis. Monoclonal antibodies now available for the identification and isolation of specific human T-lymphocyte subpopulations reveal a decreased proportion of circulating T3+ cells and T8+ suppressor T cells with a selective increase in the ratio of T4 to T8 cells. In patients who have outgrown their atopic dermatitis, the proportion of circulating T/B cells returns to normal. Elevated levels of serum IgE are found in over 80% of children with atopic disorders. In experimental animals, selective elimination of suppressor T cells has resulted in an elevation in IgE responses. Although it is not clear that this association is established in humans, it seems probable that the defect in IgE is related to abnormal T-cell function. This combination of abnormalities can also be found in the Wiskott-Aldrich syndrome, the hyper-IgE syndrome and in thymic-alymphoplasia.

The adenyl cyclase system is also disordered in atopic dermatitis, possibly via a fundamental abnormality in the activity of phosphodiesterase.

Epidemiology

Children have the highest prevalence of atopic dermatitis, with an estimated seven cases per thousand population in the United States (Johnson, 1977). The association with other allergic manifestations is compelling. In a prospective study by Halpern et al (1973), atopic dermatitis occurred in one-third of the children with a personal or family history of allergic rhinitis or asthma. In this study of 1753 infants, 4.3% had developed symptoms by age 7 years, although others have reported a much earlier onset in the majority of patients, and occasionally, the findings may present within the first month of life.

Table 18.1
Morphologic Varieties of Cutaneous Lesions in Atopic Dermatitis [1]

Morphologic Variety of Lesion	Aggravating or Causative Factor(s)
Erythematous papules and erythema	"Irritation"
Follicular eczema (follicular papules)	"Irritation"
Lichenification	Chronic friction
Linear erosions	Self-mutilation
Dry, lackluster skin	Barrier function defect (?) Ichthyosis vulgaris
Fissured palms/soles	Barrier function defect (?)
Hypo- and hyperpigmentation	Post inflammatory change
Vesicles, pustules, crusting	Herpes simplex, *Staphylococcus aureus, Candida*
Exfoliative erythroderma	Atopic dermatitis "out of control" (irritation, infection, withdrawal of systemic steroids, etc)

[1]From Leung DYM: In Fitzpatrick TB (ed): *Dermatology in General Medicine*, 3rd edition. New York, McGraw Hill, 1986.

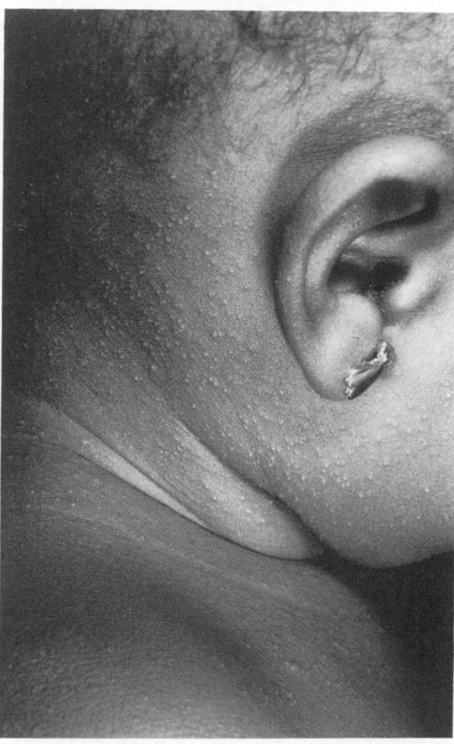

Figure 18.23. Atopic dermatitis in an 11-month-old black female infant. This follicular dermatitis reaction is the first manifestation of atopic dermatitis in infancy.

Natural History

Individuals with atopic dermatitis experience intense and severe itching. In young children, itching is aggravated by further scratching and ensuing secondary infection. During the initial eruption, follicular papules are the predominant lesions, usually occurring in clusters, mainly on the exposed portions of the body (Fig. 18.23). There is a predilection for involvement in areas of flexion such as the antecubital and popliteal fossae. With rubbing or scratching, the dome-shaped papules break down and serous crusts form. The lesions come and go, often in response to irritant factors. Interestingly, however, the diaper area of infants is usually spared, perhaps due to protection from external irritant factors. During the healing phase, lichenification is characteristic. This reaction of thickened skin with exaggerated linear markings is most prevalent in the areas where the lesions have been chronic, such as in the extremities and the flexural creases, where scratching and rubbing occurred (Figs. 18.24 and 18.25).

The disorder may be affected by seasonal changes. Thus, some individuals have greater difficulty during the winter because of excessive dryness, whereas others have relapses during the summer in association with excessive humidity and sweating. In contrast, some individuals actually improve during the summer, which may be the result of increased exposure to the sun.

The majority of individuals who have atopic dermatitis will have their first attack by 5 years of age, but the problem has been noted, although very rarely, to have an onset as late as 30 years of age. The course is extremely variable between individuals and quite unpredictable. No laboratory findings are of prognostic value in this regard.

Several other conditions have been observed in individuals with atopic dermatitis. Thus, cataracts have been reported in as many as 21% of patients with severe atopic dermatitis, but are rarely found in children. These probably are related to both atopy and the use of steroids on a chronic basis. Some individuals have a geographic tongue and a higher than expected incidence

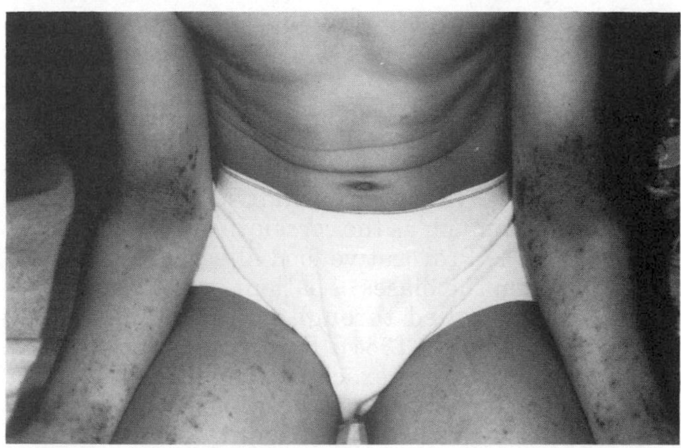

Figure 18.24. Atopic dermatitis in a 6-year-old white male. Note the flexural accentuation and lichenification and scattered folliculitis of the arms and thighs.

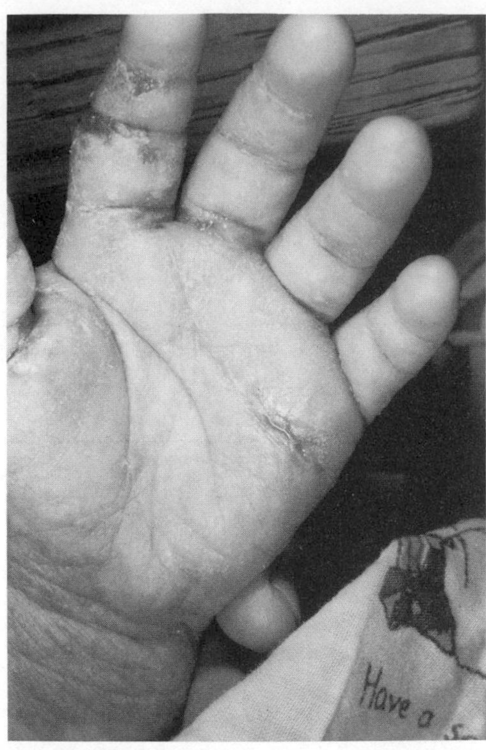

Figure 18.25. Atopic dermatitis in a 4-year-old white female. Note the weeping and crusting, manifestations of staphylococcal superinfection.

of ulcerative colitis and celiac disease has been noted in patients with atopic dermatitis. Ichthyosis vulgaris is commonly associated with this disorder; about 50% of patients with ichthyosis vulgaris have some manifestation of atopy.

Diagnosis

A complete history of eczema, allergic rhinitis, and asthma in the family is a necessary first step. The initiating events in exacerbations in the patient may be ascertained by history. Past therapies should be elicited and evaluated.

Both IgE and blood eosinophil levels may be elevated during the course of atopic dermatitis, although not in all instances. Moreover, the abnormalities of the T cells are not invariable and their measurements should be considered investigational at this time. There are no pathognomonic lesions, even by electron microscopy.

Routine skin testing for allergies is not recommended in the evaluation of individuals with atopic dermatitis inasmuch as the correlation with symptoms is only 40–70%. Provocative food allergies are best ascertained when the biases of patient, parents, and physician are controlled through "blinded" challenges (Sampson and Jolie, 1984). Food may aggravate the dermatitis; a history of exacerbation within an hour of challenge is usually obtained. Elimination diets are not recommended in the routine treatment of atopic dermatitis, unless there is a strong history of increased symptoms with certain foods.

An eruption that resembles atopic dermatitis can be a part of more serious systemic diagnosis. The Wiskott-Aldrich syndrome is an X-linked recessive disorder with skin findings indistinguishable from those of individuals with atopic dermatitis. An abnormal depression in platelets distinguishes this more severe condition that is also associated with recurrent bacterial infections.

Hyperimmunoglobulin E syndrome is characterized by the more markedly elevated IgE levels and recurrent infections in those patients. Essential fatty acid deficiencies may produce some lesions similar to those found in atopic dermatitis.

Nearly half of the patients with phenylketonuria have a dermatitis which may be indistinguishable from atopic dermatitis, but appropriate dietary management is associated with the disappearance of the skin lesion.

Psoriasis, decarboxylase deficiency, prolidase deficiency, seborrheic dermatitis, candidiasis, severe combined immune deficiency syndrome, and histiocytosis X may be confused with atopic dermatitis during infancy but are distinguished by other clinical findings and biopsy.

Treatment

Therapy depends on the stage of disease. Follicular eczema (papular dermatitis) is treated with steroid ointments with a view toward identifying irritating factors. Pustular eruptions should be evaluated for *S. aureus,* herpes simplex, and vaccinia. Staphylococcal pustulosis and eruptions that are weeping and crusting are treated with multiple warm baths and systemic antistaphylococcal therapy. Antihistamines have a variable benefit in reducing itching. Habitual scratching may require behavioral therapy.

Possible allergens should be identified by history and eliminated if they appear to relate to the onset of lesions. Some physicians advocate use of systemic antihistamines, but excessive doses are associated with drowsiness or hyperexcitability. Appropriate doses are useful during periods of excessive scratching, particularly during the early evening or at night. Topical antihistamines and anesthetics should be avoided because they can be sensitizing by themselves. Systemic corticosteroids also should be avoided. Many other agents have been tried, but none are particularly satisfactory. In the most severe cases, hospitalization will be required.

CONTROVERSY

The extent to which elimination diets are appropriate to evaluate the role of potential allergens is a subject of controversy. It has been observed that breastfed infants are less likely to have symptomatic eczema during the first 6 months of life, but later elimination of cow's milk is not predictably associated with an improvement even in these very young infants. Some feel that the early introduction of solid foods (before age 4 months) has a deleterious effect, but others have taken exception to that point of view. Even when children with a positive family history have been fed prospectively with breast milk or soy milk they have been found to develop eczema.

Prognosis

The prognosis is exceedingly variable but, in general, the disease remits in 3–5 years. There are very few longitudinal studies. Most individuals report 40–50% recovery by age 15 years. Vickers in 1980 had a more optimistic note; among 2000 children, 90% were clear at a 15-year follow-up.

ERYTHEMA MULTIFORME

Erythema multiforme is a hypersensitivity reaction to infection, drugs, or toxic substances. The skin lesions can present at any site, but most commonly on exterior surfaces of extremities. They may be macular, papular, or urticarial initially, and become vesicobullous and even hemorrhagic. The lesions appear in clusters for about 3 weeks, then heal without scarring. When they involve two or more mucous membranes, as is the case in about 25% of patients, the term erythema multiforme major is applicable (formerly Stevens-Johnson syndrome).

The illnesses associated with erythema multiforme include many infections (herpes, mycoplasma, coxsackie, influenza, tuberculosis, hemolytic streptococci, etc) and drugs (penicillin, hydantoin, barbiturates, aspirin, etc). Erythema multiforme has been described with collagen diseases, radiation therapy, and many allergens.

Diagnosis

Skin biopsy will show intraepidermal edema and vesicles in the epidermal basal layer. Lymphocytic infiltration may be present in the dermis.

Treatment

Treatment or removal of the underlying cause is essential. If extensive and painful, systemic corticosteroid therapy (prednisone, 1–2 mg/kg/day) has been used, although there are no good studies to support its efficacy. It is contraindicated if herpetic eye lesions are present.

Prognosis

In general, the disorder is mild and self-limited, although it may be recurrent in about 20% of children. When the disorder is systemic, lesions may be found in conjunctivae, nares, mouth, anorectal area, vagina, or urethra. They have been described in larynx, bronchi, gastrointestinal tract, and bladder in fatal cases. The mortality may be 5–10%.

ERYTHEMA NODOSUM

Erythema nodosum is a hypersensitivity reaction that is expressed by the appearance of painful, raised, red hot nodules 1–3 cm in diameter, most commonly over the shins, but sometimes over all extremities and buttocks.

The lesions appear in crops over an extended period of up to 6 weeks. They persist as red to violet nodules for 1–2 weeks, then gradually fade to a brown hue.

A careful search for systemic infection may reveal the trigger for the inflammatory response in the skin. Streptococcal infections are the most common in children. Tuberculosis, sarcoidosis, histoplasmosis, coccidiomycosis inflammatory bowel disease, and drugs, including birth control pills, are also likely offenders.

Treatment

Bed rest, salicylates, and other nonsteroidal anti-inflammatory agents may provide relief. The lesions are self-limited and therapy should be directed to the underlying condition.

URTICARIA (HIVES)

Urticaria is a localized, raised wheal or welt that can be very small or extensive, with one lesion coalescing with another.

The lesions are produced when an antigen interacts with mast-cell or basophil-cell IgE to promote histamine release. The lesion is caused by vasodilatation that stimulates an axon reflex to produce the so-called wheal and flare.

Urticaria can result from IgE release or other mechanisms that are not understood. For example, physical factors such as pressure or cold can produce urticaria. Some individuals experience urticaria from inhalation of pollens, or in association with infections.

Treatment

Urticaria occurs in most everyone at sometime, and is usually self-limited. In severe situations, epinephrine gives relief of itching. Cyproheptadine is especially helpful in prophylaxis of cold urticaria.

REFERENCES

Halpern SR, Sellars WA, Johnson RB, et al: Development of childhood allergy in infants fed breast, soy or cow milk. *J Allergy Clin Immunol* 51:139, 1973.

Johnson ML: Prevalence of dermatologic disease among persons 1–74 years of age: United States. National Center for Health Statistics, January 26, 1977.

Leung DYM, Bhan AK, Schneeberger E, et al: Characterization of the mononuclear cell infiltrate in atopic dermatitis using monoclonal antibodies. *J Allergy Clin Immunol* 71:47, 1983.

Leung DYM, Rhodes AR, Geha RS: Atopic dermatitis. In: Fitzpatrick TB (ed): *Dermatology in General Medicine,* 3rd edition. New York, McGraw Hill, 1986.

Sampson HA, Jolie PL: Increased plasma histamine concentrations after food challenges in children with atopic dermatitis. *N Engl J Med* 311:372, 1984.

Vickers CFH: The natural history of atopic eczema. *Acta Dermatol Vener (Stockholm)* (Suppl) 92:113, 1980.

Photosensitivity

6

Definition

Diseases induced by or aggravated by light are designated disorders of photosensitivity.

Basic Science

Less than 1% of all solar radiation is in the ultraviolet spectrum (290–400 mm), and it is the radiation between 290 and 320 nm that most potently produces erythema. The rate at which ultraviolet rays can injure skin depends on latitude, time of day, and environmental pollution. Window glass blocks ultraviolet radiation below 320 nm. Fair-skinned individuals are more susceptible to sun damage (acute and chronic) than are dark-skinned ones.

Sensitivity to visible and ultraviolet radiation may be associated with inherited conditions (see Table 18.2) and may also be acquired, i.e., during the administration of thiazide diuretics, sulfonamide compounds, and some of the tetracycline derivatives. Photosensitivity may be induced locally by exposure to certain agents, i.e., psoralen-containing substances such as meadow grass, parsnips, and limes.

SUNBURN

Definition

Sunburn can range from mild erythema to blisters, which are followed by desquamation (peeling). Excessive sunburn can lead to irreversible degeneration of collagen and, in some individuals, to skin cancer.

Natural History

Erythema appears 2–4 hours after exposure to ultraviolet light, and redness reaches a peak 10–24 hours later. Fading begins in about 48 hours.

Table 18.2
Conditions Characterized by Photosensitivity

Xeroderma pigmentosum	Autosomal recessive
Hartnup disease	Autosomal recessive
Bloom syndrome	Autosomal recessive
Ataxia telangiectasia	Autosomal recessive
Cockayne syndrome	Autosomal recessive
Pellagra	Nicotinamide deficiency
Erythropoietic porphyria	Autosomal dominant
Solar urticaria	
Lupus erythematosus	

Treatment

Cool tap water or Burow compresses (aluminum acetate) provide local relief. Topical steroids such as 1.0% hydrocortisone are sometimes helpful, but systemic corticosteroids should be avoided.

Prevention

Chemical sunscreens that contain paraminobenzoic acid are widely used when exposure to strong sunlight cannot be avoided or when a tan is desired. The compounds, which penetrate the stratum corneum, are graded by a "sun protection factor" (SPF) of 2–30 (a designation of 15 indicates the user can tolerate sunlight 15 times longer than would be possible without it). Daily use over a long period is inadvisable because the drug can accumulate in the skin. Waterproof opaque make-up is a satisfactory alternative.

The best prevention is avoidance, or exposure for short periods that can be lengthened as melanin (browning) occurs. Infants should be protected completely from bright sunlight or have, at the most, very brief exposures. It should be remembered that the sun can burn even on a cloudy day.

ERYTHROPOIETIC PORPHYRIA

Erythropoietic porphyria usually presents in early childhood and is characterized by persistent photosensitivity to visible light (410 nm).

The initial manifestation may be the observation that the diaper is stained pink from uroporphyrin I in the urine, which is a photosensitizer. Individuals with erythropoietic porphyria are at risk even when visible light penetrates window glass, so that exposed parts of the body, especially face and hands can become ulcerated and even mutilated.

The autosomal recessive condition is very rare, but is probably underreported. Of these patients, 90% have a severe hemolytic anemia and often splenomegaly, which occasionally requires splenectomy.

Erythropoietic protoporphyria (EPP) is an autosomal dominant disease which presents in childhood with painful and edematous erythema that develops within minutes of exposure to sunlight, even through window glass (410 nm). The diagnosis depends on observation of fluorescence in the red blood cells through a fluorescent microscope, and detection of protoporphyrins in stool. Treatment with betacarotene orally up to 180 mg/day, although it produces carotenemia, is effective for some patients.

XERODERMA PIGMENTOSA

This autosomal recessive disease is very rare, estimated to occur in 1 in every 250,000 births. About one-half of the affected individuals become sensitive to sunlight in early infancy and develop atypical solar lentigines even before age 2 years. The skin can become dry, scaly, hypopigmented, and even atrophic. Malignant melanomas, squamous cell carcinomas, ocular squamous cell carcinomas, actinic keratinoses, and severe actinic damage are common in this condition.

Cultured skin fibroblasts have a diminished ability to repair DNA damaged by short-wave (300–320 nm) ultraviolet light. This is presumably due to an inborn error of endonuclease metabolism in these unfortunate families. The diagnosis can be made by examination of the cultured fibroblast, and thus, prenatal diagnosis is possible.

The only therapy is to avoid exposure to ultraviolet light. Long hair, protective clothing, glasses, and sunscreens are recommended from early infancy.

COCKAYNE SYNDROME (TRISOMY 10)

This syndrome is characterized by light sensitivity and telangiectasia in addition to dwarfism. It is recessively inherited and very rare. There is a 4:1 male-female predominance. The onset of premature aging may be as early as the second year of life and the disorder progresses with optic degeneration, deafness, and mental retardation. The skin becomes atrophic with striae and scalp and body hair are sparse. The disease can be distinguished from progeria, which it resembles, by its normal content of plasma lipids.

BLOOM SYNDROME (CONGENITAL TELANGIECTACTIC ERYTHEMA)

This autosomal recessive disorder, which occurs predominantly in Jewish male children, presents in the first weeks of life with photosensitivity, especially in the face and upper extremities. The children are dwarfed and age prematurely.

The danger in this syndrome is the development of malignant tumors early in life. Extensive chromosomal breakage is found and there are abnormal chromosome configurations in up to 15% of cells. Defects in humoral and cellular immune function predispose these infants to lethal infection.

ATAXIA TELANGIECTASIA

Vascular abnormalities of the cerebellum and skin are evident in this autosomal recessive disease. Ataxia may be evident as soon as the child walks, but telangiectasia appears between ages 3 and 6 years on sun-exposed skin and in the conjunctivae. Growth is retarded. Eventually the skin becomes tight, red, and has a scaly dermatitis.

The condition is associated with low serum IgA and occasionally low IgE. α-Fetoprotein levels are elevated. Delayed hypersensitivity is depressed.

Ataxia telangiectasia is characterized by fragile chromosomes which show increased breakage when exposed to x-rays. The course is slowly progressive with death usually in early adulthood from infection or malignancy (especially brain tumor or lymphoma).

HARTNUP DISEASE

Hartnup disease is an inborn error of metabolism characterized by aminoaciduria and indole excretion. It is autosomal recessive and manifests between ages 3 and 9 years with rough, red, eczematous patches on surfaces exposed to light or heat. Acute dermatitis with blisters may follow exposure to sunlight. Glossitis and gastrointestinal symptoms are common. Tryptophan transport in the jejunum and the kidney is impaired in this disorder.

The symptoms resemble those of pellagra and, in both instances, are thought to be related to a deficiency in nicotinamide. Mental retardation and cerebellar ataxia are prominent features of Hartnup disease (see pp. 97).

Treatment is avoidance of sunlight and oral nicotinamide therapy.

REFERENCES

Longridge NS: Audiological assessment of deafness associated with xeroderma pigmentosa. *J Laryngol Otol* 90:539, 1976.

McKinnon PJ: Ataxia telangiectasia: An inherited disorder of ionizing-radiation sensitivity in man. Progress in the elucidation of the underlying biochemical defect. *Hum Genet* 75:197, 1987.

Scaly Lesions (Disorders of Epidermis) 7

PSORIASIS

Definition

Psoriasis is a chronic disorder of heightened epidermal turnover. Sharply demarcated plaques with a silvery scale may appear anywhere and recur throughout life.

Basic Science

The basic cause of psoriasis is unknown. Its principal manifestation is an accelerated turnover of epidermis so that excess cells and scale accumulate in patches.

Epidemiology

This common skin disorder has a multifactoral inheritance pattern. About one-half of the patients have a positive family history. It is estimated that 1–3% of the population has psoriasis, and about one-third of them had their first symptoms during adolescence (Solomon and Esterly, 1978).

Natural History

The onset may be in infancy or childhood but, more commonly, the disorder manifests first in patients in their teens or 20s. Exposure to sunlight (but not sunburn) usually tends to make lesions resolve. Lesions occur at any site, but classically they involve scalp, knees, elbows, gluteal cleft, and genitalia. Erythematous plaques with sharply demarcated, irregular borders are characteristic. As the epidermis accumulates, it appears silvery and flaky. Careful removal of the thick silvery scale may result in pinpoint bleeding (Fig. 18.26) because a thinned epidermis overlies a vascular papillary dermis. New lesions may appear at sites of trauma (Koebner phenomenon).

A variant, guttate psoriasis, is an eruption of many small lesions identical to the more familiar plaques. It may follow viral or streptococcal infections, or even sunburn. If psoriasis becomes "out of control," it may lead to exfoliative dermatitis.

Exacerbation and remissions are characteristic and unpredictable. Precipitating factors include streptococcal infections, poison ivy, insect bites, chemical irritation, trauma, and other skin conditions, such as acne and pityriasis. About 7% of adult psoriatic patients have arthritis, which can be very severe, with bone destruction around joints. Spondylitis and sacroiliitis can be the major manifestations.

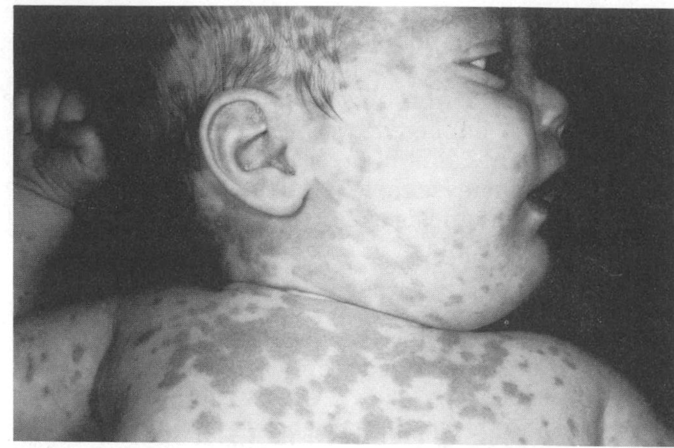

Figure 18.26. Psoriasis in a 4-month-old white male presenting with generalized "fixed" red papules and plaque.

Diagnosis

When psoriasis presents in the diaper area, it may be difficult to distinguish from seborrheic dermatitis or irritative dermatitis or candidiasis except by subtle morphologic features or biopsy (Fig. 18.27). The stratum corneum is thickened and epidermis is hyperplastic. The dermis shows vascular proliferation and an inflammatory infiltrate. Deep pitting of nails occurs in 20% of patients.

Treatment

Some individuals improve with exposure to ultraviolet light, provided that it is not intense enough to

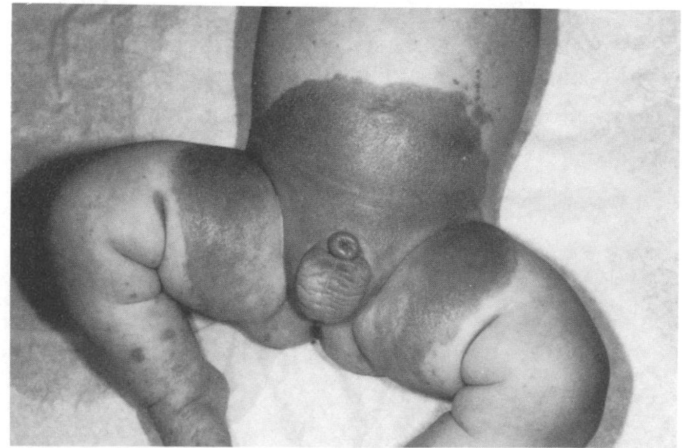

Figure 18.27. Psoriasis in a 4-month-old white male (same patient as shown in Fig. 18.26).

produce sunburn. Now widely used for psoriasis, mycosis fungoides, and other inflammatory disorders in adults, psoralens (sun sensitizers) and long-wave ultraviolet radiation (320–400 nm, peak 365 nm) in combination can produce remission. This relatively recent approach has not been evaluated for long-term effects over 7 years, (Stern, 1986; Reusch and Christophers, 1986). Because of an increased incidence of severe actinic damage, keratocanthoses, atypical pigmented lesions, and squamous cell cancers, this therapy is not approved for children.

Etretinate, a synthetic retinoid and vitamin A derivate, is effective in patients with severe recalcitrant psoriasis. Known to be a potent teratogen, etretinate is contraindicated in pregnancy (FDA, 1986). Since the half-life of the drug is several years, it should not be given to females of child-bearing age.

CASE ILLUSTRATION (abstracted from Lawlor F, Peiris S: *Br J Dermatol* 112:585,1985)

A 1.75-kg infant was delivered at 34 weeks' gestation to Bangladeshi parents. She was the 12th child born to unrelated parents who had lost four fetuses from severe icthyosis (harlequin fetus). She appeared at birth to be encased in cracked, thickened skin separated by glazed red surfaces. She was immobile. The nose was flattened, the ears underdeveloped and bound down, and the eyes were occluded by severe ectropion and eclabium.

A skin biopsy showed marked hyperkeratosis, a normal granular layer, and irregular acanthosis.

Local skin care consisted of humidified environment at 33°C, twice daily baths with bath oil and chlorhexidine, followed by application of liquid paraffin in 50% soft white paraffin every 2 hours. Saline-soaked pads were applied to both eyes.

At age 2 days, 1 mg of etretinate was given by nasogastric tube twice daily. Initially, progress was described as slow, but gradually, the scales split and peeled off and new ones formed that were paler and less yellow. By 20 weeks, she had improved markedly, with a "dramatic reversal" of ectropion and improvement in the shape of nose and ears.

COMMENT

This first documented use of etretinate in a harlequin fetus is encouraging because the longest known survivor previously was 9 months. It is sufficiently encouraging to warrent further use in infants with this distressing and fatal illness.

Topical tar preparations or steroids are useful in some instances. Tar shampoos are recommended for scalp lesions, followed by application of a steroid solution. Systemic corticosteroid therapy is not recommended in the treatment of psoriasis. Systemic therapy with methotrexate is rarely indicated for children and should not be given without consultation with a dermatologist.

For a moving and insightful description of living with psoriasis, we recommend John Updike's personal history, "At War with my Skin", *The New Yorker*, September 2, 1985.

ICHTHYOSIS

The ichthyosiform dermatoses are rare inherited disorders; the most common form, ichthyosis vulgaris (prevalence about 1 in 300) is autosomal dominant and all other forms are autosomal recessive, except for a single X-linked variant which is associated with a deficiency of steroid sulfatase.

The dermatoses may be severe (and even fatal) in the first days of life, as in harlequin fetus, or milder, as in "collodion baby" who sheds the collodion-like skin and remains normal thereafter.

If the diagnosis is not obvious from the condition of the skin, a skin biopsy may be helpful but it should be interpreted by an expert dermatologist or dermatopathologist. A normal or increased cell turnover may be present, which aids categorization.

Treatment

Treatment for scale retention in X-linked icthyosis vulgaris, is keratolysis to remove the scale. 13-cis-Retinoic acid is a treatment for those ichthyosiform dermatoses with increased turnover. Long-term treatment is inappropriate because of side effects. It is contraindicated in pregnancy because it is a potent teratogen. Successful treatment of one infant resulted by using 20 weeks of oral etretinate 1 mg twice daily. Relapse followed cessation of therapy (Lawlor and Peiris, 1985).

REFERENCES

Food and Drug Administration: Etretinate approved. *FDA Drug Bulletin* 16:16, 1986.

Lawlor F, Peiris S: Harlequin fetus successfully treated with etretinate. *Br J Dermatol* 112:585, 1985.

Reusch M, Christophers E: Psoriasis: A continuing challenge for phototherapy. *Curr Probl Dermatol* 15:219, 1986.

Solomon LM, Esterly NB, Loeffel ED: *Adolescent Dermatology*. Philadelphia, WB Saunders, 1978.

Stern RS: Long-term use of psoralens and ultraviolet A for psoriasis: Evidence for efficacy and cost savings. *J Am Acad Dermatol* 14:520, 1986.

Hair

8

Every complete physical examination should include consideration of the quality and quantity of hair and its distribution. Changes in color or fragility may be hallmarks of other diseases. Hair that is unusual can be examined effectively under a dissecting microscope, with and without a polarizing lens. Amino acid analysis and electron microscopy also may be useful.

HYPERTRICHOSIS (TOO MUCH HAIR)

The amount of hair present in adults is greater in individuals of Mediterranean origin than in those from other geographic areas. Hair over the extremities is naturally sparse in orientals. Thus, the diagnosis of excess hair should take into consideration the ethnic background of the patient.

Hair growth is abnormal in some congenital disorders such as in the Cornelia De Lange syndrome, trisomy 18, and ring chromosome E. Rarely is a significant abnormality of the hair an isolated defect. Thus, it is a part of several well-recognized syndromes. This is exemplified in Menkes steely-hair disease, which is a disorder of copper metabolism characterized by significant developmental delay and convulsions. The hair is sparse, hypopigmented, and the shafts break easily, leaving short ends that feel like steel wool. The hair shaft is twisted and quite characteristic when examined under the microscope (see also pp. 974).

Generalized hypertrichosis is seen in many CNS disorders such as encephalitis or multiple sclerosis.

Hirsutism may be secondary to endocrine abnormalities including adrenal hyperplasia and Cushing syndrome. It is also a feature of the Stein-Leventhal syndrome and other ovarian tumors. Testosterone and other anabolic steroids that produce virilization can also cause hirsutism.

Diagnosis

The evaluation of hirsute young girls should be directed toward a search for an androgen-secreting neoplasm in adrenal or ovary, or congenital adrenal hyperplasia, or Cushing syndrome (Table 18.3). An elevation in serum testosterone or DHEA-sulfate levels occur with androgen-secreting tumors. Ultrasonography or CT scans of ovaries and adrenals are often diagnostic.

Treatment

Specific treatment for underlying disorders such as resection of a neoplasm or discontinuance of a drug can reverse hirsutism.

If 21-hydroxylase deficiency is excluded, a single bedtime dose of 0.5 mg dexamethasone can suppress serum testosterone in adolescent girls with hirsutism on the basis of adrogen excess. In some patients, hirsutism regressed. Others required oral contraceptives to suppress ovulation (Emans et al, 1988).

Table 18.3
Hirsutism in Association with Androgen Excess in Adolescence

Congenital adrenal hyperplasia
Cushing syndrome
Adrenal neoplasma
Polycystic ovaries
Ovarian neoplasms
Incomplete testicular feminization
Acromegaly
Porphyria
Drug-induced
Phenytoin
Danazol
Androgenic steroids

HYPOTRICHOSIS

The normal scalp has about 100,000 hairs, 90% of which are growing, and 10% resting or falling out. The growth phase averages 1000 days and the resting phase before the hair falls out averages 100 days. An average rate of hair loss is 50–100 hairs/day. The normal rate of growth is 10 mm/month. Loss of hair can be the result of a variety of reasons (see Table 18.4).

Baldness in males is well-known and is genetically determined. It can begin in young adults as frontal recession and occipital thinning, and then progress to other areas or remain stationary. Complete loss of scalp hair occurs when hair cycles are synchronized, sometimes in the face of surgical shock, weight loss, or after a high fever. The most common cause of acute baldness in the 1980s is chemotherapy or radiation for malig-

Table 18.4
Some Causes of Hair Loss

Hereditary baldness
Ectodermal dysplasias
Infection
Tinea capitis
Severe infections with high fever
Chronic inflammatory conditions (atopic dermatitis)
Radiation
Some toxins and heavy metals (thallium, coumarin, heparin)
Alopecia areata (family history in about 20%)
Autoimmune thyroiditis, Addison disease
Excessive traction

nant disease. In this instance, loss is diffuse 1–3 weeks after beginning treatment. Most of the disorders associated with loss of hair are reversible; however, occasionally, in the rare case of loss of hair after high fever, it may be irreversible.

Alopecia areata is an acute loss of patches of hair most commonly in individuals under 25 years of age. This condition is usually of unknown etiology but can occur with vitiligo and sometimes autoimmune thyroid disease. The hair loss can be complete in areas several centimeters in diameter or hair can be easily removed by pulling gently at the periphery of an active lesion. When the areas are small and the duration short, full recovery is likely. Eyebrow and eyelash involvement, extensive loss, younger age, and nail involvement are bad prognostic signs. At the end of 1 year, one-third of patients are worse, one-third better, and one-third unchanged. Available effective therapy (albeit dangerous) includes systemic corticosteroids, psoralen-ultraviolet-light treatment (PUVA, not for children under 12 years), and topical minoxidal. The disease has a genetic predisposition, with positive family history in 20% of cases.

Excessive traction applied to hair by tight braids may be associated with subsequent hair loss. The problem is seen most often in black girls who may have tightly plaited hair over long periods of time. The baldness usually reverses.

Prognosis

If the insult that caused hair loss was an isolated event, after 4–6 weeks regrowth can be expected. If the cause is malnutrition and hypovitaminosis, the alopecia develops gradually and regrowth depends on restoration of adequate nutrition. Focal alopecia at birth may occur at the site of nevi, hemangiomas, or aplasia cutis. Such hair problems cannot be treated.

Diffuse alopecia at birth, or failure of hair growth in childhood is most often the result of congenital hair shaft abnormalities. Ectodermal dysplasia and congenital hypothyroidism are possible underlying conditions.

REFERENCES

Datloff J, Esterly NB: A system for sorting out pediatric alopecia. *Contemp Pediatr* Oct:13, 1986.

Emans SJ, Grace E, Woods ER: Treatment with dexamethasone of androgen excess in adolescent patients. *J Pediatr* 112:821, 1988.

Stroud JD: Hair loss in children. *Pediatr Clin North Am* 30:641, 1983.

GENERAL REFERENCES

Rasmussen JE (ed): Symposium on Pediatric Dermatology. *Pediatr Clin North Am* 30:417, 1983.

Solomon LM, Esterly NB: *Neonatal Dermatology*. Philadelphia, WB Saunders, 1973.

Solomon LM, Esterly NB, Loeffel ED: *Adolescent Dermatology*. Philadelphia, WB Saunders, 1978.

Miscellaneous Disorders 9

PITYRIASIS ROSEA

Definition

Pityriasis rosea is a common eruption without systemic involvement that lasts 2–12 weeks and is self-limited. This disorder is thought to be virus-induced, possibly by a rotavirus.

Natural History

The clinical course is characteristic; in 70% of patients, the disorder starts with a single, round, or oval "herald patch" anywhere on the body. The patch is 1–10 cm in diameter, has a raised border, and very fine peripheral scale lifting centrally on an erythematous base. Five to 10 days later, multiple, small, slightly raised pink or tan lesions appear, mostly on the trunk, but then may involve proximal extremities or face. The lesions align along cutaneous cleavage lines, especially on the torso and axillary folds. Lesions are usually asymptomatic, but may be mildly pruritic in 20% of cases. They last 2–12 weeks, and disappear without scabs or scars.

Diagnosis

The clinical course is pathognomonic, although at times the condition is confused with viral exanthems or drug eruptions. Secondary syphilis may have an identical presentation. Other possible diagnoses are psoriasis and lichen planus.

Treatment

No treatment is needed for this self-limited benign condition. Pruritis may be treated with oatmeal baths and antihistamines. In severe cases, ultraviolet light has been helpful.

Prognosis

Hypopigmentation may persist for some weeks, especially in darkly pigmented individuals.

Prevention

The condition is not likely to spread among contacts, but it is presumably infectious. Recurrences are unusual but do occur.

ACNE

Definition

Acne is a common inflammatory condition of skin characterized by pustules, inflamed nodules, and, in the most severe forms, superficial pus-filled cysts.

Basic Science

The initial process that leads to acne starts 1–2 years before the onset of puberty from androgen stimulation of the sebaceous glands. The follicles may become obstructed by abnormal keratinization of the lining epidermal cells and form a comedone or "whitehead." With continued formation of keratin, the follicular wall ruptures and releases free fatty acids and sebum which presumably inflame the surrounding dermis. The organisms most commonly associated with the lesions are *Propionibacterium acnes* and *Staphylococcus epidermis*. The bacteria are also thought to be important in promoting inflammation.

Neonatal acne results from hormonal stimulation of sebaceous glands that have not involuted to their childhood immature state.

Epidemiology and Natural History

Neonatal acne presents as typical raised pustular lesions occurring in the neonatal period. All lesions are at the same stage at the same time. The lesions are usually on the face and shoulders, and sometimes the back.

Infantile acne may occur in the first month of life, especially in males, with lesions confined to the face. A history of severe acne in parents is common in this condition.

Adolescent acne appears with the onset of puberty, at 8–10 years of age. Eventually it is estimated that 85% of adolescents will have some acne on the face, shoulders, and back, if acne is defined by the presence of comedones. A tendency to acne may persist to the late 30s or early 40s, or even later.

Drug-induced acne may occur at any age in response to glucocorticoids, androgens, hydantoin, and isoniazid. The lesions may occur on the face and shoulders, but also extend to the trunk and extremities. The lesions in steroid-induced acne (folliculitis) are usually in the same stage of development.

Diagnosis

Superficial acne is characterized by comedones (whiteheads if closed, blackheads if open). Papules are red, owing to inflammation and they may become pustular or cystic. In severe cystic acne, lesions extend more deeply into the skin and form collections which may lead to severe scarring (pitted, hypertrophic, even keloidal).

Treatment

In patients with moderate to severe acne, the face is usually oily and several washes each day with soap and water (but not abrasives or astringents) are recommended. Sunlight and ultraviolet radiation are helpful drying agents. The best nonprescription topical agent is 5% benzoyl peroxide, an antimicrobial that is also comedolytic. Retinoic acid cream is keratolytic at a concentration of 0.05% or 0.1%. Individuals using the topical cream should avoid the sun. Oral tetracycline, 500–1000 mg/day may be required until a response is seen, after which it should be decreased to lowest amount that protects from recurrence while using intensive topical therapy. If the patient is pregnant, or the response to tetracycline is disappointing, erythromycin in similar doses may be effective.

For nodulocystic acne or extensive disease that is refractory to simple measures, oral isotretinoin, approved in 1982, may be indicated. It is estimated that over 600,000 patients have been treated with this drug since 1982 with gratifying clinical results that persist after discontinuation of a 4- to 5-month course. Less obvious benefit has been observed for acne-related skin disorders such as Gram-negative folliculitis. Variable results have been seen with psoriasis and other scaling disorders (Pochi, 1985). Because this agent has been associated with a 25-fold increase in serious congenital malformations if taken in the first trimester of pregnancy, it is contraindicated during pregnancy and, indeed, in any female at risk of pregnancy (Lammer et al, 1985). The drug has also some unpleasant side effects such as dry eyes and nose, reversible hair loss, and increases in mean levels of triglycerides and low-density lipoprotein cholesterol. Consultation with a dermatologist is appropriate if the child with acne is a candidate for isotretinoin. The risks, benefits, and potential side effects require that treatment be individualized (Chaulker et al, 1987).

X-radiation is effective in temporarily reducing sebaceous gland size, but long-term side effects of X-radiation and the availability of newer agents make radiation outmoded.

Prevention

Little evidence supports dietary changes as a mean of prevention of acne. If, on the other hand, some individuals relate an exacerbation to certain foods, a trial of avoidance is appropriate.

Washing the face gently several times a day, and washing oily hair frequently makes sense, although the extent of benefit is not clear.

Exposure to sunlight sufficient to give a light burn has been found useful, although excessive exposure with peeling is not helpful. If an individual is using topical retinoic acid, sunlight should be avoided.

WARTS

Definition

Warts are epidermal tumors induced by human papilloma viruses.

Epidemiology

The incidence is not known, but the condition is very common in children and tends to be recurrent.

Natural History

The incubation period is variable, depending on size of inoculum of virus, site of infection, and host defenses, but the average is about 3 months. The usual sites for common warts are hands and feet. Other viral types may induce warts in the perianal and genital region (condyloma acuminatum), and may involve the larynx (see laryngeal papillomatosis). About 20–30% of common warts regress spontaneously within 6 months, and 50% regress within a year (Bunney, 1977). Common warts appear in groups and can continue to arise at different sites. Condylomata acuminata and laryngeal warts are much more indolent (see pp. 1199).

Diagnosis

Diagnosis is evident on inspection. Lesions consist of flesh-colored papules which, on magnification, display punctate capillaries over the surface, many of which are thrombosed.

Treatment

Usually no treatment is indicated for asymptomatic children. Topical liquid nitrogen applied every 2–3 weeks will form small blisters and hasten disappearance. For common warts, topical preparations of salicylic acid (17.5%) and lactic acid (17.5%) in flexible collodion have a cure rate of 70% at 12 weeks. (For treatment of laryngeal papillomas see Bauer, 1982).

Prevention

Warts are not highly contagious, but can be spread to moist areas by direct contact. Genital spread among sexually active adults is known to occur (Oriel, 1982). Perianal and genital warts in young children may indicate sexual abuse (or inoculation through an infected vagina for very small children or infants).

SCABIES

Definition

Scabies is the result of an infestation of the skin by a mite (sarcoptes scabiei, subspecies hominis).

Epidemiology and Natural History

Scabies is one of the most widespread infestations among children worldwide. It is most common among individuals living in crowded conditions, and is highly contagious. Epidemics are said to occur in 15-year cycles, but the United States has experienced endemic scabies for at least 20 years. Humans are the source of infection. In the absence of previous exposure, an interval of 2–6 weeks precedes symptoms; with earlier exposure, the interval is 1–4 days.

Diagnosis

The characteristic lesion is a linear papule, papulovesicle, or papulopustule. In older children, papules tend to be concentrated on the wrists, ankles, finger webs, buttocks, and groin, whereas, in infants, the lesions are found in any location, including face, trunk, palms, and soles. Because the lesions itch and frequently become secondarily infected when scratched by the patient, this can confuse the diagnosis.

The mite can be identified in an unscratched papule, vesicle, or burrow if scraped or shaved with a blade, and examined in 10% KOH or mineral oil under a microscope.

Treatment

One percent γ-benzene hexachloride (Lindane), is effective when applied to unbathed skin as a lotion for 8–12 hours, one time only. Transcutaneous absorption can lead to CNS toxicity in young infants. Crotamiton is an alternative in infants under 2 years and in pregnant women (Reeves, 1987). One treatment is usually sufficient. All skin-to-skin contacts (within 3 months of contact plus symptoms) should be treated. Pregnant or nursing women and premature or sick infants should be treated with 6% sulfur in petrolatum USP with daily applications for 5 days, repeated 1 week later.

DERMATOPHYTOSES (TINEA)

Definition

The designation tinea comprises a variety of fungal infections of the skin that produce characteristic scaling erythematous lesions. Species of *Trichophyton, Microsporum,* and *Epidermophyton* are the organisms most frequently involved in the infections, which are designated by the site of the lesions: thus, tinea capitis, tinea corporis, tinea cruris, tinea pedis (athlete's foot), tinea manuum (hands), and tinea unguium (nails). Tinea versicolor, so-called because of the tan or brown patches that may appear white in contrast to suntanned (hyperpigmented) skin, lesions may be found on the face, trunk or extremities.

Basic Science

Dermatophytes are limited to keratinized layers of skin, hair, and nails and do not usually invade below the epidermis. Serum has a fungistatic activity, so that disseminated infection is rare except in immunocompromised hosts. An allergic "id" reaction, presumably mediated by cellular factors and/or antibody, occurs in some patients with weeping forms of tinea. Spontaneous cure and relative resistance of children to subsequent infections are associated with a delayed type hypersensitivity.

Epidemiology

Tinea pedis (athlete's foot) is the most common of the dermatophytoses. It is rare before age 7 years, but by age 20 years about 20% of the population has had at least one episode of tinea pedis.

Natural History

Tinea capitis starts as a scaling maculopapule, or pustule, with crusting at the base of a hair follicle, and spreads peripherally. Eventually, loss of hair results in patches of alopecia, which can be extensive. One form of dermatophyte infection of the scalp is called black dot since the hairs break at the scalp surface, and there is no scaling or redness (Figs. 18.28 and 18.29).

Tinea pedis, which is most common in adolescents, involves the webs of the toes and/or nails. The severity and distribution of lesions depend on the type of fungus involved. Lesions may consist of redness, scaling, red papulae, vesicles, bullae, and pustules. Intense itching is common.

Infections in some patients tend to become chronic, with or without treatment. The natural course of tinea capitis is gradual spread of lesions for 3–4 months, a refractory period of 4 months to several years, and then gradual spontaneous resolution. In the process of untreated infection of the scalp, permanent hair loss from scarring of the hair follicles may occur.

Tinea versicolor typically causes scaly oral macules about 5–10 mm in diameter. They may be hypo- or hyperpigmented and mildly pruritic. Warm, humid conditions encourage growth.

Diagnosis

The clinical presentation of tinea is usually so characteristic that the diagnosis can be strongly suspected, except when intense inflammation is present.

The mainstays of definitive diagnosis are examination of scrapings of scale and their culture. The Wood lamp, which emits filtered ultraviolet light, will reveal infected hair shafts as blue and green fluorescence for the *Microsporum* species and for *Trichophyton schoenleinii*. The most common organism currently causing tinea capitis, *T. tonsurans,* does not fluoresce, nor does tinea corporis.

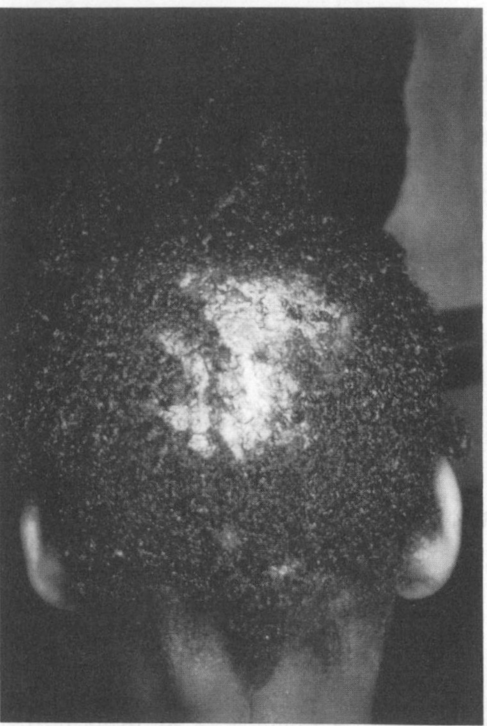

Figure 18.28. Tinea capitis due to *Trichophyton tonsurans* in a 7-year-old black male child, presenting as a crusted and weeping plaque.

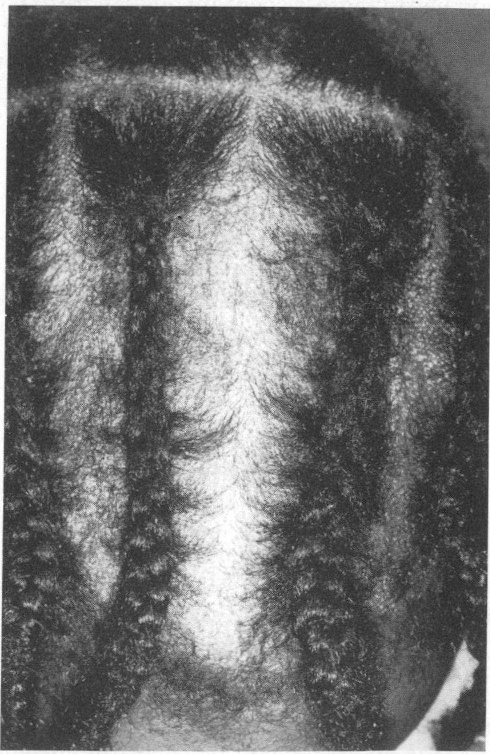

Figure 18.29. Tinea capitis due to *Trichophyton tonsurans* in a 10-year-old black female youngster, presenting as a diffuse "seborrheic dermatitis." A proper diagnosis requires scrapings and/or culture for the organism.

A KOH preparation (1–2 drops of 10–20% KOH) on a glass slide is useful to detect fungal elements, such as mycelia and spores, under a microscope. Because the KOH is used to digest the keratin, 5–10 minutes is adequate to wait to analyze skin scrapings, 15–30 minutes for hair, and up to 24 hours for nails. A negative scraping does not necessarily exclude infection, however.

Cultures on Sabouraud media with cycloheximide may be needed to identify the fungus. Most dermatophytes require 4–6 weeks to yield a positive culture. Tinea versicolor *(Pityrosporum orbiculare)* requires mineral oil on top of routine mycologic media to grow. It takes several weeks to grow, while *Candida albicans* will grow in 48 hours.

Treatment

Treatment of tinea depends on the location of the lesions to some extent, but the disorders may recur, as described below.

TINEA CAPITIS

These lesions are treated with oral griseofulvin microcrystalline (10 mg/kg/24 hours) for 8–12 weeks. Topical antifungal therapy alone is usually ineffective. Topical selenium sulfide in a 2.5% solution applied every other day will reduce infectivity of tinea capitis.

TINEA PEDIS

Local treatment with miconazole or chlotrimazole is usually curative. Careful drying of toes will retard reinfection. Recurrences are common if occlusive shoes are worn, thus increasing moist surfaces. Moist infections of the toe web spaces are usually superimposed with Gram-negative bacteria and will not respond to topical antifungal agents. Drying preparations such as aluminum chloride in alcohol are required for 5–7 days before topical antifungal therapy is effective.

TINEA UNGUIUM

The treatment of fungal infection of nails is disappointing. Prolonged (up to a year) griseofulvin and topical agents help in some instances. Cure can be expected to occur in 50% of cases after 6 months of therapy, and relapse occurs in 50% of "those cured." Blood counts and liver function tests should be monitored in individuals on prolonged systemic therapy with griseofulvin.

TINEA VERSICOLOR

Treatment with a 2.5% selenium sulfide shampoo, left on the lesion for 10–15 minutes before rinsing, daily for several weeks is usually effective.

REFERENCES

Bauer DJ: Treatment of plantar warts with acyclovir. *Am J Med* 73:313, 1982.

Bunney MH: The treatment of viral warts. *Drugs* 13:445, 1977.

Chaulker DK, Lesher JL Jr, Smith JG Jr, et al: Efficacy of topical isotretinoin 0.05% gel in acne vulgaris: Results of a multicenter, double-blind investigation. *J Am Acad Dermatol* 17:251, 1987

Dicken CH: Retinoids: A review. *J Am Acad Dermatol* 11:541, 1984.

Lammer EJ, Chen DT, Hoar RM, et al: Retinoic acid embryopathy. *N Engl J Med* 313:837, 1985.

Oriel JD: Genital warts. *Sex Transm Dis* 8:326, 1982.

Pochi PE: Isotretinoin for acne: the experience broadens. Editorial. *N Engl J Med* 313:1013, 1985.

Reeves JRT: Head lice and scabies in children. *Pediatr Infect Dis* 6:598,1987.

Solomon LM, Fahrner L, West DP: Gamma benzene hexachloride toxicity. *Arch Dermatol* 113:353, 1977.

MARY ELLEN AVERY

Consultants
Arthur Rhodes
Rita Berman

Section 19

Otolaryngology

Pediatric otolaryngology is now a recognized subspecialty of otolaryngology and, unquestionably, deserves special emphasis in a textbook of pediatrics. We have tried to orient this section in a way that will be helpful to the general pediatrician, whose practice is likely to be weighted with patients who have disorders of ears, nose, and throat. It is estimated that between 25 and 50% of all visits to the pediatrician include problems (mostly infections) of these organs. Because the complaint is usually localized anatomically, the problems are considered by region. This section is in no way comprehensive; embryology, pathophysiology, and surgical techniques are not discussed. The interested reader is referred to the standard textbooks in pediatric otolaryngology and dentistry.

APPROACH TO THE HEARING-IMPAIRED CHILD

Parental suspicion that a child does not hear must always be taken seriously. Unfortunately, delays in diagnosis are common and frustrating to parents, physicians, and patients alike. Significant hearing impairment is present in approximately 50,000 children of school age in the United States; congenital deafness occurs in about 1/1000 live births although this number should decrease with wide use of rubella immunization.

The early signs of hearing impairment may be a delay in speech development, or unresponsiveness to ordinary auditory stimuli. No child is too young for evaluation of auditory-evoked potentials by electroencephalography. In our institution, all high-risk infants and all infants or children who have had meningitis are tested by evoked potentials and conventional audiometry. As many as 16% of survivors of meningitis have some degree of permanent hearing loss (Dodge et al, 1984). Low birth weight infants may have abnormal tests at the time of hospital discharge and normal tests 3 months later. The rate of abnormality at 3 months was 2.3% in Robert's series (1982) of infants who received neonatal intensive care. Occasionally an infant may have a normal auditory brain stem response as a newborn, but have significant hearing loss at 1 year of age (Nield et al, 1986).

Detection of hearing impairment should be made as early as possible. For that reason, a number of risk factors have been identified to pinpoint the population that should be tested. Because many infants with known risk factors are not being tested, it would be appropriate to post the list in every intensive care nursery or infants' ward (Table 19.1).

The most widely used test is pure-tone audiometry. Electric response audiometry is preferable and, in experienced hands, is reproducible and accurate. A repeat test is desirable about 3 months later. The test measures only the peripheral auditory system. If the infant has normal tests, but still does not seem to hear, cortical auditory dysfunction may be present.

Any infant or child who has a loss detected by repeat audiometry 3 months after the initial illness or after discharge from intensive care should have a full evaluation that measures precochlear, cochlear, retrocochlear, midbrain, and cortical function.

REMEDIAL APPROACHES TO THE HEARING-IMPAIRED CHILD

Delay in acquisition of language is the major consequence of deafness in infancy. Once a careful eval-

Table 19.1
Risk Factors for Hearing Loss in Infancy [1]

Family history of childhood impairment
Often associated with other malformations especially cranial and skeletal defects
Low birth weight especially under 1500 g
Sensorineural hearing loss is estimated in 2% of survivors of neonatal intensive care
Perinatal infections, especially the TORCH group
Toxoplasmosis, rubella, cytomegalovirus, herpes, and syphilis
Anatomic malformations of head and neck
Indirect hyperbilirubinemia at levels above those for which exchange transfusion is recommended
Bacterial meningitis, especially *H. influenzae* type B and *S. pneumoniae*
Ototoxicity, especially with aminoglycosides (essential to follow serum levels in individuals being treated)
Severe asphyxia with damage to cochlear nuclei
Chronic serous otitis media (reversible)

[1] Adapted from Report of Task Force on Childhood Hearing Impairment, National Health and Welfare, Ottawa, Canada, December, 1984.

uation has been undertaken, alternative methods of communication should be instituted as soon as possible.

Vision, hearing, and touch are all important in the development of language. Loss of hearing can be compensated for by gaining the infant's visual attention when speaking with slow clear enunciation. If appropriate, the infant should have hearing aids to maximize limited hearing.

Formal teaching of speech is usually delayed until about age 5 years, after which time the child requires help from a trained speech therapist together with understanding and well-motivated family or other caretakers.

Hearing-impaired parents may use sign language and wish their child to learn it as well (Groce, 1985). The American sign language, known as Amesian, uses hand configuration, movement and position to represent a concept rather than a word. The syntax differs from English and it may be difficult for the child to acquire both forms of communication at the same time.

The pediatrician has a pivotal role in establishing the diagnosis, referral to an otolaryngologist, and ongoing emotional support to the family. Referral to organizations prepared to help hearing-impaired children is very important. Examples are Gallaudet College, 7th Street and Florida Avenue, Washington, DC, and the Alexander Graham Bell Association for the Deaf, 3417 Volta Place, Washington, DC, 20007.

REFERENCES

Bernard PA: Freedom from ototoxicity in aminoglycoside treated neonates: A mistaken notion. *Laryngoscope* 12:1985, 1981.

Dodge PR, Dairs H, Feigin RD, et al: Prospective evaluation of hearing impairment as a sequela of acute bacterial meningitis. *N Engl J Med* 311:869, 1984.

Fischer TJ: The pediatrician and the deaf child: Perspectives of a pediatrician-parent. *Pediatrics* 67:313, 1981.

Groce NE: "Everyone here spoke sign language." Hereditary Deafness on Martha's Vineyard. Cambridge, MA, Harvard University Press, 1985.

Kaplan SL, Catlin FI, Weaver T, et al: Onset of hearing loss in children with bacterial meningitis. *Pediatrics* 73:575, 1984.

Nield TA, Schrier S, Ramos AD, et al: Unexpected hearing loss in high risk infants. *Pediatrics* 78:417, 1986.

Report of a Task Force on Childhood Hearing Impairment, National Health and Welfare, Ottawa, Canada, December 1984.

Roberts JL, Davis H, Phon GL, et al: Auditory brainstem responses in preterm neonates: Maturation and follow-up. *J Pediatr* 101:257, 1982.

Inner Ear Disorders

1

SENSORINEURAL HEARING LOSS

Definition

Sensorineural hearing loss refers to dysfunction in the cochlea, cochlear nuclei, or the central perception of hearing. It can be congenital or acquired and is irreversible. The degree of hearing loss can range from mild to total.

Epidemiology

The incidence of hearing loss in newborn infants is about 1/1000 population, but as high as 2–3% in infants in intensive care units. Congenital hearing loss accounts for about 20% of deafness in children (Ruben and Rozycki, 1971; Konigsmark, 1969) (Fig. 19.1).

Natural History

Hereditary conditions that may be associated with congenital sensorineural hearing loss include albinism, Waardenburg syndrome, Alpert syndrome, craniosynostoses, Cockayne syndrome, and others (Table 19.2).

Congenital infections can result in damage to the CNS auditory centers. The so-called TORCHES group is most common (*toxoplasmosis, rubella, cytomegalovirus, herpes,* and *syphilis*). Bilirubin, especially in sick premature infants, can enter cells in the basal ganglia and produce injury (kernicterus). The most common predisposing event was maternal-fetal blood group incompatibility. The routine identification of Rh-negative mothers during pregnancy, and use of high-titer anti-Rh D globulin given to the mother at the time of delivery prevent development of anti-D antibodies in

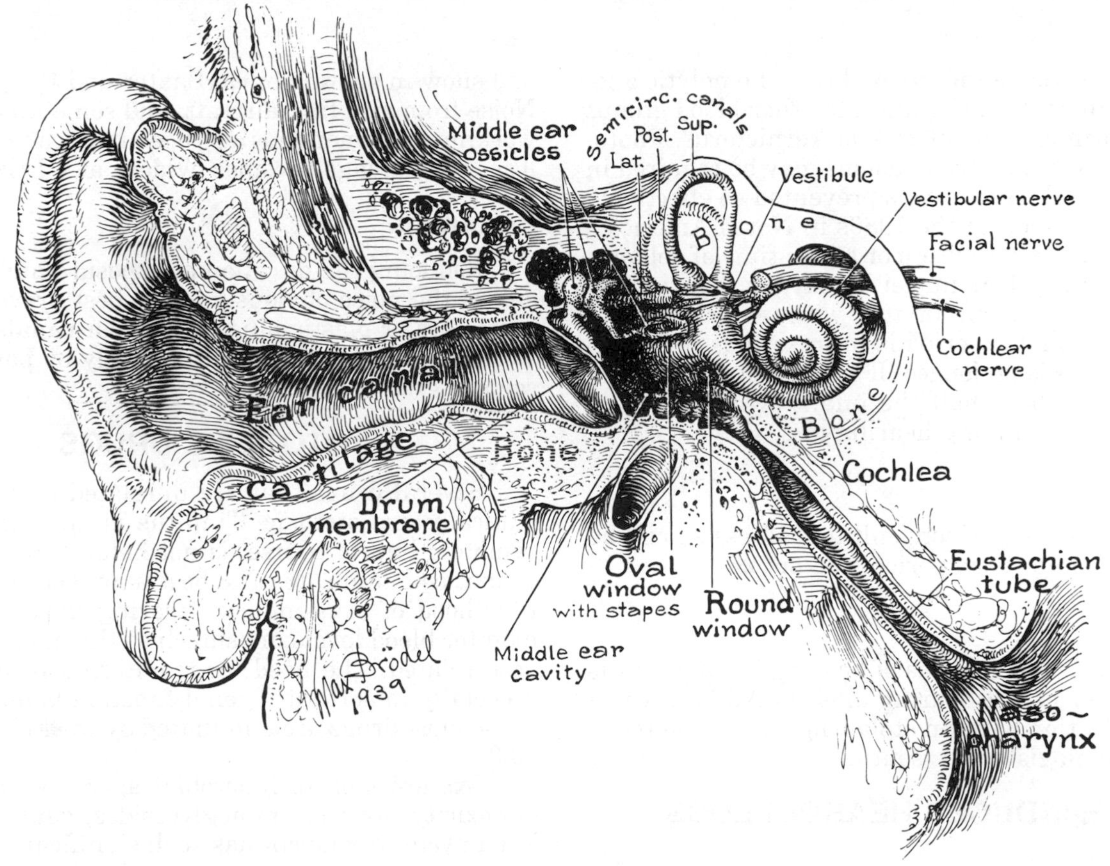

Figure 19.1. This famous drawing by the late Max Brödel of Johns Hopkins demonstrates the anatomical relationships of external, middle, and inner ear in a way neither photographs nor words can equal.

Table 19.2
Some Physical Abnormalities That May Be Associated with Deafness [1]

	Abnormality	Disease or Syndrome	Type of Hearing Loss		Conductive
			Sensorineural		
Skull	Macrocephaly	Osteopetrosis	X		X
	Abnormal shape	Apert	X	*or*	X
		Crouzon			X
	Persistent fontanelle	Cleidocranial dysostosis	X		
Hair	White forelock, heterochromia of iris	Waardenburg	X		
Face	Prominence of frontal bone	Hurler			X
	Flattened cheeks	Treacher-Collins			X
	Facial paralysis strabismus	Mobius			X
Eyes	Cataracts	Rubella	X		
	Retinitis pigmentosa	Laurence-Moon-Bardet-Biedl	X		
Nose	Saddle	Congenital syphilis	X		
Mouth	Cleft lip and palate	Trisomy 18	X	*or*	X
		Pierre Robin	X	*and*	X
Neck	Short neck	Klippel-Feil	X	*and*	X
	Webbing	Turner	X	*and*	X
Skin	Depigmentation	Albinism	X		
	Inability to sweat	Ectodermal dysplasia	X		
	Neurofibromatosis	von Recklinghausen	X		

[1]Modified from Jaffee BF (ed): *Hearing Loss in Children: A Comprehensive Text.* Baltimore, University Park Press, 1977.

most instances. Some infants will have hemolytic anemia from maternal sensitization to other blood groups and will continue to be at risk of kernicterus. Phototherapy and exchange transfusions may be required in such instances. Kernicterus is prevented so effectively that it is rarely seen in the 1980s in North America.

Severe asphyxia in utero or at the time of delivery can injure the cochlear nuclei by oxygen deprivation. Hypoxic-ischemic brain injury, with associated seizures in the neonatal period is most serious if the duration of seizures is prolonged. If symptoms persist more than 36 hours, about half the infants will have neurologic residua, including hearing loss.

Diagnosis

Any child at risk of congenital deafness should be screened in the newborn period (see pp. 26).

Treatment

As soon as the diagnosis of hearing impairment is made the early use of hearing aids should be encouraged. Consultation with an otolaryngologist and referral to an audiologist are essential.

NOISE-INDUCED HEARING LOSS

Definition

Prolonged exposure to any intense noise can lead to significant sensorineural hearing loss. For example, hearing loss was documented among the Inuit people in the Arctic who traveled long distances across rock and snow in snowmobiles (Baxter and Rjskjaer, 1979). Noise from gun fire, aircraft, and some kinds of woodworking equipment has also been implicated in hearing loss. The damage becomes evident at 4 kHz.

Prevention

Reducing the duration of exposure and the intensity of the noise obviously is the best prevention. Ear protectors or plastic plugs in the ear canals should be worn in all noisy settings, especially by patients with some degree of deafness.

OTOTOXIC DRUGS

Several drugs that are unrelated chemically and clinically are ototoxic. Tinnitus is an early warning symptom but, of course, is not helpful in infants who cannot communicate. The best approach to lessen the likelihood of drug-induced hearing impairment is to monitor blood levels, inasmuch as the injury is usually dose related. The need for monitoring blood levels is especially important if renal function is impaired, because most drugs are eliminated by the kidneys (Table 19.3).

Examples of antimicrobial agents with potential ototoxicity are the aminoglycosides, gentamicin, and kanamycin. Neomycin has such significant ototoxicity that it is rarely given parenterally. Vancomycin and erythromycin can produce permanent hearing loss. It can be used by the oral route or topically because it is poorly absorbed. Streptomycin can injure the vestibular apparatus and, for that reason, is rarely prescribed.

Table 19.3
Potentially Ototoxic Drugs [1]

Aminoglycosides
Neomycin—most toxic of all antibiotics; rarely indicated, and then only by mouth because it is poorly absorbed
Streptomycin—damages vestibular portion of inner ear, and may produce permanent deafness
Gentamicin—rarely toxic at serum levels 4–8 μg/ml; measured 1 hour after a dose
Amikacin—desired serum level 10–25 μg/ml
Diuretics
Furosemide (maximum dose is 4 mg/kg/day); hearing loss is unusual and mostly transient
Ethacrynic acid—rarely used in children
Others (rarely used in infants)
Quinine
Salicylates—usual dose 65–100 mg/kg/day in four to six doses.

[1] Note: Renal impairment predisposes to elevated blood levels of most ototoxic drugs. If possible, hearing should be measured before starting a long course of potentially ototoxic drugs.

Dihydrostreptomycin is no longer recommended because it has even greater ototoxicity. Diuretics such as ethacrynic acid and furosemide are potentially ototoxic. Other drugs that may produce tinnitus are salicylates and quinine.

LABYRINTHITIS

Definition

Disorders of the inner ear are rare in children, but can present as dizziness, tinnitus, or sudden loss of hearing.

Epidemiology

Although there are no systematic studies to evaluate incidence, all forms of acquired inner ear disease are unusual before adulthood.

Natural History

Labyrinthitis, which is characterized by severe vertigo and nystagmus, can be the consequence of untreated or partially treated purulent otitis media. It can also be a complication of meningitis and may contribute to loss of hearing during and sometimes after acute bacterial meningitis. It can result in complete hearing loss.

Trauma to the temporal bone may also produce symptoms of vertigo or unsteadiness. Any patient with symptoms after such injury should have a neuro-otologic examination and radiographic investigation for fractures. Chronic vertigo can be the result of subtle damage to the oval or round windows and requires more extensive investigation.

Diagnosis

If the diagnosis of labyrinthitis is suspected by the history and findings, the patient must be referred to an otolaryngologist.

In the absence of purulent otitis or any other abnormal findings on physical examination, recurrent dizzy spells suggest the possibility of benign paroxysmal vertigo of childhood (Koenigsberger et al, 1968). Tinnitus and deafness are absent, which distinguishes this self-limited disorder from labyrinthitis. Caloric tests may be abnormal.

Vertigo with loss of consciousness can occur with epilepsy.

Trauma to the temporal bone may also produce vertigo or unsteadiness. Any patient with symptoms after such an injury should have a neuro-otologic examination and radiographic investigation for fractures. Chronic vertigo can result from subtle damage to the oval or round windows and requires more extensive investigation.

For discussion of other disorders of the inner ear, or for discussion of Meniere's disease or the differential diagnosis of sudden deafness from sensorineural hearing loss, the reader is referred to textbooks of otolaryngology.

REFERENCES

Baxter JD, Rjskjaer C: A Greenland-Baffin Zone Project. *J Otolaryngol* 8:315, 1979.

Koenigsberger MR, Chutorian AM, Gold AP, et al: Benign paroxysmal vertigo of childhood. *Neurology* 18:301, 1968.

Konigsmark BW: Hereditary deafness in man. *N Engl J Med* 281:731, 1969.

Ruben RJ, Rozycki DL: Clinical aspects of genetic deafness. *Ann Otol Rhinol Laryngol* 80:255, 1971.

Middle and Outer Ear Disorders

2

ACUTE OTITIS MEDIA WITH EFFUSION (SUPPURATIVE OTITIS MEDIA)

Definition

Purulent infection in the middle ear is designated acute otitis media with effusion.

Epidemiology

Approximately one-third of a practicing pediatrician's time is devoted to otitis media. When purulent fluid is in the middle ear, the disorder is considered to be suppurative. For reasons that are not clear, purulent otitis media is especially prevalent among Inuit and Indian children, and Australian aboriginals.

Natural History

Infection in the middle ear is a complication of upper respiratory tract inflammation. Occlusion of the eustachian tube by adenoidal enlargement or chronic inflammation favors effusion and infection in the middle ear. In some instances, otitis is a complication of sinusitis in which purulent material may enter the eustachian tube during forceful nose blowing. Traumatic perforations of the tympanic membrane permit direct entry of pathogenic organisms.

Bacteria are thought to be responsible for 80–85% of episodes of suppurative otitis media. The most common organisms are *Streptococcus pneumoniae, Haemophilus influenzae,* or β-hemolytic streptococci. In young children noninvasive *H. influenzae* are most commonly found. In the first 6 weeks of life, Shurin et al (1978) reported *S. pneumoniae, Neisseria catarrhalis, H. influenzae, Enterobacteriaceae,* and *Staphylococcus aureus* as most commonly recovered bacteria, but noted that in 43% of infants, no pathogenic bacteria were recovered.

Antecedent upper respiratory infection is followed after about a week by temperature elevation, pain in the ear, decreased feeding, and occasionally vomiting and diarrhea.

Diagnosis

Pneumatic otoscopy is the mainstay of diagnosis of middle ear effusion. The tympanic membrane is thickened and dull, landmarks are lost, and occasionally it bulges outward. Mobility is decreased. The membrane may be red but redness alone is not diagnostic of infection or effusion, inasmuch as it may be associated with elevated temperature or even vigorous crying (Fig. 19.2*A* and *B*).

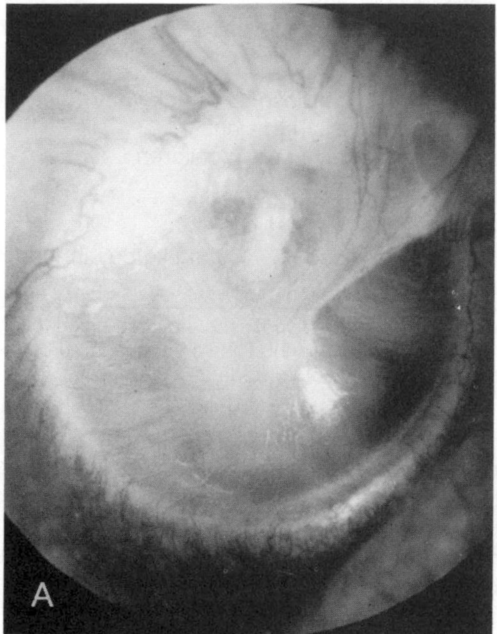

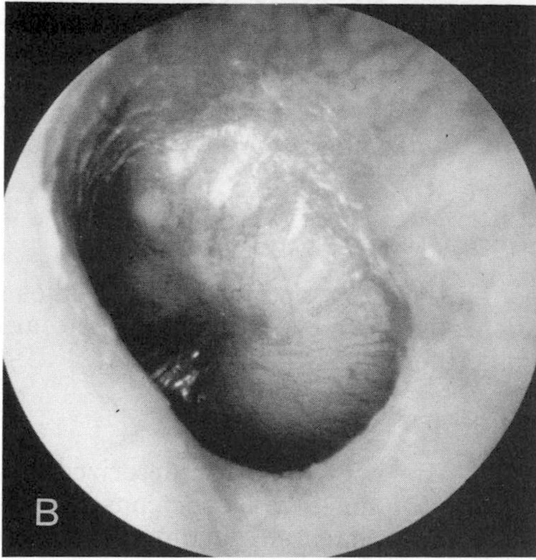

Figure 19.2. A. Normal tympanic membrane (right ear); note the landmarks with the handle of the malleus clearly outlined. The light reflex is sharply outlined. *B.* Bulging and injected tympanic membrane (left ear) with loss of landmarks and blurred light reflex. (Courtesy of Dr. G. Healy.)

Tympanometry has the advantage of providing an objective record of compliance of the tympanic membrane and is often used to confirm otoscopic findings.

If culture is required, as in situations in which otitis developed while the infant was being treated with antibiotics for other reasons, or if the drum is bulging, tympanocentesis is appropriate. After the external canal is cleansed with an organic iodine solution or alcohol, the infant or child should be restrained and an 18 gauge spinal needle should be inserted through the inferior part of the membrane to aspirate material for culture.

Treatment

The initial drug is usually oral amoxicillin 50–100 mg/kg/day in three or four divided doses for 2 weeks. The dose for newborn infants is 30–40 mg/kg/day. In areas where β-lactamase-producing strains of *Haemophilus* are prevalent, erythromycin-sulfonamide or amoxicillin/clavulanate potassium is preferable. If purulent material is obtained by myringotomy or from the deep portion of the external canal, Gram stain, culture, sensitivities, and appropriate choice of antibiotic can be based on the results. If the infant is allergic to penicillin, trimethoprim sulfamethoxazole can be used.

Prevention

Immunization with *H. influenzae* polysaccharide may reduce the incidence of otitis media with that organism. In general, adequate nutrition and good oral hygiene are associated with less otitis media. Reduction in exposure to upper respiratory tract infection would be helpful although, admittedly, this is impractical in childhood.

Holding the infant during feeding, rather than giving him a bottle when he is lying down has been found to be helpful.

In otitis-prone children, chemoprophylaxis with amoxicillin at 10 mg/kg twice a day (or 20 mg/kg at bedtime), or sulfasoxazole 25 mg/kg twice a day is appropriate during the season when respiratory diseases are at their height. If otitis occurs while the child is on prophylaxis, some physicians recommend use of tympanostomy tubes (Gebhart, 1981; see pp. 1180 for controversy about tubes.) Chemoprophylaxis is also indicated in children who are immunodeficient and prone to recurrent otitis media.

CASE ILLUSTRATION

An infant of 6 weeks had a temperature of 38.5°C, was irritable, anorectic, and had watery stools. On examination a red bulging immobile right ear drum was found. The rest of the examination was unremarkable.

QUESTIONS AND COMMENTS

Should a myringotomy be performed?

The answers are unclear. When tympanocentesis was carried out in a group of infants under 6 weeks of age, coliform organisms were found in 18%, no pathogens were found in 39%, and common upper respiratory tract organisms were identified in the remainder. More importantly, other illnesses were often found, including pneumonia, meningitis, conjunctivitis, and omphalitis (Tetzlaff et al, 1977). We recommend blood culture and a trial of antibiotics before tympanocentesis. Hospitalization may be desirable depending on how severely the infant is affected and whether intravenous fluids are needed: only if the fever and otitis persist would we perform a myringotomy. If coliform organisms are predominant on smear, intravenous aminoglycosides should be given.

If a child is febrile and crying, can a red tympanic membrane be present without underlying infection?

We think so, as we have seen red dull tympanic membranes, without loss of landmarks, return to normal overnight without treatment. Nevertheless, systematic documentation of the appearance of the membrane is required for a definitive answer probably with tympanocentesis. Even then variations in observer diagnostic rates could obscure the issue (Thibodeau and Berwick, 1980).

What are the criteria for chemoprophylaxis?

Again, we are unaware of relevant studies on this point. Persistent and recurrent episodes may be confused. If, however, a child has persistent symptoms or more than three episodes within 16 weeks, we would consider further work-up. Chronic adenoiditis, sinusitis, mastoiditis, or underlying immune deficiencies should be ruled out before initiating chemoprophylaxis.

Are oral decongestants of value during an acute episode to clear edema in the eustachian tube orifice?

The use of antihistamines does not reduce the incidence of acute otitis media with effusion (Cantekin et al, 1983).

CHRONIC OTITIS MEDIA WITH EFFUSION (SEROUS OR SECRETORY OTITIS MEDIA)

Definition

Chronic otitis media with effusion is a secretory condition in the middle ear chamber.

Epidemiology

Residual effusion of some degree follows acute otitis in nearly half the cases. Spontaneous resolution by 2 months is the rule. Persistent serous or mucoid otitis media occurs in 90% of children with cleft palate and in increased incidence in cystic fibrosis and Down syndrome.

Natural History

Persistent fluid in the ear, which may promote recurrent infection, is usually the result of poor ventilation through the eustachian tube. Forceful nose blowing, and aspiration of milk when an infant is fed in a supine position have been incriminated in the pathogenesis of chronic recurrent ear infections.

The mean duration of effusion in the study of Gates (1987) was 27–51 weeks depending on the intervention.

Diagnosis

Painless hearing loss of 15–30 dB is the cardinal symptom. The tympanic membrane is dull and retracted, with reduced mobility. Air bubbles may be visualized as the condition is improving.

Conductive hearing loss is present, often more on one side. Impedance or acoustic tympanometry is useful to measure mobility of the tympanic membrane, but pneumatic otoscopy is often adequate (Teele and Teele, 1984). A tuning fork (256 cps) on the forehead will be best heard in the affected ear (Weber test).

Treatment

In the past, repeated courses of decongestants were prescribed, with no clear benefit. Oral decongestants and antihistamines have not been shown to be effective in controlled trials (1983). Viable bacteria may be present in what was traditionally considered as sterile fluid. Antimicrobial therapy has been found to be effective. In a study of children between ages 2 and 5 years with otitis media with effusion present for longer than 6 weeks, Healy reported an improved outcome when trimethoprim sulfamethoxazole (8 and 40 mg/kg/day) were given in two divided doses daily for 4 weeks (Healy, 1984). Referral to an otolaryngologist often led to a recommendation for adenoidectomy. Because the condition is self-limited, some support for these interventions seemed inevitable.

CONTROVERSY

In the early 1950s surgery to insert drainage tubes in the middle ear was advocated and subsequently was widely accepted. It is estimated now that almost one million children per year in the United States have tubes or grommets placed in their ears to lessen likelihood of cholesteatoma and hearing loss. The tubes are usually extruded spontaneously 6–12 months after insertion.

Controlled studies of unilateral tube placement in children with bilateral otitis have now shown no lasting benefit from insertion of the tube; nor was there improvement from including adenoidectomy. However, Gates et al (1987) reported a 47% reduction in time with recurrent effusion in patients who had an adenoidectomy and placement of tympanostomy tubes compared with myringotomy alone. The largest treatment differences were in the first year of the prospective study. The study included children 4–8 years. In the series described by Brown et al (1978), some thickening of the tympanic membrane 5 years later was observed, apparently resulting from presence of the tube.

Because evidence for long-term benefit of drainage tubes is lacking, the question remains whether there is any short-term benefit. Teele et al (1984) followed 205 children with middle ear effusions. This cohort, followed from birth, could be examined at age 3 years with standardized tests of speech and language. These children who had had prolonged periods of middle ear effusion, especially in the first 6–12 months of life, had poorer scores than those without a history of middle ear disease. Hearing loss with effusion has been well documented; these studies suggest it is sufficient to interfere with the timing of acquisition of language. Nevertheless, there is not sufficient evidence to determine if such children catch up or remain language deficient.

In children with repaired palatal clefts chronic otitis media with effusion is unremitting. Hubbard et al (1985) reported that, at age 30 months, verbal performance, IQ tests, and psychosocial indices were normal with or without early placement of tympanostomy tubes.

Current criteria at The Children's Hospital, Boston, for placement of ear tubes are: (1) conductive hearing loss of greater than 15 dB present for more than 12 weeks with persisting effusion, (2) high negative pressure (retraction of tympanic membrane), and (3) recurrent episodes of acute otitis media with effusion unresponsive to antimicrobial therapy.

CHRONIC SUPPURATIVE OTITIS MEDIA

Definition

Chronic inflammation of the middle ear and mastoid with perforated tympanic membrane with or without cholesteatoma is defined as chronic suppurative otitis media. In general, chronic refers to otorrhea for over 6 weeks.

Epidemiology

This complication of otitis media can occur at any age in childhood, although it is uncommon.

Natural History

Persistent otorrhea through a perforation of the tympanic membrane or a tympanostomy tube can occur with secondary infection. *Pseudomonas* is most common, and *Staphylococcus aureus* and diphtheroids are often present. Twenty-three species of microorganisms were isolated from ears of 36 children by Kenna and Bluestone (1986).

Diagnosis

The diagnosis is established when suppuration persists in children with otitis. Culture of the exudate with sensitivity determination to antibiotics is required to guide therapy.

Treatment

Several weeks of optimal antibiotic therapy is often effective. If cholesteatoma is present, surgical excision is needed.

COMPLICATIONS OF OTITIS MEDIA—MASTOIDITIS

Definition

Mastoiditis is an inflammation of the lining of the air cells within the mastoid complex.

Epidemiology

The disorder is so unusual since the advent and wide use of antibiotics that it may be overlooked and diagnosis may be delayed. Thus, there are no satisfactory current figures for incidence. The disorder is unusual before age 2 years when air cells first begin to develop in the mastoid bone.

Natural History

The infection is almost always a complication of acute purulent otitis media. Infection of the mastoid can lead to abscess formation with rupture into the meninges; thus, there is about a 10% risk of meningitis being a complication of mastoiditis. Sometimes, in the face of dehydration and mastoiditis, dural sinus thrombosis can occur. There can also be an extension of infection to the petrous ridge of the temporal bone. The organisms most commonly associated are *S. pneumoniae, S. pyogenes,* and *S. aureus* and less commonly, *Pseudomonas* and mycobacteria.

Diagnosis

The patient usually has had recent acute purulent otitis media and then complains of postauricular pain and has an increase in temperature. The mastoid area is often tender and sometimes fluctuant; occasionally, the skin is indurated and red. As the infection spreads, there can be sufficient postauricular swelling to move the pinna forward.

The diagnosis is a clinical one but it can be confirmed by radiographic evidence of diffuse clouding of the mastoid cells. In the late stages true osteomyelitis may develop, with destruction of the bone and resorption of the mastoid air cells.

Treatment

Initial treatment consists of administration of high doses of intravenous antibiotics to cover a wide spectrum of organisms. If, however, there is an extensive infection, immediate surgery to drain the infected area is appropriate. The condition should be treated as an osteomyelitis and oral antibiotics should be continued for 4–6 weeks after the acute symptoms have resolved.

CASE ILLUSTRATION

A 13-year-old boy had a 3-week history of left otitis media and pharyngitis treated with courses of antibiotics. He remained symptomatic and complained of pain in his ear, vomiting, and a stiff neck.

On presentation he was delirious, with a temperature of 39°C. The left tympanic membrane was bulging and there was some left mastoid tenderness. A tympanocentesis produced purulent fluid, but no organisms were identified on Gram stain. A lumbar puncture showed 900 white blood cells, 87% lymphocytes, glucose 60, protein 66, and also a negative Gram stain. Ampicillin and chloramphenicol were instituted, based on a presumptive diagnosis of partially treated meningitis. On the second hospital day, he developed a left lateral gaze nystagmus and a CT scan was performed. Opacification of the mastoid air cells on the left was demonstrated adjacent to a posterior fossa brain abscess. Upon aspiration of pus from the abscess, the patient improved. That material was also Gram-stain negative. He recovered completely after 6 weeks on intravenous antibiotics.

QUESTIONS AND COMMENTS

What should have alerted the physicians to the possibility of mastoiditis or brain abscess?

In retrospect, an otitis would be unlikely to persist for 3 weeks with several courses of antibiotics unless there was an infected focus inaccessible to antibiotics. The most common focus would be the mastoid. Antibiotics presumably had some effect inasmuch as no organisms were cultured either from the middle ear or from the spinal fluid in this youngster.

Would radiographs of the sinus and mastoid have been of value in this instance?

Presumably, the diagnosis of mastoiditis might have been made with plain radiographs of the mastoid at an earlier stage. By the time the child was admitted to the hospital with cells in the spinal fluid, a CT scan was mandatory to rule out the possibility of abscess or dural sinus thrombosis. In this case, therefore, mastoid radiographs would have been redundant because they would have confirmed the mastoiditis, but might not have aroused suspicion as to the brain abscess.

Do you have any criticism of the management of this patient?

In retrospect, the CT scan should have been done before the lumbar puncture because, if abscess was a possibility, increased intracranial pressure could have produced herniation of the medulla.

BAROTITIS

Definition

Barotitis is defined as pain in the middle ear from sudden changes in barometric pressure. An acute serous effusion can occur and persist for several days.

Epidemiology

The symptoms are produced by an increase in pressure in the oropharynx relative to that in the middle ear as caused by sudden changes in pressure, such as in an airplane or even by rapid descent in an elevator. Thus, the incidence of this disorder is very high.

Natural History

Any condition that narrows the eustachian tube predisposes to poor communication between middle ear and oropharynx. Thus, a mild upper respiratory infection is commonly present in symptomatic individuals.

Diagnosis

The sudden onset of pain in the middle ear under conditions where there are sudden changes in pressure confirms the diagnosis. Serous effusion and a hemorrhagic tympanic membrane may be seen by otoscopy.

Prevention and Treatment

Swallowing and yawning are time honored means of prevention and treatment. Use of a nasal inhaler to provide immediate decongestion is helpful in the presence of an upper respiratory infection.

CHOLESTEATOMA

Definition

Cholesteatomas (or keratoma) are congenital or acquired accumulations of keratin surrounded by connective tissue. They may occur in the middle ear, within layers of tympanic membrane, or in the mastoid. They may enlarge and erode middle ear or intracranial structures even though they are histologically benign.

Epidemiology

According to the studies of Schwartz et al (1984), congenital cholesteatomas occur most commonly in young children, mean age 4.7 years. The incidence is unknown. Acquired cholesteatoma, secondary to chronic middle ear disease, may occur at any age.

Natural History

The etiology is not always clear. Some cholesteatomas result from "epithelial rests" in the middle ear cleft. Intramembranous collections of epithelial cells may appear as pearl-like cysts behind an intact tympanic membrane. They are often seen in association with recurrent otitis media, although it is not clear whether they are the consequence of it. In a survey by Schwartz et al (1984) of 35 membranous cholesteatomas in 34 children, six of these children had no documented prior otitis media.

Acquired cholesteatomas are the result of epithelial debris trapped in the middle ear space. They are thought to be the consequence of chronic eustachian tube dysfunction. The resultant negative pressure injures the retracted tympanic membrane which sloughs squamous epithelium. Cholesteatomas may follow chronic perforation of the tympanic membrane.

Diagnosis

Improved recognition of this condition depends on greater use of pneumotoscopy with an airtight halogen-illuminated otoscope. A white or yellowish mass can be seen behind the translucent tympanic membrane, or a pearl white cyst may be evident in the membrane. Careful examination of the entire ear drum, with special attention to the posterior-superior quadrant should be a part of the examination of every child.

Chronic recurrent otorrhea or brownish crusting around a tympanic membrane should alert the examiner to this condition. CT scans of the temporal bone may reveal otherwise undetected lesions. Hearing may be normal or decreased.

Treatment

In both congenital and acquired cholesteatomas, excision is necessary. Recurrences of intramembranous lesions are rare. Complete resection of lesions in the middle ear may be difficult, however, in which case the cholesteatoma may recur.

OTITIS EXTERNA

Definition

Otitis externa is an inflammation of the lining of the external ear canals.

Epidemiology and Natural History

The most common cause of otitis externa is the accumulation of water in the ear of swimmers, hence the appellation "swimmer's ear." Swimmers in fresh water are particularly prone to this disorder. The patient presents with exquisite pain in the ear, sometimes accompanied by itching. The most modest amount of pressure on the tragus can elicit severe pain. The ear canal is grossly swollen and usually squamous debris is present. There may also be some compromise of hearing.

Otitis externa may also occur in association with generalized eczema, which can involve the ear canal as well as the external ear. Sometimes this becomes secondarily infected and can be confused with purulent otitis media and both conditions may be present as is commonly the case in patients with histiocytosis X. Superinfections with *S. aureus* or *P. aeruginosa* are common under these circumstances.

Finally, otitis externa can result from trauma associated with inept attempts to remove wax from the ear or the use of poorly fitted ear plugs in swimming.

Diagnosis

The diagnosis is made on inspection, particularly if the patient has been swimming or has an injury to the external canal. The hallmark is extreme pain when the pinna is retracted, in association with an inflamed ear canal which is frequently filled with squamous debris.

Treatment

Gentle rinsing with a weak acetic acid solution or warm half-strength white vinegar can remove external debris. Hydrocortisone drops (1%) further reduce the swelling and allow penetration of a local antibiotic, such as neomycin and polymyxin. Cortisporin, an antibiotic-corticosteroid mixture, given three times a day is effective against most of the contaminating bacteria.

Prevention

Those children who seem predisposed to the problem may have some relief from instillation of 2–3 drops of a 1:1 mixture of white vinegar and 70% ethyl alcohol into their ears before and after swimming. The mixture is hygroscopic and keeps the canal dry.

REFERENCES

Bluestone C, Stool S: *Pediatric Otolaryngology*. Philadelphia, WB Saunders, 1983.

Brown M, Richards SH: Grommets and glue ear: A five year follow-up of a controlled trial. *J Ray Soc Med* 71:353, 1978.

Cantekin EI, Mandel EM, Bluestone CD, et al: Lack of efficacy of a decongestant-antihistamine combination for otitis media with effusion "secretory" otitis media in children. *N Engl J Med* 308:297, 1983.

English GM: Choosing the right therapy for acute otitis media. *J Respir Dis* 6:93, 1985.

Gates GA, Avery CA, Prihoda TJ, et al: Effectiveness of adenoidectomy and tympanostomy tubes in the treatment of chronic otitis media. *N Engl J Med* 317:1444, 1987.

Gebhart DE: Tympanostomy tubes in the otitis prone child. *Laryngoscope* 91:849, 1981.

Hawkins DB, et al: Acute mastoiditis in children: A review of 54 cases. *Laryngoscope* 93:568, 1983.

Healy GB: Antimicrobial therapy of chronic otitis media with effusion. *Int J Pediatr Otorhinolaryngol* 8:13, 1984.

Healy GB, Friedman J, DiTroia J: Ataxia and hearing loss secondary to perilymphatic fistula. *Pediatrics* 61:238, 1978.

Healy GB, Smith HG: Current concepts in the management of otitis media with effusion. *Am J Otolaryngol* 2:138, 1981.

Healy GB, Teele DW: The microbiology of middle ear effusions in children. *Laryngoscope* 87:1472, 1977.

Hubbard TW, Paradise JL, McWilliams BJ, et al: Consequences of unremitting middle ear disease in early life. *N Engl J Med* 312:1529, 1985.

Kenna MA, Bluestone CD: Microbiology of chronic suppurative otitis media in children. *Pediatr Infect Dis* 5:223, 1986.

Lampe RM, Weir MR, Spier J, et al: Acoustic reflectometry in the detection of audible ear effusion. *Pediatrics* 76:75, 1985.

Manning P, Avery ME, Ross A: Purulent otitis media: Differences between populations in different environments. *Pediatrics* 53:135, 1974.

Marcy SM: Prevention of respiratory infections. *Pediatr Infect Dis* 4:442, 1985.

McCracken GH: Selection of antimicrobial agents for treatment of acute otitis media with effusion. *Pediatr Infect Dis J* 6:985, 1987.

Paradise JL, Rogers KD: On otitis media, child development, and tympanostomy tubes: New answers or old questions. *Pediatrics* 77:88, 1986

Perrin JM, Charney E, MacWhinney JD, et al: Sulfisoxazole as chemoprophylaxis for recurrent otitis media: A double-blind crossover study in pediatric practice. *N Engl J Med* 291:664, 1974.

Schmitt BD, Berman S: Ear, nose and throat. In Kempe H, Silver H, O'Brien D (eds): *Current Pediatric Diagnosis and Treatment*, 8th edition. Los Altos, CA, Lange Medical Publications, 1984.

Schwartz RH, Grundfast KM, Feldman B, et al: Cholesteatoma medial to an intact tympanic membrane in 34 young children. *Pediatrics* 74:236, 1984.

Schwartz RH, Puglise J, Rodriguez, WJ: Sulphamethoxazole prophylaxis in the otitis-prone child. *Arch Dis Child* 57:590, 1982.

Shurin PA, Howie VM, Pelton SI, et al: Bacterial etiology of otitis media during the first six weeks of life. *J Pediatr* 92:893, 1978.

Stickler GB: The attack on the tympanic membrane. *Pediatrics* 74:291, 1984.

Teele DW, Teele J: Detection of middle ear effusion by acoustic reflectometry. *J Pediatr* 104:832, 1984.

Teele DW, Klein JO, Rosner BA: Otitis media with effusion during the first three years of life and development of speech and language. *Pediatrics* 74:282, 1984.

Tetzlaff TR, Ashworth C, Nelson JD: Otitis media in children less than 12 weeks of age. *Pediatrics* 59:827, 1977.

Thibodeau LA, Berwick DM: Variation in rates of diagnosis of acute otitis media. *J Med Educ* 55:1021, 1980.

Venezio FR, et al: Complications of mastoiditis with special emphasis on venus sinus thrombosis. *J Pediatr* 101:509, 1982.

Nose and Sinus Disorders

3

EPISTAXIS

Definition

Except for infants, bleeding from the nose is a universal experience from trauma, infection, bleeding disorders, or vascular malformations or tumors.

Epidemiology

Because the nose is a very vascular structure, almost every child has had isolated nose bleeds. Recurrent nosebleeds are less common, but incidence is not known.

Natural History

The anterior part of the nasal septum (Kiesselbach area) is very vascular and prone to bleed from minor trauma such as picking the nose, or even forceful blowing, especially if infection is present.

Associated problems that may aggravate epistaxis are allergic nasal mucosa or telangiectasis in the anterior septum.

Bleeding disorders may present with nosebleeds that persist in spite of packing. Excessive or prolonged epistaxis is characteristic of hemophilia, von Willebrand disease, or any condition in which thrombocytopenia is common, such as leukemia.

Aspirin, even in usual doses, can interfere with platelet aggregation and prolong bleeding.

Rarely, tumors of the nasopharynx, such as angiofibroma may present with bleeding, more often into the pharynx than through the nose. The lesion is most frequent in adolescent males.

Treatment

For mild nosebleeds, the nose should be pinched for about 10 minutes, with the patient leaning forward to prevent swallowing blood. Gentle blowing to remove clots may help, and 0.25% Neo-Synephrine on a pledget inserted into the nostril will produce vasoconstriction. In unusual cases, referral to an otolaryngologist for a posterior pack is appropriate.

OBSTRUCTIVE INFLAMMATION—ALLERGIC RHINITIS

Definition

Chronic or episodic inflammation of the nasal mucosa can lead to watery discharge and nasal obstruction, a condition defined as allergic rhinitis.

Basic Science

Allergic rhinitis is an overreaction of a normal defense against inhalation of irritants. It is associated with eosinophilia in the peripheral blood and nasal secretions, and immunoglobulin E levels are elevated. It is often associated with other manifestations of atopy, such as eczema in infancy.

Natural History

Allergic rhinitis is common in childhood and is characterized by itching and paroxysmal sneezing, as well as a watery discharge. It may be seasonal or year round. Often, the intraorbital area in affected children appears sunken and dark. The condition may be aggravated by excessive use of nasal vasoconstrictors.

Diagnosis

Eosinophil counts in nasal secretions and blood are helpful, but levels are not always increased. Serum IgE may be elevated many fold. RAST tests (radioallergosorbent) are often positive for dust and grasses.

The condition should be distinguished from rhinorrhea of CSF, in that there is clear discharge in the absence of allergic manifestations such as itching or sneezing. The diagnosis is confirmed by measuring glucose in the nasal discharge. It is higher in spinal fluid than in nasal discharge.

Treatment

Use of topical steroid nasal sprays and avoidance of known allergens and cigarette smoke are the first lines of treatment. Some success has been reported with cromolyn sodium (4% solution) (Cohan et al, 1976). A new antihistamine, terfenadine, is under study for individuals over age 12 years. Preliminary reports describe efficacy with fewer side effects, such as sedation (FDA Drug Bulletin, 1985).

CHOANAL ATRESIA

Definition

Choanal atresia, the most common form of nasal obstruction in the newborn, is the result of unilateral or bilateral membranous or bony obstruction in the posterior nares.

Basic Science

The obstruction is most often a bony plate but may be a thin membrane. It has a multifactorial inheritance pattern, with the risk of recurrence about 5%. The condition is thought to result from a defect in the nasal-palatal processes that disturbs the movement of embyronic neural crest cells to the nasal region (Hengerer and Strome, 1982). Associated malformations include Treacher-Collins syndrome, palatal abnormalities, colobomas, tracheoesophageal fistula, and congenital heart disease (Hall, 1979).

Epidemiology

The condition is unilateral in about 20–40% of infants and, as such, it is seldom diagnosed in the newborn period. When bilateral, however, at least 75% of the infants have one other anomaly according to Kaplan (1985).

Natural History

With complete obstruction, the infant may be in severe respiratory distress at birth.

Choanal atresia may be part of the CHARGE association of anomalies, and this mnemonic may be helpful as a reminder of the other associated components: **C** = coloboma, **H** = heart disease, **A** = atresia choanae, **R** = retarded growth, and/or CNS problems, **G** = genital hypoplasia in males, **E** = malformations of pinnae and deafness.

According to Kaplan, who reviewed The Children's Hospital (Boston) experience with 41 patients, more than one-third had some postnatal growth retardation, 21% had structural heart disease, and 21% were deaf. Coloboma and blocked tear ducts were present in 10%.

Diagnosis

The inability to pass a catheter through the nares suggests the diagnosis. A few drops of methylene blue instilled into the nares can be seen in the pharynx if obstruction is not complete. A CT scan delineates the extent of the lesion.

Treatment

An oral airway should be secured as soon as nasal obstruction is suspected. Gavage feedings are necessary. If the bony obstruction is less than 1-mm thick, transnasal resection with the CO_2 laser is effective in the first hours of life. More dense bone requires a transpalatal approach to repair. The air passages will require stenting for a few weeks (Healy et al, 1978; Stahl and Jurkiewicz, 1985).

Prognosis

With prompt recognition, repair, and skillful nursing, the prognosis is excellent. The long-term outlook depends upon the severity of associated malformations.

DEVIATED SEPTUM

Deviation of the nasal septum may be congenital and sometimes is associated with other malformations, such as cleft lip and palate. More commonly, the septum is deviated because of trauma and may obstruct a nasal passage. In the past, surgery was deferred until age 14 or 15 years when the bones of the face are fully formed. If obstruction is severe, surgical correction can be undertaken after the age of 3 years (Healy, 1986).

FOREIGN BODIES

Toddlers often explore body cavities, particularly the nose. Food, crayons, beads, stones, and a variety of other objects can be inserted far enough into the nose that they are not easily expelled by sneezing. In time, mucosal irritation and swelling follow and infection is not uncommon. Indeed, a foul-smelling purulent unilateral nasal discharge should suggest the presence of a foreign body until proven otherwise.

The diagnosis can often be made on examination with a nasoscope or an otoscope. Usually, the object can be seen and removed under topical anesthesia. If the child does not cooperate, general anesthesia may be preferable to reduce the risk of aspiration.

REFERENCES

Cohan RH, Bloom FL, Rhoades RB, et al: Treatment of perennial allergic rhinitis with cromolyn sodium. *J Allergy Clin Immunol* 58:121, 1976.

Food and Drug Administration: Terfenadine approved for allergic rhinitis. *FDA Drug Bull* 15:20, 1985.

Hall BD: Choanal atresia and associated multiple anomalies. *Pediatrics* 95:395, 1979.

Healy G: An approach to the nasal septum in children. *Laryngoscope* 96:1239, 1986.

Healy G, McGill T, Jako GJ, et al: Management of choanal atresia with the carbon dioxide laser. *Ann Otol Rhinol Laryngol* 87:658, 1978.

Hengerer AS, Strome M: Choanal atresia. *J Laryngol Otol* 92:913, 1982.

Kaplan LC: Choanal atresia and its associated anomalies. Further support for the CHARGE association. *Int J Pediatr Otorhinolaryngol* 8:237, 1985.

Stahl RS, Jurkiewicz MJ: Congenital posterior choanal atresia. *Pediatrics* 76:429, 1985.

SINUSITIS

Definition

Sinusitis is an inflammation of the mucosal lining of the paranasal sinuses.

Basic Science

Only the ethmoid and maxillary sinuses are present at birth. The sphenoid sinuses remain underdeveloped until about 6 years of age and the frontal sinuses do not begin their development until after the second year of life, and become significant at age 5 or 6 years.

The maxillary and frontal sinuses communicate with the nose below the middle turbinates in the middle meatus. The sphenoid sinus and the posterior ethmoid sinus openings are below the superior turbinates. The sinuses are lined by ciliated columnar epithelium with many goblet cells. The cells are covered with mucus which is propelled by the cilia toward the respective openings in the turbinates.

The paranasal sinuses are analogous in some respects to the middle ear inasmuch as both communicate with the nasopharynx through small openings that are subject to occlusion by edema associated with upper respiratory infection. Likewise, the habit of forceful blowing of the nose tends to move infected material from the nose through the passageways into the sinuses or middle ear. (Sniffing has the opposite effect. Sniffing lowers pressure in the nasal cavities with respect to that in the sinuses and helps expel mucus from the sinuses.)

Epidemiology

The diagnosis of sinusitis is not always clear and, hence, incidence is not well known. In general, it is a complication of the common cold and seems to be more common in allergic children, those with chronic ear infections, and in patients with ciliary dysfunction, as well as cystic fibrosis.

Individuals with immune deficiency conditions are prone to sinusitis. A recently recognized subset of children with recurrent sinopulmonary infections have selective IgG subclass deficiencies (Umetsu et al, 1985). They were not identified by any clinically distinguishing features from other children with recurrent upper and lower respiratory tract infections. Twenty affected children were found on laboratory investigation of immunoglobulins among an allergy and chest clinic population of 2800 new patients seen over 3 years. Recognition of this syndrome is important because this group of patients will be improved by antibiotic prophylaxis and gammaglobulin replacement.

Sinusitis is also more common among individuals who spend a lot of time swimming, particularly in sea water or chlorinated pools with excessive diving, water can enter the sinuses and establish infection.

Natural History

The diagnosis of sinusitis is very difficult in young children where the involvement is most likely to be in the ethmoid and maxillary areas. There is usually an upper respiratory tract infection, followed by persistent nasal discharge which is frequently purulent. If fever occurs and nasal discharge persists, the possibility of sinusitis should be considered. Periorbital swelling is common.

In older children, the same sequence of events can occur, but frontal sinuses may be involved and headache is a more prominent complaint. Sinus tenderness is also more common in older children. Evidence of free purulent material in the pharynx suggests drainage from infected sinuses. The course of the disease depends on whether appropriate antibiotics have been prescribed during the illness. The most common organisms found in sinusitis in children include streptococci and *H. influenzae*; *S. aureus* ranks third as an etiological agent in sinusitis.

Diagnosis

The diagnosis of sinusitis depends primarily on clinical evaluation in children.

CONTROVERSY

The value of radiographs in diagnosis of sinusitis is disputed. One group concludes that radiographic examination of sinuses has little validity in children under 6 years of age, and is of limited value in the 6- to 14-year age group. In an extensive evaluation of radiographic changes and clinical symptoms, Shopfner and Rossi (1973) found sinus opacity present in 57% of children without symptoms of sinusitis or upper respiratory infection, and in 75% of children with upper respiratory infection but no fever, erythema, edema, or pain or tenderness over the sinuses. When clinical signs were present, the radiographs were abnormal but, as the authors noted, in those individuals the radiographs did not add anything of diagnostic or therapeutic importance. They further noted no difference in radiographic findings between children identified as having allergic sinusitis and asymptomatic children. Apparently most upper respiratory infections involve the sinus mucosa in children, but do not cause symptoms.

The study by Shopfner and Rossi has been criticized for lack of a correlation of clinical findings with radiographs and failure to include a normal population. Kovatch et al (1984) attempted to clarify the situation in a prospective evaluation of a group of children who had skull films for evaluation of problems unrelated to infection, such as trauma, skull growth, and craniosynostosis. They conducted an examination of the ears, nose, and throat and noted whether crying had occurred within 30 minutes of the radiographic examination. In this study of 112 children aged 5 days to 16 years, evidence of respiratory inflammation was found in 53% of them. They noted that, in children under 1 year of age, the radiographs did not correlate with physical findings (crying did not appear to cloud the sinuses). After 1 year of age, abnormal maxillary sinus radiographs were infrequent; between 1 and 16 years of age, only 7% of those without symptoms or physical findings had abnormal radiographs. Of those with symptoms and physical findings (14 children), four had normal films, eight were abnormal, and two had minor abnormalities. (Abnormal was defined as complete or partial opacification, or an air-fluid level, or 4 mm or greater of mucous membrane thickening.)

The lack of relationship between pneumatization of the maxillary sinus and symptoms in children was documented in 191 Nigerian children by Odita et al (1986).

The significance of these observations is that recommendations for therapy often depend on radiographic assessments. It is important to recognize the presence of false-positive and false-negative radiographic findings. Our view is that clinical symptoms of high fever and a purulent nasal discharge or protracted respiratory symptoms of cough for more than

10 days that is attributed to postnasal discharge is indication for a course of ampicillin, amoxicillin, or in areas with resistant *H. influenzae,* either amoxicillin/clavulanate potassium, trimethoprim-sulfamethoxazole, or erythromycin-sulfasoxale is appropriate until symptoms subside. We do not feel confident in interpreting the radiographic findings as a basis for therapy and, thus, seldom request studies in children under age 6 years. Exceptions, of course, occur when upper respiratory symptoms are severe and persistent in a younger age group or in the presence of retro-orbital abscess. Opacification of sinuses and fluid levels are probably indicative of infection and prompt us to treat for about 2 weeks or refer to an otolaryngologist to consider drainage.

Culture of secretions from the middle meatus of both nostrils is the best way to assess which bacteria are pathogenic.

Treatment

Antibiotics appropriate to cover *H. influenzae* and streptococci are the first line of treatment. The drug should be continued for a minimum of 2 weeks and, if there is no response, reculture is important. Nasal topical decongestants are often used. Severe pain or high fever is a mandate for consultation with an ear, nose, and throat specialist to have ENT consultation and consideration of antral puncture or culture.

Untreated sinusitis can extend to involve the meninges, the bone, and the cavernous sinus. Epidural, brain, and orbital abscesses have been described.

Prevention

It is useful to teach children not to blow their noses forcefully but to sniff and spit or swallow instead. If swimming appears to be a factor in promoting the condition, a change in swimming habits should be undertaken.

REFERENCES

Kovatch AL, Wald ER, Ledesma-Medina J, et al: Maxillary sinus radiographs in children with nonrespiratory complaints. *Pediatrics* 73:306, 1984.

Odita JC, Akamaguna AI, Ogisi FO, et al: Pneumatisation of the maxillary sinus in normal and symptomatic children. *Pediatr Radiol* 16:368, 1986.

Shopfner CE, Rossi JO: Roentgen evaluation of the paranasal sinuses in children. *AJR* 118:176, 1973.

Umetsu DT, Ambrosino DM, Quinti I, et al: Recurrent sinopulmonary infection and impaired antibody response to bacterial capsular polysaccharide antigen in children with selective IgG-subclass deficiency. *N Engl J Med* 313:1247, 1985.

Wald ER: Acute sinusitis in children. *Pediatr Infect Dis* 2:61, 1983.

Mouth, Face, and Pharynx Disorders 4

ORAL MUCOSA—APHTHOUS ULCERS

Definition

The most common lesions of the oral mucosa are aphthous ulcers or canker sores. These are recurrent minor ulcers with an erythematous rim. They occur in clusters.

Epidemiology

Aphthous ulcers have a nearly universal incidence.

Natural History

Although the cause is unknown, outbreaks of canker sores occur most commonly when an individual is under stress. The painful period lasts 3–4 days and the sores disappear by 7–10 days. The lesions are raised, usually red, but sometimes gray or white.

Diagnosis

Differentiation from herpes simplex and oral pemphigus may be difficult, except by observing the location of the lesions; aphthous stomatitis rarely occurs in the hard palate or gums which are the prime areas for oral herpes.

Treatment

No specific therapy exists. Sucking ice before eating is helpful, as is avoidance of acid foods.

HERPETIC STOMATITIS

The lesions of herpetic stomatitis (herpes I infection; see Section 7) are very similar to those of the recurrent aphthous ulcers. Infants and children with herpetic diseases, however, are likely to have high fevers, diffusely inflamed mucosa, painful cervical lymph nodes, and malaise. The lesions are usually found in the lips, but they may extend into the posterior pharynx.

Epidemiology

The most extensive study was conducted in Yugoslavia by Juretic (1966) on 3278 cases of primary oral herpes among nearly 19,000 children. In that study, 10–15% of all children had herpetic gingivostomatitis by age 9 years, with most cases between ages 2–3 years, and no cases in infants under 6 months.

Natural History

The incubation period averaged 6 days, with a range of 2–12 days. Although stomatitis is most common, keratitis can occur with type 1 infection. The prodromal period is characterized by itching, then the appearance of small vesicles on an erythematous base. Clusters of 0.5- to 1.5-cm lesions tend to coalesce. Healing usually starts after 3–5 days and is complete in 7–10 days.

Diagnosis

Tissue culture is the most sensitive and specific test. The results can be known within 24 hours, although with low titer they may take 7 days. The Tzanck test is a rapid method in which scrapings from the lesion are stained with Giemsa or Wright stain for the presence of multinucleated giant cells. Direct electron microscopy can reveal the organism, although it is not specific.

Treatment

Usually no antimicrobial therapy is required in this self-limited infection. Frequent sips of bland liquids to maintain hydration are important. With extensive involvement, intravenous hydration may be required.

Acyclovir is available for intravenous, topical and oral use, but no trials for therapy of primary oral herpes have been reported. Topical acyclovir for recurrent oral infections has been disappointing.

CLEFT LIP AND/OR PALATE

Definition

Cleft lip may be only a small notch on one side of the lip or a complete opening into the floor of the nasal cavity. Clefts are most frequent on the left side but may be bilateral and involve the alveolar ridge. Cleft palate may be an isolated lesion of the uvula or extend the length of the soft and hard palates. When associated with a cleft lip, the defect can extend into one or both nasal cavities.

Basic Science

The defects occur during the second month of pregnancy when the maxillary process normally fuses with the nasomedial process. The cause is unknown, although multifactional inheritance is clearly present. The risk of recurrence of cleft lip and palate in siblings is about 4% and recurrence of cleft lip alone is about 3%. Offspring of affected individuals have a 6.2% risk of cleft palate and a 3.5% risk of cleft lip and palate combined. Identical twins are both affected 20–60% of the time. Cleft lip with or without cleft palate is more common in males. Cleft palate alone is more frequently seen in females (Carter, 1969).

Epidemiology

About 1/800–1000 infants has either a cleft lip, cleft palate, or both. Thirty percent of all infants with clefts also have congenital heart disease. Other associated malformations include all forms of trisomy syndromes and spina bifida.

Diagnosis

The defects are evident at birth and should be described fully at the first physical examination. A careful search for other anomalies is always indicated.

Treatment

Initially, discussion with the family about the subsequent course of events should be undertaken with an experienced plastic surgeon. Pediatric concerns include provision of adequate nutrition with softened nipples with enlarged openings or gavage feedings. Surgical closure of the cleft lip is usually done as soon as the infant is stabilized and gaining weight (within the first month). Cleft palates are usually closed about 5–6 months. Later, correction of nasal deformities, occlusal problems, and midface alignment can be performed as needed.

Chronic serous otitis media is uniformly present in association with cleft palate and ventilation tubes are inserted at the time of closure of the lip.

Follow-up should include evaluation of speech and hearing and orthodontic management.

PALATAL GROOVES

Palatal grooves are depressions in the hard palate that result from prolonged orotracheal intubation in low birth weight infants. More than half of infants under 1000 g birth weight were found to have palatal grooves of more than 5 mm in depth by Molteni and Bumstead (1986). No relationship to the hardness of the tube was found, but the longer the intubation the more likely the lesion.

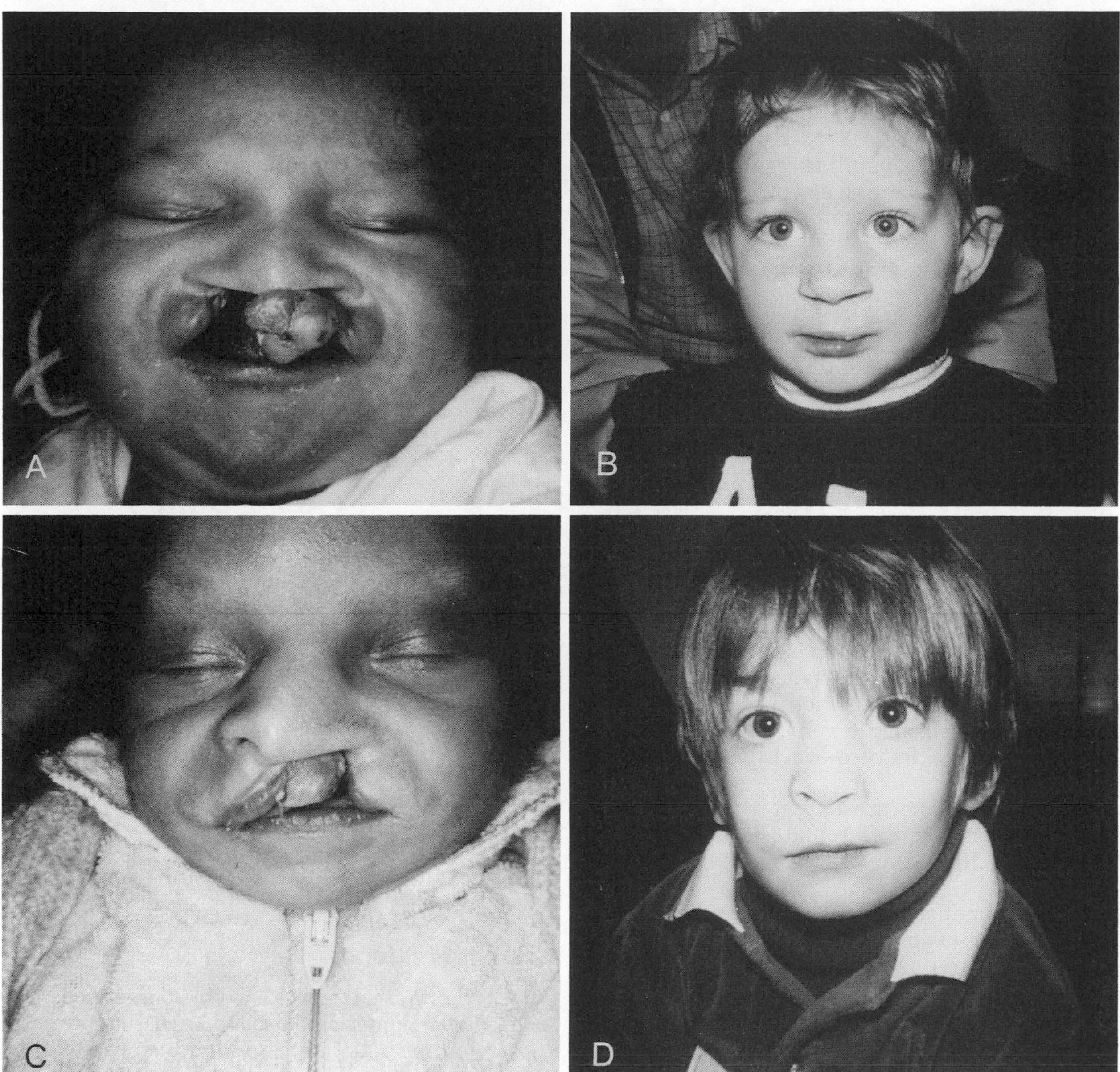

Figure 19.3. **A.** Bilateral cleft lip and palate, age 6 days. **B.** Status post staped lip repair and palate repair within the first year of life (age 2 years). **C.** Complete cleft of left lip and palate (11 days old). **D.** Status post cleft lip repair at 1 month and cleft palate repair at age 1 year. (Photograph at age 3 years). Photographs courtesy of Dr. George H. Gifford Jr.

TONGUE

Inspection of the tongue is a routine and important part of a complete physical examination.

Embryology

The tongue is first seen by the third week of gestation. The anterior portion is covered by ectoderm; the posterior portion by endoderm. At the junction of the two zones, an invagination becomes the thyroglossal duct.

Failure of migration of embryonic thyroid may leave thyroid follicles in the body of the tongue, or the gland itself at the base of the tongue (Santiago et al, 1985). Occasionally a nodule appears at the foramen cecum which may enlarge in adolescence.

MIGRATORY GLOSSITIS (GEOGRAPHIC TONGUE)

An unusual condition of unknown etiology is loss of papillae of the tongue in irregular areas. Sometimes these appear as red areas surrounded by a thin white margin. The lesions sometimes enlarge and coalesce, but eventually they heal spontaneously in weeks or months. They may recur in other sites. No treatment is required.

STRAWBERRY TONGUE (GLOSSITIS)

The filiform papillae are shed, leaving the fungiform papillae raised and reddened. This is characteristic of scarlet fever, but it can occur in other febrile illnesses.

Absence of fungiform papillae resulting in a tongue that appears homogeneous and smooth is characteristic of Riley-Day syndrome or dysatonomia.

MACROGLOSSIA

A tongue so large it will not fit into the oral cavity and prevents dental occlusion is designated as macroglossia. (Relative macroglossia is defined as a normal size tongue in an undersized oral cavity, as occurs in Pierre Robin syndrome or trisomy 21.)

All conditions associated with macroglossia are rare. Less than 100 cases of Beckwith-Wiedemann syndrome, one form of macroglossia, have been reported since the original description in 1964.

Beckwith-Wiedemann syndrome is characterized by macroglossia, exomphalos, hemibody hypertrophy, and islet cell hyperplasia. Polycythemia, mild microcephaly, renal medullary dysplasia, earlobe creases, and facial nevus flammeus are also observed.

Several conditions are clearly associated with macroglossia. One is advanced hypothyroidism in which the tongue is included in the generalized myxedema; macroglossia is also a feature of acromegaly (see pp. 828).

Macroglossia can be present in glycogen storage disease, amyloidosis, neurofibromatosis, and some parasitic infections. Rhabdomyosarcomas have been described.

The diagnosis depends on the presence of associated features. For example, of major significance in Beckwith-Wiedemann syndrome is the profound sustained hypoglycemia.

Other lesions that occur on the tongue are lipomas, cystic hygromas, papillomas and dermoid cysts, and lingual tonsils. Lingual thyroid can be distinguished from these other rare lesions by scintigraphy.

Treatment

Macroglossia may require surgical correction, which should be carried out in the first year of life, before speech develops. Rizer et al (1985) consider 7 months an appropriate age and discuss operative approaches.

TONGUE TIE

Definition

Tongue tie is a condition in which the maxillary labial frenulum is attached closely to the crest of the alveolar ridge.

Epidemiology

Less than 1% of frenulas that are labeled tongue tie cause any difficulty or require excision.

Natural History

All newborn infants have a relatively close attachment of the labial frenulum to the alveolar ridge that recedes as the primary teeth erupt. In a few infants, the frenulum seems unusually prominent and may cause a notch in the tip of the tongue (ankyloglossia); however, no difficulty in sucking or swallowing occurs.

Diagnosis and Treatment

No clear guidelines distinguish an abnormal frenulum from a normal one. If at 1–2 years of age, as speech develops, it appears that the tongue is not normally mobile, simple lysis of the frenulum can be undertaken.

FACIAL BONES
Caffey Disease (Infantile Cortical Hyperostosis)

Definition

Caffey disease is a swelling of the shafts of bones of infants usually under 6 months of age, with fever and irritability. The disease is benign and of unknown cause.

Epidemiology

This extraordinary condition was seen commonly in the 1950s, but has been seen less and less often ever since. Nonetheless, it still exists and has a characteristic age of predilection and presentation.

Natural History

The illness is apparently a spontaneous hyperplasia of the subperiosteal bone with some edema of the surrounding soft tissues. Mandibles are affected most frequently, followed by clavicles, scapulae, and ribs, but occasionally the long bone and even the metatarsals may be involved. Systemic signs include persistent fever, often as high as 40°C, and diminution of activity probably associated with pain. There is tenderness over the affected bone, and the infants are often miserable.

Laboratory findings reveal a leukocytosis and an elevated sedimentation rate, but no specific serological changes have been identified, nor have any microorganisms been found to be associated with this condition. The course is unpredictable, with exacerbations, remissions, and regression sometimes occurring within 1–2 months but, in other cases, taking place over several years. Corticosteroids have been found effective in relieving symptoms during exacerbation, but long-term corticosteroid therapy is ill advised.

Treatment

There is no specific treatment except for the use of corticosteroids during acute febrile episodes to provide some alleviation of symptoms. The importance of this disorder is to recognize its existence and not confuse it with more serious bone disorders such as tumors.

Prognosis

Once the disease has resolved, it does not recur.

TEMPOROMANDIBULAR JOINT DYSFUNCTION (TMJ SYNDROME)

Definition

The combination of subluxation and inflammation of the temporomandibular joint is known as temporomandibular joint dysfunction or TMJ syndrome and is an important cause of facial pain in children.

Basic Science

An asymmetry, malocclusion, or grinding of teeth can put unusual stress on the temporomandibular joints, with resulting pathology (Ahliu and Ko, 1985).

Epidemiology

The problem is most common in individuals with craniofacial disorders or malocclusion, but may also occur in stressful situations in which grinding of teeth occurs in sleep. It is probably underdiagnosed.

Natural History

Subjective clicking (what the child feels), snapping, or pain on opening the mouth are early signs of TMJ pathology. The disorder is likely to be progressive and to cause injury to condyles and, later, may cause partial or complete ankylosis. As a consequence of ankylosis the mandible fails to grow and there is progressive facial asymmetry (Dibbets et al, 1985).

Diagnosis

Preauricular or ear pain and tenderness over the joint are characteristic. Sometimes a click can be felt by the examiner as the bone slips when the mouth is opened or closed. CT scans of the joint are essential to evaluate bone damage.

Treatment

Consultation with an orthodontist and an oral surgeon with experience with this condition is essential. Realignment of the teeth may be sufficient, but some children will require surgical correction. Since as many as one-third of patients have primary psychopathology, including depression, eating disorders, anxiety, and conversion, psychiatric evaluation is appropriate (Belfer and Kaban, 1982).

HYPOPLASIA OF MANDIBLE

Definition

Bilateral hypoplasia of the mandible (Pierre Robin syndrome) is a congenital defect that tends to be less conspicuous with age. Less severe mandibular hypoplasia in association with other craniofacial abnormalities is seen in Treacher-Collins' syndrome.

Epidemiology

In a review of experience in Glasgow, Scotland, Dykes et al (1985) reported on 59 cases seen over 27 years, with an estimated incidence of 1/8500 live births.

Natural History

Infants with mandibular hypoplasia may be asymptomatic or have obstructed airways from the relative oversize of the tongue (micrognathia, glossoptosis, and respiratory obstruction). Feeding may be complicated by cleft palate which is present in 60% and is part of the Robin triad (micrognathia, glossoptosis, and cleft palate).

If airway obstruction is sufficient to raise carbon dioxide tensions, pulmonary hypertension can evolve. If recognized, intubation or tracheostomy provides immediate relief.

In time, growth of the mandible occurs and the problems become less severe. In general, infants who required intubation have been successfully extubated in 2–4 months.

Treatment

Expert nursing care is the key to treatment of these infants. The prevention of aspiration requires care with feedings. Various splints and other mechanical devices have had some successes but also some failures. Individualization is the key to successful attempts to achieve oral feeding without aspiration. Gavage feeding is, of course, an alternative, but should be accompanied by use of a pacifier for oral stimulation.

Prognosis

The mandible grows with the rest of the face, so that the profile is usually normal by 4–6 years.

MANDIBULAR DYSOSTOSIS (TREACHER-COLLINS SYNDROME)

Definition

This autosomal dominant constellation of malformations also occurs in a sporadic form (60%). The features are defective eyes, ears, and mandibles. One of the most characteristic features (present in 75%) is a notch at the junction of the outer and middle thirds of the lower eyelid. Ears may be malformed in many ways, and over one-third of infants have conductive deafness. High arched palate and choanal atresia may occur. Affected infants may hypoventilate and have cyanotic spells. Excessive mucus is common. Mental deficiency is not a feature of Treacher-Collins syndrome.

Treatment

Initially, feeding difficulties may be present and require a similar approach as that for Pierre Robin syndrome. Hearing testing and operative treatment of a stenotic auditory meatus may be appropriate. Later, plastic surgeons can often improve the child's general appearance.

GOLDENHAR SYNDROME

Diagnosis

The central features of this syndrome (also called oculoauriculovertebral syndrome) are malar hypoplasia, mandibular hypoplasia, incomplete external auricle often with conductive deafness and abnormalties in the atlas and cervical or thoracic vertebrae. Most cases are sporadic. Intelligence is usually normal; about 13% have IQs below 85.

Treatment

Hearing testing in early infancy is mandatory so hearing aids can be used if needed. Reconstructive surgery may be appropriate for the facial deformities.

DISEASES OF TONSILS AND ADENOIDS

Definition

Acute edema and erythema, and sometimes purulent exudates and abscesses may develop in the crypts of the adenoids (near the eustachian orifice of the nasopharynx) and the tonsils on the anterior fauces of the pharynx. Lymphoid tissue is distributed on the posterior pharyngeal wall and under the tongue, but not as masses of nodes with crypts such as compose the palatine adenoids and faucial tonsils.

Basic Science

Tonsils and adenoids are usually inapparent in early infancy, but gradually undergo hypertrophy and hyperplasia to reach their relatively greatest mass between 2 and 5 years. Their location is such that they are exposed to inspired air and food, and whatever antigens may be carried in either one. These tissues are part of the bursal system of immunity and consist mostly of B cells. Their contribution to acquired immunity must be considerable, although the relative proportion is not known. In severe combined immune deficiency syndrome, absence of lymphoid tissue and plasma cells is associated with profound depression of B- and T-cell function. In children who had tonsillectomy and adenoidectomy, the risk of bulbar polio was enhanced. These epidemiologic observations support the concept that pharyngeal lymphoid tissue acts as a local defense mechanism (Ogra, 1971).

Epidemiology

Inasmuch as criteria for enlarged or chronically infected tonsils and adenoids are not uniform, the incidence of a "pathologic condition" of these tissues is not known. The perception that tonsils and/or adenoids deserve removal can be assumed from the approximately 400,000 operations carried out in the United States each year.

Natural History

The anatomy and location of tonsils and adenoids are such that they are exposed to pathogens and their function is to entrap and neutralize them. Excessive exposure can lead to microabscesses in the crypts, with chronic or recurrent infection. The manifestations of infection can be a sore throat or peritonsillar abscess. Chronic infection of adenoids predisposes to otitis media. Enlargement of either lymphoid mass can cause obstruction of the upper airway.

Diagnosis

Chronic infection can present as anorexia, failure to gain weight, low grade fever or recurrent sore throats with high fever. Hypertrophy can be considerable and lead to mouth breathing, or even upper airway obstruction, CO_2 retention, sleep apnea, and rarely, cor pulmonale (Brouilette et al, 1984).

The question of how many episodes of tonsillitis are excessive is not settled. Paradise et al (1978) examined the reliability of histories of recurrent throat infections and concluded that undocumented histories do not forecast subsequent experience.

Persistent anterior and posterior cervical adenopathy in the absence of generalized lymphadenopathy is evidence of chronic or recurrent infection. Inspection of the tonsils is of limited help during an acute episode. Persistent enlargement with exudate in the crypts carries greater significance, especially when associated with hyperemia of the surrounding tissues.

Cultures of the surface of the tonsils are often misleading. Rosen et al (1977) compared surface cultures with cultures from the interior of tonsils obtained surgically. Pathogens differed between the two sites in 48% of cases.

Treatment

Courses of penicillin or amoxicillin are indicated for recurrent tonsillitis and adenoiditis. If these do not reduce the frequency or severity of episodes, consultation with an otolaryngologist is indicated.

SUGGESTED CRITERIA FOR TONSILLECTOMY/ ADENOIDECTOMY

Mandatory. Evidence of upper airway obstruction from hypertrophied tonsils mandates tonsillectomy/adenoidectomy.

Advisable. If the child is over age 5 years with at least five documented episodes of tonsillitis per year, the procedure is advisable. Other indications are:

Major sleep disturbances, apneic spells, snoring, restlessness (Lind and Lindell, 1982).
Difficulty swallowing.
Mouth breathing when awake from chronic nasal obstruction.
Anorexia, poor weight gain, low grade fevers, and cervical adenitis (with no other underlying cause).
Recurrent or persistent otitis (adenoidectomy).
Peritonsillar abscess.
Altered speech attributable to enlarged tonsils.
Biopsy for suspected tumor.

WHAT TONSILLECTOMY AND/OR ADENOIDECTOMY WILL NOT DO

The number of upper respiratory infections will not be reduced significantly, nor will nasal allergy be diminished. Mouth breathing and snoring may persist. No evidence supports the contention that tonsillectomy lessens recurrence of rheumatic fever.

Complications of Tonsillitis

Definition

Extension of tonsillar infection can take place in the surrounding tissues and is called peritonsillar abscess or quinsy. The retropharyngeal nodes drain both the adenoids and the nasopharynx and can become chronically infected. This is known as retropharyngeal abscess.

Epidemiology

These complications of tonsillitis are usually caused by beta hemolytic streptococci which are sensitive to penicillin. Consequently, the widespread use of antibiotics to treat streptococcal pharyngitis has been associated with less suppuration in the peritonsillar or retropharyngeal spaces.

Natural History

Peritonsillar cellulitis and abscess are characterized by an extremely sore throat and often high fever. If the condition is untreated, it may lead to significant swelling and even occlusion of the oral pharynx. The child may have trismus, dysphagia, and drooling.

Retropharyngeal abscess is virtually limited to infants in the first 2 years of life. The characteristic findings are fever, hyperextension of the neck, dysphagia, and noisy respirations. There is prominence of the infected pharyngeal wall but the swelling is almost always unilateral.

Diagnosis

The combinations of signs and symptoms of these infectious complications of tonsillitis and adenoiditis render the diagnosis obvious on physical examination. The prompt initiation of intravenous antibiotic therapy if the lesions are suppurative is necessary. In addition, an otolaryngologist should be consulted about possible aspiration or drainage of the abscess.

QUESTIONS AND COMMENTS

A child of 2½ years has enlarged tonsils and three documented streptococcal infections within the past 6 months. Is tonsillectomy indicated?

We recommend chemoprophylaxis for streptococcal infection for patients at this age. Rarely is tonsillectomy indicated or helpful before age 3 years except in cases of sleep apnea. Benefits in terms of a reduction in sore throat episodes is greatest in those over age 7 years (Paradise et al, 1984).

A child is scheduled for tonsillectomy and adenoidectomy and develops a sore throat and temperature of 38.5°C on the eve of the operation. What should be done?

The answer to the question remains controversial. Some surgeons will advise that, because they operate to drain abscesses, why not remove abscessed tonsils regardless of the presence of fever? Pediatricians may want to minimize any chance of extension of infection, and are more willing to postpone an elective procedure until the fever has subsided for 2–3 weeks. Some anesthesiologists avoid anesthesia in febrile infants because of a possible greater risk of laryngeal edema. Other considerations are the nuisance and expense of hospitalization and the anxiety engendered by delay.

We do not have the answers. Our pediatric practice is to treat with oral penicillin for 10 days, and reschedule the procedure in about 2 weeks.

Should tonsils and adenoids be removed in ambulatory surgical settings?

We are reluctant to take this procedure lightly. Even with careful preoperative attention to the general health of the child, including a history of bleeding tendencies, we sometimes encounter postoperative bleeding within the first 24 hours, and often administer intravenous fluids to children unwilling to swallow because their throats are sore. We continue to recommend admission the day of the procedure, and defer discharge until at least 24 hours after it.

What are possible complications of the operation?

Anesthetic risks in experienced hands are negligible. Hemorrhage may occur in the first postoperative hours, or 1 week later. Persistent sore throat and dysphagia may require intravenous fluids. The mean duration of postoperative sore throat is 5 days. Although the psychological impact of hospitalization can be distressing, it can be lessened by allowing a parent to "room-in" and by careful preparation of the child before operation. Full discussion of forthcoming events and their probable duration is appropriate at the level of the child's understanding.

Acute Cervical Adenoiditis

Definition

Acute cervical adenoiditis involves the lymph nodes that drain various regions of the head and neck.

Natural History

In young children, palpable anterior and posterior cervical nodes are normal, but usually they are small and moderately firm, often characterized as "shotty." Enlargement of a group of nodes with tenderness may follow an acute attack of tonsillitis or adenoiditis. If a single node or a group of nodes continues to grow and is associated with fever, it is likely to suppurate unless appropriate antibiotics are initiated early enough. The persistence of a large node or group of nodes after antibiotic therapy raises the possibility of a diverse group of conditions that should be considered. These include any of the following: infectious mononucleosis (although generalized lymphadenopathy would be more likely in that case); tularemia, which can present with cervical adenoiditis, if the patient has been in contact with wild rabbits; cat scratch fever, which is usually associated with a papule at the site of scratch with swollen and tender regional nodes; tuberculosis or one of the atypical mycobacteria disorders, which can present with enlarged cervical nodes. A tuberculin test is appropriate in any instance of persistent cervical adenopathy.

In the 1970s in Japan, an unusual form of lymphadenopathy with a characteristic pathology was described. Termed histiocytic necrotizing lymphadenitis (Kikuchi disease), subsequently it has been recognized in the United States with increasing frequency so that 30 cases (21 United States residents) were reported by Turner et al in 1983.

The disorder occurs most frequently in young women who have painless well-circumscribed cervical lymphadenophathy with or without fever. On biopsy, the nodes show histiocytes, macrophages, and cytotoxic suppressor T lymphocytes in the necrotic areas. Aggregates of large mononuclear cells have been described, with few neutrophils or plasma cells. The condition is benign, but has been misdiagnosed as malignant lymphoma.

Treatment

Penicillin is the antibiotic of choice and it should be given for 10 days to eliminate the most likely organisms (beta hemolytic streptococci). If the node is fluctuant, it should be incised and drained. If it is known to be tuberculous, total excision is preferable.

A persistent enlarging node should raise suspicion of malignancy. A thorough examination of the mucous membranes of the nasopharynx, thus, is required and consideration should also be given to the possibility that a cervical node is the first manifestation of leukemia or lymphoma.

REFERENCES

Ahliu JH, Ko CM: Functional disorders of the stomatognathic system. Part I. A review. *J Pedodont* 9:179, 1985.
Belfer ML, Kaban LB: Temporomandibular joint dysfunction with facial pain in children. *Pediatrics* 69:564, 1982.
Braham RL, Morris ME: *Textbook of Pediatric Dentistry,* 2nd edition. Baltimore, Williams & Wilkins, 1985.
Brouilette R, Hanson D, David R, et al: A diagnostic approach to suspected obstructive sleep apnea in children. *J Pediatr* 105:10, 1984.
Carter CO: Genetics of common disorders. *Br Med Bull* 25:52, 1969.
Dibbets J, Van der Weele L, Uildriks AK: Symptoms of TMJ dysfunction. Indicators of growth patterns? *J Pedodont* 9:265, 1985.
Dykes EH, Raine PAM, Arthur DS, et al: Pierre Robin syndrome and pulmonary hypertension. *J Pediatr Surg* 40:49, 1985.
Fraser FC: The genetics of cleft lip and cleft palate. *Am J Hum Genet* 22:336, 1970.
Handelman SL, Leverett DH, Iker HP: Longitudinal radiographic evaluation of the progress of caries under sealants. *J Pedodont* 9:119, 1985.
Jersaty RM: Pierre Robin syndrome. *Am J Dis Child* 117:710, 1969.
Juretic M: Natural history of herpetic infection. *Helv Paediatr Acta* 21:356, 1966.
Levin LS: Genetic disease in children. In Forrester DJ, Waggoner ML, Fleming J (eds): *Pediatric Dental Medicine.* Philadelphia, Lea & Febiger, 1981.
Lind MG, Lindell BPW: Tonsillar hyperplasia in children: a cause of obstructive sleep apneas, CO_2 retention, and retarded growth. *Arch Otolaryngol* 108:650, 1982.
Mellow DH, Richardson JE, Douglas DM: Goldenhar's syndrome—oculoauriculo-vertebral dysplasia. *Arch Dis Child* 48:537, 1973.
Molteni RA, Bumstead DH: Development and severity of palatal groove in orally intubated infants. *Am J Dis Child* 140:357, 1986.
O'Donnell JP, Cohen MM: Dental care for the institutionalized retarded individual. *J Pedodont* 9:3, 1985.
Ogra PL: Effect of tonsillectomy and adenoidectomy on nasopharyngeal antibody responses to poliovirus. *N Engl J Med* 284:59, 1971.
Paradise JL, Bluestone CD, Bachman RZ, et al: Efficacy of tonsillectomy for recurrent throat infections in severely affected children. *N Engl J Med* 310:674, 1984.
Paradise JL, Bluestone CD, Bachman RZ, et al: History of recurrent sore throat as an indication for tonsillectomy. Predictive limitations of histories that are undocumented. *N Engl J Med* 298:409, 1978.
Pillemer FG, Masek BJ, Kaban LB: Temporomandibular joint dysfunction and facial pain in children: An approach to diagnosis and treatment. *Pediatrics* 80:565, 1987.
Rizer FM, Schechter GL, Richardson MA: Macroglossia-etiologic considerations and management techniques. *Int J Pediatr Otorhinolaryngol* 8:225, 1985.
Rosen G, Samuel J, Vered I: Surface tonsillar microflora versus deep tonsillar microflora in recurrent acute tonsillitis. *J Laryngol Otol* 91:911, 1977.
Santiago W, Rybak LP, Bass RM: Thyroglossal duct cyst of the tongue. *J Otolaryngol* 14:4, 1985.
Smith DW: *Recognizable Patterns of Human Malformation.* 3rd edition. Philadelphia, WB Saunders, 1982.
Stool SE: Tonsillectomy and adenoidectomy: When they are warranted? *J Respir Dis* 6:11, 1985.
Turner RR, Martin J, Dorfman RF: Necrotizing lymphadenitis. A study of 30 cases. *Am J Surg Pathol* 7:115, 1983.

Upper Airway Disorders

5

APPROACH TO A CHILD WITH STRIDOR

Stridor or an audible inspiratory sound, sometimes called crowing respiration, is one of the most common clinical abnormalities among infants and children. The condition may arise from problems within or near the larynx, the trachea, or within the CNS.

Simple congenital laryngeal stridor is one of the most common findings in infants. In this condition, sometimes called laryngomalacia, persistent noisy inspirations are noted at birth or at least shortly thereafter (for example, the parent usually comments on the symptoms at the first monthly visit to the pediatrician). The diagnosis is suggested when the sound is altered by change of position and is usually intensified when the infant is supine. The reason for the stridor has been convincingly demonstrated radiographically by Dunbar who showed that when the infant was in the supine position, horizontal beam lateral views of the neck showed anterior-inferior displacement and vibration of the aryepiglottic folds on inspiration (Dunbar, 1970). Simple congenital laryngeal stridor usually disappears between 16 and 18 months of age and requires no treatment. In one follow-up study, it had resolved in all patients by age 4 years, although limitation to inspiratory airflow was detectable on flow-volume studies at 8–16 years of age (Macfarlane et al, 1985).

Other problems that are more serious are also fortunately less common. For example, laryngeal webs which are usually glottic in location can cause an obstruction at the level of the true cords. This is manifest as difficult inspiration with the first breath, and if it is not recognized on laryngoscopy and treated immediately, obstruction and death can follow. Recognition of this problem and perforation of an obstructing web can be lifesaving.

Laryngoceles, which may arise from the branchial arches located within the mucous lining of the larynx, may also represent an important cause of obstruction.

Extrinsic obstruction of the upper airway, anomalies of the great vessels, particularly a right aortic arch or a double aortic arch, can compress the airways and produce respiratory symptoms that may be present at birth or appear in the weeks thereafter. Characteristically, wheezing is more prominent than stridor, although many of the infants have noisy inspiration during sleep. Feeding is likely to accentuate the respiratory noises and may stimulate a paroxysmal cough. A severely affected baby prefers to lie with his head sharply extended presumably to lessen compression on the trachea.

STRIDOR IN OLDER CHILDREN

Episodic stridor in older children is most commonly associated with croup, otherwise known as laryngotracheitis (see pp. 1196). In children 1–5 years, epiglottitis is the most common cause of stridor (see pp. 1197). Older children with persistent stridor should always be referred to an otolaryngologist for careful direct laryngoscopy. Laryngeal papillomas are one of the important causes of persistent stridor but cysts and laryngoceles or even foreign bodies may also require expert treatment and removal.

Persistent stridor can also be the consequence of subglottic stenosis that may be acquired from chronic intubation. Some of the extrinsic masses that cause stridor in the newborn may also cause persistent stridor in later years (Jones et al, 1981).

PARALYSIS OF VOCAL CORDS

Paralysis of the vocal cords may be bilateral, in which case it is almost invariably central in origin, or unilateral. Probably because the recurrent laryngeal nerve on the left side arises low in the neck and its course is longer and more vulnerable to injury, unilateral paralysis is almost always left-sided. Infants with unilateral vocal cord paralysis are characteristically hoarse or even aphonic. Stridor is almost universal and is characteristically inspiratory with deep thoracic retraction. Infants with bilateral paralysis may have a normal cry.

Treatment

The treatment of vocal cord paralysis must be directed toward the underlying cause. In older children, it is possible to carry out some surgical plication which may help speech. In instances where respiratory distress is present, tracheotomy may be necessary.

REFERENCES

Dunbar JS: Upper respiratory tract obstruction in infants and children. *AJR* 109:227, 1970.

Jones R, Bodnar A, Roan Y: Subglottic stenosis in newborn intensive care graduates. *Am J Dis Child* 135:367, 1981.

Macfarlane PI, Olinsky A, Phelan PD: Proximal airway function at 8 to 16 years after laryngomalacia: Follow-up using flow-volume loop studies. *J Pediatr* 107:216, 1985.

Tucker JA, Tucker GF, Vidic B: Clinical correlation of anomalies of supraglottic larynx with a staged sequence of normal human laryngeal development. *Ann Otol Rhinol Laryngol* 87:636, 1978.

CROUP (LARYNGOTRACHEITIS)

Definition

Croup is the common word for an inflammatory reaction of the area of the larynx and trachea. This can result from multiple causes, which can be infectious and mechanical as well as allergic (angioneurotic edema). In this section, acute laryngotracheitis is discussed.

Basic Science

Apparently the initial infection is within the upper air passages and spreads to the nasal and pharyngeal epithelial surfaces and eventually to the larynx. Marked edema is observed, with cellular infiltration of histiocytes, lymphocytes, plasma cells, and polys.

Epidemiology

Croup is almost exclusively a disorder of children under 4 years of age, and is more common in boys than girls. It tends to occur in outbreaks every 3 years in late fall or early winter in the temperate zones. These outbreaks reflect community-wide prevalence of parainfluenza 1 and 2 or influenza A or B outbreaks. Croup can occur at any season, however, because it is associated with a number of viruses that can cause common colds including rhinoviruses as well as adenoviruses. In older children, croup may be due to influenza, mycoplasma, or associated with bacterial tracheitis (Liston et al, 1983). About 3–5% of children in a temperate climate will experience croup.

Natural History

The initial symptoms are usually those of a cold with low grade fever. Often at night the child wakens with a barking cough and difficulty associated with inspiration. The child may have a hoarse voice, stridor, and is likely to be apprehensive. If respiratory distress is severe, the child may become hypoxic and restless, with an increase in heart rate. These are ominous signs and should stimulate an immediate contact with a physician, preferably in an emergency room where intubation or tracheostomy could be carried out. In the severely affected youngsters, the illness usually lasts about 1 week.

Diagnosis

Laboratory study is not very helpful. The white count may or may not be elevated. A posteroanterior radiograph is diagnostic because it can show the subglottic narrowing that is the hallmark of acute laryngitis (Fig. 19.4*A* and *B*).

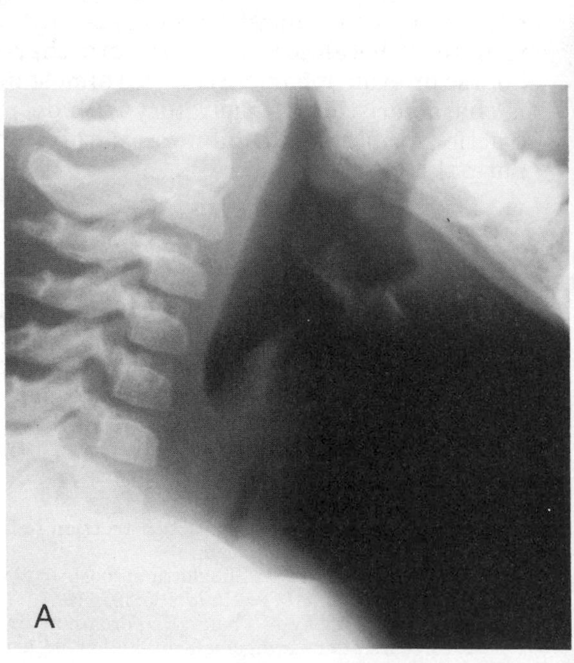

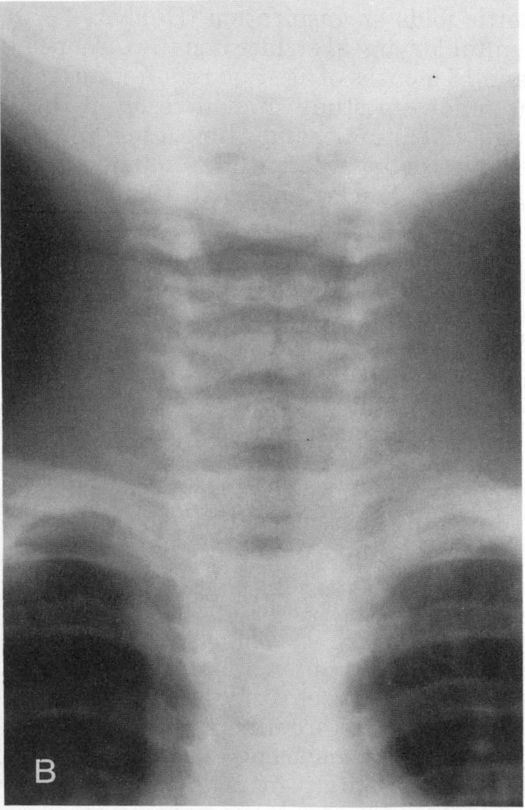

Figure 19.4 A and **B.** Patients with croup typically have a barking cough. Occasionally, there is confusion as to whether or not the patient with respiratory distress has epiglottitis or croup. This lateral film (**A**) of the airway in a patient with croup shows normal epiglottis, dilated laryngeal ventricle, and narrowing of the subglottic airway. The anteroposterior view (**B**) shows a "steeple" configuration of the trachea just inferior to the larynx, which is typical of croup.

Treatment

The treatment of acute laryngotracheitis continues to be controversial, partly because of the unpredictable nature of the disease which can sometimes be mild and self-limited and, at other times, is fulminant and severe. Inasmuch as the children with airway obstruction almost always breathe through their mouths, they will bring dry air into the inflamed epithelial surfaces and further aggravate the condition. Thus, mist therapy has been advocated in this condition. Some physicians find that cold mist is helpful whereas others find hot steam more efficacious, but it is not clear that there is an optimal temperature for the mist. In a prospective controlled study, Bourchier et al (1984) found no benefit from high humidity compared to room air. It seems appropriate to provide moisture at a temperature that makes the child comfortable.

The greatest controversy concerns the use of corticosteroids. Publications that support their use are as numerous as those that do not (Leipzig et al, 1979; Koren et al, 1983). Most infants improve with rest and mist therapy long before corticosteroids have a chance to affect the disease. If respiratory obstruction is severe, intubation or tracheostomy is indicated. Because some of the episodes of croup are associated with adenoviruses that can cause fatal pneumonia, suppression of host defenses with corticosteroids may be ill-advised.

Because the majority of cases of laryngotracheitis are associated with viral illnesses for which no known antibiotic is effective, antibiotic therapy is not useful. If the infant has an associated otitis media or pneumonia, however, the possibility of secondary infection is significant and antibiotics may be advisable.

The inhalation of racemic epinephrine has its advocates. It certainly should not be used on an outpatient basis inasmuch as significant rebound may follow an immediate improvement. In a hospitalized child with a severe episode, use of racemic epinephrine may be helpful while preparations are being made for intubation or tracheostomy. Occasionally, tracheostomy can be avoided with continued use of racemic epinephrine (Taussig et al, 1975).

If obstruction is severe, insertion of an airway may be necessary. If edema is severe, a tracheostomy may be required, although it is a rare event.

Prevention

There is no known prevention.

Spasmodic Croup

A variant of croup which also occurs in association with upper respiratory tract infections has been entitled spasmodic croup to distinguish it from laryngotracheitis. In spasmodic croup, there is noninflammatory edema in the submucosa of the trachea, but no involvement of the larynx. The problem tends to occur in families and to be self-limited, but characteristically recurs. The attacks are of sudden onset, respond well to the administration of mist, and no other therapy is indicated.

Bacterial Tracheitis

An increasing problem is purulent tracheitis, which sometimes follows viral-associated croup or occurs postextubation. Lethargy, leukocytosis, and stridor are the major findings in infants and older children. On laryngoscopy, purulent secretions are found with an intensely inflamed trachea. *Staphylococcus aureus* and *Haemophilus influenzae* are the most frequently found organisms. Treatment should be initiated immediately with aspiration of purulent material through bronchoscopy, tracheostomy if needed, and intravenous antibiotics. Tracheal stenosis has occurred after tracheitis in infants (Rojas and Flanigan, 1986).

REFERENCES

Bourchier D, et al: Humidification in viral croup. *Austr Paediatr J* 20:289, 1984.

Friedman E, Jorgensen K, Healy GB, et al: Bacterial tracheitis—2 year experience. *Laryngoscope* 95:9, 1985.

Koren G, Frand M, Barzilay Z, et al: Corticosteroid treatment of laryngo tracheitis versus spasmodic croup in children. *Am J Dis Child* 137:941, 1983.

Leipzig B, Oski FA, Cummings CW, et al: A prospective randomized study to determine the efficacy of steroids in treatment of croup. *J Pediatr* 96:194, 1979.

Liston SL, Gehrz RC, Siegel LG, et al: Bacterial tracheitis. *Am J Dis Child* 137:764, 1983.

Rojas J, Flanigan TH: Postintubation tracheitis in the newborn. *Pediatr Infect Dis* 5:714, 1986.

Taussig LM, Castro O, Beaudry PH, et al: Treatment of laryngotracheobronchitis (croup): Use of intermittent posture pressure breathing with racemic epinephrine. *Am J Dis Child* 29:790, 1975.

EPIGLOTTITIS (SUPRAGLOTTITIS)

Definition

Epiglottitis is an acute usually severe edema of the epiglottis associated almost always with bacteremia from *H. influenzae* type B infection. Rarely, respiratory viruses and group A and C streptococci have been associated with epiglottitis.

Basic Science

The leaf-like epiglottis is attached to the anterior surface of the thyroid cartilage and arches slightly posteriorly. It is covered by stratified squamous epithelium over the anterior surface and respiratory epithelium over the posterior surface. The aryepiglottic folds arise from the epiglottis and extend posteriorly to the paired arytenoid cartilages.

The soft tissues of the epiglottis can become markedly edematous. During inspiration the inflamed supraglottic ring can obscure the laryngeal inlet. During expiration the larynx is open.

Infection is characterized by a transient bacteremia, and later antibody production.

Epidemiology

The condition can occur at any age from newborns to the elderly, but about 75% of patients are between 1 and 5 years of age, and thus, on the average, these patients are slightly older than those who have acute laryngotracheitis (croup). Epiglottitis accounts for about 10% of all laryngeal infections.

The disease is most common in the winter, but can be seen in any season.

Natural History

The onset of epiglottitis is usually abrupt, and generally follows a mild respiratory tract infection. Early signs of epiglottitis include: anxiety on the part of the patient with inspiratory effort and hyperextension of the neck and protrusion of the chin. Drooling is a very important symptom because dysphagia is present and there is often a profound sore throat. The majority of children have temperatures of 39–40°C. Epiglottitis may be associated with extrapulmonary infection, such as otitis, pneumonia, and meningitis (Molteni, 1976).

Diagnosis

Usually the peripheral blood count is increased with an elevation of polymorphonuclear cells. The most important procedure if the diagnosis is in doubt is a lateral radiograph of the neck (Fig. 19.5) with the patient in an upright position so that soft tissues can be delineated. The hypopharynx is dilated from inspiratory effort and a thickened mass of tissue can be seen in the area of the epiglottis. Direct visualization with a laryngoscope is to be discouraged because, not infrequently, the child resists the procedure and may have respiratory depression. Restraining a child in a supine position and insertion of a tongue depressor can lead to airway obstruction. Radiographic evidence is usually sufficient to establish the diagnosis.

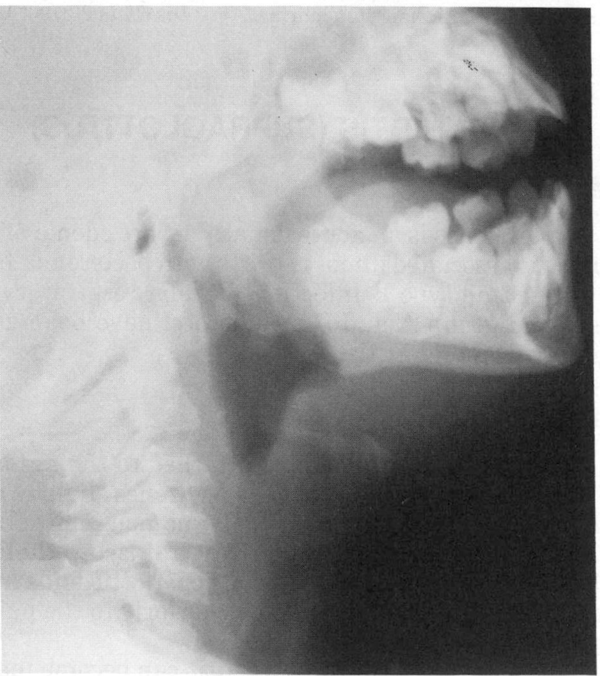

Figure 19.5. This 1½-year-old presented with drooling, respiratory distress, and high fever. Lateral radiograph shows typical features of epiglottitis with a swollen epiglottis partially obliterating the valleculae. The hyoid bone is a good marker for locating the base of the epiglottis.

Etiological diagnosis can be made on the basis of detection of the capsular antigen of *H. influenzae* type B. This can be detected by using a sensitive latex particle agglutination assay, and a positive test is assurance of *H. influenzae* infection. Blood cultures are positive in most cases early in the disease.

Treatment

Epiglottitis should always be considered an emergency and hospitalization or continual observation in an ambulatory setting is essential. The disease can progress very rapidly to complete airway obstruction and the ability to intubate or carry out tracheostomy can be life-saving. Which steps are required and in which order depend on assessment of the severity of the illness. Usually children are placed in a mist tent with added oxygen, although there has been no controlled trial to demonstrate the benefit of mist. Humidified oxygen is probably more appropriate for those children who are hypoxic. On the other hand, if the child is having inspiratory difficulty, elective intubation carried out in an operating room by a trained individual establishes the airway immediately and has been the most common way of managing severe epiglottitis. The mean time of intubation is about 48 hours although many children can be safely extubated by 36 hours. For infants from 6 months to 2 years of age, a nasotracheal tube (size 3.5 mm) is appropriate and for children 3–5 years of age, a 4-mm tube is appropriate.

Chloramphenicol, administered as early as possible, is the drug of choice because some strains of *H. influenzae* are resistant to ampicillin (up to 40% have been described). Intravenous antibiotics are rarely required for more than 3 days. The total duration of therapy is usually 7 days.

Prognosis

The mortality from acute epiglottitis is about 2% of cases. Death results from airway obstruction, or meningitis in association with bacteremia (Bates, 1979; Bass et al, 1985).

Prevention

Use of hemophilus type B vaccine should reduce the incidence of epiglottitis in children over age 2 years.

Early diagnosis in the presence of drooling and apprehension and prompt referral for intubation or tracheostomy can be life-saving. The interval between onset of respiratory symptoms and death may be as short as 4 hours (Bass et al, 1985).

LARYNGEAL WEBS

Definition

Laryngeal webs (and stenosis) are membranous obstructions (or narrowing) at the level of the cords or just above or below them, which may be partial or complete.

Basic Science

Webs result from incomplete recanalization of the primitive laryngeal airway in the seventh to tenth week of gestation.

Epidemiology

Webs are rare, with an occurrence of approximately 1/10,000 births. Congenital subglottic stenosis is also rare. About 10% of infants will have associated malformations. An autosomal dominant pattern of inheritance was reported in four families (Baker and Savetsky, 1966).

Natural History

A complete web prevents the first breath, and only awareness of this possibility with immediate inspection and perforation of the web is compatible with life. With the more common partial webs, an infant has a weak cry and labored respirations.

Diagnosis

Direct inspection of the larynx is required. Radiographs of the neck are helpful in delineating the symmetric narrowing of the subglottic air column.

Treatment

If the membrane can be penetrated adequately, endotracheal intubation for some days is appropriate. If it cannot be penetrated, emergency tracheostomy is mandatory until the web can be surgically excised.

Prognosis

A high-pitched, weak voice may persist even after the web is perforated.

LARYNGOTRACHEOESOPHAGEAL CLEFT

Definition

This congenital defect is a failure of dorsal fusion of cricoid lamina, between the posterior laryngeal wall, and sometimes, the trachea and the esophagus. A more severe form of the anomaly is a persistent esophagotrachea, which is not compatible with life (Griscom, 1966).

Epidemiology

As of 1974, only 34 such infants had been described in the literature (Burroughs and Leape, 1974). They have been described in sibships of double first cousins (Phelan et al, 1973).

Natural History

Infants with this condition may resemble those with an H-type tracheoesophageal fistula. Aspiration of liquids, with impairment of phonation, suggests the diagnosis. In other cases, the vocal cords function, but at some phases of respiration and swallowing, liquid can enter the airway through the cleft.

Diagnosis

Small clefts may be very difficult to see even with the use of contrast materials in radiographic studies, because aspiration may be intermittent. Likewise, they can be overlooked even on careful laryngoscopy if the midline structures are opposed.

Treatment

Operative repair is necessary if continued aspiration is a problem. Alternatively, gavage feedings or gastrostomy to bypass the lesion will allow time for the larynx to grow. In some instances, as the child grows and, perhaps, learns responses, aspiration is no longer a problem.

Prognosis

The outlook depends on the extent of the cleft and the degree of involvement of the vocal cords.

PAPILLOMATOSIS

Definition

Respiratory (laryngeal) papilloma is a histologically benign tumor with a propensity to spread and recur. It grows rapidly, is noninvasive, and consists of a connective tissue stalk covered with stratified squamous epithelium.

Basic Science

Respiratory papillomas have been noted to occur with cutaneous lesions, generally described as warts, which they resemble. As early as 1923, it became possible to transplant papillomas leading to the suspicion of a viral etiology. Virus-like particles have been observed with electron microscopy. Presumably the human papilloma virus (HPV) is the etiological agent and has been found to have as many as 12 different serotypes.

Many children with papillomatosis have mothers with a history of genital warts (condyloma acuminatum) during pregnancy. Human papilloma virus has been demonstrated in both laryngeal papilloma and maternal condyloma (Quick et al, 1980).

Epidemiology

Recurrent respiratory papillomatosis is the most common tumor of the larynx in childhood. Papillomas have been identified in the newborn but, for the most part, appear years later, with 29% having their onset before 5 years of age and 40% appearing before 16 years. There is apparently no difference in incidence by race or sex.

Natural History

By far the most common site of involvement is the larynx, but lesions may occur in the tracheobronchial tree, lung, palate, nasopharynx, or even the lips (Borkowsky et al, 1984). The presenting complaint with laryngeal papillomas is almost always stridor. When the lesion spreads into the intrathoracic trachea, however, the manifestations may mimic asthma. The propensity of the lesion to have exacerbations and remissions further accentuates the similarities to asthma.

Microscopically, the papillomas consist of vascular connective tissue cores covered by stratifed squamous epithelium. There is usually no invasion of the basement membrane and there are no histological differences between the tumors found in children and adults.

Diagnosis

On laryngoscopy the tumor appears as a regular nodular mass, pink or red, of variable size. Usually many small nodules, a few millimeters in diameter, merge into masses that occlude the larynx. They are friable and prone to bleed (Fig. 19.6).

Treatment

Laser therapy is the treatment of choice for respiratory papilloma (Strong et al, 1976). The aim of therapy is total ablation of all visible lesions, with the hope that the host immune system can suppress reappearance. Spontaneous remissions are possible, but recurrences are common (Steinberg et al, 1983). Careful follow-up of these patients is essential. In general, a disease-free interval of 1 year augurs well for complete remission. Furthermore, regression frequently occurs at puberty, and during pregnancy, which suggests some hormonal regulation.

Laser therapy may have some complications, including edema, after excessive laryngeal manipulation. Webs may occur at the site of excision and require further surgery or tracheostomy.

CONTROVERSY

Many other attempts to reduce these lesions have been suggested, such as cautery, radiation, and steroid hormones. None is efficacious and many are dangerous. Radiotherapy in particular is contraindicated.

The possibility that the causative agent is a virus has led to use of antiviral agents, including interferon (McCabe and Clark, 1983). The use of a dialyzable leukocyte extract (transfer factor) was reported in 1975 by Quick who induced a remission in one patient by transfer factor derived from the mother and in another patient by transfer factor from a person who was cured of laryngeal papillomatosis. The tumors regressed and the lymphocyte infiltration was demonstrated in the regressing tumors. The rationale is that this disease may be caused by maternal transmission of a papova-like virus and that antigen-specific antiviral immunotherapy might be useful.

Prevention

The association of maternal vaginal lesions with juvenile disease raises the question of acquisition during vaginal birth. The virus-like particles on the surface of the lesion could be aspirated by the infant with the first breath, lie dormant, and be triggered to develop by minor trauma or infection later. If this scenario is correct, delivery by cesarean section would be indicated if maternal condylomas are present in the vagina. No systematic evaluation of this approach has been reported.

CASE ILLUSTRATION

The parents of a 2-year-old female consulted their pediatrician because of a 3-week history of gradual worsening hoarseness. This was not associated with dysphagia, cough, stridor, or respiratory distress. Physical examination was essentially normal including clear lung fields as well as a normal pharyngeal examination. A diagnosis of laryngitis was made and the parents were reassured. Over the next 2 weeks, the hoarseness worsened and the parents were advised to have the child sleep with humidification during the night.

One week later, the parents began to note that the child was short of breath with exertion but again no stridor was evident. At this point, a diagnosis of vocal nodules was made and the parents were advised to encourage the child to diminish voice use. Over the next few days, however, shortness of breath increased and, therefore, an otolaryngologist was consulted.

At this time, a lateral neck radiograph revealed diffuse loss of definition in the area of the vocal cords and the question of a mass in this location was raised. Because of this, a direct laryngoscopy was performed and laryngeal papillomas were found.

It is of interest to note that there was a maternal history of vaginal condylomata present at the time of delivery of this youngster.

COMMENT

This case stresses several points, including the gradual worsening of hoarseness which is classic for this disease, as well as the onset of shortness of breath. Many patients do not have stridor and, therefore, this may mislead the physician into thinking the problem is simple laryngitis or, at most, vocal nodules. It stresses the importance of obtaining a lateral neck radiograph if hoarseness worsens and especially if it becomes associated with any respiratory symptoms.

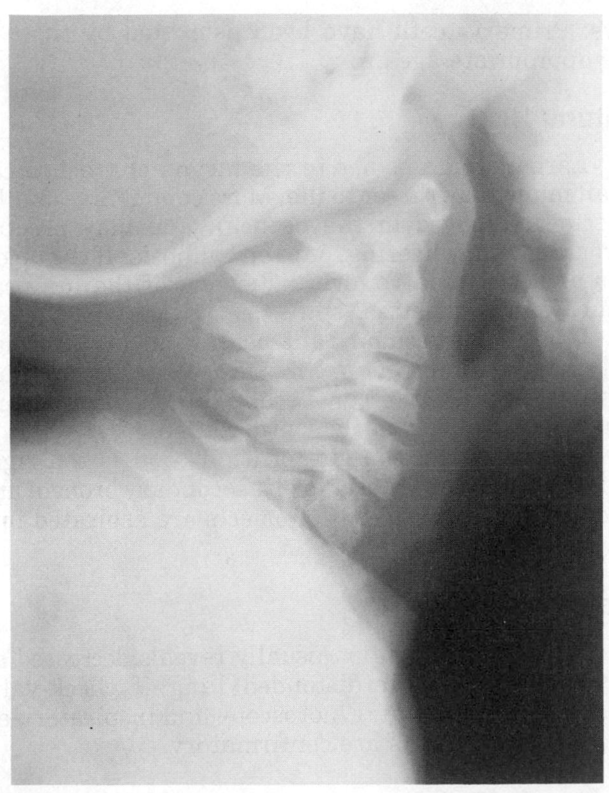

Figure 19.6. Papillomatosis. Lateral view of the neck shows multiple filling defects in the air column that are from multiple papillomata. Caused by viral infection, these masses are now treated by laser removal.

SUBGLOTTIC HEMANGIOMA

Definition

Subglottic hemangioma is a tumor of blood vessels that usually presents in the first 6 months of life as stridor, and can be life-threatening.

Epidemiology

The incidence of subglottic hemangiomas is not known.

Natural History

The pathogenesis of hemangiomas is not known. They occur most commonly in the head and neck, usually arising from a small nodule present at birth, but often overlooked. Rapid growth in the first weeks of life is the rule (see pp. 1148). Subglottic hemangiomas are usually solitary capillary hemangiomas and, in about one-half of the cases, are associated with the most common cutaneous hemangiomas. Occasionally, hemangioma-lymphangiomas of the cavernous type in the neck can extend into the upper airway.

Diagnosis

The diagnosis is suggested by the gradual onset of biphasic stridor associated with respiratory difficulty. The symptoms can progress then wane, and the diagnosis should be considered in any infant with recurrent croup. On laryngoscopy, the lesion is a smooth compressible mass which may extend around the lateral wall of the subglottic space. Because it is covered with respiratory mucosa, it may not appear red.

Treatment

The treatment of choice is use of a CO_2 laser which may give complete remission or require several applications. Humidification is required in the postoperative period to avoid crusting of the raw mucosal surface (Healy et al, 1980; 1984). Radiation is contraindicated. Corticosteroids cause regression in some instances and deserve a trial if laser therapy is not available.

SUBGLOTTIC STENOSIS

Definition

Subglottic stenosis is a narrowing of the subglottic larynx which may be extrinsic or intrinsic, congenital or acquired.

Epidemiology

Acquired subglottic stenosis is increasingly common as a consequence of long-term intubation in newborn infants in intensive care. Of 100 cases reported by Cotton (1984) seen over a decade, 92 were acquired mostly from prolonged intubation, five were congenital, and three had dystrophic cartilage. Our experience is similar. Of 65 patients with subglottic stenosis, 63 had acquired disease.

Diagnosis

Individuals with subglottic narrowing from any cause usually have some inspiratory stridor and, occasionally, an audible expiration as well. Plain radiographs of the upper airway are often sufficient to delineate the region of narrowing. Direct laryngoscopy and bronchoscopy by a trained observer will provide further information.

Treatment

Mild degrees of stenosis may not require treatment. If the individual has episodes of acute shortness of breath sufficient to suggest consideration of tracheostomy, operative repair of the stenosis may be beneficial. Some cases have responded to treatment with CO_2 laser (Healy, 1982), and others to cryotherapy (Rodgers et al, 1983). Increasing experience with an anterior laryngotracheal split with division of the posterior plate of the cricoid is promising (Seid and Canty, 1985).

Occasionally, the stenotic area is short enough to permit resection and reanastomosis (Sorensen and Holsteen, 1984).

Prevention

The incidence of complications from intubation apparently varies considerably among centers. In one study, Donn and Blane (1985) reported that they had fewer problems when the endotracheal tube was inserted by the oral route, so that movement within the trachea was reduced. They advocated use of a 2.5-mm constant diameter polyvinylchloride tube. Others have found the nasotracheal route to be preferable and have had few complications.

TRACHEOMEGALY

Definition

Tracheomegaly is an increase in tracheal diameter above normal. No precise numerical increase is agreed upon but, in general, abnormalities are said to exist when dimensions are more than 2 standard deviations from the mean.

Natural History

Prolonged mechanical ventilation in preterm infants has been associated with an increase in width and volume of the trachea (Bhutani et al, 1986). The consequences and natural history of this phenomenon deserve further study. At the least, it is evident that dead space ventilation is increased.

Diagnosis

The diagnosis depends on careful radiographic evaluation of the trachea.

Treatment

No data are available.

Prognosis

Tracheomegaly has been noted in some children at age 7 years who had been on ventilators as infants (Wohl ME, personal communication).

ASPIRATION OF FOREIGN BODIES

Definition

Aspiration of any material not naturally present that persists in trachea (or bronchi) is considered as aspiration of a foreign body.

Epidemiology

Aspiration occurs commonly in all individuals, but usually coughing or other maneuvers dislodge the offending body. The persistence of a foreign body in the airway is less common, but remains a major problem particularly in toddlers who explore their environment by tasting an enormous variety of objects. Peanuts are the leading offenders, followed by apple skin and a wide variety of inorganic objects such as pins, buttons, and toys. Primary teeth have been aspirated by those in the appropriate age group.

Natural History

Large foreign bodies in the larynx or trachea can be an immediate threat to life. More commonly, smaller objects are lodged in the bronchi, and may produce chronic cough, wheezing, or even cyanosis. If the object acts as a check-valve, overdistention of the lung can occur, with mediastinal shift.

If there has been no frank aspiration, but a foreign body has been inhaled (such as grasses) a chronic suppurative process can occur. Localized bronchiectasis and lung abscess may cause a septic course.

The most common site of aspiration is the right main bronchus and, more rarely, secondary bronchi and trachea. About two-thirds of objects are aspirated into the right side.

Diagnosis

Physical examination usually reveals decreased air exchange in the overdistended lung if check-valve mechanism is present. Fluoroscopy and inspiratory-expiratory radiographs are confirmatory.

Treatment

In a life-threatening situation, if the child cannot expel the object by coughing, the Heimlich maneuver (1975) can be used. If that is unsuccessful, prompt endoscopy is mandatory. If there is movement of air around the foreign object, it should be removed through a rigid bronchoscope. (Flexible bronchoscopes should not be used because the instruments available do not permit ventilation.) Only rarely is thoracotomy required. If the airway is inflamed, culture and antibiotics are appropriate. Corticosteroids for 24–48 hours can be helpful if the inflammatory response is severe.

Prevention

Aspects of prevention include "babyproofing" the child's environment by removing all objects that could be aspirated. In particular, nuts and open safety pins should not be within reach of toddlers.

Parents and babysitters should recognize the symptoms of aspiration and know the route to the nearest hospital emergency room that is equipped to carry out endoscopy.

REFERENCES

Baker DC, Savetsky L: Congenital partial atresia of the larynx. *Laryngoscope* 76:616, 1966.

Bass JW, Fajardo E, Brien JH, et al: Sudden death due to acute epiglottitis. *Pediatr Infect Dis* 4:447, 1985.

Bates JR: Epiglottitis: Diagnosis and treatment. *Pediatr Rev* 1:173, 1979.

Bhutani VK, Ritchie WG, Shaffer TH: Acquired tracheomegaly in very preterm infants. *Am J Dis Child* 140:449, 1986.

Blazer S, Naveh Y, Friedman A: Foreign body in the airway. A review of 200 cases. *Am J Dis Child* 134:68, 1980.

Borkowsky W, Martin D, Lawrence HS: Juvenile laryngeal papillomatosis with pulmonary spread. *Am J Dis Child* 138:667, 1984.

Burroughs N, Leape LL: Laryngotracheoesophageal cleft: Report of a case successfully treated and review of the literature. *Pediatrics* 53:516,1974.

Cotton RT: Pediatric laryngotracheal stenosis. *J Pediatr Surg* 19:699, 1984.

Donn SM, Blane CE: Endotracheal tube movement in preterm neonate: Oral versus nasal intubation. *Ann Otol Rhinol Laryngol* 94:18, 1985.

Griscom, NT: Persistent esophagotrachea: The most severe form of laryngotracheoesophageal cleft. *AJR* 97:211, 1966.

Healy GB: An experimental model for the endoscopic correction of subglottic stenosis with clinical implications. *Laryngoscope* 92:1103, 1982.

Healy GB, Fearon B, French R, et al: Treatment of subglottic hemangioma with the carbon dioxide laser. *Laryngoscope* 90:809, 1980.

Healy GB, McGill T: CO_2 laser in subglottic hemangioma—An update. *Ann Otol Rhinol Laryngol* 93:270, 1984.

Heimlich JH: A life-saving maneuver to prevent food choking. *JAMA* 234:398, 1975.

Marshak G, Grundfest: Subglottic stenosis. *Pediatr Clin North Am* 28:941, 1981.

McCabe BF, Clark KF: Interferon and laryngeal papillomatosis. *Ann Otol Rhinol Laryngol* 92:2-7, 1983.

Molteni RA: Epiglottitis: Incidence of extraepiglottitic infection: Report of 72 cases and review of the literature. *Pediatrics* 58:526, 1976.

Phelan PD, Stocks JG, Williams HE, et al: Familial occurrence of congenital laryngeal clefts. *Arch Dis Child* 48:275, 1973.

Quick CA, Behrens HW, Brinton-Darnell M, et al: Treatment of papillomatosis of the larynx with transfer factors. *Ann Otol* 84:597, 1975.

Quick CA, Krzyzek RA, Watts SL, et al: Relationship between condylomata and laryngeal papillomata. *Ann Otol Rhinol Laryngol* 89:467, 1980.

Rodgers BM, Moazam F, Talbert JL: Endotracheal cryotherapy in the treatment of refractory airway strictures. *Ann Thorac Surg* 35:52, 1983.

Seid AB, Canty TG: The anterior cricoid split procedure for the management of subglottic stenosis in infants and children. *J Pediatr Surg* 20:388, 1985.

Shann FA, Phelan PD, Stocks JG, et al: Prolonged nasotracheal intubation of tracheostomy in acute laryngotracheobronchitis and epiglottitis. *Austral Pediatr J* 11:212, 1975.

Sorensen HR, Holsteen V: Resection of congenital stenosis of the trachea in an infant. *Acta Paediatr Scand* 73:141, 1984.

Steinberg BM, Topp WC, Schneider PS, et al: Laryngeal papillomavirus infection during clinical remission. *N Engl J Med* 308:1261, 1983.

Strong MS, Vaughan CV, Healy GB, et al: Recurrent respiratory papillomatosis; management with CO_2 laser. *Ann Otol Rhinol Laryngol* 85:508, 1976.

Svensson G: Foreign bodies in the tracheobronchial tree. Special reference to experience in 92 children. *Int J Pediatr Otorhinolaryngol* 8:243, 1985.

MARY ELLEN AVERY

Consultant
Gerald B. Healy

Section 20

Ophthalmology

Approach to a Child with Visual Problems

1

Definition

Impairment in vision in infants and children may result from many causes. Of first importance is its detection.

Basic Science

Newborn infants, even those born as early as 28 weeks, respond to changes in illumination and can fix on certain objects. Although it cannot be measured directly, visual acuity is estimated to be about 20/600 at term. Three techniques, optokinetic nystagmus, preferential looking (PL), and visually evoked potential (VEP) have been used to assess visual acuity between birth and 6 months. All three demonstrate that visual acuity increases during that time. Because the different techniques involve different neural pathways, comparison between them may prove important (Dobson and Teller, 1978). Almost from birth, the infant will fix on objects, in particular, mother's face. By 8–10 weeks most infants will follow a moving object through a 180° arc. Visual acuity improves rapidly. With the use of operant preferential looking Mayer and Dobson (1982) showed that visual acuity for black and white square gratings improved from 6.3 minutes of arc in 5-month-old infants to 0.94 minutes of arc in 4-year-old children. The mean acuity of the 4- to 5-year-old children was not statistically different from that of adults, and by 5 years of age it is assumed to be close to that of adults.

Examination

Inspection of the cornea, the iris and pupils, clarity of lens and vitreous, and appearance of the retina should be a part of every well child check-up. If the child cannot fix, and the gaze wanders, or if a constant strabismus is present, referral to an ophthalmologist is appropriate at any age.

A more formal evaluation of visual acuity can be made with use of vision cards or charts. Color vision testing can be done with suitable color plates. Pupillary reactivity should be noted. Ocular motility can be noted on inspection, and strabismus can be detected with the cover-uncover test. (For recommendations on vision screening by the American Academy of Pediatrics, see Shea et al, 1986.)

The lacrimal apparatus is evaluated by looking at moisture of the cornea, ability to tear, and appearance of the lacrimal sac. Lids and conjunctivae should be inspected for inflammation.

Funduscopic examination is difficult in a newborn infant or an uncooperative child. At least a red reflex,

Table 20.1
Gross Motor Items and Age Achieved by Blind (Child Development Project) and Sighted (Bayley) [1]

Item	Age Range [2]		Median Age		Difference in Median Age
	Sighted	Blind	Sighted	Blind	
Elevates self by arms, prone [3]	0.7–5.0	4.5–9.5	2.1	8.75	6.65
Sits alone momentarily	4.0–8.0	5.0–8.5	5.3	6.75	1.45
Rolls from back to stomach [3]	4.0–10.0	4.5–9.5	6.4	7.25	.85
Sits alone steadily	5.0–9.0	6.5–9.5	6.6	8.00	1.40
Raises self to sitting position [3]	6.0–11.0	9.5–15.5	8.3	11.00	2.70
Stands up by furniture (pulls up to stand) [3]	6.0–12.0	9.5–15.0	8.6	13.00	4.40
Stepping movements (walks hands held) [3, 4]	6.0–12.0	8.0–11.5	8.8	10.75	1.95
Stands alone [4]	9.0–16.0	9.0–15.5	11.0	13.00	2.00
Walks alone, three steps [3]	9.0–17.0	11.5–19.0	11.7	15.25	3.55
[Walks alone, across room] [3]	[11.3–14.3]	12.0–20.5	[12.11]	19.25	7.15

[1]Adapted from Adelson E, Fraiberg S: *Insights from the Blind*. New York, Basic Books, Inc, 1977, p. 204. Reproduced with permission from Levine et al: *Developmental Behavioral Pediatrics*. Philadelphia, WB Saunders, 1983.
[2]All ages given in months. Ages rounded to nearest half month. Three cases corrected for 3 months' prematurity. Age range includes 5–95% of Bayley sample, 25–90% of Denver sample, and 10–90% of Child Development Project sample.
[3]One child had not achieved by 2 years.
[4]Not observed for one child prior to walking alone.
[ ]: Item from Denver Developmental Screening Test.

which reflects clarity of lens and vitreous, and a normal retina, can be noted in most instances. Full dilatation of the pupil, and use of indirect ophthalmoscopy is needed to examine the entire fundus.

Slit-lamp examinations and tonometry are usually performed by ophthalmologists.

Treatment (See also under specific conditions)

Once visual impairment is discovered, and a thorough search for underlying causes is completed, the paramount question concerns meeting the ongoing needs of the child.

TOTAL LOSS OF VISION

Significant delays in gross motor development, including prehension and locomotion, can be expected in the absence of vision (Table 20.1). Introduction of paired auditory-tactile cues can sustain contact with the environment and arouse interest. The talking book program is a successful alternative to Braille. Special schooling and access to aids for the blind are important.

PARTIAL LOSS OF VISION

Most visually impaired children can be helped significantly by appropriate glasses, hand lenses, bright light on printed matter, and enlarged type.

Community resources vary greatly. Pediatricians should advocate the need for library resources for the blind and special programs in schools. Contact should be made with the local school district's committee on the handicapped, and state Departments of Social Services and Health.

REFERENCES

Dobson V, Teller DY: Visual acuity in human infants: A review and comparison of behavioral and electrophysiological studies. *Vision Res* 18:1469, 1978.

Mayer DL, Dobson V: Visual acuity development in infants and young children, as assessed by operant preferential looking. *Vision Res* 22:1141, 1982.

Shea WW, Committee on Practice and Ambulatory Medicine: Vision screening and eye examination in children. *Pediatrics* 77:918, 1986.

Approach to Eye Movement Disorders: Strabismus (Squint, Cross-eye) 2

Definition

Strabismus is misalignment of the visual axes. It may be evident in any field of gaze, may be intermittent or constant, and may be present with near or far fixation or both. (The word means to squint or to look obliquely.)

Basic Science

Heredity has a role in pathogenesis of strabismus, but the etiology of nonparalytic strabismus is unknown. Accommodative convergence plays a role in etiology associated with significant degrees of hyperopia. Some strabismus is termed congenital, although it has not been established that the onset is in the first months of life. Asymmetrical refractive errors can give rise to preferential use of one eye, which in turn results in loss of vision and sometimes misalignment of the other.

Visual development in infancy proceeds rapidly, with evidence of accommodation and binocular vision by 6 months of age. This fact has prompted advice to identify strabismus early, and treat as soon as it is identified, preferably before 2 years of age. Treatment of early onset strabismus after 3–4 years may improve vision and alignment, but binocular vision with stereopsis is seldom achieved.

Epidemiology

It is estimated that about 2–5% of the population has some degree of strabismus, and some amblyopia (Table 20.2). About 60,000 eye muscle operations are performed each year in the United States (Gammon et al, 1985).

Natural History

The most common strabismus in the first year is esotropia in which the eyes are convergent. Exotropia

Table 20.2
Summary of Eye Problems Referred to Ophthalmology Department, The Children's Hospital, Boston, 1966–1986

Strabismus	13747
Refractive errors beyond usual range	8582
Amblyopia	5000
Cataracts	1540
Nasolacrimal duct obstruction	1084
Ptosis	859
Uveitis	470

is more often discovered after 1 year of age and is intermittent. Acquired esotropia may become apparent at the time of a febrile illness or other stress. The strabismus can be monocular or alternating, depending on visual fixation. Only those infants with monocular fixation are candidates for strabismic amblyopia.

Diagnosis

The cover-uncover test is most widely used by pediatricians (Fig. 20.1). The child fixes on a distant target, and the examiner alternately covers and uncovers each eye in turn. If there is esotropia (internal deviation of one eye), the deviating eye will move outward as the fixating eye is covered. If there is exotropia, the deviating eye will move inward. The procedure should be repeated with fixation on a close object such as a small photograph. Any abnormality of gaze determined by the cover test or evident on inspection warrants referral to an ophthalmologist.

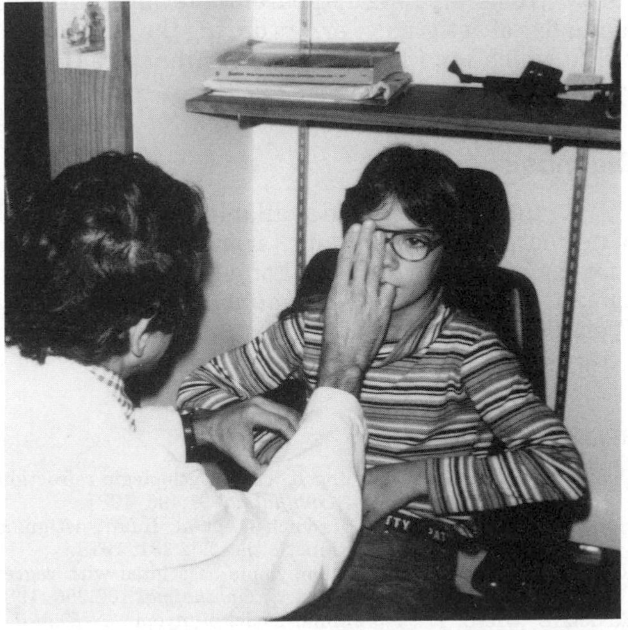

Figure 20.1. Cover-uncover test for strabismus (courtesy Dr. Richard Robb).

CASE ILLUSTRATION

An 8-year-old girl was noted to have crossed eyes in the first month of life. She had been a full-term baby and was in good general health. On ophthalmological examination at 7 months of age she had a large right esotropia, preferred to fix with the left eye, and had incomplete abduction of either eye. There was no important refractive error, and both eyes were anatomically normal.

The left eye was patched for varying parts of each day over the next 9 months, until the fixation pattern became alternating. During this same period the abduction of both eyes improved. At 18 months of age a recession of the right medial rectus muscle and resection of the right lateral rectus muscle was carried out to improve the ocular alignment.

After the operation, a moderate esotropia remained and it became apparent that there was an imbalance of the oblique muscles of both eyes as well. The alternating fixation pattern continued. At 3½ years of age, the left medial rectus muscle was recessed and the left lateral rectus muscle was resected. Both inferior oblique muscles were weakened by a myectomy near their insertion to the globe.

After the second strabismus operation a small, somewhat variable esotropia remained. Glasses were prescribed for a small amount of farsightedness, and these further reduced the residual deviation. Visual acuity could be measured, first with picture cards and then with E symbols, and was 20/30 in each eye. The oblique muscle imbalance was no longer apparent.

By 7 years of age, the glasses were being worn with less interest. A repeat refraction revealed a reduction in the amount of farsightedness to an insignificant level, so the glasses were discontinued. There was now some preference for fixation with the left eye, and on tests for binocular vision the right eye was suppressed.

Currently, at 8 years of age, the vision in the right eye is 20/25 and in the left eye 20/20. The residual esotropia is small enough to be cosmetically inapparent. Both eyes remain anatomically normal and there is a full range of ocular motility. No binocular vision is demonstrable.

Failure of one or both eyes to move fully in all directions suggests paralytic strabismus and requires a thorough workup to uncover the cause of the paretic muscle, whether of long-standing or recent origin.

Treatment

Refractive errors require corrective glasses. Any degree of visual loss should be managed by patching the better eye to stimulate use of the impaired one. Misalignment is usually corrected by using glasses to correct farsightedness or by surgery on the eye muscles. Recently, injection of botulinum toxin to paralyze a muscle has been used in selected cases of strabismus (Magoon, 1984, 1987; Gammon et al, 1985). Most pediatric ophthalmologists advise surgical relief of muscle imbalance.

CONTROVERSY

The management of congenital esotropia is controversial. Advocates of early surgical correction (6 months of age) argue that the chances for binocular vision are enhanced. However, the data presented have been retrospective and selected. Some infants with esotropia in the first year of life will recover spontaneously. The case presentation above represents our current approach to the problem including patching for amblyopia and surgery to realign the eyes when the deviation is found to be stable (Robb et al, 1987).

REFERENCES

Gammon JA, Gemmill M, Tiggers J, et al: Botulinum toxin chemodenervation treatment of strabismus. *J Pediatr Ophthalmol Strabis* 22:221, 1985.

Magoon EH: Botulinum toxin chemo-denervation for strabismus in infants and children. *J Pediatr Ophthalmol Strabis* 21:110, 1984.

Magoon E, Scott AB: Botulinum toxin chemodenervation in infants and children: An alternative to incisional strabismus surgery. *J Pediatr* 110:719, 1987.

Nelson LB: *Pediatric Ophthalmology*. Philadelphia, WB Saunders, 1984.

Reinecke RD: Current concepts in ophthalmology. Strabismus. *N Engl J Med* 300:1139, 1979.

Robb RM, Rodier DW: The variable clinical characteristics and course of early infantile esotropia *J Pediatr Ophthalmol Strabis* 24:276, 1987.

Refractive Errors 3

Definition

The refractive status of the eye depends on its anterior to posterior length, corneal curvature, and the power of the lens. When light is focused anterior to the retina, it is called myopia or nearsightedness. When light is focused behind the retina, it is called hyperopia or farsightedness. Astigmatism is a refractive error, which is caused by irregularities in the shape of the cornea or the lens.

Basic Science

Studies on full-term infants have shown that nearly three-quarters of them are hyperopic and about 25% are myopic. The hyperopia tends to increase until approximately 7 years of age and then tends to decline.

The causes of myopia have been under intensive study for a number of years with little consensus as to the pathogenesis of this condition. In extensive animal studies, Raviola and Wiesel (1985) have found that axial myopia can be induced in infant monkeys by lid fusion. The elongation of the eye appears to be due to an alteration of the visual input and is mediated by the nervous system (Raviola and Wiesel, 1985).

Epidemiology

It is estimated that about 25% of the American population is nearsighted. Variable degrees of myopia and astigmatism are common among premature infants. About 70% will have more than 1 diopter of astigmatism (Dobson et al, 1981). This is especially so among those who have had the retinopathy of prematurity (Kushner, 1982). Apparently term children have a number of astigmatic errors during the first 6 months of life which tend to decrease after that age (Howland et al, 1978).

Diagnosis

A number of tests are available to assess the ability of newborns to discriminate various forms and to measure their refractive status. For a full discussion of this subject, see Robb RM: *Ophthalmology for the Pediatric Practitioner*. Boston, Little, Brown & Co., 1981, pp. 1-10.

REFERENCES

Dobson V, Fulton AB, Manning K, et al: Cycloplegic refractions of premature infants. *Am J Ophthalmol* 91:490, 1981.

Howland HC, Atkinson J, Braddick O, et al: Infant astigmatism measured by photorefraction. *Science* 202:331, 1978.

Kushner BJ: Strabismus and ambylopia associated with regressed retinopathy of prematurity. *Arch Ophthalmol* 100:256, 1982.

Raviola E, Wiesel TN: An animal model of myopia. *N Engl J Med* 312, 1609, 1985.

Robb RM: *Ophthalmology for the Pediatric Practitioner*. Boston, Little, Brown & Co., 1981, pp. 1–10.

Retinal Disorders

4

RETINOPATHY OF PREMATURITY

Retrolental Fibroplasia

Definition

Retinopathy of prematurity is an injury to the immature retina mediated by relative or absolute hyperoxia. If mild, it is potentially reversible. If severe, retinal detachment and retrolental scar tissue can result in blindness. Termed retrolental fibroplasia when first described by Terry in 1942, it is evident that that name applies only to the late cicatricial changes, which are rare. It is more appropriate to describe all phases of the disorder as retinopathy of prematurity.

Basic Science

The lesion begins in the vessels of the developing eye. The earliest phase is peripheral vasoconstriction. The resulting ischemic injury is followed by vascular proliferation that promotes eruption of vessels into the vitreous. Spontaneous regression occurs in about 80% of the infants, but some have residual scarring that can lead to retinal detachment.

The role of oxygen in causing retrolental fibroplasia is not disputed (Patz et al, 1953). Questions remain, however, as to why the retinal vessels are susceptible to oxygen and whether associations other than prematurity may predispose a particular infant to retinopathy, at a given concentration of oxygen, which is not harmful to another. Very sick and very low birth weight infants are at greatest risk.

An observation well known to those who have studied newborn kittens in high oxygen was that the young animals appeared to tolerate high concentrations better than the older ones. A possible reason is that oxygen-tolerant newborn animals show a rapid increase in levels of all enzymes that detoxify oxygen radicals. Adult animals lack the ability to increase levels of "antioxidant enzymes" such as superoxide dismutase, catalase, and glutathione peroxidase. Presumably, similar events occur in the premature human infant. Even so, the eye is the vulnerable organ in the infant because of its incomplete vascularization.

Epidemiology

Once the association with high oxygen was noted, the ambient oxygen supplied to premature infants was reduced and, in the mid-1950s, fewer cases of retrolental fibroplasia were found. However, severe oxygen restriction, to less than 40%, which was widely used regardless of the condition of the infant, was found to be associated with increased neonatal mortality (Avery and Oppenheimer, 1960). It was recognized subsequently that the oxygen levels in the blood rather than the ambient gases were crucial in terms of injury to the developing retinal vessels. This required serial measurements of oxygen tension in the blood of the infant. Once micromethods for measuring partial pressure of oxygen in blood and continuous transcutaneous monitoring were available, the infants could be maintained in an appropriate range of oxygenation by regulating the inspired mixture. Hyperoxia, thus, could be prevented.

The trend for survival of ever smaller infants has increased significantly the number of infants at risk of retinopathy of prematurity. Some infants of very low birth weight have developed lesions while breathing room air (Yamanouchi et al, 1981). Apparently the relative hyperoxia of room air compared to that within the uterus can be sufficient to cause periods of vasoconstriction. Some signs of retinopathy are found in 40–70% of survivors with birth weight under 1000 g. In the experience of Petersen at The Children's Hospital, Boston, from 1979–1981, almost 10% of preterm infants had some retinopathy of prematurity but only three were blind and all three were born after fewer than 27 weeks of gestation (Petersen, 1981).

Natural History

The staging of retinopathy of prematurity is described in "An International Classification of Retinopathy of Prematurity" published in 1984. The earliest sign is a demarcation line, which is a thin but definite structure that separates the avascular retina anteriorly from the more vascularized posterior retina. Abnormal branching of vessels can be seen leading up to the line of demarcation. Stage 2 is called a ridge and represents a growth of the demarcation line which extends out of the plane of the retina. The ridge may change from white to pink as vessels extend to it from the plane of the retina. In stage 3, the ridge shows extraretinal fibrovascular proliferation. The proliferating tissue is found mostly in the posterior aspect of the ridge causing a ragged appearance, or it may be posterior to the ridge but not necessarily connected with it, sometimes extending into the vitreous perpendicular to the plane of the retina. Stage 4 represents unequivocal detachment of the retina which may be caused by an effusion of fluid or traction, or both (Fig. 20.2). About 75% of infants in stage 3 progress to stage 4 with loss of vision (Reisner et al, 1985).

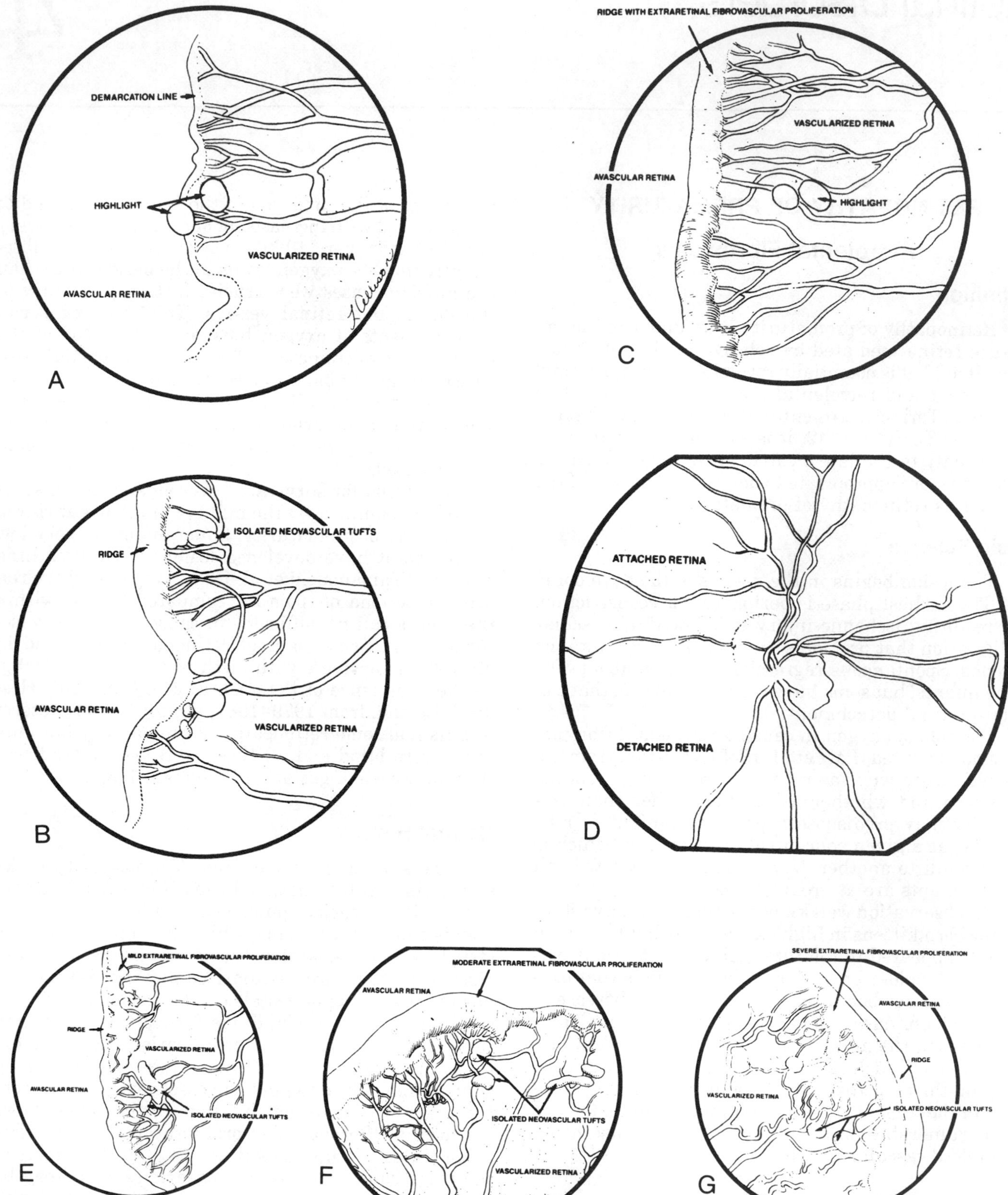

Figure 20.2. Line drawings of stages 1–4 retinal lesions in retinopathy of prematurity. **A**. Stage 1. **B**. Stage 2. **C**. Stage 3. **D**. Stage 4. **E**. Mild stage 3. **F**. Moderate stage 3. **G**. Severe stage 3. Reproduced with permission from Patz A: An international classification of retinopathy of prematurity. *Pediatrics* 74:127, 1984).

The lesions are usually first evident at several weeks of postnatal age (between 32 and 38 weeks' postconceptual age), during the time the infant is receiving oxygen, but may only be visible by indirect ophthalmoscopy carried out by a trained observer. The more obvious changes are apparent long after oxygen has been discontinued, between 4 and 8 weeks of age, and may progress after that period even in room air.

Diagnosis

All infants of less than 36 weeks' gestation or less than 2000 g birth weight who have received oxygen therapy, and all infants less than 1000 g at birth even if they have not received oxygen therapy, should have an eye examination with indirect ophthalmoscopy between 4 and 8 weeks postnatally, with follow-up every 2–3 weeks if there is active disease. The active stages of the disease are so characteristic that no other disorder would be considered. The advanced critical stage may present as a white pupil, which requires differentiation from retinoblastoma, hyperplastic vitreous, congenital cataracts, and a variety of other disorders, including all those with retinal detachment.

Treatment

Attempts to reduce oxygen toxicity to the immature retina have included use of prenatal glucocorticoids, which are known to accelerate maturation of the pulmonary surfactant system, and may affect antioxidant enzymes as well. No convincing evidence of efficacy has been reported. Another approach is administration of vitamin E with the hope that it will scavenge oxygen-free radicals in the lung and the retina, inasmuch as vitamin E levels are known to be low in preterm infants. No convincing evidence of efficacy of vitamin E has been reported to date (Phelps et al, 1987). Infants with immature retinas or those with signs of retinopathy should not receive iron supplements unless iron deficiency anemia is documented, since iron interferes with vitamin E metabolism.

CONTROVERSY

Attempts at laser therapy and cryosurgery have been undertaken. Some encouraging observations were reported by Reisner et al (1985) on the use of cryotherapy on the avascular part of the retina if the infant had mild to moderate fibrovascular proliferation with posterior-pole tortuosity and dilatation of iris vessels.

CASE ILLUSTRATION (courtesy of Dr. Richard Robb)

This prematurely born boy was delivered 24 hours after spontaneous rupture of the fetal membranes at 26 weeks of gestation. Birth weight was 850 g, and Apgar scores were 5 at both 1 and 5 minutes. There were initial respiratory retractions, but these cleared and his respiratory status was satisfactory until apneic spells began at 4 days of age. He was intubated and maintained on artificial ventilation for approximately 36 hours, after which he was rapidly weaned from the ventilator. Inspired O_2 levels were maintained between 30 and 40% for the first 4 weeks, but thereafter the patient was placed in room air. Numerous capillary Po_2 levels were mostly between 40 and 60 mm Hg, with a high of 83 mm Hg on only one occasion. A blood culture at birth grew *Escherichia coli,* and this was treated with intravenous ampicillin and kanamycin for 2 weeks, after which repeat blood cultures were negative.

An eye examination at 1 month of age, with dilated pupils and indirect ophthalmoscopy, showed a white demarcation line between vascular and avascular retina in the temporal periphery of both eyes, and in the left eye there was some dilatation of the temporal retinal vessels. No retinal hemorrhages were seen and the vitreous was clear. The patient gained weight steadily and was discharged from the hospital at 3 months of age, weighing 2220 g.

At 6 months of age, a follow-up eye examination revealed shallowing of the anterior chamber of the left eye. There was a left esotropia and, whereas the right eye followed visual stimuli, the left had no definite visual fixation and the pupillary reaction to light was poor. In the fundi, there was a dense fibrovascular band extending from the left optic disc to the temporal periphery, elevating the whole temporal retina toward the lens; in the right eye the retina was flat but there was dragging of the disc and retina temporally toward a peripheral mound of fibrovascular tissue at the ora serrata.

A number of subsequent eye examinations showed little change until 1½ years of age, when the left eye became infected and apparently painful, with a hazy cornea. The child was admitted to the hospital and, under anesthesia, the pressure of the left eye was markedly elevated. The left anterior chamber was extremely shallow and the anterior chamber angle appeared closed. Surgery was performed to remove the lens and to create several iridectomies. A white mass could be seen lying behind the plane of the lens. The right eye had a normal pressure, a shallow but formed anterior chamber, and temporal dragging of the optic disc as seen on earlier examinations.

Postoperatively, the pressure of the left eye dropped to normal levels, but the eye lost all light perception. The right eye remained anatomically unchanged, and at 7 years of age the vision in the right eye is 20/100 with a glass correction for oblique astigmatism. The patient can read 6–8 words at close distances and occasionally uses a bar magnifier or a monocular telescope. He is an avid reader, but the speed and range of his schoolwork are somewhat limited by his reduced vision.

The aim is to induce involution of neovascularization (Topilow et al, 1985). A preliminary report of a multicenter randomized evaluation of cryotherapy on one eye versus no therapy supported the efficacy and safety of transcleral cryotherapy to the avascular retina. Further follow-up will be needed to assess long-term benefits (Cryotherapy Cooperative Group, 1988).

Vitamin E has been advocated as an antioxidant, but a prospective randomized clinical trial failed to show that plasma levels maintained at 3.0–3.5 mg/dl were beneficial (Phelps et al, 1987).

The question of whether bright lights to which low birth weight infants may be exposed in intensive care nurseries could promote retinopathy has long been debated. In a sequential study, Glass et al (1985) reported suggestive evidence that light could be dangerous. Methodologic problems in their study are of concern, and the question must remain open, especially for very low birth weight infants.

Prevention

Children who had retinopathy of prematurity as infants may have late complications (Kalina, 1980). All such children should be followed regularly by an ophthalmologist. Myopia, strabismus, and amblyopia are common; late retinal detachments are rare, but do occur. Retinal pigmentation and vitreous membranes may persist.

Because therapy is limited, prevention is crucial. Meticulous monitoring of ambient oxygen tension in the incubator and transcutaneous oxygen measurements in the baby are now standard aspects of intensive care of low birth weight infants. Such measurements recorded continuously permit adjustment of the inspired oxygen to maintain normoxemia. In general, the range that satisfies metabolic demands is 50–80 mm Hg. In very sick infants in whom poor perfusion of the skin is evident, transcutaneous monitoring is inadequate and intermittent blood sampling for blood gas measurement is necessary.

RETINAL DEGENERATION

A form of retinal degeneration in infancy is known as Leber congenital amaurosis, a recessively inherited condition with severe visual loss from the time of birth that progresses to blindness. The fundus may be normal or have hazy granular pigmentation. In time, the pigmentation becomes more prominent and the optic discs are pale. The diagnosis can be established by depressed electroretinogram responses.

Retinal degeneration of later onset may be seen in abetalipoproteinemia, Laurence-Moon-Bardet-Biedl syndrome, and Refsum disease (elevated phytanic acid and polyneuritis). All these disorders have a recessive pattern of inheritance (see also pp. 965).

RETINITIS PIGMENTOSA

This term refers to a group of disorders characterized by progressive degeneration of rods and cones, and the pigmented epithelium of the retina. It occurs in 1/4000–1/20,000 individuals and may have an autosomal dominant, recessive or sex-linked inheritance. The onset may be in early childhood, but decreased vision is often not apparent until the second or third decade. On ophthalmoscopic examination, the retinal vessels are attenuated, clumps of pigment appear, especially in the periphery, and the optic nerve is pale. The electroretinogram is diagnostic. The condition is associated with a wide variety of systemic diseases, which may be of overriding importance in prognosis.

SPHINGOLIPIDOSES

Tay-Sachs disease (Gm_2 gangliosidosis) is characterized by abnormal accumulation of opaque gangliosides in the cells of the retina that surround the fovea, which appears as a cherry red spot by about 6 weeks of age. The course is one of progressive neurologic deterioration, and eventually blindness from optic atrophy in the first years of life.

Niemann-Pick disease has a cherry red fovea similar to that in Tay-Sachs disease. Sphingomyelin and cholesterol are stored in brain and retina, and many other tissues so that hepatosplenomegaly and bone marrow depression occur. The cornea may become opacified and there may be a brown discoloration of the anterior lens epithelium from stored lipids.

JUVENILE MACULAR DEGENERATION (STARGARDT DISEASE)

This rare disorder of unknown etiology presents with visual diminution between ages 6 and 20 years. It is inherited as an autosomal recessive disorder.

RETINOBLASTOMA (see also Section 9)

This potentially lethal malignant tumor can be treated successfully if recognized early. Most cases are sporadic, but it may be inherited as an autosomal dominant condition in about 40% of patients. All bilateral tumors must be considered heritable, even without a family history of disease. The heritable tendency is governed by a locus on the long arm of chromosome 13 (Dryja et al, 1984). The prognosis for retinoblastoma depends on the following findings, based on a review of 1531 patients (Abramson et al, 1985).

—Survival with bilateral disease is worse than that in unilateral disease.
—After 5 years, death is more likely from a second tumor than from metastatic retinoblastoma. Fifty percent of patients are dead by 25 years and 59% are dead 35 years after diagnosis.
—Death from metastatic retinoblastoma in unilateral disease occurs within 4 years of diagnosis.

The average age of diagnosis is 12 months for bilateral disease and 24–30 months for unilateral disease. The white reflex is often noted first by a parent, and should stimulate immediate referral to an ophthalmologist. Other signs are strabismus, painful eye with glaucoma, and visual loss. There is a high incidence of second nonocular (mostly sarcomas) tumors (>60%) in the hereditary form of retinoblastoma.

Survival with metastatic disease is rare, but it has been reported after aggressive chemotherapy (Petersen et al, 1987).

DIABETIC RETINOPATHY

Definition

Diabetic retinopathy is a progressive vascular lesion that produces recurrent hemorrhages, occlusion of retinal capillaries, and infarction and may lead to vitreous scarring and retinal detachment.

Basic Science and Natural History

The initial lesions are capillary microaneurysms, often located in the macular area. Later, occlusion of capillaries produces soft or "cotton-wool" exudates. As the disease advances, vitreous hemorrhages occur with visual loss that may improve as the blood is resorbed. Retinal edema and cysts appear, and may produce holes in the inner retinal layers. In some instances, retinal vascular proliferation occurs. Progressive visual loss is caused by hemorrhage and by retinal detachment. Glaucoma and cataracts can develop.

Epidemiology

Among juvenile diabetics, about 10% will have retinopathy 5–9 years after onset of diabetes, 50% by 15 years, and 80–90% by 25 years. With maturity onset diabetes, 30% have retinopathy after 5 years.

Diagnosis

All diabetics should have periodic eye examinations by an ophthalmologist who is familiar with the ocular changes in that disorder. Rapid changes in refraction can occur if blood sugar levels fluctuate. Cataracts may develop in addition to the retinal lesions.

Treatment and Prevention

Most complications of diabetes relate to hyperglycemia. Control of blood glucose is the best way to defer ocular complications, although some will develop in nearly all long-standing cases.

There is now some clearly effective therapy for diabetic retinopathy by diffuse "spot" photocoagulation of the retina.

REFERENCES

Abramson DH, Ellsworth RM, Grumbach N, et al: Retinoblastoma: Survival age at detection and comparison 1914–58, 1958–83. *J Pediatr Ophthalmol Strabis* 22:246, 1985.

Ashton N, Ward B, Serpell G: Role of oxygen in the genesis of retrolental fibroplasia; a preliminary report. *Br J Ophthalmol* 37:513, 1953.

Avery ME, Oppenheimer EH: Recent increase in mortality from hyaline membrane disease. *J Pediatr* 57:553, 1960.

Cryotherapy for retinopathy of prematurity cooperation group: Multicenter trial of cryotherapy for retinopathy of prematurity: Preliminary results. *Pediatrics* 81:697, 1988.

Dryja TP, Cavenee W, White R, et al: Homozygosity of chromosome 13 in retinoblastoma. *N Engl J Med* 310:550, 1984.

Frank RN: In: Ryan SJ, Smith RE (eds): *Selected Topics on the Eye in Systemic Disease.* New York, Grune & Stratton, 1974, p. 65.

Frauenfelder FT, LaBraico JM, Meyer SM: Adverse ocular reactions possibly associated with isoretretinoin. *Am J Ophthalmol* 100:534, 1985.

Glass P, Avery GB, Subramanian KNS, et al: Effect of bright light in the hospital nursery on the incidence of retinopathy of prematurity. *N Engl J Med* 313:401, 1985.

Kalina RE: Treatment of retrolental fibroplasia: Therapeutic review. *Surv Ophthalmol* 24:229, 1980.

Kinsey VE, et al: PaO_2 levels and retrolental fibroplasia; a report of the cooperative study. *Pediatrics* 60:655, 1977.

Kolata G: Blindness of prematurity unexplained. *Science* 231:20, 1986.

Lucey JL, Dangman B: A reexamination of the role of oxygen in retrolental fibroplasia. *Pediatrics* 73:82, 1984.

McPherson AR, Hittner HM, Kretzer FL: *Retinopathy of Prematurity—Current Concepts and Controversies.* Philadelphia, BC Decker Inc., 1986.

Nelson LB: *Pediatric Ophthalmology.* Philadelphia, WB Saunders, 1984, p. 149.

Patz A, Eastham A, Higginbotham DH, et al: Oxygen studies in retrolental fibroplasia in experimental animals. *Am J Ophthalmol* 36:1511, 1953.

Petersen RA: Six years' experience with retrolental fibroplasia in the Joint Program in Neonatology, Harvard Medical School Syllabus: Retinopathy of prematurity conference, Washington, DC, Dec. 4–6, 1981.

Petersen RA, Friend SH, Albert DM: Prolonged survival of a child with metastatic retinoblastoma. *J Pediatr Ophthalmol Strabis* 24:247, 1987.

Phelps DL, Rosenbaum A, Isenberg SJ, et al: Tocopherol efficacy and safety for preventing retinopathy of prematurity: A randomized, controlled, double-masked trial. *Pediatrics* 79:489, 1987.

Purohit DM, Ellison RC, Zierler S, et al: Risk factors for retrolental fibroplasia: Experience with 3025 premature infants. *Pediatrics* 76:339, 1985.

Reisner SH, Amir J, Shohat M, et al: Retinopathy of prematurity: Incidence and treatment. *Arch Dis Child* 60:698, 1985.

Shohat M, Reisner SH, Krikler R, et al: Retinopathy of prematurity: Incidence and risk factors. *Pediatrics* 72:159, 1983.

Silverman WA: *Retrolental Fibroplasia: A Modern Parable.* New York, Grune & Stratton, 1980.

Special Article: An international classfication of retinopathy of prematurity. *Pediatrics* 74:127, 1984.

Tassman W: Management of retinopathy of prematurity. *Ophthalmology* 92:995, 1985.

Terry TL: Extreme prematurity and fibroblastic overgrowth of persistent vascular sheath behind each crystalline lens; preliminary report. *Am J Ophthalmol* 25:203, 1942.

Topilow HW, Ackerman AL, Wang FM: The treatment of advanced retinopathy of prematurity by cryotherapy and scleral buckling surgery. *Ophthalmology* 92:379, 1985.

Yamanouchi I, Igarashi I, Ouchi E: Incidence and severity of retinopathy of prematurity in low birth weight infants monitored by continuous transcutaneous oxygen monitoring. Syllabus: Retinopathy of prematurity conferences, Vol 11, Washington, DC, Dec. 4–6, 1981, p 505.

Cataracts 5

Definition

A cataract is an opacity in the lens that limits vision.

Epidemiology

True congenital cataracts are rare, and may not be detected at birth. Indeed in the series of Burns and Jones (1985), it was the mother who most often first noticed the cataracts. Acquired cataracts are found in many storage diseases, and can be drug-induced or follow trauma (Table 20.3).

Table 20.3
Some Conditions Associated with Cataracts in Children

I.	Genetic-Mendelian Dominant (mostly) or recessive (rarely)
II.	Chromosome disorders Trisomy 13, 18, 21 Turner syndrome
III.	Congenital infections (Rubella, syphilis, toxoplasmosis)
IV.	Metabolic disorders Galactosemia Lowe syndrome Diabetes mellitus Alport syndrome Hypoparathyroidism Pseudohypoparathyroidism
V.	Systemic diseases Smith-Lemli-Opitz syndrome Rubenstein-Taybi syndrome Potter syndrome Myotonic dystrophy and others
VI.	Dermatologic disorders Ectodermal dysplasia Atopic dermatitis Congenital icthyosis
VII.	Craniofacial disorders Crouzon syndrome Apert syndrome Oxycephaly
VIII.	Persistent hyperplastic vitreous
IX.	Trauma; ionizing radiation
X.	Prolonged corticosterioid therapy
XI.	Secondary to other intraocular pathology (retrolental fibroplasia, uveitis)

CASE ILLUSTRATION

A girl was the final child born to parents with a significant family history of childhood cataracts. The mother, maternal grandfather, and two maternal aunts had had cataracts requiring surgery in infancy. The girl's cataracts were found by her pediatrician at 2 months of age. There was pendular nystagmus and poor visual fixation in both eyes. The fundi could not be visualized because of dense central lens opacities. The pupils dilated only to 5 mm with cycloplegic drops.

The left cataract was aspirated at 4 months of age and the right cataract at 5 months of age. Full-sector iridectomies were made at the time of surgery because of the poor pupillary dilatation. The posterior capsule of the lens was left intact at the time of initial surgery, but this was later incised in both eyes when it became thickened and opaque.

Some crossing of the eyes (esotropia) became apparent after the first cataract extraction. After the second cataract had been removed, a preference for fixation with the right eye developed. Aphakic contact lenses were prescribed and the right eye was patched part time. Cataract glasses were also made available, and by 1 year of age either glasses or contact lenses were worn most of the time.

By 3½ years of age, visual acuity could be measured at 5/30 in each eye. (Normal acuity at this age would be 20/30.) A variable esotropia remained, and for approximately 2 years the fixation pattern seemed to be alternating. By 5½ years of age, a preference for fixation with the left eye had developed, and the nystagmus was noted to be more marked in the right eye. Visual acuity was measured in the right eye at 20/200 and in the left eye at 20/100. Part-time patching was begun on the left eye. By 8 years of age, the visual acuity had improved to 20/80 in the left eye, but remained 20/200 in the right. Nystagmus was still a limiting factor in achieving better vision. The esotropia had become less noticeable. Glasses were worn more than contact lenses, and with the bifocal segment newspaper print could be read at 6 inches. Patching was discontinued because it was frustrating to the patient and did not appear to improve the vision.

COMMENT

A complete history should include questions about vision in family members. If congenital cataracts are present in the family, careful evaluation of the infant's eyes is mandatory; the earlier the diagnosis and treatment, the better the outlook for vision.

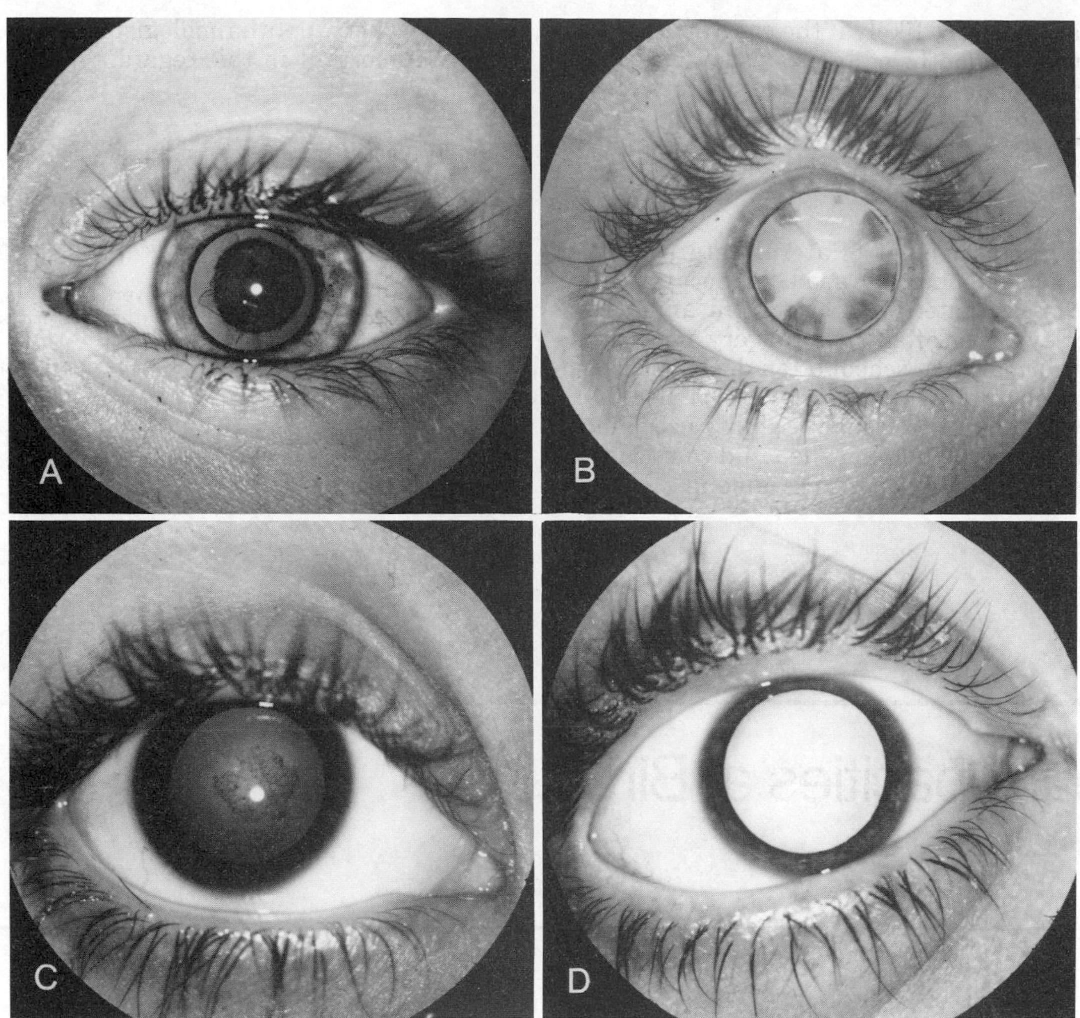

Figure 20.3. **A**. Lamellar cataract, etiology unknown. **B.** Cataract in a child with hypoparathyroidism. **C.** Cataract in a child on long-term corticosteroid therapy for nephrosis. **D.** Normal fundus. The lens will appear red and no opacities are evident.

In more than half of the children who present with congenital cataracts, there is a positive family history, mostly showing autosomal dominant inheritance, but occasionally autosomal recessive. When sporadic congenital cataracts occur, the chance of their appearance in subsequent siblings is about 1/40.

Natural History

Congenital cataracts are frequently bilateral. They are associated with other ophthalmic abnormalities including nystagmus, microphthalmus, rubella syndrome, Lowe syndrome, and mental retardation of unknown etiology. Galactosemia is another recognized cause of a characteristic kind of congenital cataract (Winder et al, 1983).

Cataracts can be induced by long-term high-dose corticosteroid therapy, but fortunately they do not often reduce vision to an important degree. Cataracts that develop very early in steroid therapy may disappear after the drug is discontinued (Forman et al, 1977).

Monocular congenital cataracts often occur in an eye that is slightly smaller than the normal fellow eye. In this case it may be associated with persistence of the primary vitreous or some remnant of the embryonic hyaloid system.

Diagnosis

Early symptoms may be photophobia, or lack of visual attention. The diagnosis is often apparent on inspection of a white pupil. *Checking the red reflex with the direct ophthalmoscope is the most important and useful diagnostic maneuver.* A less dense cataract presents as a hazy lens; sometimes they are not clear enough to allow an image to be formed on the retina. In most circumstances there is significant loss of vision. Nystagmus, of a searching type, indicates severe loss of vision (Fig. 20.3*A*-*D*).

Treatment

Surgical removal of a monocular congenital cataract should be undertaken soon after diagnosis because visual deprivation is very likely if the cataracts are left untreated beyond 4 months of age. Contact lenses can be used, but if not tolerated, eye glasses have been prescribed even for infants (Robb et al, 1987).

Prognosis

With early treatment of bilateral cataracts, the outlook for vision is generally good. Monocular cataracts tend to be associated with persistent amblyopia in the involved eye, even after early surgery and optical correction. Performance in school often depends on the existence of other medical conditions (see Table 20.3).

Parents of children with visual disability need much guidance with respect to helping the child compensate for loss of visual input. Cooperation among pediatricians, teachers, ophthalmologists, and parents groups is very important in this regard.

REFERENCES

Burns EC, Jones RB: Long-term management of congenital cataracts. *Arch Dis Child* 60:322, 1985.

Calhoun JH: Cataracts in children. *Pediatr Clin North Am* 30:1061, 1983.

Calhoun JH: In: *Nelson Pediatric Ophthalmology*. Philadelphia, WB Saunders, 1984.

Forman AR, Loreta JA, Tina LV: Reversibility of corticosteroid-associated cataracts in children with nephrotic syndrome. *Am J Ophthalmol* 84:75, 1977.

Robb RM, Mayer DL, Moore BD: Results of early treatment of unilateral congenital cataracts. *J Pediatr Ophthalmol Strabis* 24:178, 1987.

Winder AF, Claringbold LJ, Jones RB, et al: Partial galactose disorders in families with premature cataracts. *Arch Dis Child* 58:362, 1983.

Corneal Opacities at Birth 6

CONGENITAL GLAUCOMA

Definition

Glaucoma, an increase in intraocular pressure, may be present at birth as a result of a developmental anomaly of the eye. It can accompany a number of systemic disorders.

Basic Science

Whenever intraocular pressure rises there is a danger of permanent injury to the optic disc and cornea. The cornea becomes edematous and hazy. When Descemet's membrane tears, irregular corneal opacities may appear.

Ocular anomalies that are sometimes associated with congenital glaucoma are adhesions between iris and cornea, aniridia, persistent hyperplastic primary vitreous, and retinoblastoma.

Among systemic disorders in which congenital glaucoma can occur are Sturge-Weber syndrome with hemangiomatous involvement of the upper eyelid (unilateral), neurofibromatosis, Lowe syndrome (oculocerebrorenal syndrome), and congenital rubella. Glaucoma can complicate the anterior uveitis seen in about 15% of children with juvenile rheumatoid arthritis. Prolonged use of topical steroid eyedrops can produce glaucoma, which usually reverses when the medication is discontinued.

Glaucoma may be mistakenly diagnosed in the presence of corneal clouding from other conditions such as Hurler or Scheie syndromes. In these conditions, mucopolysaccharides may deposit in the cornea. Occasionally forceps injury at the time of delivery may lead to unilateral corneal opacification.

Epidemiology

The condition is rare, except in certain epidemics such as rubella. It can be inherited, sometimes in an autosomal recessive manner (1 of 4 chance of occurrence in siblings) or a multifactoral manner, about 5% risk of repeat. About 65% of patients are boys. Occurrence with aniridia, Sturge-Weber syndrome, and neurofibromatosis implies an inheritance pattern of those diseases.

Natural History

The earliest sign may be excessive tearing, which can be confused with a blocked nasolacrimal duct. Pho-

CASE ILLUSTRATION

A 3-day-old girl was found by her pediatrician to have enlarged, hazy corneas in both eyes. The child had been born at term, weighing 3400 g, and there was no family history of serious eye disease. On closer examination it appeared that the right cornea was slightly larger and hazier than the left. The pupil in the right eye looked larger than in the left, but details of the iris and lens were hard to see through the hazy cornea.

An ophthalmologist was consulted and an examination under anesthesia was arranged. At 10 days of age the ocular pressures under anesthesia were 24 mm Hg in the right eye and 21 mm Hg in the left. Normal pressures under these circumstances would be 10–12 mm Hg. The corneal diameters were 12.25 mm and 11.25 mm, well above the 10-mm horizontal diameter of a normal newborn cornea, and both corneas were hazy. Glaucoma surgery on the trabecular meshwork was performed in the right eye at 10 days of age and in the left eye 1 week later. Postoperative pressures under anesthesia 1 month later were between 10 and 14 mm Hg, and the corneas had begun to clear, especially in the left eye. On the right there was a persistent central corneal opacity, which could still be detected at 3 years of age, despite ocular pressures that continued to be in the normal range. There was bilateral pendular nystagmus and a reluctance to fix with the right eye.

The corneal diameters increased to 12.75 mm in each eye by 11 months of age and remained at that size over the next year. Corneal clarity improved to the point that the optic discs could be seen in both eyes with the direct ophthalmoscope, and both discs appeared to be healthy with normal-sized physiological cups and good color. The right eye began to cross about 1 year of age. Subsequent refraction revealed a large myopic refractive error in that eye, whereas there was only a small astigmatic error in the left eye. Visual fixation was poor in the right eye and attempts to patch the left eye were unsuccessful.

At 3½ years of age the vision in the better left eye was 5/30 with picture cards. Normal vision at this age would be 20/30. There continued to be eccentric fixation in the right eye. The right pupil could now be seen to be larger than the left and there was anomalous iris stromal thinning temporally along with distortion of the pigment at the pupillary border. Ocular pressures with topical anesthesia were 17–18 mm Hg (normal = <20 mm Hg) in both eyes, and by gonioscopy the surgically created openings could be seen in the trabecular meshwork. The child tended to hold her head turned slightly to the left in order to fix with the better left eye in adduction, the position in which nystagmus was least marked.

tophobia, and enlargement of cornea with edema appear later. The sometimes very large eyes are termed buphthalmos or "ox-eye." Late signs are more severe manifestations of early ones and may lead to blindness.

Diagnosis

Corneal haze should be taken seriously, and a thorough medical and ophthalmologic investigation undertaken (Fig. 20.4). If it is accompanied by increased intraocular pressure (above 15 mm Hg—usually determined at the time of an examination under anesthesia), surgical correction is usually indicated.

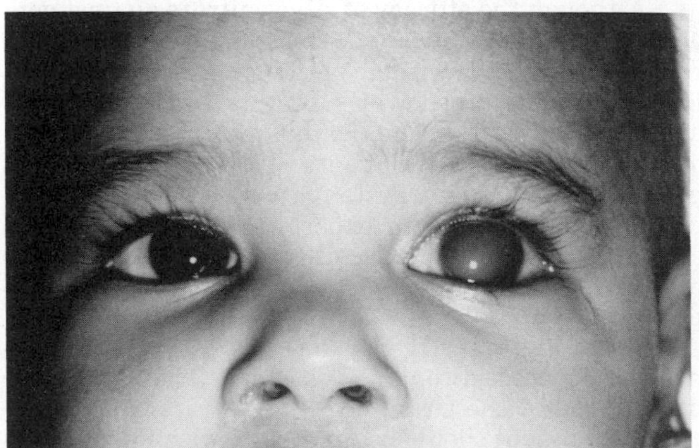

Figure 20.4. Note enlarged, hazy cornea suggestive of congenital glaucoma in left eye. The right eye is normal (courtesy Dr. Richard Robb).

Prognosis

Optic nerve atrophy is the most serious sequel to untreated glaucoma. Myopia and corneal opacity contribute to permanent disability. The outlook for good vision depends on early diagnosis and prompt treatment.

Prevention

Inspection of the cornea and lens is an essential component of every physical examination. Early treatment can save vision.

OTHER CORNEAL OPACITIES

Corneal inflammation can occur from infectious agents, such as herpes simplex, herpes zoster, mumps, or cystinosis. Some of the mucopolysaccharidoses such as Hurler's are associated with accumulation of metabolites throughout most regions of the eyes, including cornea, sclera, iris, and retina.

Injury at any age, including during birth, can lead to permanent clouding of the cornea.

REFERENCES

Nelson LB: *Pediatric Ophthalmology.* Philadelphia, WB Saunders, 1984, pp 113–121.

Walton DS: Glaucoma in infants and children. In: Harley RD (ed): *Pediatric Ophthalmology,* 2nd edition. Philadelphia, WB Saunders, 1983.

Infections: Conjunctivitis

7

Definition

Conjunctivitis is inflammation of conjunctiva, a thin mucous membrane that lines the posterior surface of the lids and the bulbar portion of the eyeball except for the cornea. Inflammation can occur from chemical or mechanical injury, or viral or bacterial infection.

Basic Science

The eye is exposed to atmosphere, but relatively resistant to injury because of blinking, and the flushing mechanism of tears that contain a lysozyme.

Infection can occur with a wide variety of organisms. In a prospective comparison of 55 infants with purulent conjunctivitis and 60 healthy control infants, Sandstrom et al (1984) in Seattle identified the pathogens associated with the purulent response. They found that *Chlamydia, Haemophilus* species, *Staphylococcus aureus, Enterococci,* and *Streptococcus pneumoniae* were most commonly associated with purulent conjunctivitis. Most of these organisms can be seen in uninfected controls, albeit at a much lower frequency. The range of organisms was very wide indeed and included many that are not usually considered pathogenic, although they may be in the newborn period. Among these are *S. epidermidis* and several *Neisseria* species.

In the Seattle experience, the age of onset of the conjunctivitis ranged from 2–6 days. Neither the age of onset nor the severity of the lesion correlated with the presence of a given pathogen; thus, identification requires Wright and Gram stains for the presence of white cells and organisms followed by culture to verify the presence of the putative pathogen.

In children, sticky lids are commonly the result of low grade infection with *S. aureus, Haemophilus* species, or *Pneumococcus*. Involvement of the conjunctivae can lead to inflammation, commonly designated "pink eye."

Viral conjunctivitis may occur as an isolated event or may be part of an upper respiratory infection or systemic viral infection such as measles. The discharge is watery rather than purulent as in bacterial infection.

Vernal conjunctivitis is a type of allergic conjunctivitis, often worse in spring and summer.

Natural History

The most common cause of irritation of conjunctivae of newborn infants is a reaction to the topical silver nitrate solution used for prophylaxis against the gonococcus. This mild, self-limited chemical conjunctivitis is thought to occur in about 90% of infants so treated and is most prominent within the first 6 hours of life, receding thereafter (Nishida and Risemberg, 1975).

At the present time, when many infants leave the hospital 1–2 days after birth, most bacterial conjunctivitis makes itself manifest after discharge. The types of organisms that can be recovered will vary from place to place and may depend on the facilities available to identify the offending agent. For example, for many years the presence of *Chlamydia trachomatis,* the most common cause, was overlooked simply because the necessary techniques of culture were not employed.

The most feared form of conjunctivitis in the newborn is caused by gonococcus because that agent is capable of producing corneal ulceration, perforation, and even loss of vision.

Neisseria gonorrhoeae is transmitted to the infant on passage through the genital canal. The onset of the infection is early, often within the first 2–3 days after birth and almost always before 5 days. Initially there is lid swelling, then edema, then a serous exudate followed by a purulent one (see pp. 1068).

Diagnosis

History of exposure to *Gonococcus* or *Chlamydia* is important. Culture of maternal vagina and of conjunctival scrapings from newborns is advised. Conjunctival scrapings can be examined by Gram or Giemsa stains, and cultured on chocolate agar or Thayer-Martin media (Table 20.4). Diagnostic features of conjunctivitis, from other causes are also in Table 20.4.

Treatment

Although the efficacy of silver nitrate against gonococcus is without question, there has been continual reassessment of the wisdom of inducing a chemical conjunctivitis in normal newborn infants. Nonetheless, the alternative use of antibiotics has the possible hazard of sensitization to those agents. Although this has not been confirmed in any systematic study, the potential risk is sufficient to lead experts to conclude that 1% silver nitrate solution in a single dose wax ampule is probably the safest and most effective approach to prophylaxis.

There is great urgency in establishing the diagnosis of gonococcal conjunctivitis and Gram stain will usually reveal the Gram-negative intracellular diplococci. Treatment should begin at once with intravenous crystalline penicillin, 50,000 units/kg body weight/day in two divided doses for at least 7 days. It is tempting to use topical agents, but they do not appear to be ef-

Table 20.4
Differential Diagnostic Features of Conjunctivitis

Agent	Onset	Resolves	Comment
$AgNO_3$	Several hours after instillation	24–36 hours	$AgNO_3$ effective against gonococcus but not *Chlamydia*
Bacterial gonococcus	2–4 days after birth	In days with treatment	Marked purulent discharge and edema
Chlamydia	5–12 days after birth	Days to a few weeks	Mild mucopurulent discharge, basophilic intracytoplasmic inclusions in scrapings; may be associated with pneumonia (later onset)
Other bacteria	Any time	In days with treatment	Mild "sticky lids" to acute purulent inflammation, one or both eyes
Viral	Any time, initially in one eye	4 days to 2 weeks	May be associated with corneal changes
Herpes simplex	Any time, unilateral	About 1 week or may be recurrent	Often associated with skin lesions, steroids contraindicated
Allergic	In association with other symptoms most common in spring	As allergies resolved—about 1 week	Itching followed by mild redness and tearing; "ropy" secretions; cobblestone papillae in vernal type

fective. Local hygiene to the affected eye is appropriate. Because the infant acquired the disease from the mother, her treatment is the responsibility of the pediatrician and obstetrician together. If the patient is resistant to penicillin, kanamycin or cefuroxime can be administered.

Most bacterial infections, (including *Chlamydia*), can be treated with topical ointments. In infants with *Chlamydia,* however, systemic erythromycin should be considered because of the likelihood of pneumonia occurring at any time in the first few months of life. For Gram-negative organisms, gentamicin ophthalmic solution four times daily is effective.

No specific therapy is effective for viral conjunctivitis. If herpes simplex is identified and the lesion is progressive, systemic treatment with adenosine arabinoside or acyclovir is appropriate. Referral to an ophthalmologist is essential for slit-lamp evaluation and advice on local care. Steroids should be avoided because they can exacerbate the infection.

REFERENCES

Nishida KI, Risemberg HM: Silver nitrate ophthalmic solution and chemical conjunctivitis. *Pediatrics* 56:368, 1975.

Sandstrom KI, Bell TA, Chandler JW, et al: Microbial causes of neonatal conjunctivitis. *J Pediatr* 105:706, 1984.

Uveitis (Chronic Intraocular Inflammation) 8

Definition

All or part of the uveal tract can be inflamed. Iritis, cyclitis, or choroiditis designate the involved regions. Cells can enter the aqueous humor and be seen by slit-lamp examination. Alternatively, cells can adhere to the posterior corneal surface to produce keratic precipitates (KP). Adhesions may also form as posterior synechiae between the iris and the lens. In choroiditis, inflammatory cells accumulate and may destroy patches of retina and choroid, leaving white areas that can be seen by direct ophthalmoscopy.

DISORDERS

Iridocyclitis (anterior uveitis) occurs in about 15% of patients with *juvenile rheumatoid arthritis* and in some patients with *Kawasaki syndrome*. It is occasionally seen in tuberculosis, sarcoidosis, ulcerative colitis, and rarely in acute viral illnesses.

Posterior uveitis is most commonly caused by congenital toxoplasmosis, which can also cause intracranial calcifications. Choreoretinitis is present in about 80% of diagnosed cases, and is usually bilateral. The diagnosis is most often made when one eye deviates, and a funduscopic examination is undertaken.

Infection with *Toxoplasma goudii* occurs in about 1/1000 births in the United States (Wilson et al 1980). However, only 10% of infected infants are symptomatic in the newborn period. In a prospective 20-year follow-up of 11 congenitally infected children in The Netherlands, new eye lesions appeared as late as 18 years of age. Thus, careful follow-up is mandatory (Koppe et al 1986). (For a discussion of therapy of toxoplasmosis, see pp. 1135.)

Treatment of uveitis is with cycloplegics to lessen the incidence of synechiae and topical steroid to suppress inflammation. The hazard of prolonged exposure to topical steroids is that they can produce glaucoma and cataracts. Serial slit-lamp examinations are required to assess disease activity and monitor effects of therapy.

Prenatal diagnosis of fetal infection was accomplished by a group in Paris on 39 of 42 fetuses. Diagnosis depended on identification of maternal infection followed by culture of fetal blood and amniotic fluid, testing of fetal blood for toxoplasma-specific IgM, and ultrasound examination of fetal brain. All mothers were treated with spiramycin throughout pregnancy (Daffos et al, 1988).

REFERENCES

Burns JC, Joffe L, Sargent R, et al: Anterior uveitis in Kawasaki syndrome. *Pediatr Infect Dis* 4:258, 1985.

Daffos F, Forestier F, Capella-Pavlovsky M, et al: Prenatal management of 746 pregnancies at risk for congenital toxoplasmosis. *N Engl J Med* 318:271, 1988.

Desmonts G, Couvreur J: Congenital toxoplasmosis. A prospective study of 378 pregnancies. *N Engl J Med* 290:1110, 1974.

Koppe JG, Loewer-Sieger DH, deRoever-Bonnet H: Results of 20-year follow-up of congenital toxoplasmosis. *Lancet* 1:254, 1986.

Wilson CB, Remington JS, Stagno S, et al: Development of adverse sequelae in children born with subclinical congenital toxoplasma infection. *Pediatrics* 66:767, 1980.

Wolf MD, Lichter PR, Ragsdate CG: Prognostic factors in the uveitis of juvenile rheumatoid arthritis. *Ophthalmology* 94:1242, 1987.

Periorbital and Orbital Cellulitis

9

Definition

Infection around the eye, including lid and adjacent tissues is termed periorbital cellulitis. It is nearly always unilateral. Infection that extends into the orbit (beyond the fascia that separates orbit from eyelids) is often associated with proptosis and is termed orbital cellulitis. A rapidly spreading infection such as erysipelas involves both areas.

Basic Science

Infection can involve the eye by spread from sinuses into the orbit, or from adjacent skin lesions or trauma (usually periorbital). The most common organism in children under the age of 3 years is *Haemophilus influenzae* type B, which is often spread by hematogenous routes. In older children, periorbital infections are most commonly *Staphylococcus aureus,* but a wide variety of other organisms including fungi can be involved, especially after trauma.

Epidemiology

Periorbital infection occurred in 85% and orbital in 15% of a series of infants hospitalized for eye infections (Gellady et al, 1978). The incidence of infection is not known.

Natural History

Periorbital cellulitis causes lid edema and, often, conjunctivitis. Extraocular movements and vision are normal. Surrounding skin may be involved, with a purplish discoloration, but pain is not prominent. With orbital infection there may be pain and limitation of ocular movements and proptosis. Vision is usually normal. If untreated, cavernous sinus thrombosis, papilledema, and loss of vision can occur.

Diagnosis

Diagnosis is made by inspection. The specific organism responsible may be identified by blood culture (especially *H. influenzae*) or by smear of purulent material. If sinus involvement is suspected, appropriate radiographs should be obtained and sinus drainage may be indicated. In a serial study of traumatic infections, Gellady et al (1978) found β-hemolytic streptococci accounted for 23% of infections and *S. aureus* accounted for another 18%.

Treatment

Mild periorbital infection can be treated with oral antibiotics. If swelling and redness are marked or progressive, and orbital infection is considered possible, hospitalization for intravenous antibiotics is appropriate. Because *H. influenzae* or *S. aureus* are the most likely organisms, intravenous penicillinase-resistant penicillin and chloramphenicol are indicated. Treatment should continue until complete resolution occurs, which is usually in a few days in periorbital infection, but longer (7–10 days) in orbital infection.

REFERENCE

Gellady AM, Shulman ST, Ayoub EM: Periorbital and orbital cellulitis in children. *Pediatrics* 61:272, 1978.

Eyelid Disorders 10

Definition

Anomalies of eyelids include a series of malformations acquired during development, as part of a number of syndromes that affect multiple organs or as a result of injury.

Basic Science

Eyelids consist of four layers: conjunctiva, tarsus, muscle, and skin. Their lubricating and blinking actions are essential to pump tears and foreign bodies from the eye.

TYPES OF ANOMALIES

Eyelids can be part of other constellations of malformations. Colobomas (missing portions of lids) are found in Goldenhar and Treacher Collins syndromes. Fusion of eyelids, termed ankyloblepharon may occur near the inner or outer canthus and represents a developmental anomaly. Downward sloping of palpebral fissures occurs in Treacher Collins syndrome and upward sloping in Down syndrome. Ptosis of upper lid may be bilateral, unilateral, and inherited as an autosomal dominant.

Ectropion or turning out of entire lid margin occurs either as a congenital condition or is acquired from eyelid scarring. Entropion of the eyelid can cause irritation and scarring from rubbing of the lashes against the eye.

Epidemiology

All anomalies of eyelids are rare. Ptosis is the most common of them.

Natural History

If the malformation causes the eyelid to obscure vision, or puts the cornea at risk of exposure, loss of vision or corneal injury will occur.

Diagnosis

Early recognition and referral to an ophthalmologist or surgeon specializing in craniofacial surgery can lead to excellent results and preservation of vision.

Treatment

Partial ptosis is usually not treated surgically before the age of 4–5 years. Other conditions are very rare, and generalizations about treatment are inappropriate; each child must be evaluated in terms of relative risks and advantages of operation (Fig. 20.5*A* and *B*).

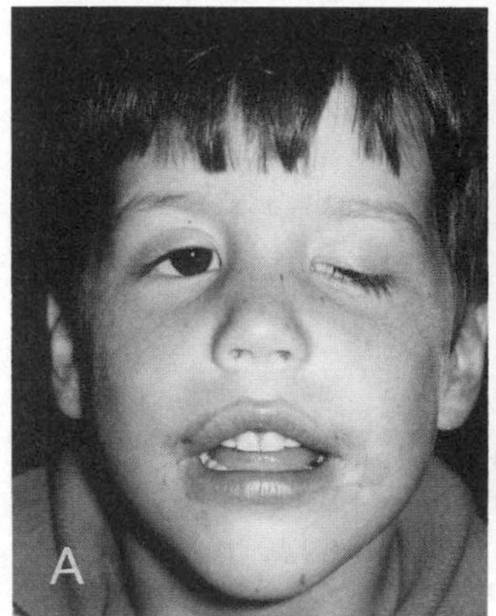

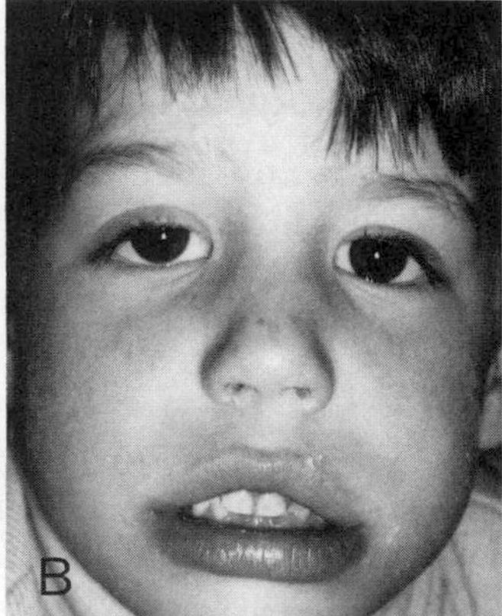

Figure 20.5. Congenital ptosis preoperative (**A**) and postoperative (**B**) (courtesy Dr. Richard Robb).

REFERENCE

Crawford JS: Congenital eyelid anomalies in children. *J Pediatr Ophthalmol Strabis* 21:140, 1984.

Nasolacrimal Duct Obstruction

11

Definition

Obstruction of the nasolacrimal duct can prevent tears from entering the nasopharynx. Usually the obstruction is caused by an imperforate membrane at the nasal end of the duct.

Epidemiology

This is a common abnormality estimated to occur in 1.75–6.0% of newborn infants.

Natural History

Persistent tearing is often first noticed by crusting of the eyelashes. The tears spill over the lower lid and often the eye and surrounding tissues are chronically moist. The condition is usually associated with low-grade infection. The obstruction tends to resolve spontaneously over several months. Up to 80% may clear between 3 and 8 months of age (Petersen and Robb, 1978).

Diagnosis

The diagnosis is suggested by tearing and discharge from an early age in the presence of a white and quiet eye. Pressure over the nasolacrimal sac may produce some mucoid material emerging from the puncta.

Nasolacrimal duct obstruction should be distinguished from lacrimal hypersecretion. Some children with normal lacrimal ducts produce excessive tears intermittently in response to stress. The condition is self-limited (Clarke et al, 1987).

Treatment

Persistence of the obstruction for 8 or more months has generally been thought to be an indication for probing, because most spontaneous improvement has taken place by that time (Nelson et al, 1985). Earlier probing is advocated by some (Baker, 1985). If there is any mucopurulent discharge present, some ophthalmologists recommend the use of topical erythromycin.

Prognosis

The long-term outlook is excellent. The high rate of spontaneous resolution and the success of probing for those that do not resolve means that few children are left with persistent tearing. More extensive surgery is possible if simple probing is not curative.

REFERENCES

Baker JD: Treatment of congenital nasolacrimal system obstruction. *J Pediatr Ophthalmol Strabis* 22:36, 1985.

Clarke WN, Bastianelli F, Noel LP: Lacrimal hypersecretion in children. *J Pediatr Ophthalmol Strabis* 24:204, 1987.

Nelson LB, Calhoun JH, Menduke H: Medical management of congenital nasolacrimal duct obstruction. *Pediatrics* 76:172, 1985.

Petersen RA, Robb RM: The natural course of congenital obstruction of the nasolacrimal duct. *J Pediatr Ophthalmol Strabis* 15:246, 1978.

Robb RM: Treatment of congenital nasolacrimal system obstruction. *J Pediatr Ophthalmol Strabis* 22:36, 1985.

MARY ELLEN AVERY

Consultant
Richard Robb

Section 21

Dentistry

The primary dentition forms the basis for the size and shape of the permanent dental arches. Failure to maintain optimal dental health in both the primary and permanent dentitions can result not only in the loss of function, but also in the impairment of general health or the exacerbation of existing disease.

Children may be seen by a dentist before the eruption of primary teeth, but routine visits should start no later than age 2 years. At the initial dental visit, oral examination, formal instruction on oral hygiene techniques, dietary counseling, and fluoride recommendations are given to the parent(s). Radiographs may be taken when pathology is suspected, when eruption patterns are in question, or periodically to detect caries. Fluoride applications and follow-up examinations are generally repeated semiannually after tooth eruption, but may be more frequent depending on caries experience and treatment needs.

The pediatrician should assess symmetry of the face and alveolar ridges, observe the buccal and vestibular spaces, and note the eruption pattern and quality of the teeth. Cleaning of the dentition begins with the cleaning of the gum pads in the newborn by use of a moist face cloth or gauze pad. Plaque removal must be initiated with the eruption of the first tooth.

Fluoride supplementation should begin at or shortly after birth for children living in *suboptimally* fluoridated areas (see Table 21.1). Adequate fluoride intake is the single most effective method for caries reduction and assuring it in early childhood either through the food chain or through dietary supplementation remains a major responsibility of the pediatrician and the pediatric dentist. Fluorosis (see Anomalies of Tooth Structure) is the most common consequence of excessive ingestion of fluoride and has been observed with increasing frequency in recent years. Fluorosis is characterized by brown staining and hypoplasia of enamel in its most acute form, or as white opacities (marblized enamel) in its milder form (Glenn et al, 1984).

Early medical visits are the best opportunities to teach the importance of oral health and its relation to our general health. Referral to a pediatric dentist who specializes in the care of children should be considered, because the practitioner who routinely treats children more readily understands their developmental status and recognizes pediatric dental problems. Handicapped children or children whose behavior is a problem can best be managed by the pediatric dentist who has been trained in methods of behavioral modification, in the use of conscious sedation techniques and in the utilization of the surgical operating suite and general anesthesia in the hospital setting. Complex management and complex dental treatment alike are indications for referral to the pediatric dentist (O'Donnell and Cohen, 1985).

Table 21.1
Supplemental Fluoride Dosage Schedule [1]

Age (yr)	Supplement of Fluoride (mg) — Concentration of Fluoride in Water (ppm) 0–0.3	0.3–0.7	0.7
Birth–2	0.25	0.	0
2–3	0.50	0.25	0
3–14	1.00	0.50	0

[1] From: Protocol for fluoride therapy. *Pediatr Dent* 7:338–339, 1985.

Disorders of Oral Hard Tissues—Dentition

1

ANOMALIES OF TOOTH ERUPTION

Definition

Tooth eruption refers to the general phenomenon of tooth movement from the early developmental stage to the establishment of the tooth's position in full occlusion.

Natural History

Primary teeth develop by the 12th week of embryonic life. Calcification begins about 14 weeks. Permanent teeth are developed starting at the 4th or 5th month. The normal chronology of eruption and shedding is shown in Tables 21.2 and 21.3. Wide variation exists among individuals. In general, only poor correlation exists between dental age and bone age or chronological age (Grahnan and Grahnan, 1961; Lunt and Law, 1974).

Diagnosis

Because the range of variation in normal eruption time for both the primary and permanent dentitions is so broad, it is often difficult to determine when any specific individual lies outside the norm. When gross variations in timing and/or atypical clinical findings exist, however, a pathologic disorder should be considered.

The presence of a tooth at birth (natal tooth) or eruption within the first 2 months after birth (neonatal tooth) occurs in about 1/1400 live births (Kates et al, 1984). In 95% of these cases, the teeth are normal primary mandibular central incisors and are believed to have erupted prematurely because of an ectopic location of the tooth germ within the alveolar bone. If possible, these teeth should be left in place and allowed to develop a normal attachment to the bone. Natal or neonatal teeth should be removed only if they are extremely mobile inasmuch as it is then unlikely that they will gain a normal reattachment and/or they interfere with nursing. Almost half of the natal and neonatal teeth will be lost within the first 4 months of life; if they survive beyond this period they are likely to be retained as normal primary teeth. Natal teeth have been associated with various congenital anomalies such as chondroectodermal dysplasia and Ellis-van Creveld syndrome.

Generalized accelerated eruption of the primary permanent dentition is rare, but can be a result of a systemic endocrine disturbance, e.g., hyperthyroidism or precocious puberty. In addition, early eruption can

Table 21.2
Chronology of Eruption of the Primary and Permanent Dentition

	Maxillary	Mandible
Primary[1]		
Central incisor	10 (8-12)	8 (6-10)
Lateral incisor	11 (9-13)	13 (10-16)
Canine	19 (16-22)	20 (17-23)
First molar	16 (13-19 boys) (14-19 girls)	16 (14-18)
Second molar	29 (25-33)	27 (23-31)
Permanent[2]		
Central incisor	7-7.5	6-6.5
Lateral incisor	8-8.5	7.2-7.7
Canine	11-11.6	9.7-10.2
First premolar	10-10.3	10-10.7
Second premolar	10.7-11.2	10.7-11.5
First molar	6-6.3	6-6.2
Second molar	12.2-12.7	11.7-12
Third molar	20.5	20-20.5

[1]Eruption: mean age in months + 1 SD; from Lunt RC, Law DB: *J Am Dent Assoc* 89:878, 1974.
[2]Eruption: mean age in years; from Burdi AR. The development and eruption of the human dentitions. In: Forrester DJ, Wagoner ML, Fleming J (eds): *Pediatric Dental Medicine*. Chapter 5, Philadelphia, Lea & Febiger, 1981.

Table 21.3
Sequence of Primary Tooth Exfoliation

			Mean Age (year.month)	
Rank	Mandibular Arch	Maxillary Arch	Boys	Girls
First	Central incisors		6.0	5.7
Second		Central incisors	6.10	6.7
Third	Lateral incisors		7.2	6.10
Fourth		Lateral incisors	7.10	7.5
Fifth	Canines		10.5	9.7
Sixth	First molars		10.8	10.2
Seventh		First molars	10.11	10.6
Eighth		Canines	11.3	10.7
Ninth	Second molars	Second molars	11.9	11.5

[1]Ages are for right side of mouth; however, exfoliation is generally bilaterally symmetrical. From Ripa LW, Lesks GS, Sposato AL, et al: Chronology and sequence of exfoliation of primary teeth. *J Am Dent Assoc* 105:641, 1982.

be seen in hemifacial hypertrophy and in the affected areas of the dental arch in Sturge-Weber syndrome. Premature or accelerated eruption of an individual permanent tooth is usually the result of an infection and premature loss of its preceding primary tooth but can also be due to acrodynia, histiocytosis, hypophosphatasia or Papillon-Levere syndrome.

A generalized delayed eruption of the primary or permanent dentition can have a variety of systemic causes, including prematurity and/or low birth weight, severe malnutrition, hypothyroidism, hypopituitarism, rickets, as well as several entities such as Down syndrome, cleidocranial or craniofacial dysostosis, and hemifacial atrophy. Local factors may also result in a delay or even total failure of eruption of individual teeth; such factors include crowding of the dental arch, disturbances of morphologic tooth development (e.g., peg laterals), abnormal placement of the tooth bud within the alveolar bone (rotations), cysts or odontoma formation around the developing tooth and presence of supernumerary teeth or malformed primary teeth (e.g., fusion).

The ectopic eruption of teeth is not unusual and is most commonly seen in the early mixed dentition when crowding exists. In these cases, the mandibular incisors often will erupt ectopically, most frequently lingual to the primary incisors. The deflection of erupting succedaneous teeth can also occur in other areas, such as the canine/premolar region, when the dental arch may be too small, or when primary teeth are lost prematurely. Ectopic eruption can also be the result of some of the same factors that cause localized delayed eruption (see above). Even the agenesis of teeth may cause abnormal paths of eruption of adjacent teeth.

The total failure of tooth eruption, i.e., impaction, can result from many of the same causes as delayed or ectopic eruption; in the most severe cases, a tooth may be prevented from erupting because of a physical barrier. Although any tooth may become impacted, those most commonly impacted are the third molars (wisdom teeth) and the permanent maxillary canines.

It is not uncommon for one or more primary molars to appear to be "submerging" into the alveolar bone. This phenomenon, which is clinically detectable when the teeth appear at a level lower than the height of the surrounding teeth, is due to ankylosis of a portion of the root of the primary tooth to the surrounding bone, probably because the periodontal ligament is altered or damaged. This prevents the tooth from continuing to "erupt passively" with vertical growth of the alveolar bone, and the adjacent teeth appear to "submerge." There is a familial tendency for submergence of teeth and it is probably an inherited trait.

Treatment

Treatment of delayed eruption, ectopic eruption, or impaction is directed at removing the physical barrier interfering with eruption, usually accomplished through orthodontics, surgery, or a combination of the two. If a submerging tooth causes the surrounding teeth to tip over and there is loss in arch length, treatment may involve extraction of the offending tooth, followed by placement of a space maintainer to prevent tooth movement and space loss.

Prognosis

The prognosis for anomalies of eruption is good if early diagnosis is made. If left undetected and untreated, these teeth may cause damage to the adjacent teeth or require complex surgical removal.

Prevention

Early intervention with surgery and/or orthodontic care can often prevent delayed or ectopic eruptions as well as impaction of teeth.

ANOMALIES OF TOOTH MORPHOLOGY

Definition

Anomalies of tooth morphology include developmental disturbances in which the teeth are normal in structure, but tooth morphology has been altered at an early stage of development. This includes anomalies of tooth number, size, and shape.

Basic Science

The primitive tooth-forming tissue called the dental lamina can be identified as early as the 6th week of gestation. The dental lamina is derived embryologically from neural crest cells and appears in the epithelial thickening at the lateral margins of the stomodeum. Individual tooth development is initiated at specific sites along the dental lamina. Odontogenesis, or tooth development, proceeds from this early prenatal beginning well into adolescence. Control of these developmental phenomena appears to be multifactorial, primarily polygenetic, with some environmental influence. Numerous etiologies can affect odontogenesis at any one or multiple stages; these include genetic or chromosomal abnormalities; inborn errors of metabolism; irradiation; fever; immunizations; allergies; infection (viral and bacterial, local, or systemic); nutritional deficiencies; cerebral palsy (neonatal anoxia); endocrinopathies; and mechanical trauma.

Epidemiology

The most commonly missing teeth are the permanent third molars, maxillary lateral incisors, and the second premolars. Agenesis has been reported to occur with varied frequency depending on the population studied. Hypodontia of the permanent dentition is so common as to be considered a variant of normal. Frequency estimates for the agenesis of various teeth range from 2.3–9.6% of the population (excluding third molars). Congenital absence of primary teeth is less common and is usually limited to the incisor region. Hyperdontia of the permanent dentition (supernumerary teeth) is not uncommon and occurs in 1–3% of the Caucasian population. Hyperdontia of the primary dentition usually in the maxillary incisor region occurs in about 0.5% of the population (Grahnan and Grahnan, 1961).

Natural History

Anomalies of tooth number, agenesis (missing teeth), or supernumerary teeth (more than the normal complement of teeth) are genetically controlled. Before eruption, the absence (or presence) of a specific tooth may only be confirmed radiographically. When a primary tooth is missing, its succedaneous permanent tooth is also congenitally absent. Existence of more than one congenitally missing tooth, i.e., oligodontia, suggests the possibility of a genetic disorder. Oligodontia can be associated with such disorders as Down syndrome, incontinentia pigmenti, Ellis-van Creveld syndrome, the oral-facial-digital syndromes, and anhidrotic ectodermal dysplasia. Total absence of teeth or anodontia has been observed with ectodermal dysplasia (Fig. 21.1). In patients with cleft lip and/or palate, congenitally missing teeth in the area of clefting are common. In many of these entities, the teeth are often morphologically abnormal as well; the incisors may be small and conically shaped. Environmental influences such as radiation and viral infections (e.g., rubella) also can cause hypodontia.

Anomalies in Tooth Number

Diagnosis

The most frequently occurring permanent supernumerary tooth is the so-called "mesiodens," which is located at or near the midline of the incisor region in the maxilla and is usually conically shaped. Most often, mesiodens fail to erupt and, thus, prevent the normal eruption of one or more of the surrounding permanent maxillary central incisors (usually between ages 6 and 8 years). Multiple supernumerary teeth are associated with such syndromes as cleidocranial dysostosis, Gardner syndrome, Hallermann-Streiff syndrome, and the oral-facial-digital syndromes. Patients with cleft lip and/or palate often have primary and/or permanent supernumerary teeth in the area of the clefting.

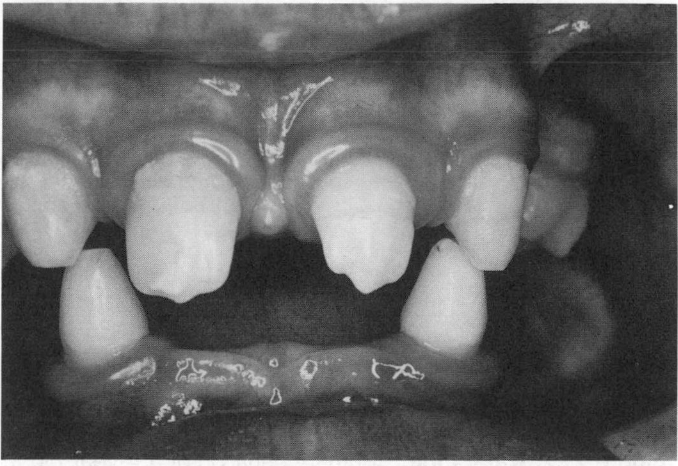

Figure 21.1. Ectodermal Dysplasia. Early mixed dentition of an 8-year-old boy with anhydrotic ectodermal dysplasia. Note multiple congenitally missing primary and permanent teeth, and conical morphology. A combination of orthodontic and prosthetic dental management will be necessary to restore this dentition cosmetically and functionally.

Treatment

If normal tooth eruption is impeded, removal of the supernumerary tooth or teeth may be necessary to allow normal eruption and alignment of adjacent teeth. If eruption is not impeded, the supernumerary tooth should be removed at age 10–12 years when all teeth in the vicinity are fully developed.

Anomalies of Size and Shape

Diagnosis

Morphologic variations in size and shape of teeth are not uncommon. The teeth that are most frequently congenitally absent, i.e., the permanent maxillary lateral incisors, second premolars, and third molars, also are most likely to show morphologic variation. The maxillary lateral incisor may be small and conical, i.e., "peg-shaped." Teeth present in the area of clefting of the alveolar ridges in cleft lip and/or palate patients are often conically shaped. Generalized microdontia and morphologic abnormalities of the dentition are rare, but they may be present in such entities as ectodermal dysplasia, congenital rubella, Down syndrome, and incontinentia pigmenti. In these disorders, the molars often appear "mulberry-like" in shape while the incisors are conically shaped.

Generalized macrodontia, or abnormally large teeth have been associated with pituitary gigantism and hemihypertrophy, both of which are rare. Macrodontia of individual teeth is also rare and should not be confused with "fused teeth."

Cojoined teeth may appear in both the primary and permanent dentitions. Three variations of cojoined teeth exist; gemination, twinning, and/or fusion. Gemination is an abortive attempt by a single tooth bud to divide. The extent of invagination of the tooth bud will determine the amount of cleavage or notching of a single crown. Twinning occurs when the abnormal cleavage of a tooth bud is complete and a supernumerary tooth is created, which is a mirror image of its adjacent partner tooth. Fusion is the embryologic union of discrete tooth germs and is more common in the primary dentition than in the permanent dentition. Fusion results in a reduced number of teeth in the dental arch and is not uncommon in the maxillary and mandibular lateral incisor/canine regions.

Other morphologic abnormalities that are not uncommon include shovel-shaped incisors among the Asian races and an extrapalatal cusp on the maxillary permanent molars or cusp of Carabelli in the general population.

Treatment

Treatment of these morphologic abnormalities consists of appropriate surgery and/or restorative reconstruction of the malformed tooth.

Prevention

Because numerous causes exist, there is no single basic approach to prevention. Recognition and treatment of preventable insults can help to decrease the effect on odontogenesis. Once a morphologic anomaly is noted, intervention can help prevent complex sequelae.

ANOMALIES OF TOOTH STRUCTURE

Definition

Anomalies of tooth structure include abnormalities of the hard tissues of the teeth, i.e., enamel and dentin.

Basic Science

The outer 2–3 mm of a tooth consist of enamel, which in its mature state is highly mineralized, containing 96–98% inorganic substance. Dentin, a yellowish-white hard dental tissue, lies under the enamel and constitutes the main portion of the tooth. The internal surface of the dentin forms the walls of the pulp chamber. Because the pulpal tissues extend into the dentinal matrix, dentin is considered a vital tissue. Dentin is 75% inorganic with the remainder organic tissue. Both hard tissues are formed through the deposition of incremental concentric layers of extracellular organic matrix (apposition) followed by mineralization (calcification) of this matrix. The inorganic matrix of both dentin and enamel is primarily hydroxyapatite, which is laid down either concomitantly with or immediately after formation of the organic matrix.

Natural History

The deposition of the concentric layers of the dental hard tissues is normally extremely regular and interference with its development may be clinically evident in various abnormalities of tooth structure. Thus, the location and extent of the structural defects can serve as a chronologic marker indicating the time and extent of the insult both pre- and postnatally.

Anomalies of Enamel Development

Diagnosis

These disorders include the incomplete or defective formation of the enamel of teeth. The defect can be localized to one tooth or occur in all teeth, indicating a systemic insult. Within a single tooth, the hypoplastic defect can be localized to one area as evidenced by grooves, pits, or depressed areas of enamel. The color may be normal, yellow, or even brown depending on the source of the insult. Hypoplasia may appear linear, encircling the tooth or teeth horizontally, thus indicating a developmental effect limited to a short period of time (Fig. 21.6, pp. 1238). The exact location of the defect on the crown can help to identify the approximate date of the insult (Cohen and Diner, 1970). In the most severe and prolonged disturbances (genetic or systemic), the enamel may be totally defective in both primary and permanent teeth.

Most primary teeth show a small area of arrested calcification of the enamel corresponding to the time of birth. This neonatal line is usually observable only microscopically; however, trauma associated with birth, such as anoxia, prematurity, and/or nutritional deficiencies, may cause a clinically detectable enamel defect. In these cases, the neonatal line appears as a linear hypoplastic defect in the middle third of the primary maxillary central incisors and incisal third of the lateral incisors (Fig. 21.2). Nutritional deficiencies can also result in defective enamel formation, particularly vitamin D deficiency, although vitamin A and C deficiencies have also been implicated as have deficiencies in calcium, phosphorus, magnesium, and protein. The exanthematous diseases, such as chickenpox, measles, and scarlet fever, as well as any febrile disease, can cause enamel hypoplasia. Bacterial infections, such as congenital syphilis, and viral infections, such as rubella, have been associated with specific structural defects as well as morphologic defects of the enamel. Trauma to and/or infection of primary teeth can result in a hypoplastic defect to succedaneous teeth. Irradiation of at least 1500 rads to developing tooth germs will arrest their development at the stage corresponding to the time of insult, which can result in complete agenesis of the teeth, incomplete tooth formation, microdontia, altered crown morphology, and hypoplastic defects. Drug intoxication can also interfere with enamel formation, e.g., fluorosis and hypervitaminosis D. Genetic factors are responsible for amelogenesis imperfecta, an inherited hypoplastic defect of enamel which involves the entire enamel of all teeth to different degrees.

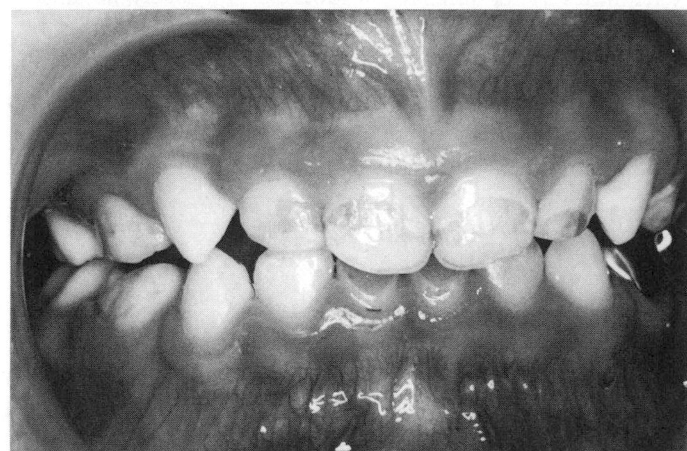

Figure 21.2. Natal Line. Primary dentition of a 4-year-old female who was born in Colombia, South America. Note the broad band of hypoplastic enamel of the maxillary central and lateral incisors, as well as the mandibular central incisors, referred to as the natal line, corresponding to those portions of the primary teeth calcifying perinatally. Nutritional deprivation during tooth formation may result in dysplastic enamel.

Treatment

Treatment of hypoplastic defects involves cosmetic and functional restoration of the defective enamel. Various dental restorative materials, such as composite resins, acrylic, porcelain and, in posterior teeth, various metal restorations such as stainless steel, nonprecious metal, or gold are used to restore defective teeth. Techniques such as bonding, veneering, or full coverage of the affected teeth are utilized in application of these materials.

Anomalies of Dentin Development

Diagnosis

Defects of dentin development can be grouped into those that are primary diseases of dentin itself (e.g., dentinogenesis imperfecta and dentin dysplasia) and those in which the dentinal defect is associated with defects of other tissue systems (e.g., vitamin D-resistant rickets). Dentinogenesis imperfecta (also commonly known as hereditary opalescent dentin) is an inherited defect which occurs in both the primary and permanent dentition, and is reported in about 1 in 8000 individuals. Dentinogenesis imperfecta may be associated with osteogenesis imperfecta; in the latter disorder, the primary teeth are affected in 80% of patients, and only 35% of patients show effects on the permanent dentition. Soon after these teeth erupt, the enamel chips away from the defective dentin, resulting in rapid wear of the teeth, which appear opalescent, almost amber-like. Dentin dysplasia is similar to dentinogenesis imperfecta. It affects both the primary and permanent dentition and clinically is characterized by early loosening and premature exfoliation. In vitamin D-resistant rickets, the dentin is defective, resulting in loss of vitality and abscess formation with draining fistulas commonly seen in the primary dentition. The enamel is normal, in contrast to vitamin D-dependent rickets where enamel is also defective. Dentinal defects also can be associated with other diseases, such as Albright hereditary osteodystrophy, generalized calcinosis, and Ehlers-Danlos syndrome and, indeed, may be the first overt symptoms of these systemic disorders.

Treatment

Treatment of dentinal defects consists of early recognition and prophylactic restoration of the posterior teeth with full crowns of prefabricated stainless steel for primary and precious metal/porcelain for permanent posterior teeth. Cosmetic restoration of the anterior teeth is accomplished with resins, acrylics, porcelain veneers or full crowns.

Staining of Teeth

Diagnosis

Intrinsic staining of the dental hard tissues can be caused either by changes in the structure or thickness of dental hard tissues or by coloring agents taken up by these tissues during their formation. Structural changes that occur in dental fluorosis can result in a white discoloration of the enamel, i.e., enamel opacities, which also occur in a small percentage of the general population even without fluoride exposure. If the fluorosis is severe, the enamel appears "mottled," i.e., yellow to brown and hypoplastic.

Pathologic changes in the pulp of teeth can result in a uniform discoloration of the crown; e.g., gray indicating hemorrhage or necrosis, yellow indicating calcification, or pink indicating resorption. The dental hard tissues also can be intrinsically discolored by endogenous coloring agents that are incorporated into their structure during development; e.g., erythroblastosis fetalis (bluish-green to yellow, brown, or black), biliary atresia (green), congenital porphyria (pinkish-brown), and tetracycline ingestion (gray-brown, yellow, or brown depending on which group was ingested). If taken during pregnancy and the first 3 months of age, chlortetracyclines discolor deciduous teeth; permanent teeth are discolored when drugs are given between birth and 6 years.

Intrinsic staining of enamel and/or dentin should be distinguished from extrinsic staining of accumulated plaque on the enamel surface. Among the causes of extrinsic staining are: the effects of chromogenic bacteria of the oral cavity (which most commonly stain the plaque green, although brown, black, or orange stains can occur); various foods, beverages, and tobacco; and metallic compounds, such as iron supplements which often stain plaque gray-black.

Treatment

Extrinsic staining is best treated by professional dental prophylaxis and can be prevented by meticulous oral hygiene. Intrinsic staining is more difficult to remove and requires specialized bleaching techniques (external or internal) or cosmetic veneering on restorations.

DENTAL CARIES

Definition

Dental caries is an infectious disease of tooth structural elements, the outcome of which is progressive destruction of tooth substance. This is a result of metabolic products of microorganisms interacting with plaque on tooth surfaces and the inorganic and organic components of enamel, dentin, and/or cementum.

Basic Science

Dental plaque, the soft noncalcified deposit that adheres to tooth surfaces, is associated with the carious process. Plaque consists of bacteria (its major component) and other insoluble products, such as salivary proteins, desquamated epithelial cells and trapped food particles. Plaque accumulates on tooth surfaces when a sticky, thin, absorbent salivary coating called the acquired enamel pellicle coats the enamel. Indigenous oral microorganisms are then transported to the tooth surfaces via saliva and attach to the enamel pellicle. The bacteria of the oral cavity that can colonize the tooth surfaces are those which produce extracellular polysaccharides, thus allowing the bacteria to adhere to the smooth tooth surfaces as well as to one another. *Streptococcus mutans* is the organism most consistently implicated in the caries process. Other organisms in plaque, however, such as lactobacilli, are acidogenic and can cause caries. Many of these bacteria are anaerobic, thus, the ingested dietary carbohydrates are incompletely oxidized and produce acid rather than carbon dioxide and water. The acid production results in a significant decrease in the local pH (to below 5) of the plaque on the tooth surface, thus favoring demineralization of enamel. Because the acid products cannot easily diffuse out of the polysaccharide matrix, nor can the salivary buffers easily reach deep into the plaque, the low pH is maintained until stimulated saliva acts as a buffer and neutralization occurs, usually in about 30 minutes. The normally high pH and high ion content of saliva favors remineralization of enamel providing a natural protective mechanism against decay.

Unfortunately, frequent ingestion of fermentable carbohydrates allows demineralization of enamel for significant periods of time, which eventually leads to dental decay. Sucrose is the chief offender although other carbohydrates, such as fructose and glucose, are also cariogenic. The form of the food (which affects how long it is retained in the mouth), the frequency of intake, and the sucrose content of the diet are strongly correlated to dental caries.

Epidemiology

According to a 1979–1980 National Institute of Dental Research survey, only 36.6% of the 43.5 million United States children between 5 and 17 years of age were estimated to be free from caries (1981). By contrast, 7.7% of these children had nine or more decayed, missing, or filled (DMF) teeth. By the age of 5 years, children had an average of four decayed or filled *primary* tooth surfaces. By age 12 years, United States children had an average of four decayed, missing, or filled *permanent* tooth surfaces and this number rose to 11 by age 17 years. Females had a slightly higher caries prevalence than had males at all ages and rural communities had a higher prevalence of caries (probably due to the absence of water fluoridation).

Natural History

Dental decay is initiated on the smooth surfaces of teeth and in their developmental pits and fissures. If left untreated, caries progresses from a small white spot on the surface of the enamel to a cavitation of the tooth structure. This progressive softening and staining of the tooth structure continues through the enamel and enters the dentin. Because dentin contains less inorganic material than does enamel, caries progresses more rapidly within dentin. The rate of progress depends on the thickness of enamel and dentin (which varies from tooth to tooth) as well as on other factors, such as diet, oral hygiene practices, and genetic susceptibility. Once the carious process approaches the pulpal tissues, clinical symptoms may be present. Pulpal hyperemia and inflammation will develop, and if left untreated, will result in irreversible pulpal degeneration. A periapical infection will eventually develop leading to formation of an acute or chronic dental alveolar abscess, which can then extend through the alveolar bone into the soft tissue fascial planes of the face and/or neck resulting in cellulitis.

Diagnosis

Dental caries can be diagnosed by clinical examination, radiographic interpretation, and/or symptoms. Small carious lesions appear early as a white spot on the enamel surface, but are not readily detectable radiographically and are not symptomatic. As the lesion progresses and cavitation begins, the lesion may appear yellow-brownish, may be evident as a radiolucent area radiograhically and often becomes symptomatic, showing sensitivity to dietary sweets and/or thermal changes in the oral cavity. This sharp lancing pain is dentinal in origin and usually lasts only while the stimulus is present. Once the lesion has reached deeply into the dentin and approaches the pulp, signs and symptoms of pulpitis will become evident. During the initial phases, sensitivity to chemical and/or thermal stimulus may last beyond the stimulation. As infection of the pulp progresses, the pain becomes spontaneous and is described as dull and throbbing. Clinically, the tooth may become mobile within the alveolar socket and/or sensitive to percussion, indicating edema of the periodontal ligament surrounding the root. A radiolucent area may appear on radiographs around the apex of the root or between the roots of primary teeth indicating extension of the infection into the surrounding bone. The periapical infection can then move laterally through the alveolar bone and soft tissues and establish purulent drainage through a fistula, i.e., a chronic alveolar abscess. If the progress of the infection is apical and drainage is not spontaneously established, an acute alveolar abscess may develop. Clinically, this may appear as a swelling in the mucobuccal fold next to the offending tooth which usually is exquisitely tender to percussion and chewing. Infection can then spread through the fascial planes and develop into a cellulitis involving the face and/or neck regions. Localized lymphadenopathy is usually evident together with systemic signs and symptoms including malaise and fever.

In many cases, the carious process may be insidious and the symptoms may not be severe enough to compel the individual to seek professional care.

Treatment

The goals in the treatment of dental caries include the halting of the tooth destruction, prevention of the progress of the decay into the pulpal tissues, and restoration of the tooth to its original form and size. Incipient carious lesions may be arrested by changing the balance of the carious process toward remineralization. This can be accomplished by practicing ideal oral hygiene, decreasing the sucrose intake, and by the use of various topical fluoride applications. Once frank cavitation of the enamel occurs, the decay must be removed mechanically. Local anesthesia is required to prevent stimulation of the sensitive dentin during caries removal. This is especially important for children who are usually unable to tolerate extensive excavation for long periods of time. If the child is very young (under 4 years of age) nitrous oxide/oxygen sedation along with local anesthesia may be required to allay apprehension.

Currently, silver amalgam is primarily used in the restoration of posterior teeth and tooth-colored resinous materials are used in anterior teeth. Resinous materials, however, are being developed for use in posterior teeth. If the caries destruction involves a large portion of the tooth, crowns covering the entire tooth may be indicated in order to prevent further breakdown. Stainless steel is generally used for crowning primary teeth, while gold, porcelain, or combinations of these are used on mature permanent teeth.

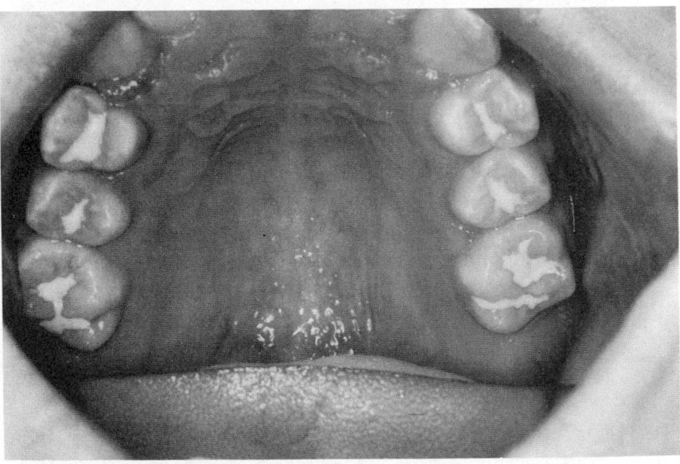

Figure 21.3. Sealants. Permanent dentition of an 11-year-old female with pit and fissure sealant applied to the maxillary first molars and premolars. The individual had deep anatomical fissures of the occlusal surfaces of these teeth. In order to "seal" these developmental grooves, a bonding technique was utilized to retain this white, resinous material. Clinical studies have shown significant long-term caries reduction with this technique.

Prevention

Dental caries is a preventable disease. Systemic fluoride therapy initiated at birth via water fluoridation or systemic fluoride supplementation decreases dental decay on the smooth surface of the teeth by about 60% (see pp. 34). Topical fluoride agents in the form of dentrifices, rinses, and gels can further decrease the incidence of caries activity by as much as 30%, although this figure is somewhat lower in optimally fluoridated communities.

The chewing surfaces of teeth are the most susceptible to decay and the least benefited by fluoride therapy. The single application and bonding of resinous materials to "seal" the developmental grooves of these surfaces (Fig. 21.3) have reduced caries between 80 and 100% after 2 years (Ripa, 1980). Although the effectiveness of sealants decreases slightly with time, they remain about 60% effective after their initial application. Moreover, if sealants are partially or totally lost, they can be reapplied. Sealants are most frequently used on the first and second permanent molars, but primary molars, permanent premolars, and others with developmental defects can be sealed if they appear caries-prone (Handelman et al, 1985).

Limiting the intake of dietary sugars can decrease dental caries significantly. A dietary analysis is helpful in identifying poor dietary habits for both patients and their parents so that more appropriate foods can be substituted for those with a high sugar content.

The practice of good oral hygiene plays a significant role in the prevention of dental caries. Children should be assisted in toothbrushing as teeth erupt. Only when children achieve adequate dexterity and interest (ages 6–8 years) should parental assistance give way to parental supervision. Flossing should be instituted when teeth develop contacts (usually after age 3–4 years). Brushing and flossing before bedtime is of paramount importance, as caries activity is higher at night when salivary flow decreases. Brushing in the morning as well as after meals or snacks is also beneficial. Modification of eating habits to avoid between-meal carbohydrates is recommended. Fruits, cheese, or nuts are preferable (Shaw, 1987).

CONTROVERSY

The effectiveness and necessity of prenatal fluoride supplementation remain controversial. As early as 1966, the U.S. Food and Drug Administration banned the advertising and marketing of fluoride products that claim caries-preventive benefits when ingested as a prenatal supplement. This ban was based on equivocal studies showing their effectiveness. Recently, there has been renewed interest in use of prenatal supplements. In several studies, virtually all children whose mothers had ingested fluorides during pregnancy were caries-free (Glenn et al, 1984). Although remarkable, these studies have been criticized for small sample size and lack of adequately matched control groups.

The need for fluoride supplementation of exclusively breast-fed children in fluoridated communities is also controversial. Because these children are not receiving any substantial amounts of fluoridated water, it has been recommended that supplemental fluoride be given to them, but no definitive trials exist demonstrating the necessity for this supplementation. Satisfactory reduction in the incidence of caries can probably be accomplished even without fluoride supplementation in the initial few months of life. Moreover, breast milk does contain small amounts of fluoride, ranging from trace amounts to two-tenths of a part per million depending on assay method.

NEW DEVELOPMENTS

For the past several years, research on animal and human populations has been underway to develop an oral caries vaccine. Antibodies to *S. mutans* can be induced through oral administration of freeze-dried serotype C (the most prevalent form of *S. mutans* found in humans). While this approach has been shown to reduce the number of organisms, as yet no reduction of caries activity has been demonstrated.

Disorders of Oral Soft Tissues 2

DEVELOPMENTAL ANOMALIES

Definition

Developmental anomalies of the oral soft tissues are present at birth or arise from formative tissues. They are usually evident before the dentition is fully developed and functional. These include several innocuous neonatal anomalies, such as Bohn nodules, Epstein pearls, and dental lamina cysts. Of more concern in the natal period is the congenital epulis and neuroectodermal tumor, i.e., a tumor of neural crest origin occurring on the alveolar ridges in newborns and infants.

Some developmental anomalies are not evident until after the neonatal period. Cysts such as follicular or dentigerous cysts arise from the developmental sac surrounding teeth. Midpalatal cysts have their origin early in embryonic development, but are not evident until they are revealed by dental radiographs or until problems arise in tooth eruption. Finally, the so-called eruption cyst, although not a true cyst, appears as a raised bluish area overlying teeth just before they erupt.

Epidemiology

Nodular anomalies such as Bohn nodules and Epstein pearls are common in newborns and may be found in as many as 80% of infants examined within 24 hours of birth (Fromm, 1967). Dental lamina cysts are found less frequently, usually along the crest of the alveolar ridges. They may be bilateral or quadrilateral. Congenital epulis and neuroectodermal tumors are found infrequently.

Eruption cysts/hematomas are frequently present, although infrequently observed (Fig. 21.4). Because they are painless, usually occur within 48 hours of eruption and disappear on eruption, they may go unnoticed. Occasionally, the emergence of tooth cusps may stimulate hypertrophy of the dental sac tissue which may then focus attention on those areas. Follicular, dentigerous, and midpalatal cysts are true cysts but are unusual.

Natural History

Nonpathogenic anomalies of dental soft tissues are painless and usually resolve without interference. Dental lamina cysts disappear during the first several weeks of life. Eruption cysts are usually present just before tooth eruption and resolve without treatment as the tooth emerges. Congenital epulis and neuroectodermal tumors continue to enlarge producing a problem by space occupied and, for the neuroectodermal tumor, by invasion.

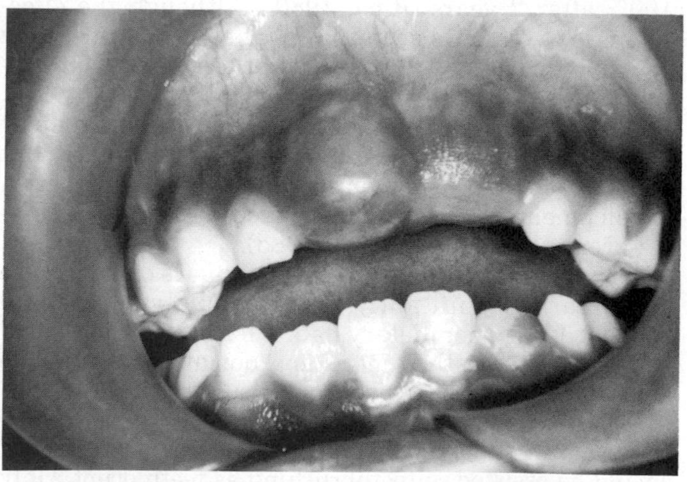

Figure 21.4. Eruption Hematoma. This 7-year-old black female presents with a gingival hematoma over an erupting maxillary right permanent central incisor. It is not uncommon to find bleeding into the developmental sac surrounding the tooth just before eruption.

Midpalatal, follicular, and dentigerous cysts have the potential for further degeneration, neoplastic change, and enlargement. These sequelae may cause displacement of other structures, expansion, or increase the susceptibility to bony fracture.

Diagnosis

Intraoral changes on the oral mucosa or on the alveolar ridges in the newborn are easily observed and identified. The differentiation between Bohn nodules and Epstein pearls is based on location, inasmuch as they may be histologically similar. Dental lamina cysts occur on the crests of the alveolar ridges.

Eruption hematomas or cysts occur with tooth eruption and are usually not present for more than 48 hours. They are raised, soft and bluish, and correspond chronologically to the age-appropriate eruption of teeth. Follicular and dentigerous cysts should be suspected when teeth fail to erupt and these and midpalatal cysts require radiographic examination for diagnosis. The presence of tumors of the alveolar ridge is obvious on examination either within the oral cavity or by their expansion of the alveolar ridges. These conditions are diagnosed after biopsy and radiographic examination.

Treatment

No treatment is necessary for Epstein pearls, Bohn nodules, dental lamina cysts, or eruption cysts/hematomas. Dental lamina cysts may exist for several weeks or months but fluids are absorbed and cystic areas disappear. There is usually no disturbance of feeding or function.

Congenital epulis and neuroectodermal tumors of childhood must be excised to prevent interference with oral growth and development. Recurrence in both cases is unusual.

The follicular, dentigerous, and midpalatal cysts or, indeed, any impediment to tooth eruption, also should be surgically removed and the erupting tooth exposed. Care must be taken to remove epithelial lining of the cyst to prevent recurrence. In some cases, unerupted teeth must be surgically exposed and guided into position by orthodontic measures.

Prevention

Unerupted or retained primary teeth and supernumerary teeth may be removed and malpositioned permanent teeth may be surgically exposed and guided to normal positions. Eruption patterns should be closely observed along with any changes in contour of the oral soft tissues. Dental radiographs obtained when aberrations in eruption are suspected may identify the presence of cysts or other impediments to eruption.

DISORDERS OF THE PERIODONTIUM

Definition

The periodontium is composed of the hard and soft tissues that surround and support the dentition. It includes both the attached and unattached or free gingivae, alveolar bone, and the periodontal ligament which connects the tooth root and alveolar bone. Whereas dental caries and malocclusions comprise the bulk of dental problems in childhood, the major cause of tooth loss after the age of 30 years is chronic destructive periodontal disease.

Basic Science

Both dental plaque, the soft noncalcified deposits that adhere to tooth surfaces, and dental caries are associated with periodontal disease. The accumulation of plaque on the tooth allows the proliferation of bacterial colonies. If not removed, plaque becomes calcified, forming calculus (often referred to as tartar). The combination of calculus, bacteria, and their toxins initiate inflammation of the gingiva. Inflammation and the associated infiltration of lymphocytes and intracellular fluids cause the tissues to lose their contour as fluid accumulates in the normal sulcus between tooth and gum (normally 1–3 mm deep). The normal tight collar of attached gingiva around the neck of the tooth migrates apically, increasing the sulcular depth to more than 3 mm. This pathologic sulcus is referred to as a pocket and contains cellular debris, bacteria, and extracellular fluids. Inflammation can then spread to include the surrounding alveolar bone. The gingival attachment and alveolar bone continue to migrate apically down the root surface. As the disease progresses, bony support for the tooth is decreased and the teeth become increasingly mobile. Occasionally, there are acute exacerbations of this chronic inflammation with development of acute periodontal abscesses.

Localized pericoronal gingivitis (pericoronitis) may occur around the crown of erupting teeth. This is caused by irritation from eruption and collection of bacteria and food debris under receding gingiva. It may be complicated by crowding or angulations which prevent full and normal eruption.

Mucogingival problems occur as a result of abnormal placement of the tooth within the alveolar ridge, crowding of the dentition, frenal influence, and shallow vestibular space. Crowding, a common occurrence in the early mixed dentition stage, may result in labial positioning of lower anterior teeth and in inadequate bone and tissue support. Similarly, a shallow vestibule, particularly in the anterior areas of the mouth, may result in excessive tension on the attached gingiva.

Frenal pathology usually involves the maxillary labial frenum, occasionally the labial or lingual frenum in the mandible, and rarely, other frenal attachments. The frena are the attachments of perioral and extraoral muscle to alveolar bone which become less conspicuously attached to the alveolar ridge with increasing chronologic age, owing to the growth of the alveolar ridge or minor trauma. Occasionally, the frena are quite prominent and apical repositioning does not occur to a large extent, creating tension on the gingival tissues surrounding the tooth. This frenal tension may gradually pull the attached gingiva away from the tooth or be responsible for a separation of teeth called a diastema.

Periodontitis in children is usually the result of predisposition to a juvenile form of periodontitis, systemic disease, or stress-related acute-onset periodontal disease. Generalized disease as a result of neglect and periodontitis are usually long-term problems manifest in the early adult years, although causative factors may be present during childhood (Newman, 1981).

Juvenile periodontitis (formerly referred to as periodontosis) is a form of periodontal disease which may result in a very rapid destruction of gingival attachment and bone in the incisor and molar areas of pre- and early adolescent children. Earlier considered to be a result of a genetic defect, it is now thought to be a bacterial infection characterized microbiologically by the presence of Gram-negative flora. Immunologic studies have found evidence of reduced white cell function in patients and their siblings. It may be so severe as to mimic late stages of chronic destructive periodontal disease in adults and becomes obvious because of looseness of teeth, fetid odor, and soft tissue symptoms typical of chronic infection.

Gingival hyperplasia may occur as a result of diphenylhydantoin (Dilantin) or cyclosporin therapy in the absence of significant local irritants (Fig. 21.5). It is related to dosage and may be controlled by fastidious oral hygiene techniques and reduced drug levels. The tissues appear firm, pink, and fibrotic. Inflammatory elements are usually confined to marginal areas.

Systemic diseases, such as hematologic and cardiac disease, may manifest themselves in gingival changes. Enlargement of local vessels, extravasation of cellular elements, and multiple hemorrhagic sites are found in the gingivae of patients with these systemic diseases. The gingival response is exacerbated by local degenerative changes of simple periodontal disease.

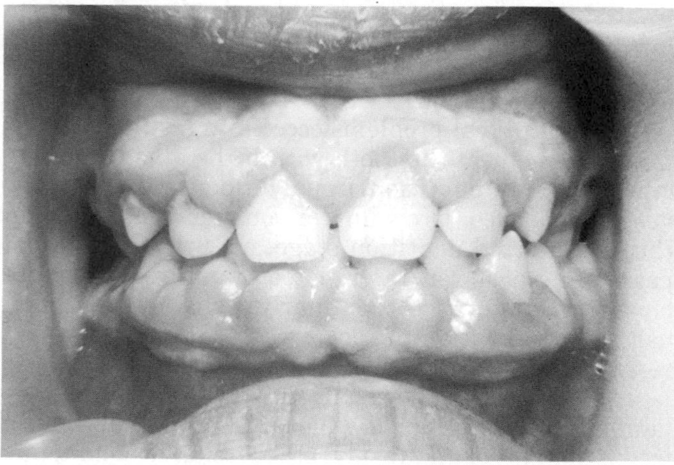

Figure 21.5. Dilantin Hyperplasia. This 9-year-old male exhibits mild to moderate gingival hyperplasia. The patient has grand mal seizures which are being controlled with diphenylhydantoin. The poor oral hygiene by the patient is a significant contributing factor to the gingival response which can be minimized with improved plaque control. Progression of this hyperplasia might indicate surgical removal of the excessive tissues if it interferes with function. The hyperplasia will resolve if drug therapy is stopped.

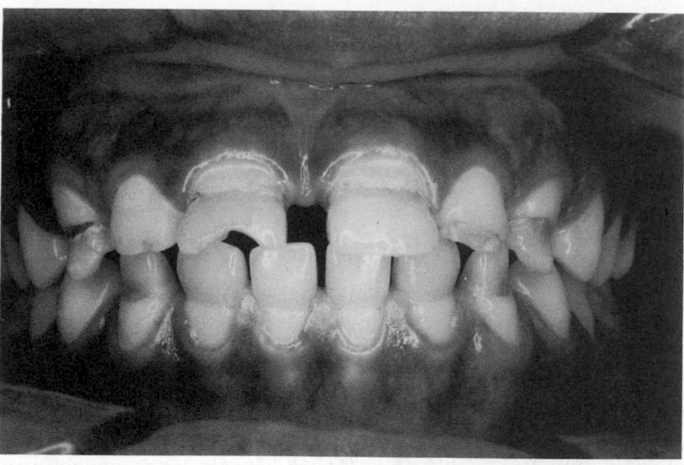

Figure 21.6. Linear Hypoplasia. Permanent dentition of a 14-year-old female exhibiting linear hypoplasia of the anterior teeth. Onset of acute glomerulonephritis at age 2 years interfered with ameloblastic activity resulting in band of hypoplastic enamel on all teeth calcifying at that time. The locations of the dysplastic enamel act as a marker of the systemic insult.

Stress and metabolic imbalance may be predisposing factors to acute necrotizing ulcerative gingivitis (ANUG), an acute form of periodontal disease usually limited to adolescents and young adults. Microscopically, fusiform spirochetes are found in cellular tissues and fluids. Decreased tissue resistance may allow microorganisms normally present in the mouth to become pathogenic.

Epidemiology

In the survey conducted by the United States Department of Health and Human Services, it was noted that 92% of all United States school children have mild to moderate gingival inflammation and 3% of 1.4 million children had severe gingival conditions warranting treatment. The report concluded that most children would benefit from improved oral hygiene procedures at home and regular dental prophylaxis (Hughes et al, 1981; Rosenblatt et al, 1983; Poulsen, 1981).

Diagnosis

After ruling out systemic disease and drug therapy as obvious causative agents, the diagnosis is related to the extent of involvement, age, and the presence of local irritating factors. Clinically, redness, swelling, loss of stippled appearance, friability and bleeding without provocation, and fetid odor are early signs of disease. Increased depth of the gingival sulcus, increased mobility of teeth, and radiographic appearance of alveolar bone loss are indicators of periodontitis. Juvenile periodontitis is characterized by looseness of incisor and molar teeth and fetid odor, but classical inflammatory signs may only become obvious late in the disease. Familial history and radiographs are important to the diagnosis (Ranney et al, 1981).

Gingival hyperplasia is typified by growth of gingival tissues, which may cover the teeth and prevent eruption. The tissues appear pink, firm, and fibrotic and inflammatory signs are secondary.

Treatment

Gingivitis responds to the removal of local irritating factors and the routine maintenance of oral hygiene. Plaque must be completely removed at least once every day at home on all surfaces of the teeth. Plaque removal is accomplished through tooth-brushing with a soft, multitufted brush and the use of dental floss on the areas between teeth. Debris and other local irritants are more likely to accumulate in the presence of crowding and irregular alignment and those conditions should be treated. Routine professional prophylaxis (at least every 6 months) is recommended to ensure proper maintenance, to clean areas missed by patient's home care, and to remove calculus.

Periodontitis requires additional treatment because deeper periodontal structures are involved. Scaling of the enamel and root (cementum) surface to remove calculus and curettage of the necrotic and inflamed marginal tissues and gingival sulci must be performed. Surgical procedures such as gingivectomy or apically repositioning flap procedures can be used in the treatment of periodontitis in children, although these are more commonly needed in the treatment of adult periodontitis.

Gingival hyperplasia may not require treatment in children as long as it does not interfere with mastication or the eruption of teeth. When these functions are drastically interrupted, surgical removal (gingivectomy) procedures for limited areas or the entire dentition are performed.

Surgical correction of mucogingival problems is usually delayed until permanent teeth have erupted. Maxillary labial frenectomy to allow closure of the space between the maxillary incisors or relieve tension on the marginal gingiva is performed usually after eruption of permanent canine teeth (ages 12–14 years) because this often closes the space spontaneously. Surgically repositioned flap and gingival graft procedures are done to produce an adequate border of attached gingiva around the permanent teeth.

Acute necrotizing ulcerative gingivitis usually responds to rest, diet, control, and local mechanical therapy.

Prognosis

The prognosis for local and generalized periodontal problems is good if the causative factors can be removed or controlled. Gingivitis is reversible, but periodontitis which progresses to the stage of alveolar bone loss may be irreversible.

Prevention

Periodontal disease is a process that can largely be prevented by aggressive oral hygiene, regular dental visits, relief of crowding of teeth, and maintenance of oral health.

Orofacial Trauma 3

Definition

Trauma to the orofacial complex can be divided into injuries to the hard tissues, i.e., teeth and/or bone and injuries to the soft tissues of the oral cavity (physical, chemical, or electrical). Soft tissue injuries consist of abrasions, lacerations, contusions, ecchymoses, hematomas and burns. Injuries to the teeth consist of fractures and displacements.

Epidemiology

Trauma to the teeth of children is very common, with reported incidences depending on the definitions of the types of injuries and population studied. According to one study, 46% of children sustained traumatic injuries to their primary and/or permanent teeth (Andreasen and Ravn, 1972). Orofacial trauma including trauma to the teeth is commonly seen in cases of child abuse with about 50% of children who are abused showing such injuries (Becker, 1978).

Natural History

The survival of an injured tooth depends on the normal reattachment of its periodontal ligament to the surrounding bone, as well as to the preservation of the vitality of its pulpal tissues. Abnormal reattachments of a tooth to its alveolar bone include resorption of the root surface, resulting in increased tooth mobility, and ankylosis of the root surface, resulting in decreased tooth mobility. These abnormal reattachments are often irreversible and can result in loss of the tooth. Devitalization and infection of the pulp may be manifested clinically as discoloration of the crown, pain, excessive mobility, and/or alveolar abscess formation. The prognosis for the long-term vitality of the pulp is usually predictable by 3 months after the traumatic incident. If the dental pulp becomes nonvital, root canal therapy is the treatment of choice.

Trauma to the primary teeth can cause damage to the succedaneous teeth, such as hypoplastic defects of the crown (Turner hypoplasia), root deformities, and/or disturbances of eruption (accelerated, delayed, and/or ectopic).

Diagnosis and Treatment

Fractures of teeth are classified by the extent of the lost tooth structure. Class I fractures involve only the enamel of the tooth and treatment consists of smoothing the rough edges or restoring the fracture by utilizing the bonding of a tooth-colored resin material to the fractured site. Class II fractures involve the dentin as well as enamel, causing the tooth to be sensitive to thermal changes when the exposed dentin is stimulated. A tooth sustaining a class II fracture must be treated immediately after the accident so that exposed dentin will be covered and irritation of the pulpal tissues diminished. The tooth can be restored completely at a later time by bonding a resin to the fracture site. Class III fractures extend into the pulpal tissues and also require immediate attention. Pulpal therapy (partial or total root canal treatment) should be instituted to avoid necrosis of the pulp and eventual alveolar abscess formation. Again, restoration of the involved tooth is accomplished later. Root fractures are usually diagnosed radiographically; clinically, the tooth may appear excessively mobile. The fractured segments must be stabilized with a splint which is fabricated by bonding the involved tooth to the adjacent uninvolved teeth. Splints should remain in place for several months and root canal therapy may be necessary if there is necrosis of the pulp (Needleman, 1982).

Other injuries to the teeth include: (1) concussion—an injury to the tooth resulting only in edema and/or inflammation of the periodontal ligament, evident clinically by tenderness of the tooth to percussion; (2) subluxation—an injury in which a tooth is not displaced but is mobile within its socket; (3) luxation—the tooth is displaced from its socket (either intruded, extruded and/or laterally displaced); and (4) avulsion—the tooth is totally displaced from its socket. The goal of treatment of displacement injuries is normal reattachment of the periodontal ligament of the tooth to the alveolar bone. This is best accomplished through reduction and stabilization of the tooth, ideal oral hygiene of the surrounding soft tissues, and minimizing chewing with the involved tooth or teeth. Normal reattachment is usually complete at 3 weeks and the prognosis for pulpal survival can be made at about 3 months after trauma. Permanent teeth that are avulsed should be reimplanted immediately. Prognosis is based on the extra-alveolar period inasmuch as the cells of the periodontal ligament usually are unable to survive for more than 60 minutes out of their socket. Immediate reimplantation at the site of the injury is vital to minimize this extra-alveolar period. If this is not possible, the tooth should be stored in milk, saline, or in the oral cavity of the patient to maintain vitality of the ligament. Once reimplantation is complete, stabilization and root canal therapy are required.

Prognosis

Prognosis for the avulsed tooth is favorable if the reimplantation has been completed within 60 minutes of the avulsion or if the tooth has been stored in the appropriate medium before reimplantation. If the extra-alveolar period is greater than 60 minutes, and the periodontal ligament is allowed to dry, prognosis is extremely poor. More than 90% of these teeth become ankylosed, which is not reversible, and eventually require extraction. *Avulsed primary teeth should not be reimplanted* because complex treatment is contraindicated for young children, the primary incisors are not important within the developing dental arch, and there is risk of infection on the developing permanent dentition. The prognosis of other tooth injuries depends on the extent and type of injury, but is generally good if prompt and appropriate treatment is rendered.

Prevention

Children who are involved in contact sports, who are accident-prone, or who have protrusive maxillary incisors should seek preventive dental care. Early orthodontic care can often reduce severe protrusion of the maxillary incisors and render trauma to these teeth less likely. The fitting of protective mouth guards also can decrease trauma significantly to the orofacial complex. Mouth guards of a vinyl material can be adapted at home by softening a stock-variety in boiling water or may be custom-made from impressions of the dental arch.

Disorders of Mastication

4

MALOCCLUSION

Definition

Occlusion refers to the relationship of the maxillary and mandibular teeth when the jaws are closed and to the relationship of the teeth within each jaw. A malocclusion may occur not only as a result of anomalies of tooth morphology and position, but also from bony or skeletal abnormalities, soft tissue anomalies, and functional problems, such as swallowing and sucking.

Basic Science

Individual tooth positions are a function of the space available within each jaw and the size of the teeth. Some spacing between primary teeth is more likely to provide adequate space for the larger permanent teeth and, therefore, proper alignment within each dental arch (Pederson et al, 1978).

Genetic influence is a strong determinant of the positions of the maxilla and mandible as well as other facial bones. Malocclusions may be skeletal in origin rather than determined by the dentition. Underdevelopment of the maxilla and nasal bones may result in a midface deficiency reflected as "relative" mandibular prognathism, whereas overdevelopment of the same bones may appear as a maxillary prognathism. Similarly, the mandible may be over- or underdeveloped.

Epidemiology

Prevalence of malocclusion varies among races, sexes, socioeconomic backgrounds, and age (Goyit et al, 1984). Based on surveys by the United States Department of Health, Education and Welfare, 75% of children and almost 90% of the adolescents in a representative sampling of United States' children had some form of malocclusion, with 5.5% of the young children and 16% of the adolescents requiring urgent care (Kelly et al, 1973; 1977). In addition, a large percentage of observed malocclusions, while not related to functional disharmonies or severe aesthetic problems, would still benefit from treatment.

Natural History

A number of etiologic factors have been identified in the development of malocclusion. These include heredity, premature loss of teeth, anomalies of tooth morphology and eruption, digit or pacifier sucking, tongue habits and position, and airway obstruction.

Sucking habits normally persist for several years. Malocclusions in the primary dentition from these habits often will resolve spontaneously if children abandon them by the time of eruption of the permanent teeth. Persistence of sucking habits into the mixed dentition stage is more likely to cause occlusal abnormalities requiring orthodontic intervention.

Severe dental caries resulting in cavitation of the primary teeth or loss of tooth contact and subsequent tipping and drifting of teeth results in less space available for the permanent dentition. Inadequate space for alignment is further compromised by the eruption of the first permanent molar which places an anterior component of force on the primary dentition.

Airway obstruction can cause postural changes and functional influences on the developing face and dentition. The typical "adenoidal" facies include mouth breathing, protrusion of both anterior maxillary and mandibular teeth, and narrowing of the dental arches.

Diagnosis

A comprehensive evaluation of occlusion should be based on several factors: molar relationship, crown angulation, crown inclination, rotations, contacts, and occlusal plan (Andrews, 1972).

Examination, dental radiographs, facial photographs, and diagnostic casts of the teeth are necessary in diagnosing orthodontic problems. Radiographs are taken to determine the health of individual teeth and supporting bone, the presence or absence of permanent teeth, and skeletal/dental relationships. Cephalometric radiographs and their analysis help in determining whether a malocclusion is dental or skeletal in origin as well as the relationship between the dentition and the skeletal structures. Dental casts are used to predict the adequacy of space for the permanent dentition as well as to provide a record of the occlusion. Actual projection of growth patterns and their influence on the malocclusion and treatment are not yet possible, but computer programs aimed toward that goal are being developed.

Treatment

Orthodontic treatment may be functional, which selectively influences the growth of certain bones, or orthodontic, which affects the position of teeth. Diagnostic findings may indicate the need for removal of permanent teeth to obtain needed space in severely crowded dentitions. Tooth movement may be accomplished with removable or fixed appliances. Fixed appliances allow better control and permit finite adjustments of angulation and position. Removable appliances are used for limited treatment after orthodontic alignment or to influence growth patterns.

Treatment may be divided into preventive, interceptive, and corrective. Preventive treatment may be accomplished early and often in the primary dentition, and includes caries control, space maintenance, and habit control. Habits which persist and result in malocclusion may be treated by appliances which discourage sucking or tongue movements. Posterior cross bites may be successfully treated before the eruption of first permanent molars.

Interceptive treatment usually begins in the mixed dentition. Developing problems are treated to create more favorable positions of the teeth or facial bones. Crowding and rotations of permanent teeth, for example, may be reduced by decreasing the width of the primary canines or by their removal.

Corrective treatment refers to the definitive correction of malocclusions which cannot be completed until the permanent dentition has fully erupted. Definitive orthodontic care generally starts earlier for girls (ages 9–11 years) than for boys (ages 12–14 years) due to eruption differences. The wearing of retainers to prevent relapse after multibanded therapy is customary for indefinite periods of time.

Prevention

Control of oral habits is a common concern. Many parents and physicians encourage the use of pacifiers to discourage digit sucking, although no evidence exists to suggest fewer malocclusions as a result of their use. Some evidence suggests, however, that resilient air-filled pacifers result in greater malocclusion because of their reactive force after compression. Thumb-sucking, on the other hand, may be more difficult to curtail because of the gratification to both the digit and palate. As social contacts broaden, sucking habits usually disappear. For ideal dental development, all sucking habits should cease before the eruption of the permanent maxillary central incisors (Popovich and Thompson, 1973).

Prognosis

A definitive correction, with teeth properly angulated and in contact, is stable and usually will not relapse. Eruption of third molars (wisdom teeth) has been implicated in late crowding after treatment. Supporting evidence for this theory is limited and function, wear, and loss of tooth structure in later years is more likely the cause of late crowding.

CONTROVERSY

Considerable debate exists over timing of treatment and appropriate training level of the dentist performing orthodontic care. Advocates of early treatment point to the flexibility in the young child, the opportunity to take advantage of growth patterns, and the stability resulting from early alignment of teeth. Proponents of more conventional timing, i.e., adolescence, point out that most treatment cannot be completed until the eruption of permanent dentition is complete. Principles of prevention would seem to support early intervention when possible, because, in many cases, the development of more complex malocclusions can be avoided.

BRUXISM

Definition

Bruxism is defined as the habitual grinding of the teeth with enough force so as to be audible and cause visible wear of the teeth.

Basic Science

Bruxism can be attributed to stress and/or occlusal disharmonies. It can be a response to psychologic stress and seems to occur more frequently in tense children.

In malocclusions, bruxism may be triggered by occlusal disharmonies such as cross bites and deep bites. Moreover, bruxism may place unusual strain on the muscles of mastication and may result in temporomandibular joint symptoms. In the absence of malocclusions and specific causes, the habit is considered to be annoying but transient. It is not unusual to see occlusal wear patterns on primary teeth in the absence of pathologic periodontal response.

Epidemiology

Parental reports of bruxism based on "nocturnal noise" are very common in 3- to 6-year-old children, but become less frequent as children mature.

Natural History

Nocturnal noise and wear on facets are indications of early bruxism in children. If the habit persists to the adult dentition, the possibility of a psychologic basis or the presence of occlusal irregularities exists. The likelihood of periodontal disease or degenerative changes of the temporomandibular joint increases, the longer the habit continues.

Diagnosis

Diagnosis is based on reports from parents or observation of occlusal wear pattern by the dentist or health care provider. Occasionally, children complain of dental pain or joint and muscle pain (see TMJ pain and dysfunction syndrome) and these findings warrant a more thorough pursuit of the causative agents (pp. 1191).

Treatment

Treatment is usually not necessary in young children unless there are dental, muscular, or joint symptoms. An occlusal splint or "night guard" may be constructed and worn at night to keep the teeth from contact with opposing teeth. These splints are thin, interarch wafer-like outlines of the bite which eliminate occlusal triggering mechanisms by preventing the teeth from interdigitating when the patient is at rest.

Prevention

Bruxism may occur in any child. Focal issues causing tension in children should be alleviated and timely interceptive treatment for developing occlusal problems should be practiced.

REFERENCES

Andreasen JO, Ravn JJ: Epidemiology of traumatic dental injuries to primary and permanent teeth in a Danish population sample. *Int J Oral Surg* 1:235, 1972.

Andrews LF: Six keys to normal occlusion. *Am J Orthodont* 62:296, 1972.

Becker DB, Needleman HL, Kotelchuck M: Child abuse and dentistry: Orofacial trauma and its recognition by dentists. *J Am Dent Assoc* 97:24, 1978.

Braham RL, Morris ME: *Textbook of Pediatric Dentistry,* 2nd edition. Baltimore, Williams & Wilkins, 1985.

Burdi AR: The development and eruption of the human dentitions. In Forrester DJ, Wagoner ML, Fleming J (eds): *Pediatric Dental Medicine*, Chapter 5, Philadelphia, Lea & Febiger, 1981.

Cohen HJ, Diner H: The significance of developmental dental enamel defects in neurological diagnosis. *Pediatrics* 46:737, 1970.

Fromm A: Epstein's pearls, Bohn's nodules and inclusion-cysts of the oral cavity. *J Dent Child* 34:275, 1967.

Glenn FB, Glenn WD, Duncan RC: Prenatal fluoride tablet supplementation and the fluoride content of teeth. *J Dent Child* 51:344, 1984.

Goyit E, Lieberman M, Eini R, et al: Prevalence of mandibular dysfunction in 10–18 year old Israeli school children. *J Oral Rehabil* 4:307, 1984.

Grahnan H, Grahnan L: Numerical variations in primary dentition and their correlation with permanent dentition. *Odontol Rev* 12:348, 1961.

Handelman SL, Leverett DH, Iker HP: Longitudinal radiographic evaluation of the progress of caries under sealants. *J Pedodont* 9:119, 1985.

Hughes JT, Rozier RG, Bawden JW: A survey of periodontal disease in a state population—an emphasis on children. Special Issue. *Pediatr Dent* 3:114, 1981.

Kates GA, Needleman HL, Holmes LB: Natal and neonatal teeth: A clinical study. *J Am Dent Assoc* 109:441, 1984.

Kelly JE, et al: An assessment of the occlusion of teeth of youths 12–17 years. Vital Health Statistics, Series 11, no. 162, 1–65, Washington, DC, DHEW, Gant Printing Services, February, 1977.

Kelly JE, Sanchez M, Van Kirk LE: An assessment of the occlusion of the teeth of children 6–9 years. Vital Health Statistics, Series 11, no. 130, Washington, DC, DHEW, Gant Printing Services, 1973.

Levin LS: Genetic disease in children. In: Forrester DJ, Waggoner ML, Fleming J(eds): *Pediatric Dental Medicine.* Philadelphia, Lea & Febiger, 1981.

Lunt RC, Law DB: A review of the chronology of calcification of deciduous teeth. *J Am Dent Assoc* 89:599, 1974.

National Institute of Dental Research: The prevalence of dental caries in the United States in children 1979–1980. The National Dental Caries Prevalence Survey, NIH pub no. 82–2245, Bethesda, MD, US NIH, 1981.

Needleman HL: Management of injuries to anterior primary teeth. *J Mass Dent Soc* 31:5, 1982.

Newman MG: Localized juvenile periodontitis (periodontosis). Special Issue. *Pediatr Dent* 3:121, 1981.

O'Donnell JP, Cohen MM: Dental care for the institutionalized retarded individual. *J Pedodont* 9:3, 1985.

Pederson J, Stensgaard K, Millsen B: Prevalence of malocclusion in relation to premature loss of primary teeth. *Comm Dent Oral Epid* 6:204, 1978.

Pinborg JJ: Pathology of the dental hard tissues. In: *Abnormalities of Tooth Morphology*. Chap 1, Philadelphia, WB Saunders, 1970.

Popovich F, Thompson GW: Thumb and finger sucking: Its relation to malocclusion. *Am J Orthodont* 63:148, 1973.

Poulsen S: Epidemiology and indices of gingival and periodontal disease. Special Issue. *Pediatr Dent* 3:82, 1981.

Ranney RR, Debski BF, Tew JG: Pathogenesis of gingivitis and periodontal disease in children and young adults. Special Issue. *Pediatr Dent* 3:89, 1981.

Ripa LW: Occlusal sealants: Rationale and review of clinical trials. *Int Dent J* 30:127, 1980.

Ripa LW, Leske GS, Sposato AL, et al: Chronology and sequence of exfoliation of primary teeth. *J Am Dent Assoc* 105:641, 1982.

Rosenblatt GM, Alongi JA, Deasy MJ: Periodontal disease in children. *Clin Prev Dent* 5:17–20, 1983.

Shaw JH: Causes and control of dental caries. *N Engl J Med* 317:996, 1987.

STEPHEN SHUSTERMAN
HOWARD NEEDLEMAN

Section 22

Rheumatology

Introduction 1

Definition

The rheumatic diseases are a group of disorders that share the common property of inflammation of connective tissues throughout the body. This inflammatory process is characteristically chronic or recurrent and is of unknown cause. Immunologic aberrations of the host are frequently associated with these disorders. Because the musculoskeletal system is made up predominantly of connective tissues, the rheumatic diseases all share the property of prominent musculoskeletal involvement. These diseases include *acute rheumatic fever, juvenile rheumatoid arthritis (JRA), ankylosing spondylitis* and the *spondyloarthropathies, systemic lupus erythematosus, dermatomyositis,* various *vasculitis syndromes* (of which Schönlein-Henoch vasculitis and Kawasaki disease are of particular importance in children), *scleroderma,* and a number of less common conditions including mixed connective tissue disease and *fasciitis.* Although there are few if any diagnostic tests for any of these conditions, they usually appear as distinct entities, each being identified by a characteristic pattern of organ system involvement. *Acute rheumatic fever* is a poststreptococcal state best characterized by inflammation of the endocardium of the heart, resulting in valvular carditis. The diseases called *juvenile rheumatoid arthritis* are all characterized by chronic inflammation of synovial tissues; several different diseases are included under this umbrella term. *Ankylosing spondylitis* and the *spondyloarthropathies* are characterized by chronic synovitis and inflammation of connective tissues around bones and joints which affect the axial skeleton more than the peripheral joints. *Systemic lupus erythematosus* is a multisystem disease characterized by inflammation in a number of organs and by the presence of a number of host immunologic aberrations. *Dermatomyositis* is characterized by inflammation of skeletal muscle and skin, resulting in myositis and a distinctive skin rash. The various vasculitis syndromes are characterized by inflammation of blood vessels of various sizes; *Henoch-Schönlein vasculitis* is a disease of inflammation of very small blood vessels, whereas *Kawasaki disease* is a febrile illness that is associated with inflammation of large coronary vessels and other large blood vessels. *Scleroderma* is characterized by fibrosis of skin and subcutaneous tissue and of internal organs; this disease can exist in localized cutaneous forms or as a systemic disease. *Mixed connective tissue disease* is a multisystem overlap disease which is characterized by the presence of a certain antinuclear antibody reactive with ribonucleoprotein. *Fasciitis* is a condition resulting from inflammation of fascial tissues. The rheumatic diseases often affect many organ systems, and sometimes overlapping symptoms and signs make precise identification of the particular disease difficult.

Basic Science

The basic causes of the inflammation that characterize the rheumatic diseases and the explanation for mechanisms that perpetuate the chronicity of this inflammatory process remain to be found. Various laboratory observations over the years have led to the idea that these diseases are in some way caused by "autoimmunity"; however, the situation appears to be more complicated than one of simple autoimmunity. Recent findings suggest that several factors are interrelated in the causation of at least some of the rheumatic diseases: genetic predisposition, exposure to environmental agents, and aberrant host immune responses.

ABERRANT IMMUNE RESPONSES

It has been known for several years that a number of "autoantibodies," that is, antibodies that react with various body constituents, are present in some of the rheumatic disease states. The most commonly measured of these autoantibodies are the rheumatoid factors, antibodies that react with IgG immunoglobulin, and the antinuclear antibodies, a family of antibodies that react with various constituents of cell nuclei. *Rheumatoid factors* are generally detected by agglutination tests, such as the latex agglutination test which primarily detects antibodies of the IgM class. IgM antibodies to IgG immunoglobulin are termed classic rheumatoid factors and provide an excellent laboratory marker for classic adult rheumatoid arthritis. Rheumatoid factors are in no way diagnostic of rheumatoid arthritis, however; they also occur in a number of other disease states including various chronic infectious diseases and certain malignancies. The *antinuclear antibodies* are commonly measured by indirect immunofluorescence with frozen tissue sections or cultures of cells as substrate; this method measures antinuclear antibodies of various specificities and provides the best screening test. Antinuclear antibody tests are most always positive in patients with systemic lupus erythematosus; however, antinuclear antibodies are not specific for lupus, being found also in a number of other rheumatic disease states, in various infectious diseases, and in association with ingestion of a number of commonly used drugs. Other methods can detect different kinds of antinuclear antibodies. Measurement of antibodies reactive with DNA is useful in following the course of lupus, and measurement of antibodies reactive with ribonucleoprotein (RNP) is useful in diagnosis of mixed connective tissue disease. The lupus erythematosus cell preparation is a rather insensitive method for measuring a particular antinuclear antibody which reacts with deoxyribonucleoprotein and is uniformly found in lupus, but also in other disease states. The lupus erythematosus cell is of historical interest since its discovery opened the way to the discovery of antinuclear antibodies; however, this test has been superseded by the more sensitive fluorescent antinuclear antibody test.

A number of other autoantibodies can be measured in human beings. *The Coombs test* detects antibodies reactive with red blood cells and, thus, is helpful in evaluating possible hemolytic anemia. Antibodies to platelets can be measured in idiopathic thrombocytopenic purpura, and antibodies to granulocytes and lymphocytes can be demonstrated in disease states such as systemic lupus. Antibodies reactive with thyroid tissue can be found in autoimmune thyroiditis, those reactive with gastric cells in pernicious anemia, and those reactive with smooth muscle in chronic active hepatitis and certain viral infections.

With the exception of antibodies directed to single tissues (such as red cells, platelets and white cells) no autoantibody has yet been clearly shown to cause direct destruction of host tissues. However, some autoantibodies, notably the antinuclear antibodies and rheumatoid factors, may cause tissue damage through the formation of immune complexes with their respective antigens. These *immune complexes* circulate, lodge in certain tissues, activate the complement system, and cause secondary inflammation and tissue destruction. This mechanism has been shown to be very important in systemic lupus erythematosus where DNA and antibodies reactive with DNA cause much of the tissue damage in important involved systems, such as nephritis from kidney damage. Immune complexes of rheumatoid factors and immunoglobulin have been shown to cause certain manifestations of seropositive rheumatoid arthritis, notably rheumatoid vasculitis. Although various techniques can be used to measure immune complexes in the serum in a number of the rheumatic diseases, such tests are neither diagnostic nor specific and appear to be of limited usefulness in evaluating the activity or course of disease. Serum hemolytic complement and some of its components can be measured; lowered levels of complement are indicative of active immune complex disease and hence, the activity of the disease lupus erythematosus. Such tests are not diagnostic, however.

Arthritis and other rheumatic disease states have been associated with a number of immunodeficiency syndromes, including hypogammaglobulinemia and the Wiskott-Aldrich syndrome; individuals with these conditions may have chronic or recurrent arthritis which closely resembles JRA. A disease state reminiscent of dermatomyositis has also been described in hypogammaglobulinemia; this illness appears to be a result of direct viral myositis in an immunocompromised host. Maternal carriers of chronic granulomatous disease have an increased prevalence of discoid and mild lupus. One family with a granulocyte defect has been described with a disease resembling rheumatoid arthritis. Deficiencies of various complement components, including C2, C4, and C7, C8, and Cl esterase inhibitor have been associated with various rheumatic disease states, most commonly systemic lupus. The most common deficiency is C2, that results from a genetically determined deficiency in C2 gene expression (Cole et al, 1985). Reasons for these associations of rheumatic diseases with immunodeficiency states remain to be found. Infectious agents in immunocompromised hosts may play a role as in the dermatomyositis-like syndrome in hypogammaglobulinemia. It is probable that an intact immune system is central to control of the inflammatory process, and that chronic inflammation may result from immunodeficiency. Abnormal immune responses have been described in systemic lupus erythematosus, with a deficiency in the regulatory mechanisms of T cells and an overexuberance of the B cell system. It is not yet known whether these abnormal immune mechanisms antedate the disease or are secondary manifestations. It is known that antibodies reactive with lymphocytes exist in lupus; whether or not these lymphocytotoxic antibodies play a role in impairing immune function remains to be clarified.

GENETIC PREDISPOSITION

A *genetic predisposition* has been shown for a number of rheumatic diseases. Although none of these diseases is inherited by simple Mendelian inheritance, increased familial incidence of disease has been observed in ankylosing spondylitis and the other spondyloarthropathies, in systemic lupus erythematosus, in classic adult rheumatoid arthritis, and in three of the subgroups of JRA (rheumatoid factor-positive disease, pauciarticular disease type I, and pauciarticular disease type II). Associations of rheumatic diseases with various HLA antigens have been made for the spondyloathropathies (HLA-B27), classic adult rheumatoid arthritis and seropositive juvenile rheumatoid arthritis (HLA DR4) (Nepom et al, 1984), pauciarticular JRA type I (HLA-DRW8, W6 and 5), and pauciarticular JRA type II (HLA-B27). There are also HLA associations for systemic lupus erythematosus (HLA-B8, DR3, HLA-DR2) and dermatomyositis (HLA-B8-DR3). These HLA associations point to genetic predisposition to disease, although the HLA antigens themselves are clearly not the disease genes nor do they alone cause disease. Also suggesting genetic predisposition to disease are racial predilections of systemic lupus erythematosus (more common in blacks and other dark-skinned races), the spondyloarthropathies (virtually absent in Japanese and other Orientals, more common in certain native American tribes than in whites), and Kawasaki disease (apparent predilection for Japanese). It can also be argued, however, that racial differences reflect environmental differences rather than genetic predisposition to disease (Schoenfeld and Schwartz, 1984).

ENVIRONMENTAL AGENTS

A number of interesting models demonstrate that environmental agents can cause rheumatic disease in predisposed hosts. Of most interest are various infectious agents. One of the best examples is the occurrence of Reiter syndrome in persons with HLA-B27 after they contract infections with *Shigella*. A similar situation exists with the reactive arthritis occurring after intestinal infections with organisms such as *Salmonella, Shigella, Campylobacter,* or *Yersinia enterocolitica*; given these infections, individuals with HLA-B27 may have related arthritis, while those without this genetic marker do not have this complication. Infectious agents are also associated with other rheumatic disease states, notably, acute rheumatic fever that follows group A β streptococcal pharyngitis. A number of infectious diseases can themselves be associated with rheumatic manifestations. Examples are the prodrome resembling systemic onset JRA which can precede hepatitis B infection and the arthritis of SBE (immune complex phenomena), the pauciarticular arthritis of Lyme disease (a direct synovial infection with the spirochete B. Bingdorfini), and the arthritis of infections with meningococcus, gonococcus, *H. influenzae*, rubella, EB virus, and mycoplasma which may result from either direct synovial infection with the causative organisms or which may be sterile (reactive).

LABORATORY STUDIES

A multitude of laboratory tests can be performed in evaluating a patient for the rheumatic diseases. The usefulness of some of these tests is summarized in Table 22.1. The most important tests are, in fact, those used in excluding other conditions that may mimic rheumatic diseases; these tests include the old standbys, such as complete blood counts, tests for infectious diseases, and appropriate radiographs, bone scans, and biopsies. The rheumatoid factors, antinuclear antibodies, other autoantibodies, and HLA antigens are of interest in classifying types of disease but none is diagnostic of any one disease. Tests such as complement and antibodies to DNA may be useful in following the course of disease such as lupus. The main diagnostic tools for childhood rheumatic diseases remain the careful history and physical examination.

Table 22.1
Laboratory Tests in Rheumatic Diseases

Rheumatoid factors:
- Classification of juvenile rheumatoid arthritis

Antinuclear antibody:
- Diagnosis of SLE (DNP, DNA, Sm, etc.)
- Diagnosis of MCTD (RNP)
- Course of SLE (DNA)
- Classification of JRA (?Specificity)

HLA:
- Chiefly for research interest
- B27: Spondyloarthropathies

Complement:
- Course of SLE
- Evidence of immune complex disease

Acute phase reactants, serum proteins:
- Minor role in following disease course

Blood counts:
- Suspicion of malignancy

Culture:
- Infectious disease studies:

Radiographs, bone scans:
- Underlying bony abnormalities (infection, trauma, malignancy, congenital or genetic conditions)

Biopsies:
- Confirm clinical impression of tissue involvement and permit classification in some instances; diagnosis of malignancy

Epidemiology

There are no very compelling studies concerning incidence and prevalence of rheumatic diseases affecting children. In the context of chronic childhood illnesses, the rheumatic diseases seem to occur in numbers similar to childhood diabetes, childhood renal disease, congenital heart disease, childhood malignancies and cystic fibrosis. Because childhood rheumatic diseases are relatively rare, the absence of specific diagnostic laboratory tests, and the reliance on careful and expert physical evaluation for diagnosis, epidemiologic studies of these diseases are difficult to perform. Two recent studies addressing the epidemiology of JRA in the United States, one in Rochester, Minnesota, and one in Rochester, New York, have suggested prevalence figures of about 1/1000 children (Gewanter et al, 1983; Towner et al, 1983). The Arthritis Foundation has used the figure that a quarter of a million American children are affected with JRA. Most rheumatic disease specialists consider that there are an equal number of children affected by other rheumatic diseases. Until recent years, care for children with rheumatic diseases has been fragmented and there have been few centers where large groups of children have been registered. With the advent of comprehensive rheumatic disease clinics for children, most experts agree that pediatric rheumatology clinics attract as many patients as many commonly emphasized pediatric subspecialties. In such clinics, lupus and dermatomyositis in children are about one-tenth as common as JRA; Henoch-Schönlein vasculitis is a relatively common condition, and scleroderma and other types of vasculitis are quite rare in children. Recent epidemics have brought Kawasaki disease into medical prominence, although the occurrence of cases tends to be episodic and sporadic in the United States. Acute rheumatic fever used to be the most important of the rheumatic diseases affecting children in the United States and in other parts of the world; it remains common in many underdeveloped parts of the world today, and has been rare in the United States and other industrial countries in recent years, although since 1985 several outbreaks have been reported (Veasy et al, 1987).

Differential Diagnosis of Childhood Rheumatic Diseases

Because there are no clear diagnostic tests for the rheumatic diseases, thoughtful differential diagnosis is particularly important. A number of nonrheumatic disorders can cause inflammation of connective tissues with resulting symptoms and signs reflecting connective tissue inflammation in various parts of the body (Cassidy, 1986). Such conditions can closely mimic rheumatic diseases (Table 22.2). Infectious diseases can cause rheumatic complaints. Infectious agents are directly present in the synovium in patients with bacterial arthritis, mycobacterial arthritis, Lyme disease, and certain types of viral arthritis. Arthritis without the presence of infectious agents in affected joints can be found associated with immune complex arthritis (for example, the arthritis of subacute bacterial endocarditis), reactive arthritis (sterile arthritis secondary to gastrointestinal infections with *Salmonella, Shigella, Campylobacter,* and *Yersinia)* and the "sympathetic" joint effusions of adjacent osteomyolitis. Needless to say, children with infectious diseases may have fevers, malaise, rashes and other nonspecific indications of systemic disease, which can also closely mimic rheumatic diseases.

Any one of the childhood malignancies can result in "arthritis" and rheumatic disease-like states. This arthritis is most often the result of infiltrations of malignant cells into the periosteum, joint capsule, and periarticular tissues rather than direct involvement of synovial tissue with malignancy. These conditions are often quite painful, and severe joint pain should always be a tip-off to malignancy as the cause of arthritis. Childhood malignancies associated with rheumatic complaints include leukemia, neuroblastoma, histiocytosis, Hodgkin disease, and lymphoma. Other malignancies can cause joint complaints by direct involvement of bones and joints; these include rhabdomyosarcoma, osteogenic sarcoma, Ewing sarcoma, and other primary bone tumors. Clues to malignancy include soft tissue or bony swellings, severe pain, severe illness, abnormalities in peripheral blood counts (leukopenia, abnormal white cell forms, extremely high white counts, thrombocytopenia, anemia), and radiographic findings of metaphyseal rarefaction, periostitis, lytic bone lesions, or soft tissue masses. A host of noninflammatory conditions also can result in rheumatic complaints. Among these are trauma (including bone fractures), the avascular necrosis syndromes, Legg-Perthes disease (femoral head), Kohler disease (tarsal navicular), Freiberg disease (metatarsal heads), the chondromalacia patella syndrome, slipped capital femoral epiphysis, osteochondritis dissecans, toxic synovitis, various genetic or congenital conditions affecting the musculoskeletal system, hematologic disorders (hemophilia, sickle cell disease), idiopathic limb pains (growing pains), reflex sympathetic dystrophy syndrome, and psychogenic rheumatism.

These various conditions can usually be sorted out by a careful history and physical examination along with appropriate laboratory tests. As pointed out in the preceding section, the laboratory can be helpful in differential diagnosis, particularly in excluding the conditions noted above. A diagnosis of rheumatic disease should never be considered established until these various possibilities have been at least considered and excluded in the mind of the physician.

Table 22.2
Disorders Mimicking Rheumatic Diseases in Children

Infectious diseases
Septic arthritis
Osteomyelitis
Viral arthritis
Lyme disease
Reactive arthritis
"Toxic synovitis"
Malignancies
Leukemia
Neuroblastoma
Osteogenic sarcoma
Others
Noninflammatory conditions
Trauma
Avascular necrosis
Chondromalacia patella
Genetic-congenital conditions
Idiopathic limb pains
Reflex sympathetic dystrophy
Psychogenic rheumatism
Miscellaneous

Individual Diseases

2

ACUTE RHEUMATIC FEVER

This important rheumatic disease is potentially fatal and is still a leading cause of death among older children in a number of underdeveloped countries today. For reasons poorly understood, but probably at least partially related to better socioeconomic conditions and treatment of streptococcal pharyngitis with antibiotics, rheumatic fever (see p. 386) has been very rare in the United States in recent years. Recent reports, however, suggest that this disease may be appearing again in the United States (Veasy et al, 1987; CDC, 1988).

Rheumatic fever requires prior infection with group A β streptococci. The most characteristic involvement is with the endocardium, which results in valvular carditis. Other disease manifestations include arthritis, rash (erythema marginatum), subcutaneous nodules, chorea (Sydenham chorea), and nonspecific findings such as fever and malaise. Attacks of rheumatic fever are generally self-limited (weeks to months duration); a few observers have supported the concept of chronic rheumatic fever. Attacks may recur if further streptococcal infections are permitted. Treatment consists of anti-inflammatory drugs during the active bouts of disease and prevention of streptococcal infection with prophylactic penicillin.

JUVENILE RHEUMATOID ARTHRITIS

Definition

Juvenile rheumatoid arthritis (JRA) is not a single disease, but rather a group of conditions or diseases that are characterized by the presence of chronic synovitis in children (Table 22.3). Various names have been applied to this condition in recent years; the term JRA remains the official designation in the United States (Schaller, 1980).

The arthritis results from chronic synovial inflammation of unknown cause. Affected joints are swollen and may be painful, limited in motion, warm, and occasionally erythematous. Synovitis may persist for months, or even years, without causing joint destruction; however, in some patients damage to cartilage, subchondral bone, and other joint structures may result. Juvenile rheumatoid arthritis is also associated with a number of extra-articular manifestations. Both the patterns and severity of joint disease and the types of extra-articular manifestations differ in the various disease subgroups. These subgroups also differ in other important characteristics such as age at disease onset, sex of affected patients, genetic predisposition and prognosis. As noted previously, three of the five subgroups of JRA have HLA associations that indicate genetic predispositions.

Clinical Manifestations

SYSTEMIC ONSET JRA

This subgroup includes about 20% of children with JRA, affects boys slightly more than girls, and can begin at any age. The disease is characterized by dramatic extra-articular manifestations, which are usually the presenting manifestations of disease. These include high intermittent fevers (greater than 103° F) that occur once or twice daily and are often associated with shaking chills, and an evanescent erythematous rash, which is maximal during periods of fever and which may occur in scratch marks (isomorphic or Koebner response), hepatomegaly (which may be associated with mildly abnormal liver function studies), splenomegaly, lymphadenopathy, pericarditis, occasional myocarditis, pleuritis, abdominal pain and peritonitis, anemia, and leukocytosis. The most characteristic findings are fever (present in all patients by definition) and the rash (present in about 95% of patients); other findings occur in more than half of patients. The systemic complaints are usually self-limited to a period of about 6 months, regardless of therapy. Recurrences may occur months or years later in disease. The systemic manifestations are rarely fatal, particularly with the availability of corticosteroid therapy; occasionally severe pericarditis or myocarditis or severe anemia may be life-threatening and demand acute corticosteroid therapy.

Patients with systemic onset JRA may have arthralgia, myalgia or transient arthritis at the beginning of the disease; definitive diagnosis, however, requires that chronic (more than 6 consecutive weeks) arthritis must be documented. The arthritis nearly always takes the form of polyarticular disease, affecting multiple joints both large and small. There is a predilection for midcarpal and midtarsal joints, resulting in dramatic dorsal swelling of the wrists and ankles. A few children with the systemic manifestations of JRA never develop lasting arthritis; in such individuals the diagnosis of possible or probable systemic onset JRA is appropriate.

Rheumatoid Factor-Negative Polyarthritis. This subgroup includes about 25% of children with JRA, affects girls more than boys, and can begin at any age. Affected children have arthritis affecting multiple joints both large and small, without either the systemic manifestations of systemic disease or positive tests for rheu-

Table 22.3
Subgroups of Juvenile Rheumatoid Arthritis[1]

Subgroup	Ratio of Girls to Boys	Time of Onset	Pattern of Arthritis	Immunogenetics	Extra-articular Manifestations	Prognosis
Systemic onset	8/10	Any age	Any joints	ANA negative; RF negative; HLA-?	High fever, rash, organomegaly, polyserositis, leukocytosis	20% severe arthritis
Polyarticular: rheumatoid factor-negative	8/1	Any age	Any joints	ANA 25%; RF negative; HLA-?	Low-grade fever, mild anemia, malaise	10% severe arthritis
Polyarticular: rheumatoid factor-positive	6/1	Late childhood	Any joints	ANA 75%; RF 100%; HLA-DR4	Mild fever, anemia, malaise, rheumatoid nodules	>50% severe arthritis
Pauciarticular: early childhood onset	7/1	Early childhood	Scattered joints, predominantly large joints; hips and sacroiliac joints spared	ANA 60%; RF negative; HLA-DRW8, -DR5, -DRW6	Few constitutional complaints; chronic iridocyclitis in 30–40%	20% develop polyarthritis; some incur ocular damage from iridocyclitis
Pauciarticular: late childhood onset	1/10	Late childhood	Scattered large joints; hip girdle and sacroiliac involvement common	ANA negative; RF negative, HLA-B27	Few constitutional complaints; acute iridocyclitis in 5–10%	Some will develop spondyloarthropathy

[1] ANA = Antinuclear antibodies; RF = rheumatoid factor.

matoid factors. Disease may begin at any age; indeed about 20% of adults with rheumatoid arthritis have this condition. The arthritis is frequently mild.

Rheumatoid Factor-Positive Polyarthritis. This condition is the childhood equivalent of classic adult rheumatoid arthritis, includes about 5% of children with JRA, and rarely begins before the eighth birthday. Rheumatoid factors in high titer are present from the beginning of disease and remain consistently present throughout the disease. Multiple joints, both large and small are affected. The arthritis is often severe, with joint destruction occurring with the first year of disease. Subcutaneous rheumatoid nodules are present over pressure points, and occasionally rheumatoid vasculitis, Felty syndrome (splenomegaly and leukopenia), and Sjögren syndrome (parotitis, dry mouth, dry eyes) are associated.

Pauciarticular JRA Type I. This condition appears to be distinctive to childhood, generally begins before the fifth birthday, and includes about 40% of children with JRA. Girls are affected more often than are boys. Arthritis may affect one or more joints, generally large joints, with an asymmetrical distribution. Knees, ankles, and elbows are most often affected; hips are generally spared. One in three affected children will develop chronic iridocyclitis; this insidious eye disorder results from inflammation of the iris and ciliary body, is characteristically unassociated with early symptoms or signs, and may cause significant ocular damage and loss of vision. Iridocyclitis may begin as long as 10 years after the onset of disease, and is not necessarily related to active joint disease.

Pauciarticular JRA Type II. This type of arthritis is closely related to the spondyloarthropathies, and accounts for about 15% of what is called JRA. Boys are predominantly affected and the disease usually begins in children older than 8 years. A family history of ankylosing spondylitis or one of the other spondyloarthropathies is common; indeed, such conditions often evolve from pauciarticular disease type II over a period of years. Affected patients have arthritis in a few joints, most often those of the lower extremities; hips are often affected. Arthritis may be acute and episodic or chronic and relatively indolent. Patients may have sacroiliitis that is silent and detectable only by radiographs or acutely symptomatic. Extra-articular features include acute iridocyclitis and occasional fever. Features of the spondyloarthropathies (limited back motion, features of Reiter syndrome, or inflammatory bowel disease) may appear during the course of disease (see next section).

Natural History

Taken together, at least 75% of children with JRA will eventually enter remissions and become functional adults without significant lasting disease disability. The natural history of JRA can be understood better by considering individual subgroups. The fever and other systemic manifestations of systemic onset disease generally run a self-limited course of about 6 months' duration; bouts of systemic disease may recur but rarely do so after children reach adulthood. Children with *systemic onset disease* develop seronegative polyarthritis which can be quite severe and which often outlasts the period of systemic complaints; about 25% of these children will incur severe joint damage. This arthritis may remain active into the adult years. *Rheumatoid factor-negative polyarthritis* can be chronic, but is often mild and may not result in extensive subjoint destruction. On the other hand, *rheumatoid factor-positive disease,* the childhood equivalent of classic adult rheumatoid arthritis, is usually severe, with early joint destruction and significant potential disability. *Pauciarticular JRA type I* remains mild and is limited to a few joints in about 80% of affected children; however, in about 20%, additional joint involvement occurs over the years and the resulting polyarthritis may be quite severe. One of three children with pauciarticular disease type I will develop a chronic insidious iridocyclitis over the first 10 years of disease; this eye disease can cause ocular damage and visual loss leading to significant permanent disability. The natural history for children with *pauciarticular disease type II* is not known with certainty; some appear to enter long remissions, while others appear to develop features of chronic spondyloarthropathy.

Diagnosis

Diagnosis of JRA rests on the demonstration of objective synovitis (signaled by joint swelling or a combination of joint pain, loss of motion, and swelling or redness; onset during the childhood years [before the 17th birthday in the United States]), the exclusion of other nonrheumatic conditions (considered in the differential diagnosis section above) and other rheumatic diseases (Table 22.4). Classification of subgroups depends on the clinical findings described above. There are no diagnostic laboratory tests. Anemia and leukocytosis may be present (particularly in systemic onset disease) and acute phase reactants are often present during periods of active disease (elevated sedimentation rates, positive C-reactive proteins). Urinalyses are normal. Liver function studies may be mildly abnormal in systemic onset disease and in children receiving salicylate therapy. Antinuclear antibodies may be found in seronegative polyarthritis, rheumatoid factor-positive polyarthritis, and particularly in pauciarticular disease type I. Rheumatoid factors are found only in rheumatoid factor-positive polyarthritis.

Serum immunoglobulin levels may be elevated, although serum complement levels are normal and antibodies to DNA are not detected. Radiographs may show evidence of joint destruction in late and severe disease; such changes are fairly characteristic of rheumatoid arthritis. Radiographs and electrocardiograms may also show evidence of pleuritis and pericarditis.

Table 22.4
Criteria for Juvenile Rheumatoid Arthritis[1]

1. Objective arthritis in 1 or more joints for 6 or more consecutive weeks. Arthritis is defined as swelling of a joint or limitation of motion with heat, pain or tenderness. (Pain or tenderness alone is not sufficient for a diagnosis of arthritis.)
2. Onset before 17th birthday
3. Exclusion of other known causes of arthritis/arthropathy:
   A. Other rheumatic diseases
   B. Infectious arthritis
   C. Inflammatory bowel disease
   D. Neoplastic diseases including leukemia
   E. Nonrheumatic conditions of bones and joints
   F. Hematologic diseases
   G. Psychogenic rheumatism
   H. Miscellaneous causes

[1] Adapted from JRA Criteria Subcommittee of the American Rheumatism Association.

Treatment

The first important step in therapy is accurate diagnosis and identification of problems in the individual patient. Potential problems include systemic complaints, active joint disease, existing disabilities, ocular disease, growth retardation, and psychosocial disability. Since the etiology and pathogenesis of chronic arthritis are poorly understood, treatment remains symptomatic, not curative. Drug therapy is used to reduce the inflammatory response as much as possible, and physical and occupational therapy are essential to restore and preserve musculoskeletal function. Great care must be taken to treat the whole child in the context of the family and environment, to promote normal growth and development, and to avoid the problems of psychogenic invalidism.

Salicylates remain the mainstay of drug therapy for JRA. Salicylates are generally given three or four times a day; blood levels of about 20 mg/dl (no higher than 30 mg/dl) are considered optimal for disease control. Doses of 100 mg/kg/day for children up to 25 kg are generally adequate to achieve such levels; total daily doses of 2400–3600 mg/day are usually sufficient for older children. Salicylates should generally be given with food; liver function should be monitored occasionally. There has been recent concern over the development of Reye syndrome in children receiving salicylates; the drug should be discontinued after known exposure to varicella or influenza, since instances are known (although very rare) of children with JRA receiving aspirin who have developed Reye syndrome. A number of alternative drugs to salicylates are lumped together under the term nonsteroidal anti-inflammatory drugs (NSAIDs); of these only tolmetin (Tolectin) is currently labeled for use by children in the United States. None of the other NSAIDs has been shown to be superior to aspirin in double blinded studies; however, some are believed to have a useful role in the treatment of arthritis in adults, particularly in the treatment of spondyloarthropathies.

For children with severe arthritis who do not respond to an adequate trial of salicylates or other nonsteroidal agents (generally a trial of 3–6 months is required), slow acting agents may be considered. Of these, gold is the most frequently used (Brewer et al, 1980). Gold therapy has traditionally consisted of weekly injections of either gold sodium thiomalate (Myochrysine) or gold thioglucose (Solganal). Injections are started with a low test dose and increased to a weekly maintenance dose of 1 mg/kg. A course of gold is generally given for 6 months; if patients respond, dramatic improvement usually occurs within that time. Side-effects are potentially severe and patients must be carefully monitored particularly before each injection. These include skin rashes, mucosal lesions, bone marrow suppression (leukopenia, thrombocytopenia, anemia), and proteinuria or hematuria. The drug should not be given if there is any question of toxicity. Oral gold is available in the form of auranofin; this drug has been tested in children and has been found to be effective, although perhaps less so than injectible gold (Giannini et al, 1983). The side effects are similar, as is the required monitoring. Antimalarials in the form of hydroxychloroquine have been considered remittive agents; however, a double blinded study did not show their efficacy in JRA (Brewer et al, 1986). Side-effects are potentially severe; these drugs are deposited in pigmented tissues, including the retina of the eye and may cause permanent retinal damage if not carefully monitored. D-Penicillamine has also been considered a remittive agent; however, this drug was not shown to be effective in children in a single double blinded study, although there have been claims made for its efficacy in uncontrolled trials (Brewer et al, 1986).

It is unfortunate that corticosteroids, the most potent anti-inflammatory agents we know, have so many serious side effects that their usefulness in treating JRA is minimal. They are clearly the agents of choice in severe systemic disease which is life-threatening and in iridocyclitis if topical steroid therapy is not sufficient. In systemic JRA, the doses should be reasonably high, sufficient to control the systemic manifestations quickly, and the duration of therapy as short as possible (weeks to months). In severe iridocyclitis the doses should be sufficient to control the ocular inflammation as monitored by slit-lamp examinations in the hands of an experienced ophthalmologist; at times alternate-day therapy is sufficient.

CONTROVERSY

The role of corticosteroids in therapy of the joint disease of JRA remains a subject of some controversy. Many observers feel that the side effects of steroids greatly outweigh their potential benefit in most children, particularly since it seems clear that the drugs do not themselves cure arthritis but simply suppress the symptoms. If steroids are used for joint manifestations, they should be used in the lowest possible doses and for the shortest possible times.

Other drugs have been suggested in the therapy of JRA, but no definitive studies have proved their efficacy. Methotrexate has been widely touted as an effective agent in adults with rheumatoid arthritis; a controlled study is currently underway in children (Furst and Kremer, 1988). Cyclophosphamide and azathioprine have been used to treat adults with rheumatoid arthritis, but there are no controlled studies in children. Obviously the long-term side effects are of concern, particularly regarding possible induction of malignancy and interference with reproductive capacity.

Other Aspects of Therapy

Physical and occupational therapy are essential components of therapy. The aims of therapy are to preserve and increase range of motion in the joints and the strength of supporting muscle groups. The overall function of the child is also evaluated, and tasks that are difficult, such as climbing stairs or writing, are specifically addressed. Children with severe disabilities may require hospitalization for intensive therapy. All children with significant joint involvement should be on a daily home program of physical therapy which, after appropriate teaching, can be supervised by the parents. Splinting may be useful for preserving or regaining joint motion, and heat in the form of a hot morning bath or more concentrated heat of paraffin baths for hands may be useful in loosening affected joints. Prolonged immobilization of joints in plaster is generally contraindicated.

Orthopedists can be valuable allies in the care of children with JRA. Several types of surgical procedures are possible. Synovectomy, the removal of inflamed synovium from selected joints, was at one time touted as a curative procedure. However, this operation appears to have limited usefulness in JRA. Replacement of damaged joints is a procedure that offers great promise in the rehabilitation of older children who have been severely damaged; considerable experience has been gained with total hip and total knee replacements in teenage patients and the results appear to be good (Ruddlesdin et al, 1986). There is much less experience with the replacement of other joints. Unfortunately, because of the problems of growth, joint replacements are not routinely available for younger children. A third type of procedure, that of soft tissue release around joints with severe flexion contractures not amenable to physical therapy, remains somewhat experimental but has potential benefit. Such procedures must be accompanied by intensive physical therapy.

Other health professionals who may be important to the care of children with JRA are ophthalmologists (who should be knowledgeable about iridocyclitis and skillful with slit-lamp examinations on young children), pediatric nurses, social workers, psychiatrists, and the child's school teachers and parents. The family pediatrician or family physician is extremely important in the coordination of care. As in any kind of childhood illness, the optimal care of the child with JRA requires the cooperation of a number of specialists, and is sometimes best handled at tertiary referral centers where all the required services are available and coordinated.

Prognosis

With early diagnosis and appropriate therapy, the prognosis for most children with JRA is good. The systemic complaints of systemic onset JRA are nearly always controllable with nonsteroidal agents or with corticosteroids if needed. At least 75% of children with systemic onset JRA will end up in good physical condition; about 25%, however, have severe seronegative arthritis, which may result in disability. Children with seronegative polyarthritis often do well; between 80% and 90% of them escape without permanent significant joint damage, although the disease itself may be chronic. Children with seropositive arthritis do not generally fare so well; more than 50% experience joint damage and disability within the first years of disease even with the best forms of therapy currently available. Eighty percent of children with pauciarticular disease type I have mild arthritis which remains limited to few joints; 20% later develop multiple joint involvement and may have severe arthritis. One-third will have iridocyclitis; it appears that with early detection by regular slit-lamp examinations and early therapy ocular damage can often be prevented. The overall prognosis for chil-

CASE ILLUSTRATION

A 14-year-old boy with JRA came to the emergency room complaining of chest pain.

At age 2 years he was ill for 7 weeks with malaise, daily spiking fevers as high as 104°F, an evanescent macular rash, and several tender swollen joints. A diagnosis of JRA was made and he was treated briefly with salicylates and then started on prednisone to which he responded dramatically. During the subsequent years he has had four exacerbations of his disease, characterized by diffuse arthralgias and rash, which have responded to short courses of either aspirin or prednisone. For the past 3 years he has been asymptomatic on no medications.

Six days before this admission, he developed pain in the neck, shoulders, arms, and legs and had a fever. One day before admission a macular skin rash developed over his shoulders, and at that time he began to experience chest pain in the retrosternal area. The pain radiated to the shoulder and was especially severe when he was supine.

On physical examination, he had a temperature of 37.8° C, heart rate 140 beats/min, respiratory rate 24 breaths/min, blood pressure 130/90 mm Hg with a pulsus paradoxus. There was no jugular venous distension. The precordium was hyperactive and a grade II/VI midsystolic flow murmur was heard along the left lower sternal border. A friction rub was present intermittently. The liver was not enlarged, although the spleen tip was palpable. There was no significant abdominal tenderness. He had severe arthralgia in multiple joints, and loss of motion in both wrists and his cervical spine.

Laboratory investigation revealed a white count of 27,300 mm^3 with a left shift (72% polys, 11% bands), hematocrit 39%, sedimentation rate 106 mm/hr. Three blood cultures were sterile, and the tuberculin test was negative. Viral studies subsequently proved to be negative. An ECG showed some slight but nonspecific ST-T wave changes. A chest radiograph revealed a mildly enlarged cardiac silouette. This was confirmed with an echocardiogram which showed a small pericardial effusion; myocardial contractility was normal. Joint films revealed old changes in the carpal bones and fusion of C2-C3, both consistent with the previous diagnosis of JRA.

During hospitalization he was treated with high doses of salicylates for 5 days, but the fever and chest pain persisted, and the pericardial effusion increased in size. He subsequently responded to prednisone therapy, and was discharged asymptomatic. The prednisone was slowly tapered over several months while the patient was maintained on salicylate therapy.

QUESTIONS AND COMMENTS

Can one be assured that the pericarditis is on the basis of the underlying collagen vascular disease or should one consider other diagnostic possibilities?

About 30% of patients with systemic onset JRA will, at some time, have pericardial involvement; thus, the most likely diagnosis was pericarditis on that basis. Infectious diseases must always be considered, particularly if corticosteroid therapy is to be used. In this boy, blood cultures were sterile and the tuberculin test negative. In some instances, a pericardial tap might be required to exclude bacterial pericarditis; in this boy clinical judgment did not mandate that invasive procedure. A number of viral agents such as EBV, cytomegalovirus and enteroviruses can also cause pericarditis and might be sought in the evaluation.

What is the most appropriate way to diagnose pericardial effusion?

Echocardiograms are the most valuable studies. When patients with JRA without any pericardial symptoms have been examined by echocardiograms, about one-third of them have been found to have evidence of pericardial disease during clinical exacerbations of their arthritis. In many of these individuals, ECGs and chest films were within normal limits.

What is the prognosis?

In general, pericarditis in association with JRA responds within 1–2 days to steroid therapy and the outlook is excellent. Constrictive pericarditis occur only very rarely in these patients, and cardiac tamponade is very unusual.

dren with pauciarticular disease type II is not currently known. Many appear to do well, but some will later have chronic spondyloarthropathy.

SPONDYLOARTHROPATHIES

Definition

The spondyloarthropathies are a group of disorders characterized by chronic or recurrent arthritis that typically affects the spine and axial joints with or without the occurrence of peripheral arthritis. These conditions include ankylosing spondylitis, Reiter syndrome, the spondylitis of inflammatory bowel disease and psoriasis, reactive arthritis, the enthesopathy syndromes, and pauciarticular JRA type II. A few individuals with only acute iridocyclitis also cluster with this group of disorders. These conditions share the common properties of male preponderance, seronegativity for both antinuclear antibodies and rheumatoid factors, familial clustering, and associations with HLA B27 (Jacobs et al, 1982). Onset is rarely before age 8 years.

Natural History

Ankylosing spondylitis is the prototype disease of this group. This disease may begin in one of two ways: pain and stiffness in the hips, hip girdles, or back or peripheral arthritis generally affecting a few large joints, particularly of the lower extremities. In children, the disease most frequently begins with peripheral arthritis; hence, many of these patients have been relegated to the category previously described as pauciarticular JRA type II. The peripheral arthritis may be acute and very painful, or may be more indolent. Bouts of arthritis are often transient and recurrent, although some patients have chronic arthritis from the onset. Occasionally spinal involvement is apparent early in disease, manifest as pain, stiffness, and loss of motion in the back. The lower back is generally affected first, with later involvement of the spine in an ascending fashion. Limited flexion of the lumbar spine can be measured objectively on physical examination. Occasionally chest expansion is decreased early in disease because of involvement of costovertebral joints. Stiffness of the neck may also be present, although this usually occurs late in disease. Patients with ankylosing spondylitis may have bouts of inflammation of sites of attachment of tendons and ligaments to bone (enteropathy); heel pain from Achilles tendonitis is particularly common. A few patients have constitutional symptoms of malaise and weight loss. Episodes of acute iridocyclitis are occasionally associated; these are heralded by photophobia, redness, and eye pain and are generally self-limited, without causing permanent eye damage.

Reiter syndrome occurs at times in young children, but more often in older ones; this condition has been considered rare in childhood. Affected children usually present with bouts of peripheral arthritis, generally resembling pauciarticular JRA type II. Associated findings necessary for diagnosis include conjunctivitis or acute iritis and urethritis manifest either by genitourinary symptoms or abnormal urinalysis. Skin rashes and mucosal lesions (keratoderma blennorrhagica, balanitis, and mouth ulcers) may be associated. Fever, sometimes high, is common (Rosenberg and Petty, 1979).

Inflammatory bowel disease, both ulcerative colitis and Crohn disease, may be associated with a peripheral arthritis which is generally benign and resembles pauciarticular JRA type II. Bouts of peripheral arthritis generally parallel the activity of the underlying bowel disease. This type of arthritis is not associated with HLA-B27 or with subsequent ankylosing spondylitis. A small percentage of children with inflammatory bowel disease have a type of spondyloarthropathy that closely resembles ankylosing spondylitis, which is associated with HLA-B 27, and which is sometimes progressive regardless of control of the underlying bowel disease (Lindsley and Schaller, 1974).

Psoriasis and arthritis can coexist in some children; either the psoriasis or the arthritis may be the initial event. In the majority of affected children, the arthritis is peripheral, either pauciarticular or polyarticular in nature. This peripheral arthritis is not associated with HLA-B27 or with spondylitis. A few children with psoriatic arthritis, however, do have HLA-B27-associated arthritis that resembles ankylosing spondylitis (Shore and Ansell, 1982).

In *reactive arthritis,* pauciarticular arthritis, generally considered to be transient, occurs after gastrointestinal infections with *Shigella, Salmonella, Yersinia enterocolitica,* or *Campylobacter* in individuals who are genetically predisposed; such individuals have HLA-B27 (Keat, 1983).

In enthesopathy, transient and recurrent bouts of inflammation occur at sites where tendons and ligaments attach to bone; bouts of enthesopathy may be associated with peripheral arthritis or with the axial arthritis of spondylitis. Enthesopathy is common in all of the spondyloarthropic conditions.

COURSE

Ankylosing spondylitis and the spondyloarthropathies may be progressive or may show surprisingly long remissions without further disease progression. The peripheral arthritis of pauciarticular JRA type II and of all of the spondyloarthropathies is often acute and transient, with symptom-free intervals of months or years between attacks. It seems likely that many individuals with spondyloarthropathy have mild disease that does not progress and which, in fact, often remains unrecognized. Some affected individuals have progressive disease that can cause disability. Causes of disability in ankylosing spondylitis are related to severe spinal immobility and deformity, severe hip disease, and rarely to severe peripheral arthritis. Reiter syndrome also can be associated with disabling peripheral arthritis. Psoriatic arthritis is sometimes quite disabling because of destruction of peripheral joints.

Diagnosis

Diagnosis of the spondyloarthropathies rests on recognition of the above patterns of arthritis, along with any features that would permit designation of more specific conditions such as Reiter syndrome. There are no specific laboratory abnormalities, although anemia, slightly elevated white counts, elevated sedimentation rates, and the presence of other acute phase reactants are frequently associated with bouts of active disease. Ninety to 95% of individuals with ankylosing spondylitis and slightly lower percentages of individuals with the other forms of spondyloarthropathy can be found to have HLA-B27. The presence of HLA-B27 itself is not a diagnostic test for these diseases, however, since only about 10% of individuals with HLA-B27 ever have any rheumatic disorders. Demonstration of sacroiliitis by radiography is essential for the diagnosis of ankylosing spondylitis, as is demonstration of limited mobility of the lumbodorsal spine. Radiographic changes in the spine occur later in disease and are also diagnostic; these include calcification of paraspinal ligaments with bridging of vertebral bodies resulting in the so-called bamboo spine. Diagnosis of Reiter syndrome requires demonstration of the triad of arthritis, ocular findings, and genitourinary findings; the designation partial Reiter syndrome has come into use in some circles for patients who have only peripheral arthritis characteristic of pauciarticular JRA type II.

Treatment

Treatment rests on the use of nonsteroidal anti-inflammatory drugs as described for JRA, and physical therapy. Physical therapy should be geared to preservation of normal spinal alignment and normal strength of paravertebral and abdominal and neck muscles. Therapy for peripheral arthritis is similar to that of pauciarticular JRA type II. Occasionally experts have recommended the use of drugs such as antimalarials and gold in the therapy of spondyloarthropathy. Methotrexate has also been tried on an experimental basis. There is little role for steroids in the therapy of ankylosing spondylitis and the other spondyloarthropathies, although they may be used for treatment of underlying conditions, such as inflammatory bowel disease.

Prognosis

The prognosis for the majority of patients with spondyloarthropathy is quite good. The long-term prognosis for children with spondyloarthropathy is not accurately known. It is clear that some children will have ankylosing spondylitis in the future, and it has been suggested that early onset of ankylosing spondylitis may be associated with severe hip disease. The prognosis for childhood-onset Reiter syndrome and psoriatic arthritis has been described as good; however, long-term studies are not yet available. Even in progressive ankylosing spondylitis, with maintenance of good spinal alignment and good peripheral musculoskeletal function, the overall functional outcome can be satisfactory.

SYSTEMIC LUPUS ERYTHEMATOSUS

Definition

Systemic lupus erythematosus (SLE) is a chronic rheumatic disease that characteristically involves many organ systems and is associated with serologic aberrations, particularly with the presence of antinuclear antibodies. SLE is primarily a disease of young adult women; about 15% of cases begin during the childhood years. When lupus begins before puberty, the sex ratio includes relatively more males; after the age of puberty the sex ratio of patients with lupus is about nine girls for one boy. Discoid lupus is a form of disease that is considered to be limited to the skin without systemic manifestations; affected persons may have positive tests for antinuclear antibodies and other serologic abnormalities. This form of disease is unusual in children. Lupus is sometimes familial and genetic markers within the HLA system have been demonstrated (Nepom and Schaller, 1984).

Natural History

Most children with lupus have SLE with involvement of multiple organ systems (Table 22.5). Most affected children are clinically ill with malaise and fever; the fever may take any pattern, either low grade or high, either intermittent or sustained. The only individually clinically distinctive manifestation of lupus is the facial butterfly rash which occurs perhaps in half of the patients. Other cutaneous manifestations include maculopapular lesions on the palms, soles, and extremities; various polymorphic rashes anywhere on the body;

Table 22.5
Systemic Lupus Erythematosus:

Childhood-Onset: Disease Manifestations	
Malaise	96%
Cutaneous abnormalities	96%
Hematological abnormalities	91%
Fever	84%
Nephritis	84%
Musculoskeletal complaints	82%
Pleural/pulmonary disease	67%
Hepatosplenomegaly and/or lymphadenopathy	58%
Neurological disease	49%
Cardiac abnormalities	42%
Weight loss/growth retardation	38%
Hypertension	33%
Ocular abnormalities	31%
Gastrointestinal symptoms	29%
Raynaud	13%

and purpura. Involvement of hair follicles can lead to generalized or localized alopecia. Mucosal ulcers, particularly in the mouth and pharynx, are also common. Hematologic abnormalities include leukopenia, anemia (often with a positive Coombs test), and thrombocytopenia. The majority of children with SLE have overt nephritis with hematuria, proteinuria, or both; occasionally the nephrotic syndrome is the presenting manifestation. Hypertension may occur as a concomitant of renal disease, as may renal failure; these are generally later manifestations of disease. Musculoskeletal complaints are common early in lupus; arthritis or arthralgia, often transient but occasionally chronic, is the most common. Avascular necrosis of the femoral heads or other juxta-articular bones may be a cause of joint pain. Myalgia or myositis may also occur. Pleuritis and pericarditis are common; these are generally mild but painful. Pulmonary disease in the form of interstitial pneumonia, pulmonary hemorrhage, or pulmonary fibrosis are potentially severe manifestations of disease; pulmonary infections must always be excluded. Hepatosplenomegaly and lymphadenopathy are common; occasionally a picture of mild hepatitis may be related to liver involvement. Neurologic diseases can be manifest in many ways; seizures, cerebral dysfunction or psychosis, strokes, peripheral neuropathy, or transverse myelitis. Cardiac abnormalities other than pericarditis include myocarditis and endocarditis (Libman-Sacks); endocarditis can cause changing heart murmurs, but rarely causes valvular dysfunction. The most frequent ocular abnormalities are small cotton wool exudates (cytoid bodies) in the retina, which are not associated with symptoms. Iritis, episcleritis, or Sjögren syndrome may also occur. Many forms of gastrointestinal symptoms may be associated; the most severe is vasculitis with bowel necrosis or perforation. Raynaud phenomenon occurs in a few patients.

COURSE

The course of untreated SLE in children is usually relentless, with progressive organ system involvement. Indeed, it appears that before the advent of modern treatment regimes the majority of children with this disease died, with infections, acute uncontrolled lupus involving multiple organ systems, renal failure, and hypertension being common fatal manifestations. Since the advent of corticosteroids and treatment protocols including corticosteroids and some of the cytotoxic drugs, and the realization that tests such as serum hemolytic complement and DNA antibodies provide reasonable parameters for judging disease activity, survival has improved greatly. Most centers with experience in the therapy of childhood lupus now report 5-year survivals of at least 95%. The disease usually remains chronic, however, with recurring manifestations involving various organ systems. Pulmonary disease, myocardial infarction, and CNS disease remain troublesome late complications, and occasionally control of the acute disease manifestations is difficult. Infections related to the disease itself and also related to therapy remain a major problem.

Diagnosis

The diagnosis of lupus rests on the recognition of the multisystem disease and the associated serologic abnormalities. Only the butterfly rash is clinically distinctive, and this does not occur in all patients. The combination of abnormalities in a number of organ systems should be sufficient to raise suspicion of this disease. For all practical purposes, all patients with lupus have positive tests for antinuclear antibodies by the fluorescent antinuclear antibody technique. Lupus erythematosus cells may also be found, although this method is a much less sensitive way of detecting antinuclear antibodies. The presence of antibodies to DNA and lowered serum hemolytic complement levels is also highly suggestive of SLE; such studies indicate the presence of active immune complex disease and are useful in following the course of disease. A number of complement component deficiencies have been associated with systemic lupus (Agnello, 1978). Other laboratory abnormalities suggestive of lupus include leukopenia, anemia, thrombocytopenia, the presence of antibodies to platelets, positive Coombs test, positive tests for rheumatoid factors, false-positive serology for syphilis, and elevated serum immunoglobulin levels. Circulating anticoagulants may be present. Abnormal urinalyses indicative of renal involvement should also raise the suspicion of SLE in any child with arthritis or other rheumatic complaints; renal function studies may also be abnormal. Radiographic and ECHO studies may be helpful in uncovering evidence of pericarditis or pleuritis, and studies such as EEGs, spinal taps, brain scans, and ECGs may also provide evidence of specific organ involvement. Biopsies and histologic evaluation of tissue are rarely necessary for diagnosis of SLE, although renal biopsies are commonly done to gauge the extent and severity of nephritis.

Treatment

The treatment of lupus is difficult and should be geared to disease manifestations and severity of disease in the individual patient. Hence, the first step in therapy is an accurate evaluation of the individual patient with regard to organ systems involved, severity of involvement, and presence or absence of active immune complex disease as perhaps best gauged by clinical manifestations and serum levels of hemolytic complement and DNA antibodies. For mild lupus without major organ involvement, potentially life-threatening manifestations, or evidence of active immune complex disease, symptomatic therapy with nonsteroidal agents or perhaps antimalarials may suffice. However, patients require careful follow-up for evidence of worsening disease. Unfortunately, the vast majority of children with SLE have potentially life-threatening organ involvement and also have evidence of active immune complex disease. For such patients, initial therapy with high doses of corticosteroids, usually in split daily dosage, are required to control both clinical manifestations of the disease and serologic evidence of active immune complex disease. When initial disease control is achieved, some observers switch to alternate-day high steroid doses; some continue with daily steroid regimens. In some patients in whom disease cannot be controlled with steroid therapy alone, additional drugs such as azathioprine, chlorambucil, or cyclophosphamide are added. There are no well-controlled studies of such agents in children, nor any agreement as to which is optimal. Recent experience suggests that intravenous cytoxan therapy may be associated with control of difficult disease. In acute life-threatening disease, measures such as high intravenous pulses of corticosteroids or even high intravenous doses of drugs such as cyclophosphamide have been used. Therapy of severe lupus is best managed by a specialist cognizant of the manifestations and the dangers of this disease. Close and careful follow-up is always required. Needless to say, the drug regimens mentioned above are often associated with severe side effects—those of chronic corticosteroid administration or the long-term effects of the various cytotoxic agents.

Patient education and counseling are crucial aspects of therapy. Children with potentially fatal illnesses need firm support in continuing the growth and development necessary to childhood and teenage years. A number of consultants may be important to the ad-

CASE ILLUSTRATION

A 9-year-old girl presented with a history of persistent fevers over a 4-week period. She was in her usual state of excellent health until 6 months before presentation when she experienced the onset of leg pains involving the soles of feet, ankles, shins and knees bilaterally. The pains were worse on waking and resulted in her missing a total of 25 days of school before the summer months. A physical examination done at the time of presentation of these symptoms was felt to be normal. She received physical therapy and became symptom-free over the summer vacation months. In the fall upon return to school she developed a fever and was found to have a urinary tract infection. At that time her hematocrit was 29% and sedimentation rate was 35 min/hr. She was treated with a 10-day course of amoxicillin with resolution of her urinary symptoms. However, toward the end of the course she broke out in a generalized itchy rash and again developed the onset of fevers persisting in the range of 102° F with recurrent extremity pain. There was an undocumented weight loss, but an otherwise negative review of systems.

On physical examination she appeared ill with a temperature of 103° F and tachycardia of 122. Her blood pressure was 114/60 mm Hg. The examination was notable for apthous mouth ulcers and a spleen palpable 2 cm below the left costal margin. Her joints were tender and painful on motion, but not swollen. There were no heart murmurs heard.

Laboratory values showed a hematocrit of 28%, with a mean corpuscular volume of 79μm^3, white blood count of 3000mm^3, with 79% polys, 13% lymphs, 6% monos, 2% eos, and platelet count 105,000. Reticulocyte count was 0.2%, sedimentation rate was 53 mm/hr. Urinalysis showed a specific gravity of 1.031, pH of 5.0, 3+ protein, 50–60 red blood cells, and 2–4 white blood cells per high power field, and small numbers of red cell and granular casts. BUN was 32mg/dl, creatinine 1.1 mg/kg, calcium 9.0 mg/dl, phosphorus 4.2 mg/dl.

QUESTION AND COMMENT

What is the differential diagnosis in this patient, and what further diagnostic work-up is indicated?

This patient presented with fever of unknown origin and a multisystem disease with chronic arthralgias, nephritis, and anemia, leukopenia, and thrombocytopenia. The possibility of subacute bacterial endocarditis was raised, although while fevers, nephritis, arthralgias, and anemia are consistent with this diagnosis, the absence of cardiac findings and the time course lasting over 6 months were not. Epstein-Barr infection or other viral infections were also considered possible although subsequent serologic studies were negative and the coexistence of nephritis would be unusual. Malignancy can also be considered given the arthralgia and cytopenia; a bone marrow examination was equally unremarkable except for a paucity of red blood cell precursors but no infiltrative cells.

Finally, rheumatologic disorders must be considered. Given the patients multisystem involvement, SLE was believed to be the most likely diagnosis. Although systemic JRA was considered, it was thought that this was not consistent with the patient's presentation of a nephritis. Blood was therefore sent for antinuclear antibody, anti-DNA antibodies, and serum complement analysis. The fluorescent ANA test was positive in high titers, as was the test for antibodies to DNA. The total serum hemolytic complement was greatly lowered, consistent with the immune complex disease of active SLE. The patient fulfilled the criteria for SLE, having 4 of the 11 items needed (positive anti-DNA, oral mucous lesions, arthritis, and nephritis).

As pediatricians, we tend to think of SLE as an adult disease. As many as 20% of patients with newly diagnosed lupus are under 16 years of age. Patients who present in childhood or early adolescence usually have evidence of multisystem disease, as was true with this patient. Malaise, rashes, hematologic abnormalities, fever, arthritis or arthralgia, nephritis, serositis, hepatosplenomegaly, and neurologic disorders are all frequent manifestations of childhood lupus (see Table 22.5). Classification of the renal lesion may be helpful in judging ultimate prognosis. This patient underwent a renal biopsy; histopathology revealed only mild mesangial and focal changes. The patient was treated with high dose corticoid steroid therapy and demonstrated dramatic improvement in her disease symptomatology over the next several weeks. Her DNA antibody levels fell to normal and her serum complement rose to normal levels within 7 weeks. She continues to do well 5 years after presentation, on low doses of prednisone; her serologic studies have remained normal.

equate care of children with lupus. These include nephrologists, ophthalmologists, and physical and occupational therapists. Careful, long-term follow-up by one physician who is designated as the primary physician is essential.

Prognosis

With early diagnosis and vigorous therapy, the 5-year survival now approaches 95% for children with SLE. Nevertheless, the disease remains chronic and troublesome, and individual patients need careful medical surveillance and usually require long periods of drug therapy.

Troublesome late complications such as myocardial infarctions can be unexpected causes of death.

Young women with lupus are at risk of having infants with the neonatal lupus syndrome or with congenital heart block; the exact risks of these occurrences have yet to be defined. It is now known that an unknown percentage of infants with the neonatal lupus syndrome will themselves have SLE years later (Chameides et al, 1977).

NEONATAL LUPUS SYNDROME

Definition

Infants of mothers with clinical or laboratory stigmata of lupus, Sjögren syndrome, or certain "undifferentiated" rheumatic disease may have at birth either clinical or laboratory stigmata of lupus or congenital heart block (Chameides et al, 1977; Harley et al, 1985). These phenomena are thought to be related to the transplacental passage of maternal antinuclear antibodies, most notably those directed against the nuclear antigens Ro (SSA) and La (SSB). Most of these phenomena disappear with the clearance of maternal autoantibodies during the latter part of the first year of life; however, the cardiac damage, in the form of congenital heart block, is permanent.

Natural History

The most common of the neonatal lupus phenomena are serologic abnormalities resulting from transplacental maternal autoantibodies, including the presence of circulating antinuclear antibodies and antibodies reactive with specific nuclear antigens. Leukopenia, hemolytic anemia, and thrombocytopenia may occur if there is transplacental passage of maternal antibodies reactive with these blood cells. Babies exhibiting these phenomena generally appear well, unless of course hemolytic anemia or thrombocytopenia are clinically significant. These serologic findings disappear before the first birthday.

The most frequent clinical manifestation of neonatal lupus is a rash which histologically resembles discoid lupus. This rash becomes apparent within hours or days of birth. Erythematous discoid lesions may affect the face, trunk, or limbs. These lesions generally clear by 6–9 months of age, and are presumably related to some transplacental factor which has not yet been identified. Occasionally babies show manifestations of systemic illness including hepatosplenomegaly and fever; however, the babies are usually clinically well.

Congenital heart block has been strongly associated with the presence of maternal antibody reactive with Ro (SSA) or La (SSB). Heart block may occur with or without other stigmata of neonatal lupus. Complete congenital heart block is detectable in utero as bradycardia and has been noted as early as the second trimester of pregnancy. It is not known whether incomplete heart block may also be part of this spectrum. A minority of affected children have other associated congenital heart defects, and some have been found to have endocardial fibroelastosis. Available pathologic specimens have shown multiple lesions of the connective tissue of the conduction system; immunoglobulin and complement deposits have been described in cardiac tissues from neonates who had died, suggesting that immune mechanisms may underlie this damage to fetal conduction system (Litsey et al, 1985). It has been suggested, but not proven, that some infants have additional myocardial involvement.

The transplacental serologic abnormalities, the discoid rash, and any attendant constitutional symptoms resolve before the first birthday, coincident with decay in transplacentally acquired maternal antibody. The congenital heart block, however, is permanent. True systemic lupus erythematus beginning in the neonatal period or the first year of life is exceptionally rare. Three case reports within recent years have described systemic lupus occurring later in life in individuals previously affected with the neonatal lupus syndrome; the true future risk of children with neonatal lupus for lupus later in life remains to be determined. Indeed, it is conceivable that familial predisposition to lupus may be the determining factor rather than the occurrence of the neonatal lupus syndrome.

Diagnosis and Treatment

Diagnosis of the neonatal lupus syndrome rests upon recognition of the discoid rash or complete congenital heart block plus the presence of maternal and transplacental antibodies to Ro or La, or upon identification of other serologic abnormalities in the infant consistent with lupus and also present in the mother. Therapy for the discoid rash is generally symptomatic; topical steroids may be helpful if the rash is severe. Rarely, specific therapy for thrombocytopenia or hemolytic anemia may be required. There is no specific therapy for congenital heart block; pacemaker implantation may be necessary. Any associated congenital cardiac defects require appropriate management.

CONTROVERSY

Some controversy has arisen over the possibility of "preventive" intrauterine therapy for infants carried by mothers with known antibodies to Ro and La. Proposed therapy has included treatment of the pregnant mother with anti-inflammatory drugs and plasmapheresis (Buyon et al, 1987). There is no good evidence, however, that such therapy is either warranted or effective; indeed, it is not certain that the transplacental antibody alone is responsible for the heart defects.

Prognosis

A few infants have developed adult lupus or juvenile arthritis or Sjögren syndrome. In the absence of complete heart block which may be fatal, the prognosis for life is excellent.

DERMATOMYOSITIS

Definition and Epidemiology

Dermatomyositis is a chronic rheumatic disease characterized by inflammation of striated muscle and a characteristic skin rash (Bowyer et al, 1983; Crowe et al, 1982). This disease is rare before the third or fourth year of life and affects boys and girls in about equal proportions. Although a genetic predisposition has been shown (association with HLA-B8-DR3), the disease rarely affects multiple first degree relatives in the same family.

Natural History

Both cutaneous manifestations and myositis are generally present early in disease. Occasionally the skin rash precedes the occurrence of myositis; rarely the myositis precedes the skin rash. The skin lesions are characteristic: there is a violaceous erythema of the upper eyelids and sometimes of the butterfly area; sometimes the butterfly rash can resemble that of lupus. Periorbital edema or even facial edema may be associated. There are violaceous lesions, sometimes with scaliness and patches of vitiligo, on extensor surfaces of the extremities, most characteristically the knuckles and dorsal surfaces of the finger joints, the elbows, the knees, and the medial malleoli. Occasionally violaceous lesions occur on the skin in the upper trunk area (shawl distribution) and other parts of the body. These skin lesions are chronic and often persist after resolution of the myositis. Occasionally necrotic skin lesions occur, particularly in the axillary, genital, and neck areas.

The myositis affects predominantly proximal limb girdle muscles and the muscles of the neck, perispinal, and abdominal areas. Onset is usually insidious, manifest by weakness and progressive loss of function. Occasionally patients have acute onset, with weakness and pain and swelling of affected muscles. Rarely facial and limb swelling are sufficient to resemble the generalized edema of such conditions as the nephrotic syndrome.

Underlying the lesions of dermatomyositis is a vasculitis of small blood vessels. This vasculitis can affect the gastrointestinal tract at any level, with various gastrointestinal symptoms and occasionally severe complications such as perforation of the gut. Involvement of muscles of deglutition and respiration may lead to problems with handling of secretions, aspiration, and respiratory insufficiency. Rarely the disease can affect other organ systems as well. Patients may have low grade fever and malaise. Calcinosis can occur as a late manifestation of disease, generally in patients who have not received adequate therapy.

Before the advent of corticosteroid therapy, as many as 50% of children with dermatomyositis died of their disease within the first 1 or 2 years of illness; causes of death were usually related to the respiratory insufficiency or vasculitis of the gastrointestinal tract. Of the children who survived, as many as half had significant musculoskeletal disability related to the myositis. The major period of disease activity for most affected patients appeared to be of about 2 years' duration.

Diagnosis

The diagnosis is generally clinical and rests on appreciation of the characteristic skin rash and the association of myositis. Occasionally, the skin rash may resemble that of SLE or mixed connective tissue disease; however, these diseases can be distinguished on laboratory and clinical grounds. The recognition of myositis is based on physical examination, which shows proximal muscle weakness. Electromyograms can be helpful in confirming myositis, showing a combined pattern of neuropathic and myopathic changes. Muscle biopsy is rarely necessary for diagnosis, although the histology is quite characteristic. There is a relatively noninflammatory vasculitis of the smallest blood vessels; intimal swelling and occlusion of small vessels is the most characteristic finding. Mild perivascular inflammation occurs, as well as necrosis, loss, and some inflammatory changes in scattered muscle fibers. Similar vasculitic changes have been described in other organs as well (Crowe et al, 1982).

Laboratory studies that are helpful include measurement of serum levels of enzymes that are found in muscle (creatinine phosphokinase, transaminases, aldolase, lactic dehydrogenase); although these tests are not specific for dermatomyositis, elevations are consistent with myositis and provide a convenient measurement with which to follow disease activity. Sedimentation rates may be normal or elevated with active disease and there are no characteristic changes in the complete blood count. Antinuclear antibody and rheumatoid factor tests may be positive or negative. Rarely myocardial involvement occurs as witnessed by abnormal ECGs. Radiographs late in disease may show evidence of calcinosis.

Treatment

Therapy rests on early dignosis and complete evaluation of the individual patient. It is of particular importance to seek any evident involvement of palatal respiratory muscles, any respiratory insufficiency, or any myocardial or gastrointestinal involvement. Prompt early treatment with large doses of corticosteroids (2–3 mg/kg/day in split doses) usually results in control of disease, as evidenced by improving clinical condition and return of elevated muscle enzyme levels to normal within a few weeks. Physical and occupational therapy are also important; such measures preserve muscle function and prevent the appearance of flexion contractures. Patients with potential respiratory problems need careful monitoring. If there are problems with palatal function or swallowing, soft diets should be instituted and the patient should be observed carefully. Occasionally, respiratory assistance is required. Gastrointestinal vasculitis generally responds to therapy of the disease; any episodes of severe abdominal pain should be promptly evaluated by a surgeon.

Occasionally, patients have severe disease that does not respond to corticosteroids; in such instances therapy with high dose pulse intravenous steroids or with the addition of drugs such as methotrexate, azathioprine or cytoxan has been considered effective in a few cases.

Prognosis

With early diagnosis and adequate therapy, the prognosis is good for the vast majority of patients. In our experience 90% of children treated early and optimally will go into remission and remain well. Occasionally, disease recurs years later and patients require second courses of therapy. In a few patients the disease seems to become chronic; in our experience this occurs when diagnosis and, thus, adequate treatment have been delayed. Causes of death include respiratory failure, aspiration or inability to handle secretions, gastrointestinal disease with perforation and resulting complications, or rare myocardial failure or arrythmias. Severe calcinosis can be a late concomitant of disease, which in itself can be very crippling. Calcinosis appears to occur most often in children who do not receive adequate early therapy (Bowyer et al, 1983).

VASCULITIS SYNDROMES

The vasculitis syndromes are a group of disorders related to inflammation of blood vessels. Distinctive clinical pictures depend on the size and site of involved vessels. These conditions include Takayasu arteritis (vasculitis of the aorta and the largest blood vessels), polyarteritis nodosa (vasculitis of medium sized blood vessels), variants of polyarteritis nodosa (including Wegener granulomatosis, infantile polyarteritis, and Kawasaki disease), and Henoch-Schönlein vasculitis (inflammation of the smallest blood vessels). Of these conditions, Henoch-Schönlein vasculitis with its distinctive picture of rash, arthralgia or arthritis, angioedema, abdominal pain, and nephritis, is the most frequently encountered in pediatrics; this disease is discussed in Section 8. Kawasaki disease is also of importance in pediatrics; this febrile illness is associated with vasculitis of large coronary vessels and other large central vessels in at least 30% of affected children. This condition, probably identical with what has been called infantile polyarteritis, is unique to pediatrics and unique in its distribution of vasculitis. It is discussed in Section 17.

RARE VASCULITIS SYNDROMES IN CHILDHOOD

Polyarteritis Nodosa

Polyarteritis nodosa is a serious illness, manifest by multisystem disease which reflects the pattern of inflammation of medium sized blood vessels throughout the body. Frequent disease manifestations include fever, vasculitic skin rashes, arthralgia or arthritis, nodular lesions, abdominal pain, renal disease, hypertension, central nervous system disease, peripheral neuropathy, pulmonary disease, cardiac disease, and ocular involvement. There are no diagnostic laboratory studies other than biopsy evidence of vascular changes in affected vessels. Laboratory studies are not specific; tests for antinuclear antibodies and rheumatoid factors and other autoantibodies are generally negative. Of recent interest has been the realization that the syndrome of polyarteritis nodosa can result from hepatitis B infection, probably by an immune complex mechanism which affects vessel walls; polyarteritis has also followed streptococcal infections and serous otitis media. Antecedent causes are unknown in the majority of cases, however. Untreated, this disease is progressive and potentially fatal. Vigorous therapy with corticosteroids or agents such as cyclophosphamide has been successful in some patients (Fauci et al, 1979).

WEGENER GRANULOMATOSIS

In this condition, systemic necrotizing vasculitis is associated with necrotizing granulomas of the upper and lower respiratory tracts (Hall et al, 1985a; Bernhard et al, 1986). Respiratory tract granulomas may result in chronic rhinitis and nasal perforation, chronic sinusitis, or chronic pulmonary disease. The vasculitis resembles that of polyarteritis nodosa clinically, and is often severe and rapidly progressive. Clinical manifestations include sinusitis, chronic rhinitis, or chronic pulmonary disease combined with any of the manifestations of severe systemic vasculitis. Renal disease is frequently severe and progressive. There are no diagnostic laboratory tests other than biopsy evidence of necrotizing vasculitis, combined with characteristic giant cell granulomas of the respiratory tract. This disease has rarely been reported in children. Untreated, the disease is potentially fatal; treatment with steroids and cyclophosphamide may be successful and even curative (Fauci et al, 1983).

TAKAYASU DISEASE

This condition,resulting from inflammation of the aorta and the largest blood vessels, is exceedingly rare in the United States but does affect children in other parts of the world, particularly in the Asian countries (Hall et al, 1985b). Antecedent causes for this type of vasculitis are unknown; associations with tuberculosis have been suggested. Clinical manifestations include fever, hypertension (related to occlusion of the renal vessels), hypertensive encephalopathy, renal failure, weak or absent pulses in the upper extremities (hence the designation "pulseless disease"), neurologic disturbances (related to decreased blood flow to the brain), visual complaints, and assorted rheumatic complaints. There are no specific laboratory studies other than arteriographic demonstrations of vascular involvement or histologic evidence of vasculitis. The natural history of this disorder is variable; the disease progresses rapidly in some patients and pursues a benign and chronic course in others. In severe disease, vigorous treatment with anti-inflammatory or immunosuppressive agents should be tried. Attention must be paid to controlling hypertension, seizures, and cardiac failure. Surgery to alleviate vascular occlusion may be required.

SCLERODERMA

Scleroderma is perhaps the oddest of the rheumatic diseases and is characterized by fibrosis rather than by inflammation. Two forms exist: cutaneous and systemic. The cutaneous forms of scleroderma include morphea, with patches of cutaneous and subcutaneous fibrosis, and linear scleroderma, with lines of cutaneous and subcutaneous fibrosis. Cutaneous scleroderma is clinically distinctive and rarely requires biopsy for diagnosis. Abnormalities in immunologic tests such as presence of antinuclear antibodies, rheumatoid factors, and elevated immunogloulin may be associated; the meaning of these abnormal tests is not understood. Children with cutaneous scleroderma rarely if ever develop systemic disease. Cutaneous involvement may, however, cause significant musculoskeletal crippling should entire limbs or tissues around joints be affected. In systemic disease (called systemic sclerosis), Raynaud phenomenon is always present and is usually the first manifestation of disease. Fingertip ulcers and loss of distal phalanges may occur over the years. Fibrosis of skin and subcutaneous tissues occurs in a generalized fashion, affecting the distal extremities and the face in the earliest forms of disease. Fibrosis also affects internal organs, including the gastrointestinal tract (esophageal and bowel dysfunction and dysmotility), the heart (pericarditis or myocardial fibrosis), and the lungs (pulmonary fibrosis). Renal involvement is manifest by hypertension rather than by the usual findings of nephritis. The systemic forms of the disease may be relentlessly progressive and potentially fatal. Systemic sclerosis is quite rare in children (Suarez-Almazor et al, 1985).

There are no proven effective means of therapy for either form of the disease, although many drugs have been tried. Topical corticosteroids are often used for cutaneous forms of the disease. Therapy with penicillamine has been proposed for severe cutaneous disease and for systemic sclerosis. Corticosteroid therapy has been proposed for forms of disease where significant amounts of edema are present and the process is thought to be acute. Physical and occupational therapy are important for the maintenance of good musculoskeletal function, and appropriate management of Raynaud phenomenon is required if this is troublesome.

MIXED CONNECTIVE TISSUE DISEASE AND FASCIITIS

These two recently described rheumatic disease syndromes are rare in children. Mixed connective tissue disease is an overlap syndrome combining features of JRA, SLE, dermatomyositis, and scleroderma (Oetgen et al, 1981). It has also been defined on the basis of a particular kind of antinuclear antibody, antibody to ribonucleoprotein (RNP). This antibody is first detected as high-titer antinuclear antibody with a speckled pattern; specific studies can then define the presence of antibody to RNP. This condition was first described as a separate disease that was amenable to therapy with corticosteroids. However, longer experience has shown that antibody to RNP is found also in other rheumatic disease states and that this condition is not always easily controlled with steroid therapy. Many observers consider this condition to be a form of SLE. Children with antibody to RNP often have Raynaud phenomenon and severe musculoskeletal disease; involvement of other organs consistent with SLE has also been observed. Therapy is geared to control of musculoskeletal complaints and organ involvement as present in the individual patient. Corticosteroid therapy is often required.

Fasciitis is characterized by primary inflammation of fascial tissues. Eosinophilia, either in the affected tissues or the blood, is often associated. This condition may be amenable to therapy with corticosteriods. Fasciitis, at times, occurs in an isolated form and may have a good prognosis. At other times, fasciitis appears to be a component of scleroderma. Fasciitis in children may be associated with apparent arthritis and lack of motion in small joints of the hands and wrists.

There is no extensive long-term experience or prognostic information available about these conditions in the childhood years.

REFERENCES

Agnello V: Complement deficiency states. *Medicine* 57:1, 1978.

Allen DM, Diamond LK, Howell DA: Anaphylactoid purpura in children (Schönlein-Henoch syndrome): Review with a follow-up of the renal complications. *Am J Dis Child* 99:833, 1960.

Bernhard JD, Mark EJ: In Case Records of the Massachusetts General Hospital. Wegener's granulomatosis. *N Engl J Med* 314:1170, 1986.

Bernstein B, Takahashi M, Hanson V: Cardiac involvement in juvenile rheumatoid arthritis. *J Pediatr* 85:313, 1974.

Bowyer SL, Blane CE, Sullivan DB, et al: Childhood dermatomyositis: Factors predicting functional outcome and development of dystrophic calcification. *J Pediatr* 103:882, 1983.

Brewer EJ, Giannini EH, Barkley E: Gold therapy in the management of juvenile rheumatoid arthritis. *Arthritis Rheum* 23:404, 1980.

Brewer EJ, Giannini EH, Kuzmina N, et al: Penicillamine and hydroxychloroquine in the treatment of severe juvenile rheumatoid arthritis. *N Engl J Med* 314:1270, 1986.

Buyon JP, Swersky SH, Fox HE, et al: Intrauterine therapy for presumptive fetal myocarditis with acquired heart block due to systemic lupus erythematosus. *Arthritis Rheum* 30:44,1987.

Cassidy JT: Miscellaneous conditions associated with arthritis in children *Pediatr Clin North Am* 33:1033, 1986.

CDC: Acute rheumatic fever at a Navy training center—San Diego, Calif. *MMWR* 37:101, 1988.

Chameides L, Truex RC, Vetter V, et al: Association of maternal systemic lupus erythematosus with congenital complete heart block. *N Engl J Med* 297:1204, 1977.

Cole S, Whitehead AS, Auerbach HS, et al: The molecular basis for genetic deficiency of the second component of human complement. *N Engl J Med* 313:1, 1985.

Crowe WE, Bove KE, Levinson JE, et al: Clinical and pathogenetic implications of histopathology in childhood polydermatomyositis. *Arthritis Rheum* 25:126, 1982.

Fauci AS, Haynes BF, Katz P: Wegener's granulomatosis: Prospective clinical and therapeutic experience with 85 patients for 21 years. *Ann Intern Med* 98:76, 1983.

Furst DE, Kremer JM: Methotrexate in rheumatoid arthritis, *Arthritis Rheum* 31:305, 1988.

Gewanter HL, Roghmann KJ, Baum J: The prevalence of juvenile arthritis. *Arthritis Rheum* 26:599, 1983.

Giannini EH, Brewer EJ, Person DA: Auranofin in the treatment of juvenile rheumatoid arthritis. *J Pediatr* 102:138, 1983.

Glidden RS, Mantzouranis EC, Borel Y: Systemic lupus erythematosus in childhood: Clinical manifestations and improved survival in fifty-five patients. *Clin Immunol Immunopathol* 29:196, 1983.

Hall SL, Miller LC, Duggan E, et al: Wegener granulomatosis in pediatric patients. *J Pediatr* 106:739, 1985a.

Hall S, Barr W, Lie JT, et al: Takayasu arteritis: A study of 32 North American patients. *Medicine* 64:89, 1985b.

Harley JB, Kaine JL, Fox OF, et al: Ro(SS-A) antibody and antigen in a patient with congenital complete heart block. *Arthritis Rheum* 28:12:1321, 1985.

Jacobs JC, Berdon WE, Johnston AD: HLA-B27 associated spondyloarthritis and enthesopathy in childhood: Clinical, pathologic, and radiographic observations in 58 patients. *J Pediatr* 100:521, 1982.

Kawasaki T, Kosaki F, Okawa S, et al: A new infantile acute febrile mucocutaneous lymph node syndrome (MLNS) prevailing in Japan. *Pediatrics* 54:271, 1974.

Keat A: Reiter's syndrome and reactive arthritis in perspective. *N Engl J Med* 309:1606, 1983.

King KK, et al: Clinical spectrum of SLE in childhood. *Arthritis Rheumatol* 20:287, 1977.

Lindsley SB, Schaller JG: Arthritis associated with inflammatory bowel disease in children. *J Pediatr* 84:16, 1974.

Litsey SE, Noonan JA, O'Connor WN, et al: Maternal connective tissue disease and congenital heart block. *N Engl J Med* 312:98, 1985.

Marin-Garcia J, Sheridan R, Hanissian AS: Echocardiographic detection of early cardiac involvement in juvenile rheumatoid arthritis. *Pediatrics* 73:394, 1984.

Nepom, BS, Nepom GT, Mickelson E, et al: Specific HLA-DR4-associated histocompatibility molecules characterized patients with sero-positive juvenile rheumatoid arthritis. *J Clin Invest* 74:287, 1984.

Nepom BS, Schaller JG: Childhood systemic lupus erythematosus. In Cohen AS (ed): *Progress in Clinical Rheumatology I*. Florida, Grune & Stratton, Inc. 1984, pp. 33–69.

Newburger JW, Takahashi M, Burns JC, et al: The treatment of Kawasaki syndrome with intravenous gamma globulin. *N Engl J Med* 315:342, 1986.

Oetgen WJ, Boice JA, Lawless OJ: Mixed connective tissue disease in children and adolescents. *Pediatrics* 67:333, 1981.

Rosenberg AM, Petty RE: Reiter's disease in children. *Am J Dis Child* 133:394, 1979.

Ruddlesdin C, Ansell BM, Arden GP, et al: Total hip replacement in children with juvenile chronic arthritis *J Bone Joint Surg* (Br) 68:218,1986.

Rush PJ, Shore A, Inman R, et al: Arthritis associated with *Haemophilus influenzae* meningitis: Septic or reactive? *J Pediatr* 109:412, 1986.

Schaller JG: Chronic salicylate administration in juvenile rheumatoid arthritis: Aspirin "hepatitis" and its clinical significance. *Pediatrics* 62(suppl):916, 1978.

Schaller JG: Juvenile rheumatoid arthritis. *Pediatr Rev* 2:163, 1980.

Schaller J, Bitnun S, Wedgwood RJ: Ankylosing spondylitis with childhood onset. *J Pediatr* 74:505, 1969.

Schoenfeld Y, Schwartz RS: Immunologic and genetic factors in autoimmune diseases. *N Engl J Med* 311:1019, 1984.

Shore A, Ansell BM: Juvenile psoriatic arthritis—an analysis of 60 cases. *J Pediatr* 100:529, 1982.

Suarez-Almazor ME, Cataggio LJ, Maldonado-Cocco JA, et al: Juvenile progressive systemic sclerosis: Clinical and serologic findings. *Arthritis Rheum* 28:699, 1985.

Towner SR, Michet CJ, O'Fallon WM, et al: The epidemiology of juvenile arthritis in Rochester, Minnesota 1960-1979. *Arthritis Rheum* 26:1208, 1983.

Veasy LG, Wiedmeier SE, Osmond GS, et al: Resurgence of acute rheumatic fever in the intermountain areas of the United States. *N Engl J Med* 316:421, 1987.

JANE G. SCHALLER

Section 23

Orthopedics

Structure and function are closely related in the musculoskeletal system of the child. Most pediatric orthopedic problems are straightforward in diagnosis, and their treatment is based on simple mechanical and physiologic principles. Therefore, a basic knowledge of musculoskeletal structure and physiology is an important aid in the primary care of pediatric orthopedic problems. Also helpful is a familiarity with normal motor development and with the usual patterns of skeletal growth.

ORTHOPEDIC EXAMINATION

The evaluation of the musculoskeletal system is only a part of a complete examination of the child. In performing this examination, the amount of information gained can be optimized in subtle ways. For example, in orthopedics, the most useful information about how a child normally walks or stands may be obtained in those moments before and after the formal examination when the child is unaware of the examiner's scrutiny. If possible, the child should be observed when walking down the hall to the examining room, and after he is dressed and leaving. No matter how localized the complaint appears, a thorough physical examination should be carried out. This means undressing the child sufficiently to get a look at the whole of the trunk and limbs. Palpation of the area in question as well as assessment of active and passive range of motion is mandatory. Observing the child's posture as well as watching the child stand, walk, jump and run, comprise a very important part of a complete evaluation.

INVESTIGATIONS

Clinical measurements are important. For example, a tape measure is needed to measure leg lengths accurately (best done from the anterior superior iliac spine to the medial malleolus on each side), and to measure thigh and calf circumferences to check for atrophy. A goniometer is required to measure accurately the range of motion of joints. Photographs can be most helpful in documenting abnormal shapes.

IMAGING

The assessment of an orthopedic problem often is facilitated by special studies, supplementing and confirming clinical observations. These include plain radiographs, CT scans, bone scans, ultrasonography, or magnetic resonance imaging (MRI).

Despite the new developments in imaging, there is still a clear role for the traditional plain radiograph in assessing children with trauma, infection, neoplasms, and anomalies.

In evaluating nontraumatic hip disorders, it is usually best to request an anteroposterior and frog lateral view of the pelvis centered over the hips so that both sides can be compared on the same film. In evaluating spinal deformities, a full length standing or sitting posteroanterior spinal radiograph is needed. A lateral view is not needed unless a specific sagittal deformity, such as hyperkyphosis, hyperlordosis, or spondylolisthesis is suspected.

Bone scintigraphy or "bone scan" can be uniquely helpful in localizing certain inflammatory and neoplastic conditions of bones and joints. Nevertheless, because the scan is only sensitive to regional blood flow and bone turnover, it is a nonspecific test. Scans using technetium 99m-tagged agents are standard. Together with a plain radiograph, a bone scan may allow an experienced interpreter to distinguish septic arthritis from cellulitis or osteomyelitis.

Ultrasonography is gaining increasing use in evaluating the musculoskeletal system. Its most important current use is in the diagnosis of unstable or dislocated hips in children less than 3 months of age, a time when plain radiographs are subject to significant numbers of false-positive and -negative evaluations. It is useful also for identifying cysts and/or soft tissue tumors. Doppler imaging helps to assess vascular injury associated with fractures and traumatic amputations.

CT allows a cross-sectional view of bones, joints, and soft tissues. Spinal fractures, soft tissue and bony tumors, and femoral anteversion are particularly well defined on CT scanning.

MRI has a unique application in diagnosing certain metabolic and anatomic alterations in the musculoskeletal system. Unfortunately, it is still expensive, not universally obtainable, and experimental in many of its applications.

Approach to the Child With a Limp

1

Definition

A limp represents an abnormality of gait that can be due to many different problems.

Basic Science

Determining the origin of a child's limp requires an understanding of the mechanics of normal gait. Gait is composed of a stance phase and a swing phase. The stance phase, normally 60% of the gait cycle, starts with the "heel strike" and ends with lifting the "toe off" the ground. If, for example, there is pain on weight-bearing in the foot, knee, or hip, the stance phase will be shortened. The swing phase begins with the "toe off" and continues with the foot in the air until the "heel strike" recurs. If the child has limited motion at the hip joint, (e.g., secondary to tight hamstrings), the swing phase would be shortened, with forward elevation of the pelvis to gain more clearance for a stiff hip or knee.

Special types of limps include the following:

1. Gluteus medius limp (Trendelenburg gait or abductor lurch). Because of weakened hip abductors, the child is forced to lean into or swing the upper trunk in the direction of the involved hip during the stance phase to prevent loss of balance. This gait pattern is often seen in congenital hip dislocation.
2. Gluteus maximus limp. Conditions that cause proximal muscle weakness (such as Duchenne muscular dystrophy, spinal muscular atrophy, or poliomyelitis) result in hyperextension of the trunk and pelvis over the hips to keep the center of gravity posterior to the hip joint.
3. Quadriceps femoris limp. Weakness in this muscle results in a visible hyperextension of the knee during the stance phase particularly when the child climbs stairs.
4. Steppage gait. Children who are unable to dorsiflex the foot must lift the ipsilateral knee higher to clear the foot during the swing phase of gait. In addition, there is no clear heel strike as the child begins the stance phase; the entire sole of the foot makes contact with the ground at once, rather than the normal progression from heel strike to foot flat.

Natural History

Occasionally, a child may acquire a limp in imitation of adults or to feign illness. Such limps change over time, are usually transient, and are readily distinguished from those secondary to pathologic causes.

Acute onset of limp in association with fever requires that osteomyelitis and septic arthritis be ruled out. Usually the child can localize the pain to the hip or knee and appropriate radiographic and radionuclide studies are carried out to evaluate the child.

A painful hip or knee in an afebrile child commonly signals trauma. A pathological fracture through a cyst or other lesion is seen occasionally. Bleeding into joints in hemophiliacs was common before the availablility of Factor VIII.

A chronic limp can be secondary to a leg length difference, congential coxa vara, spastic hemiplegias, Legg-Perthes disease, myopathies, and neuropathies, including poliomyelitis. The nature of the gait will depend on the muscle groups affected.

In general, when evaluating the child with a limp, it is important to try to determine if it is secondary to a short leg, a stiff joint, weak muscles, or pain, (Hensinger, 1986).

Diagnosis

In addition to time course and association with pain, the age of the limping child can also be useful. For example, in an infant or toddler, infection or trauma are common causes of limp, whereas in the preschool- and school-age child, toxic synovitis or Legg-Perthes disease are more common. In the adolescent, slipped capital femoral epiphysis, or a patellofemoral problem are more likely etiologies of a limp.

The key to examining children who limp is to observe their gait, focusing on the different areas of the lower extremities with each cycle while the child walks on a flat surface as well as up a set of stairs. The child's shoes should be examined for areas of abnormal wear. The joints of the lower extremities and back should be examined thoroughly. Leg lengths should be carefully measured (e.g., if a dislocated hip is considered) as should the thigh or calf circumferences if muscle atrophy or hypertrophy is suspected. A careful neurologic examination is also useful. The Trendelenburg test, asking the child to stand on one foot and observing the pelvis, will rule out hip abductor weakness.

The evaluation of the child with a limp may require extensive imaging studies and is best accomplished in consultation with pediatric orthopedists and radiologists.

Imaging begins with radiographic examination of the lower extremities, usually including radiographs of the joints above and below the area of interest. If an inflammatory process is suspected, a bone scan may be the next test of choice, as findings may not appear on plain radiographs until later. The scan may also be useful for identifying osteoid osteomas, osteonecrosis (early Legg-Perthes disease), or a bony infarct secondary to sickle cell disease. More invasive tests or other imaging procedures should be discussed in consultation with an orthopedist and/or radiologist. If a septic joint is suspected, this requires prompt needle aspiration and possible open drainage.

Foot Disorders

2

POSITIONAL DEFORMATION

Natural History

The most common finding in the first days of life is deformation of the feet from intrauterine positioning. Usually gentle flexion of the limbs will allow resumption of intrauterine posture and demonstrate clearly how the "positional" abnormality developed.

While an abnormality involving the feet usually represents a local process, it may also signal a more systemic disease, for example, spina bifida. Friedreich ataxia, Charcot-Marie-Tooth disease, Duchenne muscular dystrophy, spinal cord and brain tumors may initially present with foot deformities and reconfirm the need for an extensive general physical and neurologic examination.

Common foot deformities in infants are: (1) a calcaneovalgus foot (pointed up and outward), (2) metatarsus varus, and (3) talipes equinovarus or clubfoot (pointed down and inward). It is important to be able to distinguish among these three in the neonatal period. This is best done by observing the shape of the infant's feet and viewing them from the side and the bottom. The alignment of the heel (varus-deviated medially versus valgus-deviated laterally) should be viewed from behind.

Clubfoot (Equinovarus Deformity)

Definition

The term clubfoot is used to describe a number of abnormalities, the most prominent of which is a rigid equinovarus posture. The foot is plantar flexed at the ankle (in equinus) and the forefoot curves in (is in varus). Severe cases are thought to be malformations rather than deformations (positional defect) (Turco, 1981).

Epidemiology

Clubfoot occurs in 1/700 live births. A nonidiopathic type occurs commonly with neuromuscular problems such as arthrogryposis or spinal dysraphism. Clubfoot can be familial, with a sibling risk of 3–8%.

Treatment

Serial casting by a pediatric orthopedist is often effective treatment and is begun in the first days of life, when the infant's ligaments remain lax because of presence of maternal hormones. About 30% of feet will be normal after some months of casting; 70% will require some surgery, usually to release muscles and restore a more normal alignment. Following surgery, serial casts are required for 8–12 weeks, with splinting at night for several more months.

Prognosis

Treatment is very effective, although some calf atrophy and mild (1–2 cm) limb shortening is characteristic of this disease with or without surgery. The goal is to create a foot that will fit into regular shoes. Further surgery is often needed in late childhood, because of the dysplastic nature of the defect, and also to correct residual deformities.

Congenital Vertical Talus (Rocker-Bottom Foot)

Definition

The medial aspect of the foot is convex, and the head of the talus is palpable on the plantar medial aspect of the foot. The foot viewed from the lateral aspect resembles a rocker; both the forefoot and hindfoot are higher than the midfoot. This is a rigid dysplastic deformity associated with extensive muscular contractures.

Epidemiology

Rocker-bottom feet are characteristic of trisomy 18, but may be found in association with other deformities, such as arthrogryposis or spina bifida, as well as an isolated deformity.

Diagnosis

Vertical talus is similar to calcaneovalgus, although the vertical talus foot also has a tight heel cord while the calcaneovalgus does not.

Treatment

Although manipulation and casting can be tried, surgery is often the treatment of choice (Clark et al, 1977).

Calcaneovalgus Foot

Definition

This defect represents a deformation or positional abnormality in which a laterally deviated foot folds up against the anterolateral surface of the tibia.

Treatment

This defect usually resolves spontaneously and rapidly or after simple stretching of the dorsal tendons and ligaments with each diaper change. Rarely is the deformation so severe as to need casting.

Metatarsus Adductus (Varus)

Definition

This defect also represents a deformation or intrauterine positional abnormality. It is characterized by a varus mildly supinated deviation of the forefoot at the tarso-metatarsal joints, with the heel in neutral or slight valgus.

Epidemiology

It occurs in 1/1000 births and has an increased familial incidence. Five to 10% of patients will also have congenital dysplasia of the hip.

Treatment

Stretching exercises are the mainstay of initial treatment. The heel is stabilized and then the forefoot is stretched laterally for 5 seconds several times with each diaper change. Usually, improvement is seen by age 2 months.

If there is no improvement by 2 months of age, referral to an orthopedist is indicated to assess the need for serial casting. Usually straight-last shoes are required after a period of manipulation and serial casting. In the older child, surgery is often needed to correct the deformity.

Prognosis

Untreated persistent metatarsus adductus may be associated with common adult foot problems including bunions and calluses of the toes. In more than 80% of patients, however, the condition will resolve spontaneously. Metatarsus adductus is not a progressive deformity (Bordelon, 1983).

Pes Planus (Flat Feet)

Definition

A flat foot results from loss of the longitudinal arch of the foot. The heel is often in slight valgus giving the foot a pronated appearance. Most flat foot deformities are flexible and reflect generalized ligamentous laxity. A stiff flat foot suggests mechanical problems and the patient should be referred to an orthopedist.

Diagnosis

With the onset of weight-bearing, many toddlers appear to lose the curvature of the midplantar arch. The feet should be examined with the child sitting on the edge of a table or chair with feet dangling, or in a tip-toe position. If the foot has a normal arch, no treatment is required since this represents the benign flexible type.

If the non-weight-bearing foot does not assume a normal arch, referral to an orthopedist for diagnosis and treatment is appropriate. Rigid flat feet can be seen in association with mild cerebral palsy and some muscular dystrophies. A stiff and painful flat foot may occur secondary to trauma, bone tumors, occult infection, foreign body, or tarsal coalition and again the child should be referred to an orthopedist. In addition, radiographs should be taken of the painful flat foot (Cowell and Elenon, 1983).

Treatment

Various treatments can be used for flexible flat feet, including arch pads in the shoes, a medial heel wedge, or, in severe cases, a molded plastic insert to hold the foot in a neutral position inside the shoe. This, in turn, will prolong shoe wear, prevent overstretching of ligaments, and perhaps relieve the fatigue and discomfort attributed to flat feet with increased activity. They will not, however, cure the deformity or change the natural history of the flat feet. Surgery can help the very rare symptomatic child for whom orthotics are not helpful (Bordelon, 1983).

CONTROVERSY

Although corrective shoes are widely recommended, in a study of 98 children who wore such shoes for 3 years, no improvement in the flat feet was found (Staheli, 1980; Wenger et al, 1986).

Intoeing

Definition

The forepart of the foot is turned medially, as in metatarsus adductus or talipes equinovarus; the whole foot turns inward, as in internal tibial torsion; or the whole lower limb turns inward, as in internal torsion or femoral anteversion. An inward deviation of the foot with gait of more than 10° is cause for a careful examination of the child to determine its source.

Epidemiology

Some degree of intoeing is almost universal in toddlers, and is the most common complaint concerning the lower extremities in children.

While metatarsus adductus is most common in infancy, tibial torsion is evident beginning shortly after the child starts walking and femoral anteversion predominates in the 3- to 7-year-old age group.

Diagnosis

Intoeing can originate anywhere from the spine to the foot. The differential diagnosis of intoeing can almost always be determined by a careful physical examination. Intoeing present at rest (static) should be distinguished from that which is present only in gait (dynamic). Bony malalignment is the most common cause of static intoeing. Muscle imbalance is probably the main factor contributing to dynamic intoeing.

While examining the child's gait, if the patellae and the feet point in the same direction, any torsional problem present is in the femur (femoral torsion). If the feet and knees point in different directions, the rotational problem is distal to the knee (tibial torsion). The lateral malleolus should lie 10–15° posterior to the medial malleolus in the older child and adult. Frequently up to age 4 years but occasionally up to age 7 years some residual internal tibial torsion is common and the two malleoli will lie in the frontal plane.

A kidney-shaped sole of the foot with a deep medial crease should suggest metatarsus adductus, as discussed previously. Tibial torsion can be identified by a "thigh-foot" angle less than 10°. The thigh-foot angle can be noted with the child prone on the table and knees flexed to 90°. An imaginary line is drawn through the axis of the femur and another from midpoint of the heel to the toes. The angle formed by the intersection of these two lines is usually between 10 and 30°, with the foot turned out relative to the thigh. With internal tibial torsion, the foot is turned inward with relation to the thigh, and the lateral malleolus appears to lie in the same plane or anterior to the medial malleolus.

Finally, the hip should be examined for internal and external rotation. If internal rotation is greater than 70° in association with limited external rotation, it is likely to be due to femoral anteversion.

Treatment

No treatment is required for flexible metatarsus varus or internal tibial torsion, which are normal in newborn infants. The bones become normally aligned as the infant begins to walk so that tibial torsion disappears by 18–24 months in most children, and by age 6 years in nearly all. Night-splinting treatment with a Dennis-Browne Bar may be indicated, if (1) the deformity is severe, (2) there is a strong family history, and (3) the child sleeps prone in a knee-chest position. Children over 18 months of age usually will not tolerate the bar. Only rarely is femoral anteversion persistent beyond age 5 years, and if so, consultation and referral to an orthopedist are important. Derotation osteotomies of the femur could be considered between the ages of 6 and 10 years for persistent and symptomatic femoral anteversion. There is, however, no evidence that persistent femoral anteversion progresses to degenerative arthritis and any persistent functional disability in adulthood is rare.

Knee Disorders

3

Approach to Evaluation

The evaluation of knee problems in children begins with a careful examination, focusing on symmetry and alignment in stance and gait and inspection (for muscle atrophy, effusion, or soft-tissue swelling) and palpation (for effusions or tenderness). In addition, mobility (both active and passive range of motion) and stability of the joints of the lower extremity must be assessed. The collateral ligaments of the knee can be tested for medial and lateral ligamentous laxity by stressing one side of the knee while applying counterpressure to the opposite side. Cruciate ligamentous laxity is tested by the Lachman and drawer tests, in which the knee is flexed 30° or 90°, respectively, and the anterior and posterior laxity of the knee is assessed. If excessive sliding motion is obtained, a cruciate ligament injury should be suspected. A meniscal tear can be detected with the McMurray test, in which the knee is extended from full flexion with the tibia rotated first laterally and then medially. While rotating, lateral and medial bending stress is also applied, and if the meniscus is damaged, a 'snapping' or 'clicking' sound is heard at the joint line. A negative test, however, does not rule out a tear. Finally, no knee examination is complete without a careful examination of the hips as well since knee pain may be the only complaint in patients presenting with primary hip disease (Smith, 1986).

Specific knee problems follow:

Genu Valgus (Knock-knee)

During normal development, the legs tend to be bowed for the first 18–36 months, to shift to genu valgus between 30 and 60 months, and then assume the normal about 5–8° valgus after the age of 5–6 years (Salenius and Wankka, 1975).

Definition

Genu valgus is considered pathologic only when the intermedial malleolar distance exceeds 10 cm with the femoral condyles together. At maturity, there should be no more than 7° of valgus across the knee joint. Slight genu valgus is normal in females, in association with their wider pelvis.

Natural History

Conditions that may produce pathologic genu valgus include a hereditary tendency, or traumatic or metabolic processes that disturb the growth plates around the knee (fracture, rickets, etc). Apparent pseudo knock-knees are seen with fat thighs, hypotonia, and increased joint laxity.

Diagnosis

The pathologic diagnosis is best confirmed radiographically, with knees and feet pointing straight ahead to assure accurate angle measurement. Mild external tibial torsion also often accompanies this defect.

Treatment

Severe genu valgus persisting into adolescence requires operative repair to prevent degenerative arthritis in the knee. There is no role for corrective shoes. Patients with physiologic knock-knee deformities generally require no treatment as they outgrow this problem.

Genu Varus (Bowlegs)

Definition

Genu varus exists when the knees are over 10 cm apart when the malleoli are together. Most genu varus is physiologic in infancy and resolves spontaneously by age 2 years. Internal tibial torsion often accompanies this defect. No amount of varus is normal in the knee at maturity. Varus deformity in the adult knee predisposes to degenerative arthritis.

Diagnosis

Radiographs of the limbs are appropriate to document the degree and location of the deformity and demonstrate the presence of metabolic bone disease (such as rickets) or Blount disease (tibia vara).

Treatment

Idiopathic genu varus usually resolves, but if it persists into adolescence, then either lateral physeal arrest or osteomy should be considered. In infants with greater than 15° of bowing a Denis-Browne bar with a knee wrap may be useful during sleep to speed correction by increasing pressure on the lateral side of the knee to slow lateral growth. In Blount disease, osteotomy of proximal tibia and fibula may be required after age 2 years and may need to be repeated more than once.

PAINFUL KNEE DISORDERS

Knee pain is common (especially in the adolescent) and may result from mechanical disorders of the knee (especially patellofemoral), systemic disorders (such as arthritis), or from referred pain from the hip.

Congenital Discoid Lateral Meniscus

Lateral joint line pain associated with popping or snapping may be due to a discoid lateral meniscus, the abnormal thickness of which creates a mechanical derangement. Not all discoid menisci are painful. Arthroscopy can be diagnostic and curative by excision of the meniscus to prevent degenerative arthritis.

Popliteal Cyst

Popliteal or Baker cysts form posteriorly at the medial head of the gastrocnemius or at the semimembranous muscle insertion; these cysts are filled with synovial fluid. They are benign and usually resolve spontaneously. Only if painful should they be excised. More than one-third will recur postoperatively. Needle aspiration is rarely curative.

Osgood-Schlatter Disease

Definition

Painful swelling of the tibial tubercle in adolescents is called Osgood-Schlätter disease. The condition is most common in 10- to 15-year-old athletic males. It is probably an overuse syndrome resulting from the repetitive contraction of the quadriceps muscle which produces a stress avulsion fracture of the tibial tubercle.

Diagnosis

The tibial tubercle of one or both legs may be prominent and tender. Contraction of the quadriceps produces pain at the site of attachment of its infrapatellar ligament to the tibial tubercle. Radiographs may be normal or may show apparent fragmentation of the tubercle, soft-tissue swelling, and blurring of the infrapatellar ligament.

Treatment

The symptoms will usually abate with rest over 2–3 weeks. Ice and acetaminophen may be useful. A knee immobilizer, crutches, or cast may rarely be required. The radiographic fragmentation may persist until the epiphysis fuses with the metaphysis of the tibia. Some prominence of the tubercle persists after maturity in at least 25% of patients, although symptoms almost always abate at the end of growth.

Osteochondritis Dissecans (Epiphyseal Ischemic Necrosis)

Definition

This is a disease of joints in which a small portion of the subchondral bone becomes avascular. The lateral portion of the medial femoral condyle is affected most commonly.

Epidemiology

The disorder occurs most frequently in adolescent males and is thought to be the result of repetitive microtrauma. It is bilateral in about 10% of patients. Constitutional factors (heredity and endocrine dysfunction) are common (Mubaraić and Carroll, 1981).

Diagnosis

The earliest symptom might be a vague persistent ache. Localized tenderness of the femoral condyle may be the only early sign. Locking of the knee (fixed in either flexion or extension) is characteristic if the fragment of ischemic bone and overlying cartilage comes loose from the condyle. Radiographs are diagnostic. The lesion is usually present on the lateral aspect of the femoral condyle and is best seen on a tunnel view (Fig. 23.1).

Treatment

If the knee is not locked, activity need only be restricted to a level of tolerance and quadriceps exercises should be encouraged. A bivalved cast may help in most symptomatic cases. If the fragment becomes loose, arthroscopy is required to remove the fragment and to drill the bed to promote revascularization. Sometimes, especially with large or incompletely displaced fragments, they can be internally fixed with pins rather than resected in an attempt to get them to heal in place (Guhl, 1982).

Subluxation of Patella

Definition

The patella may subluxate (partially dislocate) or dislocate entirely laterally, out of the femoral trochleal groove.

Epidemiology

Patellar subluxation commonly occurs between ages 10 and 25 years and is three times as frequent in females.

Diagnosis

The child with loose ligaments (especially in Down syndrome) or a valgus (knock-knee) malalignment may experience the patella "popping" laterally, but it often returns to the normal position with extension of the knee. A mild effusion may be present. A history of trauma may or may not be present. Tenderness along the medial side of the patella is usual, where the supporting ligaments are stretched. The so-called apprehension or Fairbank sign is pathognomonic of patellar instability: laterally directed pressure on the medial side of the patella causes the patient to have a worried expression and contract the quadriceps, thereby ex-

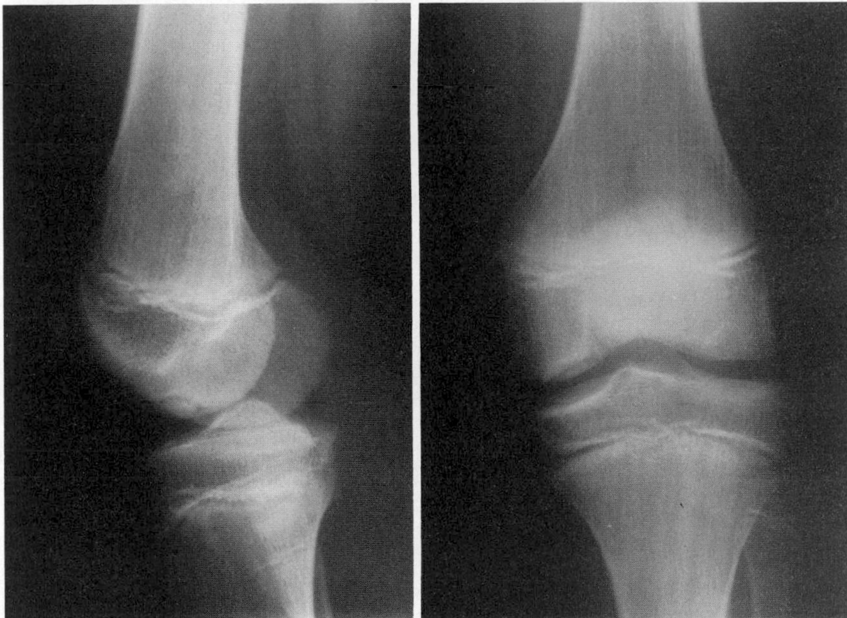

Figure 23.1. This 15-year-old boy had pain in the knee, which prompted these radiographs. Osteochondritis dissecans involving the lateral femoral condyle. The lesion is probably aseptic necrosis of the subchondral bone, which then affects the overlying cartilage. Trauma may be the initiating factor. If the fragment of bone and cartilage detaches, it becomes a "joint mouse," interfering with normal motion at the knee, and must be removed.

tending the knee and pulling the patella medially and stabilizing it against dislocation. If complete dislocation occurs, the knee will remain locked in flexion, with a concavity noted anteriorly. Radiographic examination is crucial to check for the possibility of loose patella or fragments from a femoral condylar fracture resulting from the dislocation.

Treatment

Quadriceps-strengthening exercises should be prescribed for subluxation. Immobilization for 4–6 weeks may be needed for acute traumatic dislocation. Only rarely is surgical realignment or repair indicated (Griffin, 1978).

Hip Disorders 4

CONGENITAL DISLOCATION OF THE HIP

Definition

Congenital instability of the hip is a spectrum of disease. It ranges from mild subluxability of the femoral head in response to pushing and pulling on the ipsilateral flexed knee (an almost-normal finding in the newborn) to a frank dislocation of the femoral head out of the acetabulum. A dislocatable hip is one in which the femoral head can be pushed out of the acetabulum, with spontaneous reduction occurring thereafter. This type of hip, by definition, lies in a normal location at rest. A very different entity is the truly dislocated hip, which lies with the femoral head outside the acetabulum at rest. The truly dislocated hip usually can be reduced in the newborn easily with a gentle flexion and abduction maneuver. If reduction can thus be achieved in the truly dislocated hip, the dislocation is termed reducible. If no reduction, thus, can be achieved of a known dislocated hip, then it is termed irreducible.

Basic Science

The pathoanatomy in the congenitally unstable hip usually is related to pathologic laxity of the hip joint capsule. The influence of maternal hormones render the capsular ligaments lax around the time of birth. In addition, the neonate's femoral head is relatively large compared to the relatively small size and shallow contour of the socket. If these factors coexist with any other neonatal condition tending to destabilize the hips, (breech position, relatively small uterus, or oligohydramnios, all of which reduce the normal mobility of the hip joint in utero), clinically significant instability of the hips becomes much more likely.

In so-called idiopathic dislocation, the migration of the femoral head out of the acetabulum is thought to take place very late in gestation or around the time of birth. The so-called teratologic hip dislocation is believed to occur much earlier in prenatal development. Teratologic dislocations are usually irreducible at birth, with stiffness and contracture present even in the neonate. Such severe dislocations often are associated with more widespread musculoskeletal disorders, such as arthrogryposis or chromosomal abnormalities.

Epidemiology

The prevalence of a dislocatable hip is perhaps 2–5% of all infants depending on the vigor of the examiner, the time after birth at which the evaluation is done, and the gene pool from which the baby comes. There is a strong genetic predisposition to congenital hip instability. The prevalence of frank dislocation is about 1/800 live births in North America. Idiopathic congenital hip instability is very uncommon among blacks. It is more common in females, and more common if another member of the family has been affected.

Diagnosis

The examination of the newborn's hips is straightforward but requires some patience and attention to detail. The child should be positioned supine on a firm surface. The infant should be relaxed and both the infant and the examiner's hands should be warm. Gentleness is the rule or a subtle instability may be missed.

The hips and knees are flexed to 90°. With the hips abducted 45°, the hip to be examined is grasped with the examiner's thumb in the groin and the long finger on the greater trochanter. The first part of the examination consists of bringing the knee toward the midline, adducting the hip, as the examiner's thumb pushes posteriorly and laterally on the inner side of the thigh in an attempt to see whether the femoral head can be pushed backward out of the acetabulum. This is the Barlow provocative test for dislocatability. The second part of the evaluation consists of abducting the hip by pushing the knee outward, while the examiner's long finger lifts forward on the greater trochanter. This is the Ortolani test. If a click or clunk is felt as the femoral head slips over the back edge of the socket into the acetabulum during the Ortolani test, this is presumptive evidence that the hip was dislocated.

These manual tests are extremely important and are far better than a radiograph of the newborn child. They should be repeated frequently in the first 6 months of life, since almost half are not detected with the first examination (Asher, 1986). Ultrasonography is also useful in early infancy, both for initial diagnosis and for following the response of an unstable hip to treatment. With ultrasonography, the cartilaginous outlines of the femoral head and acetabulum can be seen, and the stability of the joint readily assessed (Graf, 1983; Zieger, 1986).

Dislocation of a hip in the newborn usually is unaccompanied by any apparent shortening of the extremity or contracture. There may be asymmetry of the gluteal folds, but such secondary signs tend to develop only after weeks of dislocation.

Treatment

Dynamic splinting in a position of stability virtually guarantees successful treatment of the idiopathic dislocation if the diagnosis is made within the first few days of life. Triple diapers are the traditional remedy but they probably do not maintain the flexed and abducted position securely enough to be both safe for the circulation to the femoral head and successful in achieving and maintaining its reduction. The Pavlik harness is the splinting method of choice for the newborn with a frank dislocation. Having the child lie prone as much as possible is probably almost as important as the harness itself, and, indeed, prone positioning may be treatment enough for the dislocatable, but not dislocated hip. The Pavlik harness holds the leg in a flexed and abducted position (jockey position) but it allows some movement of the leg, which protects the circulation without overly jeopardizing stability (Ramsay et al, 1976). Diaper changes can be made without removing the harness and it should be kept on day and night. Frequent follow-up is needed to ensure that a reduction has been achieved and is being maintained. After the newborn period, the hip requires as much time in the harness after a reduction has been achieved as the age of the child was at the time the reduction was achieved. In the newborn, usually 2–4 weeks of treatment is required. In other words, a dislocated hip that is diagnosed at age 2 weeks, in which a reduction is immediately achieved at that time by application of a Pavlik harness, will usually require 2–4 weeks for stabilization. The infant usually is weaned gradually from the harness rather than being removed abruptly.

Prognosis

Orthopedic follow-up of a dislocated hip should continue through skeletal maturity. Even the most apparently successful early treatment of a congenital hip dislocation can occasionally lead to a growth disturbance that manifests itself only in adolescence. Among 23,000 newborns treated within 2 days of birth with abduction splints (6 weeks for dislocatable, 12 weeks for dislocated hips) only five infants required further orthopedic therapy. None had avascular necrosis (Dunn et al, 1985).

There is progressive functional disability in gait associated with the untreated dislocation or subluxation. Crippling osteoarthritis before middle age is the rule without treatment.

LEGG-CALVÉ-PERTHES DISEASE

Definition

Pain in or about the hip or the knee in a growing child with typical radiographic abnormalities of the femoral head is considered Legg-Calvé-Perthes disease. It is an idiopathic process characterized by repeated ischemic insults to the proximal femoral epiphysis.

Epidemiology

The disorder affects mostly boys ages 3–11 years. It is familial in 10–20% of cases. Ninety percent of cases have delayed bone age. Rarely are blacks affected by this disorder and there is a five times increased incidence in low birth weight males (Chung, 1986).

Natural History and Diagnosis

Pain in the hip (or referred to the medial thigh or knee) and a resultant limp can be present for up to 1 year before diagnosis. Limp and pain are aggravated by activity. Clinical examination demonstrates variable loss of internal rotation and abduction, with an antalgic gait. Classification of the disorder is radiographic, with the earliest stage an apparent increase in joint space due to a temporary cessation of growth of the bony epiphysis. Later, a lucent subchondral crack, "the crescent sign" may appear in the femoral head, indicating the portion of head rendered ischemic. The femoral capital epiphyseal center may then become flattened and relatively dense. With repair, new bone is formed over an interval of 2–3 years. The aim of treatment is to prevent the cartilaginous portion of the head from flattening. Blood supply is always restored to the epiphysis, but if growth is significantly disturbed and the articular surface becomes deformed, osteoarthritis is likely in middle age (Stulberg et al, 1981; McAnderson and Weinstein, 1984).

Pain in the hip or knee associated with limp in a child of appropriate age demands a thorough work-up. An isotopic bone scan may show decreased uptake in the femoral head, before the plain radiographic views show the characteristic changes.

The differential diagnosis in the synovial (early) stage of the disease includes a septic hip, and occasionally, patients who go on to develop the syndrome of Legg-Calvé-Perthes disease are hospitalized for aspiration and culture of their synovial fluid.

Treatment

The overall goal of therapy is to prevent progressive deformity of the femoral head.

If less than 50% of the epiphysis is ischemic, there is little risk of head deformation and treatment may be symptomatic physiotherapy, crutches, and rest as needed.

If more than 50% of the epiphysis is involved in the disease process, the risk of deformation is great. In this case, "containment" of the femoral head, burying the head deep inside the acetabulum by either bracing in abduction or surgery, seems to improve the prognosis. Bracing is noninvasive, but is restrictive and it may be required for 2–4 years to be effective. Surgery is invasive, but yields immediate results. Either approach carries a good long-term prognosis, although if the femoral head is already flattened at the time of diagnosis, degenerative arthritis can occur in the adult (Stulberg et al, 1981).

SLIPPED CAPITAL FEMORAL EPIPHYSIS

Definition

The capital femoral epiphysis slips posteromedially off the metaphysis as a result of a shearing failure of the cartilaginous growth plate in the proximal femur. It may occur in an acute form, sometimes associated with trauma, or in a very chronic atraumatic form (at least 75% of patients; Weinstein, 1984).

Epidemiology

This disorder, although usually unilateral, is bilateral in 20–40% of cases. It occurs most frequently in obese adolescents, usually boys, 10–16 years of age. The annual incidence in adolescents ranges from 2.8–10.1/100,000 (Chung, 1986). The combination of widening and weakening of a growth plate by the growth spurt, and associated increased body weight, leads to the mechanical failure of the physis.

Diagnosis

A limp is almost universal. Some pain, usually in the ipsilateral thigh, knee, or groin, is common. Hip abduction and internal rotation are limited and may be painful. As the affected hip is flexed, the leg falls out into external rotation and abduction. Hip radiographs are diagnostic, particularly the frog lateral view (Fig. 23.2). A bone scan may demonstrate increased uptake at the epiphyseal plate if the plain radiographs are inconclusive.

Treatment

Surgical treatment is urgent to prevent further slipping of the epiphysis. The child should not be allowed to bear weight even en route to the hospital. This

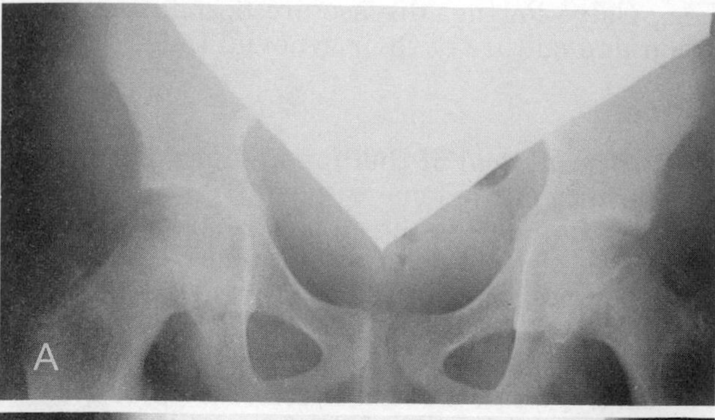

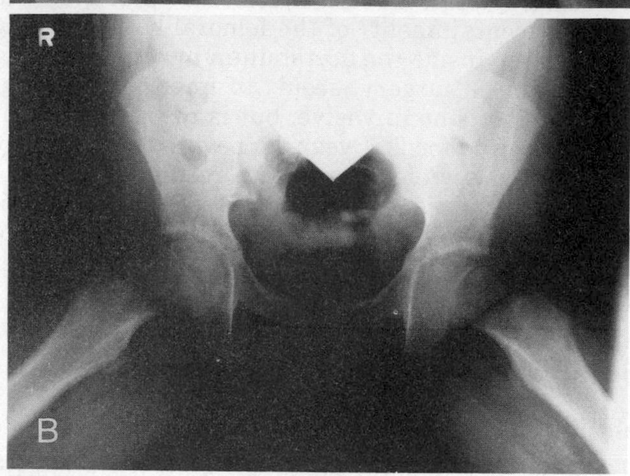

Figure 23.2. Slipped capital femoral epiphysis. This rather chubby 11-year-old girl was brought to the emergency room complaining of pain in the left hip. Her anteroposterior radiograph **(A)** showed subtle widening of the growth plate. The frog-leg view **(B)** shows definite medial slip of the capital femoral epiphysis on the left. Obese children beginning their growth spurt are prone to this injury. Treatment consists of pinning the epiphysis with two or three screws.

is a growth plate fracture and must be stabilized by insertion of pins into the neck of the femur across the epiphyseal cartilage into the femoral head. If considerable deformity or displacement is present, an out-toeing gait with limp and late arthritis may follow. Therefore, a severe case should have some form of realignment, not necessarily at the time of presentation, in addition to pinning. The blood supply to the femoral head is fragile in this condition, and both avascular necrosis and chondrolysis (articular cartilage necrosis) of the femoral head and acetabulum are hazards of overzealous realignment. Osteoarthritis is rare, even in severe cases, unless there has been avascular necrosis or chondrolysis.

Shoulder Disorders 5

Children and adolescents are remarkably free from disorders of the shoulder joint and region other than fractures. Bursitis and inflammatory conditions are almost unknown except in the setting of overuse syndrome, which can occasionally occur in competitive swimmers. Rest, appropriate stretching and strengthening, and appropriate changes in training programs will usually lead to resolution of these overuse syndromes.

Fractures in the region are rather common, occurring particularly in proximal humerus and clavicle.

CLAVICLE FRACTURES

Clavicular fractures are extremely common, and, owing to both the great capabilities of the clavicle to remodel and the great tolerance in shoulder girdle function to moderate degrees of deformity, rarely require reduction maneuvers. Moderate improvement in the deformity of a severely displaced fracture can usually be achieved by use of a figure-of-eight splint. Three weeks is sufficient for immobilization of most clavicle fractures, although return to sports should be restricted for several additional weeks, particularly in adolescents.

HUMERAL FRACTURES

Proximal humeral fractures also have great capacity for remodelling, particularly those fractures through the growth plate, as 80% of the growth of the humerus occurs at the proximal physis (Fig. 23.3). Disturbances of longitudinal growth are extremely rare, even though these injuries frequently extend through the growth plate. The spherical shape of the humeral head allows accommodation for considerable angular deformity through the fracture. With nearly completely displaced physeal injuries, reduction maneuvers may be appropriate and occasionally may need to be followed by immobilization for 2–3 weeks in an airplane splint in a salute position or in a statue of liberty-type spica cast.

BONE CYSTS OF PROXIMAL HUMERUS

Definition

One subgroup of proximal humeral fractures deserves special mention, i.e., the pathologic fractures through bone cysts. Simple bone cysts, which are by definition benign, are very common in the proximal humerus and may be the sight of repeated fractures. While as many as 20% of these cysts will heal after a fracture, if the cyst fails to heal after an initial fracture, consideration will be given to treatment, both to encourage healing and to reduce the incidence of future pathologic fractures.

Diagnosis and Treatment

The first choice in treating the cyst itself is to allow the fracture to heal, and to see if the cyst will heal on its own. If healing does not occur, the cyst should be aspirated; clear light yellow fluid will confirm the diagnosis. The fluid should always be sent for pathologic examination. Instillation of methylprednisolone at the time of the aspiration can hasten healing in as many as 50–60% of patients (Scaglietti et al, 1982). Further steroid injections (up to three) lead to a cure in as many as 90% of the patients. Hence, surgical curettage and packing of the cyst with bone graft are rarely necessary. Since open curettage and packing of the cyst constitute a rather large operative procedure, the noninvasive steroid technique is preferable.

DISLOCATIONS

Dislocation of the head of the humerus anteriorly and inferiorly out of the glenoid humeral joint is common in the young adult and adolescent but is extremely rare in childhood. Such dislocations which almost always are traumatic, should be treated with gentle manipulative closed reduction and immobilization for 2–4 weeks in a sling and swathe, depending on the circumstances of the injury. A small subgroup of older children and adolescents comprises habitual or vol-

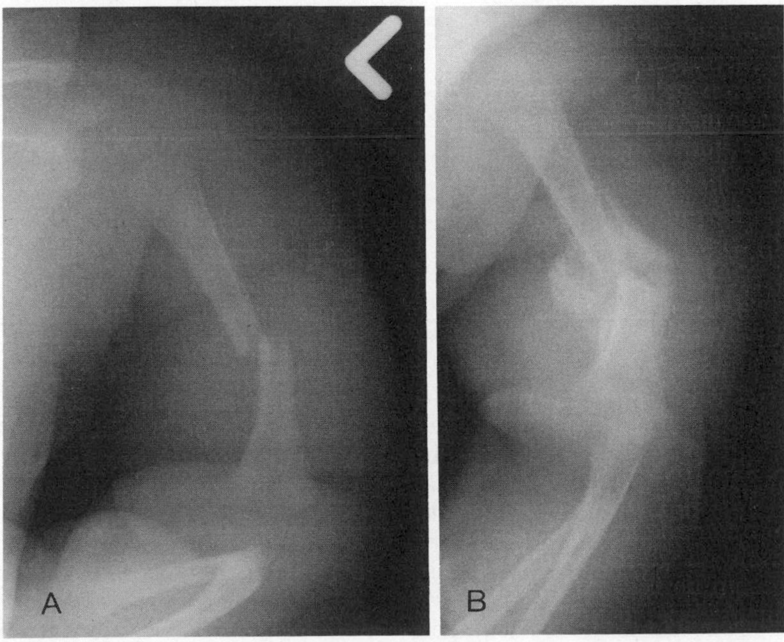

Figure 23.3. This fractured humerus **(A)** was identified after a difficult delivery when the baby was noted to move only the right arm and to have swelling on the left. Two weeks later, there is exuberant callus formation around the fracture site as well as periosteal new bone **(B)**.

CASE ILLUSTRATION

A 1½-year-old infant was brought in by his parents who were afraid that they may have broken his right shoulder, since he no longer was raising or using his right forearm. He was previously well until his mother pulled him by the wrist out of the sandbox earlier that day, when he would not get out himself. On examination, his right elbow was flexed and his forearm was pronated. The child held his arm "clamped" to his side. Any attempt to touch, let alone move, his arm or forearm resulted in his crying although no localized area of swelling, erythema, or pain could be detected.

QUESTION AND COMMENT

Has this child broken his shoulder? If not, what else may have occurred and how should it be treated?

Shoulder injuries are extremely rare in young children, and, in this case, it was not the shoulder but the elbow that was abnormal. This child was presenting with a transient subluxation of the radial head associated with a slipping of the annular ligament normally surrounding the radial neck proximally. It is a condition also referred to as a "pulled" or "nursemaid's" elbow and is common in the toddler and preschool-age child. Radiographs are usually normal since the annular ligament caught between joint surfaces of the radial head and capitellum is radiolucent.

Treatment involves a maneuver in which the elbow is extended with one hand and then flexed while fully supinating the forearm with the other hand. When gentle thumb pressure is placed over the patient's radial head, a palpable pop is felt as 90° of flexion is passed. Use of the arm usually returns within several minutes. A repeat injury probably requires that the arm be splinted in supination for a few days, whereas an initial injury usually requires no immobilization.

untary dislocators (Rowe et al, 1973). Surgery in such cases is usually not indicated. Rather attention should be directed at instructing the child not to perform the dislocation maneuver, together with an aggressive physical therapy program to strengthen the shoulder muscles.

SHOULDER DEFORMITIES

Sprengel deformity or congenital elevation of the scapula results from failure of normal descent of the scapula during gestation (Carson et al, 1981). It is unilateral in two-thirds of cases. These children appear to have fuller and shorter necks and have torticollis. Limitation of shoulder abduction and forward flexion are the major disabilities. Surgical release of the scapula is a major operation and is indicated only in severe cases. It is usually performed between ages 3 and 5 years since there is an increased risk of brachial plexus injury from clavicular compression or stretching if a severe case is left untreated.

Spinal Disorders 6

The spine has important supportive and protective functions for neurologic and visceral structures. Abnormalities in spinal structure and function, therefore, can have dire consequences if not diagnosed and treated appropriately. Many spinal deformities can be progressive, and many are not particularly obvious in their early stages when management may be the easiest. Screening school children for scoliosis is now required in at least nine states, and is endorsed by the American Academy of Orthopaedic Surgeons.

CONGENITAL DEFORMITIES

Definition

Congenital deformities of the spine are defined as those due to anomalous vertebral development (Winter, 1983). These congenital anomalies can be classified either as defects of segmentation or of formation, or some combination of the two. Further classification of congenital deformities involves specifying the pattern of the deformity (scoliosis [lateral curvature], kyphosis and lordosis [sagittal plane curvature], or a combination), as well as specifying the area of the spine involved.

Myelodysplasia (Neural Tube Defects)

Definition

Myelodysplasia (see also pp. 719), spinal dysraphism, and spina bifida are all terms relating to a wide spectrum of abnormalities in development of the bony spinal column, its neural contents, or both. Usually these terms indicate some degree of failure of the bony spine to complete its embryologic closure posteriorly, which usually occurs last in the caudal regions of the vertebral column (see also Section 12).

The mildest form of myelodysplasia is, therefore, spina bifida occulta, a usually insignificant failure of the posterior laminae of a vertebra (usually L5) to fuse in the midline. More severe degrees of spina bifida may occur, often at multiple levels, and, when severe, are usually associated with some dysplasia of the neural elements within.

In the so-called meningocele, failure of fusion of the posterior elements of the spine results in herniation of intact meninges. In this condition, the skin is usually intact. Neurologic function is often normal. If a posterior lumbar or lumbosacral mass associated with the meningocele is symptomatic, neurosurgical and plastic surgical reconstruction is often feasible.

Basic Science

True myelomeningocele defines a condition where not only the bony elements are dysraphic and incompletely formed, but the meninges and contained neural elements are dysplastic as well. Myelomeningocele has a high association with Arnold-Chiari malformation and secondary hydrocephalus, as well as with greatly disturbed or absent neurologic function distal to the level of the myelomeningocele. The lumbar level is most commonly involved, but the condition can be found from the sacrum to as high as the cervical region.

In myelomeningocele, the distal motor disturbance is classically a flaccid paralysis, but varying degrees of spasticity can sometimes occur. Depending on the level of neurological disturbance, muscle imbalance may be present, leading to contractures and deformities of the lower extremities. Scoliosis, and occasionally a very severe form of kyphosis, are found in association with higher lesions.

Treatment

Treatment of the patient who has an open myelomeningocele involves a multidisciplinary team approach from birth. Most of these patients have multiple problems and require attention from orthopedists, neurosurgeons, and urologists, as well as from pediatricians. Although there is general agreement that patients with low lesions should have closure of their sac soon after birth (with corresponding aggressive treatment thereafter), the treatment of patients with high lesions remains to some extent controversial.

To a large extent, the patients ultimate maximal level of function can be correlated with the level of the spinal cord at which their lesion lies. Specifically, the higher the lesion, the more handicapped the patient will be. Although, in general, myelomeningocele represents a static condition, tethering of the dysplastic neural elements distally can lead to progressive loss of function during growth. Neurosurgical consultation about the approach to hydrocephalus is essential.

Prognosis

If early closure of a meningomyelocele is not undertaken, the mortality is 85–90% within 10 years. When early closure has been undertaken along with treatment of hydrocephalus, the mortality is 50% within 10 years. Renal failure is a common major complication. Of the survivors, about half are ambulatory. The IQ can be normal, but many patients have some degree of mental deficiency.

Genetic counseling should be undertaken to advise on risk of recurrence in a sibling. In Great Britain, the risk is about 5%; in other populations, it has been reported as low as 1.4%. Prenatal diagnosis with measurements of α-fetoprotein and ultrasonographic examination of the fetus can provide useful information in subsequent pregnancies (Volpe, 1981; see pp. 785).

CERVICAL SPINE ABNORMALITIES

Torticollis (Wry Neck)

Definition

Torticollis is unilateral shortening of the sternocleidomastoid muscle, on the side of the lowered ear. The common and rather benign congenital muscular torticollis can be found in as many as 1% of live births (Canale et al, 1982). It is usually a deformation or molding syndrome, not surprisingly associated often with congenital hip instability and metatarsus adductus.

Some degree of flattening of the head (plagiocephaly) may be found in this condition. Torticollis may also be a presenting finding in bony abnormalities of the cervical region, and any torticollis that does not seem to be improving should be evaluated radiographically.

Treatment

Although most cases respond well to gentle stretching exercises of the sternocleidomastoid, persisting asymmetry of head posture beyond 12 months should probably be treated by surgical release of the tight sternocleidomastoid, in order to prevent permanent asymmetry of the face and head, and even, in very severe cases, visual disturbances.

Klippel-Feil Syndrome

Definition

The so-called Klippel-Feil syndrome describes any condition with congenital fusion of cervical vertebrae.

Diagnosis

In the classical syndrome, the children have a short neck, limited cervical motion, a low hairline, and any of multiple other deformities. Radiographs may show a reduction in number as well as fusion of cervical vertebrae. Scoliosis or kyphosis are found in nearly two-thirds of the cases. Sprengel deformity occurs in one-third of the cases. Genitourinary abnormalities and auditory disturbances occur in more than 30%, and cardiac lesions occur in one-sixth of the cases.

Treatment

Most patients require no treatment, although a long segment of fused cervical vertebrae may lead to some instability above and below the fused segment.

CONGENITAL CERVICAL INSTABILITY

Diagnosis

Congenital cervical instability is rarely found, although certain syndromes should alert the pediatrician to its probable presence. Certain dwarfing conditions, particularly Morquio disease and spondyloepiphyseal dysplasia, frequently have associated odontoid hypoplasia. In Down syndrome, Cl-C2 instability occurs in perhaps 10–15%, due in this case to laxity of the transverse atlantal ligaments. Cervical instability may be diagnosed radiographically on lateral flexion/extension views of the cervical spine and may be suspected in infants with unexplained disturbances of tone, either increased or decreased.

CONGENITAL SCOLIOSIS

Definition

Congenital lateral deviation of the spine can occur from a failure either of formation or of segmentation of the bony elements. While mild degrees of congenital scoliosis are inconsequential, severe degrees can cause not only cardiopulmonary problems but also neurologic compromise.

Natural History

The natural history of congenital scoliosis depends more on the anatomic lesion than on the initial degree of severity. Specifically, the so-called unilateral unsegmented bar (fusion of adjacent asymmetric vertebrae) has the worst prognosis, since continuing growth opposite the bar leads to inexorable deformation. Multiple unbalanced hemivertebrae also carry a poor prognosis.

Diagnosis

Congenital scoliosis should be suspected when any asymmetry of shoulders, ribs, or trunk rotation is seen. In addition, midline defects of the back, such as dimples, cystic masses, sinus tracts, hairy patches or hemangiomata should raise suspicion of scoliosis (Table 23.1).

As many as 40% of children with congenital scoliosis will have genitourinary anomalies that are often occult. This is related to the fact that the genitourinary system and spine go through their major embryologic development at the same time. An evaluation of the kidneys by ultrasonography is appropriate in any child with a spinal abnormality.

Treatment

As many as 50% of patients with congenital scoliosis may require a spinal fusion to halt progressive deformity. Others may stabilize with bracing alone because of compensatory curves above and below the involved segment. While some period of observation is always in order to assess the character of deformity, these patients need to be followed closely for progression as well.

Table 23.1
Conditions Sometimes Associated with Scoliosis

Idiopathic scoliosis (about 65% of cases)
Congenital skeletal abnormalities (15% of cases)
- Vertebral anomalies with or without neurotopic defect
- Rib fusion

Neuromuscular disease
- Cerebral palsy
- Spinocerebellar degeneration
- Syringomyelia
- Spinal cord tumors
- Spinal cord injury
- Poliomyelitis
- Progressive muscle atrophy (Werdnig-Hoffmann)
- Dysautonomia (Riley-Day)

Myopathy
- Muscular dystrophy
- Myotonia congenita (Thomsen disease)
- Arthrogryposis

Neurofibromatosis (5% of cases)
Mesenchymal disease
- Marfan
- Ehlers-Danlos
- Rheumatoid arthritis

Irradiation and other injury
Osteochondrodystrophies
- Morquio disease
- Diastrophic dwarfism

Osteomyelitis
Metabolic disorders
- Osteogenesis imperfecta
- Rickets
- Hemocystinuria

Spondylolisthesis
- Congenital anomalies of the sacrum

Prognosis

The patient with congenital scoliosis does not have a normal prognosis for spinal growth. Allowing continuing spinal growth and progressive deformity to develop in part of the spine will not result in more longitudinal growth. While congenital spinal deformities in the central parts of the spine can be compensated for to some extent by the normal segments above and below, at either end of the spine, relatively small congenital deformities can be quite devastating. Cervical or low lumbar deformities, therefore, require early treatment with bracing.

Congenital Kyphosis

Definition

Congenital kyphosis is a failure of formation or of segmentation of the anterior elements of the bony spine.

Treatment

This group of deformities has a high potential for causing neurologic compromise and any degree of progression should probably be treated by spinal fusion. Mild-to-moderate amounts of kyphosis (up to 50°) can usually be treated by a fusion of the posterior portions of the spine alone, but more severe degrees of kyphosis may require anterior and posterior fusions. Prevention of neurologic loss is crucial in congenital kyphosis, because once neurologic loss occurs, return of function, even with extensive decompressions, is unusual. Bracing is ineffective and is not indicated.

Caudal Spinal Agenesis

Definition

This syndrome involves agenesis of the sacrum, lumbar spine, or lumbosacral articulations. Absence of the corresponding motor units is usual, although sensation is often intact. No clear etiology has been discovered, although maternal diabetes has been associated with more than 20% of cases.

Diagnosis

The child with caudal spinal dysgenesis has a clinical presentation with varying degrees of flexion and abduction contractures of the hips, flexion deformities of the knees, and a very dysplastic pelvis, with hypoplasia or aplasia of the gluteal cleft. Associated problems often include gastrointestinal and genitourinary abnormalities in addition to a neurogenic bladder.

Treatment

Treatment of these patients presents difficulties similar to those found in severe myelodysplasia and a similar multidisciplinary team approach is recommended. Extensive surgery and use of orthotic devices are often necessary to maximize the functional level of these children. Long leg braces with boots are helpful for household ambulation. Most affected children will be wheelchair-bound, however.

ACQUIRED SPINAL ABNORMALITIES

Hyperlordosis

Definition

Hyperlordosis or "swayback," an accentuation of the expected amount of lumbar lordosis, is perhaps most common in prepubertal girls, especially in blacks. Contracture of the hip flexors is sometimes associated, as is hamstring tightness and, occasionally, tightness of the lumbar fascia. A coincident thoracic hyperkyphosis is often noted.

Diagnosis

Diagnosis is confirmed with a full length standing lateral radiograph. Spondylolisthesis, thoracic hyperkyphosis, or femoral anteversion must be ruled out.

Treatment

The treatment of choice for simple hyperlordosis is a physical therapy program that stresses postural awareness, strengthening of the abdominal musculature, and stretching of any associated contractures. Rarely, a lumbar brace may be needed if exercise fails.

Hyperkyphosis

Some degree of kyphosis or round back in the thoracic spine and of lordosis in the lumbar spine is normal. A significant amount of curvature is abnormal, however; it may either be the cause or effect of altered spinal mechanics. Thoracic hyperkyphosis is most common in the adolescent. No congenital varieties have been noted in the literature.

In the adolescent, there are two major types of hyperkyphosis. One is termed postural roundback, in which there is definite clinical deformity, sometimes leading to stiffness and back pain (although this is rare). In postural roundback, there are no abnormalities of the vertebral end-plate seen on the standing face full length lateral radiograph. It is rarely associated with neurologic deficits.

The second type of hyperkyphosis is Scheuermann disease, defined as hyperkyphosis associated with vertebral end-plate abnormalities and greater than 5° of anterior wedging in at least three vertebrae. It is thought to be due to relative osteopenia of vertebral end-plates. Nearly half of the patients with Scheuermann disease have back pain on presentation, in marked contrast to the usual patient with postural roundback.

Epidemiology

About 4% of school-age children have hyperkyphosis.

Treatment

In both conditions, the initial treatment consists of either observation alone for mild cases or physical therapy in the form of postural awareness and correction. The postural awareness and physical therapy program consists of antilordotic lumbar exercises and simultaneous thoracic hyperextension exercises. Deformities not responding to a physical therapy program or curves greater than 20–30° (up to 50°) often require orthotic treatment in the form of a modified Milwaukee brace. This brace, when needed, is usually effective when worn 12–16 hours a day for at least 1–2 years. Bracing programs are successful only if the degree of deformity is not too severe, if accompanied by a physical therapy program, and if there is enough growth remaining to induce compensatory correction. Since the thoracic spine finishes its growth later than do other portions of the spine, orthotic treatment may succeed in correcting thoracic hyperkyphosis through the midteenage years.

For patients in whom the deformity is severe (greater than 50°), consideration should be given to surgery rather than bracing. Patients whose deformities or symptoms have been unresponsive to bracing, or patients with severe deformities who have finished growth, should definitely have the details of surgery explained to them. The natural history of severe adolescent hyperkyphosis is for slowly progressive deformity throughout life, with probable thoracic and lumbar discomfort. Surgical correction is reliable, provides satisfactory reduction of deformity, and is low in risk. While it involves stiffening of a significant portion of the spine through surgical fusion, these patients for whom surgery is a consideration already have a stiff spine, and for them the trade-off is an excellent one.

Idiopathic Scoliosis

Definition

Idiopathic scoliosis, an acquired lateral curvature of the spine, is, in its most common North American form, largely a genetic disease of adolescent females (Wynne-Davies, 1968). It involves a significant rotatory deformity as well as lateral curvature of the spine. Minor degrees of scoliosis are insignificant both functionally and cosmetically. Large degrees may have both cosmetic and functional consequences, in terms of cardiopulmonary compromise with severe thoracic curves, and in terms of disturbed lumbar mechanics and low back pain with severe lumbar curves.

Epidemiology

Although scoliosis is common if small curves are included (at least 3% of adults have curves of 10° or more), only about three patients per 1000 have a degree of spinal deformity that requires treatment (Rogala et al, 1978).

Natural History

Idiopathic scoliosis can be divided into types by age, with the infantile type defined as having onset before age 3 years, the juvenile type has onset between ages 3 and 9 years and the adolescent type has onset (or discovery) at age 10 years or more.

Infantile idiopathic scoliosis is much more common in Europe and Great Britain than in North America. The infantile type is different from other types of idiopathic scoliosis, in that spontaneous resolution of the deformity occurs in at least 75% of cases.

Diagnosis

Measurement of the rib/vertebral angle difference on progressive radiographs has been found to be extremely helpful in predicting the natural history of infantile scoliosis.

Treatment

Since curves presenting with more than 30° of scoliosis have a poorer prognosis than do smaller ones, rib/vertebral angle difference notwithstanding, a bracing program is recommended. Spinal fusion may be necessary in the rare very progressive case, but it is to be avoided if at all possible because of loss of spine growth that follows lengthy fusions in a very young spine.

Diagnosis

Juvenile idiopathic scoliosis and the *adolescent* type are similar and will be considered together. For an appropriate screening examination, the patient, with torso unclad, must be observed from behind. The patient stands with feet together, with back to the examiner, looking straight ahead, with arms relaxed at the side. The examiner checks for the following points: (1) asymmetric shoulder levels, (2) scapular asymmetry, (3) asymmetry of waistline or flank contour, (4) asymmetric distances from the arms to the trunk, (5) a palpable curve in the alignment of the spinous processes, and most important, (6) asymmetric prominence of one side of the thoracic or lumbar regions of the trunk on forward bend (Fig. 23.4).

Pain is rare, and indeed, if it is present, diagnosis other than idiopathic scoliosis should be considered, and urgent referral made.

Screening for spinal deformity in children is often carried out at school, and school screening is mandatory in many developed countries. Because scoliosis is usually asymptomatic, yet may have severe consequences if not appropriately treated, the spine should be examined as part of the annual physical examination (Berwick, 1984).

If scoliosis with a curvature greater than 25° is suspected after the suggested screening examination, orthopedic referral should be made. Since scoliosis is a physical finding rather than a definitive diagnosis, a careful history and neurologic examination should ac-

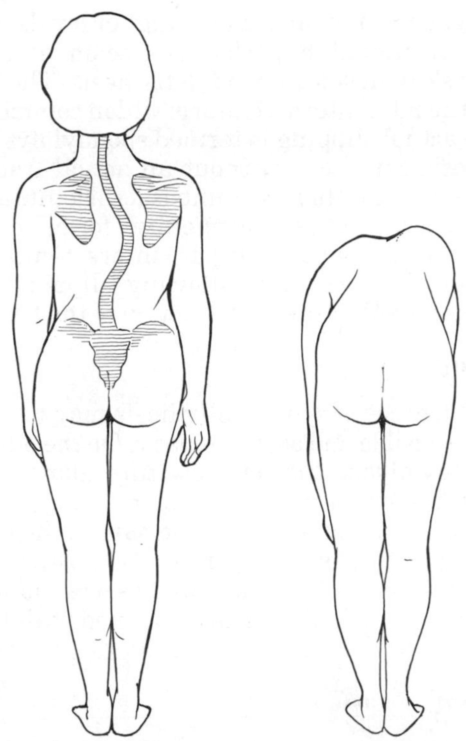

Figure 23.4. The spine is best examined by inspection of the child upright and bending forward from the waist with arms extended as illustrated.

company the orthopedic evaluation. Although radiographs will often be necessary to quantify the deformity in a patient referred after a positive screening examination, nonradiographic means (inclinometer, moire fringe photography) may be used in the place of radiographs to assess and follow some smaller curves. If radiographs are to be taken, a standing, full length posteroanterior radiograph of the entire spine should be obtained. Lateral radiographs and bending films should be taken only with special indications and never for initial screening.

Treatment

Patients with mild deformity, who are not in need of active treatment, can be followed by their primary care givers. Currently, few patients with stable idiopathic curves under 25° are believed to require braces; patients who are still growing and have curves progressing to 25° or diagnosed at more than 25°, should be referred to an orthopedist specializing in spinal disorders (Moe, 1980).

Treatment of progressive spinal deformity with neuromuscular stimulation, spinal orthoses, and surgical stabilization has been shown to be effective. Although multiple other modalities such as physiotherapy, traction, and manipulation have been tried, none have been shown to be effective in altering the natural history of progressive spinal deformity either singly or in combination.

The rationale for treating progressive idiopathic scoliosis in the growing child usually is not to take care of the current symptomatic problem, but much more often to prevent future problems. Although many curvatures in adolescents are displeasing cosmetically, almost none are symptomatic. Since idiopathic scoliosis is almost always painless during childhood, any child with scoliosis and pain should be referred immediately to rule out infection or neoplasia.

In general, the younger the child and the greater the size of the curve, the greater is the risk of progression. As a rough rule, curves under 25° of idiopathic type are seldom actively treated. Curves between 25 and 40° in immature patients are usually treated with a brace or neuromuscular stimulation. These nonsurgical forms of treatment usually are continued until growth in the deformed part of the spine is complete, as measured both radiographically and clinically. Braces are usually worn between 16 and 20 hours a day, and neuromuscular stimulation, when used, is performed only at night.

Surgery is usually restricted to the idiopathic curves greater than 40–50°. The advantages of surgical correction of idiopathic curves includes greater reduction in deformity than with nonsurgical means, a more reliable outcome, and often, less immobilization during the treatment program. Many surgical treatment programs now involve immobilization after surgery in only a very light brace, or sometimes without a brace. Restriction of activities for 6–12 months following surgery is the rule. A disadvantage of surgery is that the straightened part of the spine is permanently stiffened. Other disadvantages include surgical risks, which are rare, but may cause significant morbidity. These include infection, failure of the fusion to become solid, and neurological damage (risk well under 1/2500).

Prognosis

Curves in the lumbar region interfere with low back mechanics and are associated with an increased risk of low back pain in later life. In general, curves that remain under 40° at the end of growth will tend not to progress further, while those over 50° will tend to be progressive.

CONTROVERSY

It was formerly thought that (a) regardless of the size of the curve, progression would stop once growth of the spine had stopped; (b) a scoliotic curve was only a cosmetic problem; (c) nonsurgical treatment was conservative, whereas surgical treatment was not. All of these myths about scoliosis have largely been dispelled.

Neuromuscular Scoliosis

Various neuromuscular diseases, ranging from classic poliomyelitis, to the muscular dystrophies, cerebral palsy, myelodysplasia, dysautonomia, and many others, are important causes of progressive spinal deformity.

Treatment

In general, patients with neuromuscular diseases tolerate bracing treatment less well than do patients with idiopathic spinal deformity, and results of bracing are less successful. Hence, many cases of neuromuscular scoliosis should be considered for surgical stabilization at smaller degrees of deformity than idiopathic cases.

The usual patient with neuromuscular scoliosis who undergoes surgical fusion is treated with rigid internal fixation, in the form of very strong rods, hooks, and wires, so that external fixation following the surgery can be minimized. In patients in whom the quality of bone is very poor (in myelodysplasia in particular), postoperative orthotic treatment can rarely be dispensed with entirely.

Spondylolisthesis

Definition

Spondylolisthesis refers to a forward slipping of one vertebral body on the body below. It occurs only if there has been structural weakening or failure, sometimes in the form of a fracture, in the posterior elements, usually in the pars interarticularis. It may have a frankly traumatic cause, as in gymnasts or football players, who suffer repetitive microtrauma in the form of hyperextension maneuvers to the lower spine. There is, in addition, a strong genetic predisposition. Most cases occur, however, without any clear antecedent trauma. The most common location for spondylolisthesis to occur in the immature individual is at L5, where the vertebral body slips forward on the sacrum. The condition is significantly less common at L4, and exceedingly uncommon at much higher levels. Patients with constitutional hyperlordosis seem at some increased risk to develop spondylolisthesis. The fracture through the pars interarticularis which commonly precedes the actual slipping is termed spondylolysis. Spondylolisthesis can occur without an actual fracture, in situations where either the lumbosacral joints and discs are dysplastic, so-called "congenital form," or in conditions where the bone of the pars interarticularis itself is structurally abnormal, allowing slipping forward without either a fracture or disruption of the facet joints.

Diagnosis

Mild degrees of spondylolisthesis may be both cosmetically invisible and asymptomatic. On the other hand, even spondylolysis, the pars fracture alone, can give rise to severe symptoms on occasion.

The presentation may include pain in the low back, buttocks, and thighs, a hyperlordotic posture or even a palpable "step off" at the lumbosacral junction in severe cases. The diagnosis is confirmed with plain radiographs.

Treatment

Asymptomatic patients are followed closely for evidence of increased slippage, while nonoperative supportive treatment (bed rest, anti-inflammatory agents, and even a cast or brace) can be tried for a symptomatic patient. Refractory pain, greater than 50% slippage, or gait abnormality will usually require surgical fusion of the involved vertebral bodies.

Prognosis

More than 95% of patients will return to a normal active lifestyle following surgical fusion.

Congenital Limb Abnormalities 7

ARTHROGRYPOSIS

Definition

Arthrogryposis multiplex congenita refers to fixed contractures of multiple joints present at birth.

Basic Science

Arthrogryposis can result from any condition that limits intrauterine movement. Thus, oligohydramnios, myopathies, and disorders of anterior horn cells can lead to arthrogryposis. The degree of involvement can vary greatly.

Epidemiology

The disorders are usually sporadic and not associated with familial clubfoot or congenital dislocation of the hip. Nevertheless, a child with arthrogryposis not infrequently has clubfeet or congenitally dislocated hips (Wynne-Davies et al, 1981). Contractures of the temporomandibular joint occur in about 25% (Hageman and Willemse, 1983).

Diagnosis and Treatment

The diagnosis is descriptive, based on observation of fixed joints present at birth. A search for etiology may require nerve or muscle biopsy, electromyography, MRI and other tests. The approach to treatment is the same as that described for cerebral palsy. Treatment requires early initiation of active and passive range of motion exercises for involved joints. Use of orthotics and surgical procedures are common, although recurrences of joint disabilities are frequent despite these interventions.

Prognosis

The outlook for the patient with these joint deformities depends on the extent of disease and the availability of expert orthopedic care and physical therapy. These children are usually of normal intelligence and usually have a normal life span despite their joint abnormalities. About 10% have malformations of the CNS and mental retardation.

The most immediate need is to discuss the situation fully with the parents, whose initial shock may be profound. If the infant is normal in all other respects, which is usually the case, the family can be reassured about the possibility of the child coping well with the handicap, and the availability of prostheses. Furthermore, anxiety about a recurrence in another pregnancy can be allayed. The lesion is not a congenital malformation but rather an intrauterine accident that is most unlikely to recur in subsequent pregnancies.

CONGENITAL AMPUTATIONS

Infants can be born with amputations of extremities at any level. Usually the remaining limb ends in a healed stump. Although in a given situation the cause can only be speculated, amniotic bands can constrain a developing limb and compromise the circulation, with necrosis and separation of the distal limb. Oligohydramnios and clubfeet are associated findings.

PHOCOMELIA

Definition

Phocomelia refers to partial or total absence of limbs with some normal or abnormal terminal fingers and nails. It is an example of a reduction malformation rather than an amputation.

Basic Science

Only rare sporadic cases of phocomelia were reported before an epidemic which occurred in association with maternal ingestion of thalidomide at a critical period between the 40th and 47th day of pregnancy. Apparently, the drug interfered with limb development, but did not interfere with the genetic program for hand or foot development (Lenz, 1962; Taussig, 1962).

Diagnosis

The gross limb deformities are evident at birth, and may be associated with malformations in other systems (McBride, 1961).

Treatment

Treatment requires construction of orthopedic appliances and devices to facilitate function. These require the skills of an orthopedist.

FINGERS AND TOES

Polydactyly

Polydactyly, extra digits, are frequent events and commonly inherited as an autosomal dominant trait. Skin tags at the level of the fifth or first digits can be readily removed with a suture tied tightly around their base. After a few days, the necrotic tag will slough. If bone or cartilage are present, removal is deferred for a few months in order to assess more adequately the amount of tissue that must be removed. Surgery is usually performed between age 6 months to 1 year when the cartilage and bony structures can be better defined radiographically.

Syndactyly

Syndactyly, or fusion of adjacent fingers, requires surgical separation since allowing fusion to persist may promote later loss of function in the affected joints. Syndactyly of the toes generally requires no treatment.

Skeletal Dysplasias 8

Definition

Skeletal dysplasias, or chondrodystrophies, are generally characterized by disproportionate short stature with an associated skeletal disorder. Best known among the more than 100 distinct dysplasias are achondrodysplasia (short limbs) and Morquio disease (short trunk), under which rubric most of the others are grouped.

An international classification divides skeletal dysplasias into osteochondrodysplasias (abnormalities of cartilage and bone growth) and dysostoses (malformations of individual bones). Osteochondrodysplasias may be apparent at birth or become apparent later in life (Rimoin and Sillence, 1982).

Many of the skeletal dysplasias have craniofacial anomalies, with some bones more likely to be involved than others. The mandible is spared in achondroplasia, for example.

Basic Science

Histologic and biochemical studies of bones have made possible a correlation of specific defects with the clinical syndromes. The rapid increase in research on the chemistry of collagen and proteoglycans is making possible clearer delineation of the types of skeletal dysplasias.

Diagnosis

Prenatal diagnosis by ultrasonography is possible in a number of disorders, including achondrogenesis, asphyxiating thoracic dystrophy, osteogenesis imperfecta, and thanatophoric dysplasia. For the most part, diagnosis cannot be verified before midgestation, but occasionally, it is possible to have prognostic information from radiographs in time for the mother to opt for termination of pregnancy. Since the basic defect in most skeletal dysplasia is unknown (except in osteogenesis imperfecta), earlier diagnosis is not feasible.

An International Skeletal Dysplasia Registry exists at: Cedars-Sinai Medical Center, 8700 Beverly Boulevard, Los Angeles CA 90048, (213)855-4461.

ACHONDROPLASIA

Definition

Achondroplasia refers to a group of disorders in which the trunk is within the range of normal size at birth, but the limbs are short, especially the proximal segments. The head may be large and, in time, shows a prominent forehead, depressed nasal bridge, and prominent mandible. The foramen magnum is small and mild ventricular dilatation is common.

Epidemiology

The condition occurs in about 1/1000 births. The inheritance is autosomal dominant, with a high rate of spontaneous mutations since about 80% of affected infants are born to normal patients (Prockop and Kivirikko, 1984).

Natural History

The infants may be hypotonic and slow in motor development, but usually catch up by age 2 years. Intelligence is usually normal. Achrondroplastic infants are at increased risk of sudden unexplained death (Pauli et al, 1984).

Treatment of Orthopedic Aspects of Achondroplasia

Patients with achondroplasia may develop certain well-defined orthopedic problems. Probably the most dramatic is that of a gibbus or severe kyphotic deformity at the thoracolumbar junction. It develops in less than 10% of patients, but when it occurs it is relentlessly progressive and is associated with paraplegia unless stabilized by spinal fusion. An anterior interbody fusion is usually required. The diagnosis is usually obvious in retrospect, but since these patients are often stocky, it may be missed in its early stages when treatment is relatively easy. All children with achondroplasia should, therefore, have standing lateral radiographs of their spine some time in their first years of life. The diagnosis of potential gibbus deformity is usually possible by age 3 or 4 years.

A second orthopedic problem relates to the hyperlordosis and spinal stenosis which is universal in achondroplasts. The distance between the pedicles in the achondroplastic lumbar spine is much less than normal, even though achondroplasts have a relatively normal length trunk. This reduced intrapedicular distance, along with thick laminae and ligamentum flavum, greatly reduces the volume of the spinal canal and jeopardizes the integrity of the spinal cord and cauda equina. Most achondroplasts develop some symptoms in middle age from spinal stenosis. If the symptoms are progressive, extensive decompressive laminectomies are required. This procedure is rarely necessary in the child, although bracing of progressive lordotic deformities in the achondroplastic child may diminish the incidence of symptomatic spinal stenosis later on.

Tibia vara is a very frequent abnormality in achondroplasts. It is associated with relative overgrowth of the fibula, and sometimes epiphysiodesis of the fibula is carried out in an effort to equalize the length of the tibia and fibula. It remains uncertain whether epiphysiodesis of the fibula will prevent progression of tibia vara. A valgus osteotomy may be necessary if a varus deformity of the tibia is progressive and threatens knee function. Bracing is usually ineffective for this problem.

Dwarfism occurs universally in the achondroplastic syndrome. This is a short limbed type of dwarfism due to dysfunction of the physeal growth cartilage. Limbs can be lengthened although the surgery is extensive, and its indication is extremely controversial. Nevertheless, methods of long bone lengthening are improving and several centers are participating in prospective limited trials employing multiple surgical lengthenings of long bones in achondroplastic patients.

Thanataphoric Dwarfism

This condition is characterized by extreme shortening of extremities, hydrocephalus, and a narrow thorax. The condition is not familial. The cause is most likely a dominant mutation.

Respiratory distress is evident shortly after delivery and death usually follows quickly.

MORQUIO SYNDROME (MUCOPOLYSACCHARIDOSIS IV)

Definition

Children with a disproportionately short trunk, abnormal vertebrae, lax ligaments and dysplastic acetabula are considered to have Morquio syndrome (see also pp. 979).

Natural History

The observation of a relatively short trunk in comparison with extremities is usually made between 18 months and 2 years because of knock knees, waddling gait, pectus carinatum, and generalized joint laxity. Growth is stunted. With time, the lower limbs become proportionately shorter secondary to increasing genu valgus and abnormal physeal growth. In later childhood, heart and lung problems result from progressive spinal curvature. Deafness and hepatomegaly are often present.

Diagnosis

With slit-lamp examination fine corneal opacities are seen. The teeth may be gray. Keratosulfates are present in urine, hence, its inclusion as a mucopolysaccharidosis.

Radiographs of the spine show platyspondyly and characteristic anterior, central beaking of the vertebrae.

Treatment

While no direct treatment of the enzyme deficiency is possible in Morquio syndrome, orthopedic attention can be given to some of the secondary problems. Odontoid hypoplasia is common and is frequently associated with dangerous upper cervical instability. If instability of C1 and C2 is diagnosed by flexion-extension views, the upper cervical spine should be stabilized by surgical fusion.

Major mechanical problems often arise in the lower extremities in patients with Morquio syndrome. Osteotomies are occasionally required around the hips and knees to correct progressive deformities.

Prognosis

Death usually occurs in early adulthood.

HURLER SYNDROME (MUCOPOLYSACCHARIDOSIS I-H)

Definition

Hurler syndrome (see also pp. 979) is an autosomal recessive disorder sometimes called gargoylism because of a characteristic facies (thickened lips, coarse hair, wide nostrils).

Natural History

The infants may appear normal, but by 2–3 years it is evident that growth is impaired, and mental function deteriorates. Flexion contractures develop and walking is impaired. Blindness and deafness may occur. Both the liver and spleen are involved. Corneal opacities may be seen on slit-lamp examination.

Diagnosis

The facies and habitus are suggestive of this storage disease. Excretion of heparitin sulfate and dermatan sulfate are increased in urine. Spinal radiographs show characteristic beaking of the vertebrae, particularly in the thoracolumbar region.

Treatment and Prognosis

Supportive care is the only treatment available. These children usually die before adolescence.

Infections 9

SEPTIC ARTHRITIS

Definition

Septic arthritis is infection within the joint capsule, and commonly is associated with an adjacent osteomyelitis.

Basic Science

Septic arthritis occurs both as a primary and secondary event. In the primary form, exactly how bacteria invade the joint space remains unclear as of 1987. In the secondary form, i.e., secondary to adjacent osteomyelitis, it appears that bacteremia alone is not sufficient to cause the arthritis, but that another precursor, such as localized trauma to the area may be required as well. The organisms enter the metaphysis via the blood stream lodging in the sinusoidal loops beneath the epiphyseal plate where phagocytic function is diminished. Once infection starts, it proceeds into the subperiosteal space through the porous metaphyseal cortex and enters the joint capsule producing a septic arthritis. With elevation of the periosteum, the underlying bone is deprived of its blood supply and characteristic radiologic changes of osteomyelitis develop. Once established in the joint, bacteria will cause the release of synovial collagenase which, in conjunction with lysosomal enzymes, will destroy the articular surface (Morrisey, 1986).

Epidemiology

Eighty percent of cases involve the joints of the lower extremity, and two-thirds occur before age 3 years. Streptococci and *Escherichia coli* are the most common organisms in newborns, *Haemophilus influenzae* is the most common in children up to age 2 years, and staphylococci are most common in older children (Marks, 1985).

Diagnosis

Long-term complications of a septic joint are related to delay in diagnosis as well as inadequacy of treatment. A swollen, painful, erythematous joint should be considered septic arthritis until proven otherwise. The diagnosis depends on aspiration of purulent fluid from the joint, elevated sedimentation rate and identification of the organism by smear and culture. Bacteremia is common. The earliest radiographic change is widening of the joint space, with joint destruction being a late finding. The bone scan may be less helpful than it is in osteomyelitis.

Treatment

Aspiration should be done as soon as possible to make an accurate diagnosis. In hip infections, surgical drainage is an emergency because of the possible compromise of the fragile blood supply to the femoral head by a tense effusion (aspiration always is inadequate for a septic hip). Systemic antibiotics are required. Instillation of antibiotics into the infected joint is not only unnecessary (high penetration is achieved by intravenous medications), but unwise (toxic to cartilage in high doses). Open drainage with irrigation of the purulent joint with saline or Ringer solution should follow a diagnostic aspiration. In a major joint, this reduces the concentration of chondrolytic bacterial and white cell enzymes in the joint. In septic knees, repeated joint aspirations in conjunction with antibiotic treatment can be elected. If the white blood cell count in the joint fluid decreases and the clinical picture is improving, continuing therapy with antibiotics may be satisfactory. If the child remains toxic, or the joint fluid is persistently purulent, surgical drainage of the joint is required. Recovery of joint function is achieved by gradual resumption of motion. Splints, crutches, and physical therapy may be needed temporarily.

Prognosis

Prompt diagnosis, aspiration, and appropriate chemotherapy usually lead to complete resolution of the infection. Failure to treat promptly can lead to destruction of the joint, ankylosis, and resultant disability, particularly of the hip joint.

DISCITIS

Definition

Discitis is an inflammation, usually infectious, in the intervertebral disc space.

Epidemiology

Sixty percent of disc space infections occur in children under age 6 years. The most common site is the lumbar region, and the organism most frequently recovered on aspiration is *S. aureus*.

Diagnosis

The child may present with a complaint of pain which may be intermittent and severe. Less often, the child will present with a limp, or in younger children, refusal to walk. Tenderness to percussion of the involved vertebra's spinous process localizes the lesion. Fever may be present, but an elevated white blood count is unusual. The erythrocyte sedimentation rate is elevated, often for weeks or even months.

Radionuclide scans may be positive before changes are seen on radiographs. Narrowing of the disc space and irregular erosions of the end-plate are typical plain radiographic findings.

A tuberculin test is essential, since tuberculous infection can have the same presentation.

If the child is toxic, aspiration of the involved disc space under fluoroscopy or CT monitoring may be necessary to make a definite bacteriologic diagnosis.

Treatment

Immobilization of the spine with body cast or brace alone almost always leads to complete resolution. Aspiration of the space is advocated by some physicians, but considered unnecessary by others. Since the most likely organism is *S. aureus,* we advocate 4 weeks of therapy with an antistaphylococcal antibiotic. Whether to administer the drug orally or intravenously should be individualized on the basis of severity of symptoms, and systemic responses such as fever or a high white blood count. In general, these children can remain semiambulatory in their casts or braces and receive their antibiotics orally, assuming adequate blood levels can be maintained.

OSTEOMYELITIS

Definition

Osteomyelitis is an infection of bone.

Basic Science

Bacteria enter the bone usually via hematogenous spread, often in the setting of local trauma, localizing beneath the epiphyseal plate where blood flow is sluggish in the venous system and phagocytic activity is diminished. Once this metaphyseal osteitis is established, the bacteria gain access to the subperiosteal space, elevating it off the underlying cortex depriving it of its blood supply. This produces a dead bone fragment or a sequestrum. New bone forms from the elevated periosteum, creating an involucrum. In young infants who lack epiphyseal plates, the ends of long bones may be destroyed by an adjacent osteomyelitis, the femoral head being particularly vulnerable.

Epidemiology

Osteomyelitis is most common between ages 1 and 12 years with a four to one preponderance in males. It can occur in newborn infants and in individuals of any age in association with trauma or decubitus ulcers. Individuals at greatest risk are those with injuries, or those with conditions that can lead to bacteremia. Osteomyelitis is most common in the metaphyses of long bones, particularly the distal femur and proximal tibia.

Natural History

In newborn infants, staphylococci, group B streptococci, and Gram-negative bacteria are commonly associated with osteomyelitis. The initial infection may be acquired directly through a heel stick or traumatic femoral venipuncture, or in association with cephalohematoma, and rarely, emboli from an infected umbilical artery catheter. Bacteria enter the circulation and establish foci of infection in the metaphyseal regions of long bones.

In older children, injuries such as puncture wounds in the feet, animal bites, and lacerations may be the portal of entry of bacteria. More frequently, no primary focus is recognized.

Osteomyelitis requires prompt diagnosis and treatment to prevent disabling bone and joint destruction.

Diagnosis

The initial symptoms may be pain, local tenderness, and fever. Swelling, redness, and decreased movement point to the site of infection. Sterile effusions in the adjacent joint are common.

Radiographic changes in the soft tissues can be detected within 4 days, and bony changes are usually evident within 5 days in newborns and 10–14 days in older children. Blood cultures are positive in the bacteremic stage of infection. Radionuclide scans with technetium or gallium may be abnormal before changes are evident on plain radiographs. False-positives can occur after trauma so caution is required in their interpretation. The most accurate means of identifying the cause is aspiration of purulent material from the subperiosteal space. A blood culture should be taken in addition to this aspiration, as up to 50% are positive.

Treatment

Antibiotics should be initiated as soon as cultures are obtained. Some guidance can come from a Gram stain. Antibiotics are initially chosen based on the most likely organism and coverage is subsequently refined when the culture results are available. Since staphylococci are most commonly involved, a drug such as oxacillin is given intravenously.

If there is a poor response to chemotherapy, or radiographic evidence of osteolysis or abscess formation, or if the symptoms have been present for 10 days or more, surgical drainage of the lesion will be required, in addition to antimicrobial therapy for the child. Surgical debridement removes necrotic tissue, decompresses the medullary space, and improves the ability of antibiotics to reach remaining vascularized tissue.

The duration of therapy is a matter of some debate. In general, at least 6–8 weeks is considered essential, with a longer period if signs or symptoms persist. The infection can be treated orally if adequate drug absorption is documented by blood levels. A serum concentration of at least 8 times the minimum bactericidal concentration is advised. Oral medication requires assurance of compliance and careful monitoring of the clinical response (Anderson et al, 1981).

Chronic osteomyelitis may require several months of therapy, or even longer, depending on the extent of infection, the organism, and the response to surgical and medical treatment. Tuberculous infections require at least 6 months of therapy with isoniazid and rifampin.

Splinting of the infected region may be required for relief of pain initially, although passive motion should be initiated as soon as tolerable. Once the pain subsides, we encourage gradual rehabilitation and ambulation, limiting only vigorous exercise initially.

Prognosis

Early treatment with effective antibiotics usually leads to complete resolution. In a longitudinal study of over 200 children, only nine had long-term sequelae (Anderson et al, 1981). The greatest danger in infants less than 1 year old is that infection may involve the growth plate and result in limb shortening. After age 18 months, vessels do not cross the growth plate, and it acts as a barrier to infection.

Chronic Recurrent Multifocal Osteomyelitis

Definition

The name of this condition not only defines the disorder, but includes most of what is known about it.

Epidemiology

First described in 1972, only 31 cases have been reported in the literature through 1986. The disease may well not be new, and may be under-reported. It does, however, have enough features to warrant a name that distinguishes it from the much more common bacterial osteomyelitis. All the reported cases have had their onset within the first two decades of life, the oldest patient being 16 years of age. The natural course of the disease is variable from a few months to 5 years.

Natural History

The presenting symptoms will depend on which bone is involved, and often the lesion is identified by pain and local swelling. The youngsters are rarely sick, although they may have local discomfort. They are usually afebrile. The bones most likely to be involved include the vertebrae which can collapse or become sclerotic, and the metaphyseal ends of long bones such as the tibia.

Diagnosis

Radiographs may show punched out lesions or lesions with surrounding sclerosis. They may progress to involve most of a bone or remain localized to the metaphyseal ends of the long bones. The lesions are rarely seen in the skull, which distinguishes them from eosinophilic granuloma. The only evidence of inflammation is the sustained elevation of the erythrocyte sedimentation rate. Usually the peripheral blood count is normal as are calcium, phosphorus, and alkaline phosphatase (Fig. 23.5; Giedion et al, 1972).

Histologic examination reveals a granuloma composed of histiocytes, but eosinophils and giant cells are rarely present. Necrotic bone spicules are surrounded by the granulomatous tissue. All attempts to identify an organism by culture or special staining techniques have failed. There is no pathognomonic diagnostic test.

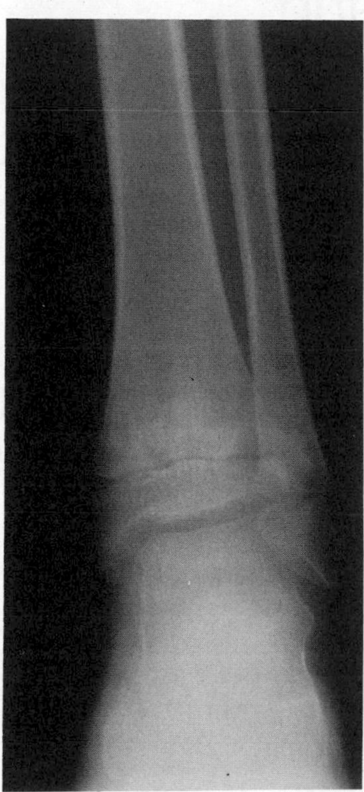

Figure 23.5. Radiograph of bone lesions in the 9-year-old girl described in the case illustration with relapsing multifocal osteomyelitis. The lesions cannot be distinguished from bacterial osteomyelitis on radiographs. The diagnosis requires biopsy to identify the granulomatous lesions.

Diagnosis involves biopsy and is by exclusion of other conditions such as bacterial osteomyelitis or eosinophilic granuloma (Kasser, 1986).

Treatment

There has been no response to antibiotics or steroids. It is important to know that these lesions tend to heal over a period of months to years.

CASE ILLUSTRATION

A 9-year-old Puerto Rican girl with multiple bone lesions first developed lymphadenopathy in January, 1984. She had pain and swelling over the dorsum of her right foot without fever or history of injury. A radiograph was interpreted as consistent with osteomyelitis of the right second metatarsal. She was treated with a cast and antibiotics, but failed to improve over a course of a month. Two months later, she had right Achilles tendinitis and was put in a cast again. The following month she had low back pain and on X-ray showed a nearly total collapse of a thoracic vertebra. Repeat radiographic studies in September, 1984 showed a lytic lesion in the left distal tibial metaphysis which, in retrospect, had been present since June of 1984 (Fig. 23.5).

The physical examination was unremarkable except for slight warmth and swelling over the left ankle. All the laboratory studies were within normal limits except for the elevated erythrocyte sedimentation rate. Extensive evaluation of her immune system failed to show any evidence of B-cell or T-cell dysfunction. She had a positive monilia skin test and a negative tuberculin test.

She was diagnosed as having chronic relapsing multifocal osteomyelitis when a pathologic examination of the lesion in the lower tibia failed to reveal any specific findings other than necrotic bone spicules and surrounding granuloma. Over the subsequent 2 years the lesion in the lower end of the tibia spread to include most of the tibia, but she remained asymptomatic and has been normally active. The other lesions have healed although she continues to have a collapsed thoracic vertebra.

COMMENT

This rare condition acts like a chronic infection; however, no organism has been identified after exhaustive searches. The importance of considering this diagnosis is that the disorder is self-limited and has not been seen in adults. Thus, it is inappropriate to treat with antibiotics or steroids (both of which have been tried and found not to be helpful). (Case illustration courtesy of Drs. John Emans, Harry Kozakewich, and Leisure Yu, radiograph courtesy of Dr. Robert Wilkinson).

Hereditary Disorders of Collagen and Bone Metabolism

10

A group of disorders of collagen structure have major clinical problems that are best discussed in a section in orthopedics (osteogenesis imperfecta, Ehlers-Danlos disease, Marfan syndrome). Others are more pertinent to dermatologists (dystrophic epidermolysis bullosa, keloids) and one is of importance to neurologists, berry aneurysms of the circle of Willis. Biochemists have unravelled some of the mysteries, and molecular biologists are making progress that portends prenatal diagnosis. For further review, the reader is referred to Pope and Nicholls, 1987; and Canalis, 1983.

MARFAN SYNDROME (ARACHNODACTYLY)

Definition

Marfan syndrome (see pp. 753) is a disorder of connective tissue with skeletal, ocular, and cardiovascular abnormalities. The nature of the basic defect is unknown.

Epidemiology

About 20,000 Americans (in a population of 240,000,000) are affected. It is an autosomal dominant disorder with variable expression (Sisk et al, 1983).

Natural History

Individuals with this disorder are tall and slender, with disproportionately long extremities usually from excessive length of distal bones. The arm span exceeds the height. Excessive growth of ribs is responsible for pectus excavatum or pigeon breast deformities.

With age, the laxity of the ligaments becomes a more significant problem, with weakness of joint capsules and recurrent dislocations of hips and patella. Subluxation of the lens, myopia, and retinal detachment may occur. Strabismus and nystagmus are prominent.

The cardiovascular abnormalities include dilatation of the ascending aorta which may be present in early childhood. Mitral valve regurgitation is the main cause of morbidity in childhood. Aortic dilatation can lead to regurgitation and heart failure. Aortic rupture is a hazard in adolescence, particularly among basketball and volleyball players (Gott et al, 1986).

Orthopedic problems sometimes occurring with Marfan syndrome include scoliosis and spondylolisthesis. Severe flat feet are almost always present, but rarely need direct treatment.

The scoliosis and spondylolisthesis can be rapidly progressive and when present, usually require surgical treatment in the form of correction with internal fixation devices and stabilization by intervertebral fusion.

Treatment

Propranolol can retard the enlargement of the aorta (Pyeritz, 1983). In individuals with damaged aortas, a graft can replace both the aortic valve and the dilated aorta.

Prognosis

The outlook is much improved by prophylactic surgery to prevent ruptured aortic aneurysms. For those patients who wish to keep abreast of current research, contact the National Marfan Association, 382 Main Street, Fort Washington, NY 11050.

OSTEOGENESIS IMPERFECTA

Definition

Osteogenesis imperfecta is a connective tissue disease characterized by abnormal collagen in bones, ligaments, skin, eyes, and ears. At least four distinct syndromes can be delineated among a group of disorders characterized clinically by increased radiolucency and fragility of bones. Type I osteogenesis imperfecta is characterized by brittle bones, blue sclerae, and hearing impairment. Type II is the most severe form and is usually fatal in utero. Prenatal ultrasonography may show shortened limbs from multiple fractures. The rare type III is recessive. It is distinguished from type II radiographically. Sclerae are normal. Type IV is an autosomal dominant disorder, with bone fragility, but normal hearing and sclerae. Other variants include infants with distinctive dysmorphic features including proptosis and hydrocephalus (Smith et al, 1983; Cole and Carpenter, 1987).

Basic Science

Collagen fibers in the bony matrix are abnormal on histologic examination. Abnormalities in type I collagen result from structural gene abnormalities that have been identified by linkage studies (Sykes et al, 1986). It is now clear that the most lethal form of the disease with fractures in utero can be inherited both as an autosomal dominant and recessive. Prenatal diagnosis for this type of osteogenesis imperfecta is now possible.

Natural History

The course depends on the frequency and severity of fractures. Severely affected infants can develop a flail chest and often die soon after birth. Linear growth is impaired because of reduced height of vertebral bodies. Tibial bowing as well as distortion of the pelvis and skull may occur. Scoliosis is common and often is evident by age 6 years. If the curvature reaches 30–40°, spinal fusion is necessary (Renshaw, 1986).

Diagnosis

The disorder must be distinguished from Morquio disease and other causes of dwarfism. The osteoporosis and predisposition to fractures are characteristic. Hands and feet are usually spared.

Blue sclerae and deafness may be present. The teeth are yellow and transparent (dentinogenesis imperfecta).

It is essential to consider this diagnosis in the differential of multiple fractures from child abuse.

Treatment

Orthopedic management is directed to specific fractures. Intramedullary rods are sometimes used to correct severe long bone deformity and protect against further fractures before the end of growth, since nonunion is more common in adults. Spinal fusions are often required for progressive scoliosis.

Prognosis

The prognosis is variable, from 90% fatality within the first day of life in the most severe form, to no significant symptoms in the milder forms (Sillence et al, 1984).

OSTEOPETROSIS (ALBERS-SCHONBERG DISEASE)

Definition

Osteopetrosis is characterized by dense bones throughout the entire skeleton and progressive anemia. Extramedullary erythropoiesis leads to hepatosplenomegaly. Narrowing of the optic foramina leads to optic atrophy.

Basic Science

Osteopetrosis occurs when abnormal chondroid tissue persists and has a high uptake of calcium. Intestinal absorption of calcium is increased. The basic abnormalities that lead to these "marble bones" are unknown.

The anemia results in part from the physical loss of marrow space, although this explanation may be too simplistic. A generalized mesenchymal disease may affect both bone and its marrow.

Epidemiology

The condition, if lethal in infancy, is inherited as an autosomal recessive. Parental consanguinity has been reported. Another form with onset later in life is inherited as a dominant, and is much less severe than the infantile form. Occasionally patients are identified only on routine screening of the family of an affected individual.

Natural History

Infants affected early in life show growth failure, ocular disturbances, which may be the first symptoms as vision is impaired progressively, anemia, and hepatosplenomegaly. The skull is often larger than normal and hydrocephalus may be present. Death occurs in the first years of life.

Diagnosis

The radiographic finding of generalized increase in skeletal density establishes the diagnosis. The findings are particularly characteristic in the phalanges. The base of the skull is very dense, but the cranial vault is normal in early life. Later, a "hair-on-end" appearance develops as anemia becomes more severe.

Treatment

In severe cases, bone marrow transplantation should be undertaken early if vision is to be preserved (Ballet et al, 1977). High doses of calcitriol (up to 32 μg/day) have been helpful in about half the patients treated (Key et al, 1984; personal communication, 1988). Thyroidectomy, to remove calcitonin-secreting cells, has not been effective.

EHLERS-DANLOS SYNDROME

Definition

Ehlers-Danlos syndrome comprises a heterogeneous group of inborn errors of collagen metabolism that lead to hyperelasticity of the skin, hypermotility of joints, short stature, and small widely spaced teeth. Ocular and cardiac involvement is present in some patients.

Basic Science

At least 10 clinical syndromes are described, but in only five of them have biochemical defects been identified. Only half of the patients fit into one of the 10 designated categories, which illustrates the wide range of phenotypic expression of collagen disorders.

The most common, and mildest forms are types I, II, and III, all autosomal dominant and all with an unknown biochemical defect. Ultrastructural studies show disorganization of collagen fibers. Some, or perhaps all types have a deficiency in production of type III collagen (see Table 23.2).

Table 23.2
Categories of Inborn Errors of Collagen Metabolism (Ehlers-Danlos Syndrome)[1]

Category	Mode of Inheritance	Defect	Clinical Characteristics
Type I	Autosomal dominant		Mild, disorganization of collagen fibers
Type II	Autosomal dominant or recessive		As type I, but ecchymoses prominent
Type III	Autosomal dominant		As type I, except scar formation is normal
Type IV	Autosomal dominant or recessive	Collagen Type III deficient in tissues	Risk for rupture of major blood vessels
Type V	X-linked recessive		As type II, but severe mitral regurgitation may occur
Type VI (ocular-scoliotic form)	Autosomal recessive	Deficiency of lysyl hydroxylase	Extreme joint hyperextensibility; scleral and corneal fragility
Type VII	Dominant or recessive	Defective conversion of procollagen to collagen	Extreme joint laxity, e.g., loose congenital hip dislocation
Type VIII	Autosomal dominant		Severe periodontitis and early loss of teeth
Type IX (occipital horn syndrome)	X-linked recessive	Altered copper metabolism leading to lysyl oxidase deficiency	Skeletal abnormalities, exostoses in occipital area of skull
Type X	Autosomal recessive	Deficient plasma fibronectin	Hypermobility of small joints; marked bruising tendency

[1]This is the current status of our information on these disorders. Only with further understanding of collagen metabolism will the disorders be more specifically characterized.

Treatment

The fragility of the skin leads to easy bruising and bleeding, poor wound healing, and dehiscence of surgical wounds. Hence, great care must be taken to avoid injury. No means of enhancing healing ability is known.

Patients should be followed by an ophthalmologist since microcornia, retinal detachment, and subluxation of the lens can occur and may require treatment.

Cardiac consultation is important because of the tendency toward mitral valve insufficiency, and, in some patients, dissecting aneurysms of the aorta.

Prognosis

No intervention is available to alter the underlying disorder. The prognosis depends on the severity of manifestations and the supportive care available. Genetic counseling is appropriate.

Approach to Back Pain in Children and Adolescents

11

While back pain is a rather common complaint in the adult population, it is relatively rare before adolescence. When back pain does occur in the immature patient, it is much more likely to have its origin in a significant diagnosable pathologic lesion than in the adult, where sprains, strains, and degenerative changes are the usual etiology. A specific etiology for spinal symptoms should, therefore, be sought very aggressively when back pain occurs in a pediatric or adolescent practice. Neoplasms, infections, and major mechanical disorders are to be ruled out before a diagnosis of strain, sprain, or rarely, a functional or hysterical disorder can be made reliably. These last diagnoses are made by exclusion.

Diagnosis

In back pain, as in any other orthopedic problem, the diagnosis begins with the history. Location of the pain, character, duration, associated symptoms, exacerbating or ameliorating factors are all to be sought. Very acute onset suggests an infectious cause, although neoplasms can often be subclinical until an unknown factor precipitates recognizable symptoms.

The physical examination of the patient with back pain focuses very carefully on the posture, particularly flexibility or rigidity of the involved part of the spine, as well as local tenderness. Movements that reproduce the pain may be helpful in diagnosis. A careful neurologic examination is essential.

Plain radiographs of the area under suspicion are also essential and should be done in two planes. Coned down views or tomograms may be helpful if plain radiographs are inconclusive. Other more sophisticated imaging methods, such as radionuclide bone scans (to detect abnormalities in local blood flow) are helpful in detecting fractures, infections, and tumors. CAT scan or magnetic resonance imaging (useful for spinal cord and surrounding soft-tissue abnormalities) may be necessary and helpful. CBC, sedimentation rate, and urinalysis should precede any imaging studies because genitourinary pathology can sometimes present as back pain. A collagen vascular laboratory work-up also may be useful.

Neoplasms

Diagnosis and Treatment

Spinal neoplasms classically present with rather constant pain that may be worse at night. Rigidity, secondary to muscle spasm of the involved area of the spine is often present, as are neurologic deficits, particularly if the neoplasm is within the neural canal rather than primarily intraosseous. The neurologic deficit may be quite peripheral, manifesting itself as a foot deformity, or as a sphincter disturbance. Of the bony lesions, among the more common is an osteoid osteoma (which classically presents with night pain that is dramatically relieved by aspirin). It is extremely well visualized on technetium bone scans and is often located in the pedicle or lateral lamina. An osteoid osteoma is often associated with a painful scoliosis, which usually resolves dramatically upon excision of this benign lesion.

Eosinophilic granuloma is another benign neoplasm often found in the spine, which may or may not be evident on bone scan, and which often leads to dramatic collapse of the involved vertebra called "vertebra plana." Over time, and with support of the spine in a brace or cast, the vertebral body will usually reconstitute itself, at least partially. Low-dose radiotherapy may be helpful in selected cases. Eosinophilic granuloma is often found in multiple sites so that a skeletal survey is necessary.

Intradural tumors have a very variable presentation, but all are much more likely to present with a frank neurologic deficit than are the primarily intraosseous tumors. Whereas the intraosseous lesions may be amenable to needle biopsy, intradural tumors usually require surgical exploration for definitive diagnosis and treatment. Often, this is a combined approach with neurosurgery and orthopedics.

Infections

The most common type of spinal infection in the child or adolescent is discitis, which in the immature spine seems to be the equivalent of vertebral osteomyelitis in adults. About two-thirds of these intervertebral disc space infections occur in children under the age of 7 years, most commonly in the thoracolumbar junctional area and below. A reluctance to walk, an even greater reluctance to flex the lumbar spine, and local tenderness to percussion are classic findings. The bone scan is typically abnormal and plain radiographs show diminution in the height of the involved disc space. In early stages, the only laboratory abnormality may be an elevated sedimentation rate, and while plain radiographs may be normal, the bone scan is usually quite "hot" in the involved area. Aspiration is indicated only in the complicated case. Rest and immobilization of the involved portion of the spine are usually curative, although some physicians recommend a course of antistaphylococcal antibiotics.

Mechanical Back Pain

The most common causes of mechanical back pain in the immature child are Scheuermann disease, spondylolisthesis, and herniated intervertebral disc. Scheuermann disease is characterized by hyperkyphosis associated with structural vertebral changes. It is diagnosable by physical examination and radiographs, because of the classic thoracic hyperkyphosis, vertebral end-plate irregularity, and hence, wedging of the involved vertebral bodies. Treatment involves physical therapy, occasionally bracing, and rarely surgery.

Spondylolisthesis, consisting of a slippage forward of a lower lumbar vertebra on the one below, is usually found in a hyperlordotic individual. The classic physical findings include pain on hyperextension of the lumbar spine. A standing lateral radiograph of the lumbosacral junction is usually diagnostic. Spondylolysis, a linear fracture in the pars interverticularis is discussed on page 1284.

Treatment of symptomatic spondylolisthesis consists of bracing and abdominal muscular strengthening at the least, and surgical stabilization by lumbosacral fusion at the most.

A protruding intervertebral disc is very rare in children but, occasionally, occurs in the teenager. Its presentation and treatment are exactly the same as those in the adult. Chronic low back ache not due to any of the above causes may, occasionally, be noted in the child who is obese or has poor posture. It will often respond to a postural correction and physical therapy program.

Hysterical Back Pain

A rare child may complain of back pain and yet no organic cause can be found. The back may be a locus for a conversion reaction in children, as it can be in adults. This is usually associated with an unusual affect. Treatment here is obviously nonorthopedic and is directed to the etiologic factors as determined by an extensive psychosocial evaluation.

Musculoskeletal Injuries 12

The adage that "every child falls every day" makes it important for every pediatrician to have some familiarity with patterns and consequences of injury to the musculoskeletal system.

The long bones of a growing child are different from those of an adult in two major ways: first, the presence of open cartilaginous growth plates, (the physes), and second, in the greater elasticity of the bones as well as the soft tissues, when compared with the adult's. The presence of open growth plates gives the child's bone a ready mechanism for remodeling even considerable deformity with growth. On the other hand, if a fracture involves the growth plate, deformity from subsequently unbalanced growth can occur. Any discussion of pediatric bony injuries must, therefore, discuss injuries to the growth plate. In general, children's fractures heal much more rapidly than do similarly located fractures in an adult. Bending, buckling, or greenstick-type fractures, which are common in children, are rare in adults. Stiffness, which is often found following adult bone injuries, is rare after an uncomplicated fracture in a child.

FRACTURES

Definition

Fractures can be classified according to location, configuration, and character of deformity. The location of a fracture is described as physeal (involving the growth plate), metaphyseal, or diaphyseal. Growth plate injuries are of such importance that they are usually described by a special classification, the Salter-Harris system (Fig. 23.6). They constitute 15–20% of major long bone fractures in children (Shapiro, 1987).

A description of fractures by their physical configuration and manner of deformation of the bone ends is important in communicating with a specialist.

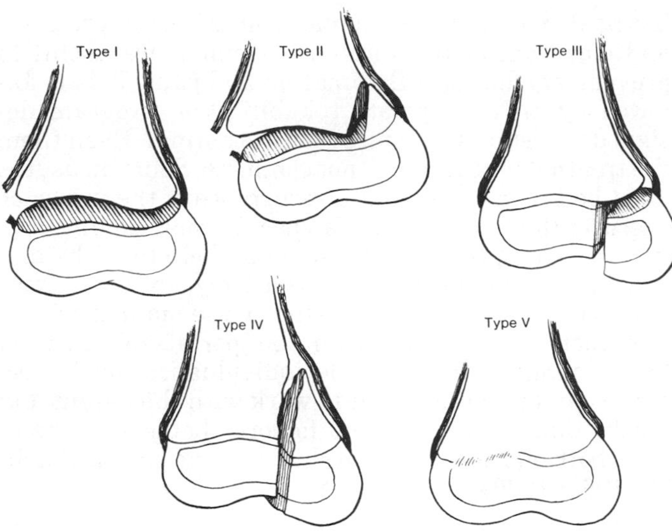

Figure 23.6. Diagram of the Salter classification of epiphyseal plate injuries. Type I is the least severe, and prognosis for growth disturbance worsens from I to IV. Reproduced with permission from Fleischer G, Ludwig S: *Textbook ok of Pediatric Emergency Medicine*. Baltimore, Williams & Wilkins, 1983, p. 955.

Fractures of the Physis (Growth Plate)

The physis (epiphyseal plate) is the cartilaginous, relatively transverse, growth plate that is responsible for longitudinal growth in a long bone. It is mitosis in the columns of cartilage cells in the growth plate, with subsequent conversion of the daughter cartilage cells to bone; that provides for longitudinal growth. Hence, any vascular or mechanical disturbance to the growth plate may interrupt orderly longitudinal growth. This often occurs in a child under the circumstances in which a ligament sprain would occur in an adult, because the cartilaginous growth plate is weaker than the child's adjacent ligaments, and because the growth plate is located at the level of attachment of the supporting ligaments in many joints. In general, children do not suffer ligament sprains, and what often looks like a ligament sprain in a child is often a displaced or undisplaced growth plate fracture (Shapiro, 1987).

Evaluation of Fractures and Sprains

Diagnosis

The clinical examination of the injured part should usually begin with the normal side if an injured extremity is being evaluated. This provides some basis for comparison. Circulation, neurologic function, stability, and deformity should be assessed before appropriate radiographs are ordered. In certain circumstances, it may be necessary to obtain a radiograph of the normal side for comparison. This is particularly true around the hip or elbow, where the many epiphyseal lines may be confusing. In cases of obvious injury, for both comfort and protection, an injured part should be splinted before radiographic studies. Biplanar films need to be obtained and, in general, the joint above and below the area of interest should be visualized on a radiograph.

Treatment of Fractures

After evaluation, the treatment of a fracture involves several decisions. It is necessary to determine: first, whether the position of the fracture is acceptable as found, or whether some formal reduction of the fracture is required; second, how much immobilization is needed to ensure both comfort and appropriate healing; and third, what is the appropriate follow-up and length of immobilization? These decisions should be made either by the orthopedist or in conjunction with the orthopedist.

In general, circular casts should be applied only by an orthopedist. Any circular cast applied for either a fracture or a sprain should probably be checked at the initial treating facility after 12–24 hours. At the time of primary treatment, clear follow-up plans should be made.

Children with epiphyseal fractures may have growth arrest identified several years later, and hence, should be followed through puberty. If growth is arrested, consultation with an orthopedist is essential since lengthening the involved bone is possible.

SPRAINS

Sprains are injuries to ligaments, which may be partial or complete. Sprains are *extremely rare* in children, because the ligaments are attached close to growth plates. Under traumatic conditions that, in an adult, would lead to a ligament sprain, a fracture of the growth plate will usually occur in a child. Therefore, tenderness and swelling in the area of a ligament in a child with an open growth plate is to be considered a growth plate fracture until proven otherwise.

STRAINS

Strains result from overstretching some part of a muscle-tendon unit.

SPORTS MEDICINE

Injuries to the child's musculoskeletal system incurred during participation in sports are, in general, no different from injuries suffered in any other type of activity. Certain so-called overuse syndromes, from repetitive microtrauma to musculoskeletal structures, may be more common under the stresses of certain sports than with more generalized activity. These overuse syndromes tend to occur in the knees or feet with running sports, and in the dominant arm with throwing or serving sports (most often in the elbow, occasionally in the shoulder).

The knee is the most frequently injured joint in football and skiing. Eighty percent of knee injuries in skiing involve rupture of the anterior cruciate ligament. Failure to diagnose and treat this injury can lead to a tendency for the knee to give way during pivoting motions, tearing the meniscus with subsequent pain and swelling. (For a review of knee injuries, see Zarins and Adams, 1988.)

Diagnosis and Treatment

A careful history will often reveal that an activity has been taken up without any preceding conditioning program. The history is often crucial in diagnosing the problem, when no signs or symptoms may be present at the time of the examination. Radiographs are often negative. Arthroscopy is an important tool in diagnosis, particularly in the case of a torn anterior cruciate ligament in the knee. Treatment of any injury, whether sports-related or not, cannot be satisfactory until an accurate diagnosis is reached. Once the diagnosis is made, rest is certainly necessary until the injured part has healed. In addition, application of ice, compression, and elevation of the injured extremity are useful to prevent worsening inflammation and pain. This is followed by an appropriate rehabilitation program designed to restore the injured part to normal. Even then, the treatment program is not complete. Some measures must be taken to prevent a recurrence of the injury or overuse; this may require a specific conditioning program to strengthen the athlete and help to withstand the rigors of competition. Alternatively, and sometimes necessary, the level of competition, the manner of participation in the sport, or even the sport itself may need to be changed. Considerable individualization is necessary, and it is important to work with the parent and coach. Finally, psychologic factors should be considered, both on the part of the child and the parent (Micheli, 1983; 1986).

Cerebral Palsy 13

While cerebral palsy is, by definition, a nonprogressive neurologic condition of varied etiology, the orthopedic problems can change considerably with growth and development and, therefore, appear progressive. A relatively new problem in pediatric orthopedics, certainly one that is an increasing challenge, is the management of the adolescent and young adult with residual deformities secondary to neurologic (cerebral palsy and other) problems for which the patient may or may not have had previous surgery. This population is steadily increasing in size as the care for newborn and young children improves.

Cerebral palsy can be classified neurophysiologically or anatomically. Neurophysiologically, patients may exhibit spasticity and rigidity, indicating pyramidal tract damage; they may exhibit signs of dyskinetic movements, indicating extrapyramidal system damage; or they may exhibit signs of both. Anatomically, cerebral palsy may be classified as involving the total body (quadriparesis); primarily lower extremity (diplegia); or one-half of the body, with the upper extremity involved more frequently than the lower (hemiparesis). Patients with both arms affected more than the lower extremities are classified as bilateral hemiparetics. Generally with hemiparesis, the upper extremities are involved more than the lower and if this is not the case, then chances are the patient represents an asymptomatic quadriparetic.

In children with the spastic type of cerebral palsy, hypertonicity of particular muscles in the upper and lower extremities leads to characteristic posturing and gait abnormalities, and to joint contractures, all of which may be helped by orthopedic intervention, in attempts to balance the muscle forces across the joints and either progressively stretch out or release contractures. Surgery in such patients is only a small part of their care, as an ongoing program of stretching or possibly bracing is needed to maintain the improvement.

Cerebral palsy patients with movement disorders are perhaps the most unpredictable subjects for any orthopedic intervention. Associated problems related to sensation, mental retardation, as well as seizures can complicate orthopedic management.

Approach to Treatment

In general, the orthopedic treatment of patients with cerebral palsy should be oriented toward a goal. Maintaining or working toward the child's ability to communicate, carry out normal activities, and retain mobility are primary goals of management. Generally, parents or therapists involved with the child will determine what specific problems are interfering with the child's progress and if they are amenable to stretching with serial casts, release, or bracing. In general, procedures are directed toward maintaining maximal joint motion and achieving muscle balance across involved joints. In the absence of bony deformity, soft tissue procedures (release and transfer) may be helpful. If both bony deformity and muscle imbalance are present, surgery must be directed at both.

HIP

Hip problems in the form of subluxation and dislocation are relatively common in cerebral palsy patients. The prevalence of these problems is generally related to the severity of involvement, i.e., hip dislocation is uncommon in ambulatory patients but may occur in 50–75% of quadriplegic bed care patients. Scoliosis and pelvic obliquity, are frequent concomitants of hip dislocation and subluxation. Whether scoliosis, pelvic obliquity and hip instability are directly related is under debate. About 50% of hip dislocations are painful. Generally with $< 30\%$ of hip abduction associated with increasing hip flexion contractures, soft tissue should be released around the hip. If done early, such releases can be very effective in maintaining the hip in the socket. In the older child, reduction of a unilaterally dislocated hip decreases the chance for the development of pain and pelvic obliquity in adulthood. In established painful dislocations in nonambulatory patients, a proximal femoral resection at the level of the lesser trochanter is probably the treatment of choice.

LOWER LIMBS

Perhaps one of the most common problems is tightness of the lower limb muscles producing a toe-toe gait secondary to equinus deformity of the ankle. This may be associated with varus or valgus of the hindfoot or it may be the primary problem. Physical therapy and bracing programs are the first line of treatment. If these fail, appropriate muscle lengthening, or transfer, and/or other orthopedic procedures may be needed to balance the forces about the foot and ankle in an effort to achieve a plantigrade foot.

UPPER LIMBS

Involvement of the upper extremity in cerebral palsy can be quite varied. The goals of treatment directed at the upper extremity include correcting the deformity, achieving muscle balance, and stabilizing joints in an effort to optimize grasp, release and prehension. An approach to upper extremity problems in cerebral palsy must be thoughtful and individualized. Patients with spastic quadripresis or hemiparesis are most likely to benefit from surgical intervention. Tests are designed to determine the level of cognition (intelligence), the child's ability to place the hand in space, and sensation. Evaluating patients with involvement of the upper extremities is directed at determining the presence of joint contracture, tendon-muscle contracture, and increased tone in muscles. Surgical procedures are directed at lengthening or transfering muscles to strengthen weakened antagonists and, thus, stabilize the joints and improve function.

SPINE

Spinal deformity and pelvic obliquity constitute another major problem. The prevalence of spinal curvature in patients with cerebral palsy varies from 5–65% in different groups studied and parallels the degree of neurologic involvement. Spinal curvature may be aggravated by gravitational forces when patients are propped in a sitting position, as well as by persistent primitive reflexes.

Spasticity and the degree of neurologic involvement appear to be the two next most important risk factors for spinal curvature to develop. Indications for surgical intervention include progression of curvature, pain, and compromised pulmonary function. Surgical treatment frequently will involve a circumferential fusion via a staged anterior fusion, followed by posterior spinal instrumentation and fusion. These patients are difficult to manage and the complication rate from balance problems, pressure sores, pseudoarthrosis, and infections is high. Progression of spinal deformity may continue despite the attainment of skeletal maturity; therefore, older children and adults need prolonged observation for the development and progression of spinal deformity.

REFERENCES

Anderson JR, Scobie WG, Watt B: The treatment of acute osteomyelitis in children: A ten year experience. *J Antimicrob Chemother* 7:43, 1981.

Asher MA: Screening for congenital dislocation of the hip, scoliosis, and other abnormalities affecting the musculoskeletal system. *Pediatr Clin North Am* 33:1335, 1986.

Ballet JJ, Gtiscelli C, Coutris C, et al: Bone marrow transplantation in osteopetrosis. *Lancet* 2:1137, 1977.

Baron R, Gertner JM, Lang R, et al: Increased bone turnover with decreased bone formation by osteoblasts in children with osteogenesis imperfecta tarda. *Pediatr Res* 17:204, 1983.

Berwick DM: Scoliosis screening. *Pediatr Rev* 5:238, 1984.

Bordelon FL: Hypermobile flatfeet in children: Evaluation and treatment. *Clin Orthop* 181:7, 1983.

Boyer DW, Mickleson MR, Ponsetti IV: Slipped capital femoral epiphysis: Long-term follow-up study of 121 patients. *J Bone Joint Surg* 63:85, 1981.

Canale ST, Griffin DW, Hubbard CN: Congenital muscular torticollis. A long-term followup. *J Bone Joint Surg* 64:810, 1982.

Canalis E: Hormonal and local regulation of bone formation. *Endocr Rev* 4:67, 1983.

Carson WG, Lovell WW, Whitesides TE Jr: Congenital elevation of the scapula. Surgical correction by the Woodward procedure. *J Bone Joint Surg* 63:1199, 1981.

Chung SMK: Diseases of the developing hip joint. *Pediatr Clin North Am* 33:1457, 1986.

Clark MW, D'Ambrosia RD, Ferguson AB: Congenital vertical talus treatment by open reduction and navicular excision. *J Bone Joint Surg* 59:816, 1977.

Cole DEC, Carpenter TO: Bone fragility, craniosynostosis, ocular proptosis, hydrocephalus, and distinctive facial features: A newly recognized type of osteogenesis imperfecta. *J Pediatr* 110:76, 1987.

Cowell HR, Elenon V: Rigid painful flatfoot secondary to tarsal coalition. *Clin Orthop* 177:54, 1983.

Dunn PM, Evans RE, Thearle MJ, et al: Congenital dislocation of the hip: early and late diagnosis and management compared. *Arch Dis Child* 60:407, 1985.

Emery AEH, Rimoin DL: The chondrodysplasias. In *Principles and Practice of Medical Genetics*. Vol. 2. New York, Churchill Livingstone, 1983.

Giedion A, Holthusen W, Masel LF, et al: Subacute and chronic "symmetrical" osteomyelitis. *Ann Radiol* (Paris) 15:329, 1972.

Gott VL, Pyeritz RE, Magovern GJ, et al: Surgical treatment of aneurysms of the ascending aorta in Marfan syndrome. *N Engl J Med* 314:1070, 1986.

Graf R: Diagnosis of congenital hip joint dislocation by ultrasonography. *J Pediatr Orthop* 3:354, 1983.

Griffin PP: Recurrent obstruction and subluxation of the patella. In Lovell WW, Winter RB (eds): *Pediatric Orthopedics*. Philadelphia, Lippincott, 1978, pp. 894-898.

Guhl J: Arthroscopic treatment of osteochondritis dissecans. *Clin Orthop* 167:65, 1982.

Hageman C, Willemse J: Arthrogryposis multiplex congenita. Review with comment. *Neuropediatrics* 14:6, 1983.

Hensinger RN: Limp. *Pediatr Clin North Am* 33:1355, 1986.

Kasser JR: In Case Records of the Massachusetts General Hospital. *N Engl J Med* 315:178, 1986.

Keim H: *The Adolescent Spine,* 2nd edition. New York, Springer Verlag, 1982.

Key L, Carnes D, Cole S, et al: Treatment of congenital osteoporosis with high-dose calcitriol. *N Engl J Med* 310:409, 1984.

King HA: Evaluating the child with back pain. *Pediatr Clin North Am* 33:1489, 1986.

Lenz W: Thalidomide and congenital abnormalities. *Lancet* 1:45, 1962.

Levine A, Drennan J: Physiologic bowing and tibia vara. *J Bone Joint Surg* 64:1158, 1982.

Marks MI: *Pediatric Infectious Diseases for the Practitioner.* New York, Springer Verlag, 1985.

McAnderson M, Weinstein S: A long-term follow-up of Legg-Calve-Perthes disease. *J Bone Joint Surg* 66:860, 1984.

McBride WG: Thalidomide and congenital abnormalities. *Lancet* 2:1358, 1961.

McKay DW: New concept of an approach to clubfoot treatment. I. Principles and morbid anatomy. *J Pediatr Orthop* 2:347, 1980.

McKay DW: New concept of an approach to clubfoot treatment. II. Correction. *J Pediatr Orthop* 3:10, 1983.

Menislaus MB: *The Orthopaedic Management of Spina Bifida Cystica,* 2nd edition. New York, Churchill Livingstone, 1980.

Micheli L: Sports injuries commonly incurred by amateurs. *J Musculoskel Med* 3:13, 1986.

Micheli L: Overuse injuries in children's sports: The growth factor *Orthop Clin North Am* 14:337, 1983.

Moe JH: Modern concepts of treatment of spinal deformities in children and adults. *Clin Orthop* 150:137, 1980.

Morrissy RT, Shore SL: Bone and joint sepsis. *Pediatr Clin North Am* 33:1551, 1986.

Mubaraic SJ, Carroll NC: Juvenile osteochondritis dissecans of the knee: Etiology. *Clin Orthop* 157:200, 1981.

Pauli RM, Scott C, Wassman ER, et al: Apnea and sudden unexpected death in infants with achondroplasia. *J Pediatr* 104:342, 1984.

Pope FM, Nicholls AC: Molecular abnormalities of collagen in human disease. *Arch Dis Child* 62:523, 1987.

Prockop DJ, Kivirikko KI: Heritable diseases of collagen. *N Engl J Med* 311:376, 1984.

Pyeritz RE: Propranolol retards aortic root dilatation in Marfan syndrome. *Circulation* 68(Suppl 3):111, 1983.

Ramsay PL, Lassor S, MacEwen GD: Congenital dislocation of the hip: Use of the Pavlik harness in the child during the first 6 months of life. *J Bone Joint Surg* 58:1000, 1976.

Renshaw TS: *Pediatric Orthopedics*. Philadelphia, WB Saunders, 1986.

Rimoin DL, Sillence DO: The skeletal dysplasias: Nomenclature, classification and clinical evaluation. In Akesson WH, Bornstein P, Glimcher M (eds): *Heritable Disorders of Connective Tissue.* St. Louis, CV Mosby, 27:324, 1982.

Rockwood, et al (eds): *Fractures in Children.* Vol. 3. Philadelphia, Lippincott, 1984.

Rogala EJ Drummond DS, Guir J: Scoliosis: Incidence and natural history, a prospective epidemiological study. *J Bone Joint Surg* 60:173, 1978.

Rowe CR, Pierce DS, Clark JG, et al: Voluntary dislocation of the shoulder. *J Bone Joint Surg* 55:445, 1973.

Salenius P, Wankka J: The development of the tibiofemoral angle in children. *J Bone Joint Surg* 57:253, 1975.

Scaglietti O, Marchetti PG, Bartolozzi P, et al: Final results in the treatment of bone cysts with methylprednisolone acetate (depomedrol). *Clin Orthop* 165:33, 1982.

Shapiro F: Epiphyseal disorders. *N Engl J Med* 317:1702, 1987.

Sillence DO, Barlow KK, Garber AP, et al: Osteogenesis imperfecta type II. Delineation of the phenotype with reference to genetic heterogeneity. *Am J Med Genet* 17:407, 1984.

Sisk HE, Zahkak G, Pyeritz RE: The Marfan syndrome in early childhood: Analysis of 15 patients diagnosed at less than 4 years of age. *Am J Cardiol* 52:353, 1983.

Smith R, Francis MJO, Houghton OR: *The Brittle Bone Syndrome: Osteogenesis Imperfecta.* London, Butterworths, 1983, pp. 1–218.

Smith JB: Knee problems in children. *Pediatr Clin North Am* 33:1439, 1986.

Staheli L: Corrective shoes for children: A survey of current practice. *Pediatrics* 65:13, 1980.

Staheli L: Torsional deformity. *Pediatr Clin North Am* 33:1373, 1986.

Stulberg SD, Cooperman DR, Wallensten R: The natural history of Legg-Perthes Disease. *J Bone Joint Surg* 63:1095, 1981.

Sykes B, Wordsworth P, Ogilvie D, et al: Osteogenesis imperfecta is linked to both type I collagen structural genes. *Lancet* 2:69, 1986.

Taussig HB: A study of the German outbreak of phocomelia. *JAMA* 180:1106, 1962.

Turco VJ: *Clubfoot.* New York, Churchill Livingstone, 1981.

Volpe JJ: *Neurology of the Newborn.* Philadelphia, WB Saunders, 1981, p 9.

Weinstein SV: Slipped capital femoral epiphysis. *AAOS Instr Courses Lectures* 33:310, 1984. St Louis, CV Mosby, 1984.

Weinstein UN: Idiopathic scoliosis. Long-term follow-up and prognosis in untreated patients. *J Bone Joint Surg* 63:702, 1981.

Wenger DR, Leach J: Foot deformities in infants and children. *Pediatr Clin North Am* 33:1411, 1986.

Wenger D, Mauldin D, Speck G, et al: The effect of corrective shoes and inserts on flexible flat foot: A prospective randomized trial. Presented at the Pediatric Orthopaedic Society of North America, Boston, May 1986.

Winter RB: *Congenital Deformities of the Spine.* New York, Thieme-Stratton, 1983.

Wynne-Davies R: Familial (idiopathic) scoliosis. A family survey. *J Bone Joint Surg* 50-B:24, 1968.

Wynne-Davies R, Williams PF, O'Connor JCB: The 1960 epidemic of arthrogryposis multiplex congenita. *J Bone Joint Surg* 63B:76, 1981.

Zarins B, Adams M: Knee injuries in sports. *N Engl J Med* 318:950, 1988.

Zieger M: Ultrasound of the infant hip. *Pediatr Radiol* 16:483, 1986.

MICHAEL MILLIS
MARY ELLEN AVERY
LEWIS R. FIRST

Consultants
Frank Rand and Kenneth R. First

Section 24

Childhood Injuries

Introduction

1

Injuries are the most common and serious threat to a child's health, surpassing cancer, congenital defects, and all the infectious diseases in morbidity and mortality. Each year more than 22,000 children in the United States die from injury-related causes, making trauma the leading cause of death outside the neonatal period. Indeed, 20% of all children will sustain at least one injury requiring medical attention each year and 17% of all pediatric hospitalizations are injury-related. These childhood injuries exact an extraordinary price from society not only in direct health care utilization costs, inconvenience, and time lost from work or school, but also in terms of human suffering, disability, and loss of future productivity.

This section is intended to provide only brief overviews of some of the more common pediatric injuries. Because of space limitations, some important causes of childhood injuries, such as motor vehicles and guns, are not discussed specifically. The reader is referred to emergency medicine and surgical texts for further details of the principles of emergency and long-term management of these and other types of injury.

Definition

The study of both "injury" and injury "severity" has been hampered by imprecise definition and misclassification. While the nosology of specific injuries has improved, the lack of detail about the circumstances surrounding the injury often makes it difficult retrospectively to reconstruct what happened and assign causation. The International Classification of Disease (ICD, 9th ed., revised 1981) provides a standard classification for the major types of childhood injuries. Even within this comprehensive attempt at identifying injuries, there is a lack of consensus as to what constitutes a traumatic event. For example, while some might consider "food poisoning" a toxic ingestion and, therefore, an injury, most clinicians classify it as an infectious disease caused, for example, by Salmonella or Clostridia.

The term "accident" has fallen into disfavor since it connotes an "act of God" responsibility for an event over which we have no control. Whereas an accident cannot be prevented, an injury often can. Haddon defines an injury as:

> "an energy (e.g., chemical, mechanical, thermal, electrical, etc) transfer from a hazardous agent to a susceptible host in a conducive environment (physical and social) such that the host sustains physical damage."

Injuries can be classified according to many different dimensions depending on this interaction of *agent, host,* and *environment* dynamically over time. One categorization of injury uses circumstance (i.e., motor vehicle injuries, falls, occupational injuries, housefires, etc) or physical seriousness (e.g., injuries with residua, injuries requiring hospitalization vs. trivial injuries or "near-misses"). Another classification invokes intentionality. Intentional injuries result from interpersonal or self-inflicted violence and include homicides, assaults, suicide, child abuse, and sexual abuse or rape. Unintentional injuries include those from natural or manmade disasters and encompass motor vehicle injuries, fires, poisonings, etc. Clearly in pediatrics there is considerable overlap and uncertainty in such definitions and a spectrum of intentionality in the production of an injury.

Epidemiology

The number of children injured in the United States each year is staggering. In 1978, 839,000 children were injured by home structural products; 625,000 were injured by furniture and fixtures; 147,000 were injured by falling down stairs; 28,000 suffered lacerations from broken windows; 55,000 were injured by sharp coffee tables; and 20,000 were injured in bathtubs and showers (Rivara, 1982). In 1985, poison control centers nationwide handled over 1,400,000 poisoning-related calls, the majority of which concerned children (CDC, 1985). One of 12 children under the age of 6 years will require hospital treatment for a fall; and 1 of 50 teenagers is injured annually as a motor vehicle occupant (Guyer and Gallagher, 1985). Death rates are shown in Table 24.1.

Injuries occurring to populations in aggregate are nonrandomly assorted. For many injury types, the child's developmental and chronologic age influence the degree of high or low risk. For infants and small children, caretaker supervision and anticipation of dangerous situations are of paramount importance in the prevention of an injury; whereas for the older child, knowledge of safety and injury avoidance assumes greater importance. The preschooler suffers 2 times as many falls, 4 times as many burns, 7 times as many foreign body choking episodes, and 10 times as many poisonings than do older children and adolescents (Guyer and Gallagher, 1985). Sports and bicycle injuries are much more common among adolescents than among younger children.

INJURY CONTROL AND PREVENTION

While it is arguable whether or not every minor incident producing an injury to a child can be prevented, most clinicians agree much childhood trauma

Table 24.1
Injury Deaths, United States, 1980[1]

Injury Type	Less than 1 year old	1–4	5–14	15–19	Total
Motor Vehicle					
Occupant	218	493	1122	7246	9079
Pedestrian	13	435	1005	757	2210
Motorcycle	1	8	120	788	917
Pedal Cycle	0	16	387	159	562
Other	20	264	285	480	1049
Total	252	1216	2919	9430	13817
Bicycle	0	4	25	10	39
Burn	177	735	535	348	1795
Drowning	91	693	795	1012	2591
Choking/Suffocation	439	214	205	131	989
Foreign Body	1	4	2	2	9
Poison	22	83	52	293	450
Falls	44	111	89	209	453
Other	140	253	602	824	1819
Total	1166	3313	5224	12,259	21,962

[1]Source: National Center for Health Statistics.

is preventable. If the circumstances surrounding the interaction of the *host, hazardous agent,* and *conducive environment* components do not reach the necessary threshold of hazard, either the injury will not occur or the child may escape a "near miss" situation and not be harmed. Such instances happen every day and may, in fact, be important in helping children learn how to ensure their own safety by avoiding such hazards in the future.

Haddon and Baker (1981) have introduced the concept of prevention of injuries as an intervention during the pre-event, event, or postevent phase of injury production that modifies the interaction of the three factors (agent, host, environment) involved in time and space so that the threshold to injury is never reached. The reader is offered examples of such prevention strategies during the categorical discussion of the prevention of specific injury types in the chapters to follow.

REFERENCES

Baker SP, O'Neill B, Karpf RS: *The Injury Fact Book.* Lexington MA, Lexington Books, 1984.

CDC Update: Childhood poisonings—United States. *MMWR* 34:117, 1985.

Guyer B, Gallagher S: An approach to the epidemiology of childhood injuries. *Pediatr Clin North Am* 32:5, 1985.

Haddon W Jr, Baker SP: Injury Control. In Clark D, MacMahon B (eds): *Preventive and Community Medicine.* Boston, Little Brown & Co., 1981.

Margolis L, Kotch J, Lacey J. Children in alcohol-related motor vehicle crashes. *Pediatrics* 77:870, 1986.

Rivara F: Preventing childhood injuries. *12th Ross Roundtable Report,* 13, 1982.

Children with Repeated Injuries

2

Definition

No single definition of an injury-repeating or "accident-prone" child has been accepted. Some clinicians consider a child with two or more injuries requiring medical attention within a 12-month interval to be an injury repeater.

Epidemiology

For most types of injuries males outnumber females across all age ranges and socioeconomic groups. Injuries are also sorted by age and developmental considerations. For example, the peak age range for childhood poisoning occurs at 18–36 months, whereas for bicycle injuries it is at 5–8 years old. Risk-taking behavior seems to characterize special groups. For example, both the injury rate and the hospitalization rate for injuries among juvenile delinquents in detention are much higher than are those of their noninstitutionalized peers (Woolf and Funk, 1985).

Although the prevalence of recurrent injury episodes in children is unknown, we recently reviewed the records of 317 children under 36 months old followed in a hospital-based well child clinic who had sustained one injury and found 60 of them (19%) had a record of previous trauma requiring medical attention.

Natural History

Families of injury repeaters may be more disorganized and socially isolated than are others. They are often under considerable daily stress and the injuries occur around peak periods of distraction when supervision of the children may be minimal. Often the physical environment where these children play is unsafe. Injury repeaters have been characterized behaviorally as hyperactive, aggressive, and risk-taking. Sobel and Margolis (1965) could find no increased numbers of hazards in the homes of poison repeaters versus controls but did observe such children to be more active and negativistic. They suggest such children are engaged in a power struggle with their parents and that such ingesting behavior represents a bid for attention (Sobel and Margolis, 1965).

CASE ILLUSTRATION

A.C. was born to a 34-year-old married Cape Verdian woman with three other children at home. Both parents worked and the children were cared for by an elderly grandmother. During his first year, A.C. received regular well child care and all his immunizations. However, during his second year the child's mother returned to work full-time and only one well child visit was recorded. At 16 months of age, A.C. was seen in the emergency clinic for ingestion of baby powder. At 27 months of age, he was again seen for a question of a foreign body in his finger. Three months later, he was seen in the clinic having sustained a fracture of the radius and ulna subsequent to a fall down a flight of stairs. Four months later, he tripped while running away from a falling ladder outside his home and suffered a fractured left tibia, a scalp hematoma, a small parieto-occipital skull fracture, and a small epidural hematoma. The child was hospitalized for observation and a child abuse report was filed. State social workers could not substantiate the report since there was no evidence of abuse or neglect at the home and, in their view, the child merely had a series of unfortunate "accidents." The mother independently rearranged her work schedule to provide more supervision for A.C. and also was considering daycare as an option.

QUESTIONS AND COMMENTS

Why were social services personnel not involved with this family sooner?

Hospital staff considered each injury to this child as an isolated accident, out of the context of family or social considerations. Treated as a "snapshot" instead of as part of a "movie" of a child's interaction with his environment, such incidents represent opportunities to intervene which are lost. Also many social services agencies lack the personnel and expertise to address the needs of families with children who are nonintentional injury repeaters. Priority for their resources is necessarily given to those families where there is a clear-cut history of intentional abuse.

How could this child's injuries have been prevented?

The physician who sees injured children should be alert to the circumstances surrounding the injury and also to the child's previous history of trauma. Families of preschool injury repeaters often need intense counseling about childproofing the home, reporting safety violations to a landlord or public health authorities, arranging for appropriate supervision for the child, and understanding better the child's developmental stage, his motor capabilities and curiosity, and his behavioral style.

Treatment and Prevention

Parents should be counseled routinely by health care providers about safety provisions in the home. The Injury Prevention Program (TIPP) is one such format developed by the American Academy of Pediatrics. Families with toddlers should be forewarned about the child's developmental capabilities and the necessity for adequate supervision. Parents of injury-repeating children may require special counseling on parenting skills and a safety inspection of the house; other social and psychologic support needs should be explored.

REFERENCES

American Academy of Pediatrics: *The Injury Prevention Program.* Elk Grove Village, Illinois, 1983.

Jones J: The child accident repeater. *Clin Pediatr* 19:284, 1980.

Meyer R, Roelofs H, Bluestone J, et al: Accidental injury to the preschool child. *J Pediatr* 63:95, 1963.

Sobel R, Margolis J: Repetitive poisoning in children: A psychosocial study. *Pediatrics* 35:641, 1965.

Woolf A, Funk S: Epidemiology of trauma in a population of incarcerated youth. *Pediatrics* 75:463, 1985.

Child Abuse 3

Definition

By child abuse, we mean any form of physical maltreatment of children. By the term "neglect" we mean also some of the aspects of emotional deprivation that can have physical consequences.

Epidemiology

Because of these imprecise definitions, the true prevalence of child abuse has been difficult to ascertain. With the passage of state laws that mandate reporting of suspicious injuries or neglectful situations, a more accurate estimate of prevalence has been possible. Whereas in 1969 a national study by Gil revealed 6000 reported cases, by 1978 it was estimated that more than 600,000 reports were filed annually.

Diagnosis

The differential diagnosis of child abuse is exceedingly important. Other causes of dermatologic lesions or an increased susceptibility to injury, such as bleeding diatheses, osteogenesis imperfecta, systemic lupus erythematosus, Ehlers-Danlos syndrome, or underlying neoplasm, have been confused with child abuse.

A strong suspicion of abuse and neglect is always needed in the initial evaluation of a child's failure to thrive or injuries; however, a cautious approach is advised since hasty conclusions can also be damaging to the child.

It is well to keep in mind some of the recognized risk factors for abuse. Family stressors have been strongly associated with physical and emotional abuse of the child. Some of these originate in the child as in the temperamentally difficult or mentally retarded or autistic child. Some are social situational stressors that relate to parental discord, poverty, social isolation, unemployment, alcoholism, and adverse parent/child relationships such as in a punitive style of child rearing. Low birth weight infants appear to be at increased risk for abuse, which may be related to the failure to develop appropriate maternal-infant bonding in the nursery setting. Parent-originating stressors follow from low self-esteem, a history of abuse when the parent was a child, depression, substance abuse, or ignorance of correct child-rearing methods. The maltreatment may occur only once, but is more likely to be repetitive.

Objectives in the Initial Family Interview

Newberger suggests the initial interview with the family in which child abuse or neglect is suspected should have the following five objectives:

1. Understand the historical and medical antecedents of the injury and assess the plausibility of the report.
2. Determine the dimensions of the risk to the child so as to decide whether immediate separation is necessary.

3. Gather the past medical history of the child and the family.
4. Form a relationship with the family that will be supportive and encourage their participation in subsequent diagnostic and therapeutic work with social workers, psychologists, and others.
5. File a case report and explain to other protective services the means taken to protect the child.

Treatment

Child abuse and neglect are medical conditions of complex determinants requiring a multidisciplinary approach to management. The physician should retain the role as gatekeeper for diagnostic assessment and management plans. He should serve as the medical liaison and advocate to the family in accordance with the best interests of the child and coordinate a team of specialists, who may include social workers, psychologists, psychiatrists, therapists, lawyers, and others, in planning short- and long-term future management objectives. Training in advocacy should also include a familiarity with the state child abuse reporting laws as well as the correct approach to the gathering of information that may be crucial to future case disposition. Familiarity with the role of an expert witness in court proceedings is also part of such advocacy.

SEXUAL ABUSE

An increasing awareness of the extent of sexual abuse of small children has been a startling development in the United States in recent years. Episodes of sexual abuse in daycare centers have been highly publicized and shocking to most pediatricians. Such incidents have undermined parental confidence in trusting the care of their children to others.

Here also, precise definitions are difficult. Sometimes the child might be exposed to sexual stimulation inappropriate for the occasion or for the child's role in the family, or inadvertent overstepping of the boundaries of a loving caress may "shade" into sexual abuse. Forced genital contact or even rape occurs with children with an unknown incidence. When sexual abuse is inflicted by a parent or sibling it is defined as incest. By far the most frequent relationship is father-daughter. The generally accepted definitions of rape and sexual abuse are:

Rape. Rape includes coitus, sodomy, and/or unnatural sexual acts without consent.

Sexual Misuse. This refers to sexual activity or the stimulation of a child which is inappropriate because of the child's immature age, level of psychosexual development, or role within the family.

When sexual misuse or abuse is suspected, the clinician must mobilize a multidisciplinary team of nursing, social services, and psychiatric specialists. Some members of the team should be summoned urgently if the family appears to be having an acute emotional crisis, if the child is bleeding or complaining of pain, or if the child is actively hiding from an assailant.

A history from a parent or other reliable informant should be gathered. Details of past assaults, the circumstances of the present episode, whether or not there was penetration, symptoms (e.g., dysuria, vaginal discharge, bleeding, pain, nightmares, enuresis, etc) and,

CASE ILLUSTRATION

A 22-month-old white male infant was referred to the emergency clinics by his pediatrician for blood work. He was entirely well until 3 days before presentation when he reportedly awakened from his nap with a bump on the left forehead. Skull films taken at the local hospital were normal. Over the next several days the bruise became purple and he also developed ecchymoses around the eyes. The mother also reported bruising of his left great toe and over his back. She also felt the child had been increasingly "clumsy" over the past several days. There was no history of viral prodrome, trauma, seizures, nausea or vomiting, or lethargy. There was no family history of a bleeding diathesis; however, the mother did feel perhaps this child bruised easily, even during infancy.

On physical examination the child was playful, with normal vital signs. A prominent 2-cm mass on the forehead was bluish-purple. Ecchymoses were present along the inner canthus of both eyes. The rest of the skin examination was remarkable for scattered ecchymoses on the lower extremities. There were no petechiae or purpura. The neurologic examination was normal. The CBC was normal with a Hct = 40.5%; WBC = 15,200/mm^3; platelets = 306,000/mm^3. Prothrombin time, fibrinogen levels, factor VIII and factor IX levels were normal. The urinalysis was normal. The child was suspected to have an inherited bleeding disorder or an occult tumor, and further studies were scheduled. When the family failed to keep a clinic follow-up appointment, they were referred to social services. At that time, the father admitted to the physical abuse of the child, and no further hematologic investigation was thought necessary.

QUESTION AND COMMENT

How could child abuse have been diagnosed earlier in this case?

The diagnosis of child abuse is an emotional and distressing one for physicians and families alike. The most common manifestation of abuse is a skin lesion (e.g., bruise, burn, scrape, laceration). In this case the absence of an alternative adequate explanation for the child's bruises, even after an extensive work-up for a bleeding disorder, should have suggested careful re-evaluation of the social situation. More often than not child abuse is a subtle diagnosis, requiring the diagnostic acumen of a perceptive and rigorous clinician.

for adolescent women, a menstruation and contraception history are important. A careful, sensitive interview should be conducted with the child alone, with use of the easiest methods of communication, such as doll-play, crayons and paper, pictures, or toys.

The physician should carefully document the history and physical findings in the medical record. All specimens and washings become evidence and should be carefully sealed and stored in a safe place in case they are needed in future court proceedings. State social services should be immediately notified by telephone and a written report filed with them in a timely fashion. The physician, in conjunction with the child abuse team, must determine whether or not the child is at further risk and should be hospitalized or placed in temporary foster care. Finally a plan for follow-up social services, psychiatric, and medical care should be formulated.

REFERENCES

Bittner S, Newberger E: Pediatric understanding of child abuse and neglect. *Pediatr Rev* 2:197, 1981.

Gil D: Unraveling child abuse. *Am J Orthopsychiatry* 45:346, 1975.

Johnson C, Showers J: Injury variables in child abuse. *Child Abuse Neglect* 9:207, 1985.

Kempe C: Sexual abuse; the 1977 C. Anderson Aldrich Lecture. *Pediatrics* 62:382, 1978.

Taylor L, Newberger E: Child abuse in the international year of the child. *N Engl J Med* 301:1205, 1979.

Pediatric Resuscitation Techniques 4

MANAGEMENT OF THE SEVERELY INJURED CHILD

The immediate management of the severely injured patient should include cardiopulmonary resuscitation (CPR), when necessary, with immediate administration of oxygen and continuous reassessment of his cardiorespiratory status. The victim should have his temperature monitored and then be kept warm to avoid more vasoconstriction, acidosis, and shock. A nasogastric tube should be inserted to empty the stomach and thereby avoid vomiting, aspiration, or gastric distention from air-swallowing. Intubation and ventilatory assistance (as detailed below in advanced cardiac life support) may be necessary to forestall respiratory failure. Insertion of a catheter into venous circulation secures access for fluid and drug administration. Arterial blood gases should be assessed and acid-base disturbances corrected when necessary. Arterial catheterization may be necessary for continuous monitoring of blood gases and cardiac function. Catheterization of the urinary tract facilitates collection of a urine sample for analysis and also allows accurate monitoring of urinary output. Fluid input and output should be monitored as well as shifts in electrolytes and other metabolites. The patient's blood should be typed and cross-matched should transfusions be necessary. The patient should be stabilized and then transported to a regional trauma center staffed with personnel expert in the management of the complex medical problems of the pediatric patient who is severely injured.

Although the principles of CPR in children are generally the same as those for the adult, certain unique considerations pertain. The guidelines for pediatric CPR as per the American Heart Association were announced in 1986 for implementation in 1987. (The reader is referred to Section 4, Neonatology for information on resuscitation of the newborn.) The principles of CPR of a child can be divided into basic life support (BLS) skills, suitable for the lay person, and advanced cardiac life support (ACLS) skills for the health professional.

Basic Life Support

Basic life support (BLS) is directed at (1) the prevention of respiratory and cardiac arrest through prompt diagnosis and management and (2) the treatment of cardiopulmonary arrest where there is no specialized equipment or medications Table 24.2.

The physician first assesses the patient's state of consciousness by gently shaking him or calling his name. The patient should not be moved unless he is in imminent danger of further injury; he is positioned supine on a hard surface if resuscitation is contemplated. The admonition to keep the neck stable if head and neck injuries are suspected is repeated. The physician then sends a witness or fellow rescuer to call for help and

Table 24.2
Steps in Pediatric Resuscitation

1. Determine responsiveness
2. Call for help
3. Position the victim
4. Open the airway
5. Determine breathing
6. Breathe for the victim
7. Assess circulation
8. Perform chest compressions
9. Coordinate compressions/breathing

activate the Emergency Medical Services (EMS) system. Inability to access an advanced life support team after 4 or 5 minutes of resuscitation will increase the risk of mortality and worsen neurologic morbidity from the hypoxic insult.

The physician then follows the "ABCs" of resuscitation:

1. Airway
2. Breathing
3. Circulation

The airway is opened by clearing the mouth of visible dirt, blood, broken teeth and debris and then lifting the chin and jaw forward placing two or three fingers at each angle of the jaw (jaw thrust). This removes the tongue from obstructing the airway. Hyperextension of the neck is not recommended since it may lead to compression of the child's soft tracheal cartilage. Therefore, the head is placed in a neutral or "sniffing" position.

The rescuer then inspects the chest for movement, listens for gasping, and feels for evidence of exhaled air from the victim's mouth. If he determines the patient is in respiratory arrest, the physician takes a deep breath, forms a seal with his mouth over the mouth of the victim (or, in the case of an infant, over both the nose and the mouth), and exhales hard enough to produce chest wall movement in the victim. Two good breaths are attempted.

If no chest wall movement is noted, then airway obstruction should be suspected. If the child is older than 1 year of age, abdominal thrusts upward from below the xyphoid process (the Heimlich maneuver) should be administered (see Chapter on Foreign Bodies). If the child is an infant (less than 1 year old) then back blows at the midscapular level followed by upward chest thrusts (pushing upward over the lower third of the sternum) should be tried to dislodge a foreign body and reopen the airway. If unsuccessful, the process should be repeated until help arrives or the airway is patent. There is no purpose doing chest compressions if oxygen cannot be delivered to the blood.

If there is chest wall movement, the rescuer feels for the victim's carotid, brachial, or femoral pulse. If the patient is in cardiac arrest, the rescurer places one hand two finger-breadths above the xiphoid notch with the heel of the palm resting on the sternum. In an infant, the index and middle finger are placed over the sternum one finger breadth below the nipple line. The physician compresses the sternum to a depth where the pulsations can be felt by palpating the femoral artery. Compression/relaxation phases should be approximately of equal duration such that 80–100 beats/minute are delivered in an adult, 100 in a child, and at least 120 in an infant.

Chest compressions should never be attempted in the absence of rescue breathing. In children with one rescuer, the manuevers should be synchronized at a rate of five compressions for each breath; in adults, the ratio is 15 compressions to two breaths. If two rescuers are present, the ratio is 5:1 regardless of age. The chest compresser should pause after five compressions to allow a good breath to be given and then cycle again. At the end of each minute or so, the chest compressions/rescue breathing cycle should be interrupted to assess the patient for evidence of success at restoring endogenous cardiopulmonary function. Once the decision to start CPR is made, it should be continued until the patient is successfully breathing on his own or until expert help arrives for the implementation of ACLS.

The decision to stop CPR is a difficult one in the best of circumstances; patients with seeming irreversible and overwhelming injuries have gone on to make remarkable recoveries. It is almost impossible to judge the potential for recovery in many types of injury (for example, coma from drug overdoses, submersion injuries, smoke inhalation, and hypothermic trauma). Unless the physician can judge with confidence that all hope for recovery is lost, the patient must be presumed salvageable and CPR continued until a more careful assessment can be carried out in the controlled circumstances of a hospital's emergency room or intensive care center.

Advanced Cardiac Life Support

Advanced Cardiac Life Support (ACLS) consists of BLS and adjunctive therapies related to: (1) respiratory support, (2) cardiac stabilization, (3) fluids infusion and monitoring, and (4) postresuscitation support. One physician knowledgeable in ACLS is designated as the leader of the team. He directs the progress of the resuscitative effort making judgments about the timing and choice of drugs, fluids, and other therapeutic modalities. Another member of the team records the time and details of all therapies administered to the patient. Other team members may be assigned to the stabilization of the airway, acquisition of access to the circulatory system, blood drawing, etc. The team must operate with a concerted and efficient effort; onlookers and other personnel without ACLS assignments must be excluded from the scene of resuscitation to minimize confusion.

Respiratory Support

Rescue breathing is replaced with oxygen administration by a bag and tight-fitting circular mask. If there is no spontaneous respiratory effort and the chest does not move with mask ventilation, or if there is a need to protect the airway from aspiration, the patient should be intubated. Endotracheal intubation is performed with an uncuffed tube in children less than 8 years old. The premature infant will take a 2.5 mm endotracheal tube (ET) whereas the full-term newborn ET tube size is usually 3.5–4.0 mm. The size of the ET tube (in millimeters internal diameter) in the older child can be calculated by the equation:

$$ET = \frac{16 + \text{age (in years)}}{4}$$

The child's head is slightly extended and the neck is flexed during laryngoscopy for proper visualization of the vocal cords. The physician must remember the child's trachea is relatively short (5–7 cm); the tendency to intubate too far can result in perforation or unilateral bronchus intubation with the danger of pneumothorax. Bilateral breath sounds should be auscultated before the ET tube is secured and a chest radiograph should be obtained to ensure proper placement.

Cardiac Stabilization

The common pediatric resuscitation drugs are shown in Table 24.3.

Epinephrine is an adrenergic agent with a pronounced vasoconstrictive effect which promotes blood flow to and oxygenation of the heart. In addition, epinephrine has inotropic properties increasing the heartbeat strength and improving cardiac output. It may be given every 5–10 minutes as necessary during resuscitative efforts.

Atropine is a vagolytic agent which accelerates the heartbeat and facilitates atrioventricular conduction. It can be useful in situations of vagally mediated bradycardia, bradycardia with AV block, or ventricular asystole.

Large volumes of bicarbonate and/or dextrose-containing solutions can cause osmotic imbalances at the blood-brain interface resulting in brain damage and poor neurologic outcomes. Thus, both should be used judiciously and only with supporting metabolic data in pediatric resuscitations.

Catecholamines, such as dopamine and dobutamine, are important adjuncts used to support the blood pressure and circulation in hypotensive situations where there is poor perfusion. Conversely, nitroprusside is used emergently to treat malignant hypertensive crises.

Isoproterenol is a pure β-adrenergic agonist which has both chronotropic and inotropic cardiac effects and can be used in bradycardia syndromes. However, intravenous drips of epinephrine have similar actions on the heart and peripheral perfusion without isoproterenol's adverse effect of peripheral vasodilation.

Defibrillation employs an electric current across the heart to effect simultaneous depolarization of myocardial cells such that a new, synchronous rhythm can be established. Typically, the pediatric cardioversion dose is 2–6 joules (watt-seconds)/kg for ventricular fibrillation and 0.5–2.0 joules/kg for ventricular tachycardia.

Cardioversion dosages for atrial arrhthymias are started at about 20 joules and raised incrementally should further cardioversion attempts be necessary.

Lidocaine is the first line drug for the management of most pediatric arrhythmias commonly manifested during resuscitative efforts. It is used for ventricular ectopy, ventricular tachycardia, and ventricular fibrillation. Its use as a bolus must be followed up by the administration of a continuous intravenous drip in order to achieve stability of normal sinus rhythm.

Bretyllium has complex actions which can convert ventricular fibrillation to a sinus rhythm or render the heart engaged in refractory ventricular fibrillation more susceptible to defibrillation. It is useful when lidocaine and defibrillation fail.

Fluid Infusion and Monitoring

Table 24.4 presents fluid doses appropriate for use in pediatric resuscitations.

Administration of both colloid and crystalloid solutions is the mainstay of resuscitative efforts to improve perfusion and treat shock. Saline solutions or Ringers lactate should be employed until the patient's fluid reqirements can be more completely evaluated. The general rule of replacing what the patient has lost should be followed; fluid and electrolytes should be monitored both during and after the resuscitation event.

Table 24.3
Drugs Used In Resuscitation[1]

Drug	Dose	Preparation	Route[2]	Indication
Atropine	0.03 mg/kg	0.4 mg/cc	IV/IC/IM/ETT	Bradycardia
Bicarbonate	1–2 mEq/kg	1 mEq/cc	IV/IC	Metabolic acidosis
Calcium	10 mg/kg	CaCl:27 mg/cc CaGluc:9 mg/cc	IV/IC	Increase vasomotor tone for positive inotropy
Dextrose	8 mg/kg/minute	10% in water	IV	Hypoglycemia
Dopamine	2–20 μg/kg/minute	40 mg/cc	IV	Hypotension
Epinephrine	0.1 cc/kg	1:10,000	IV/IC/ETT	Asystole, bradycardia, hypotension
Isoproterenol	0.17 μg/kg/minute	0.2 mg/cc	IV	Hypotension
Lidocaine	1 mg/kg	100 mg/10 cc	IV/IC/ETT	Ventricular arrhythmias
Naloxone	0.01 mg/kg	0.4 mg/cc	IV	Opiate intoxication

[1]The Committee on Drugs of the American Academy of Pediatrics guideline for emergency drug dose appeared in *Pediatrics* 81:462, 1988. The recommendations in Table 24.3 (above) differ slightly from the Academy recommendations.
[2]Abbreviations: IV = intravenous; IC = intracardiac; IM = intramuscular; ETT = via endotracheal tube.

Table 24.4
Fluids Used In Pediatric Resuscitation

Maintenance fluids:	4 cc/kg/hr (first 10 kg) 2 cc/kg/hr (next 10 kg) 1 cc/kg/hr (each kg thereafter)
Hypovolemic shock:	10–20 cc/kg bolus isotonic solution
Maintenance electrolytes:	Na^+ = 2–5 mEq/kg/day K^+ = 2–3 mEq/kg/day

Postresuscitation Care

Despite its most valiant efforts, CPR is not the ultimate solution to preventing childhood morbidity and mortality. A recent follow-up study of 30 patients who required CPR on arrival to a pediatric emergency room resulted in eight survivors, all of them neurologically devastated (O'Rourke, 1986). Thus, efforts to prevent childhood injuries and promote childhood safety inside and outside the home continue to be the mainstay responsible for saving the most lives.

REFERENCES

1985 Conference on Cardiopulmonary Resuscitation (CPR) and Emergency Cardiac Care (ECC). Standards and guidelines for cardiopulmonary resuscitation (CPR) and emergency cardiac care (ECC). *JAMA* 255:2905, 1986.

Committee on Traumas, American College of Surgeons. Advanced Trauma Life Support Course. Instructor's Manual. 1984.

O'Rourke PP: Outcome of children who are apneic and pulseless in the emergency room. *Crit Care Med* 14:466, 1986.

Drowning 5

Definition

Drowning can be defined as death from suffocation by immersion in water, with or without aspiration, within the first 24 hours of the immersion. Near-drowning requires survival for at least 24 hours.

Epidemiology

Submersion injuries are the third most common cause of nonintentional injury mortality in the United States, accounting for 6000 nonboat-related deaths, 1200 boat-related drownings, and 1000 suicides annually. Males outnumber females 12:1 for boat-related drownings and 5:1 for non-boat drownings.

The overall drowning death rate has a bimodal peak incidence greater for children under age 5 years and in adolescence; 33% of non-boat related drownings were among children under 5 years old. Most drowning deaths in young children occur when they fall into water in or near their own homes; each year about 250 children (1–4 years old) drown in bathtubs (Fig. 24.1).

The second peak of drownings in adolescence reflects the association of this injury with recreational watercraft and swimming and diving activities. Indeed 66% of drownings occur during May through August and 40% occur on the weekends; swimming pools, ponds, quarries, lakes, rivers, and reservoirs are the usual sites of such incidents. It is estimated that about one-third of drowning victims are adequate swimmers who overexert themselves by attempting to swim long distances or are involved in boating accidents where life-preservers were not available.

Natural History

The major effect of submersion is lack of oxygen. When immersed in water, the initial response is breath-holding; ultimately 10% of humans die during this period without actually aspirating fluid. In experimental situations, it can be demonstrated that, with occlusion of the airway, the rate of fall of arterial oxygen tension is about 50% after 1 minute but only 10% after 3 minutes (or about 10 mm Hg after 3 minutes and 4 mm Hg after 5 minutes of airway obstruction). The rate of rise of carbon dioxide, on the other hand, is only 6 mm Hg/minute and the fall in pH about 0.05 unit/minute.

If the drowning victim aspirates, obviously the effects on the lung depend on the nature of the aspirated material. Some of the changes in pulmonary function are clearly reflex inasmuch as very small amounts of water may significantly decrease lung compliance (Halmagyi and Colebatch, 1962). From various exper-

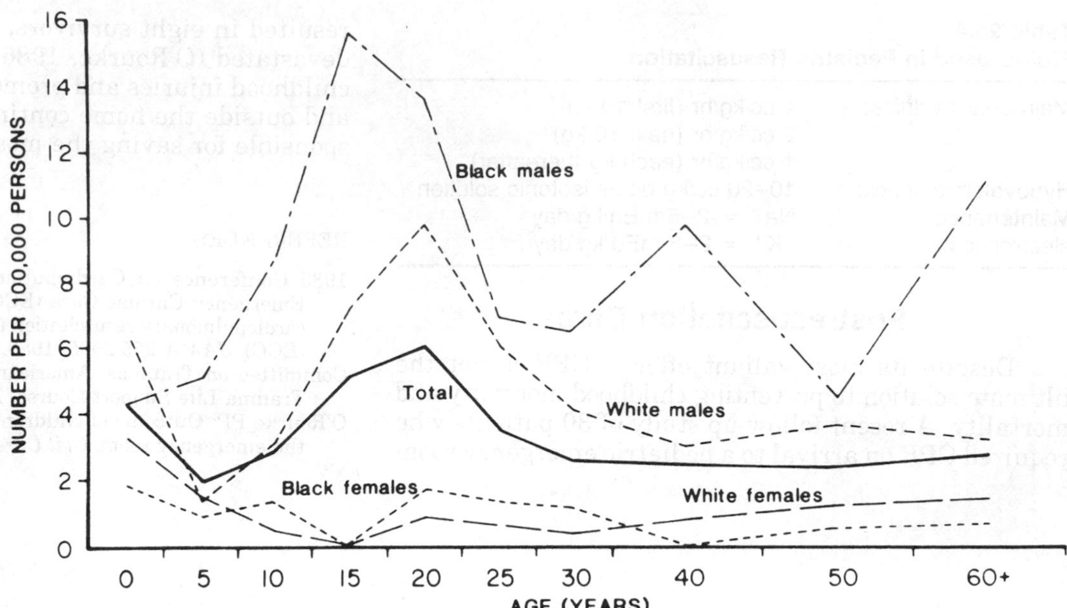

Figure 24.1 Drowning rates, by age, race, and sex in Georgia, 1981–1983. (CDC: *MMWR* 34:281, 1985).

imental studies, it appears that the aspiration of water initiates a parasympathetic reflex which, in turn, produces airway closure. The effects are only temporary, however, and it is assumed that with aspiration, water itself can pose a problem. For example, sea water is hypertonic so that lung volume may be further compromised by pulmonary edema and sometimes hemorrhage. When experimental animals aspirate fresh water, on the other hand, significant amounts of fluid are not found in the lungs, presumably because of rapid absorption of the hypoosmolar water. With significant aspiration of any kind of fluid the pulmonary surfactant may be altered so that the alveoli become unstable; the resulting atelectasis causes intrapulmonary shunting and severe hypoxemia.

Treatment

The aim of therapy is to overcome hypoxia as soon as possible. It is urgent to initiate resuscitation in order to overcome a rapidly falling oxygen tension. In most circumstances this can be achieved most effectively by mouth-to-mouth or mouth-to-nose ventilation. The resuscitator should first inspect the airway, remove any visible foreign objects from the mouth, and support the airway by elevating the jaw and soft tissues. There is little to be gained from trying to drain water from the lungs. If the patient does not have an effective heart beat, closed chest cardiac massage should be instituted once the airway has been established.

After initial resuscitative efforts, the patient may breathe spontaneously, but later show signs of deterioration. It is important to stay with the patient and make supplemental oxygen available as soon as possible. If the hypoxemia is persistent, even with ventilation, it may be necessary to intubate the patient so that continuous distending airway pressure can be applied to treat atelectasis and pulmonary edema. This can dramatically improve ventilation-to-perfusion ratios and greatly increase oxygenation at the same inspired oxygen tension. In some patients continuous distending airway pressure may be obtained by the use of a mask.

Most patients who have been hypoxic have a significant metabolic acidosis, but this can be corrected with maintenance fluid support. It is rare to have sufficient absorption of fresh water for hemolysis, but serial hematocrit determinations are appropriate if that seems to be a possibility. Serial determinations of arterial blood gases, electrocardiographic monitoring, and urinary output determinations are indicated in most patients who are brought to the hospital. Intra-arterial catheters facilitate frequent blood sampling. Only if metabolic acidosis supervenes would it be appropriate to administer sodium bicarbonate, and even then it should never be administered as a bolus because of the possibility of transient hypernatremia.

The patient with severe hypoxia is at considerable risk for cerebral edema. If the patient is on a ventilator, reduction of the P_{CO_2} to about 30 mm Hg and elevation of the head to a 30–45° angle, can lessen the severity of cerebral edema. Hypothermia has been advocated to decrease the requirement for cerebral oxygen but is useful only if the hypothermia effect occurs before hypoxia.

CONTROVERSY

Some physicians have advocated the use of steroids or prophylactic broad spectrum antibiotics to treat victims of near-drowning. Experimental studies with aspirated hydrochloric acid or significant amounts of fresh water have not shown any beneficial effects of steroids. Modell (1980) reported that a retrospective review of records of 121 near-drowning victims failed to demonstrate any beneficial effects of corticosteroids. He advocates culturing pulmonary flora daily and treating with antibiotics only if infection supervenes to avoid

CASE ILLUSTRATION

M.C. was a 5-year-old white child in good health until she fell into a fresh water river, was swept downstream and fell over a 10-foot dam onto ice which broke under her. She was pulled out after about 20 minutes of submersion and resuscitated. On arrival at the local emergency clinic, she was found to be cyanotic, pulseless, and apneic with fixed and dilated pupils, a temperature of 79.9°F, and a flat EEG. She was resuscitated with intracardiac epinephrine and cardioversion; and stabilized with an intravenous lidocaine drip, calcium, dopamine, sodium bicarbonate, decadron, and mannitol. Vigorous rewarming with nasogastric and peritoneal lavage succeeded in bringing the core temperature to 98.2°F. An initial arterial gas: pH = 6.78, Pco_2 = 166 mm Hg, Po_2 = 37 mm Hg was corrected to pH = 7.25, Pco_2 = 35 mm Hg, and Po_2 = 144 mm Hg by assisted ventilation with Fio_2 = 100%. Diffuse alveolar infiltrates consistent with adult respiratory distress syndrome were apparent bilaterally on chest radiograph; a head CT scan showed a small right occipitoparietal subgaleal hematoma. A subarachnoid bolt was placed to monitor intracranial pressure; increased pressure was treated with fluid restriction, furosemide, mannitol, hypothermia, steroids, hyperventilation, and a nembutal drip.

This patient was weaned from the ventilator 19 days after admission, although repeated aspiration episodes and the development of aspiration pneumonias forced placement of a tracheostomy to protect her airway from further aspiration. A gastrostomy was also placed to facilitate her nutrition. Her increased intracranial pressure resolved slowly over a 10-day period and her clinical neurologic examination improved only to the stage of showing random spontaneous movements with posturing and increased tone. Major motor seizures occurred 3 weeks after admission and were controlled with anticonvulsants; an EEG showed disorganization with low-amplitude delta waves predominating. The child was transferred to a chronic care facility for further convalescence.

QUESTION AND COMMENT

How would you manage her cerebral edema?

The patient with severe hypoxia is at increased risk for cerebral edema. If the patient is on a ventilator, reduction of the Pco_2 to about 30 mm Hg can lessen the severity of the cerebral edema. Moreover, an adequate cerebral perfusion pressure (mean arterial pressure minus intracranial pressure) must be maintained. This can be done with fluid resuscitation and diuretics if the mean systemic pressure is adequate. Hypothermia has been advocated to reduce cerebral oxygen requirements, as have pharmacologic doses of steroids, although few controlled studies are available to evaluate these interventions. There is no proof that barbiturates help in reducing the effects of cerebral edema in drowning injury.

the overgrowth of resistant organisms such as *Pseudomonas*.

Prognosis

Irrespective of their state at the scene of the accident, the outlook for normal survival of individuals who arrive at the hospital awake or drowsy is excellent if intensive pulmonary and cardiac care is available. Of patients who were comatose when they arrived in the emergency room, 73% of adults survived with apparently normal brain function, but the remaining died. In contrast, 44% of children survived with normal brain function, about 17% had incapacitating brain damage, and 39% died (Modell et al, 1980). If the patient arrives at the intensive care unit flaccid and unresponsive, the outlook is grim. In one series from Los Angeles, Allman et al (1986) reported that of 37 children in flaccid coma, 26 died and 11 survived in a vegetative state. Of 24 children in coma but with reflexes (Glasgow Coma Score >3), half survived intact, 25% survived in a vegetative state, and 25% died (Table 24.5).

Strategies for the prevention of childhood drowning include the teaching of the following water survival skills to all youngsters: knowing how to swim, taking proper precautions when diving, knowing the rules of boating safety, and knowing the use of essential safety equipment in the water. Parents should be warned to supervise bathtime for toddlers; and private and public swimming pools should be childproofed with locks and barriers.

Other preventive strategies include public advocacy for the drainage of abandoned quarries and for safety improvements for public areas that include bodies of water. Swimming pool construction, alcohol availability near recreational bodies of water, and the use of recreational watercraft could also be better regu-

Table 24.5
The Glasgow Coma Scale[1]

Eye Opening	Best Motor Response	Best Verbal Response
4 Spontaneously	6 Follows commands	5 Oriented
3 To voice	5 Localized painful stimulus	4 Confused
2 To pain	4 Complex arm movement	3 Inappropriate words
1 None	3 Reflex flexor posturing	2 Incomprehensible sounds
	2 Reflex extensor posturing	1 None
	1 Flaccid	

[1]From Teasdale G, Jennett B: *Lancet* 2:81, 1974.

lated. The responsiveness of emergency medical support systems for the retrieval and resuscitation of drowning victims could be improved. Finally, boats and other watercraft could be redesigned to function at lower speeds and improve their safety features.

REFERENCES

Allman FD, Nelson WB, Pacentine GA, et al: Outcome following cardiopulmonary resuscitation in severe pediatric near-drowning. *Am J Dis Child* 140:571, 1986.

Baker SP, O'Neill B, Karpf RS: *The Injury Fact Book.* Chapter 13. Lexington MA, Lexington Books, D.C. Heath Co, 1984.

CDC: Aquatic deaths and injuries—United States. *MMWR* 31:417, 1982.

CDC: Drownings—Georgia 1981–1983. *MMWR* 34:281, 1985.

Dietz PE, Baker SP: Drowning: Epidemiology and prevention. *Am J Public Health* 64:303, 1974.

Halmagyi DFJ, Colebatch HJH: Reflex airway reaction to fluid aspiration. *J Appl Physiol* 17:787, 1962.

Modell JH, Graves SA, Kuck EJ: Near drowning: Correlation of level of consciousness and survival. *Can Anesth Soc J* 27:211, 1980.

Modell JH: Drowning. In Staub NC, Taylor AE (eds): *Edema.* New York, Raven Press, 1984.

Nussbaum E: Prognostic variables in nearly drowned comatose children. *Am J Dis Child* 139:1058, 1985.

Spyker DA: Submersion injury. *Pediatr Clin North Am* 32:113, 1985.

Animal Bites

6

Definition

An animal bite of consequence takes place when the skin is broken, most commonly as a minor laceration or puncture wound. In this chapter, we will consider only those wounds produced by the dog, cat, and snakes.

Basic Science

About 5% of dog bites and 20–50% of cat bites become infected. This discrepancy is thought to be related to the tearing and crush injury caused by a dog, which is easily debrided and often open and superficial; whereas the cat bite is more like a puncture wound, driving a septic inoculum possibly several centimeters into deep, unaerated tissues.

A number of studies have documented the normal flora of the mouth and throat of dogs, with various species of *Streptococcus* predominating. Many other organisms, including Gram-negative aerobes are also identified including *Pasteurella multocida.* The carrier rate for that organism is estimated to be 50% for dogs and 67% for cats. Interestingly, this organism is more often implicated in infections after cat bites than after dog bites, perhaps related to the pathogenicity of the strains carried by each animal.

Streptococcus, coagulase-negative *Staphylococcus,* and *Staphylococcus aureus* are other common pathogens encountered in animal bites. DF2 Bacillus, which is part of the dog's normal flora and grows slowly in blood cultures, also can produce disease. The organism has produced symmetric peripheral purpura and a generalized Schwartzman reaction most commonly in asplenic patients, but in others as well (Barza, 1986). Other organisms, including *Bacteroides* and *Blastomyces dermatitidis,* have been implicated in case reports of dog bites.

Rabies virus, formerly the scourge of man and animals alike, has been virtually eradicated as a public health problem for domesticated animals with the institution of an aggressive active immunization program in the United States. Rabies is still encountered in nocturnal foxes, skunks, bats, raccoons, and wild dogs in the Southwestern parts of the United States (see pp. 1046).

Epidemiology

Animal bites are a worldwide problem of major dimensions, with an estimated 3½ million bites occurring each year in the United States. Children 5–14 years old are at greatest risk, accounting for almost 50% of this type of injury. Males are bitten more than twice as frequently as are females and 90% of bites are caused by dogs and 10% by cats. Contrary to popular belief, the dogs usually involved are owned by the family of the victim or by a neighbor; strays account for very few of the reported cases (Elliot et al, 1985).

Diagnosis

The diagnosis is usually obvious inasmuch as the victim complains of the wound. The signs of infection, however, usually become apparent 24–72 hours later. Particularly dangerous are puncture wounds that may heal superficially and encapsulate some virulent organisms. Redness, swelling, and tenderness may develop with extension through the subcutaneous space and by way of lymphatics. Occasionally, with deeper infections, fasciitis or osteomyelitis may appear but may not be clinically evident until several weeks or even months after the initial injury.

Treatment

With prompt cleansing of the wound, most bites can be closed primarily with tape or loose sutures to allow drainage if infection occurs. Nevertheless, many dog bites result in jagged irregular wounds with associated crush injury and devitalized tissue making primary closure contraindicated with the exception of a jagged facial bite for cosmetic reasons. Close monitoring and follow-up during healing is an important aspect of management. Tetanus prophylaxis should be given if the individual has not received a recent booster.

No single antibiotic can eradicate all of the possible pathogens that may be associated with a dog or cat bite. If the wound has not been previously cleaned, it is appropriate to culture the site. In most instances, the specific pathogen causing the infection is not identified and treatment with a bactericidal agent, directed against the more common aerobes and anaerobes (usually penicillin), is indicated. Alternately, amoxicillin with clavulinic acid has been recommended for broad spectrum treatment of animal bite injuries. If response to this empiric therapy is poor, definitive identification of a culture should be aggressively pursued.

CONTROVERSY

Controversy exists concerning the use of rabies vaccine or rabies immunoglobulin. The need for rabies prophylaxis depends on the likelihood of rabies being present in the environment where the bite took place as well as in the individual animal. Most domestic pets are safe. Zoonotic reservoirs of rabies include bats, skunks, and other wild animals which are responsible for a small proportion of the number of bites presenting to the pediatrician. In an area where no rabid animals have been known to exist for a number of years, it seems inappropriate for a pediatrician to consider rabies prophylaxis. Nevertheless, it is a prudent recommendation that the offending animal be quarantined and monitored for 21 days for signs of illness (see pp. 1047).

Prevention

Children should be educated with respect to appropriate behavior around family pets as well as strange animals. In most instances the child incites the animal to bite, rather than the other way around. All dogs and cats should be immunized every other year for rabies, beginning at 9–12 months of age. Also immunocompromised individuals, who are known to tolerate infections poorly, should receive antibiotic prophylaxis after an animal bite.

SNAKE BITES

Although snake bites are common, only about 1 in 5 are poisonous, and of the estimated 8000 bites from poisonous snakes that occur in the United States each year, fewer than 20 are fatal.

The major species of poisonous snakes in the United States are the *Crotilidae* (pit vipers), which include rattlesnakes, copperheads, and cottonmouths and the *Elapidae*, which include coral snakes. *Crotilidae* account for almost all venomous bites in the country; these snakes are characterized by a triangular-shaped

CASE ILLUSTRATION

AD is a 2½-year-old girl who was bitten on the face by a neighbor's dog. Physical examination revealed two larger lacerations approximately 3 cm in length extending vertically down the left forehead to include the left eyelid. The eye itself was spared. A separate horizontal bite, also about 3 cm long was present in the region of the left zygoma.

The child was admitted and received 2 days of intravenous penicillin and a total 7-day course of antibiotics. She continued to complain of left eye pain and nightmares 3 months after the event.

QUESTIONS AND COMMENTS

How should the facial bites be managed?

Due to the possibility of scarring, the wounds were cleansed and closed with 6–0 nylon sutures. The sutures used for this child were thin, 6–0 monofilament, which are less likely to heal with thick scarring. However, it is recommended that plastic surgery consultants be involved in such cases. Photographs may also be helpful in following the course of scarring. In some patients, reconstructive surgery may be necessary.

Can topical therapy help?

Use of a topical ointment containing povidone-iodine or bacitracin is acceptable adjunctive therapy. If the lesions are red or painful and oozing 2 or 3 days after suturing, it may be necessary to remove the sutures which can serve, in wick-like fashion, as a continuing conduit of infection to the deeper tissues.

What about this child's nightmares?

Such terrifying events may leave a child with fears and emotional "baggage" often overlooked in the concern over physical injury. Careful explanations and reassurance by parents are important to the healing process; a child's excessive fears may present clinically as phobias, night terrors, or regression in previously attained developmental milestones. Such signposts of distress may require short-term directed psychotherapy.

head, pits between the eyes and nostrils, retractible fangs, and, in the case of rattlers, the bony rattle at the end of the snake. Coral snakes have bright yellow, black, and red rings, a rounded snout, and small, rather ineffectual fangs.

Diagnosis

A history of a bite with evidence of scratches or a puncture wound on the skin is suggestive. Swelling is the most prominent and diagnostic physical finding and may progress within minutes to involve an entire extremity. Venoms also variably produce local pain or burning, ecchymoses, bullae, and skin necrosis. Systemic signs such as diaphoresis, oral paresthesias, muscle fasciculations, weakness, and shock may develop within minutes. Disseminated intravascular coagulation may supervene. Untreated volume depletion, hemolysis, and shock may lead to cardiac arrhythmias, renal failure, and death. Coral snake venoms specifically may produce little local pain but a rapidly progressive respiratory depression due to bulbar paralysis. This respiratory failure may progress to cardiovascular collapse and death.

Treatment

Local cleansing of the wound and checking on the child's immunization status is sufficient for harmless snake bites. If the bite is from a poisonous snake, immobilization of the affected body part and transport of the patient to a medical facility are of paramount importance. All patients with suspected envenomations should be hospitalized at least for observation for 18-24 hours.

First aid measures include the placement of a constriction band (not a tourniquet) just proximal to the bite. The use of suction through 1-cm linear incisions through the fang wounds remains of uncertain value but is perhaps useful if performed within 5 minutes of the bite.

At the medical facility, a determination of the necessity for antivenin must be made depending on the severity of the bite and subsequent clinical manifestations. Polyvalent antivenin, given after appropriate intradermal hypersensitivity testing, is most effective when administered within the first 4 hours after a bite, but may have value as late as 24 hours after envenomation. Tetanus immunization and penicillin prophylaxis are recommended because of the potential for wound contamination. Late scarring may require surgical revision. Edrophonium (Tensilson), an anticholinesterase drug, is effective in treating the neurotoxic effects of Asian cobras (Watt et al, 1986).

Prevention

Knowledge of the likelihood of snake bite should be sufficient to wear protective clothing such as boots, long pants, long sleeves, and gloves, especially when rock climbing or walking through brush. Hands should be kept out of dark crevices or cracks in rocks where snakes hide. Children should not hike alone, since a companion can usually summon help.

REFERENCES

Barza MJ: Case records of the Massachusetts General Hospital. *N Engl J Med* 315:241, 1986.

Carithers H: Mammalian bites of children. *Am J Dis Child* 95:150, 1958.

CDC: ACIP Recommendations: Rabies Prevention. *MMWR* 29:265, 1980.

CDC: ACIP Recommendations: Diphtheria tetanus pertussis, guidelines for vaccine prophylaxis and other preventive measures. *MMWR* 30:392, 1981.

Christopher D, Rodning C: *Crotalidae* envenomation. *South Med J* 79:159, 1986.

Elliot DL, Tolle SW, Goldberg L, et al: Pet-associated illness. *N Engl J Med* 313:985, 1985.

Gnann JW, Bressler GS, Bodet CA, et al: Human blastomycosis after a dog bite. *Ann Intern Med* 98:48, 1983.

Marcy SM: Infections due to dog and cat bites. *Pediatr Infect Dis* 1:351, 1982.

Russell FE, Picchioni AL: Snake venom poisoning. *Clin Toxicol Consult* 5:73, 1983.

Sprenger TR, Bailey WJ: Snakebite treatment in the United States: A review. *Int J Dermatol* 25:479, 1986.

Watt G, Theakston RD, Hayes CG, et al: Positive response to edrophonium in patients with neurotoxic envenoming by cobras *(Naja naja philippinensis)*. A placebo-controlled study. *N Engl J Med* 315:1444, 1986.

Foreign Body Injuries 7

Definition

Foreign body injuries are defined as secondary effects from the oral ingestion and/or aspiration of a foreign body, its insertion in another body orifice, or its placement in either the eye or the skin.

Epidemiology

Foreign bodies that come to medical attention include those inserted by young children into an ear canal, nose, or vaginal orifice. Small objects such as peanuts, beads, erasers, crayons, small toy parts, etc are the more common offenders. Occasionally an insect, such as a fly, maggot or roach, can also find refuge in an ear canal.

More dangerous are those foreign bodies that are ingested and/or aspirated such as balloons, small balls, or marbles.

Diagnosis

Foreign bodies can go undetected for days or weeks until the chronic irritation and inflammatory response cause secondary symptoms. If objects are inserted into the ear canal or nose, the presenting complaint may be that the child has a foul, rather musty odor that a parent mistakes for bad breath. The low-grade inflammatory reaction may produce a chronic, thick greenish or yellowish purulent discharge from the orifice as well. The surrounding mucosa is irritated and red and often the object itself is obscured by debris clogging the entrance. The foreign body may be lodged high in the back of the canal and can be readily discovered by a speculum examination of the orifice after the debris is removed.

The ingested foreign body is more difficult to detect. Often the diagnosis relies on a witness to the event. In the case of a coin or other radiopaque object, radiographic examinations of the neck, chest, and abdomen can be used serially to follow the progress of the object through the gastrointestinal tract. With normal intestinal motility, most objects smaller than a quarter will pass through in about 3 days. Radiographic examination becomes particularly important with objects that may obstruct or perforate the intestinal lumen. Some foreign bodies themselves contain toxins that can damage the mucosa or cause systemic injury. Ingestion of button batteries can injure the intestine by spilling a corrosive alkali such as potassium hydroxide and/or a poisonous agent such as mercuric salts into the intestine.

The aspirated foreign body can produce a variety of clinical symptoms from the immediate emergency of cyanosis, aphonia, and collapse associated with acute asphyxiation to chronic wheezing or cough with unilateral air-trapping, which may persist undetected or be misdiagnosed as asthma for months.

Treatment

Foreign bodies in the ear, nose, vaginal orifice, or rectum should be removed under controlled circumstances with use of proper equipment. The Magill forceps, bayonet forceps, or Kelly clamp are particularly effective when skillfully employed by personnel trained in their use. Insects present in the ear canal can be most easily removed by the instillation of mineral oil or viscous xylocaine into the canal to float out the live insect or its dead body parts. The primary care physician must use judgment when determining which foreign bodies can be easily extracted and which require more cautious approach. Many such objects look deceptively easy to ensnare, but may, in fact, be dislodged only with great difficulty and at some risk of damage to delicate structures nearby. Some foreign bodies require removal in the operating room under light anesthesia by a trained otolaryngologist, gynecologist, or general surgeon.

Ingested or inhaled foreign bodies require a substantially different approach. In an emergency choking episode, where the subject is cyanotic and cannot speak or breathe, the rescuer must promptly embrace the victim from behind with his fist midline under the xiphoid process of the sternum clasped to the other hand. He should then deliver a series of four to six firm upward thrusts toward the sternal notch (i.e., the Heimlich maneuver). A child may require only one hand rather than two to generate sufficient force. An infant less than 1 year of age requires chest thrusts and back blows at the midscapular level rather than abdominal thrusts to avoid unnecessary trauma to liver and spleen. These maneuvers force air from the lungs in sufficient velocity and volume to create an artificial cough that will dislodge and expel a foreign body completely blocking the airway.

If the adult or child victim is unconscious, the rescuer can apply the Heimlich maneuver by kneeling over the victim with the heel of hand on the midline abdomen just above the umbilicus and the other hand on top of the first. He should then press into the abdomen with a quick upward thrust.

Where the choking victim suffers only partial blockage of the airway and is breathing, it is best to

CASE ILLUSTRATION

A.L. is a 2½-year-old child seen in the emergency clinics with a 2-week history of fever, coryza, and possible streptococcal throat infection treated with erythromycin. On the eighth day of therapy, 2 days before admission, the child choked on a piece of gum which was pulled from his mouth. He had four to six episodes of paroxysmal coughing and then had a 36-hour progressive course of decreased appetite, decreased activity, increased listlessness, and increased cough. No voice change, stridor, or wheezing was noted. On the day of admission the patient developed a temperature of 102° F, tachypnea, abdominal pain, and difficulty breathing. Physical examination revealed fever, respiratory rate of 52/minute, perioral cyanosis, and decreased breath sounds in the left lung field. Blood gases showed a pH = 7.36, Po_2 = 54 mm Hg, and Pco_2 = 35 mm Hg. Complete blood count was remarkable only for WBC = 14,900/mm^3 with 77% PMNs, 6% bands, 11% lymphs, 4% monos, and 2% eos. A chest radiograph revealed a complete opacification of the left lung field with blurred diaphragm margins and a tracheal shift to the left. The patient received intravenous antibiotics and glucocorticoids and was taken to the operating room where multiple gum plugs were visualized in the left lower bronchus and lingular bronchus forming an anatomic "cast" of the bronchial tree. The gum plugs were removed at bronchoscopy.

The patient was treated with penicillin at 50,000 units/kg/day orally for 7 days as well as chest physiotherapy and made an uneventful recovery.

QUESTIONS AND COMMENTS

Why were steroids used in the management of an aspirated foreign body?

The use of steroids in aspiration pneumonias of any kind is controversial. The hope is that steroids will decrease inflammatory injury to the lung parenchyma, but there are no controlled studies of its efficacy in shortening the course of disease or improving functional outcome. In this case it was thought that steroids might decrease peribronchial swelling and edema. Postoperatively, theophyllin bronchodilators were also given as well as a full 10-day course of broad spectrum antibiotics.

What are the residual effects of an aspirated foreign body?

It is anticipated this child would make a full recovery. However, retained foreign bodies in the lungs may later provide the nidus for abscess formation, recurrent pneumonia, or chronic symptoms, such as cough or unilateral wheezing so that close pulmonary monitoring and follow-up are important.

allow his own repetitive cough to clear the foreign object. Those with poor air exchange or a weak cough or who are cyanotic should be managed as though suffering from complete obstruction.

In the past, blind finger sweeps were recommended to dislodge a foreign body from the airway. However, there is concern that this maneuver may work adversely to implant the foreign body more securely into the airway, in that the index finger may inadvertently push the protruding foreign body even further into the airway to obstruct it completely. Hence, blind finger sweeps are no longer recommended in the 1986 CPR guidelines.

REFERENCES

Blazer S, Naveh Y, Friedman A: Foreign body in the airway. *Am J Dis Child* 134:68, 1980.

Campbell D, Cotton E, Lilly J: A dual approach to tracheobronchial foreign bodies in children. *Surgery* 91:178, 1982.

Filston H: Foreign body aspiration in children: Recognition and safe management. *North Carolina Med J* 40:79, 1979.

Greensher J, Aronow R, Bass J, et al: Revised first aid for the choking child. *Pediatrics* 78:177, 1986.

National Conference on Cardiopulmonary Resuscitation (CPR) & Emergency Cardiac Care (ECC): Standards and guidelines for cardiopulmonary resuscitation (CPR) and emergency cardiac care (ECC). *JAMA* 255:2905, 1986.

Burns and Smoke Inhalation

8

Definition

A burn can be defined as a transfer of thermal, chemical, radiation or electric energy from a hazardous agent to the child such that there is damage to the epithelial or mucosal surfaces. In flame-related injury, pulmonary damage is often associated with direct thermal injury or smoke inhalation damage to the respiratory passages and the lungs. Smoke inhalation is a most dangerous and, indeed, life-threatening hazard associated with fires, accounting for more than 50% of fire-related deaths. This chapter covers thermal burns caused by fire, hot liquid, or hot surfaces and also injuries resulting from smoke inhalation.

Epidemiology

Burns are second only to motor vehicle-related trauma as the major cause of injury-related mortality and morbidity among children in the United States. The most common causes of house fires are smoldering cigarettes on upholstered furniture or mattresses; kerosene heaters and other vented space heaters used unsafely are also implicated commonly.

For all ages, hot water scalds are the leading cause of all hospital admissions for burns, with clothing ignition the second leading cause.

Diagnosis

THERMAL BURNS

Advances in our understanding of the pathophysiology of thermal burns within the past 10–15 years have led to improved medical management, with an attendant decline in mortality and morbidity from this type of injury. The extent of injury is measured by the extent of surface area burned and by the depth of the burn and associated thermal injury to the lungs. In children the proportionately greater surface area of the head makes the rule of 9's surface area calculation inaccurate and a surface body map suitable for infants and children should be substituted (Figs. 24.2 and 24.3).

Burns are classified as either partial thickness or full thickness. Table 24.6 gives the criteria for determining the depth of a thermal burn.

Full thickness burns of more than 15% body surface area are generally considered serious and are best treated, at least initially, in the hospital setting. Larger burns, 50% of body surface area or more, are most appropriately treated in one of the more than 200 specialized burn units around the country. In children, any burn of the hands, feet, or perineum usually will require hospitalization to ensure adequate burn care and to prevent joint contractures. Criteria for the evaluation of the burned patient are given in Table 24.7.

Often the extent of burn injury may not be fully appreciated until after careful debridement and a complete examination of the patient. Electrical burns in particular may present with trivial entrance and exit wounds but with severe deep tissue necrosis.

Flame injuries in the vicinity of the head and neck may be associated with extensive damage to the respiratory passages and lungs from burns and smoke inhalation. Respiratory involvement is diagnosed by edema of the face and oropharynx, singed nasal hairs, carbon particles in the sputum, and stridorous, positional breathing.

SMOKE INHALATION

Smoke inhalation is a most dangerous and indeed life-threatening hazard associated with fires, that accounts for more than 50% of fire-related deaths. The toxicity of smoke is related to its concentration, composition, and the length and type of exposure of the victim. Because of the complexity of our environment, the smoke associated with most fires is a complex mixture of particulate matter and noxious gases derived from wood, plastics, and an assortment of synthetic materials. Most smoke contains considerable amounts of carbon monoxide as well as various amounts of cyanide (from polyurethane, nylon, and other synthetics), nitrates (from polyacrylonitriles and other synthetics), hydrogen chloride (from chlorinated acrylics and polyvinyl chloride), sulfur dioxide, acrolein (an aldehyde formed from cellulose-containing materials such as wood and cotton), and other toxic chemicals.

Particulate matter and chemical irritation can produce bronchospasm and respiratory obstruction along with an inflammatory reaction with edema and sloughing of cellular debris into the peribronchiolar area leading to a bronchiolitis obliterans or an "adult type" respiratory distress syndrome with hyaline membrane formation. Such effects produce ventilation-perfusion mismatching and areas of atelectasis contributing to hypoxemia and acidosis. Membrane damage may lead to leakage of interstitial fluid and a delayed onset pulmonary edema. In severe cases, the alveoli may be involved directly or by superinfection such that bronchopneumonia occurs.

Finally, agents such as chlorine, sulfur dioxide, nitrous compounds, and others may have a sensitizing effect on the victim, inducing allergic manifestations such as bronchospasm, chest tightness, and edema formation.

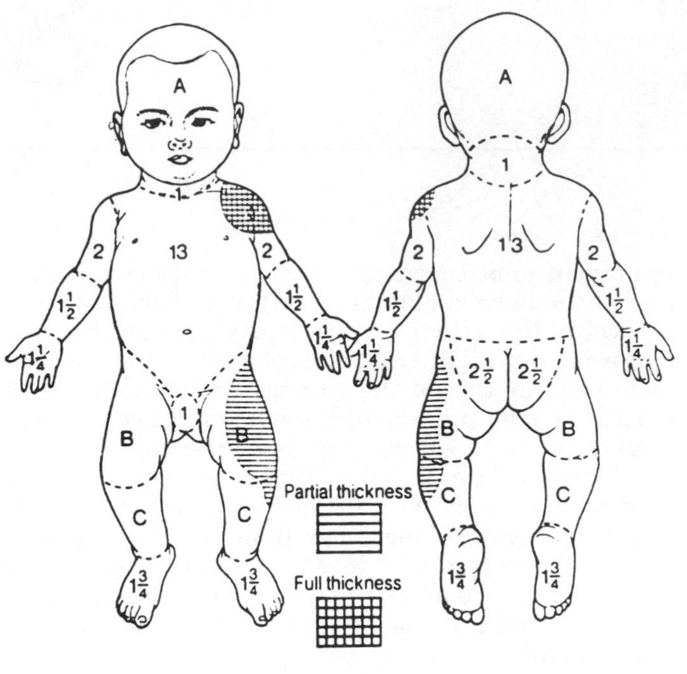

Approximate percentage of whole body surface

Area	Newborn	Age 1	Age 5
A = Half of head	9.50%	8.50%	6.50%
B = Half of one thigh	2.75	3.25	4.00
C = Half of one lower leg	2.50	2.50	2.75

Figure 24.2. Percentage of body surface area in infant burn victims.

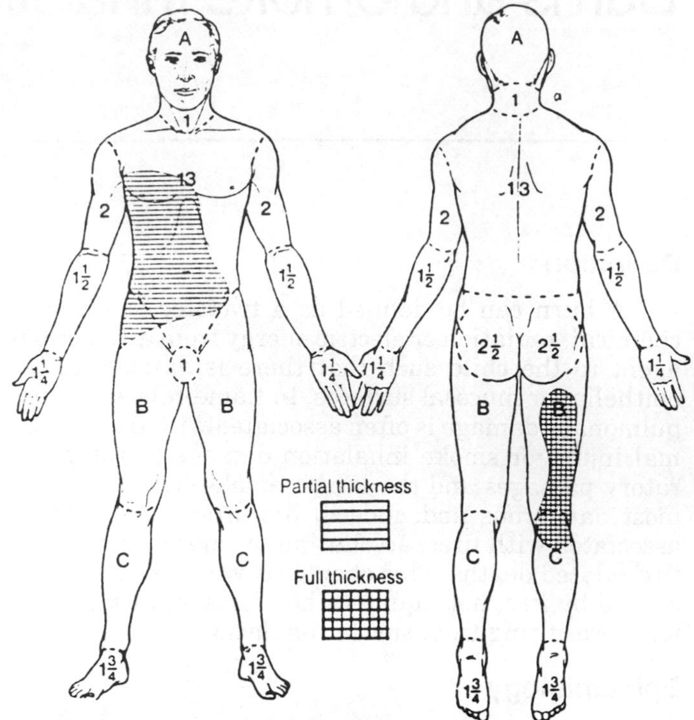

Approximate percentage of whole body surface

Area	Age 10	Age 15	Adult
A = Half of head	5.50%	4.50%	3.50%
B = Half of one thigh	4.50	4.50	4.25
C = Half of one lower leg	3.00	3.25	3.50

Figure 24.3. Percentage of body surface area in adult burn victims.

The victim of smoke-related injury will not necessarily have symptoms or signs of direct burns. Indeed, the signs of smoke injury may be delayed as much as 24 hours after the exposure, so that hospital admission and careful observation of individuals at high risk for smoke inhalation are wise even if they are asymptomatic.

Respiratory or central nervous system symptoms related to hypoxemia are typical. The victim may have a dry cough, wheezing, retractions, cyanosis, and other signs of respiratory distress and may be stuporous or lapse into coma.

Diagnosis and Treatment

THERMAL BURNS

Rapid assessment of burn and other injuries and immediate attention to cardiopulmonary resuscitation are the important first goals for rescuers of major burn victims.

Large fluid losses from the denuded integument can be anticipated; *rehydration should begin as soon as possible.* If fluid losses are extensive, hospitalization for volume expansion is necessary. Both colloid and crystalloid treatments have their proponents for the prevention of shock and electrolyte imbalance. Initially fluids are replaced with a nondextrose-containing solution such as Ringers lactate (administration of half of the 24-hour total volume in the first 8 hours at a rate of 4 ml/kg/% burn) with urinary monitoring to keep output greater than 1 ml/kg/hour.

The burned skin, if less than 20% of body surface area, should be bathed in cold water as soon as possible or wrapped lightly with cold soaks. Otherwise burns should just be wrapped in dry sterile sheets. No ointments should be applied until the wound is carefully

Table 24.6
Criteria for the Depth of Burns

Skin Destruction	Degree	Appearance	Sensation
1. Partial thickness (epidermal)	1st	Erythema	Normal
2. Deep partial thickness (dermal)	2nd	Red to grey-brown with blisters	Reduced
3. Full thickness (subdermal)	3rd	Scald: grey-white Flame: brown-black	Absent

Table 24.7
Hospital Admission Evaluation of Burned Patients

1. Burn evaluation	
Major:	>20% 2nd degree burns
	>10% 3rd degree burns
Moderate:	10–20% 2nd degree burns
	2–10% 3rd degree burns
Minor:	<10% 2nd degree burns
	<2% 3rd degree burns
2. Burn type and location	
>5% Burns in child < 2 years old	
Serious burns involving face, genitals, hands, or feet	
Electrical burns	
3. Other injuries	
Associated abdominal trauma, fractures, etc.	
Evidence for smoke inhalation	

inspected and cleansed. In extensive burns, debridement is best accomplished in the operating room. After debridement, lubricated gauze and/or silver sulfadiazine or another antibacterial topical agent can be applied as a dressing. Blisters are kept intact whenever possible. Tetanus vaccine is given if there is no history of recent immunization.

Advances in burn management include the use of temporary artificial coverings, which compensate for the lost barrier function of the skin. Skin grafting is accomplished over a period of weeks to months and may require prolonged convalescence and physical therapy. Psychologic supports for the burn patient and his family are also an important aspect of the complete management of this injury.

Penicillin (30,000–50,000 unit/kg/day orally) is often given for 48 hours to hospitalized burn patients to prevent superinfection with *Streptococcus*. If the patient has evidence of infection, cultures should dictate the choice of antibiotic.

Prevention

Home hot water should not exceed 50°C to lessen the likelihood of scalding.

Parents should inspect heat sources in the home and create barriers around grates or radiators with hot surfaces. Space heaters should only be used according to the manufacturer's recommendations and should be inaccessible to the toddler. All homes should be equipped with working smoke detectors and fire extinguishers; families should draw an escape route and practice an escape from fire in the home. The first aid burn principles of: (1) drop and roll; (2) apply cold water; and (3) crawl under smoke, should be part of the anticipatory guidance by pediatricians for all families in their practice.

SMOKE INHALATION

Whenever significant smoke exposure is suspected after a fire, the victim should be given oxygen, stabilized, and examined for burns or other injuries, triaged to medical services, and hospitalized at least overnight for observation. Close monitoring of vital signs and consciousness is advisable, with determinations of blood gases, cyanide and carboxyhemoglobin concentrations. Radiographic evidence of lung damage may lag behind clinical findings for some hours.

Indications for intubation include: (1) evidence for progressive oropharyngeal obstruction; (2) laryngeal obstruction; (3) difficulty in handling secretions; and (4) progressive respiratory insufficiency. A tracheostomy may be required to stabilize the airway for some patients.

Close attention should be paid to the patient's fluid, electrolyte, and acid-base balance. In severely injured patients, who are at considerable risk of developing pulmonary insufficiency or pulmonary edema, central venous and arterial catheterization may be anticipated so that fluid status can be accurately assessed.

Supportive therapy should include bronchodilators such as aerosolized sympathomimetics or intravenous theophylline preparations and correction of hypoxemia. Steroids, systemic or aerosolized, may be helpful in the treatment of refractory bronchospasm. Carbon monoxide poisoning should be treated as described in Section 25.

REFERENCES

Baker S, O'Neill B, Karpf R: Burns and fire deaths. In *The Injury Fact Book*. Chap 12, Lexington MA, Lexington Books, 1984.

Cohen M, Guzzardi L: Inhalation of products of combustion. *Ann Emerg Med* 12:628, 1983.

Crapo R: Smoke inhalation injuries. *JAMA* 246:1694, 1981.

Demling R: Burns. *N Engl J Med* 313:1389, 1985.

Libber G, Slayton D: Childhood burns reconsidered: The child, the family, and the burn injury. *J Trauma* 24:245, 1984.

McLoughlin E, Crawford J: Burns. *Pediatr Clin North Am* 32:61, 1985.

Mellins R, Park S: Respiratory complications of smoke inhalation in victims of fires. *J Pediatr* 87:1, 1975.

O'Neill J: Evaluation and treatment of the burned child. *Pediatr Clin North Am* 22:407, 1975.

Shirani KZ, Moylan JA, Pruitt BA: Diagnosis and treatment of inhalation injury in burn patients. In Loke J (ed): *Pathophysiology and Treatment of Inhalation Injuries*. New York, Marcel Dekker, Inc., 1988.

Heat-Induced Illness

9

Definition

Overheating is defined as any environmental condition that leads to an elevation of body temperature. Five major heat-induced illnesses are described: heat edema, heat cramps, heat syncope, heat exhaustion, and heatstroke.

Natural History

For infants, the likelihood of heat exhaustion is greatest in warm, humid environments in association with overdressing and exercise. Infants overdressed, under blankets, and near radiators are at risk, as are those left in closed automobiles in direct sunlight.

For older children and adolescents, heat exhaustion is greatest in situations of strenuous activity without gradual acclimation to a warm environment. Twice-a-day football practices with helmets and shoulder pads in August; midday parade marching in full uniforms on the 4th of July; 5-mile road races at noon on a sweltering summer day, are all examples.

Factors that predispose to heat-induced injury include inadequate fluid and salt intake to counterbalance losses via sweating. Chronic illnesses that predispose to heat injury include cystic fibrosis (sodium chloride loss), congenital heart disease (impaired ability to increase cardiac output), diabetes mellitus and insipidus (increased water loss), familial dysautonomia (temperature instability), cerebral palsy (central hyperthermia and impaired thirst), and either malnutrition or obesity.

Diagnosis

Heat injury represents a spectrum from the relatively benign conditions of heat edema, heat syncope, and heat cramps to the more severe heat exhaustion and heatstroke. The first three conditions are heralded by increased sweating, flushed appearance, fatigue, tachycardia, and muscle cramps and are readily reversed by cessation of extreme activity and removal to a cooler environment.

Heat exhaustion has been divided into hypertonic and hypotonic forms. In hypertonic heat exhaustion, which is more common, the strenuously exercising individual has a normal intake of salt (via diet), but a reduced fluid intake such that the excretion of hypotonic sweat results in a state of hypernatremic dehydration. Symptoms include extreme thirst, impaired cognition, anxiety, fatigue, excessive sweating, and raised body temperature. Hypotonic heat exhaustion occurs when copious sweating losses are replaced by large amounts of water intake such that total body sodium is depleted. Symptoms are more subtle and include headache, cramps, weakness, confusion, vomiting, and diarrhea.

Heatstroke is defined by the triad of severe hyperthermia, coma, and anhidrosis. Agitation and seizures can also occur. Coagulation necrosis, shock, and rhabdomyolysis make this a systemic disease: cardiac, renal, and hepatic failure occur. Electrolyte and acid-base derangements are quite common and hypokalemia or metabolic acidosis may be present. Disseminated intravascular coagulation is less common and is associated with a very poor prognosis.

Treatment

Rapid cooling is essential in heat-associated injury and can be facilitated by removal of the patient to a cool environment or a tub of cold water. The patient should be undressed; direct application of "iced" towels or sheets and use of a fan to enhance evaporative cooling will result in the lowering of core body temperature. The extremities should be massaged to promote circulation. Oral electrolyte solutions including readily available soft drinks, or intravenous solutions if the patient is confused or comatose and at risk for aspiration should be offered to promote rehydration.

Prognosis

Untreated heat injury can progress rapidly to heatstroke with serious renal, hepatic, and neurologic consequences; the condition can be fatal.

Prevention

Clearly, this is one condition that can be avoided with the proper precautions. Mothers should be aware of leaving infants exposed to overheated conditions in automobiles or at the beach. Older children and adolescents should acclimate themselves to a warm environment slowly, over several weeks, before undertaking strenuous exercise. Repletion of body fluids and salt is important.

REFERENCES

Clowes GHA, O'Donnell TF: Heat stroke. *N Engl J Med* 291:564, 1974.

Danks DM, Webb DW, Allen J: Heat illness in infants and young children. *Br Med J* 2:287, 1962.

Knochel JP: Environmental heat illness. *Arch Intern Med* 133:841, 1974.

Rosenstein BJ: The twin perils of heat exhaustion and heatstroke. *Contemp Pediatr* 3:46, 1986.

Smith NJ: The prevention of heat disorders in sports. *Am J Dis Child* 138:786, 1984.

Hypothermia

10

Definition

Hypothermia is defined as cooling the body's core temperature to injurious levels. Frostbite occurs when body parts are chilled to the point of freezing with the formation of ice crystals in the epidermis and dermis.

Basic Science

At core temperatures below 94° F (34.5°C), the body can no longer maintain homeostasis through mechanisms such as shivering, muscular activity, and peripheral vasoconstriction. Severe hypothermia leads to accelerating heat loss and affects the medullary respiratory center, cerebration, and cardiovascular function resulting in hypovolemic shock, acidosis, and electrolyte and other metabolic abnormalities.

Frostbite occurs when excessive heat loss to local tissues allows ice crystals to form in extracellular spaces with extraction of cell water and consequent cellular desiccation. The pathogenesis of injury consists of two states: (1) freezing—structural damage by ice, protein denaturation, pH changes, loss of cellular integrity, mitochondrial damage in muscle cells, and damage to blood vessel capillaries; and (2) thawing—with red blood cell aggregation and stasis, venous thrombosis, tissue edema and ischemic damage, blood vessel collapse, increased tissue compartment pressure, and regional tissue death and necrosis.

Epidemiology

Inadequate housing, old age, alcohol consumption, and temporarily incapacitating diseases, such as seizures and diabetes, are predisposing factors to hypothermia. In children and adolescents, winter sports, camping, and other outdoor activities with inattention to or inexperience with cold survival can increase the risk of cold injury.

Diagnosis

As the body temperature falls below 90° F (32.2°C), most patients begin to experience CNS depression. Symptoms include excessive fatigue, confused thinking, combativeness, and an inappropriate sense of well-being. "Paradoxical undressing" has been described in some patients during which, because of a failure of peripheral vasoconstriction, patients experience a sense of warmth prompting them in a confused state to take clothes off. Frostbitten extremities may appear grey or white and pulseless.

Sinus bradycardia, ventricular arrhythmias, and cardiovascular instability are common. The ECG may demonstrate a characteristic "J" wave following the QRS complex. Atrial or ventricular fibrillation may be spontaneous or may accompany rough handling or uncontrolled rewarming. Children and adolescents who are hypothermic more often experience asystole than do adults who are more likely to manifest fibrillation.

Victims who are discovered after prolonged hypothermia may appear dead because of the depression of vital body functions. Pupils may be fixed and dilated, muscles rigid, and respirations shallow or seemingly absent. A pulse may not be detectable. All hypothermia victims should be presumed alive unless repeated resuscitation attempts after rewarming are unsuccessful.

Prognosis has been directly correlated with the degree of hypothermia and method of rewarming and is adversely affected by the presence of other underlying medical conditions such as diabetes, sepsis, or uremia.

Treatment

Management of patients in the field includes the protection of the victim from further cold injury. In patients with rectal temperatures greater than 33° C , gradual body warming by blankets or baths at a rate of 1–2°F per hour is usually safe. Warm humidified air may also be useful. Rapid uncontrolled rewarming may send a bolus of peripheral cold, acidotic blood to the heart provoking lethal arrhythmias. Dehydration can be treated with a solution of normal saline and glucose until urinary function is established and electrolyte abnormalities are known. Often during rewarming, damage to peripheral tissues releases large amounts of potassium which aggravates cardiac irritability. Monitoring of acid-base and respiratory status, cardiac function, and fluid-electrolyte and renal status should be undertaken in an intensive care setting during the rewarming process.

Active internal rewarming may consist of warm humidified oxygen, intravenous fluids, rectal lavage, peritoneal lavage with warm fluids, extracorporeal blood rewarming, and/or hemodialysis. These methods are useful for patients with prolonged hypothermia with core body temperatures of less than 33°C and persistent, severe cardiac disturbances. No study has proven one method better than another although peritoneal lavage and extracorporeal bypass are the quickest and most efficient methods of rewarming. The arrhythmias in these patients are difficult to control and often resolve spontaneously with rewarming.

Frostbitten body parts should be protected to avoid further trauma or pressure and should be thawed in a bath at 38–41° C only when the core temperature is greater than 37°C. Skin blebs should be left intact if they appear blue or black. Superficial blisters that are pink or white should be opened since these contain thromboxane, a potent prostaglandin that stimulates white blood cell and platelet aggregation and, hence, enhances inflammation and thrombosis. Open wounds or blisters secondary to freezing should be covered with aloe ointments and ibuprofen (prostaglandin-inhibitors) administered orally to counteract the effect of the thromboxane (Heggers et al, 1987). Other specialized procedures, such as escharotomy, debridement, fasciotomy, sympathectomy, skin grafting, or amputation, may be necessary and require surgical expertise and consultation. Plasma volume expanders, anticoagulants, vasodilators, and antitetanus immunization also have a role in therapy.

Prevention

The prevention of cold injury depends on anticipation of wintery conditions and knowledge of cold survival skills. Adequate protection when outdoors should always be a concern of parents and children living in cold climates. Adverse weather conditions must dictate precautions against unexpected prolonged exposure to the cold. Many families living in cold climates store extra blankets, food rations, and other equipment in their vehicles as insurance against an unexpected mechanical breakdown in cold weather.

REFERENCES

Treatment of Hypothermia. *Med Lett* 25:9, 1983.

Danal DF, Pozos RS, Auerbach PS et al: Multicenter hypothermia survey. *Ann Emerg Med* 16:1042, 1987.

Heggers JP, Robson MC, Manavalen K: Experimental and clinical observations on frostbite. *Ann Emerg Med* 16:1056, 1987.

Mills W: Summary of treatment of the cold injured patient. *Alaska Med* 25:29, 1983.

Reuler JB: Hypothermia: Pathophysiology, clinical settings, and management. *Ann Intern Med* 89:519, 1978.

Robinson M, Seward PH: Environmental hypothermia in children. *Pediatr Emerg Care* 2:254, 1986.

Sofer S, Yagupsky P, et al: Improved outcome of hypothermic infants. *Pediatr Emerg Care* 2:211, 1986.

Southwick F, Dalglish P: Recovery after prolonged asystolic cardiac arrest in profound hypothermia. *JAMA* 243:1250, 1980.

Welton D, Mattox K, Miller R, et al: Treatment of profound hypothermia. *JAMA* 240:2291, 1978.

Head Trauma 11

Definition

Any blow to the head that causes injury, immediate or delayed, is known as head trauma.

If loss of consciousness occurs without anatomic brain injury, the condition is called a concussion. If the patient has a focal neurologic examination with either a prolonged episode of unconsciousness or serious alterations in level of consciousness, he is said to have had a contusion. The frontal and temporal lobes are frequent sites for contusions following an injury to the occipital region.

The most common types of intracranial hemorrhages are those due to meningeal injuries. There are three major types of meningeal hemorrhage.

1. *Epidural hemorrhage*. This type of bleed is usually due to a tear in the middle meningeal artery. It is exceedingly rare in children and is often associated with linear skull fractures over the parietal or temporal areas that intersect the artery. It is characterized by loss of consciousness followed by a lucid interval accompanied by headache and/or lethargy, and then a return to loss of consciousness along with a hemiparesis on the side opposite the bleed, as well as an ipsilaterally fixed and dilated pupil. Prognosis is excellent if surgical evacuation and repair is immediate.
2. *Subdural hematoma*. This hemorrhagic episode is usually due to venous bleeding and is slower to appear. It is usually associated with underlying brain injury and is, therefore, associated with significant morbidity, if not mortality, even if the hematoma can be evacuated quickly.
3. *Subarachnoid hemorrhage*. This type of bleed is characterized by meningeal signs (stiff neck, headache, photophobia) and hemorrhagic CSF. It usually requires no treatment other than bed rest and

observation (and radiographic elimination of cervical spine injury which can mimic it).

The other types of intracranial bleeds are those within the brain itself. Intraventricular and intracerebellar hemorrhages, for example, are associated with very high mortality rates. Diagnosis is by careful neurologic examination and CT scan.

Basic Science

The brain is cushioned by layers of meninges, the CSF, and a rigid, thick cranial vault. In head trauma, the brain is exposed to a transfer of mechanical energy as a result of sharp acceleration-deceleration forces resulting in a "coup" injury as it is driven to make an impact on one wall of the cranial vault and a "contracoup" injury as, within milliseconds, force vectors drive it backward onto the opposite wall. The injury sustained is related to direct (crush and contusion) damage to tissues and shearing, stretching stresses on vessels and nerves. Injury can also be related to indirect damage from laceration and entrapment of vessels, nerve, or cortex by the fracture of overlying bony structures. Finally, injury can also be caused by compression of tissues due to increased intracranial pressure secondary to cerebral edema, subdural or extradural bleeding, or, as a late sequela, hydrocephalus.

Epidemiology

Head trauma is responsible for about 250,000 hospitalizations of children each year in the United States. About 4000 die annually from head trauma. The most common cause of head injury in childhood is a vertical fall. The clinician frequently hears the story of an infant who rolled off the bed while the parents were not looking, tumbled down a few stairs, or fell while in a "baby walker." Most often, these injuries are trivial and many can be handled by telephone triage. More severe head injuries, however, are caused by motor vehicle-related incidents (e.g., collisions, automobile-bicycle injuries, automobile-pedestrian injuries, motorcycle-related trauma, etc). It is these circumstances that place head trauma at the head of the list of injuries causing long-term neurologic sequelae or death. Retrospective studies of younger children and infants hospitalized with nonmotor vehicle-related head injuries have revealed child abuse to be commonly implicated in such cases (Hobbs, 1984).

Natural History

The natural history of head trauma in children is most often inconsequential if the blow was trivial. Nevertheless, the consequences of misdiagnosis of severe head injury can be fatal if an unrecognized, expanding subdural hematoma produces increased intracranial pressure, herniation, and brain stem compromise. Within this spectrum of outcomes, a number of complications can occur.

The most common sequela observed in head injury is a "postconcussion syndrome" of vague headaches, dizziness, and poor memory or concentration lasting for days to months. Such effects are nonspecific and are believed to be self-limited. Longer term cognitive, developmental, and neurologic deficits, however, termed "acquired post-traumatic cerebral palsy," are also observed secondary to brain damage associated with head trauma. The more severe the head injury, as measured by duration of coma or amnesia, the more likely a child is to suffer such cognitive and developmental effects. Deficits in perceptuomotor skills are most often observed, although speech disturbances, poor memory, and attentional defects are also described. Progress in school is occasionally poor, but gradual slow recovery is more common.

Other complications of head trauma have been observed in children. Seizures may be late in onset and difficult to control. In cases of concussion or more severe head trauma (contusion), with or without skull fracture, 7% of children in one controlled study (Vartiainen et al, 1985) suffered sensorineural hearing loss that resolved spontaneously in only 33% of cases. Conductive hearing loss also occurs, mostly in association with a longitudinal fracture of the temporal bone, which causes hemotympanum and/or disruption of the ossicular chain.

A communicating hydrocephalus is sometimes seen resulting from impairment of CSF resorption as a consequence of subarachnoid bleeding in the acute phase. The patient with behavioral changes, altered consciousness, or chronic headaches weeks after an episode of head trauma should be evaluated for increased intracranial pressure due to a communicating hydrocephalus or the effects of a chronic subdural hematoma or cerebral abscess.

Disruption of the cribriform plate with fistula formation and chronic leakage of CSF is another late complication of head trauma. A clear rhinorrhea is seen clinically and recurrent meningitis can occur unless the structural defect is diagnosed and corrected surgically.

Uncommonly, damage to the hypothalamus may cause diabetes insipidus, diagnosed by the presence of progressively rising serum sodium and osmolarity with inappropriately low urinary sodium and osmolarity values. Other neuroendocrinologic effects, such as the onset of precocious puberty, are reported to occur rarely after extremely severe head trauma.

Transient anosmia is commonly seen after head trauma and other cranial nerve damage may be sustained according to the area of the injury. Facial nerve palsy or impairment of visual acuity may be related to injury to the seventh or optic nerves, respectively, and may require surgical intervention.

Diagnosis

Head trauma can result in a medical emergency and must always be assessed and managed carefully and conservatively. The history of circumstances surrounding the event is of obvious importance. Although nausea and vomiting, sweating, and irritability portend a more serious prognosis in adults, they are common signs and symptoms in children even with minor injuries. A rapid but complete physical and neurologic examination can provide baseline measures upon which to gauge later improvement or deterioration. The Glasgow Coma Scale has replaced other, more imprecise qualitative measures of consciousness and is presented in Table 24.5 (pp. 1313).

This scale is quite reliable and also useful in the prognosis of head trauma, with Glasgow Scale total scores of less than 7 indicating a high risk of permanent and serious neurologic damage.

Any child who reports loss of consciousness for a minimum of 5 minutes regardless of having a nonfocal symmetric neurologic examination should be admitted to the hospital overnight for observation. The persistence of amnesia is also an indication for admission despite perhaps a shorter period of loss of consciousness. One should always err on the conservative side of "admit and observe" if there is any concern for potential neurologic injury. Contusions rarely require surgery unless delayed hemorrhage occurs in the localized area of injury. Such patients should be admitted for at least 24 and usually 48 hours to observe for such bleeding.

Treatment

First aid for a child with serious head trauma includes protecting him from further insult, resuscitation and stabilization, and transport for further assessment and treatment. The neck should be supported and the head held in neutral position to prevent aggravation of possible cervical spine injury. The airway should be cleared and resuscitation carried out when necessary. A quick assessment for other seriously injured body parts is important as well. Bleeding from head wounds should be stopped by direct compression.

When the child has been safely transported to medical care, further treatment is possible. The question of which studies to perform often provokes controversy. Masters et al (1988) have tried to define criteria for radiographic imaging in head trauma patients. Those patients who are over 2 years of age and are asymptomatic, complain only of headache or dizziness, or have only a scalp laceration, hematoma, abrasion, or contusion are considered at "low" risk for head injury and do not require a skull film or CT scan. Patients at "high" risk for head injury include those children with depressed levels of consciousness, focal neurologic signs, penetrating skull injury, or palpable depressed fractures, and require an emergency CT examination and neuorosurgical consultation.

Those patients at "moderate" risk are less well defined. They include children less than 2 years old with more than "trivial" injury, those with changing levels of consciousness while under close observation, or those with persistent vomiting following the injury, facial injury and/or multiple trauma, suspected child or substance abuse, or evidence of basilar or possible skull fracture on examination. In the "moderate risk" category both a skull series and CT scan may be beneficial. Magnetic resonance imaging promises to be increasingly valuable as more experience is obtained.

Other studies are rarely indicated. A lumbar puncture is contraindicated in the face of increased intracranial pressure. Subdural taps may be needed to remove fluid if shown by x-rays or ultrasonography. A maximum of 15 ml may be removed without aspiration (Rosman, 1986).

If cerebral edema is suspected, intravenous mannitol (1 g/kg intravenously) to promote an osmotic diuresis and corticosteroids (dexamethasone, 3 mg/kg intravenously every 6 hours) to reduce swelling are usually given. The child should receive no fluids by mouth because of the risk of aspiration of vomitus. Intravenous fluids should be infused at about half maintenance requirements so that cerebral edema is minimized. Both input and output should be carefully monitored with serial measurement of serum/urinary electrolytes and osmolarity since both the syndrome of inappropriate antidiuretic hormone (SIADH) and diabetes insipidus are associated complications of head trauma. Arterial and central venous pressures should be monitored. Signs of transtentorial herniation or rapidly increasing intracranial pressure must be managed as emergencies by surgical decompression and the introduction of direct pressure monitoring devices. Forced hyperventilation can also be used to lower the brain's metabolic and oxygen needs, reduce intracranial pressure, and protect the brain from further injury.

Prevention

Clinicians should be aware that most serious head trauma in early childhood is related to the intentional circumstances of child abuse; social services interventions are necessary in such cases to prevent the recurrence of more deadly injuries. Anticipatory guidance should include discussion of age-related hazards.

REFERENCES

Chadwick O: Psychological sequelae of head injury in children. *Dev Med Child Neurol* 27:69, 1985.

Hobbs C: Skull fracture and the diagnosis of abuse. *Arch Dis Child* 59:246, 1984.

Jamison D, Kaye H: Accidental head injury in childhood. *Arch Dis Child* 49:376, 1974.

Jennett B, Teasdale G, Braakman R, et al: Predicting outcome in individual patients after severe head injury. *Lancet* 1:1031, 1976.

Masters SJ, McClean PM, Arcarese JS, et al: Skull X-ray examinations after head trauma. *N Engl J Med* 316:84, 1987.

Rosman NP: Pediatric emergencies: Managing acute head trauma. *Contemp Pediatr* 3:24, 1986.

Vartiainen E, Karjalainen S, Karja J: Auditory disorders following head injury in children. *Acta Otolaryngol* (Stockholm) 99:529, 1985.

ALAN WOOLF

LEWIS R. FIRST

Section 25

Toxicology

Overview

1

Childhood poisonings continue to be an important public health problem. With the increasing sophistication of everyday life has come the expanded use of toxic agents in the workplace, in schools, at home, and in the environment. The public has heightened awareness and concern about both new and traditional environmental toxins, including radioactive wastes, organic and inorganic pollutants of the air, land, and water, food additives, and prescription and nonprescription drugs. Pediatricians are commonly queried by parents as to what substances may be teratogens or can be passed in toxic amounts to their infants by breast-feeding, which medications have significant toxic side-effects, and what measures can guard against a household poisoning. Clinicians must understand the principles of management of acute poisoning, and be vigilant to "subtle" poisonings—that is, iatrogenic overdoses, drug-drug interactions, variability in drug metabolism, and the hazards of chronic drug overdose. In this chapter, we give a brief overview of important principles in the definition, prevention, and management of childhood poisonings generally and discuss the principles of management for some of the more common, specific hazardous agents in childhood poisonings.

Definition

A poisoning can be defined as an energy transfer from a hazardous agent to a susceptible host. For our purposes, the type of energy transferred is usually chemical, although radiant energy is also responsible for some types of poisoning-associated injuries. At the molecular level, toxins exert a spectrum of effects which disrupt membranes, interfere with the function of specific organelles, or initiate a cascade of inflammatory immunologic responses indirectly causing tissue damage.

Basic Science

The pharmacologic properties of the toxic agent can help the clinician plan rational management in overdose situations. The mechanisms of absorption and pharmacokinetics (serum half-life and elimination rate) may be important clues to the duration of symptoms and when they are to be expected to reach a peak. The volume of distribution (V_d) refers to the percentage of body mass in which a drug or agent is dispersed. Drugs that are protein-bound and water-soluble will have a low V_d approximately equivalent to that of body water (0.6 L/kg body weight) and will be amenable to such procedures as osmotic dialysis or forced diuresis. Lipophilic agents will be sequestered into fatty tissues, will have a large V_d, and will less readily be dialyzed or undergo diuresis. Finally, the metabolism and the route of endogenous elimination (e.g., pulmonary, hepatic, enteroenteric, renal) of a specific agent or its active metabolites will be important in planning management.

Epidemiology

Poison Control Centers in the United States handle over 1,500,000 poison-related calls annually, many of them concerning childhood poisoning incidents. Despite a dramatic fall in the number of childhood drug exposures associated with child-resistant closure packaging regulations (Walton, 1982), over 110,000 children under 5 years of age were treated for toxic exposures in 1983 and 14% of them required hospitalization (CDC, 1984).

The nonrandom occurrences of poisonings depend upon: (1) intrinsic properties of the hazardous agent; (2) behavioral and developmental characteristics of the child; and (3) environmental conditions conducive to a poisoning incident.

The dangerousness of the agent depends on both its toxicity and the exposure characteristics. Aspects of intrinsic toxicity include: (1) the pathogenesis of the injury it induces; (2) whether the number of toxin molecules required to produce the injury fits a "one-hit" or threshold model; (3) whether there is a lag time between exposure and the onset of clinical toxicity; and (4) distribution, storage, metabolism, and elimination characteristics of the agent in this particular patient. The exposure variables important in the injury production from a poison include: (1) the duration of the exposure; (2) the type of the exposure; (3) the dose of the agent absorbed; (4) whether there is a repetitive exposure; (5) whether there is a cumulative effect; and (6) susceptibility of the particular patient to the particular agent.

Studies of the behavioral and developmental characteristics of children at high risk for repetitive poisoning incidents disclose that they tend to be somewhat socially immature, negativistic, hyperactive and adventuresome, and aggressive. Pica and excessive oral behavior are common characteristics of such children. Sobel and Margolis (1963) have demonstrated that children who repeatedly poison themselves are often locked in a power struggle with their parents, such that the parent-child interaction appears dysfunctional.

Other studies have characterized physical and social environments conducive to a poisoning incident. Childhood poison-repeaters often come from disorganized or single parent families with poor supervision, frequent moves, and/or substandard housing. Other susceptible families may be socially isolated or stressed by physical or psychiatric illness. Many out-of-home poisonings have been traced to grandparents' homes where a number of prescribed medications are present, but the measures for storing them safely are not.

Diagnosis

The diagnosis of a poisoning injury requires a careful history which should include: (1) the age and approximate weight of the victim; (2) if the diagnosis is by telephone, a reliable means of ensuring contact with the caller (e.g., address, telephone number), (3) all sources of environmental exposure (the label on the container should be read to the physician); (4) the time and duration of exposure; (5) the amount of a suspected poison ingested or otherwise contacted; (6) witnesses to the incident(s); (7) a temporal documentation of the development of any symptoms and signs; and (8) therapies tried so far. The telephone triage of potential poisonings depends on the pediatrician's judgment as to the seriousness of the event; the principle of "do no harm" should always be foremost in consideration. The clinician should make use of the regional poison control center in his area for specific advice about all poisonings; if he believes the child should be seen, he should remind parents to bring to the emergency clinic the container the poison was in.

On examination, particular attention should be paid to pulse and respiration, blood pressure and evidence for orthostasis, body temperature, skin manifestations, unusual breath or urine odors, pupillary size and reactivity, and other CNS signs. Common symptoms and signs are presented in Tables 25.1 and 25.2. Polypharmacy overdoses should be anticipated in suicide attempts or drug abuse cases. Toxic exposures should always be suspected in patients who present with an altered state of consciousness or are comatose without evident cause.

A clinical toxicology laboratory can aid in the diagnosis of an unknown poison; other laboratory screen-

Table 25.1
Common Poisonings[1]

Toxic Agent	Manifestations of Poisoning
Atropine, LSD	Agitation, hallucination, dilated pupils, dry skin, fever
Amphetamines	Argumentativeness, diarrhea, dilated pupils, tachycardia, sweating
Narcotics	Slow respirations, pinpoint pupils, coma
Organophosphates	Salivation, lacrimation, miosis, increased urination
Barbiturates, tranquilizers	Nystagmus, ataxia, slurred speech, hypotension, bradycardia
Phenothiazines	Torticollis, oculogyric crisis, ataxia, tachycardia
Tricyclic antidepressants	Coma, convulsions, arrhythmias

[1]Reproduced with permission from Mofenson H, Greensher J: The unknown poisoning. *Pediatrics* 54:336, 1974.

Table 25.2
Common Signs of Poisoning[1]

Physical Sign	Characteristic Poisons
Abdominal colic	Lead, arsenic, mushrooms, drug withdrawal, food poisoning
Arrhythmias	Tricyclic antidepressants, cocaine, amphetamines, theophylline
Ataxia	Phenytoin, benzodiazepines, sedatives
Bradycardia	Digitalis, opiates, organophosphates
Breath odors	Acetone: acetone, alcohol, salicylate Almonds: cyanide Sweet: acetone, ether Oil of wintergreen: methyl salicylate Garlic: arsenic, organophosphates Violets: turpentine
Constipation	Anticholinergics, lead, narcotics
Cyanosis	Aniline, cyanide, smoke inhalation, many CNS depressants
Diaphoresis	Amphetamines, salicylates, cocaine, mushrooms, LSD
Diarrhea	Organophosphates, food poisoning
Dry mouth	Amphetamines, narcotics, anticholinergics
Hallucinations	LSD, phencyclidine, cocaine, mescaline, alcohol withdrawal
Hypertension	Amphetamines, tricyclic antidepressants, nicotine, sympathomimetics
Hyperthermia	Amphetamines, anesthetic agents, salicylates, phencyclidine
Hypotension	Antihypertensives, opiates, phenothiazines, cyanide
Hypothermia	Carbon monoxide, opiates, barbiturates, phenothiazines
Jaundice	Fava beans, carbon tetrachloride, acetaminophen (late)
Metabolic acidosis	Methanol, salicylates, iron, ethylene glycol, toluene
Miosis	Narcotics, organophosphates, phenothiazines
Mydriasis	Atropine, LSD, cocaine, tricyclic antidepressants, amphetamines, belladonna, sympathomimetics
Psychosis	LSD, phencyclidine, anticholinergics
Purpura	Salicylates, snake or spider bite, anticoagulants
Salivation	Mercury, strychnine, organophosphates
Seizures, coma	Amphetamines, phencyclidine, tricyclic antidepressants, phenothiazines, alcohol, cyanide, withdrawal syndrome, strychnine, organophosphates, lead, salicylates, camphor, boric acid
Tachycardia	Alcohol, caffeine, cannibis, amphetamines, cocaine, anticholinergics
Tachypnea	Alcohol, methanol, ethylene glycol, carbon monoxide, hydrocarbons, cocaine

[1]Modified from Mofenson HC, Greensher J: The unknown poisoning. *Pediatrics* 54:336, 1974.

ing tests can be done at the bedside. Most emergency toxicology laboratories are capable of a battery of specific assays ("toxic screens") which include: salicylates, barbiturates, alcohol, acetaminophen, nonbarbiturate hypnotics, tricyclic antidepressants, amphetamines, benzodiazepines, and phenothiazines. The more specific the information a clinician can provide based on clinical history and examination, the more helpful the laboratory can be in identifying the agent. Urine, blood, gastric washings, and vomitus are commonly sent for analysis; a reasonable turn-around time for emergency screenings is about 4 hours, although poisons requiring unusual or complicated methods may take longer. A negative toxic screen certainly does not rule out a toxic exposure.

The clinician can examine serum or urine samples for the evidence of hypoglycemia, glycosuria, or acetone. Chocolate-colored blood indicates significant methemoglobinemia. The 10% ferric chloride test on 2–3 ml of boiled and cooled urine can reveal phenothiazines (purplish color change intensified with 2–3 drops of sulfuric acid), mellaril (blue), and salicylates (burgundy-red).

Other potentially important diagnostic tests for given clinical situations include blood gases, a complete blood count and smear, serum electrolyte and glucose determinations, liver function tests, coagulation studies, and carboxyhemoglobin levels. An abdominal radiograph may show recent lead, iron, or other heavy metal ingestion or confirm a suspected ileus secondary to an anticholinergic ingestion. A chest radiograph and ECG can help diagnose suspected pneumonia or cardiac involvement.

Treatment

The mainstays of therapy once a poisoning has occurred are as follows: (1) reduce absorption of the poison; (2) administer specific therapies (antidotes), if any; (3) increase clearance of the poison; (4) provide whatever supportive therapy is needed; and (5) maintain the airway.

DECONTAMINATION

Initial efforts are directed at effective decontamination to reduce the concentration of the hazardous agent in the body. Oral decontamination is effected by having the patient vomit; when given with supplemental fluids, syrup of ipecac at a dose of 30 ml for adults, 15 ml for children, or 10 ml for infants over 9 months of age usually produces emesis within 20–30 minutes. The dose of ipecac may be repeated but it must be removed along with the poison by lavage if it has not induced emesis after two doses. It should not be given to patients who have ingested caustics or hydrocarbons, or those with a changing state of consciousness where there is an increased risk of aspiration.

Alternatively gastric lavage with use of a 16–32F red rubber catheter modified by cutting additional holes at 2-cm intervals from the tip, has been shown to be effective (Tandberg et al, 1986). The patient is placed in the left lateral decubitus position, the upper abdomen is manually agitated to promote resuspension of particulate matter, and room temperature normal saline is repeatedly instilled and withdrawn. Tandberg et al reported recovery rates of up to 45% of the tracer tablets ingested by volunteer adults as opposed to only a 28% recovery rate by ipecac emesis. There is still considerable controversy, however, as to whether ipecac or lavage is more effective in children.

A third effective modality is adsorption of the poison by orally administered activated charcoal. The engineering of superfine particles of activated charcoal has increased the effectiveness of this agent by increasing the surface area and thereby its adsorption potential; 1 g of activated charcoal may have a surface area as much as 1600 m^2. It has been shown to lower dramatically the acetaminophen, aspirin, and tricyclic antidepressant levels. The dose of activated charcoal, dissolved in water, is about 1 g/kg body weight for children and up to 50 g for an adult. Besides its ability to decrease the gastrointestinal absorption of toxic agents by adsorption and removal, activated charcoal also causes "gastrointestinal dialysis," promoting the clearance of certain dialyzable poisons and disrupting their enterohepatic or enteroenteric cycles. In this way, the concentration of the poison in the intestinal fluid is kept near zero such that there is an "infinite sink" effect moving the poison across the semipermeable gastrointestinal blood vessel cell membranes down the concentration gradient into the intestinal lumen, where it is adsorbed by charcoal and removed from contact with the patient (Pond, 1986). Only those poisons with characteristics that facilitate such a dialysis mechanism (i.e., nonprotein-bound, nonionized, small volume of distribution, low endogenous clearance) are appropriate. Moreover, charcoal may adsorb potential antidotes or other therapeutic agents (e.g., ipecac, anticonvulsants, antibiotics). Its effectiveness as a dialysis agent may be compromised if gastrointestinal motility is reduced (e.g., anticholinergic overdoses) or gastrointestinal blood flow is diminished (e.g., shock). Table 25.3 presents some of the poisons for which activated charcoal is an effective adsorbent.

SPECIFIC ANTIDOTES

Most poisons do not have specific systemic antidotes. For those poisons that do, the mechanisms of action range from competitive binding at the cellular level or promotion of enzymatic degradation processes to chelation or antigen-antibody binding and immunologic inactivation of the toxic agent. Some examples of specific antidotes are given in Table 25.4.

ELIMINATION MEASURES

The promotion of endogenous clearance mechanisms also decreases the serum concentration of poisons. Thus, poisons are removed from the circulation by metabolic, renal, hepatic, gastrointestinal, and pulmonary mechanisms. Such strategies as the alkalinization of urine for salicylate or phenobarbital poisoning,

Table 25.3
Selected Poisons Effectively Adsorbed by Activated Charcoal

Acetaminophen
Amphetamines
Barbiturates
Chlordane
Cocaine
Digitalis
Dilantin
Opium
Oxalates
Phenothiazines
Parathion
Primaquine
Penicillin
Phenol
Phenylpropanolamine
Quinine
Salicylates
Salicylamide
Strychnine
Sulfonamides
Theophylline
Tricyclic antidepressants

Adapted from Corby and Decker: *Pediatrics* 54:324, 1974, with permission of publisher.

Table 25.4
Specific Systemic Antidotes for Selected Poisons

Poison	Antidote
Acetaminophen	Acetylcysteine
Carbon monoxide	Oxygen
Cyanide	Amyl nitrate, sodium thiosulfate
Digoxin	Digoxin fab fragments
Nitrites, nitrates	Methylene blue
Narcotics	Naloxone
Anticholinergics	Physostigmine
Carbamates	2-PAM (Pralidoxime)
Methanol, ethylene glycol	Ethanol
Iron	Deferoxamine
Arsenic, mercury	Dimercaprol
Coumadin	Vitamin K_1
Heparin	Protamine sulfate
Phenothiazines	Diphenhydramine

acidification diuresis for amphetamines, strychnine, quinine, or phencyclidine, forced diuresis with mannitol or furosemide, gastrointestinal catharsis with magnesium citrate, or sorbitol, hyperventilation, and the induction of enzymatic processes that inactivate or conjugate bioactive species of a poison may be variably useful as adjunctive measures in the management of selected poisonings. Exogenous clearance therapies, such as extracorporeal charcoal hemoperfusion, peritoneal or hemodialysis, exchange transfusion, and plasmapheresis are of practical or, at least, theoretical benefit for selected serious overdoses.

Poisoning Prevention

General concepts of injury prevention were discussed previously in Childhood Injuries, Section 24. Efforts in poison prevention can also be divided into: *primary poisoning prevention*: efforts to decrease the exposure of all people generally to hazardous substances in the environment; *secondary poisoning prevention*: those efforts that separate the host from specific hazardous agents so that no injury can occur; and finally, *tertiary poisoning prevention*: those efforts that reduce excess morbidity and prevent mortality once an injury has already taken place. Legislation requiring the use of child-resistant containers on prescription drugs and hazardous household products or limiting the concentration of caustic agents available as household cleaners (secondary prevention measure) are examples of effective poisoning prevention. Studies have demonstrated the regionalization of Poison Control Centers across the country has dramatically reduced the mortality and morbidity from poisonings by facilitating accurate and effective triage and management of the patient after a poisoning has taken place (tertiary prevention). These passive measures require little effort on the part of parents or children to make them work. It is less evident whether health education requiring active behavioral changes on the part of parents or children, such as education with respect to poison recognition and avoidance, safe storage at home, readiness, and appropriate first response in case of a poisoning incident, are truly effective in decreasing the incidence or severity of poisonings. Nonetheless, we continue to advocate health education to prevent poisoning.

REFERENCES

Chafee-Bahamou C, Lacouture PG, Lovejoy FH: Risk assessment of ipecac in the home. *Pediatrics* 75:1105, 1985.

CDC: Poisoning among young children—United States. *MMWR* 33:129, 1984.

Fergusson D, Horwood L, Beautrais A, et al: A controlled field trial of a poisoning prevention method. *Pediatrics* 69:515, 1982.

Haddad L, Winchester J: *Clinical Management of Poisoning and Drug Overdose*. Philadelphia, WB Saunders, 1983.

Mofenson HC, Greensher J: The unknown poison. *Pediatrics* 54:336, 1974.

Pond S: Role of repeated oral doses of activated charcoal in clinical toxicology. *Med Toxicol* 1:3, 1986.

Sobel R, Margolis J: Repetitive poisoning in children: A psychosocial study. *Pediatrics* 35:641, 1965.

Tandberg D, Diven B, Mcleod J: Ipecac-induced emesis versus gastric lavage: A controlled study in normal adults. *Am J Emerg Med* 4:205, 1986.

Walton W: An evaluation of the poison prevention packaging act. *Pediatrics* 69:363, 1982.

Acetaminophen Overdose

2

Definition

Amino-para-acetaminophen (APAP) is the most commonly used pediatric analgesic/antipyretic in the United States and is an ingredient in over 300 prescription and over-the-counter medications. Acute toxicity occurs when an adult ingests more than 10–20 g or a 2-year-old ingests more than 2 g. Alternatively, a nomogram can be used to relate a probable toxic dose to the APAP serum level at any specific time after ingestion; a toxic level is $\geq$ 200 μg/ml 4 hours post-ingestion.

Basic Science

There are three pathways for acetaminophen metabolism in the human: 25% of APAP is excreted unchanged, 71% is conjugated as the nontoxic glucuronide or sulfated derivative in the liver, and 4% is metabolized via the cytochrome P-450 mixed oxidase system in the liver, which utilizes glutathione to produce APAP-mercapturate. If glutathione stores are depleted by a large amount of available substrate as occurs in an acute ingestion, an intermediary reactive metabolite forms in excess, binds to liver cell proteins, and causes damage. Concurrent alcohol ingestion is protective in such instances as alcohol competes for the cytochrome P-450 system; drugs that induce the cytochrome P-450 system, such as phenobarbital, will predictably exacerbate APAP's toxic effects. Some studies suggest younger children divert a larger percentage of APAP to the glucuronide and sulfate conjugation pathways and are, therefore, relatively less susceptible to injurious effects of comparable doses of APAP.

Natural History

Clinical symptoms are insidious and nonspecific. Nausea, vomiting, hypothermia, diaphoresis, and anorexia occur in stage 1 about 7–14 hours after ingestion. By stage 2 at 24–48 hours these symptoms have resolved and liver damage, with elevated enzymes, bilirubin, and abnormal clotting studies occurs. Liver damage reaches a peak at 72–96 hours (stage 3) and recovery (stage 4) ensues by 7–8 days after ingestion.

Diagnosis

The diagnosis is easily confused with infectious hepatitis or Reye syndrome in a younger child, unless a careful history of previous medication use is taken. α-1-Antitrypsin deficiency also enters the differential diagnosis.

In suicide gestures or unclear circumstances, the diagnosis of polydrug ingestion must be considered and a toxic screen ordered. Plasma levels of APAP should always be obtained, but no sooner than 4 hours post-ingestion so that peak levels will not be underestimated. A plot of acetaminophen plasma levels versus time from ingestion gives a basis for the calculation of plasma levels associated with probable hepatic toxicity. Levels over 200 μg/ml 4 hours after ingestion, or over 50 μg/ml 12 hours after ingestion are associated with probable hepatic toxicity.

CASE ILLUSTRATION

A 15-year-old adolescent girl swallowed an unknown quantity of tablets from a nearly full 60-tablet bottle of APAP (325 mg acetaminophen/tablet) between 8:00 and 10:00 PM the evening before admission. Within 1 hour, she began to vomit but could not recall if tablets were in the vomitus. She went to school the following day without telling anyone of the incident, was noted to be in some distress by a teacher, and confessed the ingestion stating she was despondent over a fight with her boyfriend. In the emergency clinic, an acetaminophen level of 108 μg/ml was found at about 14 hours after ingestion. The physical examination was remarkable only for the patient's inappropriate elevated affect at the idea of being hospitalized. Liver function tests, blood gases, electrolytes, clotting studies, and blood glucose were normal at admission. NAC was administered at 140 mg/kg by mouth as a loading dose and then 70 mg/kg at 4-hour intervals for a total of 18 doses. By 36 hours postingestion, SGOT = 313 U/L, LDH = 296 U/L; by 60 hours SGOT = 688 U/L, SGPT = 2111 U/L, LDH = 109 U/L, ammonia = 106 mg/dl. By 110 hours postingestion, SGOT = 125 U/L, SGPT = 992 U/L, LDH = 109 U/L, ammonia = 67 mg/dl. The patient remained clinically asymptomatic and later received intensive psychiatric intervention.

QUESTION AND COMMENT

Why is the time factor particularly crucial in APAP overdose?

The antidote, NAC, must be given no later than 16 hours after ingestion to be effective in preventing liver cell damage from the reactive intermediary metabolite. NAC is nontoxic and can be administered when a toxic dose has been taken even before serum levels are known. However, most authorities suggest giving NAC even 24 hours postingestion, to give the patient the benefit of the doubt.

Treatment

Gastric decontamination should be attempted with ipecac and/or gastric lavage through a large bore catheter. If administration of the antidote, n-acetylcysteine (NAC), is delayed, 30–50 g of activated charcoal for a child and 100 g for an adult should be administered. Oral NAC should be given empirically if it is close to 16 hours after ingestion or if the serum APAP levels will not be available before that time. Repeated vomiting of NAC requires use of a nasoduodenal tube to facilitate antidote delivery.

CONTROVERSY

Hemodialysis has been recommended in massive overdoses of APAP although whether it is necessary for children is controversial since there are few known instances of long-term liver damage.

Use of NAC is not recommended in newborns; instead, exchange transfusion has been attempted with apparently satisfactory results.

Charcoal will bind acetaminophen 5- to 10-fold in excess by weight. Some authors suggest, however, that it may also interfere with the beneficial effects of NAC and should be avoided if that compound is available immediately.

Prognosis

The prognosis for children is excellent; long-term hepatic residua are almost unknown. For adults with massive overdose or a delay in therapy, there is a chance of chronic hepatitis or cirrhosis and the prognosis is more guarded.

REFERENCES

Levy G, Houston JB: Effect of activated charcoal on acetaminophen absorption. *Pediatrics* 58:432, 1976.

Peterson RG, Rumack BH: Age as a variable in acetaminophen overdose. *Arch Intern Med* 141:390, 1981.

Rumack BH, Peterson RC, Koch GG, et al: Acetaminophen overdose, 662 cases with evaluation of oral acetylcystein treatment. *Arch Intern Med* 141:380, 1981.

Rumack BH: Acetaminophen overdose in children and adolescents. *Pediatr Clin North Am* 33:691, 1986.

Substance Abuse 3

Definition

Substance abuse can be defined as the intentional introduction of a drug into the body for stimulation and pleasure. The spectrum of substance abuse extends from experimentation to "recreational" use to more habitual and dependent use. Besides the direct toxic effects of the drug, indirect effects on the health of the adolescent are just as important. Drug and alcohol use are implicated in many adolescent motor vehicle accidents, violent and aggressive behavior resulting in delinquency or homicide, suicide attempts, and poor school performance. Although many psychologic and social ramifications of such behavior exist, this chapter focuses on the toxicologic properties of a sample of the most commonly abused substances. The reader is referred to Section 2 for additional information on the psychiatric implications of drug abuse, and Section 4 for perinatal effects (Braude et al, 1987).

Epidemiology

Substance abuse is increasingly becoming a pediatric concern. Whereas previous efforts at curbing drug use were directed at college-aged students and young adults, experimentation now occurs in late childhood and early adolescence.

In a 1985 survey of high school seniors, 54% had used marijuana at some time, and 4.9% used it daily. Cocaine use in the past year was 13% among members of the high school class of 1985 (Kozel and Adams, 1986).

Diagnosis and Management

The diagnosis and management of substance abuse cases can be complicated by the erratic behavior of a patient under the influence of drugs who also is often mistrustful of health care workers and may not readily volunteer information. Suicidal patients may resist treatment and give misleading and unreliable information about what drugs they took. Polypharmacy and adulterated street drugs make the interpretation of clinical findings difficult (Table 25.5; see pp. 182).

Toxic screens of blood, urine, vomitus, and gastric washings can aid detection of opiates, phenothiazines, amphetamines, barbiturates, antidepressants, ethanol, phencyclidine, and some sedative-hypnotics; they should be routinely ordered on any child or adolescent presenting with an unexplained change in consciousness or other symptoms that might be compatible with drug use. The reader is referred to the first chapter in this section for further details in the management of the unknown poisoning. The diagnosis and management of representative drug abuse syndromes is presented below.

OPIATES

Although opiate use is uncommon in children and adolescents, appropriate management of a patient suffering from acute or chronic opiate effects or the abstinence syndrome requires recognition of the medical and toxicologic implications of these drugs.

This class of drugs inhibits CNS and peripheral pain receptors to produce impressive analgesic effects. Depression of the CNS is manifested by drowsiness or coma, suppression of the cough reflex, hypothermia, hypotension, and pupillary constriction. Constipation, secondary amenorrhea, and increased vagal tone with bradyarrhythmias, atrial and ventricular premature contractions, and heart block are also seen. The typical withdrawal syndrome is associated with anxiety, yawning, lacrimation, rhinorrhea, mydriasis, nausea, vomiting, myalgias, and hypertension.

Heroin street use puts the adolescent at high risk for a number of medical complications related both to the pharmacologic effects of the drug and to the route of administration. Street heroin is usually only 1–5% pure and is often cut with toxic agents such as talc, quinine, procaine, strychnine, or phencyclidine. Nasal inhalation ("snorting") can result in necrosis of the septum. Subcutaneous, intradermal, and intramuscular injection of diluted heroin ("skin-popping") is associated with scarring, cellulitis ("puffy hand syndrome"), and abscess formation. Intravenous use ("mainlining") is associated with thrombophlebitis, inadvertent foreign body introduction, and embolization phenomena. Needles or other drug paraphernalia shared among addicts may account for the spread of human immunodeficiency virus. Hepatitis, spread in a similar fashion, is also endemic among addicts. Death may be due to a pharmacologic overdose, an allergic-type reaction, synergism of multiple drug effects, pulmonary edema, fatal arrhythmias, and/or septic/embolic complications.

Treatment

Treatment of the acute opiate overdose relies on naloxone (1.2–2.0 mg intravenously). The patient should be carefully monitored with repeated doses of naloxone given as necessary to control symptoms. In overdoses of methadone, such monitoring may be necessary for up to 72 hours. Detoxification may be safely accomplished by stabilizing the patient clinically with dependence-equivalent doses of methadone and then slowly weaning him over a number of days by tapering the doses.

STIMULANTS

Amphetamines

Acute signs of amphetamine abuse include dilated pupils, tachycardia, and insomnia. Chronic use is associated with weight loss, anxiety, and suicidal behavior. Both amphetamine overdose and abstinence syndromes are associated with an hallucinatory state marked by aggression and paranoia. Treatment includes abrupt discontinuation of abuse, sedatives, and a quiet controlled environment.

Cocaine

Cocaine, also known on the street as "nose," "coke," or "flake," is a white powdery drug processed from the leaves of Erythroxylon Coca trees native to Bolivia and Peru. It can be further refined by heating and extraction, called "free basing," into a thick brownish liquid. This residue can be further purified and dried into the brownish-white nuggets called "crack." The drug can be absorbed from mucous membranes, by ingestion, by injection of the aqueous solution, or by smoking the free-based derivative. Usually the street drug has been cut with additives such as sugar or novocaine to reduce its potency and increase the seller's profit. Often it is used with other substances to heighten or prolong its effects. Intravenous use of cocaine and heroin together, known as "speedballing," has grown in popularity.

The illicit use of cocaine, by nasal inhalation ("snorting"), injection, or smoking, results in its systemic effects. The habitual snorting of cocaine produces vasoconstriction of the nasal septum with eventual scab formation and perforation. The drug's CNS effects are similar to those of amphetamines with the user appearing agitated, hyperactive, and euphoric. The "high" is of short duration, less than 20 minutes, followed by negative sensations of depression. Chronic users or those with advanced toxicity associated with poisoning by the drug may experience paranoia, emotional lability, seizures, and even tactile ("cocaine bugs") or visual ("snow lights") hallucinations. Chronic users may develop behavioral changes including confused thinking, restlessness, mild agitation, paranoia, and repetitive behaviors such as scratching or lip-biting. Nausea, vomiting, and diarrhea are other common side effects. Withdrawal from heavy use may precipitate extreme paranoia, depression, irritability, or suicidal ideation. The risk of cardiovascular effects is present for both the one-time and the experienced user. Because of its vasoconstrictive effects, cocaine can cause angina, dysrhythmias, myocardial infarction with constriction band

Table 25.5
Symptoms and Signs of Drug Abuse[1]

Drug	Acute Intoxication and Overdose	Withdrawal Syndrome
Hallucinogens		
LSD[2]; psilocybin; mescaline; PCP[3]; STP[4]	Pupils dilated (normal or small with PCP); BP elevated; heart rate increased; tendon reflexes hyperactive; temperature elevated; face flushed; euphoria, anxiety or panic; paranoid thought disorder; sensorium often clear; affect inappropriate; illusions; time and visual distortions; visual hallucinations; depersonalization; with PCP cyclic coma or extreme hyperactivity, drooling, blank stare, mutism, amnesia, analgesia, nystagmus (sometimes vertical), gait ataxia, muscle rigidity, impulsive, often violent, behavior, rarely intracranial hemorrhage	None
Cannabis Group		
Marijuana; hashish; THC[5]; hash oil	Pupils unchanged; conjunctiva injected; BP decreased on standing; heart rate increased; increased appetite; euphoria, anxiety; sensorium often clear, dreamy, fantasy state; time-space distortions; hallucinations rare	Nonspecific symptoms including anorexia, nausea, insomnia, restlessness, irritability
Narcotics		
Heroin; morphine; codeine; meperidine; methadone; hydromorphone; opium; pentazocine; propoxyphene	Pupils constricted (may be dilated with meperidine or extreme hypoxia); respiration depressed to absent with cyanosis; BP decreased, sometimes shock; temperature reduced; reflexes dimished to absent; stupor or coma; pulmonary edema; constipation; convulsions with propoxyphene or meperidine	Pupils dilated; pulse rapid; goose-flesh; muscle jerks; "flu" syndrome; vomiting, diarrhea; tremulousness, yawning, "yen sleep"
CNS Sedatives		
Barbiturates; chlordiazepoxide; diazepam; flurazepam; glutethimide; meprobamate; methaqualone; others	Pupils usually unchanged or small (but dilated with glutethimide or in severe poisoning); BP decreased, sometimes shock; respiration depressed; tendon reflexes depressed; drowsiness or coma; nystagmus; confusion; ataxia, slurred speech, delirium; convulsions or hyper-irritability with methaqualone overdosage; serious poisoning rare with benzodiazepines alone	Tremulousness; insomnia; sweating; fever, clonic blink reflex; cardiovascular collapse; agitation; delirium; hallucinations; disorientation; late convulsions; fever; shock
CNS Stimulants		
Amphetamines; cocaine; methylphenidate; phenmetrazine; phenylpropanolamine; most anti-obesity drugs	Pupils dilated and reactive; respiration shallow; BP elevated; heart rate increased; tendon reflexes hyperactive; temperature elevated; cardiac arrhythmias; dry mouth; sweating; tremors; sensorium hyperacute or confused; paranoid ideation; hallucinations; impulsivity; hyperactivity; stereotypy; convulsions; coma; exhaustion	Muscular aches; abdominal pain; chills, tremors, voracious hunger; prolonged sleep, lack of energy; profound psychologic depression, sometimes suicidal
Anticholinergics		
Atropine; belladonna; henbane; scopolamine; trihexyphenidyl; benztropine mesylate; tricyclic antidepressants	Pupils dilated and fixed; heart rate increased; temperature elevated; decreased bowel sounds; drowsiness or coma; flushed, dry skin and mucous membranes; sensorium clouded; amnesia; disorientation, visual hallucinations; body image alterations; confusion	Gastrointestinal and musculoskeletal symptoms, mania and delirium after tricyclic antidepressant withdrawal

[1]Reproduced with permission from *Med Lett* 27:77, 1985. Mixed intoxications produce complex combinations of signs and symptoms.
[2]LSD (d-lysergic acid diethylamide)
[3]PCP (phencyclidine)
[4]STP (2, 5-dimethoxy-4-methylamphetamine)
[5]THC (delta-9-tetrahydrocannabinol)

necrosis, and sudden death. Related increases in pulse and blood pressure can cause acute heart failure or stroke.

Treatment of cocaine toxicity usually requires only supportive care and reassurance. Diazepam can be used for extreme anxiety or seizures; antiarrhythmic agents and antihypertensives may also be necessary.

HALLUCINOGENS

Marijuana

Marijuana (cannabis, "joint," "reefer," "hashish") is the most commonly used illicit drug in the United States. When smoked or ingested, the effects of the active component (tetrahydrocannabinol) of this easily grown plant include cardiovascular and CNS changes. The most marked physiologic change induced by cannabis is an increase in pulse rate. Dilation of peripheral vessels is responsible for the "red eye" conjunctivitis commonly associated with its use. The CNS effects include mild euphoric behavior, a sense of temporal disintegration, drowsiness, and deterioration in reaction time and motor coordination. There has been recent concern that marijuana contaminated with herbicides such as paraquat can produce irreversible restrictive pulmonary disease. Marijuana may also sometimes harbor salmonellae which can result in diarrhea. Marijuana cigarettes laced with phencyclidine or cocaine may produce more erratic and violent behavior.

Lysergic Acid Diethylamide (LSD)

LSD ("acid") has waned somewhat in its popularity among youth but is still a significant problem. It is the archetype for a number of different chemicals, plants, and mushrooms with hallucinatory properties, including psilocybin, mescaline, peyote, etc. Acute effects include visual and auditory hallucinations, disorganized or confused thinking, temporal disintegration, and preoccupation with internal or external stimuli. Chronic effects include changes in personality, LSD-induced psychosis, visual and/or auditory flashbacks, and other behavioral disturbances. LSD has teratogenic potential by inducing breaks in chromosomal DNA. Treatment consists mostly of "talking down" the patient in a quiet and controlled environment. Sedatives such as diazepam or chlorpromazine are sometimes necessary to treat panic attacks ("bad trips").

Phencyclidine

Phencyclidine ("PCP," "angel dust") has many of the hallucinatory properties of LSD, but more often it is associated with feelings of paranoia and aggression with consequent violent behavior. Patients have committed suicide or homicide under the influence of PCP. Unlike the treatment of LSD overdoses, PCP users should not be "talked down" as this is liable to increase their feelings of persecution and may lead to even more violent outbursts. Observation of the patient in a quiet environment is suggested with treatment of seizures by intravenous diazepam and of severe agitation with haloperidol or diazepam.

SEDATIVE-HYPNOTICS

Barbiturates

Barbiturates are used clinically for their sedative and anticonvulsant properties. Their CNS effects include a "disinhibition euphoria," drowsiness, slurred speech, slowed reaction time, ataxia, delirium, confusion, and, in overdose, convulsions and coma. Other physiologic effects include pupillary constriction, hypotension, and respiratory depression or apnea. Behavioral effects include disregard for personal appearance, paranoid thought processes, disinhibited aggressiveness or sexual behavior, labile mood swings, and suicidal thoughts. Barbiturate addiction remains relatively rare among adolescents. Chronic barbiturate use may cause progression of the signs and behavior described above, with additional neurologic effects including nystagmus, vertigo, diplopia, decreased deep tendon reflexes, and hypotonia. Withdrawal symptoms and signs may be heralded by delirium or convulsions, and may include sweating, shivering, and loss of short-term memory.

Treatment of acute barbiturate overdose includes CPR when necessary. Where the patient is comatose, a cuffed endotracheal tube should be used and oxygen administered. Once the airway is established and aspiration can be prevented, gastric lavage, repetitive doses of activated charcoal, and catharsis with an instilled agent such as sodium sulfate are standard decontamination procedures. Supportive therapy with fluids and vasopressors is indicated to maintain hydration and blood pressure; continuous monitoring in an intensive care setting is advisable. Forced diuresis and alkalinization of the urine are of value with longer-acting barbiturate overdoses. Treatment of the barbiturate abstinence syndrome requires phenobarbital to establish the tolerance level and stabilize the patient; the phenobarbital is then weaned over a 10-day period by constant decrements in dosage.

Glutethimide (Doriden)

Glutethimide, although first advertised as a sedative alternative to barbiturates without the danger of side-effects or addiction, has been shown to be both dangerous in overdose and capable of producing a dependency syndrome. At recommended doses its main effect is to induce sleep within 20–30 minutes by depressing the central and autonomic nervous systems. Toxic effects of an overdose include anticholinergic effects, convulsions, hypotensive shock, and coma. The abstinence syndrome includes hypertension, tremulousness, delirium, and convulsions. The mortality rate of toxic combinations of glutethimide and alcohol may be as high as 87%. Treatment includes decontamination with ipecac and then lavage and repetitive activated charcoal administration. Supportive care with monitoring of fluid status and the judicious use of vasopressors to support blood pressure is recommended. Hemodialysis has been shown to remove excess drug but its clinical utility has been questioned.

Benzodiazepines

Benzodiazepines include diazepam (Valium), chlordiazepoxide (Librium), lorazepam (Ativan), flurazepam (Dalmane). The benzodiazepines are among the most frequently prescribed antianxiety and hypnotic medications. Selected drugs within this group also have anticonvulsant and muscle relaxant effects. The toxic effects of these drugs alone are uncommon but include drowsiness, ataxia, weakness, and coma. An abstinence syndrome of agitation, anxiety and muscle spasm has been recently described in long-term users. In combination with alcohol or other depressants, the benzodiazepines can produce CNS depression and respiratory arrest.

INHALANTS

Glue and Hydrocarbon Sniffing

Several types of commercially available adhesive glues contain volatile compounds that cause giddiness and lightheadedness when inhaled in concentrated amounts. Gasoline or solvents, such as toluene, can also cause a brief "high" when inhaled in a plastic bag or enclosed space. Such practices, common among early adolescents and preadolescents, are associated with dangerous side effects on the heart, brain, and liver. Cardiac arrhythmias and sudden death have been reported from sniffing halogenated hydrocarbons. CNS damage with seizures, coma, and encephalopathy has also been observed. Toluene, carbon tetrachloride, and other solvents can also cause chemical hepatitis leading to cirrhosis as well as acute renal failure and coagulopathies.

Nitrites

Butyl and isobutyl nitrites, common ingredients in room deodorizers, and amyl nitrite inhalers are abused chiefly by homosexuals in attempts to prolong sexual erection and orgasm. These agents cause clinically significant cyanosis and methemoglobinemia resulting in headaches, shortness of breath, and other symptoms of hypoxia. Diagnosis is suspected by the chocolate appearance of blood and confirmed by elevated blood levels of methemoglobin (normally $< 1\%$). Treatment consists of administration of oxygen and intravenous methylene blue at 1 mg/kg body weight.

TOBACCO

Cigarette smoking is usually initiated in the preadolescent or adolescent child so that a history of dependency is often established by early adulthood. Cigarette smoke contains a complex array of gaseous and particulate chemical toxins that are associated with important long-term clinical effects including chronic bronchitis and lung cancer. Smokers have chronically elevated levels of carbon monoxide in their blood. Nicotine, one active ingredient in smoke, is associated with cardiovascular and sympathetic nervous system effects including hypertension, flushing, and precipitation of angina.

Snuff and chewing tobacco have become increasingly popular among adolescents. In a survey in Wisconsin, 22% of senior high school boys were regular users of smokeless tobacco (CDC, 1986). A strong association has been reported between snuff use and oral cancer. Potent carcinogens, aromatic hydrocarbons, radiation-emitting polonium, and nitrosamines are found in currently available snuff. Buccal or gingival mucosa tissue may show alterations in color, texture, contour and leukoplakia, a white wrinkled patch on the oral mucosa which is a precancerous lesion. Blisters or other lesions may appear on the lips or gums. Exposure to nicotine is comparable to that from cigarettes. Thus, those who use smokeless tobacco are at increased risk of hypertension, peripheral vascular disease, and increased fetal morbidity and mortality. Prevention of this significant health risk is of high priority and is hindered by the commercial endorsement of products by professional athletes who indulge during competition (Connolly et al, 1986).

ALCOHOL

Alcohol is the leading substance of abuse in the United States. Its effects in children and adolescents are similar to those in adults and include feelings of giddiness, irrational behavior, impaired judgment and reaction time, and drowsiness. Hypoglycemia is the notable effect in infants and young children. Acute gastritis, pancreatitis, and CNS depression may be side effects in adolescents. Alcohol dependency is increasingly common among early adolescents, although liver damage is rarely documented and is reversible if alcohol intake is prohibited thereafter.

REFERENCES

Braude MC, Szeto HH, Kuhn CM, et al: Perinatal effects of drugs of abuse (symposium summary) *Fed Proc* 46:2446, 1987.

CDC: Use of smokeless tobacco—Wisconsin. *MMWR* 35:641, 1986.

Connolly GN, Winn DM, Hecht SS, et al: The reemergence of smokeless tobacco. *N Engl J Med* 314:1020, 1986.

Fish S, DaCamara C: Glutethimide. *Clin Toxicol Rev* 9:1, 1986.

Khantzian EJ, McKenna GJ: Acute toxic and withdrawal reactions associated with drug use and abuse. *Ann Intern Med* 90:361, 1979.

Kozel NF, Adams EH: Epidemiology of drug abuse: An overview. *Science* 234:970, 1986.

Kulberg A: Substance abuse: Clinical identification and management. *Pediatr Clin North Am* 33:325, 1986.

Diagnosis and management of acute drug abuse actions. *Med Lett* 25:85, 1983.

Lead Poisoning (Plumbism)

4

Definition

Lead poisoning is present when venous whole blood levels are over 25 μg/dl or erythrocyte protoporphyrin (EP) is greater than 35 μg/dl. This definition does not require the presence of symptoms.

Basic Science

Children absorb more lead and are more sensitive to its effects than are adults. Whereas adults may absorb 10% of ingested lead, children absorb up to 50%. Moreover, the coexistence of protein, iron, or calcium deficiencies may enhance the uptake of lead and may also potentiate its toxic effects in children. Lead is stored in the blood, the soft tissues (liver and kidneys) and the bones. While more than 94% of the total body burden of lead in adults is sequestered in bone, in children, because of their lack of hard dense bone tissue, only about 64% of body lead is stored there. This leaves a higher percentage of lead in the blood and soft tissues, the compartments considered responsible for lead's acute toxic effects.

The target organs affected by lead in high concentrations include the hematopoietic system, the kidneys, and the central nervous system (CNS). Lead is a biochemical poison that interferes with cellular enzymes, membrane function, and oxidative metabolism. At levels as low as 10 μg/dl, lead inhibits red blood cell d-amino levulinic acid dehydrase (dALA-D), which is important for the conjugation of levulinic acid into porphobilinogen in the heme synthesis pathway. The accumulation of free protoporphyrin in red cells ensues; a hypochromic, microcytic anemia also develops from disordered heme synthesis. Lead also acts on brain adenylate cyclase, affecting oxidative metabolism at blood levels as low as 20 μg/dl. It interferes with mitochondrial membrane function in red cells and the cytochrome P-450 system of oxidative metabolism in liver cells.

Epidemiology

Approximately 4% of United States children 6 months to 5 years of age have elevated blood lead levels (≥ 30 μg/dl; Mahaffey et al, 1982). The ideal lead level would be 0. The prevalence of elevated blood lead levels is 12% in black children and 2% in whites. Lead is ubiquitous in the environment; being present in the air, principally due to automobile exhaust, and also contaminating many city water supplies. Ingestion of lead primarily occurs among toddlers 1–3 years old who are oral in their development and demonstrate pica behaviors (the ingestion of nonfood items). Lead-based paint or plaster found in older houses and peeling from the walls is the most common source. Sandblasting can increase absorption of lead by aerosol. Dime-sized chips of lead-based paint may contain as much as 100 mg of lead. Sometimes significant exposure can occur from the ingestion of lead-containing soil, newsprint, or household dust. Even dirty workclothes from parents who are exposed to lead at smelters or in battery or paint factories can pose a health hazard to their children (Baker et al, 1977). Rarely, acid fruit juices kept in ceramic pitchers with lead paint glazes can leach enough lead into the juice to cause acute, and even fatal, poisoning. Burning car batteries can cause massive lead intoxication from the inhalation of fumes. More commonly, repetitive ingestion of small doses of lead leads to asymptomatic lead intoxication. The prevalence is highest among the urban poor; plumbism is often associated with malnutrition, failure to thrive, and/or other nutrient deficiencies (e.g., calcium, vitamin D, zinc, iron).

Diagnosis

Table 25.6 summarizes the clinical findings in mild, moderate, and severe lead poisoning.

Although the free erythrocyte protoporphyrin level (FEP) is a good screening device for asymptomatic lead poisoning, iron deficiency, porphyria, and other disorders of disrupted heme synthesis may also give elevated FEP values. Moreover, there is a lag time of 7–14 days before ingested lead is reflected as an increase in the serum FEP value. In asymptomatic children, elevated FEP levels (greater than 35 μg/dl and often in the 500- to 750-μg/dl range) should be confirmed by a whole blood lead determination (greater than 25 μg/dl in children). The diagnosis is supported by the finding of the recent ingestion of lead paint chips in an abdominal radiograph, disturbed osteogenesis or so-called "lead lines" in the metaphyseal area of long bone and pelvic films, and/or basophilic stippling of red cells with the hypochromic, microcytic anemia on blood smear. Asymptomatic exposure to chronic low levels of lead has been linked to hyperactivity, irritability, disturbed learning, and fine-motor dysfunction in children (Needleman et al, 1979).

Symptomatic lead poisoning without encephalopathy is characterized by anorexia, lethargy, sporadic vomiting and acute intermittent abdominal pain, constipation, and listlessness. Renal toxicity is occasionally seen, mimicking the Fanconi syndrome of hyperaminoaciduria, glycosuria, and hyperphosphaturia, all of which are potentially reversible. Clinical findings are often associated with blood lead levels

Table 25.6
Clinical and Laboratory Evidence of Lead Intoxication[1]

Mild	Moderate	Severe
Clinical		
Lead exposure, usually to soil or dust	Probably paint exposure	Pica for paint
Asymptomatic	Predisposing iron deficiency	Secondary iron deficiency
May be predisposing iron deficiency	Positive family history	Abdominal pain, irritability, lethargy, fever, hepatosplenomegaly
Cognitive sequelae	Usually asymptomatic	Ataxia, seizures, coma, increased intracranial pressure, neurological sequelae
	Loss of appetite and behavior changes	
	Behavioral and cognitive sequelae	
Laboratory		
Lead levels in whole blood 25–49 μg/dl	Lead levels 49–79 μg/dl	Lead levels ≥ 80 μg/ml
EP in whole blood 35–125 μg/dl	EP in whole blood 125–250 μg/dl	EP levels > 250 μg/dl
KUB and knee x-rays usually negative	KUB x-rays negative	KUB x-rays positive
Serum iron/iron-binding capacity ≤ 16 μg/ml	Knee x-rays positive	Knee films positive
Serum ferritin < 40 μg/ml	Serum iron/iron-binding capacity ≤ 16%	Serum iron/iron-binding capacity ≤ 16%
CBC normal	Ferritin < 20 μg/dl	Ferritin < 10 μg/dl
Lead mobilization test: ≤ 1 μg Pb/mg EDTA/24 hours	CBC shows mild anemia	CBC shows basophilic stippling, anemia
	Lead mobilization test: ≅1 μg Pb/mg EDTA/24 hours	Decreased nerve conduction time
		CT scan shows increased intracranial pressure
		Aminoaciduria, glycosuria
		Lead mobilization test: > 1 μg Pb/mg EDTA/24 hours

[1]Reproduced with permission from Graef J, Cone TE: *Manual of Pediatric Therapeutics*, 3rd edition, Boston, Little, Brown & Co, 1985.

greater than 70 μg/dl but may be seen at lower levels as well.

Lead encephalopathy is characterized by abnormal irritability and changed behaviors, the subtle loss of recently acquired motor skills, ataxia, alternating lucidity and delirium, seizures, and coma. The differential diagnosis includes infectious and other toxic causes of altered consciousness, other medical and surgical causes of the acute abdomen, and porphyria. Increased intracranial pressure precludes diagnosis by lumbar puncture; the diagnosis is confirmed by the discovery of blood lead levels above 70 μg/dl (often greater than 100 μg/dl).

Treatment

The treatment of plumbism depends on the child's total lead burden, the duration and dose of the exposure, the presence of clinical symptoms, and social considerations. Chemical chelation, which depletes body tissues and enhances excretion of lead, is the mainstay of therapy. 2,3-Dimercapto-1-propanol (British antilewisite, BAL) and calcium sodium edathamil (CaNaEDTA) are the chelators of choice in lead poisoning. Penicillamine, although approved only as an investigational drug for use in children, also has value as the only oral agent capable of increasing the excretion of lead.

TREATMENT OF ASYMPTOMATIC CHILDREN

If a child is asymptomatic and the blood lead is 25–50 μg/dl with an FEP > 35 μg/dl, the decision to treat should be based on a CaNaEDTA provocation test. In this test, the urinary excretion of lead is divided by the amount of CaNaEDTA given to obtain a "lead excretion ratio." If this index is greater than 0.7, the test is positive and a 5-day chelation regimen as described below is given. If the test is > 0.6 but < 0.7, 3 days of chelation should be administered and the test repeated in 2–3 months. Therapy is designed to reduce blood lead levels to less than 25 μg/dl; blood lead should be monitored biweekly to monthly and a 5-day chelation cycle repeated should elevated lead levels recur. Renal, hepatic, and electrolyte values should be monitored during therapy; and treatment of concurrent iron deficiencies should be undertaken to depress lead absorption through the gut.

ENVIRONMENTAL MANAGEMENT AND FOLLOW-UP SURVEILLANCE

Management of confirmed cases of childhood lead poisoning must include removal of lead from the child's environment as well as chelation therapy. The reintroduction of a treated child into the same lead-containing environment will only result in a recurrence of the plumbism; therefore all cases should be reported to public health authorities. Lead poisoning has been associated with poor families living in dilapidated housing who may be mobile and difficult to reach, which complicates treatment compliance and follow-up care. Surveillance of urban areas dominated by pre-World War 2 housing in poor condition should be mandated and provisions for the removal of lead should be legislated without penalty to the family or landlord. Parents must be vigilant in their attempts to curb the child's pica behaviors. Follow-up tracking and blood lead determinations of a child who has been treated for lead poisoning should continue at weekly intervals after chelation therapy for the first month, at monthly intervals over the next 6 months, and every 3 months until the child is 6 years old.

REFERENCES

Baker E, Folland D, Taylor T, et al: Lead poisoning in children of lead workers. *N Engl J Med* 296:260, 1977.

CDC: Lead poisoning-associated death from Asian Indian folk remedies—Florida. *MMWR* 33:643, 1984.

Chisolm J: Management of increased lead absorption and lead poisoning in children. *N Engl J Med* 289:1016, 1973.

Committee on Environmental Hazards: Statement on Child Lead Poisoning. *Pediatrics* 79:457, 1987.

Landrigan PJ, Graef JW: Pediatric lead poisoning in 1987: The silent epidemic continues. *Pediatrics* 79:582, 1987.

Lansdown R, Yule W: *Lead Toxicity: History and Environmental Impact.* Baltimore, Johns Hopkins University Press, 1986.

Mahaffey KR, Annest JL, Roberts J, et al: National estimates of blood lead levels. United States 1976-1980: Association with selected demographic and socioeconomic factors. *N Engl J Med* 307:573, 1982.

Needleman H, Gunnoe C, Leviton A, et al: Deficits in psychologic and classroom performance of children with elevated dentine lead levels. *N Engl J Med* 300:689, 1979.

Piomelli S, Rosen JF, Chisolm JJ, et al: Management of childhood lead poisoning. *J Pediatr* 105:523, 1984.

Salicylate Poisoning (Salicylism) 5

Definition

Acute salicylism occurs at ingested doses of aspirin greater than 150 mg/kg. Chronic salicylism occurs in children who take large doses of aspirin daily (e.g., for arthritis) and suffer untoward effects from changes in dosage or from side effects of the drug. An association between prior ingestion of salicylates for viral syndromes and later development of the Reye hepatoencephalopathy in children has also recently been documented.

Basic Science

Salicylate in overdose is a potent cellular toxin. It uncouples oxidative phosphorylation, interferes with the Krebs cycle and carbohydrate metabolism, and stimulates the central respiratory center. These actions drive an inefficient and raised cellular metabolism, induce hyperglycemia or hypoglycemia, cause hyperventilation, and promote the accumulation of organic acids in the blood. The resulting acidemia raises the level of the nonionized species of salicylate, which facilitates penetration of the drug across cellular membranes and into brain where it damages neurons and lowers cerebral glucose levels. Salicylates also interfere with prostaglandins and platelet-associated enzymes, contributing to platelet dysfunction and a bleeding diathesis. Local irritative effects on gastric mucosa can contribute to abdominal pain, bleeding, and gastritis.

Epidemiology

Despite a decline in incidence in recent years, attributable to the use of child-resistant containers and packaging regulations concerning the number and strength of aspirin tablets in bottles, salicylates are still an important cause of accidental childhood and intentional adolescent poisoning. The Poison Prevention Packaging Safety Act of 1972 resulted in a 56% decline in the incidence of acute aspirin ingestions over the next 6 years and a 72% decline in the number of salicylate-related deaths over the same period. Nevertheless, salicylate poisonings are commonly seen in children whose parents (or physicians) incorrectly calculate the therapeutic dosage. Aspirin overdose, often in combination with other analgesics or alcohol, is also a common vehicle for suicide gestures by adolescents.

Diagnosis

Symptoms of salicylate poisoning depend on the dose taken, the weight of the child, and whether the poisoning is acute or is the result of a chronic therapeutic overdosage. Doses less than 150 mg/kg are not usually associated with toxicity; 150- to 300-mg/kg doses produce mild to moderate toxicity; 300–500 mg/kg are life-threatening. The clinician should first obtain an accurate history of the ingestion, perform a physical examination with particular attention to the respiratory and neurologic systems and vital signs, and draw blood for a salicylate level. Blood levels fall after 6 hours.

Levels of 50 mg/dl or higher and the presence of symptoms are generally indications for hospitalization of the child. The usual clinical manifestations of acute salicylism are referable to the respiratory, gastrointestinal, and central nervous systems.

Deep, rapid (Kussmaul type) respirations, an increased body temperature, nausea, and vomiting are among the first symptoms. Although respiratory alkalosis has been described in experimental situations, the development of a metabolic acidosis with a normal or increased anion gap is clinically more important in children. Hypokalemia, hyper- or hyponatremia, and hypoprothrombinemia are common. Direct toxic effects on liver and kidney function are sometimes seen.

An altered consciousness, lethargy, seizures, or coma reflect cerebral edema and serious toxicity. Progressive neurologic deterioration in the face of decreasing serum salicylate levels 24–48 hours after ingestion has been attributed to entrapment of nonionized salicylate molecules in the cerebrospinal fluid when the blood pH has been alkalinized to enhance clearance of the ionized species. Disproportionately higher cerebral salicylate levels cause subsequent disrupted cellular metabolism, lowered cerebral glucose levels, and brain swelling (Dove and Jones, 1982).

While dehydration is the rule, direct effects of salicylate on lung vessels and tissue fluid/ion shifts can cause fluid retention and precipitate pulmonary edema in up to 10% of cases of salicylate intoxication (Fisher et al, 1985). Thus, central venous monitoring and careful fluid calculations are important aspects of the management of serious poisonings.

Treatment

Since there is no specific antidote for salicylate, treatment is generally supportive. Decontamination with ipecac and/or gastric lavage with 5% sodium bicarbonate solution and administration of activated charcoal and catharsis are all recommended to prevent further drug absorption.

Since acidosis facilitates entry of salicylates into the brain, it must be aggressively corrected with sodium bicarbonate. Salicylates are cleared from the body by renal (75%) and oxidation (25%) processes. Alkalinization of the urine (2–3 mEq/kg sodium bicarbonate every 4–6 hours) and forced diuresis can improve clearance of the drug. Raising the urinary ph > 7.5 can lower the salicylate half-life from 24–36 to 6–8 hours. Monitoring of electrolytes, acid-base balance, glucose levels, calcium levels, and input/output adequacy is important. Supplemental potassium and glucose should be given based on laboratory abnormalities and daily requirements.

Prolonged prothrombin times should be corrected with vitamin K. Hyperthermia should be treated with cooling blankets or sponging. Mannitol (1 g/kg of a 20% solution intravenously) and dexamethasone (2–3 mg every 6 hours intravenously) may be necessary should signs of cerebral edema occur.

Doses of aspirin in excess of 500 mg/kg and evidence of CNS dysfunction (i.e., seizures or coma) or shock are indications for the use of peritoneal or hemodialysis to enhance clearance.

REFERENCES

Done A: Salicylate intoxication: Significance of measurements of salicylate in blood in cases of acute ingestion. *Pediatrics* 26:800, 1960.

Dove D, Jones T: Delayed coma associated with salicylate intoxication. *J Pediatr* 100:493, 1982.

Fisher C, Albertson T, Foulke G: Salicylate induced pulmonary edema: Clinical characteristics in children. *Am J Emerg Med* 3:33, 1985.

Henry J, Volans G: Analgesic poisoning I: Salicylates. *Br Med J* 289:820, 1984.

Hill J: Salicylate intoxication. *N Engl J Med* 288:1110, 1973.

Pierce A: Salicylate poisoning. *Pediatrics* 54:342, 1974.

Snodgrass W: Salicylate toxicity. *Pediatr Clin North Am* 33:381, 1986.

Caustic Ingestions

6

Definition

Caustic materials include acids and alkali that are capable of eroding mucous membranes.

Basic Science

The chemical action of an alkaline agent on a mucosal surface results in liquefaction necrosis which continues to penetrate into the deeper layers of tissue. By contrast, burns with an acidic agent produce coagulation necrosis which prevents such deeper penetration. Both types of chemical burns are associated with an exuberant inflammatory response with later granulation, organization and fibroblast response, and scarring.

Epidemiology

Caustic ingestions account for an estimated 5000–15,000 injuries in the United States annually. These poisonings most frequently occur in toddlers 12–36 months old and involve household products, including alkalis (such as lye, ammonia, Clinitest tablets, oven cleaners, and liquid drain cleaners containing sodium or potassium hydroxide) and acids (such as battery acid, toilet bowl cleaners, swimming pool cleaners, photographic chemicals, and furniture stripping agents). "Button"-type batteries commonly used in portable radios and cameras also contain a 40–45% solution of potassium hydroxide as an electrolyte. Once ingested, such batteries can corrode, come apart, or leak the alkaline chemical, causing burns along the gastrointestinal tract.

Natural History

Between 8 and 20% of children with a history of caustic agent ingestion but no evidence of oropharyngeal burns will be found to have esophageal lesions at endoscopy.

Although either acid or alkali can cause severe burns, strictures, a rare occurrence overall, are more commonly associated with alkali ingestions. The natural history of the injury is: (1) an acute phase with dysphagia lasting about 3 days; (2) an intermediate phase of resolution of symptoms lasting 2–3 weeks; and finally (3) a chronic, obstructive phase with return of the dysphagia and occasional progression to obstruction. Other complications include esophageal ulceration and rupture, gastrointestinal ulceration, secondary arterial rupture and exsanguination, and a completely dysfunctional esophagus as well as perforation, mediastinitis, pericarditis, chemical gastritis and peritonitis, pulmonary edema, and laryngeal obstruction.

Diagnosis

Commonly, victims of caustic ingestions have specific symptoms or signs including vomiting, refusal to drink, excessive drooling, rise in temperature, stridor, dysphagia, and/or abdominal pains. Neither clinical symptoms nor the presence or absence of oropharyngeal lesions can predict the presence of esophageal lesions and whether strictures will form.

CASE ILLUSTRATION

O.G. was a 15-month-old male who, when playing, found a can of "Red Devil Lye" in his home and drank an unknown quantity. The child spat out some material and was taken to the local hospital. He did not vomit; however, his lips and mouth were erythematous and had begun to swell within 30 minutes of the ingestion. On further evaluation he was noted to have tachypnea, copious oral secretions, swelling of the oral mucosa, superficial burns of the oropharynx, and mildly stridorous breathing. A chest radiograph was normal. He was immediately taken to the operating room where laryngoscopy, esophagoscopy, and nasotracheal intubation were performed. A silk suture was placed from the gastrostomy site up through the esophagus for future retrograde dilatations. The lye ingestion had caused grade 2 and 3 burns of the lips, gingiva, hard and soft palate, epiglottis, hypopharynx, entire esophagus, and cardiac region of the stomach. Steroids and antibiotics were instituted; the edema subsided over the next few days. The child developed a high fever on the fourth hospital day and a repeat chest radiograph showed bilateral upper lobe infiltrates consistent with aspiration pneumonia and air leaks. A chest tube was placed and intravenous antibiotics were continued. The child's condition steadily improved over the following 2 weeks and extubation was successful. Retrograde bougienage was begun daily for 2 weeks and continued twice weekly over a 3-month period. An adequate esophageal lumen admitting a 40F bougie was achieved, there was no evidence of further stricture formation, and therapy was discontinued with careful monitoring of the child over the following 3 years.

QUESTION AND COMMENT

How could such a massive burn result from a brief ingestion?

Liquid lye cleansers have been concentrated so that their high specific gravity pulls them through water "down to where the clogged drain is." Unfortunately this high specific gravity also pulls them farther through the gastrointestinal tract, exposing a larger mucosal surface to their more concentrated corrosive burning effects.

Treatment

The patient should be moved to the operating room for esophagoscopy as soon as the diagnosis of caustic ingestion is confirmed. He should not be allowed to vomit; attempts at decontamination or neutralization of the agent in the gastrointestinal tract are counterproductive. The objectives of therapy are to prevent stricture formation, treat complications, treat strictures, and reconstruct a severely dysfunctional esophagus. The prevention of strictures is accomplished by the use of graduated, weighted bougies to dilate the esophagus manually until healing has taken place. Oral feeding is circumvented by placement of a gastrostomy or by parenteral nutrition. Antibiotics are used to treat secondary infections. When esophageal injury is so severe as to preclude its eventual functional recovery, reconstruction with colonic transplants or a fashioned gastroesophageal tube has been recommended.

CONTROVERSY

The use of steroids in the initial management of caustic ingestions has been the subject of considerable debate. While some clinicians believe steroids limit the inflammatory reaction, decrease granulation tissue formation, and facilitate healing with less scarring, there are few experimental studies to support such impressions.

REFERENCES

Ashcraft KW, Padula RD: The effect of dilute corrosives on the esophagus. *Pediatrics* 53:226, 1974.

Crain EF, Gershel JC, Mezey AP: Caustic ingestions. *Am J Dis Child* 138:863, 1984.

Gaudreault P, Parent M, McGuigan MA, et al: Predictability of esophageal injury from signs and symptoms: A study of caustic ingestion in 378 children. *Pediatrics* 71:767, 1983.

Hawkins DB, Demeter MJ, Barnett TE: Caustic ingestion: Controversies in management: A review of 214 cases. *Laryngoscope* 90:98, 1980.

Rothstein FC: Caustic injuries to the esophagus in children. *Pediatr Clin North Am* 33:665, 1986.

Temple DM, McNeese MC: Hazards of battery ingestion. *Pediatrics* 71:100, 1985.

Acute Iron Overdose 7

Definition

An iron overdose is significant if the child swallows more than 30 mg/kg of elemental iron. Most proprietary formulations contain ferrous sulfate, which is 20% elemental iron by weight. Although the severity of the poisoning with this agent is variable, depending on host factors as well as the amount of iron ingested, doses in excess of 40 mg/kg are of concern and doses greater than 250–300 mg/kg are often lethal.

Basic Science

The ferrous ion is absorbed in the duodenum and jejunum, oxidized to the ferric ion, and bound to the storage protein, ferritin. It is released into the plasma, bound by transferrin, and carried to hematopoietic sites within the marrow. Of the 4–5 g of total body iron, only about 1 mg is lost daily from the intestinal tract, the skin, or the urinary tract. With overdoses, the total iron binding capacity (TIBC) of the storage proteins is exceeded and iron circulates in the plasma in its free form. It is this unbound iron which causes systemic toxicity.

Iron absorbed in overdose has a profound peripheral vasodilatory effect which causes venous pooling, a compensatory increase in peripheral vascular resistance, decreased tissue perfusion, and metabolic acidosis. Eventually decreased cardiac output supervenes and, in conjunction with plasma loss due to increased vascular permeability, this leads to hypovolemic shock.

Besides these cardiovascular effects, iron is scavenged by the liver and deposited in parenchymal cells. It is thought that the ferrous form is taken up preferentially by the mitochondria where it causes damage by acting as an "electron sink" during its oxidation, interfering with the electron transport system, uncoupling oxidative phosphorylation, and decreasing ATP production. This loss of respiratory control by the mitochondria leads eventually to cell death.

Metabolic acidosis is primarily due to the conversion of the ferrous to the ferric ion. Also, interference with the Krebs cycle and the induction of anaerobic metabolism lead to accumulation of lactic and organic acids with resultant acidemia.

Epidemiology

Over 2000 cases of iron poisoning occur in the United States annually; Banner and Tong (1986) report ferrous sulfate tablets and multivitamins with iron remain among the top 10 substances ingested by children under the age of 5 years.

Diagnosis

Five physiologic alterations form the basis for the clinical manifestations of iron poisoning: hemorrhagic necrosis of the gastrointestinal tract, shock, metabolic acidosis, coagulation defects, and hepatocellular damage.

The sequelae of severe acute iron poisoning can be organized temporally into the four stages summarized in Table 25.7.

About 30% of patients with iron ingestion will have radiopaque pills visible by abdominal film; a negative radiograph does not, however, rule out the diagnosis. Although serum iron levels will usually be elevated more than the TIBC and concentrations greater than 500 ug/dl are almost always associated with severe poisoning, serum iron levels are variably related to the time since ingestion, type of iron preparation ingested, rate of absorption, and rate of elimination. Indeed, serum iron levels may be normal in cases of severe poisoning.

Table 25.7
The Clinical Stages of Acute Iron Poisoning[1]

Stage 1 (1–6 hours postingestion)
- A. Symptoms
  1. Nausea and vomiting
  2. Abdominal pain
  3. Respiratory distress
- B. Signs
  1. Dehydration
  2. Increased respiratory and heart rates
  3. Melena, bloody diarrhea
  4. Hemorrhagic gastritis
  5. Lethargy, irritability
  6. Shock and coma (poor prognostic signs)
- C. Laboratory Confirmation
  1. Elevated Fe > TIBC and Ferritin
  2. Peripheral leukocytosis
  3. Hyperglycemia
  4. Radiographic shock lung
  5. Positive abdominal scout film

Stage 2 (4–12 hours postingestion)
- Stabilization, Deceptive Improvement

Stage 3 (12–48 hours postingestion)
- A. Signs
  1. Shock and circulatory collapse
  2. Metabolic acidosis and hypoperfusion syndromes
  3. Coma
  4. Jaundice and hepatic failure
  5. Bleeding
  6. Renal failure
- B. Laboratory
  1. Normal serum Fe
  2. Elevated SGOT and SGPT levels
  3. Elevated bilirubin
  4. Hypoglycemia
  5. Prolonged clotting time, hypofibrinogenemia

Stage 4 (late sequelae)
- A. Pyloric or antral stenosis
- B. Stricture formation
- C. Hepatic cirrhosis
- D. CNS damage

[1]Adapted from Jacobs J, Greene H, Gendel B: *N Engl J Med* 273:1125, 1965.

Treatment

If the patient has swallowed less than 20 mg/kg of elemental iron, he can be safely observed without intervention. If ingestion is greater than 20 mg/kg, the patient's stomach should be evacuated by emesis induced by ipecac. The vomitus should be inspected and tested for evidence of iron or blood. Contraindications to emesis, however, include the onset of bloody diarrhea and/or abdominal pain, hematemesis, convulsions, or coma.

Gastric lavage with isotonic sodium bicarbonate is recommended. Since iron may be in a sustained release form or may congeal on the wall of the stomach as a bezoar-type mass, vigorous lavage even some hours postingestion is recommended.

In the absence of a reliable serum iron determination, or when the serum iron is normal, but a severe poisoning is nevertheless suspected, a provocative chelation test can be performed by giving the subject 25–50 mg/kg (maximum 1 g) of deferoxamine intramuscularly. Vin rosé-colored urine indicates a positive test.

Therapeutic deferoxamine can be given up to 90 mg/kg intramuscularly every 8 hours for three doses or 1 g STAT, 500 mg every 4 hours for two doses, and then 500 mg every 4–12 hours as necessary. All doses are intramuscular; this regimen is only recommended if there is no evidence of acidosis, coma, or shock. Therapy should be continued until the urine no longer has a vin rosé color or until the serum iron level falls below the total iron-binding capacity (TIBC).

If there is evidence of acidosis, coma, or shock, deferoxamine can be given intravenously *slowly* up to 90 mg/kg at an infusion rate < 15 mg/kg/hour. Rapid infusion of deferoxamine causes hypotension. Other more uncommon side effects include rash, urticaria, anaphylaxis, and cataracts.

Close observation of the patient in an intensive care setting is imperative in severe iron poisoning. Frequent vital signs, the administration of large volumes of intravenous crystalloid and colloid fluids to maintain perfusion, close monitoring of fluid input and output, and serial measurements of serum glucose, iron, liver

CASE ILLUSTRATION

An 18-month-old was completely well until he ingested 49 iron sulfate tablets (325 mg each; total dose = 16 g ferrous sulfate, 3.2 g elemental iron or, in this 10 kg infant, a dose of 320 mg/kg). The mother induced vomiting with ipecac, and diarrhea was noted. Two hours later the child appeared cold, pale, and lethargic and was transported by ambulance to the emergency clinic. He had a BP = 72/palpation and a thready pulse = 150 beats/minute. The neurologic examination revealed a child with a Glasgow coma score = 8, withdrawal to pain, +3 reflexes, and downgoing toes. The serum iron level 4 hours after ingestion was 12,000 μg/dl with a TIBC = 3162 μg/dl. The child received 2 g deferoxamine in sodium bicarbonate per nasogastric tube and 12.5 mg/kg iv deferoxamine over the first hour with a continuing drip thereafter at 10–20 mg/kg/hour for 3 days tapered to 1 mg/kg/hour over the following 4 days. The serum iron determinations decreased to serum iron = 222 μg/dl by day 4 with a TIBC = 880 μg/dl. Other laboratory values included a Hct = 43%, WBC count = 35,000 (20P, 3B, 70L, 7M), PT = 36/12.5 sec, PTT = 100/32.4 sec, SGOT = 535 U/L, and SGPT = 460 U/L. All corrected by the third hospital day after administration of fresh frozen plasma, packed RBCs, and intravenous fluids at twice maintenance with sodium bicarbonate. Central venous pressure monitoring was also instituted; intubation was not required. The urine remained an orangish-brown color for the first 72 hours after admission. On day 7, the patient experienced respiratory distress; a chest radiograph showed bilateral pneumothoraces and chest tubes were inserted. Pneumonia with pleural effusion was treated with antibiotics and showed gradual resolution over the next 10 days; cultures of the blood, urine, and cerebrospinal fluid remained negative. The child was discharged on no medications 18 days after admission with no further complications.

QUESTIONS AND COMMENTS

Were this child's respiratory complications related to iron toxicity?

The lipid peroxidation produced by iron can affect other cell membranes besides those in the liver. Lung edema and damage are infrequent but well-recognized complications.

Why was deferoxamine continued for 7 days?

Deferoxamine is a highly selective chelator of iron ions with a serum half-life of 1 hour. About 8.5 mg of ferric iron can be bound by 100 mg deferoxamine. The duration of chelation therapy is a source of controversy in iron poisoning. Some clinicians taper deferoxamine when the urine color returns to normal. Others are guided by the clinical appearance of the patient, in addition to the urinary findings, and continue deferoxamine 24 hours after the resolution of all symptoms and signs of toxicity.

function tests, electrolytes, and acid-base balance are important aspects of the total management of the patient. The overgrowth of colonic pathogens, especially *Yersinia enterocolitica*, can complicate the clinical course of the patient with iron intoxication. The clinician must be vigilant for signs of sepsis or colitis and treat with appropriate antibiotics when such infections become evident.

CONTROVERSIES

Although sodium phosphate lavage and instillation were previously recommended to decrease gastrointestinal absorption of iron through the formation of the relatively insoluble ferrous phosphate, enhanced phosphate absorption with subsequent hyperphosphatemia, hypocalcemia, and hypertonic dehydration have led clinicians to question the usefulness of this modality in the management of iron overdose.

While dialysis and exchange transfusion have been recommended as last resorts for severe overdose, there is no proof of their efficacy.

REFERENCES

Banner W, Tong T: Iron poisoning. *Pediatr Clin North Am* 33:393, 1986.

James J: Acute iron poisoning: Assessment of severity and prognosis. *J Pediatr* 77:117, 1970.

Moeschlin S, Schnider U: Treatment of primary and secondary hemochromatosis and acute iron poisoning with a new, potent iron-eliminating agent (desferrioxamine-B). *N Engl J Med* 269:57, 1963.

Robotham J, Lietman P: Acute iron poisoning. *Am J Dis Child* 134:875, 1980.

Whitten C, Brough A: The pathophysiology of acute iron poisoning. *Clin Toxicol* 4:585, 1971.

Stinging Insect Hypersensitivity

8

Definition

Insects of the order *Hymenoptera*: bees (family: *Apidae*) or wasps, yellow jackets, and hornets (family: *Vespidae*) produce most of the serious stings. This chapter will concentrate on allergic reactions to stings from these insects. The reader is referred to other texts for a fuller discussion of scorpion stings and injuries from other stinging animals. Nonvenomous animal bites and snake bites are discussed in Section 24.

Basic Science

The venom from stinging insects contains allergens which interact with IgE antibodies fixed to mast cell and basophil membranes to cause the release of a variety of vasoactive substances including histamine, other biogenic amines, serotonin, and acetyl-CoA. These substances mediate the subsequent inflammatory response that results in damage to tissues and vessels and the severity of the clinical response.

Epidemiology

Although the prevalence of insect allergies in the general population as reported in the literature is between 0.4 and 0.8%, researchers indicate that fully 20% of adults may give evidence of sensitivity either by history of an untoward reaction to a sting or by the positivity of venom-specific skin tests. There is no evidence that insect allergy is an inherited phenomenon although males are affected more often than are females. Atopic individuals are no more at risk for allergic reactions to insect stings than are others; and spontaneous loss of reactivity does occur and is not uncommon in children.

Diagnosis

The reaction to an insect sting can be one of the five general types listed in Table 25.8.

Victims of insect stings who manifest only local or large local reactions can be collectively designated nonsystemic reactors. Clinical variability is common in the reactivity of any individual to a sting. This depends on the species of the offending insect and also unknown and variable biochemical and physiologic as well as immunologic host factors. Fortunately systemic reactions among children are milder than those of adults and there is less risk of life-threatening symptoms. The availability of hymenoptera venom-specific antigen has increased both the sensitivity and specificity of skin testing which can accurately distinguish those who are truly allergic to stings and who may benefit from immunotherapy (Hunt et al, 1976; Golden et al, 1981).

The radioallergosorbent test (RAST) measures serum venom IgE antibody levels; these levels reach a peak 3–6 weeks after a sting reaction. RAST results are in accord with venom-specific skin testing results in 80% of cases. However, the RAST may be falsely negative and should never be the sole basis for clinical decisions regarding the utility of immunotherapy.

Treatment

Local reactions to insect stings are best managed with cold compresses and oral antihistamines. The stinger, often left embedded in the skin after a honeybee sting, should be carefully extracted since squeezing the stinger may express more venom into the tissues. Occasionally, cellulitis may complicate a local reaction several days after the sting of a scavenger bee or wasp and should be treated with a cephalosporin or semi-

Table 25.8
Reactions to Insect Stings[1]

Local
1. Redness and pain or itching at the site
2. Swelling less than 10 centimeters

Large local
1. Pain, redness, warmth and swelling at the site of the sting
2. Extension of swelling greater than 10 centimeters but contiguous
3. May involve contiguous joints

Generalized non-life-threatening immediate reactions
1. Type I immediate anaphylaxis within 2 hours of the sting
2. Swelling greater than 10 centimeters
3. Extension of swelling to noncontiguous body areas
4. Pruritic urticaria
5. Angioedema of lips, eyelids, ears

Generalized life-threatening immediate reactions
1. Type I immediate anaphylaxis within 2 hours of the sting
2. Swelling and cutaneous manifestations described above and:
3. Laryngeal edema and laryngospasm or
4. Hypotensive shock or
5. Wheezing, bronchospasm, and dyspnea or
6. Loss of consciousness

Unusual delayed reactions
1. Nephrosis
2. Thrombocytopenia
3. Other coagulopathies
4. Vasculitides
5. Neuritis, transverse myelitis
6. Encephalopathy
7. Type III delayed hypersensitivity (serum sickness)

[1]Adapted from a lecture by Dr. Rebecca Buckley.

synthetic penicillin at 30–50 mg/kg/day after appropriate cultures are obtained.

Systemic reactions should be treated by establishing an adequate airway and administering subcutaneous aqueous epinephrine (1:1000 dilution) at 0.01 ml/kg to a maximum of 0.3 ml/injection. Heart rate and rhythm should be monitored. Shock should be managed by establishing a central line and infusing a crystalloid solution at 20 ml/kg. Systemic vasopressors may also be necessary to maintain blood pressure. Urticaria will usually respond to subcutaneous epinephrine or intramuscular antihistamine injection. Bronchospasm and respiratory distress can be treated with oxygen as necessary and inhaled nebulized sympathomimetics.

Venom immunotherapy has been shown to be effective in modulating the IgE-mediated inflammatory response from insect stings within weeks of the onset of therapy, presumably by inducing elevated levels of venom-specific blocking IgG antibodies. These high-titer blocking antibodies prevent the venom protein/mast cell membrane-fixed IgE interaction which starts the inflammatory cascade of events. Successful therapy is defined as that which induces a total lack of systemic reactions to stings. Those with positive skin tests to specific hymenoptera venoms, with or without the presence of specific serum IgE antibodies (a positive RAST test), and a positive clinical history of a life-threatening systemic reaction should be considered as candidates for desensitization by periodic injection with skin test-specific venoms. Such immunotherapy can decrease the chances of a severe reaction to a future sting from 60% to less than 5%.

CONTROVERSIES

Systemic corticosteroids are frequently used for systemic reactions although there are no controlled trials of their efficacy.

Whether venom immunotherapy should be routinely advised for children with large local reactions or non-life-threatening systemic reactions is controversial. This prophylactic treatment is expensive, inconvenient, and may necessitate monthly injections for an indefinite period of time to maintain its efficacy. Its short-term and long-term toxic side effects are not entirely known. Untreated children at risk for a systemic reaction (as judged by clinical history and venom skin testing) may in fact only react to a future sting 15% of the time. In a study of 263 children followed longitudinally there was no evidence of progression from large local reactions or non-life-threatening reactions to life-threatening reactions in those allergic children unprotected by immunotherapy who later had accidental stings (Schuberth et al, 1983).

Prevention

Campers with insect allergies should avoid clothing with floral prints or bright colors and perfumes that attract bees. Areas where hornets or wasps are abundant, such as near trash cans or hives, should also be avoided. Yellow jackets are ground nesting and often feed off fallen fruit in orchards or spoiled fruit in trash bins. Protective clothing and shoes should be worn. There are commercially available insect-allergy kits which contain an autoinjector of epinephrine. Such a kit can be life-saving when an anaphylactic response to a sting occurs in a setting where there is no immediately available medical care. Those with a history of life-threatening reactions should wear "Medi-Alert" identification.

REFERENCES

Chipps B, Valentine M, Kegey-Sobotka A, et al: Diagnosis and treatment of anaphylactic reactions to *Hymenoptera* stings in children. *J Pediatr* 97:177, 1980.

Golden D, Langlois J, Valentine M, et al: Treatment failures with whole-body extract therapy of insect sting allergy. *JAMA* 246:2460, 1981.

Graft D, Schuberth K: *Hymenoptera* allergy in children. *Pediatr Clin North Am* 30:873, 1983.

Hunt K, Valentine M, Sobotka A, et al: A controlled trial of immunotherapy in insect hypersensitivity. *N Engl J Med* 299:157, 1978.

Hunt K, Valentine M, Sobotka A, et al: Diagnosis of allergy to stinging insects by skin testing with *Hymenoptera* venoms. *Ann Intern Med* 85:56, 1976.

Schuberth K, Lichtenstein L, Kagey-Sobotka A, et al: An epidemiologic study of insect allergy in children. I. Characteristics of the disease. *J Pediatr* 100:546, 1982.

Schuberth K, Lichtenstein L, Kagey-Sobotka A, et al: Epidemiologic study of insect allergy in children. II. Effect of accidental stings in allergic children. *J Pediatr* 102:361, 1983.

Yunginger J: Advances in the diagnosis and treatment of stinging insect allergy. *Pediatrics* 67:325, 1981.

Tricyclic Antidepressant Toxicity 9

Definition

The tricyclic antidepressants (TCAs) structurally are a class of sedative drugs having a seven-membered central ring surrounded by two benzene rings. They are similar to phenothiazines, carbamazepine (Tegretol), and other drugs having a three-ringed nucleus, but are unique in their substituted tertiary amine side-chain which is metabolized to the pharmacologically active secondary amine structure. They include imipramine, amitriptyline, and others.

Basic Science

The TCAs are lipid-soluble and extensively tissue- and protein-bound providing a considerable reservoir for their slow release into plasma. The serum half-life varies between 24 and 76 hours or even longer in overdose situations. In addition, their anticholinergic effects interfere with gastrointestinal peristalsis and slow down absorption. These properties of TCAs account for the most variable serum half-lives (24–96 hours) and metabolic rates of elimination of any drug studied. Elimination is via hydroxylation, demethylation, and conjugation by liver enzymes and excretion by enterohepatic and renal routes.

The drug's major toxic effects are directed toward the cardiac and central nervous systems. Many symptoms are attributable to central and peripheral anticholinergic actions of TCAs as well as their sedative effects. In addition, these agents interfere with the "amine pump" at presynaptic nerve junctions, allowing an accumulation of aminergic neurotransmitters (e.g., serotonin and norepinephrine). Such increased concentrations of neurotransmitters can presumably alleviate depression but may also contribute a variety of symptoms listed in Tables 25.1 and 25.2.

The cardiotoxicity of TCAs is attributable to their anticholinergic properties as well as a sympathomimetic effect by preventing reuptake of norepinephrine into adrenergic neurons resulting in a sinus tachycardia. TCAs also exert direct quinidine-like effects on myocardial tissue with stabilization of membranes, depression of contractility, and reduced coronary blood flow. TCAs can interfere with the ATP-mediated sodium/potassium pump depleting sodium channels and slowing conduction in the His-Purkinje and ventricular conduction system. This action is, in itself, dysrhythmogenic by allowing re-entrant rhythms (Table 25.9).

Epidemiology

TCAs are commonly prescribed for adult depression and, in pediatrics, also for hyperkinesis, school phobia, and sleep disorders. The therapeutic/toxic ratio for TCAs is very narrow in both children and adults. These agents are the single class of drugs accounting for most of the serious poisonings in the United States (25% of all serious overdoses) and have a mortality rate of 3%. Petit and Biggs (1977) suggest the recent expanded use of TCAs for the treatment of depression in adolescents may give these susceptible teenagers the means to carry suicide attempts to completion.

Diagnosis

The erratic release of TCAs into the blood stream contributes to their unpredictable toxic effects. Patients may appear well for hours after an ingestion and then develop serious or fatal arrhythmias or seizures. The new onset of symptoms has been noted as late as 2–3 days after ingestion; ECG abnormalities may persist as long as 6 or 7 days, although most subside within 24 hours. Serum TCA levels are only helpful at a given moment since they fluctuate unpredictably, and thus, do not indicate the steady state, nor aid prediction of the clinical outcome. Serum drug levels above 1000 ng/ml are associated often with a significant overdose. However, Boehnert and Lovejoy (1985) studied 49 cases of TCA overdoses and concluded the maximal duration

Table 25.9
Clinical Signs of Tricyclic Antidepressant Overdose

- Central nervous system effects
  - Altered sensorium, agitation
  - Coma
  - Grand mal seizures
  - Pyramidal signs (clonus, Babinski, hyperreflexia)
  - Myoclonic twitches
- Cardiovascular effects and ECG changes
  - Hypotension
  - Cardiogenic failure
  - T wave, ST segment changes
  - Widened QRS duration
  - Atrioventricular conduction defects
    - Bundle branch block
    - Bigeminy
    - Trigeminy
    - Complete block
  - Supraventricular tachyarrhythmias
  - Ventricular tachycardia
  - Ventricular fibrillation
  - Electromechanical dissociation
  - Asystole

of the QRS complex on a 12-lead electrocardiogram obtained within 6 hours of ingestion could accurately classify those patients at increased risk for seizures (QRS > 0.10 second) and cardiac arrhythmias (QRS > 0.16 second), whereas the serum TCA level could predict neither complication.

Patients with significant ingestions may lapse into coma or suffer major motor seizures. Cardiovascular complications include hypotension, congestive failure, intraventricular conduction defects, ventricular arrhythmias, and asystole. Common ventricular arrhythmias include short runs of ventricular tachycardia, prolonged bigeminy or trigeminy, idioventricular rhythms, and ventricular fibrillation. Table 25.9 presents the common clinical findings in TCA overdose.

Treatment

Effective oral decontamination is pivotal in the treatment of suspected TCA overdoses. Evacuation in the alert patient by ipecac and/or lavage should be followed by repetitive doses of oral activated charcoal (1 g/kg body weight) at 4-hour intervals until the serum drug level is below 500 ng/ml. Patients with an altered sensorium or in coma should be intubated to protect against aspiration and should not receive ipecac. Catharsis with 300 ml of magnesium citrate every 4 hours is also recommended.

Serum TCA levels should be obtained; and vomitus and/or gastric contents should be inspected for pill fragments before body fluids are sent for analysis to confirm the diagnosis. Regardless of serum drug level, patients in whom significant TCA poisoning is suspected should be admitted, preferably to an intensive care unit, for continuous cardiac and CNS monitoring for at least 24 hours. A precautionary indwelling venous line should be established along with other supportive measures. Since hypokalemia and acidosis are frequent concomitants of overdose situations as well as respiratory problems, frequent monitoring of both blood gases and serum electrolytes is advisable with correction of metabolic abnormalities using sodium bicarbonate and/or potassium chloride solutions.

Anticonvulsants such as diazepam (Valium) are recommended for the treatment of seizures. Since seizures may be precipitated by the patient's agitated state, a quiet environment and the avoidance of unnecessary noxious stimuli are recommended.

An intravenous lidocaine drip at 25–50 μg/kg/minute is the preferred first-line therapy for the onset of arrhythmias. Phenytoin (Dilantin) and bicarbonate have also been successfully used to prevent cardiac rhythm disturbances. Emergency pacing may be necessary for bradyarrhythmias or advanced degrees of atrioventricular block. Pressors are indicated for hypotension.

Because TCAs bind extensively to tissue and proteins and are lipophilic, such decontamination methods as forced diuresis or peritoneal or hemodialysis are useless.

REFERENCES

Boehnart MT, Lovejoy FH: Value of the QRS duration versus the serum drug level in predicting seizures and ventricular arrhythmias after an acute overdose of tricyclic antidepressants. *N Engl J Med* 313:474, 1985.

Braden NJ, Jackson JE, Walson PD: Tricyclic antidepressant overdose. *Pediatr Clin North Am* 33:287, 1986.

Hollister L: Tricyclic antidepressants. *N Engl J Med* 299:1106 and 299:1168, 1977.

Manoguerra A, Weaver L: Poisoning with tricyclic antidepressant drugs. *Clin Toxicol* 10:149, 1977.

Petit J, Biggs J: Tricyclic antidepressant overdoses in adolescent patients. *Pediatrics* 59:283, 1977.

Sasyniuk B, Jhamandas V, Valois M: Experimental amitriptyline intoxication: Treatment of cardiac toxicity with sodium bicarbonate. *Ann Emerg Med* 15:1052, 1986.

Uhl J: Phenytoin: The drug of choice in tricyclic antidepressant overdose? *Ann Emerg Med* 10:270, 1981.

Carbon Monoxide Poisoning 10

Definition

Carbon monoxide (CO) is a colorless, odorless gas heavier than air which is a combustion product present in many types of smoke and exhausts. The severity of CO poisoning varies with the CO concentration absorbed, the activity level of the victim, and the duration of exposure.

Basic Science

Dissolved CO in the blood displaces oxygen from hemoglobin with the formation of carboxyhemoglobin (COHb), which results in a shift to the left in the oxygen dissociation curve of hemoglobin, decreased unloading of oxygen, and tissue hypoxia. The consequences of this hypoxia include tissue ischemia, a metabolic acidosis and lactic acidosis, cellular damage with leakage from cellular membranes, and adrenergic stimulation with a relative hyperglycemia.

CO can also pass from the blood to extravascular tissues where it causes direct damage at the cellular level by excluding oxygen from the cytochrome oxidase a3 enzyme of cellular respiration. Such effects can be delayed in onset beyond the period of acute exposure, may occur despite relatively low plasma COHb levels, and may be responsible for the delayed neuropsychiatric effects observed in these patients.

Epidemiology

CO poisoning is most frequently a result of accidental exposures, attempted suicide, or inhalation with other combustion products in smoke inhalation injuries. It is the single agent responsible for almost half of the fatal poisonings occurring annually in the United States. Because mild cases may be mistaken for "flu"-like syndromes, it is likely that the incidence of CO poisoning is much greater than is currently reported. It is rarely a pure poison and many victims will have been exposed to other noxious fumes and gases. The most common sources of exposure include fires, automobile exhausts, faulty furnaces, gas or propane space heaters, charcoal burners, or engines used improperly in enclosed spaces. Also, methylene chloride, present in most paint strippers, is converted to CO after absorption through the skin.

Diagnosis

The victim of CO poisoning will most often complain of flu-like symptoms of weakness and fatigue, nausea and vomiting, dizziness, and headaches. The classical "cherry red" hue of mucous membranes is not always present. Those organs most sensitive to ischemia (i.e., heart and brain) are most often affected. Tachyarrhythmias are seen and, in adults with underlying heart disease, there is a risk of angina or myocardial infarction. Cardiac arrest can occur in severe poisoning. Neurologic symptoms and signs predominate, however, and are most important in prognosis. In addition to confusion and dizziness, many patients suffer hypertonia, hyperreflexia, visual disturbances and decreased mental acuity. Loss of consciousness and seizures are associated with a worse prognosis.

CO poisoning not infrequently produces a neuropsychiatric syndrome days to weeks after apparent recovery, the causes of which are unclear. Symptoms and signs may include cogwheeling and muscular rigidity, incontinence, Parkinsonian-type effects, cortical blindness, aphasia, apraxia, hallucinations, and chronic cognitive effects.

The diagnosis rests on a circumstantial history of exposure to smoke or noxious gases and the altered neurologic examination of the patient. It can be confirmed by laboratory measurement of COHb levels in the blood. While very high COHb levels (greater than 20%) indicate a dangerous exposure, COHb levels in general do not correlate with clinical findings or prognosis; some patients with COHb levels less than 5% may present with the acute or delayed neurologic syndromes described above. The differential diagnosis in severe cases includes other causes of coma, cerebral edema, or cardiac arrhythmias, ischemia or arrest. As noted previously, mild cases are likely to be mistaken for viral syndromes.

Treatment

Once the diagnosis of CO poisoning is suspected, the patient should be given 100% oxygen at a flow of 10 liters through a plastic rebreather mask with as tight a seal as possible. Close monitoring of the patient's vital signs and neurologic status is essential. Administration of 100% oxygen can shorten the half-life of CO dissolved in the blood from 320 minutes in room air to 80 minutes.

Hyperbaric oxygen at 3 atmospheres can further reduce the COHb half-life to 23 minutes. Severe exposures (as evidenced by duration of exposure and the presence of neurologic or cardiac symptoms and signs) should be triaged to centers where hyperbaric oxygen at 3–4 atmospheres pressure is available. Since neurologic symptoms may occur or recur hours to days after a period of relative improvement, observation of the patient for several days after exposure is recommended.

REFERENCES

Kindwall E: Hyperbaric treatment of carbon monoxide poisoning. *Ann Emerg Med* 14:1233, 1985.

Mathieu D, Nolf M, Durocher A, et al: Acute carbon monoxide poisoning risk of late sequelae and treatment by hyperbaric oxygen. *Clin Toxicol* 23:315, 1985.

Norkool D, Kirkpatrick J: Treatment of acute carbon monoxide poisoning with hyperbaric oxygen: A review of 115 cases. *Ann Emerg Med* 14:1168, 1985.

ALAN WOOLF

Appendices

Appendix A

To save space, the following abbreviations are used:

ACTH	adrenocorticotrophic hormone
ALL	acute lymphocytic leukemia
AML	acute myeloid leukemia
BUN	blood urea nitrogen
C	centigrade
CT	computed tomography
CAT	computerized axial tomography
CNS	central nervous system
CSF	cerebrospinal fluid
dl	deciliter
DNA	deoxyribonucleic acid
EEG	electroencephalogram
ECG	electrocardiogram
EMG	electromyogram
EOS	eosinophils
ESR	erythrocyte sedimentation rate
g	gram
GI	gastrointestinal
Hb	hemoglobin
Hct	hematocrit
Ig	immunoglobulin
im	intramuscular
iv	intravenous
kg	kilogram
lymphs	lymphocytes
L	liter
MCV	mean corpuscular volume
mEq/L	milliequivalents per liter
mg	milligram
ml	milliliter
mm Hg	millimeters of mercury
mMole	millimoles
mOsmol	milliosmoles
mRNA	messenger ribonucleic acid
monos	monocytes
MRI	magnetic resonance imaging
polys	polymorphonuclear leukocytes
PT	prothrombin time
PTT	partial thromboplastin time
RBC	red blood cell
Rh	rhesus
RNA	ribonucleic acid
rT_3	reverse triiodothyronine
sp. gr.	specific gravity
TSH	thyroid stimulating hormone
T_4	thyroxine
T_3	triiodothyronine
WBC	white blood count

Appendix B

Table B.1
Temperature Equivalents

Celsius	Fahrenheit	Celsius	Fahrenheit
34.0	93.2	38.6	101.4
34.2	93.6	38.8	101.8
34.4	93.9	39.0	102.2
34.6	94.3	39.2	102.5
34.8	94.6	39.4	102.9
35.0	95.0	39.6	103.2
35.2	95.4	39.8	103.6
35.4	95.7	40.0	104.0
35.6	96.1	40.2	104.3
35.8	96.4	40.4	104.7
36.0	96.8	40.6	105.1
36.2	97.1	40.8	105.4
36.4	97.5	41.0	105.8
36.6	97.8	41.2	106.1
36.8	98.2	41.4	106.5
37.0	98.6	41.6	106.8
37.2	98.9	41.8	107.2
37.4	99.3	42.0	107.6
37.6	99.6	42.2	108.0
37.8	100.0	42.4	108.3
38.0	100.4	42.6	108.7
38.2	100.7	42.8	109.0
38.4	101.1	43.0	109.4

To convert Celsius to Fahrenheit

$9/5 \times \text{Temperature} + 32$

Example: To convert 40° Celsius to Fahrenheit
$9/5 \times 40 = 72 + 32 = 104°$ Fahrenheit

To convert Fahrenheit to Celsius

$(\text{Temperature minus } 32) \times 5/9$

Example: To convert 98.6° Fahrenheit to Celsius
$98.6 - 32 = 66.6 \times 5/9 = 37°$ Celsius

Table B.2
Conversion of Pounds and Ounces to Grams

Ounces	1 lb	2 lb	3 lb	4 lb	5 lb	6 lb	7 lb	8 lb
	Grams							
0	454	907	1361	1814	2268	2722	3175	3629
1	482	936	1389	1843	2296	2750	3204	3657
2	510	964	1418	1871	2325	2778	3232	3686
3	539	992	1446	1899	2353	2807	3260	3714
4	567	1021	1474	1928	2381	2835	3289	3742
5	595	1049	1503	1956	2410	2863	3317	3771
6	624	1077	1531	1985	2438	2892	3345	3799
7	652	1106	1559	2013	2466	2920	3374	3827
8	680	1134	1588	2041	2495	2948	3402	3856
9	709	1162	1616	2070	2523	2977	3430	3884
10	737	1191	1644	2098	2552	3005	3459	3912
11	765	1219	1673	2126	2580	3033	3487	3941
12	794	1247	1701	2155	2608	3062	3515	3969
13	822	1276	1729	2183	2637	3090	3544	3997
14	851	1304	1758	2211	2665	3119	3572	4026
15	879	1332	1786	2240	2693	3147	3600	4054

Table B.3
Conversion of Inches to Centimeters

Inches	cm	Inches	cm	Inches	cm
10	25.40	15	38.10	20	50.80
10½	26.67	15½	39.37	20½	52.07
11	27.94	16	40.64	21	53.34
11½	29.21	16½	41.91	21½	54.61
12	30.48	17	43.18	22	55.88
12½	31.75	17½	44.45	22½	57.15
13	33.02	18	45.72	23	58.42
13½	34.29	18½	46.99	23½	56.69
14	35.56	19	48.26	24	60.96
14½	36.83	19½	49.53		

Appendix C

Table C.1[1]
Blood, Plasma, or Serum Values

Determination	Reference Range: Conventional	Reference Range: SI	Minimal ml Required	Note	Method
Acetoacetate plus acetone	Negative		1-B		Behre: *J Lab Clin Med* 13:770, 1928 (modified)
Aldolase	1.3–8.2 U/L	22–137 nMol sec^{-1}/L	2-S	Use unhemolyzed serum	Beisenherz et al: *Z Naturforsch* 86:555, 1963
Ammonia	12–55 μMol/L	12–55 μmol/L	2-B	Collect in heparinized tube; deliver *immediately* packed in ice	Da Fonseca-Wolheim: *J Clin Chem Clin Biochem* 11:421, 1973
Amylase	4–25 units/ml	4–25 arb. unit	1-S		Zinterhofer et al: *Clin Chim Acta* 43:5, 1973
Ascorbic acid	0.4–1.5 mg/dl	23–85 μMol/L	7-B	Collect in heparinized tube before any food is given	Roe, Kuether: *J Biol Chem* 147:399, 1943
Bilirubin	Direct: up to 0.4 mg/dl. Total: up to 1.0 mg/dl	Up to 7 μMol/L Up to 17 μMol/L	1-S		Gambino: Standard Methods *Clin Chem* 5:55, 1965
Blood volume	8.5–9.0% of body weight in kg	80–85 ml/kg			Isotope dilution technique with ^{131}I albumin
Calcium	8.5–10.5 mg/dl (slightly higher in children)	2.1–2.6 mMol/L	1-S		Spectrophotometry using cresolphthalein complexone
Carbon dioxide content	24–30 mEq/L	24–30 mMol/L	1-S	Fill tube to top	By CO_2 electrode
Carbamazepine	4.0–12.0 μg/ml	17–51 μMol/L			Liquid chromatography
Carbon monoxide	Less than 5% of total hemoglobin		3-B	Fill tube to top	Multi-wavelength spectrophotometry
Carotenoids	0.8–4.0 μg/ml	1.5–7.4 μMol/L	3-S	Vitamin A may be done on same specimen	Natelson: *Microtechniques of Clinical Chemistry*, 2nd ed., 1961, p. 454
Ceruloplasmin	27–37 mg/dl	1.8–2.5 μMol/L	2-S		Ravin: *J Lab Clin Med* 58:161, 1961
Chloramphenicol	10–20 μg/ml	31–62 μMol/L	0.2-S		Liquid chromatography
Chloride	100–106 mEq/L	100–106 mMol/L	1-S		Cotlove: Standard Methods *Clin Chem* 3:81, 1961
CK isoenzymes	5% Mb or less		0.2-S		Electrophoresis
Copper	Total: 100–200 μg/dl	16–31 μMol/L	1-S		Atomic-absorption spectrophotometry
Creatine kinase (CK)	Female: 10–79 U/L Male: 17–148 U/L	167–1317 nMol · sec^{-1}/L 283–2467 nMol · sec^{-1}/L	1-S		Szasz: *Clin Chem* 22:650, 1976
Creatinine	0.6–1.5 mg/dl	53–133 μMol/L	1-S		Fabiny, Ertingshausen: *Clin Chem* 17:696, 1971
Ethanol	0 mg/dl	0 mMol/L	2-B	Collect in oxalate and refrigerate	Gas–liquid chromatography
Glucose	Fasting: 70–110 mg/dl	3.9–5.6 mMol/L	1-P	Collect with oxalate–fluoride mixture	Bergmeyer: *Methods of Enzymatic Analysis*, 1965, p. 117
Iron	50–150 μg/dl (higher in males)	9.0–26.9 μMol/L	1-S		Spectrophotometry using Ferrozine
Iron-binding capacity	250–410 μg/dl	44.8–73.4 μMol/L	1-S		Spectrophotometry using Ferrozine

Table C.1 (Continued)
Blood, Plasma, or Serum Values

Determination	Reference Range: Conventional	Reference Range: SI	Minimal ml Required	Note	Method
Lactic acid	0.6–1.8 mEq/L	0.6–1.8 mMol/L	2-B	Collect with oxalate–fluoride; deliver immediately packed in ice	Hadjivassiliou, Rieder: *Clin Chim Acta* 19:357, 1968
Lactic dehydrogenase	45–90 U/L	750–1500 nMol · sec^{-1}/L	1-S	Unsuitable if hemolyzed	Gay, McComb, Bowers: *Clin Chem* 14:740, 1968
Lead	50 μg/dl or less	Up to 2.4 μMol/L	2-B	Collect with oxalate–fluoride mixture	Berman: *Atom Absorp Newslett* 3:9, 1964 (modified)
Lipase	2 units/ml or less	Up to 2 arb. unit	1-S		Zinterhofer: *Clin Chim Acta* 44:173, 1973
Lipids					
Cholesterol	120–220 mg/dl	3.10–5.69 mMol/L	1-S	Fasting	Siedel: *J Clin Chem Clin Biochem* 19:838, 1981
Triglycerides	40–150 mg/dl	0.4–1.5 g/L	1-S	Fasting	Ziegenhorn: *Clin Chem* 21:1627, 1975
Lipoprotein electrophoresis (LEP)			2-S	Fasting, do not freeze serum	Lees, Hatch: *J Lab Clin Med* 61:518, 1963
Lithium	0.5–1.5 mEq/L	0.5–1.5 mMol/L	1-S		Pybus, Bowers: *Clin Chem* 16:139, 1970
Magnesium	1.5–2.0 mEq/L	0.8–1.3 mMol/L	1-S		Willis: *Clin Chem* 11:251, 1965 (modified)
5′ Nucleotidase	1–11 U/L	17–183 nMol · sec^{-1}/L	1-S		Arkesteijn: *J Clin Chem Clin Biochem* 14:155, 1976
Osmolality	280–296 mOsm/kg water	280–296 mMol/kg	1-S		Osmometry using freezing-point depression
Oxygen saturation (arterial)	96–100%	0.96–1.00	3-B	Deliver in sealed heparinized syringe packed in ice	Gordy, Drabkin: *J Biol Chem* 227:285, 1957
P_{CO_2}	35–45 mm Hg	4.7–6.0 kPa	2-B	Collect and deliver in sealed heparinized syringe	By CO_2 electrode
pH	7.35–7.45	Same	2-B	Collect without stasis in sealed heparinized syringe; deliver packed in ice	Glass electrode
P_{O_2}	75–100 mm Hg (dependent on age) while breathing room air Above 500 mm Hg while on 100% O_2	10.0–13.3 kPa	2-B		Oxygen electrode
Phenobarbital	15–50 μg/ml	65–215 μMol/L	1-S		Liquid chromatography
Phenytoin (Dilantin)	5–20 μg/ml	20–80 μMol/L	1-S		Liquid chromatography
Phosphatase (acid)	Male—Total: 0.13–0.63 sigma U/ml Female—total: 0.01–0.56 sigma U/ml Prostatic: 0–0.5 Fishman–Lerner U/dl	36–175 nMol · sec^{-1}/L 2.8–156 nMol · sec^{-1}/L		Must always be drawn just before analysis or stored as frozen serum; avoid hemolysis	Bessey et al: *J Biol Chem* 164:321, 1946 Babson et al: *Clin Chim Acta* 13:264, 1966
Phosphatase (alkaline)	13–39 U/L, infants and adolescents up to 104 U/L	217–650 nMol · sec^{-1}/L; up to 1.26 μMol · sec^{-1}/L	1-S		Stevens, Thomas: *Clin Chim Acta* 37:541, 1972
Phosphorus (inorganic)	3.0–4.5 mg/dl (infants in first year up to 6.0 mg/dl	1.0–1.5 mMol/L	1-S		Daly, Ertingshausen: *Clin Chem* 18:263, 1972
Potassium	3.5–5.0 mEq/L	3.5–5.0 mMol/L	1-S	Serum must be separated promptly from cells	Ion-selective electrode
Primidone (Mysoline)	4–12 μg/ml	18–55 μMol/L	1-S		Enzyme immunoassay

Table C.1 (Continued)
Blood, Plasma, or Serum Values

Determination	Reference Range: Conventional	Reference Range: SI	Minimal ml Required	Note	Method
Procainamide	4–10 μg/ml	17–42 μMol/L	1-S		Liquid chromatography
Protein: Total	6.0–8.4 g/dl	60–84 g/L	1-S		Weichselbaum: *Am J Clin Pathol* 16:40, 1946
Albumin	3.5–5.0 g/dl	35–50 g/L	1-S		Doumas et al: *Clin Chim Acta* 31:87, 1971
Globulin	2.3–3.5 g/dl	23–35 g/L		Globulin equals total protein minus albumin	
Electrophoresis	(% of total protein)		1-S	Quantitation by densitometry	Kunkel, Tiselius: *J Gen Physiol* 35:89, 1951
Albumin	52–68				
Globulin:					
α_1	4.2–7.2				Durrum: *J Am Chem Soc* 72:2943, 1950
α_2	6.8–12				
β	9.3–15				
γ	13–23				
Pyruvic acid	0–0.11 mEq/L	0–0.11 mMol/L	2-B	Collect with oxalate fluoride. Deliver immediately packed in ice	Hadjivassiliou, Rieder: *Clin Chim Acta* 19:357, 1968
Quinidine	1.2–4.0 μg/ml	3.7–12.3 μMol/L	1-S		Liquid chromatography
Salicylate:	0		2-P		Keller: *Am J Clin Pathol* 17:415, 1947
Therapeutic	20–25 mg/dl; 25–30 mg/dl to age 10 years 3 hours postdose	1.4–1.8 mMol/L 1.8–2.2 mMol/L			
Sodium	135–145 mEq/L	135–145 mMol/L	1-S		Ion-selective electrode
Sulfonamide	5–15 mg/dl		2-P		Bratton, Marshall: *J Biol Chem* 128:537, 1939
Transaminase, SGOT (aspartate amino-transferase)	7–27 U/L	117–450 nMol · sec^{-1}/L	1-S		Karmen et al: *J Clin Invest* 34:126, 1955
Transaminase, SGPT (alanine amino-transferase)	1–21 U/L	17–350 nMol · sec^{-1}/L	1-S		Henry et al: *Am J Clin Pathol* 34:381, 1960
Urea nitrogen (BUN)	8–25 mg/dl	2.9–8.9 mMol/L	1-S		Paulson et al: *Clin Chem* 17:644, 1971
Uric acid	3.0–7.0 mg/dl	0.18–0.42 mMol/L	1-S		Spectrophotometry using uricase
Vitamin A	0.15–0.6 μg/ml	0.5–2.1 μMol/L	3-S		Natelson: *Microtechniques of Clinical Chemistry*, 2nd ed. 1961, p. 451

Table C.2[1]
Urine Values

Determination	Reference Range: Conventional	Reference Range: SI	Minimal Quantity Required	Note	Method
Acetone plus acetoacetate (quantitative)	0	0 mg/L	2 ml		Behre: *J Lab Clin Med* 13:770, 1928
Amylase	24–76 units/ml	24–76 arb. unit			Zinterhofer et al: *Clin Chim Acta* 43:5, 1973
Calcium	300 mg/day or less	7.5 mMol/day or less	24-hour specimen	Collect in special bottle with 10 ml of concentrated HCl	Atomic-absorption spectrophotometry
Catecholamines	Epinephrine: under 20 μg/day Norepinephrine: under 100 μg/day	<109 nMol/day <590 nMol/day	24-hour specimen	Should be collected with 10 ml of concentrated HCl (pH should be between 2.0 and 3.0)	Fluorometry
Chorionic gonadotropin	0	0 arb. unit	1st morning void		Immunologic technique
Copper	0–100 μg/day	0–1.6 μMol/day	24-hour specimen		Atomic-absorption spectrophotometry
Coproporphyrin	50–250 μg/day Children under 80 lb (36 kg): 0–75 μg/day	80–380 nMol/day 0–115 nMol/day	24-hour specimen	Collect with 5 g of sodium carbonate	Schwartz: *J Lab Clin Med* 37:843, 1951 With: *Scand J Clin Lab Invest* 7:193, 1955
Creatine	Under 100 mg/day or less than 6% of creatinine. In pregnancy: up to 12%. In children under 1 year may equal creatinine. In older children: up to 30% of creatinine.	<0.75 mMol/day	24-hour specimen	Also order creatinine	Folin: *Laboratory Manual of Biological Chemistry*, 5th ed., 1933, p. 163
Creatinine	15–25 mg/kg of body weight/day	0.13–0.22 mMol · kg^{-1}/day	24-hour specimen		Fabiny, Ertingshausen: *Clin Chem* 17:696, 1971
Cystine or cysteine	0	0	10 ml	Qualitative	Hawk et al: *Practical Physiological Chemistry*, 13th ed., 1954, p. 141
Hemoglobin and myoglobin	0		Freshly voided sample	Chemical examination with benzidine	Spectroscopy
5-Hydroxyindoleacetic acid	2–9 mg/day (women lower than men)	10–45 μMol/day	24-hour specimen	Collect with 10 ml of concentrated HCl	Sjoerdsma et al: *JAMA* 159:397, 1955
Lead	0.08 μg/ml or 120 μg/day or less	0.39 μMol/L or less	24-hour specimen		Willis: *Anal Chem* 34:614, 1962 (modified)
Phosphorus (inorganic)	Varies with intake; average, 1 g/day	32 mMol/day	24-hour specimen	Collect with 10 ml of concentrated HCl	Daly, Ertingshausen: *Clin Chem* 18:263, 1972
Porphobilinogen	0	0	10 ml	Use freshly voided urine	Watson, Schwartz: *Proc Soc Exp Biol Med* 47:393, 1941
Protein:					
Quantitative	<150 mg/24 hours	<0.15 g/day	24-hour specimen		Meulmans: *Clin Chim Acta* 5:757, 1951
Steroids:					
17-Ketosteroids (per day)	Age / Male / Female 10 / 1–4 mg / 1–4 mg 20 / 6–21 / 4–16 30 / 8–26 / 4–14 50 / 5–18 / 3–9 70 / 2–10 / 1–7	μMol/day (Male) / μMol/day (Female) 3–14 / 3–14 21–73 / 14–56 28–90 / 14–49 17–62 / 10–31 7–35 / 3–24	24-hour specimen	Not valid if patient is receiving meprobamate	Vestergaard: *Acta Endocrinol* 8:193, 1951. Normal values taken from Hamburger: *Acta Endocrinol* 1:19, 1948

Table C.2 (Continued)
Urine Values

Determination	Reference Range Conventional	Reference Range SI	Minimal Quantity Required	Note	Method
17-Hydroxysteroids	3–8 mg/day (women lower than men)	8–22 μMol/day as tetrahydrocortisol	24-hour specimen	Keep cold; chlorpromazine and related drugs interfere with assay	Epstein: *Clin Chim Acta* 7:735, 1962
Sugar: Quantitative glucose	0	0 mMol/L	24-hour or other timed specimen		Stein. In: Bergmeyer: *Methods of Enzymatic Analysis*, 1965, p. 117
Urobilinogen	Up to 1.0 Ehrlich U	To 1.0 arb. unit	2-hour sample (1–3 PM)		Watson et al: *Am J Clin Pathol* 15:605, 1944
Uroporphyrin	0–30 μg/day	<37 nMol/day	See Coproporphyrin		Schwartz et al: *Proc Soc Exp Biol Med* 79:463, 1952
Vanilmandelic acid (VMA)	Up to 9 mg/24 hour	Up to 45 μMol/day	24-hour specimen	Collect as for catecholamines	Pisano et al: *Clin Chim Acta* 7:285, 1962

Table C.3[1]
Special Endocrine Tests: Steroid Hormones

Determination	Reference Range Conventional	Reference Range SI	Minimal ml Required	Note	Method
Aldosterone	Excretion: 5–19 μg/24 hours	14–53 nMol/day	5/day	Keep specimen cold	Bayard et al: *J Clin Endocrinol Metabol* 31:507, 1970
	Supine: 48±29 pg/ml	133±80 pMol/L	3-S, P	Fasting, at rest, 210-mEq sodium diet	Poulson et al: *Clin Immunol Immunopathol* 2:373, 1974
	Upright (2 hours): 65±23 pg/ml	180±64 pMol/L		Upright, 2 hours, 210-mEq sodium diet	
	Supine: 107±45 pg/ml	279±125 pMol/L		Fasting, at rest, 110-mEq sodium diet	
	Upright (2 hours): 239±123 pg/ml	663±341 pMol/L		Upright, 2 hour, 110-mEq sodium diet	
	Supine: 175±75 pg/ml	485±208 pMol/L		Fasting, at rest, 10-mEq sodium diet	
	Upright (2 hours): 532±228 pg/ml	1476±632 pMol/L		Upright, 2 hour, 10-mEq sodium diet	
Cortisol	8 AM: 5–25 μg/dl	0.14–0.69 μMol/L	1-P	Fasting	Catt, Tregear: *Science* 158:1670, 1967
	8 PM: Below 10 μg/dl	0–0.28 μMol/L	1-P	At rest	
	4-hour ACTH test: 30–45 μg/dl	0.83–1.24 μMol/L	1-P	20 U ACTH, IV per 4 hours	
	Overight suppression test: Below 5 μg/dl	0.14 nMol/L	1-P	8 AM sample after 0.5 mg dexamethasone by mouth at midnight	
	Excretion: 20–70 μg/24 hour	55–193 nMol/day	2/day	Keep specimen cold	

Table C.3 (Continued)
Special Endocrine Tests: Steroid Hormones

Determination	Reference Range: Conventional	Reference Range: SI	Minimal ml Required	Note	Method
Dehydro-epiandrosterone (DHEA)	Male: 0.5–5.5 ng/ml				Sekihara, Ohsawa: *Steroids* 24:317, 1974
	Female:				
	1.4–8.0 ng/ml	4.9–28 nMol/L		Adult	
	0.3–4.5 ng/ml	1.0–15.6 nMol/L		Postmenopausal	
Dehydro-epiandrosterone sulfate (DHEA-S)	Male:		2-S, P		Buster, Abraham: *Anal Lett* 5:543, 1972
	151–446 μg/dl	3.9–11.4 μMol/L			
	Female:				
	84–433 μg/dl	2.2–11.1 μMol/L		Adult	
	1.7–177 μg/dl	0.04–4.5 μMol/L		Postmenopausal	
11-Deoxycortisol	Responsive: Over 7.5 μg/dl	>0.22 μMol/L	1-P	8 AM sample, preceded by 4.5 g of metyrapone by mouth per 24 hours or by single does of 2.5 g by mouth at midnight	Mahajan et al: *Steroids* 20:609, 1972
Estradiol	Male: <50 pg/ml	<184 pMol/L	5-S, P		Mikhail et al: *Steroids* 15:333, 1970
	Female: 23–361 pg/ml	84–1325 pMol/L		Adult	
	<30 pg/ml	<110 pMol/L		Postmenopausal	
	<20 pg/ml	<73 pMol/L		Prepubertal	
Progesterone	Male: <1.0 ng/ml	<3.2 nMol/L	5-S, P		Furuyama, Nugent: *Steroids* 17:663, 1971
	Female:				
	0.2–0.6 ng/ml	0.6–1.9 nMol/L		Follicular phase	
	0.3–3.5 ng/ml	0.95–11 nMol/L		Midcycle peak	
	6.5–32.2 ng/ml	21–102 nMol/L		Postovulatory	
Testosterone	Adult male:		1-P	AM sample	Catt, Tregear: *Science* 158:1670, 1967
	300–1100 ng/dl	10.4–38.1 nMol/L			
	Adolescent male:				
	Over 100 ng/dl	>3.5 nMol/L			
	Female:				
	25–90 ng/dl	0.87–3.12 nMol/L			
Unbound testosterone	Adult male:		2-P	AM sample	Forest et al: *Steroids* 12:323, 1968
	3.06–24.0 ng/dl	106–832 pMol/L			
	Adult female:				
	0.09–1.28 ng/dl	3.1–44.4 pMol/L			

Table C.4[1]
Special Endocrine Tests: Polypeptide Hormones

Determination	Reference Range: Conventional	Reference Range: SI	Minimal ml Required	Note	Method
Adrenocorticotropin (ACTH)	15–70 pg/ml	3.3–15.4 pMol/L	5-P	Place specimen on ice and send promptly to laboratory. Use EDTA tube only.	Gonzales: *Clin Chem* 26:1228, 1980
Alpha subunit	<0.5–2.5 ng/ml	<0.4–2.0 nMol/L	2-S	Adult male or female	Kourides et al: *Endocrinology* 94:1411, 1974
	<0.5–5.0 ng/ml	<0.4–4.0 nMol/L		Postmenopausal female	
Calcitonin	Male: 0–14 pg/ml	0–4.1 pMol/L	5-S	Test done only on known or suspected cases of medullary carcinoma of the thyroid	Deftos et al: *Metabolism* 20:1129, 1971
	Female: 0–28 pg/ml	0–8.2 pMol/L			Deftos et al: *Metabolism* 20:428, 1971
	>100 pg/ml in medullary carcinoma	>29.3 pMol/L			
Follicle-stimulating hormone (FSH)	Male: 3–18 mU/ml	3–18 arb. unit	5-S, P	Same sample may be used for LH	Midgley: *J Clin Endocrinol Metab* 27:295, 1967
	Female: 4.6–22.4 mU/ml	4.6–22.4 arb. unit		Pre- or post-ovulatory	
	13–41 mU/ml	13–41 arb. unit		Mid-cycle peak	
	30–170 mU/ml	30–170 arb. unit		Post-menopausal	
Growth hormone	Below 5 ng/ml	<233 pMol/L	1-S	Fasting, at rest	Glick et al: *Nature* 199:784, 1963
	Children: Over 10 ng/ml	>465 pMol/L		After exercise	

Table C.4 (Continued)
Special Endocrine Tests: Polypeptide Hormones

Determination	Reference Range: Conventional	Reference Range: SI	Minimal ml Required	Note	Method
	Male: Below 5 ng/ml	<233 pMol/L			
	Female: Up to 30 ng/ml	0–1395 pMol/L			
	Male: Below 5 ng/ml	<233 pMol/L		After glucose load	
	Female: Below 5 ng/ml	<233 pMol/L			
Insulin	6–26 μU/ml	43–187 pMol/L	1-S	Fasting	Morgan, Lazarow: *Proc Soc Exp Biol Med* 110:29, 1962
	Below 20 μU/ml	<144 pMol/L		During hypoglycemia	
	Up to 150 μU/ml	0–1078 pMol/L		After glucose load	
Luteinizing hormone (LH)	Male: 3–18 mU/ml	3–18 arb. unit	5-S, P	Same sample may be used for FSH	Odell et al: *J Clin Invest* 46:248, 1967
	Female:				
	2.4–34.5 mU/ml	2.4–34.5 arb. unit		Pre- or post-ovulatory	
	43–187 mU/ml	43–187 arb. unit		Mid-cycle peak	
	30–150 mU/ml	30–150 arb. unit		Post-menopausal	
Parathyroid hormone	<25 pg/ml	<2.94 pMol/L	5-P	Keep blood on ice, or plasma must be frozen if it is to be sent any distance; a.m. sample	Stewart et al: *N Engl J Med* 306:1136, 1982
Prolactin	2–15 ng/ml	0.08–6.0 nMol/L	2-S		Sinha et al: *J Clin Endocrinol Metabol* 36:509, 1973
Renin activity	Supine: 1.1 ± 0.8 ng/ml/hour	0.9 ± 0.6 nMol/L/hour	4-P	EDTA tubes, on ice, normal diet	Haber et al: *J Clin Endocrinol Metabol* 29:1349, 1969
	Upright: 1.9 ± 1.7 ng/ml/hour	1.5 ± 1.3 nMol/L/hour			
	Supine: 2.7 ± 1.8 ng/ml/hour	2.1 ± 1.4 nMol/L/hour		Low-sodium diet	
	Upright: 6.6 ± 2.5 ng/ml/hour	5.1 ± 1.9 nMol/L/hour			
	Diuretics: 10.0 ± 3.7 ng/ml/hour	7.7 ± 2.9 nMol/L/hour		Low-sodium diet	
Somatomedin C (Sm-C, IGF-1)	0.08–2.8 U/ml	0.08–2.8 arb. unit	2-P	EDTA plasma	Furlanetto et al: *J Clin Invest* 60:648, 1977
				Prepubertal	
	0.9–5.9 U/ml	0.9–5.9 arb. unit		During puberty	
	0.34–1.9 U/ml	0.34–1.9 arb. unit		Adult males	
	0.45–2.2 U/ml	0.45–2.2 arb. unit		Adult females	

Table C.5[1]
Special Endocrine Tests: Thyroid Hormones

Determination	Reference Range: Conventional	Reference Range: SI	Minimal ml Required	Note	Method
Thyroid-stimulating hormone (TSH)	0.5–0.5 μU/ml	0.5–5.0 arb. unit	2-S		Ridgway et al: *J Clin Invest* 52:2785, 1973
Thyroxine-binding globulin capacity	15–25 μg T_4/100 ml	193–322 nMol/L	2-S		Levy et al: *J Clin Endocrinol Metabol* 32:372, 1971
Total triiodothyronine (T_3)	75–195 ng/dl	1.16–3.00 nMol/L	2-S		Larsen et al: *J Clin Invest* 51:1939, 1972
Reverse triiodothyronine (rT3)	13–53 ng/ml	0.2–0.8 nMol/L	2-S		Cooper et al: *J Clin Endocrinol Metabol* 54:101, 1982
Total thyroxine by RIA (T_4)	4–12 μg/dl	52–154 nMol/L	1-S		Chopra: *J Clin Endocrinol Metabol* 34:938, 1972
T_3 resin uptake	25–35%	0.25–0.35	2-S		Taybearn et al: *J Nucl Med* 8:739, 1967
Free thyroxine index (FT_4I)	1–4		2-S		Sarin, Anderson: *Arch Intern Med* 126:631, 1970

Table C.6[1]
Vitamin D Derivatives

Determination	Reference Range: Conventional	Reference Range: SI	Minimal ml Required	Note	Method
1,25-Dihydroxy-vitamin D	26–65 pg/ml	62–155 pMol/L	1-S		Reinhardt et al: *J Clin Endocrinol Metabol* 58:91, 1984
25-Hydroxy-vitamin D	8–55 ng/ml	19.4–137 nMol/L	1-S		Preece et al: *Clin Chim Acta* 54:235, 1974

Table C.7[1]
Hematologic Values

Determination	Reference Range: Conventional	Reference Range: SI	Minimal ml Required	Note	Method
Coagulation factors:					
Factor I (fibrinogen)	0.15–0.35 g/dl	4.0–10.0 μMol/L	4.5-P	Collect in Vacutainer containing sodium citrate	Ratnoff, Menzies: *J Lab Clin Med* 37:316, 1951
Factor II (prothrombin)	60–140%	0.60–1.40	4.5-P	Collect in plastic tubes with 3.8% sodium citrate	Owren, Aas: *Scand J Clin Lab Invest* 3:201, 1951
Factor V (accelerator globulin)	60–140%	0.60–1.40	4.5-P	Collect as in factor II determination	Lewis, Ware: *Proc Soc Exp Biol Med* 84:640, 1953
Factor VII-X (proconvertin-Stuart)	70–130%	0.70–1.30	4.5-P	Collect as in factor II determination	Same as factor II
Factor X (Stuart factor)	70–130%	0.70–1.30	4.5-P	Collect as in factor II determination	Bachman et al: *Thromb Diath Haemorrh* 2:29, 1958
Factor VIII (antihemophilic globulin)	50–200%	0.50–2.0	4.5-P	Collect as in factor II determination	Tocantins, Kazal: *Blood Coagulation, Hemorrhage and Thrombosis*, 2nd ed., 1964
Factor IX (plasma thromboplastic cofactor)	60–140%	0.60–1.40	4.5-P	Collect as in factor II determination	*Idem*
Factor XI (plasma thromboplastic antecedent)	60–140%	0.60–1.40	4.5-P	Collect as in factor II determination	*Idem*
Factor XII (Hageman factor)	60–140%	0.60–1.40	4.5-P	Collect as in factor II determination	*Idem*
Coagulation Screening tests:					
Bleeding time (Simplate)	3–9.5 min	180–570 sec			Simplate Bleeding Time Device (General Diagnostics)
Prothrombin time	Less than 2-sec deviation from control	Less than 2-sec deviation from control	4.5-P	Collect in Vacutainer containing 3.8% sodium citrate	Colman et al: *Am J Clin Pathol* 64:108, 1975
Partial thromboplastin time (activated)	25–38 sec	25–38 sec	4.5-P	Collect in Vacutainer containing 3.8% sodium citrate	Babson, Babson: *Am J Clin Pathol* 62:856, 1974
Whole-blood clot lysis	No clot lysis in 24 hr	0/day	2.0-whole blood	Collect in sterile tube and incubate at 37°C	Page, Culver: *Syllabus, Laboratory Examination and Clinical Diagnosis*, 1960, p. 207
Fibrinolytic studies:					
Euglobin lysis	No lysis in 2 hr	0/2 hr	4.5-P	Collect as in factor II determination	Sherry et al: *J Clin Invest* 38:810, 1959
Fibrinogen split products	Negative reaction at >1:4 dilution	0 (at 1:4 dilution)	4.5-S	Collect in special tube containing thrombin and epsilon aminocaproic acid	Carvalho: *Am J Clin Pathol* 62:107, 1974

Table C.7 (Continued)
Hematologic Values

Determination	Reference Range: Conventional	Reference Range: SI	Minimal ml Required	Note	Method
Thrombin time	Control ±5 sec	Control ±5 sec	4.5-P	Collect as in factor II determination	Stefanini, Dameshek: *Hemorrhagic Disorders*, 1962, p. 492
"Complete" blood count:					
Hematocrit	Male: 45–52% Female: 37–48%	Male: 0.45–0.52 Female: 0.37–0.48	1-B	Use EDTA as anticoagulant; the seven listed tests are performed automatically on the Ortho ELT 800, which directly determines cell counts, hemoglobin (as the cyanmethemoglobin derivative), and MCV and computes hematocrit, MCH, and MCHC	
Hemoglobin	Male: 13–18 g/dl Female: 12–16 g/dl	Male: 8.1–11.2 mMol/L Female: 7.4–9.9 mMol/L			
Leukocyte count	4300–10,800/mm^3	4.3–10.8 $\times 10^9$/L			
Erythrocyte count	4.2–5.9 million/mm^3	4.2–5.9 $\times 10^{12}$/L			
Mean corpuscular volume (MCV)	86–98 μm^3/cell	86–98 fl			
Mean corpuscular hemoglobin (MCH)	27–32 pg/RBC	1.7–2.0 pg/cell			
Mean corpuscular hemoglobin concentration (MCHC)	32–36%	0.32–0.36			
Erythrocyte sedimentation rate	Male: 1–13 mm/hr Female: 1–20 mm/hr	Male: 1–13 mm/hr Female: 1–20 mm/hr	5-B	Use EDTA as anticoagulant	Modified Westergren method. Gambino et al: *Am J Clin Pathol* 35:173, 1965
Erythrocyte enzymes:					
Glucose-6-phosphate dehydrogenase	5–15 U/g Hb	5–15 U/g	9-B	Use special anticoagulant (ACD solution)	Beck: *J Biol Chem* 232:251, 1958
Pyruvate kinase	13–17 U/g Hb	13–17 U/g	8-B	Use special anticoagulant (ACD solution)	Beutler: *Red Cell Metabolism*, 2nd ed., 1975, p. 60
Ferritin (serum)					
Iron deficiency	0–12 ng/ml 13–20 Borderline	0–4.8 nMol/L 5.2–8 nMol/L Borderline			Addison et al: *J Clin Pathol* 25:326, 1972
Iron excess	>400 ng/L	>160 nMol/L			
Folic acid					
Normal	>3.3 ng/ml	>7.3 nMol/L	1-S		Waxman, Schreiber: *Blood* 42:281, 1973
Borderline	2.5–3.2 ng/ml	5.75–7.39 nMol/L	1-S		
Haptoglobin	40–336 mg/dl	0.4–3.36 g/L	1-S		Behring Diagnostic Reagent Kit
Hemoglobin studies:					
Electrophoresis for abnormal hemoglobin			5-B	Collect with anticoagulant	Singer: *Am J Med* 18:633, 1955
Electrophoresis for A_2 hemoglobin	3.0%	0.015–0.035	5-B	Use oxalate as anticoagulant	Abraham: *Hemoglobin* 1: 27, 1976
Borderline	0.3–3.5%	0.03–0.035			
Hemoglobin F (fetal hemoglobin)	Less than 2%	<0.02	5-B	Collect with anticoagulant	Maile: *Laboratory Medicine—Hematology*, 2nd ed., 1962, p. 845
Hemoglobin, met- and sulf-	0	0	5-B	Use heparin as anticoagulant	Michel, Harris: *J Lab Clin Med* 29:445, 1940
Serum hemoglobin	2–3 mg/dl	1.2–1.9 μMol/L	2-S		Hunter et al: *Am J Clin Pathol* 20:429, 1950

Table C.7 (Continued)
Hematologic Values

Determination	Reference Range: Conventional	Reference Range: SI	Minimal ml Required	Note	Method
Thermolabile hemoglobin	0	0	1-B	Any anticoagulent	Dacie et al: *Br J Haematol* 10:388, 1964
Lupus anticoagulant	0	0	4.5-P	Collect as in factor II determination	Boxer et al: *Arthritis Rheum* 19:1244, 1976
LE (lupus erythematosus) preparation:					
Method I	0	0	5-B	Use heparin as anticoagulant	Hargraves et al: *Proc Staff Meet Mayo Clin* 24:234, 1949
Method II	0	0	5-B	Use defibrinated blood	Barnes et al: *J Invest Dermatol* 14:397, 1950
Leukocyte alkaline phosphatase:			20-Isolated blood leukocytes	Special handling of blood necessary	Valentine, Beck: *J Lab Clin Med* 38:39, 1951
Qualitative method	Males: 33–188 U Females (off contraceptive pill): 30–160 U	33–188 U 30–160 U	Smear-B		Kaplow: *Am J Clin Pathol* 39:439, 1963
Muramidase	Serum, 3–7 μg/ml Urine, 0–2 μg/ml	3–7 mg/L 0–2 mg/L	1-S 1-U		Osserman, Lawlor: *J Exp Med* 124:921, 1966
Osmotic fragility of erythrocytes	Increased if hemolysis occurs in over 0.5% NaCl; decreased if hemolysis is incomplete in 0.3% NaCl		5-B	Use heparin as anticoagulant	Beutler. In: Williams et al (eds): *Hematology*, McGraw-Hill, 1972, p. 1375
Peroxide hemolysis	Less than 10%	0.10	6-B	Use EDTA as anticoagulant	Gordon et al: *Am J Dis Child* 90:669, 1955
Platelet count	150,000–350,000/mm³	$150–350 \times 10^9$/L	0.5-B	Use EDTA as anticoagulant; counts are performed on Clay Adams Ultraflow; when counts are low, results are confirmed by hand counting	(Hand count): Brecher et al: *Am J Clin Pathol* 23:15, 1955
Platelet function tests:					
Clot retraction	50–100%/2 hour	0.50–1.00/2 hour	4.5-P	Collect as in factor II determination	Benthaus: *Thromb Diath Haemorrh* 3:311, 1959
Platelet aggregation	Full response to ADP, epinephrine, and collagen	1.0	18-P	Collect as in factor II determination	Born: *Nature* 194:927, 1962
Platelet factor 3	33–57 sec	33–57 sec	4.5-P	Collect as in factor II determination	Rabiner, Hrodek: *J Clin Invest* 47:901, 1968
Reticulocyte count	0.5–2.5% red cells	0.005–0.025	0.1-B		Brecher: *Am J Clin Pathol* 19:895, 1949
Vitamin B_{12} Borderline	205–876 pg/ml 140–204 pg/ml	150–674 pMol/L 102.6–149 pMol/L	12-S		*Difco Manual*, 9th ed., 1953, p. 221 (modified)

Table C.8[1]
Cerebrospinal Fluid Values

Determination	Reference Range Conventional	SI	Minimal ml Required	Note	Method
Bilirubin	0	0	2		See Blood Bilirubin (adapted)
Cell count	0–5 mononuclear cells		0.5		
Chloride	120–130 mEq/L	120–130 mMol/L	0.5		See Blood Chloride
Colloidal gold	0000000000–0001222111	Same	0.1		Wuth, Faupel: *Bull Johns Hopkins Hosp* 40:297, 1927
Albumin	Mean: 29.5 mg/dl ±2 SD: 11–48 mg/dl	0.295 g/L ±2 SD: 0.11–0.48	2.5		Mancini et al: *Immunochemistry* 2:235, 1965
IgG	Mean: 4/3 mg/dl ±2 SD: 0–8.6 mg/dl	0.043 g/L ±2 SD: 0–0.086			
Glucose	50–75 mg/dl	2.8–4.2 mMol/L	0.5		See Blood Glucose
Pressure (initial)	70–180 mm of water	70–180 arb. unit			
Protein:					
Lumbar	15–45 mg/dl	0.15–0.45 g/L	1		Meulmans: *Clin Chim Acta* 5:757, 1960
Cisternal	15–25 mg/dl	0.15–0.25 g/L	1		
Ventricular	5–15 mg/dl	0.05–0.15 g/L	1		

Table C.9[1]
Miscellaneous Values

Determination	Reference Range Conventional	SI	Minimal ml Required	Note	Method
Carcinoembryonic antigen (CEA)	0–2.5 ng/ml	0–2.5 μg/L	20-P	Must be sent on ice	Hansen et al: *J Clin Res* 19:143, 1971
Chylous fluid				Use fresh specimen	Todd et al: *Clinical Diagnosis*, 12th ed., 1953, p. 624
Digitoxin	17±6 ng/ml	22±7.8 nMol/L	1-S	Medication with digitoxin or digitalis	Smith, Butler, Haber: *N Engl J Med* 281:1212, 1969
Digoxin	1.2±0.4 ng/ml	1.54±0.5 nMol/L	1-S	Medication with digoxin 0.25 mg per day	Smith, Haber: *J Clin Invest* 49:2377, 1970
	1.5±0.4 ng/ml	1.92±0.5 nMol/L	1-S	Medication with digoxin 0.5 mg per day	
Duodenal drainage				pH should be in proper range with minimal amount of gastric juice	
pH (urine)	5–7	5–7			
Gastric analysis	Basal:				Marks: *Gastroenterology* 41:599, 1961
	Females: 2.0±1.8 mEq/hour	0.6±0.5 μMol/sec			
	Males: 3.0±2.0 mEq/hour	0.8±0.6 μMol/sec			
	Maximal (after histalog or gastrin):				
	Females: 16±5 mEq/hour	4.4±1.4 μMol/sec			
	Males: 23±5 mEq/hour	6.4±1.4 μMol/sec			
Gastrin-I	0–200 pg/ml	0–95 pMol/L	4-P	Heparinized sample	Dent et al: *Ann Surg* 176:360, 1972
Immunologic tests:					
α-fetoprotein	Undetectable in normal adults		2-S		

Table C.9 (Continued)
Miscellaneous Values

Determination	Reference Range: Conventional	SI	Minimal ml Required	Note	Method
α-1-antitrypsin	85–213 mg/dl	0.85–2.13 g/L	10-B		Nephelometric assay
Rheumatoid factor	<60 IU/ml		10 ml clotted blood	Fasting sample preferred	Nephelometric assay
Antinuclear antibodies	Negative at a 1:8 dilution of serum		2-S	Send to laboratory promptly	Immunofluorescence assay
Anti-DNA antibodies	Negative at a 1:10 dilution of serum		2-S		*Crithidia lucilliae* assay
Antibodies to Sm and RNP (ENA)	None detected		10 ml clotted blood		Double diffusion
Antibodies to SS-A (Ro) and SS-B (La)	None detected		10 ml clotted blood		Double diffusion
Autoantibodies to:					
Thyroid colloid and microsomal antigens	Negative at a 1:10 dilution of serum		2-S	Low titers in some elderly normal women	Doniach, Bottazzo, Drexhage: The autoimmune endocrinopathies. In: Lachmann, Peters (eds): *Clinical Aspects of Immunology*, Vol. 2, Oxford: Blackwell Scientific, 1982, p. 903
Gastric parietal cells	Negative at a 1:20 dilution of serum		2-S		
Smooth muscle	Negative at a 1:20 dilution of serum		2-S		
Mitochondria	Negative at a 1:20 dilution of serum		2-S		
Interstitial cells of the testes	Negative at a 1:10 dilution of serum		2-S		
Skeletal muscle	Negative at a 1:60 dilution of serum		2-S		
Adrenal gland	Negative at a 1:10 dilution of serum		2-S		Doniach et al: *Protocol of Autoimmunity Laboratories*. London: Middlesex Medical School
Bence Jones protein	No Bence Jones protein detected in a 50-fold concentrate of urine		50-U		
Complement, total hemolytic	150–250 U/ml		10-B	Must be sent on ice	Hook, Muschel: *Proc Soc Exp Biol Med* 117:292, 1964
Cryoprecipitable proteins	None detected	0 arb. unit	10-S	Collect and transport at 37°C	Barr et al: *Ann Intern Med* 32:6, 1950 (modified)
C3	Range, 83–177 mg/dl	0.83–1.77 g/L	2-S		Nephelometric assay
C4	Range, 15–45 mg/dl	0.15–0.45 g/L	2-S		Nephelometric assay
Factor B	12–30 mg/dl		5 ml clotted blood		Nephelometric assay
C1 esterase inhibitor	13.2–24 mg/dl		5 ml clotted blood		Nephelometric assay
Hemoglobin A_{1c}	3.8–6.4%	0.038–0.064	5-P	Send EDTA tube on ice promptly to laboratory	Nathan et al: *Clin Chem* 28:512, 1982
Hypersensitivity pneumonitis screen	No antibodies to those antigens assayed		5 ml clotted blood		Double diffusion

Table C.9 (Continued)
Miscellaneous Values

Determination	Reference Range: Conventional	Reference Range: SI	Minimal ml Required	Note	Method
Immunoglobulins:					
IgG	639–1349 mg/dl	6.39–13.49 g/L	2-S		
IgA	70–312 mg/dl	0.7–3.12 g/L	2-S		
IgM	86–352 mg/dl	0.86–3.52 g/L	2-S		
Viscosity	1.4–1.8 relative viscosity units		10-B	Expressed as the relative viscosity of serum compared with water	Barth: Viscosimetry of serum in relation to the serum globulins. In: Sunderman, Sunderman (eds): *Serum Proteins and the Dysproteinemias*, 1964, p. 102
Iontophoresis	Children: 0–40 mEq sodium/L Adults: 0–60 mEq sodium/L	0–40 mMol/L 0–60 mMol/L		Value given in terms of sodium	Gibson, Cooke: *Pediatrics* 23:545, 1959
Propranolol (includes bioactive 4-OH metabolite)	100–300 ng/ml	386–1158 nMol/L	1-S	Obtain blood sample 4 hr after last dose of beta-blocking agent	M.G.H. method of Rockson, Homcy, Haber: by radio-immunoassay
Stool fat	Less than 5 g in 24 hr or less than 4% of measured fat intake in 3-day period	<5 g/day	24-hr or 3-day speci-men		Jover et al: *J Lab Clin Med* 59:878, 1962
Stool nitrogen	Less than 2 g/day or 10% of urinary nitrogen	<2 g/day	24-hr or 3-day speci-men		Peters, Van Slyke: *Quantitative Clinical Chemistry*, Vol. 2 (Methods), 1932, p. 353
Synovial fluid:					
Glucose	Not less than 20 mg/100 ml lower than simultaneously drawn blood sugar	See Blood Glucose	1 ml of fresh fluid	Collect with oxalate–fluoride mixture	See Blood Glucose
D-Xylose absorption	5–8 g/5 hr in urine; 40 mg/dl in blood 2 hr after ingestion of 25 g of D-xylose	33–53 mMol/day 2.7 mMol/L	5-U 5-B	For directions see Benson et al: *N Engl J Med* 256:335, 1957	Roe, Rice: *J Biol Chem* 173:507, 1948

[1]Reproduced with permission from *The New England Journal of Medicine* 314:39–49, 1986 and 315:1606, 1986.

Table C.10
Update of Normal Reference Laboratory Values: Case Records of the Massachusetts General Hospital

Blood, Plasma, or Serum Values

Determination	Reference Range Conventional	SI
Amylase	53–123 U/L	884–2050 nMol · sec^{-1}/L
Ceruloplasmin	23–43 mg/dl	1.5–2.9 μMol/L
Chloride	100–108 mMol/L	100–108 mMol/L
Copper	Total: 70–150 μg/dl	11–24 μMol/L
Lactic acid	0.5–2.2 mMol/L	0.5–2.2 mMol/L
Lipase	4–24 U/dl	667–4001 nMol · sec^{-1}/L
Phosphatase (acid)		
Prostatic (delete male and female)	0–0.8 U/L	0–13.3 nMol · sec^{-1}/L
Salicylate	100–200 mg/L	724–1448 μMol/L

Urine Values

Determination	Reference Range Conventional	SI
Amylase	0–375 U/L	0–6251 nMol · sec^{-1}/L
Protein:		
Quantitative	<165 mg/24 hr	<0.16 g/24 hr

Miscellaneous Values

Determination	Reference Range Conventional	SI
Digitoxin	9–25 μg/L	11.8–32.8 nMol/L
Digoxin (delete propranolol)	0.9–2.0 ng/ml	1.15–2.56 nMol/L

Index

Page numbers in *italics* denote figures; those followed by "t" denote tables

C

H

I

P